SEVENTH EDITION

# GLENN'S UROLOGIC SURGERY

*Editors*

**Sam D. Graham, Jr., MD**
Urologic Specialists of Virginia
Medical Director
Thomas Johns Hospital
Richmond, Virginia

**Thomas E. Keane, MD**
Professor and Chair
Department of Urology
Medical University of South Carolina
Charleston, South Carolina

*Consultant Editor*

James F. Glenn, MD, DSc, FACS, FRCS

*Associate Editors*

Charles B. Brendler, MD
Marc Goldstein, MD, DSc (hon)
Leonard G. Gomella, MD, FACS
E. Ann Gormley, MD
Thomas W. Jarrett, MD
Gerald H. Jordan, MD, FACS, FAAP
Jerome P. Richie, MD
Randall G. Rowland, MD, PhD
H. Gil Rushton, MD
Urs E. Studer, MD

Wolters Kluwer | Lippincott Williams & Wilkins
Health

Philadelphia • Baltimore • New York • London
Buenos Aires • Hong Kong • Sydney • Tokyo

*Acquisitions Editor:* Brian Brown
*Product Manager:* Ryan Shaw/Erika Kors
*Senior Manufacturing Manager:* Benjamin Rivera
*Marketing Manager:* Lisa Parry
*Creative Director:* Doug Smock
*Production Service:* Macmillan Publishing Solutions


**530 Walnut Street**
**Philadelphia, PA 19106 USA**
**LWW.com**



Printed in China

---

**Library of Congress Cataloging-in-Publication Data**

Glenn's urologic surgery / editors, Sam D. Graham Jr., Thomas E. Keane ; consultant editor, James F. Glenn ; associate editors, Charles B. Brendler . . . [et al.].—7th ed.
p. ; cm.
Includes bibliographical references and index.
ISBN 978-0-7817-9141-0 (alk. paper)
1. Genitourinary organs—Surgery. I. Graham, Sam D. II. Keane, Thomas E. III. Glenn, James F. (James Francis), 1928- IV. Title: Urologic surgery.
[DNLM: 1. Urogenital Surgical Procedures. 2. Female Urogenital Diseases—surgery. 3. Male Urogenital Diseases—surgery. WJ 168 G559 2010]
RD571.U75 2010
617.4'6059—dc22

2009029905

---



10 9 8 7 6 5 4 3 2 1

CCS0909

# CONTENTS


*Editors* xi
*Contributors* xiii
*Remembrances* xxvii
*Preface* xxix

SECTION I ■ ADRENAL, RENAL, URETER, PELVIS 1
*Jerome P. Richie*

Chapter 1 **Anatomy of the Adrenal Glands, Kidney, Ureter, and Pelvis** 1
*Ricardo Beduschi, Unyime O. Nseyo, and Sam D. Graham, Jr.*

Chapter 2 **Partial Nephrectomy** 6
*Samir S. Taneja*

Chapter 3 **Radical Nephrectomy** 14
*Michael S. Cookson and Sam S. Chang*

Chapter 4 **Intracaval Tumors** 23
*Viraj A. Master and Fray F. Marshall*

Chapter 5 **Transplant Nephrectomy** 32
*Sanjaya Kumar*

Chapter 6 **Renovascular Disease** 36
*John A. Libertino and Chad Wotkowicz*

Chapter 7 **Anatrophic Nephrolithotomy** 45
*Elizabeth J. Anoia, Michael L. Paik, and Martin I. Resnick*

Chapter 8 **Renal and Retroperitoneal Abscesses** 51
*Davis P. Viprakasit and Anthony J. Schaeffer*

Chapter 9 **Renal Trauma** 58
*Jill C. Buckley and Jack W. McAninch*

Chapter 10 **Renal Allotransplantation** 65
*John W. McGillicuddy, Justin D. Ellett, and Kenneth D. Chavin*

Chapter 11 **Ureteral Complications Following Renal Transplantation** 71
*Rodney J. Taylor*

Chapter 12 **Renal Autotransplantation** 76
*Venkatesh Krishnamurthi and David A. Goldfarb*

SECTION II ■ BLADDER 85
*Charles B. Brendler*

Chapter 13 **Anatomy of the Bladder** 85
*Clinton W. Collins and Adam P. Klausner*

Chapter 14 **Simple and Partial Cystectomy** 92
*Jonathan C. Picard and J. Nathaniel Hamilton*

Chapter 15 **Radical Cystectomy in Men** 97
*Mohamed A. Ghonheim*

Chapter 16 **Radical Cystectomy in Women** 104
*Alon Z. Weizer and Cheryl T. Lee*

Chapter 17 **Bladder Diverticulectomy** 113
*Michael S. Cookson and Sam S. Chang*

Chapter 18 **Bladder Augmentation** 118
*Anne Pelletier Cameron, R. Duane Cespedes, and Edward J. McGuire*

Chapter 19 **Management of the Distal Ureter for Nephroureterectomy** 125
*J. Stuart Wolf, Jr.*

Chapter 20 **Vesicovaginal Fistula** 130
*Helen G. Zafirakis and O. Lenaine Westney*

Chapter 21 **Enterovesical and Rectourethral Fistulas** 137
*Kenneth W. Angermeier, Aaron J. Milbank, and Eric A. Klein*

Chapter 22 **Vesical Trauma and Hemorrhage** 143
*Kamal S. Pohar and Robert R. Bahnson*

Chapter 23 **Interstitial Cystitis/Painful Bladder Syndrome** 150
*Michael S. Ingber and Kenneth M. Peters*

SECTION III ■ PROSTATE 163
*Randall G. Rowland*

Chapter 24 **Anatomy of the Prostate** 163
*Sam D. Graham, Jr.*

Chapter 25 **Surgery for Benign Prostatic Hypertrophy** 166
*Brian R. Matlaga and James E. Lingeman*

Chapter 26 **Prostatic Imaging and Biopsy** 175
*Frances M. Martin, William T. Conner, and Randall G. Rowland*

Chapter 27 **Pelvic Lymphadenectomy** 179
*Michelle L. Ramírez, Raj S. Pruthi, Joon-Ha Ok, and Ralph W. deVere-White*

Chapter 28 **Open Radical Retropubic Prostatectomy** 186
*Misop Han and William J. Catalona*

Chapter 29 **Radical Perineal Prostatectomy** 194
*Sam D. Graham, Jr., Jeffrey C. Lou, and Thomas E. Keane*

Chapter 30 **Brachytherapy for Localized Prostate Cancer** 202
*John A. Fortney, A. Jason Zauls, and David T. Marshall*

SECTION IV ■ URETHRA 211
*E. Ann Gormley*

Chapter 31 **Anatomy of the Urethra** 211
*E. Ann Gormley*

Chapter 32 **Female Urethral Diverticulum** 214
*Ahmed M. El-Zawahry and Eric S. Rovner*

Chapter 33 **Reconstruction of the Female Urethra** 220
*Jerry G. Blaivas and Rajveer S. Purohit*

Chapter 34 **Surgical Management of the Incompetent Bladder Outlet in the Patient with a Neurogenic Bladder** 228
*Alienor S. Gilchrist, Gary E. Lemack, and Philippe E. Zimmern*

| | | |
|---|---|---|
| Chapter 35 | **Surgery for Urethral Stricture Disease**<br>*Jack R. Walter and George D. Webster* | 236 |
| Chapter 36 | **Surgery for Urethral Trauma Including Urethral Disruption**<br>*Jack W. McAninch and Bryan B. Voelzke* | 245 |
| Chapter 37 | **Carcinoma of the Female Urethra**<br>*Peter L. Steinberg and William Bihrle III* | 252 |
| Chapter 38 | **Carcinoma of the Male Urethra**<br>*Peter L. Steinberg and William Bihrle III* | 257 |
| Chapter 39 | **Injectable Therapies for Incontinence in Women**<br>*Rodney Appell* | 263 |
| Chapter 40 | **Pubovaginal Fascial Slings**<br>*Anne Pelletier Cameron, Christina Lewicky-Gaupp, and Edward J. McGuire* | 271 |
| Chapter 41 | **Synthetic Midurethral Retropubic Slings**<br>*Bhavin N. Patel and Gopal H. Badlani* | 278 |
| Chapter 42 | **The Transobturator Approach to the Midurethral Sling**<br>*Paul Hanissian and James Whiteside* | 282 |
| Chapter 43 | **Abdominal Retropubic Approaches for Female Incontinence**<br>*Leslie M. Rickey* | 288 |
| Chapter 44 | **The Artificial Urinary Sphincter**<br>*Helen Zafirakis and O. Lenaine Westney* | 292 |
| Chapter 45 | **The Male Sling for Postprostatectomy Incontinence: Current Concepts and Controversies**<br>*Craig V. Comiter* | 299 |
| Chapter 46 | **Sacral Neuromodulation**<br>*Sarah E. McAchran, Raymond R. Rackley, and Sandip Vasavada* | 305 |
| Chapter 47 | **Surgical Treatment of Pelvic Organ Prolapse: Anatomy of the Pelvic Floor**<br>*Ariana L. Smith, Ja-Hong Kim, and Shlomo Raz* | 311 |
| Chapter 48 | **Vaginal Hysterectomy for Uterine Prolapse**<br>*Ja-Hong Kim, Ariana L. Smith, and Shlomo Raz* | 318 |
| Chapter 49 | **Cystocele and Anterior Vaginal Prolapse**<br>*Melissa R. Kaufman, Harriette M. Scarpero, and Roger R. Dmochowski* | 326 |
| Chapter 50 | **Transvaginal Repair of Apical Prolapse**<br>*Katie N. Ballert and Victor W. Nitti* | 335 |
| Chapter 51 | **Posterior Vaginal Prolapse Repair**<br>*Lior Lowenstein and Elizabeth R. Mueller* | 343 |
| Chapter 52 | **Abdominal Sacral Colpopexy**<br>*J. Christian Winters and Scott Delacroix, Jr.* | 349 |
| SECTION V ■<br>*Marc Goldstein* | VAS DEFERENS, SEMINAL VESICLE, TESTIS | 355 |
| Chapter 53 | **Anatomy of the Epididymis, Vas Deferens, and Seminal Vesicle**<br>*Howard H. Kim and Marc Goldstein* | 355 |
| Chapter 54 | **Seminal Vesicle and Ejaculatory Duct Surgery**<br>*Jay I. Sandlow* | 361 |
| Chapter 55 | **Vasectomy**<br>*Douglas G. Stein* | 372 |

| | | |
|---|---|---|
| Chapter 56 | **Vasoepididymostomy**<br>*Peter T. K. Chan* | 379 |
| Chapter 57 | **Vasovasostomy**<br>*Marc Goldstein and Howard H. Kim* | 387 |
| Chapter 58 | **Microsurgical Varicocelectomy**<br>*Armand Zini and Ziv Maianski* | 397 |
| Chapter 59 | **Testis Biopsy and Testicular Sperm Extraction (TESE)**<br>*Peter N. Schlegel* | 401 |
| Chapter 60A | **Epididymal Sperm Aspiration**<br>*Cigdem Tanrikut and Marc Goldstein* | 407 |
| Chapter 60B | **Epididymectomy**<br>*David M. Nudell and Larry I. Lipshultz* | 410 |
| Chapter 61 | **Ejaculation Induction Procedures: Penile Vibratory Stimulation and Electroejaculation**<br>*Dana A. Ohl, Susanne A. Quallich, Jens Sønksen, Nancy L. Brackett, and Charles M. Lynne* | 412 |
| Chapter 62 | **Anatomy of the Testis**<br>*Howard H. Kim and Marc Goldstein* | 419 |
| Chapter 63 | **Simple Orchiectomy**<br>*Brett S. Carver and Sherri M. Donat* | 428 |
| Chapter 64 | **Inguinal Orchiectomy**<br>*David A. Swanson* | 433 |
| Chapter 65 | **Organ-Preserving Surgery in Testicular Tumors**<br>*Axel Heidenreich* | 438 |
| Chapter 66 | **Retroperitoneal Lymphadenectomy**<br>*Michael Leveridge and Michael A. S. Jewett* | 442 |
| Chapter 67 | **Torsion of the Testicle**<br>*Blake W. Moore and Harry P. Koo* | 448 |
| Chapter 68 | **Scrotal Trauma and Reconstruction**<br>*Timothy O. Davies and Gerald H. Jordan* | 453 |

SECTION VI ■ PENIS AND SCROTUM 465
*Gerald H. Jordan*

| | | |
|---|---|---|
| Chapter 69 | **Anatomy of the Penis and Scrotum**<br>*Sam D. Graham, Jr.* | 465 |
| Chapter 70 | **Partial and Total Penectomy in the Management of Invasive Squamous Cell Carcinoma of the Penis**<br>*Antonio Puras Baez and Alex M. Acosta Miranda* | 467 |
| Chapter 71 | **Inguinal Lymphadenectomy for Penile Carcinoma**<br>*Shahin Tabatabaei and W. Scott McDougal* | 473 |
| Chapter 72 | **Surgical Treatment of Peyronie Disease**<br>*Uri Gur and Gerald H. Jordan* | 481 |
| Chapter 73 | **Priapism**<br>*Trinity J. Bivalacqua and Arthur L. Burnett* | 487 |
| Chapter 74 | **Penile Prosthesis Implantation**<br>*Culley C. Carson* | 492 |

Chapter 75 **Penile Venous Surgery** 499
*Audrey C. Rhee, Mark R. Licht, and Ronald W. Lewis*

Chapter 76 **Microvascular Arterial Bypass Surgery for Erectile Dysfunction** 505
*Irwin Goldstein and Martin Bastuba*

Chapter 77 **Penile Trauma** 514
*Daniel I. Rosenstein, Allen F. Morey, and Jack W. McAninch*

Chapter 78 **Penile Replantation** 519
*Uri Gur and Gerald H. Jordan*

Chapter 79 **Varicocele: General Considerations** 523
*Carin V. Hopps and Marc Goldstein*

Chapter 80 **Hydrocele and Spermatocele** 528
*John A. Nesbitt*

Chapter 81 **Congenital Curvature** 532
*Timothy O. Davies and Kurt A. McCammon*

Chapter 82 **Reconstruction of the Penis for Complications of Penile Enhancement Surgery** 537
*Gary J. Alter*

SECTION VII ■ URINARY DIVERSION 545
*Urs E. Studer*

Chapter 83 **Ileal Conduit Urinary Diversion** 545
*Michael C. Lee and Eric A. Klein*

Chapter 84 **Transverse Colonic Conduit** 549
*Margit Fisch, Rudolf Hohenfellner, Raimund Stein, and Joachim W. Thüroff*

Chapter 85 **Managing the Patient with Orthotopic Bladder Substitution** 555
*Urs E. Studer and N. Bhatta-Dhar*

Chapter 86 **Orthotopic Urinary Diversion Using an Ileal Low-Pressure Reservoir with an Afferent Tubular Segment** 561
*Stephan Jeschke and Urs E. Studer*

Chapter 87 **Ileal Neobladder** 566
*Richard E. Hautmann*

Chapter 88 **The Padua Ileal Bladder** 574
*Francesco Pagano and Pierfrancesco Bassi*

Chapter 89 **The T-Pouch Ileal Neobladder** 578
*John P. Stein and Donald G. Skinner*

Chapter 90 **Colonic Orthotopic Bladder Substitution** 586
*Joachim W. Thüroff and Ludger Franzaring*

Chapter 91 **Continent Catheterizable Reservoir Made from Ileum** 594
*Hassan Abol-Enein and Mohamed A. Ghoneim*

Chapter 92 **Continent Catheterizable Reservoir Made from Colon** 599
*Hubertus Riedmiller and Elmar W. Gerharz*

Chapter 93 **Ureterosigmoidostomy: Mainz Pouch II** 610
*Margit Fisch, Rudolf Hohenfellner, Jörg Schede, and Joachim W. Thüroff*

Chapter 94 **Palliative Urinary Diversion** 618
*Burkhard Ubrig and Stephan Roth*

SECTION VIII ■ PEDIATRIC 623
*H. Gil Rushton*

Chapter 95 **Neuroblastoma** 623
*W. Robert DeFoor, Jr., Pramod P. Reddy, and Curtis A. Sheldon*

Chapter 96 **Wilms Tumor** 628
*Sarah Conley and Michael L. Ritchey*

Chapter 97 **Renal Fusion and Ectopia** 634
*Ross M. Decter*

Chapter 98 **Transureteroureterostomy** 643
*H. Gil Rushton*

Chapter 99 **Pyeloplasty** 647
*Evan J. Kass and Kevin M. Feber*

Chapter 100 **Megaureter** 649
*J. Christopher Austin and Douglas A. Canning*

Chapter 101 **Prune Belly (Triad) Syndrome** 654
*David B. Joseph*

Chapter 102 **Childhood Rhabdomyosarcoma** 662
*Hsi-Yang Wu and Howard M. Snyder III*

Chapter 103 **Vesicoureteral Reflux** 665
*Mark R. Zaontz*

Chapter 104 **Endoscopic Treatment of Vesicoureteral Reflux** 676
*Wolfgang H. Cerwinka and Andrew J. Kirsch*

Chapter 105 **Ureteroceles** 681
*Richard N. Yu, Chester J. Koh, and David A. Diamond*

Chapter 106 **Urachal Anomalies and Related Umbilical Disorders** 684
*Leslie T. McQuiston and Anthony A. Caldamone*

Chapter 107 **Vesical Neck Reconstruction** 689
*John C. Pope IV and John H. Makari*

Chapter 108 **Surgery for Posterior Urethral Valves** 697
*Rosalia Misseri and Kenneth I. Glassberg*

Chapter 109 **Hypospadias** 703
*Laurence S. Baskin*

Chapter 110 **Complete Primary Repair for Exstrophy** 711
*Richard W. Grady*

Chapter 111 **Bladder Exstrophy and Epispadias** 722
*Thomas E. Novak and John P. Gearhart*

Chapter 112 **Congenital Anomalies of the Scrotum** 731
*Sean T. Corbett and David R. Roth*

Chapter 113 **Pediatric Cryptorchidism, Hydroceles, and Hernias** 735
*Kenneth G. Nepple and Christopher S. Cooper*

Chapter 114 **Laparoscopic Management of the Undescended Testicle** 742
*Danielle D. Sweeney, Michael C. Ost, and Steven G. Docimo*

Chapter 115 **Pediatric Laparoscopic Pyeloplasty** 752
*Pasquale Casale and Walid A. Farhat*

Chapter 116 **Pediatric Laparoscopic Nephrectomy and Partial Nephrectomy** 757
*Glenn M. Cannon, Jr., and Richard S. Lee*

| | | |
|---|---|---|
| Chapter 117 | **Urogenital Sinus and Cloacal Anomalies**<br>*Jeffrey A. Leslie and Richard C. Rink* | 761 |
| Chapter 118 | **Surgery to Correct Ambiguous Genitalia (46XX Disorder of Sexual Development)**<br>*Anthony J. Casale* | 769 |
| Chapter 119 | **Circumcision**<br>*Irene M. McAleer and George W. Kaplan* | 778 |
| Chapter 120 | **Augmentation Cystoplasty in Children**<br>*Hans G. Pohl* | 783 |
| Chapter 121 | **The Mitrofanoff Procedure in Pediatric Urinary Tract Reconstruction**<br>*Mark P. Cain* | 793 |

SECTION IX ■ LAPARASCOPIC 801
*Leonard G. Gomella*

| | | |
|---|---|---|
| Chapter 122 | **Basic Principles of Laparoscopy: Transperitoneal, Extraperitoneal, and Hand-Assisted Techniques**<br>*Gaurav Bandi and Leonard G. Gomella* | 801 |
| Chapter 123 | **Laparoscopic Pelvic and Retroperitoneal Lymph Node Dissection**<br>*Howard N. Winfield and William J. Badger* | 811 |
| Chapter 124 | **Laparoscopic Nephrectomy and Partial Nephrectomy**<br>*James A. Brown* | 819 |
| Chapter 125 | **Laparoscopic Nephroureterectomy**<br>*Scott G. Hubosky and Michael D. Fabrizio* | 830 |
| Chapter 126 | **Laparoscopic Renal Procedures: Renal Cystectomy, Biopsy, and Nephropexy**<br>*Chad A. LaGrange and Stephen E. Strup* | 837 |
| Chapter 127 | **Laparoscopic Ablation of Small Renal Masses**<br>*Ilia S. Zeltser and David E. McGinnis* | 842 |
| Chapter 128 | **Donor Nephrectomy: Laparoscopic Techniques**<br>*Erik P. Castle, Rafael Nunez, Costas D. Lallas, and Paul E. Andrews* | 846 |
| Chapter 129 | **Laparoscopic and Robotically Assisted Pyeloplasty in Adults**<br>*Kristofer R. Wagner and Thomas W. Jarrett* | 853 |
| Chapter 130 | **Laparoscopic Adrenalectomy**<br>*Arvin K. George and Louis R. Kavoussi* | 859 |
| Chapter 131 | **Laparoscopic and Robotic Radical Prostatectomy**<br>*Costas D. Lallas and Edouard J. Trabulsi* | 867 |
| Chapter 132 | **Laparoscopic Management of Lymphoceles**<br>*Sean P. Hedican and Stephen Y. Nakada* | 879 |
| Chapter 133 | **Laparoscopic Bladder Procedures: Radical Cystectomy, Partial Cystectomy, Urachal Excision, Diverticulectomy**<br>*Sebastien Crouzet, Georges-Pascal Haber, and Inderbir S. Gill* | 885 |
| Chapter 134 | **Laparoscopic Bladder Neck Suspension**<br>*Richard W. Graham* | 892 |
| Chapter 135 | **Miscellaneous Laparoscopic Urologic Procedures: Calculus, Varicocele, Ureterolysis**<br>*Gordon L. Fifer and Raju Thomas* | 897 |

SECTION X ■ NEW FRONTIERS 905
*Thomas W. Jarrett*

**Chapter 136** **Tissue-Engineering Strategies for Urogenital Repair** 905
*Anthony Atala*

**Chapter 137** **Image-Guided Therapy: Current Practice and Future Directions** 913
*Peter Pinto and Hal B. Hooper*

**Chapter 138** **Robotic Surgery** 919
*David Canes and Mihir M. Desai*

**Chapter 139** **Energy Sources in Urology** 926
*Moses M. Kim and Richard E. Link*

***Index*** 937

# EDITORS

## Editors

**Sam D. Graham, Jr., MD**
Urologic Specialists of Virginia
Medical Director, Thomas Johns Hospital
Richmond, Virginia

**Thomas E. Keane, MD**
Professor and Chair
Department of Urology
Medical University of South Carolina
Charleston, South Carolina

## Consultant Editor

**James F. Glenn, MD, DSc, FACS, FRCS†**
Professor of Surgery
Department of Surgery
Division of Urology
University of Kentucky Medical Center
Lexington, Kentucky

## Associate Editors

**Charles B. Brendler, MD**
Professor and Chief
Section of Urology
University of Chicago Hospitals
Chicago, Illinois
Section: Ureter and Pelvis

**Marc Goldstein, MD, DSc (hon)**
Mathew P. Hardy Distinguished Professor
Cornell Institute for Reproductive Medicine and Urology
Surgeon-in-Chief, Male Reproductive Medicine and Surgery
New York-Presbyterian/Weill Cornell Medical Center
New York, New York
Section: Vas Deferens, Seminal Vesicle, Testis

**Leonard G. Gomella, MD, FACS**
The Bernard W. Godwin Professor of Prostate Cancer
Chairman, Department of Urology
Thomas Jefferson University
Associate Director of Clinical Affairs
Jefferson Kimmel Cancer Center
Philadelphia, Pennsylvania
Section: Laparoscopic Surgery

**E. Ann Gormley, MD**
Professor of Surgery (Urology)
Section of Urology
Department of Surgery
Dartmouth Medical School
Hanover, New Hampshire
Urologist
Section of Urology, Department of Surgery
Dartmouth-Hitchcock Medical Center
Lebanon, New Hampshire
Section: Urethra

**Thomas W. Jarrett, MD**
Professor and Chairman
Department of Urology
George Washington University Medical Center
Washington, DC

**Gerald H. Jordan, MD, FACS, FAAP**
Professor of Urology
Eastern Virginia Medical School
Director of Adult Reconstructive Surgery
The Devine Center for Genitourinary Reconstruction
Sentara Norfolk General Hospital
Devine-Fiveash Urology, Ltd.
Norfolk, Virginia
Section: Penis and Scrotum

**Jerome P. Richie, MD**
Chief, Division of Urology
Brigham and Women's Hospital
Harvard Medical School
Boston, Massachusetts
Section: Adrenal and Renal

**Randall G. Rowland, MD, PhD**
Professor and Chief of Surgery (Urology)
Program Director (Urology)
University of Kentucky College of Medicine
Lexington, Kentucky
Section: Prostate

†Deceased

**H. Gil Rushton, MD**
Department of Urology
George Washington University
Chairman, Urology
Children's National Medical Center
Washington, DC
Section: Pediatric

**Urs E. Studer, MD**
Professor and Chairman
Department of Urology
University Hospital Bern
Bern, Switzerland
Section: Urinary Diversion

# CONTRIBUTORS

**Hassan Abol-Enein MD, PhD**
Professor
Department of Urology
Faculty of Medicine, Mansoura University
Director
Department of Urology
Urology and Nephrology Center
Mansoura, Egypt
Chapter 91

**Alex M. Acosta Miranda, MD**
Assistant Professor
Department of Urology
University of Puerto Rico School of Medicine
Staff Urologist
San Juan Veterans Affairs Hospital
San Juan, Puerto Rico
Chapter 70

**Gary J. Alter, MD**
Assistant Clinical Professor
Division of Plastic Surgery
University of California
Los Angeles, California
Chapter 82

**Paul E. Andrews, MD**
Professor of Urology
Mayo Clinic
Phoenix, Arizona
Chapter 128

**Kenneth W. Angermeier, MD**
Center for Genitourinary Reconstruction
Glickman Urological and Kidney Institute
Cleveland Clinic
Cleveland, Ohio
Chapter 21

**Elizabeth J. Anoia, MD**
Urology Health Specialists, LLC
Abington, Pennsylvania
Chapter 7

**Rodney Appell, MD†**
Vanguard Urology
Houston, Texas
Chapter 39

**Anthony Atala, MD**
William H. Boyce Professor and Chair
Department of Urology
Director
Wake Forest Institute for Regenerative Medicine
Winston-Salem, North Carolina
Chapter 136

**J. Christopher Austin, MD, FAAP, FACS**
Associate Professor, Pediatric Urology
University of Iowa Hospitals and Clinics
Iowa City, Iowa
Chapter 100

**William J. Badger, MD**
Endourology Fellow
The University of Iowa
Department of Urology
Iowa City, Iowa
Chapter 123

**Gopal H. Badlani, MD, FACS**
Professor, Vice Chair of Clinical Affairs
Department of Urology
Wake Forest University School of Medicine
Wake Forest University/Baptist Medical Center
Winston Salem, North Carolina
Chapter 41

**Robert R. Bahnson, MD, FACS**
The Dave Longaberger Chair in Urology
Professor and Chairman
Department of Urology
Ohio State University
Columbus, Ohio
Chapter 22

**Katie N. Ballert, MD**
Assistant Professor of Urology
Department of Surgery
Attending Surgeon
Department of Surgery, Division of Urology
University of Kentucky
Lexington, Kentucky
Chapter 50

**Gaurav Bandi, MD**
Assistant Professor
Department of Urology
Thomas Jefferson University
Philadelphia, Pennsylvania
Chapter 122

†Deceased

**Laurence S. Baskin, MD**
Professor of Urology
University of California San Francisco
Chief, Pediatric Urology
Department of Urology
UCSF Children's Medical Center
San Francisco, California
Chapter 109

**Pierfrancesco Bassi, MD**
Chief and Chairman
Department of Urology
Catholic University School of Medicine
Rome, Italy
Chapter 88

**Martin Bastuba, MD**
Male Fertility Specialists
San Diego, California
Chapter 76

**Ricardo Beduschi, MD**
Chapter 1

**William Bihrle, III, MD**
Associate Professor, Surgery
Dartmouth Medical School
Section Chief, Urology
Dartmouth-Hitchcock Medical Center
Lebanon, New Hampshire
Chapters 37 and 38

**Trinity J. Bivalacqua, MD, PhD**
Assistant Professor of Urology
The James Buchanan Brady Urological Institute
Johns Hopkins Hospital
Baltimore, Maryland
Chapter 73

**Jerry G. Blaivas, MD**
Clinical Professor
Department of Urology
Weill Cornell Medical College
Attending
Department of Urology
New York Presbyterian Hospital
New York, New York
Chapter 33

**Nancy L. Brackett, PhD, HCLD**
Associate Professor
Neurological Surgery and Urology
University of Miami Miller School of Medicine
Miami, Florida
Chapter 61

**James A. Brown, MD**
Associate Professor
Head, Section of Urologic Oncology
Division of Urology
Medical College of Georgia
Augusta, Georgia
Chapter 124

**Jill C. Buckley, MD**
Assistant Professor
Department of Urology
Tufts University School of Medicine
Lahey Clinic Medical Center
Burlington, Massachusetts
Chapter 9

**Arthur L. Burnett, MD, MBA, FACS**
Patrick C. Walsh Professor
Department of Urology
Johns Hopkins University
Johns Hopkins Hospital
Baltimore, Maryland
Chapter 73

**Mark P. Cain, MD, FAAP**
Professor of Urology
Department of Urology
Indiana University
Division of Urology
Riley Hospital for Children
Indianapolis, Indiana
Chapter 121

**Anthony A. Caldamone, MD**
University Urology Associates
Providence, Rhode Island
Chapter 106

**Anne Pelletier Cameron, MD**
Assistant Professor
Clinical Lecturer
Department of Urology
University of Michigan
Ann Arbor, Michigan
Chapters 18 and 40

**David Canes, MD**
Lahey Institute of Urology
Parkland Medical Center
Derry, New Hampshire
Chapter 138

**Douglas A. Canning, MD**
Division of Urology,
Children's Hospital of Philadelphia
Philadelphia, Pennsylvania
Chapter 100

**Glenn M. Cannon Jr., MD**
Fellow, Pediatric Urology
Harvard Medical School
Department of Urology
Boston, Massachusetts
Chapter 116

**Brett S. Carver, MD**
Assistant Member
Department of Surgery
Assistant Attending
Department of Surgery
Memorial Sloan-Kettering Cancer Center
New York, New York
Chapter 63

**Culley C. Carson, MD**
Rhodes Distinguished Professor
Chief of Urology
University of North Carolina
Chapel Hill, North Carolina
Chapter 74

**Anthony J. Casale, MD**
Department of Urology
University of Louisville School of Medicine
Louisville, Kentucky
Chapter 118

**Pasquale Casale, MD**
Assistant Professor of Urology in Surgery,
University of Pennsylvania
Children's Hospital of Philadelphia
Philadelphia, Pennsylvania
Chapter 115

**Erik P. Castle, MD**
Associate Professor of Urology
Urologic Oncology
Laparoscopic and Robotic Urology
Mayo Clinic
Phoenix, Arizona
Chapter 128

**William J. Catalona, MD**
Northwestern University
Feinberg School of Medicine
Chicago, Illinois
Chapter 28

**Wolfgang H. Cerwinka, MD**
Clinical Instructor
Department of Urology
Emory University School of Medicine
Attending Physician
Department of Pediatric Urology
Children's Healthcare of Atlanta
Atlanta, Georgia
Chapter 104

**R. Duane Cespedes, MD**
Director, Female Urology
Wilford Hall Medical Center
Lackland AFB, Texas
Chapter 18

**Peter T. K. Chan, MD, CM, MSc, FRCS(C), FACS**
Associate Professor
Department of Surgery
McGill University
Director of Male Reproductive Medicine
Department of Urology
McGill University Health Center
Montreal, Quebec, Canada
Chapter 56

**Sam S. Chang, MD, FACS**
Associate Professor
Department of Urologic Surgery
Vanderbilt University
Department of Urologic Surgery
Vanderbilt University Medical Center
Nashville, Tennessee
Chapters 3 and 17

**Kenneth D. Chavin, MD**
Professor of Surgery, Microbiology, and Immunology
Department of Surgery
Medical University of South Carolina
Charleston, South Carolina
Chapter 10

**Clinton W. Collins, MD**
Chief Resident, Division of Urology
Virginia Commonwealth University School of Medicine
Richmond, Virginia
Chapter 13

**Craig V. Comiter, MD**
Associate Professor
Department of Urology
Stanford University Medical School
Stanford, California
Associate Professor
Department of Urology
Stanford Hospital and Clinics
Palo Alto, California
Chapter 45

**Sarah Conley, MD**
Resident
Department of Urology
Mayo Clinic
Phoenix, Arizona
Chapter 96

**William T. Conner, MD**
Division of Urology
University of Kentucky Medical Center
Lexington, Kentucky
Chapter 26

**Michael S. Cookson, MD, FACS**
Professor
Department of Urologic Surgery
Vanderbilt University Medical Center
Nashville, Tennessee
Chapters 3 and 17

**Christopher S. Cooper, MD**
Professor
Department of Urology
University of Iowa
Associate Dean for Student Affairs and Curriculum
University of Iowa Carver College of Medicine
Director, Pediatric Urology
Children's Hospital of Iowa
Iowa City, Iowa
Chapter 113

**Sean T. Corbett, MD**
Assistant Professor of Urology
University of Virginia Health System
Charlottesville, Virginia
Chapter 112

**Sebastien Crouzet, MD**
Glickman Urological and Kidney Institute
Cleveland Clinic
Cleveland, Ohio
Chapter 133

**Mihir M. Desai, MD**
Director, Stevan B. Streem Center for Endourology
Glickman Urological and Kidney Institute
Cleveland Clinic
Cleveland, Ohio
Chapter 138

**Timothy O. Davies, MD**
Instructor, Adult and Pediatric Reconstructive Fellow
Department of Urology
Eastern Virginia Medical School
Norfolk, Virginia
Chapters 68 and 81

**Ross M. Decter, MD**
Associate Professor of Surgery
Department of Surgery
Milton S. Hershey Medical Center
Penn State College of Medicine
Hershey, Pennsylvania
Chapter 97

**W. Robert DeFoor, Jr., MD, MPH**
Associate Professor
Division of Pediatric Urology
Cincinnati Children's Hospital
Cincinnati, Ohio
Chapter 95

**Scott Delacroix, Jr., MD**
Department of Urologic Surgery
Ochsner Clinic Foundation
New Orleans, Louisiana
Chapter 52

**Ralph W. deVere-White, MD**
Department of Urology and Cancer Center
University of California at Davis
Sacramento, California
Chapter 27

**Nivedita Bhatta-Dhar, MD**
Assistant Professor of Urology
Wayne State University School of Medicine
Detroit, Michigan
Chapter 85

**David A. Diamond, MD**
Professor
Department of Urological Surgery
Harvard Medical School
Associate
Department of Urology
Children's Hospital
Boston, Massachusetts
Chapter 105

**Roger R. Dmochowski, MD**
Professor
Department of Urologic Surgery
Vanderbilt University
Director, Vanderbilt Continence Center
Department of Urologic Surgery
Vanderbilt Medical Center
Nashville, Tennessee
Chapter 49

**Steven G. Docimo, MD**
Professor of Urology, Director Pediatric Urology
Department of Urology
University of Pittsburgh School of Medicine
Vice President, Medical Affairs and Chief Medical Officer
Department of Medical Affairs
Children's Hospital of Pittsburgh of UPMC
Pittsburgh, Pennsylvania
Chapter 114

**Sherri M. Donat, MD, FACS**
Associate Professor
Department of Urology
Weill Medical College of Cornell University
Associate Attending Surgeon
Dept of Surgery/Division of Urology
Memorial Sloan-Kettering Cancer Center
New York, New York
Chapter 63

**Ahmed M. El-Zawahry, MD**
Resident in Urology
Department of Urology
Medical University of South Carolina
Charleston, South Carolina
Chapter 32

**Justin D. Ellett, PhD**
Student
Department of Microbiology/Immunology
Surgery, Division of Transplant
Medical University of South Carolina
Charleston, South Carolina
Chapter 10

**Michael D. Fabrizio, MD, FACS**
Associate Professor
Department of Urology
Eastern Virginia Medical School
Sentara Medical Group
Department of Urology
Sentara Norfolk General Hospital
Norfolk, Virginia
Chapter 125

**Walid A. Farhat, MD**
Associate Professor
Department of Surgery
University of Toronto
Pediatric Urologist
Department of Urology
Hospital for Sick Children
Toronto, Ontario
Chapter 115

**Kevin M. Feber, MD**
Pediatric Urologist
William Beaumount Children's Hospital
Royal Oak, Michigan
Chapter 99

**Gordon L. Fifer, MD**
Department of Urology
Tulane University Health Sciences Center
New Orleans, Louisiana
Chapter 135

**Margit Fisch, MD, FEBV, FEAEV**
Professor of Urology
Department of Urology and Pediatric Urology
Center of Operative Medicine
University of Hamburg
Director, Department of Urology and Pediatric Urology
UKE University Clinic Eppendorf
Hamburg, Germany
Chapters 84 and 93

**John A. Fortney, MD**
Medical University of South Carolina
Charleston, South Carolina
Chapter 30

**Ludgar Franzaring, MD**
Chapter 90

**John P. Gearhart, MD**
Professor and Director of Pediatric Urology
Department of Urology
Johns Hopkins University School of Medicine
Baltimore, Maryland
Chapter 111

**Arvin K. George, MD**
Resident Physician
The Smith Institute of Urology
North Shore-Long Island Jewish Health System
New Hyde Park, New York
Chapter 130

**Elmar W. Gerharz, MD**
Department of Urology and Pediatric Urology
Julius Maximilians-University Medical School
Würzburg, Germany
Chapter 92

**Mohamed A. Ghoneim, MD**
Professor of Urology
Department of Urology
Nephrology Center
Mansoura, Egypt
Chapter 91

**Alienor S. Gilchrist, MD**
Resident in Urology, Department of Urology
University of Texas Southwestern Medical Center
Dallas, Texas
Chapter 34

**Inderbir S. Gill, MD, MCh**
Chair, Department of Urology
USC Institute of Urology
Keck School of Medicine
Los Angeles, California
Chapter 133

**Kenneth I. Glassberg, MD, FAAP, FACS**
Director, Division of Pediatric Urology
Morgan Stanley Children's Hospital of New York-Presbyterian
Professor of Neurology, Columbia University
College of Physicians and Surgeons
New York, New York
Chapter 108

**David A. Goldfarb, MD**
Professor of Surgery
Glickman Urological and Kidney Institute
Cleveland Clinic Lerner College of Medicine
Director, Center for Renal Transplantations
Department of Urology
Cleveland Clinic
Cleveland, Ohio
Chapter 12

**Irwin Goldstein, MD**
Clinical Professor
Department of Urology
University of California, San Diego
Director
Department of Sexual Medicine
Alvarado Hospital
San Diego, California
Chapter 76

**Marc Goldstein, MD, DSc (hon)**
Matthew P. Hardy Distinguished Professor
Cornell Institute for Reproductive Medicine and Urology
Surgeon-in-Chief, Male Reproductive
Medicine and Surgery
New York-Presbyterian/Weill Cornell Medical Center
New York, New York
Chapters 53, 57, 60A, 62, and 79

**Leonard G. Gomella, MD, FACS**
The Bernard W. Godwin Professor of Prostate Cancer
Chairman, Department of Urology
Thomas Jefferson University
Associate Director of Clinical Affairs
Jefferson Kimmel Cancer Center
Philadelphia, Pennsylvania
Chapter 122

**E. Ann Gormley, MD**
Professor of Surgery (Urology)
Section of Urology
Department of Surgery
Dartmouth Medical School
Hanover, New Hampshire
Urologist
Section of Urology, Department of Surgery
Dartmouth-Hitchcock Medical Center
Lebanon, New Hampshire
Chapter 31

**Richard W. Grady, MD**
Associate Professor of Urology
The University of Washington School of Medicine
Children's Hospital and Regional Medical Center
Seattle, Washington
Chapter 110

**Richard W. Graham, MD, FACS**
Urologic Specialists of Virginia
Richmond, Virginia
Chapter 134

**Sam D. Graham, Jr., MD**
Urologic Specialists of Virginia
Medical Director, Thomas Johns Hospital
Richmond, Virginia
Chapters 1, 24, 29, and 69

**Uri Gur, MD**
Fellow, Adult and Pediatric Reconstructive Urology
Eastern Virginia Medical School
Norfolk, Virginia
Chapters 72 and 78

**Georges-Pascal Haber, MD**
Section of Laparoscopic and Robotic Surgery
Glickman Urological and Kidney Institute
The Cleveland Clinic Foundation
Cleveland, Ohio
Chapter 133

**J. Nathaniel Hamilton, MD**
Resident Physician
Department of Urology
Medical University of South Carolina
Charleston, South Carolina
Chapter 14

**Misop Han, MD**
John Hopkins University
School of Medicine
Baltimore, Maryland
Chapter 28

**Paul Hanissian, MD**
Assistant Professor
Department of Obstetrics and Gynecology
Dartmouth Medical School
Hanover, New Hampshire
Department of Obstetrics and Gynecology
Dartmouth-Hitchcock Medical Center
Lebanon, New Hampshire
Chapter 42

**Richard E. Hautmann, MD, MD (hon)**
Professor of Urology
Department of Urology
University of Ulm Medical Faculty
Chief of Department of Urology
Urologische Universitasklinik
Ulm, Germany
Chapter 87

**Sean P. Hedican, MD**
Associate Professor
Department of Urology
University of Wisconsin School of Medicine
and Public Health
Madison, Wisconsin
Chapter 132

**Axel Heidenreich, MD**
Professor and Chairman of Urology
Department of Urology
RWTH University Aachen
Aachen, Germany
Chapter 65

**Rudolf Hohenfellner, MD**
Professor of Urology
Department of Urology
Emer. Director
Mainz Medical School
Mainz, Germany
Chapters 84 and 93

**Hal B. Hooper, MD**
Resident
Department of Urology
Georgetown University Hospital
Washington, DC
Chapter 137

**Carin V. Hopps, MD**
Clinical Assistant Professor of Urology
Medical University of Ohio
Toledo, Ohio
Chapter 79

**Scott G. Hubosky, MD**
Assistant Professor of Urology
Thomas Jefferson University Hospital
Philadelphia, Pennsylvania
Chapter 125

**Michael S. Ingber, MD**
Clinical Fellow
Glickman Urological and Kidney Institute
Cleveland Clinic
Cleveland, Ohio
Chapter 23

**Thomas W. Jarrett, MD**
Professor and Chairman
Department of Urology
George Washington University Medical Center
Washington, DC
Chapter 129

**Stephan Jeschke, MD**
University of Bern
Department of Urology
Inselspital
Bern, Switzerland
Chapter 86

**Michael A. S. Jewett, MD, FRCSC, FACS**
Professor of Surgery (Urology)
Department of Oncology
University of Toronto
Farquharson Clinical Research Chair in Oncology
Division of Urology, Department of Surgical Oncology
Princess Margaret Hospital, University Health
Toronto, Ontario, Canada
Chapter 66

**Gerald H. Jordan, MD, FACS, FAAP**
Professor of Urology
Eastern Virginia Medical School
Director of Adult Reconstructive Surgery
The Devine Center for Genitourinary Reconstruction
Sentara Norfolk General Hospital
Devine-Fiveash Urology, Ltd.
Norfolk, Virginia
Chapters 68, 72 and 78

**David B. Joseph, MD, FACS, FAAP**
Professor of Surgery
Department of Surgery
University of Alabama at Birmingham
School of Medicine
Chief of Pediatric Urology
Department of Surgery
Children's Hospital
Birmingham, Alabama
Chapter 101

**George W. Kaplan, MD**
Clinical Professor
Department of Surgery (Urology) and Pediatrics
University of California at San Diego School of Medicine
Chief Department of Urology
Rady Children's Hospital San Diego
San Diego, California
Chapter 119

**Evan J. Kass, MD, FAAP, FACS**
Chief of Pediatric Urology
Department of Urology
William Beaumont Children's Hospital
Rouaz Oak, Michigan
Chapter 99

**Melissa R. Kaufman, MD, PhD**
Assistant Professor
Vanderbilt University, Department of Urologic Surgery
Nashville, Tennessee
Chapter 49

**Louis R. Kavoussi, MD**
Chairman and Waldbaum Professor of Urology
Smith Institute for Urology
Hofstra University School of Medicine
North Shore-LIJ Health System
Long Island, New York
Chapter 130

**Thomas E. Keane, MD**
Professor and Chair
Department of Urology
Medical University of South Carolina
Charleston, South Carolina
Chapter 29

**Howard H. Kim, MD**
Fellow and Instructor
Department of Reproductive
Medicine and Urology
Weill Cornell Medical College
Assistant
Department of Urology
New York-Presbyterian/Weill Cornell
Medical Center
New York, New York
Chapters 53, 57 and 62

**Ja-Hong Kim, MD**
Department of Urology
University of California
Los Angeles, California
Chapters 47 and 48

**Moses M. Kim, MD**
Scoot Department of Urology
Baylor College of Medicine
Houston, Texas
Chapter 139

**Andrew J. Kirsch, MD, FAAP, FACS**
Clinical Professor of Urology
Department of Pediatric Urology
Children's Healthcare of Atlanta
Emory University School of Medicine
Atlanta, Georgia
Chapter 104

**Adam P. Klausner, MD**
Associate Professor, Division of Urology
Virginia Commonwealth University School of Medicine
Richmond, Virginia
Chapter 13

**Eric A. Klein, MD**
Chairman
Glickman Urological and Kidney Institute
Professor of Surgery
Cleveland Clinic Lerner College of Medicine
Cleveland, Ohio
Chapters 21 and 83

**Chester J. Koh, MD, FAAP**
Division of Pediatric Urology
Childrens Hospital Los Angeles
Los Angeles, California
Chapter 105

**Harry P. Koo, MD, FAAP, FACS**
Barbara and William Thalhimer Professor
Division of Urology
Virginia Commonwealth University School of Medicine
Chairman of Urology
Division of Urology/Department of Surgery
VCU Medical Center-Medical College of Virginia
Richmond, Virginia
Chapter 67

**Venkatesh Krishnamurthi, MD**
Glickman Urological and Kidney Institute
Cleveland Clinic
Cleveland, Ohio
Chapter 12

**Sanjaya Kumar, MD, MPH**
President and Chief Medical Officer
Quantros, Inc.
Milpitas, California
Chapter 5

**Chad A. LaGrange, MD**
Assistant Professor
Department of Surgery
University of Nebraska
Omaha, Nebraska
Chapter 126

**Costas D. Lallas, MD, FACS**
Assistant Professor
Department of Urology
Thomas Jefferson University
Assistant Professor
Department of Urology
Jefferson Kimmel Cancer Center
Philadelphia, Pennsylvania
Chapters 128 and 131

**Cheryl T. Lee, MD**
Associate Professor
Department of Urology
University of Michigan
Ann Arbor, Michigan
Chapter 16

**Michael C. Lee, MD**
Resident Physician
Glickman Urological and Kidney Institute
Cleveland Clinic
Cleveland, Ohio
Chapter 83

**Richard S. Lee, MD**
Urology Resident
University of Washington
Seattle, Washington
Chapter 116

**Gary E. Lemack, MD**
Professor and Residency Program Director
Department of Urology
University of Texas Southwestern Medical Center
Dallas, Texas
Chapter 34

**Jeffrey A. Leslie, MD**
Assistant Professor
Department of Urology and Pediatrics
University of Texas Health Science Center at San Antonio
Pediatric Urologist
Department of Urology
Christus Santa Rosa Children's Hospital
San Antonio, Texas
Chapter 117

**Michael Leveridge, MD, FRCSC**
Clinical Fellow-Urologic Oncology
Division of Urology
University of Toronto
Clinical Fellow-Urologic Oncology
Department of Surgical Oncology
Division of Urology
University Health Network
Princess Margaret Hospital
Toronto, Ontario
Chapter 66

**Christina Lewicky-Gaupp, MD**
Urogynecology Fellow
Department of Obstetrics and Gynecology
University of Michigan
Ann Arbor, Michigan
Chapter 40

**Ronald W. Lewis, MD**
Medical College of Georgia
Augusta, Georgia
Chapter 75

**John A. Libertino, MD**
Professor
Department of Urology
Tufts University School of Medicine
Boston, Massachusetts
Chair
Institute of Urology
Lahey Clinic Medical Center
Burlington, Massachusetts
Chapter 6

**Mark R. Licht, MD**
Urology Associates of South Florida
Boca Raton, Florida
Chapter 75

**James E. Lingeman, MD**
Director of Research
Department of Urology
Methodist Hospital Institute for Kidney Stone Disease
Indianapolis, Indiana
Chapter 25

**Richard E. Link, MD, PhD**
Associate Professor of Urology
Director, Division of Endourology and Minimally Invasive Surgery
Scott Department of Urology
Baylor College of Medicine
Houston, Texas
Chapter 139

**Larry I. Lipshultz, MD**
Professor, Scott Department of Urology
Lester and Sue Smith Chair in Reproductive Medicine
Chief, Division of Male Reproductive Medicine and Surgery
Baylor College of Medicine
Houston, Texas
Chapter 60B

**Jeffrey C. Lou, MD**
Urologic Specialists of Virginia
Richmond, Virginia
Chapter 29

**Lior Lowenstein, MD, MS**
Urogynecologist
Obstetrics and Gynecology
Ruth and Bruce Rapappport Technion School of Medicine
Rambam Medical Center
Haifa, Israel
Chapter 51

**Charles M. Lynne, MD, FACS**
Victor A. Politano Professor of Urology
University of Miami Miller School of Medicine
Miami, Florida
Chapter 61

**Ziv Maianski, MD**
Visiting Fellow
Department of Surgery, McGill University
Visiting Fellow
Department of Urology
St. Mary's Hospital
Montreal, Quebec, Canada
Chapter 58

**John H. Makari, MD, MHA, MA**
Assistant Professor
Department of Surgery, Division of Urology
University of Connecticut School of Medicine
Farmington, Connecticut
Attending Surgeon
Department of Urology
Connecticut Children's Medical Center
Hartford, Connecticut
Chapter 107

**David T. Marshall, MD, MS**
Associate Professor, Resident Training Program Director
Department of Radiation Oncology
Medical University of South Carolina
Attending Physician
Department of Radiation Oncology
Medical University Hospital
Charleston, South Carolina
Chapter 30

**Fray F. Marshall, MD**
Professor of Urology
Emory University School of Medicine
Professor and Chairman
Department of Urology, The Emory Clinic
Emory University School of Medicine
Atlanta, Georgia
Chapter 4

**Frances M. Martin, MD**
Urology Resident
The University of Kentucky
Chandler Medical Center
Lexington, Kentucky
Chapter 26

**Viraj A. Master, MD**
Assistant Professor
Urology and Winship Cancer Institute
Emory University
Attending Surgeon
Department of Urology
Emory University Hospital
Atlanta, Georgia
Chapter 4

**Brian R. Matlaga, MD**
James Buchanan Brady Urological Institute
The Johns Hopkins University School of Medicine
Baltimore, Maryland
Chapter 25

**Sarah E. McAchran, MD**
Assistant Professor
Department of Urology
UW Madison School of Medicine & Public Health
Madison, Wisconsin
Chapter 46

**Irene McAleer, MD**
Assistant Clinical Professor
Department of Pediatrics
University of California, San Francisco
Pediatric Urologist
Department of Urology
Children's Hospital Central California
Madera, California
Chapter 119

**Jack W. McAninch, MD**
Professor of Urology
Chief of Urology
San Francisco General Hospital
San Francisco, California
Chapters 9, 36 and 77

**Kurt A. McCammon, MD**
Assistant Professor and Program Director
Department of Urology
Eastern Virginia Medical School
Norfolk, Virginia
Chapter 81

**W. Scott McDougal, MD**
Walter Kerr, Jr. Professor of Urology
Department of Urology
Harvard Medical School
Chief of Urology
Department of Urology
Massachusetts General Hospital
Boston, Massachusetts
Chapter 71

**John W. McGillicuddy MD**
Assistant Professor of Surgery
Medical University of South Carolina
Charleston, South Carolina
Chapter 10

**David E. McGinnis, MD**
Clinical Assistant Professor of Urology
Thomas Jefferson University
The Bryn Mawr Urology Group
Rosemont, Pennsylvania
Chapter 127

**Edward J. McGuire, MD**
Professor
Department of Urology
University of Michigan
Ann Arbor, Michigan
Chapters 18 and 40

**Leslie T. McQuiston, MD**
Pediatric Surgery
Dartmouth-Hitchcock Medical Center
Lebanon, New Hampshire
Chapter 106

**Aaron J. Milbank, MD**
Metro Urology Robotic Surgery Center
Woodbury, Minnesota
Chapter 21

**Rosalia Misseri, MD**
Assistant Professor
Indiana University School of Medicine
Department of Urology, Riley Hospital for Children
Indianapolis, Indiana
Chapter 108

**Blake W. Moore, MD**
Division of Urology
Virginia Commonwealth University
Richmond, Virginia
Chapter 67

**Allen F. Morey, MD**
Professor of Urology
University of Texas Southwestern
Dallas, Texas
Chapter 77

**Elizabeth R. Mueller, MD, MSME**
Assistant Professor
Department of Urology and Obstetrics/Gynecology
Medical Director
Female Pelvic Medicine and Reconstructive Surgery
Loyola University Medical Center
Maywood, Illinois
Chapter 51

**Stephen Y. Nakada, MD**
The David T. Uehling Professor of Urology
Chairman, Division of Urology
UW Madison School of Medicine and Public Health
Madison, Wisconsin
Chapter 132

**Kenneth G. Nepple, MD**
Resident, Department of Urology
University of Iowa
Iowa City, Iowa
Chapter 113

**John A. Nesbitt, MD**
Attending Urologic Surgeon
Department of Surgery
T.J. Sampson Community Hospital
Glasgow, Kentucky
Chapter 80

**Victor W. Nitti, MD**
Professor and Vice Chairman
Department of Urology
New York University School of Medicine
Attending Physician
Department of Urology
NYU Langone Medical Center
New York, New York
Chapter 50

**Thomas E. Novak, MD**
Fellow, Pediatric Urology
James Buchanan Brady Urological Institute
Johns Hopkins Medical Institutions
Baltimore, Maryland
Chapter 111

**Unyime O. Nseyo, MD, FACS**
University of Florida College of Medicine
Chief, Urology Section
NF/SG Veterans Health System
Gainesville, Florida
Chapter 1

**David M. Nudell, MD**
El Camino Hospital
San Jose, California
Chapter 60B

**Rafael Nunez-Nateras, MD**
Research Fellow
Mayo Clinic
Phoenix, Arizona
Chapter 128

**Dana A. Ohl, MD**
Department of Urology
University of Michigan
Ann Arbor, Michigan
Chapter 61

**Joon-Ha Ok, MD**
Department of Urology and Cancer Center
University of California at Davis
Sacramento, California
Chapter 27

**Michael C. Ost, MD**
University of Pittsburgh Medical Center
Division of Pediatric Urology, Children's Hospital of Pittsburgh
Pittsburgh, Pennsylvania
Chapter 114

**Francesco Pagano, MD**
Professor of Urology
Venetian Institute of Molecular Medicine
Consultant
Department of Urology
S. Antonio Hospital
Padova, Italy
Chapter 88

**Michael L. Paik, MD**
Northwest Urological Associates SC
Arlington Heights, Illinois
Chapter 7

**Bhavin N. Patel, MD**
Resident
Department of Urology
Wake Forest University
Winston-Salem, North Carolina
Chapter 41

**Kenneth M. Peters, MD**
Chairman
Department of Urology
William Beaumont Hospital
Royal Oak, Michigan
Chapter 23

**Jonathan C. Picard, MD**
Assistant Professor
Department of Urology
Medical University of South Carolina
Charleston, South Carolina
Chapter 14

**Peter-Pinto, MD**
Director, Fellowship Program
Urologic Oncology Branch
National Cancer Institute
National Institutes of Health
Bethesda, Maryland
Chapter 137

**Kamal S. Pohar, MD**
Assistant Professor, Department of Urology
Ohio State University James Cancer Hospital
Louis Levy Professor of Urologic Oncology
Ohio State University
Columbus, Ohio
Chapter 22

**Hans G. Pohl, MD**
Assistant Professor, Pediatrics and Urology
George Washington University
Children's National Medical Center
Washington, DC
Chapter 120

**John C. Pope, IV, MD**
Associate Professor of Urologic Surgery and Pediatrics
Vanderbilt University Department of Urologic Surgery
Division of Pediatric Urology
Vanderbilt Children's Hospital
Nashville, Tennessee
Chapter 107

**Raj S. Pruthi, MD**
Department of Urology
University of North Carolina at Chapel Hill
Chapel Hill, North Carolina
Chapter 27

**Rajveer S. Purohit, MD**
Clinical Instructor of Urology
Weill Medical College of Cornell University
New York, New York
Chapter 33

**Antonio Puras Baez, MD, FACS**
Professor
Department of Urology
Chief, Department of Urology
University of Puerto Rico, School of Medicine
San Juan, Puerto Rico
Chapter 70

**Susanne A. Quallich, ANP-BC, NP-C, CUNP**
Andrology NP
Department of Urology
University of Michigan
Ann Arbor, Michigan
Chapter 61

**Raymond R. Rackley, MD**
Glickman Urological and Kidney Institute
Cleveland Clinic
Center for Female Pelvic Medicine
and Reconstructive Surgery
Cleveland, Ohio
Chapter 46

**Michelle L. Ramírez, MD**
Department of Urology and Cancer Center
University of California at Davis
Sacramento, California
Chapter 27

**Shlomo Raz, MD**
Professor of Urology.
UCLA School of Medicine
Chief, Pelvic Medicine and Reconstructive Urology
Los Angeles, California
Chapters 47 and 48

**Pramod P. Reddy, MD**
Associate Professor of Clinical Surgery
Cincinnati Children's Hospital Medical Center
Cincinnati, Ohio
Chapter 95

**Martin I. Resnick, MD**[†]
Department of Urology
University Hospitals School of Medicine
Case Western Reserve University
Cleveland, Ohio
Chapter 7

**Audrey C. Rhee**
Medical College of Georgia
Augusta, Georgia
Chapter 75

**Leslie M. Rickey, MD**
Assistant Professor
Division of Urology, Department of Surgery
Female Pelvic Medicine and Reconstructive Surgery
University of Maryland School of Medicine
Baltimore, Maryland
Chapter 43

**Hubertus Riedmiller, MD**
Professor and Chairman
Department of Urology and Pediatric Urology
Julius Maximilians-University Medical School
Wurzburg, Germany
Chapter 92

**Richard C. Rink, MD**
Robert A. Garrett Professor of Pediatric Urology
Chief, Pediatric Urology
James Whitcomb Riley Hospital for Children
Indiana University School of Medicine
Indianapolis, Indiana
Chapter 117

[†]Deceased

**Michael L. Ritchey, MD**
Professor of Urology, Department of Urology
Mayo Clinic College of Medicine
Chief of Surgery, Department of Urology
Phoenix Children's Hospital
Phoenix, Arizona
Chapter 96

**Daniel I. Rosenstein, MD**
Associate Chief, Department of Urology
Santa Clara Valley Medical Center
Clinical Faculty, Stanford University
San Jose, California
Chapter 77

**David R. Roth, MD**
Professor of Urology and Pediatrics
Scott Department of Urology and Department of Pediatrics
Baylor College of Medicine
Pediatric Urology Service
Texas Children's Hospital
Houston, Texas
Chapter 112

**Stephan Roth, MD**
Director
Department of Urology and Pediatric Urology
University of Witten/Herdecke
Klinikum Wuppertal
Wuppertal, Germany
Chapter 94

**Eric S. Rovner, MD**
Professor of Urology, Department of Urology
Attending, Department of Urology
Medical University of South Carolina
Charleston, South Carolina
Chapter 32

**Randall G. Rowland, MD, PhD**
Professor and Chief of Surgery (Urology)
Program Director (Urology)
University of Kentucky College of Medicine
Lexington, Kentucky
Chapter 26

**H. Gil Rushton, MD**
Department of Urology
George Washington University
Chairman, Urology
Children's National Medical Center
Washington, DC
Chapter 98

**Jay I. Sandlow, MD**
Professor and Vice-Chair
Departments of Urology and Obstetrics/Gynecology
Medical College of Wisconsin
Milwaukee, Wisconsin
Chapter 54

**Harriette M. Scarpero, MD**
Assistant Professor
Department of Urologic Surgery
Vanderbilt University Medical Center
Nashville, Tennessee
Chapter 49

**Anthony J. Schaeffer, MD**
Herman L. Kretschmer Professor
Chairman, Department of Urology
Feinberg School of Medicine
Northwestern University
Chairman, Department of Urology
Northwestern Memorial Hospital
Chicago, Illinois
Chapter 8

**Jörg Schede, MD**
Department of Urology
Mainz Medical School
Mainz, Germany
Chapter 93

**Peter N. Schlegel, MD**
Professor and Chairman
Department of Urology
Weill Cornell Medical College
Urologist in Chief, Department of Urology
New York-Presbyterian Hospital
New York, New York
Chapter 59

**Curtis A. Sheldon, MD**
Director, Urology
Professor of Surgery
University of Cincinnati College of Medicine
Cincinnati Children's Hospital Medical Center
Cincinnati, Ohio
Chapter 95

**Donald G. Skinner, MD**
Professor and Chairman, Department of Urology
USC Keck School of Medicine
Los Angeles, California
Chapter 89

**Ariana L. Smith, MD**
Fellow in Female Urology, Urodynamics and Pelvic Reconstructive Surgery
David Geffen School of Medicine, UCLA
Los Angeles, California
Chapters 47 and 48

**Howard M. Snyder, III, MD**
Professor of Urology
University of Pennsylvania
Philadelphia, Pennsylvania
Chapter 102

**Jens Sønksen, MD, PhD, DMSci**
Professor of Urology
Head, Section of Male Infertility and Microsurgery
Department of Urology, Herlev Hospital
University of Copenhagen
Copenhagen, Denmark
Chapter 61

**Douglas G. Stein, MD**
Attending Surgeon, Division of Surgical Subspecialties
University Community Hospital
Tampa, Florida
Chapter 55

**John P. Stein, MD**[†]
Associate Professor of Urology
USC Keck School of Medicine
Los Angeles, California
Chapter 89

**Raimund Stein, MD, FEAPU**
Assistant Professor of Urology
Department of Urology
Johannes Gutenberg University
Mainz, Germany
Chapter 84

**Peter L. Steinberg, MD**
Chief Resident
Section of Urology, Department of General Surgery
Dartmouth-Hitchcock Medical Center
Lebanon, New Hampshire
Chapters 37 and 38

**Stephen E. Strup, MD**
University of Kentucky
Division of Urology
Lexington, Kentucky
Chapter 126

**Urs E. Studer, MD**
Professor and Chairman
Department of Urology
University Hospital Bern
Bern, Switzerland
Chapters 85 and 86

**David A. Swanson, MD**
Clinical Professor, Department of Urology
The University of Texas MD Anderson Cancer Center
Houston, Texas
Chapter 64

**Danielle D. Sweeney, MD**
University of Pittsburgh Medical Center
Division of Pediatric Urology, Children's Hospital of Pittsburgh
Pittsburgh, Pennsylvania
Chapter 114

**Shahin Tabatabaei, MD**
Assistant Professor of Surgery
Department of Urology
Harvard Medical School
Assistant Professor of Surgery
Department of Urology
Massachusetts General Hospital
Boston, Massachusetts
Chapter 71

**Samir S. Taneja, MD**
The James M. Neissa and Janet Riha Neissa
Associate Professor of Urologic Oncology
Director, Division of Urologic Oncology
New York University
Director, Division of Urologic Oncology
NYU Langone Medical Center
New York, New York
Chapter 2

**Cigdem Tanrikut, MD**
Assistant Professor of Surgery (Urology)
Adjunct Assistant Professor of Urology and Reproductive Medicine
Harvard Medical School
Assistant in Urology, Department of Urology
Massachusetts General Hospital
Boston, Massachusetts
Weill Medical College of Cornell University
New York, New York
Chapter 60A

**Rodney J. Taylor, MD**
University of Louisville Medical Center
Louisville, Kentucky
Chapter 11

**Raju Thomas, MD**
Professor and Chair
Department of Urology
Tulane University Health Sciences Center
New Orleans, Louisiana
Chapter 135

**Joachim W. Thüroff, MD**
Professor and Chairman
Department of Urology
University Medical Center
Johannes Gutenberg University
Mainz, Germany
Chapters 84, 90 and 93

**Edouard J. Trabulsi, MD**
Associate Professor of Urology
Kimmel Cancer Center
Thomas Jefferson University
Philadelphia, Pennsylvania
Chapter 131

**Burkhard Ubrig, MD**
Department of Urology and Pediatric Urology
Witten/Herdecke University
Klinikum Wuppertal GmbH
Wuppertal, Germany
Chapter 94

**Sandip Vasavada, MD**
Associate Professor, Department of Urology
Cleveland Clinic
Cleveland, Ohio
Chapter 46

**Davis P. Viprakasit, MD**
Chief Resident, Department of Urology
Northwestern University Feinberg School of Medicine
Chicago, Illinois
Chapter 8

**Bryan B. Voelzke, MD**
Assistant Professor
Department of Urology
Harborview Medical Center and The University of Washington Medical Center
Seattle, Washington
Chapter 36

[†]Deceased

**Kristofer R. Wagner, MD**
Director of Robotic Surgery
Assistant Professor of Surgery
Division of Urology
Scott and White Health System
Texas A&M Health Science Center College of Medicine
Temple, Texas
Chapter 129

**Jack R. Walter, MD**
Duke University Medical Center
Durham, North Carolina
Chapter 35

**George D. Webster, MB, FRCS**
Professor of Urologic Surgery
Division of Urology
Duke University Medical Center
Durham, North Carolina
Chapter 35

**Alon Z. Weizer, MD, MS**
Assistant Professor
Department of Urology
University of Michigan
Ann Arbor, Michigan
Chapter 16

**O. Lenaine Westney, MD**
Associate Professor
MD Anderson Cancer Center
Houston, Texas
Chapters 20 and 44

**James Whiteside, MD**
Assistant Professor, Department of Obstetrics and Gynecology
Dartmouth Medical School
Division of Urogynecology and Reconstructive Pelvic Surgery
Dartmouth-Hitchcock Medical Center
Lebanon, New Hampshire
Chapter 42

**Howard N. Winfield, MD, FACS, FRCS(c)**
Professor of Urology and Transplantation
Department of Urology
University of Iowa
Hospitals and Clinics
Iowa City, Iowa
Chapter 123

**J. Christian Winters, MD**
Professor and Chairman
Department of Urology
Louisiana State University
New Orleans, Louisiana
Chapter 52

**J. Stuart Wolf, Jr., MD**
The David A. Bloom Professor
Department of Urology
Chief, Division of Minimally Invasive Urology
University of Michigan
Ann Arbor, Michigan
Chapter 19

**Hsi-Yang Wu, MD**
Assistant Professor of Urology
University of Pittsburgh
Children's Hospital of Pittsburgh
Pittsburgh, Pennsylvania
Chapter 102

**Chad Wotkowicz, MD**
Chief Resident
Department of Urology
Lahey Clinic
Burlington, Massachusetts
Chapter 6

**Richard N. Yu, MD**
Scott Department of Urology
Baylor College of Medicine
Houston, Texas
Chapter 105

**Helen G. Zafirakis, MD**
Fellow, Urinary Tract and Pelvic Reconstruction
MD Anderson Cancer Center
Houston, Texas
Chapters 20 and 44

**Mark R. Zaontz, MD**
Clinical Professor of Urology
Department of Urology
Temple University School of Medicine
Philadelphia, Pennsylvania
Head, Section of Pediatric Urology
Departments of Surgery and Pediatrics
Virtua Health System
Voorhees, New Jersey
Chapter 103

**A. Jason Zauls, MD**
Chapter 30

**Ilia S. Zeltser, MD**
Assistant Clinical Professor
Department of Urology
Thomas Jefferson University
Philadelphia, PA
Attending Urologist
Bryn Mawr Urology Group
Academic Urology, LLC
Rosemont, Pennsylvania
Chapter 127

**Philippe E. Zimmern, MD, FACS**
Professor
Department of Urology
UT Southwestern Medical Center
Dallas, Texas
Chapter 34

**Armand Zini, MD**
Associate Professor
Department of Surgery
McGill University
Head, Division of Urology
Department of Surgery
St. Mary's Hospital
Montreal, Quebec, Canada
Chapter 58

# REMEMBRANCES DR. JAMES FRANCIS GLENN MAY 10, 1928 – JUNE 10, 2009

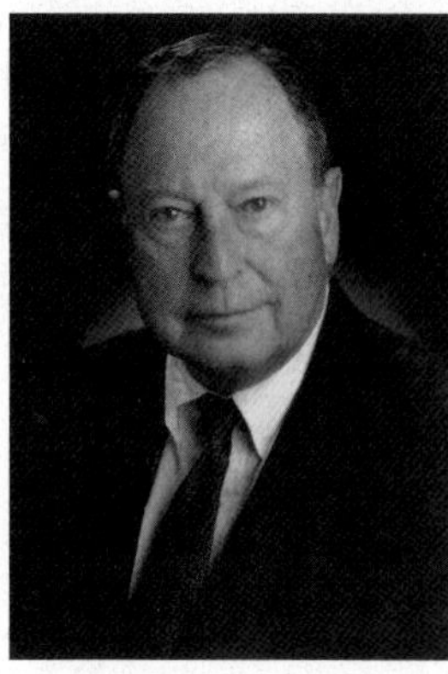

On June 10, 2009, on the eve of the publication of this Seventh Edition, the originator of this textbook, James F. Glenn, died at the age of 81 in Lexington, Kentucky. I have asked two of his closest friends and urologic colleagues, Everett Anderson and Randy Rowland, to each write their thoughts on Dr. Glenn's career. The purpose is not to delineate his curriculum vitae, which would fill another volume of this text, but to allow the reader to appreciate who Jim Glenn actually was.

For those of us who trained under him, Dr. Glenn was a mentor, a role model, and a great friend. Three personal attributes defined him: integrity, loyalty, and a principled life. He was always straightforward in his relationships with his residents, colleagues, and others with whom he worked. There was never any question as to where he stood and whether he would follow through on all that he promised. It was easy to follow someone so open, and though there may have been times when honesty was painful, Jim Glenn was always a gentleman and true to his word.

Nearly every resident, fellow, and faculty member who worked with Dr. Glenn can relate major events in his or her life on which Dr. Glenn had a significant influence, both professionally and personally. He treated all he worked with as family and was intensely loyal to all of us. Once he was your friend, you could count on him as a friend for life. Many of us who became departmental chairs and national and international leaders in urology owe him not only for the opportunities that he provided for us but also for being available and standing in when we needed help. He truly loved all of his protégées, no matter how much that love was returned by each of us.

Dr. Glenn had high expectations of his staff and residents, and though all of us on occasion did not meet his expectations, after his expression of displeasure, the incident was forgiven, and he never carried a grudge. His ultimate goal was to instill a compulsion for excellence, which he taught by example.

Finally, he lived a life that was based on principles and was unwilling to compromise those principles for political expediency. His principles were truth and excellence. He was a perpetual student; when confronted with a challenge, he gathered all the data, made a decision based on his principles, and stuck to his decision. There were no gray areas, and he never compromised his core principles. If he was assured of the rightness of his position, he delivered the message regardless of the political consequences. Although he usually tried to convince people with his great sense of humor and intelligence, in the end he remained steadfast in his beliefs. Many others would have taken the easier road, but Jim Glenn was not an ordinary man, and for that reason he will forever be a guide in our lives.

Jim Glenn was born in Lexington, Kentucky, on May 10, 1928. He attended the local university school for the first 12 years of his education and then entered the University of Rochester, where he received a BA degree in 3 years. The fast track continued with a medical degree from Duke University in 3 years. There followed a 2-year residency in General Surgery at Peter Bent Brigham Hospital and a 3-year residency in Urologic Surgery at Duke University. With a chosen career in academic medicine, he spent the next 2 years on the faculty at Yale, followed by 2 years at Bowman Gray. Four years after completing his urologic residency he returned to Duke as Chief of Urology. In 4 years he had progressed from Instructor, to Assistant Professor, to Associate Professor, to Full Professor—an unbelievable accomplishment. During his 17 years at Duke, he trained 67 residents, 12 of whom became heads of urology at other institutions.

Apart from his academic and professional achievements, Dr. Glenn was known for his warmth, good humor, and concern for his patients, house staff, and colleagues. He derived great pleasure in promoting his residents and senior staff. Dr. Glenn knew every resident's wife's name and made every resident accepted into the program quickly feel that he was now a member of the Duke urology family. Dr. Glenn entertained his "family" on many occasions at his home, and when the residency period was over, he would use his many contacts to obtain jobs for his residents in academia or private practice.

After leaving Duke, Dr. Glenn served as Dean of Emory University School of Medicine from 1980 to 1983 and then as President of Mt. Sinai School of Medicine, Medical Center, and Hospital from 1983 to 1987. Subsequently he returned to Lexington and was appointed as Professor of Surgery and then Professor Emeritus of Surgery at the University of Kentucky (UK). Dr. Glenn served as Executive Director of the Markey Cancer Center at UK from 1989 to 1993; as Associate Dean for Clinical Affairs, UK College of Medicine, and Chief of Staff, UK Hospital, from 1993 to 1995; and as Interim Chair, Department of Surgery, from 1996 to 1997.

In addition to his administrative duties at UK, Dr. Glenn maintained a close relationship with the Division of Urology.

He was especially helpful in advising the division in the "art of fundraising." With his assistance and generosity, three endowed chairs, one professorship, and two research endowments were established and funded, totaling over $9 million.

Dr. Glenn was a major contributor to advancements in both adult and pediatric urology. He was quick to recognize changing trends and to adopt the best of these in his constant quest for excellence. Dr. Glenn was a member of 37 professional societies and President of the most prestigious, including the American Association of Genitourinary Surgeons, the Clinical Society of Genitourinary Surgeons, the International Society of Urology, the Society for Pediatric Urology, the Society of Pelvic Surgeons, and the Society of University Urologists. He was elected to Alpha Omega Alpha in medical school and later became its President. He was also a past-President of the Southeastern Section and an honorary member of five sections and of the American Urological Association. His curriculum vitae includes 4 textbooks, 6 exhibits, 18 scientific movies, 37 book chapters, and 279 manuscripts. He has received the Hugh Hampton Young Award from the American Urological Association and the St. Paul's Medal for professional contributions from the British Association of Urological Surgeons. In 2007 Dr. Glenn was also awarded the Félix Guyon Medal by the Société Internationale d'Urologie in Paris for his contributions to the society.

Dr. Glenn actively supported community as well as university causes and programs, helping raise money for and contributing generously to many organizations: the St. John's Episcopal Church Building Fund, the UK Division of Urology, the Duke University Division of Urology, Transylvania University, the Bluegrass Trust for Historical Preservation, the Lexington History Museum, and Cardinal Hill Rehabilitation Hospital.

Dr. Glenn shared his wit, cheer, knowledge, and enthusiasm with all people with whom he interacted, playing a constructive role in community as well as academic organizations.

We will miss him.

*June 16, 2009*
*E. Everett Anderson, MD;*
*Sam D. Graham, MD;*
*Randall G. Rowland, MD, PhD*

# PREFACE

In 1969 when the First Edition of *Urologic Surgery* was published, the avowed purpose of the work was to present authoritative expositions of various surgical procedures, authored by acknowledged experts in the field. It was the conviction of the editors that there were atlases and textbooks that presented urology well, but there were no volumes on surgical technique, and that urology is—first and foremost—a surgical specialty.

In developing that initial effort, I was joined (and guided) by my good friend and wise mentor William H. Boyce, superb clinician, outstanding scientist, and master surgeon. Between us, we were able to recruit some of the most respected urologic surgeons to contribute to the volume. Over the years, that tradition has continued, and I am forever grateful to all of my colleagues who have given of their time, talent, and expertise to the several iterations of this book.

Having observed my 81st birthday and retired from active clinical practice, I recognize that the time has come to pass the responsibility to others, and I happily do so. Two friends—Sam D. Graham Jr., MD, Director of the Johns Cancer Center in Richmond, Virginia, and Thomas E. Keane, MD, Chairman of Urology at the Medical University of South Carolina, Charleston—have already demonstrated their proficiency in co-editing previous editions. Both Dr. Graham and Dr. Keane are products of the Duke system, as I am.

As our French friends say, "Vive urologie!"

*James F. Glenn, BA, MD, DSc, FACS, FRCS*

JEROME P. RICHIE

# CHAPTER 1 ■ ANATOMY OF THE ADRENAL GLANDS, KIDNEY, URETER, AND PELVIS

## ADRENAL

RICARDO BEDUSCHI AND UNYIME O. NSEYO

The adrenal glands are paired and located high in the retroperitoneum, on the anterior craniomedial aspect of the kidney (Figs. 1.1, 1.2, and 1.3). Their characteristic yellow color distinguishes them from the surrounding fat or pancreas. They weigh approximately 5 g, but weight and size may change significantly after prolonged illness or as the result of prolonged adrenocorticotropic hormone (ACTH) stimulation. The atrophic gland is thin and pale, and its easily recognizable hyperplasia makes it readily visible. The left adrenal gland has a semicircular or crescent shape. The right gland has an inverted pyramidal or V-shape. The adrenal gland consists of the cortex and medulla and arose from the mesoderm (cortex) and ectodermal (medulla) elements in the medial aspect of the coelomic cavity.

### Embryology

Embryologically, the ectodermal medullary elements migrate from the same primordial neural crest that gives rise to the sympathetic chain. The mesodermal cortical tissues arise from the dorsal cells of the blastema cord at the medial aspect of the mesonephric bodies. However, the ventral cells of these bodies are the origin of the interstitial cells of the testis or the theca cells of the ovary. The 8-week embryo has massive adrenals, approximately the size of the kidney, and they remain enlarged and very vascular until birth. Rapid regression occurs in the adrenal size during the first month. The large adrenal size with hypervascularity may predispose to adrenal hemorrhage in the newborn as well as misdiagnosis for Wilms tumor or neuroblastoma. The medullary tissue within the gland imparts a unique tripartite structure of the head (most medial), body, and tail (most lateral). Each adrenal gland resides within the Gerota fascia with the kidney. However, in

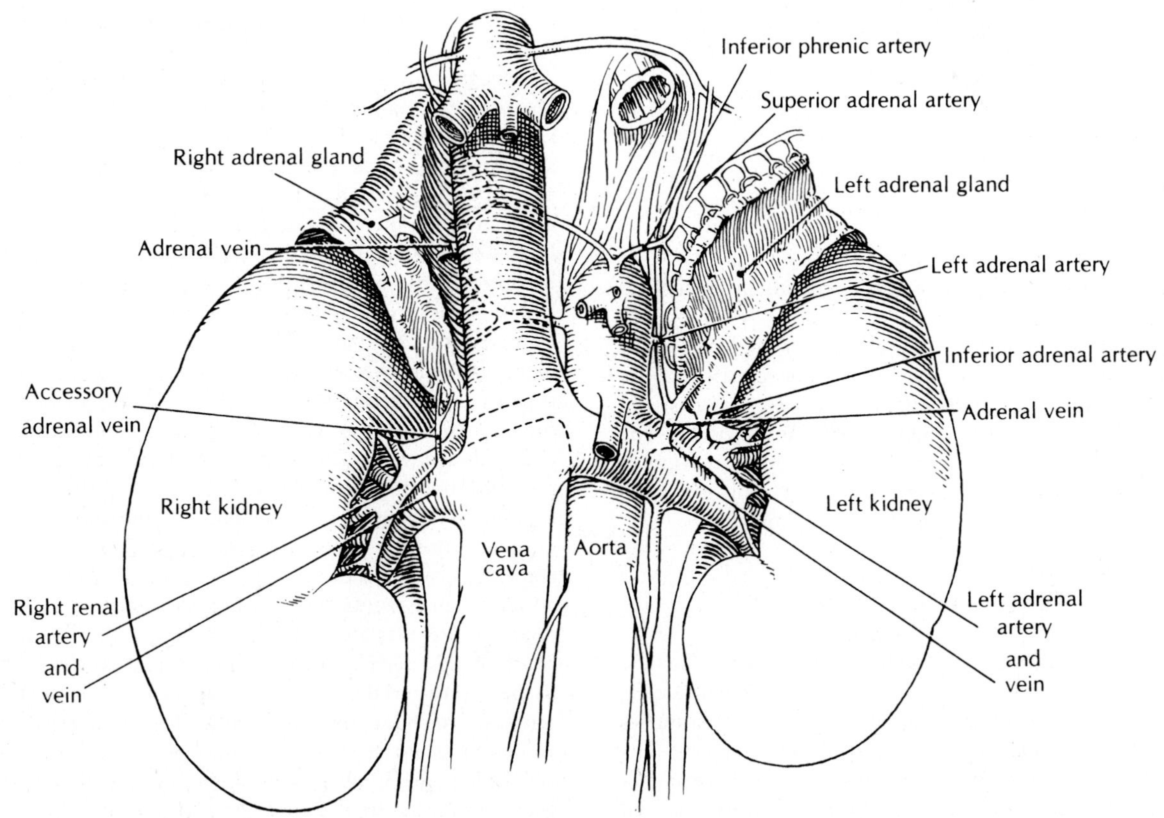


FIGURE 1.1 The anatomic relationship of the adrenal glands to the aorta and inferior vena cava. Multiple arterial vessels entering the glands indicate the rich arterial supply, while a single central adrenal vein illustrates the limited and relatively constant venous damage.

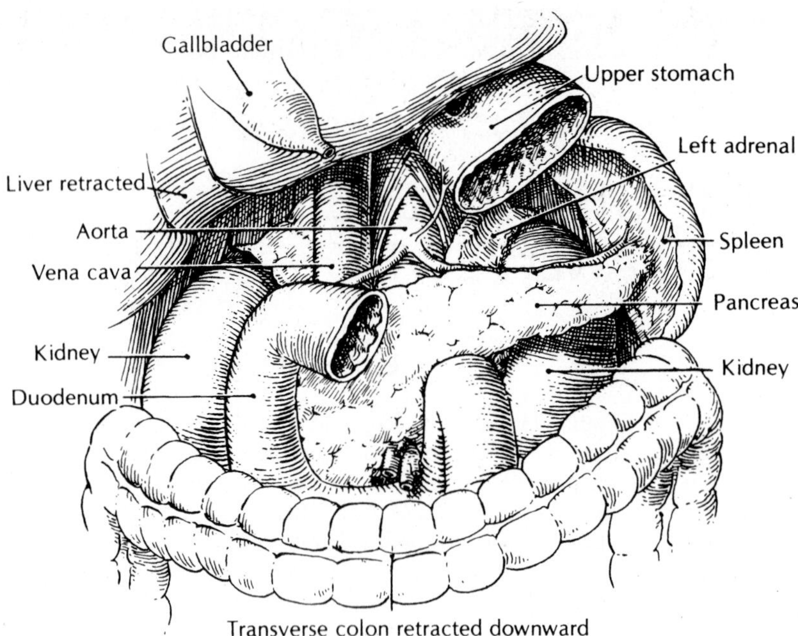


FIGURE 1.2 An anterior view of the abdomen illustrating the anatomic relationship of the adrenal glands to the surrounding gastrointestinal tract and organs.

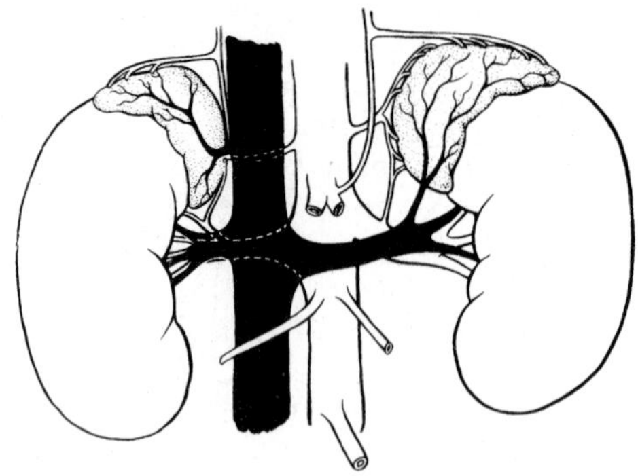

FIGURE 1.3

the case of renal ectopy, the adrenal remains in its natural position.

Ectopic adrenal tissues may develop in certain locations of the body. Although rare, they may undergo neoplastic changes or hyperplasia. Ectopic adrenal tissues in most cases consist of cortex only; rarely do they contain cortex and medulla. The embryological relationship in the urogenital ridge predisposes to adrenal ectopy in the retroperitoneum, the testis, the spermatic cord, and the region of the celiac ganglion.

## Vascular Anatomy

The arterial supply remains variable; the main sources include primarily the branches from the aorta, inferior phrenic artery, and renal artery. The multiple small-caliber arterial branches must be appreciated for hemostasis during surgery. The venous drainage, although less variable, usually represents a bigger challenge, especially during operations on large adrenal masses. The right adrenal vein is short and empties directly into the inferior vena cava (IVC) in its most posterolateral aspect. Large adrenal tumors may obscure its visualization, making identification of this vein very challenging. Bleeding from this site can be profuse and even life-threatening if not identified and controlled immediately. The left adrenal vein is much smaller than the right adrenal vein. It usually exits anteroinferiorly, draining into the ipsilateral renal vein.

## Contiguous Structures

Thorough knowledge of the anatomic relationships holds the key to preventing injury to the contiguous structures during surgical dissection (Fig. 1.2). The right adrenal gland lies superior to the upper pole of the right kidney, posterolaterally to the IVC. Dissection of the right adrenal gland is limited medially by the duodenum and superiorly by the right hepatic lobe. Access to the right adrenal gland is more easily obtained by entering the retroperitoneum behind the liver. The right hepatic lobe can be mobilized from the colon and diaphragm by transecting the triangular, coronary, and hepatocolic ligaments, allowing visualization of the right adrenal gland just superior to the upper pole of the right kidney. Mobilization of the duodenum is also required for easier identification of the right adrenal vein. This step is of special interest for large pheochromocytomas, in which early access to the adrenal vein is essential. Using the Kocher maneuver, the duodenum can be retracted medially, allowing easier access to the IVC and a complete dissection of the right adrenal vein. Once the right adrenal vein is controlled, an avascular plane can be developed toward the lateral aspect of the gland, allowing quick and bloodless removal of the gland. Attention should be paid to the main arterial trunks as well as the multiple small-caliber arteries, which can be easily controlled with electrocautery and/or surgical clips.

The left adrenal gland is usually more medial than the right gland, and it lies on the upper pole of the left kidney, just lateral to the aorta. The left adrenal gland lies in close contact with the spleen and stomach, and it is crossed on its anteroinferior surface by the body of the pancreas and the splenic artery and vein. A special technical effort must be made to prevent inadvertent injury to the tail of the pancreas and/or capsule of the spleen. Releasing the splenocolic ligament allows free mobilization of the spleen, and gentle blunt dissection allows medial mobilization of the left abdominal viscera and adequate exposure of the left adrenal gland. The left adrenal vein is usually isolated in the anteroinferior aspect of the gland, and control of this vein is usually less of a problem, with minimal blood loss (Fig. 1.3). The lowest extent of this gland is close to the renal vessel, which remains at risk of injury during adrenalectomy.

## KIDNEY

SAM D. GRAHAM, JR.

The abdominal wall is composed of three layers of muscle and fascia that are derived from the same embryonic muscle sheets as the intercostal muscles. Each muscle is covered by its own layer of deep fascia and is innervated by the intercostal nerves. The external oblique fibers are oriented anteriorly and inferiorly, attaching posteriorly to the iliac crest, and the anterior fibers attach to the linea alba in the midline (Fig. 1.4A). The internal oblique fibers are oriented anteriorly and superiorly (Fig. 1.4B). Posteriorly, the fibers of the internal oblique attach to the lower four ribs, and anteriorly they attach to the linea alba. In the upper abdomen, the internal oblique fascia splits to enclose the rectus muscle, while inferiorly the fascia only covers the rectus muscle anteriorly. The ilioinguinal and iliohypogastric nerves are found in the interior oblique fascia anterior to the internal oblique muscle. The transversus abdominis are horizontally oriented fibers that attach to the linea alba (Fig. 1.4C). The ribs are supported by the intercostal muscles and fascia as well as the costovertebral (costotransverse) ligament, which must be divided if the rib is to be retracted inferiorly (Fig. 1.5).

The kidneys are located on either side of the vertebral column in the lumbar fossa of the retroperitoneum and vary in length in adults from 11 cm to 14 cm, or from approximately 3.0 to 4.5 times the height of the second lumbar vertebrae (Fig. 1.1). The parenchyma of the kidney is covered by a thin

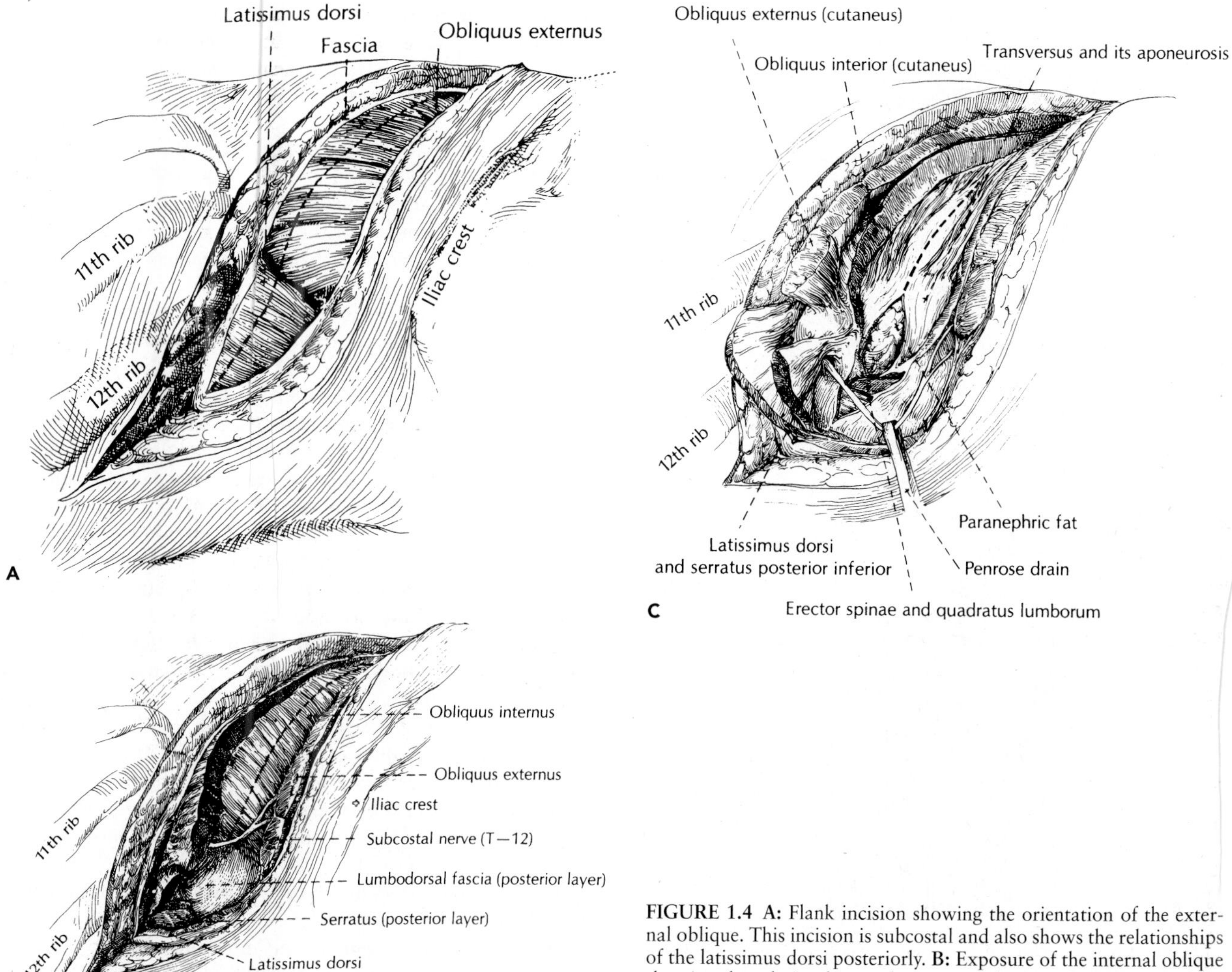


FIGURE 1.4 **A:** Flank incision showing the orientation of the external oblique. This incision is subcostal and also shows the relationships of the latissimus dorsi posteriorly. **B:** Exposure of the internal oblique showing the relationship to the intercostal nerve. **C:** Exposure of the transversus abdominis and its aponeurosis.

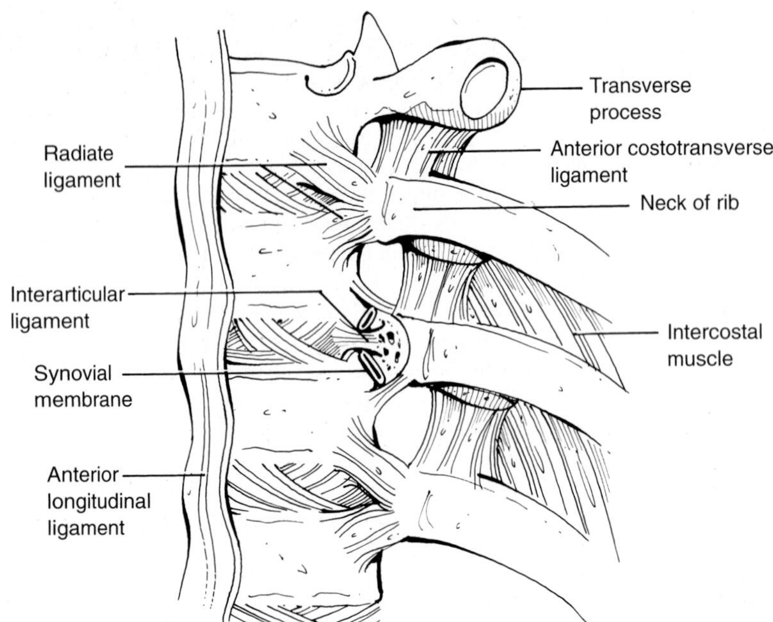


**FIGURE 1.5** Costovertebral (costotransverse) ligaments extend from the transverse process of the vertebra immediately above the rib to the neck of the rib. In order to gain exposure during a thoracolumbar or supracostal approach, this must be divided to allow the rib to rotate inferiorly.

transparent capsule, which in turn is covered by a layer of perinephric fat enclosed in a distinct layer of fascia (Gerota fascia) (Fig. 1.6). The capsule is attached to Gerota fascia by fibrous trabeculae (1). Gerota fascia is completely fused superiorly and laterally, but it is open inferiorly and to some extent medially, where it is adherent to the adventitia of the renal vessels, aorta, and inferior vena cava. Gerota fascia extends above the kidney to form a special compartment for the adrenal gland (2). Posteriorly, Gerota fascia is connected to the sheaths of the psoas and quadratus lumborum muscles by connective tissue septae. Anteriorly, Gerota fascia is closely applied to the peritoneum. On the left, the hilum of the spleen is attached to the ventral aspect of the kidney by a double layer of peritoneum known as the splenorenal ligament (2).

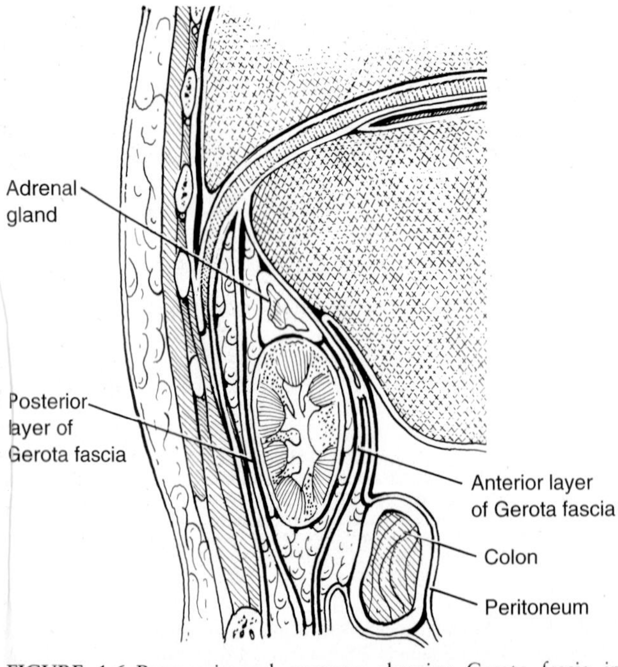

Adrenal gland
Posterior layer of Gerota fascia
Anterior layer of Gerota fascia
Colon
Peritoneum

**FIGURE 1.6** Retroperitoneal anatomy showing Gerota fascia in sagittal section.

## Vascular Anatomy

The main renal arteries are branches of the aorta emanating from the lateral portion of the aorta at approximately L-2. In general, the renal arteries divide into segmental branches at the junction of the middle and final third of their course. A single left artery most commonly lies dorsal to the renal vein, and a long right renal artery lies dorsal to the vena cava and the renal vein. Up to 35% of kidneys have an accessory renal artery, with 1.5% having more than one accessory artery (2). As the renal artery approaches the hilum, it has two branches, the inferior suprarenal (adrenal) and the ureteric arteries (Fig. 1.6). At the hilus, the main renal artery divides into an anterior and posterior branch, which further divide into segmental arteries. The kidney can be divided into four segments based upon the arterial supply (Fig. 1.7). Both the apical and basilar segmental arteries supply each respective pole of the kidney anteriorly and posteriorly. The largest segment is the anterior segment, which is supplied by two segmental arteries and extends posteriorly to the avascular plane where it meets the posterior segment (3).

The renal veins directly join the vena cava. The right renal vein is usually less than one-half the length of the left renal vein and has no significant branches. The left renal vein, however, is usually joined by the adrenal and inferior phrenic vein superiorly, the gonadal vein inferiorly, and frequently by lumbar vein(s) posteriorly (Fig. 1.8). These collaterals are of great importance in patients in whom the vena caval ligation or resection is contemplated.

The renal vein is usually the most anterior structure in the renal hilum. Posterior to the vein is the renal artery, and

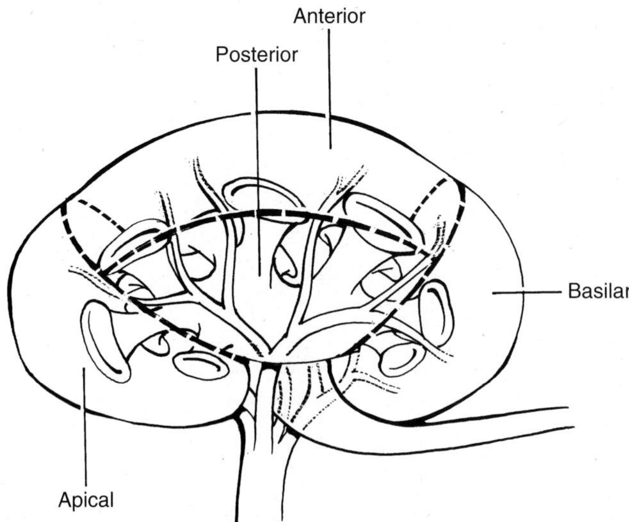


FIGURE 1.7 Segmental anatomy of the kidney. The relatively avascular plane between the anterior and posterior segments is the line of Brödel. In general, calyces tend to extend from the renal pelvis to the central mass of the segment they supply.

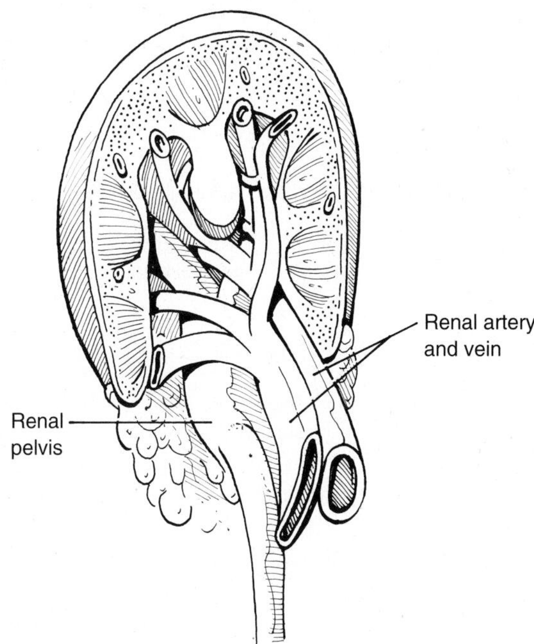


FIGURE 1.9 Transverse section of kidney showing relative anatomy of vascular structures in the renal hilum.

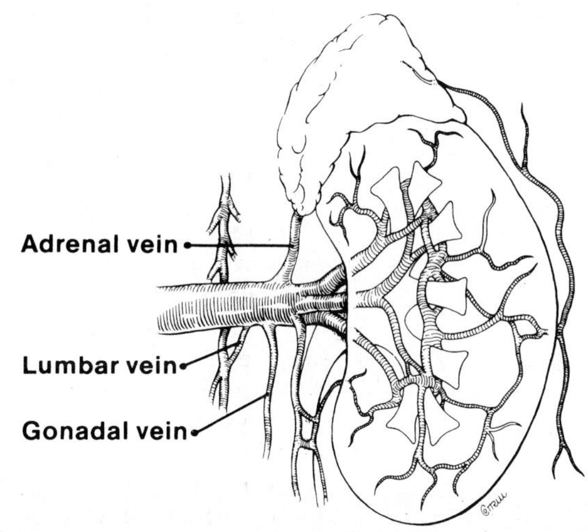


FIGURE 1.8 The complex and varied anatomy of the left renal vein. Note that there may be one or even two lumbar veins from the renal vein posteriorly, allowing alternative venous flow if the vena cava is occluded.

the most posterior structure in the hilum is the renal pelvis. The hilum is filled with fibrofatty tissue that can usually be easily dissected from these structures to allow access into the renal sinus (Fig. 1.9).

## Lymphatic Anatomy

Parenchymal and capsular lymphatics coalesce and drain into the right lumbar or paraaortic chains, respectively. These lymphatics become part of the cisterna chylae superior to the renal artery.

## Contiguous Structures (Fig. 1.10)

Posterior to the kidney lies the psoas major and quadratus lumborum muscles. Posteriorly and superiorly, the upper pole of each kidney is in contact with the diaphragm. The pleura is also adjacent to the upper poles of both kidneys, usually extending down below the level of the twelfth rib posteriorly and to the eleventh rib anteriorly (1).

Embryologically, when the gut rotates, this leaves the posterior parietal peritoneum covering the upper three-fourths of the right kidney and is directly related to the hepatorenal pouch of Morrison. The duodenum is fixed to the original peritoneal covering of the lower pole of the right kidney by fusion of the embryonic dorsal mesentery to the posterior parietal peritoneum (2). On the left, the rotation of the foregut causes a fusion of the embryonic mesogastrium with the original peritoneal covering of the upper anterior kidney, thereby causing the relationship of the left kidney to the omental bursa (2). The midportion of the left kidney loses its contact with the peritoneum due to growth of the tail of the pancreas.

Superiorly, the anteromedial surface of the right kidney is in contact with the right adrenal gland. The liver overlies the anterior two-thirds of the right kidney, and the hepatic flexure of the colon overlies the lower one-third of the right kidney. The second portion of the duodenum overlies the renal hilum. In >90% of patients, the right kidney is lower than the left (2).

The medial surface of the left kidney is also in contact with the left adrenal gland. Other structures anterior and in close approximation to the left kidney are the spleen, the tail of the pancreas, the stomach, and the splenic flexure of the colon.

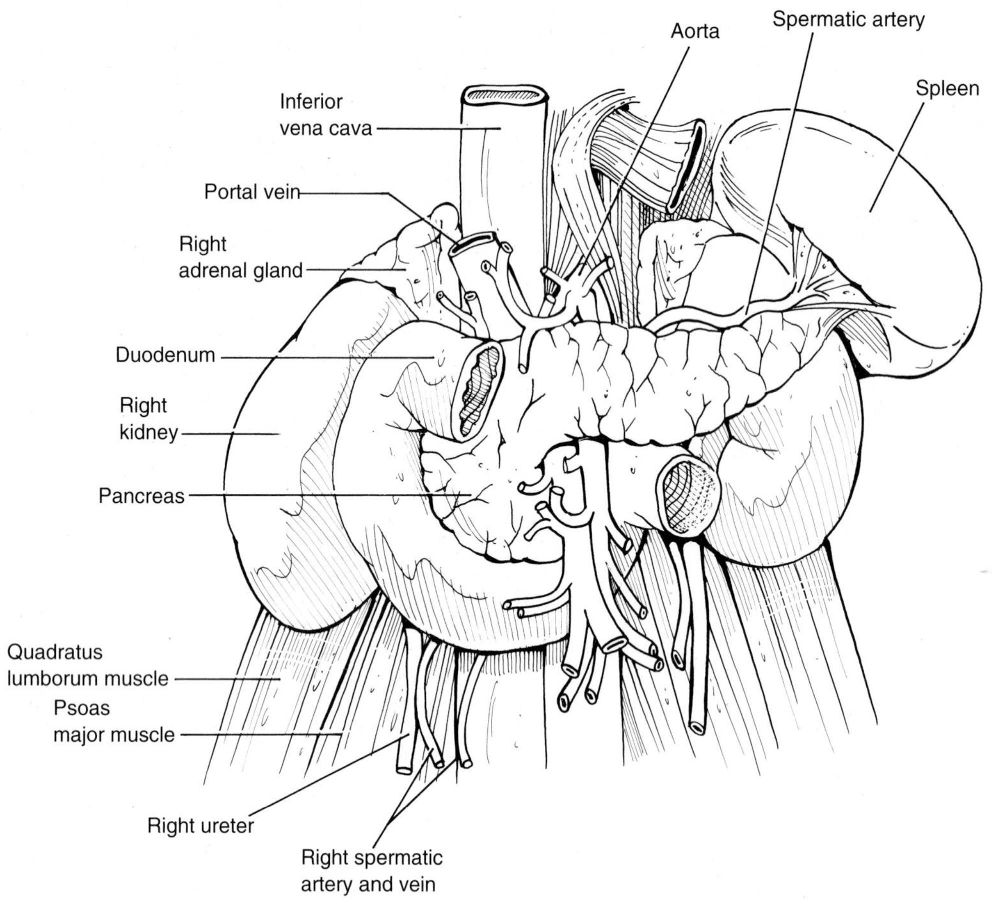


FIGURE 1.10 The kidney in relation to contiguous structures.

## *References*

1. Bergman EV, Bruns P, von Mikulicz J. *A system of practical surgery,* Vol. 5. New York: Lea Brothers, 1904. Bull WT, Foote EM, translators.
2. Healey JE Jr, Seybold WD. *A synopsis of clinical anatomy*. Philadelphia: WB Saunders, 1969.
3. Stewart BH. *Operative urology: the kidneys, adrenal glands, and retroperitoneum*. Baltimore: Williams & Wilkins, 1975.

# CHAPTER 2 ■ PARTIAL NEPHRECTOMY

SAMIR S. TANEJA

While partial nephrectomy was described over 125 years ago, its widespread use is truly confined to the last 20 years (1,2). Partial nephrectomy is utilized for a number of urologic processes, including stone disease, nonfunction within a duplicated moiety, trauma, infection, and renal tumors. Within the last 10 to 20 years, the major application of partial nephrectomy has been in the treatment of small renal tumors as an alternative to radical nephrectomy (1,2). Downward stage migration, more frequent incidental detection of tumors, better imaging techniques, and increasing surgeon comfort have led to increased utilization and expanded indications for partial nephrectomy. Despite these developments, recent surveys suggest that partial nephrectomy remains underutilized nationally in the treatment of small renal tumors.

## INDICATIONS

The primary indication for partial nephrectomy is in the resection of renal tumor. The procedure may also be performed for a nonfunctioning duplicated moiety, trauma, or stone disease, in addition to a number of less common indications. While it is acceptable to remove a solitary kidney or both kidneys if required for oncologic efficacy, in general, the presence of tumor in a solitary kidney or bilaterally is considered an absolute indication for partial nephrectomy. Likewise, cases in which radical nephrectomy would result in a need for permanent dialysis due to severe baseline azotemia should be considered absolute indication. In these cases, "absolute" implies that partial nephrectomy should be contemplated regardless of the tumor size or stage.

Relative indications include medical illnesses predisposing to renal disease, pre-existing medical renal disease, renal stones, recurrent renal infection, mild azotemia, and multifocal tumors associated with a genetic syndrome. An elective partial nephrectomy is defined as that in which the patient has none of the above risk factors, normal renal function, and a radiologically normal contralateral renal moiety. Historically, elective partial nephrectomy has been recommended only for exophytic or peripherally located tumors <4 cm in size. Much of the literature on which this recommendation was made was based upon series in which worsened oncologic outcomes were noted for central tumors and those >4 cm in size. Within these series, it is notable that many of these larger or central tumors were removed for absolute indications, potentially biasing the oncologic outcomes. As surgeons have become comfortable with the technique, indications for elective partial nephrectomy have been expanded to include central tumors and those in the T1b (4- to 7-cm) category. Thus far, there is no apparent decline in cancer control among those series reported (2).

Recent studies have suggested that partial nephrectomy may result in better long-term renal function than radical nephrectomy (3). A large cohort comparison demonstrated a higher likelihood of a glomerular filtration rate (GFR) >45 mL per minute or >60 mL per minute among those undergoing partial nephrectomy as compared to radical nephrectomy (4). Because GFR strongly correlates with the likelihood of cardiovascular mortality and other medical illnesses, in this regard partial nephrectomy may be beneficial.

## ALTERNATIVE THERAPIES

Alternative therapies to open partial nephrectomy include radical nephrectomy, laparoscopic partial nephrectomy, laparoscopic radical nephrectomy, or laparoscopic/percutaneous ablative procedures. A discussion of candidate selection for open or laparoscopic partial nephrectomy is beyond the scope of this chapter. Selection in this regard is highly dependent upon operator experience.

## SURGICAL TECHNIQUE

The technique of partial nephrectomy can be divided into renal preparation, renal incision, vascular repair and hemostasis, and collecting system reconstruction. These fundamental aspects of the operation should be considered individually in order for the surgeon to master the technique. It is most important to remember that despite the desire to preserve the kidney, partial nephrectomy for tumor is first a cancer operation, and margin control remains the primary consideration.

### Renal Preparation

In preparing a kidney for partial nephrectomy, full renal mobilization is most often necessary. The selected incisional approach can include a transperitoneal subcostal or midline incision, a thoracoabdominal incision, or an extraperitoneal flank incision, but when performing the operation through the flank, full mobilization is possible, allowing the kidney to easily stretch to the level of the skin. We have found that other advantages of the flank approach include containment of postoperative bleeding and/or urine leak, earlier resolution of ileus, and direct access to the kidney.

During renal mobilization, minimal handling of the kidney, avoidance of torque on the pedicle, and care to the position of the ureter to avoid crush injury are advisable. Rough handling can lead to subcapsular hematoma, capsule avulsion, vasospasm, and the potential for acute tubular necrosis (ATN). Destruction of the renal capsule during mobilization adds to the difficulty of reconstruction later in the operation.

When mobilizing the kidney, knowledge of variations in the renal arteriovenous anatomy is essential (Fig. 2.1). Anomalous or supernumerary renal vessels are common, and early recognition will avoid inadvertent vascular injury. We have found magnetic resonance imaging (MRI) to be useful in assessing the number and position of renal hilar vessels (5), but certainly a good computerized tomographic (CT) image should allow this as well. In resecting hilar or deep intraparenchymal tumors, a good MR or CT angiogram is advisable to understand the relationship of vessels to the tumor.

Polar renal arteries are usually divided to facilitate renal mobility as they usually feed only a small portion of the renal pole (apical branch) but may greatly limit mobility. In patients with a left-sided renal tumor and a retroaortic renal vein, hilar mobilization can be difficult, and stretching of the kidney to the skin may not be possible. As these are often secondary renal veins, division of the vein could be considered if another exists and mobility is limited. Because the renal venous anatomy has collateral parallel branches, venous branches can generally be divided to increase mobility without major sequelae.

Upon full mobilization of all hilar attachments, the renal vessels can be followed into the hilum to identify first and second segmental branchings. This may allow selective renal ischemia or arterial ligation if the tumor is located conveniently within one segment. We have found this to be rare, and more often early ligation of segmental branches results in inadequate ischemia and infarct within nonoperated areas of the kidney (Fig. 2.2). Therefore, it is generally preferable to clamp the main renal artery.

It is our preference to provide renal ischemia to facilitate renal incision and margin control, but this is certainly not uniformly necessary. Depending upon tumor location and depth, simple manual compression may be adequate to allow resection. Pitfalls of manual compression during incision include the potential for subcapsular hematoma, bleeding despite compression, poor view of the margin, destruction of the specimen, and the potential for ATN despite renal perfusion. Avoidance of renal ischemia is particularly appealing in patients at high risk of ATN due to baseline renal disease and decreased GFR, or in those with a solitary kidney in whom transient renal dysfunction could have deleterious short-term effects.

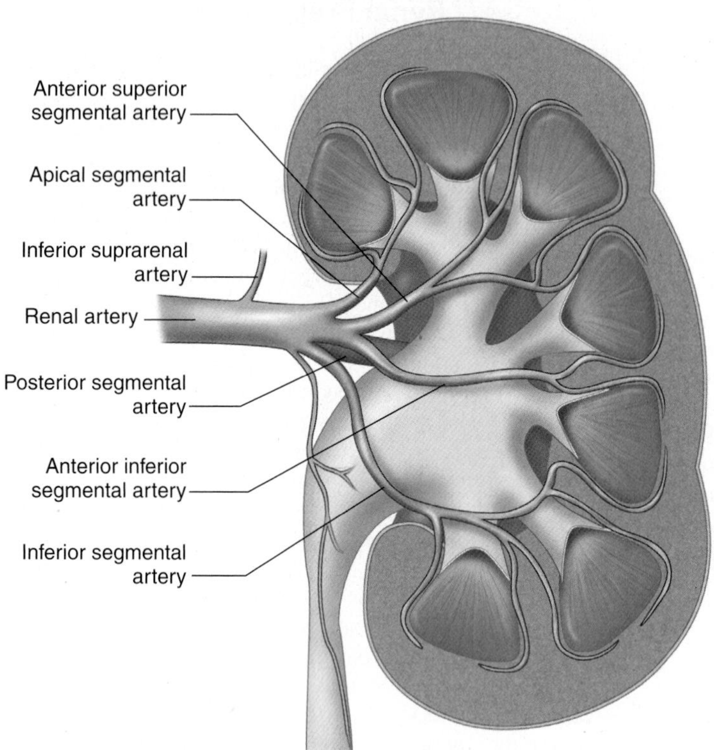


FIGURE 2.1 The renal arterial anatomy is generally predictable, with five major known segments: basilar or inferior, apical, anterior superior, anterior inferior, and posterior. Based upon the position of the tumor, a prediction can be made regarding the number of segments involved. This allows the direction and angle of the line of incision to be planned.

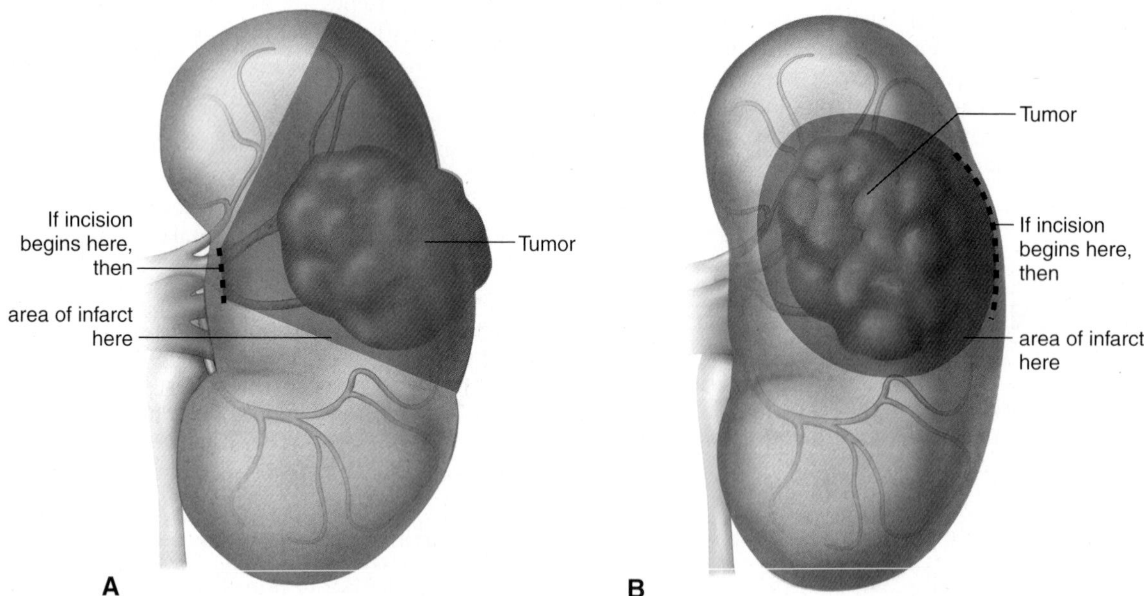


FIGURE 2.2 When incising the kidney from the hilar aspect of a tumor, particularly a tumor in the anterior or posterior segment, the incision will often result in infarct radial to the position of the tumor. Therefore, incising the kidney along the border of the tumor opposite the hilum will allow the tumor to be "lifted" from the kidney, exposing only those vessel branches that extend directly into the tumor.

We have utilized renal ischemia primarily to allow good visualization of the margin. Prior to clamping the renal artery, 12.5 g of mannitol is administered intravenously and allowed to circulate for 5 to 10 minutes. The kidney is placed in an intestinal/bowel bag and the drawstring cinched around the hilum. The closed end of the bag is cut open and filled with ice for purposes of in situ cooling. The kidney is packed in ice for 10 minutes prior to clamping the renal artery to allow surface cooling. During this time, intraoperative ultrasound may be performed to assess tumor location and plan the resection.

The renal artery is then clamped with a small spring-loaded "bulldog" clamp. We have found it unnecessary to clamp the renal vein in open partial nephrectomy, even for deep resection, as the vein is often compressed by stretch of the hilum and/or manual compression of the parenchyma. In cases of multiple arteries, it may be easier to mass-clamp the hilum with a straight or angled vascular clamp, but this may give inadequate ischemia and venous hypertension if not properly applied.

Conventional wisdom states that the kidney should be packed completely in ice for 10 to 20 minutes prior to resection in order to cool the core temperature to <20°C. As cold ischemia extends the period of safe ischemia from 30 to 40 minutes up to a theoretical 3 hours, this cooling is probably necessary for anticipated prolonged resection beyond 30 to 40 minutes. In general, it has been our preference to proceed with resection immediately upon placing the arterial clamp, while assigning a member of the operating room team to monitor and maintain the submersion of the kidney in ice throughout the resection. In using this approach, we have been able to keep the overall cold ischemia time low while maintaining adequate cooling of the parenchyma.

## Renal Incision and Margin Control

Renal incision planning is based upon position of the tumor and the arterial segment of kidney involved. For tumors lying within the anterior and posterior segment, a wedge resection technique is generally employed, whereas tumors located in the apical or basilar segments are generally managed by straight or tangential polar resection. In those cases in which the tumor lies across multiple segments, incision should be planned so as to maintain perfusion to the remaining renal segments following resection. In so doing, the surgeon minimizes the risk of renal infarct.

For tumors located in a single segment, we have generally utilized an approach of total renal ischemia. An exception to this rule might be in cases of anomalous vasculature in which multiple renal arteries are encountered. In these cases, it may not be necessary or advisable to clamp all arteries if the tumor is confined to a polar region of the kidney.

Tumor position can be best assessed by a combination of preoperative imaging and intraoperative ultrasound. Our approach with intraoperative ultrasound has been to pass the probe over the kidney in radial angles to the center of the tumor. This allows assessment of the subcortical extent of the tumor by assessing the transition from normal kidney to tumor interface in multiple planes (Fig. 2.3).

Renal incision should be carried out at a level adequate to provide a 1- to 2-cm margin of normal parenchyma. It should be noted that recent literature suggests that locoregional oncologic control is dependent upon a negative margin, and not the thickness of margin.

Nonetheless, in planning a minimum 1-cm margin, the final specimen often shows a thinner margin due to splaying and retraction of the normal parenchyma around the more dense tumor upon incision of the capsule.

For tumors that lie within 10 mm of the renal sinus, incision should be carried into visible sinus fat to ensure adequacy of margin. The same can be said for tumor within 10 mm of the collecting system. In cases of tumor abutting the collecting system, calyceal excision will usually provide an adequate margin. For those tumors invading or lying within the renal sinus fat, it is often difficult to obtain a thick margin due to

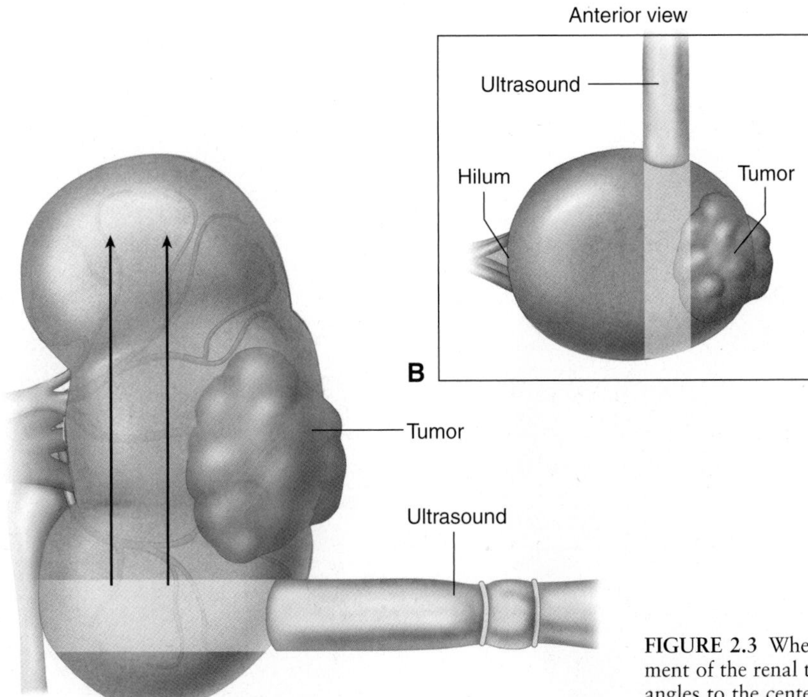


FIGURE 2.3 When performing intraoperative ultrasound for assessment of the renal tumor, the probe is passed over the kidney in radial angles to the center of the tumor. This allows assessment of the subcortical extent of the tumor in each angle, by assessing the transition from normal kidney to tumor interface in multiple planes. On the basis of this assessment, the position and line of incision are selected.

juxtaposed blood vessels. In these cases, sharp division of the surrounding sinus fat allows the surgeon to maintain a layer of normal tissue around the tumor capsule.

The technique of polar resection usually involves division of the renal parenchyma straight across the pole, or, if the tumor has an anterior or posterior lie, the incision can be carried out at a tangential angle. In polar amputation, central vascular retraction is less likely to occur upon dividing the kidney. As such, the surgeon can sharply amputate the tumor/pole with a knife or scissors. The central defect is then repaired with direct suture-ligature placement or running closure (Fig. 2.4). Alternatively, a traditional blunt separation of the parenchyma with sequential ligation and sharp incision of renal sinus structures can be carried out. This is particularly useful when attempting tangential amputation.

The technique of wedge resection within the anterior or posterior segment requires more thought on the part of the surgeon as assessing the depth and width of resection, maintaining blood supply to the opposite segment, and avoiding central vessel retraction can all pose a challenge. We have preferred a wide resection bed to bring the deepest portion of the resection up to the surface of the kidney. A narrow resection bed results in a centrally retracted, "ice cream cone" defect in which central suturing can be difficult.

The technique of wedge resection should start with a capsular incision at the leading edge of the resection. The parenchyma is gently separated with a flat instrument. We have utilized two orthopedic "freer" instruments working opposite one another to allow a well-visualized separation of the parenchyma (Fig. 2.5). Individual vessels entering the tumor specimen are identified and directly suture-ligated with 4-0 chromic catgut prior to division with tenotomy scissors.

Directed suture-ligature of vessels as they branch into the specimen avoids vessel retraction, deeper suture placement, and secondary injury to deeper vessels proximal to the branch point. Tenotomy scissors are used to divide the vessel and redirect the line of incision as needed. We have found that simple blunt division or fracturing of the parenchyma with a knife handle inevitably leads to tearing into the renal sinus structures, regardless of the tumor position. When it is necessary to traverse renal sinus structures, including the collecting system, they should be sharply divided.

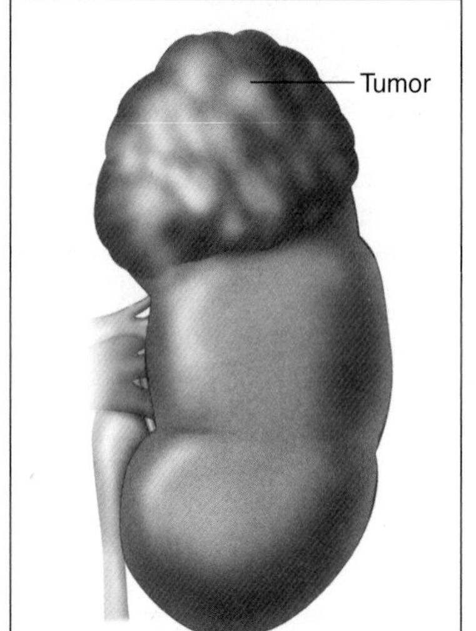


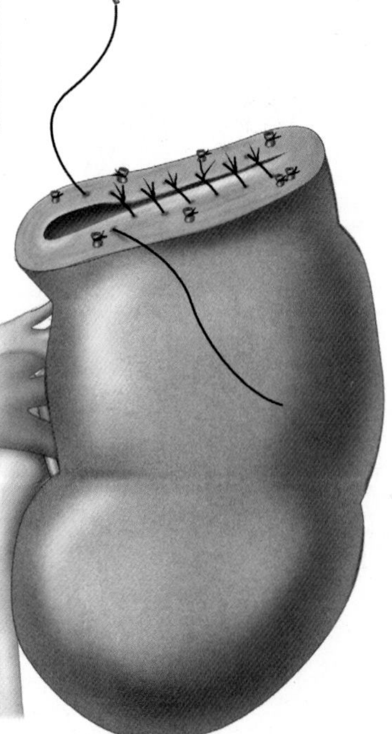


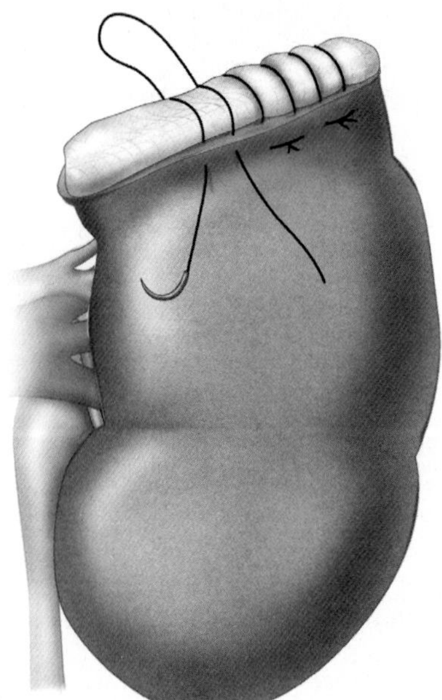


FIGURE 2.4 Polar amputation of the kidney is usually done with a flush blunt or sharp cut across the pole, allowing for a 1-to 2-cm margin of normal kidney around the tumor. Such cuts can be straight across the kidney or tangential in placement. Once the tumor has been amputated, the collecting system and central vessels are closed with interrupted absorbable sutures. A hemostatic bolster is then placed on the defect and sewn into place with horizontal mattress sutures pledgeted to the surrounding renal capsule.

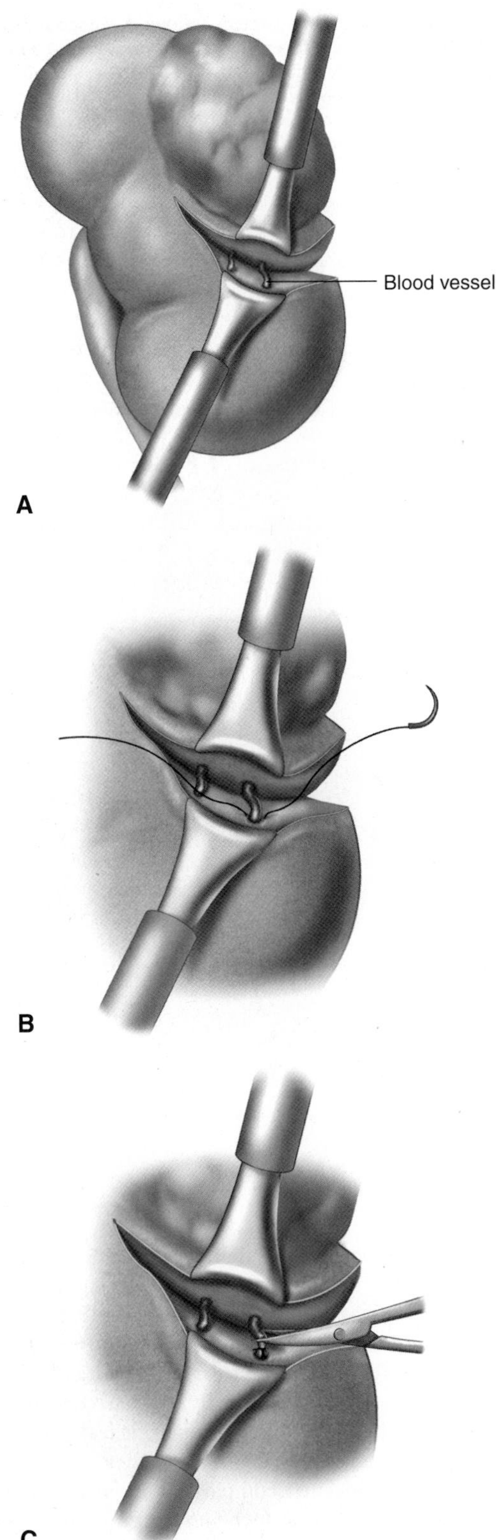


FIGURE 2.5 The technique of wedge resection should start with a capsular incision at the leading edge of the resection. The parenchyma is gently separated with a flat instrument. We have utilized two orthopedic "freer" instruments working opposite one another to allow a well-visualized separation of the parenchyma. Individual vessels entering the tumor specimen are identified and directly suture-ligated with 4-0 chromic catgut prior to division with tenotomy scissors. Directed suture-ligature of vessels as they branch into the specimen avoids vessel retraction, deeper suture placement, and secondary injury to deeper vessels proximal to the branch point.

We do not routinely employ intraoperative frozen sections to assess tumor margin. It has been suggested recently that such margins are rarely informative. Exceptions may be in the renal sinus when invasion into fat is suspected or when gross tumor violation is noted. In these cases, the presence of residual tumor in the sinus or resection bed may warrant consideration for nephrectomy.

## Renal Reconstruction

Renal reconstruction following tumor excision can be divided into vascular and collecting system repair. As these structures are juxtaposed, it is often necessary to provide simultaneous closure. Renal reconstruction usually involves three basic tenets: (a) closure of the collecting system; (b) direct suture repair of large vessels; (c) prevention of vascular retraction within the sinus; and (d) radial compression of the defect.

In the technique of wedge resection, the majority of vessels are sutured-ligated during the incision. Thus, upon removal of the arterial clamp and reperfusion, there is relatively little bleeding in most cases. Missed vessels or those partially ligated are generally directly sutured with 4-0 or 3-0 chromic catgut. It is important to note that the perfused kidney parenchyma has more turgor than the ischemic kidney and thus there is a tendency for sutures to "saw" through the parenchyma. Sutures should be placed widely across cut vessels to allow compression of the parenchyma around them. Open venous channels are usually controlled by "figure-of-eight" suture placement or, in the case of large openings, a running suture incorporating surrounding tissues for compression.

The collecting system is closed with interrupted sutures of 4-0 polyglycolic acid suture after renal perfusion has been reestablished. While running closure can be tried, tension on the collecting system opening often tears the fragile calyceal walls or creates holes along the suture line. For this reason, we have preferred a single-layer interrupted closure followed by a second layer of imbricating parenchymal sutures to reinforce the closure (Fig. 2.6). In polar resection, the collecting system and central vessels can often be closed in the same layer of interrupted sutures (Fig. 2.4), either before or after.

Following closure of the collecting system, retrograde instillation of methylene blue in the renal pelvis by a fine-gauge needle can confirm the integrity of closure and rule out additional sites of collecting system injury. After repair, the addition of a tissue adhesive layer can minimize the likelihood of leak. We have utilized a layer of Gelfoam TM (Pharmacia and Upjohn, New York) infiltrated with fibrin sealant (Tisseal, Baxter International).

A folded bolster of Surgicel TM (Johnson and Johnson, Piscataway, NJ) wrapped around fibrillar collagen (Surgicel) is placed in the defect. The kidney is then gently compressed around the bolster using horizontal mattress sutures of 4-0 chromic catgut anchored to the renal capsule as a pledget.

Following reconstruction, the kidney is returned to a normal anatomic lie with no kinking of the artery. The perinephric fat is layed over the defect and interposed between the lower-pole parenchyma and the ureter to avoid periureteral scarring. Nephropexy is only required if the kidney is notably mobile within the fossa.

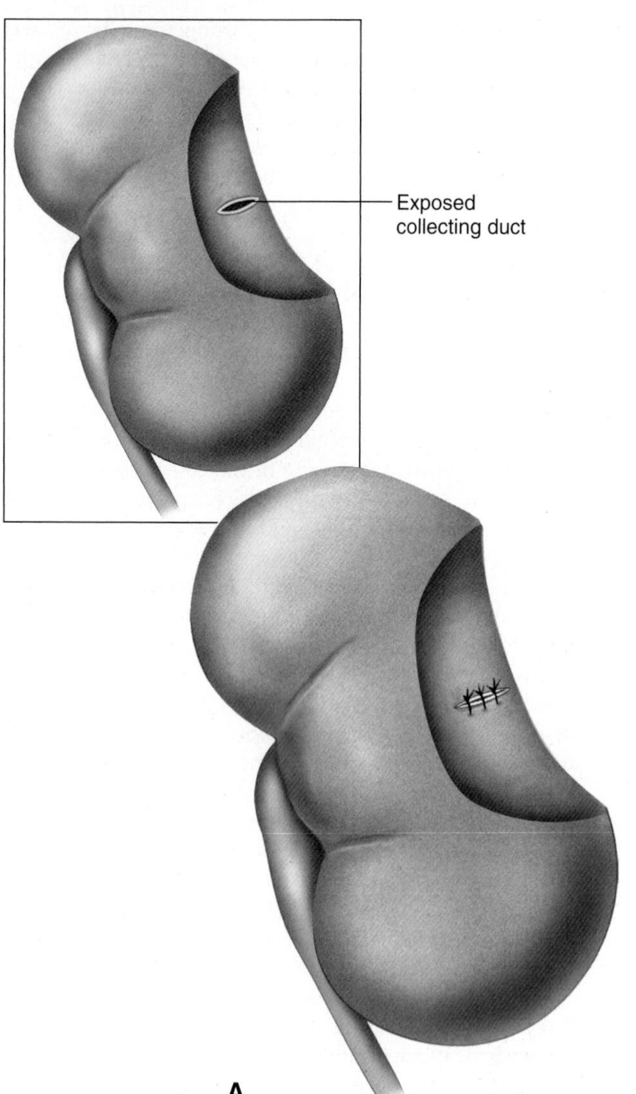


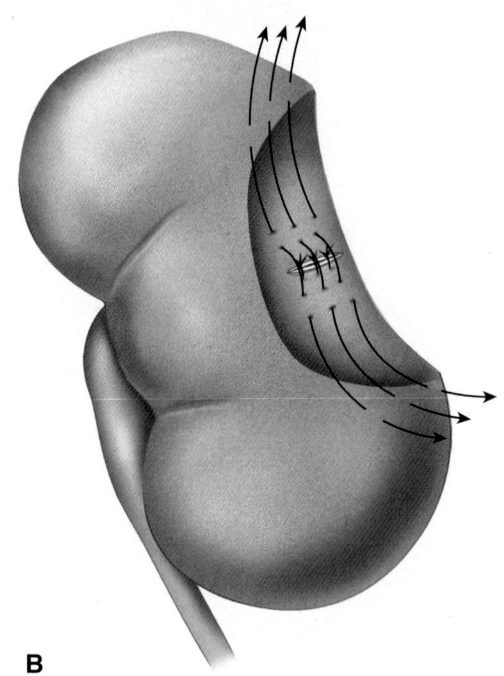


**FIGURE 2.6** Collecting system repair following wedge resection should aim for a 2-layer closure. The defect is first closed with interrupted 4-0 absorbable sutures anchored to the surrounding parenchyma. The renal parenchyma is then imbricated around the closure in a row of interrupted sutures to relieve tension on the first line. Hemostatic materials may then be used over this.

## OUTCOMES

### Complications

While partial nephrectomy is still considered by most surgeons to represent a technically challenging procedure, outcomes in recent series have suggested morbidity comparable to radical nephrectomy. Among 1,800 renal tumor resections performed between 1991 and 1998 in 123 Veterans Affairs Medical Centers, no difference in the mortality and morbidity rates between the radical and the nephron-sparing approach was observed (6). Certainly the likelihood of morbidity relates to operator experience and training.

Complications from partial nephrectomy include bleeding, urinary fistula, ureteral injury or obstruction, renal dysfunction, loss of kidney, and arteriovenous malformations. In a recent series comparing two groups of patients operated before and after 1995 (7), hemorrhage was uniformly infrequent, occurring in 1.5% and 1.2% of patients, respectively. The incidence of acute renal failure was also much less frequent (3.8% and 1%, respectively), requiring dialysis in only 2% of those operated before 1995 and in 0.6% of those treated thereafter. Urinary fistula or leak has also been a historically frequent complication in some early series, but in the same series urine leak was noted in 2.6% and 0.6% of cases before and after 1995.

In a phase III multicenter comparison of partial and radical nephrectomy, the rates of severe hemorrhage (defined as blood loss >1 L) and urinary fistula were 3.1% and 4.4%, respectively. Reoperation for complications was necessary in 4.4% of the nephron-sparing group and in 2.4% of the radical nephrectomy group (8). Complications such as arteriovenous fistula, pseudoaneurysm due to vascular injury, ureteral stricture, and renal loss are extremely rare.

Renal infarct of small portions of the kidney is common following renal reconstruction. If little perfused parenchyma is noted upon removal of the arterial clamp, vasospasm may be the culprit, and in these cases intra-arterial verapamil may improve perfusion. If the kidney is not viable, it should be removed. The general management of infarct is observation. In cases of severe hypertension due to infarcted kidney, nephrectomy should be performed.

The fundamental tenet of leak management is maximal drainage of the extrarenal collection until output diminishes. In general, a ureteral stent is not necessary unless there is evidence of ureteral obstruction, blood clots or debris within the collecting system, or a very large collecting system opening. Resolution of urine leak generally requires scarring in the potential space around the kidney during a variable time course of weeks to months. At that point the drain is slowly advanced out.

## Results

A number of studies, both open and laparoscopic, have demonstrated excellent long-term oncologic outcomes for patients undergoing partial nephrectomy. Early reports of partial nephrectomy for tumor included a large subset of patients with absolute or relative indication for surgery. Thus, recurrence-free survival often reflected survival of a nonselected population, including those with a higher tumor stage than in a contemporary elective partial nephrectomy series.

Hafez et al. (9) reviewed the Cleveland Clinic series of 485 partial nephrectomies, of which only 9% were electively performed. They reported a significant decrease in both 5-year and 10-year cancer-specific survival (CSS) for lesions >4 cm compared to those lesions <4 cm. Also observed was a statistically significant correlation between recurrence and size >4 cm. Based on these data, these authors suggested that stage T1 tumors (<7 cm) should be subdivided into T1a and T1b tumors, for those lesions <4 cm and >4 cm. In an updated study, Fergany et al. (11) reported on 10-year outcomes in 107 patients undergoing open partial nephrectomy from the same institution. Five- and 10-year CSS of 88.2% and 73%, respectively, was observed. In that series, only 10% of patients had elective indication, 50% of tumors were bilateral, and 45% were >4 cm in size. If including only the patients with tumors <4 cm, 5- and 10-year CSS improved to 98% and 95%, respectively.

A recent update of the University of California Los Angeles partial nephrectomy series (12) allows evaluation of 15-year outcomes for the procedure. Overall CSS was 98%, 96%, and 96% at 5, 10, and 15 years of follow-up, respectively. Recurrence was noted in 7%, 13%, and 13% at 5, 10, and 15 years of follow-up, but it is notable that 7% of patients had metastatic disease at time of surgery.

In a multicenter comparison of the outcomes of partial and radical nephrectomy among 1,454 patients (13), CSS was equivalent among patients undergoing partial or radical nephrectomy for either pT1a or pT1b tumor. Overall CSS at a median follow-up of 62 months was 97.8% for T1a and 93.8% for T1b tumors undergoing partial nephrectomy.

Partial nephrectomy for tumor resection is an increasingly important technique for practicing urologists to master. Oncologically, it is shown to be equivalent to radical nephrectomy for tumors <7 cm in size, and it results in quite good oncologic control for even larger tumors. The long-term benefits may be greater than initially perceived with regard to preservation of renal function and overall health. Careful preoperative imaging, knowledge of renal anatomy, attention to patient and tumor risk factors, and meticulous surgical technique are essential for achieving good surgical outcomes. Complication rates should be acceptably low if fundamental tenets of surgical technique are followed.

## *References*


1. Dash A, Vickers AJ, Schachter LR, et al. Comparison of outcomes in elective partial vs radical nephrectomy for clear cell renal cell carcinoma of 4-7 cm. *BJU Int* 2006;97:939.
2. Leibovich BC, Blute ML, Cheville JC, et al. Nephron sparing surgery for appropriately selected renal cell carcinoma between 4 and 7 cm results in outcome similar to radical nephrectomy. *J Urol* 2004;171:1066.
3. McKiernan J, Simmons R, Katz J, et al. Natural history of chronic renal insufficiency after partial and radical nephrectomy. *Urology* 2002;59:816.
4. Huang WC, Levey AS, Serio AM, et al. Chronic kidney disease after nephrectomy in patients with renal cortical tumours: a retrospective cohort study. *Lancet Oncol* 2006;7:735.
5. Huang GJ, Israel G, Berman A, et al. Preoperative renal tumor evaluation by three-dimensional magnetic resonance imaging: staging and detection of multifocality. *Urology* 2004;64:453.
6. Corman JM, Penson DF, Hur K, et al. Comparison of complications after radical and partial nephrectomy: results from the National Veterans Administration Surgical Quality Improvement Program. *BJU Int* 2000; 86:782.
7. Thompson RH, Leibovich BC, Lohse CM, et al. Complications of contemporary open nephron sparing surgery: a single institution experience. *J Urol* 2005;174:855.
8. Van Poppel H, Da Pozzo L, Albrecht W, et al. A prospective randomized EORTC intergroup phase 3 study comparing the complications of elective nephron-sparing surgery and radical nephrectomy for low-stage renal cell carcinoma. *Eur Urol* 2007;51:1606.
9. Hafez KS, Fergany AF, Novick AC. Nephron sparing surgery for localized renal cell carcinoma: impact of tumor size on patient survival, tumor recurrence and TNM staging. *J Urol* 1999;162:1930.
10. Fergany AF, Hafez KS, Novick AC. Long-term results of nephron sparing surgery for localized renal cell carcinoma: 10-year followup. *J Urol* 2000; 163:442.
11. Riggs SB, Larochelle JC, Belldegrun AS. Partial nephrectomy: a contemporary review regarding outcomes and different techniques. *Cancer J* 2008;14:302.
12. Patard JJ, Shvarts O, Lam JS, et al. Safety and efficacy of partial nephrectomy for all T1 tumors based on an international multicenter experience. *J Urol* 2004;171:2181.

# CHAPTER 3 ■ RADICAL NEPHRECTOMY

MICHAEL S. COOKSON AND SAM S. CHANG

Renal cell carcinoma (RCC) is the most common malignancy of the kidney and accounts for about 3% of all adult neoplasms. The estimated number of new cases of RCC in the United States in 2007 was 51,190 with a projected 12,890 deaths, and this incidence is expected to continue to increase as a result of the expanded use of radiographic imaging coupled with the aging population (1).

While emerging technologies such as ablative techniques may offer effective treatment for selective patients with smaller primary tumors, surgery remains the mainstay for curative treatment in the majority of patients with RCC. Furthermore, despite the expanded role of partial nephrectomy for tumors <4 cm, radical nephrectomy remains an important treatment option for most large and almost all locally advanced tumors.

The role of open radical nephrectomy in the management of RCC has changed somewhat over the last decade. Pure laparoscopic and laparoscopic hand-assisted radical nephrectomy have emerged as less morbid alternatives to open surgery in the management of low- to moderate-volume (8 to 10 cm or smaller), localized RCCs without local invasion, renal vein involvement, or lymphadenopathy (2).

However, this has placed an increased emphasis on the performance of open radical nephrectomy in a higher percentage of patients who have either comorbid illnesses or advanced tumors that preclude a minimally invasive approach. Furthermore, the beneficial impact of cytoreductive nephrectomy has increased the clinical situations in which open radical nephrectomy may be performed in the setting of metastatic disease (3).

This chapter focuses on the open surgical approach for radical nephrectomy.

## DIAGNOSIS

Typically, RCCs are characterized on computerized tomography (CT) scan by a solid parenchymal mass with a heterogeneous density and enhancement with IV contrast injection (between 15 and 40 Hounsfield units). However, despite modern imaging, some benign tumors and complex cysts may be indistinguishable from cancer and confirmed only after surgical excision. The role of percutaneous biopsy or needle aspiration in differentiating an indeterminate renal mass remains controversial and is currently used in select cases, such as in patients with known second primary tumors, suspected metastases, or lymphoma.

Clinical staging in patients suspected of RCC usually includes a contrast-enhanced CT scan of the abdomen, which may include CT angiography as well as three-dimensional reconstructions, and magnetic resonance imaging (MRI) is used on occasion, depending on the clinical scenario.

## INDICATIONS FOR SURGERY

The indication for radical nephrectomy is a clinically localized solid renal mass in a patient with a normal contralateral kidney. Patients with solitary kidneys, renal insufficiency, or bilateral renal masses should be considered candidates for nephron-sparing surgery. Increasingly, partial nephrectomy is becoming accepted for smaller T1a lesions in the "elective" setting. However, for larger lesions, radical nephrectomy remains the treatment of choice. A thorough preoperative history and physical examination should be performed before the procedure. If significant comorbidities are suspected, preoperative consultation with the appropriate physician is recommended. In an elective radical nephrectomy, the patient should be expected to physically withstand the operation, have a reasonable overall performance status, and have a 5-year life expectancy.

Radical nephrectomy in combination with immunotherapy has been demonstrated to improve survival among patients with metastatic RCC over immunotherapy alone (4). Accordingly, radical nephrectomy is being offered to an increasing number of patients with a resectable primary tumor in the setting of metastatic disease as an initial treatment strategy prior to immunotherapy. Radical nephrectomy may also be performed for palliation, such as for patients with intractable pain or life-threatening hemorrhage who fail conservative treatment despite the presence of metastases. The role of radical nephrectomy among patients with a solitary metastatic site is controversial; however, 5-year survival rates of 30% have been reported in selected patients, with best results reported in patients with solitary pulmonary metastases (2).

Although local extension of primary RCC into the perinephric fat, vena cava, or ipsilateral adrenal gland may portend a worse prognosis, in the absence of metastatic disease these factors alone should not dissuade the surgeon from attempting a radical nephrectomy. In addition, radical nephrectomy has been successfully performed in the setting of direct extension of the tumor into adjacent organs such as the liver, colon, spleen, pancreas, or psoas muscle. However, surgical removal in this setting is technically difficult and is associated with a higher morbidity and a potentially poor prognosis. Therefore, it should be attempted only after careful preparation and in cooperation with appropriate surgical consultants.

## ALTERNATIVE THERAPY

Surgery remains the only effective and potentially curative form of therapy for primary RCC. Along this line, the main challenge to radical nephrectomy in the near future appears to be from more conservative surgical approaches, including nephron-sparing surgery and minimally invasive approaches. Elective partial nephrectomy, enucleation, and wedge resection have been proven to be nearly equivalent in terms of cancer control and may afford potential advantages in terms of preserved renal function and quality of life in properly selected patients (5–7).

Radical nephrectomy is also being performed through laparoscopic approaches, including hand-assisted techniques, which again have shown equivalent cancer control and significant advantages in terms of reduced pain, shorter convalescence, and improvements in quality of life (7,8).

Open radical nephrectomy continues to play an important role in the management of RCC, and it is essential that any surgeon who employs minimally invasive techniques be well versed in its performance.

## SURGICAL TECHNIQUE

There are a variety of factors that influence the choice of incision during radical nephrectomy. These include location of the affected kidney, tumor size and characteristics, body habitus, and physician preference. There are advantages and disadvantages to each incision, and it is important to be familiar with several approaches to the kidney as no one incision is appropriate in all settings. The most commonly used incisions for radical nephrectomy are the flank, thoracoabdominal, and transabdominal (subcostal or chevron) (Fig. 3.1).

### Flank Incision

The flank approach can be advantageous for several reasons. First, it allows direct access to the retroperitoneum and kidney, and the entire procedure can often be performed in an extrapleural and extraperitoneal fashion. In addition, the incision is anatomic in that it follows the track of the intercostal nerves with minimal risk of denervation. However, in large tumors, tumors involving the upper pole, or situations where vena cava access is critical, a flank approach is often suboptimal. Although a flank approach may be performed through a subcostal incision, an eleventh- or twelfth-rib incision is superior for exposure of the upper pole and ipsilateral adrenal gland during radical nephrectomy.

The patient is positioned in the lateral decubitus position with the upper chest at about a 45-degree angle. An axillary roll is placed under the patient to cushion against pressure on the brachial plexus, and the elbows are padded to prevent ulnar nerve injury. The upper arm is draped across the body and placed on a Mayo stand or padded support. The lower leg is flexed at 90 degrees, and the upper leg is extended over one or two pillows. The kidney rest is raised and the table is flexed to elevate the flank and adjusted to make the flank horizontal to the floor. The beanbag or inflatable mattress may be helpful, and if utilized can be activated to further support the patient. The patient is then padded and secured with wide adhesive tape and safety straps.

An eleventh- or twelfth-rib incision is made based on several factors, including the kidney position, the cephalad extent of the tumor, and the patient's body habitus. A general rule is to incise over the rib so that, when extended medially, the incision will be over the renal hilum. The incision is then made off of the tip or over the rib from the posterior axillary line to the tip and extended medially as far as necessary, usually stopping short of the lateral border of the rectus abdominis (Fig. 3.2). The latissimus dorsi is divided, and the upper portion of the incision is carried down to the rib or near its tip. The incision is usually created between the ribs in the intercostal space, and additional exposure may be obtained by incising the costovertebral ligament. With larger tumors and depending on patient body habitus, a partial rib resection may be accomplished as shown in Fig. 3.3. An Alexander periosteal elevator is used to deflect the periosteum from the bone to avoid injury to the intercostal bundle located under the inferior portion of the rib. A Doyen elevator is then used to strip the periosteum from the entire undersurface of the rib to be resected. Next, a rib cutter is used to divide the proximal segment of the rib. The posterior layer of the periosteum is then incised carefully, and the pleura is protected superiorly.

Anteriorly, the external and internal oblique muscles are divided and the transversus abdominis muscle is split in the direction of its fibers, taking care not to enter the peritoneum. The peritoneum is swept medially, and the intermediate stratum of the retroperitoneal connective tissue is incised sharply to expose the perinephric space. Approaching this in a posterior

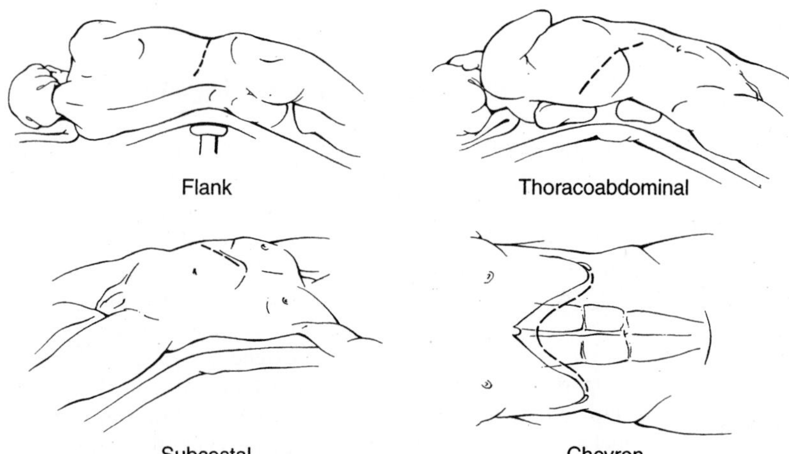


FIGURE 3.1 Types of incisions during radical nephrectomy.

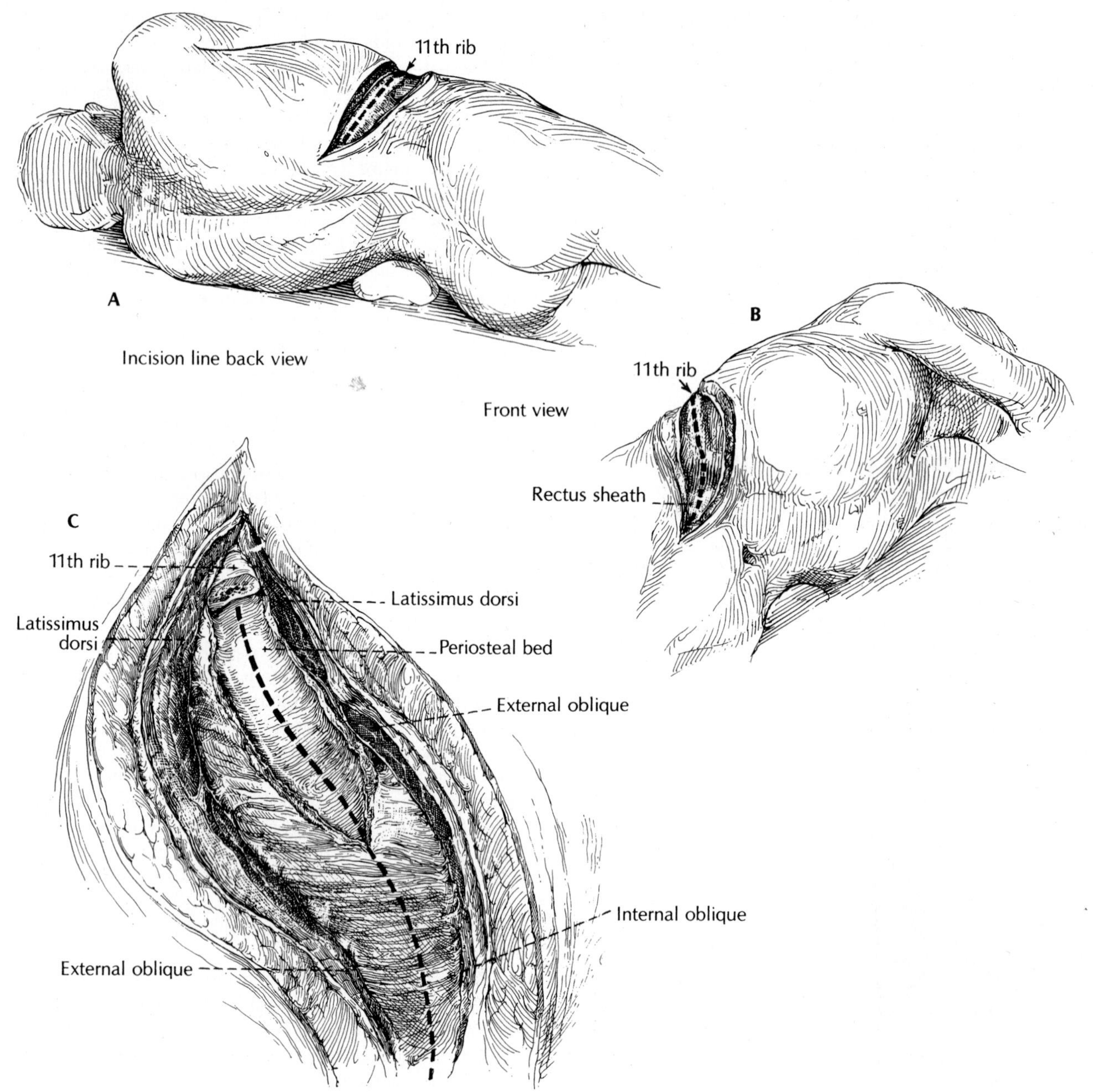


FIGURE 3.2 Technique of eleventh-rib resection. **A and B:** The incision is made over the eleventh rib. **C:** After division of the latissimus dorsi and external oblique muscles, subperiosteal resection of the rib is performed.

fashion with early identification of the psoas muscle helps keep proper orientation. A self-retaining retractor such as a Balfour, Bookwalter, or Finochietto rib spreaders helps maintain exposure. A radical nephrectomy is then performed.

The wound is closed after checking to ensure that no injury to the pleura has occurred (see complications). The table flex is released and the kidney rest is lowered. The posterior layer consisting of the fascia of the transversus abdominis and the internal oblique is closed in a running fashion with no. 1 PDS (polydioxanone suture) or Prolene. The anterior layer of external oblique fascia is closed with a running no. 1 PDS or Prolene. Alternatively, interrupted figure-of-eight sutures of no. 1 Vicryl can be used for both layers. The skin is closed in accordance with the surgeon's preference.

## Thoracoabdominal Incision

The thoracoabdominal approach allows for excellent exposure of large tumors as well as upper-pole tumors, in particular on the left. In addition, it affords easy access to the adrenal gland and thoracic cavity. The patient is positioned with the hips flat and with the break of the table located just above the iliac crest. The pelvis can be torqued up to about 30 degrees if necessary. The patient's ipsilateral shoulder is rotated 45 degrees, and the ipsilateral arm is extended over the table and properly supported on a Mayo stand or padded armrest (Fig. 3.4). It is important to properly pad all pressure points, including between the legs and the contralateral shoulder. The

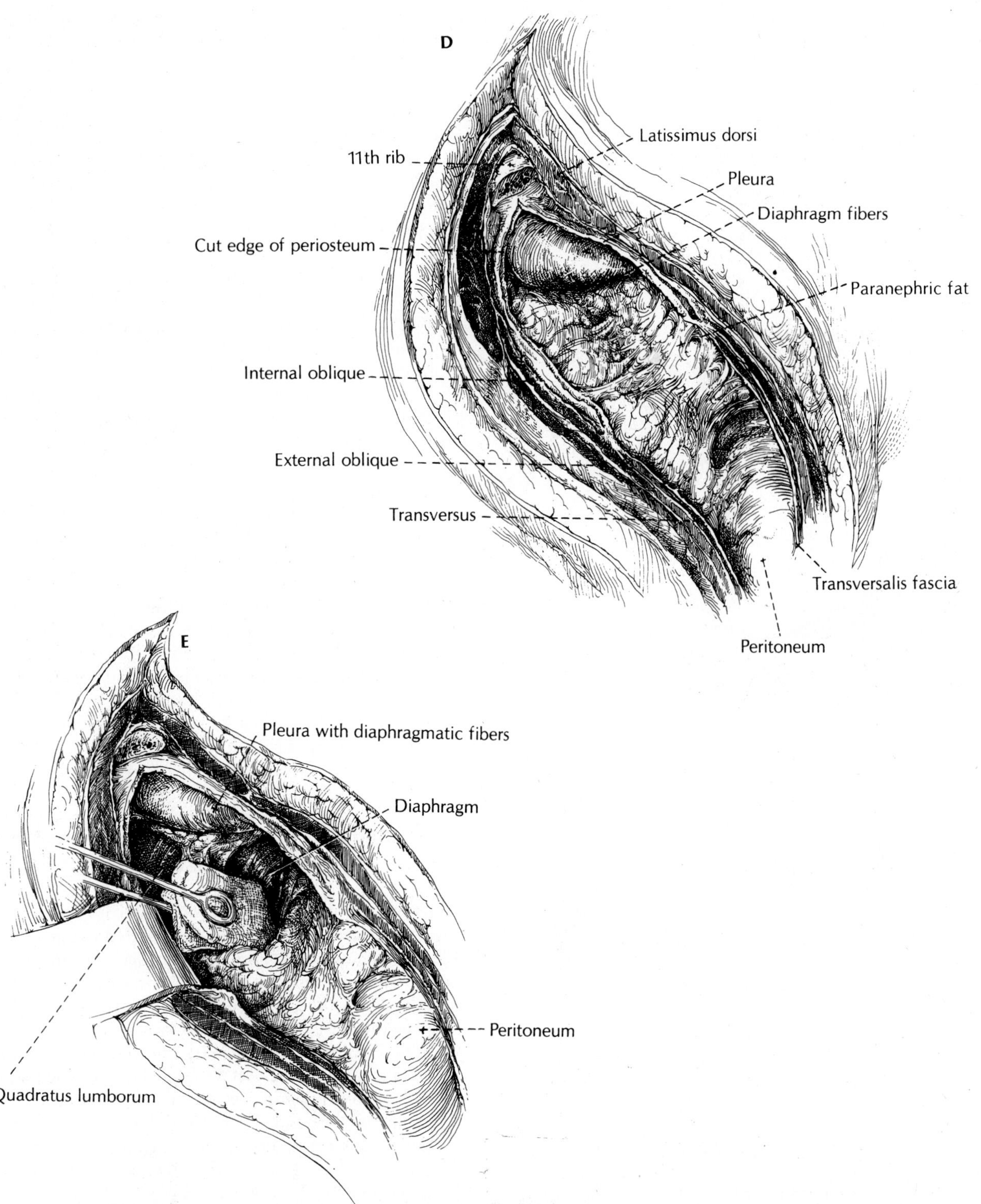


**FIGURE 3.2** Technique of eleventh-rib resection. **D:** The incision is carried through the periosteum posteriorly and the internal oblique and transversus muscles medially, exposing the paranephric space. A tongue of pleura lies in the upper portion of the wound. Diaphragmatic slips that come into view are divided, and the pleura can be retracted upward. **E:** The paranephric fat is dissected bluntly. (*continued*)

kidney rest may be elevated to accentuate the proper extension, and the break in the table is made to optimize the incision. After positioning, the patient is secured with wide adhesive tape and safety straps.

The thoracoabdominal incision is made over the bed of the eighth, ninth, or tenth rib, depending on the surgeon's preference based on patient and tumor characteristics. The incision may be made between the ribs, or a portion of the rib may be removed. The incision is made over the rib beginning at the posterior axillary line. The incision is carried medially across the costal cartilage margin to the midline and then carried down the midline to the umbilicus. Alternatively, the medial

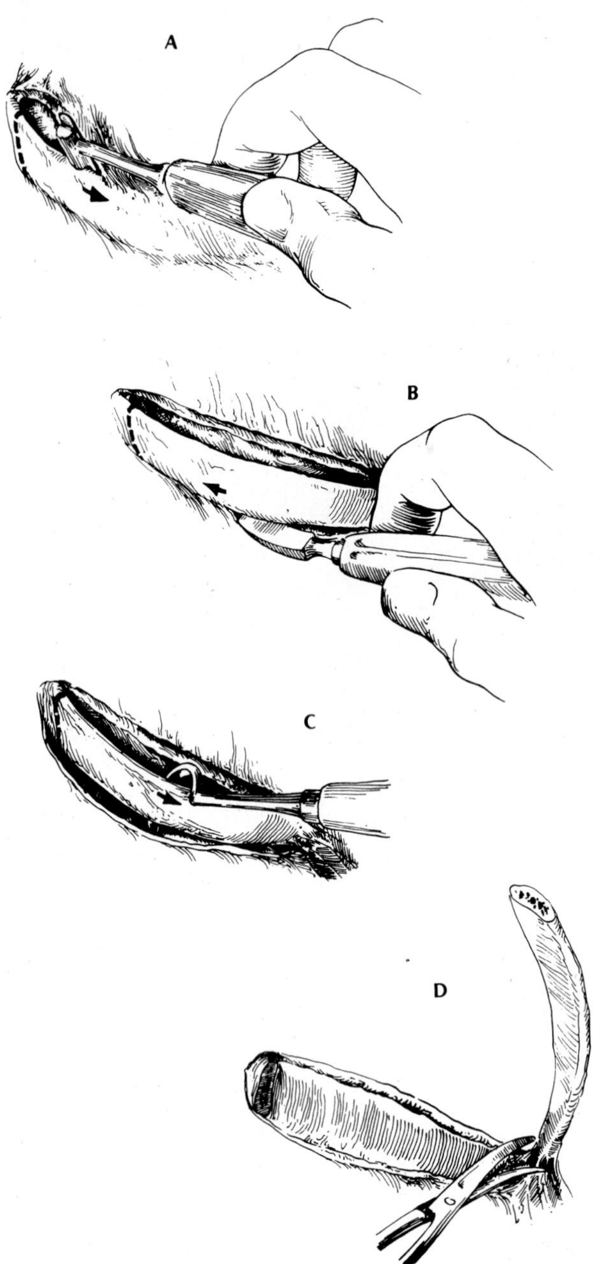


FIGURE 3.3 Rib resection technique. **A:** After exposure of the rib, the intercostal muscles are stripped from the upper and lower rib surfaces with an Alexander–Farabeuf costal periosteotome. **B:** The rib is freed from the periosteum by subperiosteal resection or from the pleura with a periosteum elevator. **C:** A Doyen costal elevator is slipped beneath the rib to free it. The proximal and distal portions of the rib are immobilized with Kocher clamps, and the rib is divided proximal to its angle with a right-angled rib cutter. **D:** The costal cartilage is cut free with scissors. The cut surface of the rib is inspected for spicules, which are removed with a rongeur and covered with bone wax.

portion of the incision may be carried across the midline or combined with a low midline to form a T-shape. The latissimus dorsi is divided, and the upper portion of the incision is carried down to the rib. At this point, a rib resection can be performed as previously described (Fig. 3.3).

The peritoneum may be entered by incising the external and internal obliques, the transversus abdominis, and the ipsilateral rectus abdominis. Next, the costochondral cartilage at the inferior portion of the upper thoracic incision is divided, and the chest is entered along the entire length of the periosteal bed. The pleural space is entered, and care should be taken not to injure the lung. The lung is protected, and the diaphragm is divided in the direction of the muscle fibers, which helps avoid injury to the phrenic nerve. A self-retaining retractor such as a Balfour, Bookwalter, or Finochietto rib spreaders is properly padded and placed to maintain exposure. A radical nephrectomy is then performed.

After completion of the radical nephrectomy, the table flex is removed and the diaphragm is closed with interrupted 2-0 permanent sutures with knots placed on the inferior (peritoneal) side. After a 20Fr to 18Fr chest tube has been inserted through a separate incision and properly positioned, the ribs are reapproximated with 2-0 absorbable sutures. The thoracic portion of the incision is closed with interrupted figure-of-eight 1-0 Vicryl sutures through all layers of the chest wall. The medial portion of the intercostal muscle closure should include at least a small portion of the diaphragm. An intercostal nerve block is administered before closure and may be accomplished by injecting approximately 10 mL of 1.0% lidocaine or 0.5% bupivacaine hydrochloride into the intercostal space of the incision and two interspaces above and below. The costal cartilage can be reapproximated with 0 chromic sutures. This is essential to prevent "clicking" of the ribs, which is oftentimes bothersome to the patient. The posterior rectus fascia, the fascia of the transversus abdominis, and the internal oblique muscles are closed with a running no. 1 PDS suture. The anterior rectus and the external oblique fascia are closed with either a running or interrupted no. 1 PDS suture. Skin closure is determined by surgeon preference. The chest tube is secured in place with a 0 silk and taped securely in place.

## Transabdominal (Chevron or Anterior Subcostal)

Anterior incisions offer several advantages, including excellent exposure of the renal pedicle and access to the entire intraperitoneal contents and contralateral retroperitoneum. With the patient in the supine position, the operative side is elevated slightly with a flank roll and the patient hyperextended to accentuate the line of incision. An incision is made from near the tip of the eleventh or twelfth rib on the ipsilateral side two finger breadths below the costal margin and extended medially to the xiphoid process. The incision is then gently curved across the midline and as far laterally as necessary for exposure up to near the tip of the contralateral eleventh rib.

On occasion, only a portion of the contralateral side will be incised just across the rectus abdominis. The incision is carried down to the anterior rectus fascia, which is then divided (Fig. 3.5). Next, the external and internal oblique fascia and muscles are divided and the fibers of the transversus abdominis split. The rectus muscle and posterior rectus sheath are divided with electrocautery by placing a straight clamp underneath and gently elevating it. The peritoneal cavity is then entered, and the falciform ligament is ligated between two Kelly clamps, divided, and ligated. To facilitate exposure, use of a self-retaining retractor such as a Bookwalter (oval or segmented) or an Omni-Flex is helpful. A radical nephrectomy is then performed.

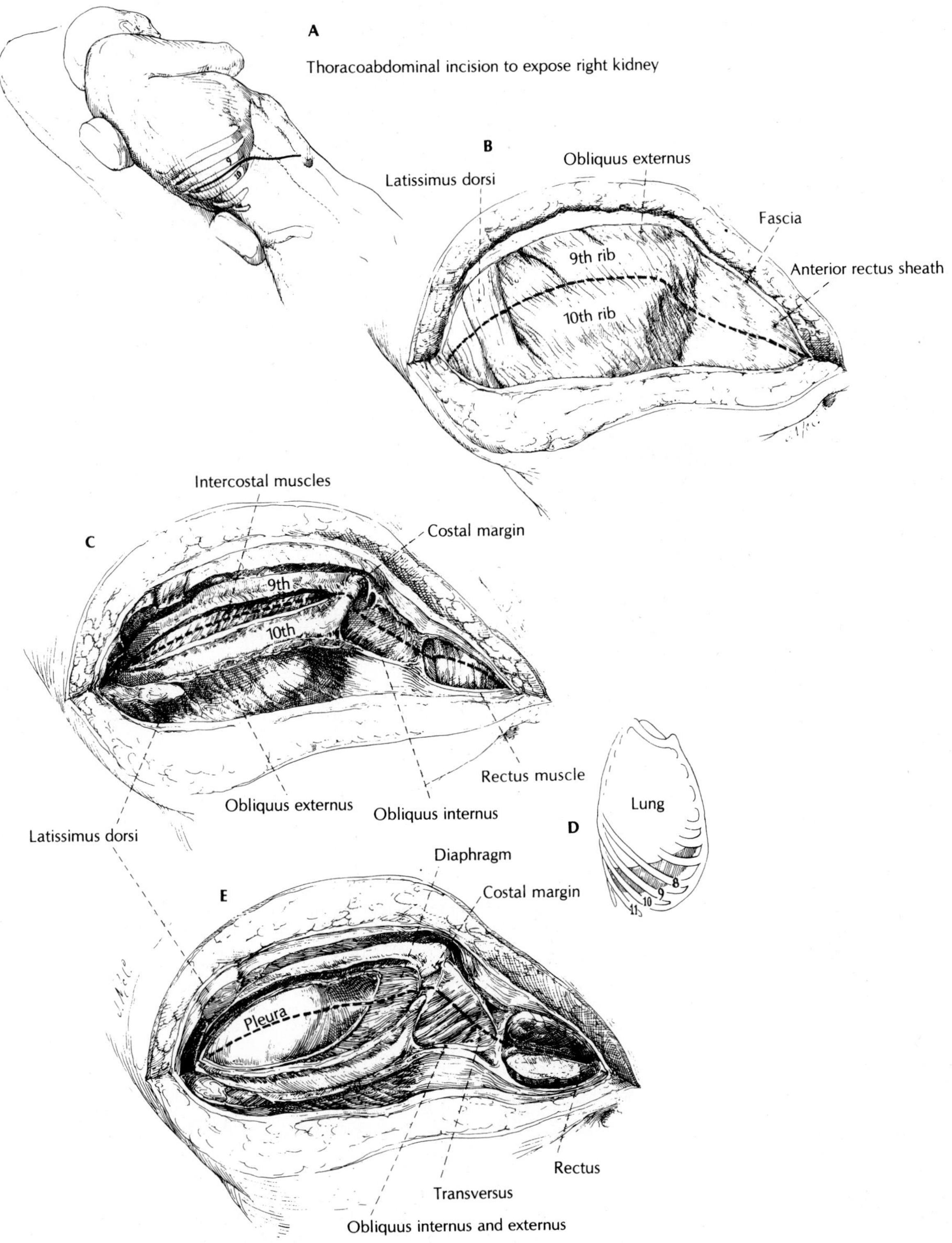


FIGURE 3.4 Thoracoabdominal incision. **A:** The patient is placed in a semirecumbent position using sandbags. If the chest is entered through the ninth intercostal space, the incision extends from the midaxillary line across the costal margin at the intercostal space to the midline or across it just above the umbilicus. **B:** The anterior rectus sheath and the external oblique and latissimus dorsi muscles are divided. **C:** The intercostal muscles parallel the direction of the three abdominal layers and are divided. The costal cartilage and the internal oblique and rectus muscles are incised. If more exposure is desired, the linea alba and opposite rectus can be divided. **D:** The pleural reflection *(shaded areas)* lies progressively closer to the costal margin in the more cephalic intercostal spaces. **E:** The pleura, reflecting as the costophrenic sinus near the costal margin, is exposed beneath the intercostal muscles. The diaphragm can be seen inferior and dorsal to the pleura. The pleura is opened with care to avoid injuring the lung, which comes into view with inspiration. After the lung is packed away gently, the diaphragmatic surface of the pleura is seen. The diaphragm is incised on its thoracic surface, avoiding the phrenic nerve.

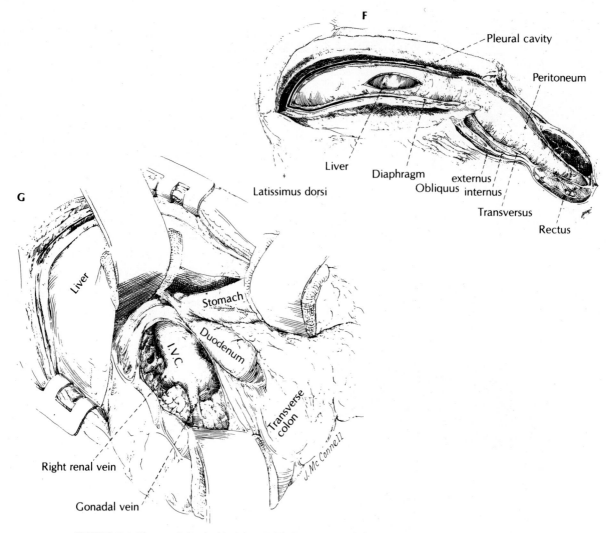

FIGURE 3.4 Thoracoabdominal incision. **F:** The transversus abdominis muscle is divided, exposing the peritoneum with the liver lying beneath it. **G:** The peritoneum is incised, and a rib-spreading retractor (Finochetto) is inserted, enabling upward displacement of the liver (or the spleen on the left) into the thoracic cavity and giving wider access to the posterior peritoneum than in an anterior abdominal incision. (*continued*)

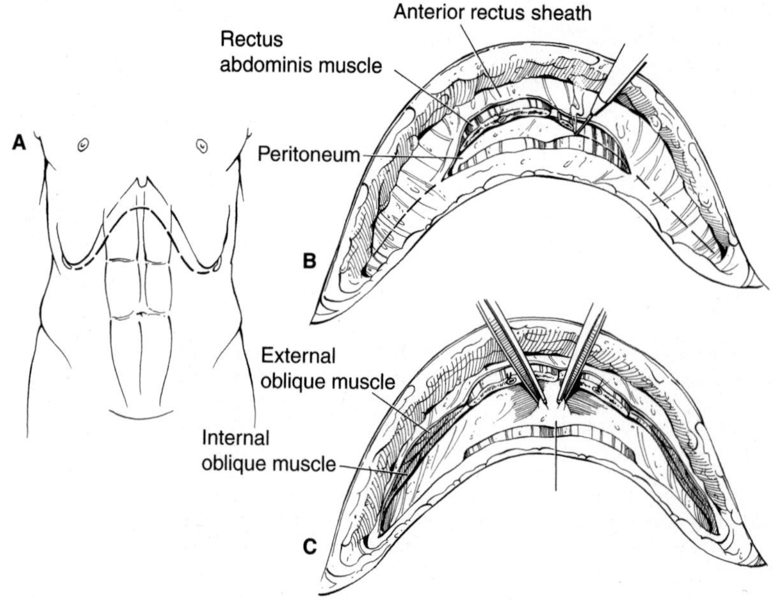


FIGURE 3.5 Transabdominal chevron incision. **A:** With the patient in the supine position and slightly hyperextended, an incision is made two finger breadths below the costal margin to just below the xiphoid process and then curved gently down across to the tip of the opposite eleventh rib. **B:** The subcutaneous tissue and the anterior rectus sheath are divided bilaterally. A Kelly or an Army-Navy retractor is insinuated under the rectus muscle, and the muscle is divided with electrocautery. **C:** The external oblique and internal oblique muscles are divided, and the transversus abdominis is split. The peritoneal cavity is entered in the midline by tenting up on the peritoneum and incising sharply with Metzenbaum scissors.

Closure of the wound is performed after the table is returned to the horizontal position. The wound is then closed in two layers. The posterior layer consisting of the fascia of the transversus abdominis and the internal oblique laterally along with the posterior rectus fascia medially is closed with two running no. 1 PDS sutures, each starting at the lateral aspect and running medially to the midline. The anterior layer of external oblique and anterior rectus fascia is closed in a similar fashion with no. 1 PDS. On occasion, it is helpful to place a U stitch of no. 1 Prolene at the apex of the chevron incision (at the location of the linea alba) before closure, including the rectus fascia on either side of the midline, securing this suture after the anterior fascia has been approximated. The skin is then closed according to the surgeon's preference.

## Radical Nephrectomy

Irrespective of the choice of incision, certain caveats are universal for the safe and successful completion of a radical nephrectomy. They include a systematic approach with careful mobilization of Gerota fascia and careful vascular control. For a flank approach, the posterior peritoneum lateral to the colon is incised along the length of the descending colon (left side) or ascending colon (right side) and reflected medially. For left-sided exposure, the lienorenal ligament is incised to mobilize the spleen cephalad. On the right side, the hepatic flexure of the colon is mobilized. The ureter is identified and encircled with a vessel loop. The gonadal vein is ligated and divided routinely on the left and when necessary on the right. The plane between the mesentery of the colon and Gerota fascia (often referred to as the gonadal space) is then developed using a combination of sharp and blunt dissection. On the right side, kocherizing the duodenum is essential and exposes the vena cava. Using blunt and/or sharp dissection with electrocautery, the retroperitoneal fat overlying the renal vessels is separated, exposing the renal hilum. It is often helpful to ligate and divide the ureter before attempting to expose the renal hilum to allow for mobilization and upward displacement of the lower pole of the kidney.

The dissection is then carried cephalad along the vena cava (right side) or aorta (left side). On the right side, the right renal vein is identified exiting from the vena cava, isolated, and encircled with a right-angle clamp and a 0 silk suture and tagged. After identification of the renal artery (exposure from the anterior approach may be enhanced by the use of a vein retractor on the renal vein), the artery is dissected free and cleaned for a distance of approximately 2 to 3 cm. With a right-angle clamp, the renal artery is encircled, and 2-0 silk ties are passed (Fig. 3.6). The sutures are then separated and tied, allowing a safe distance for division of the artery, and it is preferable to leave two ties on the aortic side. A right-angle clamp is placed under the artery to be divided and gently elevated, and the artery is cut with either a knife (no. 15 blade) or Metzenbaum scissors. The right renal vein is then ligated with two 0 silk sutures and one additional 2-0 suture ligature on the side of the vena cava.

On the left, the renal vein is isolated as it courses over the aorta. The left adrenal and gonadal veins are identified emanating from the left renal vein, and, if present, a posteriorly directed lumbar venous tributary is noted. A right-angle clamp is passed around the renal vein, followed by a 0 silk suture proximal to the tributaries, and tagged. The venous tributaries are then individually ligated and divided with 2-0 or 3-0 silk where necessary, leaving the 0 silk suture on the main renal vein tagged (Fig. 3.7). The left renal artery and vein are then ligated similarly to the technique described previously for the right side.

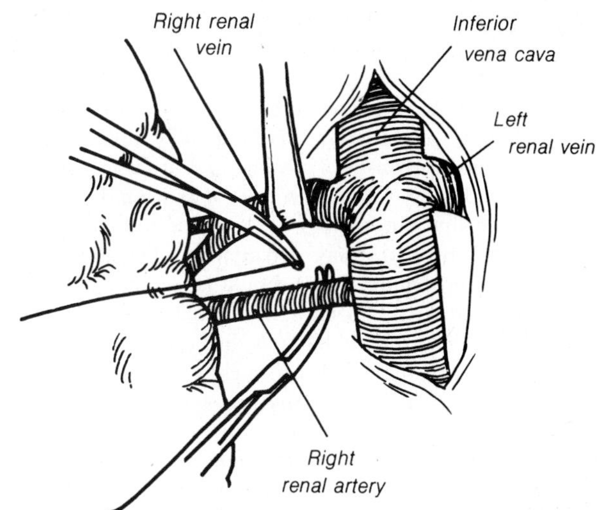


FIGURE 3.6 The right renal artery is identified by palpation beneath the vein. After identification with a right-angle clamp, the artery is cleaned in the same manner as the vein. With a right-angle clamp beneath the artery, a suture is passed on a tonsil clamp to the mouth of the right-angle clamp, and the suture is passed around the artery. (From Donohue RE. Radical nephroureterectomy for carcinoma of the renal pelvis and ureter. In: Crawford ED, Borden TA, eds. *Genitourinary cancer surgery*. Philadelphia: Lea & Febiger, 1982:101, with permission.)

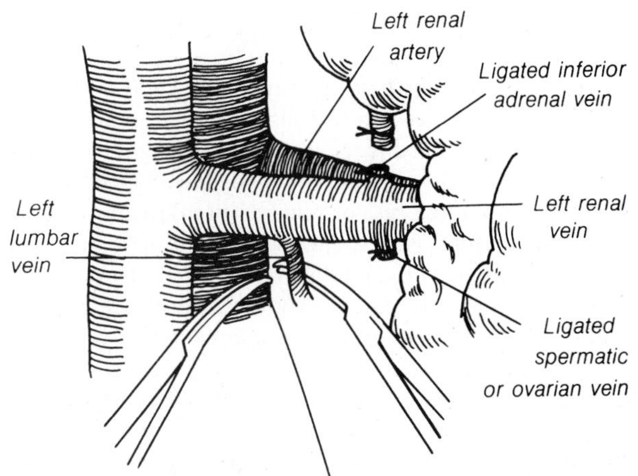


FIGURE 3.7 The same technique for ligation is employed on the left side. A suture is passed around the lumbar vein proximally and distally after the vein has been cleaned, and the vein is ligated. Sutures are passed around the main renal vein but are not tied until after the branches have been ligated. The artery is identified above the vein and cleaned, isolated, and ligated, and the proximal end is sutured with a 5-0 cardiovascular silk suture. (From Donohue RE. Radical nephroureterectomy for carcinoma of the renal pelvis and ureter. In: Crawford ED, Borden TA, eds. *Genitourinary cancer surgery*. Philadelphia: Lea & Febiger, 1982:101, with permission.)

Alternatively, a stapling device can be used to control both the renal artery and vein for either right or left-sided approaches.

Depending on the location of the tumor, prior to control of the renal hilum, Gerota fascia may be initially mobilized posteriorly and superiorly using a combination of sharp and blunt dissection, or this can follow ligation and division of the renal vessels. Small clips placed along the superior and medial border are useful to control any potential bleeding during this portion of the procedure. These should be avoided anywhere near the renal hilum as they may prove problematic if bleeding is encountered. The adrenal hilum is then dissected from caudal to cranial with the aid of either clips or straight clamps and ties. On the right side, the short posteriorly located right adrenal vein should be anticipated as it exits directly from the vena cava. When encountered, the right adrenal vein is isolated, ligated, and divided. The specimen is then delivered and meticulous hemostasis is achieved.

## OUTCOMES

### Complications

The potential for bleeding during radical nephrectomy necessitates careful patient preparation and preoperative planning to significantly reduce the chance of bleeding. Any medications that interfere with platelet function or clotting should be discontinued. A preoperative hematocrit should be obtained, and a type and screen are in general recommended. In patients with significant anemia or in those in whom significant blood loss is anticipated, a type and cross-match for possible transfusion should be performed. The patient should have either two large-bore peripheral IV lines or a central venous line to allow for rapid infusion of fluids or blood products if necessary.

Bleeding during radical nephrectomy may be from a variety of locations, including the renal hilum, collateral tumor vessels, or adjacent structures. Venous bleeding is usually the most problematic. The first maneuver is to apply direct pressure to the area of bleeding and allow for appropriate resuscitation before additional maneuvers are considered. The point of bleeding is then carefully exposed and controlled by a suture ligature. In the case of venal caval injury, pressure can be applied carefully with sponge sticks, and then an Allis or Satinsky clamp may be carefully placed; a vascular 5-0 or 6-0 Prolene suture is used to oversew the defect. Lumbar veins should be exposed by gentle retraction of the vena cava, appropriately clamped, ligated with vascular silk suture, and divided. Renal artery bleeding may be controlled by direct pressure on the aorta proximally and distally until adequate exposure can be obtained, and the artery is then ligated. Only in certain circumstances will a pedicle clamp or en bloc ligation be necessary.

Adrenal tears may result in significant hemorrhage during radical nephrectomy, in particular on the right side, where the short adrenal vein enters into the vena cava directly posterior. Control of the right adrenal vein should be attempted only after control of the vena cava, adequate exposure, and proper suction. The vein is then ligated with a 2-0 or 3-0 silk tie or vascular Prolene. Venous bleeding from a torn adrenal gland can be oversewn with a running suture or stopped by placement of surgical clips. However, removal of the ipsilateral adrenal may be the most expeditious method of controlling bleeding.

Failure to recognize a rent in the pleura during flank incision will result in a pneumothorax. Filling the flank wound with sterile water or saline and administering a deep inspiratory breath may help recognize small openings in the pleura. Small tears recognized intraoperatively can be managed by closing the pleura with a 3-0 chromic pursestring suture over a 12Fr or 14Fr Robinson catheter. Before it is removed, all air is aspirated from the pleural cavity either by suction or by placing the Robinson catheter under water and administering a deep inspiratory breath. The air is evacuated from the pleural space and the tube is removed while the pursestring suture is simultaneously tied in place. Alternatively, the Robinson catheter can be temporarily left in place with the chromic suture secured and the fascial layers closed around the catheter, which exits from the corner of the wound. Just before skin closure, after all air has been evacuated under water seal as described above, the catheter is removed. The latter technique is helpful when the pleura is attenuated or contains multiple small holes that are not easily closed. Alternatively, a 22Fr or 24Fr chest tube may be placed and left to suction and removed postoperatively.

An upright end-expiratory chest X-ray is obtained after all flank incisions to ensure that no significant pneumothorax exists. A small (usually <15%), asymptomatic pneumothorax can be followed conservatively with serial chest X-rays and oxygen therapy. In a symptomatic or large pneumothorax, aspiration of the pleural space using a needle or a central venous catheter (Seldinger technique) introduced just over the rib in the anterior fourth or fifth interspace can be therapeutic. However, if these attempts are not successful, a chest tube should be inserted and placed on suction.

Injuries to the colon during radical nephrectomy are uncommon. In locally advanced tumors suspected of extension into either the colon or mesentery, patients should undergo a mechanical and antibiotic bowel preparation. Segmental colon resection and primary anastomosis should be possible in most cases. Inadvertent injury to the colon during radical nephrectomy can usually be repaired primarily; however, in situations where there is gross spillage of fecal contents or a devascularized segment, a diverting colostomy should be considered, and a general surgery consultation is advisable. Defects in the mesentery of the colon should be closed to prevent internal herniation of peritoneal contents.

Right radical nephrectomy is also associated with the potential for injury to the duodenum and liver. The duodenum must be carefully mobilized, and care must be taken to properly pad retractors to prevent injury to the bowel and adjacent structures, including the head of the pancreas. The second portion of the duodenum may be injured during a right radical nephrectomy. Duodenal hematomas should only be observed, but rapidly enlarging hematomas will require control of the bleeding, and an intraoperative general surgery consultation should be obtained. Duodenal lacerations should be repaired in multiple layers with interrupted nonabsorbable sutures for the mucosal and serosal layers (1). When possible, an omental wrap may provide additional support, and all patients should be managed with a nasogastric tube during the postoperative period.

Bleeding from superficial liver lacerations may be controlled with Bovie electrocautery or an argon beam electrocoagulator. More significant bleeding may be repaired with absorbable horizontal mattress sutures utilizing a Surgicel or Gelfoam bolster. Deep liver lacerations, which may involve the hepatic ducts, could result in bile leakage and should be drained following repair; an intraoperative general surgical consultation is strongly recommended. Direct invasion of the liver by renal cell carcinoma is rare; however, resection including en bloc removal is possible in selected cases. If a major lobectomy or a partial hepatectomy is to be performed because of either direct extension or major hemorrhage, a general surgeon should be present to assist in its performance.

Splenic injury is one of the most common intraoperative complications during a left nephrectomy, with an incidence as high as 10% in some series. Most superficial lacerations or tears can be managed conservatively without the need for splenectomy. Although minor tears may require only some gentle pressure and the application of a Gelfoam or Surgicel bolster with spray thrombin, closure of a moderate splenic capsular tear is facilitated through the use of nonabsorbable sutures over bolsters of Surgicel. Major hemorrhage secondary to severe splenic lacerations may require splenectomy (9).

The splenic artery and vein are controlled by compressing these structures, which are located in the splenic hilum near the tail of the pancreas. Initially, this can be accomplished manually by compressing the tail of the pancreas between the thumb and forefinger. Once bleeding has been temporarily controlled, the spleen is mobilized by dividing the splenocolic and splenorenal ligaments as well as taking down the peritoneal attachments to the diaphragm. The short gastric vessels are then ligated, and the hilum of the spleen is dissected free from the tail of the pancreas. The splenic artery and vein are ligated and divided. The pancreas should be inspected closely to rule out inadvertent injury. Following splenectomy, patients will have a reduced resistance to pneumococcal organisms and should receive Pneumovax and HibTITER on a yearly basis.

## Results

Surgical excision remains the only effective and potentially curative therapy for clinically localized RCC. Pathologic staging remains the best prognostic variable in terms of patient survival, and the most commonly used staging system is the American Joint Committee on Cancer recommendations (TNM) classification (10).

The 5-year survival rate for patients with organ-confined tumors treated with radical nephrectomy for $T_1N_0M_0$ tumors is between 80% and 91%, whereas that for $T_2N_0M_0$ tumors is 68% to 92% (2). For those patients with $T_{3a}N_0M_0$ (tumor invading into the adrenal gland) and $T_{3b}N_0M_0$ (tumor invading into the renal vein) carcinomas, the 5-year survival rate is 77% and 59%, respectively. Finally, patients with node-positive disease ($N_{1\text{-}3}M_0$) have a 5-year survival rate between 5% and 30%.

## *References*


1. Jemal A, Siegel R, Ward E, et al. Cancer statistics, 2007. *CA Cancer J Clin* 2007;57(1):43–66.
2. Campbell SC, Novick AC, Bukowski R. Renal tumors. In: Wein A, ed. *Campbell-Walsh urology*, 9th ed. Philadelphia: WB Saunders, 2007: 1567–1637.
3. Flanigan RC, Mickisch G, Sylvester R, et al. Cytoreductive nephrectomy in patients with metastatic renal cancer: a combined analysis. *J Urol* 2004; 171(3):1071–1076.
4. Flanigan RC, Salmon SE, Blumenstein BA, et al. Nephrectomy followed by interferon alfa-2b compared with interferon alfa-2b alone for metastatic renal-cell cancer. *N Engl J Med* 2001;345(23):1655–1659.
5. Uzzo RG, Novick AC. Nephron sparing surgery for renal tumors: indications, techniques and outcomes. *J Urol* 2001;166:6–18.
6. Lam JS, Shvarts O, Pantuck AJ. Changing concepts in the surgical management of renal cell carcinoma. *Eur Urol* 2004;45:692–705.
7. Lesage K, Joniau S, Fransis K, et al. Comparison between open partial and radical nephrectomy for renal tumors: perioperative outcome and health-related quality of Life. *Eur Urol* 2007;51:614–620.
8. Portis AJ, Yan Y, Landman J, et al. Long-term follow-up after laparoscopic radical nephrectomy. *J Urol* 2002;167:1257–1262.
9. Naitoh J, Smith RB. Complications of renal surgery. In: Taneja SS, Smith RB, Ehrlich RM, eds. *Complications of urologic surgery: prevention and management*, 3rd ed. Philadelphia: WB Saunders, 2001:299–325.
10. American Joint Committee on Cancer. *Manual for staging of cancer*, 6th ed. Philadelphia: Lippincott Williams & Wilkins, 2002.


# CHAPTER 4 ■ INTRACAVAL TUMORS

VIRAJ A. MASTER AND FRAY F. MARSHALL

A unique feature of renal cell carcinoma (RCC) is its frequent pattern of growth intraluminally into the renal venous circulation, which is also known as venous tumor thrombus. This is the most common intracaval tumor that the urologist manages, with approximately 4% to 10% of patients having tumor extension into the muscular branches of the renal veins, with further extension into the main renal vein and then into the vena cava. The extension of thrombus is variable. Many research reports use a staging system proposed by Montie, or small variations of this system, namely: Level 0, limited to the renal vein; Level I, extending into the inferior vena cava (IVC) but <2 cm above the renal vein; Level II, >2 cm above the renal vein but under the hepatic veins; Level III, involving the intrahepatic portion of the IVC (hepatic veins) but below the diaphragm; and Level IV, extending above the diaphragm.

IVC involvement was historically considered a poor prognostic finding for RCC, but many reports have demonstrated that patients with tumor thrombi can achieve reasonable increased longevity with an aggressive surgical approach. Studies have documented approximately 45% to 70% 5-year survival rates for patients with venous tumor thrombi. There continues to be a reasonable correlation between cephalad extent of the thrombus and survival, although striking survival is observed even with suprahepatic tumor thrombus. The critical feature is that there should be an absence of nodal or metastatic disease; otherwise survival is low.

## DIAGNOSIS

The vast majority of the time, the diagnosis of an intracaval tumor is made on the basis of a cross-sectional imaging study. However, physical examination findings may sometimes be the first sign of this kind of tumor. Asymmetric leg swelling may be present. Also in men, a unilateral, acute-onset varicocele may be observed, although possibly the most sensitive sign is unintentional weight loss. CT scans of the chest, abdomen, and pelvis without and with intravenous contrast are the most commonly performed examinations. Generally, these studies demonstrate the size of the primary renal tumor and the presence, size, and rough cranial extent of the tumor thrombus. Additionally, the presence of metastatic disease can be detected. Most often MRI of the abdomen is the next examination performed. Historically, this examination has been performed to precisely locate the cranialmost extent of the tumor (Fig. 4.1). However, with advancement in MRI, this study can be powerful at detecting the number, size, and location of lumbar veins, which is critical for achieving a bloodless field (Fig. 4.1). Additionally, MRI can be highly effective at discriminating between bland thrombus (benign clot) and tumor thrombus. A bone scan should also be performed. Given the rather poor clinical course of patients with brain metastases, it is prudent to obtain brain imaging. In the modern era of advanced cross-sectional imaging, it is usually unnecessary to obtain an inferior vena cavogram. An echocardiogram, performed transthoracically or, if needed, transesophageally, is exceedingly helpful in understanding subtle issues of tumors that

A

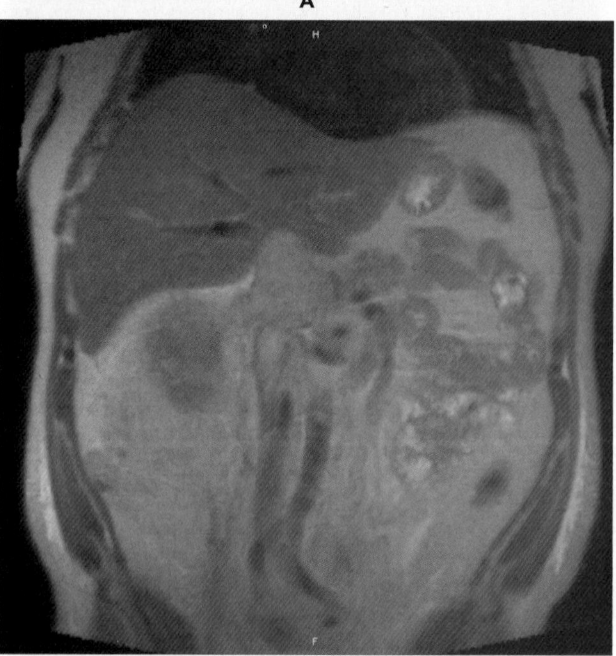

B

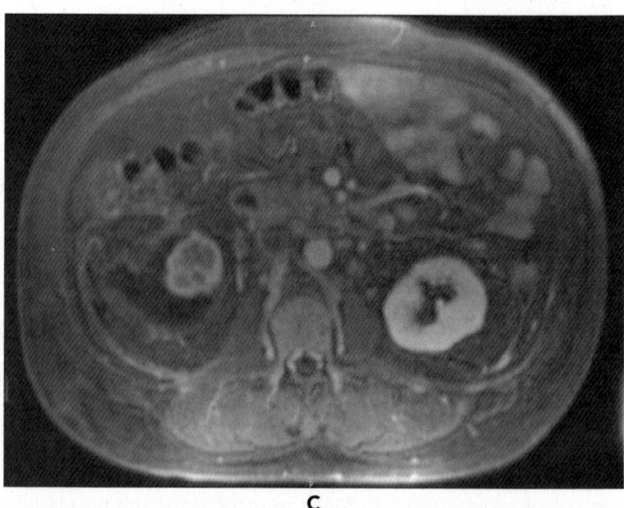

C

FIGURE 4.1 MRI is helpful in determining (A) bland thrombus versus tumor thrombus, (B) cranial extent, and (C) number and location of lumbar veins.

invade the supradiaphragmatic cava and heart. Tumors that are bulky and space-filling in the atrium will certainly require cardiac bypass for safe extraction, while those with tumor thrombus in the intrapericardial IVC or very-small-volume intracardiac tumor thrombus may be treated with an abdominal approach, sparing the patient significant morbidity. If a significant period of time has elapsed since the last imaging study and presentation to our institution (≥4 weeks), we favor repeat imaging to detect further cephalad growth of thrombus and the development of metastatic disease, as surgical management (need for bypass) may change with increasing growth.

## INDICATIONS FOR SURGERY

Historically, these challenging cases were reserved, in the main, for those fit to undergo surgery, without evidence of metastatic disease. Two general lines of evidence have emerged to expand the indications for surgery. First, the advent of the tyrosine kinase inhibitors in 2005 (sunitinb and sorafenib) and of mTOR inhibitors in 2007 (temsorilimus) provided tools to manage metastatic kidney cancer where previously therapeutic nihilism was prevalent. Second, data from the EORTC/SWOG randomized, prospective studies on the value of cytoreductive nephrectomy emerged to show that patients with good performance status, those with pulmonary-only metastatic disease burden, and those whose tumor burden was reduced by 75% after nephrectomy would benefit from cytoreductive nephrectomy (2).

Perhaps the most important issue is whom not to operate on. Patients with compromised cardiac status should be excluded. Additionally, we have observed that overall performance status is an important, sometimes subtle, clue about whom to operate on. Those patients with ECOG performance status of 0 or 1 are good candidates, while those with worse performance status have a dismal, moribund clinical course, regardless of a perfectly performed operation.

## ALTERNATIVE THERAPY

Renal cell carcinoma is classically described as a surgical disease. Neither radiation nor chemotherapy is effective as primary treatment. Since the introduction of multitargeted tyrosine kinase inhibitor medications and mTOR inhibitors, especially in patients with intracaval tumors and metastatic disease, neoadjuvant therapy may be used to potentially shrink tumors and make the operation technically easier. It may also allow for the delineation of those patients who have rapidly progressive metastatic disease and allow these patients to avoid the morbidity of an operation. This approach has not been specifically used for intracaval tumors particularly, but with locally advanced tumors with no increased risk of bleeding (3). The use of angioembolization as a means of palliation for patients with metastatic RCC has been reported in a few small case series, but it certainly will not provide a cure, and it has significant side-effects for the patient (4). Moreover, we have observed some cases of parasitization of adjacent organs after embolization, thus requiring nephrectomy down the line. Some authors have advocated for the use of preoperative embolization of the primary tumor with a view to making the operation easier. We have not noted an advantage of this approach. Metal coils can obstruct the ability to ligate the renal artery. Ethanol and/or microsphere embolization is prone to reflux from the intended site given the significant intratumor arteriovenous fistulas that occur, and indeed may cause massive systemic embolization, resulting in death.

## SURGICAL TECHNIQUE

Multidisciplinary staff communication before the case starts is critical to success. The cell-saver machine needs to be on standby if needed. In addition to a general anesthetic, a thoracic epidural can be utilized and may be effective with postoperative pain management. Alternatively, an On-Q pain pump device (I-Flow Corp, Lake Forest, CA) can replace the need for an epidural. For a thrombus at the level of the hepatic veins, transesophageal sonography is a vital tool for examining the position of the thrombus, ascertaining possible migration, and also looking at cardiac function during the case.

The patient's body habitus and extent of both the primary and intracaval tumor direct the surgical approach. For renal tumors with neoplasm extending minimally into the IVC, a supra-eleventh-rib or standard thoracoabdominal approach with rib excision is ideal (Fig. 4.2), especially in obese patients, and actually can be performed occasionally, in a completely extraperitoneal fashion. For left-sided tumors and more extensive caval tumors, an anterior incision will provide good exposure. We have used a thoracoabdominal incision extending from the tip of the scapula across the costal margin to the midline halfway between the umbilicus and the xyphoid process for right-sided tumors with intrahepatic and supradiaphragmatic intracaval tumor extension. Using this approach, the patient should be positioned with the right shoulder rotated toward the contralateral side while the hips remain in the supine position and the table is slightly extended. Although this incision provides both intra-abdominal and intrathoracic exposure and the dissection is easier for the urologist, cannulating the aortic arch for cardiopulmonary bypass is more difficult.

We typically use a median sternotomy extending into either a midline abdominal or a chevron incision when the intracaval neoplasm extends into or beyond the liver and cardiopulmonary bypass is considered (Fig. 4.3) (5). The chevron incision is useful in patients with a wide abdominal girth, in those with bulky primary tumors, and when using liver mobilization and rotation techniques to gain access to the upper retroperitoneum and chest. Although these extensive incisions provide excellent exposure, allowing for additional operations to be performed, we recommend limiting the procedure to nephrectomy and caval thrombectomy.

The patient should be widely prepared with antiseptic solution and draped to approach an extensive infra- or supradiaphragmatic tumor, and consideration should be given to preparing the neck and groin if venovenous bypass is considered. In the absence of overt metastasis, the incision is extended to include a median sternotomy, as this approach gives the best exposure.

The primary renal malignancy is approached first. For a right renal tumor, the right colon is mobilized along the line of Toldt and reflected medially to gain access to the retroperitoneum (Fig. 4.4). For significant tumors via a midline approach, incision of the root of the mesentery up to the

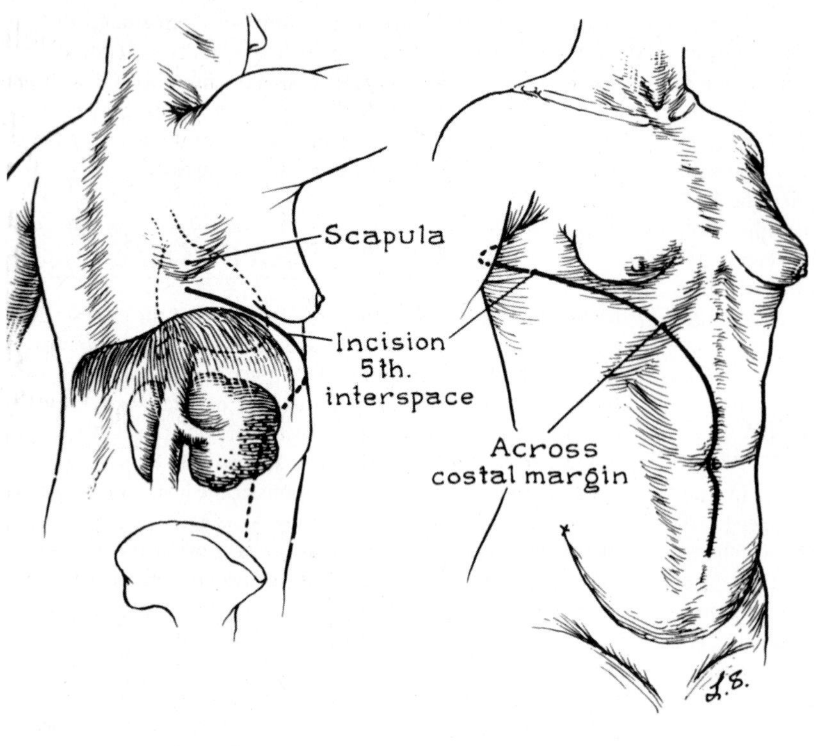


FIGURE 4.2 Thoracoabdominal incision extending from the tip of the scapula across the costal margin to the midline halfway between the umbilicus and the xyphoid process of the sternum. The shoulder is rotated by placement onto a bolster or a 3-L saline bag, but the pelvis is flat. (From Marshall FF, Reitz BA. Radical nephrectomy with excision of vena cava tumor thrombus. In: Marshall FF, ed. *Marshall's textbook of operative urology*. Philadelphia: WB Saunders, 1996:265, with permission.)

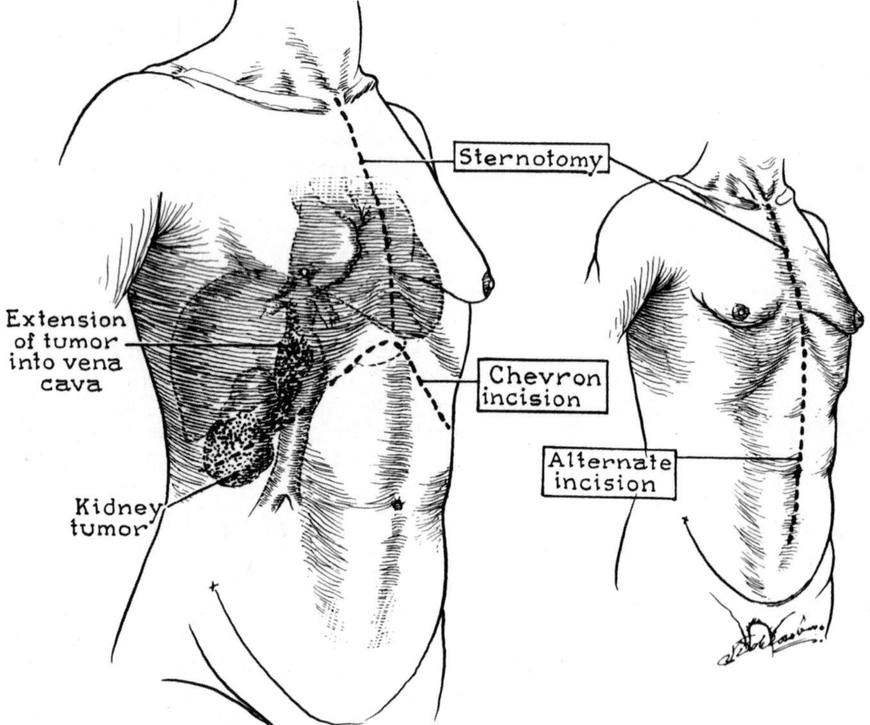


FIGURE 4.3 A midline sternotomy can be performed with a straight vertical incision or with a chevron incision extending laterally. The choice may be best made based on the body habitus of the patient. The large, obese patient is better suited to the chevron with cephalad midline extension. The acute angle of the chevron can be lessened depending on the choice of retractor. The Bookwalter retractor favors an acute angle, while the hepatic Thompson retractor favors an almost inverted-T incision. (From Marshall FF, Reitz BA. Radical nephrectomy with excision of vena cava tumor thrombus. In: Marshall FF, ed. *Marshall's textbook of operative urology*. Philadelphia: WB Saunders, 1996:265, with permission.)

Treitz ligament with placement of the bowel into an intestinal bag retracted onto the chest provides additional exposure. We tend to use the Omni-Tract retractor (Minnesota Scientific Inc.) as it provides excellent superficial and deep exposure of the surgical field. The entire kidney within the Gerota fascia is mobilized, first by a posterolateral approach developing the plane between the quadratus/psoas muscles and the Gerota fascia. After mobilizing the kidney posteriorly, the renal artery is ligated early to keep blood loss to a minimum. An even more rapid approach to the renal artery is possible using an approach popularized for renal trauma. The transverse colon is lifted superiorly and the small bowel pulled to the right. The posterior peritoneum is incised medial to the inferior mesenteric vein right on the aorta up to where the left renal vein is seen. At this point, palpation with a finger or ultrasound probe in the interaortocaval space for the right renal artery or the para-aortic space for the left renal artery will identify the artery. A small pediatric Yankaeur sucker can clear enough

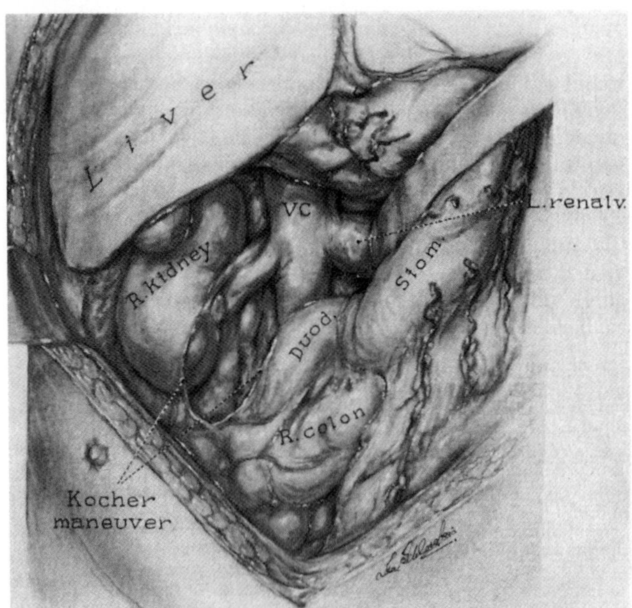


**FIGURE 4.4** Completed incision for radical nephrectomy with removal of a right-sided caval thrombus. The right colon has been widely mobilized and the cava is isolated. (From Marshall FF, Reitz BA. Radical nephrectomy with excision of vena cava tumor thrombus. In: Marshall FF, ed. *Marshall's textbook of operative urology*. Philadelphia: WB Saunders, 1996:269, with permission.)

space to allow the artery to be controlled with a clip, tie, or stapler. This move rapidly decompresses the venous back pressure and seems to allow for shrinkage of the thrombus (Fig. 4.5). Anteriorly, the mesocolon is then reflected medially from the anterior surface of the Gerota fascia until the vena cava is visualized. A Kocher maneuver provides additional medial exposure near the vena cava. Superiorly, dissection above the adrenal is undertaken using clips and the adrenal vein is ligated. Inferiorly, the kidney is mobilized along with ligation of the gonadal vein and ureter. Mobilization of the primary tumor is complete when the kidney remains attached to the vena cava by the renal vein.

A left-sided renal tumor with caval thrombus requires dissection on both sides of the abdomen to access both the vena cava and the left kidney (Fig. 4.6). A midline or chevron incision usually provides excellent exposure. The descending colon is reflected medially by incising the line of Toldt. In a dissection similar to that for a right-sided tumor, the entire kidney within the Gerota fascia is mobilized until only the left renal vein remains. For large, left-sided renal tumors, the pancreas and spleen can be mobilized to provide greater exposure of the left upper retroperitoneum (6). The ascending colon is then mobilized medially by incising the line of Toldt, and the duodenum is reflected by the Kocher maneuver. Once adequate exposure to the vena cava is obtained, the remainder of the procedure is similar to that for a right-sided renal primary tumor.

The extent of the intracaval tumor dictates the length the vena cava that needs to be isolated. Dissection should proceed directly upon the vena cava, using care to prevent potential dislodgement of caval tumor. If the intracaval tumor extends slightly beyond the ostium of the renal vein into the vena cava, a Satinsky vascular clamp can be placed on the caval sidewall beyond the tumor. This segment of caval wall can be excised with the nephrectomy specimen en bloc, and the cava can be oversewn with 4-0 polypropylene suture on a cardiovascular needle.

With a more extensive infra- or suprahepatic intracaval tumor, control of the vena cava must be obtained above and below the extent of the caval tumor thrombus, as well as the contralateral renal vein. Often, it may be advantageous to mobilize and rotate the liver to achieve additional surgical

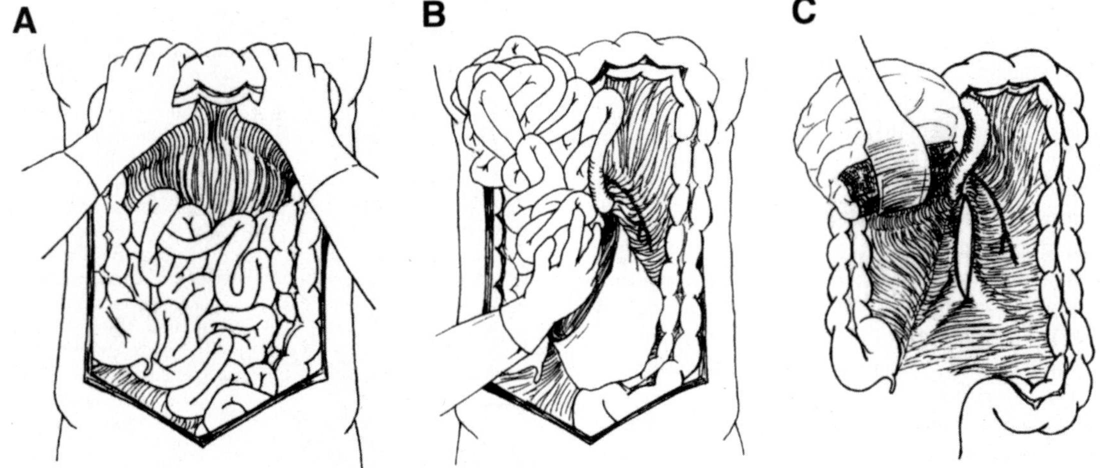


**FIGURE 4.5** Rapid exposure of the renal arteries for early proximal vascular control. This technique is widely used in renal trauma cases. **A:** After an appropriate incision is made, the first maneuver is to place the transverse colon onto the chest. **B:** The small bowel is reflected out of the body toward the right nipple. **C:** Small bowel contents are placed into a bowel bag or covered in moist laparotomy pads. The root of the small bowel mesentery should be visible, allowing for excellent visualization of the posterior peritoneal incision overlying the aorta from the ligament of Treitz to the aortic bifurcation. The posterior peritoneum is incised over the aorta medial to the inferior mesenteric vein. The left renal vein is easily visualized, and using that as a landmark, the right renal artery can be identified and controlled in the interaortocaval space, while the left renal artery may be controlled in the para-aortic space in a rapid fashion. (From Brandes SB, McAninch JW. Surgical exposure and repair of the traumatized kidney. *Atlas Urol Clin North Am* 1998:6(2):32–33, with permission.)

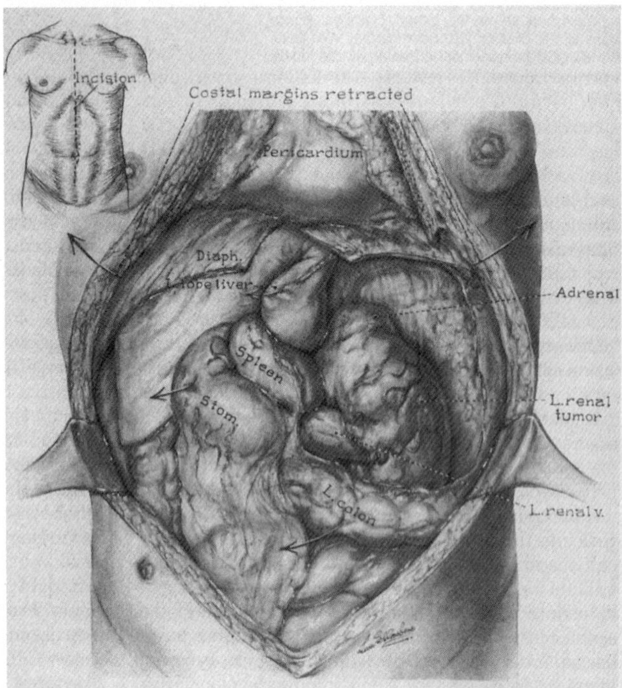


FIGURE 4.6 Completed incision for radical nephrectomy with removal of Level IV vena cava tumor thrombus with a left renal primary tumor. Note the extensive medial visceral rotation performed to safely remove the tumor for these left-sided lesions. Colon, spleen, pancreas, and stomach have all been widely mobilized. (From Marshall FF, Reitz BA. Radical nephrectomy with excision of vena cava tumor thrombus. In: Marshall FF, ed. *Marshall's textbook of operative urology*. Philadelphia: WB Saunders, 1996:268, with permission.)

exposure to the vena cava in the upper abdomen and lower chest. Several of these innovative descriptions of hepatic mobilization derive from liver transplantation techniques (6,7). To maximize surgical exposure, a bilateral subcostal incision is recommended that can be extended superiorly into a partial or conventional median sternotomy if additional exposure or cardiac bypass is necessary. The round ligament and the falciform ligament are ligated and divided to facilitate exposure of the coronary ligaments. The right and left coronary ligaments of the liver are incised, detaching the liver from the diaphragm. The posterior fold between the liver and the right kidney is incised to further mobilize the right lobe of the liver. This maneuver allows the liver to rotate medially, typically providing sufficient exposure of the suprahepatic infradiaphragmatic IVC. In addition, the hepatoduodenal and hepatogastric ligaments can be incised to expose the lesser sac. One can usually appreciate a variable number of short venous branches draining the caudate lobe into the IVC. One or more of these veins may require ligation to prevent unexpected bleeding. If these veins are short, they can be controlled using suture ligatures placed into the liver parenchyma, although a series of medium clips creating a "wall of steel" can be more rapid (Fig. 4.7). Often, mobilization and rotation of the liver will allow the surgeon direct access to the main hepatic vein and the porta hepatis, which may be controlled with a Rummel tourniquet (umbilical tape passed through a 16Fr red rubber catheter) if needed. Inferiorly, a Rummel tourniquet is placed loosely below the tumor thrombus and both renal veins. For a right-sided tumor, a Rummel tourniquet is placed loosely around a segment of the left renal vein to secure control of this vessel. Cardiopulmonary bypass can be obviated when vascular control using a vascular clamp or Rummel tourniquet can be gained above the superior extent of the tumor. Division of the diaphragm may aid in gaining vascular control above the superior extent of the tumor thrombus. It must be emphasized that minimal handling of the primary tumor and intracaval neoplasm is paramount to prevent inadvertent embolism. A Rummel tourniquet slightly tightened can be placed above the level of the caval tumor to prevent inadvertent thromboembolism.

After adequate mobilization of the vena cava superior and inferior to the tumor thrombus with ligation of any lumbar veins, all vascular clamps or Rummel tourniquets are secured. A narrow elliptical incision circumscribing the ostium of the involved renal vein is made. If the tumor is inseparable from the caval endothelium superior to the renal veins, the involved cava is excised. The renal primary and caval tumor is removed en toto under direct vision. On occasion, we have used a dental mirror to inspect the hepatic veins or a flexible cystoscope to inspect the cava to ensure complete removal of tumor. If additional verification is necessary, transesophageal echography can be used to evaluate the superior extent of the cava, or direct intraoperative sonography can be used to evaluate the extent of the cava (8).

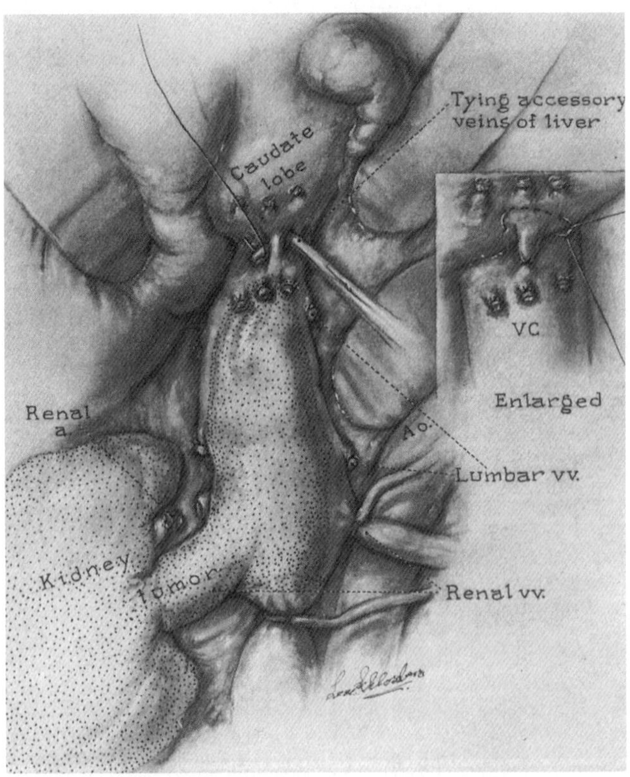


FIGURE 4.7 Ligation and division of the venous tributaries of the caudate lobe of the liver. Note that there are significant variations in the number, diameter, and location of these short caudate veins. Multiple ties or clips are required for control of these short veins. This maneuver allows for proximal control of the cava above the thrombus, or of full liver mobilization off the vena cava. (From Marshall FF, Reitz BA. Radical nephrectomy with excision of vena cava tumor thrombus. In: Marshall FF, ed. *Marshall's textbook of operative urology*. Philadelphia: WB Saunders, 1996:267, with permission.)

To close the vena cava, a 4-0 or 5-0 cardiovascular polypropylene suture on either RB-1 or SH needles is used. Before completing the cavotomy closure, the inferior tourniquet is released to allow trapped air to escape through the cavotomy site. If excision of the cava decreases the vascular diameter by >50%, reconstruction of the vena cava is recommended to prevent caval thrombosis. Initial cases of vena cava reconstruction were done using pericardium because it is less thrombogenic, although more recently prosthetic grafts have been employed. Venous drainage of the right kidney must always be preserved to prevent venous infarction. In some instances, the cava has been oversewn to prevent subsequent embolism if the thrombus below the renal veins is adherent to the caval endothelium, as is often the case with bland thrombus. Alternatively, an Adams-DeWeese clip can be placed on the IVC for this purpose. For the sake of expediency, the endovascular stapler can be used to quickly divide the vena cava.

## Abdominal Approaches to Suprahepatic and Supradiaphragmatic Thrombi (Levels III and IV)

With increasing utilization of liver transplantation worldwide, there has been a spillover of techniques with applicability to advanced retroperitoneal surgery (9). For those tumors with persistent tumor thrombus extension above the diaphragm, absolutely complete liver mobilization, followed by careful division of the central tendon of the diaphragm, entry into the pericardium, and circumferential dissection of the intrapericardial vena cava, will allow for transdiaphragmatic intrapericardial IVC control. It should be emphasized that this maneuver should be performed by those with extensive experience with the anatomy of the vena cava in the pericardium. Our experience has been that working with cardiothoracic transplant surgeons allows for the performance of this maneuver by those surgical specialists with an intimate knowledge of mediastinal anatomy, and we have not experienced problems in four such cases. That said, cardiopulmonary bypass approaches have a significantly longer track record, and many more cardiac surgeons are familiar with this approach, as outlined below.

## Cardiopulmonary Bypass, Hypothermia, and Temporary Cardiac Arrest for Level IV Thrombus

The need for cardiac bypass exists, in general, for tumor thrombi that are above the diaphragm and not obviously amenable to the techniques for abdominal access of supradiaphragmatic thrombus cases. Cardiopulmonary bypass, hypothermia, and temporary cardiac arrest greatly facilitate the resection of a suprahepatic caval thrombus (8). It is best to dissect as much of the kidney and the vena cava as possible prior to cardiac bypass. Following isolation of the renal tumor, the pericardium is opened and retracted with stay sutures. Typically, the right atrial appendage is cannulated with a 32Fr venous cannula and the aorta is cannulated with a 22Fr Bardic cannula. Heparin is then administered to maintain an activated clotting time >450 seconds. The patient is placed on bypass with flow rates maintained between 2.5 and 3.5 L per minute. A core temperature of 18°C to 20°C is attained within 30 minutes while maintaining an 8°C to 10°C gradient between the perfusion and the patient's core temperature. When a rectal temperature of 20°C is reached, the aorta is cross-clamped and 500 cc of cardioplegic solution is administered. Once cardiac arrest is achieved, bypass is terminated and the patient is temporarily exsanguinated into an oxygen reservoir. The patient's brain is protected by placing ice bags around the head. At this point, there is no anesthesia, ventilation, or circulation. To reduce the incidence of complications, circulatory arrest time is best limited to 45 minutes.

An elliptical incision is made around the ostium of the renal vein and carried superiorly along the length of the vena cava. The incision can extend into the right atrium or ventricle, depending upon the superior extent of the thrombus. Using cardiopulmonary bypass and deep hypothermic circulatory arrest, the thrombus can be removed in a bloodless field and the interior of the vena cava and heart can be inspected under direct vision (Fig. 4.8). It is not uncommon to find some degree of adherence of the tumor to the endothelium. In this case, the tumor thrombus can be "endarterectomized" from the interior of the vena cava or atrium. Reconstruction of the vena cava is as previously mentioned.

Following closure of the venacavotomy, cardiopulmonary bypass is begun. The patient is slowly warmed using a 10°C gradient between the bypass machine and a warming blanket. Mannitol (12.5 g) is given along with 1 g of calcium chloride when core temperature reaches 25°C. Electrical defibrillation is necessary if the heart does not resume spontaneous beating. Following resumption of cardiac activity, blood is returned to the patient from the oxygen reservoir. Following the rewarming process, which can take up to 1 hour, heparin is neutralized with protamine. The patient is returned to the cardiac intensive care unit intubated.

Advances in surgery have prompted investigators to describe alternatives to cardiopulmonary bypass with deep hypothermic cardiac arrest to minimize the risks associated with bypass and circulatory arrest and/or diminish the morbidity of the surgical incision. Venovenous bypass may be used as an alternative to cardiopulmonary bypass for patients with an infradiaphragmatic tumor and near occlusion of the vena cava who do not tolerate clamping of the vena cava. Test clamping of the vena cava should always be performed prior to the clamping and opening of the cava. Generally, those patients with bulky thrombus that is completely occlusive have naturally developed venous collaterals and can tolerate clamping of the cava (Fig. 4.9). Venovenous bypass avoids the risks of cardiopulmonary bypass while ensuring adequate circulation during the venacavotomy. Traditionally, to establish venovenous bypass, an incision overlying the saphenofemoral junction is made and the saphenous vein is isolated. A similar incision is made in the axilla and the axillary vein is identified. The saphenous and axillary veins are incised and cannulated with a 7-mm heparinized Gott aneurysm shunt and secured with a Rummel tourniquet. Bypass is commenced with clamping of the IVC. Following completion of the procedure, the shunts are removed, the axillary vein is reconstructed with 6-0 polypropylene, and the saphenous vein is ligated. Alternatively, with an experienced liver transplantation anesthesiologist, a large-bore venous cannula such as a Cordis (Cordis Corp, Warren, NJ), can be placed into the femoral vein and jugular vein and an adequate veno-veno bypass created.

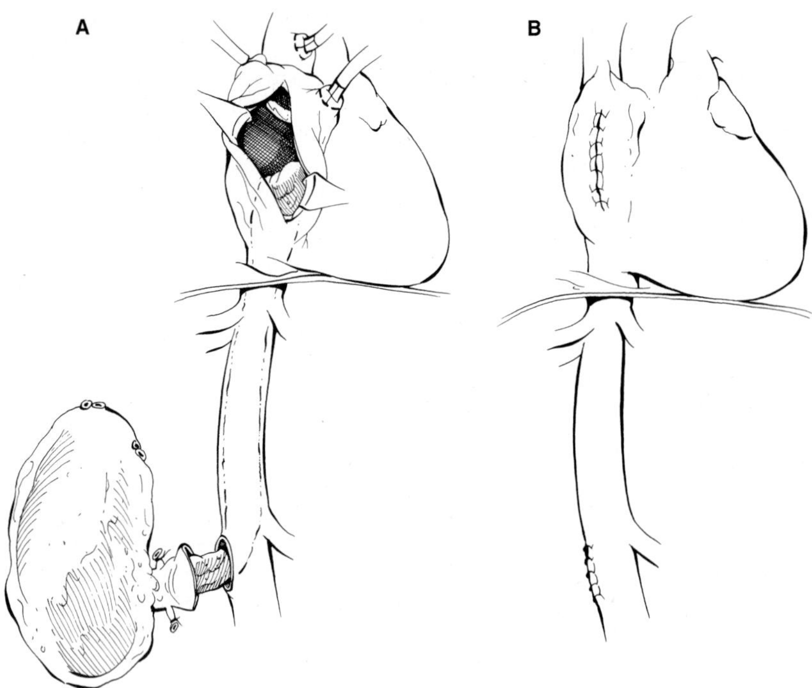


FIGURE 4.8 **A:** The ostium of the renal vein is circumferentially incised and the right atrium is opened. **B:** Following removal of the tumor thrombus, the atriotomy and vena cavatomy incisions are closed. (From Novick AC, Montie JE. Surgery for renal cell carcinoma. In Novick AC, Streem SB, Pontes JE, eds. *Stewart's operative urology*, Vol. 1, 2nd ed. Baltimore: Williams & Wilkins, 1989, with permission.)

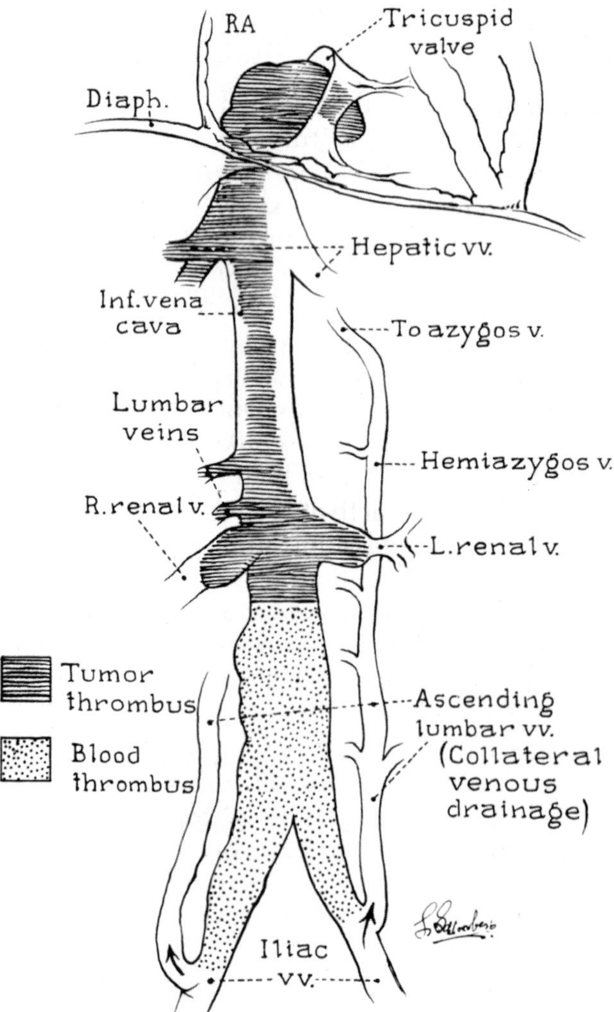


FIGURE 4.9 The vena cava can have thrombus throughout its entire extent. Below the renal vein ostia, this is generally a blood thrombus, also known as a "bland" thrombus. Attempted extraction of this thrombus is fraught with complications and is best avoided. In the setting of complete caval obstruction, the cava can actually be ligated at this point to prevent thrombus migration. Venous collaterals as shown in the figure are very well developed in this setting and will drain the lower body. From the level of the renal veins above, the thrombus is a tumor thrombus. Such thrombus has been extracted from the contralateral renal vein, lumbar veins, hepatic veins, right atrium, and right ventricle. (From Marshall FF, Reitz BA. Radical nephrectomy with excision of vena cava tumor thrombus. In: Marshall FF, ed. *Marshall's textbook of operative urology*. Philadelphia: WB Saunders, 1996:269, with permission.)

For tumors extending into the right atrium, a minimally invasive cardiac surgical approach using a right parasternal incision has been described, and extensive experience has been documented (10). This approach would enable access to the right atrium and right subclavian artery for cannulation of arterial inflow. Following isolation of the vena cava and primary renal tumor, an incision below the right clavicle is made to expose the subclavian artery. A separate incision is made from the lower segment of the third rib to the fifth rib along the right sternal border. A 3-cm segment of cartilage from the fourth and fifth ribs is resected, and the right internal thoracic artery is ligated and divided. After opening the pericardium, an 8-mm collagen-coated graft is sewn to the right subclavian artery and a venous cannula is placed into the right atrium. Following cardiopulmonary bypass, circulatory arrest, tumor excision, and decannulation, a flap of periosteum, muscle, and pleura is used to close the defect associated with this minimally invasive incision.

## OUTCOMES

The 5-year survival rates in most reported large series vary from 14% to 68% following complete surgical removal of the renal tumor and caval extension. The largest series, comprising 614 patients from the Mayo Clinic with tumor thrombus and clear cell RCC, had a 50% 5-year cancer specific survival. However, this rate significantly worsened to 15% to 20% in the presence of intercurrent lymph node involvement or distant metastatic disease, and it was further reduced to 4% if both adverse features were present. Differences in reported survival may reflect several factors, including local extension of the primary tumor, presence of lymphatic or visceral metastases, or invasion into the vascular wall. The level of caval extension correlating with survival is a matter of active and current debate in the literature. It is in general agreed that patients with metastatic disease and significant perinephric fat involvement tend to have a poorer prognosis. The majority of patients eventually dying of their disease succumb to metastases, which suggests that occult metastatic disease is frequently present at the time of surgery (11). Patients with good performance status who have tumors confined to the renal capsule and are without evidence of metastatic disease are ideal candidates for this surgery and have improved long-term survival.

## Complications

Surgery for intracaval tumors is subject to a number of complications that occur approximately 10% to 30% of the time. Certainly, over time, there is a declining incidence of complications, likely due to better patient selection and better postoperative care. For example, one large 30-year series noted a 40% decline in complications in cases done in the 1980s versus those done in the 1990s (12).

Intraoperative complications include excessive bleeding and coagulopathy. Coagulopathy is more common with prolonged cardiopulmonary bypass and cardiac arrest times. Intraoperatively, red blood cells, platelets, fresh frozen plasma, and calcium chloride are routinely administered. Furosemide and/or mannitol is given if urine output remains low. Transient hypotension can occur when clamping the vena cava. This can be managed with volume expansion. It tends to be less of a problem with bulky vena cava thrombus or completely occluded cava because this situation usually creates multiple venous collaterals. However, this difference comes at a price, as the dilated lumbar veins that drain the obstructed cava are often simultaneously large and thin-walled. Finally, embolization of a segment of tumor thrombus can be a potentially lethal intraoperative complication, and extreme care should be taken when handling the vena cava to prevent such an occurrence. Overall mortality has decreased over time but still remains present (1.5% to 7.5%).

Postoperatively, several complications can occur due to the magnitude of the surgical procedure or in those patients who also underwent the use of cardiopulmonary bypass. Potential complications include caval thrombosis, deep venous thrombosis, pulmonary embolus, postoperative bleeding, and coagulopathy. Patients may also develop hepatic dysfunction, renal failure, sepsis, or myocardial infarction. Although the modern mortality rate associated with this procedure is approximately lower over time in modern series, most patients who die of complications within the first postoperative month succumb to multisystem organ failure.

## *References*


1. Ciancio G, Livingstone AS, Soloway M. Surgical management of renal cell carcinoma with tumor thrombus in the renal and inferior vena cava: the University of Miami experience in using liver transplantation techniques. *Eur Urol* 2007:51:988.
2. Flanigan RC, Salmon SE, Blumenstein BA, et al. Nephrectomy followed by interferon alfa-2b compared with interferon alfa-2b alone for metastatic renal-cell cancer. *N Engl J Med* 2001;345:1655.
3. Margulis V, Matin SF, Tannir N, et al. Surgical morbidity associated with administration of targeted molecular therapies before cytoreductive nephrectomy or resection of locally recurrent renal cell carcinoma. *J Urol* 2008;180:94.
4. Munro NP, Woodhams S, Nawrocki JD, et al. The role of transarterial embolization in the treatment of renal cell carcinoma. *BJU Int* 2003;92:240.
5. Marshall FF, Reitz BA. Technique for removal of renal cell carcinoma with suprahepatic vena caval tumor thrombus. *Urol Clin North Am* 1986;13:551.
6. Marsh CL, Lange PH. Application of liver transplant and organ procurement techniques to difficult upper abdominal urological cases. *J Urol* 1994;151:1652.
7. Ciancio G, Hawke C, Soloway M. The use of liver transplant techniques to aid in the surgical management of urological tumors. *J Urol* 2000;164:665.
8. Marshall FF. Renal cell carcinoma with caval extension to the heart. *Urology* 1996;47:126.
9. Ciancio G, Soloway MS. Renal cell carcinoma with tumor thrombus extending above diaphragm: avoiding cardiopulmonary bypass. *Urology* 2005;66:266.
10. Wotkowicz C, Libertino JA, Sorcini A, et al. Management of renal cell carcinoma with vena cava and atrial thrombus: minimal access vs median sternotomy with circulatory arrest. *BJU Int* 2006;98:289.
11. Polascik TJ, Partin AW, Pound CR, et al. Frequent occurrence of metastatic disease in patients with renal cell carcinoma and intrahepatic or supradiaphragmatic intracaval extension treated with surgery: an outcome analysis. *Urology* 1998;52:995.
12. Blute ML, Leibovich BC, Lohse CM, et al. The Mayo Clinic experience with surgical management, complications and outcome for patients with renal cell carcinoma and venous tumour thrombus. *BJU Int* 2004;94:33.

# CHAPTER 5 ■ TRANSPLANT NEPHRECTOMY

SANJAYA KUMAR

In the United States, renal allograft survival for all transplants is 91% at 1 year and 82% at 3 years since the introduction of cyclosporine (9,13). Notwithstanding optimal immune suppression, some allografts will fail. Failed allografts frequently result in a transplant nephrectomy in similar frequency in both cadaveric and living-related transplants. The etiology and timing of graft failure play an important role in the need for transplant nephrectomy.

## DIAGNOSIS

Transplant nephrectomy is performed when the graft has failed. This may occur in the acute or chronic setting. Renal allograft rupture within days of the transplant is usually due to acute allograft rejection, renal vein thrombosis, or even acute tubular necrosis (8). Symptoms include severe allograft pain, a drop in hematocrit, and hypotension. Renal scan, Doppler ultrasound, and computerized tomography (CT) scan can help establish the diagnosis. Urgent transplant nephrectomy may be warranted under these circumstances.

In the chronic setting, graft function deteriorates slowly and the patient becomes azotemic and requires dialysis. Radiologic evaluation with Doppler ultrasound and renal scan are helpful. Renal biopsy is almost always performed to confirm rejection. Once it is confirmed that renal function is irreversible, immune suppression is tapered and sometimes completely withdrawn. The patient is placed on chronic dialysis and the need for graft nephrectomy is ascertained.

## INDICATIONS FOR SURGERY

A renal allograft may fail for several reasons. These primarily include rejection, irreversible renal vascular compromise, or significant graft sepsis. Policy regarding graft nephrectomy varies according to the transplant institution. While most failed grafts were removed in the past, the recent trend is to remove the allograft only when necessary. Further, there is some suggestion that retaining the primary graft in situ may have a protective effect on the subsequent transplant (1). Over the years, the incidence of graft nephrectomy continues to trend down. The incidence varies from 4% to 8% in some recent series (5,7,14).

Graft failure within the first few weeks following transplant is usually due to accelerated rejection or technical failure secondary to vascular compromise, and those failing within the first few months are due to irreversible acute rejection. Renal allografts rejected within the first 12 months of transplant are usually removed prophylactically regardless of the cause, even if these patients are asymptomatic (10,12,14). Significant symptoms usually develop due to the retained graft, necessitating its removal in the future. However, the policy of some centers is to remove failed transplants only when they interfere with health (7).

Graft failure that occurs 1 year after transplant is usually due to chronic rejection. Progressive withdrawal of immunosuppression may allow the patient to retain the graft in the majority (50% to 90%) of instances (4,7,10,14). Many patients, however, develop symptoms such as fever, malaise, gross hematuria, graft tenderness, and thrombocytopenia related to platelet consumption by the graft. It can be difficult to distinguish these symptoms from superimposed acute rejection or infection, and graft nephrectomy may be the only solution. Thus, the primary indication today to remove a failed graft is graft intolerance by the host after withdrawal of immunosuppression.

Rare indications for allograft nephrectomy include the development of a renal mass (11). This may involve lesions unintentionally transmitted from the donor or lesions arising in the transplant kidney. CT scan and needle biopsy help confirm the diagnosis. Intractable urinary problems such as leaks and fistulas rarely require transplant nephrectomy today. Advances in urologic endoscopy and percutaneous techniques have virtually eliminated the need for graft nephrectomy in these patients.

## ALTERNATIVE THERAPY

An alternative to graft nephrectomy is embolization of the failed allograft. The graft is embolized through femoral arterial access using coils or ethanol. The presence of multiple renal arteries is not considered a problem, although it can be technically challenging to catheterize these small arteries with their thickened intimal layer and narrow ostium. Although successful embolization has been reported in 85% of patients (3), postembolization syndrome can occur in many patients, including graft abscess and sepsis (6). These patients eventually require a nephrectomy. Graft embolization may thus be considered in patients with a failed renal graft and intolerable symptoms that do not improve with medical management and in whom transplant nephrectomy has a significant morbidity and risk of mortality.

## SURGICAL TECHNIQUE

If available, it is important to review the previous operative notes of the transplant. This will help the surgeon understand the anatomy of the vascular anastomosis and pre-empt any potential catastrophe. Patients with renal failure usually have

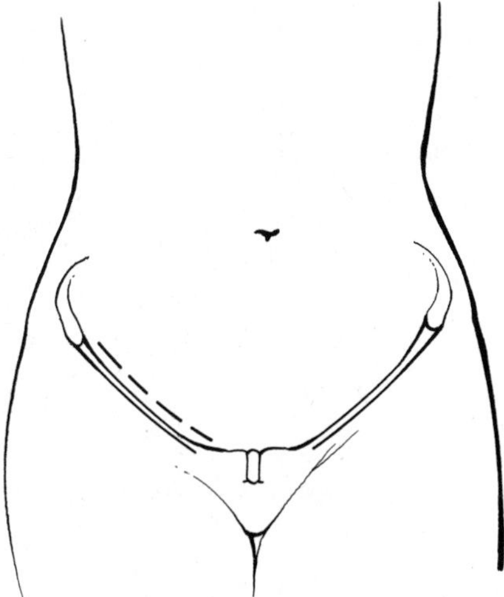

FIGURE 5.1 The patient is positioned in the supine position and the incision is made over the previous lower-quadrant transplant incision.

platelet dysfunction. Even though their coagulation parameters are normal, desmopressin (DDAVP) is usually given to improve platelet function. The adult dose of DDAVP is 0.3 μg per kg body weight.

The patient is placed in the supine position. An incision is made over the previous incision, which is usually is the lower quadrant (Fig. 5.1). The previous skin scar is excised. If the kidney is large and swollen, it may be necessary to extend the incision laterally. The external and internal oblique muscles and, in the lateral part of the incision, the transversalis are incised. As a result of previous surgery, rejection, or multiple renal biopsies, the kidney is stuck to the undersurface of the muscle, the pelvic sidewall laterally, and the peritoneum medially. The colon may drape over the entire anterior surface of the kidney. Under these circumstances, it may be easier to extend the incision laterally and enter the retroperitoneum above the superior pole of the kidney. Once the kidney has been identified, space is created in the retroperitoneum for a self-retaining retractor (e.g., Bookwalter). The relationship of the iliac vessels, bowel, and peritoneum vis-à-vis the kidney is established so as not to injure them. The kidney is identified by palpation. In cases of rejection the kidney may be large, swollen, and friable.

A decision is now made on whether to perform a subcapsular nephrectomy or to use an extracapsular approach. Depending on the degree of reaction, one may be able to perform the entire nephrectomy by staying extracapsular and removing all renal tissue. Certainly, the initial attempt can be made to perform an extracapsular nephrectomy, and as the dissection approaches the hilum or if dissection is impossible due to the inflammatory reaction, one can resort to a subcapsular approach. Extracapsular graft nephrectomy is possible when the allograft has to be removed within a few weeks of transplant. Often, the planes of dissection may be so effaced that the only recourse may be to directly enter the renal capsule and perform a subcapsular nephrectomy from the outset. Because of the increased morbidity and mortality of the extracapsular approach, many centers routinely perform a subcapsular nephrectomy when indicated in patients with chronic rejection.

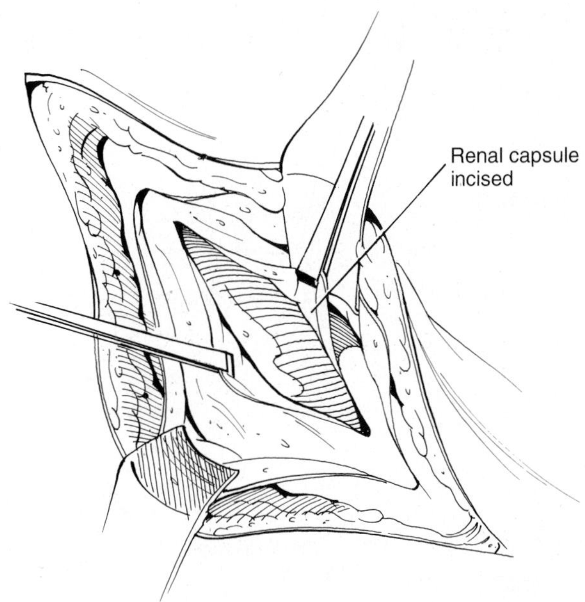


FIGURE 5.2 The incision is carried through the external and internal oblique muscles to the capsule of the kidney, where a small capsular incision is made.

Upon identifying the kidney, the renal capsule is opened with a knife (Fig. 5.2). A plane of dissection between the renal capsule and parenchyma is developed using blunt and sharp dissection. This can usually be done bluntly with a finger (Fig. 5.3). The upper and lower poles of the kidney are mobilized, inside the capsule, and delivered into the wound. Careful dissection proceeds toward the hilum, medially and laterally. The kidney is tethered at the hilum to the iliac vessels. Great caution is exercised here so as not to avulse the kidney. Bleeding from the cortical surface of the kidney is inevitable but can be controlled with pressure.

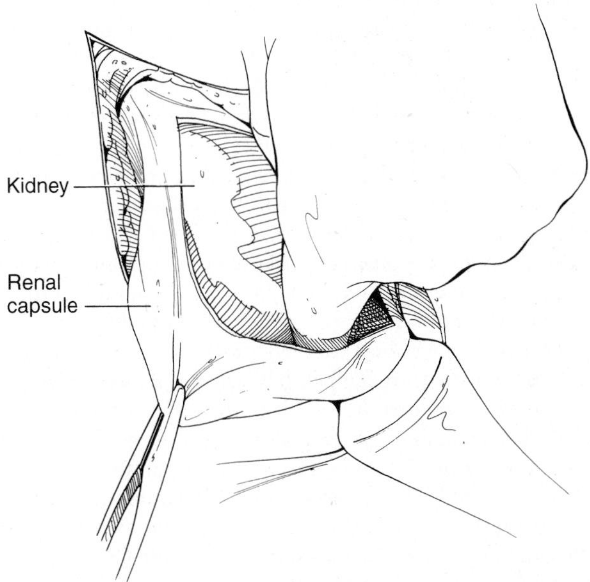


FIGURE 5.3 The renal parenchyma is enucleated subcapsularly.

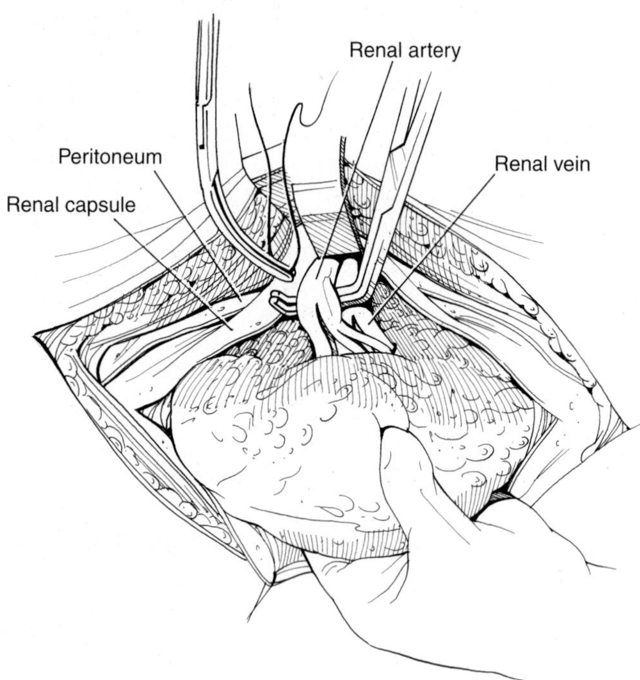


FIGURE 5.4 Intracapsular ligation of renal vessels.

Once the base of the hilum is reached, the vessels are identified and ligated. This can be done entirely intracapsularly (Fig. 5.4) or extracapsularly (Fig. 5.5). The advantage of the former is that damage to the iliac vessels is minimized. One disadvantage is that donor material may be left in situ (14). To ligate the vessels outside the capsule, the reflected capsular surface is incised either posteriorly or anteriorly. The peritoneum may be adherent to the renal hilum and iliac vessels. The vessels are carefully dissected. The renal artery and vein are suture-ligated individually (Fig. 5.6). It is easier to do this if the artery is an end-to-end hypogastric-to-renal-artery anastomosis. A permanent suture such as Prolene or silk can be used for ligation. The knot is tied down to vessels. Friable vessels can tear easily. Injuries to the iliac vein can be repaired with 5-0 Prolene. While small arterial bleeding can be controlled with a fine Prolene stitch, arterial constriction must be avoided, and larger defects therefore require repair with a synthetic graft (Fig. 5.7). Satinsky clamps are helpful in obtaining temporary vascular control. In the event that the hilum is plastered to the iliac vessel and the renal artery and vein are not identifiable, en masse ligation of the hilum may be necessary. Satinsky clamps are placed at the base of the hilum and the kidney transected distal to the clamps. The stump is oversewn with Prolene (Fig. 5.8). When performing an extremely difficult nephrectomy, it may be necessary to deliberately enter the peritoneum to gain proximal control of the iliac artery. The ureter is identified, dissected, and removed along with the graft. The surgeon may not be able to remove the entire ureter.

The wound is gently irrigated with antibiotic solution. Strict hemostasis is obtained, and the wound is closed without a drain. Bleeding from the capsule can be controlled with electrocautery or an argon beam coagulator. For additional security, Surgicel or Gelfoam soaked in thrombin can be placed on the surgical bed prior to closure. A drain is not used routinely because it can predispose to infection. The wound is closed in layers, if possible, with 0 Prolene. The skin is usually closed in a subcutaneous fashion.

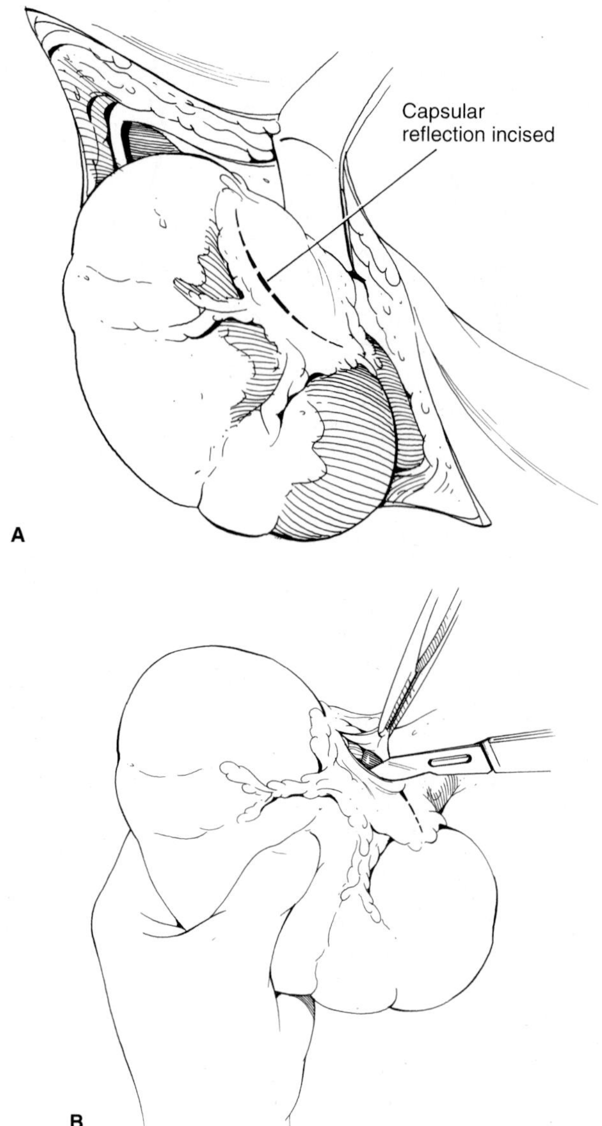


FIGURE 5.5 The hilar vessels are exposed by (**A**) making an incision close to the renal parenchyma and (**B**) incising the overlying capsule.

# OUTCOMES

## Complications

The complication rate of transplant nephrectomy in recent series is acceptable considering the dire comorbidities in this patient population. In the past, the complication rate of transplant nephrectomy was high (24% to 60%) due to underlying uremia and immunosuppression; the mortality rate is approximately 5% (5,7). With modern immunosuppressive drugs, better control of systemic factors, and anesthetic and surgical advancements, the complication rate has been reduced

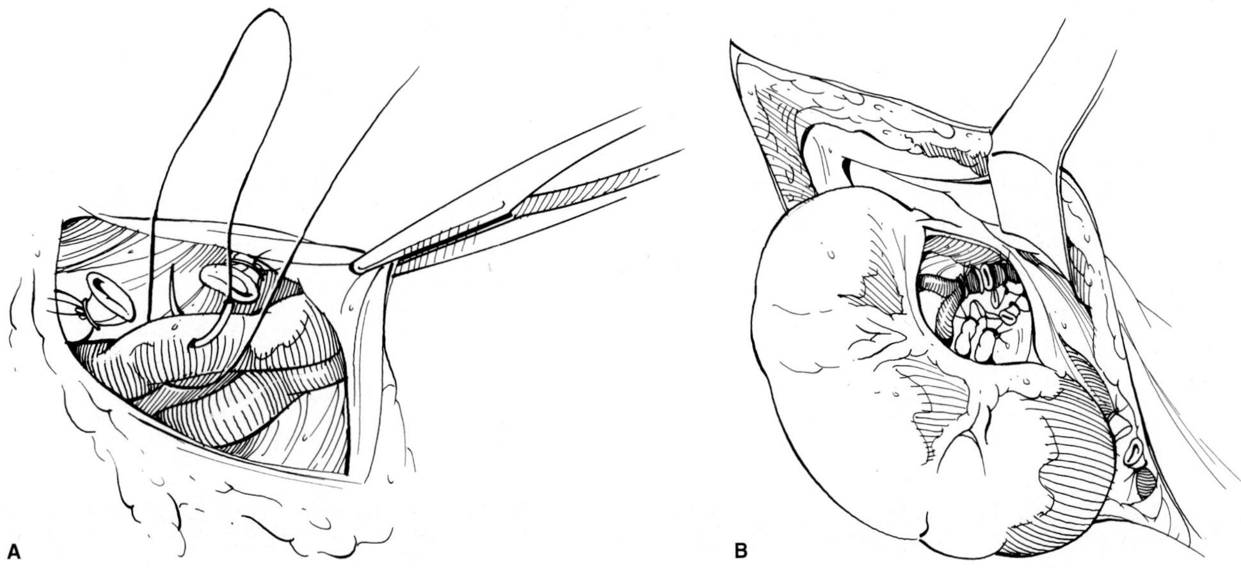


FIGURE 5.6 The renal artery and vein are (**A**) suture-ligated and (**B**) divided.

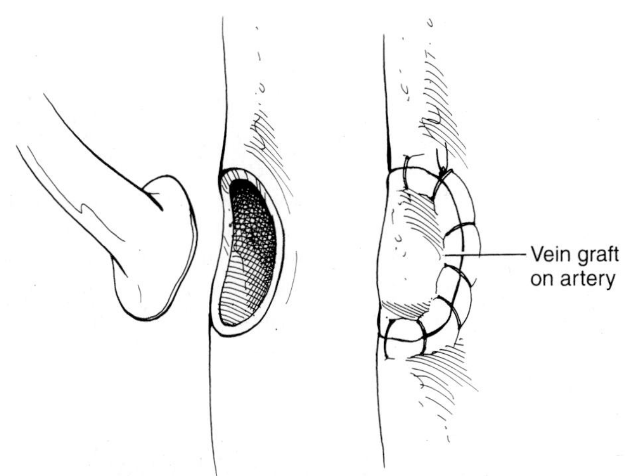


FIGURE 5.7 If the renal allograft artery is completely removed, it may be necessary to cover the defect in the iliac artery with a patch graft.

considerably. The morbidity and mortality are much higher when the nephrectomy is performed under emergent circumstances. Complications usually ensue from bleeding, infection, injury to adjacent structures, and systemic causes. Today, the overall complication rate of transplant nephrectomy for chronic rejection is about 5% and mortality is <1% (2,10,14).

## Results

Transplant nephrectomy is not necessary in all cases of transplant failure. When indicated, it can be performed successfully via an extra- or subcapsular approach. The subcapsular approach is preferred in cases of chronic rejection. Adequate preoperative patient preparation and meticulous surgical technique can minimize morbidity and mortality.

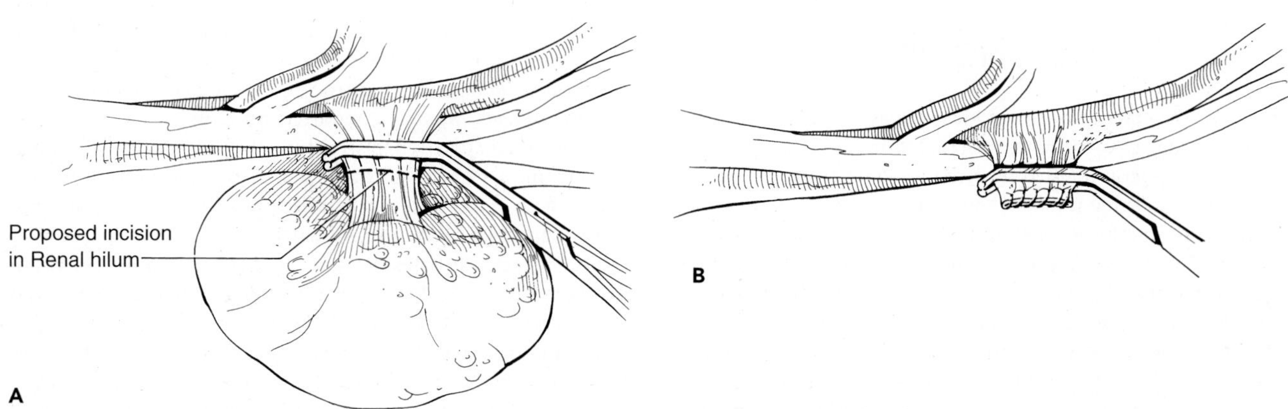


FIGURE 5.8 En masse ligation of the hilum. **A:** Satinsky clamps are placed at the base of the hilum. **B:** The kidney is transected distal to the clamps and the stump oversewn with Prolene.

## References

1. Abouljoud MS, Deiehoi MH, Hudson SL, et al. Risk factors affecting second renal transplant outcome, with special reference to primary allograft nephrectomy. *Transplantation* 1995;60:138–144.
2. Bersztel A, Wahlberg J, Gannedahl G, et al. How safe is transplant nephrectomy? A retrospective study of 107 cases. *Transplant Proc* 1995; 26:3461–3462.
3. Gonzalez-Satue L, Riera E, Franco E, et al. Percutaneous embolization of the failed renal allograft in patients with graft intolerance syndrome. *BJU Int* 2000;86:610–612.
4. Gustafsson A, Groth C, Halgrimson CG, et al. The fate of failed renal homografts retained after retransplantation. *Surg Gynecol Obstet* 1973; 137:4.
5. Koh YB, Lee IS, Moon JS, et al. Transplant nephrectomy in 927 kidney transplants. *Transplant Proc* 1996;28:1470–1476.
6. Lorenzo V, Diaz F, Perez L, et al. Ablation of irreversibly rejected renal allograft by embolization with absolute ethanol. *Am J Kidney Dis* 1993; 22:592–595.
7. O'Sullivan DC, Murphy DM, McLean P, et al. Transplant nephrectomy over 20 years: factors involved in associated morbidity and mortality. *J Urol* 1994;151;855–858.
8. Ramos M, Martins L, Henriques J, et al. Renal allograft rupture: a clinicopathologic review. *Transplant Proc* 2000;32:2597–2598.
9. Roberts CS, Lafond J, Fitts CT, et al. New patterns of transplant nephrectomy in the cyclosporine era. *J Am Coll Surg* 1994;178:59–64.
10. Rosenthal JT, Peaster ML, Laub D. The challenge of kidney transplant nephrectomy. *J Urol* 1993;149:1395–1397.
11. Rosenthal JT. Transplant nephrectomy. In: *Glenn's urologic surgery*, 5th ed. Philadelphia: Lippincott Williams & Wilkins, 1998:79–83.
12. Sharma DK, Pandey AP, Nath V, et al. Allograft nephrectomy—a 16-year experience. *Br J Urol* 1989;64;122–124.
13. United Network for Organ Sharing database: unos.org. or http://ustransplant.org/tables/K1200205-00.html.
14. Zargar MA, Kamali K. Reasons for transplant nephrectomy: a retrospective study of 60 cases. *Transplant Proc* 2001;33:2655–2656.

# CHAPTER 6 ■ RENOVASCULAR DISEASE

JOHN A. LIBERTINO AND CHAD WOTKOWICZ

The true incidence of renovascular hypertension has yet to be determined, with estimates ranging from 5% to 10% within the hypertensive population (1). Stenosis or occlusion within the renal vasculature promotes hypertension via the renin-angiotensin-aldosterone pathway, resulting in renal insufficiency and dialysis dependence over long periods of time. Improved diagnostic studies and imaging modalities have provided internists an easier means of attributing hypertension to renal lesions versus an "essential" etiology. Technological advances in minimally invasive angioplasty techniques and stenting have provided alternatives to surgical bypass in select patient populations. Despite advances in pharmacology and degrees of invasiveness, surgical revascularization remains a constant in the management of renovascular disease, especially within the atherosclerotic population. The outcomes of vascular reconstruction are tightly linked to proper preoperative evaluation, surgical planning, and sound technique.

## DIAGNOSIS

In the past, the clinician's task of identifying potentially curable patients in a safe, cost-effective, and reliable manner was difficult. A single-dose captopril test is reported by some investigators to be a reliable screening test well suited to outpatient settings. In patients with functional renal artery stenosis, angiotensin-converting enzyme (ACE) inhibitors lead to a disproportionate increase in peripheral plasma renin activity; however, baseline renal insufficiency impairs the sensitivity of this test for detecting renal artery stenosis. Renal scintigram with isotopic nephrography following the administration of captopril has also been used to diagnose renal artery stenosis. Technetium DTPA (pentetic acid) scintigraphy has a sensitivity range of 71% to 92% and a specificity range of 72% to 97% (2).

Digital venous subtraction angiography (DSA) remains a definitive and reliable screening test with sensitivity and specificity near 90% and with lower contrast exposure than conventional angiography. 3D-Gd-magnetic resonance angiography (MRA) in detecting hemodynamically significant renal artery stenosis (RAS) has been shown to be effective in the absence of accessory renal arteries. This last-mentioned technique, in addition to $CO_2$ DSA, is useful in azotemic patient populations.

## SURGICAL INDICATIONS

The last 50 years have seen a dramatic change in the management of renal artery stenosis. The first renal thromboendarterectomy was performed by Freeman in 1954 with an excellent outcome (3). The ability to restore renal function in kidneys with compromised inflow serves as a primary indication for intervention. With such a significant aging population, the indications for restoration of flow to preserve renal function will continue to grow. Percutaneous transluminal renal angioplasty was first reported by Dotter and Judkins in 1964 with equally impressive outcomes (4). Minimally invasive techniques have limited the morbidity and mortality associated with open surgery in select hypertensive populations often plagued with significant cardiac and pulmonary comorbidity. In fact, the rates of aortic and renal revascularizations decreased by 73% from 1998 to 2001, while percutaneous procedures increased by 173% (5).

Despite this trend, the basic principles and knowledge of extra-anatomic bypass techniques are essential to the urologist in training. The use of the hepatic artery, gastroduodenal artery, and other alternative procedures instead of the aortorenal saphenous vein bypass has not only reduced the morbidity and mortality of surgery but has also dramatically changed the operative potential in an expanded patient population. Equally important are the complications associated with these procedures that urologists may encounter.

The indications for angioplasty and stenting versus vascular bypass are widely variable and continue to adjust with advances in technology. Fibrous dysplasia and mid–main renal artery atherosclerosis are optimal for balloon angioplasty, while renal osteal and branch disease may be more amenable to revascularization. Renal artery aneurysms associated with hypertension can also be managed with revascularization procedures. Another strong indication for surgical repair is pregnant women with noncalcified aneurysms over 2 cm due to risk of rupture. Patients experiencing disease following balloon angioplasty are better managed surgically, as repeat angioplasty has a high complication rate. Nephrectomy may be a prudent choice in high-risk surgical patients: those with extensive branch vessel disease, nonsalvageable parenchyma, and failed arterial reconstructions.

## MEDICAL THERAPIES

Chronic azotemic renovascular disease is common in patients with atherosclerosis, whose prevalence appears to be increasing in the aging population. The pharmaceutical industry has been instrumental in the treatment of hypertension in our patient population. The advent of ACE inhibitors and angiotensinogen receptor blockers (ARB) therapy in conjunction with calcium channel blockers have improved the management of renovascular hypertension. In addition to normalizing blood pressure parameters, these medications help to retrieve renal function, as evidenced by improved glomerular filtration rates (GFRs). Despite maximal medical therapies, certain individuals will have progressive renal artery disease with associated ischemia and azotemia. Avoiding dialysis in this patient population is critical due to the inherent morbidity associated with renal replacement therapy. Identifying the group of suitable patients refractory to medical management will continue to grow in importance as the population at large grows.

## SURGICAL MANAGEMENT

### Aortorenal Bypass Graft

Bypass grafts are particularly suitable for fibrous lesions that affect the long and multiple segments of the renal artery and associated branches (Fig. 6.1). Autogenous artery (hypogastric and spleen) and autogenous saphenous veins are all options in properly selected patients. When exhausted of autogenous resources, a Dacron interposition graft may be used; however, there are concerns of thrombosis and some technical difficulty in crafting the appropriate diameter to accommodate the native renal artery. Hypogastric arteries are an excellent graft choice in the pediatric population, unlike in adults, who are often afflicted with atherosclerosis. The autologous saphenous vein remains the conduit of choice at our institution due the ease of access and size equivalence to the renal artery. The pliability of the venous versus the arterial vasculature provides for more contoured anastomoses, and the limited intima is less thrombogenic.

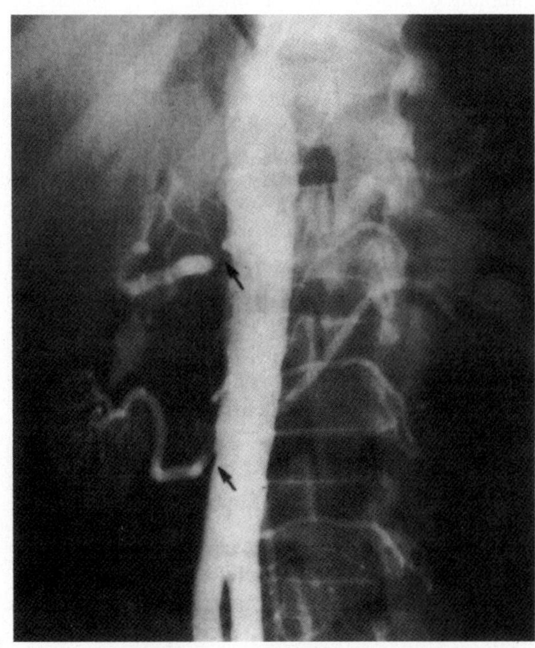


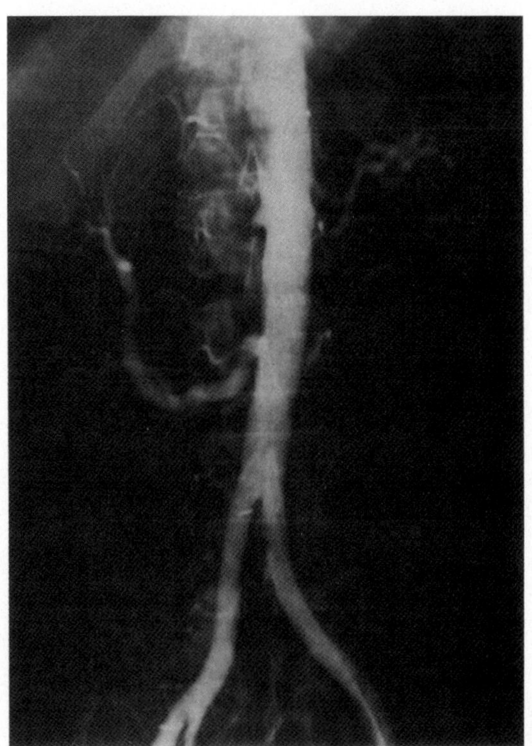


FIGURE 6.1 **A:** An aortogram shows a double right renal artery with stenoses at the ostias of both trunks. **B:** A postoperative aortogram with the vein graft making a side-to-side anastomosis to the stenotic lower renal artery and an end-to-end anastomosis to the distal stump of the upper renal artery.

## Procurement of the Saphenous Vein

The saphenous vein is initially exposed from the contralateral side, providing operative room for two surgeons and limiting operative time. Prior to the date of surgery, the saphenous vein is outlined with permanent marker and ultrasound assistance. Mobilization begins with a single incision parallel to and below the groin crease over the palpable femoral pulses and extended to the knee after the junction of the saphenous and femoral vein have been exposed. Incisions should be made over the femoral vascular complex with limited subcutaneous dissection to avoid flap devascularization (Fig. 6.2). We recommend using blunt finger dissection with a moist sponge dissector for mobilization.

In general, we harvest a 20-cm-long vein graft with an ideal outer circumference between 4 to 6 mm. Excess vein harvesting is advisable in case of technical complications and the need for revision. Venous tributaries are tied with 5-0 silk, and excess areolar tissue is dissected free, leaving the intima undisturbed.

To decrease transmural ischemia, the vein graft is left in situ until the renal vessels are mobilized. If the graft is removed inadvertently, we place in cool Ringer solution or autologous blood. The distal end of the graft is then intubated with a Marks needle and secured with a silk tie (Fig. 6.3). Dilute heparinized autologous blood is infused to dilate the vein prior to proximal transection to evaluate for untied tributaries. Once the vein is removed, the thigh incision is packed with moist gauze until the renal revision is complete to ensure that any delayed bleeding caused by systemic heparinization is identified and controlled.

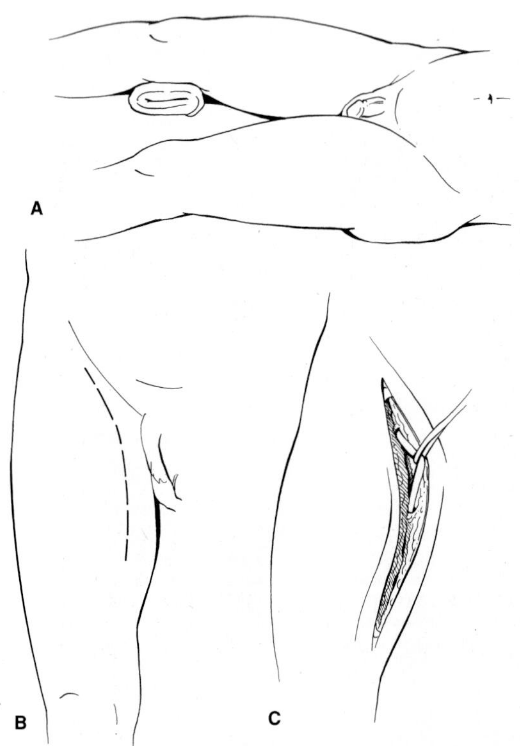


FIGURE 6.2 **A:** Position of patient for harvesting of saphenous vein graft. **B:** Line of incision of saphenous vein graft harvest. **C:** Exposure of saphenous vein.

## Insertion of the Saphenous Vein Graft

Once the renal vessels and aorta are completely mobilized, systemic heparin is given and a 30-minute window is observed prior to arterial clamping. The vein graft is next orientated to ensure proper implantation, with an end-to-end anastomosis being the preferred technique to limit nonlaminar flow associated with end-to-side reconstructions. The aorta is next palpated to locate an area free of atherosclerotic plaque for the proper location of the aortotomy.

Preoperative imaging should rule out extensive aortic atherosclerotic disease and avoid the need for plaque endarterectomy and associated emboli risk. A medium-sized DeBakey clamp is next placed on the anterolateral portion of the infrarenal aorta in a tangential manner. A vertical 13- to 16-mm aortotomy is made without excising any aortic wall or attempting to perform localized endarterectomy (Fig. 6.4).

Excision of the aortic wall is not necessary because intraluminal aortic pressure spreads the dimensions of the linear aortotomy to appropriate dimensions after the clamp is released. The vein graft is anastomosed to the aorta with 5-0 Prolene after being adequately spatulated (Fig. 6.5). A microvascular Schwartz clamp is placed on the end of the saphenous vein graft and the aorta unclamped. The graft will lie anterior to the interior vena cava on the right side and anterior to the renal vein on the left side. The graft should be relatively mobile to limit undue stress on the anastomosis; however, excess length is not recommended due to possibility of graft kinking. A second Schwartz microvascular clamp is placed on the distal main renal artery or branches. An end-to-end anastomosis is performed using 6-0 Prolene suture in a continuous or interrupted fashion, depending on the diameter of the anastomosis (Fig. 6.6). Interrupted sutures are preferable for diameters of 3 mm or less. Pediatric patients are treated with interrupted sutures to prevent a "pursestring" effect with vessel growth at a later age. Interrupted sutures should be placed at four quadrants initially to limit additional "pursestring" effects. Precision is a

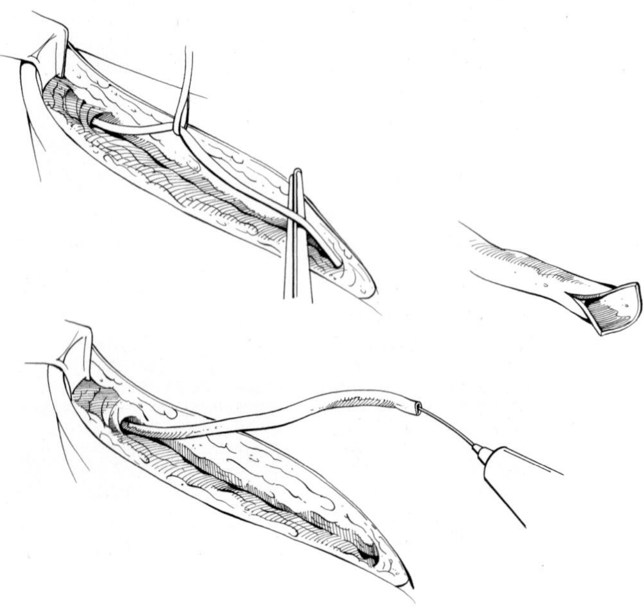

FIGURE 6.3 Harvest of saphenous vein graft.

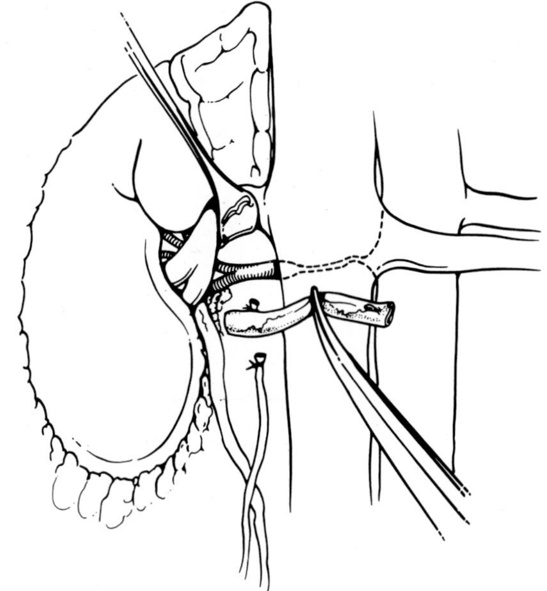

FIGURE 6.4 The bypass graft is placed along the lateral aortic wall to determine the best position for its placement. (From Novick AC, Streem SB, Pontes JE, eds. *Stewart's operative urology*. Baltimore: Williams & Wilkins, 1989, with permission.)

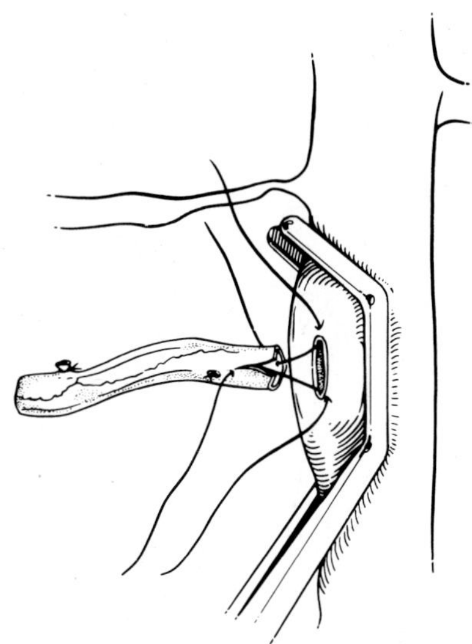

FIGURE 6.5 Following partial aortic occlusion, an oval aortotomy is made for end-to-side anastomosis with a spatulated bypass graft. (From Novick AC, Streem SB, Pontes JE, eds. *Stewart's operative urology*. Baltimore: Williams & Wilkins, 1989, with permission.)

must in placing sutures to limit unnecessary vascular trauma at the anastomosis that may impair strength or lead to intimal inflammatory reaction and narrowing of the lumen.

Once the anastomosis is complete, the bulldog clamps are removed and the anastomosis evaluated for bleeding (Fig. 6.7). Rarely may there be a need to place an additional interrupted stitch. We cannot stress enough the importance of visualization during these procedures, and we insist on the use of surgical loupes and fiberoptic lighting. In addition, the operating staff should have a wide array of equipment available due to the delicacy of these procedures. Fogarty balloons of all sizes need to be readily available in the event of a thrombus. Novice urologists should not hesitate to corroborate with a vascular surgeon in the early part of their career.

## Splenorenal Artery Bypass

The indications for splenorenal bypass include patients with diffuse atherosclerotic disease of the aorta or prior aortic surgery needing left renal artery revascularization.

Lateral and oblique angiography is essential in surgical decision making to confirm that the celiac axis is free of atherosclerotic disease. Recent advances in three-dimensional computerized tomography and magnetic resonance imaging can be implemented; however, the gold standard remains angiography because of the dynamic real-time imaging effect. Surgical exploration and intraoperative evaluation with splenic blood flow measurements can be helpful as well. Alternative bypass routes should be considered if splenic blood flow is <125 mL per minute.

A supracostal eleventh-rib incision is made, and dissection is carried along the upper border of the rib, avoiding the neurovascular complex on the underside (Fig. 6.8). The overlying latissimus dorsi, the serratus posterior inferior, and intercostal muscles are next divided with electrocautery. The next group of muscles to be divided includes the external and internal obliques and the transversus abdominis muscle. Intercostal muscle attachments are divided approximately on the distal inch of the rib until the corresponding intercostal nerve is identified and spared. This approach allows an extrapleural approach and provides excellent exposure as the rib can pivot downward in a "bucket-handle" fashion.

The plane between Gerota fascia and the adrenal gland posteriorly and the pancreas anteriorly is then entered and the splenic artery identified at the upper border of the pancreas. The investing fascia is entered and the splenic artery mobilized by a purely retroperitoneal approach. Associated pancreatic feeding vessels are isolated, ligated, and divided. A properly performed dissection should provide mobilization of the splenic artery from the hilum to the celiac access, providing a tension-free anastomosis.

After the splenic artery is mobilized, a sponge soaked with papaverine is placed on it to permit dilation. A vascular clamp is placed at the origin, and the artery is divided proximal to the bifurcation at the hilum. Splenectomy is not required because the spleen will receive blood supply from the short gastric arteries. Arterial circumference may be increased with a Fogarty catheter or Gruentzig balloon. The left kidney is approached with a posterior approach and the renal artery identified. The renal artery is ligated distal to the point of obstruction and an end-to-end anastomosis carried out with 6-0 Prolene in an interrupted or continuous fashion (Fig. 6.9). We have employed the posterior approach in over 10 patients at our institution and now prefer it to the transabdominal technique. In the rare circumstance that length is insufficient, a saphenous vein interposition graft may be required to prevent undue tension (Fig. 6.10).

## Hepatorenal Bypass Graft

The hepatic artery arises from the celiac axis and continues along the upper border of the pancreas until the portal vein

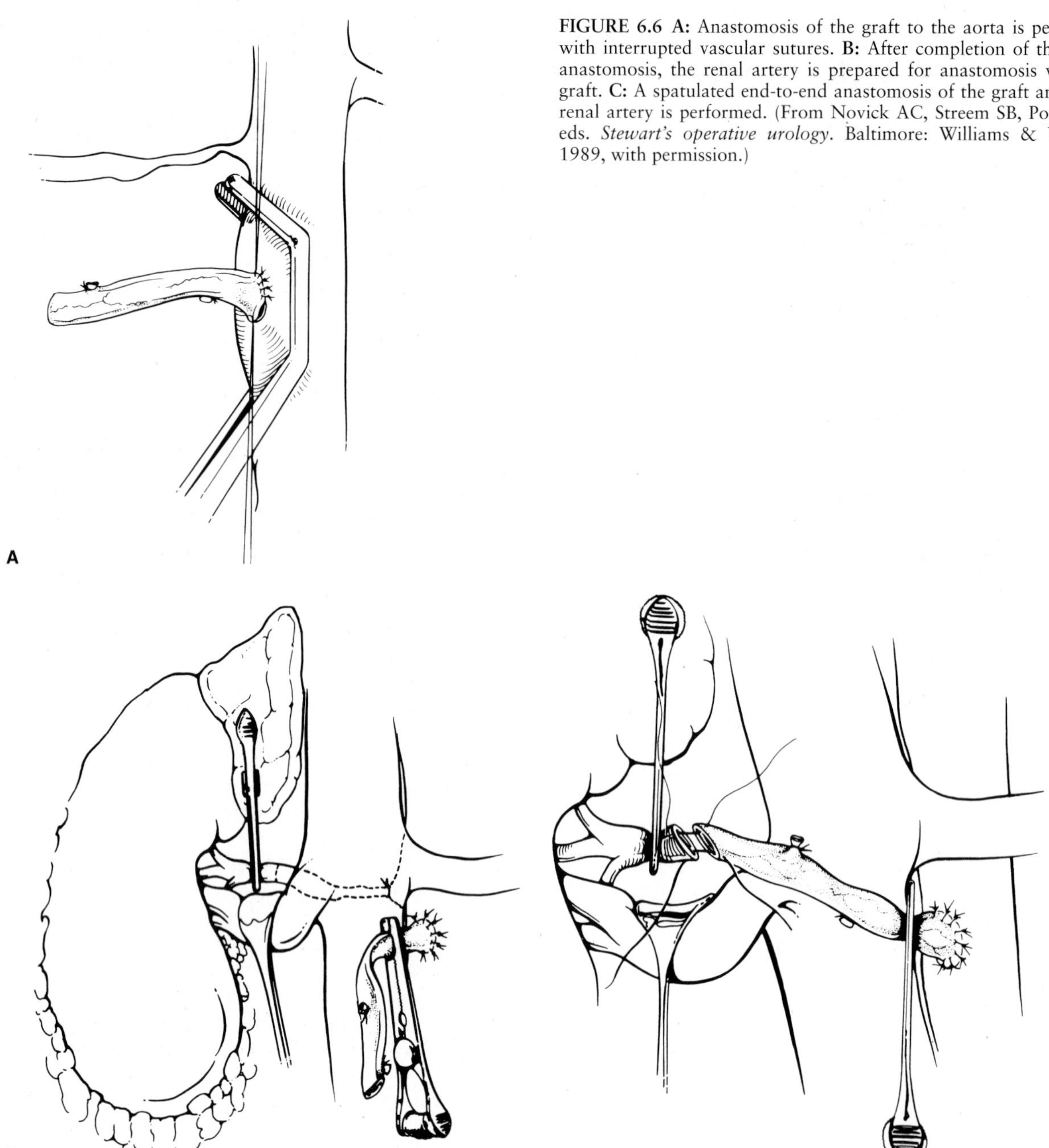


FIGURE 6.6 **A:** Anastomosis of the graft to the aorta is performed with interrupted vascular sutures. **B:** After completion of the aortic anastomosis, the renal artery is prepared for anastomosis with the graft. **C:** A spatulated end-to-end anastomosis of the graft and distal renal artery is performed. (From Novick AC, Streem SB, Ponted JE, eds. *Stewart's operative urology*. Baltimore: Williams & Wilkins, 1989, with permission.)

complex, where it branches into ascending and descending limbs. The ascending branch is a continuation of the main hepatic artery upward within the lesser omentum; it lies in front of the portal vein and to the left of the biliary tree. The descending limb forms the gastroduodenal artery. In the porta hepatis, the hepatic artery divides into the right and left hepatic branches, which supply the corresponding lobes of the liver (Fig. 6.11). The right-upper-quadrant vasculature—the hepatic artery—has marked variability in up to 48% of patients as documented in living liver donors (6). Accessory hepatic arteries provide ischemic insurance for hepatorenal bypass procedures. It is essential to identify the following arteries prior to attempting anastomosis: common hepatic, gastroduodenal, right and left hepatic arteries. In addition, the portal vein and common bile duct are isolated.

Once mobilized, the right renal artery is mobilized and the vascular clamps applied to the proximal portion of the hepatic artery and its distal branches. The gastroduodenal artery is divided and the inferior surface of the hepatic artery is mobilized from the underlying portal vein and common bile duct (Fig. 6.12). A 10- to 12-mm arteriotomy is made in the anterior inferior wall of the common hepatic artery, beginning at the ostium of the gastroduodenal artery. A reversed autogenous saphenous vein is inserted with an end-to-side anastomosis between the vein graft and hepatic artery using 6-0 Prolene suture (Fig. 6.13). A microvascular clamp is placed on the vein graft after it has been filled with heparin and after the proper alignment and length for the renal artery anastomosis has been determined. The clamps are removed from the hepatic circulation, and a small Schwartz microvascular clamp is paced on the distal renal artery.

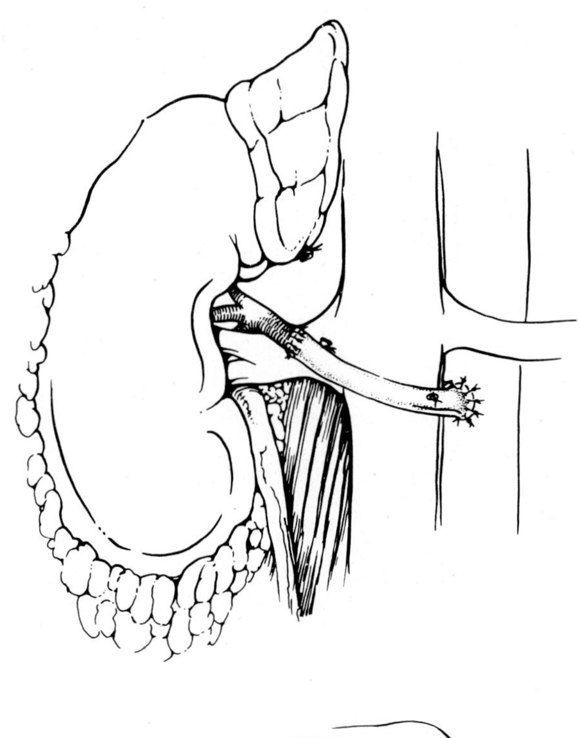

FIGURE 6.7 Completed aortorenal bypass operation. (From Novick AC, Streem SB, Pontes JE, eds. *Stewart's operative urology.* Baltimore: Williams & Wilkins, 1989, with permission.)

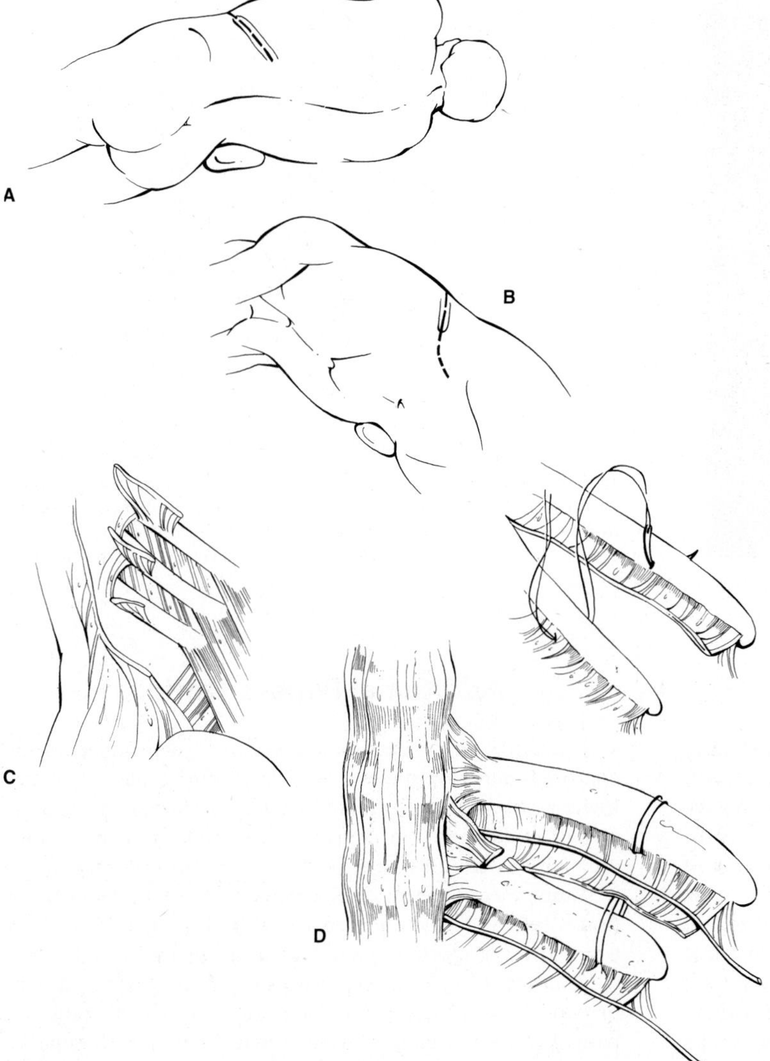


FIGURE 6.8 Supracostal eleventh-rib incision. **A:** Posterior view. **B:** Anterior view. **C:** The costovertebral ligament must be divided to allow the rib to pivot inferiorly. **D:** Closure of incision, taking care to spare the intercostal nerves. The diaphragm is not incorporated in the closure.

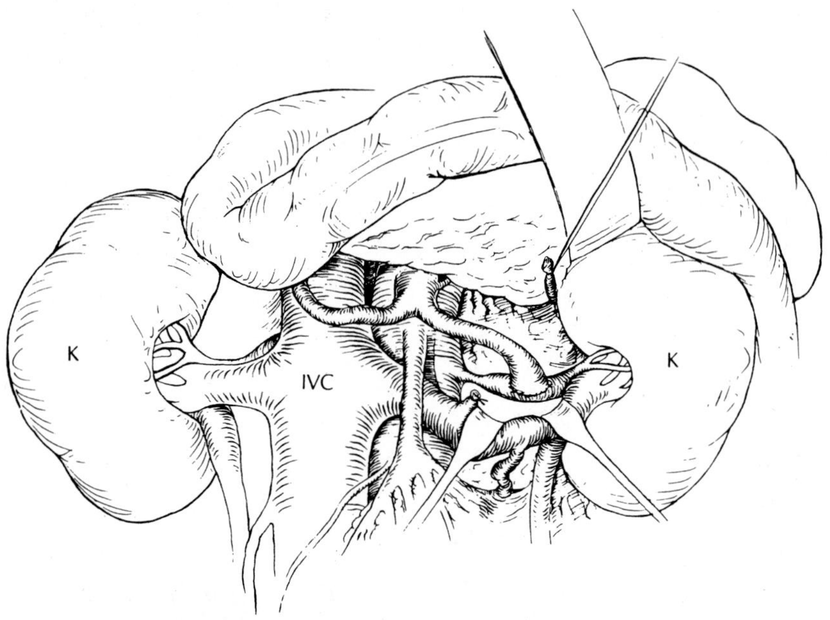


FIGURE 6.9 Technique of splenorenal bypass. Note that the pancreas is lifted cephalad to expose the splenic artery.

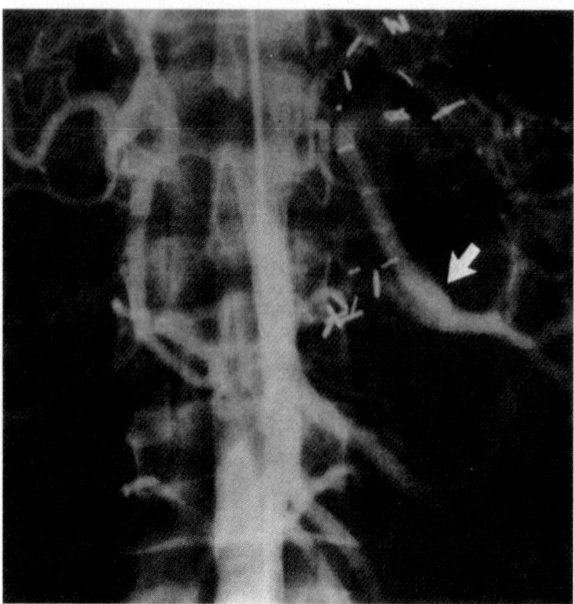

FIGURE 6.10 An aortogram shows a splenorenal end-to-side bypass.

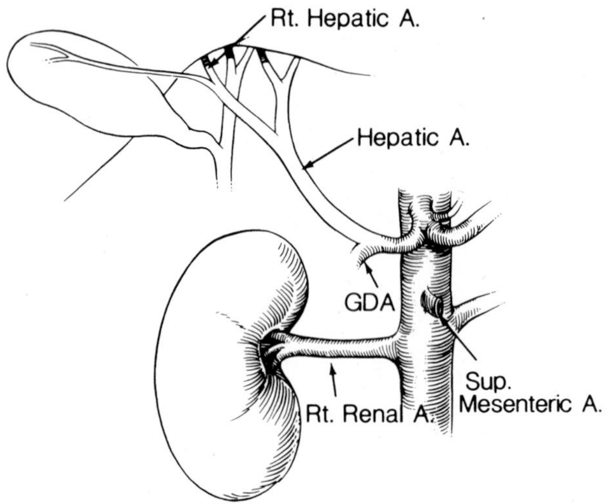


FIGURE 6.11 Normal course of the main hepatic artery and its various branches. (From Novick AC. Diminished operative risk and improved results following revascularization for atherosclerotic renal artery disease. *Urol Clin North Am* 1984;11:435, with permission.)

## Ileorenal Bypass

The presence of severe atherosclerotic disease of the aorta may preclude aortorenal bypass and requires alternative vascular bypass conduits. One option includes the ileorenal bypass, with a caveat being adequate aortic flow to that level of the common bifurcation. Our surgical approach starts with a midline abdominal incision with concomitant saphenous vein graft acquisition. The corresponding colon is mobilized to expose the ipsilateral renal vessels and the iliac bifurcation. Vessel loops are applied to the common iliac in standard fashion, and an end-to-side anastomosis is performed with an end-to-end anastomosis at the level of the renal artery using a saphenous vein graft (Fig. 6.14).

## Additional Bypass Options

Case reports from various sources vary depending on the anatomy. Superior mesenteric artery, supreceliac aorta and lower thoracic aorta bypass have been performed using autogenous saphenous vein interposition grafts. These procedures are high risk and often reserved as last resort procedures.

Simultaneous aortic replacement with renal revascularization is indicated in the presence of significant aneurysmal disease; however, morbidity and mortality are higher.

Transplant renal artery stenosis is best managed with percutaneous angioplasty. Lohr et al. reviewed 90 transplant patients with transplant stenosis. Percutaneous transluminal renal angioplasty (PTRA) intervention led to the loss of one graft

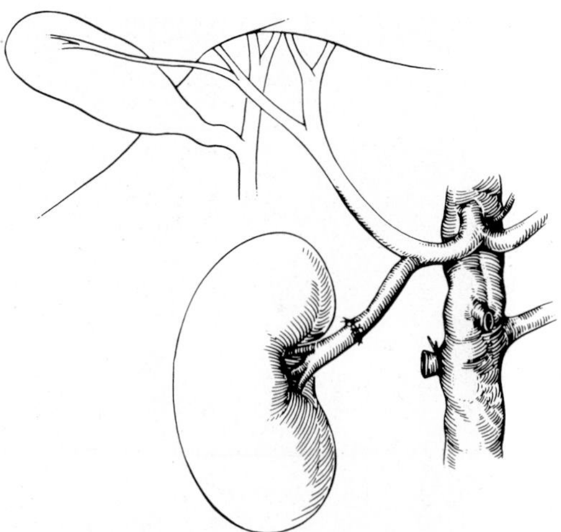

FIGURE 6.12 Hepatorenal bypass performed with an interposition saphenous graft anastomosed end-to-side to the common hepatic artery and end-to-end to the right renal artery. (From Novick AC. Diminished operative risk and improved results following revascularization for atherosclerotic renal artery disease. *Urol Clin North Am* 1984;11:435, with permission.)

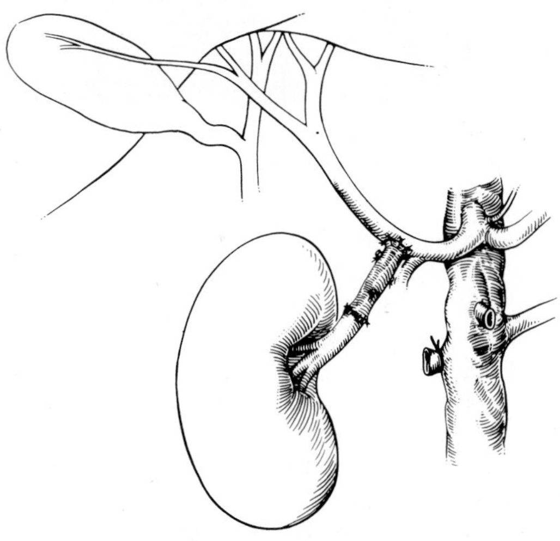

FIGURE 6.13 Use of the gastroduodenal artery to perform hepatorenal revascularization through direct end-to-end anastomosis with the right renal artery. (From Novick AC, Streem SB, Pontes JE, eds. *Stewart's operative urology*. Baltimore: Williams & Wilkins, 1989, with permission.)

and restenosis in another; however, the rates of graft loss and restenosis were 11% and 6% with open surgical repair (7).

## Renal Artery Reconstruction Using Prosthetic Grafts

Autogenous reconstruction using reversed saphenous vein grafts, arterial autografts, and transaortic endarterectomy has proven efficacious in the restoration of blood flow and renal function in numerous clinical studies. Implementation of prosthetic grafts was initially viewed with some skepticism secondary to concerns about durability and the sequelae of possible infections. A review by Paty et al. of over 400 prosthetic grafts provided excellent clinical outcomes with patency rates over 95% at the 7-year period using polytetrafluoroethylene (PTFE) grafts for primary renal arterial reconstruction and concomitant aortorenal reconstructions (8). PTFE graft size can be customized to the renal artery, and the high flow rates can retard thromogenicity.

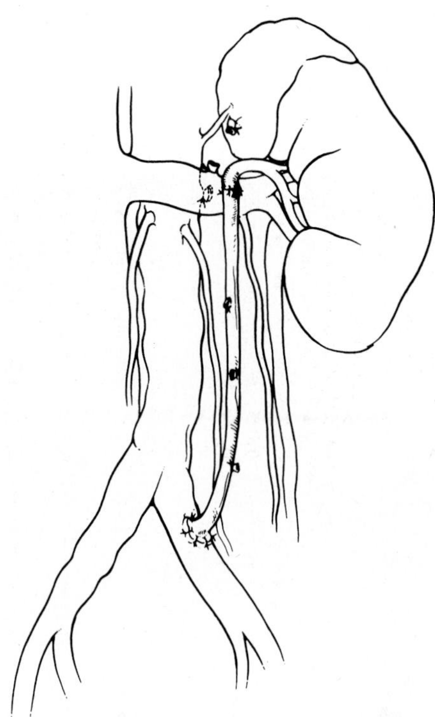

FIGURE 6.14 Ileorenal bypass with a saphenous vein graft anastomosed end-to-side to the common iliac artery and end-to-end to the renal artery. (From Novick AC, Streem SB, Pontes JE, eds. *Stewart's operative urology*. Baltimore: Williams & Wilkins, 1989, with permission.)

## Renovascular Salvage Surgery

PTRA is the preferred treatment of choice for fibroplastic and nonostial unilateral lesions sparing the anterior and posterior divisions of the renal artery. Complications can occur in the immediate postoperative period in up to 13%, with restenosis rates ranging from 15% to 25%. Lacombe et al. reviewed their experience with over 50 failed PTRAs managed via 38 in situ repairs, 10 extracorporeal repairs, and 3 nephrectomies (9). Although technically difficult, failed PTRAs are surgically correctable; however, planes of dissection are often compromised, and the increasing use of endoluminal stents precluded thromboembolectomy and reimplantation. Revisions for fibromuscular dysplasia demonstrated improved outcomes versus atherosclerosis, which tend to harbor significant inflammatory changes. These authors recommend surgical revascularization as the primary treatment in all types of arterial fibrodysplasia, citing only 17 (2.5%) postoperative occlusions in their series of 689 primary revascularizations.

## Renal Autotransplantation and Ex Vivo Bench Surgery

On rare occasions, kidneys with lesions of the renal artery or its branches are not amenable to in situ reconstruction. In

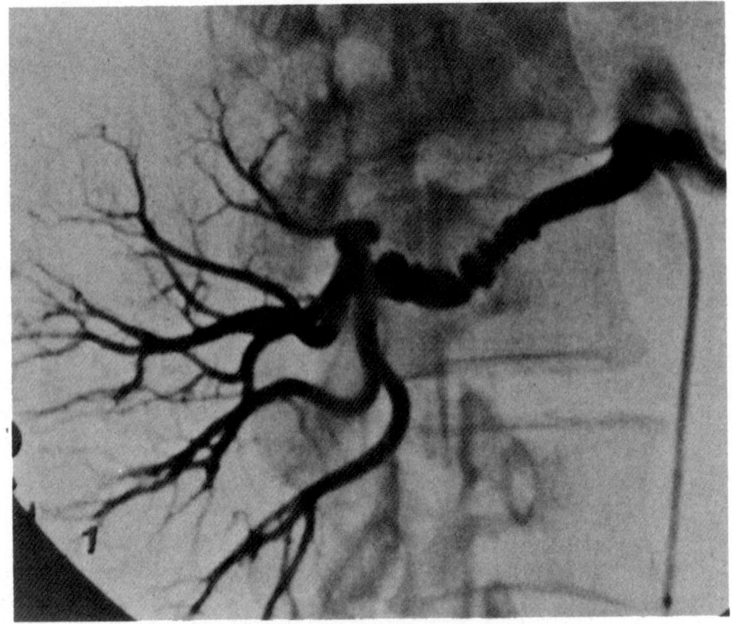


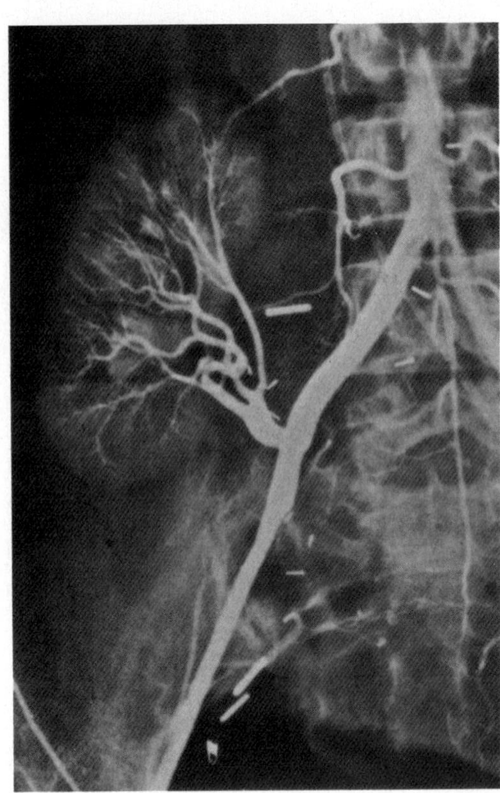


**FIGURE 6.15 A:** An arteriogram shows complex involvement of the right renal artery by disease extending into the primary branches. **B:** A postoperative arteriogram shows patent anastomoses.

these circumstances, temporary removal of the kidney, ex vivo preservation, microvascular repair (bench surgery), and autotransplantation may permit salvage. This technique should be considered in patients with traumatic arterial injuries and when disease of the major vessels extends beyond the bifurcation of the main renal artery into segmental branches, and also when multiple vessels supplying the affected kidney are repaired. Bench surgery may also be required in patients with larger aneurysms, arteriovenous fistulas, dissecting aneurysms, or malformations (Fig. 6.15). At our institution we have performed over 25 autotransplants with renovascular disease (renal artery aneurysm and renal artery stenosis) as the primary indication with over 90% success. Novick described his experience with 66 renal autotransplants with resolution of hypertension (no medical therapy) in 55 patients and improved or stable renal function in all patients (10). Taken together, these clinical outcomes support the role of renal autotransplantation and microvascular reconstruction for renovascular disease.

## SURGICAL COMPLICATIONS

Early complications include hemorrhage, graft thrombosis, distal branch vessel embolization, subintimal dissection, false aneurysm, and nephrectomy. Bleeding in the immediate postoperative period is due to surgical error often accentuated by marginal arterial wall integrity. In addition, the presence of systemic heparinization will stress the coagulation cascade and promote bleeding at suture holes from Prolene suture. We recommend the use of thrombogenic mesh to control bleeding at these anastomoses. Enlarged perihilar vessels are seen in high-grade stenosis, and cognizance of adrenal vasculature during dissection is important. Delayed bleeding may also occur with false aneurysm formation or erosion of graft anastomosis into duodenum or bowel. Infected graft suture lines may lead to delayed bleeding.

Intimal dissection can occur, and the use of a double-armed suture with needle passage from intima to adventitia can aid in decreasing the chance of dissection and associated embolization or aneurysm formation. Systemic heparinization has some prophylactic benefit for atheroemboli; however, the lower extremities need to be fully prepped in case a thromboembolectomy is warranted.

With respect to overall complications, the leading cause of morbidity and mortality in nonfibrodysplastic patients is cardiovascular in nature. This same population is afflicted with cerebrovascular comorbidities in an estimated 30%. We recommend surgical correction of these comorbidities when feasible prior to revascularization procedures.

## OUTCOMES

Balloon angioplasty is primarily used to treat mural dysplasia in a younger patient population with limited atherosclerotic disease. Using this modality, we have seen success rates of 80% to 85% at our institution. We have performed over 100 surgical revascularizations at our institute for preservation and restoration of renal function with a success rate of 85%, which is equivalent to that of our contemporary colleagues (11). In one of the largest series to date, Lawrie et al. documented improved hypertension in 82% of 919 patients observed over 6 years (12).

## *References*


1. Libertino JA. Surgery for renovascular hypertension. In: Walsh PC, Retik AB, Stamey TA, et al., eds. *Campbell's urology*, 6th ed. Philadelphia: WB Saunders, 1992:2521–2551.
2. Setaro JF, Saddler MC, Chen CC, et al. Simplified captopril renography in diagnosis and treatment of renal artery stenosis. *Hypertension* 1991;18: 289–298.
3. Freeman NE, Leeds FH, Elliott WG, et al. Thromboendarterectomy for hypertension due to renal artery occlusion. *JAMA* 1954;156(11):1077–1079.
4. Dotter CT, Judkins MP. Transluminal treatment of arteriosclerotic obstruction: description of a new technic and a preliminary report of its application. *Circulation* 1964;30:645–670.
5. Knipp BS, Dimick JB, Eliason JL, et al. Diffusion of new technology for the treatment of renovascular hypertension in the United States: surgical revascularization versus catheter-based therapy, 1988–2001. *J Vasc Surg* 2004; 40(4):717–723.
6. Hiatt JR, Gabbay J, Busutil RW. Surgical anatomy of the hepatic arteries in 1000 cases. *Ann Surg* 1994;220:50–52.
7. Lohr JW, MacDougall ML, Chonko AM, et al. Percutaneous transluminal angioplasty in transplant renal artery stenosis: experience and review of the literature. *Am J Kidney Dis* 1986;7(5):363–367.
8. Paty SK, Darling RC, Lee D, et al. Is prosthetic renal artery reconstruction a durable procedure? An analysis of 489 bypass grafts. *J Vasc Surg* 2001; 34(1):127–132.
9. Lacombe M, Ricco JB. Surgical revascularization of renal artery after complicated or failed percutaneous transluminal renal angioplasty. *J Vasc Surg* 2006;44(3):537–544.
10. Novick AC. Surgical revascularization for renal artery disease: current status. *Br J Urol Int* 2005;95 (Supp 2): 75–77.
11. Libertino JA, Bosco PJ, Ying CY, et al. Renal revascularization to preserve and restore renal function. *J Urol* 1992:147:1485–1487.
12. Lawrie GM, Morris GC, Glaeser DH, et al. Renovascular reconstruction: factors affecting long-term prognosis in 919 patients followed up to 31 years. *Am J Cardiol* 1989;63:1085–1092.


# CHAPTER 7 ■ ANATROPHIC NEPHROLITHOTOMY

ELIZABETH J. ANOIA, MICHAEL L. PAIK, AND MARTIN I. RESNICK

The treatment of nephrolithiasis has undergone a rapid evolution over the past 25 years. The introduction and refinement of extracorporeal, endourologic, and percutaneous techniques have caused a shift in the first-line management of even complex renal stones. Anatrophic nephrolithotomy is a procedure that has been used by urologists for >30 years in the removal of staghorn renal calculi. The original description of anatrophic nephrolithotomy was by Smith and Boyce in 1968 (14). The operation they described was based on the principle of placing the nephrotomy incision through a plane of the kidney that was relatively avascular. This approach would avoid damage to the renal vasculature and subsequent atrophy of the renal parenchyma, hence the term *anatrophic*. Staghorn stones are often associated with urinary tract infections, and the coexistence of these two conditions makes it difficult to eradicate either. Definitive treatment of these stones is generally advocated because of the significant morbidity and mortality associated with untreated staghorn calculi. Blandy and Singh (3) found that patient survival is reduced with untreated staghorn calculi, with a mortality rate of 28% at 10 years.

Anatrophic nephrolithotomy also involves reconstruction of the intrarenal collecting system to eliminate anatomic obstruction. Thus, this procedure would improve urinary drainage, thereby reducing the likelihood of urinary tract infection, which would prevent recurrent stone formation. Over the past 25 years, with the development of less invasive approaches such as extracorporeal shock wave lithotripsy (ESWL), percutaneous nephrolithotomy (PCNL), and ureteroscopic surgery, the role of anatrophic nephrolithotomy and other open stone operations has certainly diminished (2). The American Urologic Association Nephrolithiasis Clinical Guidelines Panel in 1994 recommended a percutaneous procedure with or without ESWL as an initial treatment for complex staghorn calculi. However, in specific situations anatrophic nephrolithotomy remains the best treatment option for renal calculi and thus has maintained an important, albeit smaller, role in the treatment of these large, complex stones.

## DIAGNOSIS

Diagnosing nephrolithiasis is based on the patient's history, physical exam, urinalysis (UA) findings, and radiographic studies. Patients may have the typical symptoms of flank pain, fever, hematuria, and dysuria or they may be asymptomatic. Physical examination may reveal costovertebral angle tenderness. The UA may show erythrocytes, leucocytes, and nitrites or bacteria if the stone is associated with an infection. The diagnosis of chronic urinary tract infection is common in patients with staghorn stones. Urine culture is often positive, and typical organisms include urea-splitting organisms such as *Proteus, Klebsiella, Providencia,* and *Pseudomonas.*

Common radiographic studies by traditionally obtained include plain abdominal radiographs, nephrotomograms, and excretory urograms to identify the stones and the collecting system and, if present, define the degree of obstruction. Retrograde pyelography is usually performed in cases of equivocal findings on excretory urography. Recently, helical nonenhanced computed tomography scanning with thin cuts of the kidneys, ureters, and bladder has become the gold standard for identifying urinary tract stones and radiolucent or poorly calcified stones. Nuclear renal scans can help determine differential renal function when such information might affect the surgical approach. Renal arteriography is usually not indicated unless there is suspicion of anomalous arterial anatomy, such as in renal fusion anomalies.

Before elective surgery, a metabolic evaluation is recommended to attempt to determine an etiology for stone formation and aid in preventing a recurrence. For instance, it is important to determine the presence of hypercalciuria, hyperuricosuria, hyperoxaluria, cystinuria, hyperparathyroidism, and renal tubular acidosis in multiple urine specimens. The measurement of serum and urine calcium, phosphorus, creatinine, uric acid, and electrolytes should be routine. A 24-hour urine collection for creatinine clearance as well as urinary calcium, phosphorus, oxalate, citrate, cystine, and uric acid is also an integral part of the workup (9).

## INDICATIONS FOR SURGERY

The indications for anatrophic nephrolithotomy have changed somewhat with advances in minimally invasive methods of treating stones. However, the inability to successfully eradicate a stone with less invasive methods remains an important indication for open stone surgery. Other relative indications include select cases of complex stone disease, especially those with a dilated collecting system, stones associated with urologic anatomic abnormalities, previous renal surgery, certain features of patient anatomy, comorbid disease, and patient preference (7,8). Specific urinary tract abnormalities account for up to 24% of open stone surgeries. These include a ureteropelvic junction (UPJ) obstruction, infundibular stenosis, calyceal diverticula, ureteral stricture, or the presence of a crossing vessel. By openly the defect can be corrected simultaneously. Patient features such as morbid obesity, limb contractures, or certain cases of transplanted kidneys may preclude proper positioning for endourologic procedures, ESWL, or percutaneous access (4). The presence of significant comorbid disease and patient preference must each be considered in choosing the best individualized treatment option.

Overall, the goals of open stone surgery should be to remove all calculi and fragments, improve urinary drainage of any obstructed intrarenal collecting system, eradicate infection, preserve and improve renal function, and prevent stone recurrence (15).

## ALTERNATIVE THERAPY

As open stone surgery accounts for <5% of treatment modalities for staghorn and other complex stones, there are now other less invasive techniques either alone or in combination that have replaced this procedure. Most staghorn calculi can now be preferentially treated with percutaneous nephrolithotomy, with or without ESWL. The stone-free rates reported vary between 50% and 87%, whereas for anatrophic nephrolithotomy stone-free rates range from 90% to 100% (7). The advantage of the former is shorter convalescent periods; the disadvantage is the possibility of requiring multiple different procedures to accomplish a stone-free state. Endoscopic therapy with holmium:YAG laser lithotripsy is reported to have an overall stone-free rate of 95% (10). ESWL monotherapy was found to have a 61% stone-free rate <10 years after its development (8). Despite impressive advances with the less invasive techniques, anatrophic nephrolithotomy remains a viable treatment option for large staghorn calculi not expected to be eliminated with a reasonable number of less invasive procedures or staghorn stones associated with anatomic abnormalities requiring open surgical correction (13).

## SURGICAL TECHNIQUE

After administration of appropriate preoperative intravenous (IV) antibiotics and induction of general anesthesia, a Foley catheter is placed. The patient is then placed in the standard flank position with elevation of the kidney rest and flexion of the operating table to achieve adequate spacing between the lower costal margin and the iliac crest. Three-inch-wide adhesive tape applied at the shoulders and hips can be used to secure the patient to the table. Adequate padding should be used to protect pressure points.

A standard flank approach is used. The incision can be placed through the bed of either the eleventh or twelfth rib, depending on the estimated position of the kidney. If a previous flank incision has been made for renal surgery, it is preferable to place the incision above the old scar, ensuring that access to the kidney can be achieved through unscarred tissue. After rib resection, when access has been gained into the retroperitoneal space, the Gerota fascia is identified overlying the kidney. The Gerota fascia is incised in a cephalad-caudal direction, which facilitates returning the kidney to its fatty pouch at the end of the operation. The kidney is then fully mobilized, and the perinephric fat is carefully dissected off the renal capsule with care taken not to disrupt the capsule. Should the capsule become inadvertently incised, it can be closed at that time with chromic catgut sutures. The kidney is now free to be suspended in the operative field by utilizing a broad tape at each pole. At this point a preliminary portable plain radiograph can be obtained.

Next is the renal hilar dissection. The main renal artery and the posterior segmental branch are approached posteriorly, carefully identified, and dissected (Fig. 7.1A). The renal pelvis and ureter should be identified but not dissected. The avascular plane, or Brödel line, can be identified by temporarily clamping the posterior segmental artery and injecting 20 mL of methylene blue intravenously. This results in the blanching of the posterior renal segment while the anterior portion turns blue, allowing identification and marking of the avascular plane (Fig. 7.1B) (6). Placing the nephrotomy incision through this plane will achieve maximal renal parenchymal preservation and minimize blood loss. The avascular plane can also be identified with the use of a Doppler stethoscope to localize the area of the kidney with minimal blood flow.

More extensive renal hilar dissection can be avoided by utilizing a modification of the original procedure described by Smith and Boyce (14). Redman et al. (11) relied on the relatively constant segmental renal vascular supply in the identification of the Brödel line. They advocated placing the incision at the expected location of the avascular plane after clamping the renal pedicle with a Satinsky clamp in an effort to prevent vasospasm of the renal artery and warm ischemia. This modification can save time and spare extensive dissection of the renal hilum. However, we continue to advocate precise identification of the avascular plane to minimize parenchymal loss.

At this point, 25 g of IV mannitol is administered. This will promote a postischemic diuresis and prevent the formation of

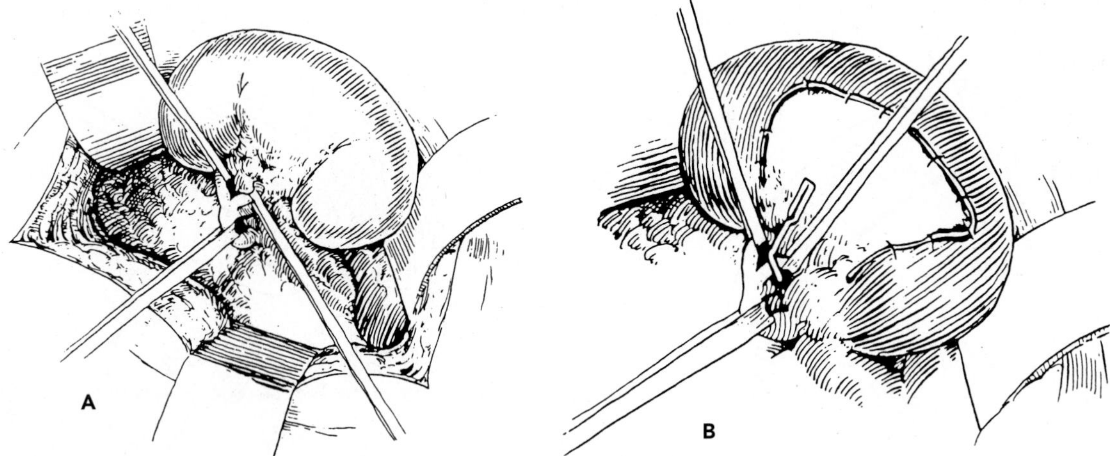


FIGURE 7.1 Anatrophic nephrolithotomy. **A:** The main renal artery and branches are isolated. **B:** The posterior segmental artery is occluded and methylene blue is administered intravenously. The resulting demarcation between pale ischemic and bluish perfused parenchyma defines a relatively avascular nephrotomy plane.

intratubular ice crystals by increasing the osmolarity of the glomerular filtrate. The main renal artery can now be occluded with an atraumatic bulldog vascular clamp (Fig. 7.2). A bowel bag or barrier drape is quickly placed around the kidney, and it is insulated from the body wall and peritoneal contents with dry gauze packs. Hypothermia is then initiated with iced saline slush covering the kidney. The kidney should be cooled for 10 to 15 minutes before the nephrotomy incision is made. This should allow achievement of a core renal temperature of 15°C to 20°C, which will allow safe ischemic times from 60 to 75 minutes and minimize renal parenchymal damage (5). The ice slush should be continuously reapplied as needed throughout the case.

The renal capsule is then incised sharply over the previously identified line, being careful to avoid extension into the upper and lower poles (Fig. 7.3). The renal parenchyma can be bluntly dissected with the back of the scalpel handle. Blunt dissection minimizes injury to the intrarenal arteries that are traversed (Fig. 7.4). Small bleeding vessels can be controlled with 4-0 or 5-0 chromic catgut figure-of-eight suture ligatures. If renal back-bleeding continues to be a problem despite these measures, the main renal vein can be occluded.

As the nephrotomy incision proceeds toward the renal hilum, the ideal location to enter the collecting system is at the base of the posterior infundibula. The intraoperative radiograph can be used as a guide to the pelvis and the base of the calyx. On occasion, with large posterior calyceal calculi, a dilated posterior calyx will be entered initially. The remainder of the collecting system can then be identified with a probe and opened. If a posterior infundibulum is entered first, the incision is then carried toward the renal pelvis (Fig. 7.5). The stone is visualized, and all ramifications of the stone are

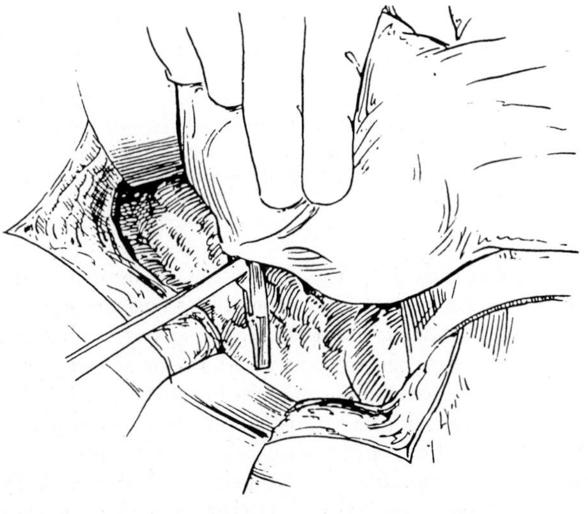

FIGURE 7.2 The main renal artery is clamped and a bowel bag or rubber dam is placed around the kidney. Dry gauze packs are placed anterior to the kidney to protect the intra-abdominal organs from hypothermia.

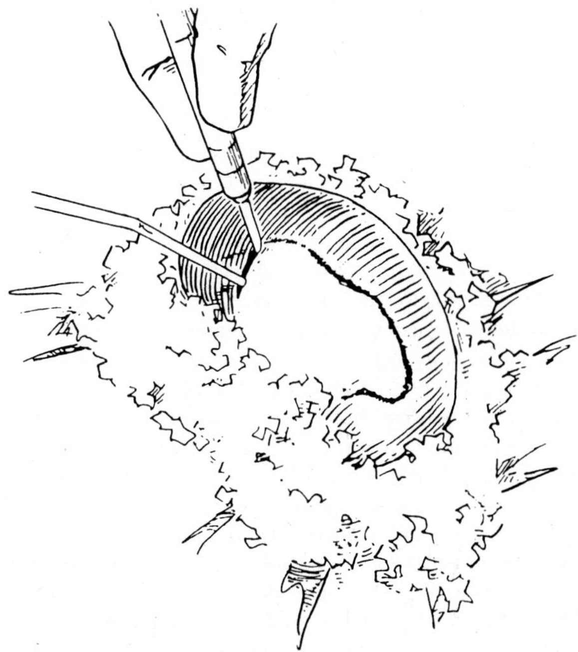

FIGURE 7.3 A superficial incision is made in the renal capsule through the avascular plane.

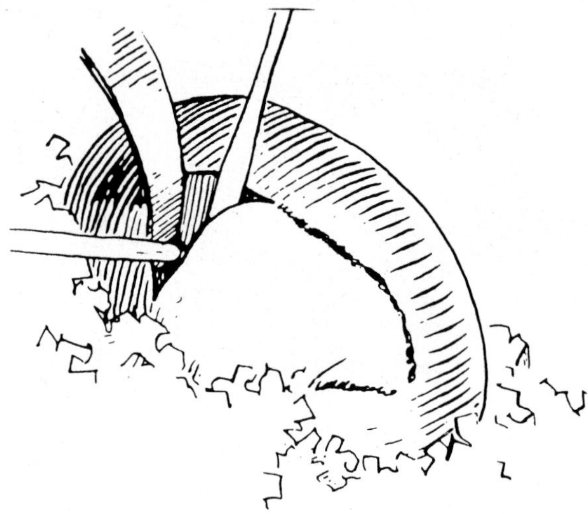

FIGURE 7.4 The parenchyma is bluntly dissected with the back of a scalpel handle. The incision closely approximates the avascular plane.

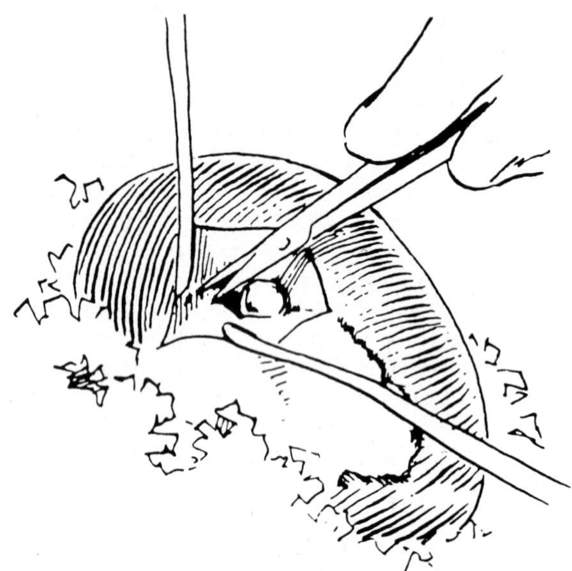

FIGURE 7.5 The collecting system is carefully incised.

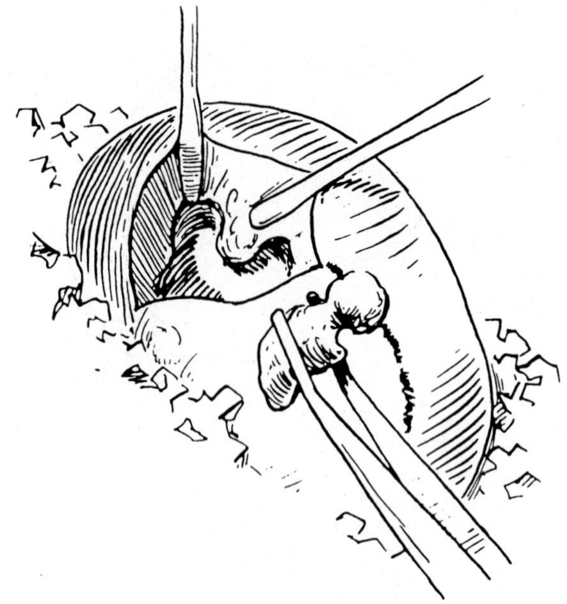

FIGURE 7.6 After the collecting system is opened, calculi are extracted and total removal is confirmed radiographically.

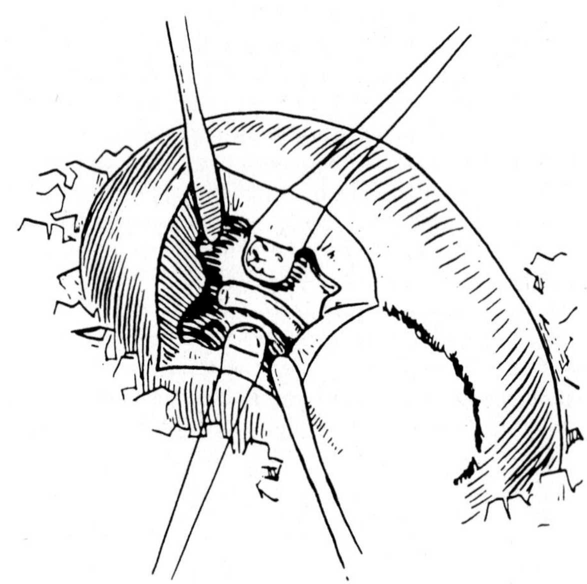

FIGURE 7.7 A ureteral stent is passed in an antegrade fashion from the pelvis to the bladder. Traction sutures are placed to mark the walls of adjacent calices before suturing them together with a running 6-0 chromic suture.

exposed by opening adjacent infundibula into the calices. To minimize stone fragmentation and retained calculi, the stone should not be manipulated or removed until all of the calyceal and infundibular extensions are appropriately identified and incised. This allows for complete visualization and mobilization of the collecting system and calculi. Ideally, the stone or stones should be removed without fragmentation; however, often it is inevitable that there will be some piecemeal extraction (Fig. 7.6). If this is necessary, a ureteral stent can be inserted to prevent stone migration during manipulation. Each calyx should be inspected for stone fragments. After removal of all stone fragments, the renal pelvis and calices are copiously irrigated with cold saline and the irrigant is aspirated. A nephroscope can be used to look for residual fragments. A plain radiograph or ultrasonography are also options. At this time, a "double-J" ureteral stent is passed from the renal pelvis into the bladder if this was not done at the time of stone manipulation (Fig. 7.7). The routine use of internal ureteral catheters is encouraged. They provide good urinary drainage, protect the freshly reconstructed collecting system, and minimize postoperative urinary extravasation. The next step in the procedure is the reconstruction of the intrarenal collecting system with correction of a coexistent anatomic abnormality if present. Infundibular stenosis or stricture that results in obstruction promoting urinary stasis and recurrent stone formation should be corrected with caliorrhaphy or calicoplasty. The former is the repair of a single narrowed calyx, achieved by incising the calyx along its appropriate margin (anterior margin for posterior calices and posterior margin for anterior

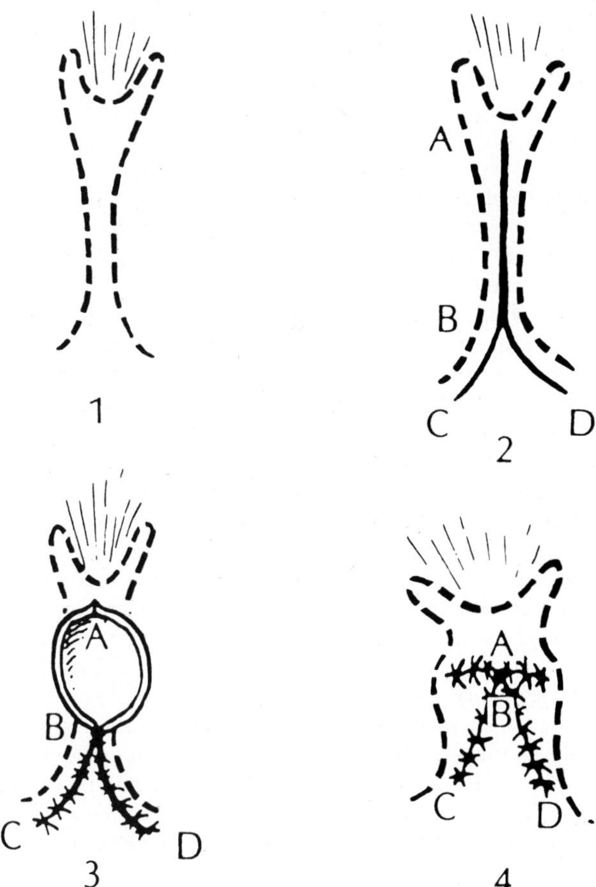


FIGURE 7.8 Technique of repairing strictured infundibula. **1:** Narrowed elongated infundibulum. **2:** Incision into calyx forms an inverted Y. **3:** Pelvic flap is advanced into infundibulotomy. **4:** Incision in calyx is closed transversely.

calices) and suturing those margins to the renal pelvis, resulting in a shorter, wider calyx (Fig. 7.8). The infundibulum can also be incised longitudinally and then closed transversely in a Heineke-Mikulicz fashion. Calicoplasty is the repair of adjacent stenotic calices by suturing the adjacent walls of the neighboring calices, thus forming a single structure (Figs. 7.9 and 7.10). All intrarenal reconstructive suturing should be accomplished with 5-0 or 6-0 chromic catgut sutures. When suturing the mucosal edges, it is important to avoid incorporation of underlying interlobular arteries, thus preventing ischemia.

The renal pelvis is then closed, first with reinforcing corner sutures and then with a running 6-0 chromic catgut suture (Fig. 7.11). The arterial clamp is briefly released to identify parenchymal bleeding points, and hemostasis is obtained with 4-0 or 5-0 chromic catgut figure-of-eight suture ligatures before closing the renal capsule. The renal capsule is closed with a running lock stitch of 4-0 chromic catgut suture (Fig. 7.12), or mattress sutures over bolsters can be used. After the capsule is closed and adequate hemostasis has been achieved, the slush surrounding the kidney is removed and the renal artery unclamped. The kidney is observed for good hemostasis and return of pink color and good turgor after unclamping. It is then returned into the Gerota fascia, and the kidney and proximal ureter are covered with some perirenal fat to minimize the postoperative scar formation. If the Gerota fascia is unavailable because of prior surgery, omentum can be mobilized

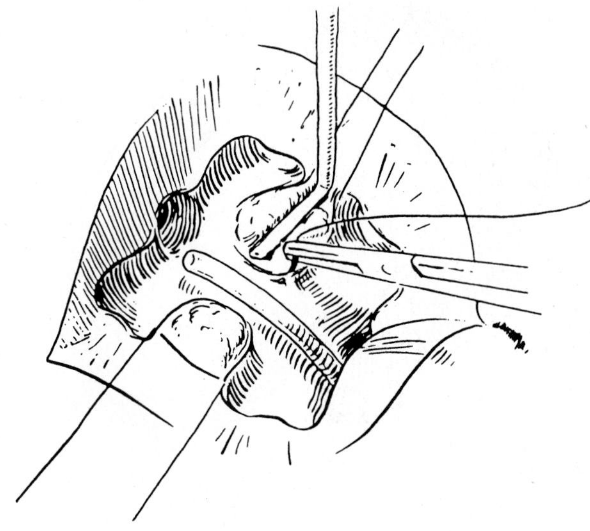

FIGURE 7.9 Adjacent infundibula are sutured together starting in the renal pelvis. Peripelvic fat is depressed during this closure.

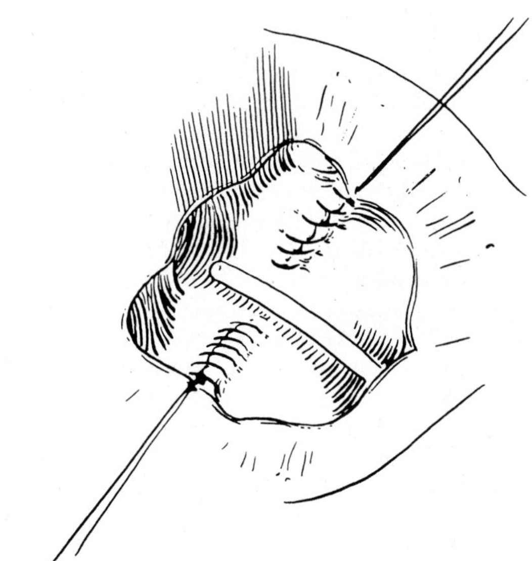

FIGURE 7.10 The collecting system is completely reconstructed.

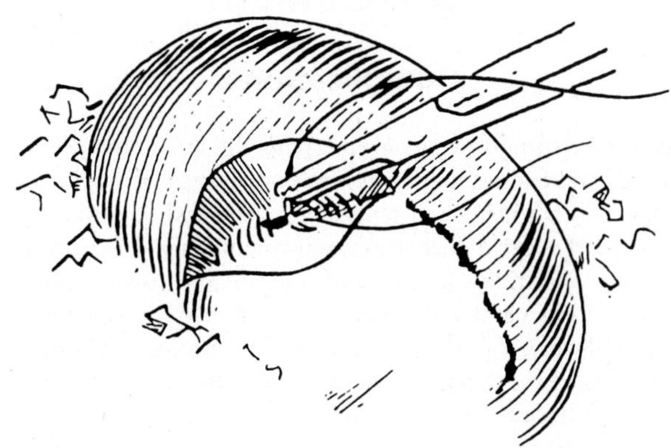

FIGURE 7.11 The renal pelvis is closed with a running 6-0 chromic suture.

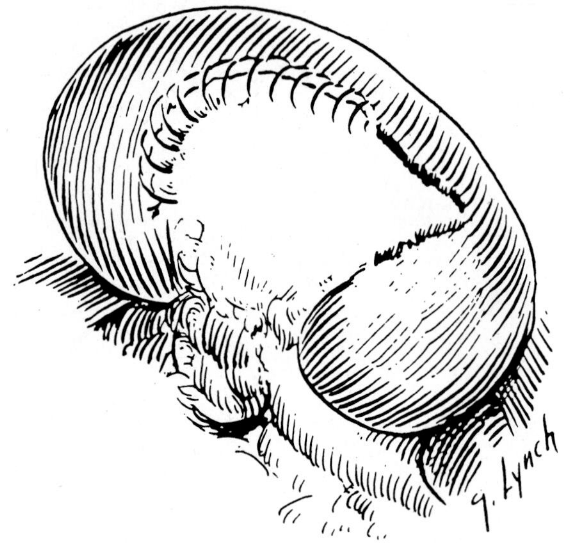

FIGURE 7.12 The renal capsule is closed with a running locking 4-0 chromic suture.

through a peritoneal opening and wrapped around these structures. The peritoneal opening should be sutured to the omentum to prevent herniation of the abdominal viscera.

A Penrose or suction-type drain is placed within the Gerota fascia and brought out through a separate stab incision. This drain is left in place until minimal drainage occurs, usually by the third or fourth postoperative day. Nephrostomy tubes are in general avoided because of their potential for causing infection or further renal damage. The flank musculature and skin are closed in the standard fashion.

Postoperative management after anatrophic nephrolithotomy should follow the same principles that guide management after other major operations. Intravenous fluids are maintained to achieve brisk urine output and until the patient is able to tolerate a clear liquid diet. Broad-spectrum IV antibiotics are administered perioperatively and continued postoperatively for 5 to 7 days. Antibiotic coverage is guided by preoperative urine culture and sensitivity results. The ureteral stent is removed cystoscopically at approximately 7 days postoperatively in uncomplicated cases. A urine culture is checked for persistence of infection.

# OUTCOMES

## Complications

Pulmonary complications are perhaps the most common following anatrophic nephrolithotomy, especially atelectasis. Patients with a history of pulmonary disease should likely undergo preoperative evaluation with pulmonary function testing and initiation of vigorous pulmonary toilet prior to surgery. Postoperatively, patients should be encouraged to breathe deeply, and use of an incentive spirometer should be routine. Early ambulation will also be beneficial.

Pneumothorax should occur in fewer than 5% of patients (15). A patient with a history of pyelonephritis or previous renal surgery is at increased risk. Inadvertent opening of the pleura, usually during incision and resection of a rib, should be readily identified intraoperatively. The defect should be closed immediately with a running chromic catgut suture. The lung is hyperinflated just before the final suture is placed to ensure re-expansion of the lung. Chest tubes are not routinely used but may be necessary if any question remains regarding the reliability of the pleural closure. A chest radiograph should be obtained in the recovery room for any patient who undergoes repair of a pleural defect. Pulmonary embolism remains a potential complication of any major surgery. Routine use of elastic support hose and sequential compression stockings can lower the risk of deep venous thrombosis. Encouragement of early ambulation is also an important preventative measure. Significant postoperative renal hemorrhage should occur in fewer than 10% of patients. Assimos et al. (1) reported an incidence of 6.4%. Bleeding usually occurs immediately or about 1 week postoperatively. Extensive intrarenal reconstruction, older age, worse renal function, and presence of blood dyscrasias were found to be significant risk factors. Slow bleeding will usually resolve on its own; management includes correction of any bleeding abnormalities and replacement with blood products as necessary. Oral ε-aminocaproic acid can be successful in certain cases. Bleeding that is brisk or cannot be adequately treated conservatively will require a more aggressive approach. A renal arteriogram can help identify the lesion, and an attempt at arteriographic embolization can be considered. Re-exploration may be required in the remainder of the cases, with reinstitution of hypothermia and suture ligation of the bleeding vessel(s). Persistent hematuria 1 to 4 weeks postoperatively should alert the clinician to the possibility of renal arteriovenous fistula formation or a false aneurysm (1). Urinary extravasation should occur infrequently with the routine use of perinephric drains and ureteral catheter drainage. Should drainage recur or persist following removal of the drain and/or ureteral stent, replacement of the ureteral stent should be considered to decompress the system and relieve any obstruction. Other possible complications resulting from arterial clamping include renal injury and hypertension.

## Results

When performed for appropriate indications and with meticulous technique, anatrophic nephrolithotomy can achieve successful removal of all calculi, preservation of renal function, improved urinary drainage, and eradication of infection. Stone-free rates >90% should be achieved. Stone recurrence rates following anatrophic nephrolithotomy have been reported from 5% to 30% (15). Recurrent calculi usually form in those with persistent urinary tract infections, persistent urinary drainage impairment, and previously unidentified or refractory metabolic disturbances (12).

For large, complex staghorn calculi, especially those associated with some anatomic abnormality leading to impaired urinary drainage, anatrophic nephrolithotomy remains a first-line treatment. This modality achieves comparable or better stone-free rates and the achievement of a stone-free state with a single operative procedure. In the long term, treatment of these staghorn calculi with anatrophic nephrolithotomy should preserve renal function in the involved kidney and, in a majority of patients, eradicate stone disease and chronic urinary infection.

## References

1. Assimos DG, Boyce WH, Harrison LH, et al. Postoperative anatrophic nephrolithotomy bleeding. *J Urol* 1986;135:1153–1156.
2. Assimos DG, Boyce WH, Harrison LH, et al. The role of open stone surgery since extracorporeal shock wave lithotripsy. *J Urol* 1989;142: 263–267.
3. Blandy JP, Singh M. The case for a more aggressive approach to staghorn stones. *J Urol* 1976;115:505–506.
4. Caldwell TC, Burns JR. Current operative management of urinary calculi after renal transplantation. *J Urol* 1988;140:1360–1363.
5. McDougal WS. Renal perfusion/reperfusion injuries. *J Urol* 1988;140: 1325–1330.
6. Myers RP. Brödel's line. *Surg Gynecol Obstet* 1971;132:424–426.
7. Paik ML, Resnick MI. Is there a role for open stone surgery? *Urol Clin North Am* 2000;27:323–331.
8. Paik ML, Wainstein MA, Spirnak JP, et al. Current indications for open stone surgery in the treatment of renal and ureteral calculi. *J Urol* 1998; 159:374–379.
9. Parks JH, Goldfisher E, Asplin JR. A single 24-hour urine collection is inadequate for the medical evaluation of nephrolithiasis. *J Urol* 2002;167: 1607–1612.
10. Razvi HA, Dendstedt JD, Chun SS, et al. Intracorporeal lithotripsy with the holmium:YAG laser. *J Urol* 1996;156:912.
11. Redman JF, Bissada NK, Harper DL. Anatrophic nephrolithotomy: experience with a simplification of the Smith and Boyce technique. *J Urol* 1979; 122:595–597.
12. Russell JM, Harrison LH, Boyce WH. Recurrent urolithiasis following anatrophic nephrolithotomy. *J Urol* 1981;125:471–474.
13. Segura JW, Preminger GM, Assimos DG, et al. Nephrolithiasis Clinical Guidelines Panel summary report on the management of staghorn calculi. *J Urol* 1994;151:1648–1651.
14. Smith MJV, Boyce WH. Anatrophic nephrotomy and plastic calyorrhaphy. *J Urol* 1968;99:521–527.
15. Spirnak JP, Resnick MI. Anatrophic nephrolithotomy. *Urol Clin North Am* 1983;10:665–675.

# CHAPTER 8 ■ RENAL AND RETROPERITONEAL ABSCESSES

DAVIS P. VIPRAKASIT AND ANTHONY J. SCHAEFFER

## INTRODUCTION

Renal and retroperitoneal abscesses are uncommon clinical entities that often pose a significant diagnostic challenge. Nonspecific signs and symptoms frequently lead to a delay in diagnosis and treatment. Early experiences reported mortality rates approaching 50%. In contemporary series with improved diagnostic imaging allowing early recognition and treatment, mortality rates of <15% are noted. However, continued significant morbidity is associated with these insidious disease processes. An understanding of the anatomy of the retroperitoneal space is essential for classification, timely diagnosis, and management of renal and retroperitoneal abscesses.

The retroperitoneal space is bounded by the posterior parietal peritoneum and transversalis fascia (Figs. 8.1 and 8.2). It is divided into the perirenal space and the pararenal space. The perirenal space surrounds the renal capsule and capsular artery and is bounded by the renal (Gerota) fascia. The anterior and posterior leaves of Gerota fascia fuse above the adrenal gland, becoming continuous with the diaphragmatic fascia. A thinner, more variable layer meets between the adrenal gland and the kidney. Laterally, the fascial layers join to form the lateroconal fascia, which becomes continuous with the posterior parietal peritoneum. Medially, the posterior layer fuses with the psoas muscle fascia and the anterior layer fuses with the connective tissue surrounding the great vessels and organs of the anterior retroperitoneum (i.e., the pancreas, duodenum, and colon). Because the perirenal space rarely crosses the midline, perirenal abscesses usually remain unilateral. Inferiorly, the Gerota fascial layers do not fuse, but become continuous with the psoas and ureteral coverings (11). This opening inferiorly allows the spread of perirenal infections to the pararenal space, pelvis, psoas muscle, and in some cases, contralateral retroperitoneum.

The pararenal space is divided into two compartments: the anterior compartment, which is bounded by the posterior parietal peritoneum and the anterior Gerota fascia, and the posterior compartment, which is bounded by the posterior Gerota fascia and transversalis fascia. Because the anterior pararenal space extends across the midline, infections arising in one space may become bilateral. The posterior pararenal space does not cross the midline, and infection within it remains unilateral. The retrofascial compartment lies posterior to the transversalis fascia. It is important only in the development of the rare retrofascial abscess from abscesses of the psoas, iliacus, and quadratus muscles.

The term "renal abscess" includes a wide range of abscesses arising from within or around the kidney. An intrarenal abscess is an abscess located within the renal parenchyma or on the renal capsule between the renal parenchyma and capsular artery. A perirenal abscess arises within Gerota fascia external to the capsular artery. A pararenal abscess is located outside of Gerota fascia within the pararenal space (Table 8.1).

### Renal Tuberculosis

Renal tuberculosis is caused by hematogenous dissemination from an infected source elsewhere in the body. Though both kidneys are seeded with tuberculosis bacilli in 90% of cases, clinical renal tuberculosis is usually unilateral. The initial lesion involves the renal cortex, and if they fail to heal spontaneously,

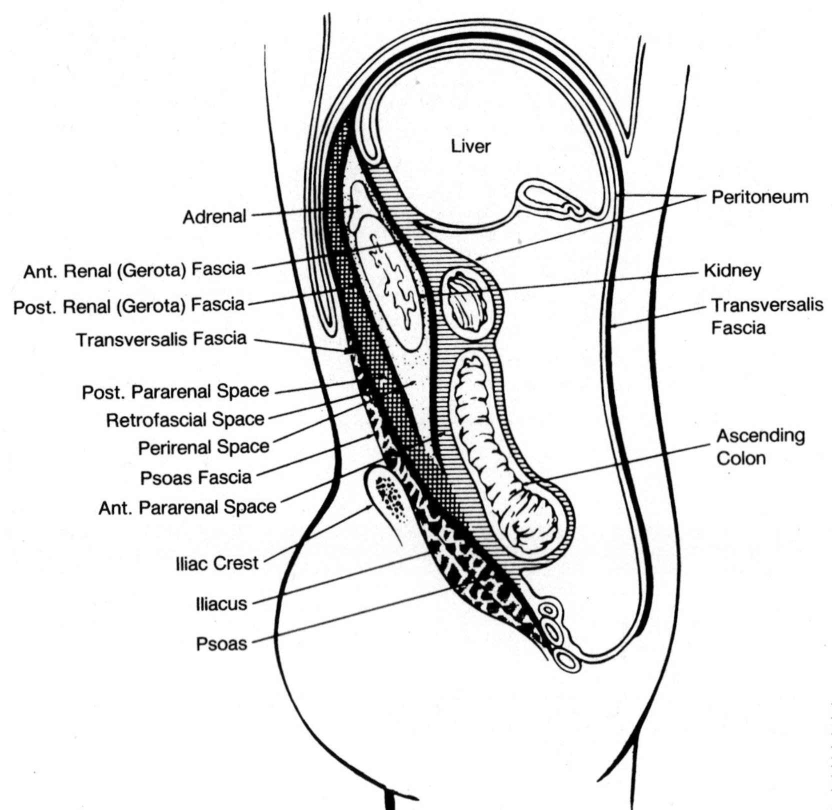


FIGURE 8.1 Right sagittal view showing the anterior pararenal, perirenal, posterior pararenal, and retrofascial spaces. (From Simons GW, Sty JR, Starshak RJ. Retroperitoneal and retrofascial abscess. *J Bone Joint Surg* 1983;65A:1041, reprinted with permission from The Journal of Bone and Joint Surgery, Inc.)

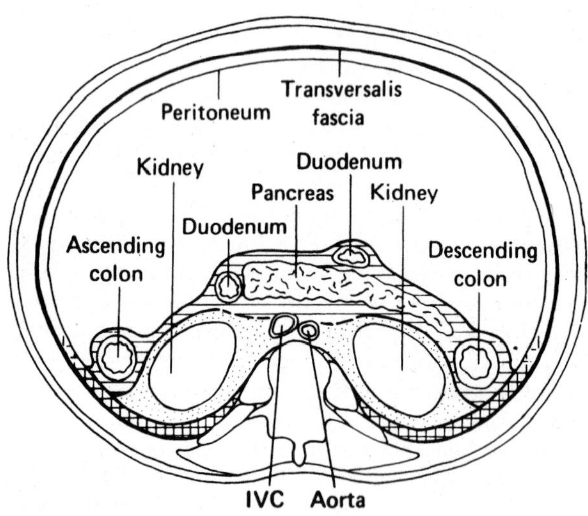


FIGURE 8.2 The three retroperitoneal compartments. The striped and crosshatched areas correspond to the perirenal and posterior pararenal space, respectively. (From Meyers MA. Dynamic radiology of the abdomen. In: *Normal and pathologic anatomy*, 2nd ed. New York: Springer-Verlag, 1982:107–110, with kind permission of Springer Science and Business Media.)

the lesions may progress slowly and remain asymptomatic for 10 to 40 years. As the lesions progress, caseous necrosis and parenchymal cavitation occur with fibrous walls that resemble solid mass lesions. Once cavities form, spontaneous healing is rare and destructive lesions ensue, with spread of the infection to the renal pelvis, resulting in a pyonephroticlike "putty" kidney and development of a parenchymal or perinephric abscess.

### Echinococcus

Echinococcosis is a benign parasitic infection caused by the larval growth of the canine tapeworm *Echinococcus granulosus.* Echinococcal or hydatid cysts occur in the kidney in 3% of patients with this disease. The hydatid cyst gradually develops at a rate of about 1 cm per year and is usually solitary and located in the cortex. The hydatid cyst is composed of a parasitic membrane that is surrounded by a nonparasitic pericyst membrane due to the resultant reactive renal tissue.

## DIAGNOSIS

The diagnosis of renal and retroperitoneal abscesses requires a high index of suspicion, as they typically present with insidious, nonspecific signs and symptoms. The physical findings often do not correlate with the severity of disease (4,10). Many contemporary studies show that only one-third of patients are correctly diagnosed at the time of hospital admission, with an average delay in diagnosis of 3 to 4 days (10). Presenting symptoms may include any combination of fever, chills, abdominal or flank pain, irritative voiding symptoms, nausea, vomiting, lethargy, or weight loss. Patients with renal and retroperitoneal abscesses more often have a longer duration of symptoms as compared with patients with pyelonephritis. The

TABLE 8.1

CHARACTERISTICS OF RENAL ANDRETROPERITONEAL ABCESSES

| Site | Source | Organism | Cofactors | Treatment |
|---|---|---|---|---|
| Cortical intrarenal | Hematogenous | *Staphylococcus aureus* and other gram positives | IV drug use and immunocompromised patients | Antibiotics |
| Intrarenal | Urinary tract | Gram negative Anaerobe (2) (*Escherichia coli, Proteus, Klebsiella*), immunocompromised (opportunistic organisms, including *Candida albicans, Aspergillus, Torulopsis glabrata*) (12,13) | Pyelonephritis with reflux, obstruction, (calculous disease) (16) or immunocompromised patient | Antibiotics + drainage, +/− nephrectomy if non-functional kidney or progressive infection |
| Perirenal | Intrarenal abscess or pyonephrosis eroding into perirenal space | Gram negative (*Escherichia coli, Proteus, Klebsiella*) | Often localizes to the lower pole kidney | Antibiotics + drainage, +/− nephrectomy if non-functional kidney or progressive infection |
| Posterior pararenal | Spinal infections, perirenal abscesses, or anterior pararenal abscesses | | | Antibiotics + drainage, +/− nephrectomy if non-functional kidney or progressive infection |
| Anterior pararenal | Gastrointestinal (colon, appendix, pancreas, duodenum) | Mixture including *Escherichia coli* and anaerobes | | Antibiotics + drainage, +/− nephrectomy if non-functional kidney or progressive infection |

majority of patients diagnosed with renal and retroperitoneal abscesses have underlying, predisposing medical conditions. These include diabetes mellitus, urinary tract calculi, previous urologic surgery, urinary tract obstruction, polycystic kidney disease, malignancy, and immunosuppression.

A palpable flank or abdominal mass is present in about one-third of cases. The mass may be better appreciated by examination of the patient in the knee–chest position. There may also be signs of psoas muscle irritation with flexion of the thigh.

Laboratory tests are helpful but nondiagnostic. Leukocytosis, elevated serum creatinine, and pyuria are common. In up to 30% of gram-negative abscesses, the abscess does not involve the collecting system and urine cultures are frequently negative. Positive urine cultures will generally correlate with blood cultures in the setting of retrograde gram-negative abscesses. In abscesses secondary to gram-positive organisms, however, the urine culture and blood culture may reflect different isolates. Overall, positive urine cultures coincide with culture results from the abscess in only 40% of cases, and the microorganisms isolated in positive blood cultures are similar to those in the abscess culture in 60% of cases.

Computerized tomography (CT) of the abdomen and pelvis with intravenous contrast remains the radiographic study of choice and can precisely localize and detect an abscess <2 cm in size, thereby determining the type of intervention and its anatomic approach. The presence of gas within a lesion is pathognomonic for an abscess. Additional CT findings characteristic of an abscess include a mass with low attenuation, rim enhancement of the abscess wall after contrast, obliteration of tissue planes, and displacement of surrounding structures. Other studies that may be used include ultrasonography or magnetic resonance imaging (MRI).

## INDICATIONS FOR SURGERY

Renal and retroperitoneal abscesses are generally lethal if untreated. Therapeutic options include antimicrobial therapy alone or in combination with percutaneous catheter drainage or open surgical drainage. Nephrectomy is typically reserved for those with nonfunctioning kidneys. If a perinephric abscess is due to long-standing obstruction and there is no functioning renal tissue, a nephrectomy at the time of drainage is theoretically attractive. Initially, however, drainage of the abscess should be performed as the primary procedure, with nephrectomy performed at a later date if necessary. Patients are frequently too ill for prolonged general anesthesia and surgical manipulation. After drainage of the abscess, removal of obstruction, and appropriate antimicrobial therapy, many kidneys may regain sufficient function to obviate future nephrectomy. Nephrectomy, if indicated, can be performed using a standard simple open nephrectomy approach or as a subcapsular nephrectomy. A small renal abscess confined to one pole of the kidney may be managed by partial nephrectomy. If the infection extends beyond the apparent line of cleavage, however, it is essential to remove all infection, and the line of excision should extend through healthy tissue. If multiple abscesses are present, internal drainage is difficult and nephrectomy may be required.

Antimicrobial therapy should be instituted after the urine has been Gram stained and urine and blood cultures have been obtained. Broad-spectrum coverage should be guided by the presumptive diagnosis and the presumed pathogen. A third-generation cephalosporin or an aminoglycoside for gram-negative rods and ampicillin for gram-positive cocci are preferred. Intravenous piperacillin/tazobactam may be used in patients with renal insufficiency. Anaerobic coverage with a drug such as clindamycin is warranted when Gram stain reveals a polymicrobial flora or when a GI source is suspected. If the abscess is suspected of staphylococcal origin, a penicillinase-resistant penicillin, such as nafcillin, should be added. Antimicrobial therapy should be re-evaluated when culture and sensitivity test results are available. Unfortunately, urine and blood cultures are frequently sterile, and empirical therapy must be modified on the basis of clinical response and changes in imaging studies.

### Renal Tuberculosis

Surgery for renal tuberculosis is reserved primarily for management of local complications, such as drainage of abscesses or tuberculous cavities or for treatment of nonfunctioning kidneys. If segmental renal damage is obvious and salvage of the kidney is possible, a drainage procedure or cavernostomy can be performed (6). Removal of a nonfunctioning kidney is usually indicated for advanced unilateral disease complicated by sepsis, hemorrhage, intractable pain, newly developed severe hypertension, suspicion of malignancy, inability to sterilize the urine with drugs alone, abscess formation with development of fistula, or inability to have appropriate follow-up (3,9,14). If surgery is warranted, it is wise to precede the operation with at least 3 weeks and preferably 3 months of a four-drug chemotherapy regimen. In adults, use of isoniazid, 300 mg per day; pyrazinamide, 20 to 25 mg per kg daily; rifampin, 600 mg per day; and ethambutol, 15 to 20 mg per kg daily is recommended unless individual drug resistance exists.

### Echinococcus

The symptoms are those of a slowly growing tumor; most patients are asymptomatic or have a dull flank pain or hematuria. Hydatiduria is pathognomonic for the disease but occurs in only 5% to 25% of cases. As a result of cyst rupture directly into the collecting system, patients exhibit passage of grapelike materials in the urine. Excretory urography typically shows a thick-walled cystic mass that is occasionally calcified. Ultrasonography and CT usually show either a unilocular or multivesicular cyst. Confirmation of the diagnosis is most reliably made by diagnostic tests using partially purified hydatid antigens in a double-diffusion test (14). Complement fixation and hemagglutination are less reliable. Diagnostic needle puncture is associated with significant risk of anaphylaxis as a result of leakage of toxic cyst contents. Cyst removal is indicated when an enlarging cyst threatens renal function or produces obstruction.

## ALTERNATIVE TREATMENT

Antimicrobial therapy as the sole treatment is an option with resolution of symptoms in a small percentage of renal abscesses depending on size, location, and other factors (1). Small intrarenal abscesses (<4 to 5 cm) may resolve if they are treated early at the carbuncle stage or have minimally liquefied through aggressive antimicrobial therapy. Similarly, antimicrobial therapy with close observation alone has been advocated in select patients with small perirenal abscesses (<3 cm) and stable patient conditions (4,10). Prolonged antimicrobial therapy without drainage is indicated only if favorable clinical response and radiological confirmation of abscess resolution indicate that therapy is effective. This form of therapy has proven more successful in children when compared to adults and least successful in immunocompromised patients. If antimicrobial therapy is not effective, prompt percutaneous or open surgical drainage of the pus is mandatory.

## SURGICAL TECHNIQUE

### Percutaneous Drainage

Most renal and retroperitoneal abscesses are treated with empirical antimicrobial therapy and immediate percutaneous drainage. With resolution of the abscess occurring at least two-thirds of the time, minimally invasive therapy eliminates operative morbidity and allows for preservation of renal tissue. In those patients with a remaining surgical indication, percutaneous drainage can help delay surgery and allow the patient's condition to be optimized. The abscess must be confirmed by CT- or ultrasonography-guided needle aspiration and must be drainable without injury to other organs. Contraindications to percutaneous puncture include coagulation disorders and calcified masses, which may indicate other processes. Immediate surgical drainage must be instituted if the procedure fails. After a multiport drainage catheter (8Fr to 12Fr) is positioned, the abscess should be drained and adequate evacuation should be confirmed by CT or ultrasonography. In the setting of abscess septation or multiloculation, multiple catheters or septal perforation during catheter placement may be utilized. The catheter should then be connected to low intermittent suction, and drainage outputs should be monitored daily. If drainage stops abruptly, occlusion of the catheter should be suspected and gentle irrigation with small amounts of normal saline performed. CT or ultrasonography should be performed periodically to monitor catheter position and size of the abscess. Direct instillation of contrast through the drainage tube may be helpful to confirm the catheter position or rule out a fistula. To avoid bacteremia, prophylactic antimicrobial coverage should be given, and the contrast should be instilled under gravity or by gentle injection. Instillation of 2,500 U of urokinase in 50 mL of normal saline on a daily basis may be successful in evacuating an organizing infected hematoma. Routine abscess irrigation with antimicrobials is of questionable benefit and may promote overgrowth of resistant bacteria. The catheter should be withdrawn gradually as the abscess cavity shrinks and the drainage decreases. The usual duration of drainage is 1 to 3 weeks. The catheter is removed when drainage stops, CT or ultrasonography confirms complete resolution, and fevers and leukocyte count normalize.

### Open Surgical Drainage

In the case of failed percutaneous therapy, open surgical drainage is usually the next step. Open surgery allows for direct anatomic evaluation and a determination of the extent of the inflammatory process. In addition, more complex pathology may be delineated, including chronic fistulas suggesting residual stone, foreign body, or persistent renal obstruction or, rarely, carcinomas that predispose a kidney to abscess formation and thus prevent a cure with only simple drainage.

For open surgical drainage, the incision should be smaller than that used for routine nephrectomy, and usually a posterior flank muscle-splitting incision below the twelfth rib is sufficient. When the retroperitoneal abscess is entered, the pus should be cultured and the space gently but thoroughly explored to ensure that all loculated cavities are drained. Thorough irrigation of the cavity is essential. Multiple Penrose drains should be inserted into the space through separate stab wounds, and the ends of the drains should be sutured to the skin and tagged with safety pins. Fascial and muscular closure may be performed with chromic catgut suture, but skin and subcutaneous tissue should be left open to prevent the formation of a secondary body wall abscess. The wound can be left to heal from within, or skin sutures may be placed and left untied for dermal approximation 5 to 7 days postoperatively after drainage has ceased. The wound should be packed with gauze and the packs changed daily. The drains should be left in place until purulent drainage has decreased, and then removed slowly over several days.

## Subcapsular Nephrectomy

When a kidney is so adherent to surrounding tissues that dissection is difficult and hazardous, a subcapsular nephrectomy is indicated. These conditions may result after multiple or chronic infections or previous operations resulting in significant fibrotic adhesions between Gerota fascia and the perirenal fat. Blunt dissection can result in tearing of structures such as the bowel wall. Sharp dissection when there is no definable tissue plane often results in lacerations of the vena cava, aorta, duodenum, spleen, and other structures. In subcapsular nephrectomy, dissection beneath the renal capsule enables one to avoid these vital structures. Subcapsular nephrectomy should not be performed for malignant disease.

The main difficulty with subcapsular nephrectomy is that the capsule is adherent to the vessels in the hilum, and one usually must go outside the capsule to ligate the renal pedicle. In this setting, the renal hilum is usually involved in the inflammatory reaction, and separate identification of the vessels is difficult.

Kidney exposure is accomplished through the flank using a twelfth-rib incision. For low-lying kidneys, a subcostal incision may be satisfactory. When the kidney is reached, the capsule is incised and freed from the underlying cortex (Fig. 8.3). To avoid damage to the duodenum or major vessels, pieces of capsule may be left behind. However, prolonged drainage can ensue, and as much of the infected tissue should be removed as possible. The capsule is stripped from the surface of the kidney and an incision is made carefully in the capsule where it is attached to the hilum (Fig. 8.4). The vessels may be protected by placing a finger in front of the pedicle when cutting the capsule. The dense apron of the capsule can usually be incised best on the anterior aspect. Controlling bleeding can be difficult in this procedure, and a harmonic scalpel or bipolar electric coagulation device may be utilized to minimize hemorrhage.

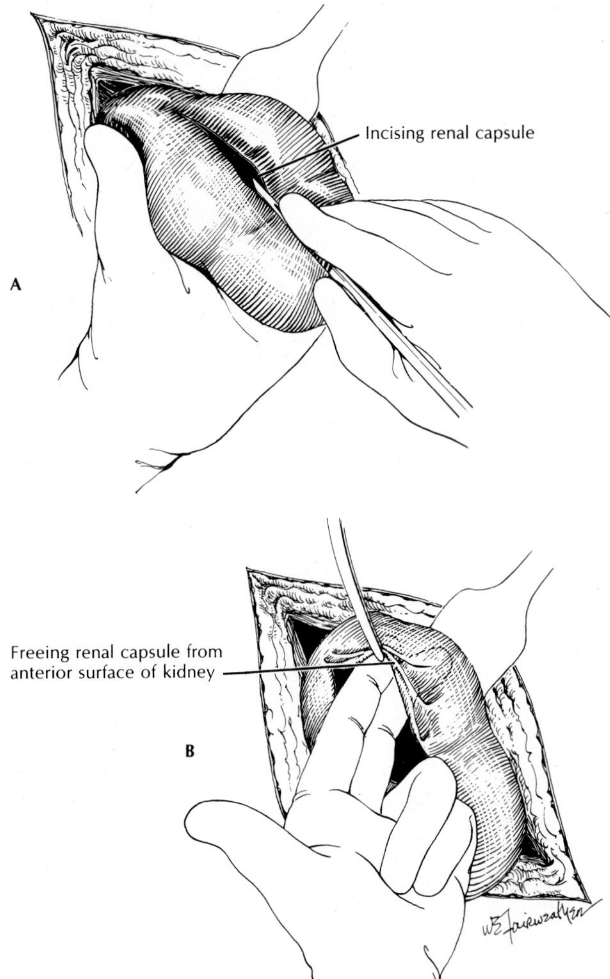


FIGURE 8.3 Subcapsular secondary nephrectomy showing freeing of the capsule from anterior surfaces of the kidney.

Frequently, all landmarks are obscured and the renal artery and vein cannot be identified. Sharp dissection is usually required, and major vessels may be entered before they are recognized. Fortunately, the dense fibrous tissue tends to prevent their retraction. Frequently, a combination of suture ligatures, clips, or a vascular load stapler can be used to divide the renal vessels. After ligation and cutting of the pedicle, the ureter is identified and cut and the distal end is ligated. If distal ureteral obstruction has caused pyonephrosis, a small, 8Fr to 10Fr red Robinson catheter may be placed in the distal ureter to allow postoperative antimicrobial irrigation. Multiple drains should be placed and brought through separate stab wounds.

## Laparoscopic Treatment of Renal Abscesses

Historically, the dense perinephric adhesions associated with renal abscess disease and the resultant high open conversion rate were relative contraindications to laparoscopic simple and subcapsular nephrectomy. However, more recent series involving laparoscopic techniques have shown feasibility in select patients with possible advantages in postoperative

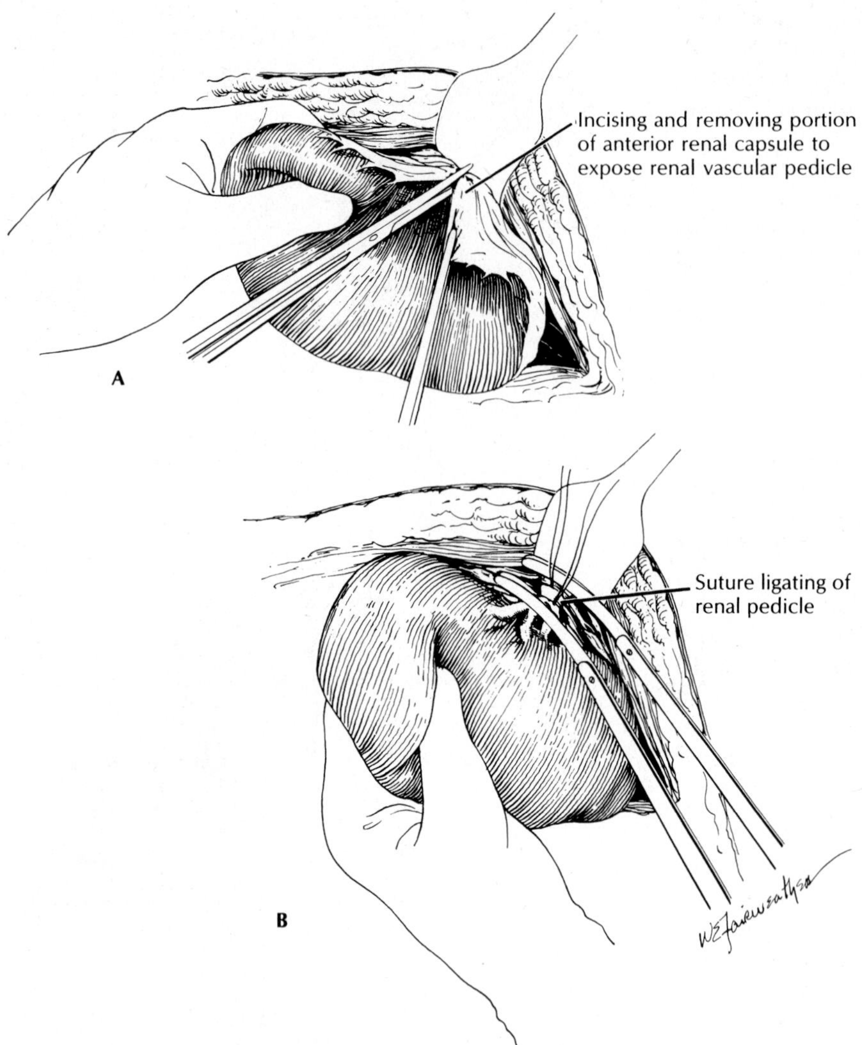


FIGURE 8.4 Subcapsular secondary nephrectomy showing incision in and removal of a portion of the renal capsule to expose and ligate the renal pedicle.

recovery and blood loss as compared to open studies. Similar to the open technique, dissociation and ligation of the renal pedicle remain the most challenging surgical step and may be facilitated with careful dissection using a harmonic or bipolar scalpel and an endoscopic linear stapler for the hilum. Given the potential to limit seeding of the peritoneum with infectious tissue, a retroperitoneal approach has been advocated. However, laparoscopic therapies remain technically challenging, and current reported experiences in the literature are small (7,17).

## Cavernostomy for Segmental Renal Tuberculosis

Renal tuberculosis sometimes results in caliceal infundibular scarring, causing a closed pyocalix abscess. In cases of sepsis, cavernostomy or unroofing of the pyocalix may be necessary. If the calyx still communicates with the renal pelvis, or if it is connected to significant functioning parenchyma, a cavernostomy should not be done as a urinary fistula or urinoma may result. To minimize wound contamination and tuberculous spread, thorough needle aspiration of purulent material and saline irrigation of the abscess cavity should be performed using a large-bore needle and syringe (Fig. 8.5). The abscess cavity is then unroofed and the edge is sutured with a running suture for hemostasis. Any unsuspected connection with the renal pelvis by an open infundibulum must be closed using 5-0 chromic catgut sutures to prevent fistula or urinoma formation. After thorough wound irrigation, multiple drains are placed and closure is undertaken. Drains are managed as previously described for perinephric abscess.

## Nephrectomy for Renal Tuberculosis

When unilateral tuberculosis causes more extensive parenchymal destruction or nonfunction, a partial or total nephrectomy, respectively, should be performed. Particular care should be taken to avoid entering the peritoneum or pleura. For partial nephrectomy, a guillotine incision is made 1 cm beyond the abscess. If the renal pedicle can be freed and the polar vessel located and occluded, the incision can be made at the line of demarcation of the ischemia. In partial nephrectomy, it is important to try to save the

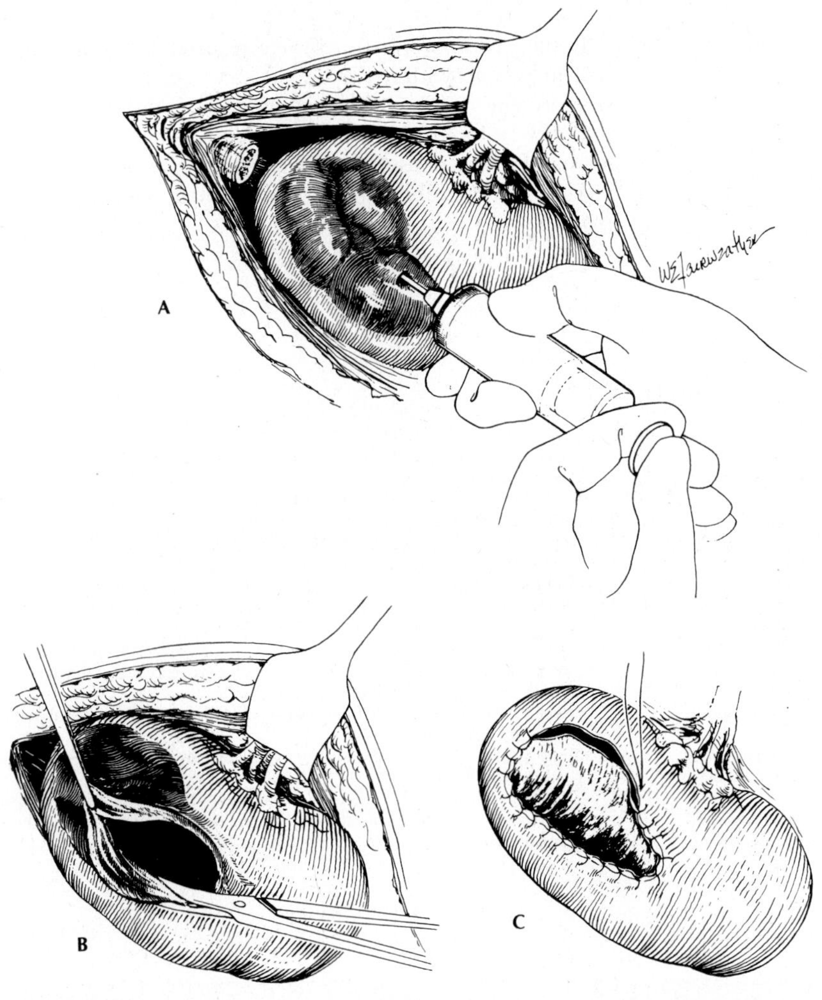


FIGURE 8.5 Cavernostomy drainage of tuberculous renal abscess. (From Hanley HG. Cavernostomy and partial nephrectomy in renal tuberculosis. *Br J Urol* 1970;42:661, with permission.)

capsule (if it is not involved with the infection) to cover the raw surface for hemostasis. Alternatively, fat can be used for hemostasis. The amputated calyx is carefully ligated with a 4-0 chromic catgut suture to prevent urinary fistula or urinoma formation.

After nephrectomy, the distal ureter can be ligated and in most cases does not need to be brought to the skin because tuberculosis of the ureteral stump generally heals with chemotherapy after nephrectomy. If renal tuberculosis is associated with severe tuberculosis cystitis, ureteral catheterization for 7 days postoperatively to minimize subsequent ureteral stump abscess formation should be considered (3).

### Resection of Echinococcal Cyst

The cyst should be removed without rupture to reduce the chance of seeding or anaphylactic-type reaction, which can prove fatal in the operating room. In cases where cyst removal is impossible because of its size or involvement of adjacent organs, marsupialization is required. Initially the cyst should be isolated with sponges, the contents aspirated, and the cyst filled with a scolicidal agent such as 30% sodium chloride, 2% formalin, or 1% iodide for about 5 minutes to kill the germinal portions. Complete evacuation of all hydatid tissue and thorough postmarsupialization irrigation are critical to preventing systemic effects. Total or partial pericystectomy can subsequently be carried out to remove the surrounding pericyst, and any open calyces can be closed. Penrose drains are left in the cystic cavity until drainage ceases. If large amounts of renal tissue have been damaged, partial or simple nephrectomy may be required.

## OUTCOMES

### Complications

Complications associated with percutaneous drainage include the formation of additional abscesses that communicate with the renal collecting system and may require temporary urinary diversion via percutaneous nephrostomy drainage to affect a cure. Sepsis, the most frequent complication of percutaneous drainage, occurs in fewer than 10% of patients. Other complications, such as transpleural puncture, vascular or enteric injury, and cutaneous fistula, are rare.

Additional complications to open or percutaneous drainage include prolonged purulent drainage, which may indicate a retained foreign body, calculus, or fistula.

## Results

Cure rates for percutaneous drainage of renal and retroperitoneal abscesses range from 60% to 90% (9,16). Multiloculated, viscous abscesses and abscesses in immunocompromised hosts are associated with lower cure rates. Large abscesses may require more than one percutaneous access procedure to completely drain them.

In the past, mortality rates were reported to be as high as 50% in patients with retroperitoneal or perinephric abscesses. More recent reports indicate a significant improvement in mortality (<15%); this is largely due to more accurate diagnosis and drainage using improved imaging techniques, more effective antimicrobial therapy, and better supportive care (4,5,10).

## *References*

1. Best CD, Terris MK, Tacker JR, et al. Clinical and radiological findings in patients with gas forming renal abscess treated conservatively. *J Urol* 1999;162:1273–1276.
2. Brook I. The role of anaerobic bacteria in perinephric and renal abscesses in children. *Pediatrics* 1994;93:261–264.
3. Carl P, Stark L. Indications for surgical management of genitourinary tuberculosis. *World J Surg* 1997;21:505–510.
4. Coelho RF, Schneider-Monteiro ED, Mesquita JL, et al. Renal and perinephric abscesses: analysis of 65 consecutive cases. *World J Surg* 2007; 31:431–436.
5. Edelstein H, McCabe RE. Perinephric abscess: modern diagnosis and treatment in 47 cases. *Medicine* 1988;67:118–131.
6. Hanley HG. Cavernostomy and partial nephrectomy in renal tuberculosis. *Br J Urol* 1970;42:661–666.
7. Hemal AK, Gupta NP, Kumar R. Comparison of retroperitoneoscopic nephrectomy with open surgery for tuberculous nonfunctioning kidneys. *J Urol* 2000;164:32–335.
8. Lambiase RE, Deyoe L, Cronan JJ, et al. Percutaneous drainage of 355 consecutive abscesses: results of primary drainage with 1-year follow-up. *Radiology* 1992;184:167–179.
9. Lorin MI, Hsu KHF, Jacob SC. Treatment of tuberculosis in children. *Pediatr Clin North Am* 1983;30:333–348.
10. Meng MV, Mario LA, McAninch JW. Current treatment and outcomes of perinephric abscesses. *J Urol* 2002;168:1337–1340.
11. Mitchell GAG. The renal fascia. *Br J Surg* 1950;37:257–266.
12. Noriega LM, Gonzalez P, Perez J, et al. [Unusual presentation of urinary tract infection in 6 cases.] *Rev Med Child* 1995;123:334–340.
13. Oda K, Inoue S, Oe H. Renal carbuncle with xanthogranulomatous change: report of a case. *Hinyokika Kiyo* 1970;16(5):211–218.
14. Schaeffer AJ. Urinary tract infections. In: Gillenwater JY, Grayhack JT, Howards SS, et al., eds. *Adult and pediatric urology*. Philadelphia: Lippincott Williams & Wilkins, 2002:211–272.
15. Siegel JF, Smith A, Moldwin R. Minimally invasive treatment of renal abscess. *J Urol* 1996;155:52–55.
16. Yoder JC, Pfister RC, Lindfors KK, et al. Pyonephrosis: imaging and intervention. *AJR Am J Roentgenol* 1983;141:735–739.
17. Zhang X, Zheng T, Ma X, et al. Comparison of retroperitoneoscopic nephrectomy versus open approaches to nonfunctioning tuberculous kidneys: a report of 44 cases. *J Urol* 2005;173:1586–1589.

# CHAPTER 9 ■ RENAL TRAUMA

JILL C. BUCKLEY AND JACK W. MCANINCH

Renal injuries occur infrequently in trauma patients, with a reported incidence between 2% and 3% (1). The vast majority of renal injuries occur as a result of blunt trauma, are grades I to III, and can be managed nonoperatively (1,2). Penetrating renal trauma usually occurs in conjunction with other intra-abdominal injuries where urgent laparotomy is performed. Grade V renal injuries by definition represent life-threatening renal injuries that require operative exploration and often nephrectomy. Grade IV renal injuries represent the most controversial management issue in renal trauma care. Many blunt and penetrating grade IV renal injuries can be successfully managed nonoperatively if the patient has been appropriated staged with computerized tomography (CT) and can be closely monitored in an intensive care unit (ICU) (3). If radiographic renal staging is not available or the patient requires immediate abdominal laparotomy for an associated nonurologic injury, renal exploration is indicated after obtaining an intraoperative single-shot intravenous pyelogram (IVP). In hemodynamically stable patients, renal reconstruction at the time of laparotomy provides excellent functional results in the majority of cases (4). The goal of all renal trauma care is preservation of enough functioning nephron mass to avoid end-stage renal failure. Nephrectomy is reserved for a life threatening injury where damage control is necessary.

## DIAGNOSIS

As with all trauma situations, the patient should undergo an acute assessment and resuscitation as defined by the American Association for the Surgery of Trauma (AAST). The hemodynamic stability of the patient will determine if an immediate operative exploration is required versus radiographic CT staging. The type of trauma (blunt versus penetrating), mechanism of injury (e.g. deceleration injury), physical examination (presence of a rib fracture or spinous process fracture, abdominal or flank tenderness, flank ecchymosis, etc.), associated nonurologic injuries, hemodynamics, and degree of hematuria are important to obtain in the initial assessment. If gross hematuria is not present, a urine dipstick analysis or formal urine analysis should be performed to detect microscopic hematuria. The degree of hematuria does not correlate with the degree of renal injury but is useful in guiding the initial emergency department assessment.

## IMAGING

All penetrating trauma should undergo CT radiographic imaging. Any patient sustaining a blunt trauma injury with a positive physical examination, a deceleration injury, gross hematuria, microscopic hematuria in the setting of hypotension (systolic blood presure <90 mmHg in the field or in the emergency department), or serial decreasing hematocrits should undergo radiographic CT imaging to stage the renal injury (1,5). Triple-phase CT radiographic imaging allows detailed staging of the renal injury by evaluating the renal hilum, parenchyma, collecting system, and surrounding tissue, as well as detecting other intra-abdominal injuries. It is important to obtain delayed images to document that the collecting system is intact, with contrast passing down into the distal ureter without extravasation (6).

In pediatric trauma patients, special attention should be given to the degree of microscopic hematuria present, as this alone may warrant CT radiographic imaging. Children are often able to maintain their hemodynamics despite underlying hypovolemia; thus blood pressure readings can be falsely reassuring. Unlike with the adult patient, isolated significant microscopic hematuria defined as >50 red blood cells per high-powered field should prompt radiographic CT imaging (7,8). As stated above, the type of trauma (blunt versus penetrating), mechanism of injury (e.g. deceleration injury), physical examination (presence of a rib fracture or spinous process fracture, abdominal or flank tenderness, flank ecchymosis, etc.), and associated nonurologic injuries in hemodynamic stable children should all undergo radiographic CT staging of the renal injury.

If immediate laparotomy is required, a single-shot IVP should be performed in the operating room. A bolus IV injection of 2 cc per kg of radiographic contrast is given followed by a 10-minute plain film of the abdomen and pelvis. It is critical to document a functioning contralateral kidney should a nephrectomy be required of the injured renal unit. With a normal single-shot intraoperative IVP demonstrating two intact renal units and a nonexpanding retroperitoneal hematoma, exploration can be avoided (9).

## MANAGEMENT

Management of the injured kidney is based on consideration of the patient's mechanism of injury, hemodynamic stability, associated injuries, and accurate radiographic staging of the injury (1). The vast majority of blunt traumatic renal injuries are clinically insignificant. Fewer than 2% of patients with blunt renal trauma require renal exploration (1,2) (Fig. 9.1).

Historically, all penetrating abdominal injuries underwent laparotomy. Now, with improved diagnostic radiographic imaging, many intra-abdominal and renal injuries can be staged and managed with nonoperative active surveillance in ICUs

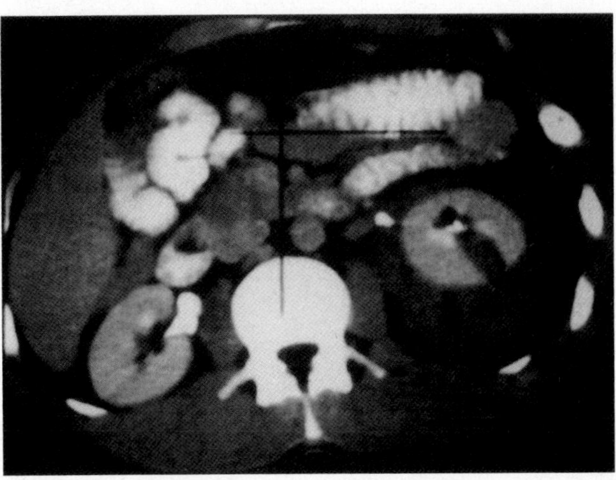

FIGURE 9.1 Abdominal computerized tomography (CT) reveals left renal laceration after blunt trauma (grade III). Even major renal lacerations occurring after blunt trauma are usually amenable to nonoperative management. Renal CT provides detailed information regarding the depth of laceration, size of perirenal hematoma, tissue viability, urinary extravasation, and status of the contralateral kidney.

combined with repeat imaging (3,10). If conservative management is chosen, it is the responsibility of the treating physician to document a stable or improving situation through clinical parameters and repeat imaging. All patients who sustain a major renal trauma should be admitted to the ICU for serial hematocrits, placed on bedrest, and have repeat CT imaging performed 48 hours after the initial staging CT scan or earlier if there is a significant change in their clinical course (3). Active surveillance ensures appropriate management either by demonstrating resolution of the renal injury or by prompting intervention, such as ureteral stent placement for nonresolving urinary extravasation or angioembolization of a segmental artery for persistent arterial extravasation (11,12). In all cases of severe renal injury, nonoperative management should only occur after radiographic CT renal staging in hemodynamically stable patients with close peritraumatic monitoring.

## ANGIOEMBOLIZATION

The minimally invasive technique of angioembolization along with radiographic CT imaging has led to a dramatic shift in trauma care in large urban centers where interventional radiology expertise is available. A clear role has emerged for selective segmental arterial embolization in a subset of severe renal injuries to control significant bleeding (13,14). Renal hilar injuries are life-threatening and require immediate operative exploration (15). As with all severe renal injuries, selection is critical for successful management, along with having available and capable interventional radiologists or trained vascular or trauma surgeons. Indications include non–life-threatening bleeding isolated to a segmental renal artery or vein in the setting of an expanding perirenal hematoma or refractory hypovolemia (>3 units of blood transfusion). The embolized vessel is typically a segmental artery, as venous bleeding will often tamponade provided Gerota fascia is still intact (Fig. 9.2). Embolization will lead to nephron loss and should be restricted to active arterial extravasation. Selective embolization has

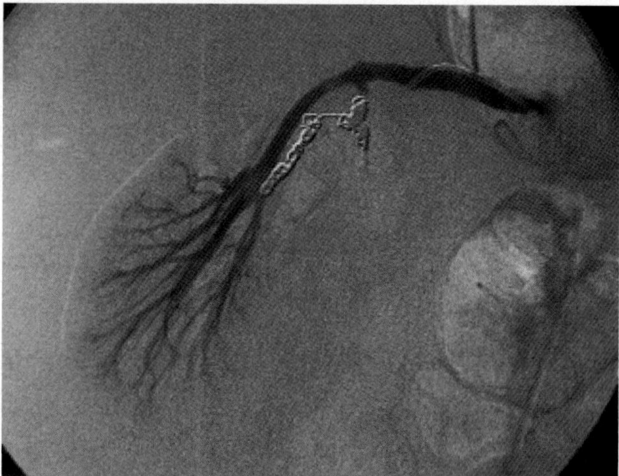

FIGURE 9.2 Angioembolization of active segmental arterial extravasation.

demonstrated excellent preservation of the remaining kidney for not only renal trauma injuries but also for symptomatic angiomyolipomas, spontaneous perirenal bleeds, pseudoaneurysms, and iatrogenic renal vascular injuries and has resulted in shorter hospital stays, decreased pain, and fewer complications by avoiding open exploration (14,16,17). Endovascular procedures will continue to expand their role in the acute trauma setting as comfort and experience with these minimally invasive techniques grow.

## INDICATIONS FOR RENAL EXPLORATION

An absolute indication for renal exploration is life-threatening hemorrhage from a severely injured renal unit. Relative indications for operative exploration include ureteropelvic junction disruption, extensive nonviable renal parenchyma with urinary extravasation, incomplete radiographic staging, and limited observational facilities (Table 9.1). In the setting of a concomitant exploratory laparotomy by the trauma surgeons, our preference is to formally explore and reconstruct any significant renal injury (grade III or greater) in a hemodynamically stable patient. Minimal time is added to the operation, and outcomes are excellent (4). Successful reconstruction can be undertaken despite spillage from bowel injury, pancreatic injury, or other associated injuries (18).

In both blunt and penetrating isolated severe renal trauma (no other significant intra-abdominal injuries), selective management is employed to determine if exploration is indicated based on the hemodynamics of the patient, radiographic CT staging of the renal injury, and clinical assessment (3,19). In our large series of grade IV renal injuries, 28% were isolated kidney injuries, 42% underwent exploration, and the remaining 58% were managed nonoperatively. Persistent bleeding requiring multiple blood transfusions was the primary indication for renal exploration (average transfusion requirement of 8.5 U packed red blood cells (prbc)). Our guidelines for intervention are hemodynamic instability causing severe hypotension and shock, a rapidly expanding renal hematoma, persistent hemodynamic instability despite 3 U prbc, and clinical decompensation (3). Renal salvage rates were high (>85%) for both operative and nonoperative management, demonstrating the utility and importance of selective management.

**TABLE 9.1**

INDICATIONS FOR RENAL EXPLORATION

| ABSOLUTE |
|---|
| Expanding renal hematoma |
| Pulsatile hematoma |
| Complete ureteropelvic junction disruption |
| **RELATIVE** |
| Urinary extravasation associated with nonviable tissue |
| Large area of nonviable renal parenchyma |
| Significant arterial extravasation[a] |
| Incomplete staging |

[a]Interventional radiology is not available or is unable to control the bleeding.

## NEPHRECTOMY

Nephrectomy should be reserved for critically ill patients during a damage control situation and/or renal pedicle avulsions that require complex vascular reconstruction. Critical to document in those acute settings is a functioning contralateral kidney with a single-shot IVP. These patients are often in shock, have high injury severity scores, receive large volumes of blood transfusions, and overall experience a high mortality rate. As stated by Nash et al., "It is not the exploration that results in the nephrectomy but the injury itself" (20).

## SURGICAL TECHNIQUE

Renal exploration in the trauma setting should be carried out through a standard midline abdominal incision (Fig. 9.3). This approach provides complete access to the intra-abdominal viscera and vasculature and also gives the greatest flexibility to assess and repair a variety of genitourinary injuries. Major bleeding noted on opening the abdominal cavity should be controlled immediately with laparotomy packs followed by surgical control and repair. Associated injuries to other abdominal organs are usually addressed before examination of the kidneys if the patient is stable. The bowel, liver, spleen, pancreas, and other organs should be inspected systematically and carefully. During this period, Gerota fascia maintains its natural tamponade effect on the perinephric hematoma.

The renal vasculature is routinely isolated before entering the retroperitoneal hematoma surrounding the injured kidney. This reduces the risk of uncontrolled renal bleeding and unplanned nephrectomy (21,22). To facilitate access to the retroperitoneum, the transverse colon is lifted out of the abdomen superiorly and placed on moist laparotomy packs. The small bowel is rotated to the patient's right and extracted from the body to allow access to the great vessels. An incision is

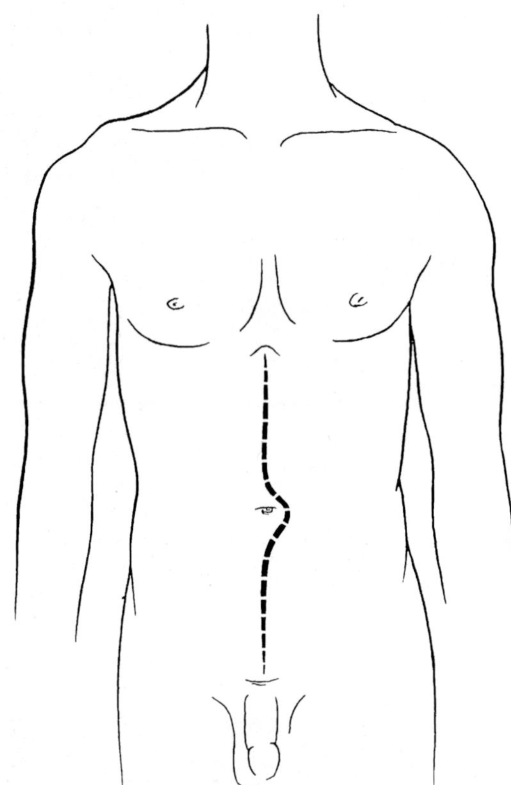

FIGURE 9.3 A midline incision provides the optimal exposure for abdominal exploration, vascular control, and repair of a variety of genitourinary injuries.

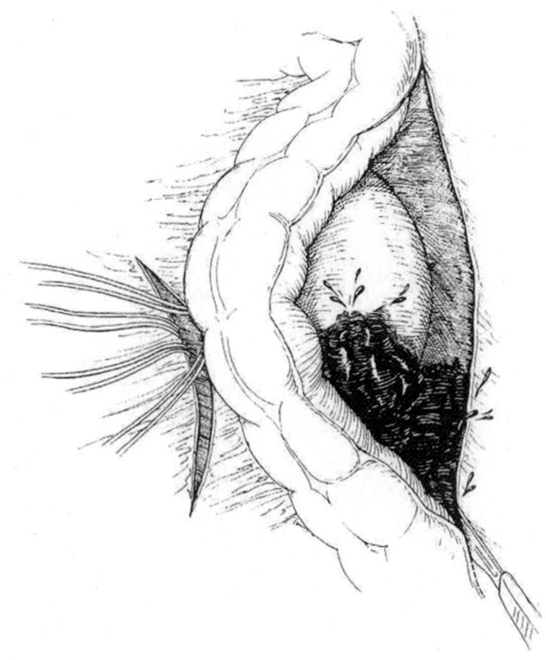

FIGURE 9.4 The colon is reflected medially to allow access to the retroperitoneum. Gerota's fascia is sharply opened.

made in the retroperitoneum over the aorta from the level of the inferior mesenteric artery to the ligament of Treitz, which can be divided for additional exposure. If a large retroperitoneal hematoma obscures the aorta, the inferior mesenteric vein is identified and the incision into the retroperitoneum is placed just medial to this important landmark. Once the aorta is identified in the lower part of the incision, it is followed superiorly to the left renal vein, which reliably crosses anteriorly. The renal arteries can be found just posterior to the left renal vein on either side of the aorta. The right renal artery can be isolated in the interaortocaval location. If it is difficult to identify the right renal artery through this approach, the second portion of the duodenum can be reflected to expose the right renal hilum. The artery is located posterior to the right renal vein.

The renal artery and vein associated with the injured renal unit are individually isolated with vessel loops. These vessels are not occluded initially unless uncontrollable bleeding is encountered. Most bleeding is successfully controlled with manual compression alone. Because the vessels are not routinely clamped, renal perfusion is continuous and warm ischemia is avoided.

Following proximal vascular control, the kidney is exposed by incising the retroperitoneum just lateral to the colon. The colon is reflected medially. Gerota's fascia is sharply opened, and the kidney is expeditiously mobilized to allow complete exposure of the renal surface (Fig. 9.4). Only after complete exposure can the extent and number of injuries be determined (Fig. 9.5/6). Maintaining the renal capsule during mobilization is important as it provides hemostasis and tensile strength for the closure. If necessary for uncontrollable hemorrhage, clamping of the previously isolated vessels can be done with vascular clamps or bulldogs.

The following principles are applied to all renal reconstructions: early vascular control, complete renal exposure, sharp debridement of nonviable tissue, oversewing of bleeding vessels for hemostasis, and watertight collecting system closure. If available, the renal capsule is loosely reapproximated over thrombin-soaked Gelfoam or another thrombogenic substance. Ideally an omental flap is placed over the reconstructed kidney for additional protection and its absorptive properties.

Major polar injuries are best approached by a polar partial nephrectomy. The kidney should be sharply debrided back to viable bleeding tissue. End vessels are individually suture-ligated with 4-0 absorbable sutures to gain hemostasis. The collecting system is then closed with a continuous watertight 4-0 absorbable suture. Methylene blue may be injected into the renal pelvis with simultaneous compression of the ureter to elucidate any leaks in the collecting system, which may then be oversewn however, oversewing is not routinely performed. The renal parenchymal defect is covered with thrombin-soaked Gelfoam or another thrombogenic bulking agent to enhance hemostasis and is covered with loosely approximated, interrupted 3-0 absorbable renal capsular sutures. If no capsule is available or the defect is too large to close primarily, an omental pedicle flap can be used to cover the defect (Fig. 9.7). Its absorbent properties and rich vascular supply make it an excellent alternative to the renal capsule. Another substance we commonly use to cover the renal defect is Vicryl mesh as it is readily available, absorbable, and can easily be tailored to the size and shape of the renal defect. A passive drain is placed, and it is removed in 48 to 72 hours after confirming closure of the collecting system.

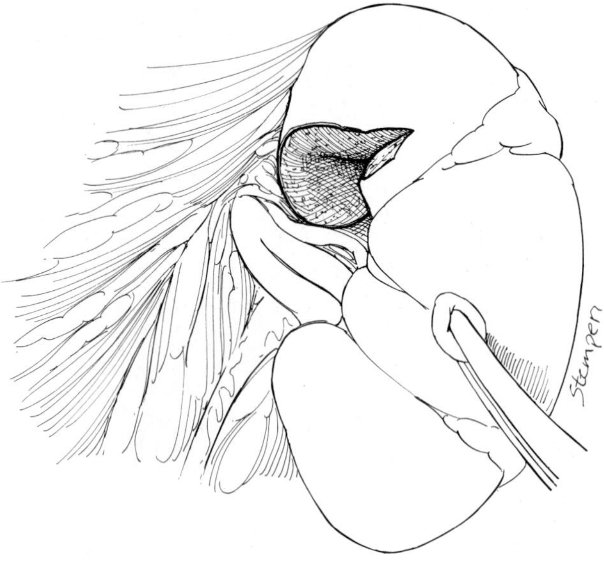


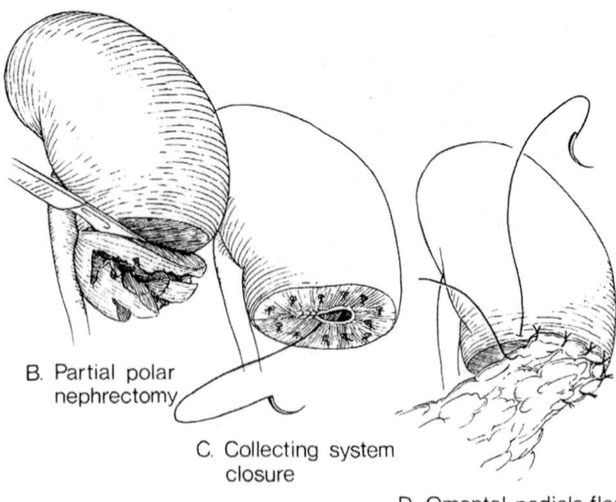


FIGURE 9.7 During a polar partial nephrectomy with reconstruction, if the renal capsule is not available for defect closure, a Vicryl mesh patch or the omentum can be used to cover the defect.

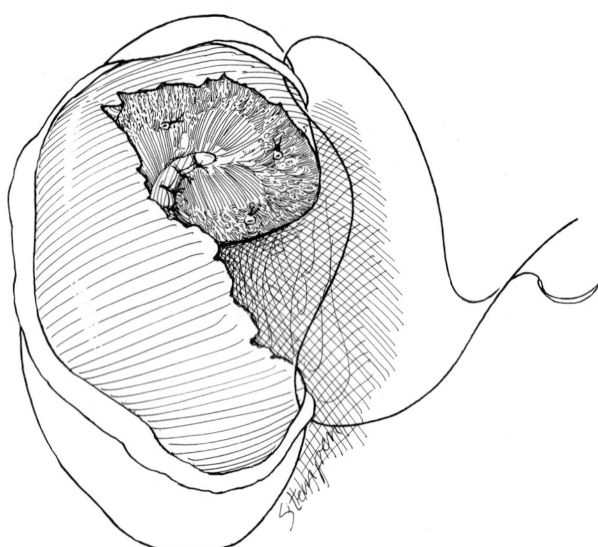

FIGURE 9.5/6 The kidney is explored. A small gunshot entrance wound on the anterior aspect of the left kidney is identified. On the posterior surface, a complex gaping exit wound is identified. Nonviable tissue is sharply debrided, segmental vessels are individually suture-ligated, and the collecting system is closed with a continuous absorbable suture. Capsular 3-0 Vicryl sutures are used to reapproximate wound edges.

Major injuries to the midportion of the kidney are best repaired by sharp wedge resection of the nonviable tissue and renorrhaphy. Devitalized tissue is sharply removed. Sites of bleeding are individually ligated with fine absorbable sutures, and the collecting system is closed with a continuous suture. Thrombin-soaked Gelfoam bolsters are placed into the defect to enhance hemostasis and reduce tension on the capsular sutures (Fig. 9.8). Interrupted absorbable 3-0 sutures are placed through the renal capsule, excluding the underlying parenchyma, as it provides no additional strength. Omentum or Vicryl mesh can be used if primary renal capsular closure cannot be achieved.

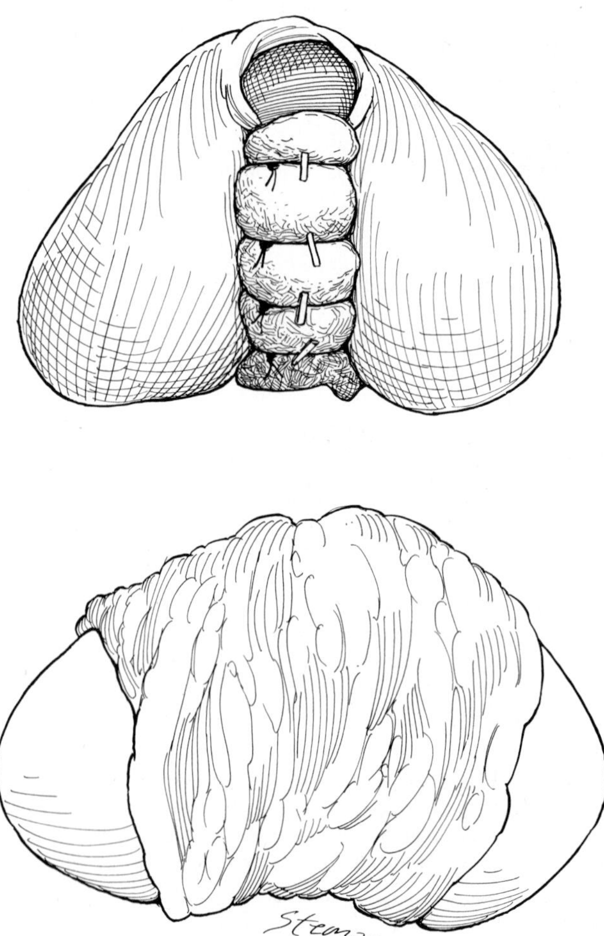


FIGURE 9.8 Closure of parenchymal defect after central renal injury. Capsular sutures of 3-0 Vicryl may be used to sew gelatin foam bolsters into the repair site. Titanium clips may be placed along the repair line to identify the area of reconstruction on subsequent imaging studies. Alternatively, if primary renal closure cannot be achieved, an omental flap may be tacked over the defect using small interrupted chromic sutures.

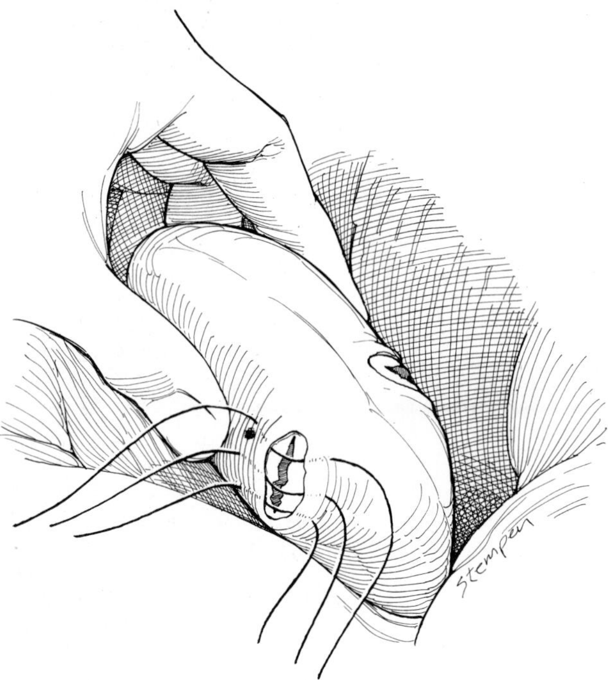

FIGURE 9.9 Technique of renorrhaphy after stab wound. Gelfoam bolsters are laid into the capsular defect, and overlying 3-0 Vicryl sutures are placed superficially to approximate the adjoining renal capsule, thus sealing the reconstructed area.

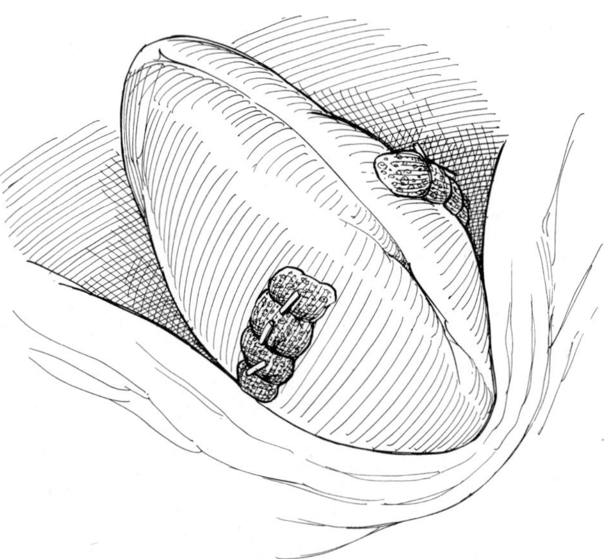

FIGURE 9.10 Completed renal reconstruction after stab wound. The entire kidney has been mobilized and evaluated for associated wounds. Titanium clips along the capsular sutures denote the area of repair.

Renal stab wounds often do not result in displaced or missing renal tissue. Frequently, entrance and exit wounds can be oversewn, and liquid thrombogenic agents such as FloSeal can be applied, resulting in excellent hemostasis (Figs. 9.9 and 9.10). Collecting system injuries that may have occurred will usually resolve with closure of the overlying parenchyma and should not be aggressively pursued. If delayed urinary extravasation is detected by a perirenal drain or radiographic imaging, a ureteral stent can be placed with anticipated collecting system closure (3,11).

## RENOVASCULAR INJURIES

Renovascular injuries are closely associated to the grade of renal injury and are a major cause of partial or total renal loss. Main renal artery or vein avulsion, in the acute trauma situation, is deemed irreparable and results in nephrectomy. Proximal control of the renal pedicle is critical in these injuries to avoid life-threatening hemorrhage. Attempts at complex hilar arterial or venous reconstruction have shown poor results and should be reserved for the solitary kidney or bilateral renal hilar injuries in a non–damage-control situation (1,19,23). If necessary, the left main renal vein can be suture-ligated with sufficient drainage through the left adrenal and gonadal vessels. Reconstruction of a partial venous or arterial hilar injury can be performed with a continuous fine nonabsorbable suture after obtaining vascular control (Fig. 9.11).

## POSTOPERATIVE CARE

Gross blood in the urine usually clears within 24 hours, and patients should be observed on bedrest until this occurs. Ambulation is resumed once the urine is clear. Routine laboratory studies are obtained. In the event of a delayed bleed, renal angiography and selective angioembolization can be utilized to control the hemorrhage. Retroperitoneal drains are normally removed within 48 to 72 hours. If drainage is excessive, an aliquot may be checked for creatinine; a level similar to that of serum suggests peritoneal fluid rather than urine. All strenuous activity is suspended for a minimum of 3 months, at which time a radiographic CT imaging study is obtained to document complete renal healing. A radionuclide study can be obtained to assess renal function.

## COMPLICATIONS

Delayed renal hemorrhage or development of an arteriovenous malformation (AVM) or pseudoaneurysm usually occurs in the acute peritrauma period and presents with flank pain and/or gross hematuria (cardiovascular issues may also develop with AVM). These situations are best managed by selective angioembolization, which is a safe and effective treatment modality. Mild to moderate urinary extravasation is rarely clinically significant and can be followed by repeat CT imaging to ensure resolution. Large urinomas can be treated with percutaneous drainage and may require a ureteral stent if repeat CT imaging demonstrates persistent or worsening urinary extravasation. Hypertension after renal trauma is classically associated with a Page kidney injury and is otherwise infrequent. Delayed nephrectomy or preferably, capsulectomy and drainage can successfully manage hypertension secondary to a Page kidney injury, as this is an anatomical compression of the renal parenchyma. Medical therapy is otherwise utilized as indicated for essential hypertension.

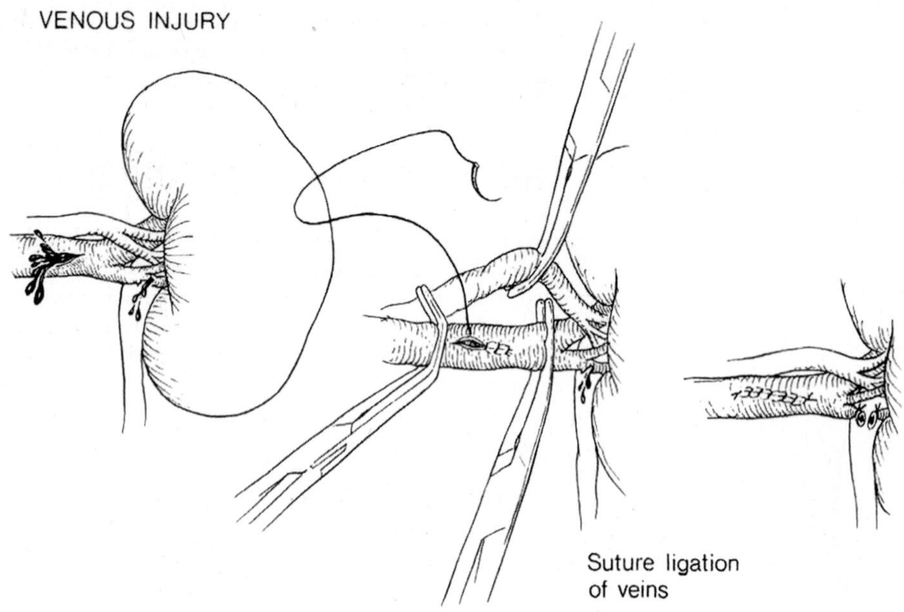


FIGURE 9.11 Repair of partial main renal vein or artery injury using a nonabsorbable continuous suture after gaining vascular control.

## SUMMARY

Radiographic CT staging, improved endovascular minimally invasive techniques, and growing experience have allowed more successful nonoperative renal trauma care to occur. Although limited, the role for renal exploration still exists in critically ill patients with potentially life-threatening hemorrhage and in those who cannot be preoperatively staged by radiographic CT imaging and observed in ICUs. If renal exploration is necessary, early vascular control and adherence to reconstructive principles will ensure high renal salvage rates.

## *References*


1. Santucci RA, Wessells H, Bartsch G, et al. Evaluation and management of renal injuries: consensus statement of the renal trauma subcommittee. *Br J Urol Int* 2004;93(7):937–954.
2. Wright JL, Nathens AB, Rivara FP, et al. Renal and extrarenal predictors of nephrectomy from the national trauma data bank. *J Urol* 2006;175(3, Pt 1):970–975; discussion 5.
3. Buckley JC, McAninch JW. Selective management of isolated and nonisolated grade IV renal injuries. *J Urol* 2006;176(6, Pt 1):2498–2502; discussion 502.
4. Wessells H, Deirmenjian J, McAninch JW. Preservation of renal function after reconstruction for trauma: quantitative assessment with radionuclide scintigraphy. *J Urol* 1997;157(5):1583–1586.
5. Miller KS, McAninch JW. Radiographic assessment of renal trauma: our 15-year experience. *J Urol* 1995;154(2, Pt 1):352–355.
6. Bretan PN Jr., McAninch JW, Federle MP, et al. Computerized tomographic staging of renal trauma: 85 consecutive cases. *J Urol* 1986;136(3): 561–565.
7. Buckley JC, McAninch JW. Pediatric renal injuries: management guidelines from a 25-year experience. *J Urol* 2004;172(2):687–690; discussion 90.
8. Morey AF, Bruce JE, McAninch JW. Efficacy of radiographic imaging in pediatric blunt renal trauma. *J Urol* 1996;156(6):2014–2018.
9. Morey AF, McAninch JW, Tiller BK. Single shot intraoperative excretory urography for the immediate evaluation of renal trauma. *J Urol* 1999;161 (4):1088–1092.
10. Demetriades D, Hadjizacharia P, Constantinou C, et al. Selective nonoperative management of penetrating abdominal solid organ injuries. *Ann Surg* 2006;244(4):620–628.
11. Alsikafi NF, McAninch JW, Elliott SP, et al. Nonoperative management outcomes of isolated urinary extravasation following renal lacerations due to external trauma. *J Urol* 2006;176(6, Pt 1):2494–2497.
12. Breyer BN, Master VA, Marder SR, et al. Endovascular management of trauma related renal artery thrombosis. *J Trauma.* 2008;64:1123–5.
13. Uflacker R, Paolini RM, Lima S. Management of traumatic hematuria by selective renal artery embolization. *J Urol* 1984;132(4):662–667.
14. Eastham JA, Wilson TG, Larsen DW, et al. Angiographic embolization of renal stab wounds. *J Urol* 1992;148(2, Pt 1):268–270.
15. Hagiwara A, Sakaki S, Goto H, et al. The role of interventional radiology in the management of blunt renal injury: a practical protocol. *J Trauma* 2001;51(3):526–531.
16. Patterson DE, Segura JW, LeRoy AJ, et al. The etiology and treatment of delayed bleeding following percutaneous lithotripsy. *J Urol* 1985;133(3): 447–451.
17. Farmer CD, Diaz-Buxo JA, Grubb WL, et al. Control of post renal biopsy hemorrhage by Gelfoam embolization. *Nephron* 1981;28(3):149–151.
18. Wessells H, McAninch JW. Effect of colon injury on the management of simultaneous renal trauma. *J Urol* 1996;155(6):1852–1856.
19. Master VA, McAninch JW. Operative management of renal injuries: parenchymal and vascular. *Urol Clin North Am* 2006;33(1):21–31, v–vi.
20. Nash PA, Bruce JE, McAninch JW. Nephrectomy for traumatic renal injuries. *J Urol* 1995;153:609–611.
21. McAninch JW, Carroll PR. Renal trauma: kidney preservation through improved vascular control—a refined approach. *J Trauma* 1982;22(4): 285–290.
22. Carroll PR, Klosterman P, McAninch JW. Early vascular control for renal trauma: a critical review. *J Urol* 1989;141(4):826–829.
23. Knudson MM, Harrison PB, Hoyt DB, et al. Outcome after major renovascular injuries: a Western trauma association multicenter report. *J Trauma* 2000;49(6):1116–1122.

# CHAPTER 10 ■ RENAL ALLOTRANSPLANTATION

JOHN W. MCGILLICUDDY, JUSTIN D. ELLETT, AND KENNETH D. CHAVIN

Successful transplantation of a kidney allograft and subsequent long-term immunosuppression management demand medical and surgical precision. The consequences of vascular, urologic, and infectious complications in renal transplantation, with their associated morbidity, mortality, and graft loss, can be devastating. Strict adherence to proper techniques and sound surgical principles, as outlined in this chapter, can reduce the incidence of these complications.

## DIAGNOSIS

Renal allotransplantation is performed as a treatment for end-stage renal disease (ESRD). Although there is no specific study required to make the diagnosis of ESRD, a thorough preoperative evaluation of the patient will include multiple studies to confirm the patient's candidacy as a transplant recipient.

## INDICATIONS FOR SURGERY

The primary indication for renal allotransplantation is ESRD requiring chronic dialysis. Some patients with poor and deteriorating renal function, but who are not yet requiring dialysis, may also be candidates. Patients need to have a creatinine clearance of <30 cc to be considered for transplantation.

Active infections and malignancies are generally considered contraindications for transplantation due to the immunosuppressive therapy that is required postoperatively. Comorbidity in other organ systems, especially cardiovascular and pulmonary, may impose operative risks or compromise long-term prognosis significantly enough to preclude transplantation. Inadequate patient motivation, commitment, compliance, psychological stability, or social support may also be contraindications.

## ALTERNATIVE THERAPY

ESRD patients may choose from the two modalities of chronic dialysis for long-term life-sustaining treatment. Hemodialysis may be done at home or at a treatment center. Peritoneal dialysis is in general performed by the patient on a continuous ambulatory or overnight schedule. Renal allotransplantation offers significant quality of life improvements and a long-term survival advantage as compared to dialysis. Studies show that patients on the kidney transplant waiting list have a death rate of 6.3 deaths per 100 patient years, which is improved to a death rate of 3.8 deaths per 100 patient years in those who were transplanted. Correspondingly, the long-term mortality risk in transplant recipients is 20% lower than those on the waiting list and 69% lower than those who remain on chronic hemodialysis (1).

## SURGICAL TECHNIQUE

The prospective transplantation recipient should be in metabolic, fluid, and electrolyte balance to avoid perioperative hyperkalemia, unstable blood pressure, pulmonary edema, dehydration, or difficult operative hemostasis associated with inadequate dialysis. When dialysis can be scheduled in advance, as with living donor transplantation, it should be performed on the day before surgery. The patient's cardiopulmonary status needs to be optimized, and central venous pressure monitoring can be useful in select patients. Swan-Ganz monitoring is rarely necessary.

The abdomen, from 2 to 3 cm above the umbilicus to below the symphysis pubica, is shaved and prepared after the induction of anesthesia and insertion of an indwelling Foley catheter. The bladder is gently distended with approximately 150 mL of a neomycin/bacitracin antibiotic solution. An alternative involves a three-way Foley catheter, allowing intraoperative bladder distention at the time of ureteroneocystostomy. Care must be taken to avoid inadvertent bladder rupture in these patients, who often have small, nondistensible bladders. Distention greatly facilitates the anterior cystostomy later in the procedure and, in addition, protects against possible wound contamination when the bladder is opened. After instillation of the antibiotic solution, the catheter is clamped. The clamp is removed after the cystotomy is created.

### Incision and Iliac Fossa Dissection

A right or left lower-quadrant curvilinear incision is created from the symphysis pubica to a point 2 cm medial to and just above the anterior superior iliac spine (Fig. 10.1A). While this is ultimately determined by surgeon preference, the implantation of a right kidney on the left side or a left kidney on the right side brings the renal pelvis anterior, simplifying re-exploration and revision should complications arise. The upper half of the incision is extended through the external oblique, internal oblique, and transversus abdominis muscles; in the lower half of the incision, the anterior rectus fascia is incised. The rectus muscle can then be dissected inferiorly to its tendinous insertion on the symphysis pubica and retracted medially. The inferior epigastric vessels are identified as they pass across the incision and are preserved if possible. An anterolateral retroperitoneal fascial plane is developed bluntly, permitting extraperitoneal entry into the iliac fossa.

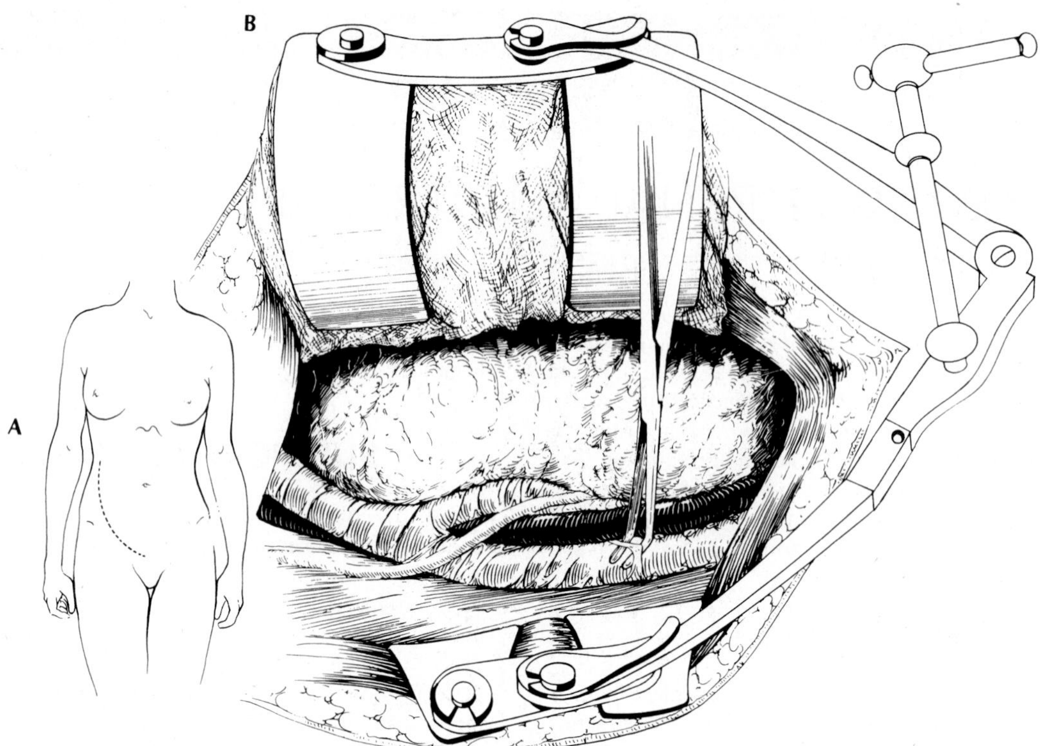


FIGURE 10.1 **A:** The incision is depicted for the right abdomen. The renal transplantation, however, can be performed on either the right or left side. **B:** The iliac vessels are best exposed with a self-retaining retractor. Sequential separation, ligation, and division of perivascular tissue containing lymphatics are essential and must precede skeletonization of the iliac vessels.

With medial retraction of the peritoneum, the spermatic cord in the male patient or the round ligament in the female patient is easily identified. Usually, cord ligation should be avoided to prevent hydrocele formation, testicular atrophy, or infertility. In women, the round ligament is divided and ligated. Further development of the extraperitoneal space in the iliac fossa is accomplished with exposure of the distal common and external iliac arteries. The insertion of a self-retaining retractor at this point ensures adequate exposure for the subsequent iliac vessel dissection and vascular anastomoses.

The dissection and skeletonization of the iliac vessels must be performed in a manner that allows secure ligation of the divided lymphatics passing along and across these vessels. Usually, this process is best approached on the superior aspect of the external iliac artery, working cephalad with a right-angle clamp toward the internal iliac artery, which crosses the internal iliac vein. In rare cases, when the donor kidney is very large or has an unusually short vein, the internal iliac artery must be sacrificed to allow sufficient mobilization of the underlying vein. The external iliac vein is similarily skeletonized as far cephalad as the vena cava if necessary. Posterior venous tributaries can be divided as necessary to permit maximum anterior mobility of the iliac vein. It is best to ligate all tributaries doubly with 2-0 or 3-0 silk in continuity before division because a double-clamping maneuver may sometimes result in injury or avulsion of a poorly accessible stump during ligation. If avulsion occurs, establishment of hemostasis risks injury to the obturator nerve. Unless the internal iliac artery already has been selected for an end-to-end allograft anastomosis, right-angle clamp dissection is used to partially skeletonize the common and external iliac arteries (Fig. 10.1B). The tissue overlying the arteries and containing the lymphatics is sequentially separated, doubly ligated with 3-0 silk, and divided, a strategy that greatly reduces the incidence of lymphocele. As with the vein, the anterior separation of tissue over the iliac artery is more easily performed in a cephalad direction.

At this point, palpation of the iliac arteries allows the surgeon to determine the most appropriate site for anastomosis. If there is moderate or severe atherosclerosis extending along the entire length of the external iliac artery, the internal iliac artery can be used for an end-to-end anastomosis. Most commonly, however, an end-to-side anastomosis of the renal artery to the external or common iliac artery is preferred as it preserves the internal iliac artery and diminishes the risks of impotency in men and gluteal or pelvic ischemia in the elderly. If the internal iliac artery is to be used, skeletonization of this vessel prepares it for end-to-end anastomosis. Before skeletonization is begun, the lymphatics on the medial aspect of the iliac bifurcation should be doubly ligated and divided. The internal iliac artery may then be clamped proximally with a Fogarty clamp and divided distal to its bifurcation with appropriate ligation of the distal stumps deep in the pelvis. The mobilized internal iliac artery is irrigated with heparinized saline solution.

## Allograft Positioning and Vascular Anastomoses

Before recipient vessel anastomotic sites are selected, placement of the allograft lateral or anterior to the iliac vessels should be considered, all anatomic factors being taken into account. The iliac vein is prepared for the end-to-side renal vein anastomosis by placement of clamps proximal and distal to the proposed venotomy. Fogarty clamps or a single broken-back Satinsky clamp usually serves this purpose well. A longitudinal incision is made on the anterior or anteromedial portion of the iliac vein segment with a no. 11 blade and extended as necessary with Potts right-angle scissors. The isolated segment of the iliac vein is irrigated with heparinized saline. After this, four 5-0 cardiovascular sutures are placed at the superior and inferior apices and at the midpoints of the medial and lateral margins of the venotomy. These sutures later are passed through corresponding points on the donor renal vein or vena cava patch for a four-quadrant, end-to-side anastomosis.

If a cadaveric kidney is used, the allograft is removed from cold storage or perfusion preservation at this point. With living-related transplantation, the flushed and cooled graft is obtained from the live donor in an adjacent operating room.

The kidney is secured in a sling containing ice slush and held in position for the vascular anastomosis by the assistant. A clamp is used to secure the sling to relieve the assistant from holding the kidney in position with the hands, which might accelerate warming or compress the kidney during the performance of the vascular anastomoses.

The previously placed sutures through the iliac vein are passed through the corresponding points of the donor renal vein or vena cava conduit and secured, bringing the renal vein into juxtaposition with the iliac vein (Fig. 10.2A). The medial and lateral sutures are retracted to separate the venotomy opening and facilitate rapid anastomosis without inadvertent suturing of the back wall. With the table rotated laterally, the superior suture is used as a running suture down the medial side of the renal vein to meet the inferior suture running up. The lateral suture line is then run in a similar fashion after the table has been rotated medially.

The external iliac artery is prepared for the end-to-side renal artery anastomosis by placement of Fogerty clamps proximal and distal to the proposed arteriotomy. This anastomosis usually is placed just cephalad to the level of the venous anastomosis. The location of clamp placement must be carefully selected so as not to disrupt existing arteriosclerotic plaques and precipitate embolization or thrombosis. A longitudinal incision is made on the anterior or anterolateral portion of the iliac artery segment with a no. 11 blade and extended as necessary with Potts right-angle scissors. If the surgeon prefers, a 4.8- or 5.6-mm aortic punch can be used to prepare an ideal oval arteriotomy. The isolated segment of the iliac artery is irrigated with heparinized saline. This anastomosis is performed with 6-0 Prolene continuous or interrupted sutures after initial fixation of the end of the renal artery to the apices of the arteriotomy, leaving one suture untied to allow for better visualization of the intima.

Less commonly, when the internal iliac artery is to be used for the arterial anastomosis, an end-to-end anastomosis is then performed with the renal artery (see Fig. 10.2B). The two vessels are positioned to allow a gentle upward curve from the iliac bifurcation to the kidney by fixing the superior and inferior arterial apices with interrupted 6-0 Prolene sutures. The anastomosis is completed with continuous or interrupted sutures. A preference for interrupted sutures instead of a running suture in this end-to-end anastomosis prevails when one needs to avoid absolutely any pursestring effect that might occur from a running suture or to achieve optimal accommodation of the two vessels to each other when a size or thickness discrepancy exists.

Upon completion of the anastomoses, the vascular clamps are released, venous clamps before arterial. Any bleeding along the line of the anastomoses is controlled with a combination of topical hemostatic agents, direct pressure, and suture repair. The sling around the kidney is removed, and any bleeding identified in the hilum or on the surface of the kidney is controlled, taking care to avoid injuring the hilar vessels. Maintenance of adequate perfusion pressure is essential and

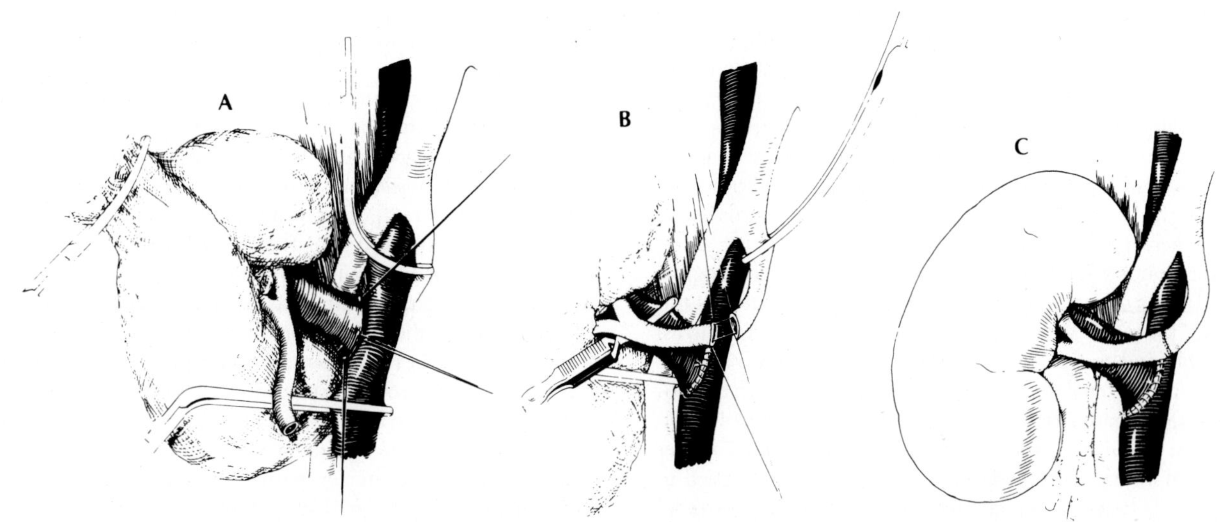


FIGURE 10.2 **A:** The renal vein is brought into exact juxtaposition with the iliac vein phlebotomy by previously placed four-quadrant sutures. A running suture anastomosis will follow. **B:** The renal artery is positioned to the end of the internal iliac artery by superior and inferior apical sutures. Subsequent placement of interrupted sutures completes the anastomosis. Note the occluding bulldog clamp on the renal vein. **C:** The completed venous and arterial anastomoses are demonstrated.

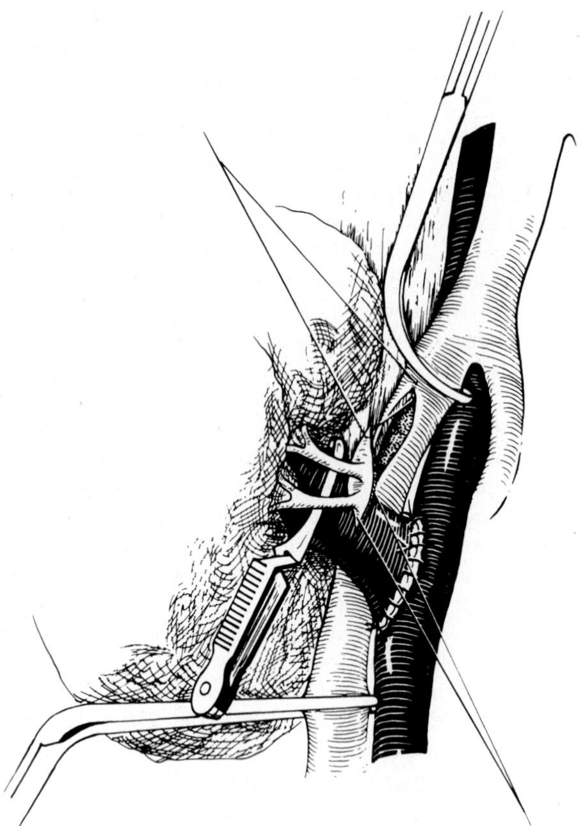

FIGURE 10.3 A donor aorta Carrel patch encompassing two renal arteries is positioned by apical sutures to an iliac arteriotomy fashioned to accommodate the length and width of the patch.

can be achieved with judicious intravenous hydration and the use of mannitol and a dopamine drip as needed.

## Multiple Renal Vessels

Although the Carrel patch may frequently be used with single arteries and veins, a cadaveric kidney with multiple renal arteries perfused through the aorta is especially well suited to an end-to-side anastomosis of a Carrel patch encompassing the multiple arteries (Fig. 10.3) (2). If the vessels are close to each other, a single Carrel patch is sufficient. The Carrel patch of donor aorta is fashioned to accommodate the multiple vessels, and its anastomosis to the common or external iliac artery is performed as previously described.

If the donor renal vessels are >2 cm apart or the allograft comes from a living donor where taking a Carrel patch is not possible, there are several strategies for arterial anastomosis: (a) double end-to-side renal arteries to iliac artery, (b) end-to-end superior renal artery to internal iliac artery with end-to-side inferior renal artery to external iliac artery, and (c) implantation of an accessory artery end-to-side into the larger main renal artery, with the larger renal artery anastomosed to the internal, external, or common iliac artery. If two renal arteries are of similar diameter, the spatulation edges of the renal arteries can be joined by the "trousers technique" with running 6-0 or 7-0 Prolene sutures to create a single bifurcating artery (2). An accessory-artery-to-main-renal-artery anastomosis should be performed with an ex vivo bench technique in cold ice slush prior to beginning implantation. Finally, some recipients have a deep inferior epigastric artery that is suitable for an end-to-end 7-0 suture interrupted anastomosis of a small lower-pole artery, which may be essential for ureteral viability (3).

## Ureteral Considerations

When the recipient urinary bladder is functional, ureteroneocystostomy is the preferred technique for establishing urinary tract continuity unless the donor ureter is absent, very short, abnormal, or damaged. Ureterectasis is not a contraindication. When the donor ureter is not suitable for reasons listed above, the recipient ureter may be used for ureteroureterostomy or ureteropyelostomy (4). If a recipient ureter is not available but the bladder is large, psoas hitch or Boari flap techniques may be used for ureteroneocystostomy or pyelocystostomy.

Some patients are prepared for kidney transplantation by creation of an ileal loop or isolated ileal stoma to divert urine from a dysfunctional or absent bladder. Other patients may come to transplantation with pre-existing bladder augmentations or continent urinary diversions utilizing ileum and colon. The nuances of techniques in these settings are beyond the scope of this discussion.

Typically, >95% of all renal transplantations are performed with various modifications of the Lich-Gregoir (5), Politano-Leadbetter (6), or Shanfield (7) techniques for allograft ureteral implantation into the bladder. In our experience, the Lich technique is appropriate in almost all cases (8). Previous filling of the bladder facilitates identification and opening of the bladder. The detrusor muscle is separated from the bladder mucosa for a length of 2 to 4 cm. A small mucosal opening is created, and the ureter is pulled down and brought into position near the site of cystotomy by gentle traction (Fig. 10.4). This avoids any excess handling of the ureter, which is important because the ureter of the transplanted kidney receives its blood supply exclusively from the renal vessel branches that course in its adventitia. In male patients, it is important to pass the ureter beneath the spermatic cord. The ureter is trimmed to an appropriate length and spatulated about 1 cm.

Two 5-0 polydioxanone sutures (PDS) are used to bring the ureteral orifice down to the cystostomy and to construct the anastomosis incorporating bladder mucosa and ureter. The ureter is routinely stented with a 6Fr, 12-cm double-J stent to reduce major ureteral complications (9). The detrusor muscle is then reapproximated over the stented ureter to provide an antireflux mechanism. Kidneys with a double ureter can also be transplanted successfully. These ureters should be dissected en bloc within their common adventitial sheath and periureteral fat so that the ureteral blood supply is protected. The technique of ureteroneocystostomy is essentially the same as with a single ureter except that the ureters are brought through together side by side in a nonconstricting tunnel. The distal end of each ureter is spatulated, and the adjacent margins are approximated with 5-0 PDS.

Rarely, situations occur in which ureteroneocystostomy unexpectedly cannot be performed and native ureters are not available. In this setting, cutaneous ureterostomy is preferred. Alternatively, an ileal loop may be created at the time of transplantation. Ureterosigmoidostomy should be avoided.

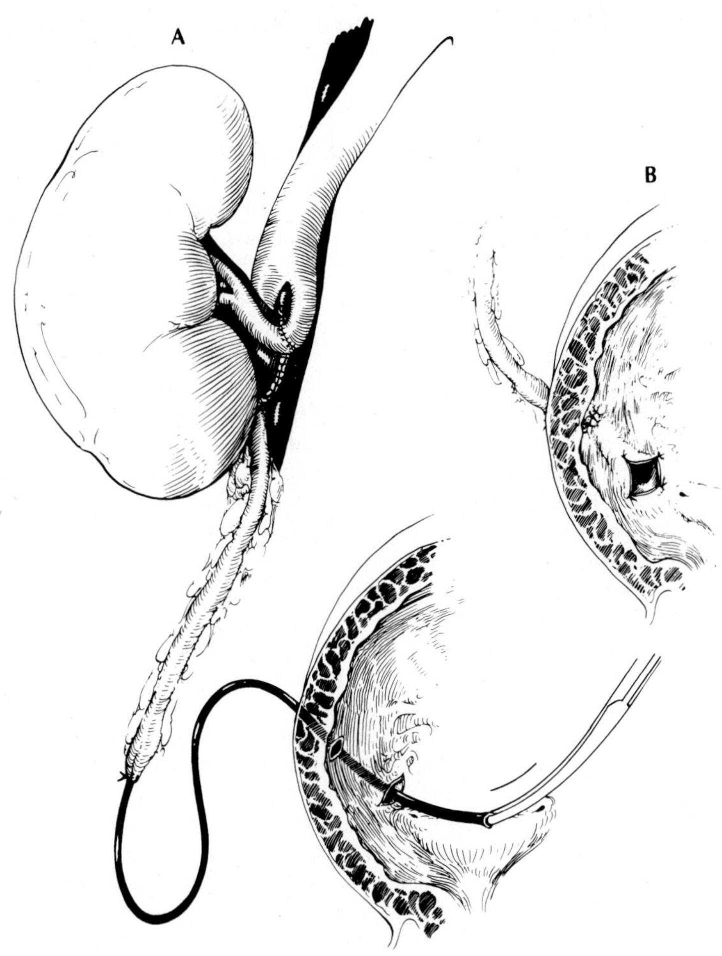


FIGURE 10.4 Ureteroneocystostomy. **A:** A small Robinson catheter or heavy silk suture with donor ureter attached is brought into the bladder through an oblique hiatus. **B:** The completed transplant ureteroneocystostomy is demonstrated. Four interrupted sutures secure the spatulated ureteral orifice.

## Pediatric Kidneys

Although en bloc transplantation of kidneys from very young children is often desirable (10), it is not necessary to transplant both kidneys from young children en bloc; each kidney can be used for a different recipient, as is the case with adult cadaveric donors, using Carrel patches of donor aorta and vena cava (Fig. 10.5) (11). A Carrel patch is mandatory in these cases because direct implantation of a small vessel into a much larger or diseased vessel may result in thrombosis or produce functional stenosis as the kidney grows. When the en bloc technique is used, the two ureters are implanted separately and stented. Pediatric kidneys have proven to be excellent donor grafts for carefully selected adults and children. Avoidance of older recipients or diabetics with advanced arteriosclerosis will minimize the potential for thrombosis. Rapid growth and hypertrophy occur in the immediate posttransplantation period. If early rejection can be avoided, these allografts achieve adult size and function in adult recipients within several weeks.

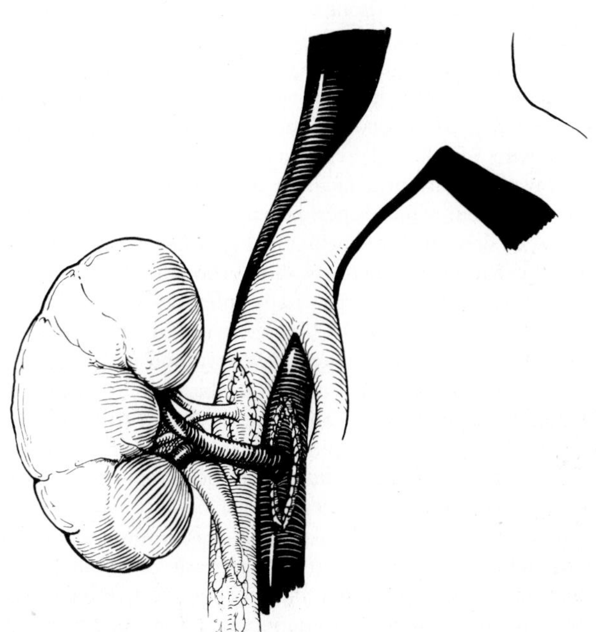

FIGURE 10.5 Small pediatric cadaver renal vessels are anastomosed to larger recipient iliac vessels using Carrel patches of donor aorta and vena cava. Note donor right kidney in right iliac fossa with renal pelvis posterior to renal vessels.

## Pediatric Transplantation

In small children, the iliac fossa is not large enough to accommodate a kidney from an adult donor, and the pelvic vessels in

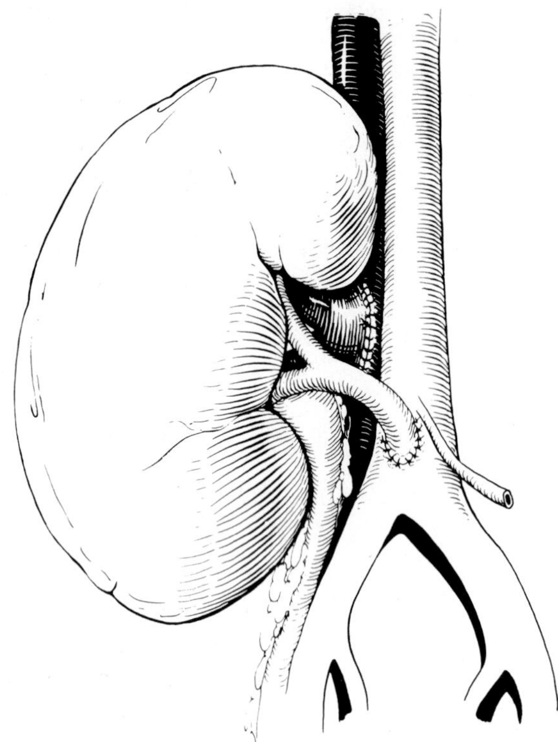

FIGURE 10.6 Anatomic relationships of an adult donor kidney in a small child are shown with renal vessel anastomoses to the inferior vena cava and aorta.

a small child are so small that the disparity between the donor renal vessels and the recipient vessels precludes the technique described for adults. In these small children, graft implantation must use the recipient aorta and vena cava, which is best accomplished through a right-sided retroperitoneal or, in children <10 kg, a transperitoneal midline abdominal incision that provides ready access to the great vessels as well as the urinary bladder. After the right colon is reflected medially, the vena cava is freed from the level of the right renal vein inferiorly to its bifurcation or beyond. Posterior lumbar veins are doubly ligated with 5-0 silk and divided as needed. Mobilization of the vena cava is important to facilitate the end-to-side anastomosis of the renal vein, which is performed with running 6-0 Prolene sutures, as described for the adult (Fig. 10.6). Performing the venous anastomosis superiorly allows room for an end-to-side anastomosis of the renal artery to the inferior abdominal aorta. Aortic mobilization should be limited to its distal portion, from the level of the inferior mesenteric artery, and including both common iliac arteries. The segment of the aorta to be used for the end-to-side renal artery anastomosis can be isolated in any number of ways, but most simply by applying a small vascular Satinsky clamp. The end-to-side anastomosis is performed with interrupted 6-0 Prolene sutures.

Important to the revascularization of an adult kidney in small children is the need to anticipate the impending consumption of several hundred milliliters of effective blood volume by the renal allograft. Initiation of volume loading before beginning the vascular anastomoses will avoid hypotension after release of the vascular clamps. Immediately after establishing circulation in the graft, the anesthesiologist must be continually attentive to the blood pressure. A dopamine drip is often necessary. The ureteral implantation is carried out as previously described.

### Wound Closure

Except in unusual cases, the space of Retzius and iliac fossa are not drained. Jackson-Pratt suction may be employed, but Penrose drains are never used. If good hemostasis has been obtained, and if the principles of implantation as outlined in this chapter have been followed, there is no need for postoperative drainage other than a urethral catheter. The optimal period of Foley catheter drainage is debatable. We prefer to remove the catheter at 72 hours unless the patient has worrisome hematuria, large diuresis, or poor bladder function, or had a technically difficult neoureterocystostomy.

In preparation for closure, the wound is thoroughly irrigated with antibiotic-containing saline. Depending on surgeon preference, a heavy absorbable or nonabsorbable suture is used to approximate transversus abdominis and internal oblique muscles in a single-layer closure; the adjacent fascia is included inferiorly at the tendinous insertion of the rectus muscle. Next, the rectus fascia anteriorly and the fascia of the external oblique are approximated in the same manner.

The subcutaneous tissue is thoroughly irrigated with saline and then may be approximated with interrupted 2-0 or 3-0 Vicryl sutures. These sutures are placed about 3 cm apart and include both edges of the Scarpa fascia and the underlying fascia. In this manner, one can obliterate dead space in the subcutaneous area in which a seroma in an immunosuppressed patient might cause dehiscence and become secondarily infected. The skin is approximated with a running 4-0 Monocryl suture in a subcuticular fashion or with surgical staples.

## OUTCOME

### Complications

Early vascular complications of kidney transplantation include arterial thrombosis, venous thrombosis, and anastomotic bleeding. These each occur in <1% of cases unless the recipient or donor vessels are diseased or small caliber. Renal or iliac artery stenosis may lead to allograft ischemia or thrombosis days or even years posttransplant in 2% to 12% of cases (12).

Urologic complications are slightly more common than vascular complications but less likely to lead to graft loss. When donor ureter and recipient bladder are normal, early ureteral necrosis, ureteral anastomotic leak, or obstruction each occur in <1% of cases. Compromised ureteral blood supply during donor nephrectomy and abnormal bladder are the most likely factors increasing these risks. Ureteral stenosis months or years posttransplant is most often a result of chronic rejection. Lymphocele occurring in 6% to 10% of transplants may be considered a urologic complication if it causes extrinsic ureteral obstruction or bladder compression. Lymphocele requires intervention posttransplant only if it becomes infected or causes pain, iliac vein compression, or allograft ureteropyelocaliectasis. Infectious, cardiovascular, metabolic, pharmacologic, and psychosocial complications of transplantation are beyond the scope of this presentation. Acute rejection superimposed on preservation injury produced irreversible failure in more than half of all cadaver donor renal allografts in the early days of transplantation. In recent years the rate of irreversible acute rejection is <10% in nearly all programs. Chronic allograft nephropathy, however, continues to contribute significantly to long-term graft loss and morbidity.

## Results

The 2007 Annual Report of the U.S. Organ Procurement and Transplantation Network documents 1-year patient survival at 98.0% and 95.8%, depending on whether the graft was from a living or cadaveric donor, respectively. It also documents 5-year allograft survival for living donor and cadaveric donor renal transplantation of 80.2% and 69.8%, respectively, as seen in Table 10.1.

TABLE 10.1

2007 ANNUAL REPORT OF THE U.S. ORGAN AND TRANSPLANTATION NETWORK AND THE SCIENTIFIC REGISTRY OF TRANSPLANT RECIPIENTS: TRANSPLANT DATA 1997 TO 2006

| | Living donor | Cadaveric donor |
|---|---|---|
| 3-mo patient survival | 99.3% | 98.3% |
| 1-yr patient survival | 98.0% | 95.8% |
| 3-yr patient survival | 94.7% | 90.1% |
| 5-yr patient survival | 90.3% | 82.8% |
| 3-mo graft survival | 97.3% | 95.3% |
| 1-yr graft survival | 95.1% | 91.3% |
| 3-yr graft survival | 88.5% | 80.9% |
| 5-yr graft survival | 80.2% | 69.8% |

From the Department of Health and Human Services, Health Resources and Services Administration, Office of Special Programs, Division of Transplantation, Rockville, MD; United Network for Organ Sharing, Richmond, VA; and University Renal Research and Education Association, Ann Arbor, MI.

## *References*


1. Wolfe RA, Ashby MA, Milford EL. Comparison of mortality in all patients on dialysis, patients on dialysis awaiting transplantation, and recipients of a first cadaveric transplant. *N Engl J Med* 1999;341:1725–1730.
2. Belzer FO, Schweizer RT, Kountz SL. Management of multiple vessels in renal transplantation. *Transplant Proc* 1972;4:639–644.
3. Merkel FK, Straus AK, Anderson O, et al. Microvascular techniques for polar artery reconstruction in kidney transplants. *Surgery* 1976;79:253.
4. Welchel JD, Cosimi AB, Young HH, et al. Pyeloureterostomy reconstruction in human renal transplantation. *Ann Surg* 1975;181:61–66.
5. Bruskewitz R, Sonneland AM, Waters RF. Extravesical ureteroplasty. *J Urol* 1979;121(5):648–649.
6. Tocci PE, Politano VA, Lynne CM. Unusual complications of transvesical ureteral reimplantation. *J Urol* 1976;115(6):731–735.
7. Texter JH Jr, Bokinsky G, Whitesell AI. Simplified experimental ureteroneocystostomy. *Urology* 1976;7(1):21–23.
8. Franz M, Klaar U, Hofbauer H. Incidence of urinary tract infections and vesicorenal reflux: a comparison between conventional and antirefluxive technique of ureter implantation. *Transplant Proc* 1992;24(6):2773–2774.
9. Wilson CH, Bhatti AA, Rix DA. Routine intraoperative ureteric stenting for kidney transplant recipients. *Cochrane Database Syst Rev* 2005;(4): CD004925.
10. Kinne DW, Spanos PK, DeShazo MM, et al. Double renal transplants from pediatric donors to adult recipients. *Am J Surg* 1974;127:292–295.
11. Salvatierra O Jr, Belzer FO. Pediatric cadaver kidneys: their use in renal transplantation. *Arch Surg* 1975;110:181–183.
12. Sebastia C, Quiroga S, Boye R. Helical CT in renal transplantation: normal findings and early and late complications. *Radiographics* 2001;21: 1103–1117.


# CHAPTER 11 ■ URETERAL COMPLICATIONS FOLLOWING RENAL TRANSPLANTATION

RODNEY J. TAYLOR

Historically, the incidence of urologic complications following kidney transplantation, manifested primarily as ureteral leaks or obstruction, was as high as 10% (1,5). These complications often resulted in significant morbidity, graft loss, and occasional patient death. Improvements in surgical techniques, immunosuppression, and methods for easily diagnosing and treating the complications have not only led to a significant decline in the rate of urologic complications to the current reported incidence of 2% to 2.5% (4,7,9) but have also resulted in lower morbidity and rare loss of a kidney or patient due to these complications. However, despite these changes, the need for diligence in diagnosing and quickly addressing complications remains as true today as in the past.

The most common cause for ureteral complications following kidney transplantation is technical error (1,5,7). Damage to the ureteral blood supply during graft recovery or transplantation may result in ureteral ischemia and subsequent leak or obstruction. Additional technical errors, such as excessive tension at the ureteroneocystostomy site or hematoma development within the tunnel, may also cause problems (4,7). With careful attention to detail, most of these problems can be minimized, especially in the early postoperative setting. Long-term or delayed ureteral obstruction may be the result of ischemic changes secondary to chronic rejection or a continuation of the spectrum of damage associated with the organ harvest and transplantation, and although not all these problems are preventable, the incidence can be markedly reduced with good surgical technique (1,4). The types of ureteral complications can be divided into ureteral leaks and ureteral obstruction.

## DIAGNOSIS

### Urinary Leaks

In current practice, most surgeons utilize an extravesical ureteroneocystostomy that uses a shorter ureter, decreasing the likelihood of ureteral ischemia, and utilizes a limited cystostomy that rarely leads to leakage from the bladder (4,10). Therefore, virtually all urinary leaks currently seen after transplantation are ureteric. The majority of these leaks that occur early after transplantation are usually present with excessive drainage from the wound, unexplained graft dysfunction, or a pelvic fluid collection. Signs and symptoms can also include fever, graft tenderness, and lower-extremity edema (8). It is critical to differentiate a suspected urinary leak from a lymphocele, as the management is entirely different.

Urinary leaks in the early postoperative period can be divided into two types according to the timing of presentation. The first usually occurs within the first 1 to 4 days and is almost always related to technical problems with the implantation. In this case, the heel of the ureter has usually retracted out of the tunnel. This is usually caused by excessive tension at the site of the anastomosis. This complication appears to be more common with extravesical ureteroneocystostomies and may be the result of too much shortening of the ureter and subsequent tension on the anastomosis when the kidney is positioned in the pelvis (8). Some investigators have recommended the use of a ureteral stent to lessen the likelihood of this complication (4,5). We recommend placing the kidney in its eventual position before deciding how much to shorten the ureter. The old adage "measure twice and cut once" applies in this circumstance.

The second type of early ureteral leak is associated with distal ureteral ischemia, which may be a consequence of injury during the donor organ recovery, technical causes such as tunnel hematoma, or distal stripping of the blood supply. This type usually presents between 5 and 10 days posttransplant (7).

Urinary leaks are often suspected because of increased drainage from the wound while at the same time associated with decreased urinary output. This is especially true in patients with limited pretransplant urine production. In patients with normal pretransplant urinary output, wound drainage and graft dysfunction are the key signs. The drainage fluid should be tested for blood urea nitrogen (BUN)/creatinine to see if it is compatible with urine. The preferred radiographic tests include an abdominal ultrasound and nuclear renal scan. A renal scan demonstrating extravasation is the most sensitive method to differentiate a urine leak from other fluid collections such as lymphoceles or hematomas (2). A cystogram should be performed if a bladder leak is suspected.

### Ureteral Obstruction

Ureteral obstruction can also be the result of ureteral ischemia but usually occurs later than ureteral leaks and usually presents as acute graft dysfunction. It may occur years after the transplant and in this situation may represent vascular injury associated not only with the technical complications but also with chronic rejection (1,7,8). The spectrum of ureteral ischemic injury extends from early necrosis and urinary leakage to delayed ureteral obstruction, presenting months to years after the actual transplantation.

Ureteral obstruction, usually manifested by graft dysfunction, requires evaluation, and again an ultrasound and nuclear renal scan are the most common screening studies. Additional radiographic studies such as a computerized tomography (CT) scan may be of assistance in some cases. With both ureteral leak and obstruction, endourologic techniques can be both diagnostic and therapeutic.

## INDICATIONS FOR SURGERY

Anything that causes graft dysfunction or results in disruption of the urinary tract in a renal transplant patient is of utmost concern and requires rapid diagnosis, control, and treatment. In the case of ureteral leakage or obstruction, the goals of treatment include careful and accurate diagnosis of the exact cause and site. To correct the leak caused by excessive tension, it is often possible to do a repeat ureteroneocystostomy as soon as the diagnosis is made. In most other cases, especially with the current techniques of extravesical reimplantation, a different operative procedure is often more suitable (5,7).

If the graft dysfunction problem has a physical cause such as a leak or an obstruction and is not associated with an acute rejection episode, then treatment is directed at stabilization of the renal function, minimization of morbidity, and restoration of the continuity and function of the urinary tract. If there is concomitant rejection, then definitive operative therapy is withheld pending the treatment of rejection (7,8).

## ALTERNATIVE THERAPY

Immediate open operative surgical intervention has been replaced, to a large extent, by early endourologic intervention (1,6–8). The placement of a percutaneous nephrostomy can divert a leak or relieve obstruction and allow more definitive diagnosis. As described by Streem, endourologic management algorithms can select patients for whom the likelihood of successful nonoperative management is good. Depending on the selection criteria, the results of management of distal ureteral leaks with stenting and a nephrostomy tube show that approximately one-third of patients do well long term and require no additional treatment. For ureteral strictures or stenoses, approximately 45% of patients, carefully selected, will avoid an open operative repair (8). For the other patients, percutaneous access can allow stabilization of renal function and a more critical assessment before open surgical repair is carried out. In a few cases, percutaneous access can offer long-term treatment with chronic stent management. This choice, in my opinion, is of limited application in most patients with a well-functioning graft because of the long-term risks (i.e., stone formation, infection, etc.) and inherent costs. However, in patients who are not operative candidates and for some patients with marginal graft function, chronic endourologic treatment can be an alternative to definitive repair (5).

## SURGICAL TECHNIQUE

There are many procedures available to restore the continuity of the urinary tract (1–3,5–7). In our experience in dealing with a difficult ureteral stenosis or a leak from significant ureteral ischemic necrosis, we favor the use of the native ureter to replace the transplant ureter. Advantages of this repair include the following: The native ureter is usually nonrefluxing, the results are reliable, there is a low likelihood of recurrence of the primary problem, and a tension-free anastomosis with good blood supply is easily attained. The focus of this operative description is on that surgical choice. Other operative alternatives include reimplantation of the ureter, Boari flap ureteral replacement, pyelovesicostomy and psoas hitch with reimplantation. As with many operative procedures, having a variety of alternatives available enhances the likelihood of a successful result.

Surgical access to the transplanted kidney and ureters (transplant and native) is usually achieved by reopening the old incision. On occasion, if extensive mobilization of transplanted kidney is anticipated or access to the contralateral native ureter is planned, a midline incision is another option (7). Surgical access to repair an early ureteral leak is usually simplified because dense fibrosis has not yet occurred, the fascial layers are easily opened, the peritoneum and its contents are freely mobilized medially and cephalad, and the kidney and ureter are identified without much difficulty. A primary repair can often be performed, and in most cases a repeat ureteroneocystostomy at a new site in the bladder is the best choice. Use of a mechanical retractor greatly simplifies exposure and allows excellent access to the pelvis. We also recommend the use of loupe magnification (2× to 3×) to enhance the repair.

If the repair has been delayed because of attempted endourologic management or because of delay in presentation or diagnosis, then access to the ureter and kidney can be much more challenging and hazardous. In these cases, mandatory preoperative preparation includes a review of the operative note, especially if the operation was performed by someone else. It is important to know whether the kidney to be operated on was the donor's right or left kidney. It is critical to know the position of the ureter and renal pelvis in relation to the renal vessels (below or above), and this depends on which kidney was used and into which side of the recipient's pelvis it was transplanted. Additional information to be sought includes the type of vascular anastomosis performed (end-to-end versus end-to-side, etc.) and whether or not the iliac vessels (especially the iliac vein) were mobilized. All of this information can help determine the likely position of the kidney in relation to the transplanted and native ureter and the anticipated ease in gaining access to these structures. Figure 11.1 demonstrates the relationship of the transplanted kidney, vessels, and ureter to the recipient's iliac vessels and ureter. Note that this figure depicts a donor left kidney on the right side, as the renal pelvis is posterior to the renal vessels.

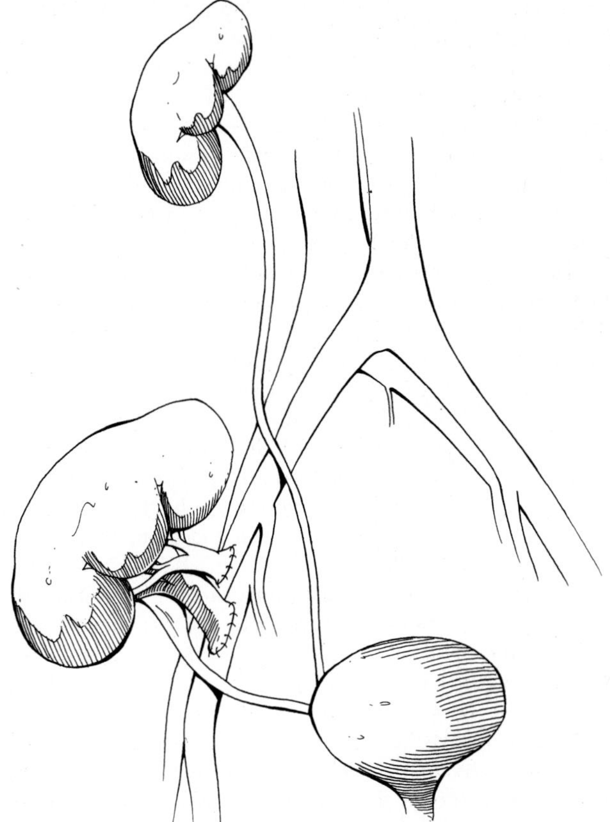

FIGURE 11.1 Relationship of the transplanted kidney and its vasculature to the recipient's iliac vessels and ureter.

In terms of the recipient, it is critical to know the status of the recipient's urinary tract. This is especially true if the recipient has a history of ureteral reflux or has undergone nephroureterectomy and might not have a suitable native ureter available to use for repair. Finally, the status of the recipient's urinary bladder in terms of capacity, compliance, and function can be important in determining which other repair options are available.

Additional preoperative preparation involves stabilization of the patient and function of the graft. It is important to delay any open operative repair until concurrent rejection episodes have been adequately treated and renal function stabilized. All patients should be treated with preoperative antibiotics based on anticipated contaminants or cultures obtained from the urine. If there is a likelihood that bowel might be needed (an unusual circumstance) to repair the urinary tract, then a full bowel preparation is indicated.

The goals of surgery are to repair the ureteral defect, re-establish continuity of the urinary system, get rid of all foreign bodies as quickly as possible, and avoid graft or patient loss. With a well-planned and executed procedure, these goals should be easily obtained in essentially all cases.

Delayed surgical repair because of attempted endourologic management, delayed diagnosis, or late presentation of obstruction can make surgical exposure of the kidney and ureter challenging. As noted earlier, access is almost always achieved through the old transplant incision, and cephalad extension of the incision is often needed in these cases because of perinephric fibrosis, the increased size of the kidney posttransplant, and the need to achieve access to the iliac vessels and native ureter. It is usually possible to extend the incision several centimeters cephalad. Additional exposure, if needed, can also be obtained by extending the inferior aspect of the incision across the midline, although this is rarely needed and should be delayed until the need presents itself.

With delayed repair, the normal tissue planes are obliterated and a dense fibrosis has occurred around the graft. This makes it easy to violate the "renal capsule" and get into significant bleeding. As a routine, it is preferable to operate from a position of "known to unknown" with good exposure. The surgeon should also plan to gain vascular control proximally and distally if it appears that the kidney may need to be mobilized to permit access to the renal pelvis. A three-way Foley catheter should always be placed into the bladder before the start of surgery to allow for irrigation and filling with an antibiotic solution.

To ensure a safe and adequate exposure, I usually open the peritoneum early in cases where there is dense fibrosis. This allows better cephalad exposure, protects the bowel, and gives good access to the bladder.

Because the transplant ureter usually crosses the external iliac vessels below the renal vessels, one should take care to avoid these structures while gaining access to the ureter. This is a critical feature of this operative procedure because exact visualization of the renal vascular structures is often difficult, and many times one is operating based on the expected, not visualized, location of these structures. In some cases a percutaneous nephrostomy tube will be placed as well as a ureteral stent. If present, the nephrostomy tube should be accessible during a procedure as injection of saline or methylene blue may aid in identifying the ureter and renal pelvis. In some cases, because of the dense fibrosis, the ureter is identified only when it is actually cut. The routine placement of a ureteral stent is of limited value in most cases because the fibrosis is so dense that it is hard to discern the presence of the catheter. If the ureter is not in dense fibrosis, then access is usually easy.

Once access to the bony pelvis is obtained, careful dissection along the lateral wall of the bladder usually leads to the ureter. Once it is identified, care must be used in mobilizing the ureter to avoid any further vascular injury. When the site of leakage and/or obstruction has been identified, the most commonly used repairs include (a) a repeat ureteroneocystostomy, (b) use of the bladder (Boari flap or bladder hitch) to help bridge the gap, or (c) use of a native ureter to perform a ureteroureterostomy or ureteropyelostomy. Repeat ureteroneocystostomies are indicated only to repair early leaks when the problem was from tension at the anastomosis or distal ureteral ischemia and a well-vascularized, minimally fibrosed ureter is present. In most circumstances, especially late, with a lot of periureteral reaction or ischemia, our preferred option is the use of the ipsilateral native ureter if it is present and of adequate caliber. If not, then a Boari flap is an excellent choice.

Access to the native ureter is obtained by identifying it as it crosses the common iliac vessels. Care must be used in mobilizing the ureter down into the pelvis to the level of the superior vesical artery to avoid injury to the ureter blood supply. The ureter is divided well above the iliac vessels, and the proximal end of the ureter is doubly ligated. In our experience of >50 cases, this has not resulted in problems of hydronephrosis with the native kidney or ureter requiring any further intervention. Figure 11.2 shows the native ureter mobilized distally and doubly ligated proximally in preparation for a ureteropyelostomy.

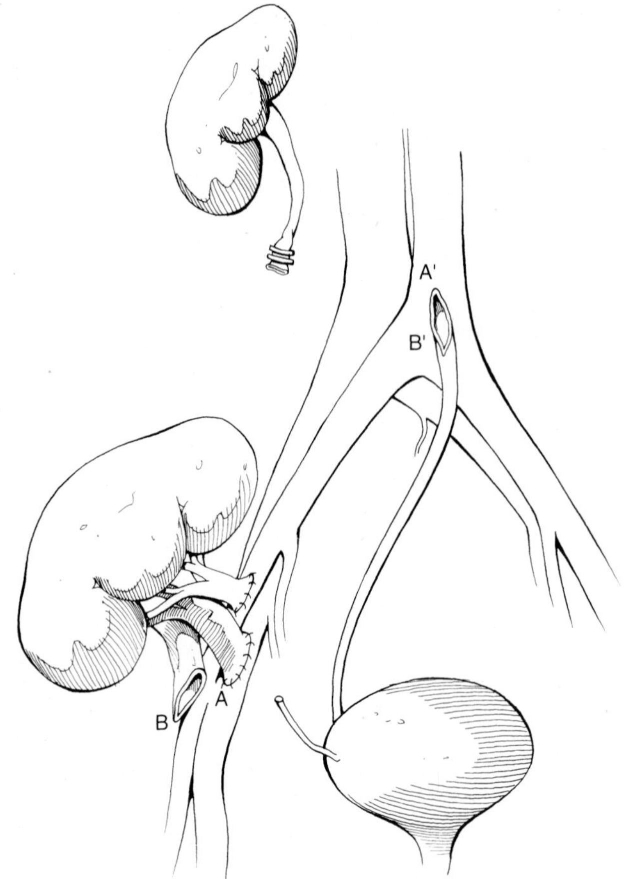


FIGURE 11.2 Mobilization of the native ureter distally with the proximal segment ligated.

The operative positioning of the native ureter depends on access to the transplant ureter and/or pelvis. In addition, whether a side-to-side ureteral anastomosis or a ureteropyelostomy is to be performed may make a difference in the exact positioning of the native ureter. All of these factors relate to the extent of fibrosis and the appearance of the transplant ureter. To prevent any additional future problems, a tension-free, widely spatulated anastomosis of well-vascularized ureter to either the transplant ureter or renal pelvis is critical (Fig. 11.3). The anastomosis is performed using 5-0 Maxon (Davis and Geck, Danbury, CT) or polydioxanone (PDS, Ethicon, Somerville, NJ) in a watertight single layer. The critical aspect is to obtain a mucosa-to-mucosa approximation to avoid tension, devascularization, and urinary leak. A 12-cm 4.7 double-J stent is routinely used on all anastomoses. The anastomosis may in addition be wrapped in omentum or peritoneal flap, if available, to decrease further the risk of leak. The wound is well irrigated with antibiotic solution, and if no preoperative infection was present, we close the wound without a drain. If there is concern about urinary leak, lymphatic leak, or possible infection, one or two Jackson–Pratt drains are indicated. The

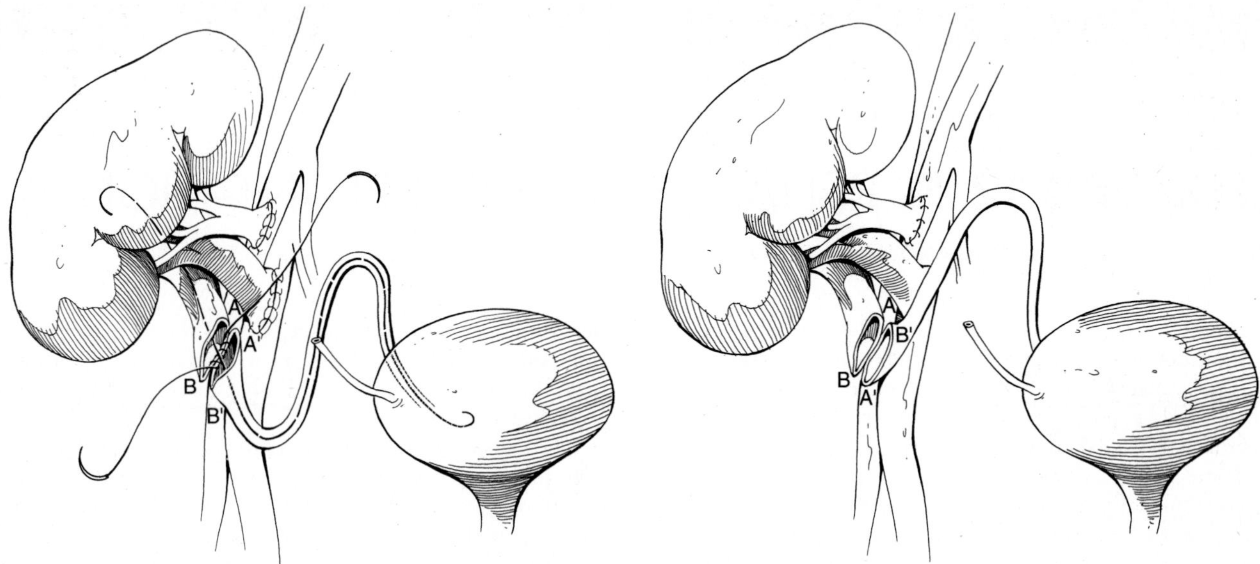


FIGURE 11.3 Anastomosis of spatulated native ureter to (**A**) transplant ureter and (**B**) transplant renal pelvis.

fascia is closed in layers with a 0 or no. 1 permanent monofilament suture. The subcutaneous tissue is not closed. The skin is usually closed with staples. A nephrostomy tube, if present, is removed at day 5 to 7 after an antegrade nephrostogram has been obtained to be sure that there is no leak. The ureteral catheter is left in for 4 to 6 weeks.

# OUTCOMES

## Complications

Complications that can occur postprocedure include infection, urinary leak, bleeding, recurrence of the stricture, and possible loss of graft. In all series, these are uncommon complications (1,7).

## Results

We have performed over 50 native-to-transplant uretero-ureterostomies or ureteropyelostomies to treat ureteral obstruction or ureteral leaks or to deal with damaged ureters at the time of the transplant. In our experience, all kidneys involved have been "salvaged" and none lost to urologic complications. There have been no significant postoperative complications and no patient deaths. We have not had to repeat any procedures in any of the patients we have treated and have not had any recurrence of either leak or stricture. As noted earlier, we routinely tie off the proximal native ureter, do not do a nephrectomy, and have not had any problems related to the native kidney. We feel that routine native nephrectomy is not indicated, and if one is ever subsequently indicated, a laparoscopic nephrectomy would be our choice.

## *References*

1. Banowsky LHW. Surgical complications of renal transplantation. In: Glenn JF, ed. *Urologic surgery*, 4th ed. Philadelphia: JB Lippincott, 1991:252–266.
2. Bretan PN Jr, Hodge E, Streem SB, et al. Diagnosis of renal transplant fistulas. *Transplant Proc* 1989;21:1962–1966.
3. Gerridzen RG. Complete ureteral replacement by Boari bladder flap after cadaveric renal transplant. *Urology* 1993;41:154–156.
4. Gibbons WS, Barr JM, Hefty TR. Complications following unstented parallel incision extravesical ureteroneocystostomy in 1,000 kidney transplants. *J Urol* 1992;148:38–40.
5. Khauli RB. Surgical aspects of renal transplantation: new approaches. *Urol Clin North Am* 1994;27:321–341.
6. Martin DC, Mims MM, Kaufman JJ, et al. The ureter in renal transplantation. *J Urol* 1969;101:680–687.
7. Rosenthal JT. Surgical management of urological complications after kidney transplantation. *Semin Urol* 1994;12:114–122.
8. Streem SB. Endourological management of urological complications following renal transplantation. *Semin Urol* 1994;12:123–133.
9. Taylor RJ, Rosenthal JT, Schwentker FN, et al. Factors in urologic complications in 400 cadaveric renal transplants. *J Urol* 1984;131:336A.
10. Thrasher JB, Temple DR, Spees EK. Extravesical versus Leadbetter-Politano ureteroneocystostomy: a comparison of urological complications in 320 renal transplants. *J Urol* 1990;144:1105–1109.

# CHAPTER 12 ■ RENAL AUTOTRANSPLANTATION

VENKATESH KRISHNAMURTHI AND DAVID A. GOLDFARB

Renal autotransplantation is usually considered a last resort in the spectrum of surgical treatment for extensive ureteral tissue loss. It is valuable for any disease where intervention on the kidney would expose it to prolonged warm ischemia resulting in permanent renal damage. This is the case for complex distal renal arterial disease and large kidney tumors where renal preservation is imperative. The basic techniques have evolved as a consequence of developments in the field of renal allotransplantation, particularly an improved understanding of renal preservation. The advantages of back-table reconstruction include optimal exposure, use of optical magnification (loupes), a bloodless surgical field, and incorporation of renal preservation techniques (intracellular flush solutions and hypothermia) (7).

## DIAGNOSIS

Since there are a variety of indications for autotransplantation, diagnostic studies will vary accordingly. Extensive ureteral loss is usually documented by computerized tomography (CT) scan, intravenous urography, retrograde urography, antegrade urography, or a combination of these imaging modalities. Complex renal vascular diseases are typically screened with CT or magnetic resonance (MR) angiography. Due to the distal nature of renal vascular disease (branch disease) amenable to autotransplant, almost all candidates may also have catheter-based arteriographic studies. Renal tumors are assessed by CT or magnetic resonance imaging (MRI). Extensive investigation is typical for the loin-pain hematuria syndrome. Patients have usually had the full spectrum of radiographic testing to assess the renal vasculature, parenchyma, and collecting system. They have also had diagnostic ureteroscopy. Most have had visceral pain blocks that have failed to provide durable pain relief.

## INDICATIONS FOR SURGERY

Autotransplantation of the kidney is an acceptable treatment option for patients with impassable proximal ureteral obstruction and extensive ureteral loss (1). Complex renal vascular lesions requiring ex vivo repair can also be successfully managed with renal autotransplantation (7).

Urinary tract disorders that require consideration for autotransplantation include proximal ureteral obstruction that cannot be managed with bladder-based methods of repair (Boari flap, with or without psoas hitch). Such repairs can rarely extend beyond the pelvic ureter. Moreover, even if bladder-based flaps can reach beyond the area of obstruction, successful re-establishment of urinary tract continuity may be compromised by excessive tension at the site of reconstruction.

The causes of proximal ureteral obstruction include multiple failed repairs of ureteropelvic junction (UPJ) obstruction (failed pyeloplasty or endoscopic repair), desmoid tumor (with or without the Gardner syndrome) obstructing the proximal ureter, and extensive ureteral stricture. Prior to pursuing autotransplantation, these patients have generally been managed with indwelling ureteral stents and/or percutaneous nephrostomy tubes. They are completely stent-dependent and often have developed recurrent episodes of pyelonephritis.

An uncommon condition that is amenable to autotransplant would be the loin-pain hematuria syndrome (2). This is characterized by flank pain with gross or microscopic hematuria for which exhaustive diagnostic testing has failed to disclose a specific etiology. Aggressive treatment is driven by the chronic pain that accompanies the syndrome.

Finally, some centers have used ex vivo back-table excision, reconstruction, and autotransplantation for large renal cancers that are not felt to be amenable to in situ repair (8,9).

## ALTERNATIVE THERAPY

An alternative to renal autotransplantation in patients with proximal ureteral obstruction is ileal ureteral substitution; however, ileal substitution may not be possible in patients with a history of extensive intestinal surgery, such as those patients with the Gardner syndrome who have undergone total proctocolectomy with ileostomy or ileal pouch creation. Additionally, the long-term consequences of intestinal interposition within the urinary tract are not completely known and must be considered when utilized in younger patients. Therefore, for patients in whom an ileal substitution does not seem favorable, autotransplantation may be the only option.

Complex renal vascular disorders are also an indication for renal autotransplantation. These are most often arterial disorders such as stenoses or aneurysms involving the segmental renal arteries and are difficult to treat with in situ methods. As an extension of the techniques routinely applied in renal allotransplantation, the renal hilum can be readily accessed while the kidney is on the "back table." Revascularization to branch vessels or excision of aneurysms deep in the hilum is much easier on the back table and thus can be accomplished satisfactorily prior to autotransplantation.

# TECHNIQUE OF RENAL AUTOTRANSPLANTATION

## Surgical Instrumentation

Renal autotransplantation is a combination of living donor nephrectomy and standard renal transplant within the same patient. A satisfactory performance of these procedures requires instrumentation to facilitate fine vascular repairs. Although the specific instrument is a matter of individual preference, instrumentation for vascular surgical procedures should include (a) noncrushing vascular clamps designed for blood vessel occlusion, (b) forceps with fine tips designed to atraumatically grasp vessel walls as well as suture needles, (c) needle holders with fine tips to grasp small needles yet prevent unwanted needle movement, and (d) an assortment of silastic vessel loops and umbilical tapes for atraumatic vessel manipulation.

Vascular clamps are manufactured in a variety of shapes and sizes. Their selection depends upon the size of the vessel to be occluded and the desired direction of vessel wall occlusion (longitudinal, transverse, or oblique). The jaws of vascular clamps should have rows of interdigitating teeth that allow vessel wall apposition without endothelial damage. Vascular clamps should be applied by compressing the jaws only to the point necessary for blood flow cessation. Overaggressive application can result in endothelial damage and subsequent dissection.

For small, delicate vessels or relatively inaccessible areas, spring-loaded (bulldog) clamps are useful devices. These also come in a variety of sizes, strengths, and shapes. Additionally, plastic varieties with soft padded jaws may be useful for extremely delicate vessels.

Vascular forceps must have tines that are in direct apposition, and the tips should be fine enough to grasp the vascular adventitia as well as a suture needle. Forceps with rows of interdigitating teeth serve to accomplish both of these purposes. In contrast, forceps designed for stable needle grasp, such as diamond jaw forceps, do not allow for reliable manipulation of tissue.

Vascular needle holders should have fine tips to grasp fine suture needles. The two common choices in vascular needle holders are a ring-handled needle holder and the spring-loaded type. Needle holder selection, again, is a matter of individual preference; however, spring-loaded needle holders generally allow for precise needle placement without large degrees of wrist rotation. Ring-handled needle holders enable a more stable needle grasp and facilitate accurate placement in deep structures or through densely calcified vessels.

To some degree, the selection of vascular suture is also a matter of individual preference. The caliber of the suture should be as fine as possible, without risking suture line disruption, to minimize bleeding through suture holes. In most cases, suture sizes between 2-0 and 7-0 will be applicable for vascular procedures in the abdomen and pelvis. At the level of the aorta, a 2-0 or 3-0 suture should suffice, and 4-0 is almost always suitable for the inferior vena cava. As one progresses to smaller vessels, including the common and external iliac arteries and veins, a 5-0 and 6-0 suture is most often satisfactory. Repair of small vessels, such as segmental renal arteries, may require a 7-0 or 8-0 suture.

Nonabsorbable sutures are most often selected for vascular procedures. Although silk suture has favorable handling and tying characteristics, its popularity has waned with the development of synthetic, nonabsorbable sutures such as polypropylene. In comparison to silk, synthetic monofilament sutures are relatively inert in tissue, have a low coefficient of friction and thereby result in less tissue drag, and tend to retain a greater amount of tensile strength over time. Vascular sutures are swaged onto fine, one-half-circle or three-eighths-circle needles. The vascular needle should be large enough to penetrate tissue yet small enough so as not to cause hemorrhage from the needle holes. A common practice in vascular repair is to use a continuous suture with needles swaged onto both ends. This construction allows for greater flexibility in accomplishing the repair (e.g., closure from both directions). In select instances, specifically that of pediatric vascular surgery, absorbable monofilament suture with a long half-life (e.g., polydioxanone suture) can be used to allow anastomotic growth.

Another essential component for autotransplantation of the kidney is retraction. We prefer to use a self-retaining, ring-based retractor system that is fixed to the table. For flank exposure, the Bookwalter retractor (Codman & Shurtleff, Inc., Raynham, Mass.) provides for excellent exposure of the kidney and renal hilum. We have modified the medium oval ring on the Bookwalter by creating a modest angle (20 to 30 degrees) along the two ends of the ring. This enables the ring to better "fit" the patient's flank during the operative procedure. A standard oval ring works very well in the iliac fossa. Lastly, for midline intraperitoneal abdominal incisions, we have utilized both the Bookwalter retractor system and the Thompson retractor (Thompson Surgical Instruments, Inc., Traverse City, Mich.). We feel that the Thompson retractor provides better exposure in more obese patients as the side bars of the retractor can be placed further from the incision. One disadvantage of this feature, however, is that the side bars tend to be closer to the operating surgeon and can be difficult to work around.

## Renal Autotransplantation: Operative Approaches

The selection of the incision for renal autotransplantation depends on (a) the patient's prior surgical history and (b) the indication for autotransplantation. When the autotransplant is being performed for urinary tract conditions (as opposed to vascular disorders), we prefer to place the kidney into the contralateral iliac fossa. This approach allows the renal pelvis and ureter to be the most superficial structures so that the urinary tract can be reaccessed without needing to dissect or retract the main renal vessels. Although the kidney can be placed in either iliac fossa through a midline intraperitoneal incision, a retroperitoneal flank donor nephrectomy works quite favorably (4). Following completion of the flank approach for the "donor" nephrectomy, the patient is placed back in the supine position, the contralateral iliac fossa is reprepped and draped, and exposure of the iliac vessels is commenced. In theory, this combination of two separate procedures may result in longer total operative time; however, this must be counterbalanced by the benefit of extraperitoneal procedures and improved exposure along both the flank and iliac operative fields.

A midline intraperitoneal approach is also quite satisfactory for renal autotransplantation. We prefer to use this technique when the autotransplant is being performed for vascular conditions, since the midline approach enables dissection of any abdominal structure. During repair of vascular disorders, arterial conduits (e.g., hypogastric artery) are often necessary for reconstruction, and these vessels can be easily exposed through a midline intraperitoneal approach. In contrast to two retroperitoneal procedures, the midline approach does require mobilization and retraction of the small bowel and colon, which may add to postoperative ileus. A transverse intraperitoneal approach is not recommended because it is very difficult to expose structures caudal to the aortic bifurcation, such as the iliac vessels.

Lastly, a laparoscopic approach has been quite effectively utilized for the donor nephrectomy portion (3,6). In order to efficiently utilize the laparoscopic approach, however, the kidney extraction incision is made over the ipsilateral iliac vessels so that the autograft can be implanted at this location. As mentioned previously, when autotransplantation is performed for urinary tract disorders, placement of the kidney in the ipsilateral iliac fossa puts the urinary tract structures in the most posterior location, which is suboptimal should further procedures become necessary.

## Technique of Flank Donor Nephrectomy

Following satisfactory induction of general endotracheal anesthesia and placement of the necessary arterial and central venous monitoring lines, a Foley catheter is placed in the bladder. The patient is then placed on his or her side with the kidney that will be operated on facing "up." The "down" leg is then bent and the "up" leg is maintained in a straight position. Pillows are placed between both legs, and the greater trochanter along the table surface is padded with egg crate mattresses. The kidney rest is maximally elevated and the table is fully flexed. This enables a maximum distance between the lower ribs and the iliac crest. An axillary roll is placed, and the arms are padded and secured to a double arm board. The patient is then adequately secured to the table prior to preparation and drape of the operative field.

We prefer to utilize an incision over the course of the eleventh rib. Although selection of the twelfth rib may be suitable in many instances, the exposure of the kidney through the bed of the eleventh rib always provides for adequate exposure of the kidney and renal hilum. Although an approach through the eleventh rib has a slightly greater chance of pleural entry, this is easily managed by evacuation of the entrained air or by placement of a thoracostomy tube. The most important aspect of flank donor nephrectomy is exposure of the renal hilum, and the disadvantage of approaching this through the twelfth rib is that the hilum may be at the most superior portion of the operative field. Additionally, exposure through the twelfth rib bed may require significant caudal retraction on the kidney during mobilization, which may add to trauma to the kidney.

After the skin is incised sharply, the subcutaneous tissue and flank musculature are divided with the electrocautery. The anterior surface of the eleventh rib is exposed, and the rib is then dissected in a subperiosteal plane. The rib can be dissected in a subperiosteal manner. Once the rib is mobilized to a suitable posterior location, it is transected. It is sometimes necessary to cauterize the cut end of the rib or obtain hemostasis with bone wax. The retroperitoneal space is then entered along the tip of the removed rib, and, once retroperitoneal entry is verified, the abdominal contents are swept off the undersurface of the flank musculature. These muscles are then further opened in the direction of the incision.

The next step in the flank exposure is mobilization of the diaphragm and pleura. The neurovascular bundle associated with the removed rib is identified and is swept inferiorly and laterally. The attachments of the periosteum and diaphragm against the adjacent lower rib are then divided sharply with the electrocautery. We prefer to continue this division all the way back to the insertion of the diaphragm on the psoas muscle, or lumbocostal arch. This allows for excellent exposure, and, by completely mobilizing the pleura and diaphragm, avoids retraction-related tears on the pleura. Finally, the kidney can be mobilized within Gerota fascia since the procedure is being done for benign conditions. Once the kidney is suitably mobilized, the self-retaining retractor can be positioned to retract everything but the kidney and associated structures.

At the time of kidney mobilization, intravenous mannitol 12.5 g is given. A second 12.5-g dose is usually given just prior to renal artery clamping. The perinephric fat is then completely removed. The renal artery and vein are skeletonized to as proximal a level as possible. The renal artery should be dissected so that an adequate length is maintained for the implantation and the diseased portion can be reconstructed; however, it is extremely important not to dissect the artery too close to the aorta, since a minimal amount of artery must be maintained for suitable control. Too short of a stump on the aorta can lead to catastrophic complications; however, too short of a stump on the kidney side can be reconstructed through a variety of techniques. One must differentiate the dissection of the renal artery during an autotransplant from that of in situ revascularization procedures. In revascularization procedures, the aorta is more accessible and may be more readily controlled, in contrast to flank exposures.

On the right side, the renal vein should be dissected all the way to the inferior vena cava (IVC), and the juxtarenal IVC must also be exposed. It is essential to mobilize the IVC posterior to the insertion of the renal vein, as the posterior wall of the IVC must be easily clamped during extraction of the kidney. On the left side, the adrenal, gonadal, and lumbar venous branches should be divided.

The ureter is dissected usually to the level of its crossing over the iliac vessel. In cases of proximal ureteral obstruction, the ureter should be dissected approximately to the level of obstruction, but more importantly, it must be dissected to only a length suitable for reimplantation. A generous amount of periureteral tissue should be maintained with the ureteral dissection. We prefer to include the gonadal vein and intervening tissue along with the ureter. In cases where the ureter is dilated due to chronic obstruction, the need to maintain an adequate amount of periureteral tissue is less important due to the development of neovascularity. The ureter is then divided above the level of the obstruction (if present), and a satisfactory diuresis is verified by observing urine flow from the cut end of the ureter.

The kidney should be palpated to ensure a turgid feel. A soft kidney with no urine production should raise concern for arterial spasm. In these situations, the kidney should not be handled, and warm saline can be placed as an initial maneuver. If the kidney turgor has not improved and the spasm has not abated after a period of several minutes, papaverine can be applied topically along the renal artery adventitia.

When the kidney is firm and there is an adequate diuresis of urine, it is acceptable to proceed with removal. Mannitol (12.5 g) is given intravenously. The renal artery is then clamped and transected and the kidney mobilized so that the renal vein is placed on stretch. The renal vein, or inferior vena cava, is then clamped, and the vein is divided sharply at a suitable location. The kidney is then passed off to a separate team, who will commence with both surface hypothermia and in situ cold perfusion.

Attention is directed toward securing the renal vessels. The renal vessels can be secured with any combination of ties, clips, or suture ligatures. Our typical practice is to place two ties with 0 silk. When two ties are not possible, we may use a single clip and oversew the renal artery stump with a 5-0 polypropylene suture. The left renal vein can be similarly controlled (Figs. 12.1 and 12.2). On the right side, however, it is essential to remove the kidney with a small (few millimeters) margin of IVC (Figs. 12.3 and 12.4). In this situation, the vena cava is closed with a 4-0 polypropylene suture. We generally place one suture at each apex and run toward the midpoint. It is not essential to run this closure in an over-and-back manner as the low-pressure venous system is unlikely to leak between the suture lines. It is also important to leave a suitable margin of vein above the clamp so the cavotomy can be safely closed. If the renal vein is inadvertently transected directly on the clamp, two options exist. One option would be to place a larger clamp below the existing clamp and to remove the first clamp. If this option is pursued, it is imperative to make sure that the second clamp is properly placed and that the walls of the vena cava are firmly apposed. Another option, which may be potentially safer, would be to reapproximate the IVC walls in a horizontal mattress fashion by

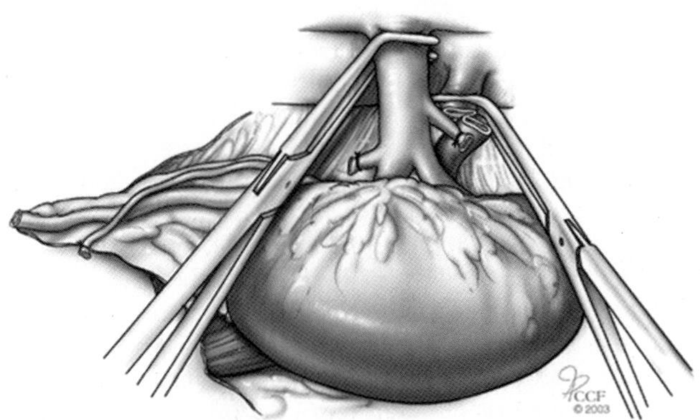


**FIGURE 12.1** Control of left renal hilum. Note that the renal vein is clamped as close to the IVC as possible.

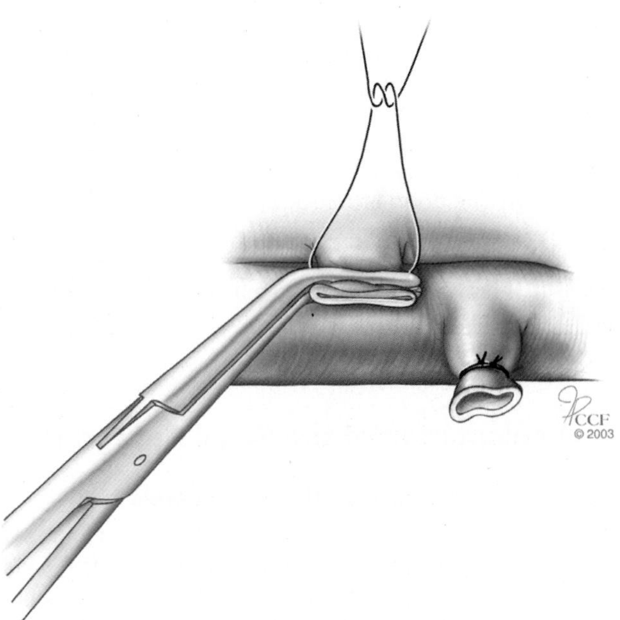


**FIGURE 12.2** A small stump of left renal artery is preserved to ensure safe ligation.

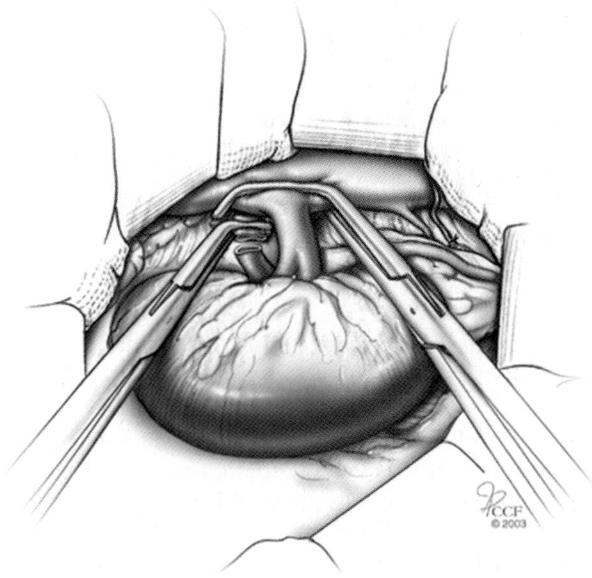


**FIGURE 12.3** Control of the renal vein includes a small cuff of IVC.

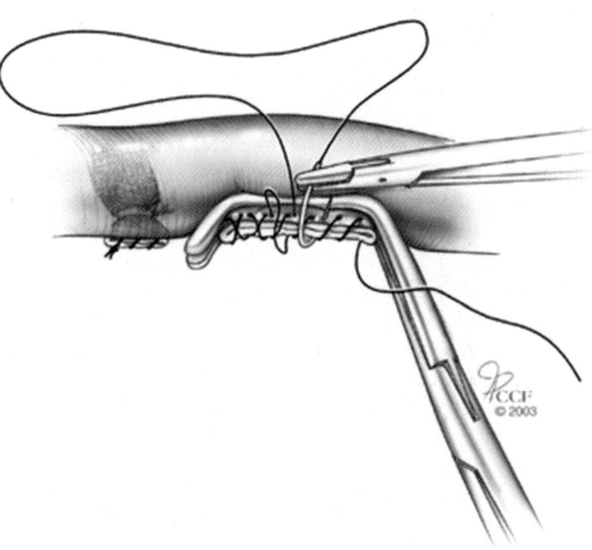


**FIGURE 12.4** Securing the IVC with a running suture.

sewing "under" the clamp. In all cases, we recommend that the vena caval clamp be released slowly so that it can be reapplied immediately should there be unexpected significant bleeding from the vena caval closure.

Once the renal vessels are secured, the operative field is irrigated and inspected for hemostasis. The retractor is then removed, and the flank musculature and fascia are closed in two layers. Following completion of the flank procedure, general anesthesia is maintained and the patient is repositioned for the renal transplant procedure.

## Donor Nephrectomy via a Midline Intraperitoneal Approach

The patient is placed in the supine position. General endotracheal anesthesia is induced. The appropriate arterial and central venous monitor lines are placed. A Foley catheter is placed in the bladder in a sterile manner. Surgical preparation should include the field from the nipples to the lower thighs. The genitalia should be shaved and prepped and covered with a sterile surgical towel. Both groins should be available for access should there be a need for saphenous vein procurement.

For renal autotransplantation, a midline incision from xiphisternum to pubic symphysis should be employed. The subcutaneous tissues and linea alba are divided with the electrocautery, and the abdominal wall can be retracted with a self-retaining retractor. It is important to ensure complete neuromuscular blockade so that the abdominal wall can be retracted maximally. For right-sided autotransplantation, we prefer to mobilize the right colon and duodenum medially to expose the entire infrarenal vena cava, left renal vein, and abdominal aorta. For left renal autotransplantation, the left colon should be mobilized medially so that the left renal vein can be accessed as it crosses over the aorta. Following mobilization, the viscera are retracted with the self-retaining retractor. The kidney can be mobilized within Gerota fascia, as mentioned previously. The ureter should be mobilized with a generous amount of periureteral tissue until the point of obstruction or to a level where it crosses the iliac vessels. When autotransplantation is being performed for vascular conditions, the ureter does not always need to be divided as the renal vascular reconstruction can be performed in a basin containing iced slush placed on the patient's abdomen. We prefer to divide the ureter so that the kidney can be taken off the operative field and exposed maximally on the back table, during which time the iliac fossa can be prepared by a separate surgical team.

With the kidney fully mobilized and the ureter divided, the renal vessels are dissected. Because cases of renal autotransplantation for vascular diseases usually involve arterial disorders, it is necessary to completely skeletonize the renal vein so that it can be mobilized away from the posterior renal artery. Accurate preoperative judgment is essential to determine the feasibility of in situ repair. However, even in cases in which in situ repair is thought to be unfeasible, intraoperative findings may dictate otherwise, and the surgeon should be prepared to reconstruct the kidney in situ. However, in cases of proximal ureteral obstruction and in cases of vascular disease requiring ex vivo repair, the kidney has to be removed and reconstructed on the back table. As previously described, the vessels are dissected as proximally as is necessary to correct the lesion. Intravenous mannitol (12.5 g) is administered. After an adequate diuresis and a firm kidney are verified, the renal artery is clamped and divided, the renal vein or IVC is clamped, and the vein is divided. The kidney is passed off to a separate team, who will commence surface hypothermia and in situ cooling. The main renal vessels are secured, and the field is inspected. As the kidney is being perfused, the iliac fossa can be prepared by a separate surgical team.

## Back-Table Preparation of the Renal Autograft

Once removed, the kidney is placed in a basin containing ice slush. The renal artery is cannulated and in situ perfusion with cold preservation solution started. Cannulation may be achieved with a large-gauge angiocatheter (14 gauge) or a metal-tipped cannulation device.

Since there is minimal ischemic time during renal autotransplantation, almost any electrolyte solution can be used to provide in situ cooling for the kidney. In our center, we routinely use a Euro-Collins solution. We prefer to perfuse the kidney with an entire volume of perfusate (approximately 1,000 mL); however, it is necessary to perfuse a kidney only until the venous effluent is clear. In cases of multiple arteries, all arterial branches need to be separately perfused as these represent end vessels to the kidney. Very small vessels may require manual perfusion with a syringe and a small-caliber (22-gauge) angiocath tip. Once the kidney has been perfused, the renal vasculature can be prepared. The renal vein should be dissected back to its segmental branches. Small venous tributaries can be ligated with silk ties and divided. Large segmental branches should be preserved, and it is imperative to maintain at least 50% of the total venous drainage of the kidney. Once the vein is skeletonized back to its segmental branches, it can be retracted away from the artery, which can then be similarly dissected. The lymphatic tissue surrounding the artery is sharply excised and secured along the segmental arterial branches. Large lymphatic trunks in this location should be secured with silk ties in order to prevent a lymph leak, particularly if the implantation of the kidney is going to be placed in a retroperitoneal location. Once the artery has been mobilized to its segmental branches, it should be ready for implantation. Any remaining perinephric fat should be removed, and we also prefer to perform a needle biopsy of the kidney at this time to provide any additional histologic information.

In cases of renal vascular disease, the renal artery should be dissected distally, beyond the level of the disease. The diseased segment of the artery or arteries should be excised, and the remaining normal artery or branch artery can be reconstructed in a variety of techniques (Fig. 12.5).

## Implantation of the Renal Autograft

### Exposure of the Iliac Vessels

As mentioned previously, the site for renal autograft implantation can be exposed by a second surgical team while the kidney is being prepared on the back table (5). A standard lower-quadrant oblique (Gibson) incision can be used to enter the retroperitoneum when two separate incisions are utilized for autotransplantation. Of particular importance with the

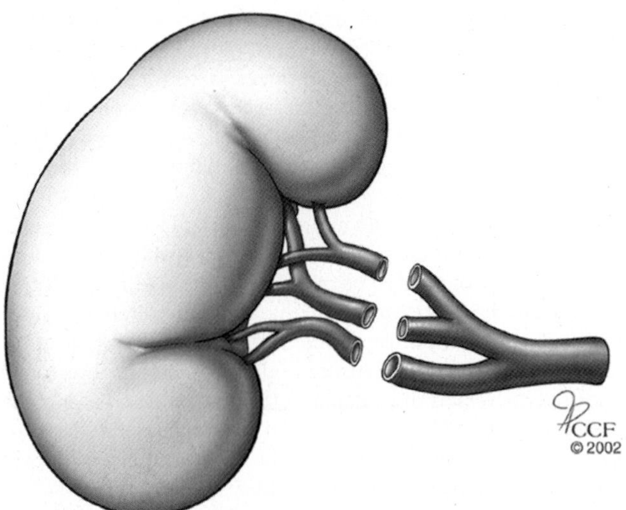


FIGURE 12.5 The native hypogastric artery can often be used as an interposition graft in complex branch renal artery repair. The hypogastric artery must be free of significant vascular disease to be useful.

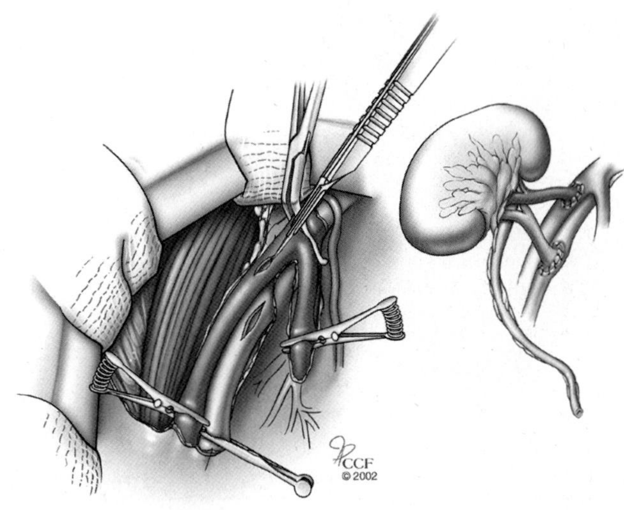


FIGURE 12.6 This figure demonstrates regional control of the external iliac artery and vein. It also shows the final appearance of the transplanted kidney.

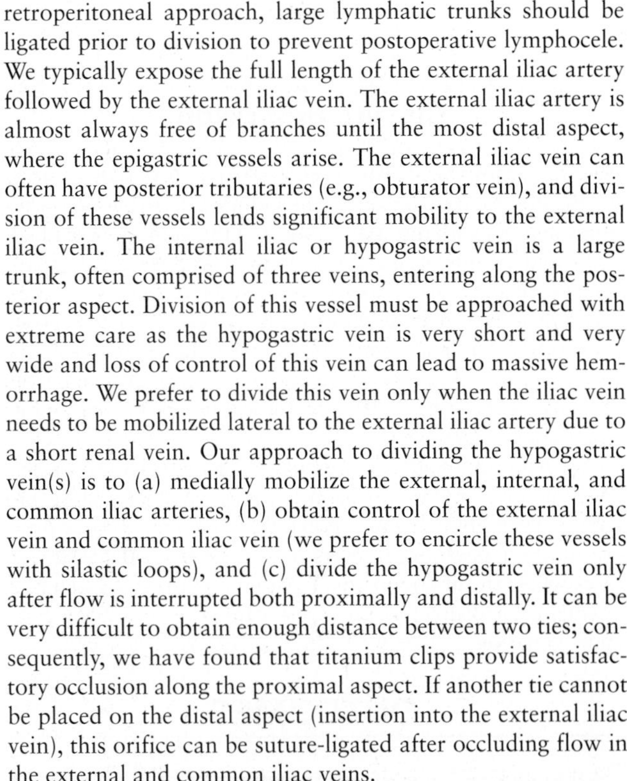

retroperitoneal approach, large lymphatic trunks should be ligated prior to division to prevent postoperative lymphocele. We typically expose the full length of the external iliac artery followed by the external iliac vein. The external iliac artery is almost always free of branches until the most distal aspect, where the epigastric vessels arise. The external iliac vein can often have posterior tributaries (e.g., obturator vein), and division of these vessels lends significant mobility to the external iliac vein. The internal iliac or hypogastric vein is a large trunk, often comprised of three veins, entering along the posterior aspect. Division of this vessel must be approached with extreme care as the hypogastric vein is very short and very wide and loss of control of this vein can lead to massive hemorrhage. We prefer to divide this vein only when the iliac vein needs to be mobilized lateral to the external iliac artery due to a short renal vein. Our approach to dividing the hypogastric vein(s) is to (a) medially mobilize the external, internal, and common iliac arteries, (b) obtain control of the external iliac vein and common iliac vein (we prefer to encircle these vessels with silastic loops), and (c) divide the hypogastric vein only after flow is interrupted both proximally and distally. It can be very difficult to obtain enough distance between two ties; consequently, we have found that titanium clips provide satisfactory occlusion along the proximal aspect. If another tie cannot be placed on the distal aspect (insertion into the external iliac vein), this orifice can be suture-ligated after occluding flow in the external and common iliac veins.

In contrast to an extraperitoneal approach, the iliac vessels can be exposed directly when using an intraperitoneal approach. Lymphatic trunks are simply cauterized, and similar exposure of the iliac vessels is obtained. Another distinction of an intraperitoneal approach is that it is often easier to expose larger vessels for implantation, specifically the common iliac artery and infrarenal vena cava. These vessels are more accessible and larger caliber, features that may facilitate renal vascular anastomoses.

Important points in selecting the target for renal autograft implantation are that (a) the vessels should be adequately mobile to allow for tension-free anastomoses to the renal artery and vein, and (b) the inflow artery should be adequately free of atherosclerotic disease. The second point deserves further elaboration in that, not only should the anastomotic site be acceptable, but the location for clamp placement should also be "soft." If there is concern over the suitability of the artery, a "softer" location should be explored both proximally and distally.

## Renal Autograft Revascularization

Revascularization of the kidney is commenced by anastomosis of the renal vein to the iliac vein (or vena cava) (Fig. 12.6). We typically occlude the iliac vein with a tangentially occluding or Satinsky-type clamp. An appropriate-length venotomy is made on the anterior wall, and the lumen is irrigated with heparinized saline. The kidney is brought into the operative field, and a continuous anastomosis is completed by first placing sutures at both apices of the venotomy and then running around each "side." For anastomosis to the iliac vein, both 5-0 and 6-0 polypropylene sutures are acceptable, and when the vena cava is used for outflow, 5-0 polypropylene is suitable.

We perform the arterial anastomosis following completion of the venous anastomosis. The iliac artery (common or external) is occluded with vascular clamps both proximally and distally. Alternatively, a single clamp (Satinsky type) can be used for arterial occlusion as well, but the disadvantage to this approach is that the artery cannot be unclamped without restoring the high-pressure antegrade flow. Following clamp control, the periadventitial tissue at the proposed site of anastomosis is sharply excised, an arteriotomy is made with a no. 11 blade, which is then further fashioned to match the caliber of the renal artery, and the lumen is irrigated with heparinized saline. We commonly use a continuous 6-0 or 7-0 polypropylene suture to complete the end-to-side anastomosis to the iliac artery.

Following completion of the vascular anastomoses, we release the venous clamp first, then the distal arterial clamp, and last the proximal areterial clamp. This allows the anastomoses to be "tested" in a low- to high-pressure direction. Once hemostasis is ensured, the operative field and kidney are bathed in warm saline solution, after which the kidney is inspected for

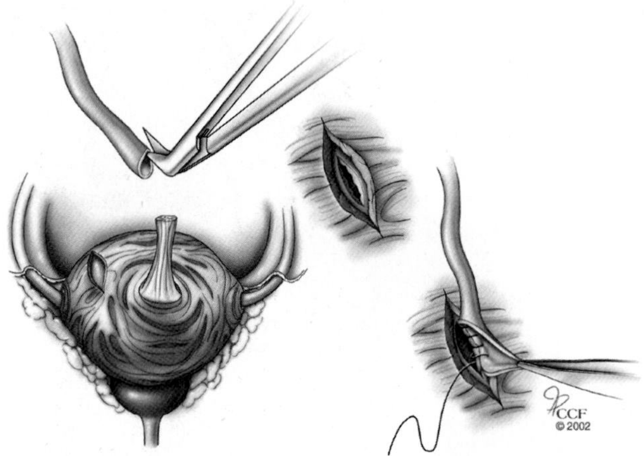


FIGURE 12.7 The location and creation of the extravesical ureteroneocystostomy is demonstrated.

uniform perfusion. The renal cortex may take several minutes to become homogenously perfused (pink-appearing), and soon after this occurs, urine production should be seen from the distal ureteral end.

### Ureteroneocystostomy

In general, we prefer to reimplant the autograft ureter in an extravesical manner (Figs. 12.7 and 12.8). We do not feel that creation of an antireflux tunnel is essential.

Unlike dialysis-dependent patients who are undergoing renal allotransplantation, nearly all patients who are undergoing autotransplantation have "normal" urine volumes and "normal" bladder capacities. The bladder, which is readily distensible, is filled by instillation of saline solution. The perivesical fat over the intended site of ureteral reimplantation is removed with electrocautery dissection. Occasionally, large veins in the perivesical fat must be ligated, for which we prefer to use absorbable suture to avoid potential migration into the anastomosis.

We then trim the ureter at an appropriate length. For renal autotransplantation, the ureter is not excessively long and, in general, does not need to be trimmed to any significant degree (1 to 2 cm at most). Additionally, unlike the ureter received with a deceased donor renal allograft, the viability of the autograft ureter can be ensured during the nephrectomy. Periureteral vessels are ligated with absorbable ties, and the ureter is spatulated for a distance of 8 to 12 mm. The detrusor musculature is then divided with the electrocautery, with care taken to avoid entering the bladder mucosa. The bladder mucosa is entered sharply, and the ureter is anchored at this site with one or two absorbable sutures placed at the "heel" and "toe" of the anastomosis, respectively. We prefer to complete the typical extravesical ureteroneocystostomy with a continuous 5-0 polydioxanone suture. Routine use of an indwelling double J stent is dependent on surgeon preference; however, if there are concerns over the integrity of the anastomosis or the viability of the ureteral end, use of a stent is recommended.

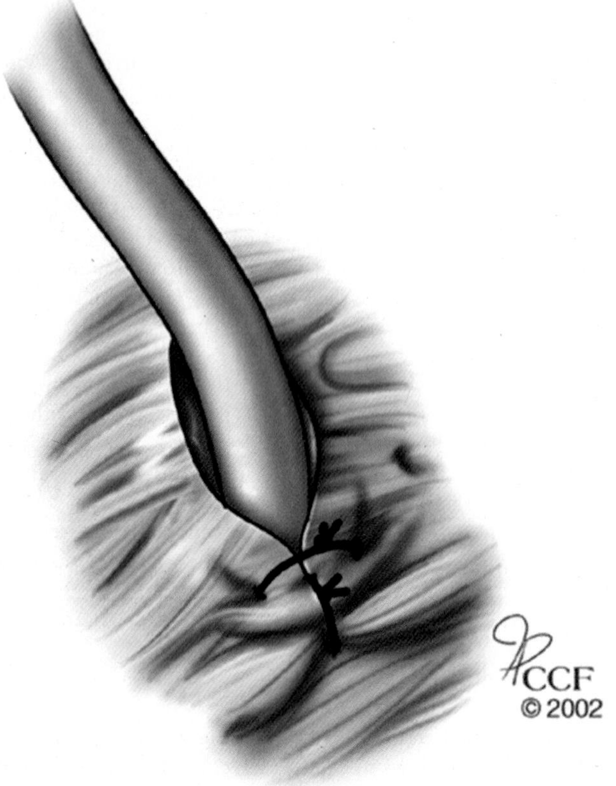


FIGURE 12.8 Final appearance of a tunneled anastomosis.

## Closure of Incision

Prior to closing the incison, we ensure an appropriate position for the kidney. In most cases, the kidney can be placed on the psoas muscle, with the lateral aspect of the kidney directed laterally and the hilum directed medially. This position places the urinary tract in a medial position, should later access be necessary. Once the kidney is positioned, cortical perfusion should be verified and the hilum should be palpated to ensure a strong arterial pulse. Additionally, satisfactory drainage from the renal vein can be ensured by the palpation of a soft, easily compressible renal vein.

We reapproximate the musculature most often in a single layer. When a midline incision is used, we always close this with a single layer of no. 1 polydioxanone or polypropylene. For most retroperitoneal incisions, one layer is satisfactory. In cases where the abdominal wall is thin and the musculature is attenuated, closure in two layers can provide adequate reapproximation.

# OUTCOMES

The end points for outcomes vary according to the indication for the procedure (ureteral obstruction, renal vascular disease, loin-pain hematuria syndrome). Preservation of the affected kidney is very high. Several reports have demonstrated >90% technical success rates for renal autotransplantation that seem durable. Understand that autotransplantation for a diseased kidney is a more complicated endeavor than renal allotransplantation. Simultaneous donor and transplantation procedures are performed on the same individual, which is an enormous physiological burden. The kidney being autotransplanted is often anatomically compromised. This is in contrast to the donor kidneys in standard allotransplantation, which are normal, and for which the reported technical loss rates are <5%.

## COMPLICATIONS

Complications of using autotransplantation may derive from the procurement of the kidney or may be related to the implantation of the kidney. The main complications arising from procurement would be bleeding and injury to adjacent viscera (colon, pancreas, spleen, liver). From the implantation portion of the procedure there may be vascular problems. The biggest concern is the potential for arterial or venous thrombosis. Attending to proper vascular technique and ensuring appropriate geometric alignment of the kidney in its final location will help prevent vessel kinking. Recipient vessel dissection or embolization is rare; nonetheless, early recognition and repair are required to avoid catastrophic limb-threatening problems. With respect to the ureter, there is potential for urine leak or obstruction. Attention to creating a tension-free anastomosis by using a ureter with a well-preserved blood supply is important. Given the diseased status of the vessels or ureter, a ureteral stent is recommended. Finally, when kidneys are autotransplanted into a retroperitoneal position, lymphocele is possible. Meticulous ligation of perivascular lymphatics will help to prevent this complication. A retroperitoneal drain for a brief period may also help avoid this complication. If a lymphocele is causing graft dysfunction, it can be drained percutaneously or surgically.

## *References*


1. Bodie B, Novick AC, Rose M, et al. Long-term results with renal autotransplantation for ureteral replacement. *J Urol* 1986;136:1187–1189.
2. Chin JL, Kloth D, Pautler SE, et al. Renal autotransplantation for the loin pain–hematuria syndrome: long-term followup of 26 cases. *J Urol* 1998; 160:1232–1236.
3. Gill IS, Uzzo RG, Hobart MG, et al. Laparoscopic retroperitoneal live donor right nephrectomy for purposes of allotransplantation and auto transplantation. *J Urol* 2000;164:1500–1504.
4. Goldfarb DA. Open donor nephrectomy. In: Novick AC, Jones JS, eds. *Operative urology at the Cleveland Clinic*. Totowa: Humana Press, 2006:111–116.
5. Goldfarb DA, Flechner SM, Modlin CS. Renal transplantation. In: Novick AC, Jones JS, eds. *Operative urology at the Cleveland Clinic*. Totowa: Humana Press, 2006:121–132.
6. Meraney AM, Gill IS, Kaouk JH, et al. Laparoscopic renal autotransplantation. *J Endourol* 2001;15:143–149.
7. Novick AC, Straffon RA, Stewart BH. Experience with extracorporeal renal operations and autotransplantation in the management of complicated urologic disorders. *Surg Gynecol Obstet* 1981;153:10–18.
8. van der Velden JJ, van Bockel JH, Zwartendijk J, et al. Long-term results of surgical treatment of renal carcinoma in solitary kidneys by extracorporeal resection and autotransplantation. *Br J Urol* 1992;69:486–490.
9. Zincke H, Sen SE. Experience with extracorporeal surgery and autotransplantation for renal cell and transitional cell cancer of the kidney. *J Urol* 1988;140:25–27.

# SECTION II ■ BLADDER

CHARLES B. BRENDLER

# CHAPTER 13 ■ ANATOMY OF THE BLADDER

CLINTON W. COLLINS AND ADAM P. KLAUSNER

## GENERAL DESCRIPTION

The bladder is a hollow, muscular retroperitoneal organ with a capacity of 400 to 500 mL in the normal adult. When empty, it is a pelvic organ, lying behind the pubic symphysis. However, when distended, it can be palpated above the pubic symphysis and can protude well into the abdomen during an episode of severe urinary retention.

## PERITONEAL RELATIONSHIPS

The peritoneum covers the superior bladder and a portion of the posterior bladder. In women, the peritoneum continues posteriorly onto the surface of the uterus and rectum, establishing the vesicouterine and rectouterine pouches, respectively (Fig. 13.1) (1). In men, the peritoneum continues along the surface of the rectum, establishing the rectovesical pouch of Douglas. The two leaves of the peritoneum embryologically coalesce to form the anterior and posterior layers of the Denonvilliers fascia (rectovesical fascia), a critical landmark in the performance of a radical retropubic prostatectomy (Fig. 13.2) (13).

### Peritoneal Folds

As seen from a typical laparascopic approach to the abdominal cavity, the anterior surface of the peritoneum has three characteristic deflections, also called folds. The midline fold is called the "median umbilical ligament," and the paired paramedian folds are called the "medial umbilical ligamants." Fortunately, the anatomy itself is less confusing than the terminology. In relation to the bladder, the median umbilical fold is the most important of these structures as it contains the urachal ligament. Attaching to the bladder anteriorly at its dome, this ligamentous structure, containing fatty and vascular tissue, tethers the bladder to the umbilicus. This stucture, which represents the obliterated urachus, contains paraumbilical veins and must be ligated when divided during surgical exposure of the bladder. The bladder muscle, also called the "detrusor," is attenuated where the urachal ligament attaches, predisposing this area to the formation of diverticuli. Retropubic and perivesical fat is present anteroinferior and lateral to the bladder.

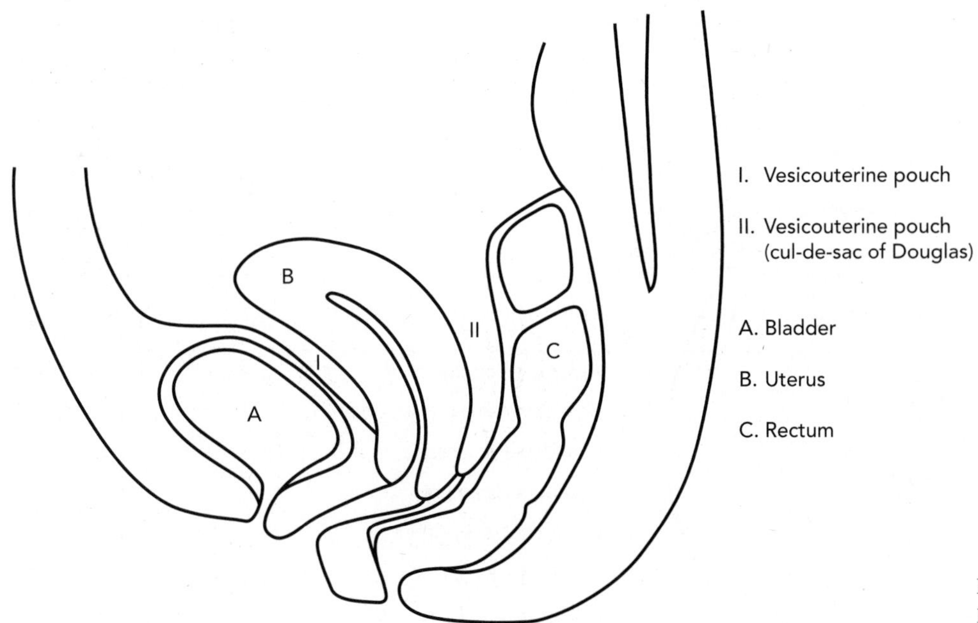


FIGURE 13.1 Sagittal view of female pouches.

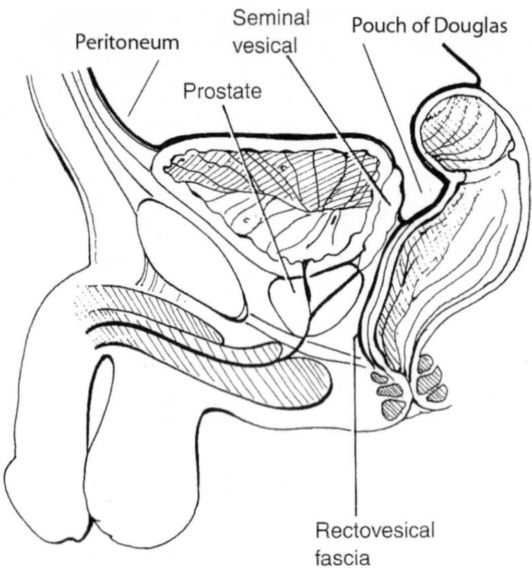


FIGURE 13.2 Lateral view of the male pelvis showing the peritoneal reflection and the pouch of Douglas.

## LIGAMENTOUS ATTACHMENTS

In the pelvis, the bladder is supported anatomically by two types of ligaments: fibroareolar (true) ligaments and peritoneal folds. True ligaments provide support for the bladder laterally via the lateral ligament of the bladder and posteriorly via the vesicovenous plexus. The lateral ligament derives from the transversalis (endopelvic) fascia as it courses over the levators and attaches the bladder to the tendinous arch of the endopelvic fascia. This ligament contains the inferior vesical and vesicodeferential arteries in the lateral extensions, as well as the pudendal plexuses of nerves and vessels. In addition, in men, this ligament contains the vasa deferentia. The posterior ligaments provide posterolateral support to the bladder. These ligaments are connective tissue condensations in which the vesicovenous plexus drains into the internal iliac veins. Peritoneal folds also connect the bladder to the pelvic sidewalls and consist of the median, medial, and lateral umbilical folds as well as the sacrogenital folds. The median umbilical fold and medial umbilical folds originate at the bladder and terminate at the umbilicus. They contain the urachus and the obliterated umbilical arteries, respectively. The lateral umbilical folds attach the bladder to the pelvic sidewalls and contain the inferior epigastric arteries. The sacrogenital folds connect the bladder to the sacrum (Fig. 13.3) (7).

The bladder is also fixed to the symphysis pubica by the pubovesical ligaments in women and the puboprostatic ligaments in men. The dorsal vein of the clitoris or penis passes between these paired ligaments. These ligaments represent an important surgical landmark as they form the anteromedial portion of the retropubic space, also called the space of Retzius. The space of Retzius is bound anteriorly by the transversalis fascia, inferiorly by the puboprostatic (pubovesical) ligaments, and infralaterally by the lateral ligaments of the bladder (Fig. 13.4).

## HISTOLOGIC STRUCTURE

The lumen of the bladder is lined by transitional epithelium, also called "urothelium." This unique epithelium is characterized by its outer layer of "umbrella cells," which are sealed closely together and communicate via tight junctions. The term *transitional* denotes the ability of these outer cells to undergo significant transitions in shape depending on the state of bladder filling. Thus, the cells are puffy and cuboidal when the bladder is empty and become flat and elongated when the bladder is distended (6). Beneath these umbrella cells, the transitional epithelium contains additional layers of cells (usually about seven) and a distinct layer of basal cells. Deep to the transitional epithelium lies the lamina propria, composed of fibroelastic connective tissue through which vessels course. Wisps of smooth muscle also course within the lamina propria, and this portion of the lamina propria is sometimes referred to as the muscularis mucosa (Fig. 13.5).

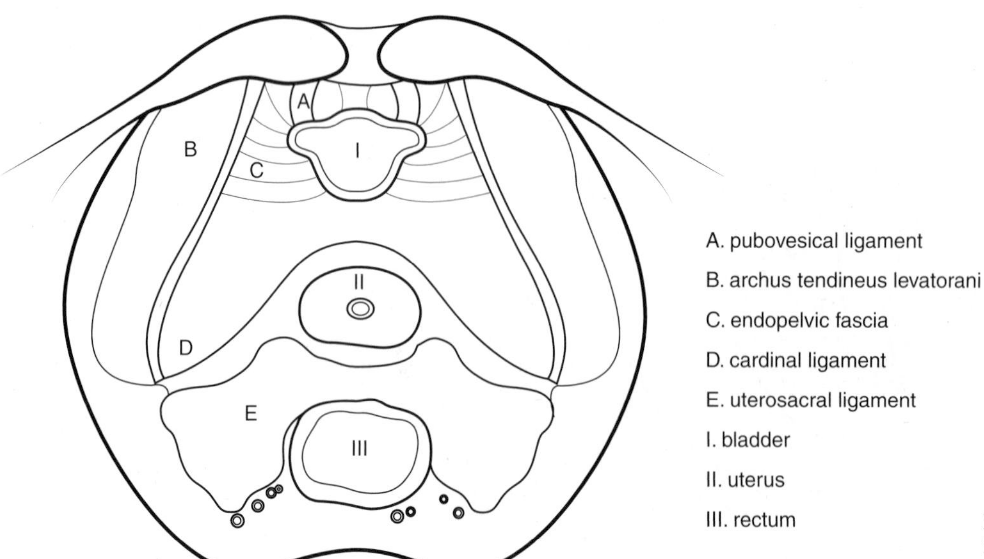


FIGURE 13.3 Axial view of the female pelvis illustrating the ligamentous supports of the bladder.

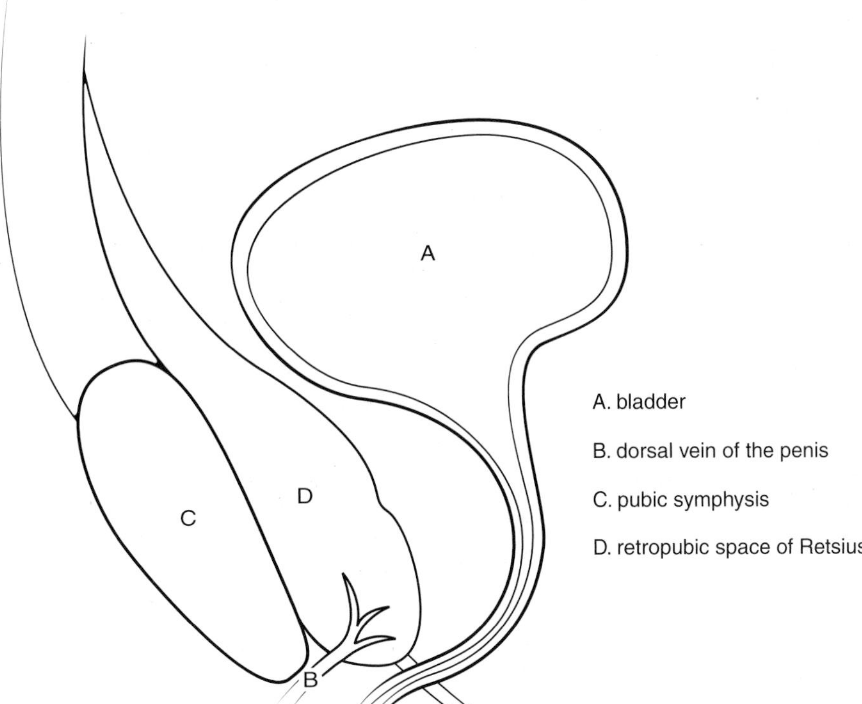


FIGURE 13.4 Lateral view of a portion of the male pelvis showing the space of Retzius. The space of Retzius is bound anteriorly by the transversalis fascia, inferiorly by the pub-oprostatic (pubovesical) ligaments, and infra-laterally by the lateral ligaments of the bladder.

The distinction between the muscularis mucosa and the muscularis propria, or true muscular layer of the bladder that lies deep to the lamina propria, is critical in the staging and prognosis of urothelial cancer. Cancer that is confined to the urothelium or lamina propria, even when surrounded by wisps of muscularis mucosa, is considered superficial disease and is mainly treated via local resection or with intravesical immuno- or chemotherapeutic agents. However, cancer that penetrates into the muscularis propria, characterized histologically by large, distinct detrusor smooth muscle bundles (Fig. 13.6), is considered invasive cancer and is treated more aggressively; it usually requires surgical removal of the entire bladder. Within the muscularis propria, detrusor smooth muscle bundles course in inner longitudinal, middle circular, and

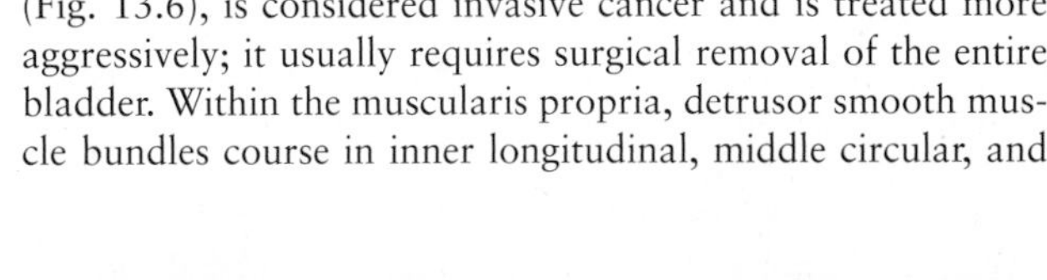

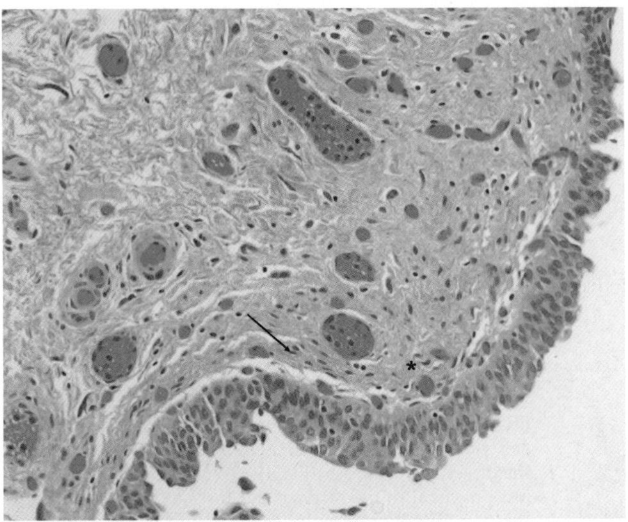

FIGURE 13.5 Microscopic cross-sectional image of normal human bladder. Note wisps of smooth muscle *(arrow)* within the lamina propria *(star)*. (Courtesy of Dr. Marigny Roberts.)

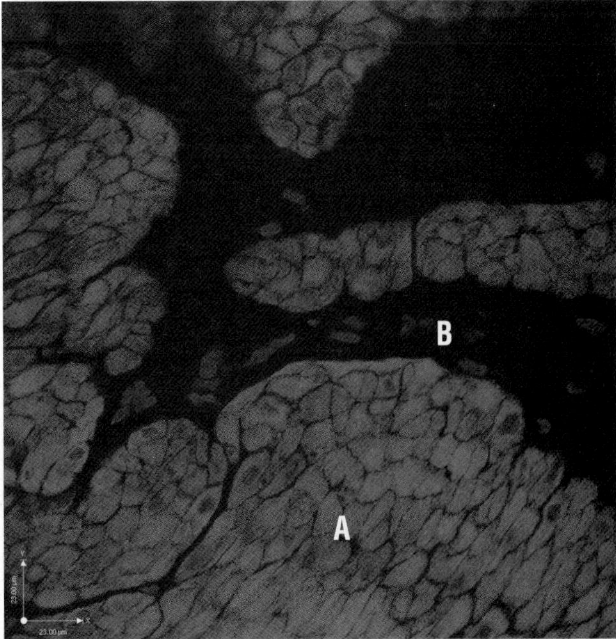


FIGURE 13.6 Confocal immunohistochemical imaging showing rabbit detrusor bundle. **A:** Densely packed hexagonal shaped detrusor smooth muscle cells. **B:** Interstitial area between smooth muscle bundles containing interstitial cells and fibroblasts.

outer longitudinal orientations. In addition, interstitial cells surround and percolate within the muscle bundles and may be important in the maintenance or modulation of bladder muscle tone (8). These muscle layers are less distinct in the upper aspect of the bladder. However, they become quite prominent at the bladder neck, although composed of finer fibers. In men, the middle layer of circular detrusor smooth muscle forms a preprostatic layer that has robust expression of alpha receptors (mainly alpha 1a) and contributes to continence at the bladder neck. Furthermore, the success in treatment of benign prostatic hypertrophy (BPH) with alpha blockers stems, in part, from a pharmacologic reduction in tone in the smooth muscle surrounding the prostate and bladder neck (2). In women, the bladder neck differs dramatically, having a less distinct middle layer of smooth muscle (1,5).

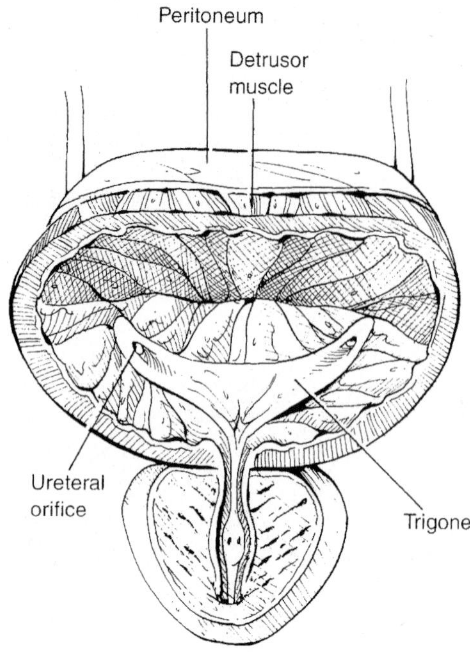


FIGURE 13.7 Anterior view of the bladder of a man opened and demonstrating intravesical anatomy. Note that the trigone continues into the prostatic urethra.

## URETEROVESICAL JUNCTION AND TRIGONE

The spiral fibers of the ureter become more longitudinally oriented near the bladder and are encased in the fibromuscular Waldeyer sheath from a distance just proximal to its entrance into the bladder wall through its course to the trigone (1,11). Obliquely, the ureters enter the bladder posteroinferiorly and course approximately 2 cm toward the ureteral orifice, narrowing as the intramural ureter is compressed by the detrusor of the bladder surrounding it. The ureter lies just beneath the bladder mucosa with a muscular layer backing (1).

A distinct landmark is formed at a triangle located between the ureteral orifices and the bladder neck, referred to as the bladder trigone. Layers of ureteral and bladder smooth muscle coalesce here as a raised ridge of tissue between the two orifices referred to as the interureteric ridge. This ridge is helpful in identifying orifices endoscopically (Fig. 13.7). The trigone is composed of three distinct layers: (a) a superficial layer derived from the longitudinal layer of ureteral smooth muscle; (b) a deep layer that is continuous from the Waldeyer sheath, inserting at the bladder neck (Fig. 13.8); and (c) the detrusor

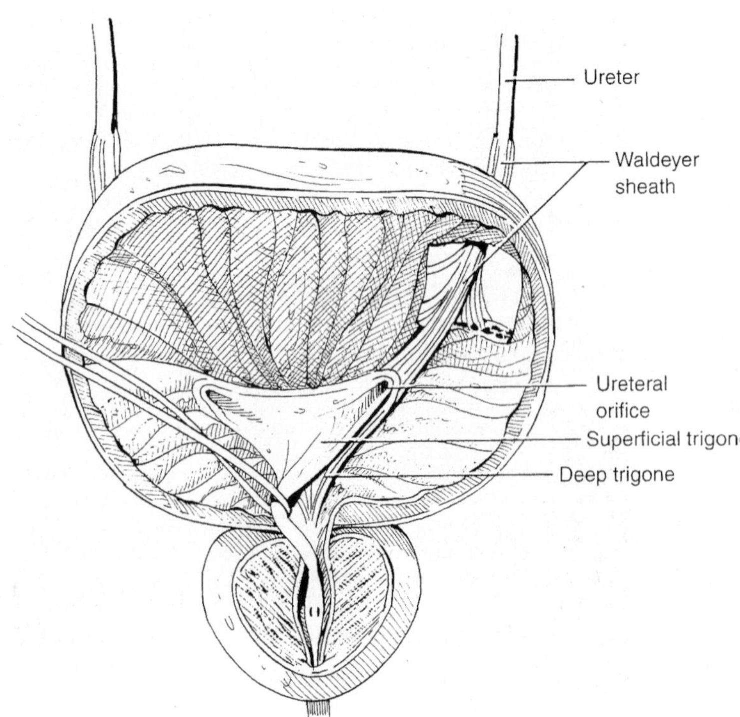


FIGURE 13.8 Lateral view of ureter as it enters the bladder via the intramural tunnel. Note that the Waldeyer sheath extends from the bladder to encase the distal ureter just proximal to the bladder and fuses to the ureteral musculature. The Waldeyer sheath is a continuation of the deep trigone and connects by a few fibers to the detrusor muscle at the ureteral hiatus.

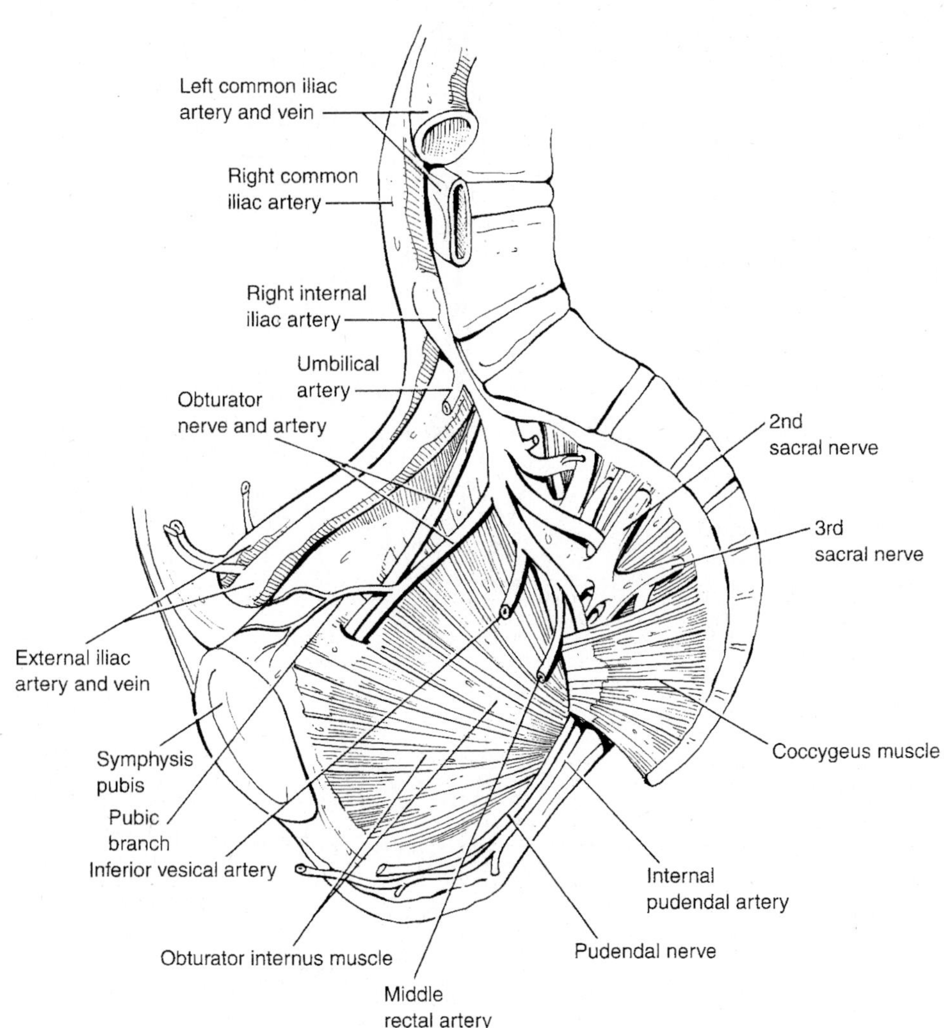


FIGURE 13.9 Lateral pelvic sidewall demonstrating the vasculature and innervation of the deep pelvis. The arterial supply of the bladder is from the superior lateral vesical artery and the inferior vesical artery enclosed in the posterior pedicle.

layer, derived from the outer longitudinal and middle circular layers of smooth muscle (1). The unique anatomic structure of the intramural ureter and trigone contributes to the intrinsic continence mechanism that prevents vesicoureteral reflux during bladder filling and voiding.

## BLOOD SUPPLY

Multiple blood vessels supply the urinary bladder; however, the exact vascular anatomy can vary somewhat between individuals. Less variable is the presence of two more distinct collections of vessels, referred to as the lateral and posterior pedicles (Fig. 13.9). In men, the lateral and posterior pedicles are also called the lateral and posterior ligaments. In women, these vascular pedicles are part of the cardinal and uterosacral ligaments. The blood vessels within these pedicles branch from the superior and inferior vesical arteries. The superior vesical artery arises from the internal iliac close to its origin from the common iliac. It can also arise as a branch from the umbilical artery, which branches off of the proximal internal iliac. The inferior vesical artery branches off of the internal iliac artery at a more distal location. However, it is important to recognize that the arterial supply to the bladder may arise from *any* portion of the internal iliac. In terms of venous drainage, veins from the bladder drain predominantly into lateral plexuses and then empty into veins within the lateral prostatic ligaments and ultimately into the internal iliac veins (1).

## INNERVATION

### Sensory Innervation

In the bladder, there are two types of sensory (afferent) nerve fibers: alpha-delta and C fibers. Alpha-delta fibers are partially myelinated and carry information to the central nervous system regarding bladder fullness and wall tension. These sensory fibers are responsible for initiating the normal voiding reflex. On the other hand, C fibers are unmyelinated nociceptive fibers that mainly carry information to the central nervous system regarding noxious or painful stimuli. Although these C fibers comprise about 70% of the total afferent nerves supplying the bladder, they are generally silent and only become sensitive during inflammation, irritation, or suprasacral spinal cord injury. Prolonged activation of C fiber afferents may be responsible for the development of pathologic voiding reflexes associated with some forms of overactive bladder.

## Motor Innervation

Motor innervation to the bladder arises from three sets of nerves: (a) the *parasympathetic* sacral (pelvic) nerve, arising from the sacral spinal cord between S2 and S4; (b) the *sympathetic* thoracolumbar (hypogastric) nerve, arising from the spinal cord between T10 and L2; and (c) the *somatic* pudendal nerve, which also arises between S2 and S4.

Preganglionic parasympathetic motor efferent fibers exit between S2 and S4 via pelvic nerves, with nerve bodies located in the sacral parasympathetic nucleus (SPN). The SPN is located in the intermediolateral region of the sacral spinal cord. Importantly, an increase in parasympathetic tone, supplied by these nerves, is the main trigger for a coordinated contraction of the detrusor muscle that leads to voiding. In the bladder body, sympathetic fibers supply beta receptors contributing to smooth muscle relaxation during filling and also synapse prejunctionally along axons of parasympathetic nerves. This anatomic relationship may allow for additional reduction of detrusor smooth muscle tone during the filling phase, a process that is likely necessary to prevent involuntary contractions and urge incontinence. The only somatic (voluntary) motor fibers in the lower urinary tract supply the external urethral sphincter, sometimes called the rhabdosphincter (9). Preganglionic somatic motor efferent fibers exit between S2 and S4 with nerve bodies located in the Onuf nucleus in the anterolateral horn of the sacral spinal cord. These somatic fibers run in the pudendal nerve, modulating striated (voluntary) urethral sphincter contraction.

## The Micturition Reflex

Sensory or "afferent" fibers from the bladder are contained in the pelvic, hypogastric, and pudendal nerves. The pelvic and pudendal nerves enter the sacral spinal cord via dorsal root ganglia, with the most prominent projection passing anterolateral toward the SPN. Afferent fibers in the hypogastric nerves also enter the spinal cord via dorsal root ganglia in the lumbar spinal cord. Afferent fibers from the external urethral sphincter pass through the Onuf nucleus in the sacral spinal cord. All of these inputs relay sensory information to the lateral pons, referred to as the pontine storage center. After processing in higher brain centers, motor signals are then relayed back through the pontine micturition center (PMC) located in the Barrington nucleus in the dorsal medial pons. These pontine centers receive input indirectly through relay neurons in the periaqueductal gray (PAG) or directly from lateral spinal tract neurons. There is also input from the cerebellum, basal ganglia, thalamus, hypothalamus, and cerebral cortex (4,12). Therefore, these PMCs are responsible for the coordination of urine storage and voiding. Thus, damage to the spinal cord between the sacral motor outflow and the PMCs leads to a characteristic pattern of neurogenic detrusor overactivity (involuntary contractions) and detrusor sphincter dyssynergia (lack of coordination between the bladder and urethral sphincter). In this situation, the coordinated spinal→ bulbo→ spinal reflex is converted to an uncoordinated spinal→ spinal reflex.

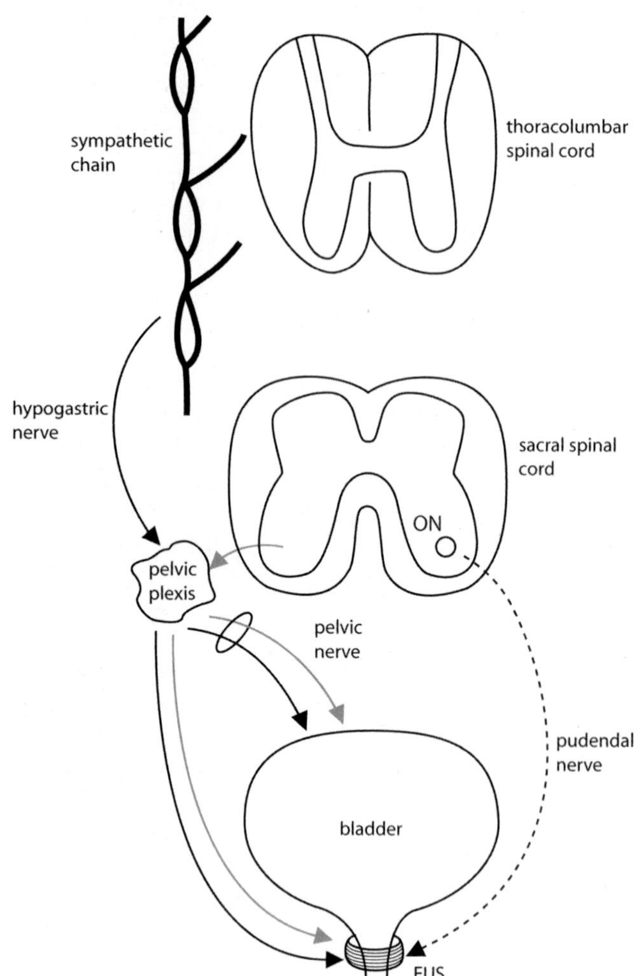


**FIGURE 13.10** Autonomic and somatic innervation of the lower urinary tract. There is extensive motor outflow to the bladder and urethral sphincter from the spinal cord. Parasympathetic outflow *(as shown in gray)* is conveyed by the pelvic nerve and leads to bladder contraction during voiding and contraction of urethral smooth muscle during filling. Sympathetic outflow originates from the thoracolumbar cord, travels in the hypogastric nerve *(as shown in black)*, and leads to bladder relaxation and bladder neck contraction during filling. Somatic outflow also originates from the sacral cord and travels via the pudendal nerve *(dashed line)*. Outflow leads to contraction of the urethral sphincter during filling and relaxation during voiding (possibly nitric oxide-mediated).

## Storage Reflex

Storage is facilitated by bladder afferent stimulation of the Onuf nucleus, which increases the tone of the external urethral sphincter via the somatic pudendal nerve. The pontine storage center, in the lateral pons, also stimulates the Onuf nucleus and the pudendal nerve output to the external urethral sphincter. Simultaneously, the hypogastric (sympathetic) nerve, receiving input from pelvic afferents, inhibits the detrusor muscle and bladder ganglia while stimulating the internal urethral sphincter (bladder neck), which has robust expression of alpha-1 receptors. As mentioned earlier, pharmacologic reduction in this bladder neck tone with alpha blockers is a mainstay for the treatment of BPH as well as detrusor-sphincter dyssynergia and other forms of voiding dysfunction (Fig. 13.10).

## Emptying Reflex

Emptying is mediated through the PMC, which stimulates parasympathetic motor or "efferent" fibers whose cell bodies are in the SPN. Parasympathetic outflow via the pelvic nerve causes detrusor contraction and inhibition of the internal sphincter (bladder neck), processes that facilitate emptying. In addition, signals from the PMC also inhibit sympathetic outflow from the hypogastric nerve, leading to relaxation of the bladder neck, a process that also facilitates emptying. Furthermore, signals from the PMC also inhibit the motor outflow to the pudendal nerve, leading to relaxation of the striated urethral sphincter, again facilitating emptying (Fig. 13.11) (10).

# LYMPHATICS

The lymphatic drainage of the bladder is to the external iliac vein, the hypogastric nodes, or the presacral promonotory.

# CONTIGUOUS STRUCTURES

In men, the bladder joins the prostate and is anterior to the seminal vesicles and ampulla of the vas deferens. In women, the bladder is in more direct contact with the pubococcygeus portion of the levator ani. Superiorly, the bladder is covered by peritoneum in both men and women. Posteriorly in women, the bladder is adjacent to the uterus and vagina. In men, the posterior bladder is adjacent to the seminal vesicles and rectum.

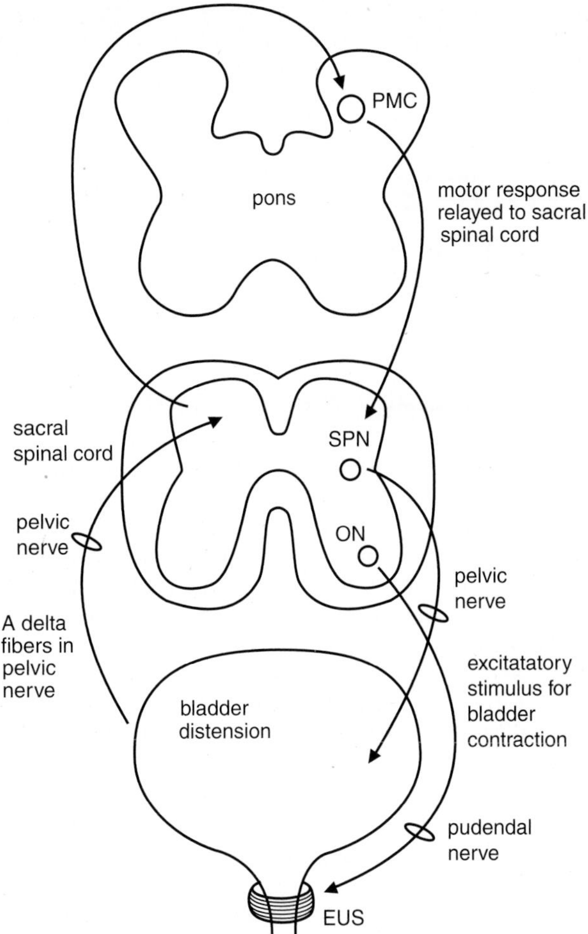


FIGURE 13.11 Micturition phase of bladder function. As shown in this diagram, micturition is stimulated by bladder distention. Sensory fibers carry information about bladder distention to the sacral spinal cord. Signals then ascend via pathways in the dorsal columns to the pontine micturition center (PMC). The PMC is the main center for coordination of lower-urinary-tract function. Information may pass through projections from the periaqueductal gray (PAG) to the PMC (3). Motor responses then relay information back to the sacral spinal cord, ultimately triggering an excitatory stimulus for bladder contraction.

## *References*

1. Brooks JD. Anatomy of lower urinary tract and male genitalia. In: Wein AJ, Kavoussi L, Novick A, et al., eds. *Campbell-Walsh urology*, 9th ed. Philadelphia: WB Saunders, 2006:56–68.
2. Caine M, Raz S, Ziegler M. Adrenergic and cholinergic receptors in the human prostate, prostatic capsule and bladder neck. *Br J Urol* 1975;47: 193–202.
3. Ding Y-Q, Wang D, Nie H, et al. Direct projections from the periaqueductal gray to pontine micturition center neurons projecting to the lumbosacral cord segments: an electron microscopic study in the rat. *Neurosci Lett* 1998;242:97–100.
4. Erickson V, Roppolo JR, Booth AM, et al. l'ranssynaptic labeling of neurons within CNS which control the bladder or penis of the cat. *Soc Neurosci Abstr* 1995;21:1872.
5. Gosling JA. The structure of the bladder and urethra in relation to function. *Urol Clin North Am* 1979;6:31–38.
6. Hicks M. The mammalian urinary bladder: an accommodating organ. *Biol Rev* 1975;50:215–246.
7. Hinman F. *Atlas of urosurgical anatomy*. Philadelphia: WB Saunders, 1993.
8. Johnston L, et al. *Am J Physiol Renal Physiol* 2008;294(3):F645–655. Epub January 2, 2008.
9. Juenemann KP, Lue TF, Schmidt RA, et al. Clinical significance of sacral and pudendal nerve anatomy. *J Urol* 1988;139(1):74–80.
10. Raz S. *Female urology*, 3rd ed. Philadelphia: WB Saunders, 2008.
11. Tanagho EA. Anatomy of the lower urinary tract. In: Walsh PC, Retik AB, Stamey TA, et al., eds. *Campbell's urology*, 6th ed. Philadelphia: WB Saunders, 1992:40–69.
12. Vizzard MA, Erickson VL, Card JP, et al. Transneuronal labelling of neurons in the adult rat brainstem and spinal cord after injection of pseudorabies virus into the urethra. *J Comp Neurol* 1995;355:629–640.
13. Weyrauch HM. *Surgery of the prostate*. Philadelphia: WB Saunders, 1959.

# CHAPTER 14 ■ SIMPLE AND PARTIAL CYSTECTOMY

JONATHAN C. PICARD AND J. NATHANIEL HAMILTON

## SIMPLE CYSTECTOMY

Simple cystectomy is performed in the setting of benign disease requiring urinary diversion or locally invasive nonurologic malignancy. Simple cystectomy involves removal of the bladder without resection of adjacent structures or performance of a formal lymph node dissection. The other pelvic organs are also left intact; to preserve sexual function, the prostate, seminal vesicles, and urethra are spared in the male patient and the uterus, anterior vagina, adnexa, and urethra are spared in the female patient. Removal of a defunctionalized bladder is often very beneficial and can prevent many complications.

### Diagnosis

Preoperative evaluation should include a complete history and physical examination. Specifically, a thorough investigation into the etiology of the voiding dysfunction, radiation treatments, prior pelvic surgeries, and all other interventions leading up to this evaluation should be performed. Biopsy should be undertaken if primary bladder malignancy is a consideration. Preoperative imaging of the abdomen and bladder are usually helpful, and we prefer a contrasted CT scan of both the abdomen and pelvis with delayed images to allow for visualization of the ureters and any abdominal or pelvic pathology that would preclude the procedure.

### Indications for Surgery

Urinary diversion is indicated for patients who have refractory conditions such as severe radiation or chemical cystitis, intractable bladder pain from interstitial cystitis, severe urinary incontinence, neurogenic bladder, extensive trauma, large vesical fistula, or recurrent pyocystis. Simple cystectomy can also be undertaken for invasive nongenitourinary cancers that are not amenable to resection with partial cystectomy.

Previous attempts at urinary diversion without concomitant simple cystectomy have led to complications in 54% to 80% of patients (1, 2, 7). Complications include pyocystis, intractable hemorrhage, severe pain or spasms, and the sensation of incomplete emptying. In these patients, the salvage cystectomy rate ranges from 20% to 30% (1, 2, 7). We therefore recommend concomitant simple cystectomy when permanent urinary diversion is undertaken.

Additionally, the risk of developing urothelial cancer of the bladder is significantly increased in patients who have received previous pelvic irradiation (relative risk = 4.6) (7). Some authors have even cited a risk for malignant degeneration in the setting of chronic irritation such as interstitial cystitis (6).

### Alternative Therapy

Radical cystoprostatectomy in men and radical cystectomy in women should be considered as alternatives to simple cystectomy in the setting of possible prostate cancer or urothelial carcinoma (UCC) and can be considered as alternatives in nonurologic malignancies that are locally invasive into the bladder or in many benign diseases of the bladder. In the majority of patients, continued observation, hyperbaric oxygen, analgesic prescription, and other symptomatic treatments are the initial options, with simple cystectomy only being offered as a final intervention in patients with refractory disease.

In patients with nonurologic malignancies that are locally invasive into the bladder, simple cystectomy can be considered if the resection can be accomplished with negative margins. Laparoscopic and robotic-assisted laparoscopic techniques are also being refined and are certainly an option for appropriately trained surgeons, despite the fact that these procedures are often difficult due to the challenges of previously irradiated fields, previous surgery, and chronic infection or inflammation.

### Surgical Technique

Simple cystectomy can be undertaken extraperitoneally to avoid abdominal adhesions due to multiple previous surgeries or radiation; however, we prefer an intraperitoneal approach as these patients also frequently require concomitant urinary diversion. Antithrombotic medication, pneumatic compression cuffs, or compression stockings should be strongly considered prior to induction of anesthesia. The patient is positioned supine on the operating room table with the anterior superior iliac spines positioned over the inferior portion of the table break or kidney rest. The table is flexed to facilitate exposure, and the bed is slightly tilted in the Trendelenburg position until the abdomen is parallel to the floor. When urethrectomy is planned, a modified lithotomy position provides improved exposure to the perineum. The abdomen and pelvis are then prepped with an antibiotic solution extending from the costal margin superiorly to the perineum, including the penis in men and the vagina in women. The patient is draped, and a Foley catheter is inserted following sterile procedures. The bladder is allowed to drain completely. Filling the bladder with 150 to 200 mL of sterile water may facilitate the dissection.

An intravenous antibiotic agent should be administered prior to skin incision. A lower midline incision extending from the umbilicus to the pubic symphysis is made using a no. 10 blade scalpel and deepened with Bovie cautery to the anterior rectus fascia. The anterior rectus fascia should be opened sharply, and the rectus abdominis muscles in the midline should then be separated to facilitate entry into the space of Retzius.

The extraperitoneal space lateral to the bladder should be bluntly developed by extending the dissection from the bladder neck cranially to the dome of the bladder. In benign conditions, incising the anterior bladder wall may facilitate the dissection. The peritoneum should be incised lateral to the bladder in a posterior direction. The ureters can often be identified as the peritoneum is divided and reflected. They should then be dissected from their surrounding attachments, with care being taken to maintain a sufficient amount of periureteral tissue. The ureteral dissection should be continued proximally and distally. In women, care must be taken to avoid the uterine artery during the distal ureteral dissection. When the superior vesical arteries are encountered crossing anterior to the distal ureters, they should be ligated with 2-0 silk ties and divided (Fig. 14.1) to allow for improved exposure of the distal ureter and maximization of the ureteral length. The ureters are then clipped close to their insertion into the bladder and divided sharply. They can be packed away to prevent injury during the remainder of the bladder dissection.

In male patients, we begin our posterior dissection several centimeters anterior to the peritoneal reflection and enter the plane between the bladder (anterior) and the vasa deferentia and seminal vesicles (posterior) (Fig. 14.2). This dissection is continued to the prostatovesical junction using a combination of blunt and sharp dissection. Attention is then returned to the anterior dissection of the prostatovesical junction. The veins overlying the prostate and bladder can be ligated with 3-0 silk suture and divided. The bladder is then drained and the Foley catheter removed. Bovie cautery is used to transect the bladder in an anterolateral direction, and the posterior bladder wall is then divided to expose the previously exposed vasa deferentia and seminal vesicles (Fig. 14.3). The lateral vascular pedicles should be readily visible and can be ligated with 2-0 silk ties and divided. At this point, the bladder should be free and can be removed. The urethra is oversewn with 3-0 Vicryl suture, and the prostatic surgical capsule is oversewn with 0 Vicryl suture (Fig. 14.4). If significant prostatic hyperplasia prevents adequate closure of the capsule, a simple prostatectomy should be considered followed by closure of the prostatic surgical capsule as previously described.

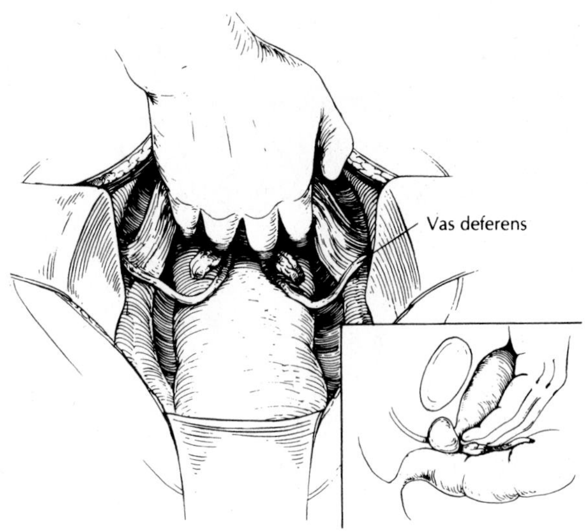


FIGURE 14.2 The plane between the bladder (anterior) and the vasa deferentia and seminal vesicles (posterior) is dissected.

In female patients, the posterior dissection begins anterior to the peritoneal reflection. The plane between the bladder and the anterior vaginal wall is entered and is developed with sharp and blunt dissection. An intravaginal sponge stick is beneficial for traction and identification of the proper planes. During this dissection the lateral pedicles are ligated with 2-0

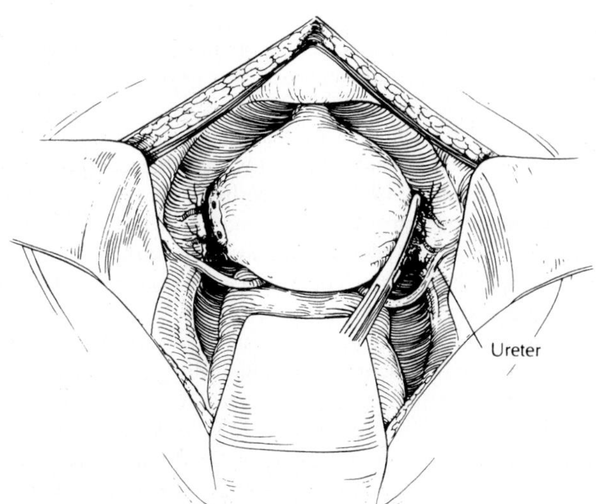


FIGURE 14.1 The vesical pedicles are clipped and divided.

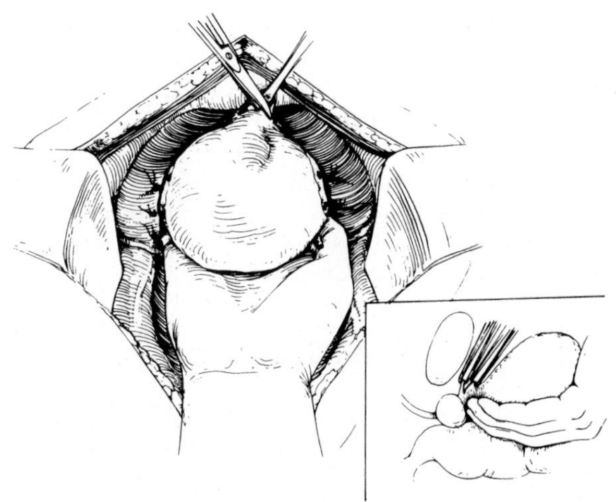

FIGURE 14.3 The bladder neck is incised anteriorly.

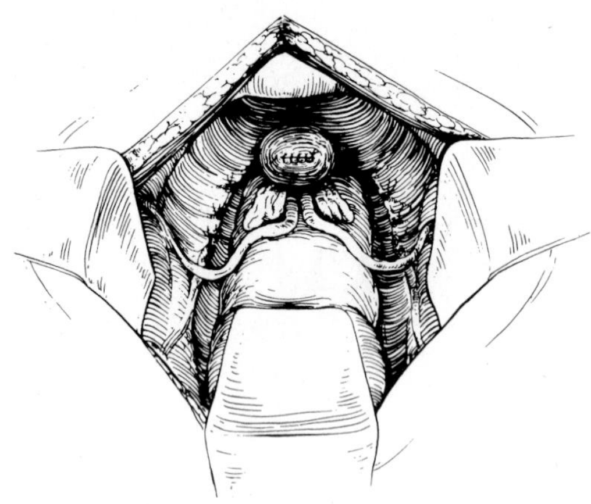

FIGURE 14.4 The bladder is removed. The urethra is oversewn. The prostatic surgical capsule is oversewn.

silk ties and divided as they are encountered. Upon reaching the bladder neck, the Foley catheter is removed and Bovie cautery is used to transect the urethra. The urethral stump is then oversewn with 3-0 Vicryl sutures. Some authors advocate complete urethrectomy including the meatus in patients who have cystectomy performed for interstitial cystitis.

After the cystectomy is complete, the wound is copiously irrigated with sterile water. A closed drainage system, such as a Jackson-Pratt or Blake drain, is almost universally placed in the pelvis because this procedure is frequently performed in the setting of chronic inflammation or infection. Attention is next turned to creation of the urinary diversion of the surgeon's choice.

The abdominal wall is closed beginning with the rectus fascia. The edges of the rectus fascia are reapproximated using a 0 looped polydioxanone (PDS) suture in a running fashion. The wound is copiously irrigated with sterile water. If there is a large amount of subcutaneous tissue, the Scarpa fascia can be reapproximated using a 3-0 or 4-0 Vicryl suture to minimize the dead space. The skin is closed with a subcuticular 4-0 Monocryl suture or skin staples.

### Outcomes

Surgical outcomes are generally very good, although the available literature is limited. One series suggested a mortality rate of 0% with no morbidities directly attributable to the cystectomy itself (2). Likely, the most important aspect of simple cystectomy is the morbidity that is prevented by removing the bladder at the time of urinary diversion. In patients not undergoing concomitant cystectomy with urinary diversion, major complications and hospitalization occur in >50% with >20% requiring a salvage operation (1, 2, 7).

### Complications

For both partial cystectomy and simple cystectomy, the usual risks associated with urologic surgeries exist, including pulmonary embolus, myocardial infarction, bleeding that requires transfusion, ileus, and wound complications such as infections or seromas. The majority of complications are related to the urinary diversion rather than the simple cystectomy itself. Although there are no data directly related to simple cystectomy, the overall complication rate of partial cystectomy is classically reported as 11% to 29%, and the complication rate for simple cystectomy is likely similar.

## PARTIAL CYSTECTOMY

Partial cystectomy is a full-thickness excision of abnormal bladder and a margin of adjacent normal bladder with the goal of preserving adequate bladder function and capacity. Traditionally, this surgery has been utilized in the management of localized urachal adenocarcinoma, an isolated UCC associated with a diverticulum, localized unifocal urothelial carcinoma in favorable locations, or in patients who are unable or unwilling to undergo radical cystectomy. This procedure offers the advantages of full-thickness resection of the diseased bladder in conjunction with a pelvic lymph node dissection for pathologic review while allowing for conservation of the native bladder and preservation of potency and continence.

### Diagnosis

Preoperative evaluation before undertaking a partial cystectomy should include a thorough history and physical examination with a focus on prior pelvic surgeries or procedures and previous bladder pathology. Cystoscopy should be performed with biopsy of the lesion for histological diagnosis. Additional mapping biopsies should be performed to confirm unifocality of the disease and to exclude carcinoma in situ. Both noncontrasted and contrasted CT scans of the abdomen and pelvis should be performed to assist with staging. Delayed images of the urinary collecting system should be performed if upper-tract UCC is a consideration. Findings such as upper-urinary-tract involvement with disease, metastatic lesions, enlarged lymph nodes >1 cm, or other pelvic pathology may preclude utilizing this procedure.

### Indications for Surgery

Partial cystectomy has emerged as the treatment of choice for localized urachal adenocarcinoma. The urachus is an embryological remnant that persists in approximately 30% of the population and is capable of malignant transformation. In this setting, open partial cystectomy or laparoscopic partial cystectomy should be undertaken with *en bloc* resection of the involved bladder with a 2-cm margin of normal tissue, umbilicus, peritoneum, and posterior rectus fascia with concomitant pelvic lymphadenectomy. The 5-year survival rate in this setting is approximately 88% (3).

In the setting of UCC, partial cystectomy is indicated only in highly selected patients with limited disease, patients who are not candidates for radical cystectomy due to comorbid conditions, and patients who refuse radical cystectomy. Selection criteria should include no history of previous urothelial cancer, localized disease that is unifocal in nature without coexisting carcinoma in situ (CIS), and disease that is present in an area of the bladder that is amenable to complete resection with a negative margin. Patients must have a bladder volume that allows for resection of the diseased site with an adjacent 2-cm margin while still maintaining adequate functional capacity with normal compliance. We do not recommend partial cystectomy if resection of the bladder neck is required.

A special circumstance exists in the patient who presents with a bladder diverticulum containing a UCC. Because of the thin, amuscular walls of the diverticulum, these lesions are often associated with higher-stage disease. Additionally, attempted transurethral resection of a UCC within a diverticulum has a higher risk of perforation. For these reasons, this pathology is particularly amenable to partial cystectomy.

Other indications for partial cystectomy include resection of nonurologic cancers in the bladder, including pheochromocytoma, paraganglioma, rhabdomyosarcoma, osteosarcoma, lymphoma, and adjacent tumors that are locally invasive into the bladder, such as invasive colorectal cancer. Partial cystectomy may also be indicated in benign diseases such as a symptomatic diverticulum.

## Alternative Therapy

Any malignant bladder tumor that is removable by partial cystectomy can also be removed by radical cystectomy, although morbidity may be increased. There have also been many advances in endoscopic tools and techniques. Some tumors may now be approached endoscopically via an aggressive transurethral approach or laparoscopically with a simple cystectomy. In regards to urothelial cancer, intravesical agents—including chemotherapy and bacille Calmette-Guérin (BCG) immunotherapeutic agents—have also been utilized to manage some of these patients. Radiotherapy and chemotherapy, alone or in combination, are also alternatives to cystectomy in the setting of muscle-invasive UCC. For many benign indications, simple cystectomy is an alternative.

## Surgical Technique

Antithrombotic medication, pneumatic compression cuffs, or compression stockings should be strongly considered prior to induction of anesthesia. The patient is positioned supine on the operating room table with the anterior superior iliac spines positioned over the inferior portion of the table break or kidney rest. The table is flexed to facilitate exposure, and the bed is tilted slightly in the Trendelenburg position until the abdomen is parallel to the floor. The abdomen and pelvis are then prepped with an antibiotic solution extending from the costal margin superiorly to the perineum, including the penis in men and the vagina in women. After the patient is draped, a Foley catheter is inserted following sterile procedures. The bladder is then allowed to drain completely. At this point, filling the bladder with 150 to 200 mL of sterile water may facilitate the dissection.

An intravenous antibiotic agent should be administered prior to skin incision. A lower midline incision from just below the umbilicus (around and including the umbilicus if for urachal adenocarcinoma) to the pubic symphysis is made using a no. 10 blade scalpel and deepened with Bovie cautery to the anterior rectus fascia. The anterior rectus fascia should be opened sharply, followed by separation of the rectus abdominis muscles in the midline to facilitate entry into the space of Retzius.

Using blunt dissection, the tissues are dissected down to the level of the bladder dome at the reflection of the peritoneum. For dome or anterior tumors, it is possible to remain extraperitoneal; however, for posterior tumors, an intraperitoneal approach is recommended.

## Extraperitoneal Partial Cystectomy

The extraperitoneal space lateral to the bladder is developed bluntly, extending from the bladder neck cranially to the dome of the bladder. The anterior aspect of the bladder is exposed to the peritoneal reflection, which is mobilized where it is readily separable. A bilateral pelvic lymph node dissection is undertaken using the bifurcation of the common iliac artery as the cranial limit, the pubic symphysis as the caudal limit, the genitofemoral nerve as the lateral limit, and the bladder as the medial limit of the dissection. All nodal tissue is dissected and sent for pathologic review. Prudent use of silk ties or titanium clips, especially at the cranial and caudal limits of the dissection, may limit the risk of lymphocele formation.

The bladder is freed from its surrounding attachments, with care being taken to preserve the perivesical fat overlying the region of interest. Blunt dissection is the primary approach, along with judicious use of cautery to minimize the risk to adjacent peritoneal contents. The superior vesical pedicle may be divided to provide adequate exposure of the resection site. This division may be performed with a LigaSure (Valleylab) device or in the traditional manner with hemostats and 2-0 silk ties. Once the bladder is freed, the area of the tumor should be localized with preoperative or intraoperative cystoscopy.

Several sutures are placed some distance from the known pathology. At this point, the bladder should be drained completely to prevent urinary spillage. The free wound edges can be covered with laparotomy pads moistened with sterile water. The bladder is incised using Bovie cautery in an area at least 2 cm away from the expected lesion. The incision is extended to allow for visualization of the pathology. The tumor is excised using Bovie cautery with a 2-cm margin on all sides, and the specimen is removed *en bloc* with the overlying perivesical fat and any adherent peritoneum (Fig. 14.5).

In general, we do not recommend this operation when ureteral reimplantation is necessary. However, in the event that a ureteral reimplantation is needed to complete the partial cystectomy, the ureter should be divided and the proximal ureter reimplanted into the bladder via the Politano-Leadbetter technique or the simple nipple reimplantation technique. A 4-0 Vicryl suture should be used for performing an interrupted ureterovesical anastomosis over a ureteral stent.

Once excision of the tumor is completed and adequate hemostasis is ensured, the bladder can be closed in two layers utilizing a running 4-0 Vicryl suture on the urothelium and a running, locking 2-0 Vicryl suture to close the muscularis layer (Fig. 14.6). Special consideration should be given to the apices of the closure because these are the most frequent sites of urinary leakage after closure. A suprapubic cystostomy is contraindicated in the setting of UCC; however, it can be considered for other pathologies. The wound is copiously irrigated with warm sterile water. A closed drainage system, such as a Jackson-Pratt drain or Blake drain, can be placed in a

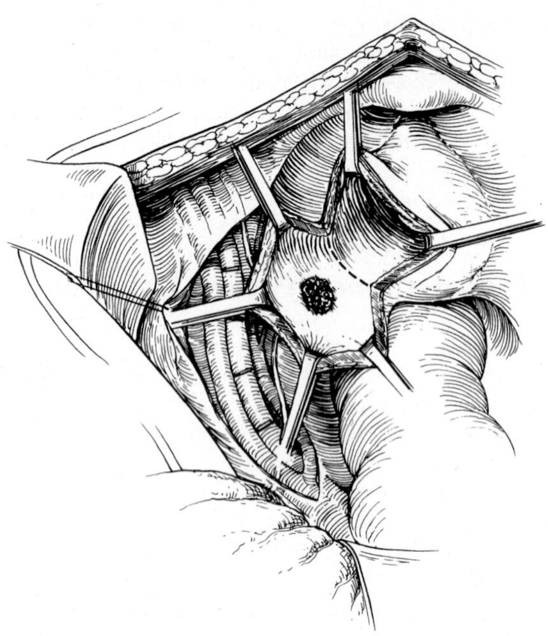

FIGURE 14.5 A 2-cm margin of normal bladder is taken around the tumor.

dependent position within the area of dissection. To minimize fistula formation, this drain should not be placed directly adjacent to the cystotomy closure. The anterior rectus fascia is reapproximated using a 0 looped PDS in a running fashion, and the wound is copiously irrigated with sterile water. If there is a large amount of subcutaneous tissue, the Scarpa fascia can be reapproximated using a 3-0 or 4-0 Vicryl suture to minimize the dead space. The skin is closed with a subcuticular 4-0 monocryl suture.

The drain is removed on postoperative day 2 or 3 or when the output is <30 mL per shift. The catheter is removed on postoperative day 7. If complete bladder healing is a concern, a low-pressure cystogram can be performed.

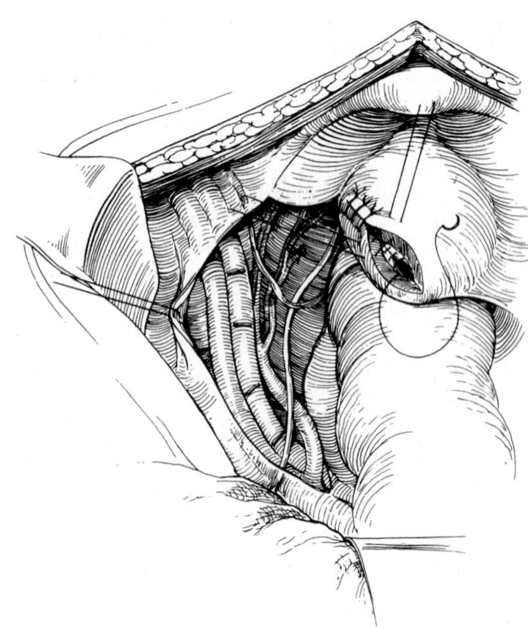

FIGURE 14.6 The bladder is closed in two layers.

## Intraperitoneal Partial Cystectomy

Partial cystectomy through an intraperitoneal approach is often necessary with tumors on the posterior bladder wall. The extraperitoneal space lateral to the bladder is bluntly developed by extending the dissection from the bladder neck cranially to the dome of the bladder. The posterior rectus sheath and peritoneum just inferior and lateral to the umbilicus are divided sharply to enter the peritoneal cavity. The bowel is retracted into the upper abdomen using a retraction system such as the Buchwalter or Omni-Tract system. Trendelenburg can be steepened to assist in packing the bowel away. The peritoneum is incised over the iliac vessels, and the node dissection is undertaken using the same landmarks as described in the extraperitoneal approach. The procedure follows the steps previously described; the posterior aspect of the bladder is freed to allow adequate exposure, and the superior vesical artery is divided as needed. The lesion is located, and stay sutures are placed some distance away from the site of disease. After the bladder dissection is complete, the bladder is drained. The bladder is then incised, and the tumor is excised with a 2-cm margin followed by bladder closure and management of the Foley catheter and drains as previously described in the extraperitoneal approach.

## Outcomes

In modern partial cystectomy series for the management of UCC, outcomes are good, with a 5-year overall survival rate of 64% to 70% and a 5-year disease-specific survival rate of 74% to 84% (4, 5, 8). However, UCC is well known for its high recurrence rates. In partial cystectomy series, recurrence rates range from 28% to 49%, with an approximate recurrence rate of 20% to 25% in locally advanced or metastatic disease. Because of this high recurrence rate, most authors agree that lifelong cystoscopy and repeat abdominal and pelvic imaging should be performed in these patients. Disease recurrence requires aggressive treatment similar to treatment for recurrence with other treatment modalities, including repeat transurethral resection, use of intravesical agents, chemotherapy and/or radiation protocols, and radical cystectomy with urinary diversion when indicated.

The success of partial cystectomy for urachal adenocarcinoma with *en bloc* resection of the urachus, umbilicus, and surrounding soft tissues with negative margins has resulted in an 88% 5-year disease-free survival rate (3). Local recurrence rates are approximately 18% with aggressive resection. Furthermore, a review of multiple small surgical series would suggest no survival benefit to radical cystectomy over extended partial cystectomy with *en bloc* resection, but a randomized trial has not been done.

## Complications

For both partial cystectomy and simple cystectomy, the usual risks associated with urologic surgeries exist, including pulmonary embolus, myocardial infarction, bleeding that requires transfusion, ileus, and wound complications such as infections or seromas. Other more specific complications include reduction of bladder capacity, urinary leakage, fistula formation, and lymphocele formation. Recurrence is a concern and is discussed previously. The overall complication rate of partial cystectomy is classically reported as 11% to 29%.

Of special consideration is the reduction in functional capacity during partial cystectomy. There are no good data to determine how much bladder capacity can be removed while still allowing good function. Preoperative urodynamic testing may be of some benefit in accurately assessing preoperative bladder capacity.

## References


1. Eigner EB, Freiha FS. The fate of the remaining bladder following supravesical diversion. *J Urol* 1990;144:31–33.
2. Fazili T, Bhat TR, Masood S, et al. Fate of the leftover bladder after supravesical urinary diversion for benign disease. *J Urol* 2006;176:620–621.
3. Herr HW, Bochner BH, Sharp D, et al. Urachal carcinoma: contemporary surgical outcomes. *J Urol* 2007;178:74–78.
4. Holzbeierlein JM, Lopez-Corona E, Bochner BH, et al. Partial cystectomy: a contemporary review of the Memorial Sloan-Kettering cancer experience and recommendations for patient selection. *J Urol* 2004; 172:878–881.
5. Kassouf W, Swanson D, Kamat AM, et al. Partial cystectomy for muscle invasive urothelial carcinoma of the bladder: a contemporary review of the M.D. Anderson Cancer Center experience. *J Urol* 2006;175:2058–2062.
6. Lamm DL, Gittes RF. Inflammatory carcinoma of the bladder and interstitial cystitis. *J Urol* 1977;117:49–51.
7. Neulander EZ, Rivera I, Eisenbrown N, et al. Simple cystectomy in patients requiring urinary diversion. *J Urol* 2000;164:1169–1172.
8. Smaldone MC, Jacobs BL, Smaldone AM, et al. Long-term results of selective partial cystectomy for invasive urothelial bladder carcinoma. *Urology* 2008;72:613–616.


# CHAPTER 15 ■ RADICAL CYSTECTOMY IN MEN

MOHAMED A. GHONHEIM

One of the first detailed operative descriptions of radical cystoprostatectomy and pelvic lymphadenectomy was probably provided by Marshall and Whitmore in 1949 (2). In the 1950s and early 1960s, the operation was attended with significant mortality and morbidity. Although more complex urinary diversions are increasingly employed, contemporary cystectomy is associated with very low mortality. Furthermore, the advent of nerve-sparing cystectomy and orthotopic bladder substitution has significantly reduced functional losses and provided many patients with good locoregional control as well as a good quality of life. The technique, herein described, is based on cumulative experience of >20 years during which >1,000 cystectomies were carried out at the Department of Urology, Mansoura University, Egypt.

## DIAGNOSIS

The diagnosis of transitional-cell carcinoma is generally made by transurethral resection of the tumor in the bladder (see Chapter 111). Once the diagnosis has been established, it is important to know the histologic stage, particularly if the tumor invades the muscularis propria. Invasion of the muscularis mucosa is not considered as constituting a muscle-invasive tumor. The clinical staging of transitional-cell carcinoma can generally be performed by abdominal and pelvic computerized tomographic (CT) scans. Occasionally radionuclide bone scans are indicated if there is either symptomatic bone pain or abnormalities on the CT scan, or if the patient has either an elevated serum calcium or alkaline phosphatase.

## INDICATIONS FOR RADICAL CYSTECTOMY IN MEN

The major indication for cystectomy in men is carcinoma of the bladder. In general, the operation is carried out for the following:

1. Patients with superficial tumors in whom endoscopic control has failed in spite of adjuvant intravesical chemo- and/or immunotherapy. Although these measures have proved effective in the management of such cases (<T1), an important minority fail. High tumor grade, multifocal lesions, diffuse carcinoma in situ, and involvement of the prostatic urethra were all reported as high-risk factors.
2. Infiltrating tumor without evidence of distant metastasis. These include tumors infiltrating the muscle layers ($P_2$, $P_{3a}$) or the perivesical fat short of the pelvic wall ($P_{3b}$). Infiltration of adjacent organs ($P_4$) or involvement of the regional lymph nodes is not considered a contraindication for the procedure.

The radical operation in men includes the removal of the bladder, its peritoneal covering, the perivesical fat, the lower ureters, the prostate, the seminal vesicles, and the vasa deferentia. In the standard procedure, as much as possible of the membranous urethra is also removed, and total urethrectomy is carried out only if there is involvement of the prostatic urethra (4).

## ALTERNATIVE THERAPY

Alternatives to radical cystectomy include local therapy, partial cystectomy, intravenous chemotherapy, radiation therapy, or a combination of chemotherapy and radiation therapy. Local therapy in invasive disease generally results in progression of the disease and death of the patient within 5 years. Systemic chemotherapy or radiation therapy is associated with a 25% 5-year survival, though the combination of the two modalities results in significant synergy, with up to 50% 5-year survival.

## SURGICAL TECHNIQUE

### Preparation of the Patient

In view of the extent of surgery and the length of the operative time, a thorough medical evaluation and anesthetic consultation are required.

Bowel preparation is necessary before surgery. If it is planned to use the small bowel, oral neomycin and a low-residue diet are all that are needed. More rigorous preparation with full bowel prep is required if the colon is utilized.

Patients with histories of thromboembolic disease or varicose veins should receive a prophylactic dose of heparin (5,000 U subcutaneously) the night before the operation and every 12 hours thereafter until ambulation. A parenteral broad-spectrum antibiotic is given just before induction of anesthesia and continued postoperatively for 3 days. The region extending from the midchest to the midthigh should be cleaned and prepared on the night before surgery.

### Anesthesia and Instrumentation

Full relaxation of the abdominal muscles by an appropriate anesthetic is necessary throughout the entire procedure. Hypotensive anesthesia would provide an additional advantage and would reduce blood loss.

The choice of instruments depends mainly on the surgeon's preference. Standard retractors of various sizes and curves as well as long curved and angled scissors are needed. Long curved clamps should also be available.

### Position and Initial Exposure

The patient is put in the supine position with a Trendelenberg tilt. Slight bending of the knees would further help in the relaxation of the abdominal muscles, facilitate retraction, and provide a wider exposure. If a total urethrectomy is planned, the patient is put in a slight lithotomy position for access to the perineum.

The surgical area to be sterilized and draped extends from the lower chest down to the root of the penis. A self-retaining catheter is introduced into the bladder and kept indwelling for its evacuation throughout the procedure.

A long, vertical, right paramedian incision extending from the symphysis pubis inferiorly to a point halfway between the umbilicus and xyphoid process of the sternum superiorly is generally employed. Alternatively, a midline incision encircling the umbilicus can also be utilized. For obese patients a lower abdominal muscle-cutting transverse incision is preferred. Under such circumstances it provides a wide and direct exposure of the pelvis.

Initially, the abdominal and pelvic cavities are explored. The growth is palpated, its degree of mobility determined, and its relation to the adjacent structures assessed. The endopelvic and aortic lymph nodes are palpated, and frozen sections are taken if necessary. The general peritoneal cavity, omentum, intestinal tract, kidney, spleen, and liver are thoroughly examined. If the decision is to proceed with the radical operation, the intestines are packed out of the pelvis, and the retropubic space is opened by blunt dissection. Any small bleeders are coagulated. This dissection is extended inferiorly and laterally until the ventral surface of the bladder and prostate are exposed. The peritoneal incision is extended inferiorly on either side of the urachal remnant. The urachal remnant is dissected off its attachment with the umbilicus and clamped. In this manner a triangular peritoneal flap with its apex pointing superiorly is raised and will be removed later en bloc with the bladder.

### Lymphadenectomy

The peritoneal incision, on either side, is extended posterolaterally along the lateral border of the external iliac and common iliac vessels up to the aortic bifurcation. The vas deferens is identified and ligated near the internal ring. The fascia on the iliopsoas is incised and reflected medially. The triangle of Marceille is exposed by retracting the common and external iliac arteries medially and dissecting the space between these vessels and the medial border of the psoas muscle (3). Dissection of the fibrolymphatic tissues in this space will expose the obturator nerve as it emerges from the medial border of the psoas muscle (Fig. 15.1). The fibrofascial sheath covering the distal half of the common iliac and the external iliac vessels is then opened and stripped medially to remove the

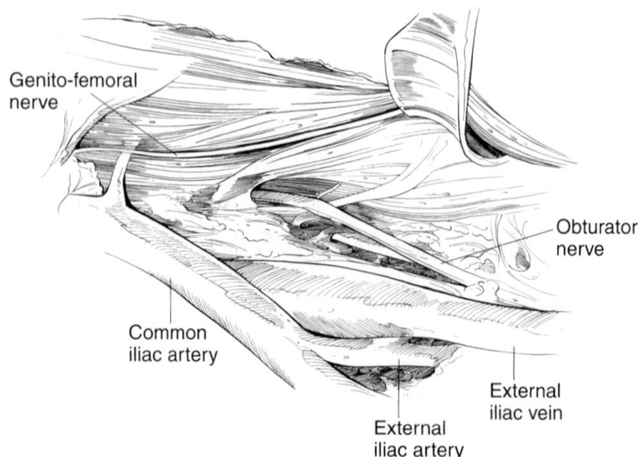


FIGURE 15.1 Dissection of the triangle of Marceille. The psoas muscle is retracted laterally and the iliac vessels medially. The obturator nerve is exposed in the floor of the triangle as it emerges from the medial border of the psoas muscle.

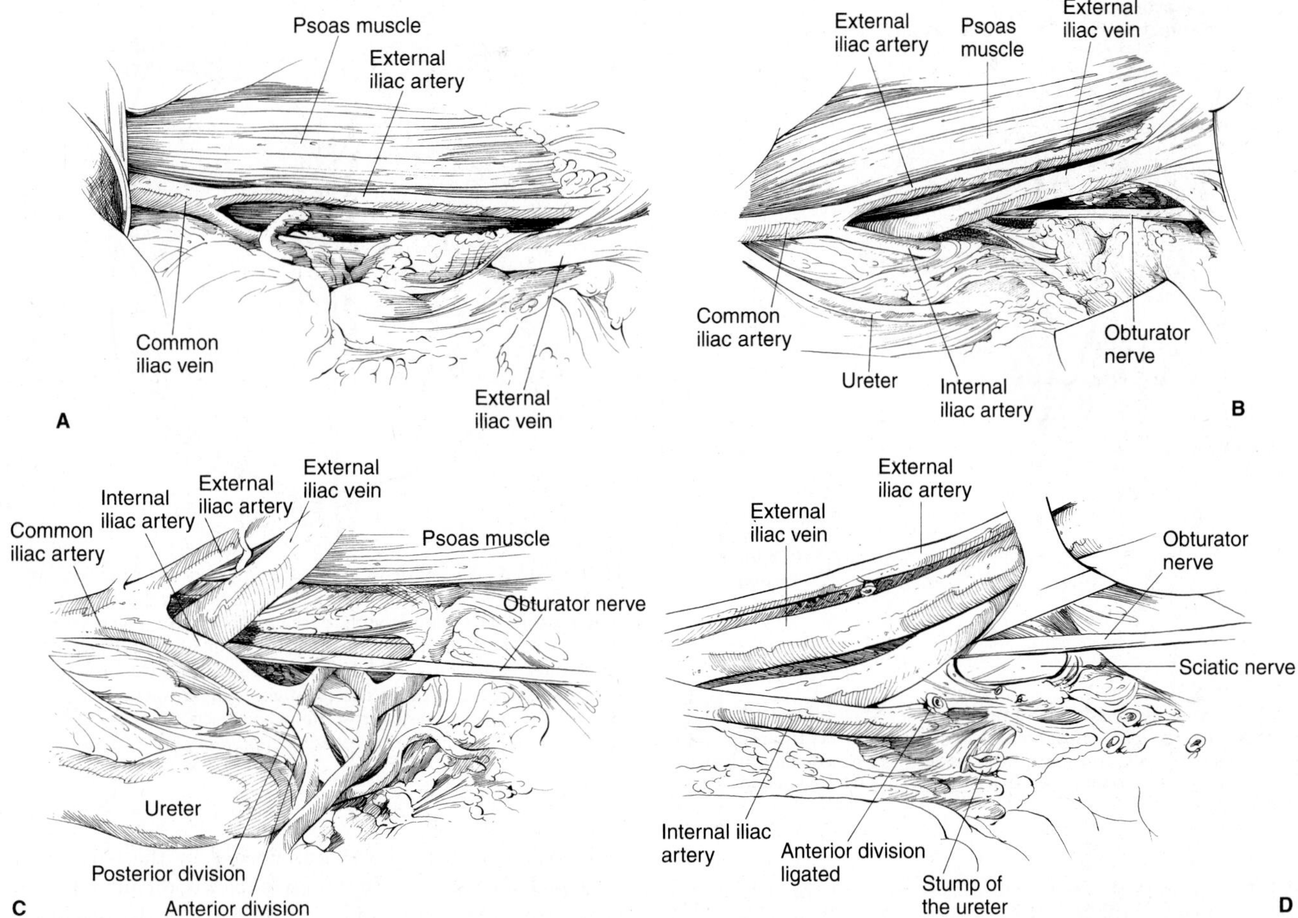


FIGURE 15.2 The lymphadenectomy. **A:** The fibroareolar tissue has been dissected from the anterior and medial aspects of the psoas major muscle. The external and common iliac arteries are exposed and skeletonized. **B:** Further dissection exposes the external vein. The obturator fossa is cleared with separation of the obturator nerve. **C:** Further dissection of the internal iliac artery and its branches prior to their control. **D:** The lateral dissection is completed. The anterior division of the internal iliac artery is divided with control of its parietal branches. The ureter is divided and the ligature on its stump is used for traction.

perivascular lymphatics and lymph nodes. The vessels are gently retracted, laterally and immediately below and medial to the cleaned external iliac vein, and the obturator space is entered. By working right on the psoas and obturator muscles, one can strip all the pelvic fascia medially without difficulty. The obturator neurovascular bundle is included in the stripped mass. The obturator nerve is identified and separated from the vessels, which are divided and ligated as they leave the pelvis through the obturator foramen. Dissection is facilitated and the operating time reduced by the use of electrocoagulation to control lymphatic and small blood vessels throughout the lymphadenectomy.

## Cystoprostatectomy

The fibrolymphatic mass is now reflected medially. The internal iliac artery is dissected free, and its anterior division is divided and ligated. The ureter is identified where it crosses the common iliac bifurcation, dissected free for 3 to 4 cm, divided, and its distal end ligated. While traction is applied on the ligated ureteric stump of the ureter, finger dissection along its posteromedial border opens the space of Denonvilliers laterally. The step greatly helps in the definition of the plane between the bladder and rectum, which will be required at a later stage in the operation. The phases of the lateral dissection are illustrated in Figure 15.2.

The endopelvic fascia on either side on the prostate is then opened by the tip of a blunt pair of scissors (Fig. 15.3). The optimal site for the creation of this opening is a white line marking the fusion of the parietal fascia lining the pelvic surface of the levator ani with the visceral fascia covering the lateral surface of the prostate. A right-angled clamp is used to lift the fascia from the underlying venous plexus, and it is further incised medially until the prostatic ligaments are reached. By blunt dissection, this plane is further developed posteriorly on either side of the prostate. Further anterior dissection is deferred to the final stages of the procedure to minimize the possibility of sudden blood losses from inadvertent injury of the prostatic venous plexus.

The specimen is now lifted ventrally by applying traction on the median umbilical ligament (urachus). The two planes

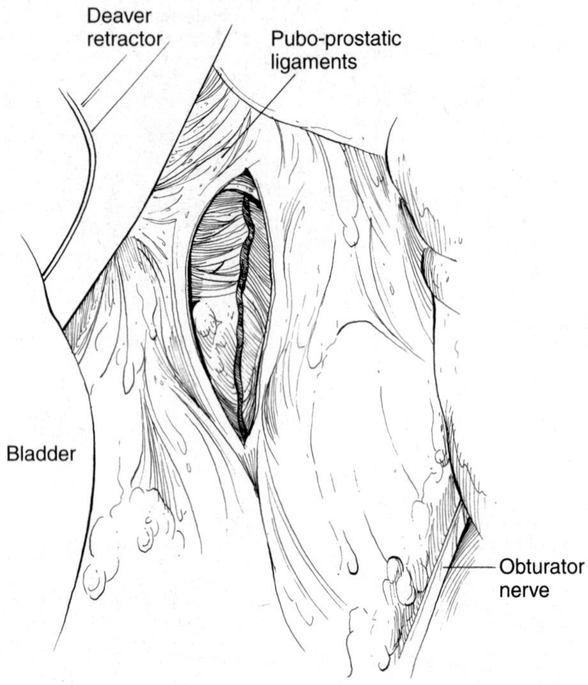


FIGURE 15.3 The bladder and prostate are retracted medially by a Deaver retractor. The reflection of the endopelvic fascia from the ventral surface of the levator ani to the prostate is opened. Blunt dissection would further develop this space and expose the lateral surface of the prostate.

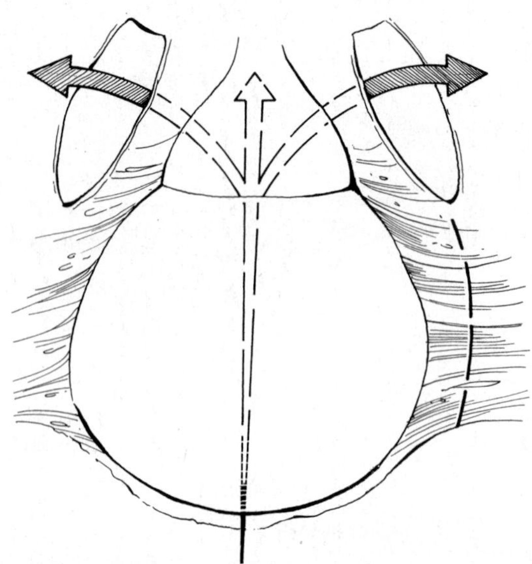

FIGURE 15.5 The cul-de-sac formed by the fusion of the two layers of the fascia of Denonvilliers is opened by the tip of a blunt pair of long scissors. Thereafter, the tip of the surgeon's forefinger would feel the apex of the prostate and the catheter in the urethra. If the forefinger is directed laterally, it will appear through the previously created openings on either side of the prostate. Thus a thick, wide, fascial band is defined (the vesicoprostatic pelvic fascia). It is divided piecemeal between clamps (*arrow and interrupted line*).

developed along the posteromedial borders of the ureter on either side are easily joined together by blunt dissection. As a result, the peritoneal reflection from the anterior surface of the rectum to the back of the bladder could be stretched and safely incised by diathermy. The potential space between the rectum posteriorly and the bladder, seminal vesicles, and prostate anteriorly is opened by blunt dissection (Fig. 15.4). As the prostatic apex is reached, this space becomes obliterated as a result of fusion of the two layers of the fascia of Denonvilliers. This cul-de-sac is opened by the blunt tip of long angled scissors. Once this is completed, the tip of the surgeon's forefinger can readily feel the apex of the prostate as well as the catheter in the urethra in the midline. Alternatively, if it is directed laterally, it will appear through the previously created openings on either side of the prostate (Fig. 15.5).

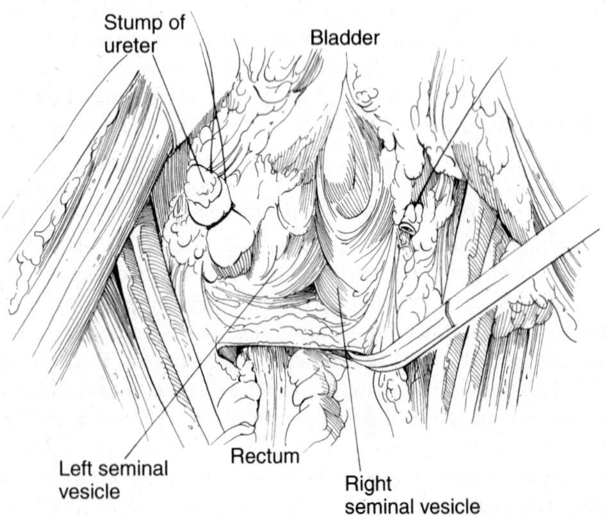


FIGURE 15.4 The peritoneum of the floor of the Douglas pouch is incised by diathermy. The space between the rectum posteriorly and the bladder and seminal vesicles anteriorly is dissected and opened.

In this manner, a thick and wide fascial band is created on either side, connecting the bladder, vesicles, and prostate anteriorly with the pararectal fascia posteriorly (the vesicoprostatopelvic fascia). This is divided piecemeal between clamps, which are underrun by 2-0 polyglactin sutures.

The bladder is now free laterally and posteriorly, and the mass is left to drop in the pelvis. Attention is now focused on the anterior and final phase of the procedure. The puboprostatic ligaments are identified by applying traction on the prostate in a cephalad and posterior direction. These ligaments are carefully severed at the point of their insertion in the pubic bone. The prostatic venous plexus is controlled by one or two sutures of 3-0 polyglactin acid placed near the prostatic apex. A transverse incision is made proximal to these sutures with a long scalpel and extended with sharp dissection by scissors, exposing the urethra, within which the catheter can be palpated (Fig. 15.6). The catheter is then withdrawn; the urethra is clamped and transected; the distal end is ligated; and the specimen is removed. Final hemostasis is achieved by inserting deep 2-0 polyglactin sutures between the edges of the levator ani muscles on either side (Fig. 15.7). No attempt is made to reperitonealize the pelvis. Two tube drains are placed in the pelvic cavity and brought out through separate incisions in the abdominal wall. The wound is closed in layers with particular attention for careful closure of the anterior rectus sheath. This is closed with interrupted sutures of nylon with the knots tied to the inside.

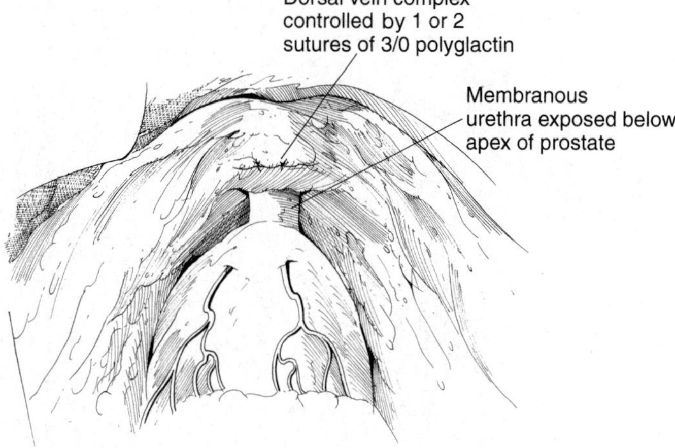


FIGURE 15.6 The puboprostatic ligament is incised and the prostatic venous complex controlled. The membranous urethra is thus exposed.

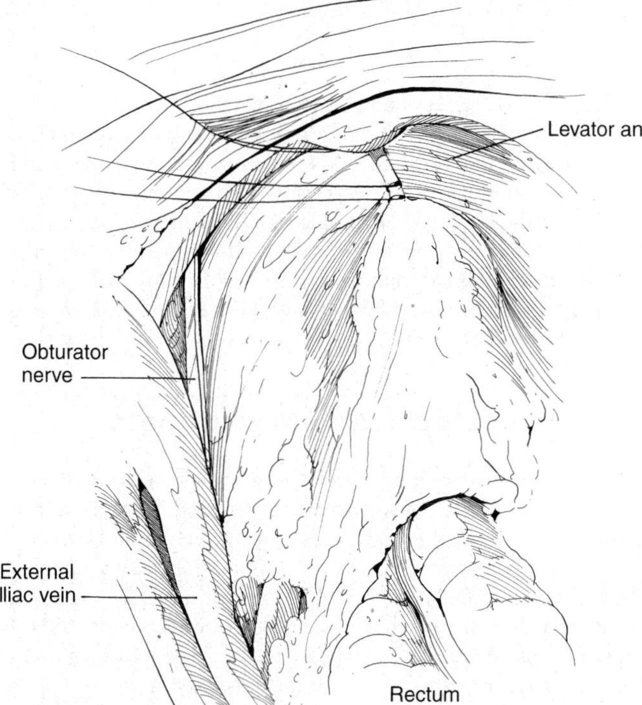


FIGURE 15.7 The specimen is removed. Final hemostasis is achieved by two to three interrupted sutures of 3-0 polyglactin between the two medial borders of the levator ani muscles.

## Variations on a Theme

### One-Stage Cystoprostatourethrectomy

Urethrectomy is indicated in a subpopulation of patients with multifocal tumors, diffuse carcinoma in situ, or tumor involving the bladder neck and/or the prostate. Following incision of the puboprostatic ligaments and control of the prostatic venous plexus described, traction is applied on the cystectomy specimen in a cephalad direction. The urethra is dissected from the urogenital diaphragm with a long pair of dissecting scissors. In this manner, 2 to 3 cm of the membranous urethra can be mobilized. The pelvis is temporarily packed with gauze, and further steps are carried out perineally without urethral transaction.

A midline incision in the perineum is usually employed. The skin, subcutaneous tissue, and bulbocavernosus muscle are incised in the midline. The Foley catheter can now be palpated in the urethra. The urethra is dissected sharply from the overlying corpora cavernosus. Further dissection is carried out in the direction of the glans penis. Traction on the urethra results in inversion on the penis, allowing dissection of the urethra as far as the coronal sulcus. The penis is then allowed to restore its normal position. The urethral meatus is circumscribed sharply, and the glans penis is incised in the midline to allow dissection of the fossa navicularis. The entire penile urethra is now free. The glans penis is reconstructed by a few sutures of interrupted 3-0 chromic catgut.

Attention is now focused on dissection of the bulbar urethra. The relatively avascular tissues ventral to the bulbar urethra and beneath the symphysis pubis are dissected first. Thus, the corresponding part that had been previously dissected in the pelvis can be reached, and the pelvic and perineal exposures joined. Dissection is further developed laterally and posteriorly with control of the bulbar urethral arteries. In this manner the urethra is freed totally, and the whole specimen is removed in one block.

### Radical Cystoprostatectomy with Orthotopic Bladder Substitution

A standard radical cystoprostatectomy is performed except that the final stages of the operation must be done with attention to detail to avoid damage to the urethra and periurethral musculature. The integrity of these structures has a central role in the functional success of orthotopic substitution. Following lymphadenectomy and control of the pedicles, the endopelvic fascia on either side of the prostate is opened by the tip of a blunt pair of scissors. A right-angled clamp is used to lift the fascia from the underlying venous plexus, and then it is further incised medially until the puboprostatic ligaments are reached. These ligaments are carefully severed at the point of their insertion in the pubic bone. The prostatic venous plexus is controlled by one or two suture ligatures of 3-0 polyglactin just distal to the vesicoprostatic junction. A transverse incision is made proximal to these sutures and extended by sharp dissection with scissors toward the apex of the prostate. The catheter is palpated in the urethra, the anterior wall of which is then incised just distal to the prostatic apex. The exposed Foley catheter is transected, clamped, and held for traction. At this point, three stay sutures of 4-0 polyglactin are placed through the urethra at the 3, 9, and 12 o'clock positions, incorporating the mucosa as well as the periurethral musculature (Fig. 15.8). These sutures prevent retraction of the urethra following its complete transection and are used later for the urethroileal anastomosis. The posterior urethral wall is then incised to expose the dorsal fibrous raphe formed by the fascia of Denonvilliers, which is lifted from the anterior surface of the rectum by a right-angled clamp and divided. The divided fascia is then included in two posterior stay sutures at the 5 and 7 o'clock positions for its later incorporation in the urethrointestinal anastomosis.

### Radical Cystoprostatectomy with Nerve Sparing

This procedure was initially described by Schlegel and Walsh (5). It can be carried out in an antegrade or a retrograde manner,

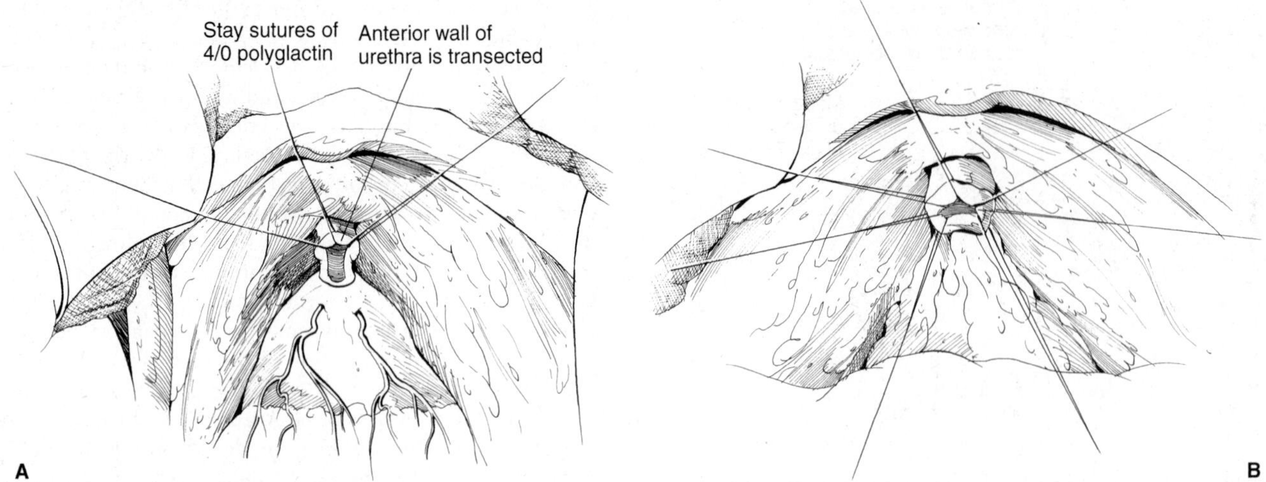


FIGURE 15.8 Preparation of the urethral stump for orthotopic substitution. **A:** The anterior wall of the urethra is transected. Three stay sutures of 4-0 polyglactin are placed through the urethra at the 3, 9, and 12 o'clock positions. **B:** Transection of the urethra is completed and further stay sutures applied. These will prevent retraction of the urethral stump and will be later used for the urethroileal anastomosis.

though in our practice we prefer the antegrade approach. During radical cystectomy there are two points where the neurovascular bundle could be injured: (a) posterolateral to the prostate and (b) behind the seminal vesicles. If the extent of the pathology allows the surgeon to avoid these areas, potency can be preserved.

Bilateral lymphadenectomy with creation of the space between the rectum posteriorly and the bladder, seminal vesicles, and prostate anteriorly is carried out as previously described. By a combination of blunt and sharp dissection, the lateral surface of the seminal vesicles is freed from the medial aspect of the vesicoprostatopelvic fascia. This allows the control of these ligaments at a more ventral plane. As a result, the neurovascular pathway behind the seminal vesicles is avoided. These pedicles are controlled by a series of simple interrupted sutures of 3-0 Vicryl. The use of heavy clamps, clips, and diathermy should be avoided. The dorsal vein complex is now controlled, and the urethra isolated carefully from the adjacent fascia. The urethra is then transected, and the Foley catheter is clamped and held for traction. The prostate can thus be elevated superiorly. A right-angle clamp is used to identify branches of the neurovascular bundle to the prostate. These are ligated and divided, freeing the prostate from all its lateral attachments.

## Prostate-Sparing Radical Cystectomy

Several authors have advocated retaining the prostate in some selected patients for whom orthotopic diversion is contemplated (6,7). It was suggested that preserving the prostate in whole or in part can circumvent problems related to continence and results in the preservation of erectile function. However, serious concerns were raised by other authorities of the possible increased oncological risks following such a procedure. In a review by Hautmann and Stein it was reported that the incidence of prostatic carcinoma in cytoprostatectomy specimens ranged between 29% and 46% and that of prostate TCC between 33% and 58% (8). In a prospective pathologic evaluation of 425 cystoprostatectomy specimens at our institution, there was histological evidence of adenocarcinoma of the prostate in 21.2% of cases and concomitant noncontiguous TCC in 6.4% (9). In view of all of these observations, we feel that the potential oncologic risks of prostate-sparing cystectomy outweigh any small and possible functional benefits. Properly conducted radical cystoprostatectomy with orthotopic substitution should remain the standard for treating invasive bladder tumors.

## Postoperative Management

Intravenous alimentation and nasogastric suction are maintained until normal bowel activity is resumed. Systemic antibiotics are continued for 3 days postoperatively. Chest exercises and physiotherapy to the lower limbs should be carried out. Subcutaneous heparin should be administered if indicated. The tube drains are removed when drainage becomes <100 mL per day. It is advisable to estimate the creatinine content of the fluid to ensure that it is not the result of a urinary leak. Patients with an ileal conduit can be discharged on the 10th to the 12th postoperative day. Following orthotopic substitution, patients are usually kept in the hospital for 3 weeks. Before discharge, a pouchography is carried out to make sure that there are no leaks from the neobladder or from the urethroileal anastomosis.

# OUTCOMES

## Complications

The two most serious complications that may occur during the procedure are excessive blood loss and rectal perforation. Sudden massive bleeding is usually venous in origin, arising from tributaries of the external iliac vein during the lymphadenectomy: the deep circumflex iliac vein laterally and an abnormal obturator vein medially. Since both are located near the inguinal ligament, good retraction, illumination, and suction are needed. A laceration of the external iliac vein is then sutured with 5-0 Prolene.

Another source of bleeding is in relation to the dorsal vein complex. Dissection of this area has to be deferred to the final phase of the procedure. This venous complex is usually injured when the puboprostatic ligaments are incised. Compression of the bleeding area by a piece of gauze (4 × 8) and the tip of a long thin blade of a Deaver retractor is necessary until the dissection of the urethra is completed. Thereafter, bleeding is controlled by one or two interrupted 3-0 sutures of polyglactin acid placed between the two medial borders of the levator ani muscles.

However, the most serious source of bleeding is from the internal iliac vein or one of its tributaries. Sudden excessive bleeding occurs from the depth of a narrow deep recess. Blind attempts to control the bleeding with clamps usually fail and result in more damage. In our experience, one has to achieve an initial temporary control by packing. One or two 4 × 8 pieces of moist gauze are sufficient. The pack is tightly and constantly compressed for a few minutes and then is left in place. The operator should proceed with further operative steps until the specimen is removed. Now, the working space is wide enough to allow manipulations under vision. The ipsilateral external iliac and common iliac veins as well as the main stem of the internal iliac artery are controlled by bulldog clamps. The gauze pack is then removed. There will still be some back bleeding, but with the help of a little suction, the bleeding vessels are readily located and easily secured by suture ligation using 4-0 silk.

The other serious intraoperative complication is rectal perforation. This usually takes place during the final phase of the operation if the space between the prostate and rectum was not adequately and completely opened. Under such circumstances, traction on the specimen will lead to tenting of the anterior wall of the rectum. Sharp dissection with scissors or application of clamps would result in an injury of the anterior wall of the rectum well below the peritoneal reflection. If this injury is recognized, the tear is meticulously repaired. The edges are trimmed and closed in two layers using 3-0 polyglactin acid: the first through and through, and the second inverting as a fascia muscular layer (Lembert technique). An omental flap is raised, brought down to the pelvis, and sutured over the repair for additional security. The pelvic cavity is then thoroughly irrigated with 1% solution of kanamycin in saline. At the end of surgery, while the patient is still under anesthesia, anal dilation is carried out up to three to four fingers to establish adequate decompression. Generally, by following these principles, one can avoid the need for a temporary proximal colostomy.

The postoperative mortality following contemporary cystectomy is 2% or less (10). The most common postoperative complication is prolonged ileus. This is treated by nasogastric suction, intravenous alimentation, and hyperalimentation if necessary. Septic complications, including abdominal and/or pelvic abscesses, wound sepsis, and septicemia, are not uncommon. These are treated by the appropriate antibiotics and drainage of the infected collection. This is best achieved by ultrasound-guided aspiration and/or insertion of a percutaneous tube drain. Wound dehiscence should be immediately repaired by proper closure using tension sutures. Urinary collections (urinoma) are drained under ultrasound guidance. If the source of leak is the ureterointestinal anastomosis, a percutaneous nephrostomy tube is inserted until healing is achieved and checked with an antegrade study.

## Results

Radical cystectomy has evolved as the standard therapeutic modality for muscle-invasive bladder cancer. It can be accomplished with very low mortality, and technical innovations with nerve sparing and orthotopic substitution can provide many patients with a good quality of life with minimal functional losses.

All contemporary series demonstrate that radical cystectomy can result in a substantial rate of cure with overall survival ranges between 48% and 53% (1,11). For low-stage tumors (<P2), the survival could be as high as 75%. With further stage progression, the survival expectancy is decreased. Radical cystectomy with pelvic lymphadenectomy also provides a survival advantage for cases with nodal disease (5-year survival in the range of 20%) (7). Evidence has also been provided that adjuvant cisplatin-based polychemotherapy improves the chances of survival among patients with advanced locoregional disease (12).

## *References*


1. Frazier HA, Robertson JE, Dodge RK, et al. The value of pathologie factors in predicting cancer-specific survival among patients treated with radical cystectomy for transitional cell carcinoma of the bladder. *Cancer* 1993;71:3993–4001.
2. Marshall VF, Whitmore WF Jr. A technique for the extension of radical surgery in the treatment of vesical cancer. *Cancer* 1949;2:424–428.
3. McGregor AL. *A synopsis of surgical anatomy*, 9th ed. Bristol: John Wright and Sons, 1963:99.
4. Schellhammer PF, Whitmore WF Jr. Transitional cell carcinoma in men having cystectomy for bladder cancer. *J Urol* 1076;115:56–60.
5. Schlegel PN, Walsh PC. Neuroanatomical approach to radical cystoprostectomy with preservation of sexual function. *J Urol* 1987;138:1402–1406.
6. Horenblas S, Meinbardt W, Ijzerman W, et al. Sexuality preserving cystectomy and neobladder: initial results. *J Urol* 2001;166:837–840.
7. Vallencien G, Abou El-Fettouh H, Cathelineaux, Baumert H, et al. Cystectomy with prostate sparing for bladder cancer in 100 patients: 10-year experience. *J Urol* 2002;168:2413–2417.
8. Hautmann RE, Stein JP. Neobladder with prostatic capsule and seminal-sparing cystectomy for bladder cancer: a step in the wrong direction. *Urol Clin North Am* 2005;32:177–185.
9. Saad M, Abdel-Rahim M, Abol-Enein H, et al. Concomitant pathology in the prostate in cystoprostatectomy specimens: a prospective study and review. *BJU Int* 2008;102.
10. Skinner DG, Crawford ED, Kaufman JJ. Complications of radical cystectomy for carcinoma of the bladder. *J Urol* 1980;123:640–643.
11. Skinner DG. Management of invasive bladder cancer: a meticulous pelvic node dissection can make a difference. *J Urol* 1982;128:34–36.
12. Soloway MS, Lopez AE, Patel J, et al. Results of radical cystectomy for transitional cell carcinoma of the bladder and the effect of chemotherapy. *Cancer* 1994;73:1926–1931.
13. Stockle M, Meyenburg W, Wallek S, et al. Adjuvant polychemotherapy of non-organ-confined bladder cancer after radical cystectomy revisited: long-term results of a controlled prospective study and further clinical experience. *J Urol* 1995;153:47–52.

# CHAPTER 16 ■ RADICAL CYSTECTOMY IN WOMEN

ALON Z. WEIZER AND CHERYL T. LEE

In 2007, 67,000 new cases of bladder cancer were diagnosed in the United States; over 17,000 occurred in women, with 4,000 dying from their disease (1). Although most urothelial carcinomas are noninvasive, up to one-third of patients present with muscle-invasive disease. In addition, 30% to 40% of patients presenting with non–muscle-invasive tumors will progress to muscle invasion. Once patients progress to muscle-invasive disease, their 5-year survival declines substantially. Radical cystectomy remains the most effective single-modality treatment for these patients and also for those with refractory non–muscle-invasive disease, with a reported 10-year survival of 70% to 80% in patients with organ-confined tumors (2). Improvements in processes of care, particularly at high-volume centers, have led to a reduction in perioperative mortality, further strengthening the role of cystectomy (3).

Historically, radical cystectomy in women has posed several technical challenges and concerns, including (a) bleeding from the paravaginal tissues and venous plexus around the urethra, which can be brisk and tedious to control; (b) an intraoperative position change for the surgeon during urethrectomy; and (c) vaginal reconstruction, which can be complex, requiring tissue flaps to maximize organ function.

More recently, additional challenges have related to female organ preservation. Radical cystectomy in women has traditionally been equated with anterior exenteration, including resection of the bladder, urethra, uterus, ovaries, and the anterior one-third of the vagina. This approach is certainly indicated for extensive posterior invasive bladder tumors at risk for reproductive organ involvement. However, tumor involvement of adjacent reproductive organs is rare, suggesting that the routine removal of female reproductive and sex organs is not necessary to achieve local cancer control (4). Moreover, the increasing attention to preserving quality of life after cancer surgery provides another incentive to spare part or all of the reproductive organs and urethra when feasible and when dictated by the diversion choice.

## INDICATIONS FOR SURGERY

Radical cystectomy is indicated for patients with muscle-invasive urothelial malignancy or non–muscle-invasive disease refractory to transurethral resection and intravesical therapy. While radical cystectomy is well accepted as a standard for patients with muscle-invasive disease, other indications for cystectomy are well supported by the literature.

### Non–Muscle-Invasive Disease

Radical cystectomy may be considered an alternative to intravesical therapy in patients with high-grade lamina-propria–invasive disease, especially in the setting of associated carcinoma in situ with the potential for improved survival benefit. The presence of additional adverse histologic features, such as mixed histology, lymphovascular invasion, inverted growth pattern, or nested variant, should also drive consideration of early cystectomy. Patients with non–muscle-invasive disease refractory to intravesical therapy (bacille Calmette-Guérin) are at significant risk of progression, and repeated courses of intravesical therapy can compromise overall survival (5); this may be due to the 30% incidence of understaging in patients with noninvasive disease.

### Intractable Local Symptoms

Radical cystectomy can be considered in patients with persistent local symptoms related to tumor or intravesical therapy side effects failing conservative management without the presence of invasive disease. This decision requires an active discussion between the physician and patient to balance the risks of surgical intervention with the impact of the symptoms on the patient's quality of life.

### Failure of Other Primary Forms of Intervention

Patients undergoing organ preservation strategies are at lifelong risk of local recurrence. These patients require surveillance and management of recurrence with transurethral resection. While some recurrences can be managed with intravesical therapies, patients with high-grade noninvasive and invasive tumors should be considered for cystectomy. In most series of patients undergoing primary chemoradiation for bladder cancer, 30% to 40% require radical cystectomy for recurrence of disease or intractable local symptoms (6).

# OTHER OPERATIVE CONSIDERATIONS

## Elderly/Multiple Medical Comorbidities

While cystectomy is readily applied to younger populations, the elderly often have limited access to radical surgery and are counseled toward nonsurgical interventions. However, cystectomy is often the best treatment option for invasive bladder cancer in the elderly who are in reasonably good health (7). Invasive bladder cancer is not an indolent disease, and death from uncontrolled urothelial carcinoma is high in the first 3 to 4 years. Thus, for a healthy 75-year-old woman, the invasive bladder cancer is her biggest health risk. Furthermore, the risk of radiation therapy and chemotherapy is substantial, with the continued need for bladder surveillance and the potential need for subsequent cystectomy in patients who have continued to age with progression of their medical comorbidities and of their bladder cancer (6). Improved perioperative care allows cystectomy to be done with a low operative mortality, supporting an expedient cystectomy as the overall safest and most effective approach (8).

## Extent of Surgery

When proceeding to definitive surgical treatment in the female bladder cancer patient, the physician should consider the woman's age, sexual function, and childbearing status in conjunction with her clinical stage. For premenopausal patients with carcinoma in situ, early invasive disease (T1), or anterior low-volume T2 disease, radical cystectomy should be performed with intent to preserve the vagina, uterus, and ovaries, potentially preserving sexual and reproductive quality of life. In addition, we must consider the need to maintain body image for women by offering continent and orthotopic diversions. Table 16.1 outlines our paradigm for the extent of surgical intervention. Indications for urinary diversion are outlined in Section 7 of this text.

# ALTERNATIVE THERAPY

Alternatives to cystectomy include observation, systemic chemotherapy, radiation therapy, or a combination of chemotherapy and radiation along with aggressive transurethral resection of the tumor. These modalities have historically been

**TABLE 16.1**

INDICATIONS FOR SURGICAL EXTENT OF RADICAL CYSTECTOMY IN WOMEN

| TYPE | EXTENT | INDICATION |
|---|---|---|
| I | Cystectomy alone<br>Preserve reproductive organs/vagina/urethra (for neobladder) | ≤ T2<br>Childbearing potential desired<br>Potentially sexually active |
| II | Cystectomy plus TAH[a]/BSO[b] (if uterus and ovaries are present)<br>Preserve vagina/urethra (for neobladder) | ≤ T2<br>Postchildbearing<br>Postmenopausal<br>Potentially sexually active |
| IIa | Cystectomy plus TAH (if organs present)<br>Preserve vagina/urethra (for neobladder) | ≤ T2<br>Postchildbearing<br>Premenopausal; grossly normal ovaries<br>Potentially sexually active |
| III | Cystectomy plus TAH/BSO (if organs present) plus anterior vaginectomy<br>Preserve urethra for neobladder | T2 or T3<br>Posterior wall tumor away from bladder neck |
| IIIa | Cystectomy plus TAH (if organs present) plus anterior vaginectomy<br>Preserve urethra for neobladder | T2 or T3<br>Posterior wall tumor away from bladder neck<br>Premenopausal; grossly normal ovaries |
| IV | Cystectomy plus TAH/BSO (if organs present) plus anterior vaginectomy and urethrectomy | T2 or T3<br>Tumor at bladder neck or urethra |
| IVa | Cystectomy plus TAH (if organs present) plus anterior vaginectomy and urethrectomy | T2 or T3<br>Tumor at bladder neck or urethra<br>Premenopausal; grossly normal ovaries |

[a]TAH, total abdominal hysterectomy.
[b]BSO, bilateral salpingo-oophorectomy.

Source: *Urinary Diversion*, 2nd ed., 2005, pg 191, Orthotopic bladder replacement in women, Cheryl T. Lee and James E. Montie, Table 20.1, with kind permission of Springer Science and Business Media.

reserved for surgically ineligible patients, those refusing surgery, or the elderly. More recently newer chemoradiation regimens have been proposed, even for non–muscle-invasive tumors, in an effort to provide greater sexual and urinary quality of life in bladder cancer patients (9).

# PREOPERATIVE CARE

Optimization of preoperative nutritional status will reduce the risk of perioperative complications. Patients are encouraged to augment their diet with protein and caloric supplements if they have anorexia or significant unintended weight loss. Although some have abandoned bowel preparation in patients with diversions utilizing small intestine (10), the current authors still prefer formal bowel preparation prior to cystectomy. In the majority of patients, preparation consists of a clear liquid diet and either GoLytely (Braintree Laboratory, Braintree, MA) or Phospho-Soda (Fleet Corporation, Lynchburg, VA) solutions on the day prior to surgery. Wound prophylaxis is achieved in the perioperative period with a second-generation cephalosporin antibiotic administered over a 24-hour period.

# SURGICAL TECHNIQUE

## Anatomic Considerations

### Female Continence

An understanding of the female continence mechanism in women is critical prior to creation of an orthotopic neobladder. There are two continence mechanisms in women (11). One is in the proximal urethra, which is innervated via the pelvic plexus that courses adjacent to the bladder neck and vagina. These nerves often are transected during a radical cystectomy. In the middle to lower third of the urethra there is an intermingling of smooth and striated muscle fibers called the rhabdosphincter muscle that is innervated via the pudendal nerves and appears to be the critical sphincter mechanism for continence in women. Because the rhabdosphincter is present in the middle to lower urethra, the entire bladder and bladder neck can be resected in a woman without compromising eventual continence. Complete resection of the bladder is necessary to minimize the transitional epithelium left in situ and thus reduce the risk of local tumor recurrence and also hypercontinence after orthotopic urinary diversion.

### Female Sexual Function

A similar pelvic plexus supporting erectile function exists in both men and women. Anterior exenteration with removal of the urethra has been shown to result in clitoral devascularization with decreased sexual arousal. In addition, resection of the vagina is often associated with disruption of the autonomic neurovascular plexus, further compounding the impact on sexuality. Preservation of all or the lateral portions of the vaginal wall as well as the urethra can avoid injury to the pelvic plexus and may reduce the impact on sexual function (12).

## Anterior Exenteration

Access to the urethra and vagina is necessary during the anterior pelvic exenteration in women. A modified lithotomy position is used with Allen, Lloyd-Davies, or Yellofin stirrups. The vagina and perineum must be well prepared with an iodine or Betadine scrub. An infraumbilical vertical midline incision gives ideal exposure; however, patient habitus or a planned extended lymph node dissection may necessitate an extension of this incision another 2 to 3 cm superiorly. The urachal remnant provides a convenient handle for traction on the bladder (Fig. 16.1). The peritoneum is divided along the lateral umbilical ligaments (Fig. 16.2), and the round ligament is clipped and divided. A self-retaining retractor, such as the Bookwalter device, will maintain exposure. The fallopian tubes and ovaries are present and nonfunctional in this predominantly postmenopausal population and thus are ultimately removed with the uterus, cervix, and anterior vagina. The gonadal vessels and suspensory ligament are divided above the ovaries (Fig. 16.3). The ureters are mobilized with substantial periureteral adventitia to preserve optimal blood supply and later divided at the bladder hiatus (Fig. 16.4). Ligation and division of the uterine and vaginal arteries branching from the hypogastric artery is usually required to accomplish this.

The lateral blood supply to the bladder and uterus is isolated as it courses from the internal iliac artery and vein. The endopelvic fascia and the perirectal "fat pad" are exposed with medial traction on the bladder and ureter. The index finger is used to bluntly develop a plane just medial to the well-defined superior vesical artery, aiming obliquely toward the perirectal tissue. This will isolate the superior vesical artery, which requires ligation. Several small associated arteries and veins are controlled with ligaclips or the Gyrus device (Gyrus ACMI, MA), thus dividing the lateral pedicle under direct vision (Fig. 16.5). Medial traction on the bladder with fingers above and below the pedicles enhances exposure.

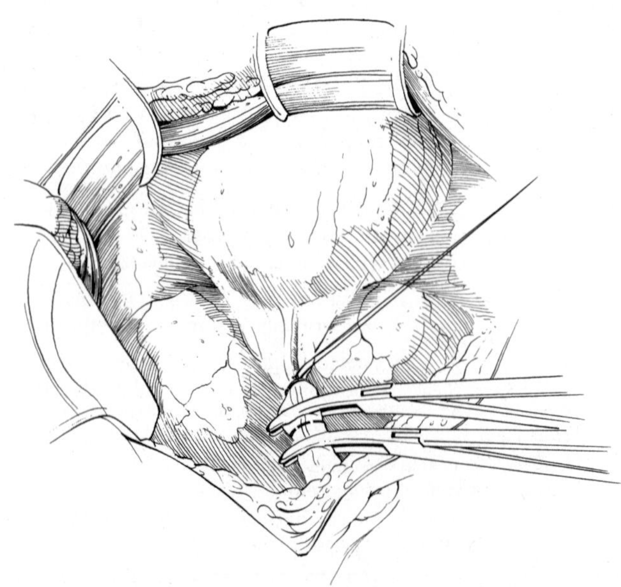

FIGURE 16.1 The urachal remnant provides a convenient handle for traction on the bladder through the case and is divided between Kelly clamps and ligated.

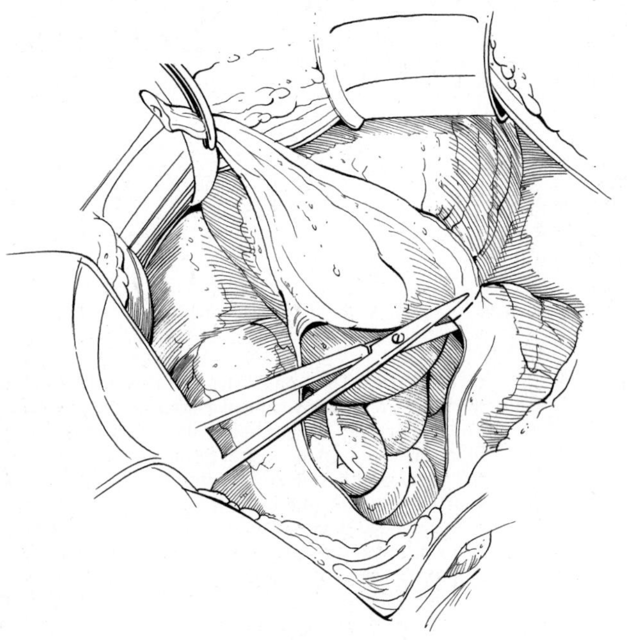

FIGURE 16.2 The division of the peritoneum follows the course of the lateral umbilical ligament until the round ligament is identified, clipped, and divided.

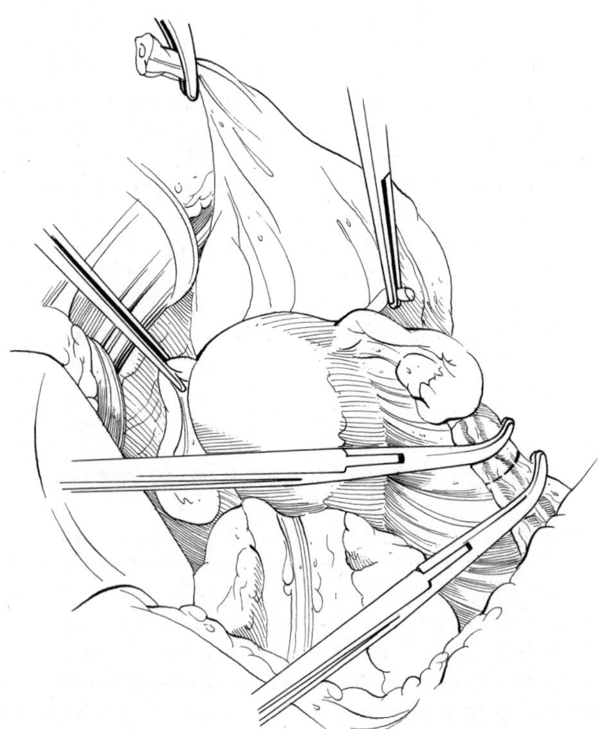

FIGURE 16.3 The fallopian tubes and ovaries, if present, are commonly removed with the uterus and bladder. The gonadal vessels, surrounded by the suspensory ligament, are divided and ligated cephalad to the ovary.

After division of the lateral pedicles on each side, the technique is modified depending on the type of extirpative procedure to be performed. In a classic anterior pelvic exenteration, the bladder, uterus, bilateral fallopian tubes and ovaries, anterior vaginal wall, and urethra are removed en bloc (Fig. 16.6).

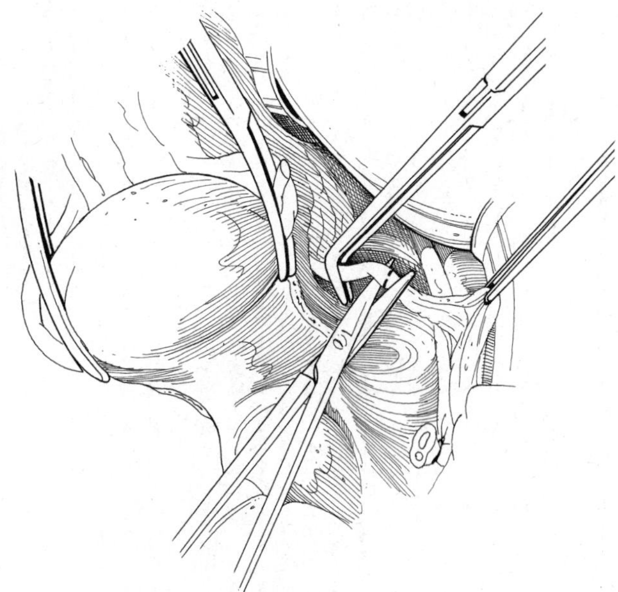

FIGURE 16.4 Each ureter is mobilized with a large amount of periureteral adventitial tissue to preserve optimal blood supply. The ureter is divided a short distance above the bladder.

This is warranted for a deeply invasive posterior bladder wall cancer. Alternatively, partial or complete preservation of the reproductive organs can be considered, especially if orthotopic urinary diversion is planned, as described below. To mobilize the anterior pelvic organs, an incision is made in the posterior peritoneum down to the rectovaginal cul-de-sac. Blunt and sharp dissection in the midline mobilizes the posterior vaginal wall; this mobility will allow the posterior vaginal wall to be rolled anteriorly away from the rectum for vaginal reconstruction.

A Betadine-soaked sponge stick is placed in the vagina, elevating the apex of the vagina just posterior to the cervix. Cautery is used to open the apex of the vagina in the midline; this incision is carried laterally down the anterior vaginal wall on each side (Fig. 16.6A–C). The Gyrus device is useful in this manuever, greatly minimizing venous bleeding from the vaginal wall. Additional bleeders from the adjacent tissue may be controlled with 2-0 Vicryl suture ligatures. This dissection is continued to the bladder neck. If cutaneous diversion is planned, the endopelvic fascia and pubovesical attachments are sharply divided and the proximal urethra is mobilized. Depending on the tumor location, a portion of the proximal urethra can be sharply dissected off of the anterior vaginal wall, which is transected at the bladder neck, leaving a portion of the anterior vaginal wall intact within the pelvis. This preserves a greater portion of the vagina and allows for an easier vaginal reconstruction later. The dissection then moves to the perineum after reasonable hemostasis has been ensured in the pelvis.

## Urethrectomy

To perform the urethrectomy, the labia are retracted laterally with suture ligatures. Army-Navy or self-retaining retractors provide exposure to the urethral meatus. An inverted

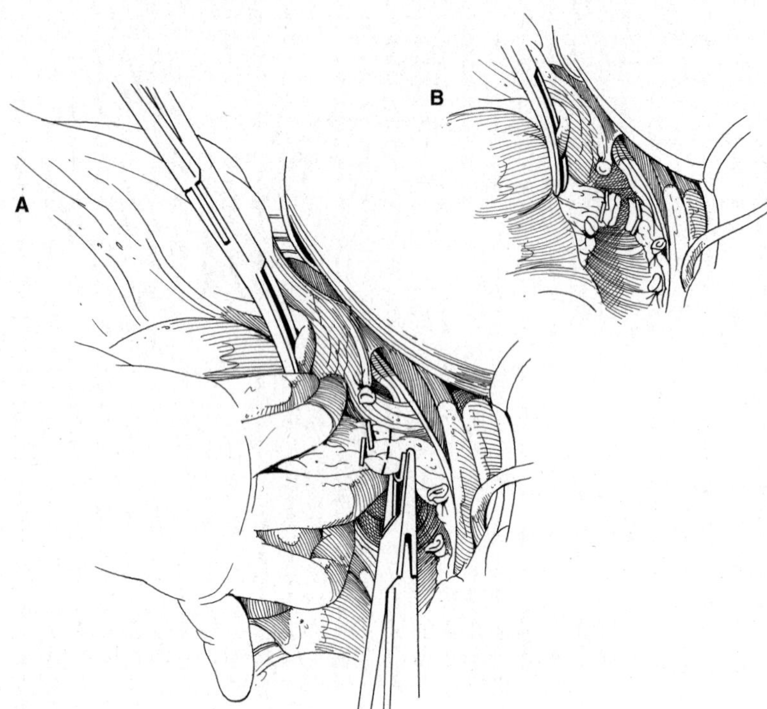


FIGURE 16.5 Division of the lateral pedicle is one of the more important technical aspects of the procedure. The endopelvic fascia should be well exposed with blunt dissection. A perirectal fat pad lying adjacent to the rectum defines the lower limit of the lateral pedicle coursing from the internal iliac vesical. Medial traction on the urachal remnant and retraction of the ureter medially allow an index finger to create a plane just medial to the origin of the superior vesical artery outlining the lateral pedicle. The caudad extent of blunt dissection is the perirectal fat tissue. **A:** The medial traction on the bladder with the surgeon's nondominant hand easily exposes the entire pedicle. **B:** The superior vesical artery is ligated, but the remainder of the small vessels can be controlled with clips on both sides.

U-shaped incision is made around the urethra (Fig. 16.7A), and the urethra is mobilized anteriorly and laterally. Returning to the pelvic approach, suture ligatures are placed in the venous plexus anterior to the urethra, analogous to control of the dorsal venous plexus in men. Further simultaneous antegrade dissection can help to direct the retrograde dissection from the perineum until there is a continuum from the pelvis to perineum. Ultimately, from the perineal approach, the anterior vaginal wall posterolateral to the urethra is divided to connect with the pelvic dissection, permitting removal of the entire specimen. Alternatively, a circumferential periurethral incision can be made, preserving a portion of the anterior vagina located posterior to the urethra (Fig. 16.7B and C). Subsequent simultaneous antegrade and retrograde dissection will allow complete urethral mobilization and excision, as noted above.

## Vaginal Reconstruction

The vagina is reconstructed by rotating the apex of the posterior vaginal wall anteriorly to create a foreshortened vagina that maintains the previous width (Fig. 16.8). A stay suture in the apex of the posterior vaginal wall brings the vaginal wall to the perineum, if a total anterior vaginectomy was required; this flap of vagina is sutured to the periurethral vaginal tissue anteriorly in the midline and then sequentially on each side. After two to three interrupted sutures are placed on each side from the perineum, additional sutures higher up on the vaginal wall are more easily placed from the pelvic exposure. A watertight closure provides optimal hemostasis of the paravaginal tissue.

If the tumor characteristics permitted partial anterior vaginectomy, and a portion of the anterior vaginal wall was preserved within the pelvis below the bladder neck, the posterior vaginal flap is apposed to this anterior stump within the pelvis (Fig. 16.8). The lateral walls are then closed sequentially from within the pelvis with running Vicryl suture. Using this approach, a circumferential urethral incision would have been used (Fig 16.7B), and the prevaginal tissues identified in the perineum would then be sutured to the retropubic tissues with running or interrupted Vicryl suture. A vaginal pack soaked in Betadine is left in the vagina for 24 hours.

## Reproductive Organ Preservation

In appropriately selected patients, all or part of the female reproductive tract can be preserved. Certainly, the age, childbearing status, and sexual function of the patient must be considered when planning radical extirpative procedures (Table 16.1). If the disease is felt to be organ-confined and located favorably, it is reasonable in young women with childbearing potential to spare the reproductive organs, since it is increasingly clear that most female organs are uninvolved by primary bladder cancer and that local recurrence is uncommon (4). When orthotopic diversion is planned in the sexually active postmenopausal woman with a tumor site away from the trigone or bladder neck, the anterior vagina should be preserved.

The surgical approach begins with a similar midline incision as described for anterior pelvic exenteration followed by the development of the extravesical space. The urachus is divided, and peritoneal flaps are developed on either side of the

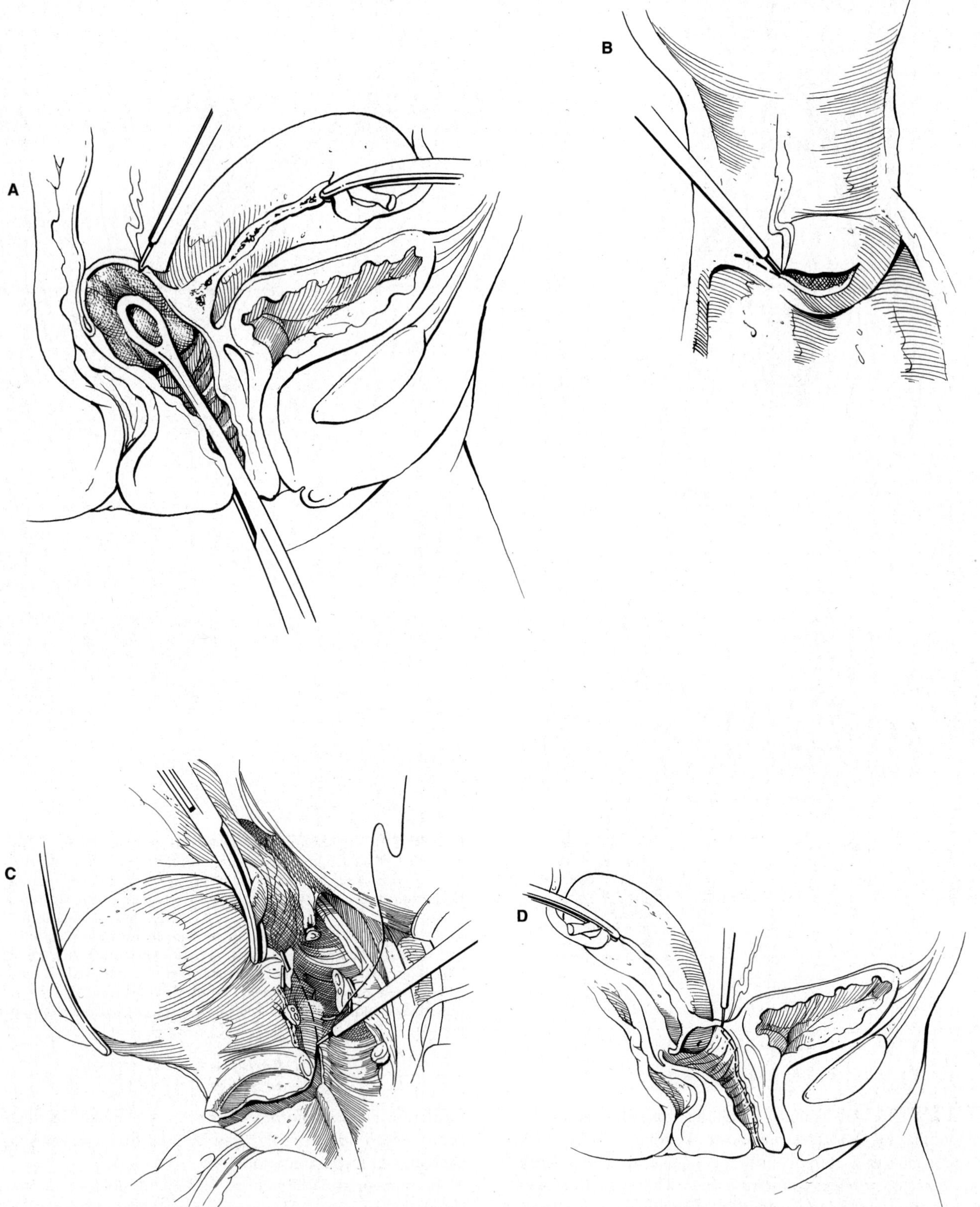


FIGURE 16.6 The classic anterior pelvic exenteration includes removal of the bladder, uterus, bilateral fallopian tubes and ovaries, anterior vaginal wall, and urethra. **A and B:** An incision is made with cautery at the apex of the vagina. This is often facilitated with a Betadine-soaked sponge stick placed in the vagina on upward traction. The incision should be as close as possible to the posterior aspect of the cervix. **C:** The incision is then carried around laterally along the anterolateral aspect of the vagina. There is commonly a rich blood supply to the lateral aspect of the vagina, and this is most easily controlled with multiple suture ligatures in a stepwise fashion. The incision stops just before the endopelvic fascia. **D:** With this dissection, the entire anterior vaginal wall, posterior bladder wall, and urethra are removed en bloc.

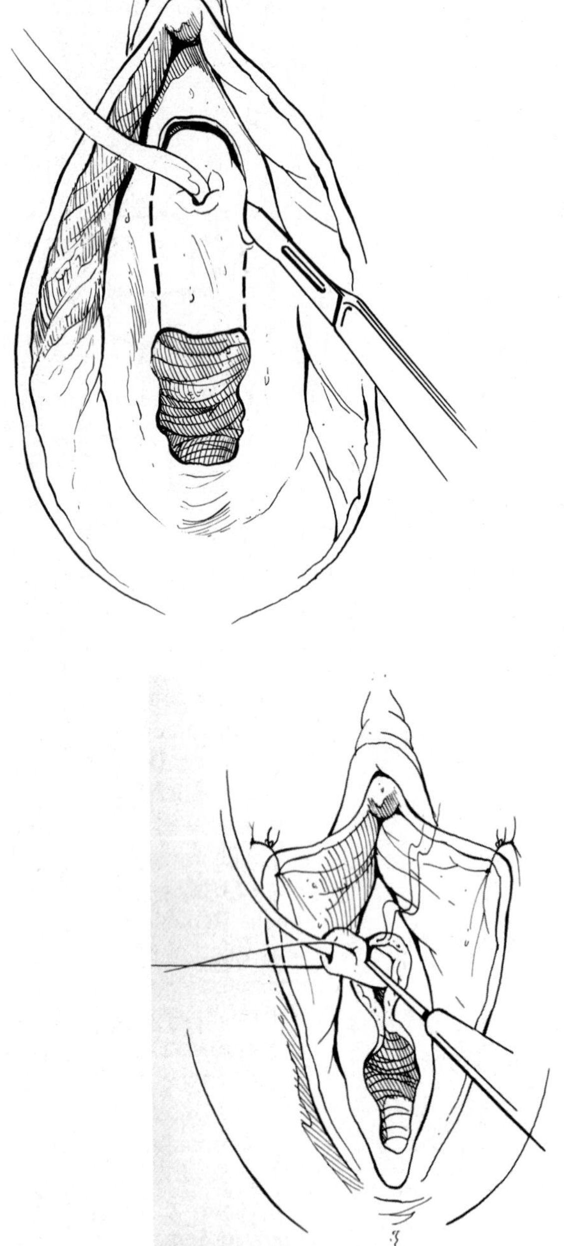


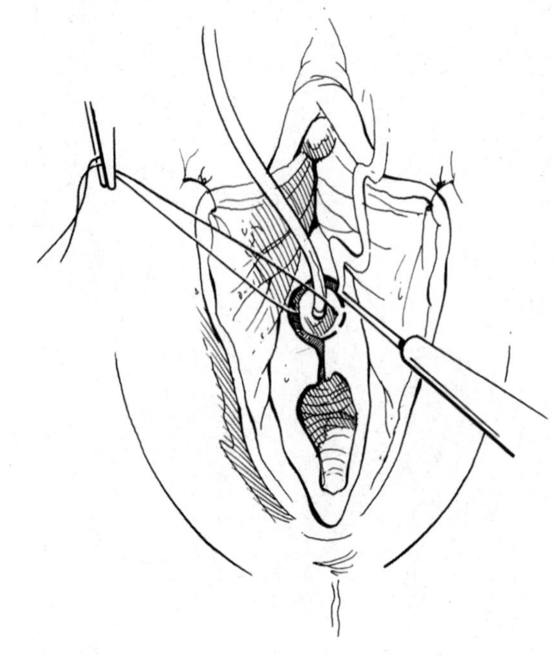


FIGURE 16.7 **A:** Attention is now turned to the perineum, where an inverted U-shaped incision is made around the urethral meatus and the anterior and lateral aspects of the urethra are mobilized. Dissection returns to the pelvic exposure, where suture ligatures are placed in the venous plexus anterior to the urethra, analogous to control of the dorsal venous complex in men. Incisions in the anterolateral vaginal wall are connected between the perineum and the pelvic dissection. The entire specimen can then be removed. **B and C:** Alternatively, a circumferential periurethral incision can be made preserving a portion of the anterior vagina located posterior to the urethra.

bladder. The round ligament is still-ligation, and the ureters are mobilized as described previously. A sponge stick is placed in the vagina to readily identify the vaginal apex and cervix and also to provide countertraction. The plane between the posterior bladder and anterior vaginal wall is developed (Fig. 16.9). This dissection must hug the anterior vaginal wall so as not to compromise the cancer surgery but also to avoid the troublesome bleeding that can be encountered when the dissection is in the wrong plane. An advantage of this approach is avoidance of the rich vascularity of the vagina, which is appreciated when the entire anterior vaginal wall is resected. During this dissection, care should be taken to avoid entry into the vagina, which could increase the risk of fistula formation when orthotopic diversion is planned. In this circumstance, an omental flap can be used to cover any significant vaginal reconstruction.

If appropriate, the uterus, fallopian tubes, and ovaries should be left in situ. This is an optimal choice for the sexually active female with low-volume or early-stage disease who has concerns about future fertility. If hysterectomy is required after vaginal-sparing surgery, a sharp incision is created at the vaginal apex and carried circumferentially around the cervix, preserving as much vaginal tissue as is feasible. The vaginal cuff is closed using 3-0 Vicryl in a continuous fashion, followed by an additional layer of 2-0 Vicryl interrupted Lembert sutures.

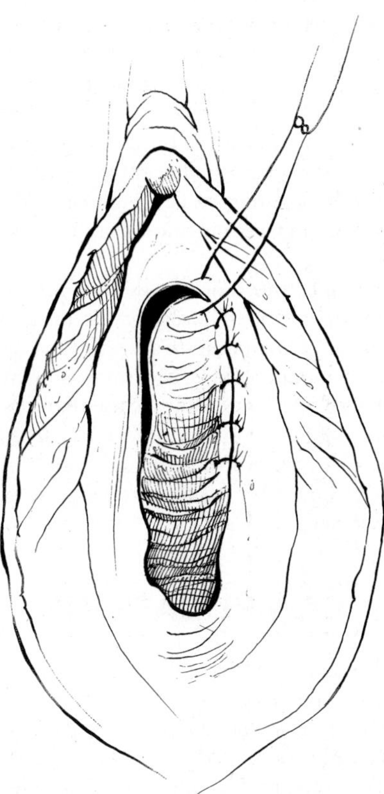

FIGURE 16.8 Several methods of closure of the vagina are feasible. One that appears to supply strong support of the pelvis uses the posterior vaginal wall as a flap to create a neovagina. This foreshortens the vagina but does not narrow it as a side-to-side closure does and thus provides for a better return of sexual function, if appropriate. A suture is placed in the apex of the posterior vaginal wall from above; this is used to bring the posterior flap of the vagina down to the perineum. Several sutures are placed from below, incorporating a full thickness of the periurethral vaginal tissue to the posterior vaginal wall flap. Sutures closer to the apex of the vagina are more easily placed from the pelvic exposure.

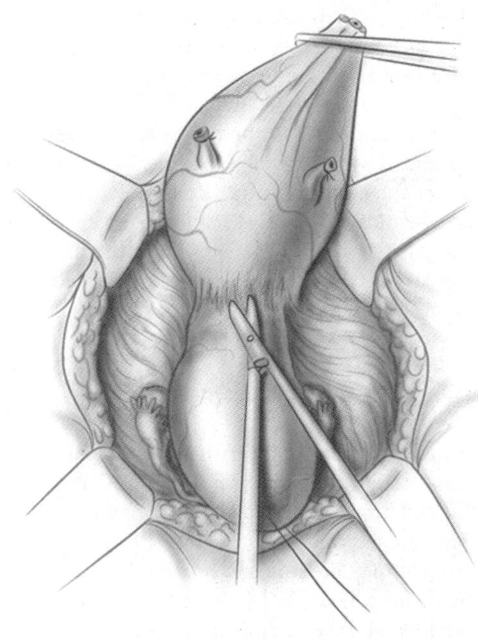

FIGURE 16.9 When partial or complete female pelvic organ preservation is planned with or without orthotopic urinary diversion, a plane is created sharply between the posterior bladder wall and anterior vagina. Care should be taken to avoid entry into the vagina as this increases the risk of fistula formation. Vaginotomies should be closed. (from Lee CT, Montie. Orthotopic bladder replacement in women. In: JE Kreder KJ, Stone AR eds. Urinary Diversion, 2nd edition. Oxfordshire, UK: Taylor and Francis, 2005: 190, with permission).

## Retrograde Dissection and Urethral-Sparing Technique

In planning for orthotopic diversion, modifications in the technique of pelvic exenteration are necessary when approaching the bladder neck and urethra. It is important to maintain the integrity of the endopelvic fascia and thus preserve the support of the external sphincter. Dissection of the lateral wall of the vagina should also be avoided to prevent injury to the neurogenic innervation of the rhabdoid sphincter. Lastly, the bladder neck must be removed entirely to minimize postoperative urinary retention.

Once the bladder has been mobilized off the vagina down to the bladder neck, fine sutures are used anteriorly in the periurethral tissue as necessary for hemostasis of the venous plexus. The urethra is amputated sharply at the junction with the bladder neck, avoiding distal mobilization or dissection of the urethra (Fig. 16.10). After the bladder has been removed, a sample of the urethra is circumferentially excised from the specimen or the urethral stump (if necessary) and sent for frozen section to ensure a negative urethral margin. Exposure is often ideal for the enterourethral anastomosis. The authors prefer six to eight fine absorbable sutures using 2-0 to 3-0 Monocryl, taking small bites on the urethra. Mobility of the intestinal reservoir to the urethra is generally not a problem in women, although it can be in men.

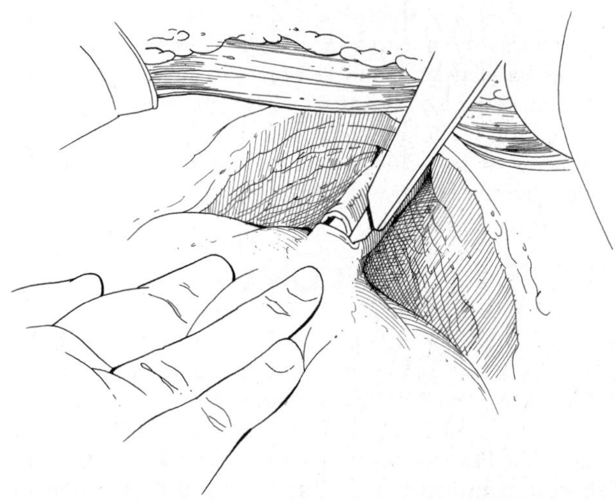

FIGURE 16.10 In the situation in which an orthotopic diversion is planned, neither the endopelvic fascia nor the anterior venous plexus is disturbed. An incision is made in the anterior urethra just distal to the junction with the bladder neck. The urethra is divided completely, and the dissection of the bladder off the anterior vaginal wall can be done in either an antegrade or retrograde fashion.

In the initial experience with orthotopic diversion, the concern for stress incontinence was such that anterior urethral fixation sutures were placed to prevent hypermobility of the urethra. This maneuver is not only unnecessary (unless documented stress incontinence from hypermobility is evident preoperatively) but is also counterproductive by contributing to increased urinary retention or "hypercontinence." A possible additional mechanism for postoperative urinary retention may be exacerbation of a pre-existing but previously insignificant cystocele. After the cystectomy, the urethra is fixed anteriorly and the patient voids by Valsalva maneuver after relaxing the external sphincter. If a cystocele is present, the increased abdominal pressure needed for voiding across the fixed urethra and bladder neck could be blunted by the cystocele.

### Postoperative Care

Establishment of a critical care pathway is useful for cystectomy patients (8). Compliance with the ideal postoperative course is difficult after cystectomy because of a high frequency of comorbid disease and complications, which may delay discharge even if they are not life-threatening. Epidural analgesia, patient-controlled analgesia, and nonsteroidal anti-inflammatory agents are useful adjuncts to provide better postoperative pain control, which translates into better pulmonary hygiene, ambulation, and return of bowel function. The authors no longer routinely utilize nasogastric decompression postoperatively, though it can be helpful intraoperatively. Overall, excellent pain control, judicious use of diuretics to combat fluid retention, and aggressive pulmonary toilet are important strategies to prevent complications. Early ambulation, intermittent compression stockings, and 5000 U of subcutaneous heparin sulfate are currently used for deep venous thrombosis prophylaxis. Routine perioperative parenteral nutrition is not necessary in the well-nourished patient; however, the clinician should consider this therapy in the early postoperative period for nutritionally debilitated patients or those likely to have prolonged ileus. In our experience, approximately 10% to 20% of patients need postoperative nutritional support.

## OUTCOMES

From July 1995 through January 2008, we have performed 1,058 cystectomies; 240 (23%) patients were women. The median age in women was 70 years old. For us, age has not been a deterrent to providing definitive treatment in a patient with a reasonable life expectancy. This is reflected by the fact that 40% of patients undergoing cystectomy at our institution are over 70 years of age, including 8% of patients over 80 years. In addition, 35% of our patients are obese (body mass index >30 kg per m$^2$), and 38% of patients have an American Society of Anesthesiologists class of 3 or higher, suggesting greater operative risk. Adding to the patient complexity are the 30% of patients receiving neoadjuvant systemic chemotherapy (most frequently consisting of gemcitabine, carboplatin, and paclitaxel), which impacts nutritional status prior to surgical intervention.

Our median operative time was 6 hours for women, which is comparable to the operative time for men; this time included anesthetic induction and reversal. Our median length of stay for women undergoing cystectomy is 8 days, reflecting our willingness to offer cystectomy to an often medically complex group of patients. Urinary diversion consisted of 57% ileal conduit, 40% orthotopic neobladder, and 3% cutaneous continent diversion, reflecting our growing use of orthotopic diversion in women.

## COMPLICATIONS

Cystectomy remains a difficult operation in men or women, with a mortality rate of 2% to 3%. Twenty percent to 30% of patients will have a complication delaying discharge. Many of the specific complications after cystectomy are a consequence of the urinary diversion. Complications from the cystectomy portion include bleeding with subsequent coagulation abnormalities and rectal injury. Pelvic bleeding can be more difficult to control in women. Since 1995, the median blood loss in women has been 1,011 cc. A rectal injury should be extremely rare in women and seen only in association with prior surgery or radiation therapy. The most frequent complications experienced in our female cystectomy series were prolonged ileus in 15% of patients, anemia in 9%, incisional complications in 5%, and dehydration or failure to thrive in 5%. Thirty-day mortality was under 1%.

The postoperative care after cystectomy requires a diligence over and above that seen with other urologic procedures. Some complications are preventable. A regimented, reproducible plan for the technique of cystectomy and diversion is enormously helpful to prevent errors during a 4- to 6-hour operation. Some complications are unavoidable, but recognition early in their evolution may drastically minimize the negative consequences, and a high index of suspicion is essential. Early recognition of a complication may prevent a cascade of other successive complications that may ultimately lead to increased morbidity or mortality.

## *References*


1. Jemal A, Siegel R, Ward E, et al. Cancer statistics, 2007. *CA Cancer J Clin* 2007;57(1):43–66.
2. Hautmann RE, Gschwend JE, de Petriconi RC, et al. Cystectomy for transitional cell carcinoma of the bladder: results of a surgery only series in the neobladder era. *J Urol* 2006;176(2):486–492; discussion 491–492.
3. Hollenbeck BK, Wei Y, Birkmeyer JD. Volume, process of care, and operative mortality for cystectomy for bladder cancer. *Urology* 2007;69(5): 871–875.
4. Chen ME, Pisters LL, Malpica A, et al. Risk of urethral, vaginal and cervical involvement in patients undergoing radical cystectomy for bladder cancer: results of a contemporary cystectomy series from M. D. Anderson Cancer Center. *J Urol* 1997;157(6):2120–2123.
5. Lambert EH, Pierorazio PM, Benson MC, et al. The increasing use of intravesical therapies for stage T1 bladder cancer coincides with decreasing survival after cystectomy. *BJU Int* 2007;100(1):33–36.
6. Holmang S, Borghede G. Early complications and survival following short-term palliative radiotherapy in invasive bladder cancer. *J Urol* 1996; 155(1):100–102.
7. Clark PE, Stein JP, Groshen SG, et al. Radical cystectomy in the elderly: comparison of clinical outcomes between younger and older patients. *Cancer* 2005;104(1):36–43.
8. Chang SS, Cookson MS, Baumgartner RG, et al. Analysis of early complications after radical cystectomy: results of a collaborative care pathway. *J Urol* 2002;167(5):2012–2016.

9. Weiss C, Wolze C, Engehausen DG, et al. Radiochemotherapy after transurethral resection for high-risk T1 bladder cancer: an alternative to intravesical therapy or early cystectomy? *J Clin Oncol* 2006;24(15): 2318–2324.
10. Shafii M, Murphy DM, Donovan MG, et al. Is mechanical bowel preparation necessary in patients undergoing cystectomy and urinary diversion? *BJU Int* 2002;89(9):879–881.
11. Colleselli K, Stenzl A, Eder R, et al. The female urethral sphincter: a morphological and topographical study. *J Urol* 1998;160(1):49–54.
12. Raina R, Pahlajani G, Khan S, et al. Female sexual dysfunction: classification, pathophysiology, and management. *Fertil Steril* 2007;88(5):1273–1284.

# CHAPTER 17 ■ BLADDER DIVERTICULECTOMY

MICHAEL S. COOKSON AND SAM S. CHANG

A bladder diverticulum is the protrusion or herniation of the bladder mucosa through the detrusor muscle fibers as a result of a structural defect in the bladder or as a secondary change due to chronic dysfunctional voiding (8). The wall of the diverticulum is composed of the following layers from inside out: mucosa, subepithelial connective tissue or lamina propria, isolated and thin muscle fibers, and adventitial tissue (Figs. 17.1 and 17.2) (7). Diverticula may be congenital or acquired, the latter developing secondary to increased intravesical pressure (5,8). The most frequent causes of increased bladder voiding pressure and the eventual formation of an acquired diverticulum are benign prostatic hyperplasia, urethral strictures, contracture of the bladder neck or urethral valves, and neurogenic voiding dysfunction, such as detrusor–sphincteric dyssynergy. The diverticula are located in the weakest points of the bladder, such as the ureteral hiatus (paraureteral or Hutch diverticulum) and both posterolateral walls (2,3,5,8).

## DIAGNOSIS

Congenital diverticula are more common in men than in women, and while they may be discovered incidentally in adulthood, the peak incidence is <10 years of age (2,8). In contrast, acquired diverticula have a peak incidence of >60 years of age and are almost exclusively found in men (5). Acquired bladder diverticula are commonly asymptomatic, although irritative and/or obstructive voiding symptoms, pelvic pain, and hematuria may arise from complications thereof, including infection, stones, obstruction, and tumor.

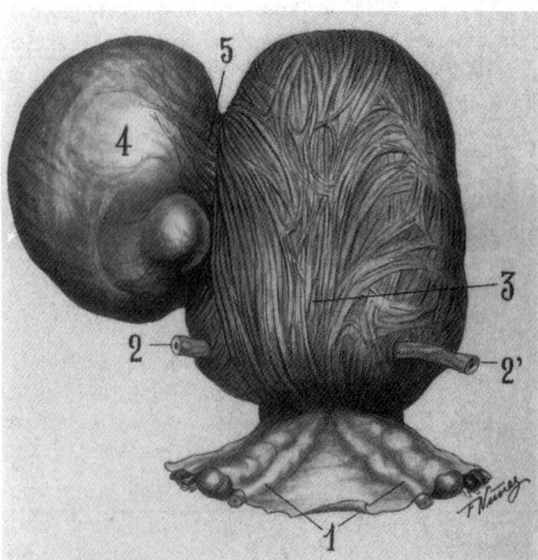


FIGURE 17.1 Posterior view of bladder and diverticulum: ampulla of vas deferens (1); ureters (2 and 2′); posterior longitudinal bundle of the outer layer of the detrusor (3); diverticulum (4); circular fibers of the middle layer of the detrusor around the diverticular neck (5).

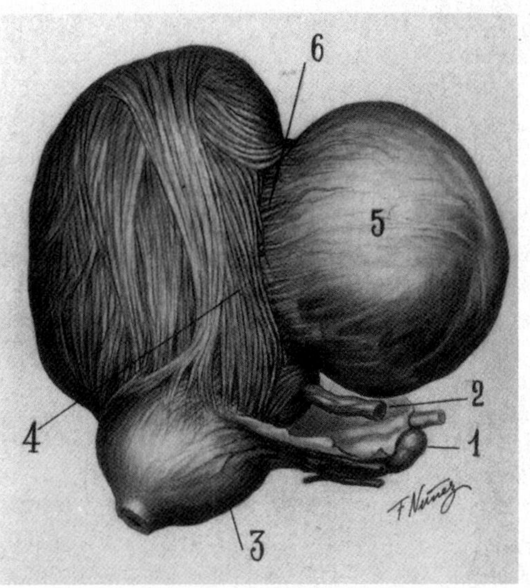


FIGURE 17.2 Lateral view of bladder and diverticulum: seminal vesical (1); ureter (2); prostate (3); anterolateral longitudinal fibers of the outer layer of the detrusor (4); diverticulum (5); fine, circularly oriented fibers around the diverticular neck (6).

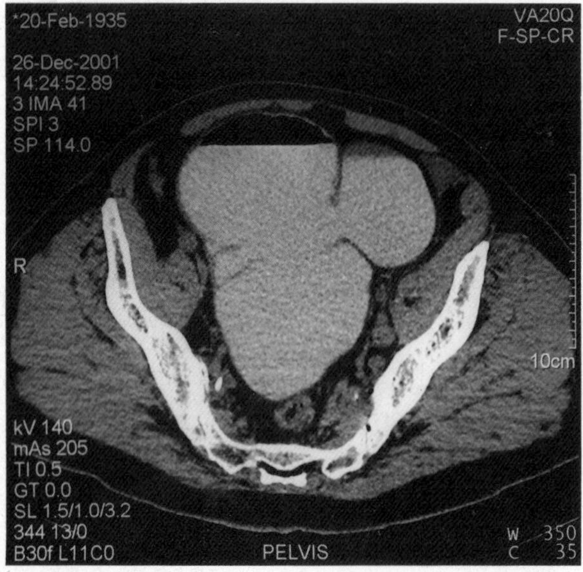


A

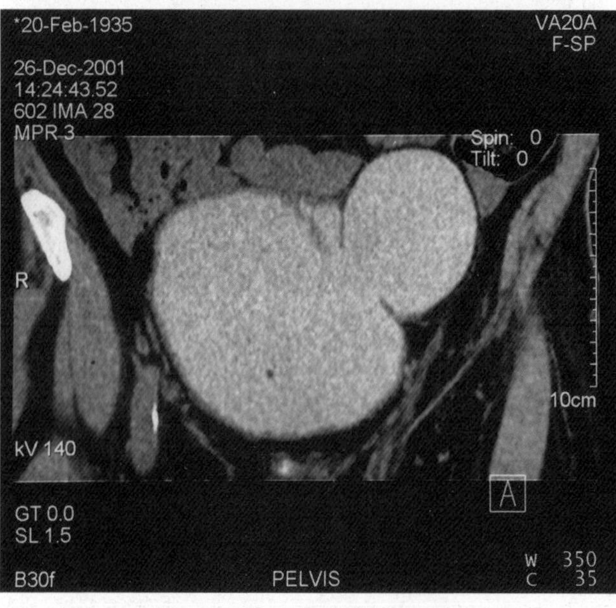


B

FIGURE 17.3 Contrast-enhanced computerized tomography scan demonstrating a large posteriorly based bladder diverticulum seen on (A) transverse and (B) sagittal images.

Given the nonspecific nature of the presenting symptoms, diverticula are most commonly diagnosed by radiographic imaging, including ultrasound, intravenous pyelogram (IVP), voiding cystourethrogram (VCUG), and contrast-enhanced computerized tomography (CT scan) (Fig. 17.3). Diverticula are also found on ultrasound of an empty and full bladder performed for the study of bladder outlet obstructive symptoms in men or repeated urinary infections in women. Cystograms obtained by IVP or through retrograde instillation of contrast medium may provide information with regard to the number, location, size, and urinary retention volume of the diverticulum. However, a VCUG with lateral, oblique, and postvoid images is important in defining the extent of the diverticulum and of particular use in congenital cases to rule out possible vesicoureteral reflux (2,8). A video urodynamics study can provide not only important anatomic information but also information regarding bladder function and voiding pressure, which may be of special interest in cases where neurogenic voiding dysfunction is suspected (8).

Cystourethroscopy should be performed to exclude urethral stricture disease and/or bladder neck contractures but is most important to rule out occult pathology such as a stone or carcinoma within the diverticulum (1). The entire surface of the diverticulum should be visualized, and the relative location of the ureteral orifices should be noted to assist in planning for any potential surgical procedure. The differential diagnosis includes "pseudodiverticular" images observed in cystograms such as bladder ears, hourglass bladder, and vesical hernias. Other diagnoses include urachal cysts, prostatic utricle cysts, or müllerian duct cysts and blind-ending bifid ureters. Other less frequent congenital anomalies should also be considered, such as vesicourachal diverticulum, incomplete bladder duplication, and septation of the bladder (2).

## INDICATIONS FOR SURGERY

Patients who have poor bladder emptying after relief of obstruction or who are unable or unwilling to undergo surgical treatment of the bladder diverticulum may be effectively treated with clean intermittent catheterization (CIC) or an indwelling catheter (8). In such patients, and in the absence of future complicating factors, surveillance of the bladder diverticulum and monitoring of the upper tracts, including renal function, may be all that is required. Importantly, long-term CIC and periodic renal ultrasound may be a viable option in these patients.

In general, the indications for surgical intervention include chronic infections, stones, and premalignant changes such as dysplasia or carcinoma in situ and frank carcinoma (8). A large diverticulum may be the cause of deficient voiding and chronic urinary infection or obstruction of the ureter and even of the posterior urethra in children, whereas a paraureteral or hiatal diverticulum is usually associated with different degrees of reflux (4,5). In addition, spontaneous diverticular rupture or complications related to the size or location of the diverticulum are indications for surgery. With the aim of improving functional voiding, we recommend the simultaneous resection of all poorly emptying bladder diverticula if the patient must undergo open prostatectomy, cystolithotomy, ureteroneocystostomy, or YV-plasty of the bladder neck. Similarly, a vesical diverticulum should never be operated on without previously or simultaneously correcting the cause, whether anatomic or functional (neurogenic bladder), of the outlet obstruction that provoked it.

Although occurring in a small subset of these patients (0.8% to 10%), urothelial carcinoma can develop within bladder diverticula at a mean age of 65 years (range, 45 to 80) (1). Approximately 75% to 80% of these tumors are urothelial carcinoma, while 20% to 25% are squamous cell carcinomas likely induced from chronic stasis of urine and infection. Because of this potential malignant risk and the fact that these tumors can be difficult to diagnose, some have advocated prophylactic diverticulectomy. Alternatively, a more conservative strategy may be offered that should include surveillance cystoscopy and urinary cytology obtained at 6- to 12-month intervals.

## ALTERNATIVE THERAPY

Many children with congenital diverticula who are asymptomatic do not require therapy, and a conservative approach has been advocated (2). Saccules and small diverticula may be treated successfully by electrocoagulation of their mucosa when the primary obstructive disease is endoscopically resolved. In addition, laparoscopic approaches to bladder diverticulum may be effective as an alternative to open surgery with the distinct advantage of shortened convalescence time (6).

## PREOPERATIVE ASSESSMENT

Aside from the laparoscopic approach, there are essentially two methods of surgical therapy: (a) transurethral resection of the diverticular neck and (b) open diverticulectomy. In either case, infection must be adequately treated prior to surgery. If the lesion is acquired due to obstruction, the obstruction must be relieved prior to repair of the diverticula to prevent recurrence and subsequent treatment failure (9). If the diverticulum is due to high detrusor pressure of neurological origin, this must also be addressed prior to surgical correction.

## SURGICAL TECHNIQUE

### Transurethral Resection

Endoscopic management may be important in the management of elderly patients, those that are not good open surgical candidates, or those with a smaller diverticulum that can be addressed at the time of a transurethral resection of the prostate (8). Transurethral resection of the neck of small to midsized diverticula in situations where the opening is not immediately impinging on the ureter is a well-recognized treatment (10). If the opening is small, a Collins knife or right-angle hooked electrode can be used to open the ostium of the diverticulum to allow for subsequent inspection of the entire diverticular wall and facilitate drainage. Transurethral resection or fulguration of the mucosa with a rollerball electrode can then be used to ablate the mucosa of the inner wall.

In the case of tumor within a bladder diverticulum, caution must be exercised. Because there is no muscular backing, transurethral resection of bladder tumors within diverticula carries a high risk of perforation. Cold-cup biopsy and fulguration may be appropriate for low-grade, low-stage tumors. The holmium laser may also be of use in this unique situation because it has a small fiber and a shallow depth of penetration (only 0.3 to 0.5 mm) and would certainly lower the risk of perforation or injury to adjacent structures. In those patients with high-grade or large diverticular carcinomas, in particular those with narrow openings in which the risk of endoscopic perforation or inadequate resection is high, open diverticulectomy/partial cystectomy or total cystectomy has been advocated.

### Open Surgical Technique

A Foley catheter is placed in the bladder on the surgically prepared field to allow for passive drainage and active filling of the bladder as needed throughout the procedure. The bladder is approached via an infraumbilical midline extraperitoneal incision, although alternatively a Gibson incision may be used. The linea of the rectus fascia is divided in the midline, along with the transversalis fascia, and the pelvis is exposed. In the case of benign bladder pathology, the dissection is carried into the space of Retzius and the anterior bladder wall and vesical neck are identified. After reflecting the peritoneum cephalad off the bladder dome, a transverse cystotomy is performed at this level. This provides better exposure of bladder contents and facilitates placement of a small self-retaining retractor and additional stay sutures. The trigone, ureteral orifices, bladder neck, and all possible diverticular orifices are clearly visualized from the bladder dome opening.

In cases of intradiverticular tumor, some have advocated the instillation of 40 mg of mitomycin C by urethral catheter before the surgery. Intraoperatively, we carefully protect the surgical field with moist, sterile towels draped around the wound to avoid possible tumor contamination during diverticulectomy. The bladder mucosa should also be thoroughly inspected to rule out papillary tumors that may have gone unnoticed on the previous endoscopic examination. The mouth of the diverticulum can also be packed with a small gauze pad to avoid or minimize potential tumor spillage.

Diverticulum excision has been described in three different approaches: extravesical; intravesical, also known as transvesical; and the intravesical and extravesical combination. The most commonly used procedures and the points of technique that we use are the following.

#### Intravesical or Transvesical Diverticulectomy

If the diverticulum is small (<2.5 cm diameter), we perform intravesicalization and eversion of its wall, grasping and tractioning its bottom gently with an Allis- or Péan-type clamp inserted through its neck. If this maneuver is performed carefully and fibrosis secondary to infection is absent, the majority of these diverticula are rapidly and easily removed. The mucosa of the everted diverticular neck is divided using electrocautery, and the defect of the bladder wall is sutured with 3-0 chromic catgut or Vicryl using separate submucosal and muscular sutures in two separate layers. In case of a saccule, a fine ligature of the neck and resection of its everted mucosa will suffice.

If this maneuver is not feasible because of peridiverticular adhesions, we proceed to sharply split the mucosa around the diverticular orifice and dissect with scissors as far as the periadventitial space. In this way, the diverticular neck remains separated from the bladder wall and is pulled toward the vesical cavity with Allis-type clamps. At the same time, the adventitial adhesions that fix the diverticular sac are freed gently with a small moist gauze and the sac is drawn into the bladder. The bladder wall is then closed as mentioned previously (Fig. 17.4).

#### Combined Intravesical and Extravesical Diverticulectomy

In a large diverticulum complicated with peridiverticulitis or in a paraureteral location, it is obligatory to place a 7Fr or 8Fr catheter into the ipsilateral ureter before dissection. This will allow for easy identification of the ureter and hopefully avoid inadvertent ureteral injury. If the dissection is extensive, a double-J ureteral catheter remains indwelling for a short

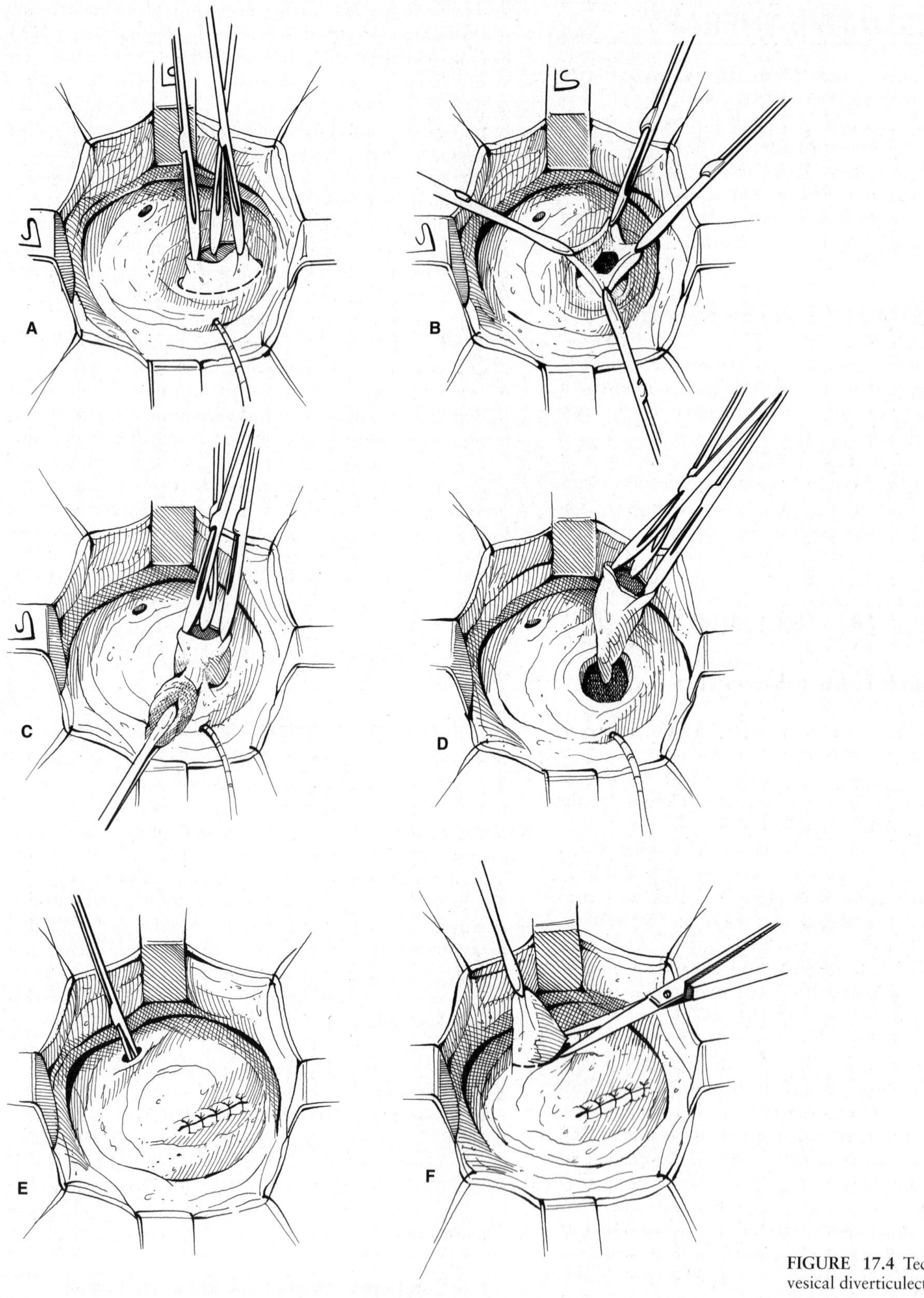


FIGURE 17.4 Technique of intravesical diverticulectomy.

period of time (usually 2 to 3 weeks). These diverticula must be excised by a combined intra- and extravesical approach, first identifying and dissecting the diverticular neck. For this, the maneuver of inserting the surgeon's index finger into the diverticulum and gently tractioning the upper face of its neck toward the surface is useful. We also recommend completely filling the diverticular sac with a moist gauze to unfold its wall and delimit its margins as accurately as possible. Dissection must begin at the diverticular neck, which is incised extravesically with electrocautery and separated from the bladder wall,

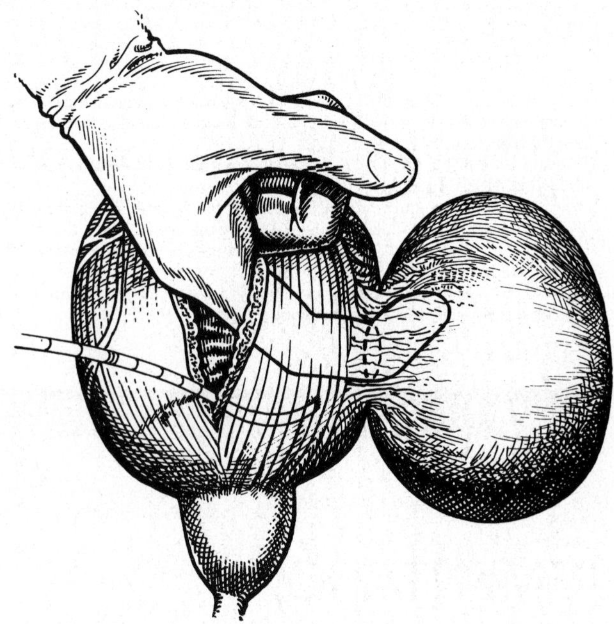

FIGURE 17.5 Procedure of combined intravesical–extravesical diverticulectomy. A finger is inserted into the bladder diverticulum from within the bladder.

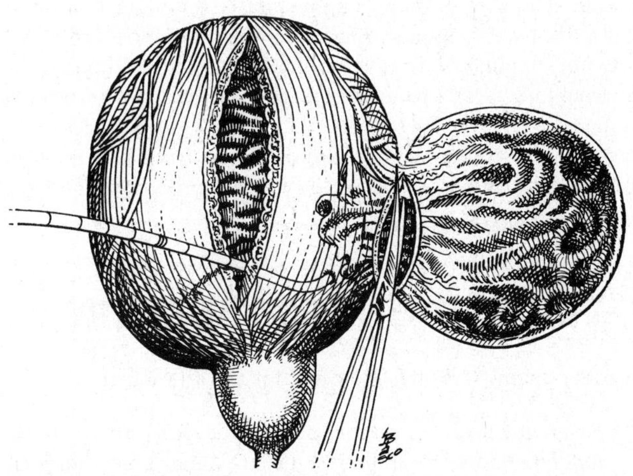

FIGURE 17.6 Procedure of combined intravesical–extravesical diverticulectomy. Once the diverticulum has been dissected, the mouth of the diverticulum is excised sharply.

whose orifice is sutured with 3-0 chromic catgut using extramucosal separate stitches (Figs. 17.5 and 17.6).

Tractioning the edges of the diverticular mouth toward the surface with Allis-type clamps allows the sac wall to be dissected from neighboring tissue with scissors and a small moist swab. It should always be borne in mind that the ureteral course may have been modified by the great diverticular volume, and the ureter may be closely adhered to its wall if repeated infectious processes have occurred. This dissection will be difficult if extensive peridiverticulitis is present, and it is more advisable simply to denude it of its mucosal lining with fine scissors or with the cutting current and the ball electrode from inside the diverticular cavity and then place a suction drain within it (first described by Pousson in 1901 and Geraghty in 1922). The bladder wall is closed with absorbable 3-0 interrupted or continuous absorbable sutures, and a two-layer closure is preferable when possible. We leave a 10Fr closed suction drain in the space of Retzius and a urethral 18Fr or 20Fr Foley catheter, which may both be removed after 5 or 6 days. For more extensive cases, those requiring large cystotomies, or in situations where there is prolonged drain output, a Foley catheter may be left in place for 10 to 14 days and a cystogram may be indicated prior to catheter removal.

## OUTCOMES

### Complications

The most serious specific complication of excision of a bladder diverticulum is an injury to the intramural or pelvic ureter during dissection of a large diverticulum. With prior placement of an ipsilateral ureteral catheter, this injury should be avoidable or at least recognizable and promptly repaired. A small ureterotomy can be easily sutured with absorbable 5-0 or 6-0 chromic or Vicryl. If the ureter has been severely damaged or its section is complete and near the vesical hiatus, the distal ureter must be abandoned, and it is preferable to carry out ureteral reimplantation following the technique of Leadbetter–Politano with or without vesical mobilization to the psoas muscle ("psoas hitch"). More extensive injuries to the ureter may require a bladder tube (Boari flap) or a transureteroureterostomy. End-to-end suture of ureteral edges must never be performed in precarious conditions because it is highly likely that it will be complicated by urinary fistula or ureteral stenosis, which will further aggravate the situation.

Other complications include urinary fistula, rectal injury, and pelvic abscess. Less serious complications include vesical urine leakage, which may cease spontaneously if the Foley catheter is maintained for additional days, providing the obstructive pathology has been resolved.

### Results

With transurethral resection, approximately one-third of these lesions are cured or significantly improved. For benign disease, an open excision of the diverticulum is in general curative for that particular lesion, although correction of the underlying cause (e.g., outlet obstruction) is required to prevent formation of additional diverticula or recurrence. In cases of diverticula involving carcinoma, the prognosis has in general been poor and attributed to the difficult and often delayed diagnosis with early escape from the confines of the bladder through the thin mucosal backing. However, more contemporary reports suggest relatively high rates of survival (about 70% 5-year survival), attributed in part to earlier detection through improved radiographic imaging and a lower threshold for cystoscopy in the presence of hematuria, coupled with early aggressive surgical treatment (1). Nevertheless, due to the relative paucity of cases, treatment recommendations for these unique situations will continue to be based largely on patient characteristics and surgeon preferences.

## *References*


1. Baniel J, Vishna T. Primary transitional cell carcinoma in vesical diverticula. *Urology* 1997;50:697.
2. Canning DA, Koo HP, Duckett JW. Anomalies of the bladder and cloaca. In: Gillenwater JY, Grayhack JT, Howards SS, et al., eds. *Adult and pediatric urology*, 3rd ed. St. Louis: Mosby–Year Book, 1996:2445.
3. Hutch JA. *Anatomy and physiology of the bladder, trigone, and urethra.* New York: Appleton Century Crofts, 1972:8.
4. Jarow JP, Brendler CB. Urinary retention caused by a large bladder diverticulum: a simple method of diverticulectomy. *J Urol* 1988;139:1260.
5. Miller A. The aetiology and treatment of diverticulum of the bladder. *Br J Urol* 1958;30:43.
6. Parra RO, Jones JP, Andrus CH, et al. Laparoscopic diverticulectomy: preliminary report of a new approach for the treatment of bladder diverticulum. *J Urol* 1992;148:869.
7. Peterson LJ, Paulson DF, Glenn JF. The histopathology of vesical diverticula. *J Urol* 1973;110:62P.
8. Rovner ES. Bladder and urethral diverticula. In: Wein A, ed. *Campbell-Walsh urology*, 9th ed. Philadelphia: WB Saunders, 2007:2361.
9. Quirinia A, Hoffmann AL. Bladder diverticula in patients with prostatism. *Int Urol Nephrol* 1993;25:243.
10. Vitale PJ, Woodside JR. Management of bladder diverticula by transurethral resection: reevaluation of an old technique. *J Urol* 1979;122:744.


# CHAPTER 18 ■ BLADDER AUGMENTATION

ANNE PELLETIER CAMERON, R. DUANE CESPEDES, AND EDWARD J. MCGUIRE

Bladder augmentation, also referred to as augmentation cystoplasty or enterocystoplasty, is the addition of tissue to the bladder to increase its capacity. The goal of this procedure is to create a large capacity and compliant bladder to achieve continence, decrease detrusor overactivity, and protect the renal units from vesicoureteric reflux and high storage pressures. The most common indication for bladder augmentation is the neurogenic bladder that has failed conservative therapy. The majority of neurogenic bladder disorders can be managed with medical therapy, but a significant minority will require augmentation cystoplasty. In the past, these patients would have been treated with an incontinent urinary diversion such as an ileal conduit. With the advent of clean intermittent catheterization (CIC) and decreased morbidity of the procedure, augmentation has almost replaced incontinent diversion as bladder management for this typically young population, resulting in great improvements in patient quality of life. Patients with incontinent diversions like ileal conduits more frequently develop urinary infections and upper-tract deterioration compared to those with a large, low-pressure reservoir employing the urethra as a continence method (1).

Most urologists are familiar with the use of ileum and prefer to use this segment for bladder reconstructions. It must be noted that each bowel segment has its own advantages and disadvantages, but none is universally superior (2).

The ileum, 25 cm from the ileocecal valve, when detubularized for augmentation, ensures low pressures, produces only a moderate amount of mucus, and results in the least metabolic disturbances of all the bowel segments. The sigmoid is low pressure if detubularized, is thicker than ileum allowing reimplantation of ureters, has a large lumen and a long mesentery, but has more mucus production and a greater risk of subsequent urinary infections.

The cecum is typically only used in conjunction with the terminal ileum. The ileocecal valve can be used as an antireflux mechanism for ureter reimplantation; however, the resulting diarrhea and malabsorption become problematic in the neurogenic population, who often only maintain fecal continence with purposeful constipation. We avoid this segment if at all possible. The stomach is used only in the event that both the small and large bowel are not suitable for augmentation. It has a thick wall and produces little mucus, but most urologists are not familiar with its mobilization, and, although the hydrochloric acid production is bactericidal, the associated hematuria-dysuria syndrome can be troublesome. The segment chosen should be based on the patient's past medical and surgical history, findings during the procedure, and the surgeon's experience (2,3).

## INDICATIONS FOR SURGERY

Bladder augmentation is indicated for the following:

1. Severe medically refractory neurogenic detrusor overactivity. This is most commonly due to spinal cord injury or spina bifida.
2. Poorly compliant bladder from neuropathic conditions secondary to pelvic radiation or intravesical chemotherapy, or bladder scarring from surgical or traumatic injury.
3. Idiopathic detrusor overactivity refractory to all therapy.
4. Prolonged bladder defunctionalization after long-term catheter drainage, cutaneous vesicostomy drainage, or bilateral cutaneous ureterostomy.
5. Inflammatory conditions such as interstitial cystitis or bilharzial or tuberculosis bladder dysfunction.
6. Patients previously diverted who are candidates for undiversion.
7. Intractable autonomic dysreflexia that is associated with detrusor hyperactivity or irritation from indwelling catheters.

Incontinence from detrusor overactivity in patients who do not suffer from identifiable neurogenic disease (i.e., idiopathic detrusor overactivity) can be an indication for augmentation cystoplasty if other treatments, including medication, sacral nerve stimulation therapy, botulinum toxin detrusor injection, and myomectomy, have failed.

Interstitial cystitis is a difficult disease to manage by any means. Treating it with augmentation cystoplasty has been disappointing unless supratrigonal cystectomy is also performed, but success with this approach has not been universal (4).

Patient selection is critical in the success of augmentation cystoplasty. Patients unwilling or unable to catheterize are not candidates for this procedure. Postoperatively, even those patients who do not have neurologic bladder dysfunction require CIC 39% to 89% of the time (3,4). We counsel all augmentation patients at our institution that they will have to self-catheterize at least temporarily after surgery. Persons with progressive neurologic or cognitive diseases, such as multiple sclerosis and dementia, may be poor augmentation candidates since their ability to perform CIC may deteriorate with time. This makes them dependent on others for catheterization, which puts them at risk for recurrent urinary tract infections (UTIs) and bladder perforation. Patients unable to self-catheterize because of their anatomy should be considered for a continent catheterizable stoma along with the augmentation.

In some instances, certain bowel segments may be unavailable because of pre-existing disease. The small bowel should not be used if extensive pelvic radiation has been performed. The large bowel is contraindicated if the patient has a history of colon cancer, diverticulitis, or ulcerative colitis. Any disease, such as Crohn disease, or prior surgery that results in a critically short or abnormal bowel is another contraindication to augmentation cystoplasty using bowel, especially if the removal of the segment will have adverse effects on bowel absorptive function.

Chronic renal failure is a relative contraindication to augmentation cystoplasty since both the ileum and colon absorb urinary solutes that may result in worsening renal function and metabolic disturbances. However, in many cases the bladder dysfunction itself is the cause of the renal deterioration, and the procedure will slow the decline in their renal function (2). In such instances gastrocystoplasty has been suggested because of the stomach's limited adverse effects on metabolic balance.

## DIAGNOSIS

The decision to perform an augmentation cystoplasty is complex and is not guided by a single test or office visit. It is a last resort once all conservative measures such as medications, clean intermittent catheterization, and minimally invasive procedures have failed. "Failure" in this context is defined as persistent incontinence, recurrent symptomatic UTIs, urosepsis, vesicoureteric reflux, or hydronephrosis. These clinical problems are common in patients with neurogenic bladder dysfunction and are all secondary to uncontrolled detrusor pressure and poor compliance. These variables are controllable with an augmentation cystoplasty.

The basic evaluation includes a urodynamic study, preferably using fluoroscopy to evaluate bladder compliance, the status of the bladder neck, and the presence of vesicoureteric reflux.

Incontinence in this population is often a complex problem. It can be a result of elevated detrusor pressures, a lack of urethral closing function, or both. Accurate assessment of urethral function in cases where the bladder is very poorly compliant or grossly hyperreflexic is difficult.

Incontinence due to an open urethra as demonstrated on upright cystogram will persist after augmentation. This condition is associated with low thoracic or lumbar spinal cord injury, myelodysplasia, long-term urethral catheter drainage, and certain pelvic surgeries, such as abdominal perineal resection or radical hysterectomy. These conditions are best treated by urethral closure at the time of the augmentation. This can be achieved with a tight pubovaginal sling, an artificial urinary sphincter, or deliberate surgical closure of the bladder neck.

Vesicoureteric reflux is also a common complication of neurogenic bladder and is almost always driven by increased bladder pressures. "Low-pressure reflux" is a condition in which reflux occurs at relatively low detrusor pressures and can be very difficult to diagnose. Our practice is to ignore reflux and augment the bladder, and the reflux in most cases resolves provided the augmentation is a low-pressure and compliant reservoir. Other authors support this stance and have found that simply augmenting the bladder resolves vesicoureteric reflux in 86% of patients, and success does not depend on the grade of reflux or the bowel segment used for augmentation (5).

## ALTERNATIVE THERAPY

Recently, several options have become available for intractable detrusor overactivity or poor compliance. Botulinum toxin injections of the detrusor have been shown to be effective in both the neurogenic and nonneurogenic populations (6). Given the procedure's low morbidity, it should be tried before augmentation cystoplasty; however, it is still not approved by many regulatory agencies. Its high cost and need for repeat injections are a barrier to its widespread use. Sacral nerve stimulation has been available since 1997 for the treatment of refractory urgency and urge incontinence of nonneurogenic etiology (7). Autoaugmentation of the bladder, also know as partial detrusor myomectomy, is the excision of the detrusor muscle over the dome and anterior wall of the bladder. This allows the bladder epithelium to distend outward, improving storage capacity and bladder compliance (8). This significantly less morbid procedure has the advantage of not incorporating any mucus-producing bowel into the bladder, the almost uniform ability to void spontaneously after the procedure, and no increased risk of malignancy. In general, patients achieve less improvement in compliance than after formal enterocystoplasty. The gains in bladder capacity and compliance in patients with neurogenic bladder are small, so the routine use of myomectomy is not recommended in these patients. We continue to use this technique, especially in younger patients with intractable idiopathic urge incontinence, with favorable results.

For patients in whom a low-pressure diversion is required but the patient is unable to self-catheterize, an ileovesicostomy, or "bladder chimney," can be a good option (9). In the neurogenic patient whose only other option is an ileal conduit, an ileovesicostomy provides the same benefits of decreasing storage pressures and eliminating urethral incontinence, but it does not involve dissection of the ureters or bladder removal, thus significantly reducing both early and late morbidity.

Laparoscopic bladder augmentation using ileum has been reported, but this technique is still under investigation (10). Other nonautologous tissues (Teflon, Silastic, human dura, Gore-Tex, bovine dura) have been utilized to augment the bladder; however, complications with the anastomosis, contracture, fistulas, infections, and stone formation have precluded their use (2). An innovative alternative is the tissue-engineered autologous bladder. A small clinical trial in children with spina bifida augmented with their own urothelial and muscle cells grown on a biodegradable bladder-shaped scaffold has promising results with little morbidity (11). Clinical trials are under way to better study this novel alternative.

## SURGICAL TECHNIQUE

Preoperatively all patients require a urine culture one week prior to the surgery date and urine sterilization with antibiotics based on sensitivities. Serum electrolytes including creatinine should be drawn at baseline for future comparison and to help dictate the segment of bowel best suited for the patient.

Patients with idiopathic detrusor overactivity should start a clear liquid diet for 2 to 3 days prior to the operative procedure. No antibiotic or mechanical bowel preparation is needed if ileum is the bowel segment to be utilized for the augmentation.

Patients with neurogenic conditions can be treated with a 3-day clear liquid diet and enemas without mechanical bowel preparation or oral antibiotics if ileum is the segment to be utilized. This bowel regime has been well supported in the general surgery literature and has been shown to be safe, even in children undergoing augmentation cystoplasty (12).

When large bowel is the segment to be used, a mechanical preparation is required along with oral antibiotics. Mechanical bowel preparation in neurogenic patients may take slightly longer than in patients with normal bowel function and should be done gently over a 2- to 3-day period.

A nasogastric tube is inserted after induction of anesthesia but is removed prior to extubation. We have eliminated the use of routine nasogastric tube drainage after bowel surgery. This is based on results of a trial showing that bowel function returns more swiftly and there are no increases in complications in neurogenic bladder patients undergoing augmentation treated without postoperative nasogastric tube drainage (13).

After preparation of the skin from xiphoid to genitalia, a urethral catheter is placed and positioned so that the bladder can be filled and emptied during the case. In general, if an anti-incontinence procedure is necessary, it is performed first.

A midline incision is the best approach for augmentation cystoplasty. A Pfannenstiel incision can be used, but it is suitable only when ileum will be used since a colonic augmentation through a Pfannenstiel incision is a rather difficult operative procedure. It should be kept in mind that occasionally it is only discovered intraoperatively that the ileum is unusable and one is forced to use colon.

After entry into the peritoneum, a self-retaining retractor is placed (the Bookwalter is our preference in the adult), and the bladder is filled with saline and identified. The peritoneum is dissected off the bladder down to the level of the trigone posteriorly (Fig. 18.1). A wide U-shaped incision is made posteriorly on the bladder starting just above the ureters, creating an anteriorly based bladder flap with a posteriorly facing opening (Fig. 18.2). This approach will allow a tension-free augmentation.

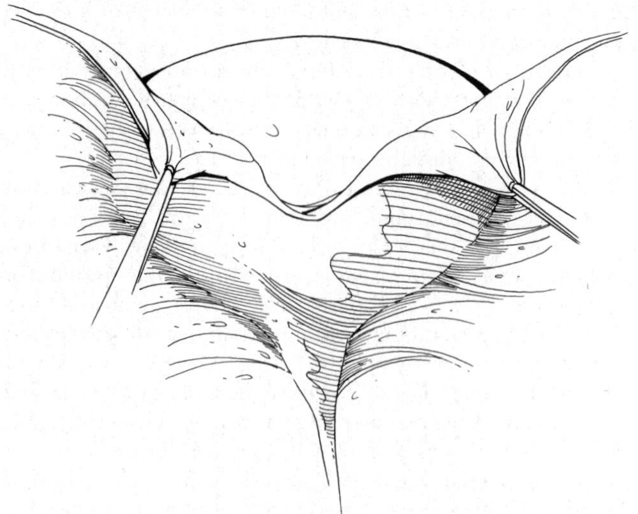

**FIGURE 18.1** The peritoneum is dissected off the posterior bladder to the level of the trigone and 2 to 3 cm above the level of the ureters.

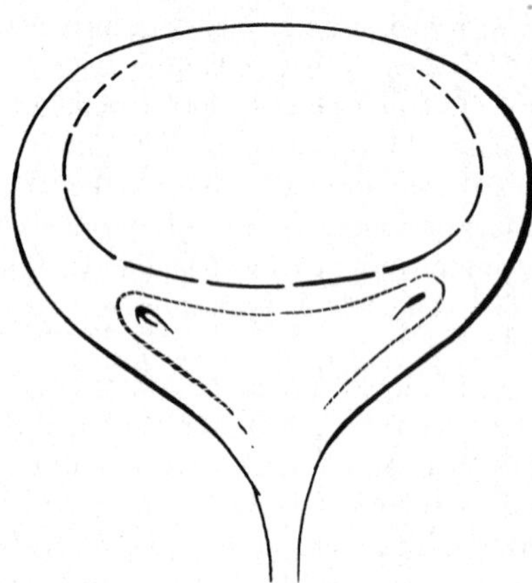

**FIGURE 18.2** A U-shaped incision is made on the bladder with the transverse portion just superior to the trigone and the limbs of the incision extending to the dome of the bladder.

A 25- to 30-cm segment of ileum at least 20 cm proximal to the ileocecal valve is selected and marked with sutures. Before harvesting the bowel, the surgeon should fold this section of ileum in two and ensure that it can easily reach the bladder without tension; if not, a new section should be selected. The mesentery is incised on either end of the 25-cm segment, and both ends of the ileum section are divided using standard stapling devices (Fig. 18.3).

The exact length of ileum required varies between individuals, but enough length should be used to allow an estimated 4 hours between catheterizations after the bowel is fully "stretched" over the ensuing months. Ileal continuity is then achieved using one of the hand-sewn or stapled techniques and the mesenteric defect closed. To prevent stone formation, the ileal ends are oversewn with running 2-0 chromic catgut to exclude the staples (Fig. 18.3), and then the antimesenteric

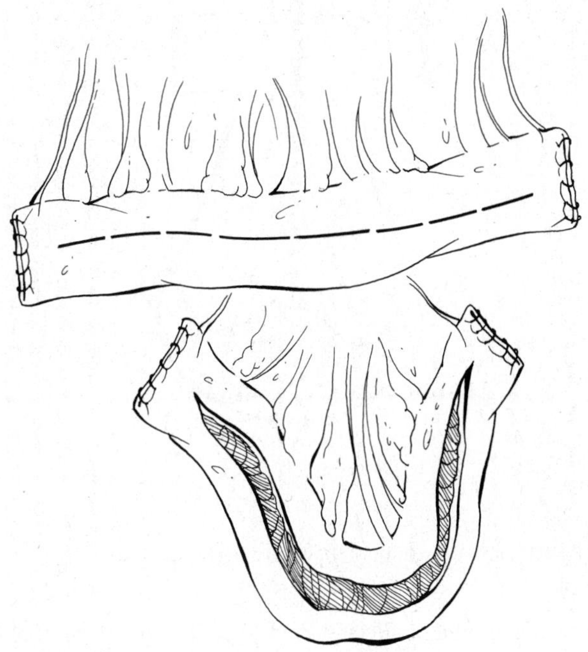

FIGURE 18.3 Approximately 15 cm proximal to the ileocecal valve, a 25-cm segment of bowel is selected, the mesentery cleared, and the segment removed using standard stapling techniques. The segment of ileum is oversewn at the ends to exclude the staples and then opened along the antimesenteric border.

surface of the bowel is opened using electrocautery. The posterior wall of the ileum is folded back on itself and sutured together using a running 2-0 delayed absorbable synthetic stitch such as Vicryl (Figs. 18.4 and 18.5). The required size of the augmentation opening on the bladder is roughly measured, and the superior, anterior wall of the ileum is partially closed with running 2-0 Vicryl to match this opening (Fig. 18.6).

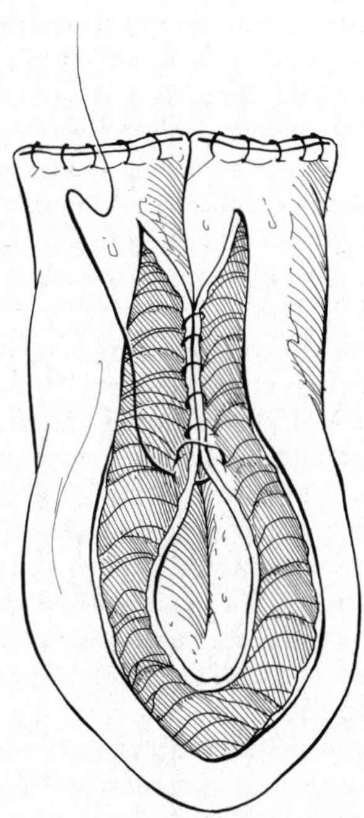

FIGURE 18.4 The ileal segment is folded, and closure of the posterior wall is initiated using a running absorbable suture.

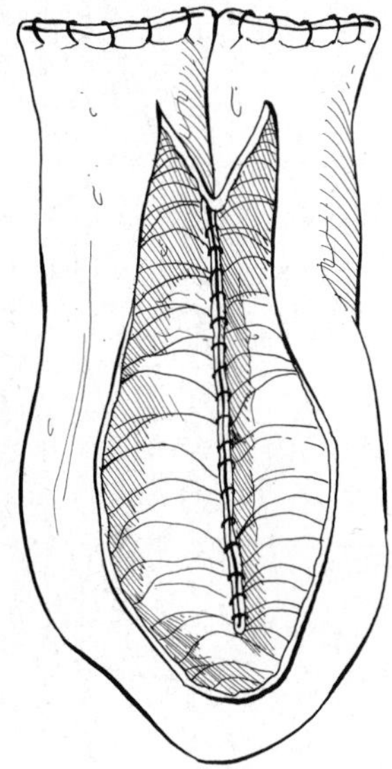

FIGURE 18.5 The posterior wall of the augment is completely closed.

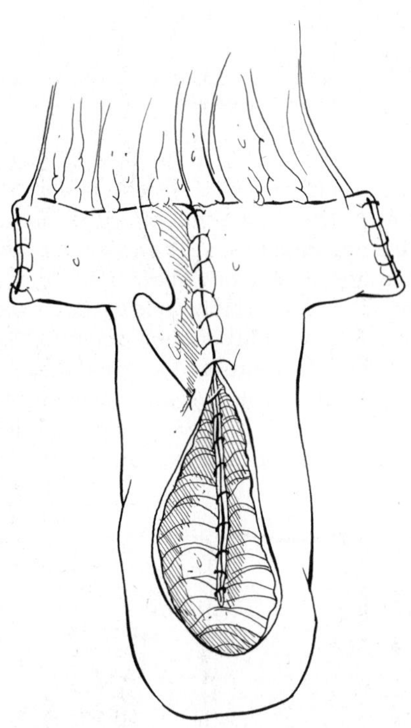

FIGURE 18.6 The superior, anterior wall of the augment is partially closed. The size of the augment opening should roughly correspond to the size of the opened bladder.

A large-bore suprapubic (SP) tube is placed through the lateral bladder wall, not the bowel segment, prior to suturing the augment onto the bladder. The SP tube allows reliable postoperative drainage and irrigation of mucus until the suture lines are healed. Alternatively, a large-bore urethral catheter can be left in place. The choice of an SP tube or a urethral catheter, or both, is surgeon dependent, although we prefer a urethral catheter since it is simpler to remove. The ileal segment is then sewn onto the opened bladder using running 2-0 Vicryl, with the initial suture placed at the most inferior

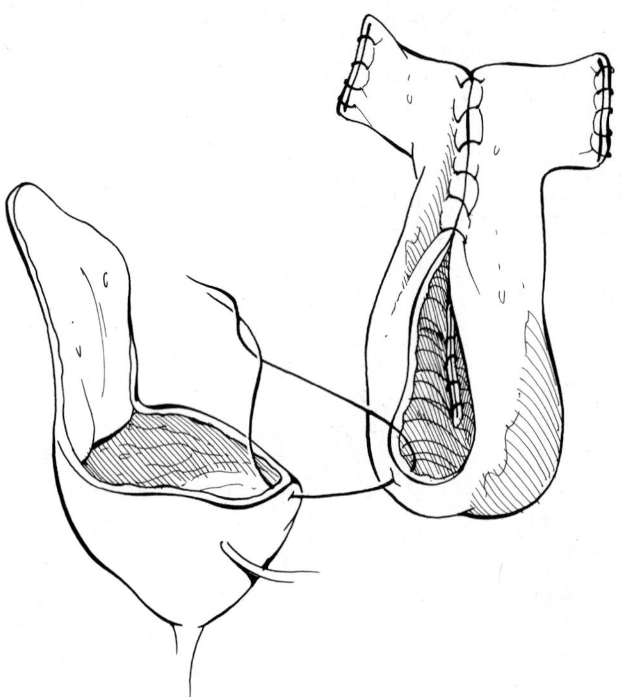

FIGURE 18.7 Initial suture placement for enterocystoplasty. Note that the bladder flap opens anteriorly.

portion of the bladder opening posteriorly (Fig. 18.7). Suture lines must be watertight and full thickness, and the bladder mucosa must oppose the bowel mucosa. Once the posterior closure is finished, the anterior closure is completed in a similar fashion (Fig. 18.8). The completed enterocystoplasty is shown in Fig. 18.9. A closed-suction drain is placed near the suture line and brought through the skin on the side opposite the SP tube. The abdomen is closed in standard fashion. If a continence procedure has been performed, it is imperative that a urethral catheter can be easily passed.

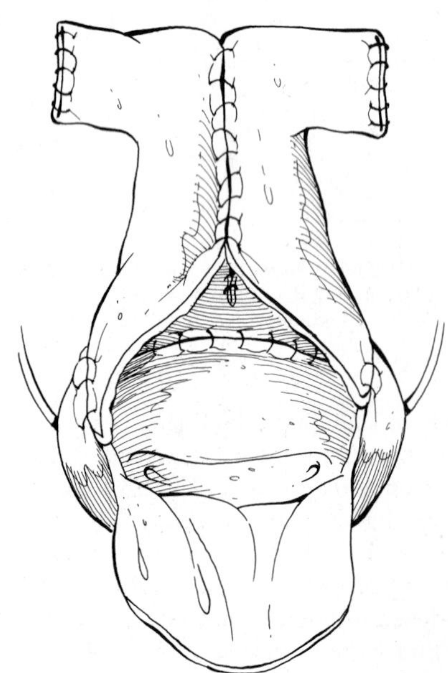

FIGURE 18.8 Closure of the anterior aspect of the enterocystoplasty.

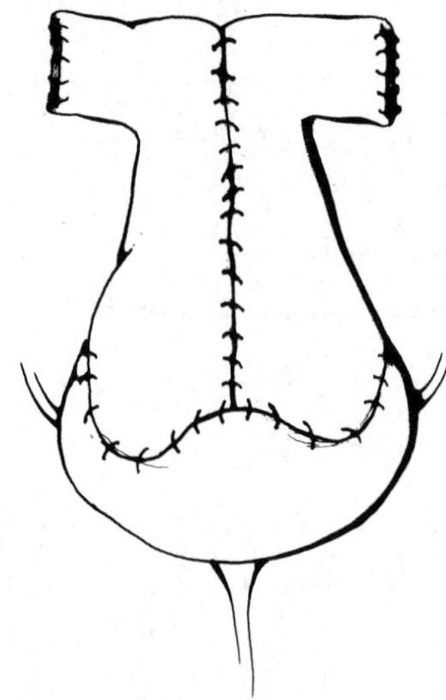

FIGURE 18.9 View of the completed enterocystoplasty.

Although this is our preferred technique, other methods of performing an augmentation exist. One such method involves splitting the bladder sagittally from just above the bladder neck and ending near the level of the ureters posteriorly to form a "clam shell" (3). A 23- to 30-cm segment of ileum is isolated and divided completely along the antimesenteric border (Fig. 18.10). The posterior wall of the augment is closed with running 2-0 Vicryl and then either anastomosed to the bladder as a "patch" or folded again and partially closed to form a "cup." A cup is especially useful if the patient's own bladder is very small, but it sometimes requires the use of up to 40 cm of bowel. In both cases, the anastomosis is started on the posterior wall until approximately one third is closed, and then the anterior wall is closed. The lateral walls are closed last, and any redundant bowel is closed to itself.

Postoperatively, fluid and electrolyte management is important due to large third-space losses and suction drainage. Although the nasogastric tube is not left in place, it is important to remember that bowel function is often deranged in the neurogenic bladder patient, and recovery of bowel motility may be significantly delayed. The abdominal drain is removed once drainage is consistently minimal. The bladder is irrigated via the catheter while in hospital and after discharge at least three times per day with 30 to 60 mL of saline to clear mucus. Typically a cystogram is performed at 2 to 3 weeks, and if no urinary extravasation is noted, the patient begins CIC. If an SP tube was originally placed, the patients can perform CIC with the SP tube clamped until proficient at CIC. At 3 to 4 weeks, the SP tube is removed and the patient continues CIC every 2 to 3 hours during the day and twice at night. It typically requires up to 6 to 12 months for the augment to stretch to full capacity, during which time more frequent CIC is necessary. This may be distressing to the patient at first. Continuing the regimen of anticholinergic therapy will help maintain native bladder compliance and maximize capacity. As capacity increases, the CIC intervals can lengthen, and, ultimately, most patients are able to wait 4 to 5 hours between catheterizations during the day and catheterize only once at night. Patients who are able to void per urethra must document consistently small postvoid residuals before CIC is stopped. In some cases, apparent early normal

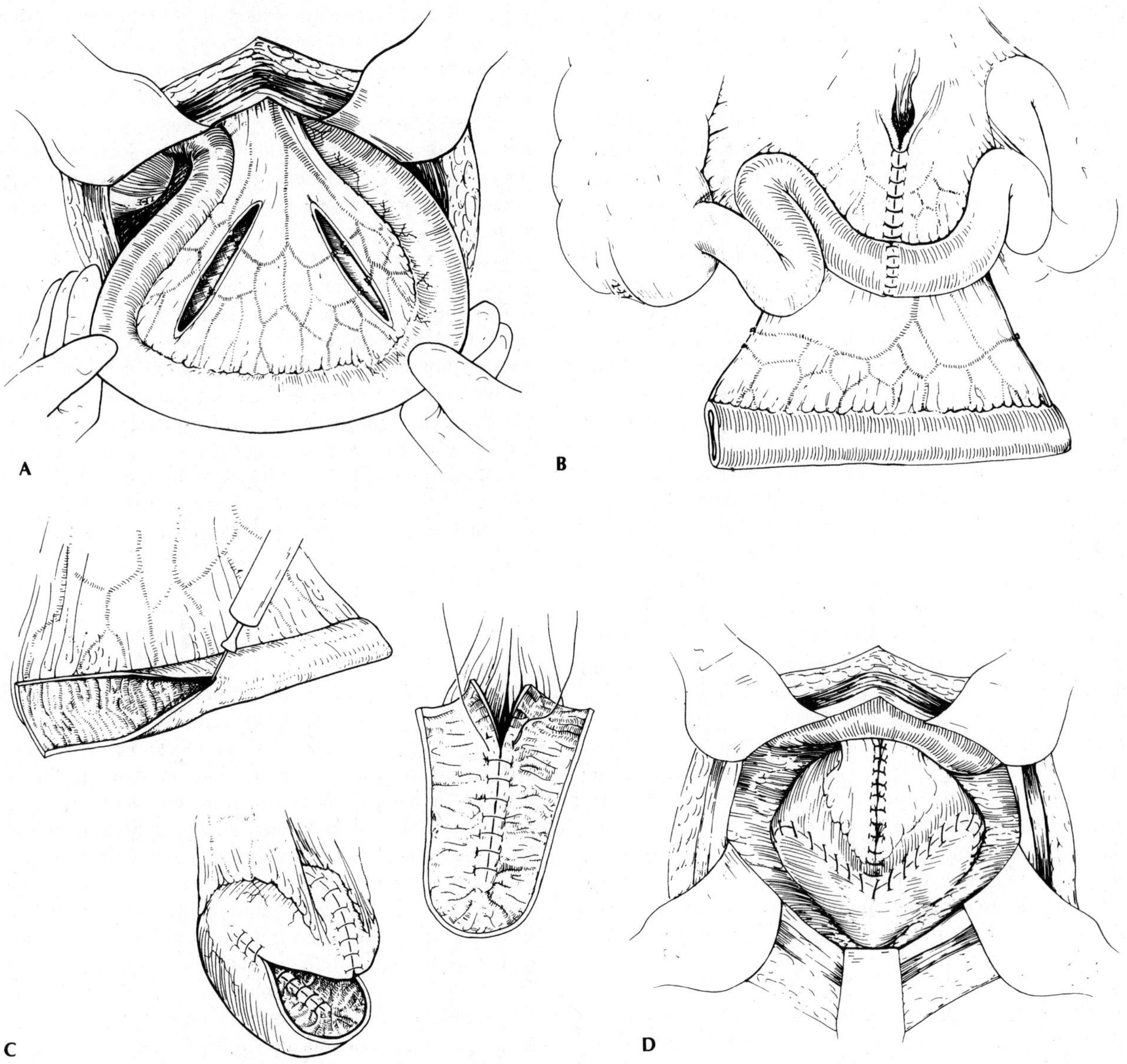


FIGURE 18.10 Augmentation cystoplasty with formation of a cup patch. **A:** Isolation of a distal ileal segment. **B and C:** Isolated ileal segment opened on antimesenteric border and double-folded to create a reservoir. **D:** Cup patch reservoir sutured to the bladder-incised sagittal plane.

voiding deteriorates over time, and in some cases the bowel segment can become overstretched and either rupture or become overly capacious and defunctionalized. Patients who are able to void postoperatively should be followed with intermittent postvoid residuals. Daily irrigation to clear mucus is essential, especially for the first few months.

Routine electrolytes, creatinine, blood urea nitrogen, and upper-tract studies should be performed at regular intervals. It is unlikely that vitamin $B_{12}$ deficiency should develop because a short ileal segment is usually used.

## COMPLICATIONS

A comprehensive long-term study of 122 patients by Flood and colleagues reported an overall 28% early and 44% late complication rate in a complex group of patients (4). Most of the complications were manageable and consisted primarily of prolonged ileus, transient urinary extravasation, or stomal problems. Surgical interventions were necessary in only 15% of patients, with stomal revisions being most common.

Small-bowel obstructions occur in approximately 3% of patients, similar to the rate reported in urinary diversions. The rate of bladder stones varies from 13% to 21% (2,4), but it has been reported to be much higher (3). Stone formation is lowest in those patients who void spontaneously but is five times higher in those who catheterize urethrally and ten times higher in those with continent cutaneous stomas (2). Stones usually form secondary to retained mucus or exposed staples as a nidus. Routine bladder irrigation, treatment of infections, and excluding staples at the time of surgery minimize stone formation.

Although patients with bacteriuria and recurring urinary infection remain as bacteriuric after augmentation as they were before the surgery, the infections and their resulting complications are ameliorated by the procedure. This results from improved control of detrusor pressure, which is the ultimate goal of treatment of any bladder dysfunction. Since bacteriuria is extremely common, especially if the patient is performing self-catheterization, routine urine culture is not helpful. Bacteriuria is only considered an infection if the patient becomes symptomatic (fever, pain, foul-smelling urine, incontinence, or increased mucus production) (3). The treatment of asymptomatic bacteriuria, unless it is a urease-splitting organism, is of no benefit and will only promote antibiotic resistance.

Reservoir perforation is perhaps the most feared complication, with reported rates of up to 6% (4). Perforation is a catastrophic event, and the patient may quickly become septic, but the presentation is variable, and patients with spinal cord injury may not present with the classic signs of an acute abdomen (3). Fortunately, fatalities are uncommon if diagnosed early. Different theories have been proposed to explain the etiology of bladder perforation. Obviously, acute trauma can rupture the augmented bladder, but the majority of perforations are nontraumatic. Infrequent catheterization, recurrent urinary infections, and bowel ischemia secondary to recurrent overdistention have all been implicated (3). Clinical suspicion of a perforation must always be high in this population, and the method of diagnosis is a cystogram both filled and post drainage. Standard treatment is open repair of the rupture, which is typically at the bowel-to-bladder junction.

Metabolic acidosis that requires bicarbonate treatment is uncommon if patients are properly selected and a reasonable length of bowel is used. Patients should be screened for this disturbance at least annually.

The development of tumors has been reported with the use of all bowel segments. Although the risk to any individual patient is small, after 5 years annual cystoscopic surveillance should be considered, especially if a colonic segment is used.

If the bladder is extremely small or the bladder incision is not generous, the "augmentation" may ultimately become no more than a large, nondraining bladder diverticulum. This complication may be manifested by recurrent urinary tract infections and can easily be identified by the classic hourglass appearance on a cystogram. Reaugmentation is the only solution to this rare problem, but prevention by creating a very large bladder opening initially (Fig. 18.2) is the key.

Augmentation cystoplasty has gained widespread use in both the pediatric and adult populations such that there are many women of reproductive age who are currently living with a bladder augmentation. There are small case series indicating an increase in pyelonephritis, ureteric dilatation or obstruction, renal deterioration, and premature labor in these women. These potential complications should be actively screened for during the pregnancy, and bacteriuria should be aggressively treated. Women with an augmentation cystoplasty alone, without any contraindications to vaginal delivery, should be allowed to deliver vaginally, thereby avoiding any possible injury to the pedicle of the augmented bowel during Caesarean section. Women who have a bladder outlet procedure along with their augmentation should be counseled about the risks and benefits of vaginal delivery versus cesarean, and if the latter is chosen, their urologists should be present for the procedure (2,3).

## RESULTS

Achieving a successful augmentation cystoplasty depends on three factors: performing the procedure for the correct indications only after exhausting all other conservative measures, proper patient selection, and good operative technique. In selected patients with neuropathic bladders requiring improved compliance and capacity, augmentation cystoplasty has a high likelihood of improving compliance and capacity and can be equally efficacious in the nonneurogenic patient with intractable bladder symptoms. An augmentation is less successful in treating the symptoms of interstitial cystitis and by itself does not guarantee continence, especially in patients with high rates of intrinsic sphincter deficiency (ISD), such as in the case of myelomeningocele and radiation cystitis, who will often require an anti-incontinence procedure.

## *References*


1. Madersbacher S, Schmidt J, Eberle JM, et al. Long-term outcome of ileal conduit diversion. *J Urol* 2003;169(3):985–990.
2. Greenwell TJ, Venn SN, Mundy AR. Augmentation cystoplasty. *Br J Urol Int* 2001;88(6):511–525.
3. Niknejad KG, Atala A. Bladder augmentation techniques in women. *Int Urogynecol J Pelvic Floor Dysfunct* 2000;11(3):156–169.
4. Flood HD, Malhotra SJ, O'Connell HE, et al. Long-term results and complications using augmentation cystoplasty in reconstructive urology. *Neurourol Urodyn* 1995;14(4):297–309.
5. Juhasz Z, Somogyi R, Vajda P, et al. Does the type of bladder augmentation influence the resolution of pre-existing vesicoureteral reflux? Urodynamic studies. *Neurourol Urodyn* 2008;27(5):412–416.
6. Kim DK, Thomas CA, Smith C, et al. The case for bladder botulinum toxin application. *Urol Clin North Am* 2006;33(4):503–510, ix.
7. van Kerrebroeck PE, van Voskuilen AC, Heesakkers JP, et al. Results of sacral neuromodulation therapy for urinary voiding dysfunction: outcomes of a prospective, worldwide clinical study. *J Urol* 2007;178(5):2029–2034.
8. Gurocak S, De Gier RP, Feitz W. Bladder augmentation without integration of intact bowel segments: critical review and future perspectives. *J Urol* 2007;177(3):839–844.
9. Tan HJ, Stoffel J, Daignault S, et al. Ileovesicostomy for adults with neurogenic bladders: complications and potential risk factors for adverse outcomes. *Neurourol Urodyn* 2008;27(3):238–243.
10. Lorenzo AJ, Cerveira J, Farhat WA. Pediatric laparoscopic ileal cystoplasty: complete intracorporeal surgical technique. *Urology* 2007;69(5):977–981.
11. Atala A, Bauer SB, Soker S, et al. Tissue-engineered autologous bladders for patients needing cystoplasty. *Lancet* 2006;367(9518):1241–1246.
12. Gundeti MS, Godbole PP, Wilcox DT. Is bowel preparation required before cystoplasty in children? *J Urol* 2006;176(4, Pt 1):1574–1576; discussion 1576–1577.
13. Erickson BA, Dorin RP, Clemens JQ. Is nasogastric tube drainage required after reconstructive surgery for neurogenic bladder dysfunction? *Urology* 2007;69(5):885–888.

# CHAPTER 19 ■ MANAGEMENT OF THE DISTAL URETER FOR NEPHROURETERECTOMY

J. STUART WOLF, JR.

The traditional therapy for urothelial cell carcinoma of the renal pelvis or ureter is nephroureterectomy, including a 1-cm cuff of bladder around the ureteral orifice. When performed using open surgery, this entails a long midline or thoracoabdominal incision or two incisions (a flank incision for the nephrectomy and a lower midline or Gibson incision for the distal ureterectomy). Because of the morbidity associated with the extension of the incision for the distal ureterectomy, alternative approaches such as the "pluck" and "intussusception" techniques were devised. The advent of laparoscopic nephroureterectomy, which further reduces morbidity by eliminating the flank incision for the renal portion of the procedure, has stimulated the development of additional minimally invasive approaches to the distal ureter. Although there is some advantage in terms of reducing the intensity and duration of convalescence with these less invasive approaches, since intact extraction of the specimen is recommended after laparoscopic nephroureterectomy (owing to the importance of pathologic staging and the propensity for urothelial carcinoma to implant into wounds), an open surgical approach to the distal ureterectomy does not necessarily mean a much larger incision than would be required for the nephrectomy portion of the case.

## DIAGNOSIS

The most common presenting symptom or sign of upper-tract urothelial tumors is hematuria, which occurs in approximately 75% of patients, and the second most common symptom or sign is flank pain, present in approximately 30% of patients (3). The subsequent evaluation entails an upper-tract imaging study with intravenous urography, computerized tomography, magnetic resonance imaging, or retrograde pyelography. Most patients will have a filling defect that suggests upper-tract urothelial tumor. Both sides of the urinary system need to be evaluated due to the potential for bilateral tumors.

The combination of urinary cytology positive for upper-tract urothelial tumor with radiographic abnormality consistent with an upper-tract urothelial tumor is adequate for diagnosis if nephroureterectomy is intended. If either cytology or imaging is not definitive, or if a nephron-sparing approach is being considered, then ureteroscopy and biopsy are recommended. In either case, cystoscopy is essential due to the high association with urothelial tumors of the bladder.

Once urothelial malignancy is diagnosed, metastatic evaluation consists of an abdominal and pelvic computerized tomogram and a chest radiograph. A bone scan is performed if there is bone pain, the alkaline phosphatase is elevated, or bony abnormalities are seen on other imaging studies. A complete blood count, serum electrolytes with creatinine, and liver function tests should also be obtained. If the creatinine is elevated, a renal scan to determine differential function may aid in decision making.

## INDICATIONS FOR SURGERY

Radical nephroureterectomy with complete distal ureterectomy is the standard therapy for upper-tract urothelial tumors, using either laparoscopic (standard or hand-assisted) or open surgical techniques. Nephrectomy without complete ureterectomy should be avoided due to a 30% incidence of recurrence in the ureteral stump (2). Patients with a positive cytology but without an identifiable lesion on imaging or ureteroscopy should be followed closely rather than undergo nephroureterectomy without a definitive diagnosis.

## ALTERNATIVE THERAPY

Endoscopic resection and fulguration are acceptable for patients with low-grade, low-stage, and small-tumor burdens. An alternative for a distal ureteral tumor is a distal ureterectomy with a ureteroneocystostomy or other reconstruction. Topical therapy with bacille Calmette-Guérin or mitomycin C may be attempted for patients with carcinoma in situ who have limited renal function or bilateral disease.

## SURGICAL TECHNIQUE

### Open Surgical Techniques

#### Intravesical Approach

Open surgical distal ureterectomy can be used in conjunction with any technique of nephrectomy. After completing the nephrectomy and proximal ureteral dissection, place the patient in the supine position, with or without flexion of the table. Insert a three-way 20Fr urethral catheter into the bladder. Make a lower midline incision, divide the rectus fascia, develop the space of Retzius, and place a self-retaining retractor. Fill the bladder with saline and then open it longitudinally between two stay sutures. Place additional stay sutures at the apices of the bladder incision. Pack the dome of the bladder with a gauze sponge, and use a bladder blade to retract the bladder dome cephalad. Insert a ureteral catheter or feeding tube in the targeted ureteral orifice and sew it in place

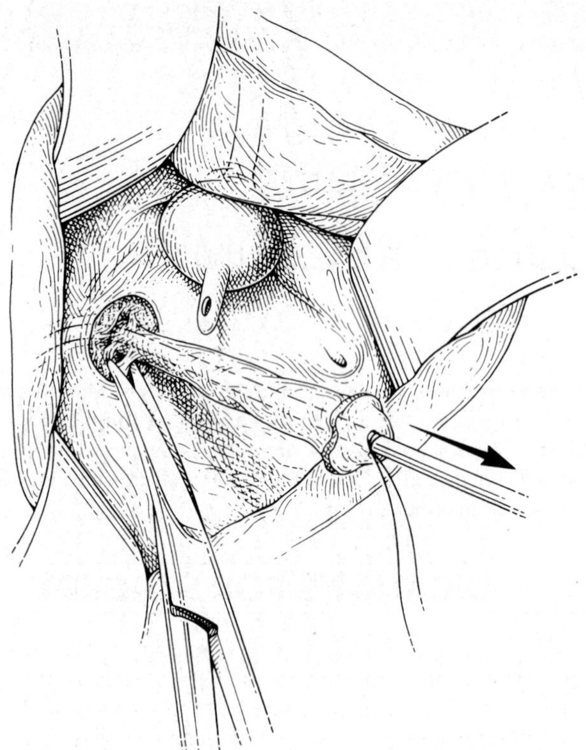

FIGURE 19.1 A ureteral catheter is secured to the ureteral orifice. Tenotomy scissors and electrocautery are used to dissect free the intramural ureter. (From Lange PH. Carcinoma of the renal pelvis and ureter. In: Glenn JF, ed. *Urologic surgery*, 4th ed. Philadelphia: JB Lippincott Co, 1991:273, with permission.)

with a 4-0 suture. Use electrocautery cutting current to incise the mucosa 1 cm around the ureteral orifice. Dissect the intramural ureter using tenotomy scissors and pinpoint electrocautery (Fig. 19.1).

Dissect the entire distal ureter free to join the point of previous dissection completed during the nephrectomy portion of the procedure. Close the posterior bladder wall in two layers (2-0 absorbable sutures for the serosa and muscle and 4-0 absorbable sutures for the mucosa), and close the anterior bladder incision similarly. Insert a pelvic drain through a separate stab incision. Leave the urethral catheter in place for 3 to 5 days. Some perform a cystogram to ensure the bladder has healed prior to removing the catheter, while others remove the catheter and perform a voiding trial.

At times, the dissection of the distal ureter may be difficult and the ureter may need to be dissected extravesically as well. This may require division of the superior vesical artery to provide access to the distal ureter.

### Extravesical Approach

A completely extravesical approach is best performed through a Gibson incision. After entering the retroperitoneal space and identifying the distal ureter, retract the bladder to the contralateral side. Divide the superior vesical artery to facilitate dissection of the distal ureter. Identify the ureteral hiatus and dissect the intramural ureter using electrocautery. Cephalad traction on the ureter will help identify the bladder mucosa. Use a right-angle clamp to secure the ureteral orifice, and then excise the ureter. Tie a 2-0 absorbable suture around the right-angle clamp to close the bladder mucosa, or use running 4-0 absorbable suture. Close a second layer over the resection site using 2-0 absorbable sutures. Manage drains and catheters as above.

## Laparoscopic Extravesical Bladder Cuff Technique (6)

This technique is similar to the open surgical extravesical approach. Place the patient in a modified flank position for transperitoneal laparoscopic nephrectomy. Using flexible cystoscopy, insert a ureteral catheter. At the conclusion of the laparoscopic nephrectomy, dissect the ureter distally and place clips on the ureter to prevent extravasation of tumor cells. Retract the ureter cephalad and continue dissecting it distally to the bladder. After inserting a 10-mm port in the lower abdomen to facilitate resection of the distal ureter, incise the bladder just anterior to the ureter using electrocautery. Upon entering the bladder, the ureteral catheter identifies the ureteral orifice. Excise the posterior portion of the bladder cuff and detach the ureter after dividing the ureteral catheter. Suture the bladder closed using laparoscopic techniques (recently, robotic assistance has been described to facilitate this step). Manage drains and catheters as above.

## Endoscopic Techniques

Except for the "pluck" procedures, all of the endoscopic techniques described in this section have been developed specifically for use in conjunction with laparoscopic nephroureterectomy. The techniques are described below in the settings in which they were initially described or are in common use at this time. The hand-assisted approach to laparoscopic nephroureterectomy may be preferable with particular techniques, as indicated below, but any approach to nephroureterectomy—laparoscopic or open surgical—can be used in conjunction with any of the following techniques, with modifications.

### Transvesical Bladder Cuff Technique: Single Port (5)

After completing a hand-assisted laparoscopic nephrectomy with the patient in the modified flank position, dissect the ureter to the bladder. Place clips on the ureter to prevent tumor spillage.

Without repositioning the patient, fill the bladder with fluid through a three-way urethral catheter. Make an incision for a 10-mm laparoscopic port in the midline, three finger breadths above the pubis. Using the surgeon's hand via the hand-assist port, push the bladder upward toward the abdominal wall. Insert a spinal needle through the incision into the bladder to ascertain proper angle and depth of entry, and then insert a 10-mm laparoscopic port directly into the bladder through the extraperitoneal space. Using a 24Fr resectoscope with a Collins knife through this port, and with the surgeon's hand alternately elevating the ipsilateral hemitrigone and retracting the ureter, incise around the ureteral orifice and intramural ureter with the Collins knife (Fig. 19.2). During the

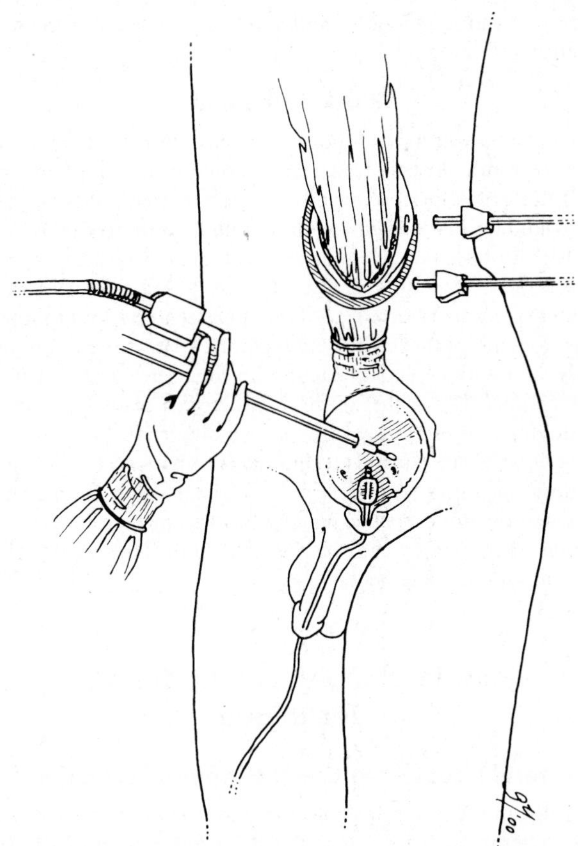

FIGURE 19.2 The surgeon's hand elevates the ipsilateral hemitrigone while the Collins knife is used to incise around the ureteral orifice. (Adapted from Gonzalez CM, Batler RA, Schoor RA, et al. A novel endoscopic approach towards resection of the distal ureter with surrounding bladder cuff during hand assisted laparoscopic nephroureterectomy. *J Urol* 2001;165:484.)

resection, controlling the height of the urethal catheter drainage bag controls the filling of the bladder. As soon as the ureter is detached, placing the drainage bag on the floor minimizes extravasation of urine and irrigant. Note that once the bladder has been opened into the retroperitoneum, it collapses quickly, so take care to keep the dissection at equal depth all around the orifice so that once the bladder collapses the ureter can be pulled free easily.

After specimen removal, remove the bladder port. Neither the port site nor the resection site needs to be closed, but placement of a pelvic drain through a laparoscopic port site is optional. The initial description of this technique includes a cystogram performed on postoperative day 7 to verify lack of extravasation prior to catheter removal, but in the author's experience with this technique the cystotomy is adequately healed by this time and a voiding trial is sufficient.

## Transurethral Bladder Cuff Technique

This technique is similar to the transvesical bladder cuff technique except that the resection is performed transurethrally, which obviates the need for placement of a transvesical port. One option is to use a flexible cystoscope with an electrocautery probe to perform the periureteral dissection (11). Another alternative is to position the patient in a combined lithotomy-semiflank position that allows simultaneous laparoscopic nephrectomy and transurethral access with a 24Fr resectoscope with a Collins knife (12).

## Transvesical Bladder Cuff Technique: Two Ports (4)

Prior to performing the nephrectomy portion of the procedure, place the patient in the lithotomy position. Perform cystoscopy to evaluate the bladder mucosa and distend the bladder. Under cystoscopic guidance, place two 5-mm balloon-tipped laparoscopic ports into the bladder just above the pubic bone on both sides of the midline, placing both ports to wall suction to prevent extravasation and overdistention of the bladder. Insert a 5-mm endoloop through the ipsilateral port, and then insert a 6Fr ureteral catheter cystoscopically into the targeted ureter. Exchange the cystoscope for a resectoscope with a Collins knife, which is used to incise around the ureteral orifice. Using a grasper inserted through the other laparoscopic port that is passed through the endoloop, retract the ureteral orifice anteriorly. After freeing up 3 to 4 cm of ureter, suspend the ureter from the anterior bladder wall with the grasper (Fig. 19.3); then remove the ureteral catheter and tighten the endoloop around the ureter to occlude the lumen.

After removing the laparoscopic ports, place a urethral catheter to gravity drainage. Perform the nephrectomy portion of the procedure after repositioning, and with cephalad traction dissect the ureter distally such that the distal ureter can be pulled into the operative space for intact removal. Again, a urethral catheter is left in place for 1 week, with the option of

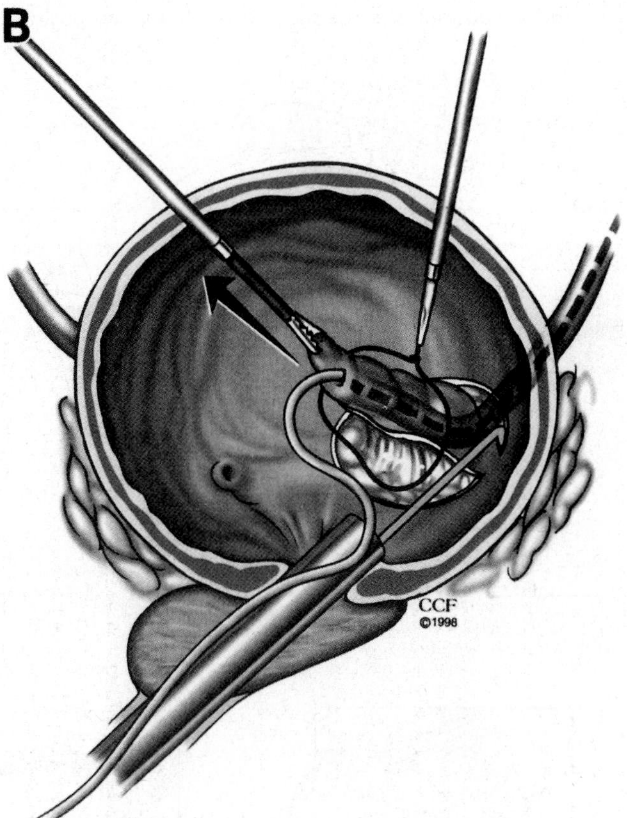


FIGURE 19.3 The Collins knife is used transurethrally while a grasper elevates the ureter and the endoloop is around the resected orifice. (Adapted from Gill IS, Soble JJ, Miller SD, et al. A novel technique for the management of the en bloc bladder cuff and distal ureter during laparoscopic nephroureterectomy. *J Urol* 1999;161:432.)

a cystogram to confirm adequate bladder healing prior to catheter removal.

### Ureteral Unroofing Technique (10)

Prior to performing the nephrectomy portion of the procedure, place the patient in the lithotomy position. Perform cystoscopy and insert a ureteral dilating balloon (5 mm diameter, 10 cm length) into the targeted intramural ureter. Inflate the balloon to 1-atm pressure with dilute contrast material using fluoroscopic guidance. Exchange the cystoscope for a resectoscope with a Collins knife, and incise the ureteral tunnel at the 12 o'clock position along the entire length of the intramural ureter. Remove the dilating balloon and use a rollerball electrode to cauterize the edges and floor of the intramural ureter. Insert a 7Fr 11.5-mm balloon occlusion catheter into the renal pelvis and inflate it at the ureteropelvic junction, to prevent urine extravasation. Connect this catheter, and a urethral catheter, to gravity drainage.

Take the patient out of the lithotomy position and perform the nephrectomy. Once completed, mobilize the distal ureter to the ureteral hiatus, dividing the superior vesical artery if necessary. Ligate and incise the remaining distal ureter and bladder cuff using an endoscopic stapler (Fig. 19.4), removing the ureteral balloon occlusion catheter just prior to engaging the stapler. Leave the urethral catheter in place for 3 to 5 days, removing it after cystography or a voiding trial demonstrates no urinary extravasation. A modification of the technique, which allows for nephrectomy to be performed before ureterectomy, is to address the distal ureter with a stapler as described above and then reposition the patient into the lithotomy position. Use a resectoscope and a rollerball to ablate the intramural ureter until the staple line is visible.

### Pluck Technique

Place the patient in the lithotomy position prior to performing nephrectomy. Insert a ureteral catheter into the targeted ureteral orifice cystoscopically. Incise the ureteral orifice and surrounding bladder cuff with a Collins knife to the level of retroperitoneal fat. Alternatively, use a loop resectoscope to resect the orifice and intramural ureter. Place a 24Fr urethral catheter to gravity drainage. Take the patient out of lithotomy position and perform the nephrectomy. Dissect the ureter distally, and with cephalad traction on the ureter detach it from the bladder. Leave the urethral catheter in place for 7 days, removing it after cystography or a voiding trial.

A modification of this technique is to pass a 7Fr, 11.5-mm balloon occlusion catheter into the renal pelvis, snugging it down at the ureteropelvic junction, to minimize urine extravasation. Mitomycin can be instilled into the renal pelvis through this catheter (9).

## Combined Open and Endoscopic Technique

### Ureteral Intussusception (Stripping) Technique (1)

Initially, in the lithotomy position, insert either a stone basket or ureteral catheter into the targeted proximal ureter. Reposition the patient and perform nephrectomy, dissecting

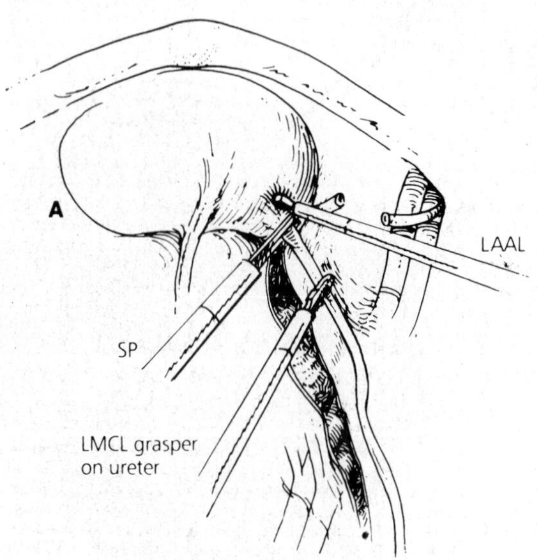


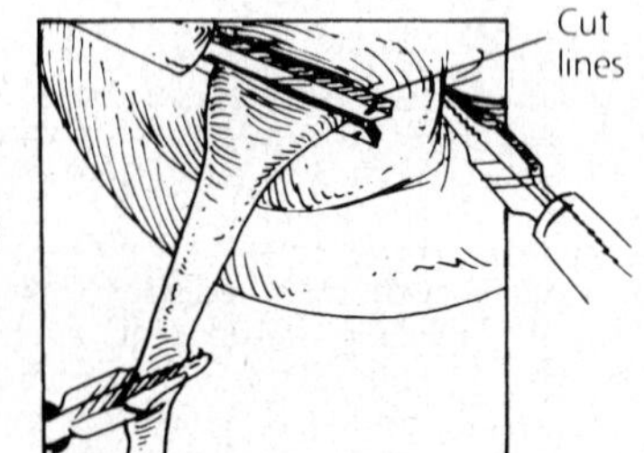


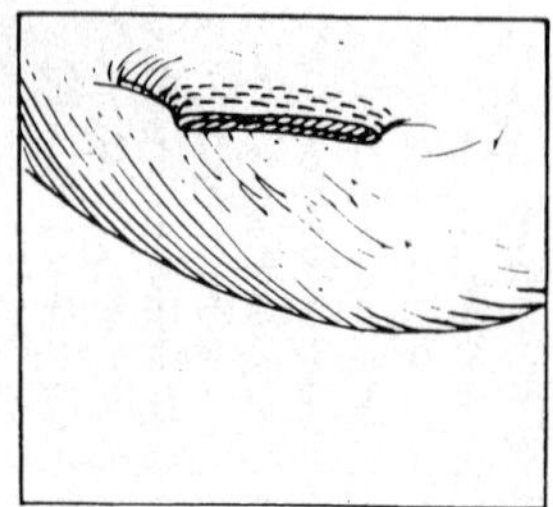


FIGURE 19.4 **A:** The endoscopic stapler is placed across the ureterovesical junction. **B:** Close-up view of the stapler across the ureterovesical junction. **C:** Staples are seen securing the bladder cuff. (Adapted from Clayman RV. Laparoscopic ureteral surgery. In: Clayman RV, McDougall EM, eds. *Laparoscopic urology*. St. Louis, MO: Quality Medical Publishers, 1993:360.)

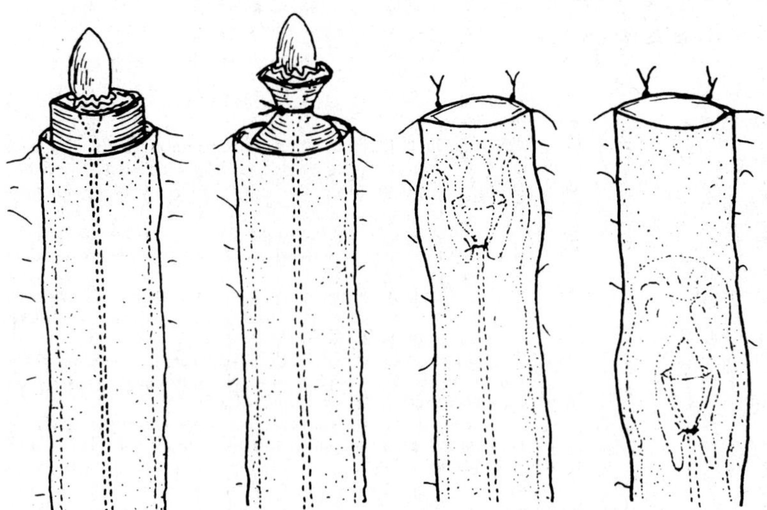

FIGURE 19.5 The proximal ureter is divided and secured to the ureteral catheter. The ureter is then intussuscepted as the catheter is removed. (Adapted from Angulo JC, Hontoria J, Sanchez-Chapado M. One incision nephroureterectomy endoscopically assisted by transurethral stripping. *Urology* 1998;52:204.)

the ureter to the pelvic brim. Clip the proximal ureter, and then divide the ureter cephalad to the basket/ureteral catheter. Advance the stone basket into the retroperitoneum and open and close it to entrap the ureteral wall, or, if a ureteral catheter has been used, tie it to the ureter with a 0-silk suture (Fig. 19.5). Apply gentle traction to the stone basket/ureteral catheter to intussuscept the ureter into the bladder (Fig. 19.6). Then use a Collins knife mounted on a resectoscope inserted transurethrally (after repositioning into the lithotomy position) to incise the bladder cuff around the intussuscepted ureter while exerting traction on the stone basket/ureteral catheter out of the urethra.

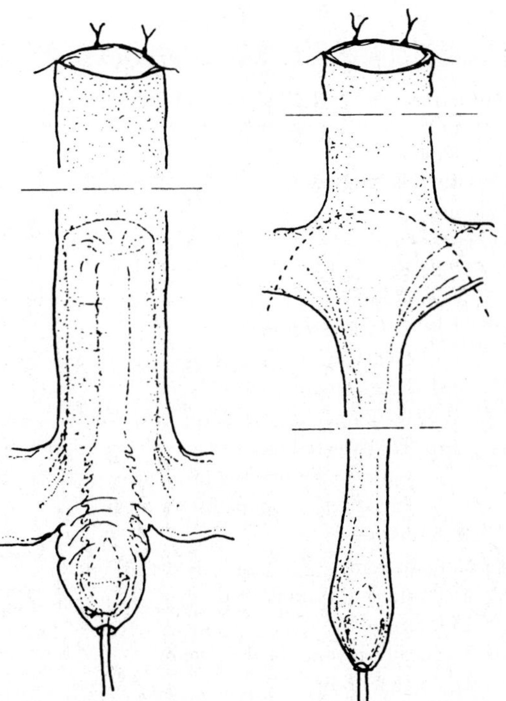

FIGURE 19.6 The catheter is retracted through the bladder wall and urethra. (Adapted from Angulo JC, Hontoria J, Sanchez-Chapado M. One incision nephroureterectomy endoscopically assisted by transurethral stripping. *Urology* 1998;52:204.)

Place a urethral catheter for 7 days, following a normal cystogram or voiding trial. This technique should not be used for distal or midureteral tumors.

## OUTCOMES

Survival after nephroureterectomy is strongly dependent on the grade and stage of the tumor (7). Five-year survival rates following a radical nephroureterectomy for low-grade tumors are 40% to 87%, compared to 0% to 33% for high-grade disease. Five-year survival estimates according to stage are as follows: stage Tis/Ta,/T1, 60% to 90%; stage T2, 43% to 75%; stage T3, 26% to 33%; stage T4/N+/M+, 0% to 5% (7).

## COMPLICATIONS

Early complications include hematuria, retroperitoneal hematoma, and retroperitoneal abscess. Ureteral intussusception may be technically unsuccessful in 10% of patients. Prolonged urinary extravasation can in general be managed conservatively with urethral catheter drainage. Although not yet reported clinically, there is the potential for calculi to form on the staple line when the ureteral unroofing technique is used, or for urothelial cells to survive in between the staples. Other factors to be considered in the choice of technique include the risk of tumor spillage, the addition of a bladder incision, the timing of the ureterectomy relative to nephrectomy, the need for repositioning, the approach to nephrectomy that is desired, and surgeon preference. Of these, the potential for tumor cell spillage is probably the most important with regard to outcome. The technique to excise the distal ureter is probably not a factor for recurrence as long as there is no spillage of tumor cells in the retroperitoneum. Of note, isolated retrovesical recurrences following "pluck" ureterectomy have been reported. There is not yet enough reported experience with the newer endoscopic techniques to allow reliable comparison of the risk of local, regional, and port site recurrences among the new techniques and the standard open surgical techniques, although one group has reported a greater intravesical recurrence rate after the intussusception technique compared to open surgical bladder cuff (8).

## References


1. Angulo JC, Hontoria J, Sanchez-Chapado M. One incision nephroureterectomy endoscopically assisted by transurethral stripping. *Urology* 1998;52: 203–207.
2. Bloom NA, Vidone RA, Lytton B. Primary carcinoma of the ureter: a report of 102 new cases. *J Urol* 1970;103:590–598.
3. Flanigan RC. Urothelial tumors of the upper urinary tract. In: Wein AJ, Kavoussi LR, Novick AC, et al., eds. *Campbell-Walsh urology*, 9th ed., Vol. 2. Philadelphia: Saunders-Elsevier, 2007:1638–1652.
4. Gill IS, Soble JJ, Miller SD, et al. A novel technique for the management of the en bloc bladder cuff and distal ureter during laparoscopic nephroureterectomy. *J Urol* 1999;161:430–434.
5. Gonzalez CM, Batler RA, Schoor RA, et al. A novel endoscopic approach towards resection of the distal ureter with surrounding bladder cuff during hand assisted laparoscopic nephroureterectomy. *J Urol* 2001;165:483–485.
6. McGinnis DE, Trabulsi EJ, Gomella LG, et al. Hand-assisted laparoscopic nephroureterectomy: description of technique. *Techniques Urol* 2001;7:7–11.
7. Sagalowsky AI, Jarrett TW. Management of urothelial tumors of the renal pelvis and ureter. In: Wein AJ, Kavoussi LR, Novick AC, et al., eds. *Campbell-Walsh urology*, 9th ed., Vol. 2. Philadelphia: Saunders-Elsevier, 2007:1653–1685.
8. Saika T, Nishiguchi J, Tsushima T, et al. Comparative study of ureteral stripping versus open ureterectomy for nephroureterectomy in patients with transitional carcinoma of the renal pelvis. *Urology* 2004;63: 848–852.
9. Seifman BD, Montie JE, Wolf JS Jr. Prospective comparison between hand-assisted laparoscopic and open surgical nephroureterectomy for urothelial carcinoma. *Urology* 2001;57:133–137.
10. Shalhav AL, Elbahnasy AM, McDougall EM, et al. Laparoscopic nephroureterectomy for upper tract transitional cell cancer: technical aspects. *J Endourol* 1998;12:345–353.
11. Vardi IY, Stern JA, Gonzalez CM, et al. Novel technique for management of distal ureter and en bloc resection of bladder cuff during hand-assisted laparoscopic nephroureterectomy. *Urology* 2006;67:89–92.
12. Wong C, Leveillee RJ. Hand-assisted laparoscopic nephroureterectomy with cystoscopic en bloc excision of the distal ureter and bladder cuff. *J Endourol* 2002;16:329–332.


# CHAPTER 20 ■ VESICOVAGINAL FISTULA

HELEN G. ZAFIRAKIS AND O. LENAINE WESTNEY

A vesicovaginal fistula (VVF) is an epithelialized or fibrous communication between the bladder and vagina. Physically, psychologically, and socially, it is a source of major distress for the patient contending with urine leakage from the vagina. Documentation of VVFs exists from as early as 1550 B.C. in the Eber papyrus of ancient Egypt (10). In 1845 James Marion Sims, considered the father of American gynecology, began his exploration into the challenges of treating the condition in Montgomery, Alabama (10). He is credited with developing the foundation of VVF repair and establishing sound surgical principles for repair of fistulas.

The causative factors leading to VVF formation can be broadly categorized into congenital and acquired (Table 20.1). The majority of cases fall into the iatrogenic and obstetric trauma subcategories. In underdeveloped countries, the leading cause of VVFs is obstetric trauma, in which prolonged labor causes ischemic pressure necrosis of the bladder and anterior vaginal wall. In contrast, obstetric trauma accounts for only 5% of VVFs in nations where modern healthcare is present. The leading cause of VVFs in industrialized countries is iatrogenic surgical trauma, accounting for 82% to 91% of VVFs. Ninety-one percent are due to gynecologic procedures, with 80% due to abdominal hysterectomy (9). The incidence of VVF after transabdominal hysterectomy is 1.0 in 1,000, as opposed to 0.2 in 1,000 after transvaginal hysterectomy. The incidence is highest (2.2 in 1,000) with laparoscopic hysterectomy (7). The most common location for a posthysterectomy VVF is the apex of the vaginal vault or "cuff" corresponding to an intravesical location just superior to the trigone (9). Theoretically, the fistula develops secondary to the unintentional inclusion of full-thickness bladder wall during closure of the vaginal cuff, an unrecognized bladder injury adjacent to the cuff suture line, or cuff abscess.

**TABLE 20.1**

**ETIOLOGIES OF VESICOVAGINAL FISTULAS**

- I. Congenital
  - A. Cloacal abnormality
- II. Acquired
  - A. Iatrogenic
    - 1. Postsurgical
      - a. Hysterectomy
      - b. Cesarean section
      - c. Dilatation and curettage
      - d. Pelvic laparoscopy
      - e. Incontinence procedure
      - f. Transvaginal biopsies
      - g. Intravescial formalin instillation
      - h. Failed vesicovaginal fistula repair
    - 2. Radiation
  - B. Noniatrogenic
    - 1. Obstetrical trauma
    - 2. Infection
    - 3. Locally advanced pelvic tumor
    - 4. Foreign body
    - 5. Pelvic trauma/fracture

Modified from Rackley RR, Appell RA. Vesicovaginal fistula: current approach. *AUA Update Series* 1998;21:161–168.

## DIAGNOSIS

Classically, the postoperative VVF presents with "continuous" urine leakage from the vagina. The time of presentation peaks at 7 to 10 days after surgery but may be variable, with some patients presenting immediately after catheter removal, ranging from 4 to 6 weeks after surgery (7). In the early postoperative period, there may also be associated ileus and abdominal pain due to intraperitoneal urine extravasation. VVFs due to pelvic irradiation usually have a delayed presentation, developing many months or years posttreatment due to progressive obliterative endarteritis causing tissue ischemia and necrosis.

The key to diagnosis of a VVF is a high suspicion. Often, a complete history and physical examination expose the pathology. In the case of less obvious fistula, a dye test is utilized to more clearly visualize the passage of fluid through the fistula. In its simplest form, a saline and dye (indigo carmine or methylene blue) mixture is instilled into the bladder via a Foley catheter while inspecting the vagina for leakage or staining of a previously placed tampon. The failure to identify any discoloration of the tampon may indicate a small fistula or ureterovaginal fistula. The second level of testing requires reinsertion of a vaginal gauze or tampon followed by administration of 5 mg indigo carmine intravenously to determine whether the source is ureteral. Dye from a ureterovaginal fistula may be present on the first gauze inspection prior to intravenous (IV) indigo carmine if there is vesicoureteral reflux, which can be determined with a voiding cystourethrogram (VCUG). An alternative to IV dye injection is oral phenazopyridine hydrochloride, but it requires several hours of lead time before examination.

All patients should have an IV pyelogram (IVP) for upper-tract evaluation. Abnormalities to look for include extravasation into the vagina or peritoneal cavity or a displaced or partially obstructed ureter. In patients with VVF, up to 25% will have hydroureteronephrosis, with 10% having a concomitant ureterovaginal fistula (6). In patients with ureteral pathology, a retrograde pyelogram is warranted to evaluate for ureterovaginal fistula if the IVP is not definitive.

Cystoscopy is performed to localize and evaluate the VVF, which often has surrounding edematous mucosa. The size and number of VVFs, their location in relation to the ureteral orifices, any lesions such as foreign bodies (i.e., sutures), tumors, and tissue quality must be noted. If there is a history of malignancy, biopsy of the VVF is indicated to rule out recurrent tumor. Vaginoscopy is performed simultaneous with cystoscopy to assess the vaginal aspect of the fistula. If IVP and retrograde pyelograms are inconclusive, then a fistulogram may be performed transvaginally.

A urodynamic study is recommended to look for other factors that may contribute to the urinary incontinence and may require surgical correction (augmentation cystoplasty, incontinence surgery) with the VVF repair simultaneously. Bladder compliance, capacity, and leak point pressure should be assessed if possible.

## INDICATIONS FOR SURGERY

The issue of how long to wait before attempting surgical repair of a VVF has long been debated. By tradition, VVF repair is delayed 3 to 6 months to allow inflammation to resolve. In cases where a VVF is due to a complicated operation or after obstetric trauma, this rationale holds true. However, independent studies by Blaivas et al. and Blandy et al. demonstrated comparable results with early (6 to 12 weeks) repair in cases related to an uncomplicated hysterectomy (1,2). Once surgical repair is decided upon, another issue that has to be considered is the approach: transvaginal, transvesical, or transabdominal. Often, the approach is the one that the surgeon is most experienced in performing. Advantages of the transvaginal approach are less blood loss, shorter hospital stay, avoidance of a laparotomy, and thus decreased morbidity. Many reserve the transabdominal approach for those patients requiring concomitant intra-abdominal surgery (ureteral reimplantation, augmentation cystoplasty) or those patients with a narrow and deep vagina causing poor exposure to the VVF. However, Dupont and Raz reported that nearly all VVFs can be accessed and repaired transvaginally (3).

## ALTERNATIVE THERAPY

Upon diagnosis, a trial of conservative therapy is started depending on fistula size. Conservative therapy consists of prolonged bladder drainage with a Foley catheter, anticholinergic agents to prevent bladder spasms, antibiotics, and estrogen if the patient is postmenopausal. Successful closure of a VVF via conservative therapy can be expected only in those 3 mm in diameter or less.

Other adjunctive minimally invasive treatments include attempts to destroy the epithelial lining of the VVF with fulguration (using electrocautery or laser) and use of occlusive substances. Since the late 1980s, glue materials have been used to treat a variety of fistulas. There are two main types of glues used to treat VVF: fibrin, which is a biologic product, and synthetic cyanoacrylic glue. Fibrin glue has the longest reported follow-up.

There have been a few small series reported on the use of fibrin glue to treat VVF that demonstrate a good success rate. Schneider et al. reported on six cases using endoscopic techniques and found a 66% closure rate using glue compared with 88% success with a traditional repair (11). Although it may involve more than one injection to treat the fistula, fibrin glue promotes healing, is biodegradable, and has been used successfully in a large variety of urologic fistulas, including those caused by irradiation.

Synthetic cyanoacrylic glue is a relatively newer product in occlusion therapy of fistulas. It polymerizes in 90 seconds once injected and can be used without difficulty in a wet environment such as the bladder; this, together with its antimicrobial properties, makes it an attractive option for the treatment of VVF. The best results are achieved in long fistulas <1 cm in diameter. Application can be performed both endovaginally and endoscopically, with the Foley catheter removal between 48 hours to 3 weeks depending on the size of the fistula. Generally, follow-up cystography is performed in 1 to 3 months.

The benefits of using occlusion therapy to treat VVFs include the ability to treat the fistula earlier rather than expecting the patient to live with the distressing symptoms of the fistula for up to 3 months while awaiting definitive surgery. Additionally, there is very low morbidity associated with using occlusion therapy; there have been no reported complications from occlusion therapy treatment of VVF, other than the occasional necessity of removing excess glue endoscopically. Importantly, it does not preclude other forms of treatment if it is unsuccessful. Although occlusion therapy appears to be safe and efficacious in selected, small VVFs, more longer-term and randomized studies are needed to evaluate its durability.

## SURGICAL TECHNIQUE

### Transvaginal Approach

The patient is placed in the dorsolithotomy position. If a narrow vagina is present or the VVF site is high lying, a Schuchardt posterolateral relaxing incision at the 4 o'clock position of the vaginal introitus and distal vaginal wall may be performed to improve exposure. A suprapubic catheter may be placed with a Lowsley retractor, and a urethral Foley catheter is placed. The labia minora are sutured to the inner thigh and a weighted vaginal speculum placed. The VVF is dilated to place an 8Fr Foley catheter. Applying gentle traction to the catheter aids in exposure and dissection of the VVF.

After submucosal injection of a vasopressin mixture (10 U per 100 mL normal saline), lidocaine with 1% epinephrine, or saline to elevate the anterior vaginal mucosa, the VVF is circumferentially incised. A posteriorly based inverted U-shaped incision is made with the apex continuous with the VVF incision (Fig. 20.1). If the VVF is situated deep in the vaginal vault, an anteriorly based U-shaped incision is utilized. The vaginal mucosa is dissected away from the perivesical fascia to form vaginal flaps anterior and posterior to the VVF (Fig. 20.2). Unless nonviable, the fistulous tract is not excised as excision enlarges the defect and risks injury to the intramural ureter. Left intact, the fistula tract also provides strength to the VVF closure, helping decrease the risk of VVF repair disruption due to bladder spasms.

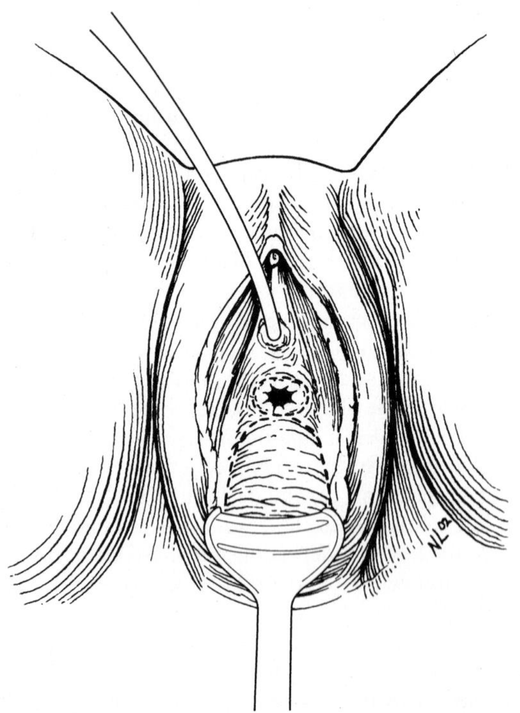

FIGURE 20.1 The apex of the vaginal inverted-U incision is continuous with the circumferential fistula incision. (Modified from Raz S, Bregg KJ, Nitti VW, et al. Transvaginal repair of vesicovaginal fistula using a peritoneal flap. *J Urol* 1993;150:56–59.)

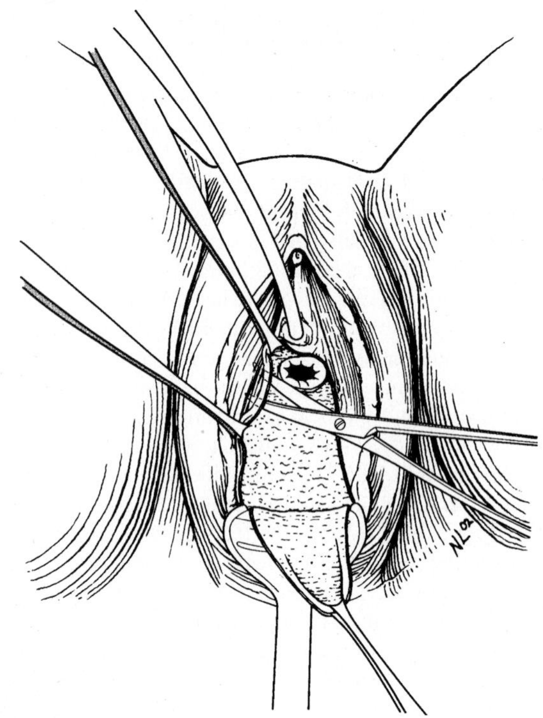

FIGURE 20.2 The vaginal mucosa is dissected away from the perivesical fascia. (Modified from Raz S, Bregg KJ, Nitti VW, et al. Transvaginal repair of vesicovaginal fistula using a peritoneal flap. *J Urol* 1993;150:56–59.)

The fistula is closed in two nonoverlapping, perpendicular layers to prevent fistula recurrence. The first layer closes the fistula with interrupted 4-0 polyglycolic acid sutures, incorporating the vaginal wall overlying the VVF, the fistula tract, and the partial thickness of the bladder wall (Fig. 20.3). The second layer, using 2-0 polyglycolic acid sutures, imbricates the perivesical fascia and the deeper musculature of the bladder over the first layer in a tension-free fashion. The repair is checked for leaks by instilling indigo carmine into the bladder. The vaginal wall is advanced over the VVF repair and closed with an interlocking, running 2-0 polyglycolic acid suture. A Betadine-soaked vaginal pack is placed.

If there is any concern about the repair, an interposing layer may be placed between the vaginal wall and bladder. The most common options are the Martius labial fat pad and the peritoneal flap. Alternative tissues include labial, vaginal wall, gluteal, and gracilis muscle flaps.

The Martius labial fat pad provides neovascularity and lymphatic drainage, fills dead space, and enhances granulation tissue formation. The flap is harvested by making a vertical incision on the labium majus; the underlying fibrofatty tissue is mobilized. The anterior portion of the graft is tied off (sacrificing the blood supply from the external pudendal artery), leaving the fibrofatty pad supplied by its posterior blood source: the posterior labial artery from the internal pudendal artery. A tunnel is developed from the vaginal incision to the labium majus; the labial fat pad is transferred through the tunnel to cover the VVF repair and secured in place with

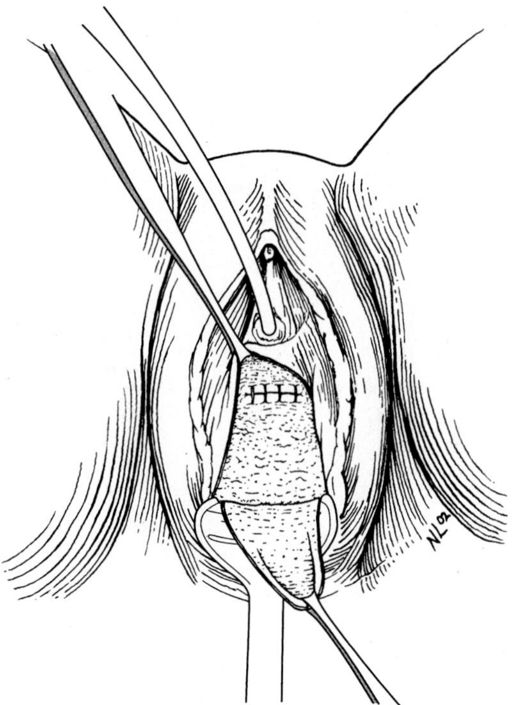

FIGURE 20.3 Closure of the first layer, including the fistulous tract and partial-thickness bladder wall. (Modified from Raz S, Bregg KJ, Nitti VW, et al. Transvaginal repair of vesicovaginal fistula using a peritoneal flap. *J Urol* 1993;150:56–59.)

interrupted 3-0 polyglycolic acid sutures (Fig. 20.4). The tunnel must be sufficiently sized to prevent constriction of the fat pad's blood supply. The labial incision is closed with a 1⁄4-in. Penrose drain in place unless the graft bed is dry (Fig. 20.5).

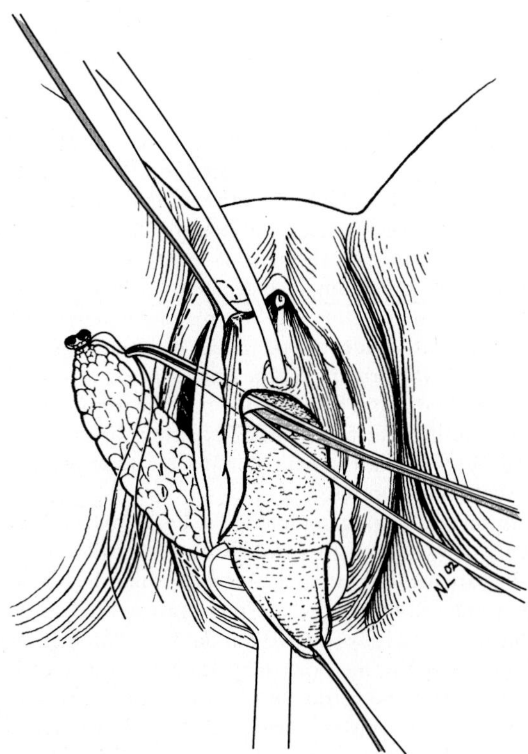

FIGURE 20.4 Using a right-angle clamp, the Martius flap is passed from the labial incision to the vaginal incision.

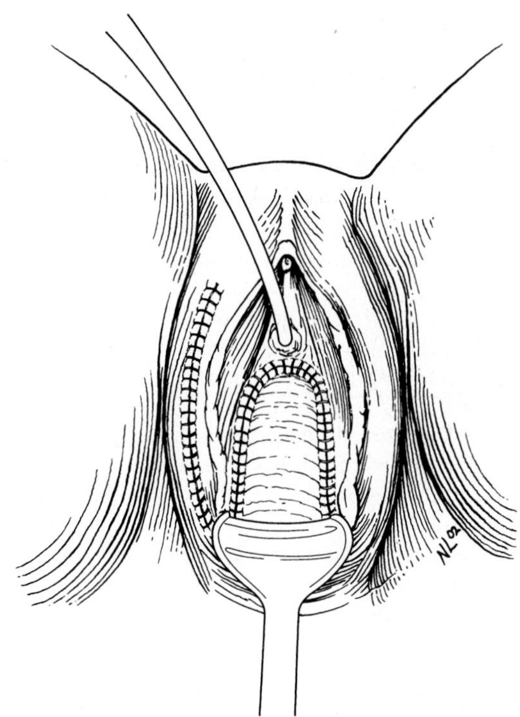

FIGURE 20.5 Closure of the labial and vaginal wall incisions.

Another effective method is peritoneal interposition as described by Dupont and Raz for routine use in fistula repair (3). With further posterior dissection of the anterior vaginal wall from the bladder, the glistening surface of the peritoneum in the anterior cul-de-sac is exposed. Without entering the intraperitoneal space, the peritoneum is mobilized from the posterior bladder wall to bring it down into the vagina and suture it over the VVF repair site (Fig. 20.6). The peritoneal flap has a 96% success rate when used in transvaginal VVF repair (4).

The vaginal pack is removed on postoperative day 1. The patient is given perioperative antibiotics and anticholinergics to prevent bladder spasms. Two weeks postoperatively the urethral catheter and suprapubic tube are removed if the

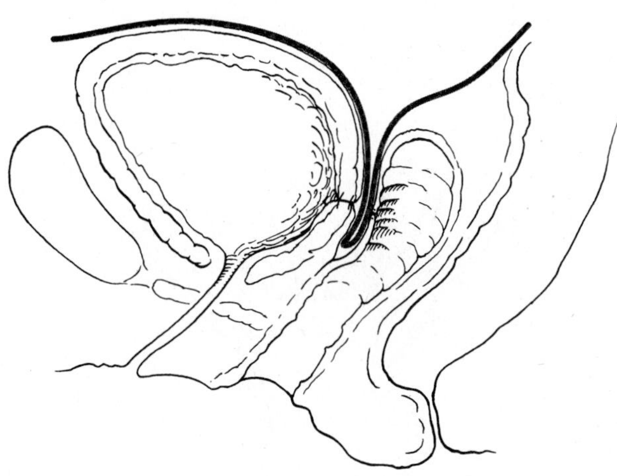

FIGURE 20.6 Interposition of the peritoneum between the bladder and vagina. (Modified from Raz S, Bregg KJ, Nitti VW, et al. Transvaginal repair of vesicovaginal fistula using a peritoneal flap. *J Urol* 1993;150:56–59.)

cystogram reveals no persistent fistula or extravasation. If a fistula is still present, bladder drainage continues for another 2 to 3 weeks and the cystogram repeated at that time.

## Transabdominal (Intraperitoneal) Approach

The patient is placed in a low lithotomy position. Cystoscopy is performed to visualize and cannulate the VVF with a 5FR to 6Fr ureteral catheter or guide wire. If unable to pass the guide wire through the VVF transvesically, it is passed from the vaginal side into the bladder, grasped cystoscopically, and brought out through the urethra.

A midline infraumbilical incision is made; the rectus muscle is split midline to enter the pelvis. The bladder is opened with a midline vertical cystotomy between two stay sutures (Fig. 20.7). The VVF is identified with the guide wire exiting its opening into the bladder. The urethral end of the guide wire is pulled into the cystotomy incision. The VVF's position in relation to the ureteral orifices is noted and the ureters are cannulated with stents, if necessary. If there is any difficulty identifying the orifices due to local inflammation, IV indigo carmine may be administered.

Entering the peritoneal cavity, the dissection along the posterior bladder wall is carried out until the guide wire traversing the VVF is palpated, indicating the junction between the vagina and bladder. With a sponge stick or endoanal sizer in the vagina to help delineate the vagina, the bladder is carefully dissected away from the vagina. Wide mobilization of the bladder and vagina to allow tension-free closure of each side of the VVF is critical. The dissection bisects the fistula tract without excising the tract extending 1.5 to 2.0 cm beyond the VVF, allowing for tension-free closure (Fig. 20.8). Using interrupted 3-0 polyglycolic acid sutures, the vaginal defect is closed in two nonoverlapping layers. The bladder defect is also closed in two nonoverlapping layers with running 4-0 polyglycolic acid and 3-0 interrupted sutures.

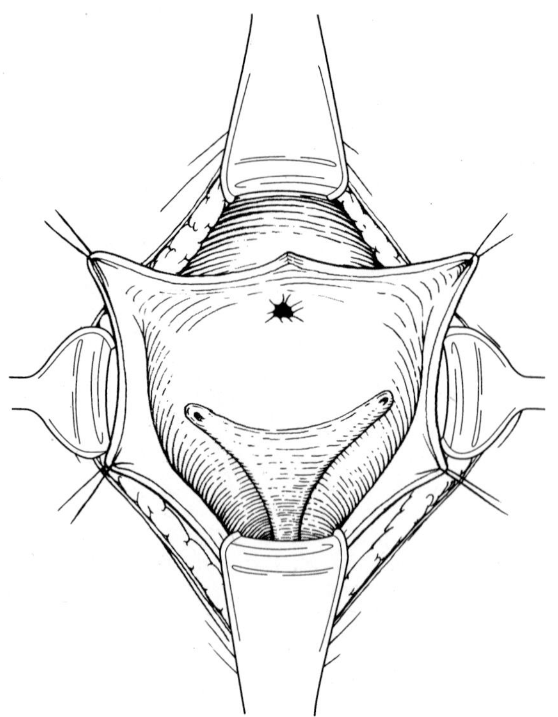

FIGURE 20.7 The bladder is opened in the midline without extending the cystotomy to the fistula.

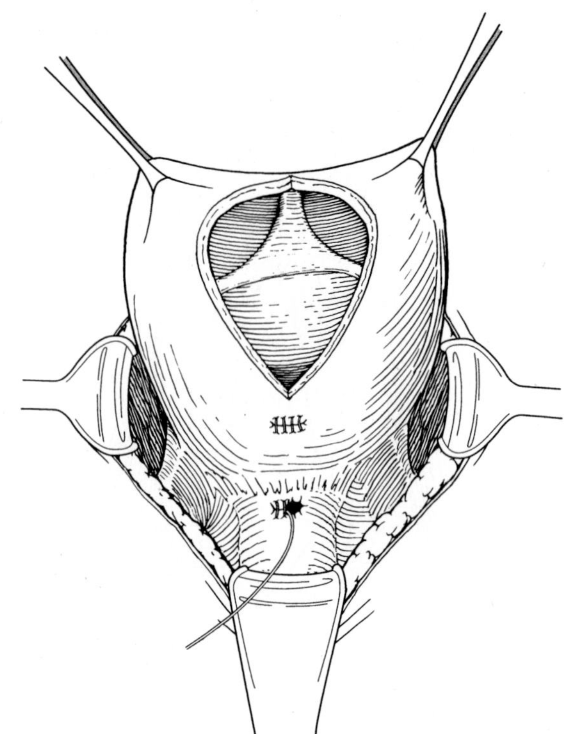

FIGURE 20.8 After dissecting between the bladder and vaginal, both defects are closed in two layers.

After the bladder and vaginal fistulous defects are closed, attention is turned to developing an omental pedicle flap to interpose between the bladder and vagina. Evans et al. recommended routine use of an interposition flap during intra-abdominal VVF repair, noting a success rate of 100% with a flap versus 63% to 67% without a flap (5). Not only does the interposition flap add an extra layer to the VVF repair to prevent recurrence, but it also increases lymphatic drainage and decreases the risk of infected fluid collection. Alternatives to omentum include lateral pelvic peritoneum, pericolic or mesenteric fat, and free bladder mucosal graft.

The omentum is identified, and an omental flap based on the more reliable right gastroepiploic artery is developed (Fig. 20.9). The flap is brought down to the pelvis and placed between the bladder and vagina, covering the fistula repair (Fig. 20.10). The graft is secured in place with interrupted 3-0 polyglycolic acid sutures.

With the VVF repair completed, a suprapubic catheter and urethral Foley catheter are placed with 5-mL balloon inflation each. In patients with prolonged large fistula, the bladder capacity is reduced due to the constant drainage. Therefore, the placement of two fully inflated balloons in combination with irritation from the incisions may lead to intensification of bladder spasms. The vertical bladder incision is closed in two layers with 2-0 polyglycolic acid sutures. A closed pelvic drain is also placed. Postoperative care is similar to that after transvaginal VVF repair.

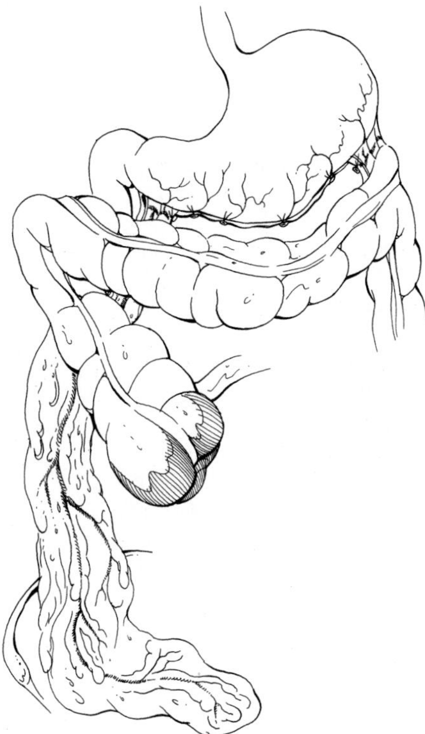

FIGURE 20.9 Development of an omental pedical flap based on the right gastroepiploic artery.

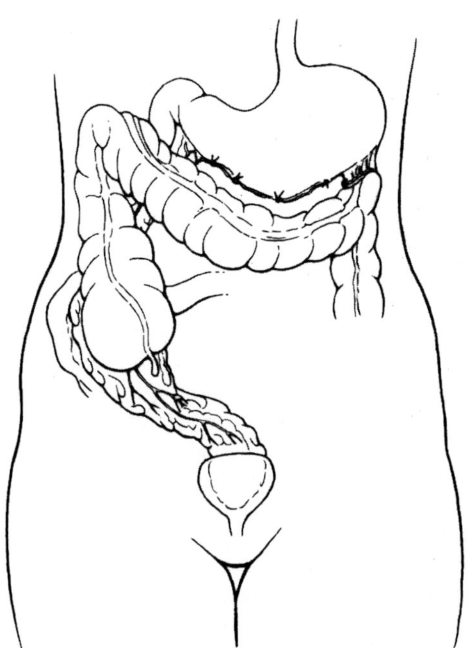

FIGURE 20.10 Placement of the distal end of the omental graft posterior to the detrusor covering the repairs.

An alternative to the above intra-abdominal technique is the standard O'Conor technique. The bladder is bivalved posteriorly from the dome to the level of the VVF. Then, the VVF is excised entirely (Figs. 20.11 through 20.13). After further dissection of the bladder from the vagina, the vaginal defect is closed in two nonopposing layers with interrupted absorbable

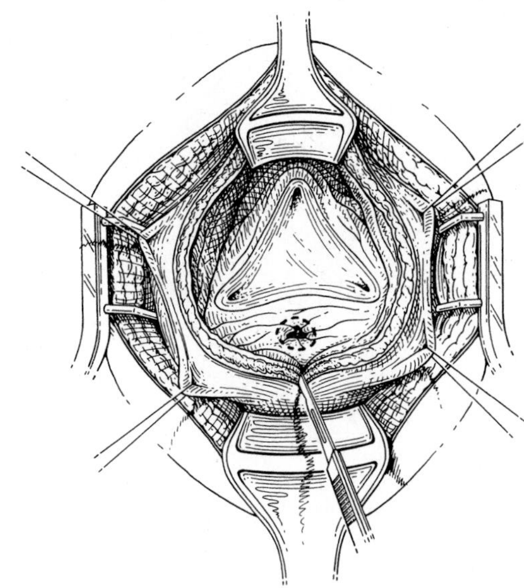

FIGURE 20.11 Cystotomy extended down to the fistula site.

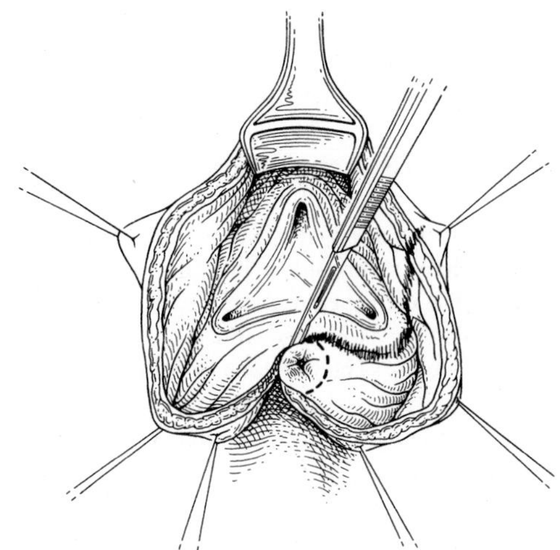

FIGURE 20.12 Circumscribing incision around the fistula.

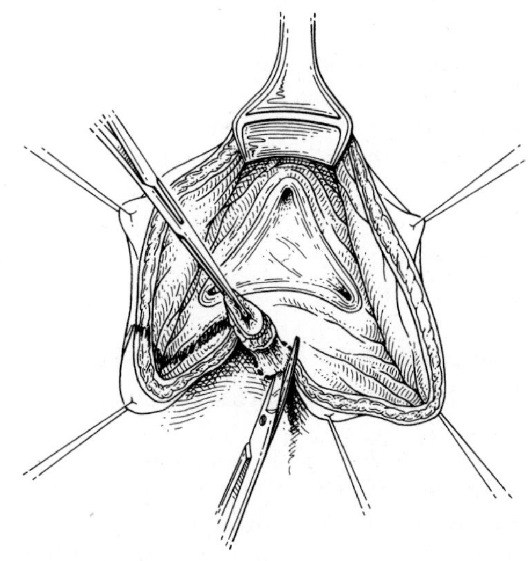

FIGURE 20.13 Sharp excision of the fistula tract.

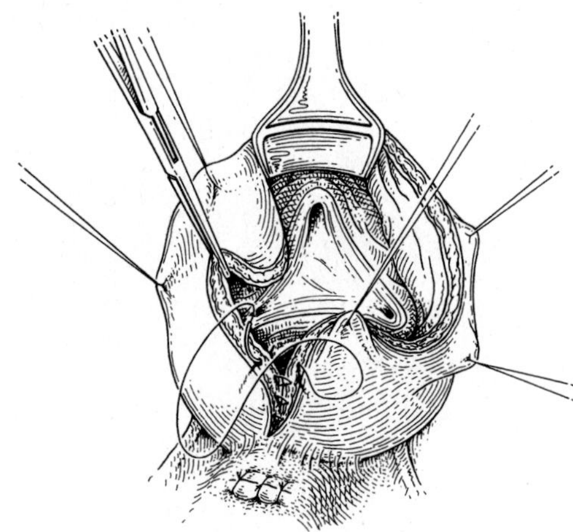

FIGURE 20.14 Relation of the cystotomy to the vaginal closure.

sutures (Fig. 20.14). An interposition flap is tacked over the vaginal closure and the bladder is closed. The first technique is slightly more difficult in that the fistula is approached posteriorly and transected between the bladder and vagina. However, the advantages are that the smaller cystotomy is separated from the repair.

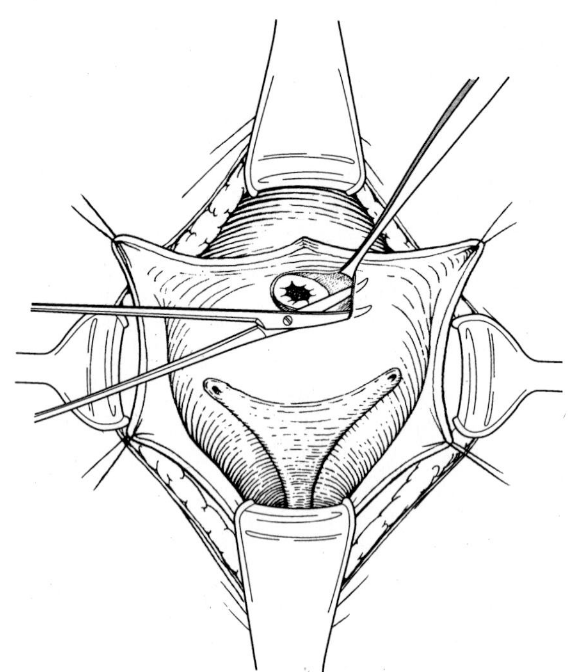

FIGURE 20.15 Transvesical development of the plane between the bladder and vaginal walls.

## Transvesical (Extraperitoneal) Approach

The advantage of this approach is that one can avoid entering the peritoneal cavity. Through a midline infraumbilical incision, the bladder is identified and opened with a midline vertical incision. The VVF is located and the ureteral orifices are cannulated with stents. The fistulous opening is circumscribed carefully with a scalpel, incising only the thickness of the bladder mucosa and staying out of the vagina. This is performed to leave the fistula tract intact, along with a 2- to 3-mm ring of bladder mucosa. With sharp dissection directed radially away from the VVF for 1 to 2 cm, the bladder is mobilized away from the vagina (Fig. 20.15). To help with exposure, a Foley catheter may be placed transvesically in the VVF for upward traction.

With interrupted 3-0 polyglycolic acid sutures, the fistula and vagina are closed together. Next, the bladder muscle is closed perpendicular to the fistula and vaginal closure, also with 3-0 polyglycolic acid sutures. Finally, the bladder mucosa is closed with running 4-0 polyglycolic acid sutures. A suprapubic cystotomy catheter and a urethral Foley catheter are placed, and the bladder is closed in two layers with 2-0 polyglycolic acid sutures. Postoperative care is similar to that previously described.

## Laparoscopic and Robot-Assisted Repair of Vesicovaginal Fistulas

The decision to repair a VVF using a transabdominal approach is controversial. High VVFs and those that lie close to the ureteric orifices, or those with failed vaginal repair, may be better served by using a transabdominal approach because of its higher success rate. This approach is, however, associated with a higher morbidity risk and longer recovery time for the patient. Also, the area of the fistula may be difficult to dissect out without performing a long cystotomy. With the development of minimally invasive surgical techniques, the laparoscope has been applied to the repair of the VVF. Its limitations have centered mostly around dissection of adhesions and fibrosis around the fistula and application of sutures in a tension-free manner. The development of robot-assisted laparoscopy has offset many of the challenges faced in the surgical repair of the VVF.

The potential benefits offered by laparoscopic and robotic repair of these fistulas include shorter recovery time, reduced morbidity, less blood loss, better cosmesis, and better visualization of the fistula area, reducing the need for extensive dissection around the fistula. The surgeon is also able to perform other concomitant procedures. As the operation is traditionally performed using a transperitoneal approach, it is easily amenable to laparoscopic techniques. The first complete transabdominal laparoscopic repair of a VVF and robotic repair of a VVF were performed in 1994 and 2005, respectively. Evidence for the efficacy and safety of this approach is based a small series of nonrandomized reports and case reports. In Sotello's series, 14 out of 15 patients were cured using the laparoscopic approach at a mean follow-up of 26 months (12).

The technical advances afforded by the laparoscopic technique include the need for a minimal cystotomy, often in a reverse tennis racquet fashion with minimal bladder mobilization and magnified anatomy such that it is easier to see the margins of the fistula. Robotic assistance has improved the fatigue factor of the surgeon and has allowed improvement in applying the tension-free sutures to the bladder and vagina. It also improves the surgeon's depth perception.

Either a four- or five-port system is used via a transabdominal approach. The fistula may be catheterized to reduce loss of pneumoperitoneum, and the bladder is catheterized after careful localization of the fistula using vaginoscopy and cystoscopy. If the fistula is close to the ureteric orifices, the ureters are cannulated also, to allow easier localization. Minimal cystotomy is performed around the fistula, and the fistula is repaired in the usual fashion. Tissue interpositioning can also be applied, usually using omentum. Average operation times run around 140 to 233 minutes, with an average length of stay of approximately 4 days. The Foley catheter is removed on days 10 to 14, preceded by cystography.

Laparoscopic and robotic techniques can be applied safely and effectively in the treatment of supratrigonal and large VVFs. This technique offers many potential benefits to the patient; however, there remains a paucity of randomized studies to quantitate its true effectiveness. It is also an evolving area, with the potential for further advances in surgical technique.

## OUTCOMES

### Complications

Clearly, the most problematic complication is recurrent or persistent fistula. The catheter is replaced for several weeks and the cystogram repeated. If the fistula fails to resolve or improve, then endoscopic evaluation—vesical and vaginal—is performed in preparation for a second procedure. For recurrent fistulas complicated by prior pelvic irradiation, a conservative approach is wise, waiting 6 to 12 months before attempting repair. Frequency, urgency, and urge incontinence in the early preoperative period are treated symptomatically with anticholinergic therapy. These, however, are expected due to bladder decompensation and trigonal/suture line irritation. Residual incontinence must be evaluated with physical examination and fluoroscopic urodynamics. Occult or de novo stress urinary incontinence occurring in 10% to 12% of patients requires separate treatment after recovery from the VVF repair. Ureteral obstruction, prolonged ileus, and bowel obstruction are uncommon.

### Results

A review of the VVF series from the last two decades demonstrates the success rate of transvaginal and transabdominal repairs to be 92.5% to 96% and 85% to 100%, respectively (1,2,4,8). Therefore, when the appropriate approach is selected based on the etiology, location, concomitant pathologies, and surgeon experience, excellent results can be expected in the great majority of patients. However, in those who have failed multiple repairs due to severe tissue compromise secondary to radiation or who have developed the end-stage detrusor, diversion may be the only alternative.

### *References*


1. Blaivas JG, Heritz DM, Romanzi LJ. Early versus late repair of vesicovaginal fistulas: vaginal and abdominal approaches. *J Urol* 1995;153:1110–1113.
2. Blandy JP, Badenoch DF, Fowler CG, et al. Early repair of iatrogenic injury to the ureter or bladder after gynecological surgery. *J Urol* 1991;146:761–765.
3. Dupont MC, Raz S. Vaginal approach to vesicovaginal fistula repair. *Urology* 1996;48:7–9.
4. Eilber KS, Rosenblum N, Rodriguez LV, et al. 10-Year experience of transvaginal vesicovaginal fistula repair utilizing a peritoneal flap. *J Urol* 2002; 167[Suppl]:202 (abst 814).
5. Evans DH, Madjar S, Politano VA, et al. Interposition flaps in transabdominal vesicovaginal fistula repairs: are they really necessary? *Urology* 2001;57:670–674.
6. Goodwin WE, Scardino PT. Vesicovaginal and ureterovaginal fistulas: a summary of 25 years of experience. *J Urol* 1980;123:370–374.
7. Harkki-Siren P, Sjoberg J, Tiitinen A. Urinary tract injuries after hysterectomy. *Obstet Gynecol* 1998;92:113–118.
8. Mondet F, Chartier-Kastler EJ, Conort P, et al. Anatomic and functional results of transperitoneal–transvesical vesicovaginal fistula repair. *Urology* 2001;58:882–886.
9. Tancer ML. Observations on prevention and management of vesicovaginal fistula after total hysterectomy. *Surg Gynecol Obstet* 1992;175:501–506.
10. Zacharin RF. A history of obstetric vesicovaginal fistula. *Aust N Z J Surg* 2000;70:851–854.
11. Schneider JA, Patel VJ, Hertel E. Closure of vesico-vaginal fistulas from the urologic viewpoint with reference to endoscopic fibrin glue technique. *Zentralbl Gynakol* 1992;114:70.
12. Sotello R, Mariano MB, Garcia-Segui A, et al. Laparoscopic repair of vesicovaginal fistula. *J Urol* 2005;173:1615–1618.


# CHAPTER 21 ■ ENTEROVESICAL AND RECTOURETHRAL FISTULAS

KENNETH W. ANGERMEIER, AARON J. MILBANK, AND ERIC A. KLEIN

An enterovesical fistula is an extra-anatomic, epithelialized connection between the intestines and the bladder. This chapter will describe the etiology, evaluation, and management of enterovesical fistulas and the less common rectourethral/rectovesical fistulas. The last half-century has seen a dramatic change in the management of enterovesical fistulas with a reduction in morbidity and mortality.

## ENTEROVESICAL FISTULAS

In unselected series, the most common etiology of enterovesical fistulas is diverticulitis. In seven series of patients with enterovesical fistulas, the etiology was diverticulitis in 53% (range, 39% to 77%). Moreover, it has been reported that

TABLE 21.1

SPECIFIC CAUSES OF VESICOENTERIC FISTULAS

| |
|---|
| **INFLAMMATORY** |
| Diverticulitis |
| Crohn disease |
| Ulcerative colitis |
| Appendiceal/pelvic abscess |
| Meckel diverticulum |
| Tuberculosis |
| Actinomycosis |
| Bladder malakoplakia |
| Colonic duplication |
| **NEOPLASTIC** |
| Carcinoma of sigmoid colon and rectum |
| Lymphomas |
| AIDS-related lymphomas |
| Carcinoma of cervix |
| Leiomyosarcoma of bladder |
| **TRAUMATIC** |
| Gunshot wounds |
| Penetrating injuries |
| Pelvic fractures |
| Transurethral or open prostatectomy |
| Vesical formalinization |
| Pelvic external beam radiation |
| Prostatic brachytherapy |
| Cryoablation of the prostate |
| Transurethral microwave thermotherapy |
| **PELVIC** |
| Gynecologic cancer |
| Foreign body |

AIDS, acquired immunodeficiency syndrome.

10% of surgically treated cases of diverticulitis are associated with a colovesical fistula. There is a significant male predominance, a finding that has been attributed to a "protective barrier" provided by the uterus and broad ligament (16).

Other common causes of enterovesical fistula are pelvic malignancy (21%) and Crohn disease (15%). Crohn disease patients tend to present at a younger age than those patients with diverticular or malignant etiologies. Radiation injury is an infrequent cause of enterovesical fistulas. Most enterovesical fistulas following pelvic radiotherapy are secondary to recurrent disease. The etiologies of enterovesical fistulas are listed in Table 21.1.

## Diagnosis

Although enterovesical fistulas are almost always secondary to extravesical pathology, the presenting symptoms are in general urinary in nature. The most common presenting symptom is pneumaturia, reported in 50% to 85% of patients, although some series report irritative voiding symptoms in as many as 71% to 93%. Fecaluria is reported in 21% to 68% of patients with enterovesical fistulas and tends to be more common with diverticular and malignant fistulas. Other symptoms include hematuria, abdominal pain, diarrhea, urinary retention, perineal pain, hematochezia, and fever. Urine in the stool is rarely reported with enterovesical fistulas; these fistulas tend to be unidirectional, with flow from the high-pressure intestinal tract to the low-pressure urinary tract.

Physical signs of enterovesical fistulas are subtle or absent. Abdominal tenderness and a palpable mass may be reported in as many as 35% and 27% of patients, respectively, and are not specific. In patients with rectal disease, a rectal mass or rectal tenderness may be present. Rarely, an enterovesical fistula may present as epididymitis. In general, physical findings are most commonly seen in patients with Crohn disease.

Urinalysis discloses pyuria, and cultures are positive in 80% to 100% of cases of enterovesical fistula. *Escherichia coli* is the most commonly identified organism, and approximately one-third to two-thirds of cultures show polymicrobial growth.

The diagnosis of an enterovesical fistula is clinical, and in some instances, despite numerous radiographic studies, the first objective demonstration of the fistula is at laparotomy. Nonetheless, numerous studies have been described to aid in the diagnosis and/or localization of fistulas. Functional studies include the charcoal test, administration of visible dyes (methylene blue, indigo carmine), and the Bourne test, in which urine voided after a barium enema is radiographed for the presence of barium. The charcoal test involves the ingestion of nonabsorbable charcoal followed by the observation of charcoaluria. Although these tests have been reported to have sensitivities of 80% to 100%, they are rarely performed because they provide no localizing anatomic information, and the information they do provide is usually evident from the patient's history.

Cystoscopy is the most common abnormal investigation in patients with enterovesical fistulas, although direct observation of a fistula is relatively unlikely. Approximately 90% of cystoscopies show at least indirect evidence of the fistula, most commonly bullous edema, and in 33% to 46% of cystoscopies the fistulous opening is identified.

Barium enema has been a commonly utilized study in the evaluation of enterovesical fistulas, with some series reporting 100% abnormal studies and fistula identification in as many as 16% to 63% of patients. Colonoscopy rarely demonstrates a fistulous tract, but the study is important in the evaluation of potentially malignant fistulas.

Computerized tomography (CT) has supplanted most of the older imaging studies in the evaluation of suspected enterovesical fistulas. Although the fistula tract may be identified in some cases, indirect evidence of the fistula, including air in the bladder, focal bladder and bowel wall thickening, and closely apposed bowel and bladder, may be present in 85% to 100% of cases. CT also provides important information in the evaluation of patients with Crohn disease and colorectal carcinoma. CT cystography in our institution has replaced many other studies, including standard cystography, intravenous pyelography (IVP), and magnetic resonance imaging (MRI).

## Indications for Surgery

Given the symptomatic nature of enterovesical fistulas and their association with recurrent urinary tract infections and sepsis, most fistulas should be addressed surgically. Over the course of the past 30 years, a one-stage operation has become the favored procedure because of reports of fewer complications and lower mortality. It has been demonstrated that a one-stage procedure may be safely performed in the setting of an abscess or purulent peritonitis provided that the inflammatory focus can be removed and the bowel anastomosis can be "quarantined from any inflammatory nest" (16). In general, diverticular disease is particularly well suited to one-stage procedures because the fistulous process is either chronic or, if acute, controllable with antibiotics.

A two-stage procedure should be considered in patients who have an obstructed bowel, have residual significant intra-abdominal inflammation, are significantly ill, and in whom a healthy anastomosis is unlikely (due to poor blood supply or tension at the anastomosis). The two stages (for colovesical fistulas) may consist of resection with the Hartmann pouch and end colostomy followed by reanastomosis or resection, anastomosis, and transverse colostomy followed by reversal of the colostomy. Fistulas secondary to radiation injury in general require multiple staged repairs and, frequently, permanent bladder and bowel diversion (10).

## Alternative Therapy

Nonoperative management may be considered in patients who are extremely debilitated. There are a few reports of spontaneous closure of fistulas with medical management. This spontaneous resolution has been reported with traumatic fistulas and in a subset of fistulas secondary to Crohn disease. Placement of bowel stents and endoscopic clipping of the colonic terminus of the fistula have also been reported for patients who are too ill to undergo open surgical procedures. Experimental evidence suggests that enterovesical fistulas, when chronic, are physiologically well tolerated (5). Amin et al. followed a cohort of four patients with diverticular colovesical fistulas who refused surgery; with 3 to 14 years of follow-up, there were no significant complications (1).

## Surgical Technique

### One-Stage Surgery

On the day prior to the operation, a mechanical bowel preparation is administered and the patient is maintained on a clear liquid diet. Gram-negative and anaerobic coverage is provided by administering a third-generation cephalosporin (ceftizoxime) and metronidazole 1 hour prior to the surgical procedure.

Most fistulas are best approached via a midline incision extending from the pubic ramus to the umbilicus (Fig. 21.1). This incision may be extended cranially as needed. Some authors prefer an infraumbilical transverse incision. The peritoneal cavity is entered and adhesiolysis is performed. The point of the fistula is identified. The remainder of the procedure is determined by the disease causing the fistula and intraoperative findings. In the setting of diverticular fistulas, the diseased colon is resected and an anastomosis is performed suturing normal bowel to normal bowel without tension and with adequate blood supply. Patients with Crohn disease often have multiple fistulas not involving the urinary tract and require multiple resections or strictureplasties. With diverticular disease, the fistula may often be "pinched off" from the bladder with curettage of the fistula tract. For malignant fistulas, the requisite oncological procedure is performed and the malignant fistula tract is excised. Partial cystectomy may be required for large or malignant fistulas; radical cystectomy is in general not required.

Closure of small bladder fistulas is not essential. Large defects should be closed in two layers using absorbable sutures. In the setting of ureteral involvement, ureteroneocystostomy may be required. Ideally, an omental flap should be interposed between the anastomosed bowel and the bladder. When an omental flap is not constructable, a peritoneal flap may be used. Suprapubic catheters and drainage of the extraperitoneal space are optional. In general, a urethral catheter is maintained until 1 week after surgery. Complete healing of the bladder defect may be confirmed with a cystogram prior to removal of the catheter. The aforementioned procedure has also been performed laparoscopically with good results.

## Outcomes

### Complications

Major complications of operative repair of enterovesical fistulas include death (0% to 5%), myocardial infarction (2% to 6%), anastomotic leak (0% to 5%), enterocutaneous fistula (0% to 1%), wound infection (0% to 21%), wound dehiscence (0% to 2%), pulmonary embolus (0% to 1%), deep vein thrombosis (0% to 1%), prolonged ileus (0% to 5%), and urine leak (0% to 3%) (4,11,15,16). One of the largest surgical series (104 patients) reported a 6.4% overall complication rate with no operative mortality (9). Significantly greater morbidity is observed in series focusing on radiation-induced and malignant fistulas (6,10).

### Results

The results of the one-stage procedure for enterovesical fistulas are very much dependent upon the etiology of the fistula. Fistula recurrence following colonic resection in patients with diverticular fistulas is virtually nonexistent (16). Following surgical intervention for Crohn disease with enterovesical fistulas, recurrent enterovesical fistulas are observed in 0% to 13% of patients (4,11). In a surgical series of 13 patients with malignant fistulas, 2 (15%) patients developed recurrent fistulas (6). In a surgical series of 13 patients with radiation-induced fistulas, 5 (39%) failed to resolve or recurred (10). It should be noted that seven of these operations were diversions or isolations; of the six patients who underwent resections, only one developed a recurrent fistula.

# RECTOURETHRAL FISTULAS

Rectourethral fistulas are rare clinical entities. The most common cause is iatrogenesis, usually incurred during prostatic or rectal surgery or following radiation. Other etiologies include congenital, infectious, and neoplastic fistulas.

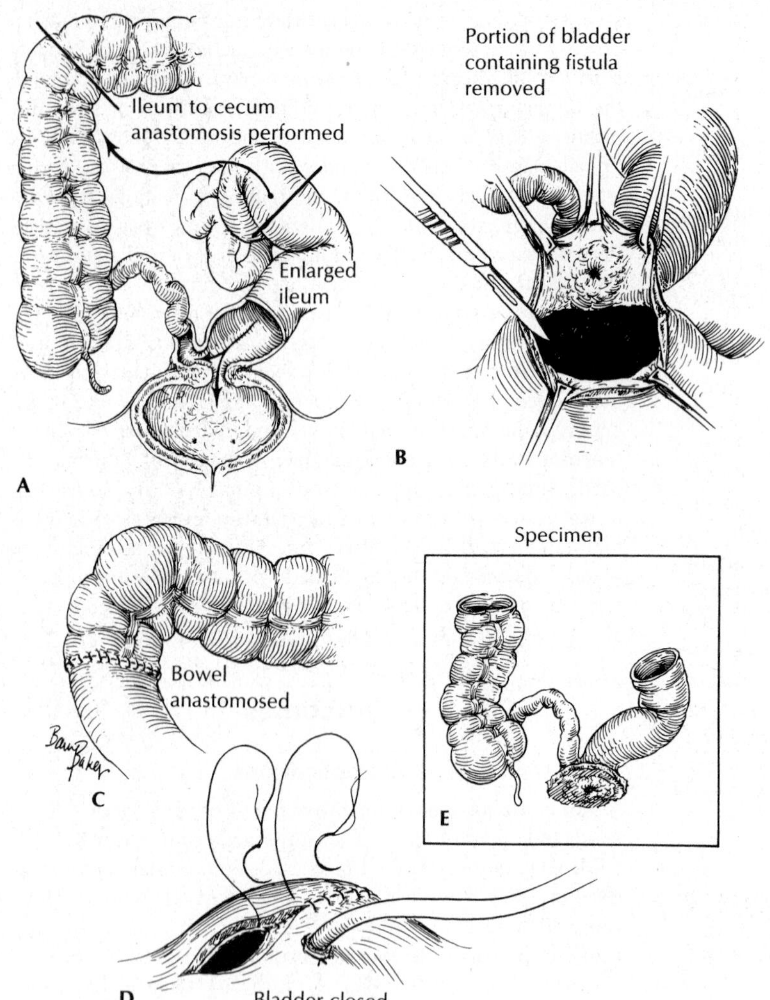


**FIGURE 21.1** Management of an enterovesical fistula using bowel resection and restitution with primary bladder closure.

## Diagnosis

Diagnosis of a rectourethral fistula is usually straightforward and suggested by the medical history. Preoperatively, antegrade and retrograde studies of the urinary tract, cystoscopy, proctoscopy, and, if indicated, anal manometry are performed to delineate the site and extent of the fistula as well as rule out distal obstruction or sphincteric incompetence. If there is clinical suspicion of disease recurrence, a biopsy should be performed.

## Indications for Surgery

Many different approaches have been proposed for the management of rectourethral fistulas. It is imperative to individualize management. There are five key factors that must be considered prior to determining the ideal approach:

1. *Sphincteric function.* In the setting of anal sphincteric incompetence, complex anal sphincter-sparing procedures should be deferred and consideration given to permanent fecal diversion. Similarly, in the setting of failure of the urinary sphincter, supravesical diversion is a valid consideration if placement of an artificial urinary sphincter is not feasible.
2. *Presence of urethral stricture or vesical neck contracture.* Coexisting urethral disease may be present in patients with rectourethral fistulas, in particular iatrogenic fistulas (surgical or radiation-induced). Distal obstruction will compromise a technically adequate repair and should be treated prior to or at the time of fistula repair.
3. *Status of adjacent tissue.* Pelvic radiation induces both delayed endothelial cell damage and damage to the connective tissue stroma of blood vessels (12). This arteritis may result in atrophy, fibrosis, and necrosis. As a result, radiation-induced fistulas in general require more extensive repairs involving interposition of omentum or muscle flaps, have higher failure rates, and on occasion require permanent diversion.
4. *Size and location of the fistula.* Whereas small distal fistulas may be effectively repaired via a transanal approach, large fistulas often require the greater exposure provided by transsphincteric, transperineal, or abdominoperineal approaches. Moreover, large defects may require the interposition of vascularized tissue (omentum or muscle flaps).
5. *Overall condition and life expectancy of the patient.*

## Surgical Therapy

Initial treatment of iatrogenic fistulas in general consists of colostomy, prolonged urinary drainage with a suprapubic catheter, and broad-spectrum antibiotics, although some authors have advocated the selective use of elemental or parenteral nutrition in lieu of bowel diversion (3). Approximately 25% of nonradiated iatrogenic fistulas will resolve with conservative management (2). For those fistulas that do not close, numerous surgical repairs have been proposed (2). In appropriate candidates, our preferred surgical approach is either transanal or posterior transanosphincteric (York–Mason) (14). Transperineal repairs allow for formal tissue interposition and are useful for large or complex fistulas. Abdominoperineal repair allows for a colonic pull-through if necessary and also for the interposition of omentum or a gracilis or rectus abdominis muscle flap. It is limited, however, by an increased risk of fecal incontinence and the morbidity of an abdominal operation. The anterior transanorectal approach (sphincter divided) and the Kraske laterosacral (sphincter not divided) approach both provide excellent exposure of the fistula; however, the former may be associated with erectile dysfunction if the plane of dissection strays from the midline, and the latter procedure risks fecal incontinence associated with denervation.

## Surgical Technique

### Transanal Approach

The procedure is performed in the prone jackknife position. A speculum is introduced into the anus and the fistula is exposed. Two alternative procedures may be performed: the fistula may be circumscribed with mobilization of the rectal mucosa in a circumferential fashion; the fistula is excised and the underlying rectal wall muscle and mucosa are closed separately. Alternatively, the mucosal dissection may be limited to the rectal wall lateral and distal to the fistula. The proximal rectal wall is then mobilized for 4 cm, thereby creating a full-thickness U-shaped flap that is pulled down over the fistula and sutured to the edge of the rectal mucosa (Fig. 21.2). A catheter is maintained for 2 to 3 weeks. The main limitation of this approach is the limited exposure, and it is best suited for small distal fistulas.

### York–Mason Approach

The York–Mason procedure is performed in a prone jackknife position with the buttocks taped laterally (14) (Fig. 21.3). A midline incision is made from the sacrococcygeal articulation to the anal verge. Prior to dividing the muscular layers of the posterior anus, matching sutures are placed on either side of the intended incision so as to allow for subsequent precise reapproximation. Each layer is marked separately and then divided. Once the sphincter is divided, the mucosa of the posterior anus and the entire posterior rectal wall are divided in midline, thereby providing excellent exposure of the fistula. The fistula is then entirely excised and any inflammatory tissue is removed. The plane between the anterior rectal wall and the urethra/bladder may then be dissected to allow sufficient mobility for closure of the rectal defect. The urethra (or bladder) is closed with absorbable sutures in either one or two layers.

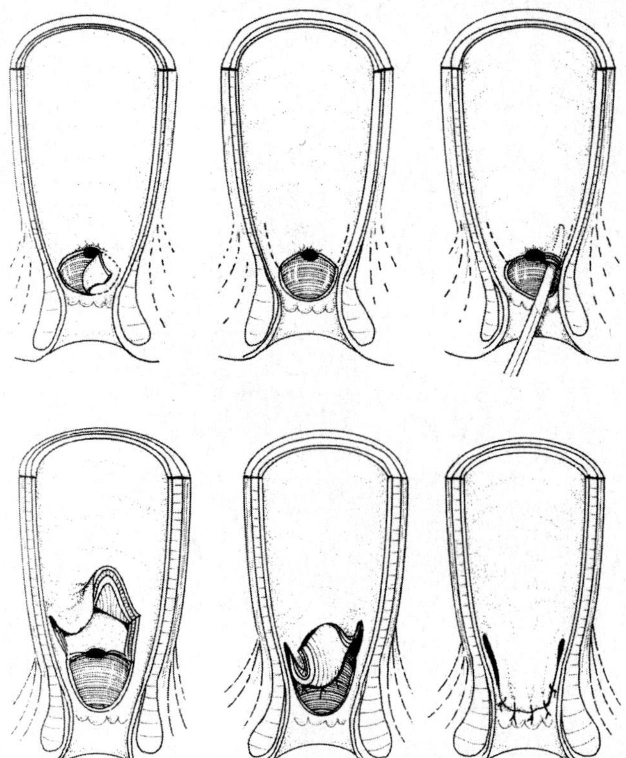

FIGURE 21.2 Through the anal canal, an ellipse of rectal mucosa is removed. A full-thickness U-shaped flap of rectal wall is elevated above the fistula. The full-thickness flap of rectal wall is brought down over the fistula and sutured in two layers to the rectal wall. (From Tiptaft RC, Motson RW, et al. Fistulae involving rectum and urethra: the place of Parks' operations. *Br J Urol* 1983; *55*:711–715, with permission.)

The rectum is closed in two layers. The posterior rectal wall and anal mucosa are then reapproximated. Finally, using the previously placed marking sutures, the anal sphincter is reapproximated in layers. Drainage of the presacral space is optional. A Foley catheter is placed and maintained for 2 to 3 weeks, at which point the absence of a leak is confirmed radiographically.

## Outcomes

### Complications

Specific complications include recurrent fistula formation, urinary and/or fecal incontinence, and erectile dysfunction.

### Results

Based upon literature reports, the York–Mason approach has become the favored repair for rectourethral fistulas not amenable to a transanal approach. There have been two relatively large series reported recently. Fengler and Abcarian performed eight York–Mason repairs for rectourethral fistulas with no recurrences and no fecal incontinence (3). Fecal diversion was performed in three of the eight patients. Stephenson and Middleton reported on 16 York–Mason repairs for rectourinary fistulas (rectovesical in 8, rectourethral in 7), with 1 recurrence and no fecal incontinence (14). The one recurrence was treated successfully with a second York–Mason procedure.

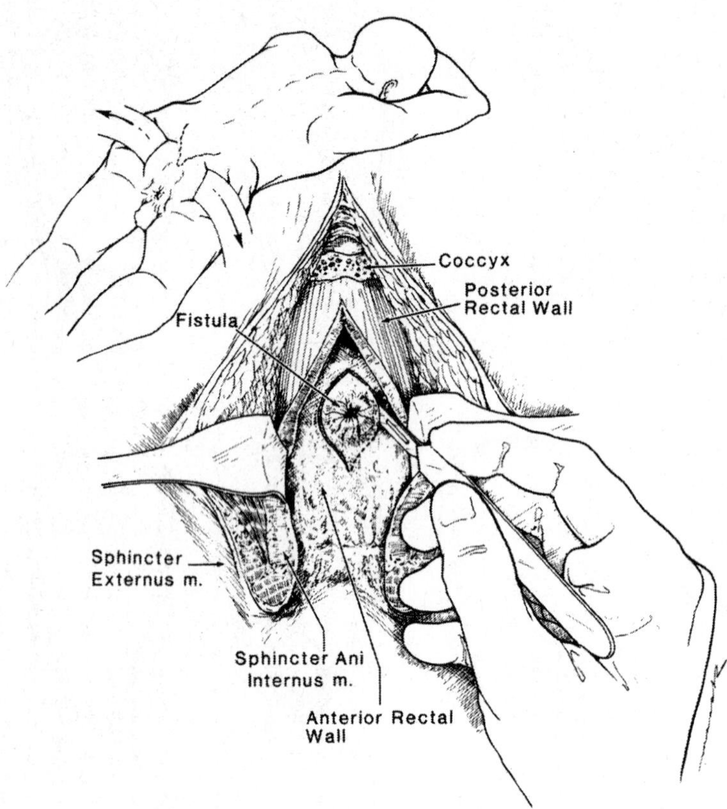


FIGURE 21.3 Posterior sagittal, transanorectal (York–Mason) approach for repair of rectourinary fistulas. The patient is placed in the prone jackknife position with tape used to displace the buttocks laterally. After division of the posterior anus and rectum, the fistula is easily identified with ample room for excision and repair. (From Stephenson RA, Middleton RG. Repair of rectourinary fistulas using a posterior sagittal transanal transrectal (modified York–Mason) approach: an update. *J Urol* 1996;155:1989–1991, with permission.)

In this series, four patients with urinary incontinence prior to the repair subsequently underwent artificial urinary sphincter placement; no patients developed urinary incontinence as a result of the repair. A diverting colostomy was used in nine of the patients.

## Surgical Reconstruction for Large or Complex Fistulas

### Preservation of Urinary or Bowel Function

Based upon the presurgical evaluation, some patients with a rectourethral fistula are candidates for surgical restoration of only one system. The most common setting would be a patient with anorectal dysfunction or sphincteric incompetence who is a candidate for permanent colostomy and urinary tract reconstruction. Urinary reconstruction is optimized by concomitant proctectomy. A small urethral fistula may be closed primarily, followed by omental mobilization to the pelvis for coverage of the area. Some fistulas too large for primary closure have been managed with omental or gracilis transposition alone (7); however, we have preferred to close the urethral defect with a buccal mucosa graft in this setting as this seems to lead to decreased urinary extravasation and more rapid healing overall. The buccal graft is buttressed with omentum or a gracilis muscle flap for optimal take.

### Preservation of Urinary and Bowel Function

In patients who are candidates for attempted preservation of both urinary and bowel function, a transperineal procedure is our preferred technique and begins with placing the patient into high lithotomy position. A very careful and meticulous dissection is then conducted in the plane between the rectum and the prostate and bladder to the level of the peritoneal reflection. The plane of dissection typically starts superior to the anal sphincter and then is carried down onto the rectum. Development of the space between the urinary tract and rectum can be quite difficult, as it is often performed in the setting of radiotherapy or previous attempts at fistula repair. Once completed, the urinary tract defect is closed primarily when feasible or patched with a buccal mucosa graft. In the setting of an associated membranous urethral stricture, a urethrotomy incision is created from the level of the fistula through the stricture into the proximal bulbous urethra. Buccal mucosa is then grafted into the resulting urethrotomy defect, with distal graft coverage using the corpus spongiosum and proximal buttressing with a gracilis muscle flap (17). The rectum is then closed and a gracilis muscle is rotated into the space between the rectum and urinary tract and anchored to the peritoneal reflection. Lateral sutures are also placed between the gracilis and the levators to ensure that its position is maintained with complete coverage of the reconstruction. Primary closure of the urethral and rectal defects with gracilis interposition was successful in 13 of 15 (87%) patients in two studies (13,18). In 2004 Zinman and colleagues reported excellent results using a transperineal approach for repair of complex rectourethral fistulas with buccal mucosa graft closure of the urethra, primary closure of the rectum, and gracilis interposition (17). We have used a similar technique in over 20 patients to date with only 1 failure of fistula closure thus far. It would seem to be most useful when the rectum and perirectal tissues are preserved well enough to allow adequate healing with primary rectal closure, as opposed to situations requiring resection of a severely diseased rectum. In these cases, we have successfully used an abdominoperineal approach in patients in whom the rectum was deemed to be too extensively damaged by radiotherapy to allow a reliable primary closure, due to either severe proctitis or extensive tissue loss (8). In these cases, proctectomy and buccal graft closure of the urethral defect were done initially in the prone jackknife position, and the patient was then placed supine for the remainder of the procedure. Turnbull–Cutait staged coloanal pull-through is then carried out via an abdominoperineal approach. We have found that simple rotation of the sigmoid mesentery anteriorly during the pull-through provides an excellent host bed for the buccal mucosa graft when omentum is not available, or if there is insufficient room in the pelvis to accommodate the omentum. This approach allows repair of large fistulas, restores fecal and urinary continuity, and eliminates a severely diseased rectum. Potentially difficult aspects of this procedure include the morbidity of an abdominal operation and the need to reposition the patient from the prone to the supine position during the case. A minor potential complication that we have encountered in two patients is the occurrence of minor rectal ectropion or prolapse that may require simple outpatient excision at a later date.

## *References*


1. Amin M, Nallinger R, et al. Conservative treatment of selected patients with colovesical fistula due to diverticulitis. *Surg Gynecol Obstet* 1984;159:442–444.
2. Elmajian DA. Surgical approaches to repair of rectourinary fistulas. *AUA Update Series* 2000;19(6):41–48.
3. Fengler SA, Abcarian H. The York Mason approach to repair of iatrogenic rectourinary fistulae. *Am J Surg* 1997;173:213–217.
4. Greenstein AJ, Sachar DB, et al. Course of enterovesical fistulas in Crohn's disease. *Am J Surg* 1984;147:788–792.
5. Heiskell CA, Vjiki GT, et al. A study of experimental colovesical fistula. *Am J Surg* 1975;129(3):316–318.
6. Holmes SA, Christmas TJ, et al. Management of colovesical fistulae associated with pelvic malignancy. *Br J Surg* 1992;79:432–434.
7. Jordan GH, Lynch DF, et al. Major rectal complications following interstitial implantation of 125-iodine for carcinoma of the prostate. *J Urol* 1985;134:1212–1214.
8. Lane BR, Stein DE, et al. Management of radiotherapy induced rectourethral fistula. *J Urol* 2006;175:1382–1387.
9. King RM, Beart RW Jr, et al. Colovesical and rectovesical fistulas. *Arch Surg* 1982;117:680–683.
10. Levenback C, Gershenson DM, et al. Enterovesical fistula following radiotherapy for gynecologic cancer. *Gynecol Oncol* 1994;52:296–300.
11. McNamara MJ, Fazio VW, et al. Surgical treatment of enterovesical fistulas in Crohn's disease. *Dis Colon Rectum* 1990;33:271–276.
12. Mundy AR. Pelvic surgery after radiotherapy. *Br J Urol* 1997;80[Suppl 1]:66–68.
13. Nyam DC, Pemberton JH. Management of iatrogenic rectourethral fistula. *Dis Colon Rectum* 1999;42:994–999.
14. Stephenson RA, Middleton RG. Repair of rectourinary fistulas using a posterior sagittal transanal transrectal (modified York–Mason) approach: an update. *J Urol* 1996;155:1989–1991.
15. Vasilevsky CA, Belliveau P, et al. Fistulas complicating diverticulitis. *Int J Colorectal Dis* 1998;13(2):57–60.
16. Woods RJ, Lavery IC, et al. Internal fistulas in diverticular disease. *Dis Colon Rectum* 1988;31:591–596.
17. Zinman L. The management of the complex recto-urethral fistula. *BJU Int* 2004;94:1212–1213.
18. Zmora O, Potenti FM, et al. Gracilis muscle transposition for iatrogenic rectourethral fistula. *Ann Surg* 2003;237:483–487.


# **CHAPTER 22** ■ VESICAL TRAUMA AND HEMORRHAGE

KAMAL S. POHAR AND ROBERT R. BAHNSON

## VESICAL TRAUMA

Vesical injury can occur as a result of blunt or penetrating trauma to the lower abdomen and pelvis. It is more commonly associated with blunt trauma such as that sustained from motor vehicle accidents, falls, blows, and during contact sports. Penetrating trauma resulting in vesical injury occurs from gunshot wounds and knife wounds. Bladder injuries can also be iatrogenic from transurethral surgery, gynecologic procedures, laparoscopy, and other intra-abdominal surgery. Bladder injury, in particular bladder rupture, is associated with pelvic fractures in 75% to 83% of patients (1). However, only 5% to 10% of patients with pelvic fractures will have associated bladder rupture (2,3). There is also a high incidence of injuries to other organs in patients with bladder rupture (3). Concomitant bladder rupture is found in 10% to 29% of patients who present with rupture of the posterior urethra, and this is the most common injury to the genitourinary tract associated with bladder rupture (1,3). The mortality rate in patients with bladder rupture ranges from 11% to 44% and is mainly attributable to other associated organ injuries.

Bladder injury occurs as three predominant types: contusion with only intramural injury and extraperitoneal or intraperitoneal bladder rupture. The exact incidence of bladder contusion is not known as it is often a diagnosis of exclusion. It is a partial-thickness tear of the bladder mucosa with ecchymosis of the bladder wall. It is often associated with a "teardrop"-shaped bladder, which occurs as a result of a compressive pelvic hematoma from a pelvic fracture (4). It is usually self-limiting and rarely requires treatment.

Traumatic extraperitoneal ruptures usually are associated with pelvic fractures (89% to 100%). Previously, the mechanism of injury was believed to be a direct perforation by a bony fragment or a disruption of the pelvic girdle. It is now generally agreed that the pelvic fracture is likely coincidental and that the bladder rupture is most often due to a direct burst injury or the shearing force of the deforming pelvic ring (5). These ruptures usually are associated with fractures of the anterior pubic arch, and they may occur from a direct laceration of the bladder by the bony fragments of the osseous pelvis. The anterolateral aspect of the bladder typically is perforated by bony spicules. Forceful disruption of the bony pelvis and/or the puboprostatic ligaments also tears the wall of the bladder. The degree of bladder injury is directly related to the severity of the fracture.

Some cases may occur by a mechanism similar to intraperitoneal bladder rupture, which is a combination of trauma and bladder overdistention. The classic cystographic finding is contrast extravasation around the base of the bladder confined to the perivesical space; flame-shaped areas of contrast extravasation are noted adjacent to the bladder. The bladder may assume a teardrop shape from compression by a pelvic hematoma. Starburst, flame-shape, and featherlike patterns also are described. Classic intraperitoneal bladder ruptures are described as large horizontal tears in the dome of the bladder. The dome is the least supported area and the only portion of the adult bladder covered by peritoneum. The mechanism of injury is a sudden large increase in intravesical pressure in a full bladder. When full, the bladder's muscle fibers are widely separated and the entire bladder wall is relatively thin, offering relatively little resistance to perforation from sudden large changes in intravesical pressure.

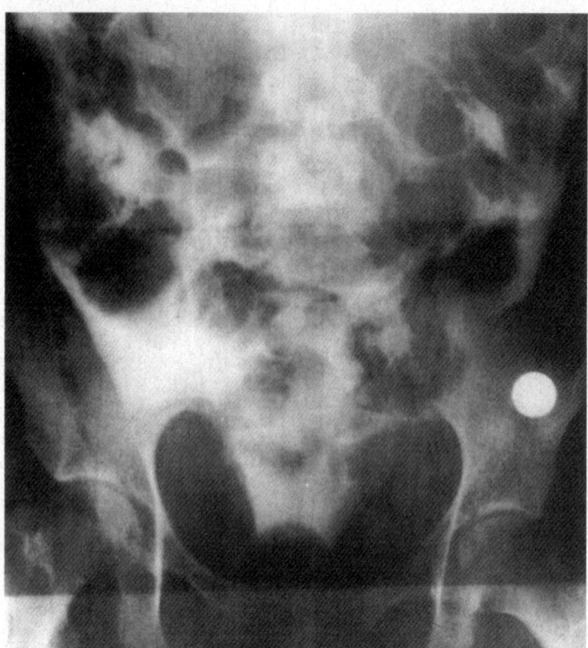

FIGURE 22.1 In intraperitoneal rupture of the bladder, free contrast within the peritoneal cavity outlines bowel loops.

## Diagnosis

Patients with bladder injury usually complain of lower abdominal pain and tenderness. Such an injury should be suspected in any patient with a pelvic fracture. Most patients with bladder trauma, including those with bladder contusions, will have gross or microscopic hematuria. Patients with contusion alone are usually able to void, whereas those with a ruptured bladder are often unable to void spontaneously. Acidosis with prerenal azotemia and elevated blood urea nitrogen is sometimes noticeable when there is a delay in diagnosis (6).

Presence of blood at the urethral meatus mandates performing a retrograde urethrogram. This is performed to rule out urethral injury before catheterization or instrumentation. If the retrograde urethrogram is normal, a urethral catheter is placed and a cystogram is obtained by plain film radiography (static), fluoroscopy (dynamic), or CT scan. The cystogram is usually normal in the presence of a bladder contusion. Intraperitoneal rupture results in ill-defined spillage of contrast into the peritoneum (Fig. 22.1). The extravasated contrast may outline loops of bowel or accumulate in the paracolic gutters, beneath the diaphragm, or over the bladder, in an hourglass pattern. Extraperitoneal rupture is seen as streaklike extravasation of contrast confined to the pelvis on retrograde cystogram (Fig. 22.2). Corriere and Sandler (7) further distinguished extraperitoneal ruptures as simple (confined to the perivesical space) or complex (extravasation into the scrotum, retroperitoneum, abdominal wall, etc.). Displacement of the bladder by a pelvic hematoma can result in a teardrop-shaped bladder on cystogram (7).

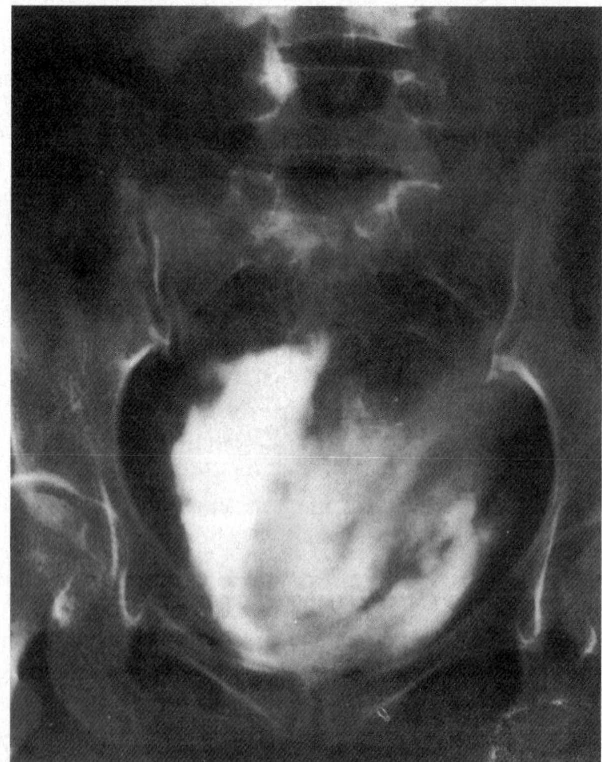

FIGURE 22.2 In extraperitoneal rupture of the bladder, contrast fills the pelvic cavity around the bladder.

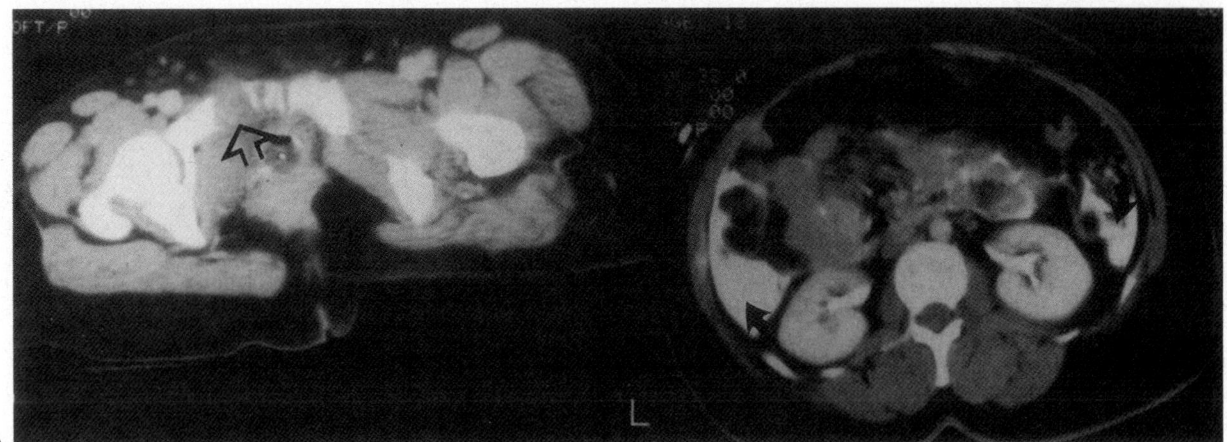

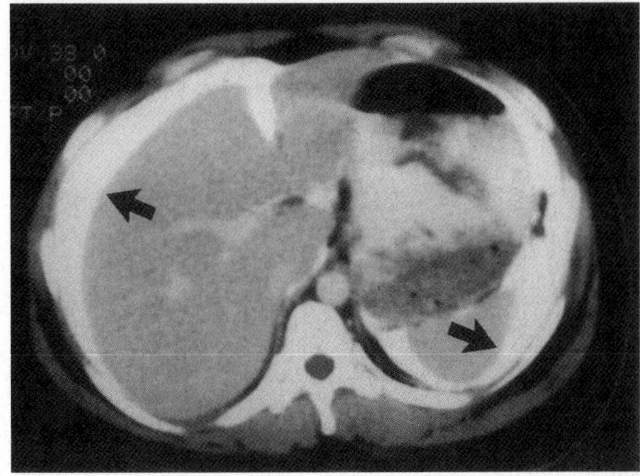

FIGURE 22.3 A CT cystogram showing evidence of intraperitoneal rupture of the bladder with extravasation around the (**A**) bladder (*arrow*), (**B**) paracolic space (*solid arrows*), and (**C**) abdominal viscera (*solid arrows*).

The most sensitive means of evaluating for the presence of bladder injury has traditionally been a cystogram performed by fluoroscopy. This is performed by obtaining a scout radiograph followed by instilling at least 250 to 400 cc of water-soluble contrast (Cystografin) in the bladder under gravity to ensure adequate distention and visualization of possible areas of rupture (1,6). One of the principal reasons for false-negative cystograms is instillation of an inadequate amount of contrast in the bladder. Static anteroposterior, oblique, or lateral films are obtained with the bladder full, and a washout film is obtained after drainage of the contrast material from the bladder. These additional films are useful in evaluating patients with posterior wall ruptures, which may be obscured in the anteroposterior view by a contrast-filled bladder. The drainage film also helps detect residual extravasation. In children the bladder is filled with contrast according to the formula, Bladder capacity = 60 cc + (30 cc × age in years).

Although it is preferable to perform the study under fluoroscopy, if clinical circumstances do not permit, a static cystogram is satisfacory with portable equipment at the bedside.

Recently, examination of a contrast-filled bladder during computerized tomography (CT) scan has been used as a method of assessing injury. This is particularly applicable in patients who first undergo abdominal CT scans to rule out suspected visceral injuries. In these situations, the ability to simultaneously evaluate the bladder would obviate the need for an additional plain-film cystogram. However, during routine abdominopelvic CT scan, the bladder may not be adequately distended to allow evaluation for rupture. The results of CT cystography improved as studies demonstrated improved sensitivity when the bladder was filled in a retrograde fashion with large volumes of contrast (250 to 500 cc) (8). Intraperitoneal bladder rupture can be distinguished from extraperitoneal rupture on CT scan. Presence of contrast around the bladder (Fig. 22.3A), in the paracolic gutters on either side (Fig. 22.3B), and around abdominal viscera such as the liver (Fig. 22.3C) indicates intraperitoneal rupture. In the case of extraperitoneal rupture, contrast extravasation is usually seen around the bladder, in the presacral space (Fig. 22.4A), and in the retroperitoneum anterior to the great vessels (Fig. 22.4B). Bladder contusions may be seen on CT scan as intramural hematomas. The recently reported improved accuracy of CT scan has resulted in CT being considered equivalent to plain-film cystography in diagnosing bladder ruptures. The accuracy of CT cystography may be significantly improved if retrograde bladder filling are performed with an adequate amount of contrast.

Intraoperatively, bladder rupture can be diagnosed by extravasation of saline, sterile milk, methylene blue, or indigo carmine, which is instilled in the bladder through a Foley catheter.

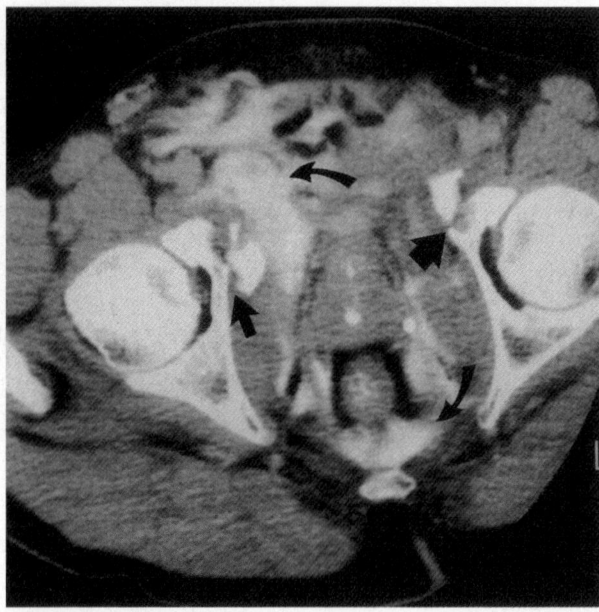


FIGURE 22.4 Extraperitoneal rupture showing contrast in the (A) presacral space (*curved arrow*), prevesical space (*open arrow*), and (B) retroperitoneum (*solid arrow*). *B*, bladder.

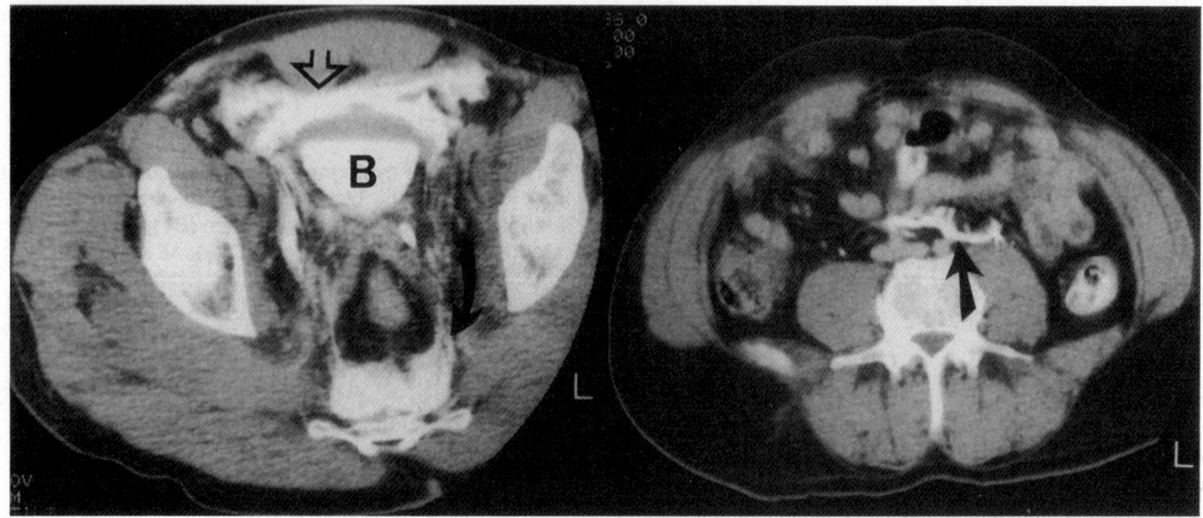


## Indications for Surgery

1. Intraperitoneal bladder rupture
2. Bladder rupture or perforation sustained during another surgical procedure
3. Extraperitoneal bladder rupture in the presence of other intra-abdominal injuries requiring surgical intervention
4. Extraperitoneal bladder rupture with the bladder being inadequately drained by urethral catheter drainage

## Alternative Therapy

Alternative treatments of bladder trauma are predominantly Foley catheter drainage, which is indicated in patients with bladder contusions and extraperitoneal extravasation. Most extraperitoneal ruptures can be managed safely with simple catheter drainage (i.e., urethral or suprapubic). The catheter is placed to drain for 7 to 10 days and a cystogram is performed. Approximately 85% of the time, the laceration is sealed and the catheter is removed for a voiding trial. Most extraperitoneal ruptures will heal within 3 weeks of catheter drainage. Most, if not all, intraperitoneal bladder ruptures require surgical exploration. These injuries do not heal with prolonged catheterization alone.

Injuries occurring during other procedures such as laparoscopic surgery may be repaired laparoscopically.

## Surgical Technique

### Intraperitoneal Bladder Rupture

Intraperitoneal bladder rupture requires immediate surgical repair. The abdomen is opened through a vertical lower midline incision, which affords better exposure and is extendable in the event a laparotomy is required. The rupture, which is usually located horizontally on the dome of the bladder, is identified. In some situations, this may require instillation of saline or colored dye in the bladder through a previously placed urethral catheter. Combined intra- and extraperitoneal rupture may coexist, and it is recommended that the opening in the bladder wall be extended to allow better visualization of the interior and bladder neck. Extraperitoneal tears can be closed from inside the bladder in two layers using running absorbable suture (3-0 chromic or polyglycolic/polyglactin acid). The intraperitoneal rupture(s) are closed in at least two layers using running 3-0 chromic or polyglycolic/polyglactin acid suture. The mucosa, muscle, and peritoneum are all closed in separate layers. The bladder is filled with saline after completion of the closure to evaluate for leaks. If any leaks are detected, they can be closed using interrupted figure-of-eight sutures.

In some situations, bony spicules that have penetrated the bladder wall may need to be removed before closure of the bladder. In cases of penetrating trauma or erosion of the bladder wall by pelvic abscess, nonviable tissue must be debrided and the edges of the perforation freshened prior to closure. In these cases, the tissue may be extremely friable, and a single-layer closure may need to be performed. The ureteral orifices should be identified and observed to ensure normal efflux of urine. This may be done after administration of IV indigo carmine to facilitate visualization. If efflux of urine is not seen, proximal ureteral obstruction, especially by fractured bony fragments, should be ruled out. This can be done by performing a retrograde or intravenous pyelogram on the operating table.

In addition to a urethral catheter, a suprapubic catheter is placed through a separate cystotomy to drain the bladder. Care must be taken not to disturb the pelvic hematoma that is invariably present. Disruption of the pelvic hematoma may give rise to significant bleeding. This can be controlled by packing the area with Gelfoam, Surgicel, or laparotomy tapes. The abdomen can be temporarily closed with the packing in place for about 24 hours; the packing is removed at the time of re-exploration. In extreme cases, angiographic embolization of the pelvic vessels may be necessary.

A 0.5-in. Penrose drain is placed adjacent to the bladder and left in place for 48 hours. In some cases, if the pelvic hematoma has not been disturbed and the bladder closure is truly watertight, drains can be omitted altogether. The abdominal fascia and skin are closed in the usual fashion.

Iatrogenic bladder injury, if suspected to have occurred during other operative procedures, should be documented by instilling methylene blue or indigo carmine in the bladder and noting any extravasation. The rupture or tear can be closed primarily in two or three layers using absorbable suture, as in other cases of rupture. Bladder perforations sustained during laparoscopic procedures can be diagnosed by noting distention of the urethral catheter drainage bag with gas (9). These injuries can be repaired as described previously by laparotomy or even laparoscopically (10).

Intravenous antibiotics are continued until hospital discharge, and the pelvic drain is removed within 48 to 72 hours of the procedure. When the follow-up cystogram confirms bladder healing, the urethral catheter is removed and a voiding trial is initiated by clamping the suprapubic catheter. The suprapubic catheter is removed when spontaneous voiding has returned.

### Extraperitoneal Bladder Rupture

Until the 1970s, extraperitoneal bladder rupture was managed as an intraperitoneal rupture. Since then several studies have demonstrated that these injuries can be managed nonoperatively (1,7). Corriere and Sandler successfully managed 41 patients with extraperitoneal bladder rupture by prolonged urethral catheterization alone. All patients healed the bladder injury spontaneously without complications (7). Since then, other studies have duplicated these results.

Isolated extraperitoneal rupture can be treated by simple urethral catheter drainage. Once urethral injury has been ruled out by means of a retrograde urethrogram, a urethral catheter is placed. The catheter is left in place for 7 to 14 days. Repeat cystograms are performed at the end of this period. If no extravasation is observed, the catheter can be removed. If any contrast extravasation is evident on the cystogram, catheter drainage is continued. Cystograms are repeated at weekly intervals until no extravasation is demonstrable. A majority of extraperitoneal ruptures treated in this manner will heal by 2 weeks, and almost all will show healing within 3 weeks.

Severe bleeding with clots or sepsis should prompt surgical exploration even in cases of extraperitoneal rupture. If patients are undergoing laparotomy for other intra-abdominal injuries, it is reasonable to repair extraperitoneal ruptures surgically.

## Outcomes

### Complications

Some patients may notice persistent urgency and increased frequency of micturition after repair of bladder ruptures. These symptoms are usually temporary and tend to subside with time. Vesical neck injuries increase the risk of subsequent incontinence, and attention should be paid to careful repair of these injuries. Infection of pelvic hematomas can result in abscess formation requiring prolonged drainage and antibiotic treatment. This can be prevented to some extent by taking care to avoid disrupting the hematoma intraoperatively. Unrecognized injury to adjacent structures can lead to subsequent vesicovaginal or vesicoenteric fistula formation. Otherwise, this complication is uncommon.

Complications such as clot retention and pseudodiverticulum formation are seen in fewer than 10% of patients treated with catheter drainage alone for extraperitoneal rupture (1,11). Significant sepsis, delayed healing, formation of bladder calculi, and vesicocutaneous fistula formation have been noted to occur in patients treated with urethral or suprapubic catheter drainage for extraperitoneal rupture (12). These patients most often had poorly functioning catheters or did not receive prophylactic antibiotics. Hence, it is important to ensure that urethral catheters are functioning adequately when used in these situations. Using a larger catheter and considering surgical intervention in 24 to 48 hours if the catheter is not functioning will reduce complications. Prophylactic antibiotics with gram-negative coverage, when administered for the duration of catheterization, will help prevent urinary tract infections.

### Results

Open repair with adequate closure of the rupture is almost uniformly successful in all patients treated in this manner, and 74% to 87% of patients managed with urethral catheter drainage for extraperitoneal rupture will show evidence of healing by 10 to 14 days (1,12). The remainder will heal with an additional 7 to 10 days of catheter drainage.

TABLE 22.1

ETIOLOGIC AGENTS FOR HEMORRHAGIC CYSTITIS

| Infectious causes | Noninfectious causes |
|---|---|
| Viral: BK virus, adenovirus, JC virus, influenza virus | Amyloidosis |
| Bacterial: *Escherichia coli*, *Staphylococcus saprophyticus*, *Proteus mirabilis*, *Klebsiella* | Radiation |
| Fungal: *Candida albicans*, *Aspergillus fumigatus*, *Cryptococcus neoformans*, *Torulopsis glabrata* | Chemicals: anilines and toluidines, pesticides (chlordimeform), ether, gentian violet, spermicidal suppositories, turpentine |
| Parasitic: *Schistosoma haematobium*, *Echinococcus granulosus* | Drugs: penicillins (carbenicillin, penicillin G, K, ticarcillin, methicillin, piperacillin), methenamine mandelate, danazol |
| | Chemotherapeutic agents: busulfan, thiotepa, cyclophosphamide, isophosphamide |

## VESICAL HEMORRHAGE

Significant bleeding from the bladder in the absence of trauma is usually associated with hemorrhagic cystitis. This can result from a variety of infectious and noninfectious etiologies. Possible etiologic factors for hemorrhagic cystitis are listed in Table 22.1. Infection-related hemorrhagic cystitis is usually treatable by addressing the underlying cause.

Radiation therapy to the prostate, bladder, or other pelvic organs can result in hemorrhagic cystitis. Initially, there is mucosal edema with submucosal hemorrhage. Chronically, radiation causes obliterative endarteritis with subsequent urothelial ischemia. Various measures, such as steroids, vitamin E, and trypsin, have proved futile in treating radiation-induced cystitis, which can manifest many years after exposure. Coating the bladder mucosa with synthetic agents such as pentosan polysulfate sodium has some beneficial effect (13). Hyperbaric oxygen therapy has also proved effective (14).

Urothelial malignancies can also cause significant bleeding, which can be controlled by transurethral resection of tumor and fulguration with electrocautery in most cases. In patients with metastatic or unresectable bladder tumors and severe hematuria, local radiation can be used to palliate the symptoms. In some cases, cystectomy or urinary diversion by means of percutaneous nephrostomy or conduit urinary diversion may be the only viable option.

A wide range of drugs and industrial toxins can also give rise to hemorrhagic cystitis. Conservative treatment with adequate hydration, bladder irrigation, and discontinuation of the causative agent will suffice as treatment for most cases.

Chemotherapeutic agents are a major cause of hemorrhagic cystitis. Busulfan, alkylating agents such as cyclophosphamide and isophosphamide, and thiotepa are commonly associated with hemorrhagic cystitis. The incidence ranges from 2% to 40%, and significant mortality rates have also been reported (15). Hemorrhagic cystitis is dose-dependent and related to the route of administration of the chemotherapeutic agent (higher with IV administration). It is more severe in dehydrated patients. Acrolein, which is a liver metabolite of cyclophosphamide, is the principal inciting agent and acts by direct contact with the bladder mucosa. Histological changes that occur in the bladder are similar to those seen with radiation and include edema, ulceration, neovascularization, hemorrhage, and necrosis. Prophylactic hydration and the use of protective agents such as N-acetyl-cysteine (Mucomyst) or 2-mercaptoethane sulfonate (mesna) can reduce the incidence of this complication. Systemic administration of Mucomyst can decrease the antineoplastic effect of cyclophosphamide and may exacerbate the hemorrhage seen with busulfan.

### Treatment of Hemorrhagic Cystitis

A practical algorithm for the management of hemorrhagic cystitis is outlined in Fig. 22.5. Mild hematuria can be managed by vigorous hydration.

Moderate hematuria can be treated with continuous saline irrigation through a Foley catheter after all clots have been evacuated. In some situations, such as with radiation cystitis, irrigation with cold saline for 24 to 48 hours may prove more effective. If hematuria persists, continuous bladder irrigation with 1% alum (potassium or ammonium aluminum sulfate) is helpful. The alum acts as an astringent and precipitates the surface proteins. Aluminum levels must be monitored, particularly in patients with renal insufficiency. Severe acidosis and encephalopathy can occur in such patients as a result of high aluminum levels. Periodic intravesical instillation of prostaglandins ($PGE_2$, $PGF_{2\alpha}$) and $PGF_{2\alpha}$ analogs (carboprost) have also proved effective. They decrease the inflammatory response and reduce the hemorrhage. They can be used prophylactically or therapeutically. Prostaglandin $E_2$ has been used in a dose of 0.75 mg in 200 cc of normal saline instilled for 4 hours. The effective dose of $PGF_{2\alpha}$ has been 1.4 mg in 200 cc of normal saline. Carboprost has been used in a dose of 0.8 mg per dL diluted in normal saline and instilled for 1 hour at 6-hour intervals; good results occurred in 62% of patients, according to one study (16). Instillation of silver nitrate (0.5% to 1.0% solution) for short periods of time followed by saline irrigation of the bladder to remove residual silver nitrate is also an effective technique.

Persistent severe hemorrhage that has not subsided despite the above-mentioned measures can be treated with intravesical instillation of carbolic acid (phenol) or 1% formalin. This requires general anesthesia. Phenol is instilled in a dose of 30 cc of a 100% solution mixed with an equal volume of glycine for 1 minute. This is washed out with 95% ethanol (60 cc) and saline to prevent methemoglobinemia. It is necessary to rule out vesicoureteral reflux by performing a voiding

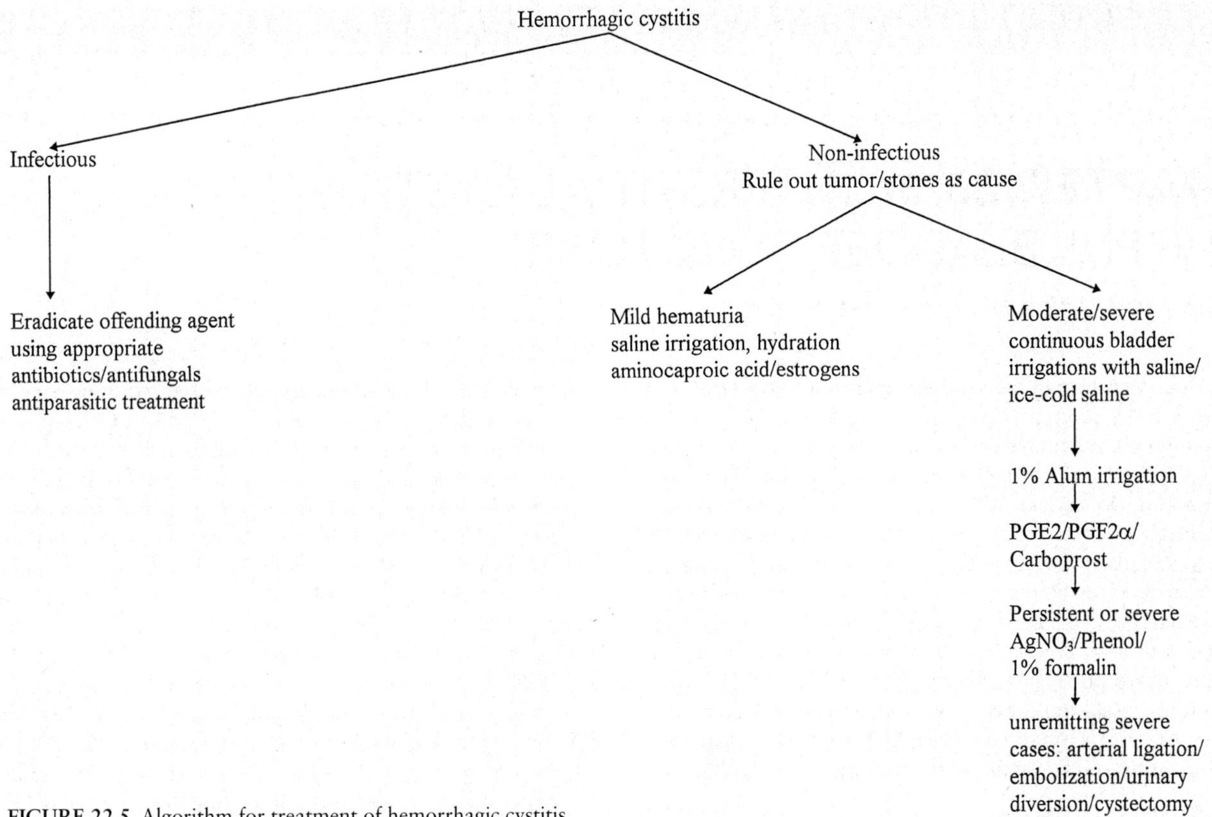


FIGURE 22.5 Algorithm for treatment of hemorrhagic cystitis.

cystourethrogram before using formalin as it can cause fibrosis and scarring of the ureters and renal pelvis. If need be, the ureters can be occluded with Fogarty balloon catheters to prevent reflux while formalin is instilled. Fifty milliliters of 1% formalin (0.37% formaldehyde) diluted with saline should be instilled for 4 to 10 minutes. This should then be washed out with saline and the saline irrigation continued for 24 hours. The external genitalia are covered with towels or Vaseline to prevent irritation.

In recalcitrant cases, use of medical antishock trousers and cryotherapy has been reported (17). Embolization of the hypogastric arteries with autologous clot, Gelfoam, coils, or ethanol can also be resorted to in such cases. This may result in temporary gluteal claudication. Open ligation of the hypogastric artery can also be performed. Supravesical urinary diversion by means of percutaneous nephrostomy tubes or ileal or sigmoid conduit urinary diversion with or without cystectomy remains a final but viable option.

## *References*


1. Cass AS, Luxenberg M. Features of 164 bladder ruptures. *J Urol* 1987;138:743.
2. Bodner DR, Selzman AA, Spirnak JP. Evaluation and treatment of bladder rupture. *Semin Urol* 1995;13:62.
3. Cass AS. Diagnostic studies in bladder rupture: indications and techniques. *Urol Clin North Am* 1989;16:267.
4. Sandler CM. Bladder trauma. In: Pollack HM, ed. *Clinical urography.* Philadelphia: WB Saunders, 1990:1505–1521.
5. Carroll PR, McAninch JW. Major bladder trauma: mechanisms of injury and a unified method of diagnosis and repair. *J Urol* 1984;132:254.
6. Peters PC. Intraperitoneal rupture of the bladder. *Urol Clin North Am* 1989;16:279.
7. Corriere JN, Sandler CM. Mechanisms of injury, patterns of extravasation and management of extraperitoneal bladder rupture due to blunt trauma. *J Urol* 1988;139:43.
8. Lis LE, Cohen AJ. CT cystography in the evaluation of bladder trauma. *J Comput Assist Tomogr* 1990;14:386.
9. Schanbacher PD, Rossi LJ, Salem MR, et al. Detection of urinary bladder perforation during laparoscopy by distension of the collection bag with carbon dioxide. *Anesthesiology* 1994;80:680–681.
10. Parra RO. Laparoscopic repair of intraperitoneal bladder perforation. *J Urol* 1994;151:1003–1005.
11. Cass AS. Diagnostic studies in bladder rupture: indications and techniques. *Urol Clin North Am* 1989;16:267.
12. Kotkin L, Koch MO. Morbidity associated with non-operative management of extraperitoneal bladder injuries. *J Trauma* 1995;38:895.
13. Parsons CL. Successful management of radiation cystitis with sodium pentosanpolysulfate. *J Urol* 1986;136:813.
14. Norkool DM, Hampson NB, Gibbons RP, et al. Hyperbaric oxygen therapy for radiation induced hemorrhagic cystitis. *J Urol* 1993;150:332.
15. Krane DM. Hemorrhagic cystitis. *AUA Update* 1992;11;lesson 31.
16. Ippoliti C, Przepiorka D, Mehra R, et al. Intravesicular carboprost for the treatment of hemorrhagic cystitis after marrow transplantation. *Urology* 1995;46:811.
17. deVries CR, Freiha FS. Hemorrhagic cystitis: a review. *J Urol* 1990;143:1.

# CHAPTER 23 ■ INTERSTITIAL CYSTITIS/ PAINFUL BLADDER SYNDROME

MICHAEL S. INGBER AND KENNETH M. PETERS

Interstitial cystitis/painful bladder syndrome (IC/PBS) is a chronic, unrelenting condition with considerable morbidity. The symptoms were first described in the early 20th century, and IC/PBS continues to be one of the most commonly missed diagnoses in urology (1). While the etiology of IC/PBS has not been clearly identified, much is now known about its characteristics and natural history. The presentation may be variable; however, the more common symptoms are urinary frequency, urgency, and pelvic pain. Until recently, IC/PBS has been considered a disease predominantly affecting women; however, more men are now being diagnosed with this disease. Men presenting with symptoms of genital or perineal pain, frequency, or dysuria are often labeled as having chronic, abacterial prostatitis; in fact, many of them suffer from IC/PBS.

## DIAGNOSIS

Before one can diagnose IC/PBS, causes that can mimic the disease must be ruled out. These include bacterial cystitis, overactive bladder, endometriosis, bladder cancer, and urethral diverticulum. Defining IC/PBS has been extremely controversial, and to date there remains considerable disagreement among experts. In 1987 and 1988 the National Institute of Diabetes and Digestive and Kidney Diseases (NIDDK) developed a research definition for IC/PBS in order to provide homogenous groups of patients that may be compared to one another in clinical studies (2). However, experts in female urology and urogynecology have found this definition to be far too restrictive, as the majority of patients with IC/PBS were being excluded. According to the International Continence Society, IC/PBS should be suspected in anyone with symptoms of suprapubic pain related to bladder filling, accompanied by urinary frequency and urgency, in the absence of urinary infection or other pathology (3). The European Society for the Study of IC/PBS (ESSIC) has developed specific diagnostic criteria that are based on a combination of urinary symptoms and bladder findings during cystoscopic evaluation.

Symptoms of IC/PBS are extremely variable and may present as mild irritative symptoms to severe symptoms refractory to all standard therapies. Treating the disease early often leads to rapid improvement in symptoms; thus, recognizing IC/PBS early so that therapy can be initiated is extremely important.

The diagnosis of IC/PBS begins with a complete history. Onset of symptoms may be days, weeks, or even months. Often patients have been clinically diagnosed with urinary tract infections despite negative cultures. Other misdiagnoses include endometriosis, fibroids, or other pelvic disorders, and some have even undergone surgery for them (4). A full dietary and fluid history is useful, as certain foods and drinks may exacerbate IC/PBS symptoms (5). A voiding diary provides objective evidence of daytime and nighttime frequency, and pain symptoms can be recorded with this as well. Sequential voiding diaries and symptom questionnaires allow one to determine the impact of various treatments for IC/PBS.

A physical examination that includes a thorough pelvic and neurological examination should be performed. The female pelvic examination should include evaluation for tenderness of the anterior vaginal wall and levator muscles, the ability to contract and relax the pelvic floor muscles, and the degree of pelvic relaxation. Urethral fullness, tenderness, or expression of pus may suggest a urethral diverticulum requiring further workup. A rectal examination can rule out any rectal abnormalities or masses, and in men the prostate should be palpated for nodules or tenderness.

A urinalysis, urine culture, and cytology should be performed to exclude active infection or evidence of carcinoma in situ. Sterile pyuria should prompt staining for acid-fast bacilli to rule out genitourinary tuberculosis. If microscopic or gross hematuria is present, a workup including CT urography, cystoscopy, and urine cytology is required in order to evaluate for bladder cancer or stone disease.

In patients with urinary urgency, frequency, or incontinence, a trial of anticholinergics may cause symptoms to subside. However, if symptoms persist, or if pelvic pain or severe dysuria is present, a cystoscopic evaluation is warranted. Interstitial cystitis was first described as a distinct ulcer seen on cystoscopic examination. This lesion is typically red, raised, and friable and can be seen during cystoscopy without hydrodistention. The lesion is difficult to distinguish from carcinoma in situ, and a biopsy with cauterization of the lesion is warranted. Only 15% to 20% of patients diagnosed with IC/PBS have an ulcer in their bladder. They are typically older and have more severe bladder-associated pain and a smaller anesthetic bladder capacity.

In patients in whom a diagnosis of IC/PBS is highly suspected, cystoscopy with hydrodistention under anesthesia may reveal petechial hemorrhages and glomerulations, which are found in over 90% of women with the syndrome. However, the presence of petechial hemorrhages alone is not diagnostic, as they can also be seen in normal men and women (6). A computerized cystometrogram may also be performed to look for uninhibited contractions and to determine the functional bladder capacity. Some investigators have suggested the use of the potassium sensitivity test (PST) to diagnose IC/PBS (7). The PST is based on the hypothesis that there is increased epithelial permeability in the bladder of IC patients. However, a significant false-positive rate exists, and many patients will eventually be diagnosed with a normal bladder (8). Additionally, 17% of women with IC/PBS may have a negative test (9). For these reasons, PST should be used only as an adjunct during evaluation and diagnosis.

## INDICATIONS FOR SURGERY

Any patient with unexplained urinary urgency, frequency, and pelvic pain is a candidate for an operative hydrodistention, which may be not only diagnostic but also therapeutic. Patients with ulcerative disease may benefit from ablation of the ulcers with cautery or laser (10).

Radical surgery for IC/PBS is rarely indicated and should be used as a last resort. Magnetic resonance imaging (MRI) of the pelvis may demonstrate a thickened, end-stage bladder that may be amenable to radical surgery (Fig. 23.1). Patients who undergo bladder augmentation or continent diversion need to be willing and able to perform clean intermittent catheterization. Additionally, patients must accept that frequency symptoms may improve but that pain may persist. Diverting the urine without removing the diseased bladder is not always sufficient to relieve the symptoms of IC/PBS. Therefore, any diversion procedure for pain should be accompanied by cystectomy (11). Finally, neuromodulation has been effective in treating refractory urinary urgency and frequency (12). Because IC/PBS is a syndrome of urgency, frequency, and pain, patients who are refractory to standard therapies would be candidates for nerve stimulation.

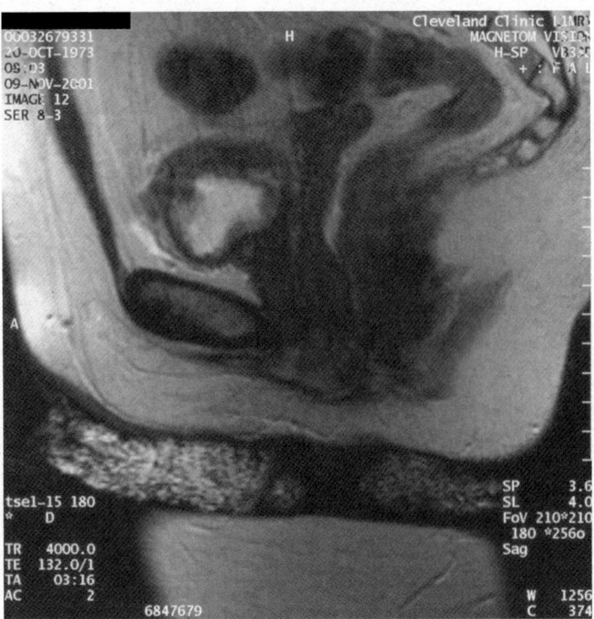


FIGURE 23.1 MRI scan of pelvis of 28-year-old woman with end-stage interstitial cystitis demonstrating a small, thickened, contracted bladder. (Courtesy of Raymond Rackley, Cleveland Clinic Foundation.)

## ALTERNATIVE THERAPY

Establishing a diagnosis of IC/PBS in itself is usually therapeutic and alleviates patient frustrations. A multimodality approach along with patient education is the most effective means of treating IC/PBS. Behavioral therapies must be stressed, such as fluid management, pelvic floor physical therapy, dietary restrictions, and relaxation therapy (13). Many patients suffer from pelvic floor spasm, which causes pelvic pain, dyspareunia, and urinary hesitancy. Treatment by a therapist knowledgeable in myofascial release techniques may be of benefit (14). Once behavioral therapy is optimized, oral medication is a reasonable first-line treatment for IC/PBS.

At the present time, the only oral therapy approved by the U.S. Food and Drug Administration (FDA) for IC/PBS is pentosan polysulfate sodium (Elmiron, Ortho-McNeil Pharmaceuticals), a glycosaminoglycan that binds tightly to the bladder mucosa. Pentosan polysulfate should be considered a first-line therapy for IC/PBS; however, because it may require several months before any clinical improvement is seen, it should not be used as a single agent for the treatment of IC/PBS. Hydroxyzine has antihistaminic and antianxiety properties and affects mast-cell degranulation, which may play a role in symptoms of IC/PBS (15). However, neither pentosan polysulfate nor hydroxyzine showed high response rates in recent clinical trials (15). Muscle relaxants such as diazepam or low-dose baclofen may be useful in women with accompanying pelvic floor spasm, although to date no major studies have been performed on these medicines. Tricyclic antidepressants such as amitriptyline or imipramine may improve symptoms due to their anticholinergic and antipain effects (16). Finally, chronic pain is recognized as a legitimate complaint and should be treated aggressively. Various narcotics and anti-inflammatories can be tried, along with nerve blocks or implantable pain pumps, to treat the severe pain that can be associated with IC/PBS. Cyclosporine has been used in some clinical trials, but results are inconclusive.

Intravesical therapies have been a mainstay in treatment for many years. Dimethyl sulfoxide (DMSO) is the only FDA-approved intravesical therapy for this disease. DMSO is a product derived from paper pulp and is mainly used as an industrial solvent. It is given in the office setting as a 50% solution in 50 mL of sterile saline. Patients rarely have side-effects, although they may complain of transient urethral pain or irritation after the first instillation, or a garliclike odor from their mouth. If effective, symptoms may resolve for months to even years (17).

Bacille Calmette-Guérin (BCG) is prepared from an attenuated strain of bovine tuberculosis bacillus, *Mycobacterium bovis*, and is given intravesically as a 50-mg dose in 50 mL saline solution. While traditionally used for treating carcinoma in situ of the bladder or low-stage urothelial carcinoma, it appeared to show promise as an intravesical agent in treating IC/PBS. In a randomized placebo-controlled clinical trial, 21% of patients responded to BCG, compared to 12% of placebo. However, the difference was not statistically significant ($p = 0.062$), and therefore this should not be offered as first-line therapy.

Other second-line agents that have been used include capsaicin, heparin, sodium oxychlorosene, and silver nitrate.

# SURGICAL TECHNIQUE

## Bladder Hydrodistention

A complete cystoscopy is performed to assess the urethra and bladder for any masses, stones, or diverticulae (Fig. 23.2). After careful inspection, the bladder is filled by gravity drainage under anesthesia at 100 cm $H_2O$ pressure to its capacity. Upward pressure with a finger along each side of the urethra is often needed to maximally distend the bladder to prevent leakage around the cystoscope. The bladder is distended until no further water will run into the bladder, and this is allowed to dwell for 2 minutes. The bladder is drained and the volume measured. The procedure is then repeated a second time.

A normal bladder will accommodate up to (or over) 1 L under a general anesthetic. On the other hand, the bladder of a patient with the ulcerative form of IC/PBS will be less compliant, often stretching to <350 mL. Typically with IC/PBS there is terminal hematuria noted when the bladder is drained. Upon reinspecting the bladder, the vast majority of patients will have glomerulations seen in all sectors of the bladder, suggestive of interstitial cystitis. Patients having the ulcerative form will have distinct inflammatory lesions on cystoscopy called Hunner ulcers, and with hydrodistention deep cracks in their bladder at the site of ulcers may occur (1) (Fig. 23.3).

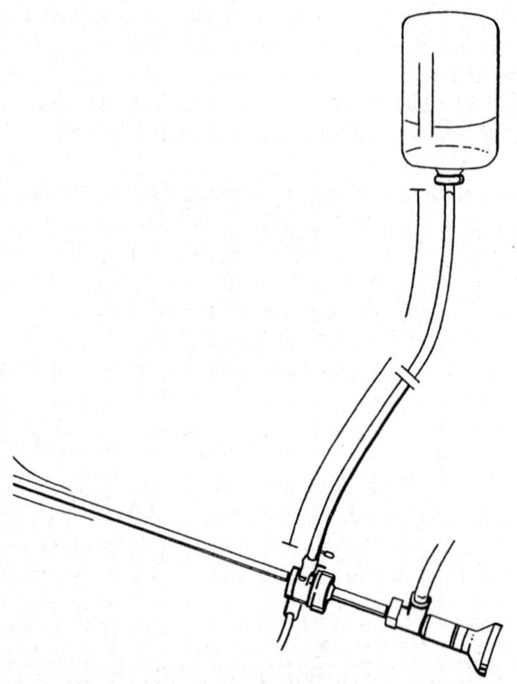

FIGURE 23.2 Hydrodistention is carried out with the irrigation bag hung 100 cm above the level of the bladder. Bladder capacity is reached when irrigant flow stops. During filling, the bladder mucosa is typically normal-appearing. After 2 minutes of distention, the bladder is drained and the capacity is measured. At the termination of bladder emptying, the irrigant fluid is often blood-tinged or grossly hemorrhagic in patients with interstitial cystitis (IC). Repeat cystoscopy will demonstrate diffuse glomerulations in all sectors of the bladder consistent with IC. Repeat hydrodistention is performed to maximally distend the bladder.

## Endoscopic Resection or Fulguration of Ulcers

Approximately 15% of IC/PBS patients comprise the ulcerative subset, and they generally have worse pain and frequency symptoms. A resectoscope with loop electrocautery can be used to resect these lesions and cauterize the base (18). Alternatively, the involved areas can be cauterized with a Bugbee electrode, ball electrode, or neodymium:YAG laser. The laser is set at 15 W with a firing duration of 1 to 3 seconds. The laser fiber is maintained in constant motion over the target, and the procedure is completed when the ulcer is completely blanched (10).

## Augmentation Cystoplasty

Simple augmentation of the bladder should only be performed if one has an operative bladder capacity with hydrodistention of <300 cc. The bladder is isolated and a posterior-based U-shaped incision is created on the anterior bladder (Fig. 23.4). A 30-cm segment of distal ileum is isolated in the standard fashion and opened along its antimesenteric border. The ileal segment is folded to create a nonperistaltic ileal patch. This is secured to the anterior bladder with running absorbable suture, effectively increasing the functional capacity of the bladder. Patients undergoing an augmentation must understand that their pelvic pain symptoms may not resolve from augmentation alone. Additionally, because the detrusor is incised, the emptying mechanism of the bladder is altered, and patients may need to perform intermittent straight catheterization to effectively empty their bladder.

## Partial Cystectomy and Substitution Cystoplasty

Supratrigonal cystectomy with enterocystoplasty is preferred over simple augmentation cystoplasty because most of the diseased bladder is removed (19) (Fig. 23.5). This technique should be reserved for patients with small bladder capacity found on hydrodistention under an anesthetic (<300 mL). Patients with a primary pain complaint are not good candidates for supratrigonal cystectomy, particularly if the pain is urethral in nature. In addition, patients should be able to perform intermittent straight catheterization and bladder irrigation in case of poor emptying or mucus formation.

The patient is placed in a supine position and a Foley catheter is placed sterilely in the bladder. The peritoneal cavity is entered through a vertical midline incision, and an appropriate segment of either large or small bowel with a mesentery long enough to reach down to the bladder is selected. The preferred bowel segments are the cecum, sigmoid colon, or ileum. The bladder is filled via the Foley catheter and divided using a clamshell technique, exposing the trigone. Ureteral catheters are

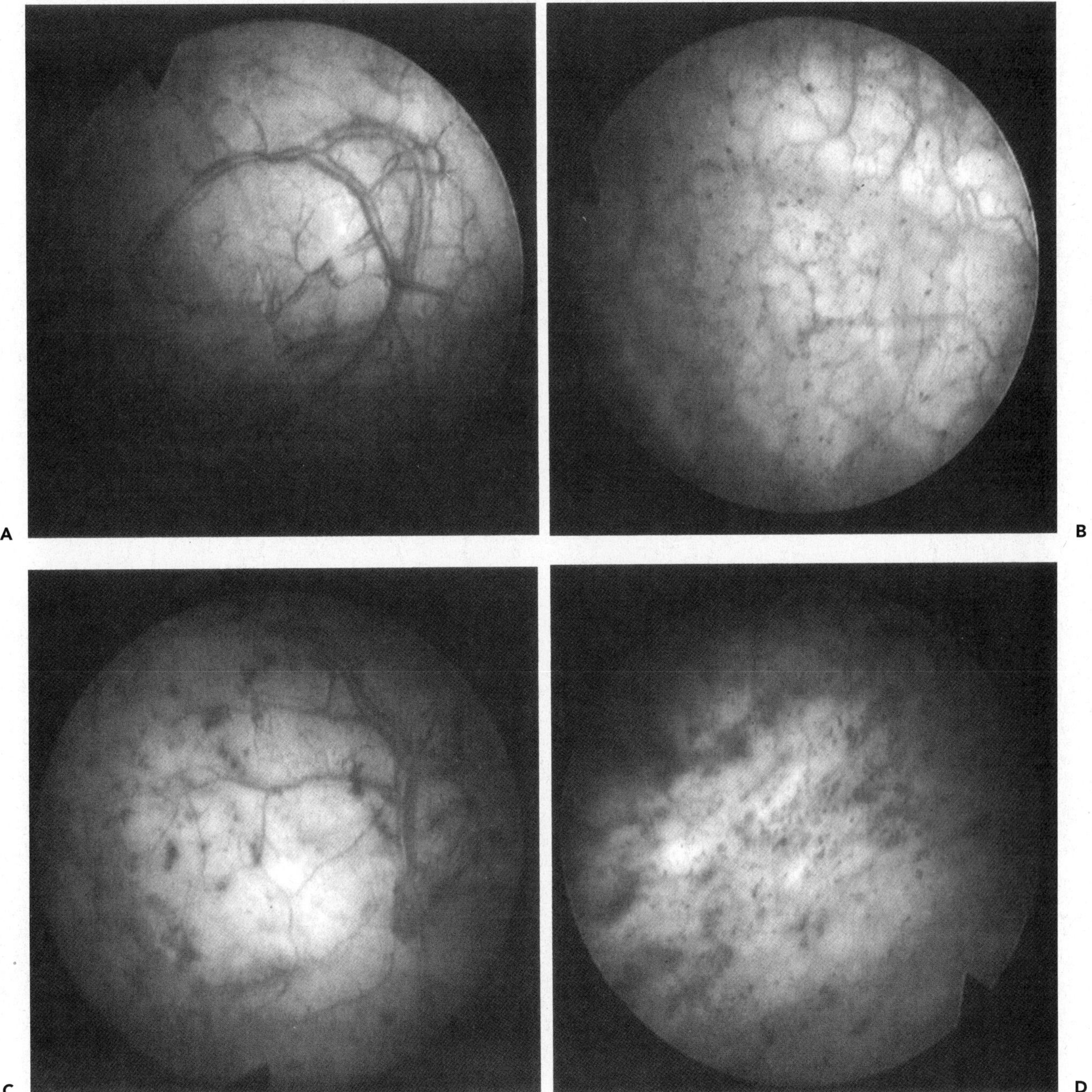


**FIGURE 23.3 A:** Normal appearance of the bladder urothelium before hydrodistention in a patient with symptoms consistent with interstitial cystitis. **B:** Same patient following hydrodistention. The urothelium is abnormal, revealing minimal to moderate glomerulation. **C:** Cystoscopic appearance of a patient with moderate glomerulations and submucosal hemorrhage. **D:** Hunner ulcer with marked hemorrhage surrounding the ulcer. This patient was successfully treated with neodymium:YAG laser ablation therapy.

placed before resection of the bladder to avoid injury to the ureters. Using electrocautery, a supratrigonal cystectomy is performed, resecting all but a 1- to 2-cm cuff of bladder that includes the trigone and bladder neck. Placing Allis clamps on the edges of the remaining bladder controls hemostasis. The vesicoenteric anastomosis is completed using a single-layer running closure of 3-0 Vicryl suture. A 22Fr Foley catheter is placed through the bowel segment and used as a suprapubic tube. Both tubes are kept to dependent drainage for 21 days, when a cystogram is performed to ensure the integrity of the anastomosis. The patient is then started on intermittent catheterization.

## Total Cystectomy with Orthotopic Neobladder or Urinary Diversion

A total cystectomy has the benefit of removing the entire diseased bladder and may be the treatment of choice for the patient with an "end-stage" bladder. The choice of performing a continent versus incontinent diversion is based mainly on patient preference. If a patient has significant urethral symptoms, an orthotopic neobladder may not be the preferred conduit. The benefits of continent diversions are obvious;

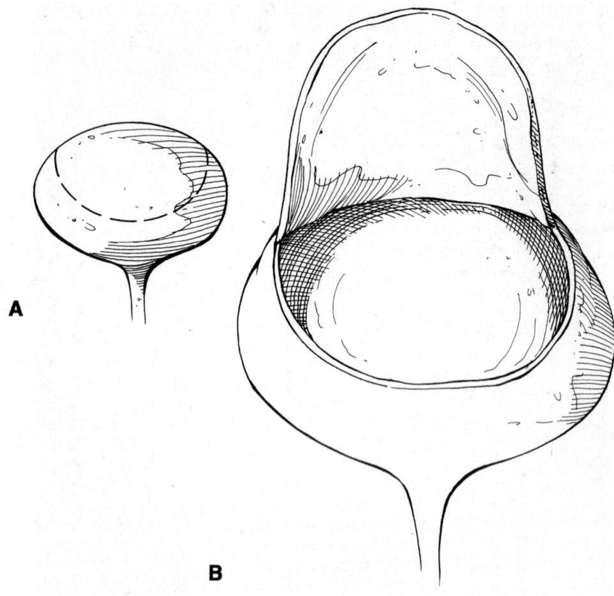


FIGURE 23.4 Ileal augmentation cystoplasty. **A:** A posterior-based U-shaped incision is created on the anterior bladder. **B:** Completion of the posterior-based bladder flap. **C:** A 30-cm segment of the distal ileum is isolated and divided along the antimesenteric border. **D:** The ileal segment is then folded and the posterior surface is closed completely with a running absorbable suture. The anterior segment is partially closed. **E:** Completed ileal bladder anastomosis.

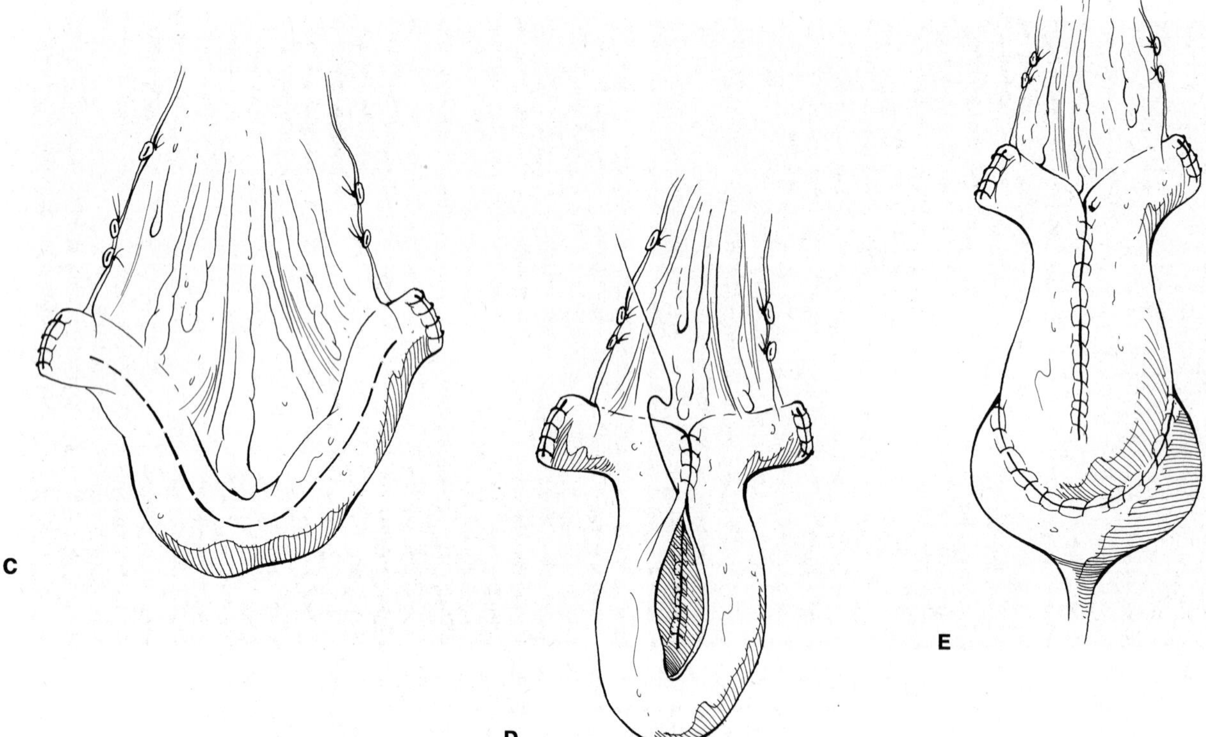


however, there have been reports of IC/PBS developing in the continent bowel segments. An informed and motivated patient would be the best candidate for a continent diversion. The techniques of cystectomy and urinary diversion, including complications, are described elsewhere.

## Sacral Nerve Stimulation

Chronic inflammation in a pelvic organ may lead to nerve upregulation to the spinal cord, affecting all pelvic structures. Sacral nerve modulation (InterStim, Medtronic, Inc, Minneapolis, MN) is approved by the FDA for urinary urgency, frequency, urge incontinence, and idiopathic urinary retention. Preoperatively, the efficacy of sacral nerve stimulation is determined by a test performed prior to placing a permanent generator. If patients experience at least a 50% improvement in their symptoms and desire a permanent implant, an implantable generator can be placed permanently in a subcutaneous pocket in the upper buttocks. Patients have an external programmer to control the degree and frequency of stimulation.

InterStim therapy has evolved since its approval in the United States in 1997. Initially, a percutaneous lead was

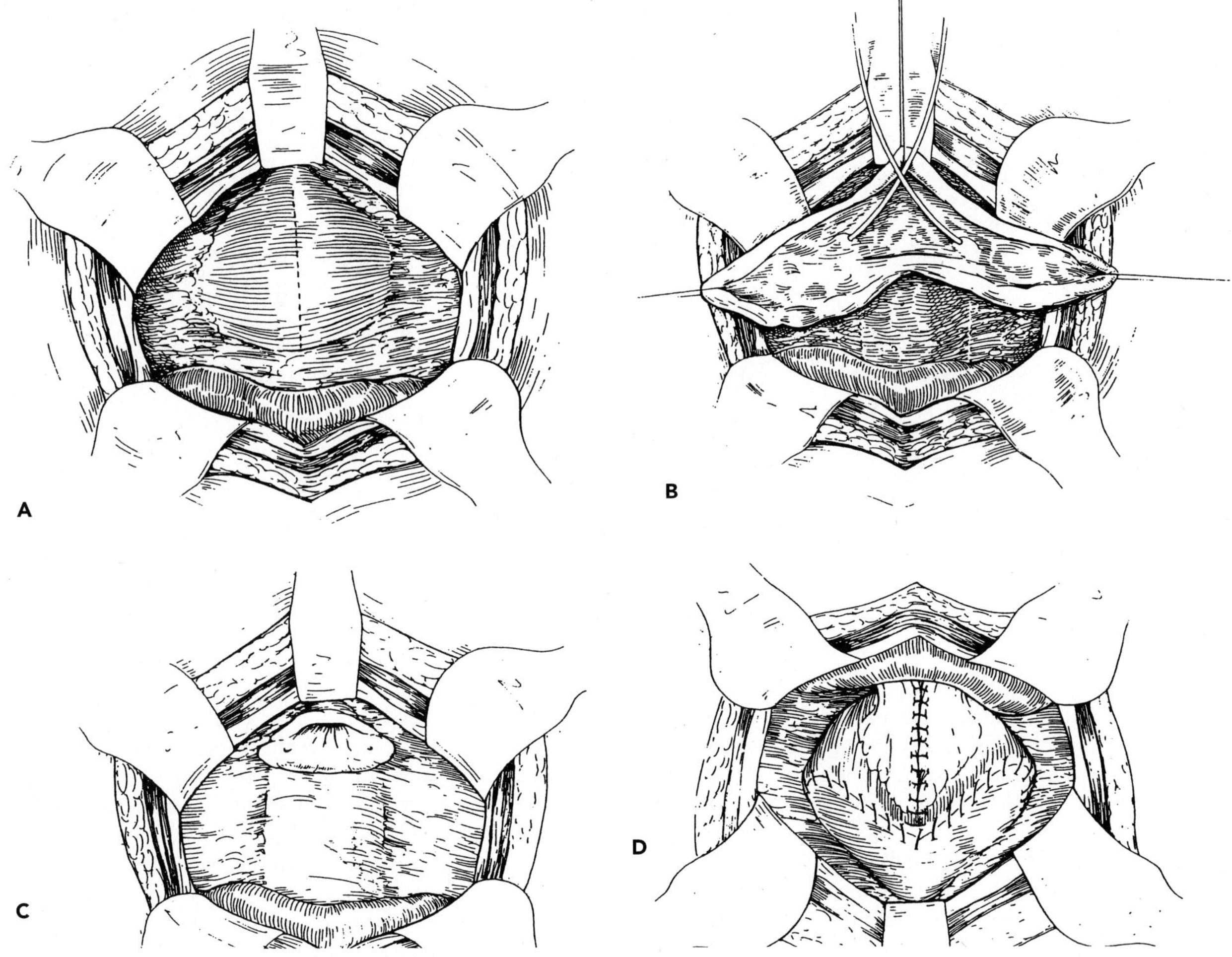


FIGURE 23.5 Technique of subtotal cystectomy and substitution cystoplasty. **A:** The bladder is being bivalved with electrocautery. **B:** View of the bladder with both ureteral orifices cannulated with ureteral catheters to avoid injury to ureters during bladder resection. **C:** Completion of subtotal cystectomy with only a small cuff of bladder remaining, which consists of the urethra, bladder neck, and trigone. **D:** Completed anastomosis of the bowel onto the bladder cuff. A Foley catheter (not shown) and a suprapubic tube are placed to ensure adequate drainage during the immediate postoperative period.

placed in the sacral foramen under local anesthetic in the office, and the lead was taped to the skin. The patient was discharged to home with an external stimulating box, and the lead was stimulated for 3 to 5 days while voiding diaries were kept. The lead was then removed, and patients responding to the test were candidates for a permanent implant that was performed in the operating room under a general anesthetic. The permanent implant was relatively complicated because it required exposing the periosteum of the sacrum, dissecting the foramen, and securing the permanent lead to the bone after testing for muscle response. This lead was then connected to an implantable pulse generator placed in a subcutaneous pocket under the upper buttocks.

Several problems were identified with the percutaneous testing/implant technique. These included migration of the percutaneous lead resulting in an inadequate test period, uncomfortable sensory response when the permanent lead was placed under a general anesthetic, the morbid nature of placing the permanent lead, and the inability to duplicate placement of the permanent lead in the identical location of the temporary percutaneous lead, resulting in a poor clinical response. The most significant advance with InterStim therapy is the introduction of a tined permanent quadripolar lead, allowing for percutaneous placement of the permanent lead for the test period. The most common procedure for InterStim therapy is a "staged implant."

## Staged Implant

The patient is given broad-spectrum antibiotic coverage, lightly sedated, and placed in the prone position on the operating room table. The lower back and buttocks are prepped and draped. Fluoroscopy is used to mark the midline of the sacrum and the inferior border of the sacral iliac junction. This intersection corresponds to the area of the S3 foramen. A mark is made 2 cm lateral and superior to this intersection, the area is infiltrated with lidocaine, and the foramen needle is advanced at a 60-degree angle into the S3 foramen with fluoroscopic guidance (Fig. 23.6). Current is applied to the needle, and the motor and sensory response is assessed. An ideal motor response is good levator ani contraction in the form of

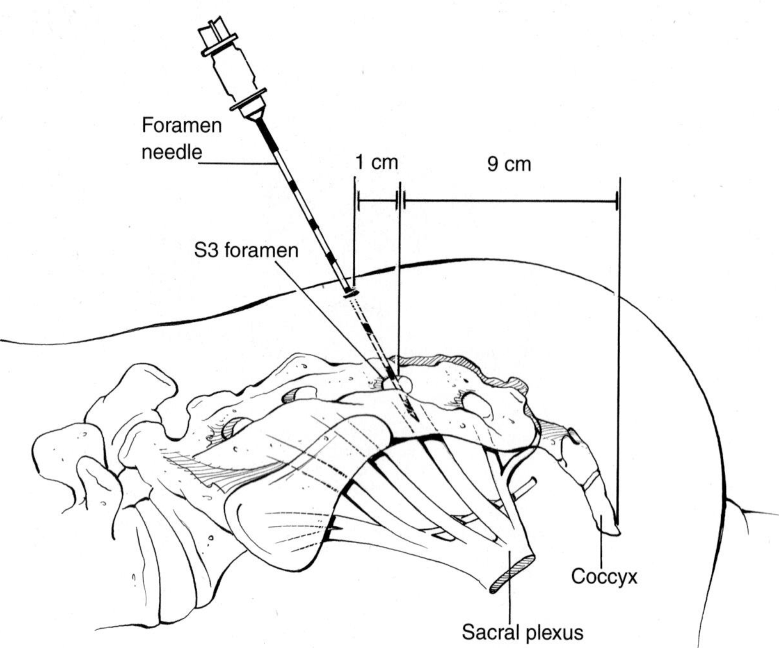


FIGURE 23.6 Insertion of a foramen needle through the S3 foramen in preparation for testing the motor and sensory responses.

anal bellows, sacral flattening, and minimal dorsiflexion of the greater toe from stimulation of the S3 portion of the medial plantar nerve. The patient should be alert enough intraoperatively to report a gentle tapping or pulsating sensation in the rectal, vaginal, or perineal region. If the stimulation is painful, the lead should be readjusted in the operating room.

To confirm S3 placement, a needle is always passed into the foramen superior to the first. Stimulation of this lead results in leg rotation consistent with S2 placement, and this ensures S3 placement of the first electrode. Next, a small skin nick is made alongside the needle, through the dermis of the skin. A directional guide wire is passed through the foramen needle, and the needle is removed. The lead introducer is advanced over the guide wire, through the dorsolumbar fascia and the foramen, and below the bone plate. The trocar is removed, and the permanent quadripolar lead is advanced through the lead introducer (Fig. 23.7). Fluoroscopy is used to confirm that all four stimulation points lie beneath the sacral bone plate. The patient remains awake and sensory, and motor responses are assessed with stimulation of each electrode. After confirming good lead placement, the lead introducer is removed under fluoroscopy, deploying the tines to secure the lead. A site on the ipsilateral upper buttocks is chosen where a future permanent generator will be placed if the patient

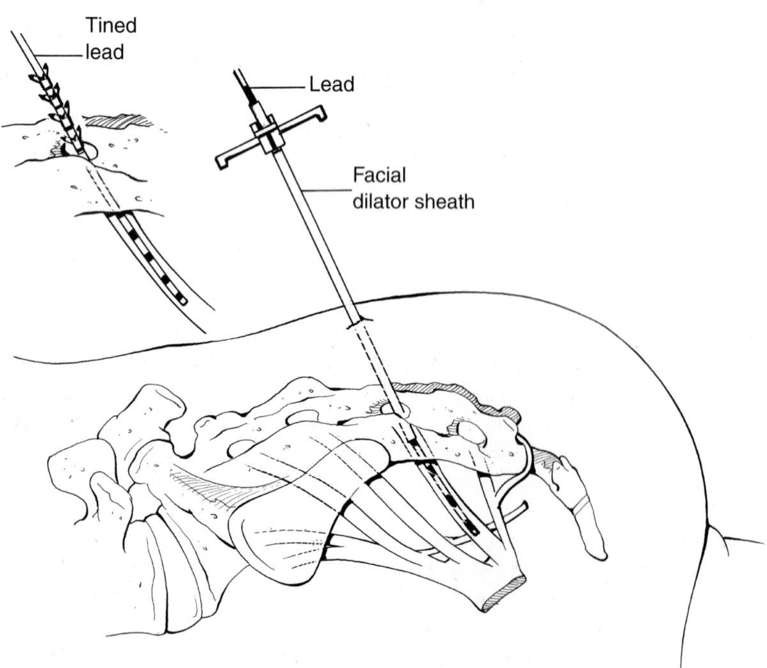


FIGURE 23.7 Stage I implant. Advancement of permanent tined lead through the lead introducer parallel to the nerve (see inset). Motor and sensory response tested and lead introducer removed, deploying the tines and securing the lead.

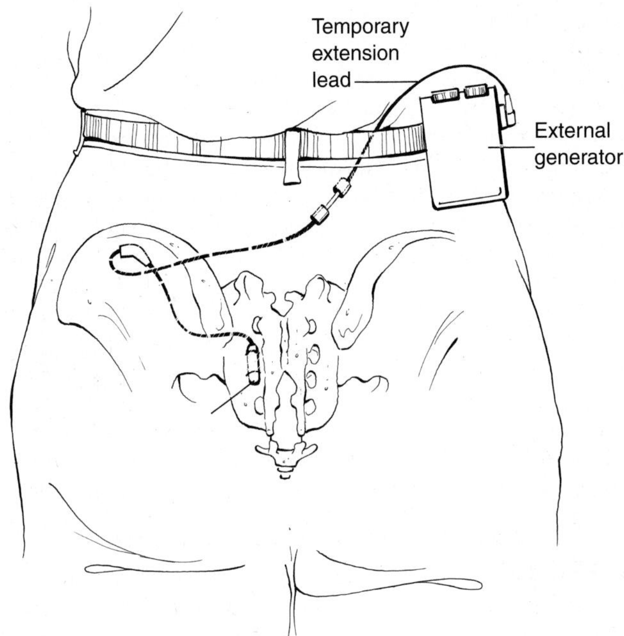


FIGURE 23.8 Stage I implant. The lead is tunneled to a small, subcutaneous pocket on the ipsilateral side. The lead is then connected to a temporary extension lead, which is tunneled to the contralateral side and externalized. The external generator is then connected to the extension lead. The patient is discharged to home, and sacral nerve stimulation is tested over a 14- to 21-day period. Voiding logs and pain scores are maintained, and the program is changed as needed to maximize the clinical response.

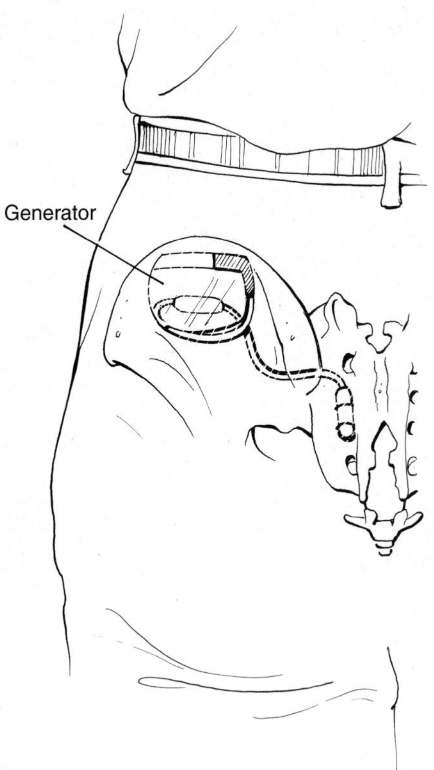


FIGURE 23.9 Stage II implant. Patients not responding to the therapy have the lead removed. Responders have the extension lead removed, the ipsilateral subcutaneous pocket extended, and the generator placed. The generator is then programmed to the settings that gave a good clinical response during the test phase.

responds to therapy. A small (2-cm) transverse incision is made and a subcutaneous pocket created. The proximal end of the lead is then tunneled to this pocket using the lead introducer. The permanent lead is then connected to a temporary extension wire, and the distal end of the wire is tunneled to the contralateral upper buttocks and externalized (Fig. 23.8).

One of four electrodes is chosen for initial outpatient stimulation, and the patient is discharged wearing the standard external generator for 2 weeks. The permanent lead allows for four different points of stimulation along the nerve. Variables such as rate, pulse width, and voltage can be adjusted by the patient with guidance from the clinician over the phone. The patient monitors voids per day, voided volume, urge scores, incontinence episodes, and pelvic pain during the 2-week test period. Responders are considered those with at least a 50% improvement in symptoms and the desire for a permanent implant based on improvement in quality of life. Nonresponders have the leads removed, and responders have a permanent generator placed. Permanent generator placement in the staged technique involves extending the incision and subcutaneous pocket in the ipsilateral buttocks, removing the temporary extension lead, and connecting the permanent generator (Fig. 23.9). At the end of the procedure, the generator is programmed to the settings to which the patient responded during the test stimulation so that there is no interruption in therapy.

Currently, a smaller generator is available that may be easier to implant and more comfortable for patients. Battery life on this smaller device is 4 years, compared to 8 years for the larger generator. Regardless, patients must be aware that they will require replacement of their generator later in life.

## Pudendal Neuromodulation

Stimulation of the pudendal nerve, as with sacral nerve stimulation, affects the sacral nerve roots of S2, S3, and S4. Multiple studies have shown inhibition of the micturition reflex with afferent pudendal stimulation, which also results in an increase in bladder capacity, and a decrease in uninhibited bladder contractions (20,21). Devices used to stimulate the pudendal nerve include InterStim and the BION device (Advanced Bionics, Valencia, CA). At the present time, however, neither of these nerve stimulation devices is FDA-approved for use at the pudendal nerve. Nevertheless, some studies have shown promise in using the pudendal nerve as a site of stimulation in patients with urinary urgency, frequency, and pelvic pain (22). The electrode is implanted along the course of the pudendal nerve toward Alcock's canal, at the level of the ischial spine. Intraoperative monitoring of EMG is used to confirm pudendal nerve stimulation. The exact technique is described elsewhere.

In a recent single-blind crossover trial, patients had both sacral and pudendal tined leads placed. Each was stimulated in random order. In responders (>50% improvement in their symptoms), the "better" lead was chosen by the patient (Fig. 23.10). Pudendal lead placement took a mean of 19.6 minutes compared to 27.4 minutes for sacral leads ($p$ = 0.039). Of 22 patients involved in the study, 17 (77%) had a permanent generator placed. The mean Interstitial Cystitis Symptom Index score decreased from 14.3 preoperatively to 10.7 at 6 months

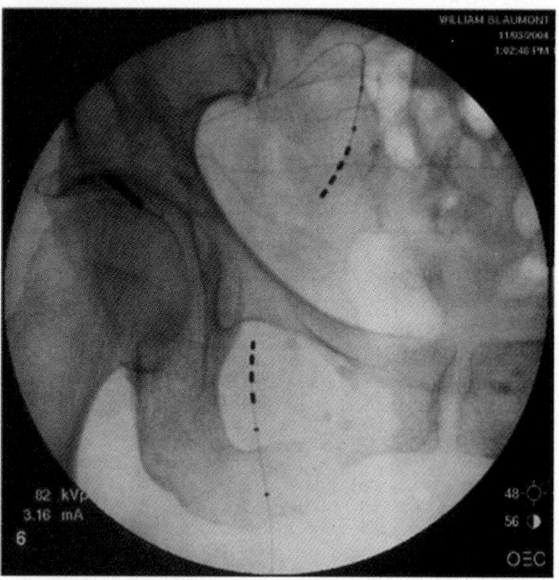


FIGURE 23.10 Postoperative photograph showing both sacral and pudendal leads in place. The pudendal lead was chosen by the majority of patients in a randomized, single-blind crossover study.

postoperatively in the sacral nerve stimulation group ($p$ = 0.03) and decreased from 15.7 to 8.6 in the pudendal group ($p$ = 0.009). The decrease in the Interstitial Cystitis Problem Index was statistically significant only for the pudendal group, with a decrease from 12.9 to 7.5 at 6 months ($p$ = 0.002). Average preoperative frequency was 24.07 per 24 hours for both groups. At 6 months, the mean total 24-hour voids decreased to 13.94 in the sacral group ($p$ = 0.001) and to 12.84 in the pudendal group ($p$ = 0.001). Mean voided volume increased from the preoperative value of 81.8 mL to 152.8 mL in the sacral group ($p$ = 0.001) and to 158.0 in the pudendal group ($p$ = 0.001). Of patients having a permanent generator placed, the majority (77%) chose to have the pudendal lead permanently implanted (22). Nevertheless, further studies with larger numbers are needed to determine if pudendal nerve stimulation is as effective or better at reducing urgency, frequency and pain symptoms than sacral stimulation.

## Posterior Tibial Nerve Stimulation

The tibial nerve arises from L4 through S3 and is a branch of the sciatic nerve. As with sacral and pudendal stimulation, it is possible to stimulate the posterior tibial nerve and modulate the innervation to the bladder, urinary sphincter, and pelvic

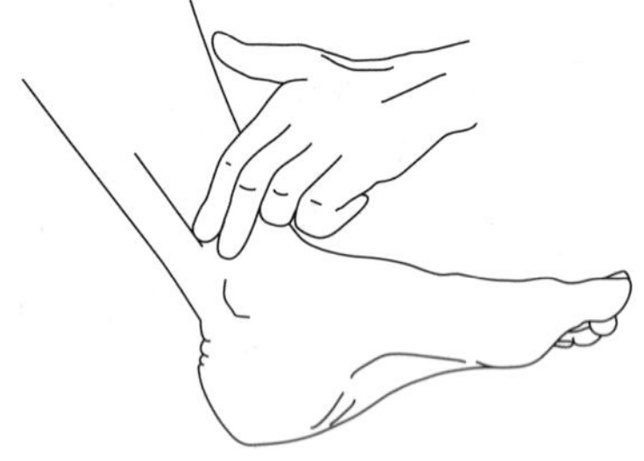

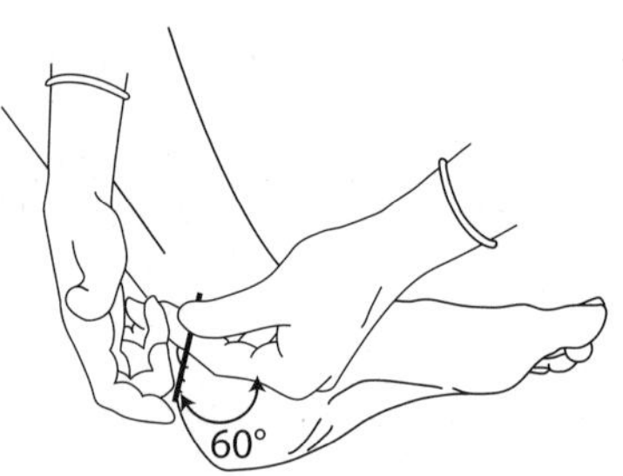


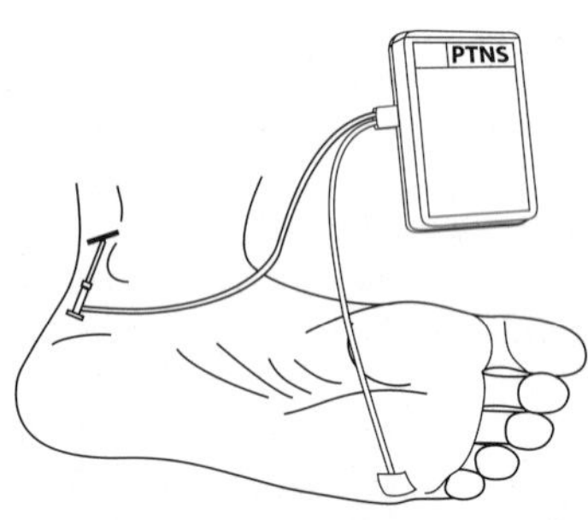


FIGURE 23.11 Neuromodulation of the posterior tibial nerve. A 34-gauge acupuncturelike needle is inserted approximately 3 to 4 cm deep to the tibial nerve for stimulation.

floor (23,24) (Fig. 23.11). The technique stimulates the posterior tibial nerve with a 34-gauge needle placed bilaterally at SP-6. The needles are placed approximately 4 cm deep at a 30-degree angle cephalad. An adhesive grounding electrode is applied on each side near the medial calcaneus. Stimulation of the posterior tibial nerve is done by an amplitude of 0.5 to 10.0 mA, with a fixed pulse width (200 μs) and frequency (20 Hz). Stimulation is applied for 30 minutes. The stimulation needs to be done on a weekly basis for 12 weeks, after which an attempt to wean treatments to once a month is tried. Unfortunately, there are no sham studies done on posterior tibial nerve stimulation for voiding dysfunction, so its use remains in question.

### Cytolysis

Bladder denervation procedures have been reported in the treatment of patients with intractable bladder pain and urinary frequency and urgency (25). Division of the posterior sacral roots, posterior rhizotomy, or division of the inferior vesical neurovascular pedicle may result in temporary improvement in urinary frequency, urgency, and pain. Ingelmann-Sundberg described a more selective denervation in which a transvaginal approach is used to resect the inferior hypogastric plexus, dividing both the sympathetic and parasympathetic fibers (25). Candidates for the transvaginal denervation are selected by first performing a subtrigonal injection of bupivacaine, which, if successful, results in significant relief of their irritative symptoms. However, with the advent of more oral therapies, along with neuromodulation, denervation is mainly mentioned in this section for its historical significance.

## OUTCOMES

### Complications

Complications of hydrodistention with or without fulguration are listed in Table 23.1. The most serious complication is bladder rupture, which should be considered if there is resumption of fluid inflow after maximally distending the bladder, return of significantly less fluid than what was instilled upon bladder drainage, or severe suprapubic or abdominal pain or distention. If a bladder rupture is suspected, an immediate cystogram should be performed. If the rupture is extraperitoneal, prolonged Foley catheter drainage is usually all that is needed to allow the rupture to heal spontaneously. If intraperitoneal leakage of contrast is seen, however, immediate exploration and repair are warranted to prevent peritonitis from urine leakage in the peritoneal cavity.

Early and late complications secondary to major bladder reconstruction are listed in Table 23.2. Persistence of IC/PBS symptoms is probably the most common and disheartening outcome for both the patient and surgeon.

The major risk of selective denervation cytolysis is ureteral injury during the vaginal dissection and is avoidable by placing ureteral catheters.

No serious, irreversible, adverse events have been reported with sacral nerve stimulation. Complications associated with InterStim are listed in Table 23.3. Reoperation occurs in approximately 25% of patients undergoing sacral nerve implantation. Causes for reoperation include sensory discomfort,

**TABLE 23.1**

**COMPLICATIONS OF BLADDER HYDRODISTENTION AND FULGURATION OF ULCERS**

| |
|---|
| Gross hematuria |
| Bladder rupture of perforation |
| Urinary tract infection |
| Exacerbation of bladder symptoms |
| Bowel perforation |

**TABLE 23.2**

**COMPLICATIONS OF MAJOR BLADDER RECONSTRUCTIVE SURGERY**

| EARLY |
|---|
| Ileus |
| Intraperitoneal abscess |
| Upper-tract obstruction |
| Thromboembolic events |
| Pneumonia |
| Wound infection |
| Cardiac events |
| Difficulty with catheterization |
| **LATE** |
| Persistence of interstitial cystitis symptoms |
| Upper-tract deterioration |
| Urolithiasis |
| Metabolic abnormalities |
| Spontaneous rupture of bowel conduit |
| Difficulty with catheterization |
| Ureteral stenosis |
| Ureteral reflux |
| Neoplasia |
| Bladder neck contracture |
| Urinary incontinence |
| Pyelonephritis/urinary tract infection |

**TABLE 23.3**

**COMPLICATIONS OF INTERSTIM NEUROMODULATION THERAPY**

| |
|---|
| Pain at generator site |
| Infection |
| Lead migration |
| Transient electric shock |
| Pain at lead site |
| Change in bowel function |
| Device malfunction |
| Change in menstrual cycle |

lead migration, device failure, pocket revision, and infection. Infection of the device requiring explantation occurs infrequently, in 5% of patients in a recent review of a large series (26). Perioperative, broad-spectrum antibiotic coverage during implantation of the lead and generator should be administered to decrease the rate of infection.

## Results

Symptoms of IC/PBS may worsen for 2 to 3 weeks after a hydrodistention. Approximately 40% to 50% of IC/PBS patients undergoing a hydrodistention will have prolonged symptom improvement. If symptoms improve significantly for at least 4 to 6 months, repeat bladder hydrodistention may be indicated. Fulguration of Hunner ulcers improves symptoms in over 80% of patients undergoing this therapy. The improvement in pain is usually seen in the first 2 to 3 days and may be long-lasting. For those who relapse, repeat fulguration of ulcers usually yields a similar response.

The more aggressive, open surgical approaches have shown good results in carefully selected patients. Relief of symptoms in patients undergoing reconstructive surgery ranges between 60% and 90%. Patients with ulcerative disease have been reported to have better results. Although a significant percentage of this highly select group of patients who undergo cystectomy will experience significant relief, there are reports of patients having persistent pelvic pain despite having no pelvic organs.

Recently, we reviewed our experience with sacral nerve modulation for refractory IC/PBS (27). When a traditional test was performed with a temporary lead, we had a test-to-implant rate of 52% versus a 94% test-to-implant rate in the staged approach. The benefit of the staged test is that the permanent lead is more programmable and can be tested for an extended period of time. If a response is found, the lead does not need to be removed prior to placing the generator, and the settings that worked on the temporary generator can be programmed into the permanent implanted neurostimulator so that there is no interruption in therapy. Twenty-six patients with refractory IC/PBS who had failed six previous treatments for their disease were implanted with a permanent generator. With a mean follow-up of 5.6 months, 96% of patients said they would undergo the implant again and would recommend the therapy to a friend. Significant improvements were seen in the number of day voids (47%) and nocturia (60%). The majority of patients reported at least a 50% improvement in frequency (72%), urgency (68%), pelvic pain (71%), pelvic pressure (67%), quality of life (76%), incontinence (69%), and vaginal pain (60%). No patients showed a >50% worsening in any symptom. The overall reoperation rate was 11.5% (3 of 26). An objective measurement of pain improvement was reported. Twenty IC/PBS patients with pelvic pain had a permanent implant placed with a median follow-up of 272 days. Seventeen of 20 (85%) used chronic narcotics prior to implant. Nineteen of 20 (95%) reported moderate or marked improvement in pain after implantation of a permanent generator. Morphine dose equivalents (MDEs) decreased from 86 mg per day to 56 mg per day (34%) ($p = 0.015$) after implant, and 24% stopped all narcotics.

In a recent prospective study, patients with symptoms of IC/PBS refractory to more conservative treatments were followed after having InterStim implanted. At 14 months follow-up, mean voided volume increased from 111 mL to 264 mL, mean daytime frequency decreased from 17.1 to 8.7, and mean nighttime voids decreased from 4.5 to 1.1. Additionally, pain and symptom scores, measured using the Interstitial Cystitis Symptom and Problem Indices, all improved. Overall, 16 of 17 patients who underwent permanent implantation (94%) had improvement in all parameters at their most recent postoperative visit (28).

## *References*


1. Hanno PM, Landis JR, Matthews-Cook Y, et al. The diagnosis of interstitial cystitis: lessons learned from the National Institutes of Health interstitial cystitis database study. *J Urol* 1999;161:553–557.
2. Hunner GL. A rare type of bladder ulcer in women: report of cases. *Boston Med Surg J* 1915;172:660–664.
3. Abrams P, Cardozo L, Fall M, et al. The standardisation of terminology in lower urinary tract function: report from the standardisation sub-committee of the International Continence Society. *Urology* 2003;61(1):37–49.
4. Ingber MS, Peters KM, Killinger KA, et al. Dilemmas in diagnosing pelvic pain: multiple pelvic surgeries common in women with interstitial cystitis. *Int Urogynecol J* 2008;19(3):341–345.
5. Gillespie LM. Interstitial cystitis and diet. In Sant GR, ed. *Interstitial cystitis.* Philadelphia: Lippincott–Raven Publishers, 1997:109–115.
6. Waxman JA, Sulak PJ, Kuehl TJ. Cystoscopic findings consistent with interstitial cystitis in normal women undergoing tubal ligation. *J Urol* 1998; 160(5):1663–1667.
7. Parsons CL. Potassium sensitivity test. *Techniques Urol* 1996;2:171–173.
8. Kuo HC. Urodynamic study and potassium sensitivity test for women with frequency-urgency syndrome and interstitial cystitis. *Urol Int* 2003;71(1): 61–65.
9. Gregoire M, Liandier F, Naud A, et al. Does the potassium stimulation test predict cystometric, cystoscopic outcome in interstitial cystitis? *J Urol* 2002; 168:556–557.
10. Rofeim O, Hom D, Freid RM, et al. Use of the neodymium:YAG laser for interstitial cystitis: a prospective study. *J Urol* 2001;166:134–136.
11. Neulander EZ, Rivera I, Eisenbrown N, et al. Simple cystectomy in patients requiring urinary diversion. *J Urol* 2000;164(4):1169–1172.
12. van Kerrebroeck PE, van Voskuilen AC, Heesakkers JP, et al. Results of sacral neuromodulation therapy for urinary voiding dysfunction: outcomes of a prospective, worldwide clinical study. *J Urol* 2007;178(5):2029–2034.
13. Chaiken DC, Blaivas JG, Blaivas ST. Behavioral therapy for the treatment of refractory interstitial cystitis. *J Urol* 1993;149(6):1445–1448.
14. Peters KM, Carrico DJ, Kalinowski SE, et al. Prevalence of pelvic floor dysfunction in patients with interstitial cystitis. *Urology* 2007;70(1): 16–18.
15. Sant GR, Propert KJ, Hanno PM, et al. Interstitial Cystitis Clinical Trials Group. A pilot clinical trial of oral pentosan polysulfate and oral hydroxyzine in patients with interstitial cystitis. *J Urol* 2003;170(3):816–817.
16. Pranikoff K, Constantino G. The use of amitriptyline in patients with urinary frequency and pain. *Urology* 1998;51[Suppl 5A]:179–181.
17. Rossberger J, Fall M, Peeker R. Critical appraisal of dimethyl sulfoxide treatment for interstitial cystitis: discomfort, side-effects and treatment outcome. *Scand J Urol Nephrol* 2005;39(1):73–77.
18. Greenberg E, Barnes R, Stewart S, et al. Transurethral resection of Hunner's ulcer. *J Urol* 1974;111(6):764–766.
19. Costello AJ, Crowe H, Agarwal D. Supratrigonal cystectomy and ileocystoplasty in management of interstitial cystitis. *Aust N Z J Surg* 2000; 70(1):34–38.
20. Light J, Vodusek D, Libby J. Inhibition of detrusor hyperreflexia by a selective electrical stimulation of the pudendal nerve. *J Urol* 1986;135:198.
21. Vodusek D, Light J, Libby J. Detrusor inhibition induced by stimulation of pudendal nerve afferents. *Neurourol Urodynam* 1986;5:381–389.
22. Peters KM, Feber KM, Bennett RC. A prospective, single-blind, randomized crossover trial of sacral vs pudendal nerve stimulation for interstitial cystitis. *BJU Int* 2007;100(4):835–839.

23. Van Balken M, Vandoninck V, Gisolf K, et al. Posterior tibial nerve stimulation as neuromodulative treatment of lower urinary tract dysfunction. *J Urol* 2001;166:914–982.
24. Vandoninck V, van Balken M, Finazzi A, et al. Posterior tibial nerve stimulation in the treatment of urge incontinence. *Neurourol Urodynam* 2003; 22:17–23.
25. Ingelmann-Sundberg A. Partial bladder denervation in the treatment of interstitial cystitis in women. In: Hanno PM, Staskin DR, Krane RJ, et al., eds. *Interstitial cystitis.* London: Springer-Verlag, 1990:189.
26. Hijaz A, Vasavada SP, Daneshgari F, et al. Complications and troubleshooting of two-stage sacral neuromodulation therapy: a single-institution experience. *Urology* 2006;68(3):533–537.
27. Peters KM, Carey JM, Karstardt DB. Sacral neuromodulation for the treatment of refractory interstitial cystitis: outcomes based on technique. *Int Urogynecol J* 2003;14:223–228.
28. Comiter CV. Sacral neuromodulation for the symptomatic treatment of refractory interstitial cystitis: a prospective study. *J Urol* 2003;169(4): 1369–1373.

# SECTION III ■ PROSTATE

RANDALL ROWLAND

# CHAPTER 24 ■ ANATOMY OF THE PROSTATE

SAM D. GRAHAM, JR.

The normal prostate is a firm, elastic organ located immediately below the bladder and resting on the superior layer of the urogenital diaphragm to which it is firmly attached. The normal adult prostate is approximately 4 cm in length and 4 to 5 cm in width. It is traversed throughout its length by the urethra and ejaculatory ducts entering at the base and terminating in the posterior prostatic urethra.

In the past the prostate has been divided into three to seven lobes. Most commonly, these segments are the two lateral lobes, a median lobe, a posterior lobe, and an anterior lobe. With the advent of ultrasound, the anatomy is now defined as a transition zone comprised of periurethral glands and a peripheral zone or true prostate. Anatomically, no true lobar anatomy exists, and the prostate has been shown to have the two concentric areas seen on ultrasound. The peripheral zone is mostly posteriorly located and is comprised of long, branched glands from which most carcinomas are thought to arrive. The central zone is comprised of submucosal glanduloductal units and short glands from which prostatic hypertrophy is thought to arise. Scattered throughout the prostate are smooth muscle fibers that are thought to be involved in ejaculation.

The prostate has a tough capsule of fibrous tissue and muscular elements that completely envelops the prostate and is densely adherent to it. This capsule is actually aglandular prostatic tissue that is connected to the acini and inseparable from the parenchyma. This is surrounded by a periprostatic fascia.

There are significant fascial investments around the prostate. The endopelvic fascia is a continuation of the endoabdominal fascia. In the pelvis, there are three parts of this fascial plane (1). The parietal layer covers the muscles lining the pelvic wall (piriformis and obturatorius internus) and continues superiorly to connect with the transversalis and iliopsoas fascias. All somatic nerves except for the obturator nerve are beneath this fascial layer. A thickening of this fascia extending from the pubis to the ischial spine is known as the arcus tendineus. The second portion of the endopelvic fascia (diaphragmatic portion) covers the two muscles on each side of the pelvis that make up the pelvis diaphragm (coccygeus and levator ani). A third (visceral) portion of the endopelvic fascia is continuous with the diaphragmatic fascia and extends upon the pelvic organs for a variable distance, blending into their fibrous coats. Anteriorly, the endopelvic fascia coalesces into the medial puboprostatic ligaments connecting the pubis to the prostatic capsule. The lateral puboprostatic ligaments extend from the superior diaphragmatic layer of the endopelvic fascia to the prostate.

Posteriorly, the prostate is invested by the two layers of Denonvilliers fascia, which embryologically is derived from the peritoneum. The posterior layer exists as the rectal fascia, while the anterior layer fuses laterally to the endopelvic and periprostatic fascia.

The urethra runs completely through the prostate, although the path is angled approximately 45 degrees at the verumontanum. The verumontanum represents the terminal end of the ejaculatory ducts as they course through the prostate from the seminal vesicles/vas deferens (Fig. 24.1). The opening in the apex of the verumontanum is known as the prostatic utricle. In addition, there are a series of ductal openings directly into the prostatic urethra from the prostatic glands. The urethra exits the prostate at the apex, and although the anatomical drawings traditionally show the apex directly on the pelvic floor, dissections during radical prostatectomies show that there is approximately a 1-cm gap from the apex to the pelvic floor.

## VASCULAR ANATOMY

The prostatic blood supply comes predominantly from the internal iliac artery and is a series of lateral pedicles, the most prominent and constant of which is the pedicle at the base of the prostate (superior prostatic artery). Additional branches may also exist, usually at the apex of the prostate (Fig. 24.2). The superior prostatic artery enters just below the bladder neck and forms two branches, one to the capsule and the other to the urethra. As patients age, the latter becomes more prominent with prostatic enlargement (2). Other sites of origin for the prostatic artery are the internal pudendal, the superior vesical, or the obturator artery.

The past 20 years have emphasized the "nerve-sparing" technique for both prostatectomy and cystectomy. This operation is actually a neurovascular-sparing technique that involves separating the neurovascular bundle from the prostate. The neurovascular bundle can be located along the posterior lateral prostate at the base of the prostate beneath the anterior layer of Denonvilliers fascia. More distally, the neurovascular bundle crosses the apex of the prostate and enters the pelvic diaphragm posterolaterally to the membranous urethra.

The venous drainage of the prostate is via the anterior venous plexus (Santorini), which is found on the anterior and lateral prostate. This plexus receives blood from the dorsal vein of the penis and empties into the hypogastric vein.

## LYMPHATIC ANATOMY

The lymphatic drainage of the prostate is predominantly along the path of the prostatic artery, with the primary nodal drop site being the obturator nodes. Other potential sites of nodal metastases include the external iliac and presacral nodes.

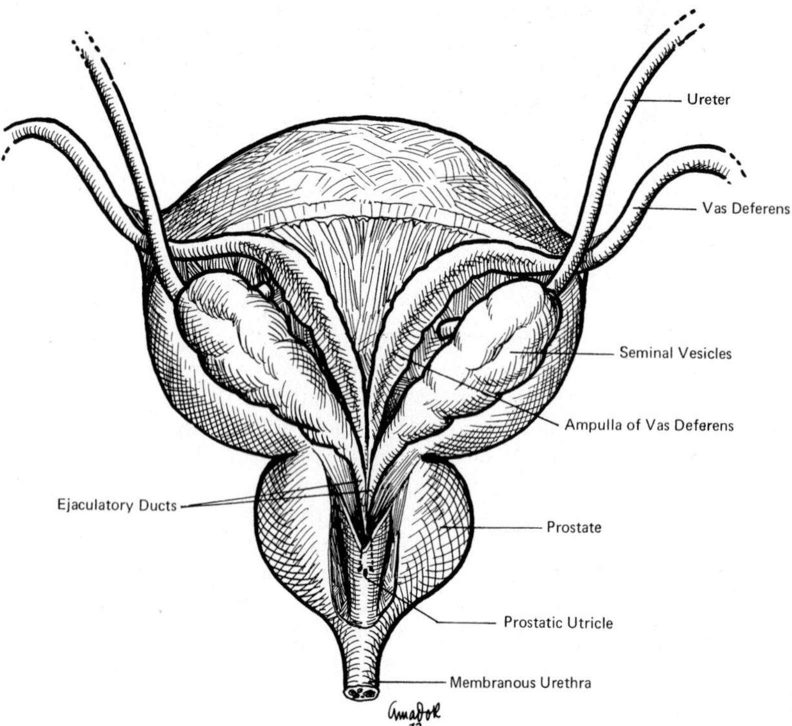


FIGURE 24.1 Relationship of the prostate and the seminal vesicles.

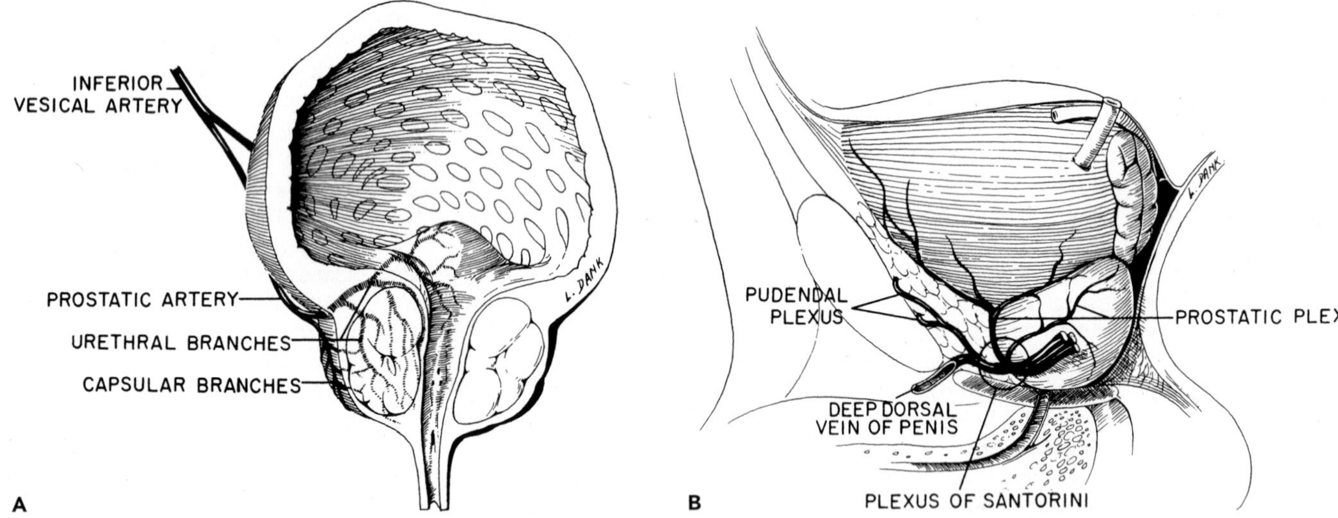


FIGURE 24.2 Vascular anatomy of the prostate. **A:** Arterial anatomy. **B:** Venous anatomy.

## NEUROANATOMY

The prostate has sympathetic, parasympathetic, and somatic innervation. The sympathetic innervation is from L1 and L2 via the superior hypogastric plexus. The parasympathetic and somatic innervation is from S2,3,4 via the inferior hypogastric plexus and pudendal nerves, respectively.

## CONTIGUOUS STRUCTURES

The prostate is inferior to the bladder and anterior to the rectum (Fig. 24.3). The perineal anatomy is a complex of muscles and tendons that comprise the pelvic floor, beginning from the skin of the perineum, the superficial (Camper) fascia and the deep (Colle) fascia. The latter is attached to the ischiopubic rami and the border of the urogenital diaphragm and is continuous with the Scarpa fascia. The most superficial pelvic musculature includes the ischiocavernosus, the bulbocavernosus, the superficial transverse perineal muscles, and the external anal sphincter (Fig. 24.4). These muscles are united in the midline as a central tendon (perineal body) and function as a single muscle. This central tendon is attached to the bulb of the rectum by fibrous bands of muscle known as the rectus urethralis (3). Beneath this layer of muscles is the deep perineal compartment that is predominantly the urogenital diaphragm, which is attached to the inferior rami of the ischia and pubis.

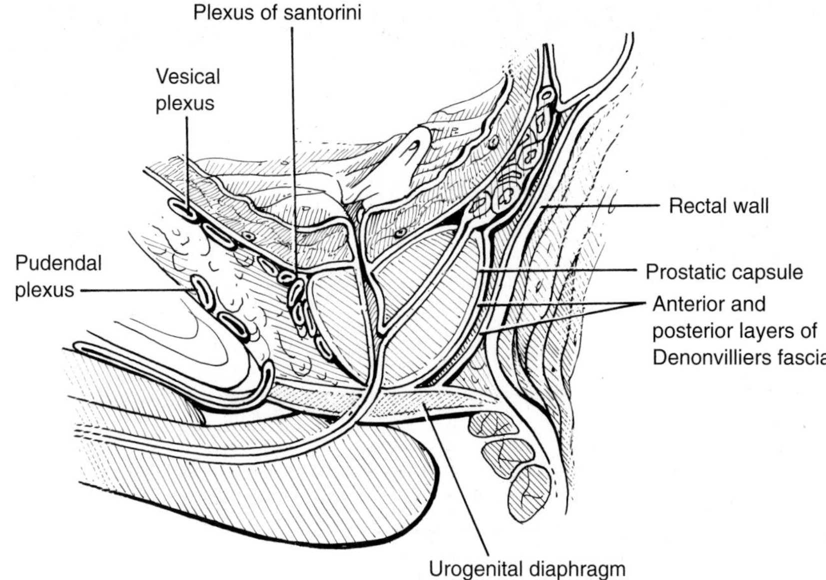


FIGURE 24.3 Relation of prostate to surrounding structures.

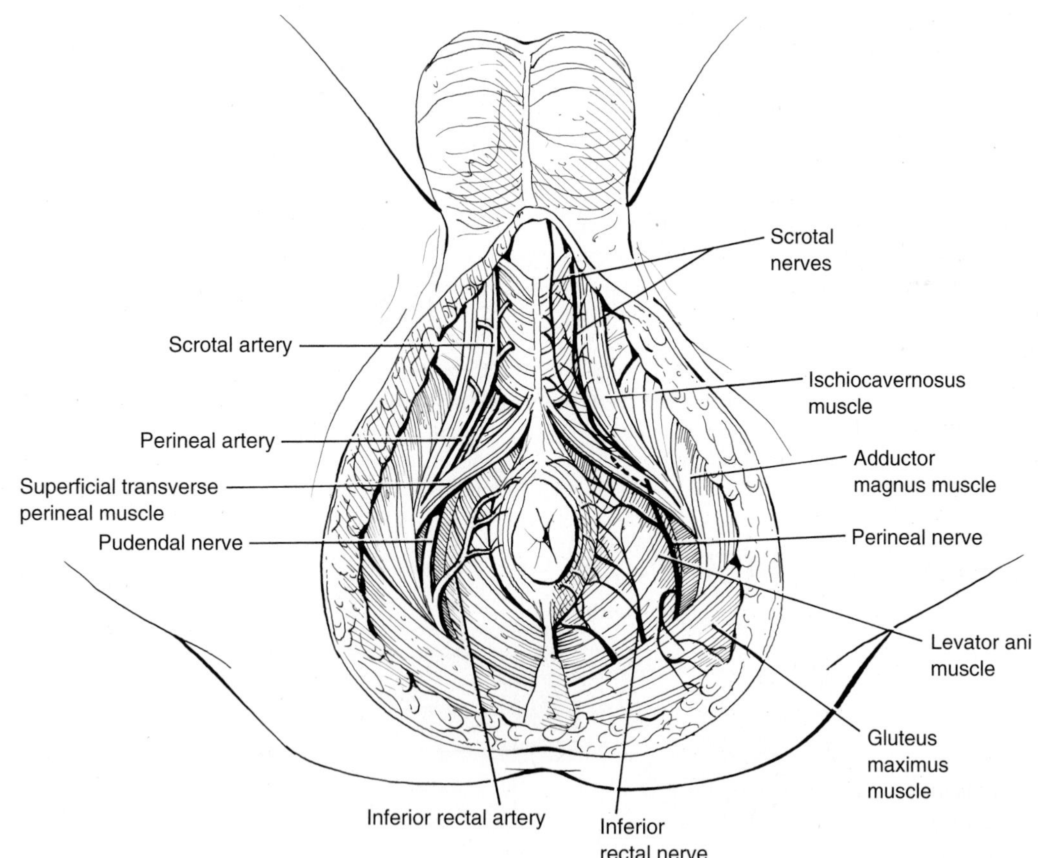


FIGURE 24.4 Pelvic nerves and musculature.

## *References*

1. Healey JE. *A synopsis of clinical anatomy.* Philadelphia: WB Saunders, 1969.
2. Brendler H. Prostatic hypertrophy and perineal surgery. In: Glenn JF, ed. *Urologic surgery*. Hagerstown, MD: Harper & Row, 1975.
3. Weyrauch HM. *Surgery of the prostate.* Philadelphia: WB Saunders, 1959.

# CHAPTER 25 ■ SURGERY FOR BENIGN PROSTATIC HYPERTROPHY

BRIAN R. MATLAGA AND JAMES E. LINGEMAN

The prevalence of benign prostatic hypertrophy (BPH) is an age-dependent phenomenon; by 60 years of age its prevalence is >50%, and by age 85 it has been reported to be as high as 90% (1). The natural history of BPH is generally considered to be one of progression, with mild symptoms becoming increasingly more bothersome over time. It has been reported that among 50-year-old men the lifetime incidence of surgical or medical intervention for BPH may be as high as 35% (1). Wasson et al. found that in a 3-year, multicenter, randomized controlled trial comparing men with moderate symptoms of BPH treated by either watchful waiting or transurethral resection of the prostate (TURP), 24% of men in the watchful waiting arm underwent surgical intervention (2).

A century ago, open suprapubic prostatectomy was considered the standard treatment of men with severe symptoms of BPH requiring removal of the adenoma. Subsequently TURP was developed and became the first significant "minimally invasive surgical procedure." More recently, a number of alternative surgical therapies have been introduced to treat men with BPH, most prominently the laser-based therapies. The American Urologic Association (AUA) convened a clinical guidelines panel that, following a meta-analysis of the published literature, determined that for patients with significant lower-urinary-tract symptoms (LUTS) due to BPH, surgical intervention is an appropriate treatment and that selection of the surgical modality should be based upon the surgeon's experience, the patient's individual prostatic anatomy, and medical comorbidities (Fig. 25.1).

## DIAGNOSIS

The AUA guidelines on the management of BPH explicitly define the appropriate evaluation of patients with LUTS, and the following recommendations are based on the meta-analytic data presented in these guidelines (Table 25.1) (3). A validated questionnaire, such as the AUA Symptom Index or the International Prostate Symptom Score (IPSS), will better quantify the effect of patients' LUTS on their quality of life.

All patients should undergo a screening urinalysis, and serum prostate specific antigen (PSA) should be measured as a screening for prostate cancer. Urinary flow-rate measures and quantification of postvoid residual urine may provide additional data, particularly for those patients with a complex medical history or those undergoing surgical therapy. A cystoscopy or transrectal ultrasound is not mandatory before a surgical treatment, but both can provide valuable information for preoperative planning.

## INDICATIONS FOR SURGERY

There are certain absolute indications for surgical treatment of BPH (Table 25.2). Typically, however, the management of patients depends on the degree of inconvenience they experience from their LUTS. The AUA clinical guidelines on BPH recommend that men who experience nonbothersome symptoms

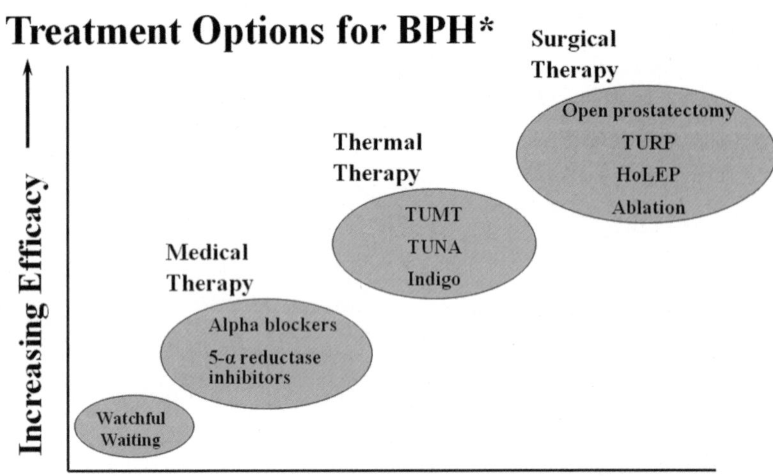


FIGURE 25.1 Treatment options for patients with BPH, as plotted with regards to increasing invasiveness and increasing efficacy.

**TABLE 25.1**

INITIAL EVALUATION OF MEN WITH LUTS

- AUA Symptom Index Questionnaire
- Medical history
  - Other causes of voiding dysfunction
  - Medical comorbidities
- Physical examination
  - Digital rectal examination
- Laboratory studies
- Urinalysis
- Serum PSA
- Diagnostic studies
  - Urinary flow rate
  - Postvoid residual urine volume
  - Cystoscopy
  - Transrectal ultrasound for prostate volume

**TABLE 25.2**

INDICATIONS FOR TREATMENT OF BPH

- Refractory urinary retention
- Persistent gross hematuria
- Bladder calculi
- Recurrent urinary tract infections
- Renal insufficiency
- Moderate or severe LUTS

of BPH should not be managed surgically. Patients with bothersome symptoms should undergo treatment, and the physician should review the benefits and risks of all approaches and interventions with the patient.

# ALTERNATIVE THERAPY

There are a number of alternative therapies besides surgery for BPH (Table 25.3).

## Watchful Waiting

Some patients experience certain mild symptoms related to BPH. For such patients, the risks may outweigh the benefits they may achieve from the therapy. With watchful waiting, patients are monitored by their urologist but do not receive any active treatment. Such patients are examined on a regular basis to monitor for progression of symptoms, when a more active intervention can be discussed.

## Medical Therapy

There are two main medical therapies for patients with symptoms of BPH: alpha-adrenergic blockers and 5 alpha reductase inhibitors. These therapies can be administered alone or in combination. Alpha blocker therapy is based on the

**TABLE 25.3**

TREATMENT OPTIONS FOR PATIENTS WITH SYMPTOMS OF BPH

- Watchful waiting
- Medical therapy
  - Alpha-adrenergic blockers
  - 5 alpha reductase inhibitors
  - Combination therapy
- Minimally invasive therapies
  - Transurethral microwave treatment
  - Transurethral needle ablation
- Surgical therapies
  - Transurethral resection of the prostate (TURP)
  - Transurethral incision of the prostate (TUIP)
  - Holmium laser enucleation of the prostate (HoLEP)
  - Laser ablation: holmium:YAG or potassium titanyl phosphate (KTP)
  - Open prostatectomy: suprapubic or retropubic

hypothesis that the symptoms of BPH are potentiated by the alpha-adrenergic–mediated contraction of prostatic smooth muscle. Five alpha reductase inhibitors block the conversion of testosterone to dihydrotestosterone, which can reduce prostate size and BPH symptoms. Both therapies have been studied extensively, and they may be most appropriately used for patients who experience mild inconvenience related to the symptoms of BPH.

## Minimally Invasive Therapy

These therapies typically are available for the treatment of patients with symptomatically bothersome BPH. Many of these minimally invasive treatments rely on the administration of high temperatures to produce coagulation necrosis of the prostate tissue. Ultimately, the goal of such hyperthermic treatment is to enlarge the prostatic fossa, similar to a surgical debulking but without the morbidity of surgery. Transurethral microwave thermotherapy (TUMT) is likely more effective than medical therapy in reducing patients' LUTS, but it is likely less effective than surgical therapy.

Transurethral needle ablation (TUNA) also affects prostate tissue by a thermal mechanism, but with this intervention heat is delivered via radiofrequency energy. A TUNA procedure involves cystoscopically placing two needles directly into the prostate by piercing the urethra and then administering radiofrequency energy that heats the prostate tissue to 100°C. As with microwave therapy devices, TUNA induces a coagulative necrosis effect. The efficacy of TUNA is comparable to that of microwave thermotherapy.

## Surgical Techniques

### Transurethral Incision of the Prostate (TUIP) and Transurethral Resection of the Prostate (TURP)

The patient is placed in a dorsal lithotomy position, with the thighs abducted to allow manipulation of the resectoscope. After sterile preparation and draping is completed, the patient's urethra is calibrated using van Buren sounds up to 30Fr. It is only necessary to calibrate the anterior urethra; excessive manipulation of the prostatic urethra may result in bleeding, which can make visualization difficult. Proper calibration is essential to reduce the risk of subsequent urethral stricture caused by the resectoscope manipulation. A 26Fr or 28Fr resectoscope is then inserted into the urethra. A 3% glycine or sorbitol solution is used for irrigation, at gravity pressure. Cutting and coagulation currents should be adjusted to the appropriate levels for the electrical generator used for the case.

If the prostate volume is small (20 g or less), the lateral lobes of the prostate are not coapting, and there is a high bladder neck or median bar present, it may be appropriate to proceed with a transurethral incision of the prostate (TUIP). The bladder should be filled via the continuous-flow resectoscope, and with a TUIP-type electrocautery knife, incisions should be created at the 5:00 and 7:00 positions. The incisions should be deepened until the capsule of the prostate is reached, and they should also be extended to just proximal to the verumontanum.

If the prostate is >20 g, or if there is a median lobe or the lateral lobes are coapting, a TURP is the more appropriate procedure to perform (Table 25.4). TURP is performed with an electrocautery loop and glycine or sorbitol irrigation. However, bipolar TURP devices have been developed that permit the resection of prostate tissue in a saline irrigant. A procedural difference between the two approaches is that when the bipolar device is used, the speed with which the loop is withdrawn through the tissue should be much slower than with the standard TURP electrocautery loop. If there is a median lobe present, resection should initially begin with this structure. In a stepwise fashion, the lobe is resected with the electrocautery loop. Resection of the median lobe is complete when bladder neck fibers are visualized. Particularly during the resection of the median lobe, care should be taken to not involve the ureteral orifices in the resection.

Following complete resection of the median lobe of the prostate, attention can be turned to resection of the lateral lobes. First, the right lobe is resected, starting at the 7:00 position, and proceeding from the bladder neck to a point just proximal to the verumontanum. Resection should be carried down to the fibers of the bladder neck and prostatic capsule. The left lobe of the prostate can be resected in a similar fashion. The surgeon should take care not to resect too deeply and perforate the capsule, as well as not to resect beyond (distal to) the verumontanum.

Following complete resection of the lateral lobes, the anterior tissue of the prostate should be inspected. If obstructing tissue is present at this location, it may be resected. The Ellik evacuator can then be used to remove the resected tissue fragments, which may be sent for pathologic analysis. The prostatic fossa should be reinspected, as oftentimes open blood vessels may become more apparent following Ellik evacuation. Hemostasis should be ensured, and a three-way Foley catheter should be placed. Continuous bladder irrigation with saline is generally necessary overnight; if bleeding persists, the Foley catheter may be placed on traction.

## Holmium Laser Enucleation of the Prostate (HoLEP)

The patient is positioned as for a TURP. A 26Fr or 28Fr resectoscope is then inserted into the urethra. The inner sheath of the resectoscope should be specially configured with a purpose-built laser bridge or laser-stabilizing catheter to minimize vibration of the laser fiber during the procedure. The 550-μm end-fire laser fiber is placed through the laser bridge or laser-stabilizing catheter. Normal saline irrigant is used during the procedure, and the resectoscope should be configured to continuous gravity flow.

Once the resectoscope has been passed via the urethra into the bladder, the ureteral orifices should be identified. The verumontanum and the external urinary sphincter should be identified and their location confirmed. If there is a significantly enlarged median lobe, it is often most expeditious to enucleate this structure first, as this maneuver will provide more room to accomplish the lateral lobe dissection (Table 25.5). To enucleate the median lobe, the holmium laser should be set at an energy of 2 J and a frequency of 50 Hz. Two sulci will be

**TABLE 25.4**

**TRANSURETHRAL INCISION OR RESECTION OF THE PROSTATE**

- Assessment of prostate
- TUIP if:
  - Prostate volume <20 cc, high bladder neck, no lateral lobe hypertrophy
  - Incisions at 5:00 position, from bladder neck to verumontanum
  - Deepen to level of prostate capsule
- TURP if:
  - Prostate volume >20 cc, coapting lateral lobes, median lobe
  - Resect median lobe, if present, first
  - If no median lobe, create groove in 6:00 position
  - Resect to bladder neck and capsular fibers
  - Resect lateral lobes in stepwise fashion, from bladder neck to verumontanum
  - Resect anterior tissue if present

**TABLE 25.5**

**HOLMIUM LASER ENUCLEATION OF PROSTATE**

- If median lobe present:
  - Create grooves in 5:00 and 7:00 positions
  - Carry down to surgical capsule
  - Join grooves just proximal to verumontanum
  - Enucleate median lobe in retrograde fashion
- Lateral lobe dissection begins just lateral to verumontanum
- Develop plane under lateral lobe, on floor of capsule
- Dissection moves anteriorly, proceeding from apex to bladder neck
- Make incision at 12:00 position
- Join anterior and lateral dissections
- Divide remaining mucosal attachments
- Once both lobes are completely enucleated, morcellation can proceed
  - Take care to always keep morcellator tip in view

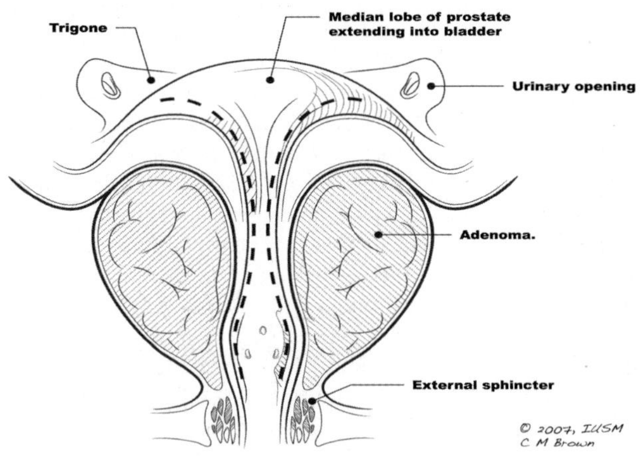


FIGURE 25.2 Cartoon representation of the architecture of the prostate and bladder neck. Dashed lines represent the 5:00 and 7:00 grooves.

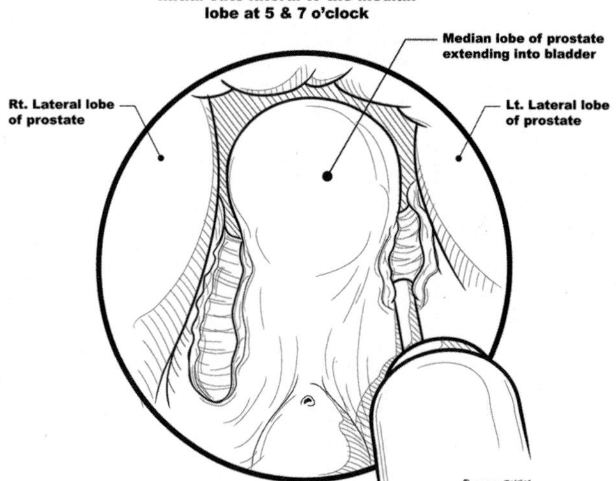


FIGURE 25.4 The 7:00 incision is subsequently developed, which isolates the median lobe.

visualized, one at the 5:00 position and the other at the 7:00 position (Fig. 25.2). Beginning at the level of the bladder neck in the 5:00 position, a groove is cut with the laser along the sulcus, from the bladder neck to a point proximal to the verumontanum (Fig. 25.3). This groove is deepened to the level of the surgical capsule. As the groove is developed, it should be undermined and widened to permit the separation of the right lateral lobe and median lobe. Once accomplished, the process should be repeated at the 7:00 position (Fig. 25.4). The final step in the enucleation of the median lobe can then be initiated at a point just prior to the verumontanum. The laser fiber is moved in a transverse fashion between the apical extent of the 5:00 and 7:00 grooves. As the distal portion of the median lobe begins to separate away from the capsule, the beak of the resectoscope should be used as a leverage point to assist in lifting the median lobe upward. The capsule will begin to slope anteriorly toward the bladder neck; careful attention to this anatomy is important, as it will prevent inadvertent undermining of the trigone. Once the dissection has reached the level of the bladder neck, the most proximal attachments of the median lobe can be divided and the entire median lobe pushed into the bladder.

Following enucleation of the median lobe, attention can be turned to the lateral lobes. If a median lobe was not present, an incision should be created at the 6:00 position, and this midline groove should extend from the bladder neck to a point just proximal to the verumontanum (Fig. 25.5). Dissection of the right lobe is initiated by incising the mucosa lateral to the verumontanum in a transverse fashion, thereby exposing the adenoma near the apex. Once the initial plane is developed under the right lobe, dissection should proceed proximally toward the bladder neck, freeing the lateral lobe from the capsular floor by moving the laser fiber in a transverse, side-to-side motion; simultaneously, the beak of the resectoscope can advance this effort by applying upward traction on the adenoma. Care should be taken not to maneuver the resectoscope into the adenoma, which will disorient the surgeon and lose the plane of enucleation.

At some point, it will become apparent that the lateral attachments of the lobe impede dissection. At this point, the surgeon should detach the lateralmost aspect of the right lobe, near the apex. During the apical dissection, the laser frequency should be changed to 40 Hz to prevent thermal injury of the

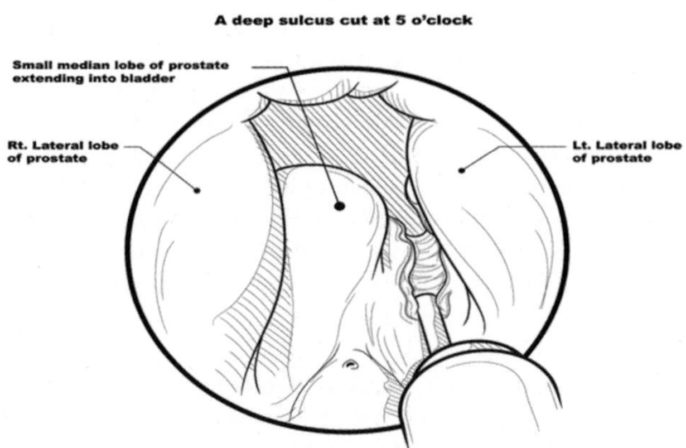


FIGURE 25.3 The 5:00 incision is created with the end-fire holmium laser fiber.

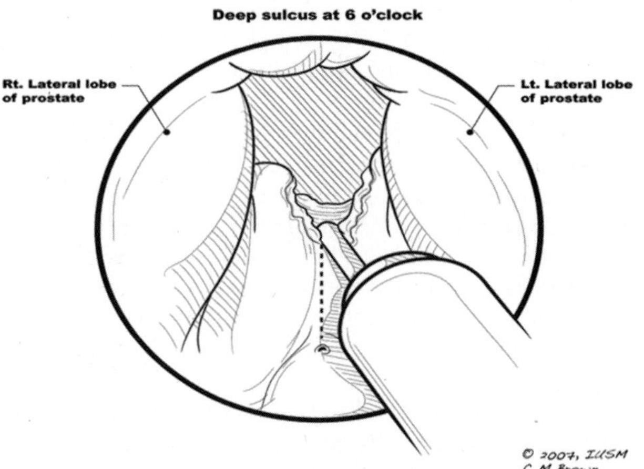


FIGURE 25.5 When no median lobe is present, a groove is created in the 6:00 position.

urinary sphincter. The surgeon should continue to dissect in this plane, staying between the apical tissue of the right lobe and the capsule by rotating the resectoscope in a clockwise direction. The lateral dissection should proceed anteriorly, and the lateral wall of the right lobe will be freed from the surgical capsule by proceeding proximally along the already defined plane. At this point, the surgeon should be rotating the resectoscope in alternating clockwise and counterclockwise directions, which causes the tip of the laser fiber to proceed in a smooth arc back and forth within the established plane. The dissection should be continued until difficulty is encountered with exposure of the plane proximally.

Attention should then be turned to the 12:00 region of the prostatic fossa, where the midline groove between the lateral lobes is located. The resectoscope is turned 180 degrees to allow the laser fiber to be positioned at the 12:00 position. The laser frequency should be readjusted to 50 Hz. Beginning at the bladder neck and proceeding distally, a groove is cut along this anterior position and should span from the bladder neck to the level of the verumontanum. The surgeon should occasionally reconfirm the location of the verumontanum by looking toward the floor to ensure that the groove is not extended too far distally. Once the groove is created, it is again widened and deepened to the level of the surgical capsule along its entire extent. The right lobe should then be enucleated from the anterior aspect of the capsule by angling the tip of the laser fiber between the adenoma and the capsule. Capsular definition is often much easier at the bladder neck, so dissection should begin at that point. The attachments between the anterior portion of the lobe and the capsule are taken down sequentially until the lateral extent of the lobe is reached. It is crucial at this stage to identify the extent of the remaining lateral attachments near the apex of the lobe. Once the junction between the planes is defined, usually by a mucosal strip or bridge, it is cut by the laser to join the planes. Laser settings are 2 J and 20 Hz during division of the mucosal strip. The surgeon can then continue the dissection proximally, at 2 J and 50 Hz, to free the lateral extent of the lobe.

At this point, the right lobe will be held only by attachments at the bladder neck level. By following this plane further laterally, any remaining attachments in this area can be freed. Finally, one should proceed under the lobe and finish dividing attachments at the floor of the capsule and the posterior bladder neck. The lobe can then be pushed into the bladder by leveraging upward with the beak of the resectoscope. With complete enucleation of the right lobe, attention should be turned to the left lobe, which is enucleated as previously described.

Once all lobes have been dissected free and pushed into the bladder, the capsular surface is then inspected carefully, and any bleeding sites should be addressed by defocusing the laser (positioning the tip of the fiber 2 to 3 mm away from the surface). A dry fossa is essential before beginning morcellation to optimize visualization and minimize the risk of bladder injury. If any residual portions of adenoma remain along the surface of the capsule, these can be easily vaporized or enucleated with the laser.

The final aspect of HoLEP is to remove the enucleated adenoma by morcellation. The inner sheath of the resectoscope, along with the laser fiber and stabilizing catheter, is removed, and the rigid offset nephroscope is then inserted into the outer resectoscope sheath. A commercially available morcellator, which is a set of hollow reciprocating blades attached to a handle apparatus, can be used for this portion of the procedure. Under direct visualization, the tip of the morcellator is inserted into the bladder and guided beneath a portion of adenoma. Once a portion of adenoma is engaged by the morcellator, it is important to keep the tip of the morcellator anteriorly within the bladder and within the visual field at all times. The morcellator shaft should be moved in and out of the working channel in small increments and rotated at times to optimize engagement of tissue. When the remaining tissue pieces are small, the surgeon should engage them with suction alone and pull them into the prostatic fossa, where morcellation can be done safely by pinning the tissue against the capsule. If difficulty is encountered in engaging these smaller pieces, an alligator forceps can be used to facilitate their removal. Lastly, an Ellik evacuator is utilized to remove any remaining pieces of adenoma or clot. A 20Fr, three-way Foley catheter is placed at the conclusion of the case with the aid of a catheter guide, and continuous bladder irrigation can be used if necessary.

## Laser Ablation of the Prostate: Holmium (Ho:YAG) and Potassium Titanyl Phosphate (KTP)

Laser ablation of the prostate employs laser energy to vaporize prostate tissue through the generation of temperatures >100°C. There are two lasers that are commonly used to ablate the prostate: the KTP laser and the Ho:YAG laser. The KTP laser is an 80-W system that generates laser energy at a wavelength of 532 nm. The laser energy of the KTP laser is preferentially absorbed by the hemoglobin pigment. The Ho:YAG laser is a 100-W system that generates laser energy at a wavelength of 2,140 nm. The holmium laser energy is preferentially absorbed by water. Despite the different inherent attributes of the laser energy sources, the fundamental techniques of laser ablation are the same for both laser types. One of the inherent limitations of all laser approaches is that laser energy will desiccate the prostate tissue, ultimately impairing the tissue ablation as the procedure proceeds. With smaller glands, this may not be a meaningful issue; however, with larger glands, tissue desiccation will impede the ablation procedure.

A side-firing laser fiber is used, with a 26Fr or 28Fr continuous-flow resectoscope configured with a laser bridge. Saline is the irrigation of choice. The resectoscope is passed into the bladder, and the locations of the ureteral orifices and verumontanum are confirmed. Laser ablation is a near contact procedure, meaning that the laser fiber should be maintained 1 to 2 mm away from the prostate tissue. The aiming beam and the side-markings of the fiber should be identified. If a median lobe is present, this structure should be addressed first. The laser fiber is placed in close approximation to the median lobe tissue, and a rotating lateral motion of the laser fiber is performed while activating the laser energy. The tissue should be vaporized in layers, with a sagittal motion of the fiber, taking care to not vaporize the trigone or ureteral orifice. If a median lobe is not present, the laser should be positioned at the bladder neck in the 7:00 position, and the tissue should be ablated with a lateral sweeping motion until the fibers of the bladder neck are visualized (Table 25.6). A groove should then be extended from the bladder neck to a point just proximal to the verumontanum. The groove should be deepened until capsular fibers are seen. A similar groove

**TABLE 25.6**

LASER ABLATION OF THE PROSTATE

- Troughs created at the 5:00 and 7:00 positions
- Direct ablation of lateral lobes
- Carried to depth of capsular fibers
- Tissue ablation moves anteriorly, proceeding from bladder neck to apex
  - To coagulate bleeding vessels, laser is defocused 2 to 3 mm away from tissue surface

should be created in the 5:00 position, and then the tissue between the grooves should be ablated.

Returning to the 5:00 position, the tissue from this location up to the 1:00 position should then be ablated with a slow, continuous sweeping motion. Again, the laser should be maintained near the tissue but not buried into the tissue. Once the lobe is ablated, the contralateral lobe from the 7:00 position to the 11:00 position should be ablated in the same fashion. Bleeding vessels, most commonly encountered at the 5:00 and 7:00 positions, can be coagulated by defocusing the laser 2 to 3 mm away from the tissue. Following ablation of the prostate tissue and assurance of hemostasis, a Foley catheter should be placed. In general, bleeding is not significant, and continuous bladder irrigation should not be required.

### Suprapubic Prostatectomy

The patient is placed in a supine position, and the lower abdomen and genitalia are prepared and draped as a surgical field. A Foley catheter is placed on the surgical field and secured into position. The initial approach is through a low midline incision, and the fascia should be opened from the umbilicus to the symphysis pubica (Table 25.7). The space

**TABLE 25.7**

OPEN SURGICAL PROSTATECTOMY

- Low midline incision
- Suprapubic
  - Cystotomy created
  - Ureteral orifices identified
  - Incision at posterior aspect of intravesical component of prostate
  - Adenoma freed from capsule with blunt digital dissection
  - Following complete removal of adenoma, bleeding vessels controlled
    - Sutures at 5:00 and 7:00 positions
  - Foley catheter and suprapubic tube, in addition to perivesical drain
- Retropubic
  - Ligation of superficial prostate capsular vessels
  - Transverse incision in midcapsule
  - Adenoma bluntly dissected away from capsule and extracted through capsulotomy
  - Hemostasis ensured, sutures placed at 5:00 and 7:00 positions
  - Foley catheter and periprostatic drain placed

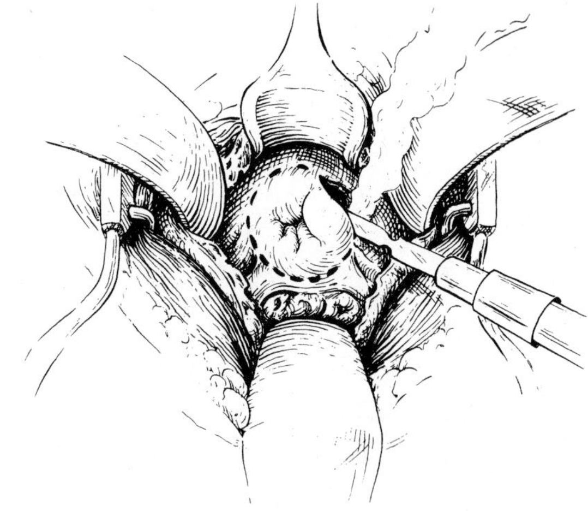

FIGURE 25.6 Incision of mucosa over the adenoma.

of Retzius is entered, perivesical fat identified, and a self-retaining retractor positioned. The bladder should be identified and cleaned of the perivesical fatty tissue. The bladder should be filled to capacity by gravity. Stay sutures should be positioned in the detrusor just to the left and right of midline, and a vertical incision in the bladder should then be created with electrocautery.

After opening the bladder, the intravesical component of the prostate should be identified. The ureteral orifices should be located, and to facilitate identification as the procedure progresses they may be cannulated with 5Fr feeding tubes. To begin the enucleation process, an incision in the posterior aspect of the intravesical component of the prostate is made with electrocautery (Fig. 25.6). Care should be taken to ensure that the incision is safely away from the ureteral orifices and trigonal region. The capsule should be sharply freed from the adenoma, and the surgeon's finger can then be used to develop the space between the adenoma and the capsule (Fig. 25.7). By moving the finger in a lateral arc, this plane is extended down to the apical aspect of the prostate. Once the adenoma is completely freed from its attachments by this blunt dissection technique, it may be removed from the surgical field (Fig. 25.8). The prostatic fascia should be packed with sponges and pressure held for 5 minutes to aid in hemostasis. Absorbable sutures, of a 2-0 size, should be placed in a figure-of-eight

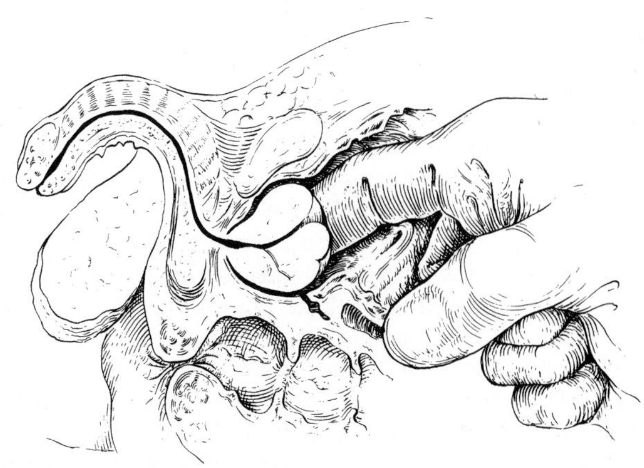

FIGURE 25.7 Digital enucleation of the adenoma.

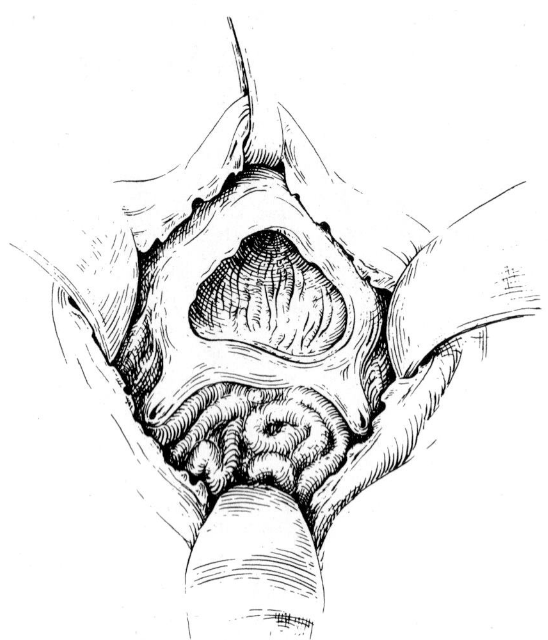

FIGURE 25.8 View of the empty prostatic fossa.

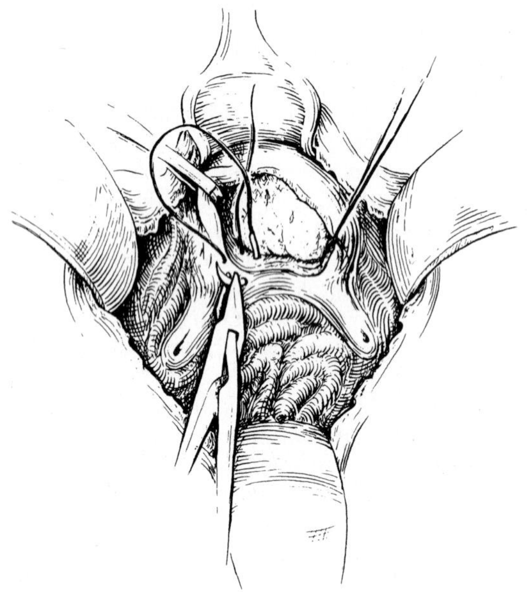

FIGURE 25.9 Hemostatic suture ligatures at the 5:00 and 7:00 positions.

fashion at the 5:00 and 7:00 positions to control any blood vessels, which are commonly encountered at these locations (Fig. 25.9). A 22Fr Foley catheter, with a 30-cc balloon, should be placed transurethrally (Fig. 25.10).

The bladder should be closed in two layers with running 3-0 and 2-0 monofilament absorbable suture. A suprapubic tube should be placed through the dome of the bladder, and the bladder closed around this tube in a pursestring fashion. A Penrose or Blake closed suction drain is then placed in the space of Retzius. The fascia is then reapproximated with no. 1 braided absorbable suture, and the skin is reapproximated with staples. The drains are sutured into place with 0 silk suture. A continuous bladder setup using the suprapubic tube

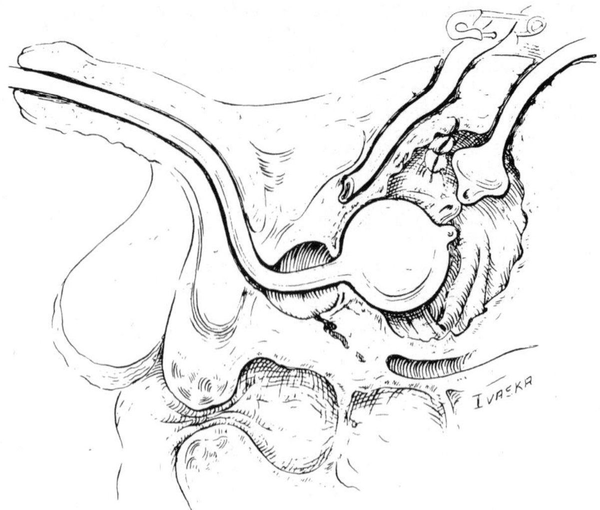


FIGURE 25.10 Foley catheter snug at the bladder neck: prevesical drain and suprapubic tube.

and the Foley catheter may be of help in maintaining patent drainage and minimizing blood clot formation.

## Retropubic Prostatectomy

The patient is placed in a supine position, and the lower abdomen and genitalia are prepared and draped as a surgical field. A Foley catheter is placed on the surgical field and secured into position. The initial approach is through a low midline incision, and the fascia should be opened from the umbilicus to the symphysis pubica. The space of Retzius is entered, perivesical fat identified, and a self-retaining retractor positioned. The fatty tissue overlying the bladder and prostatic capsule should be cleared.

At the midportion of the prostatic capsule, two 0 chromic sutures should be placed proximally and distally, to ligate the superficial blood vessels (Fig. 25.11). With electrocautery, an incision is created transversely between these two sutures

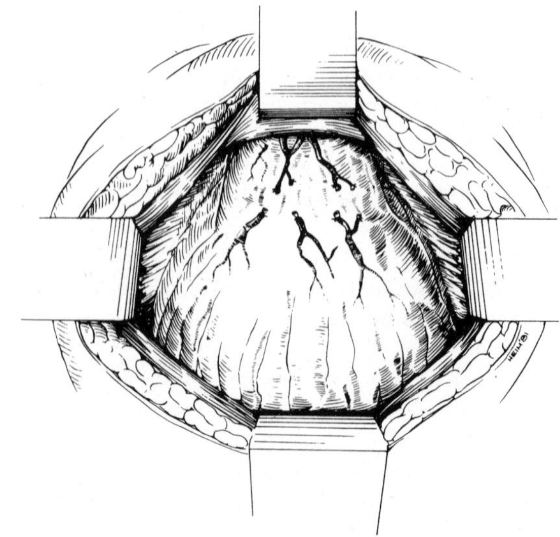

FIGURE 25.11 Ligation and division of periprostatic veins over the prostatic capsule anteriorly.

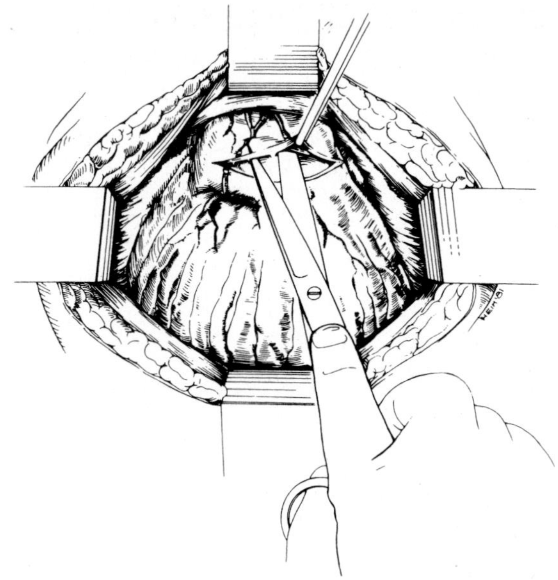

FIGURE 25.12 Transfixion sutures placed on the capsule anteriorly with an incision made transversely in the prostatic capsule.

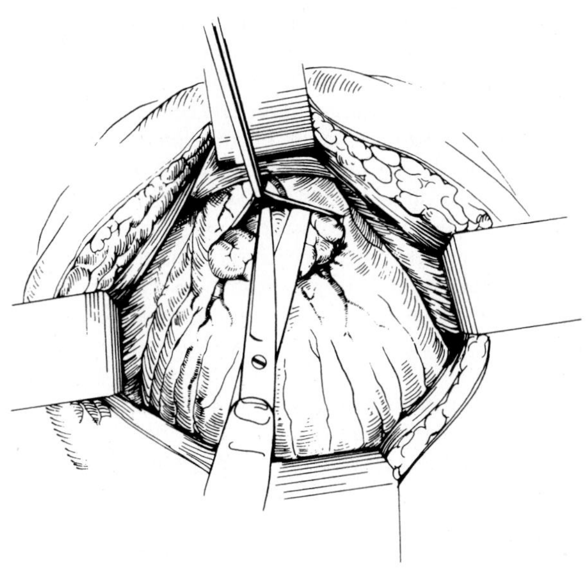

FIGURE 25.13 Continuing the dissection of the prostate of the adenoma from the prostatic capsule using Metzenbaum scissors.

(Fig. 25.12). A plane of dissection between the adenoma and the capsule should be bluntly created on either side of this incision (Fig. 25.13). The adenoma is progressively freed of its anterior, lateral, and posterior attachments with digital dissection. Following complete mobilization of the adenoma, its attachment to the membranous urethra can be sharply divided and the adenoma retrieved through the capsular incision; 2-0 chromic sutures should be placed in the 5:00 and 7:00 positions for hemostasis (Fig. 25.14). A 22Fr Foley catheter with a 30-cc balloon is placed, and the prostatic capsule is closed with 2-0 chromic sutures (Fig. 25.15). A closed suction drain is placed in the space of Retzius; the fascia should be reapproximated with no. 1 braided absorbable suture, and the skin should be reapproximated with staples.

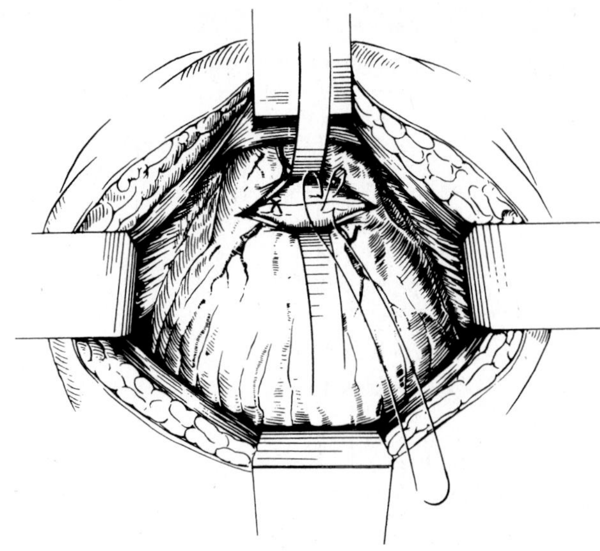

FIGURE 25.14 Figure-of-eight sutures are applied at the vesicle neck at the 5:00 and 7:00 positions to secure hemostasis.

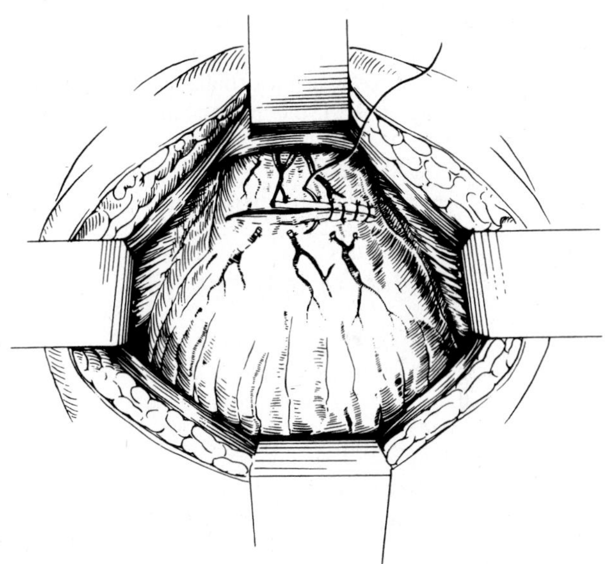

FIGURE 25.15 Closure of the incision of the prostate capsule anteriorly with interrupted chromic sutures.

## TREATMENT OUTCOMES

The ultimate assessment of the efficacy of a surgical treatment for BPH is a measure of its treatment outcome. The AUA Clinical Guidelines Panel on BPH assessed the literature on surgical therapies in order to define the treatment outcomes for particular interventions (3). TURP is considered by many to be the gold standard surgical therapy for men requiring surgical treatment of BPH. However, all surgical therapies have been reported to significantly improve patients' AUA Symptom Index; in fact, the greatest magnitude of improvement among patients undergoing surgical treatments was observed in those undergoing HoLEP (3). Similarly, all surgical therapies produced significant improvements in peak urinary flow rates; it was not possible to distinguish among the different therapies based on this outcome measure. Quality-of-life data, a measure

TABLE 25.8

PSA CHANGES FOLLOWING BPH TREATMENTS

| STUDY | TREATMENT (NUMBER OF PATIENTS) | MEAN PREOPERATIVE PSA (NG/DL) | MEAN POSTOPERATIVE PSA (NG/DL) | PERCENTAGE DECREASE IN PSA | MEAN TISSUE RESECTED (GRAMS) |
|---|---|---|---|---|---|
| Kuo, 2003 | HoLEP[a] (48) | 9.5 | 0.6 | 91.7 | 121 |
| Kim, 2004 | HoLEP[a] (10) | 6.2 | 0.9 | 85.5 | 118 |
| Ozden, 2003 | Open/TURP[b] (32) | 14.8 | 3.7 | 74.2 | N/A |
| Marks, 1996 | Open/TURP[b] (82) | 4.6 | 0.7 | 71.3 | 35 |
| Aus, 1996 | TURP[b] (190) | 6.0 | 1.9 | 69.7 | 33.5 |
| Stamey, 1987 | Open (7) | 24.1 | 1.0 | 95.6 | 88.9 |
| Stamey, 1987 | TURP[b] (73) | 7.9 | 1.3 | 83.5 | 29 |
| Te, 2006 | PVP[c] (139) | 3.5 | 2.9 | 17 | N/A |

[a]HoLEP, holmium laser enucleation of the prostate.
[b]TURP, transurethral resection of the prostate.
[c]PVP, photoselective vaporization of the prostate.

that is perhaps most important to the patient being treated, demonstrate equivalent improvements among all surgical technologies. All prostate interventions will have an effect on serum PSA. The more complete a debulking of the prostate, the greater the fall in PSA the patient should experience (Table 25.8) (4–10).

## COMPLICATIONS

### Endoscopic Surgery

One of the more common intraoperative complications for patients undergoing endoscopic surgical treatment of BPH is bleeding. Due to the continuous irrigation flow, it can often be difficult to estimate the magnitude of bleeding. When bleeding is appreciated, though, a systematic inspection of the prostatic fossa will permit identification of the source, which can then be fulgurated with cautery or coagulated with laser. If bleeding is refractory to these maneuvers, a Foley catheter placed on traction may be helpful.

Overaggressive resection may result in perforation of the prostatic capsule. Sequelae of this event may include extravasation of fluid into the retroperitoneum as well as electrolyte derangements. When a capsular perforation is encountered, it should be assessed. In the case of a small perforation, the procedure should be completed expeditiously. If a large perforation is identified, however, the procedure should be terminated. In the case of a retroperitoneal fluid collection, conservative management (catheter drainage and furosemide) is a reasonable approach, as the collections generally reabsorb spontaneously. If the perforation is extensive, however, transurethral resection (TUR) syndrome may occur, a condition brought about by intravascular absorption of hypotonic irrigating solutions, which ultimately induces a dilutional hyponatremia. Hypertension, mental confusion, and nausea and vomiting are all associated with this syndrome. TUR syndrome can be managed by diuresis and repletion with normal saline intravenous fluid or, in extreme circumstances, hypertonic (3%) saline in 100-cc boluses.

Structures in the vicinity of the prostate may be injured in the course of endoscopic surgical treatment. In some patients, the ureteral orifice may be close to the bladder neck and can be inadvertently ablated or resected. Should the ureteral orifice be injured, an attempt should be made to stent the ureter at the conclusion of the procedure. Stricture formation is the most concerning sequelae of this complication. The bladder neck may also be undermined, which can complicate the placement of a catheter at the conclusion of the procedure. In severe cases, the bladder and prostatic urethra can become completely dissociated. If the bladder neck is identified as being undermined, a Foley catheter should be placed with a catheter guide, or alternatively over a wire, to ensure proper placement.

Transient urinary incontinence or urinary retention may occur following an endoscopic prostate resection or ablation. These symptoms generally resolve in the weeks following the procedure. Permanent incontinence or retention following these procedures is exceedingly rare. All patients who undergo any of these previously described procedures will experience retrograde ejaculation and should be forewarned of this eventuality. Patients who are suffering from urinary retention prior to an intervention for BPH are at increased risk for postoperative complications (11).

### Open Surgery

Severe bleeding following open prostatectomy has been recorded to occur in up to 35% of patients; blood transfusion rates are similarly high. Urinary clot retention has been reported to occur following open prostatectomy procedures. Urinary leakage from the cystotomy is not uncommon following catheter removal, and it generally resolves within 1 to 2 days. Transient urge urinary incontinence occurs following open surgical prostatectomy, usually due to bladder instability, but this generally resolves within several weeks of surgery. Total incontinence is rare. Retrograde ejaculation occurs in all patients undergoing adenomectomy, but other effects on sexual function are rare. Postoperative bladder neck contracture may occur in up to 8% of patients undergoing open prostatectomy; its etiology is unclear. Treatment of the bladder neck contracture may require dilation or even incision of the bladder neck.

## *References*

1. Oesterling JE. Benign prostatic hyperplasia: a review of its histogenesis and natural history. *Prostate Suppl* 1996;6:67–73.
2. Wasson JH, Reda DJ, Bruskewitz RC, et al. A comparison of transurethral surgery with watchful waiting for moderate symptoms of benign prostatic hyperplasia. The Veterans Affairs Cooperative Study Group on Transurethral Resection of the Prostate. *N Engl J Med* 1995;332:75–79.
3. Roehrborn CG, Bartsch G, Kirby R, et al. Guidelines for the diagnosis and treatment of benign prostatic hyperplasia: a comparative, international overview. *Urology* 2001;58:642–650.
4. Kuo RL, Kim SC, Lingeman JE, et al. Holmium laser enucleation of prostate (HoLEP): the Methodist Hospital experience with >75 gram enucleations. *J Urol* 2003;170:149–152.
5. Kim SC, Tinmouth WW, Kuo RL, et al. Simultaneous holmium laser enucleation of prostate and upper-tract endourologic stone procedures. *J Endourol* 2004;18:971–975.
6. Ozden C, Inal G, Adsan O, et al. Detection of prostate cancer and changes in prostate-specific antigen (PSA) six months after surgery for benign prostatic hyperplasia in patients with elevated PSA. *Urol Int* 2003;71: 150–153.
7. Marks LS, Dorey FJ, Rhodes T, et al. Serum prostate specific antigen levels after transurethral resection of prostate: a longitudinal characterization in men with benign prostatic hyperplasia. *J Urol* 1996;156:1035–1039.
8. Aus G, Bergdahl S, Frosing R, et al. Reference range of prostate-specific antigen after transurethral resection of the prostate. *Urology* 1996;47: 529–531.
9. Stamey TA, Yang N, Hay AR, et al. Prostate-specific antigen as a serum marker for adenocarcinoma of the prostate. *N Engl J Med* 1987;317: 909–916.
10. Te AE, Malloy TR, Stein BS, et al. Impact of prostate-specific antigen level and prostate volume as predictors of efficacy in photoselective vaporization prostatectomy: analysis and results of an ongoing prospective multicentre study at 3 years. *BJU Int* 2006;97:1229–1233.
11. Pickard R, Emberton M, Neal DE. The management of men with acute urinary retention. National Prostatectomy Audit Steering Group. *Br J Urol* 1998;81:712–720.

# CHAPTER 26 ■ PROSTATIC IMAGING AND BIOPSY

FRANCES M. MARTIN, WILLIAM T. CONNER, AND RANDALL G. ROWLAND

Adenocarcinoma of the prostate (PC) is the most common cancer of men in the United States and Europe. Concomitant development of prostatic-specific antigen (PSA) assays and transrectal ultrasound (TRUS) provided the tools for diagnosis of PC at an earlier, and presumably more curable, stage. The transvaginal ultrasound probe was adapted to transrectal use, and the spring-loaded Biopty gun with a disposable 18-gauge needle was invented to permit ultrasound-guided biopsies (USBs) with TRUS guidance. PSA, TRUS, and USB are now the standard methods for diagnosis of PC. TRUS is an adjunct for staging PC, while PSA is the most sensitive method of evaluating response to therapy. TRUS is currently the most common method to image the prostate for initial staging, biopsy, and anatomical assessment. Ultrasound is also useful in evaluating brachytherapy and cryotherapy. Studies using three-dimensional (3-D) TRUS may show improved detection of tumor and extraglandular extension (1). Additional imaging modalities may change future management and detection.

## SCREENING AND DIAGNOSIS

Screening PSA tests are in general performed between ages 50 and 75, starting 5 years earlier in African American and high-risk men. Values up to 4 ng per mL are considered acceptable in men younger than age 60, although some laboratories consider values >2.6 ng per mL moderately elevated. PSA levels may fluctuate, and the decision for biopsy should not be based solely on one value alone. In-office screening should also include a digital rectal examination and a complete history and physical examination.

Increased PSA velocity >0.75 ng per mL per year is an indication for careful surveillance and possible biopsy. A value of >0.75 ng per mL per year requires three PSA values over a 2-year period to be statistically valid (2). PSA levels increase with age. The formula for calculating the "age-adjusted normal" is age minus 20 divided by 10. Thus, a 50-year-old man would have an age-adjusted normal of 3.0 ng per mL, while the value for a 70-year-old man would be 5.0 ng per mL. There is controversy concerning the use of the age- adjusted values, although it seems clear that this technique improves the sensitivity for cancer detection in men below age 60 (3). It is unclear if PSA velocity, PSA density, or free-to-total PSA values provide a significantly better screening test for prostate cancer. Additional markers and proteomics profiling, including prostate-specific membrane antigen (PSMA), prostate stem cell antigen (PSCA), and hepsin, are being evaluated and may provide improved screening for prostate cancer (4). Currently, PSA is the most widely used marker for screening and biopsy indication.

Both benign and malignant prostatic cells produce PSA. Infection, trauma, and ejaculation are some of the benign conditions that may cause a PSA elevation. After excluding other causes for an increased PSA, TRUS and USB are scheduled.

## INDICATIONS FOR SURGERY

The most common reasons for TRUS and USB are an elevated screening PSA or an abnormal digital rectal exam (DRE). Prior to the mid-1980s, PC was usually suspected because of an abnormal DRE. Biopsies were typically performed under spinal or general anesthesia using a digitally guided transperineal approach. With the development of PSA and TRUS with USB, the procedure became simpler, safer, more precise, and more economical.

Other indications for TRUS and USB are a suspicious prostatic nodule, asymmetry of the prostate, active surveillance, and, rarely, unexplained metastatic malignancy. TRUS without USB is used for evaluation of ejaculatory duct cysts, prostatic stones, unexplained urinary tract infection (UTI), and suspected prostatic abscess. Prostatic biopsy without TRUS is on occasion performed for very ill patients with highly suspicious prostate glands, for whom the procedure is performed at the bedside. Confirmation of the diagnosis allows prompt hormonal ablation, often with improvement in hematuria or pain. An Iowa Trumpet (©V. Mueller, McGraw Park, Illinois) allows access for the digitally guided transrectal biopsy while protecting the finger of the operator.

## ALTERNATIVE THERAPY

Not everyone who has an elevated PSA or abnormal DRE should have a prostatic biopsy. Patients should be counseled concerning the risks and benefits of both the biopsy and possible treatment. Thus, an 85-year-old man with Alzheimer's disease and no significant urinary symptoms who has an ill-advised PSA test with a result of 8 ng per mL should not have a biopsy unless there is an unusual reason. He should have another PSA in 6 months. If there is no significant change, PSA testing should be stopped.

General medical evaluation should detect anticoagulation, medications, significant cardiovascular disease, diabetes mellitus, and excessive apprehension. Any of these factors may require a change of plans for USB. Of importance, an interactive discussion with the patient should take place regarding the recommendations for or against a biopsy in light of all findings and overall health status.

## SURGICAL TECHNIQUE

Anticoagulation must be stopped before USB. Consultation with the patient's physician or cardiologist will determine if it is safe to stop oral anticoagulation 5 to 10 days in advance, depending upong the medication. If not, he is changed to a form of heparin, which is stopped for 6 to 12 hours before the biopsy. Gross hematuria and clot retention that requires a Foley catheter are more common in this group.

Antibiotics are commonly given before and after the biopsy. Regimens vary, but the usual protocol in the United States includes a full dose of a fluoroquinolone before the biopsy. Previously, routine use of antibiotics for several days after biopsy was standard. Prolonged prophylaxis can lead to resistant organisms. Single-dose regimens were evaluated to reduce this risk and support single-dose prophylaxis against infective complications (5). Patients with artificial heart valves, total joint prostheses, or implanted devices are routinely treated using standard American Heart Association guidelines. Some American urologists use cleansing rectal enemas, although there is some controversy concerning their need (6).

Some patients require monitored anesthesia care. These include those with anal stenosis, excessive apprehension, or serious cardiac arrhythmias and patients without a rectum. Oral sedatives and analgesics may be given, provided the patient has a driver to take him home.

Initial vital signs are monitored, including blood pressure and heart rate. The patient is placed in the left lateral recumbent (decubitis) position on the table in the US suite. The operator sits at a comfortable level beside the table and again explains the procedure as it is being performed. A gentle, thorough rectal examination is performed, noting significant external hemorrhoids, anal sphincter diameter and tone, and lesions in the rectum. Examination of the prostate includes specific notes concerning size, texture, tenderness, borders, fixation or mobility of the apex, symmetry, location of the midline sulcus, and the seminal vesicles. Any prostatic nodules or abnormal areas are noted.

We use a B&K Medical (Wilmington, MA) US system with either a 7.0- or 7.5-MHz endorectal probe. For the rare instances of TRUS for patients without a rectum, a 3.5- or 4.0-MHz probe is used. The TRUS probe has been prepared in advance by decontamination with glutaraldehyde solution or heated 35% peroxyacetic acid solution (STERIS) sterilization. A finger cot is placed snugly over the inflation port and inflated to exclude air bubbles, which interfere with the US image. Finally, a condom containing about 15 cc of US gel is placed over the rectal end of the probe. The US gel reduces artifacts during TRUS. The probe is lubricated and gently inserted into the rectum. Lidocaine gel (1%) may be used, if the patient is not allergic, to provide topical analgesia to the rectal wall. Inflation of the finger cot with 25 to 40 mL of water produces an acoustic window, which allows better definition of the rectal wall and prostate.

Local anesthesia has become a frequent adjunct to TRUS and USB (7). Periprostatic nerves can be blocked by injecting 5 to 10 cc of 1% lidocaine without epinephrine just lateral to the junction of the seminal vesicle and prostate on each side (Fig. 26.1). After guiding a 22-gauge, 7-in. spinal needle (Becton/Dickinson, Franklin Lakes, NJ) to the correct spot with US, and aspirating to be sure a vein has not been entered, the anesthetic is slowly injected. The area of injection expands and produces a hypoechoic image that confirms the proper location of the drug. Local anesthesia allows multiple biopsies to be taken with little discomfort for most patients. As with all procedures with conscious patients, each event must be announced in advance. Lidocaine causes the same stinging sensation in the periprostatic area that occurs with dental or other local injections. Neutralizing the lidocaine solution with alkali can prevent this, but the shelf life of the drug is significantly reduced.

The prostate is then imaged in transverse and longitudinal planes, noting areas of abnormal echogenicity, cysts, calcifications, indistinct borders, lesions of the seminal vesicles or ejaculatory ducts, and other abnormalities. Tiny corpora amylacea are easily visible and usually define the border of the transitional and peripheral zones. Bladder US can be performed if

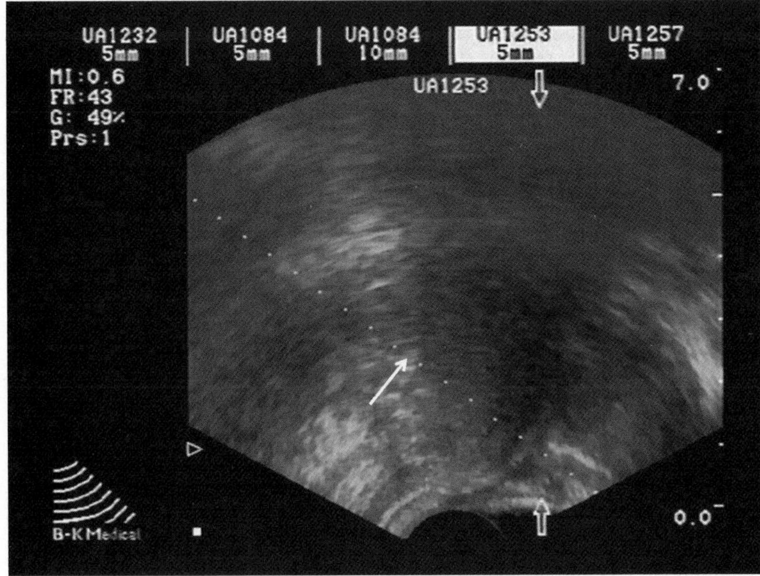


FIGURE 26.1 Prostate ultrasound. Dotted line indicates path of biopsy needle on sagittal view.

desired but is best accomplished as a suprapubic exam with a 3.5- to 4-MHz probe.

Prostatic volume is calculated using the greatest transverse, anterior–posterior, and longitudinal dimensions. Most modern TRUS machines have computer programs for computing the volume. One formula for calculating the volume of a prostate ellipse by US is as follows: height multiplied by width multiplied by length multiplied by 0.52. Images are recorded to show anatomy of the prostate and seminal vesicles, abnormalities, and prostatic volume. Digital recording of the procedure is possible. The volume of suspicious hypoechoic lesions is measured and recorded. The classical appearance of a prostate tumor is hypoechoic, but some cancers can appear isoechoic or hyperechoic. The TRUS procedure takes several minutes, enough time for the lidocaine to anesthetize the periprostatic nerves.

Biopsies are obtained with a sharp, disposable, spring-loaded 18-gauge needle, which produces a 17-mm specimen with little crush artifact. Several such needles are available. Some are completely disposable devices, whereas others use a permanent biopsy gun and disposable needles. Most brands of needles have a slightly abraded tip that makes them echogenic and easier to see. We currently use either a Bard Magnum Biopty Needle Gun with a disposable needle or a Microvasive Topnotch disposable gun and needle. The device is fired before the biopsy to familiarize the patient with the sound.

We routinely obtain 12 biopsies: lateral and medial at each base, lateral and medial at the midgland on each side, and 2 biopsies at each apex, as described by Gore et al. (8) and others. Patients who need a second biopsy because of a high suspicion of cancer will have 12 to 20 biopsies, including specimens from the transition zones (TZs) and far lateral peripheral zone. "Saturation" biopsy under anesthesia obtains up to 45 cores of tissue, although this technique is reserved for the patient who has had multiple negative biopsies and still has a suspicious PSA or rectal exam (9). The great value of TRUS is to be able to precisely sample specific areas of the prostate. Anesthetizing the urethra with lidocaine reduces the additional urethral pain with TZ biopsies but does not decrease the additional urethral bleeding. Bleeding usually stops without treatment within 24 hours.

After all biopsies are obtained and carefully labeled, the US probe is removed. A useful technique to control rectal bleeding is to roll a hand towel into a tight roll about 6 in. long and 3 in. in diameter and then have the patient sit with the towel between his ischial tuberosities for 10 minutes. This places pressure on the perineum, compressing the prostate against the symphysis pubis. Blood pressure and heart rate are again recorded. The patient sits on the table for about 10 minutes, then voids. The urine usually contains blood, especially if TZ biopsies have been obtained.

When the patient is stable and voiding well, he is given his postbiopsy instructions and allowed to leave, with a return appointment for 1 to 2 weeks depending upon the response time of the pathology department.

Instructions include the following:

1. Expect blood with urination and bowel movements for 1 to 7 days.
2. Expect blood with ejaculate for up to 6 weeks.
3. Take medications as prescribed.
4. Report temperature over 101°, passage of clots after 24 hours, persistent rectal bleeding, difficulty with urination, pain, or any other symptom that concerns him.
5. Return for discussion of the biopsy as scheduled.
6. Resume all other medications, with special instructions for anticoagulants.
7. Resume preoperative activities after 24 hours, avoiding heavy lifting or strenuous activity for 72 hours.

## OUTCOMES

### Complications

Hematuria, hematochezia, and hematospermia are expected, as mentioned above. Excessive bleeding requires evaluation and appropriate treatment. Rarely, patients require admission for bladder irrigation for urinary bleeding. Patients who are on anticoagulants on occasion require cystoscopy with fulguration of bleeding vessels. Rectal bleeding is usually minor and self-limited. If rectal bleeding is persistent or causes the hematocrit to fall, proctoscopic examination is indicated. The urologist, a general surgeon, or a gastroenterologist, depending upon the time of occurrence and the training of the physician, may perform this. Arterial or venous bleeding may be controlled with direct suture ligation or injection of epinephrine around the vessel. Hematospermia requires reassurance only. Urinary retention usually resolves unless the patient has bladder outlet obstruction, but it may require temporary catheterization.

Bacteriuria and bacteremia are fairly common but usually asymptomatic and resolve without further complications (10). Persistant rectal pain or fever >101.5°F may signal prostatic abscess or early sepsis. Isolated reports of perirectal abscess, septic shock, disseminated intravascular coagulation, and osteomyelitis are in the literature. Seeding of the biopsy tract with implantation of cancer is a theoretical complication that has been rarely reported. The biopsy technique does not interfere with radical prostatectomy, external radiation, or brachytherapy.

# ADDITIONAL IMAGING MODALITIES FOR EVALUATION OF THE PROSTATE

## Computerized Tomography (CT)

The contrast resolution of CT is ineffective in distinguishing the prostate from cancers or surrounding organs. Its use in prostate cancer detection is limited. CT can be useful in evaluating for lymphatic involvement and nodal staging, but it is based upon size criteria. It is less sensitive for bony involvement than magnetic resonance (MR) or bone scan.

## Magnetic Resonance Imaging (MRI)

Use of MRI to detect prostate cancer and locally advanced disease has provided mixed results. It provides improved anatomic visualization with better soft tissue resolution. The use of the endorectal coil may improve the specificity of MRI for detection of cancer and extraprostatic extension. Prostatitis, hemorrhage, and benign hyperplasia can mimic cancer on MRI. Studies suggest that it may be more valuable to detect local recurrence after prostatectomy (11). Newer advances, including magnetic resonance spectroscopic imaging (MRSI), may improve evaluation of tumor size, location, and extent (12). MRSI displays relative concentrations of citrate, choline, and creatinine, which are typically higher in cancer cells. Criteria for diagnosing prostate cancer are based upon choline-citrate ratios. Some authors state that combined MRI/MRSI can help stratify patients' risk by assessing the aggressiveness of the tumor biology (12).

## Positron Emission Tomography (PET)

Although PET scans have been useful in evaluating metastatic disease, the use of $^{18}$F-FDG tracer is not helpful in diagnosing or imaging localized prostate cancer. This tracer has confounding uptake in prostate cancer cells and benign prostatic hyperplasia (13). Numerous additional tracers are under investigation and may prove more useful in diagnosing prostate cancer.

## *References*

1. Garg S, Fortling B, Chadwick D, et al. Staging of prostate cancer using 3-dimensional transrectal ultrasound images: a pilot study. *J Urol* 1999; 162:1318–1321.
2. Potter SR, Carter HB. The role of prostate-specific antigen velocity in prostate cancer early detection. *Curr Urol Rep* 2000;1:15–19.
3. Polascik TJ, Oesterling JE, Partin AW. Prostate specific antigen: a decade of discovery—what have we learned and where are we going. *J Urol* 1999; 162:293–306.
4. Bradford TJ, Tomlins BA, Wang X, et al. Molecular markers of prostate cancer. *Urol Oncol: Semin Original Invest* 2006;24(6):528–551.
5. Aron M, Rajeev TP, Gupta NP. Antibiotic prophylaxis for transrectal needle biopsy of the prostate: a randomized controlled study. *BJU Int* 2000;85(6):682–685.
6. Terris MK. Letter to the Editor. *J Urol* 2002;167:2145–2146.
7. Pareek G, Armenkadas NA, Fracchia JA. Periprostatic nerve blockade for transrectal ultrasound guided biopsy of the prostate: a randomized, double-blind, placebo controlled study. *J Urol* 2001;166:894–897.
8. Gore JL, Shariat SF, Miles BJ, et al. Optimal combinations of systematic sextant and laterally directed biopsies for the detection of prostate cancer. *J Urol* 2001;165:1554–1559.
9. Stewart CS, Leibovich BC, Waver AL, et al. Prostate cancer diagnosis using a saturation needle biopsy technique after previous negative sextant biopsies. *J Urol* 2001;166:86–91.
10. Lindert KA, Kabalin JN, Terris MK. Bacteremia and bacteriuria after transrectal ultrasound guided prostate biopsy. *J Urol* 2000;164:76–80.
11. Sella T, Schwartz LH, Swindle PW, et al. Suspected local recurrence after radical prostatectomy: endorectal coil MR imaging. *Radiology* 2004; 231:379–385.
12. Hricak H. MR imaging and MR spectroscopic imaging in the pretreatment evaluation of prostate cancer. *Br J Radiol* 2005;78:S103–S111.
13. Hofer C, Laubenbacher C, Block T, et al. Fluorine-18-fluorodeoxyglucose positron emission tomography is useless for the detection of local recurrence after radical prostatectomy. *Eur Urol* 199;36:31–35.

# CHAPTER 27 ■ PELVIC LYMPHADENECTOMY

MICHELLE L. RAMÍREZ, RAJ S. PRUTHI, JOON-HA OK, AND RALPH W. DEVERE WHITE

Pelvic lymph nodes are the initial site of the spread of prostatic, bladder, and proximal urethral cancers. Tumors of the penis, scrotum, and distal urethra spread primarily to the inguinal lymph nodes but can involve the pelvic lymph nodes at a later stage. Testicular tumors rarely involve the pelvic lymph nodes unless there is massive retroperitoneal disease (retrograde spread) or a history of orchiopexy or prior pelvic procedures.

Standard practice had been that all patients undergoing radical prostatectomy undergo pelvic lymphadenectomy for staging. Currently, pelvic lymph node dissection is performed only if a patient is at significant risk for metastasis. Preoperative prostate-specific antigen (PSA), PSA kinetics, biopsy Gleason score, and clinical stage define those patients at risk for nodal metastasis. Identifying lymph node involvement is important for accurate tumor staging, prognosis, and selection of adjuvant therapy; however, the therapeutic value of lymph node removal for prostate cancer remains controversial. When cystectomy is indicated for bladder cancer, bilateral pelvic lymphadenectomy remains the standard of practice.

## PROSTATE CANCER

### Indications for Surgery

Pelvic lymphadenectomy adds modest operating room time, cost, and complication risk to a radical prostatectomy, but when performed independently, results in additional anesthetic risk and exposure to cardiopulmonary, thromboembolic, and wound complications. Several investigators have therefore attempted to identify prostate cancer patient groups in which pelvic lymphadenectomy can be omitted with an acceptable risk of understaging. By combining these criteria, patients can be grouped as low (2% to 5%), moderate (20%), and high (40%) risk categories for lymph node metastases (8). Patients at highest risk for lymph node metastases include those with a Gleason score equal to or >7 and a PSA equal to or >20 ng per mL, a Gleason score equal to or >8 and a PSA equal to or >10 ng per mL, or a PSA equal to or > 50 ng per mL (Table 27.1). Using a decision analysis, Meng and

**TABLE 27.1**

**SELECTION CRITERIA FOR PELVIC LYMPHADENECTOMY**

| PROCEDURE | CRITERIA | % OF ALL PATIENTS | % WITH POSITIVE LYMPH NODES |
|---|---|---|---|
| No lymphadenectomy[a] | PSA <10, Gleason score <7, and clinical stage <T2 | ~50% | ~2% |
| Intended retropubic prostatectomy; no laparoscopic pelvic lymphadenectomy, but open lymphadenectomy may be performed at the time of prostatectomy | PSA ≥10 or Gleason score ≥7 or clinical stage ≥T2c | ~50% | ~2% |
| Intended retropubic prostatectomy; laparoscopic pelvic lymphadenectomy may be considered | PSA ≥50 or (PSA ≥20 and Gleason score ≥7) or (PSA ≥10 and Gleason score ≥8) | ~10% | ~40% |
| Intended perineal prostatectomy; laparoscopic pelvic lymphadenectomy may be considered[b] | | | |

PSA, prostate-specific antigen.
[a]Staging lymphadenectomy does not affect outcome (PSA recurrence at 2 years). From El Galley RES, Keane TE, Petros JA, et al. Evaluation of staging lymphadenectomy in prostate cancer. *Urology* 1998;52:663–667, with permission.
[b]Pelvic lymphadenectomy has not been shown to affect the intermediate outcome. From Salomon L, Hoznek A, Lefrere-Belda MA, et al. Nondissection of the pelvic lymph nodes does not influence the results of perineal radical prostatectomy in selected patients. *Eur Urol* 2000;37:297–300, with permission.
Modified from Wolf JS. Indications, technique, and results of laparoscopic pelvic lymphadenectomy. *J Endourol* 2001;15(4):427–435, with permission.

associates have suggested that lymph node dissection is unwarranted in those with <18% risk for lymph node involvement (7). Application of the selection criteria (Table 27.1) may help to decrease the number of what at least some believe are unnecessary lymph node dissections.

We currently perform pelvic lymph node dissection concomitantly with retropubic prostatectomy in those patients with clinical T2a disease, a PSA equal to or >10 ng per mL, and/or those with high-grade tumors (biopsy Gleason score equal to or >7). Due to the stage migration, we feel that performance of lymphadenectomy as a separate procedure, that is, laparoscopically, is not cost-effective. The yield of cancerous nodes for a clinical stage T1c tumor of a Gleason sum <7 and a preoperative PSA <10 ng per mL is well within the 5% to 10% margin of error of a false-negative diagnosis at frozen section. Routine pelvic node dissection in such patients is not cost-effective regardless of technique and subjects the patient to an unnecessary procedure with possible morbidity. We no longer perform lymph node dissection prior to radiation therapy.

## Surgical Technique

The boundaries of the traditional pelvic lymph node dissection for prostate cancer include the pelvic sidewall laterally, the paravesical fascia and peritoneum medially, the genitofemoral nerve superiorly, the obturator nerve inferiorly, and the femoral canal distally (Fig. 27.1). Proximally, the dissection is carried varying distances up the common iliac artery (Figs. 27.2 and 27.3). Many urologists feel that only the obturator nodal packet need be removed, for three reasons:

1. The obturator nodes are involved in 87% of cases when lymphatic metastases are found.
2. The procedure is for staging and not therapy.
3. If radiation therapy is used for local control following surgery, patients who had an extensive lymphadenectomy have a higher incidence of scrotal or lower-limb edema.

As prophylaxis against deep venous thrombosis, patients are administered 7,500 U of subcutaneous heparin in the arm,

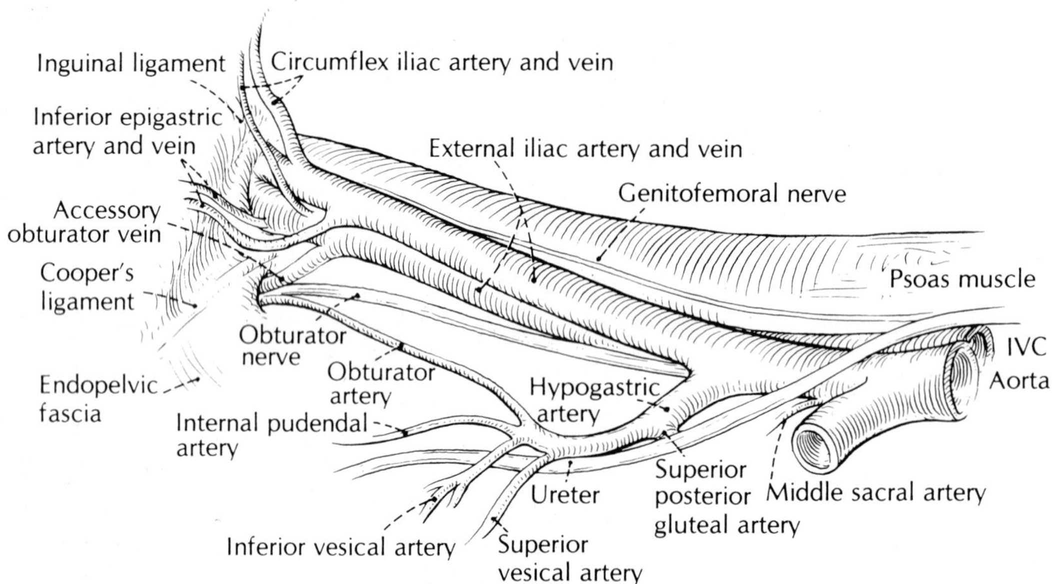


FIGURE 27.1 Right lateral pelvic wall. Anatomy of pelvic blood vessels and nerves encountered in a pelvic lymph node dissection is depicted.

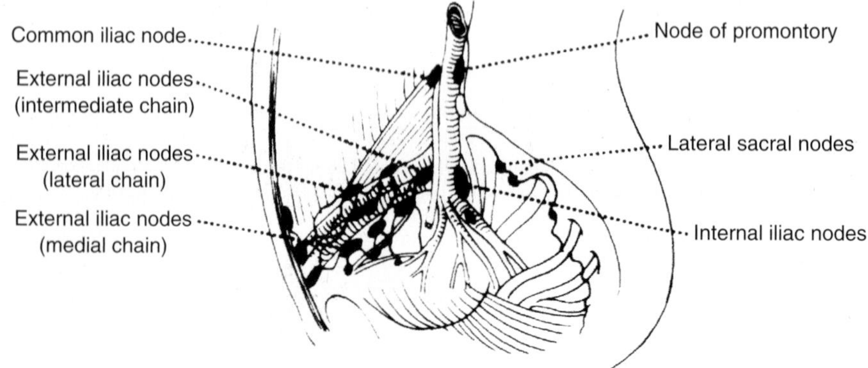


FIGURE 27.2 Incision of fibroareolar tissue loosely adherent to adventitia of the iliac artery and vein. This allows a portion of the areolar tissue to pass lateral to the iliac vessels into the obturator fossa.

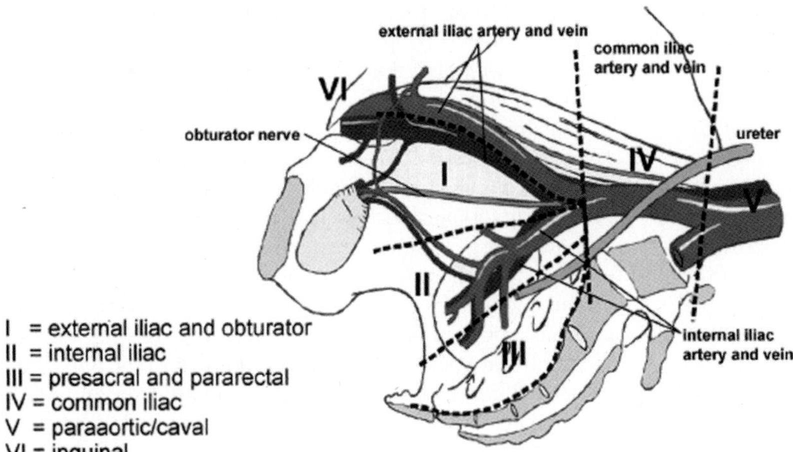


FIGURE 27.3 Boundaries of pelvic lymph node dissection subdivided into different regions. "Limited" dissection removes tissue from the obturator fossa (*region I*). "Extended" template dissection removes tissue along the major pelvic vessels (external iliac vein, obturator fossa, and internal iliac artery and vein) (*regions I and II*). The dissection is carried varying distances up the common iliac artery and vein (*region IV*). (From Mattei A, Fuechsel FG, Bhatta Dhar N, et al. The template of the primary lymphatic landing sites of the prostate should be revisited: results of a multimodality mapping study. *Eur Urol* 2008;53(1):118–125, printed with permission from Elsevier.)

which may reduce lower limb edema (1). The supine or lithotomy position may be used, although we recommend the low lithotomy position. The sacrum is positioned over the table break or a roll to allow for hyperextension of and better vision into the pelvis. The bladder is emptied using a Foley catheter. A midline incision is made from below the umbilicus to the symphysis pubica down through the anterior rectus sheath. The posterior rectus sheath is incised for 2 to 3 cm above the linea semilunaris to aid in lateral retraction of the wound. An extraperitoneal lymph node dissection is performed. If the peritoneum is entered during this incision, the defect is closed with absorbable sutures.

The transversalis fascia is sharply divided in the midline to allow lateral dissection superficial to the peritoneum, which helps avoid injury to the inferior epigastric vessels. The iliac vessels are exposed by bluntly sweeping the peritoneum superomedially. The vasa deferentia are encountered during this maneuver and may be divided. The table is tilted toward the first side for evaluation. If the prostate cancer is confined to one lobe, the dissection is begun on that side. A self-retaining retractor is applied, with care taken not to injure the inferior epigastric vessels. We use the Bookwalter retractor without the post, as it can be more quickly applied and the post can interfere with the surgeon. Other self-retaining retractors may be used.

We place the Bookwalter retractor on top of sterile towels, one on each thigh and one on the abdomen. A bladder blade and moist lap sponge are used for lateral retraction on the side of the dissection. A malleable retractor and moist lap sponge are placed on the bladder and used to retract the bladder toward the contralateral side. A third blade is placed at the apex of the incision. With these three blades, excellent visibility can be obtained.

The nodal packet is palpated to detect grossly enlarged lymph nodes. If such nodes are found, they are sent for frozen section evaluation following removal. If no enlarged nodes are palpated, we continue with the lymphadenectomy and prostatectomy and do not send the lymph nodes for frozen section.

The external iliac artery is identified, and dissection of the lymph node packet is begun over its anteromedial aspect. The correct plane of dissection is easily found here, and there are no other structures in this area to be damaged (Fig. 27.4). Blunt dissection is performed with a sponge stick, and the suction tip and smooth forceps are used to clean away adipose tissue. The dissection is brought proximally to the bifurcation of the common iliac vessels and distally to the femoral canal. The lymph node of Cloquet is the most distal aspect of the dissection. Lymphatic channels into this node and surrounding the external iliac vein are meticulously clipped and divided. We place a right-angle clamp around the lymph node packet

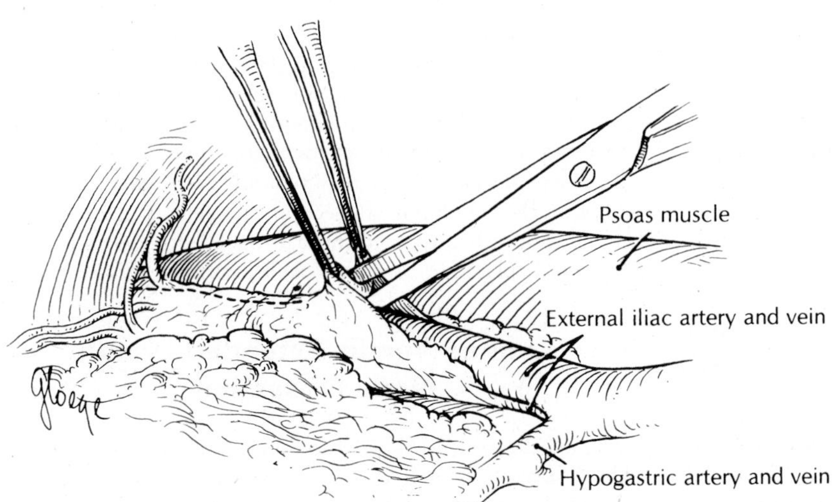


FIGURE 27.4 Correct plane of dissection is shown.

and ligate it with a 2-0 Vicryl tie. A large right-angle clip is placed below the tie. As the nodal packet is divided and swept superiorly, an accessory obturator vein may be found medial to the internal iliac artery and should be ligated (rather than clipped) and divided to avoid avulsion. Identification of this vein is necessary as damage can cause extensive bleeding.

With gentle lateral retraction of the external iliac vein, the lymph node packet is dissected off the pelvic sidewall laterally. Although a vein retractor is usually used for this maneuver, we use a peanut/Kitner dissector. Identification of the obturator nerve is essential to avoid injury as the dissection is carried into the pelvic fossa. The packet is freed from the obturator nerve and vessels. The obturator vessels are spared if they are in their usual location below the nerve. If the vessels are above the nerve or involved with the lymph node packet, it is best to ligate and divide them to prevent avulsion and bleeding. This is especially true near the femoral canal. The superior attachment of the packet is now near the internal iliac artery. Previously we used to identify and dissect out the ureter, but, in most cases, we no longer do this. To ensure the ureter is not damaged by a clip, the specimen is split over the obturator nerve, and a right-angle clip is placed over either limb of the split packet on each side of the nerve in a cranial-to-caudal fashion so that the ureter cannot accidentally be included in the clip. Additional loose attachments to the proximal hypogastric vessels are clipped and divided. The entire packet is sent to pathology as the two portions divided over the obturator nerve. The obturator fossa is irrigated with sterile saline. It had been our routine to leave a gauze sponge in the fossa for hemostasis; however, we now do this only for minimal oozing. The same dissection is then performed on the contralateral side to complete the lymph node dissection. We place one or two Jackson–Pratt drains in the pelvis postoperatively.

## Laparoscopic and Robotic Approach

In recent years laparoscopic and robotic approaches have become increasingly utilized in the surgical treatment of prostate and bladder cancers. Accordingly, the ability to perform an adequate laparoscopic pelvic lymphadenectomy is necessary, particularly at the time of the primary laparoscopic procedure.

Changes in port placement are not necessary, and the same instrumentation and setup can be used as is required for the primary surgical procedure. Instrumentation used includes broad graspers in the nondominant hand and cautery scissors in the dominant hand. Typically, we utilize nontraumatic graspers such as Hunter graspers in laparoscopic cases or fenestrated bipolar forceps in robotic cases. The surgical assistant also should be available with nontraumatic graspers and a suction irrigator.

When the lymphadenectomy is performed following a laparoscopic or robotic prostatectomy or cystectomy, the posterior peritoneum has already been incised and the retroperitoneal space exposed. If the lymph node dissection is to be performed initially, the posterior peritoneum should be incised in a cephalad-caudad direction just lateral to the medial umbilical ligament on each side. This will expose the retroperitoneal space and relevant landmarks.

The primary surgical step is to identify and expose the external iliac artery and vein by blunt dissection (e.g., with the closed scissor tips by the surgeon or with the suction irrigator by the assistant). The vein can be located lying immediately posterior and medial to the artery. It is important to dissect down to the correct fibroalveolar plane just overlying the artery and the vein. This will allow for easier and more precise dissection of the lymph node packets for the remainder of the procedure.

Our initial approach is to perform the obturator and hypogastric dissection by locating and developing the medial border of the iliac vein, thereby exposing the obturator fossa posteriorly. Typically the patient is placed in the steep Trendelenburg position and maintained relatively hypovolemic. Consequently, the iliac vein is decompressed and less prone to grasping or sharp injury. With the medial edge of the external iliac vein identified, the plane between the vein and the obturator packet can be extended down to the pubic bone distally. Blunt and sharp dissection, often with the aid of monopolar scissors, bipolar graspers, and the appropriate countertraction placed by the assistant or the surgeon's nondominant hand, can be used to facilitate retraction of the vein laterally and the obturator packet medially. With the dissection completed off the iliac vein, the nodal packet can then be dissected off the obturator nerve and vessels posteriorly. Monopolar and bipolar cautery can aid in the division of smaller lymphatic channels, and laparoscopic clips (e.g., Hemolock clips) can be used to ligate larger lymphatic channels, pedicles, and vein branches as necessary. The pubic bone and anterior surface of the obturator nerve and vessels help to mark the distal margin of the nodal packet. With the obturator packet freed and divided distally, it is peeled back in the cephalad direction to the level of the hypogastric artery while keeping the obturator nerve, medial border of the external iliac vein, and the medial umbilical ligament in clear view. The medial umbilical ligament should be retracted medially to achieve proper exposure for the hypogastric dissection.

If an extended dissection is to be performed, we begin above and along the external iliac artery. Again, it is vital to dissect down to the correct fibroalveolar plane over the artery, beginning the dissection distally. While avoiding the circumflex vein distally, all tissue between the external iliac vein and artery, as well as lymphatic tissue out to the psoas muscle and genitofemoral nerve laterally, is included. With this packet divided distally, this lymph tissue is teased and dissected in the cephalad direction with blunt and sharp dissection, occasionally with the use of monopolar and bipolar cautery. Unlike the external iliac vein, it is quite rare to encounter aberrant branches off of the artery, and this dissection is readily performed proximally up to and along the common iliac vessels. One needs to remain aware during the common iliac dissection that the ureter will be crossing over the common iliac vessels. If desired, a para-aortic dissection is achievable laparoscopically or robotically. If this dissection is anticipated, it may be necessary to place the laparoscopic or robotic ports approximately 2 cm superior or cephalad than typically positioned.

With the lymph node dissection complete, the lymph node specimen can be extracted through the 10- to 12-mm port or preferably placed in an impermeable sack and extracted.

## Limited Versus Extended Lymph Node Dissection

Though there is individual variability in lymphatic drainage, the principal location for prostate cancer lies in the pelvis, along the external and internal iliacs and in the obturator fossa. Limited dissection involves only the obturator region bounded by the external iliac artery and the obturator nerve, whereas extended dissection involves all three regions (Fig. 27.3). Extended dissection results in the resection of approximately two-thirds of all primary prostatic landing sites, compared to only one-third with a limited dissection (6). In low-risk patients, up to 7% of positive lymph nodes may be missed with limited lymph node dissection, while as high as 20% may be missed in intermediate- and high-risk patients (1). Mapping studies have also demonstrated a considerable amount of drainage to nodes along the common iliacs, in the presacral/pararectal regions, and along the aorta and vena cava as high as the origin of the inferior mesenteric artery. Using an extended template that includes the nodes along the common iliac arteries up to the ureteric crossing may remove approximately 75% of prostate primary lymphatic landing sites (6). The risk-benefit ratio may not justify a complete dissection up to the inferior mesenteric artery.

While controversy exists on the extent of lymph node dissection, evidence suggests that extended dissection improves the accuracy of surgical staging and prognosis, given that the percentage of positive lymph nodes predicts for disease progression. Data from a few retrospective analyses with long-term follow-up reveal that extended lymph node dissection may reduce the risk of disease progression and disease-specific mortality (4). Joslyn and Konety examined the Surveillance, Epidemiology and End Results (SEER) database on 1,923 patients and detected an association between the extent of lymphadenectomy and prostate cancer-specific mortality at 10 years after controlling for other variables (4). Patients undergoing excision of at least four lymph nodes (node-positive and node-negative patients) or more than ten nodes (only node-negative patients) had a lower risk of death than did those who did not undergo lymphadenectomy. The extended dissection may result in the removal of unidentified metastatic disease, explaining the potential therapeutic benefits in patients with not only positive but also negative nodes.

In contrast, several high-powered studies do not show any survival advantage, and complication rates have been reportedly higher in those undergoing extended dissection versus limited dissection. In fact, the probability of complications may increase in direct proportion to the number of lymph nodes removed and needs to be taken into account when the benefits associated with more extensive dissection are considered. A multi-institutional, randomized clinical trial is needed to determine the value of extending the boundaries of pelvic lymphadenectomy.

At this time, we do not routinely perform an extended dissection for prostate cancer; however, if indicated, it is carried out as described previously while extending the boundaries to the internal iliac vessels, bladder wall, and pelvic sidewall. Lymphatic tissue is cleared from the pubis to the bifurcation of the common iliac vessels. The lateral dissection proceeds along the external iliac vessels lateral to the circumflex vein and medial to the genitofemoral nerve as described previously. As the dissection is carried cephalad along the anterior border of the common iliac artery, any psoas branches are clipped and divided. As with the dissection for bladder cancer, the vas deferens is located over the medial umbilical ligament as it enters the internal inguinal ring and is divided. This allows exposure of the medial umbilical ligament, which is then traced back to the internal iliac artery. The medial border of dissection begins with the ureter as it crosses the common iliac artery and continues along the lateral border of the medial umbilical ligament and bladder. Large lymphatic channels are clipped and divided, and gentle traction is applied to pull lymphatic tissue from the sidewall. Posteriorly, the dissection continues deep to the obturator nodal packet to the internal iliac vessels. This packet is dissected along the obturator nerve as formerly described until the nerve passes posterior to the iliac vein, that is, the border of the lateral dissection.

## BLADDER CANCER

### Indications for Surgery

There are compelling data that regional lymphadenectomy during radical cystectomy can prolong survival in patients with locally advanced bladder cancer and should be considered the standard of care. Most urologists perform a standard bilateral pelvic lymphadenectomy (to include lymphatics as far lateral as the genitofemoral nerve) based on Skinner's early 1980s data that such a dissection can improve 5-year survival by up to 36% (11), which suggests that lymphadenectomy may have some curative potential in bladder cancer patients with limited nodal disease. Survival rates have been shown to be similar (55%) in those with minimal pelvic lymph node involvement (N1) and those without pelvic lymph node involvement if the primary cancer is organ-confined (pT0 to pT3a). Recently, a prospective, multi-institutional trial randomized 270 patients to receive neoadjuvant chemotherapy followed by radical cystectomy or radical cystectomy alone (2). Twenty-four patients forewent lymphadenectomy, 98 underwent a limited lymph node dissection (obturator nodes only), and 146 underwent a standard lymph node dissection. The 5-year survival rates for the three groups were 33%, 46%, and 60%, respectively.

The presence of positive lymph nodes in bladder cancer has therapeutic implications. If detected, some urologists forego surgery and treat with systemic therapy, whereas others favor debulking the tumor with cystectomy followed by postoperative chemotherapy. If we find grossly enlarged lymph nodes with histological evidence of metastasis, our decision to proceed with cystectomy is influenced by whether the patient received neoadjuvant chemotherapy, the bulk of local disease, and preoperative discussion with the patient. However, if the lymph nodes are grossly normal, we proceed with the radical cystectomy without sending the nodes for frozen section evaluation.

### Surgical Technique

The dissection is similar to the one described previously for prostate cancer with some differences. The incision is carried to just above the umbilicus and down to the pubic bone. We palpate the pelvic lymph nodes while remaining extraperitoneal. If no grossly enlarged nodes are palpable, the dissection becomes intraperitoneal and is performed after the cystectomy is completed, rendering the operation easier and quicker. The peritoneum is entered in midline, and inspection is performed of the intra-abdominal organs for signs of metastases. If none are found, dissection is continued by mobilizing the cecum and ascending colon. The peritoneum is incised along the white line of Toldt and the right colon is rolled medially. The right ureter is identified and freed superiorly and inferiorly. Inferiorly, this leads to the bifurcation of the iliac vessels. In freeing the peritoneum, we routinely divide the vas deferens. On the left, the peritoneum is incised lateral to the sigmoid colon, and it is reflected medially. The left ureter is identified and freed as on the right. Mobilization is aided by dividing the vas deferens.

A self-retaining retractor may be placed as described above. The bowel can easily be retracted into the upper abdomen, as it has been mobilized. The node dissection begins over either common iliac artery just proximal to the bifurcation. It is carried down the hypogastric artery to the superior vesical artery, which is identified and divided. The remainder of the lymph node dissection is similar to that for prostate cancer. Based on data demonstrating that excising and submitting lymph nodes from each site separately increases the lymph node yield and improves nodal status assessment (13), we routinely send lymph nodes from different sites separately as opposed to *en bloc* with the bladder specimen.

## Limited Versus Extended Lymph Node Dissection

There is no accepted standard for either the optimal number of lymph nodes to be removed or the surgical limits of lymph node dissection. The most common dissection includes the bifurcation of the common iliac, external and internal iliacs, and the obturator lymph nodes, and generally yields 10 to 14 nodes. Further extending the dissection to the bifurcation of the aorta, presacral, and presciatic nodes can yield >40 nodes from 13 separate nodal packets (Fig. 27.5). The surgical time is lengthened approximately 1 hour without a significant increase in complications (5).

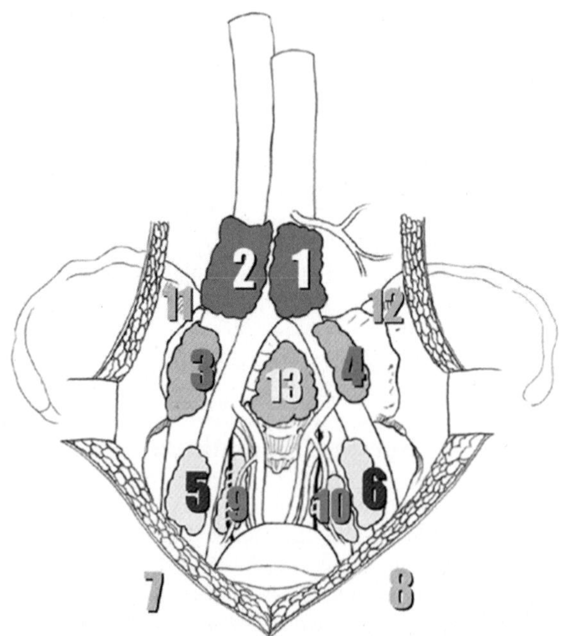


FIGURE 27.5 Total of 13 separate nodal packets: left paraaortic (1), right paracaval (2), right common iliac (3), left common iliac (4), right external iliac (5), left external iliac (6), right lymph node of Cloquet (7), left lymph node of Cloquet (8), right obturator/hypogastric (9), left obturator/hypogastric (10), right presciatic (11), left presciatic (12), presacral (13). (From Stein JP, Penson DF, Cai J, et al. Radical cystectomy with extended lymphadenectomy: evaluating separate package versus en bloc submission for node positive bladder cancer. *J Urol* 2007;177(3):876–882, with permission.)

Mapping studies have attempted to identify a pattern of anatomic distribution of metastatic lymph nodes and to demonstrate an increase in the number of positive nodes outside the boundaries of the standard dissection as the pathologic stage increases. Up to a third of patients with positive common iliac nodes will have metastases to the presacral region, which lies outside the standard template. Results from a prospective, multinational study of 290 patients with pT1G3-T4 disease revealed positive lymph nodes in 81 patients (27.9%). For analysis, three anatomic regions were identified: (I) below the bifurcation of the common iliacs, (II) between the aortic and common iliac bifurcation, and (III) between the inferior mesenteric artery and aortic bifurcation. Approximately 14% had positive nodes confined to either level I or level II. There were no skip lesions identified in level III. If level I disease was present, 57% had level II positive nodes and 31% at level III. The authors concluded that if only the obturator nodes were removed in the 81 patients, then 74.1% of the positive nodes would be left behind, potentially compromising survival.

Variation in reported 5-year survival rates (5% to 30%) in lymph-node–positive bladder cancer treated with radical cystectomy and pelvic lymph node dissection may be partly explained by the extent of the lymph node dissection. Retrospective studies suggest that recurrence-free and cancer-specific survival depend on the extent of local and regional disease and maximizing its removal. In the late 1990s, Poulsen and associates demonstrated that extending the limits of pelvic lymph node dissection from the common iliac bifurcation to the bifurcation of the aorta, along with removal of the perivesical fat containing paravesical lymph nodes, improves the recurrence-free survival rate following radical cystectomy for bladder cancer confined to the bladder wall (pT3a) (85% for <pT3a versus 64% for those with pT3b) (10). Moreover, Herr et al. reported a 92% survival rate in patients with pT2N0 disease with the removal of at least nine lymph nodes, compared to 53% survival in those who underwent less extensive dissections. Significant differences in mortality were also found among patients with pT3N0 and pT4N0 disease using the same threshold of nine lymph nodes. In those with nodal disease, a survival benefit was noted with the removal of >11 nodes (3). Similarly, Stein et al. determined that >15 lymph nodes was the cutoff point associated with a significant benefit in 5- and 10-year recurrence-free survival. They also calculated the lymph node density (ratio of positive lymph nodes to total lymph nodes) and found a density of <20% to be associated with decreasing recurrence-free survival (12).

While the extent of lymphadenectomy necessarily remains debatable and a randomized, prospective trial is needed to determine which dissection should be employed, what is not in question is that a pelvic lymph node dissection is the standard of care.

## OUTCOMES

Although pelvic lymph node dissection is usually a relatively short procedure with little morbidity, it has potential for significant complications. These can be divided into intra- and postoperative (early and late) complications (Table 27.2). Paul

**TABLE 27.2**

**COMPLICATIONS OF PELVIC LYMPHADENECTOMY**

| INTRAOPERATIVE COMPLICATIONS |
|---|
| Vascular injury |
| Ureteral injury |
| Obturator nerve injury |
| **POSTOPERATIVE COMPLICATIONS** |
| *Wound-Related* |
| Hematoma |
| Seroma |
| Wound infection |
| Wound dehiscence |
| *Non–Wound-Related* |
| Pulmonary atelectasis |
| Pneumonia |
| Myocardial infarction |
| Congestive cardiac failure |
| Prolonged lymph drainage |
| Lymphocele formation |
| Deep venous thrombosis/pulmonary embolism |
| Epididymo-orchitis |
| Urinary tract infection |
| Prolonged ileus |
| Urinary retention |
| Chronic lymphedema |

and associates (9) reported an 8.6% incidence of intraoperative complications, an 8.7% immediate postoperative wound complication incidence, and an additional 31.4% immediate non–wound-related complication rate (3). They also reviewed the complication rates reported in multiple studies. These ranged from 4% to 53% with a mean rate of 26.6% (3). Intraoperative complications can be minimized by familiarity with the pelvic anatomy and careful dissection to identify vulnerable structures. The most common vascular injury is to the accessory obturator vein. Care should be taken not to avulse the obturator vessels as they enter the pelvic foramina because they will retract caudally and ligation will be difficult. If this occurs, bone wax can be used. Significant injuries to the external iliac vessels require repair, sometimes with the aid of a vascular surgeon. Transection or avulsion of the obturator nerve leads to difficulties with adduction of the ipsilateral leg and is usually irreparable. Splitting the nodal packet as described reduces the chance of inadvertent nerve injury.

Ureteral injuries are uncommon and require repair when encountered. A problem with ureteral injuries is that they are not always identified at the time of surgery. These are often the result of a clip inadvertently being placed across the ureter. Therefore, as we now dissect out the lymph node packet, we no longer specifically look for the ureter. However, we always place a clip on the upper end of the nodal packet after splitting it over the obturator nerve in a cranial-to-caudal direction to avoid ureteral injury, identified or not. If there is any concern for ureteral injury, the ureter must be dissected out and fully visualized.

Postoperative complications include those related and unrelated to the wound. Wound infections and dehiscence are uncommon. Seroma and hematoma formation are more common and may require drainage and local wound care.

Prolonged lymph drainage and lymphocele formation may occur in 3% to 12% of patients. Prolonged drainage is treated by instilling autologous blood or Betadine solution through the preexisting drains as sclerosing agents. If Jackson–Pratt or similar drains are used, tissue will eventually grow into the drains. This has occurred twice in our experience, and in both cases a general anesthetic was required for drain removal. Although it has been reported that the use of subcutaneous heparin increases the incidence of prolonged lymph drainage, this has not been our experience. Our rate of prolonged lymph drainage and/or symptomatic lymphocele formation is <3%. Treatment of symptomatic lymphoceles varies from percutaneous drainage under radiological guidance and sclerotherapy to laparoscopic or open marsupialization into the peritoneal cavity. Although some lymphatic drainage is expected, careful dissection and meticulous ligation of lymphatic channels help minimize the risk of prolonged drainage.

Any patient with prolonged or excessive lymph drainage must be evaluated for a urinary leak. This may be done by sending a sample of the fluid for creatinine testing.

Thrombophlebitis and deep venous thrombosis are recognized complications of pelvic lymph node dissection. Although the studies are conflicting, most have shown that some method of anticoagulation, low-dose heparin, or pneumatic compression stockings are beneficial in reducing the risk of these complications. We routinely administer subcutaneous heparin preoperatively and every 8 to 12 hours postoperatively as well as use pneumatic compression stockings until the patient is discharged.

Chronic lymphedema of the lower extremities and external genitalia may occur, and this may be worsened by radiotherapy. Although extended dissections have been reported to result in improved survival rates in retrospective studies, they may be associated with increased incidence of lymphedema. The modified pelvic lymph node dissection has been a reliable way of preventing chronic lymphedema.

## ALTERNATIVE THERAPY

Pelvic lymph node dissection is currently the only definitive means of evaluating lymph node status. Enlarged lymph nodes suspicious for metastases may be identified by ultrasound, cross-sectional imaging with thin-cut computerized tomography (CT) scans, magnetic resonance imaging (MRI), and pedal lymphangiography, all of which have low sensitivity. Unless bulky disease is seen on a CT scan (1 cm), a tissue sample (e.g., by CT-guided needle aspiration core biopsy) is required for validation of a suspicious scan finding. Drawbacks with biopsy include size limitation, random sampling error, disruption of nodal architecture, low cellular yield, and need for an expert cytopathologist. While CT scans are routinely done prior to a cystectomy, we very rarely employ them prior to a radical prostatectomy.

The use of PSA alone is not a good predictor of pathological stage, as there can be significant overlap between the two variables. Costly alternatives such as radioisotopic metabolic imaging using positron emission tomography scans and tumor-directed imaging by labeled antibody scans (111In-capromab pendetide, the ProstaScint scan, Cytogen Corp., Princeton, NJ) may offer improvement in detection of nodal metastases over conventional imaging and are only indicated in high-risk patients. Methods to improve specificity, such as fusion of acquired images with three-dimensionally reconstructed MRI, are currently being investigated.

## References

1. Bader P, Burkhard FC, Markwalder R, et al. Is a limited lymph node dissection an adequate staging procedure for prostate cancer? *J Urol* 2002;168(2):514–518; discussion 518.
2. Grossman HB, Natale RB, Tangen CM, et al. Neoadjuvant chemotherapy plus cystectomy compared with cystectomy alone for locally advanced bladder cancer. *N Engl J Med* 2003;349(9):859–866.
3. Herr HW, Bochner BH, Dalbagni G, et al. Impact of the number of lymph nodes retrieved on outcome in patients with muscle invasive bladder cancer. *J Urol* 2002;167(3):1295–1298.
4. Joslyn SA, Konety BR. Impact of extent of lymphadenectomy on survival after radical prostatectomy for prostate cancer. *Urology* 2006;68(1):121–125.
5. Leissner J, Ghoneim MA, Abol-Enein H, et al. Extended radical lymphadenectomy in patients with urothelial bladder cancer: results of a prospective multicenter study. *J Urol* 2004;171(1):139–144.
6. Mattei A, Fuechsel FG, Bhatta Dhar N, et al. The template of the primary lymphatic landing sites of the prostate should be revisited: results of a multimodality mapping study. *Eur Urol* 2008;53(1):118–125.
7. Meng MV, Carroll PR. When is pelvic lymph node dissection necessary before radical prostatectomy? A decision analysis. *J Urol* 2000;164(4):1235–1240.
8. Partin AW, Kattan MW, Subong EN, et al. Combination of prostate-specific antigen, clinical stage, and Gleason score to predict pathological stage of localized prostate cancer. A multi-institutional update. *JAMA* 1997;277(18):1445–1451.
9. Paul DB, Loening SA, Narayana AS, et al. Morbidity from pelvic lymphadenectomy in staging carcinoma of the prostate. J Urol 1983;129(6):1141–1144.
10. Poulsen AL, Horn T, Steven K. Radical cystectomy: extending the limits of pelvic lymph node dissection improves survival for patients with bladder cancer confined to the bladder wall. *J Urol* 1998;160(6, Pt 1):2015–2019; discussion 2020.
11. Skinner DG. Management of invasive bladder cancer: a meticulous pelvic node dissection can make a difference. *J Urol* 1982;128(1):34–36.
12. Stein JP, Cai J, Groshen S, et al. Risk factors for patients with pelvic lymph node metastases following radical cystectomy with en bloc pelvic lymphadenectomy: concept of lymph node density. *J Urol* 2003;170(1):35–41.
13. Stein JP, Penson DF, Cai J, et al. Radical cystectomy with extended lymphadenectomy: evaluating separate package versus en bloc submission for node positive bladder cancer. *J Urol* 2007;177(3):876–881; discussion 881–882.

# CHAPTER 28 ■ OPEN RADICAL RETROPUBIC PROSTATECTOMY

MISOP HAN AND WILLIAM J. CATALONA

Over the past two decades, the management of patients with clinically localized prostate cancer has changed dramatically. Widespread screening with serum prostate-specific antigen (PSA) and digital rectal examination has allowed much earlier detection of prostate cancer (1, 2). Modification of the surgical technique of radical retropubic prostatectomy has allowed better hemostasis, improved visualization during dissection, and facilitated preservation of neurovascular bundles supplying the corpora cavernosa (3). As a result, radical prostatectomy can be performed with a high cure rate while preserving urinary and erectile function in the majority of patients. Thus, radical prostatectomy has become the most commonly performed treatment for clinically localized prostate cancer, with abundant long-term data confirming its efficacy. In this chapter, we discuss the technique, outcomes, and complications of anatomic radical retropubic prostatectomy using the senior author's surgical series, now including >5,000 anatomic radical retropubic prostatectomies as an example.

## INDICATIONS FOR SURGERY

Radical prostatectomy is indicated for men with a life expectancy of at least ten years, a completely resectable and biologically significant tumor, and no comorbidity that might make the operation unacceptably risky. Actuarial life tables can project the life expectancy of US men, and with appropriate adjustment for comorbidities, life expectancy can be estimated for the individual patient.

After confirming the likelihood of a sufficiently long life expectancy, the next step in patient selection is to identify those with potentially curable disease. Radical prostatectomy provides the best chance for cure for men whose tumor is confined to the prostate gland. Nomograms predicting the pathologic stage based on preoperative clinical and pathologic parameters have been widely used to identify patients who are likely to benefit from the surgical resection and those who are not (4). Alternatively, nomograms predicting recurrence-free survival probabilities following treatment also are sometimes useful for patients (5,6).

## ALTERNATIVE THERAPY

Alternatives to radical retropubic prostatectomy include watchful waiting/expectant management, hormonal manipulation, brachytherapy, external beam radiation therapy, and other alternative surgical approaches such as radical perineal prostatectomy and laparoscopic radical prostatectomy with or without robotic assistance.

## SURGICAL TECHNIQUE

Before the operation, a first-generation cephalosporin (or appropriate substitute, if the patient is allergic to cephalosporins) antibiotic is given intravenously. After a general endotracheal or regional anesthesia is administered, thigh-high elastic hose are placed on the patient. Sequential compression devices and prophylactic low-dose heparin are used only in patients with increased risk for thromboembolic complications. The patient is positioned with his legs on spreader bars, and the operating table is dorsiflexed with the break just above the patient's anterosuperior iliac spine (Fig. 28.1). The abdomen and genitalia are appropriately prepared and draped.

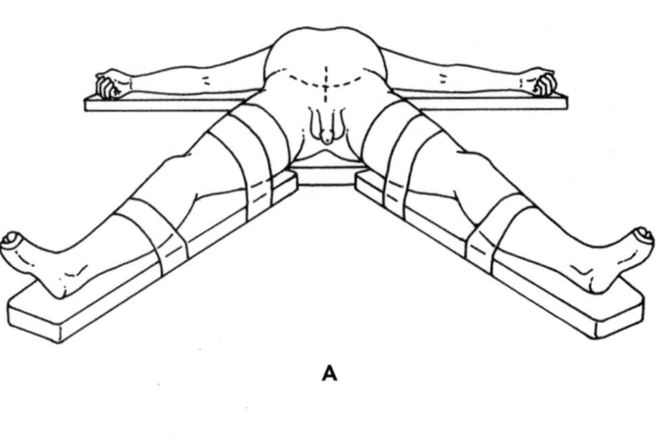

A

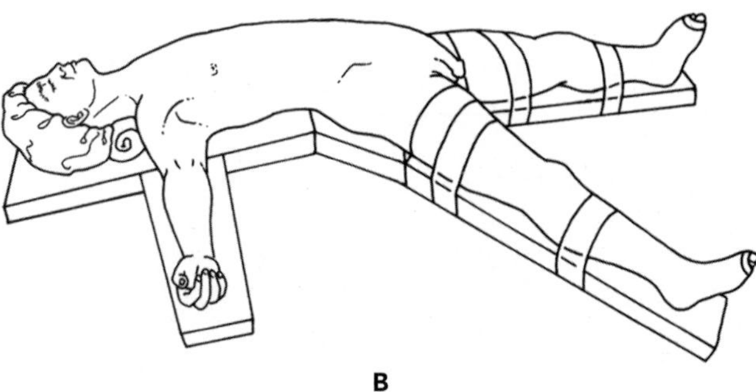

B

FIGURE 28.1 A and B: Positioning of the patient. Legs are separated on spreader bars. The operating table is flexed with the break just above the patient's anterosuperior iliac spine. (From M Han, WJ Catalona. Anatomic nerve-sparing radical retropubic prostatectomy. Chapter 29, 2005; 514–527, with permission.)

There are nine key steps in performing anatomic nerve-sparing radical prostatectomy:

1. A limited pelvic lymphadenectomy
2. Incision of the endopelvic fascia and the puboprostatic ligaments
3. Proximal and distal suture ligation, and transection of the dorsal venous complex
4. Placement of hemostatic sutures in the neurovascular bundles and the prostatic pedicles
5. Dissection of the prostate from the neurovascular bundles
6. Vascular control and transection of the prostatic pedicles
7. Transection and reconstruction of the bladder neck
8. Dissection of the seminal vesicles and ampullary portions of the vasa deferentia
9. Performance of the vesicourethral anastomosis

These steps are described in detail below with corresponding illustrations.

### 1. A Limited Pelvic Lymphadenectomy

A superficial midline (or transverse) lower abdominal incision (usually between 4 and 5 in. in length, depending upon the patient's body habitus) is made with a scalpel. The linea alba is incised and the space of Retzius is entered. Anatomic radical retropubic prostatectomy performed in the extraperitoneal space is arguably less invasive than laparoscopic and robotic prostatectomy, in which a transperitoneal approach is frequently used. By avoiding any entry into the peritoneal cavity, anatomic radical retropubic prostatectomy can be performed while minimizing the risk of injury to bowel, major vascular structures, and other adjacent organs. In addition, the cosmetic results are not significantly different between a single, limited infraumbilical incision for anatomic radical retropubic prostatectomy and multiple laparoscopic port site incisions and an incision for prostate removal during laparoscopic or robotic prostatectomy.

Taking care to avoid disrupting the lymphatic tissue lateral to the external iliac vein and to avoid compression of the vein itself, a Balfour retractor is placed. A modified pelvic lymphadenectomy is performed, removing only the lymph nodes medial to the external iliac vein. Care is taken during the lymphadenectomy to preserve any accessory arterial branches to the corpora cavernosa that arise from the distal external iliac or obturator arteries. The obturator nerve is identified and preserved. In most incidences, the patient elects to have the prostate gland removed, even if there are pelvic lymph node metastases; otherwise, the excised lymph node packet is sent for frozen section examination. If the patient elects not to have the prostate removed and there are lymph node metastases, frozen section examination of the lymph nodes is performed. If frozen sections reveal metastatic cancer, the operation is terminated. Lymphadenectomy is optional in patients who are at low risk for pelvic lymph node metastases by virtue of a low Gleason grade, low PSA, and low biopsy tumor volume.

After completing the lymphadenectomy, the adipose and areolar tissues are swept gently from the anterior surface of the prostate and the endopelvic fascia to expose the puboprostatic ligaments. Care is taken to avoid injury to the perforating branches of the Santorini plexus that pierce the

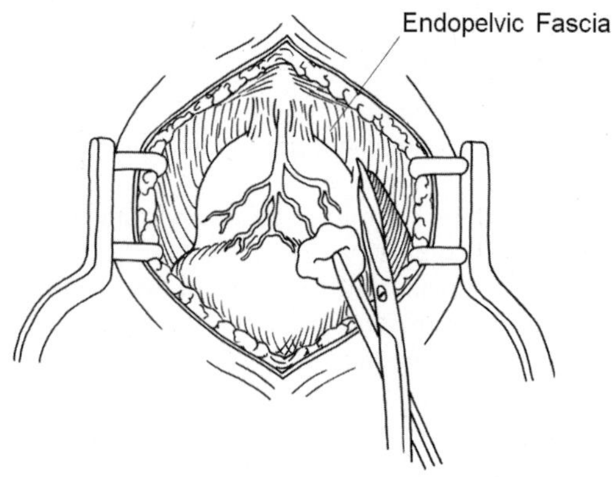


FIGURE 28.2 The endopelvic fascia is incised in the groove between the levator ani muscles and the lateral border of the prostate. (From Han, Catalona. Anatomic nerve-sparing radical retropubic prostatectomy. *Urol Oncol* 2005; 516–525, with permission.)

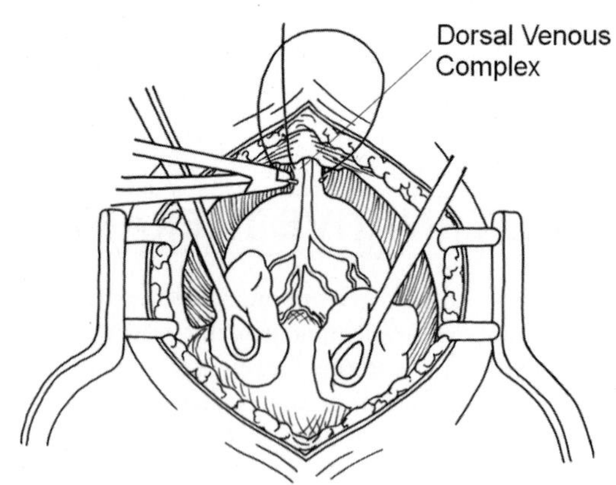


FIGURE 28.4 The dorsal venous complex is suture-ligated with a 2-0 chromic catgut suture on a CT-1 needle. (From Han, Catalona. Anatomic nerve-sparing radical retropubic prostatectomy. *Urol Oncol* 2005; 516–525, with permission.)

endopelvic fascia between the puboprostatic ligaments and pass cephalad on the anterior surface of the prostate gland and bladder.

## 2. Incision of the Endopelvic Fascia and the Puboprostatic Ligaments

The endopelvic fascia is incised in the groove between the levator ani muscles and the lateral border of the prostate (Fig. 28.2). Inside the endopelvic fascia, the lateral surface of the prostate is covered by a smooth, glistening membrane overlying the lateral portion of the Santorini plexus. Strands of the levator ani muscles are gently dissected off the prostate to the level of the urogenital diaphragm. Often, venous tributaries pass from the levator ani muscles to the prostate just lateral to the puboprostatic ligaments. These vessels are cauterized, secured with hemostatic clips, or ligated laterally; then they are clamped medially with a delicate snub-nose right-angle clamp. After the vein is transected sharply, its medial portion is ligated. When the endopelvic fascia has been opened from the base to the apex of the prostate, the superficial branch of the Santorini plexus is gently retracted medially, and the puboprostatic ligaments are placed on stretch and partially divided close to the pubic symphysis (Fig. 28.3). To avoid injuring the dorsal venous complex, care is taken not to divide the puboprostatic ligaments too medially or too far under the pubic symphysis.

## 3. Suture Ligation and Transection of the Dorsal Venous Complex

After the puboprostatic ligaments have been divided, the lateral surfaces of the urethra are palpated. The groove between the anterior surface of the urethra and the dorsal venous complex is developed with a pinching motion of the left index finger and thumb. The plane between the urethra and the dorsal venous complex is then developed gently, first with a large right-angle clamp. This facilitates tight ligation of the dorsal venous complex. After the dorsal venous complex has been ligated, it is also suture-ligated in a slightly more caudal site with a 2-0 chromic catgut suture on a CT-1 needle (Fig. 28.4). A suture ligature is also placed in the anterior surface of the prostate to reduce the back-bleeding from the Santorini plexus (Fig. 28.5).

The right-angle clamp is then passed behind the dorsal venous complex, and the jaws of the clamp are spread. The dorsal venous complex is transected with electrocautery or a

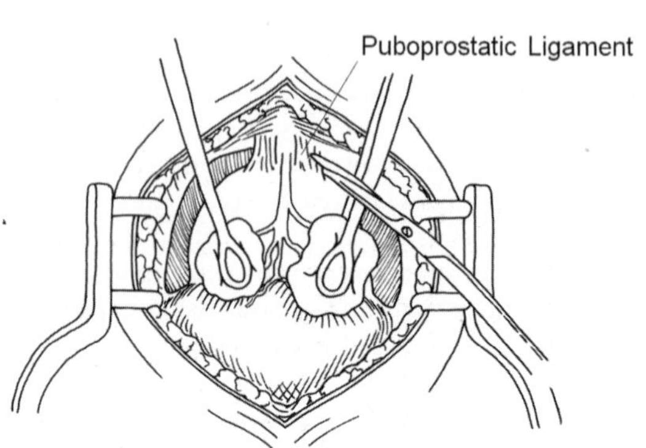


FIGURE 28.3 The puboprostatic ligaments are placed on stretch and incised. (From Han, Catalona. Anatomic nerve-sparing radical retropubic prostatectomy. *Urol Oncol* 2005;516–525, with permission.)

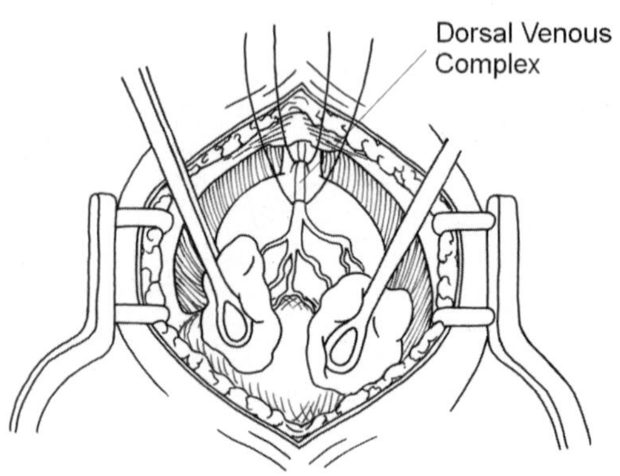


FIGURE 28.5 To reduce back-bleeding from the Santorini plexus, the cephalad aspect of the dorsal venous complex is suture–ligated. (From Han, Catalona. Anatomic nerve-sparing radical retropubic prostatectomy. *Urol Oncol* 2005;516–525, with permission.)

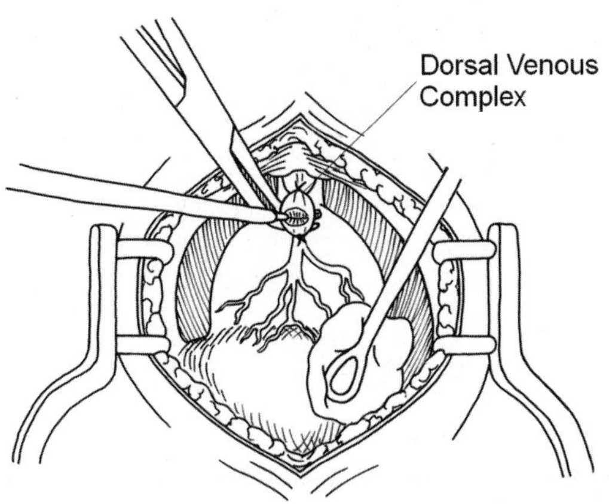


FIGURE 28.6 The dorsal venous complex is transected with a right-angle clamp jaws spread behind the complex. (From Han, Catalona. Anatomic nerve-sparing radical retropubic prostatectomy. *Urol Oncol* 2005;516–525, with permission.)

scalpel (Fig. 28.6). Back-bleeding from the dorsal venous complex is controlled with figure-of-eight 3-0 sutures. It is important to obtain good hemostasis at this time to allow the apical dissection of the prostate to be performed in a relatively bloodless field. If the dorsal venous complex ligature slips off, the complex is oversewn using a 3-0 chromic catgut suture on a 5/8-circle needle. The goal in oversewing the complex is to pass the suture just through the lateral borders of the complex itself in its anterior, middle, and posterior aspects. Wide, imprecisely placed sutures may damage the neurovascular bundles.

The anterior surface of the urethra is palpated between the neurovascular bundles. The circumurethral sphincter muscle and the anterior wall of the urethra are incised with a scalpel just distal to the apex of the prostate without dissecting around the lateral or posterior surfaces of the urethra (Figs. 28.7 and 28.8). The incision should not be carried too far laterally, or it may injure the neurovascular bundles. The urethral catheter is exposed and carefully hooked with a delicate right-angle clamp. Gentle traction on the clamp in a cephalad direction exposes the posterior urethral wall. The catheter is divided and placed on gentle cephalad traction, and the posterior urethral wall is sharply transected.

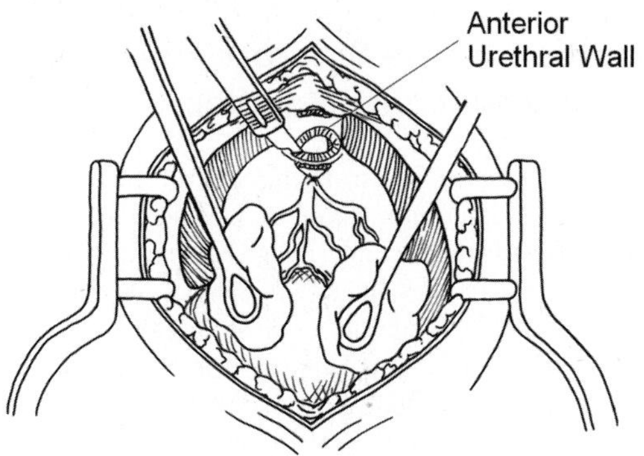


FIGURE 28.8 The anterior wall of the urethra is incised with a scalpel without dissecting around the lateral or posterior surfaces of the urethra. (From Han, Catalona. Anatomic nerve-sparing radical retropubic prostatectomy. *Urol Oncol* 2005;516–525, with permission.)

Fibromuscular bands tethering the apex of the prostate to the pelvic floor are incised using sharp dissection (Fig. 28.9). The rectourethralis muscle is incised, exposing the prerectal fat.

## 4. Placement of "Prophylactic" Hemostatic Sutures in the Neurovascular Bundles and Prostatic Pedicles

To reduce bleeding during the dissection of the neurovascular bundles and prostatic pedicles in a manner similar to that achieved with the pneumoperitoneum during laparoscopic surgery, "prophylactic" hemostatic figure-of-eight suture ligatures of 4-0 plain catgut are placed in the neurovascular bundles lateral to the prostate. Similarly, 3-0 suture ligatures are placed in the prostatic pedicles. After these sutures have been placed on both sides of the prostate, sharp, energy-free dissection can be used to dissect the neurovascular bundles from the prostate. The prophylactic hemostatic sutures are tied "softly" to avoid crushing the nerve fibers in the neurovascular bundles, and the plain catgut sutures are quickly absorbed. This technique minimizes or avoids the use of hemostatic clips and sutures that may permanently entrap the neurovascular bundles.

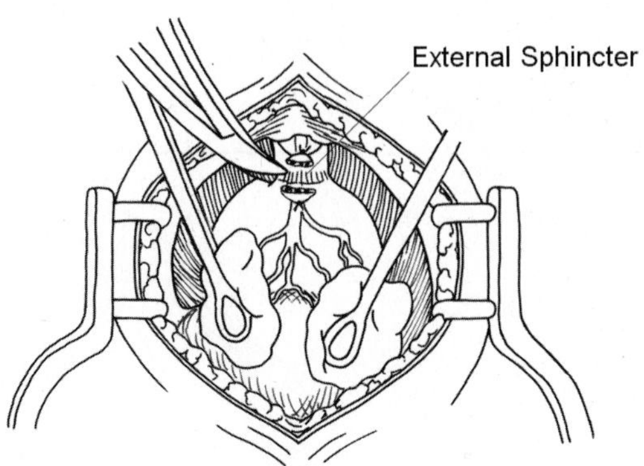


FIGURE 28.7 The circumurethral external sphincter muscle fibers are incised to expose the urethra. (From Han, Catalona. Anatomic nerve-sparing radical retropubic prostatectomy. *Urol Oncol* 2005;516–525, with permission.)

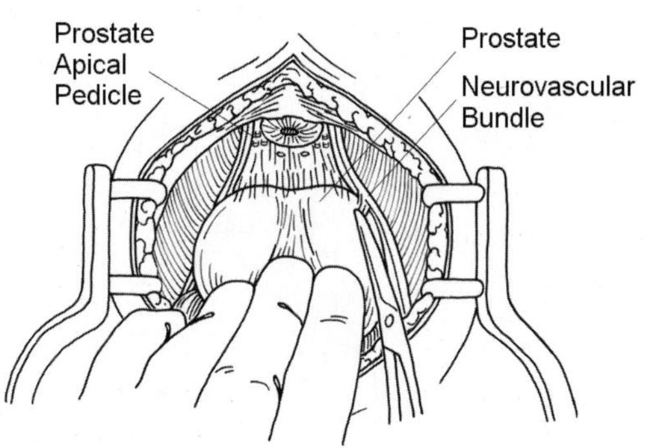


FIGURE 28.9 The apical pedicles of the prostate may require suture ligation. Fibromuscular bands tethering the apex of the prostate to the pelvic floor are incised using sharp dissection. The prostate gland is dissected from neurovascular bundles. (From Han, Catalona. Anatomic nerve-sparing radical retropubic prostatectomy. *Urol Oncol* 2005;516–525, with permission.)

## 5. Separation of the Prostate from the Neurovascular Bundles

The lateral pelvic fascia is incised from the apex of the prostate to the base. A delicate right-angle clamp may be used to elevate the lateral pelvic fascia from the underlying veins on the surface of the prostate. Recent studies suggest that high, anterior release of the neurovascular bundles is associated with improved potency rates. This maneuver must be performed carefully in patients with high-grade and high-volume disease and is sometimes difficult to perform in patients with periprostatic fibrosis or inflammatory changes. Small perforating bleeders not controlled by the prophylactic hemostatic sutures may be secured with hemoclips, ties, or ligatures to ensure adequate hemostasis. The plane between the prostate and the neurovascular bundles is developed using sharp and blunt dissection, allowing the prostate to assume a more anterior position in the pelvis.

The lateral aspect of the prostate is then dissected from the neurovascular bundles, allowing the bundles to retract laterally. In a case of extensive fibrosis, the dissection is performed only sharply to avoid tearing into the rectum with blunt dissection. The dissection is carried cephalad until the portion of the Denonvilliers fascia covering the ampullary portions of the vasa deferentia and the seminal vesicles is exposed (Fig. 28.10). The Denonvilliers fascia is incised with the cautery. The Metzenbaum scissors are then used to develop the proper plane of dissection for the prostatic vascular pedicles. If there is continued bleeding from the periurethral tissues and apical pedicles of the prostate, hemostatic sutures should be placed at this juncture to avoid continued blood loss during the remainder of the procedure.

## 6. Vascular Control and Transection of Prostatic Pedicles

The prostatic pedicles are divided by inserting the right-angle clamp medial to them, with the tip of the clamp directed almost parallel to the lateral surface of the prostate. The prostatic pedicle is ligated or hemoclipped laterally, taking care to place the tie or clip medial to the neurovascular bundle

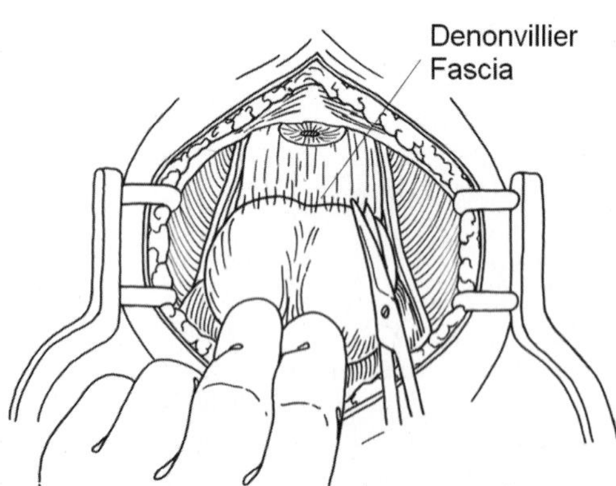


FIGURE 28.10 The dissection is carried cephalad until the portion of the Denonvilliers fascia covering the ampullary portions of the vasa deferentia and the seminal vesicles is exposed. The Denonvilliers fascia is incised with cautery to expose vascular pedicles at prostate base. (From Han, Catalona. Anatomic nerve-sparing radical retropubic prostatectomy. *Urol Oncol* 2005;516–525, with permission.)

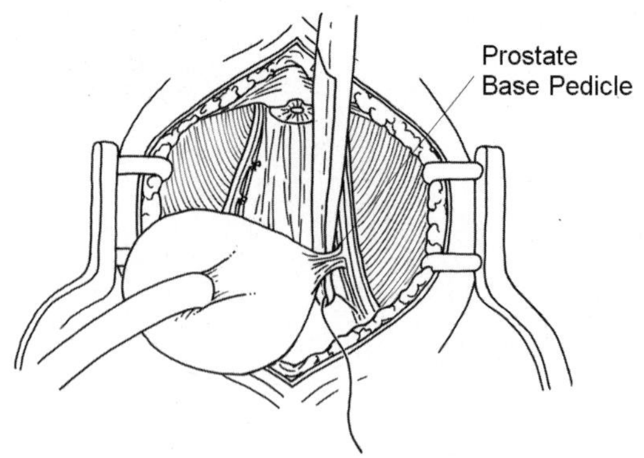


FIGURE 28.11 The prostate base pedicle is ligated or hemoclipped laterally, taking care to place the tie medial to the neurovascular bundle. (From Han, Catalona. Anatomic nerve-sparing radical retropubic prostatectomy. *Urol Oncol* 2005;516–525, with permission.)

(Fig. 28.11). The pedicle is divided close to the prostate. This dissection is performed on both sides to a point cephalad to the seminal vesicles. Care is taken when dissecting near the seminal vesicles to avoid injuring the neurovascular bundles that are situated just lateral to the seminal vesicles. The seminal vesicles are freed from the bladder base using sharp and blunt dissection, and a large right-angle clamp may be used to further develop this plane. Two hemostatic sutures of 3-0 chromic catgut are placed in the lateral bladder pedicles cephalad to the seminal vesicles, one just lateral to the prostate and another just medial to the neurovascular bundles. The lateral bladder neck fibers are then partially incised with the cautery but not through their entire thickness.

## 7. Transection and Reconstruction of the Bladder Neck

The anterior bladder neck is transected with electrocautery in the natural groove between the bladder and the prostate. The bladder neck opening is enlarged with scissors, and the catheter is pulled through and used as a tractor on the prostate (Fig. 28.12). The posterior bladder neck is incised with the

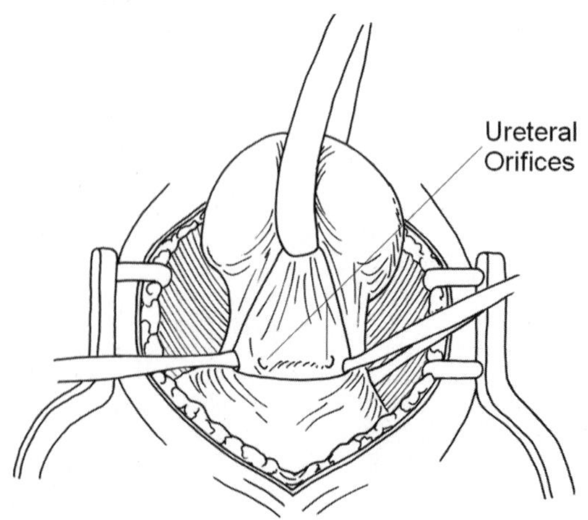


FIGURE 28.12 The anterior bladder neck is transected in the natural groove between the bladder and the prostate. The bladder neck opening is enlarged with scissors. The ureteral orifices are identified. (From Han, Catalona. Anatomic nerve-sparing radical retropubic prostatectomy. *Urol Oncol* 2005;516–525, with permission.)

cautery. The muscular attachments between the bladder and prostate are divided using electrocautery and/or hemostatic clips for hemostasis.

## 8. Dissection of Seminal Vesicles and Ampullary Portions of the Vasa Deferentia

The seminal vesicles are dissected first along their lateral edges, carrying the plane of dissection medially. Many small perforating arteries enter the lateral and terminal portions of the seminal vesicles. These are secured with small hemoclips. The ampullae are freed, using sharp and blunt dissection, and then are clipped and transected. After the seminal vesicles have been dissected to their tips and the hemoclips placed, the surgical specimen is removed. At this point, the pelvis is carefully inspected for hemostasis. Small bleeders on the neurovascular bundles may require 4-0 absorbable suture ligatures. It is important not to use the cautery for hemostasis on the neurovascular bundles, to avoid cautery injury to the cavernosal nerves. Suture ligatures of 3-0 or 4-0 absorbable material are placed in the "pockets" of the seminal vesicle pedicles on the medial aspects of the neurovascular bundles to ensure good hemostasis in this difficult-to-visualize region.

## 9. Vesicourethral Anastomosis

Reconstruction of the bladder neck begins by placing a continuous running everting suture of 3-0 chromic catgut that encompasses bladder mucosa and underlying muscle for a distance of nearly the entire anastomotic circumference (Fig. 28.13). The bladder neck is then reconstructed in a tennis racket fashion, with the handle of the racket directed posteriorly. The bladder neck closure is accomplished with a continuous 2-0 chromic catgut suture. Care should be taken to avoid compromising the ureteral orifices. The bladder neck is closed to a size of approximately 22Fr to 24Fr. Closing the bladder neck to a smaller caliber may lead to postoperative vesicourethral anastomotic stricture.

An 18Fr catheter is passed through the urethra. While an assistant exerts pressure on the perineum with a sponge forceps

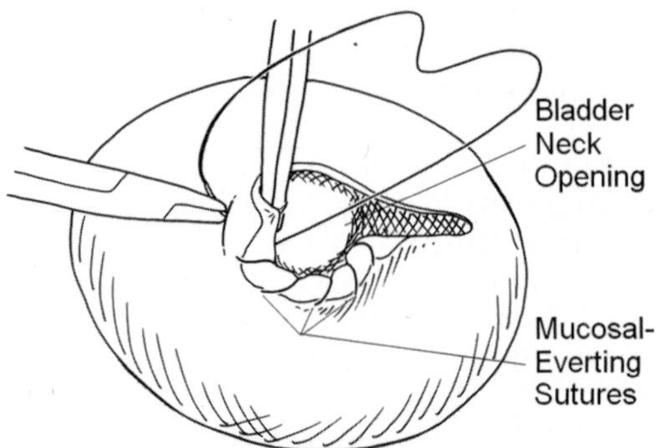


FIGURE 28.13 A continuous running mucosa-everting suture of 3-0 chromic catgut is placed for a distance of nearly the entire anastomotic circumference. (From Han, Catalona. Anatomic nerve-sparing radical retropubic prostatectomy. *Urol Oncol* 2005;516–525, with permission.)

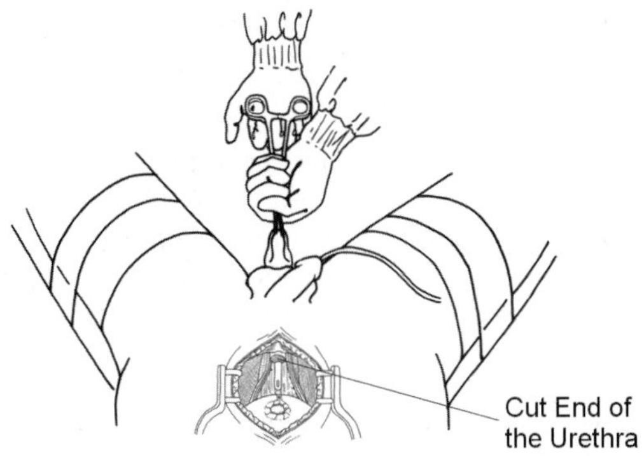


FIGURE 28.14 Perineal pressure is applied with a sponge forceps to better expose the cut end of the urethra. (From Han, Catalona. Anatomic nerve-sparing radical retropubic prostatectomy. *Urol Oncol* 2005;516–525, with permission.)

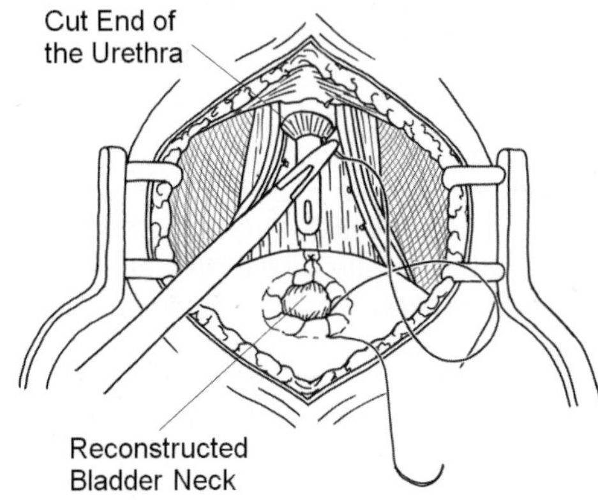


FIGURE 28.15 Double-armed 2-0 chromic catgut sutures are used for the vesicourethral anastomosis. (From Han, Catalona. Anatomic nerve-sparing radical retropubic prostatectomy. *Urol Oncol* 2005; 516–525, with permission.)

to better expose the cut end of the urethra (Fig. 28.14), double-armed 2-0 chromic catgut sutures are used for the vesicourethral anastomosis (Fig. 28.15). A 5/8-circle needle is used to place the sutures in the urethra from inside to outside, avoiding placing the suture into the neurovascular bundles. The tip of the catheter is grasped and brought out of the wound to expose the posterior lip of the cut end of the urethra. The posterior sutures are similarly placed. The anterior sutures are placed at the 10 o'clock and 2 o'clock positions, and the posterior sutures are placed at the 5 o'clock and 7 o'clock positions. In addition, a stronger 2-0 monocryl suture is placed at the 6 o'clock position to secure the most posterior aspect of the reconstructed bladder neck to the urethral stump. The other ends of the sutures containing an 1/2 circle taper point needle are placed in the corresponding positions of the bladder neck from inside to outside. These sutures encompass mucosa and muscle and exit at the edge of the mucosa. The catheter tip is placed in the bladder, and the bladder neck is guided gently toward the cut end of the urethra. The anastomotic sutures are tied carefully under direct vision. The bladder is then irrigated free of clots, and a single suction drain is placed in the pelvis and brought out the lower end of the wound. The incision is closed with no. 1 loop Maxon running sutures on the fascia, 2-0 chromic catgut suture on the subcutaneous tissue, and a 4-0 monofilament absorbable subcuticular suture on the skin. The skin incision is covered with Steri-Strips.

### Postoperative Care

Patients are ambulated with assistance once or twice on the day of surgery, 5 times on the first postoperative day, and 7 times on the second postoperative day. A clear liquid diet is given on the night of surgery, advancing to a regular diet as tolerated on the following days. A suction drain and dressing are removed, and the patient is usually discharged from the hospital on the second postoperative day. Intravenous antibiotics are discontinued after the suction drain is removed. For analgesia, ketorolac (30 to 60 mg) is given intravenously every 6 hours for the first 48 hours. It may be supplemented with acetaminophen or sparingly with morphine, as needed.

Although some claim a quicker recovery following laparoscopic surgery compared to anatomic radical retropubic prostatectomy, a recent study has shown similar low narcotic usage and patient-reported pain scores regardless of which approach was used (7). Therefore, the same clinical care pathway, without a significant difference in length of hospital stay, can be applied to patients treated by either open radical prostatectomy or laparoscopic/robot-assisted radical prostatectomy. Most patients are discharged from the hospital on the second or third postoperative day following anatomic radical retropubic prostatectomy.

Antibiotic ointment is applied to the urethral meatus around the catheter 4 to 6 times a day until catheter removal. The catheter may be removed on the seventh, tenth, or fourteenth postoperative day, depending upon the perceived amount of tension on the vesicourethral anastomosis. A cystogram is not performed before removing the catheter unless an anastomotic leak is suspected. The catheter should not be removed before 7 days, as 10% to 15% of men may experience urinary retention from edema and require recatheterization. An oral fluoroquinolone antibiotic is given 1 day before and 1 week following the catheter removal. Daily Kegel exercises are performed in four sets of ten, before the surgery and following the catheter removal until continence returns. A protective pad or diaper is used until complete urinary control is achieved. The first postoperative serum PSA level is measured 1 month after the operation.

## OUTCOMES

### Cancer Control Outcome

The most important objective of radical prostatectomy is cancer control. A rising serum PSA level is usually the earliest evidence of recurrence or progression following prostatectomy. Because follow-up data are not sufficiently mature to effectively evaluate cancer-specific survival trends, biochemical-recurrence-(detectable serum PSA)–free survival has been used frequently as a surrogate in evaluating treatment efficacy in radical retropubic prostatectomy series.

Analyses of the senior author's series recently have been reported (8). They include almost 3,500 men who underwent anatomic radical retropubic prostatectomy between 1983 and 2003, including those with adverse prognostic features. Cancer progression was defined as detectable serum PSA (>0.2 ng per mL), local recurrence, or distant metastases. With a mean follow-up of 65 months (range, 0–233), actuarial ten-year cancer progression-free survival probability was 68%. Actuarial ten-year cancer-specific and overall survival rates were 97% and 83%, respectively. Other large radical prostatectomy series have reported similar excellent results (9,10). Similar long-term oncological outcome results are not yet available in laparoscopic or robotic prostatectomy series.

### Urinary Continence Outcome

The overall urinary continence outcome following nerve-sparing radical retropubic prostatectomy was excellent in the current series. More than 93% of men achieved complete urinary continence, defined as requiring no protection for daily activities (11). The return of urinary continence was strongly associated with the age of the patient. For example, >95% of men younger than age 50 were continent following surgery. In contrast, 86% of men above age 70 were continent postoperatively. Only four men (0.2%) eventually required an artificial urinary sphincter placement for stress urinary incontinence. The relative long-term functional outcomes of laparoscopic and robotic prostatectomy methods are yet unknown.

### Erectile Function Outcome

There are several possible goals of the nerve-sparing aspect of radical retropubic prostatectomy. Patients with intact libido and erectile potency want to maintain their current quality of erections or erections sufficient for penetration with the help of oral medication, such as phosphodiesterase type 5 inhibitors. Others with poor-quality erections preoperatively might accept erections that at least offer some rigidity to provide sensory satisfaction for both sexual partners. The erectile potency in the current series was defined as an ability to maintain erections strong enough for penetration with or without the help of oral phosphodiesterase inhibitors.

The return of erectile potency following radical retropubic prostatectomy was strongly associated with the age of the patient, preoperative potency status, nerve-sparing status (bilateral versus partial sparing), and the era of surgery (1980s versus 1990s) (11). More than 75% of men younger than age 60 regained potency following bilateral nerve-sparing radical retropubic prostatectomy. In the modern era, >95% of men below age 50 recovered potency following surgery. Between 62% and 72% of men in their 60s became potent following bilateral nerve-sparing surgery. Finally, there was a significant improvement in recovery of potency in men treated in the 1990s compared to those treated in the 1980s, even after correcting for the age and nerve-sparing status. In the most favorable candidates in whom preoperative potency is normal and bilateral nerve-sparing surgery can be performed, approximately 95% in their 40s, 85% in their 50s, 75% in their 60s, and 50% in their 70s will recover erections sufficient for penetration and intercourse with or without the aid of phosphodiesterase type 5 inhibitors.

The senior author now strongly encourages patients to begin an erectile dysfunction rehabilitation program beginning 1 month postoperatively, using intracavernosal injections of Tri-Mix two to three times per week. This regimen provides excellent rigid erections with well-oxygenated arterial blood and also provides the patient with a method to return to a relatively normal sex life soon after surgery. Patients may transition to oral phosphodiesterase inhibitor therapy when spontaneous erections begin to return.

## COMPLICATIONS

With careful selection of patients and performance of necessary cardiovascular evaluation, perioperative mortality can be largely avoided. There was no intraoperative or immediate postoperative mortality in the current series.

The overall complication rate of radical prostatectomy was 9% in the current series (12). Initially, the complications occurred more commonly in older men, but the overall complication rate gradually decreased with the surgeon's experience. The most common complications of anatomic nerve-sparing radical retropubic prostatectomy included anastomotic stricture (bladder neck contracture), thromboembolic complications (deep vein thrombosis and pulmonary embolism), and postoperative inguinal hernia. In the current series, the rate of anastomotic stricture decreased from 8% in the 1980s to <1% after 1990. Similarly, a marked decrease in thromboembolic events was observed, with the rate decreasing from 3% to 1% during the past 20 years. Other rare complications (<1%) associated with radical prostatectomy included infection, lymphocele formation, neurologic deficit, and cardiovascular events.

Anastomotic stricture can be initially managed with a gentle, serial dilation. Alternatively, a careful internal urethrotomy can be performed. For a long and persistent stricture, a transurethral resection of the scar tissue cephalad to the external sphincter may be necessary. Care should be taken to avoid cutting too deeply in the posterior direction to avoid creating a fistula with the rectum. After resection, triamcinolone can be injected via a cystoscopic approach to prevent inflammatory response and subsequent, recurrent scar formation. Usually, an interval of self-catheter dilation of the anastomosis is required.

Inadvertent injury to the obturator nerve can occur during the pelvic lymphadenectomy. When a tension-free primary nerve repair is not feasible, nerve grafting can be performed utilizing either the sural nerve or the lateral antebrachial cutaneous nerve. However, even without a nerve repair, conservative management with physical therapy can compensate for the deficit, and many patients do not exhibit significant thigh adductor deficit following the injury.

An injury to the ureter can occur inadvertently during the transection of the bladder neck or the dissection of the lateral prostate pedicles. When recognized, a simple mobilization of the distal ureter and ureteroneocystostomy should be performed. The reimplanted ureter should be cannulated using a 5Fr or 8Fr pediatric feeding tube to prevent the urinary obstruction due to the edema at the reimplantation site.

Usually, a rectal injury can be repaired primarily using a multiple-layer closure. However, a diverting colostomy should be strongly considered in men with a large rectal defect, a history of pelvic radiotherapy, or long-term preoperative steroid therapy.

## *References*

1. Catalona WJ, Smith DS, Ratliff TL, et al. Measurement of prostate-specific antigen in serum as a screening test for prostate cancer. *N Engl J Med* 1991;324(17):1156–1161.
2. Han M, Partin AW, Piantadosi S, et al. Era specific biochemical recurrence-free survival following radical prostatectomy for clinically localized prostate cancer. *J Urol* 2001;166(2):416–419.
3. Walsh PC, Donker PJ. Impotence following radical prostatectomy: insight into etiology and prevention. *J Urol* 1982;128(3):492–497.
4. Makarov DV, Trock BJ, Humphreys EB, et al. Updated nomogram to predict pathologic stage of prostate cancer given prostate-specific antigen level, clinical stage, and biopsy Gleason score (Partin tables) based on cases from 2000 to 2005. *Urology* 2007;69(6):1095–1101.
5. Stephenson AJ, Scardino PT, Eastham JA, et al. Preoperative nomogram predicting the 10-year probability of prostate cancer recurrence after radical prostatectomy. *J Natl Cancer Inst* 2006;98(10):715–717.
6. Han M, Partin AW, Zahurak M, et al. Biochemical (prostate specific antigen) recurrence probability following radical prostatectomy for clinically localized prostate cancer. *J Urol* 2003;169(2):517–523.
7. Webster TM, Herrell SD, Chang SS, et al. Robotic assisted laparoscpic radical prostatectomy versus retropubic radical prostatectomy: a prospective assessment of postoperative pain. *J Urol* 2005;174:912.
8. Roehl KA, Han M, Ramos CG, et al. Cancer progression and survival rates following anatomical radical retropubic prostatectomy in 3,478 consecutive patients: long-term results. *J Urol* 2004;172(3):910–914.
9. Hull GW, Rabbani F, Abbas F, et al. Cancer control with radical prostatectomy alone in 1,000 consecutive patients. *J Urol* 2002;167(2, Pt 1): 528–534.
10. Han M, Partin AW, Pound CR, et al. Long-term biochemical disease-free and cancer-specific survival following anatomic radical retropubic prostatectomy. The 15-year Johns Hopkins experience. *Urol Clin North Am* 2001;28(3):555–565.
11. Catalona W, Roehl KA, Antenor JA. Potency, continence, complications, and survival analysis in 3,032 consecutive radical retropubic prostatectomies. *J Urol* 2002;167[Suppl 4]:625.
12. Kundu SD, Roehl KA, Eggener SE, et al. Potency, continence and complications in 3,477 consecutive radical retropubic prostatectomies. *J Urol* 2004;172(6, Pt 1 of 2):2227–2231.

# CHAPTER 29 ■ RADICAL PERINEAL PROSTATECTOMY

SAM D. GRAHAM, JR., JEFFREY C. LOU, AND THOMAS E. KEANE

Radical perineal prostatectomy, first performed in 1869 by Buchler and popularized in the United States by Young in 1903, remained the primary surgical approach to carcinoma of the prostate into the mid-1970s. With the recognition of the importance of assessing pelvic lymph nodes preoperatively and the advantage that retropubic prostatectomy offered with the concomitant pelvic node dissection, perineal prostatectomy declined in popularity for the treatment of prostate cancer. The perineal approach, however, saw a resurgence in the 1990s for several reasons: (a) the trend toward minimally invasive surgery with a focus on reducing the morbidity and therefore hospital stay of patients, (b) the advent of laparoscopic surgery for lymph node assessment, (c) the introduction of prostate-specific antigen (PSA) for screening for prostate cancer with reduction in the numbers of patients with node-positive disease, (d) algorithms that may predict patients at high risk for positive lymph nodes, and (e) increased recognition of similar results compared to all other methods of radical prostatectomy. The procedure is also associated with reduced blood loss and low morbidity, and it can be modified to incorporate the neurovascular sparing techniques for preservation of potency.

## DIAGNOSIS

All patients who are potential candidates for radical perineal prostatectomy should undergo appropriate preoperative staging to ensure that they are operable candidates; preoperative imaging is rarely required in low- to intermediate-risk patients. Methods of differentiating local versus advanced disease include digital rectal examination, transrectal ultrasonography, radionuclide bone scan, assessment of pelvic lymph nodes, and pathologic indicators of progression such as Gleason sum and other markers.

PSA screening has made a significant impact on the preoperative stage of patients with prostate cancer. Patients presenting for surgery are generally younger, healthier, and more likely to have organ-confined prostate cancer than the population treated only a decade earlier, and in many ways this attributes to the large increase in the number of radical prostatectomies done in the United States in the past decade.

Digital rectal examination has a limited role in the clinical staging of prostate cancer. It is primarily used to crudely estimate the volume of the cancer. Transrectal ultrasonography is another modality that also has limitations in assessing local disease, but combined with digital rectal examination it at least gives some gross assessment of the likelihood of extracapsular disease. Other modalities, such as transrectal magnetic resonance imaging (MRI), computerized tomography (CT) scan, and pelvic MRI, have been shown to have limited usefulness. The new generation of MRI scanners and ProstaScint scanning using fusion technology with CT or MRI have the potential to improve prostate cancer staging. Radionuclide bone scans are useful in assessing advanced bone disease but generally are not positive in patients with PSAs below 20 and no other sign of advanced disease.

For the past 20 years we have prospectively provided data that has been applied to an algorithm for the preoperative assessment of patients with prostate cancer developed through data on over 400 patients who had undergone pelvic node dissection. The current algorithm includes patients with a Gleason sum of 7, providing that the predominant pattern is 3, a low-volume cancer (T1b-c, T2a), and PSA of <10 ng per mL. Patients meeting all of these criteria have a <5% chance of positive lymph nodes, and therefore we do not routinely perform pelvic lymph node dissections (1). Patients exceeding any one of the above criteria are considered to be in the high-risk group and have undergone pelvic lymph node dissections. Using this method of assessment, our overall PSA recurrence rate from 1986 to 1993 was 24%. This compares favorably to other series of retropubic prostatectomies from that time in which all patients had a node dissection; in those series PSA recurrence rates were between 24% and 28% (2–5).

## INDICATIONS FOR SURGERY

Patients who are candidates for radical prostatectomy must have clinically organ-confined prostate cancer (T1-2). Other factors that need to be taken into consideration are the patient's life expectancy, other comorbidities, or any other factors that may affect the patient's choice. We generally do not offer a radical prostatectomy to patients who have a <10-year expectancy. Over the age of 70, we offer a radical prostatectomy only in selected cases where we feel that the benefits that can be obtained from radical prostatectomy outweigh the potential risks, particularly when compared to alternative therapies.

## ALTERNATIVE THERAPY

Alternatives to perineal prostatectomy include retropubic and laparoscopic or robot-assisted laparoscopic prostatectomies. The retropubic approach allows simultaneous node dissection and removal of larger prostate glands, though the length of hospitalization and immediate postoperative morbidity are higher in our institution. The robotically assisted laparoscopic approach allows some improvement in visualization compared to the retropubic or laparoscopic surgeries due to the magnification and three-dimensional visualization, but it has yet to show any significant advantages in terms of operative morbidity, length of stay, or reduction in long-term morbidity. There are few if any large comparisons with radical perineal prostatectomy, although results to date indicate that no significant differences exist.

Alternatives to radical prostatectomy include observation, hormonal deprivation, and radiation therapy. We do not consider either observation or hormonal deprivation to be curative; these are good options only for patients with less than a 5-year life expectancy, patients who are >70 years old with a well-differentiated cancer, and patients who are at high risk for surgery and refuse radiation. Radiation therapy, however, may be definitive and has a 5- to 10-year survival rate equivalent to that of surgery. The recurrence rates with radiation therapy are bimodal, with initial recurrences within 1 to 2 years of treatment and a delayed peak at 5 to 7 years after treatment. If the patient is young with a 15-year or longer outlook, we feel that our results would favor radical prostatectomy.

## SURGICAL TECHNIQUE

The patient is placed in an exaggerated lithotomy position (Fig. 29.1). It is important that the patient's perineum be parallel to the floor because this directly affects exposure. We use a standard operating room table with seven folded sheets under the patient's sacrum supporting the patient's entire weight. Shoulder braces are not recommended, and if a patient tends to slide off the sheets, we will place the table in a slight reverse Trendelenburg position. The patient's legs are stabilized using candy cane or Allen stirrups, again taking precautions to prevent stretching the hamstring or causing pressure on the legs.

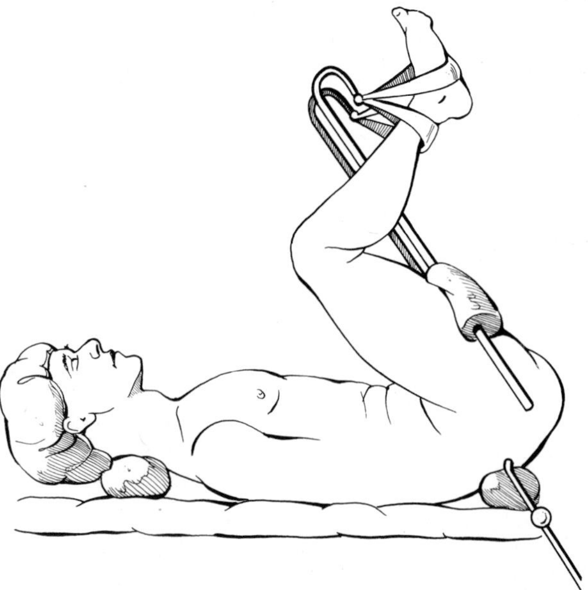

FIGURE 29.1 Positioning of the patient requires the perineum to be parallel to the floor. The sacrum supports the patient's weight, and the legs are positioned with no traction on the hamstrings. No shoulder braces are indicated.

Prior to putting the patient in position, the legs are wrapped with ACE bandages.

Five instruments are significant in assisting the surgeon for this operation. These include the Lowsley curved tractor, the Young straight prostatic tractor, a Halogen head lamp, a harmonic scalpel, and an Omni-Tract miniwishbone retractor system. The curved Lowsley tractor is used to bring the prostate up into the perineum to allow dissection against the prostate while mobilizing the rectum from the prostate. The straight Young tractor is used to manipulate the prostate laterally as well as cephalad and caudad after the membranous urethra has been divided. The Halogen head lamp is important because it allows the surgeon to aim a strong light into the operative field, which may be too deep and narrow for standard operating lights to adequately illuminate the structures. The harmonic scalpel allows coagulation and closure of vessels without transmission of electrical current, thereby reducing the risks to the neurovascular bundles. The Omni-Tract miniwishbone allows virtually unlimited retraction in any direction. We have developed a posterior weighted speculum that is compatible with the Omni-Tract (Fig. 29.2).

It should be noted that in manipulating the prostate within the pelvis, the pelvis should be viewed as a cone with the apex of the cone being the incision (Fig. 29.3). To achieve better visualization, it is sometimes necessary to actually push the

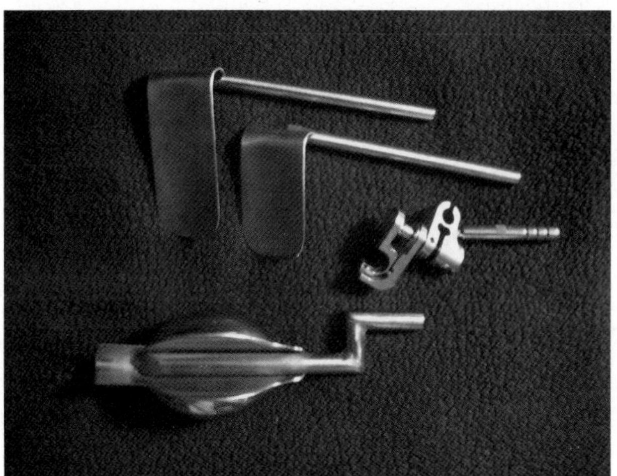

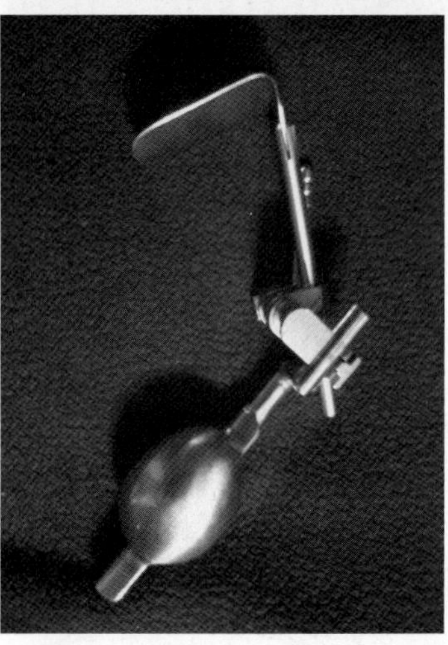

FIGURE 29.2 Posterior weighted speculum can be articulated to adapt to each patient's anatomy.

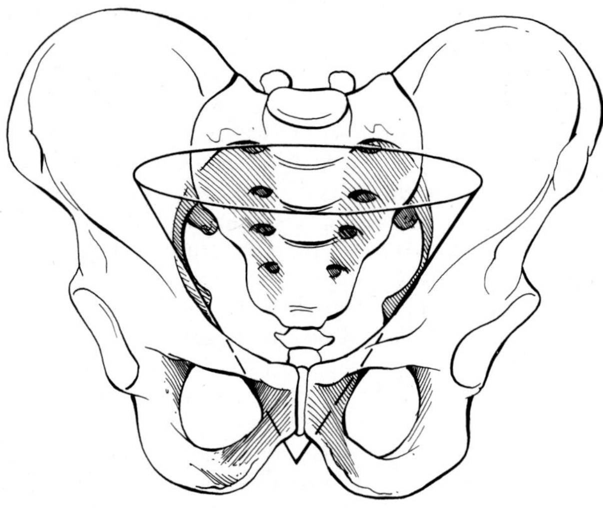

FIGURE 29.3 The bony pelvis is a cone with the apex at the incision. Better visualization can be obtained in many cases by actually pushing the prostate deeper into the pelvis.

prostate further into the pelvis. Also note that traction is not placed directly on the bulb or membranous urethra, as this will decrease the likelihood of restoration of potency and potentially affect the patient's continence postoperatively.

The incision is made from the ischial tuberosity crossing the midline at the juncture between the squamous epithelium and the mucocutaneous border of the rectum (Fig. 29.4). The incision extends posteriorly to a line equal to the posterior portion of the anus. Using sharp dissection and electrocautery, the ischiorectal fossae are entered, and using blunt dissection the central perineal tendon is identified and transected with electrocautery. At this point, we employ the Belt approach, dissecting down to the white fascia of the rectum and proceeding subsphincterically (Fig. 29.5). A transsphincteric or suprasphincteric approach is also an option. Using predominantly blunt dissection with an index finger in the rectum, the rectal sphincter and levator ani can be dissected free of the rectum with minimal bleeding (Fig. 29.6). The blades from the miniwishbone retractor are then used to retract these muscles anteriorly and laterally. With tension on these muscles and tension on the rectum, the rectourethralis is identified and divided, allowing the surgeon to dissect the rectum free of the apex of the prostate (Fig. 29.7).

In patients who are undergoing nerve-sparing surgery, the dissection is carried down to approximately 1.5 to 2.0 cm from the apex, at which point the external layer of the Denonvilliers fascia is divided and dissection is carried between the two layers of the Denonvilliers fascia (Fig. 29.8). Care is taken not to

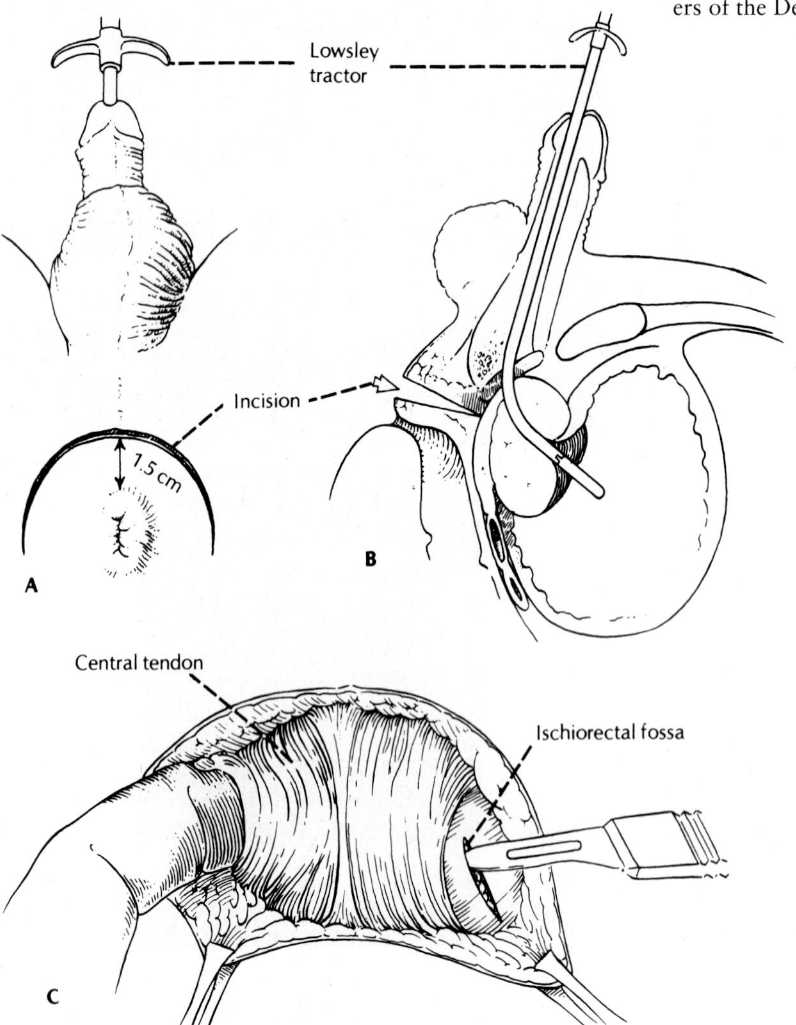


FIGURE 29.4 An inverted U-shaped incision is made in the perineum extending from ischial tuberosity to ischial tuberosity.

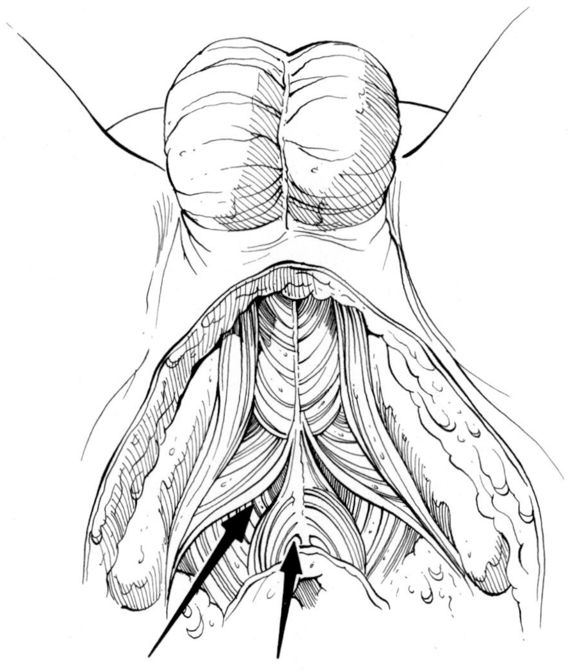

FIGURE 29.5 The dissection is carried along the rectal fascia, sparing the anal sphincter.

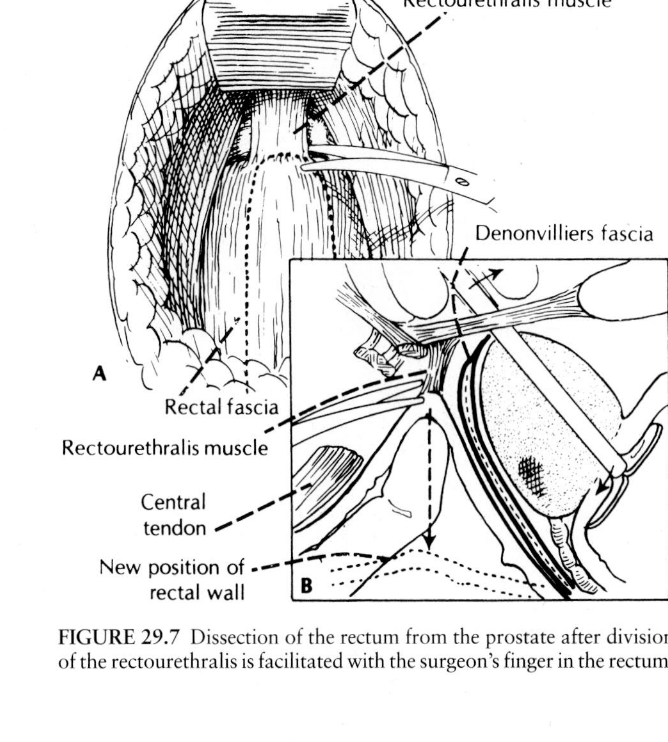


FIGURE 29.7 Dissection of the rectum from the prostate after division of the rectourethralis is facilitated with the surgeon's finger in the rectum.

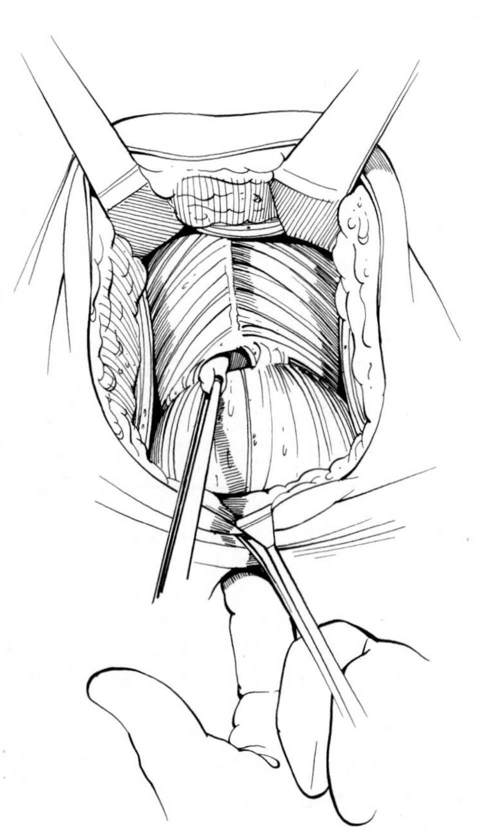

FIGURE 29.6 The Levator ani and the anal sphincter are retracted to expose the rectourethralis.

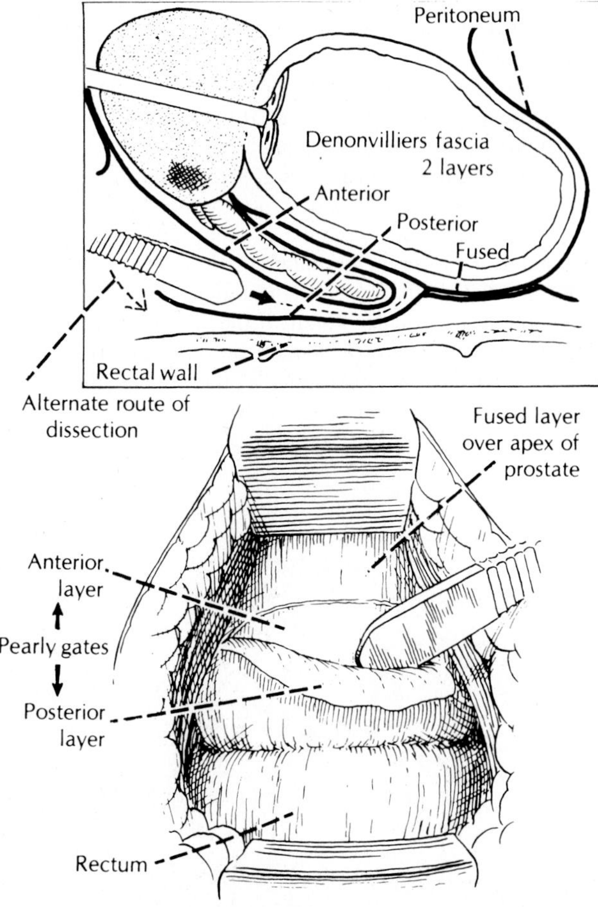


FIGURE 29.8 An incision into the posterior layer of the Denonvilliers fascia allows the dissection to continue between the two layers. For a nerve-sparing technique, this incision is made transversely 1 to 2 cm proximal to the apex of the prostate, avoiding carrying the incision into the neurovascular bundles.

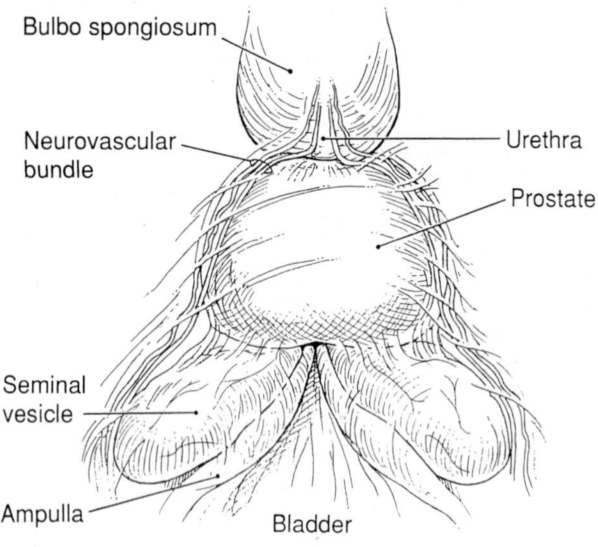


FIGURE 29.9 Anatomic view of the neurovascular bundles from the posterior view of the prostate. The vessels course along the lateral and posterior prostate and cross the apex to enter the urogenital diaphragm posterior to the membranous urethra.

damage the neurovascular bundles that course along the lateral posterior prostate on either side (Fig. 29.9).

The distal portion of the Denonvilliers fascia is then incised in the midline with scissors, and the tag is used to facilitate dissection of the neurovascular bundle from the prostate (Fig. 29.10); the inferior pedicle, if present, is then ligated and divided (Fig. 29.11). If the dissection is in any way impaired by fibrosis such that there is a potential for prostatic tissue to be left behind, the neurovascular bundle is sacrificed on that side.

It should be noted during this dissection that the neurovascular bundle actually courses across the posterior surface of the prostate at the apex and enters the urogenital diaphragm just posterior to the membranous urethra. This proximity is important in that the vesicourethral anastomosis may incorporate the neurovascular bundle if the surgeon is not precise with the placement of sutures in the posterior urethra. The retraction of the neurovascular bundle on either side thereby exposes the proximal membranous urethra.

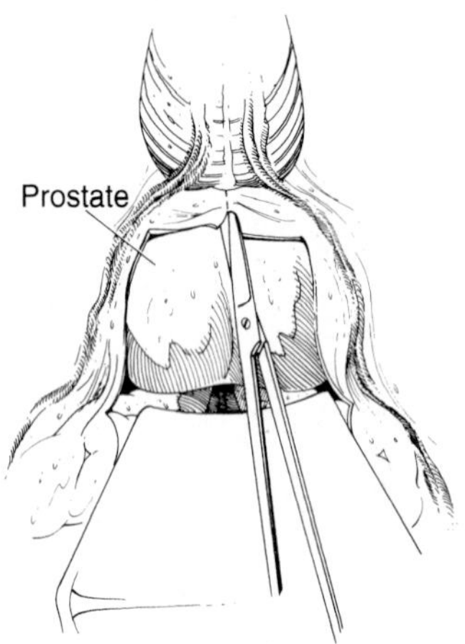


FIGURE 29.10 Incision of the distal posterior layer of the Denonvilliers fascia in the midline. This is best done *without* electrocautery if a nerve-sparing technique is planned.

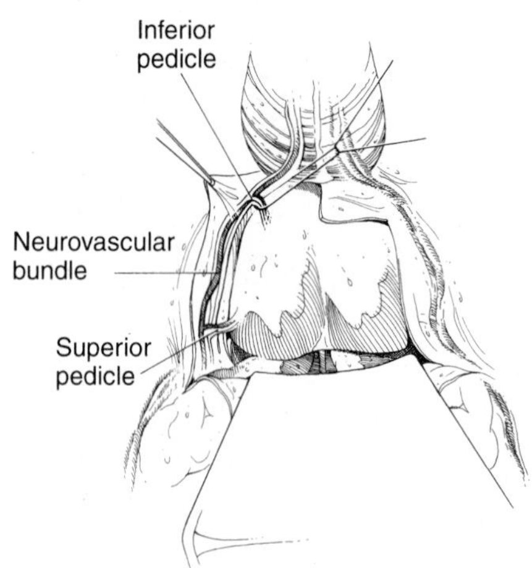


FIGURE 29.11 Using the wings of the distal posterior layer of the Denonvilliers fascia to aid in dissection, the inferior branch from the neurovascular is isolated and divided.

A right-angled clamp is placed around the membranous urethra and generally meets little resistance if one stays posterior to the endopelvic fascia (Fig. 29.12). The Lowsley tractor is removed and the membranous urethra divided. The Young tractor is then placed into the bladder through the prostatic urethra, and the endopelvic fascia is divided with the harmonic scalpel.

The anterior prostate is dissected free of the bladder. It should be noted that there are generally two small arteries that enter the prostate along the anterior bladder at 10 and 2 o'clock positions that should be cauterized and divided. The groove between the prostate and bladder is identified, and the prostate and bladder can be separated with either sharp or blunt dissection. If the plane between the prostate and bladder is not easily developed, the dissection should be performed sharply and biopsies taken of the bladder neck to ensure that there is no invasion of the bladder neck by the cancer. In patients who have had prior transurethral resections of the prostate, palpation of the blades of the Young tractor can be used to identify the bladder neck.

In most cases, there is insignificant bleeding from the dorsal venous complex in the endopelvic fascia. However, if there should be communicating veins, they may be suture-ligated using 3-0 Vicryl. The prostate is dissected from the bladder anteriorly to posteriorly to the 5 and 7 o'clock positions, respectively, on the patient's left and right, and the bladder neck is divided over the Young tractor and the Young tractor removed; a stay suture may be inserted in the bladder neck at this point (Fig. 29.13). The bladder is evacuated of any urine, and the posterior bladder neck is divided with the harmonic scalpel. The prostate is then dissected free from the posterior bladder. A plane is entered after dividing the posterior bladder neck, which is anterior to the seminal vesicles and the ampulla of the vas but posterior to the bladder. The superior pedicles lie in the lateral aspect of this plane and can be divided at this point.

Attention is then directed to the posterior surface of the prostate. The rectum is swept free of the neurovascular bundles, which also allows identification of the superior pedicles of the prostate as well as the seminal structures. The superior pedicles can be divided with the harmonic scalpel at this point,

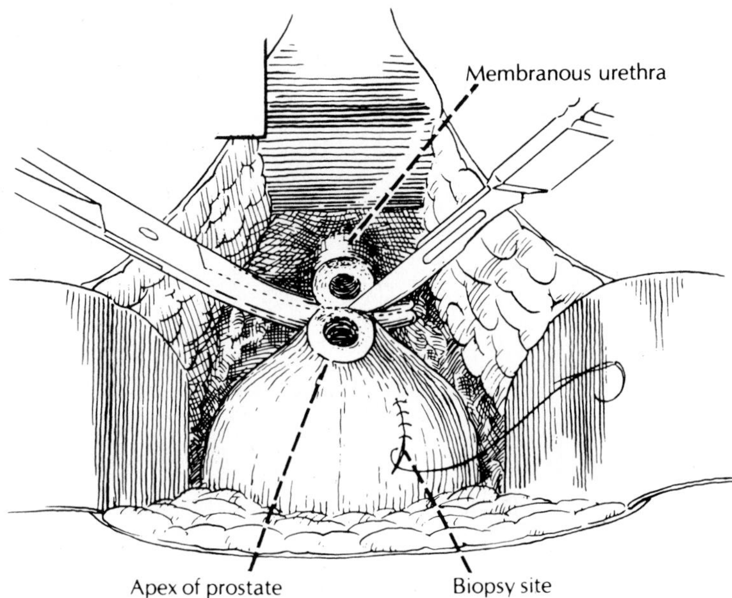


FIGURE 29.12 Division of the membranous urethra at the apex of the prostate.

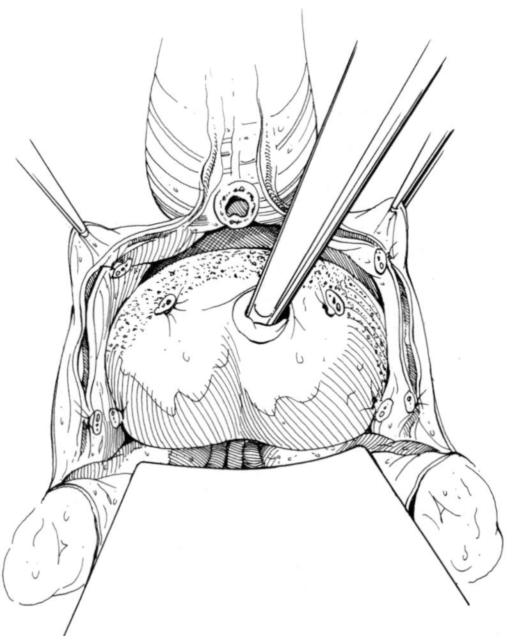

FIGURE 29.13 A Young prostatic tractor is used to manipulate the prostate and to identify the vesical neck.

if not done earlier. The seminal vesicles are dissected to their tips with blunt dissection, and the artery from the seminal vesical is divided by the harmonic scalpel. The vasa deferens are likewise divided with the harmonic scalpel. Any remaining fibrolymphatic tissue is then divided, allowing removal of the prostate.

After ensuring complete hemostasis, the bladder neck is reconstructed using 3-0 Vicryl on an SH needle beginning posteriorly to anteriorly (Fig. 29.14). This direction of the closure, beginning in the posterior bladder, is done to facilitate the closure without injury to the ureters and also to take advantage of the anatomic relationship between the bladder neck and the membranous urethra with a shorter distance being anteriorly.

The anastomosis is performed using 3-0 Vicryl simple sutures and an RB-1 controlled-release needle (Fig. 29.15). The anastomosis is performed around a 22Fr, 5-cc Foley catheter, and generally seven to eight sutures are used. Care should be taken that small portions of the membranous urethra are incorporated in the anastomosis such that the continence mechanism is left undisturbed as well as the neurovascular bundles, which contribute to potency.

The rectum is then inspected, a Foley balloon inflated, and a Penrose drain placed through the left ischiorectal fossa and a separate stab incision. The incision is closed with a 3-0 chromic gut closure. One suture is placed to reapproximate the central tendon, and the remainder of the sutures are used to close the skin in a horizontal mattress (Fig. 29.16).

Postoperatively, patients have a very low requirement for pain medication. Most patients either do not require parental pain medication or are off the parental medications within 12 to 24 hours. Average time to discharge is approximately 24 hours from the time of surgery (Table 29.1). The patient's catheter is removed on day 12. The Penrose drain is removed prior to discharge. One of the authors, Tom Keane, discharges patients and removes the catheter on day 7 (6).

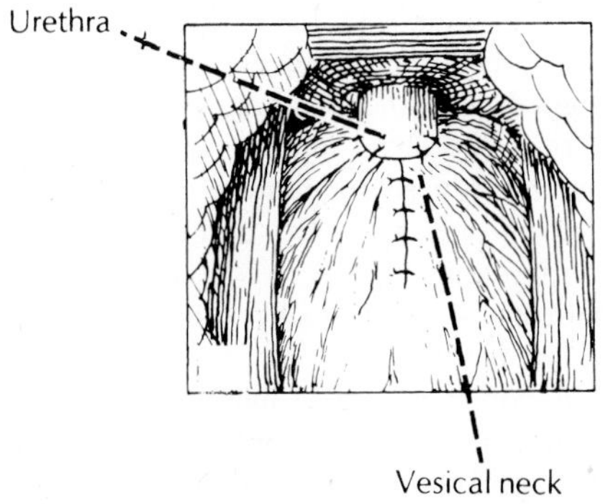


FIGURE 29.14 Reconstruction of the posterior bladder neck is carried from posterior to anterior, leaving an opening of approximately 22Fr.

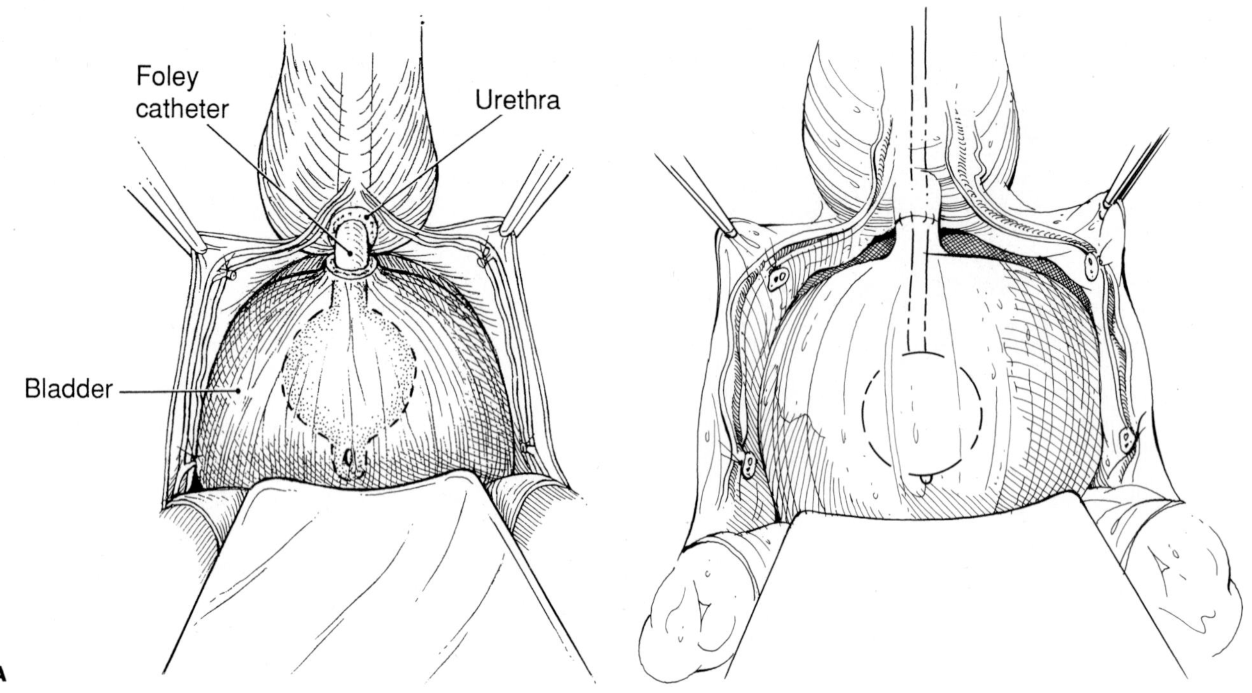


FIGURE 29.15 Anastomosis of the urethra to the bladder is performed over a 22Fr Foley catheter.

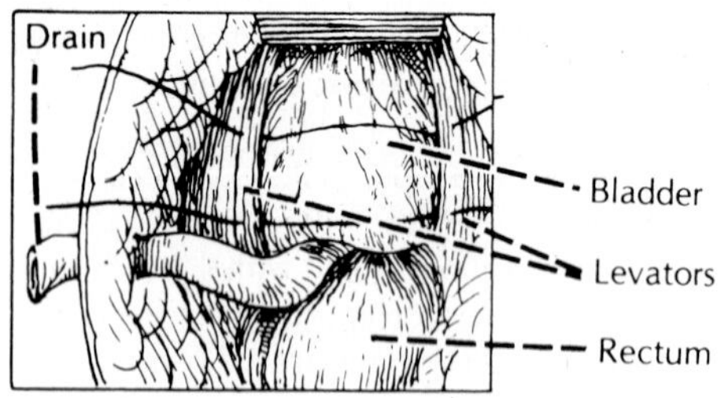


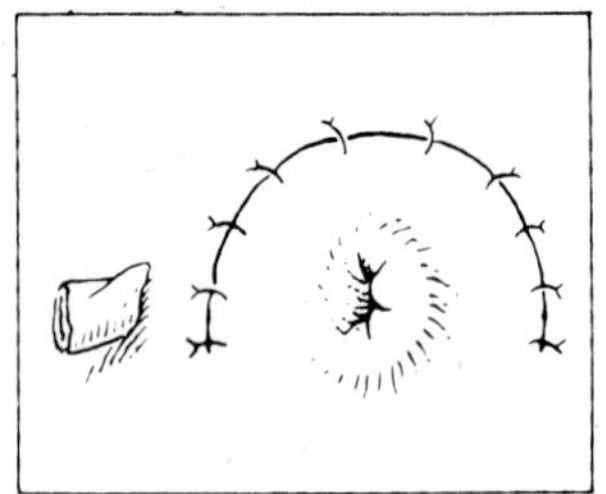

FIGURE 29.16 Closure of the incision.

# OUTCOMES

## Complications

Perioperative complications include hemorrhage, wound infection, cardiovascular complications, and rectal injury. The instance of rectal injury is <1% with current techniques and antibiotics, preoperative bowel preparation (two Fleet enemas, the night before and morning of surgery), or GoLytely and antibiotics. The rectal injury is closed primarily in two layers without the need to perform a diverting colostomy. Wound infection rates are <1%, and cardiovascular complications are approximately 1% to 2%. The average blood loss in these patients is approximately 300 to 400 cc, and our transfusion rate is <1%.

Long-term complications include incontinence and impotence. Incontinence requiring intervention such as pads, clamps, or inflatable devices occurs in 2.8% of patients. We have found that incontinence generally occurs in patients who are older, obese, and have had prior radiation therapy. Potency following nerve-sparing perineal prostatectomy is dependent upon the patient's age and preoperative status. Patients under the age of 60 who are fully potent and have both neurovascular bundles spared have approximately a 50% to 60% potency rate. Patients who are over the age of 60 have a reduced rate of potency, and we have not yet had a patient over the age of 70 who has spontaneously regained his potency. Patients who are having difficulties with potency prior to surgery and patients in whom the neurovascular bundles could not be spared will likely be impotent. We generally advocate early use of pharmacotherapy or other means of assistance in these patients.

## Results

Following radical prostatectomy, recurrence can be measured using PSA, which is exquisitely sensitive. Any patient who undergoes a radical prostatectomy can expect his PSA to fall

TABLE 29.1

POST OP ORDERS

Lab
- CBC, Basic Metabolic Panel in AM

Interventions/Treatments
- Vital signs q 4h
- I & O q shift
- Urinary catheter to bedside bag
- Leg bag at bedside upon admission to unit. Post Op day 1, staff nurse to begin leg bag teaching. Ensure that catheter remains secure at all times using catheter holder (Cath Secure)
- Dressing Changes prn
- Ace wraps to lower extremities until patient ambulatory

Activity
- Dangle at bedside evening of surgery, may get out of bed to chair
- Starting post op day 1, out of bed to chair for meals and ambulate in hall

Diet
- Clear liquids immediately post op, regular diet as tolerated

IV Fluids
- RL at 125cc/hr
- convert to heparin lock in AM

Medications
- Cefazolin 1 gram IV q 8h × 4 doses
- Gentamicin 80mg IV q 8h × 3 doses
- Morphine Sulphate 2–4 mg IV q 3h prn severe pain
- Percocet 5/325 q 3h prn pain

Respiratory
- Incentive Spirometry q 2h while awake

Patient and Family Teaching
- Review discharge instructions with patient and family on day of surgery and reinforce daily
- Instruct patient on leg bag usage, catheter care, and diet

below detectable levels. Failure to do so generally means that the patient has significant residual disease, either locally or distantly. Another group of patients will have an initial drop of their PSA to undetectable levels and then a return to measurable levels. These patients may have local and/or distant recurrence of their disease, or possibly residual malignancy. Patients who develop recurrence based upon PSA will generally manifest a clinical progression within 18 months. Additionally, if the PSA is going to rise, it will do so within 2 years in 90% of patients and within 4 years in virtually every patient. Based upon PSA, we can now predict disease recurrence earlier, allowing assessment of the outcome of radical prostatectomy within 5 years as opposed to the older data, which required a 7- to 10-year follow-up (3).

Using a clinical care pathway, we have seen better pain control, earlier ambulation, quicker short-term recovery, and earlier discharge than in patients undergoing radical retropubic prostatectomy in the same institution. This has been confirmed in other studies and will lead to a lower cost of care (2,7).

## *References*


1. El Galley RE, Keane TE, Petros JA, et al. Evaluation of staging lymphadenectomy in prostate cancer. *Urology* 1998;52:663–667.
2. Harris MJ. Radical perineal prostatectomy: cost efficient, outcome effective, minimally invasive prostate cancer management. *Eur Urol* 2003;44: 303–308; discussion 308.
3. Iselin CE, Robertson JE, Paulson DF. Radical perineal prostatectomy: oncological outcome during a 20 year period. *J Urol* 1999;161:163–168.
4. Lance RS, Freiderichs PA, Kane C, et al. A comparison of radical retropubic with perineal prostatectomy for localized prostate cancer within the Uniform Armed Services Urology Research Group. *BJU Int* 2001;87: 61–65.
5. Sullivan LD, Weir MJ, Kinahan JF, et al. A comparison of the relative merits of radical perineal and retropubic prostatectomy. *BJU Int* 2000;85: 95–100.
6. Bong GW, Ritenour CW, Osunkova AO, et al. Evaluation of modern pathological criteria for positive margins in radical prostatectomy specimens and their use for predicting biochemical recurrence. *BJU Int* 2008.
7. Weizer AZ, Silverstein AD, Young MD, et al. Prospective evaluation of pain medication requirements and recovery after radical perineal prostatectomy. *Urology* 2003;62:693–697.

# CHAPTER 30 ■ BRACHYTHERAPY FOR LOCALIZED PROSTATE CANCER

JOHN A. FORTNEY, A. JASON ZAULS, AND DAVID T. MARSHALL

The term *brachytherapy* describes the process of placing a radioactive source directly inside or in close proximity to the intended target. The use of brachytherapy in prostate cancer was first reported by Pasteau in 1913 (1), and various techniques have been explored since. Retropubic implantation of radioactive sources was used initially until the introduction of the transrectal ultrasound probe (TRUS) in the early 1980s (2). With significant advancements in ultrasound technology, ultrasound-guided transperineal prostate brachytherapy is now the accepted technique used for prostate brachytherapy and has experienced substantial growth over the last 15 years.

Brachytherapy offers several advantages over radical prostatectomy, including patient convenience, no surgical incision, decreased anesthesia requirement, minimal blood loss, rapid recovery, and less risk of incontinence. Brachytherapy also offers advantages over external beam radiation therapy (EBRT). Proper brachytherapy technique can lead to decreased radiation dose to surrounding structures, thereby limiting normal tissue morbidity. Evidence continues to accumulate stressing the importance of dose escalation in prostate cancer. In order to deliver an acceptable dose via EBRT, patients must undergo several weeks of treatment, whereas brachytherapy can be completed in one outpatient procedure. Finally, the position of the prostate and surrounding critical organs may be difficult to reproduce daily during a protracted course of treatment, which may lead to an increased dose to normal tissues or a decreased dose to the prostate.

Three isotopes ($^{125}$I, $^{103}$Pd, and $^{131}$Cs) are now available for low-dose-rate (LDR) brachytherapy. The majority of the radiation dose is delivered over 2 to 10 months, depending on which isotope is used. The timing and severity of acute side effects have been described regarding the different sources; however, no convincing evidence is available to recommend one source over another. High-dose-rate (HDR) brachytherapy has been increasingly utilized as well. Catheters are placed within the prostate as described below for LDR needles, and a dosimetric plan is developed with CT imaging and computer planning. An iridium-192 source can then be moved in and out of each catheter remotely via a robotic device. The time the radioactive source spends in each catheter and at each dwell position within each catheter can be manipulated via computer control to achieve a conformal radiotherapy plan. HDR brachytherapy typically requires a short hospital stay and two to ten treatments over a 2- to 5-day period.

## DIAGNOSIS

The diagnosis and risk-stratification of prostate cancer is via 12 to 16 core prostate biopsies following an elevated PSA or abnormal digital rectal exam. Patients with high risk of seminal vesicle involvement, such as those with clinical stage >T2a or perineural invasion seen on prostate biopsy, should undergo TRUS-guided biopsy of the seminal vesicles. Pelvic lymphadenectomy is not commonly performed for patients with low-risk disease. Patients with high risk of lymph node involvement (patients with seminal vesicle involvement, Gleason score >7, PSA >20) may benefit from laparoscopic pelvic lymph node dissection as nodal involvement changes treatment recommendations.

## INDICATIONS FOR SURGERY

When considering brachytherapy as monotherapy for prostate cancer, it is critical to carefully select patients with low-risk disease. A number of tools have been developed to aid the physician when making this selection, including the Partin tables (3) and the Roach formulas (4,5). These tools can help estimate the risk of extraprostatic extension, seminal vesicle invasion, and pelvic lymph node involvement. Recommendations have been made regarding classification of patients into low-, intermediate-, and high-risk categories as illustrated in Table 30.1. Low-risk prostate cancer can be summarized as PSA <10, Gleason score <7, and clinical stage <T2b. Other risk factors, such as PSA velocity, PSA doubling time, presence of perineural invasion or lymphovascular space invasion, and

**TABLE 30.1**

**PATIENT SELECTION FACTORS**

| | Monotherapy (Low Risk) | Combination Therapy (Intermediate to High Risk) |
|---|---|---|
| Nodule | None or small | Large or multiple |
| Gleason score | 2–6 | 7–10 |
| PSA[a] | <10 ng/mL | ≥10 ng/mL |
| Clinical stage | <T2b | ≥T2b |

[a]PSA, prostate-specific antigen.

number of cores positive on biopsy, should be considered when stratifying patients and choosing appropriate treatment modalities.

Clinical outcomes for prostate brachytherapy alone in the setting of intermediate- or high-risk disease have been conflicting. Furthermore, there is a growing body of evidence supporting the use of dose-escalated EBRT or combined androgen deprivation therapy and EBRT in this setting. Brachytherapy is often used in this situation in combination with EBRT to augment dose escalation, but it is not generally recommended as monotherapy for intermediate- or high-risk patients.

## ALTERNATIVE THERAPY

Prostate brachytherapy is an ideal treatment for men with localized, low-risk prostate cancer, but alternatives exist and may be more appropriate in certain situations. Men with high International Prostate Symptom Scores (IPSS), large prostate volume, or history of previous transurethral resection of the prostate (TURP) may tolerate EBRT or prostatectomy better than brachytherapy while achieving a similar therapeutic outcome. High IPSS before treatment predicts significant risk of severe lower urinary tract symptoms (LUTS) and acute urinary obstruction following brachytherapy (6). Similarly, large prostates have been shown to be at increased risk for urinary retention (7), although the absolute risk may still be low depending on the technique used (8). Patients with a history of prior TURP may be at increased risk for significant toxicity, including incontinence, if brachytherapy is used (9,10).

## SURGICAL TECHNIQUE

### Selection of Isotope

As noted above, three isotopes ($^{125}$I, $^{103}$Pd, and $^{131}$Cs) are currently being used for LDR prostate brachytherapy. Each delivers radiation to a volume of tissue within millimeters of each source; however, they differ in initial activity, dose rate, and half-life, as illustrated in Table 30.2. Some investigators believe $^{103}$Pd may be more effective than $^{125}$I at eradicating more rapidly proliferating tumors due to higher initial activity (20 to 25 cGy per hour and 7 to 10 cGy per hour, respectively). This belief has been propagated by convincing mathematical models and has led to the emergence of $^{131}$Cs (32 cGy per hour) as another option. However, no conclusive clinical evidence proving this theory has yet been made available, and one clinical trial has shown equivalence between $^{125}$I and $^{103}$Pd regarding PSA control at 3 years (11). The current recommended doses for the three isotopes in monotherapy and in combination with external beam therapy are shown in Table 30.3. The selection of $^{103}$Pd or $^{131}$Cs may be most appropriate in the setting of combination therapy as EBRT may be initiated sooner in the treatment paradigm after prostate brachytherapy due to earlier resolution of urinary symptoms following brachytherapy.

**TABLE 30.2**

**CHARACTERISTICS OF THE MOST COMMONLY USED PERMANENT SOURCES**

| | $^{125}$I | $^{103}$Pd | $^{131}$Cs |
|---|---|---|---|
| Half-life | 60 days | 17 days | 9.7 days |
| Initial dose rate | 8 cGy/hr | 20 cGy/hr | 32 cGy/hr |
| Average energy | 28.5 keV | 20.8 keV | 30.4 keV |
| 90% delivered | 204 days | 58 days | 33 days |

**TABLE 30.3**

**TYPICALLY PRESCRIBED MINIMUM PERIPHERAL DOSES FOR $^{125}$I AND $^{103}$PD**

| | $^{125}$I[a] | $^{103}$Pd[b] | $^{131}$Cs[c] |
|---|---|---|---|
| Monotherapy | 145–160 Gy | 125 Gy | 115 Gy |
| Combined therapy[d] | 100–110 Gy | 90–100 Gy | 85 Gy |

[a]Rivard MJ, Butler WM, Devlin PM, et al. American Brachytherapy Society recommends no change for prostate permanent implant dose prescriptions using iodine-125 or palladium-103. *Brachytherapy* 2007;6(1):34–37; Kao J, Stone NN, Lavaf A, et al. (125)I monotherapy using D90 implant doses of 180 Gy or greater. *Int J Radiat Oncol Biol Phys* 2008;70(1):96–101.
[b]Rivard MJ, Butler WM, Devlin PM, et al. American Brachytherapy Society recommends no change for prostate permanent implant dose prescriptions using iodine-125 or palladium-103. *Brachytherapy* 2007;6(1):34–37.
[c]Bice WS, Prestidge BR, Kurtzman SM, et al. Recommendations for permanent prostate brachytherapy with (131)Cs: a consensus report from the Cesium Advisory Group. *Brachytherapy* 2008;7(4):290–296.
[d]In addition to 40- to 50-Gy external beam radiation therapy.

### Treatment Planning

Prostate brachytherapy has evolved significantly over the years, and two methods now predominate: preplanned implant as popularized by the Seattle Prostate Institute and intraoperative planning as described by Stock and Stone at Mount Sinai School of Medicine (MSSM) in New York.

#### Preplanning Approach

With this approach pioneered in Seattle (12), the patient is placed in the dorsal lithotomy position (Figs. 30.1 and 30.2) and an imaging study is performed using transrectal ultrasound 1 to 2 weeks before the implant. This image data set is imported into the brachytherapy planning software and utilized to develop an optimized plan. The number of seeds ordered for the procedure is then determined from this preplan. The patient returns to the operating room (OR) on the day of the operation and is placed in position as he was on the day of planning. It is critically important that the patient is repositioned as accurately as possible. Seeds are then placed within the prostate using needles preloaded with seeds or strands of connected seeds according to the previously developed plan. Seeds may also be placed with a gun-type applicator, such as the Mick applicator (Mick Radio-Nuclear Instruments, Mount Vernon, NY),

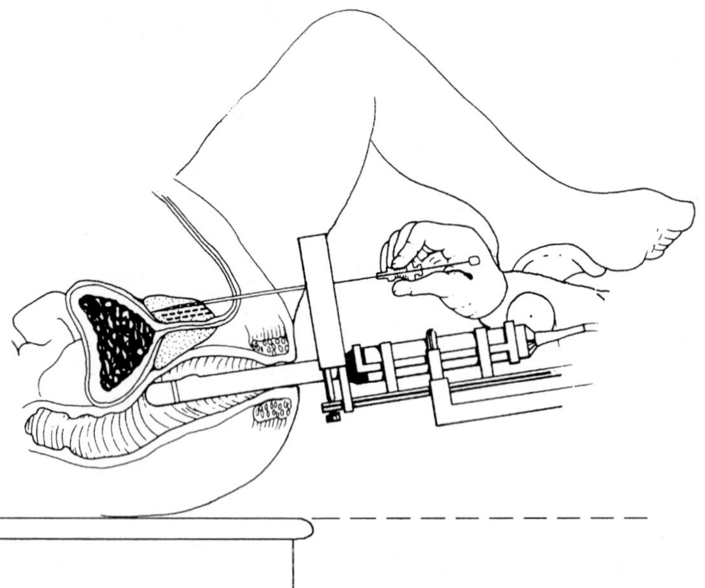

FIGURE 30.1 Schematic of the closed, ultrasound-guided implantation technique.

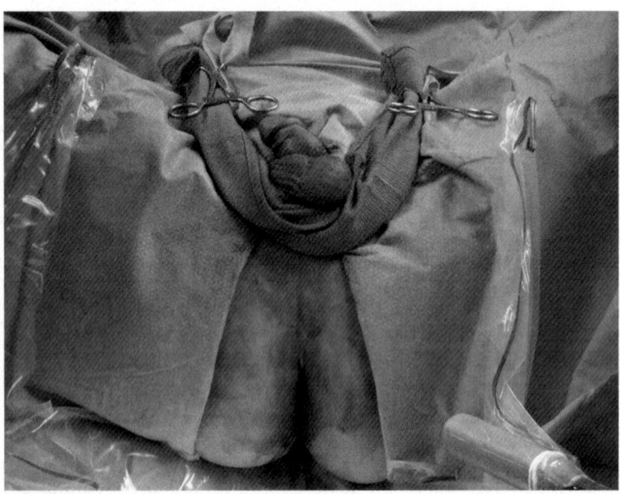

FIGURE 30.2 Patient prepared for surgery in the dorsal lithotomy position.

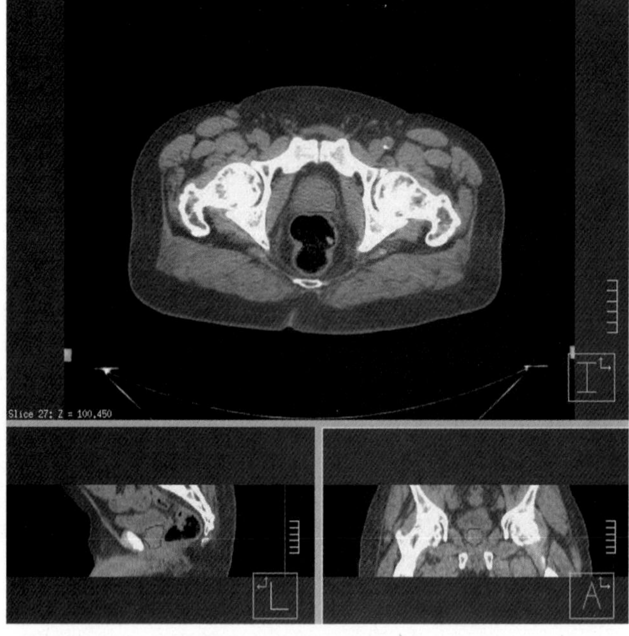


FIGURE 30.3 CT images obtained to estimate prostate volume to determine activity and number of seeds to order.

based on the planning study completed earlier. With the preplanned approach, the Mick applicator allows the practitioner to make minor adjustments to more accurately reproduce the preplanning study.

### Real-Time Intraoperative Planning Approach

With this approach developed by Stock and Stone at MSSM (13), no preplanning study is acquired; however, the prostate volume is measured via a computerized tomography (CT), magnetic resonance imaging (MRI), or TRUS study (Fig. 30.3) at some point prior to the day of the implant in order to determine how many seeds to order for the procedure. This can be the volume determined at TRUS for biopsy. The patient is then brought to the OR and placed in the dorsal lithotomy position. TRUS (Fig. 30.4) is utilized to localize the bladder, prostate, and anterior rectal wall in three-dimensional space, and these data are recorded in the intraoperative treatment planning software. An initial intraoperative plan (Figs. 30.5 and 30.6) is then developed based on a prostate volume-to-activity nomogram developed at MSSM. Needles are placed in the periphery of the prostate at approximately 1-cm intervals (Figs. 30.7 and 30.8). Once the needles are placed, images are reacquired to account for changes in size, shape, and position of the prostate that occurs with the trauma of needle placement. Longitudinal views on the TRUS are used to observe placement of the seeds into the prostate according to the intraoperative plan. Seeds are most often placed using the Mick applicator. Typically 75% of the required activity is placed in the periphery of the gland, while 25% is placed in the interior of the gland. Then needles are placed in the central portion of the gland and the Mick applicator is then used to

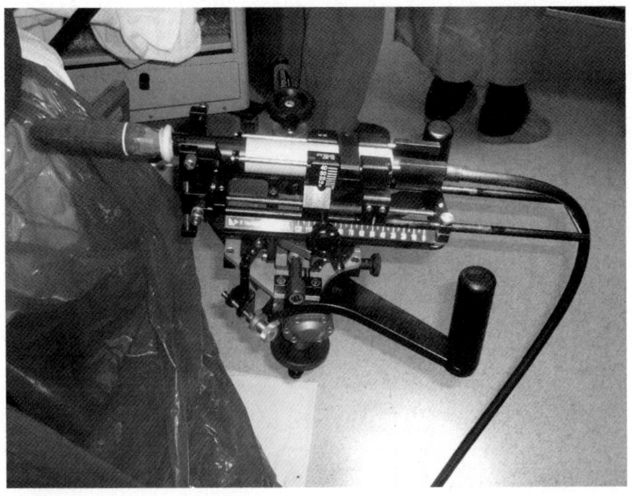

FIGURE 30.4 Transrectal ultrasound probe in ratcheting cradle/stepper.

place the remaining 25% of the required activity in the gland according to the intraoperative plan. The majority of the inner seeds are placed at the apex and base of the gland in order to "cap" the prostate. Using modern treatment planning software and TRUS, the actual seed location can be documented as the seeds are placed and the intraoperative plan can better reflect reality, allowing for dosimetric inadequacies to be detected and corrected during the procedure.

This approach offers many advantages over the previously described technique as well as some disadvantages. The most significant advantage offered by this technique is that intraoperative planning allows for real-time optimization of the plan as each seed placed in the prostate is accounted for in the planning software and the resultant isodose lines are generated. Three variables unaccounted for with the previous technique (changes in prostate size and shape with needle placement, needle deviation from planned position, and seed movement from initial placement) can be actively detected in the intraoperative treatment planning software and therefore corrected with subsequent seed deposition. Disadvantages include longer procedure duration and Mick applicator utilization, which some practitioners may find unwieldy. Although the Mick applicator requires significant operator skill, in practiced hands this applicator allows precise placement of individual seeds and significant flexibility. Some investigators have noted seed migration when seeds are placed individually in the prostate and surrounding tissues and have therefore argued for the use of stranded seeds. In fact, seeds have been observed to move significant distances and even to the lungs or other remote locations. When compared to stranded or linked seeds, single seed placement has been documented to result in increased overall seed migration (14,15). However, this has not been definitively shown to affect overall dosimetric outcome or toxicity (16–18).

### Hybrid Approach with Real-Time Planning and Linked Seeds

A novel technique has been developed and is currently being pursued at a few institutions in an attempt to combine the advantages of real-time intraoperative planning and linked seeds (19). This technique is very similar to the intraoperative technique described above; however, stranded seeds are formed in the OR at the time of implant and in response to real-time treatment planning. As before, an imaging study is obtained approximately 2 weeks before the date of implant to determine the prostate volume, and an appropriate number and activity of seeds are ordered according to nomograms developed at MSSM. On the day of implant the patient is placed in the dorsal lithotomy position and TRUS is utilized to build a three-dimensional model of the prostate, bladder, and anterior rectal wall within the treatment planning system. An initial intraoperative plan (Figs. 30.5 and 30.6) is then developed by the radiation oncologist while the urologist places needles in the periphery of the prostate at approximately 1-cm intervals (Figs. 30.7 and 30.8). Once the needles are placed, images are

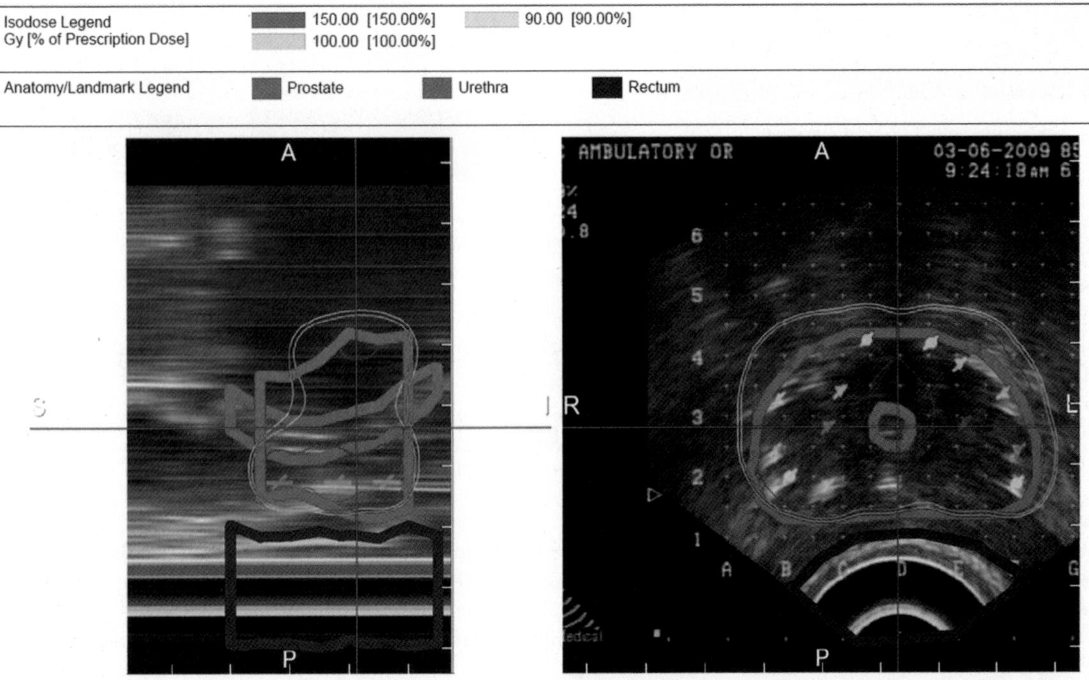


FIGURE 30.5 Treatment planning transverse and axial images of the prostate showing preliminary isodose lines for a $^{103}Pd$ implant (prescription dose = 100 Gy).

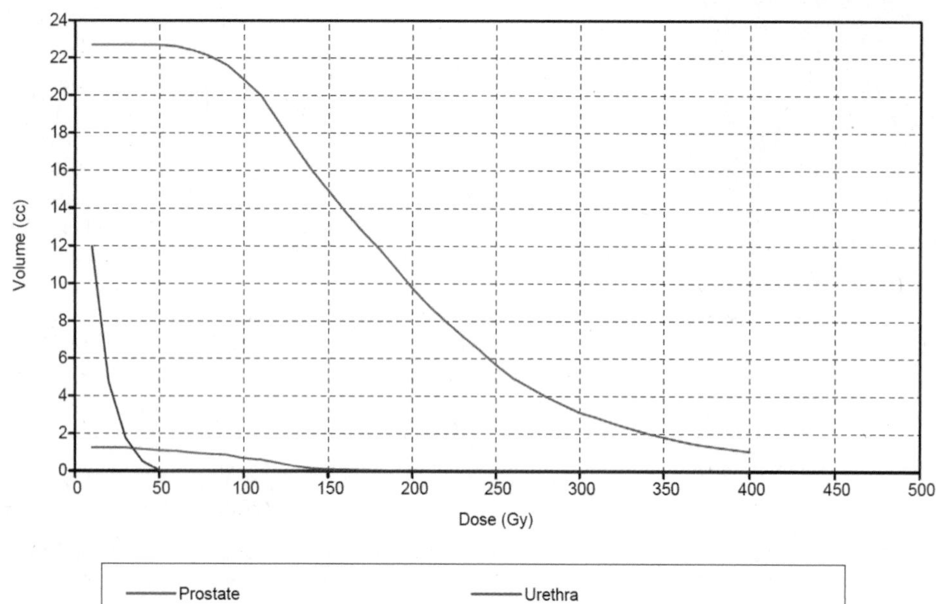


FIGURE 30.6 Dose-volume histogram for $^{103}$Pd implant depicting percentage of prescribed dose to the prostate, rectum, and urethra (prescription dose = 100 Gy).

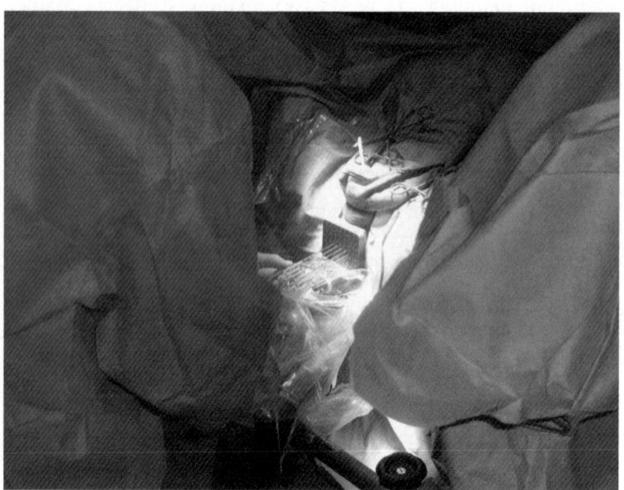

FIGURE 30.7 Operator implanting linked seeds at surgery.

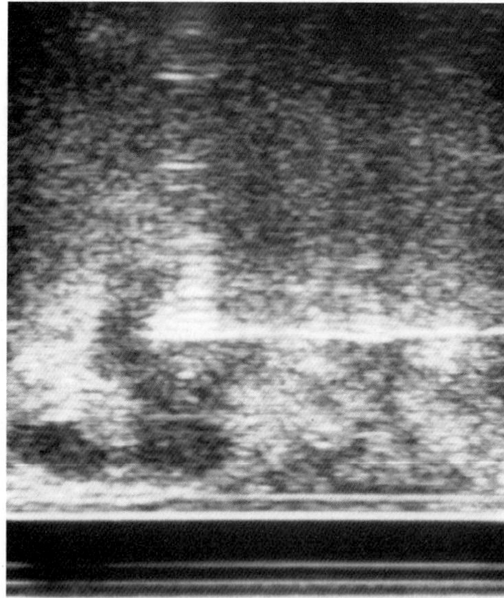

FIGURE 30.8 Sagittal ultrasound image of implant needle in the prostate preparing to place seed.

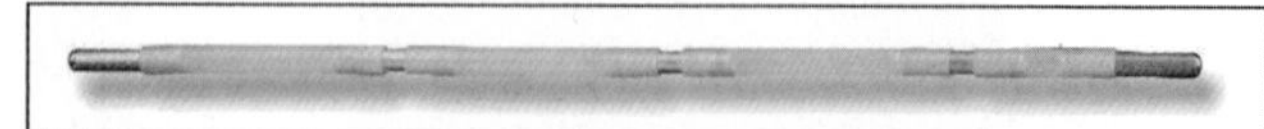

FIGURE 30.9 Custom-constructed linked seeds. Note asymmetrical seed pattern that can be constructed in the operating room according to the real-time plan.

reacquired and the plan reoptimized. Longitudinal views of each individual needle are used to calculate the distance each needle traverses through the prostate. A push-button delivery system (QuickLink, C. R. Bard, Inc., Covington, GA) is then used to construct links (Fig. 30.9) of the appropriate number of seeds for the length measured along the longitudinal path of each needle in the prostate. Each strand can be customized according to the number of seeds needed and the overall length of the needle path in the prostate via custom-sized linkers. The linked seeds are then transferred to the prostate via the appropriate needle in a manner similar to that used with a preloaded needle in a preplanned approach (Figs. 30.7 and 30.10). The process is then repeated until all peripheral seeds have been placed. The inner needles are then placed (usually five to seven). The plan is then reoptimized to determine placement of the remaining required activity. Once the plan has been approved, the remaining interior links of seeds are constructed and placed within the prostate as described previously. Preliminary data regarding this hybrid planning approach

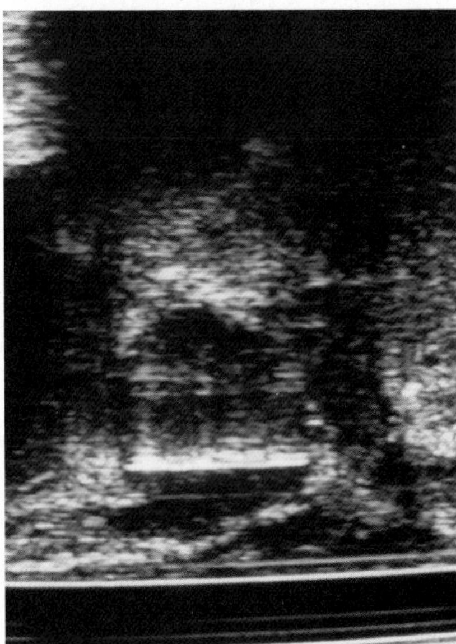

FIGURE 30.10 Ultrasound image of linked seeds in prostate after implantation.

reveal similar quality of dosimetry and OR times as compared to the traditional gun method (20).

### Postimplant Cystoscopy

Following prostate seed implantation, flexible cystoscopy is performed to verify an intact urethra and bladder wall and to account for any misplaced seeds. At the end of the procedure, C-arm radiography may also be performed to verify seed position and to document the presence or absence of loose seeds in the bladder.

### Postimplant Dosimetry

Postimplant dosimetry should be obtained at a consistent interval following prostate seed implant; however, the most appropriate interval is yet to be determined. Many institutions have patients return at 1 month following the implant for CT imaging. This image data set can then be imported into the treatment planning system, allowing for determination of dosimetric end points. Using this study, seed count should be verified, and isodose curves at 50%, 80%, 90%, 100%, 150%, and 200% of the prescribed dose should be displayed on axial images of the prostate, urethra, bladder, and rectal wall. The D90 or minimum dose delivered to 90% of the prostate as well as rectal and urethral doses should be recorded (21).

## OUTCOMES

### Complications

Immediate symptoms following brachytherapy are related to needle placement and include edema, bleeding, pain, and infection. The risk of infection can be minimized with the use of intraoperative antibiotics and a short course of postoperative antibiotics. Intraprostatic edema and bleeding may lead to urinary retention in approximately 5% to 25% of patients. Large prostate volume and an elevated pretreatment IPSS predict an increased risk of urinary retention, and some studies have shown that a short course of androgen deprivation may reduce this risk (8).

Urinary irritation may develop within 1 to 2 months after $^{125}$I implantation and within 1 to 2 weeks with $^{103}$Pd or $^{131}$Cs. These symptoms can be monitored and prospectively recorded through utilization of IPSS evaluation at each subsequent follow-up. The majority of men undergoing prostate brachytherapy will experience urinary symptoms such as increased frequency, dysuria, nocturia, and weakened stream, which can be treated symptomatically with alpha blockers and antimuscarinics. Most men will return to their baseline function at 1 to 2 years. Proctitis may also occur in approximately 15% of men and manifest as mild hematochezia typically 1 to 2 years after treatment. These symptoms can often be managed conservatively by avoiding constipation and in severe cases with argon-plasma coagulation.

Late complications associated with prostate brachytherapy include incontinence, erectile dysfunction, and the remote possibilities of severe rectal injury or secondary malignancies involving the bladder or rectum. The risk of developing incontinence is limited except for men who have undergone a previous TURP or require TURP for obstruction after brachytherapy (10).

Patients with a history of prior TURP have an approximate 20% risk of developing stress incontinence, and a post-brachytherapy TURP portends an even higher risk unless the TURP is of very limited volume. Erectile function will likely decrease in 20% to 30% of men 2 to 3 years after brachytherapy. The risk of severe rectal injury is remote but does occur in <1% of patients and can require permanent colostomy. Finally, EBRT has been associated with an absolute 1% increase in secondary malignancies of the rectum or bladder as compared to patients undergoing prostatectomy alone (22). Theoretically, prostate brachytherapy would carry a similar risk; however, this remains unproven.

### Results

Defining and subsequently reporting low-risk prostate cancer outcomes has been the subject of much debate. Unlike with prostatectomy, PSA levels rarely become undetectable following radiation therapy. Therefore, the American Society for Therapeutic Radiology and Oncology Consensus Panel issued a consensus statement in 1997 defining biochemical failure following radiation therapy for prostate cancer as three consecutive increases in PSA value. Furthermore, the date of failure has been defined as the midpoint between the postirradiation nadir PSA and the first of the three consecutive rises (23). These recommendations were subsequently revised in 2006 and defined as a PSA rise of 2 ng per mL or more above the nadir PSA with no backdating (24).

Prostate cancer outcomes have been actively studied following brachytherapy, and long-term outcomes have now been published confirming the utility of this procedure in the setting of low-risk prostate cancer. Table 30.4 summarizes four series reporting ≥10-year outcomes following brachytherapy as the sole intervention for localized prostate cancer. Freedom

**TABLE 30.4**

**LONG-TERM (>10 YEARS) BIOCHEMICAL (PSA) OUTCOMES FOR LOW-RISK DISEASE: BRACHYTHERAPY ONLY**

| Study | N | Actuarial time (yr) | Median follow-up (mo) | FFPF[a] (%) |
|---|---|---|---|---|
| Stone et al. (25) | 146 | 10 | 72 | 91 |
| Potters et al. (26)[b] | 481 | 12 | 82 | 88 |
| Grimm et al. (27) | 125 | 10 | 81 | 87 |
| Martin et al. (28) | 273 | 12 | 60 | 90 |

[a]FFPF, freedom from PSA failure.
[b]Four percent received EBRT and 23% hormonal therapy for downsizing.

from PSA failure at 10 years is approximately 90% and compares favorably with outcomes obtained from other therapeutic options such as EBRT and prostatectomy. Table 30.5 summarizes three series that combined brachytherapy and EBRT for intermediate- to high-risk prostate cancer. Long-term outcomes reveal that freedom from PSA failure at a minimum of 5 years is >75% for intermediate-risk patients and >60% for high-risk patients. Relatively early data (median follow-up of 50 months) from MSSM show promising results using brachytherapy combined with EBRT and 9 months of hormonal therapy, with 86% PSA control at 5 years for high-risk patients.

**TABLE 30.5**

**BIOCHEMICAL (PSA) OUTCOMES FOR INTERMEDIATE- TO HIGH-RISK DISEASE: BRACHYTHERAPY COMBINED WITH EXTERNAL BEAM AND/OR HORMONAL THERAPY**

| Study | N | Actuarial time (yr) | Median follow-up (mo) | FFPF[a] (%) |
|---|---|---|---|---|
| Stock et al. (29) | | 5 | 50 | |
| High-risk | 132 | | | 86 |
| Potters et al. (26) | | 12 | 82 | |
| Intermediate-risk | 554 | | | 76 |
| High-risk | 418 | | | 62 |
| Sylvester et al. (30) | | 15 | 113 | |
| Intermediate-risk | 50 | | | 80 |
| High-risk | 114 | | | 68 |

[a]FFPF, freedom from PSA failure.

## *References*


1. Pasteau O, Degrais P. The radium treatment of cancer of the prostate. *J Urol (Paris)* 1913;4(1):341–366.
2. Acher PL, Morris SL, Popert RJMP, et al. Permanent prostate brachytherapy: a century of technical evolution. *Prostate Cancer Prostatic Dis* 2006; 9(3):215–220.
3. Makarov DV, Trock BJ, Humphreys EB, et al. Updated nomogram to predict pathologic stage of prostate cancer given prostate-specific antigen level, clinical stage, and biopsy Gleason score (Partin tables) based on cases from 2000 to 2005. *Urology* 2007;69(6):1095–1101.
4. Diaz A, Roach M, Marquez C, et al. Indications for and the significance of seminal vesicle irradiation during 3D conformal radiotherapy for localized prostate cancer. *Int J Radiat Oncol Biol Phys* 1994;30(2):323–329.
5. Woo S, Kaplan I, Roach M, et al. Formula to estimate risk of pelvic lymph node metastasis from the total Gleason score for prostate cancer. *J Urol* 1988;140(2):387.
6. Crook J, McLean M, Catton C, et al. Factors influencing risk of acute urinary retention after TRUS-guided permanent prostate seed implantation. *Int J Radiat Oncol Biol Phys* 2002;52(2):453–460.
7. Niehaus A, Merrick GS, Butler WM, et al. The influence of isotope and prostate volume on urinary morbidity after prostate brachytherapy. *Int J Radiat Oncol Biol Phys* 2006;64(1):136–143.
8. Marshall D, Stone N, Stone J, et al. Hormonal therapy reduces the risk of post-implant urinary retention in symptomatic prostate cancer patients with glands larger than 50 cc. *Int J Radiat Oncol Biol Phys* 2004;60(1):S451.
9. Ragde H, Blasko JC, Grimm PD, et al. Interstitial iodine-125 radiation without adjuvant therapy in the treatment of clinically localized prostate carcinoma. *Cancer* 1997;80(3):442–453.
10. Stone NN, Stock RG. Complications following permanent prostate brachytherapy. *Eur Urol* 2002;41(4):427–433.
11. Wallner K, Merrick G, True L, et al. $^{125}$I versus $^{103}$Pd for low-risk prostate cancer: preliminary PSA outcomes from a prospective randomized multicenter trial. *Int J Radiat Oncol Biol Phys* 2003;57(5):1297–1303.
12. Grimm PD, Blasko JC, Ragde H. Ultrasound-guided transperineal implantation of iodine-125 and palladium-103 for the treatment of early-stage prostate cancer: technical concepts in planning, operative technique, and evaluation. In: *New techniques in prostate surgery*. Philadelphia: WB Saunders, 1994:113–126.
13. Stock RG, Stone NN, Wesson MF, et al. A modified technique allowing interactive ultrasound-guided three-dimensional transperineal prostate implantation. *Int J Radiat Oncol Biol Phys* 1995;32(1):219–225.
14. Kaplan ID, Meskell PM, Lieberfarb M, et al. A comparison of the precision of seeds deposited as loose seeds versus suture embedded seeds: a randomized trial. *Brachytherapy* 2004;3(1):7–9.
15. Tapen EM, Blasko JC, Grimm PD, et al. Reduction of radioactive seed embolization to the lung following prostate brachytherapy. *Int J Radiat Oncol Biol Phys* 1998;42(5):1063–1067.
16. Lin K, Lee SP, Cho JS, et al. Improvements in prostate brachytherapy dosimetry due to seed stranding. *Brachytherapy* 2007;6(1):44–48.

17. Heysek RV, Gwede CK, Torres-Roca J, et al. A dosimetric analysis of unstranded seeds versus customized stranded seeds in transperineal interstitial permanent prostate seed brachytherapy. *Brachytherapy* 2006;5(4): 244–250.
18. Fagundes HM, Keys RJ, Wojcik MF, et al. Transperineal TRUS-guided prostate brachytherapy using loose seeds versus RAPIDStrand: a dosimetric analysis. *Brachytherapy* 2004;3(3):136–140.
19. Marshall DT. Options and recent advances in permanent brachytherapy for prostate cancer. *Can J Urol* 2007;14(61):28–31.
20. Zauls J, Clarke H, Ashenafi M, et al. Permanent prostate brachytherapy using real-time dosimetry combined with intraoperatively built custom links of seeds provides equivalent dosimetric results as traditional gun applicators. *Brachytherapy* 2008;7(2):187.
21. Nag S, Bice W, Dewyngaert K, et al. The American Brachytherapy Society recommendations for permanent prostate brachytherapy postimplant dosimetric analysis. *Int J Radiat Oncol Biol Phys* 2000;46(1):221–230.
22. Brenner DJ, Curtis RE, Hall EJ, et al. Second malignancies in prostate carcinoma patients after radiotherapy compared with surgery. *Cancer* 2000; 88(2):398–406.
23. American Society for Therapeutic Radiology and Oncology Consensus Panel. Consensus statement: guidelines for PSA following radiation therapy. *Int J Radiat Oncol Biol Phys* 1997;37(5):1035–1041.
24. Roach M III, Hanks G, Thames J, et al. Defining biochemical failure following radiotherapy with or without hormonal therapy in men with clinically localized prostate cancer: recommendations of the RTOG-ASTRO Phoenix Consensus Conference. *Int J Radiat Oncol Biol Phys* 2006;65(4): 965–974.
25. Stone NN, Stock RG, Unger P. Intermediate term biochemical-free progression and local control following 125iodine brachytherapy for prostate cancer. *J Urol* 2005;173(3):803–807.
26. Potters L, Morgenstern C, Calugaru E, et al. 12-year outcomes following permanent prostate brachytherapy in patients with clinically localized prostate cancer. *J Urol* 2008;179[Suppl 5]:S20–S24.
27. Grimm PD, Blasko JC, Sylvester JE, et al. 10-year biochemical (prostate-specific antigen) control of prostate cancer with (125) I brachytherapy. *Int J Radiat Oncol Biol Phys* 2001;51(1):31–40.
28. Martin A, Roy J, Beaulieu L, et al. Permanent prostate implant using high activity seeds and inverse planning with fast simulated annealing algorithm: a 12-year Canadian experience. *Int J Radiat Oncol Biol Phys* 2007; 67(2):334–341.
29. Stock RG, Cahlon O, Cesaretti JA, et al. Combined modality treatment in the management of high-risk prostate cancer. *Int J Radiat Oncol Biol Phys* 2004;59(5):1352–1359.
30. Sylvester JE, Grimm PD, Blasko JC, et al. 15-year biochemical relapse free survival in clinical stage T1-T3 prostate cancer following combined external beam radiotherapy and brachytherapy; Seattle experience. *Int J Radiat Oncol Biol Phys* 2007;67(1):57–64.

# SECTION IV ■ URETHRA

E. ANN GORMLEY

# CHAPTER 31 ■ ANATOMY OF THE URETHRA

E. ANN GORMLEY

## FEMALE URETHRA

### Gross/Microscopic

The female urethra extends from the bladder neck to the external urethral meatus and varies in length from 3 to 5 cm. The urethra is a fibromuscular tube composed of a mucosal lining, a submucosal layer, and a muscle layer. Proximally the transitional cell mucosa is continuous with the bladder epithelium. Distally the mucosa is nonkeratinized stratified squamous epithelium (Fig. 31.1). The submucosa consists of abundant longitudinal and circular elastic fibers and contains a prominent venous system. The mucosa and submucosa act as a washer producing a seal that contributes to urethral closure pressure (1). These tissues are estrogen-dependent, and in hypoestrogenic states thinning of the tissue may result in incontinence (2). The smooth muscle layer consists of a thick sheet of longitudinally oriented fibers and a thin outer layer of circular fibers. These muscles are continuous with the bladder neck proximally and terminate distally in the subcutaneous tissue surrounding the external urethral meatus. Colleselli and others have shown in the cranial and most of the middle third of the urethra that there are three smooth muscle layers, including outer and inner longitudinal layers and a middle transverse layer (3). The density of urethral circular smooth muscle is lower in older women, which may account for the change in urethral closure pressure that is seen with increasing age (4).

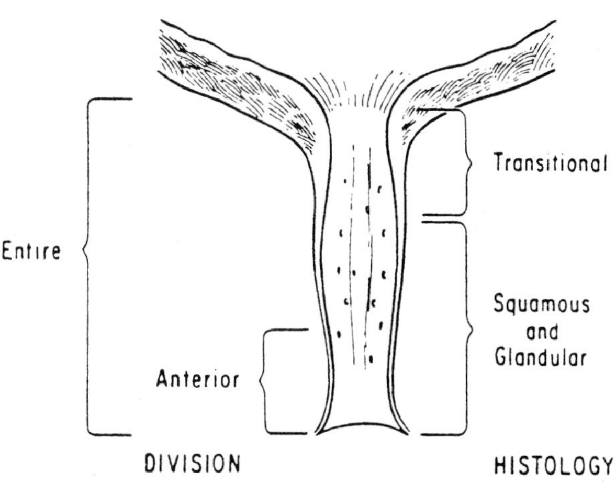


FIGURE 31.1 The female urethra.

In the distal two thirds of the urethra a layer of striated muscle, the rhabdosphincter, surrounds the smooth muscle layer, on the ventral and lateral aspects making an omegalike-shaped sphincter. The rhabdosphincter is composed of delicate Type I (slow-twitch) fibers and consists of three distinct muscles. Proximally the muscle forms a ring (sphincter urethrae) that encircles the urethra. Distally the muscle (compressor urethrae) fans out laterally along the curve of the inferior border of the pubic rami to compress the urethra against the anterior vaginal wall. At the vestibule the muscle completely surrounds the urethra and vagina to form a urethrovaginal sphincter (Fig. 31.2) (5). The three muscles work together to provide

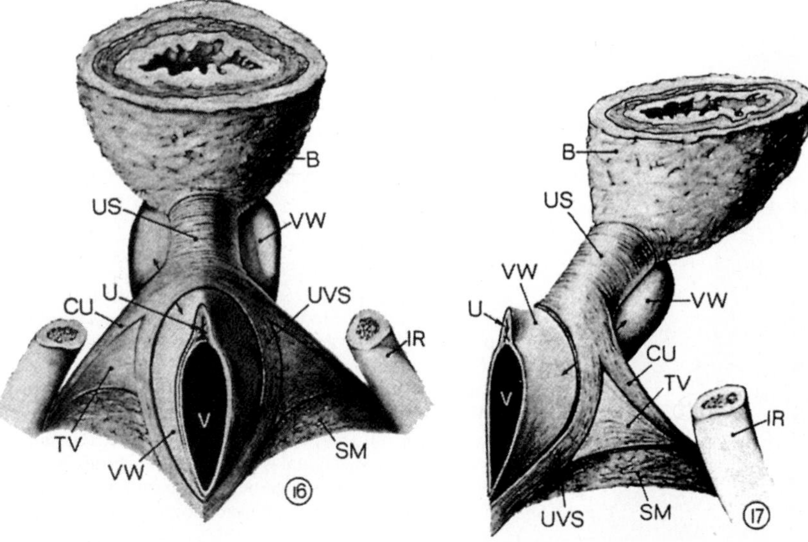


FIGURE 31.2 Striated urogenital sphincter muscle seen from below after removal of the perineal membrane and pubic bones. *US*, urethral sphincter; *UVS*, urethrovaginal sphincter; *CU*, compressor urethrae; *B*, bladder; *IR*, ischiopubic ramus; *TV*, transverse vaginae muscle; *SM*, smooth muscle; *U*, urethra; *V*, vagina; *VW*, vaginal wall. (From Oelrich TM. The striated urogenital sphincter muscle in the female. *Anat Rec* 1983; 205:223, with permission.)

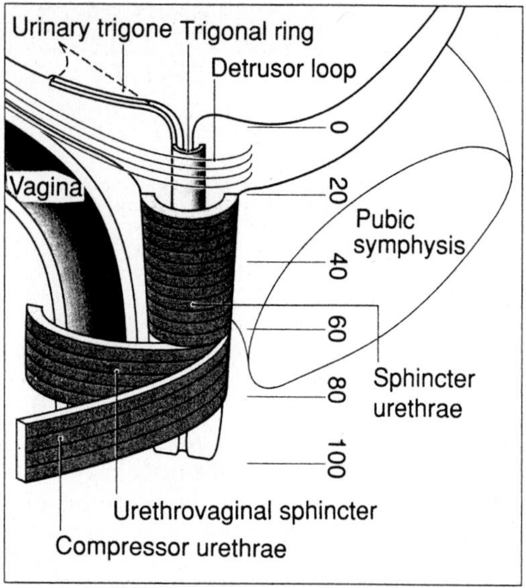


FIGURE 31.3 Location of various structures along the urethra. Note the three parts of the rhabdosphincter. (Copyright University of Michigan, 1989, with permission.)

constant urethral tone (Fig. 31.3) (6). Normally the striated sphincter plays a minimal role in resisting abdominal pressure. However, preservation of the rhabdosphincter is necessary for continence after creation of a female neobladder (3).

Paired periurethral (Skene) glands drain on either side of the midline just posterior to the urethral meatus. There are also numerous small periurethral mucous glands that open into small recesses in the mucosa.

## Vascular Anatomy

The arterial supply to the female urethra is from the urethral artery, a branch of the internal pudendal artery, which in turn is a branch of the internal iliac artery (7). The venous drainage is via the pelvic venous plexus.

## Innervation

The smooth muscle of the urethra is innervated by parasympathetic nerves. The predominant sympathetic receptors are alpha-adrenergic (8). These receptors are responsible for urethral smooth muscle contraction and possibly engorgement of the submucosal vasculature to create a watertight seal of the urethral mucosa (9). The striated muscle fibers of the external intrinsic sphincter receive innervation from the pudendal and pelvic somatic nerves (10). Both somatic and autonomic nerves to the urethra travel on the lateral walls of the vagina near the urethra. Various authors have advised against dissection in this area during transvaginal surgery to prevent development of stress urinary incontinence due to intrinsic sphincter dysfunction (11).

## Lymphatics

The lymphatic drainage of the proximal urethra is to the deep pelvic nodes. The drainage of the distal portion of the urethra is to the inguinal nodes.

## Contiguous Structures

A "hammock" of vaginal tissue supports the urethra (12). The urethral supports, also termed pubourethral ligaments, include fascial and muscular attachments to the arcus tendineus fasciae pelvis and levator ani muscles. These supports are only present in the distal third of the urethra and fix the urethra to the pubic bone. The pubovesical muscle is a separate structure that is an extension of the smooth muscle of the bladder, which extends from the detrusor muscle to the arcus tendineus fasciae pelvis and pubic bone (Fig. 31.4) (13).

Posteriorly the urethra is intimately related to the anterior surface of the vagina. The periurethral fascia is located immediately beneath the vaginal epithelium and is seen as the glistening white layer that surrounds the urethra when an incision is made in the anterior wall of the vagina. The fascia extends

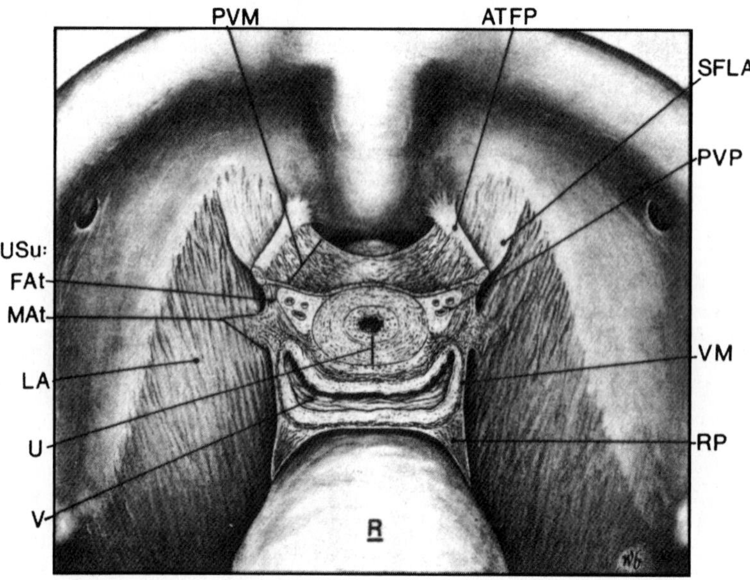


FIGURE 31.4 Cross section of the urethra (*U*), vagina (*V*), arcus tendineus fasciae pelvis (*ATFP*), and superior fascia of levator ani (*SFLA*) just below the vesical neck (drawn from cadaver dissection). Pubovesical muscles (*PVM*) lie anterior to urethra and anterior and superior to paraurethral vascular plexus (*PVP*). The urethral supports (*Usu*) (the pubourethral ligaments) attach the vagina and vaginal surface of the urethra to the levator ani muscles (*MAt*, muscular attachment) and to the superior fascia of the levator ani (*Fat*, fascial attachment). *R*, rectum; *RP*, rectal pillar; *VM*, vaginal wall muscularis. (From DeLancey JOL. The pubovesical ligament, a separate structure from the urethral supports. *Neurol Urodynam* 1989;8:53, with permission.)

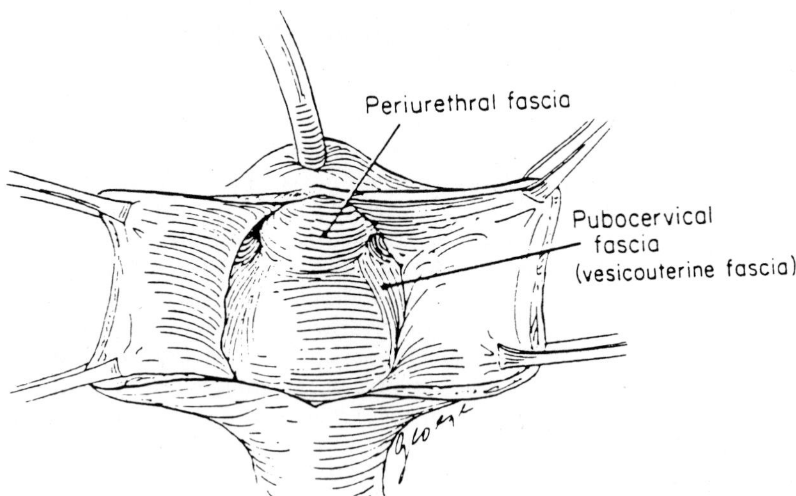


FIGURE 31.5 View of the anterior vaginal fascial support, which is found beneath the vaginal wall (shown retracted). The periurethral fascia, which forms the vaginal layer of the urethropelvic ligaments, is continuous with the pubocervical fascia proximally.

from the meatus to the bladder neck and laterally to where it fuses with the endopelvic fascia at the pubic bone (Fig 31.5).

## MALE URETHRA

### Gross/Microscopic

The posterior urethra is the portion of the urethra extending from the bladder neck through the prostate and through the urogenital diaphragm. It is divided into the prostatic urethra and the membranous urethra, which traverses the urogenital diaphragm just prior to entering the corpora spongiosa. The anterior urethra runs from the urogenital diaphragm to the tip of the glans penis and may be further divided into the bulbous urethra extending from the root of the penis to the convergence of the corpora cavernosa and the pendulous or penile urethra that traverses the pendulous portion of the penis. There is a dilation of the urethra in the area of the glans penis called the fossa navicularis (Fig. 31.6).

A number of ducts empty into the lumen of the urethra. Two to 3 cm distal to the membranous urethra the paired orifices of the Cowper glands (bulbourethral glands) are noted on the floor. On the roof of the pendulous urethra there are openings for the glands of Littre, or the submucosal urethral glands, and small recesses termed urethral lacunae. The lacuna magna is a larger lacuna in the midportion of the anterior aspect of the fossa navicularis.

The urethral epithelium varies along the length of the urethra. In the prostatic urethra the cells are transitional, whereas in the membranous urethra they are stratified columnar. The epithelium of the penile urethra is composed of pseudostratified and columnar cells. In the fossa navicularis, the epithelium is composed of stratified squamous cells.

### Vascular Anatomy

Paired bulbourethral arteries, which arise as the first of three penile branches of the internal pudendal artery, supply the urethra. The venous drainage is via the emissary veins, which drain to the circumflex branches of the deep dorsal vein of the penis.

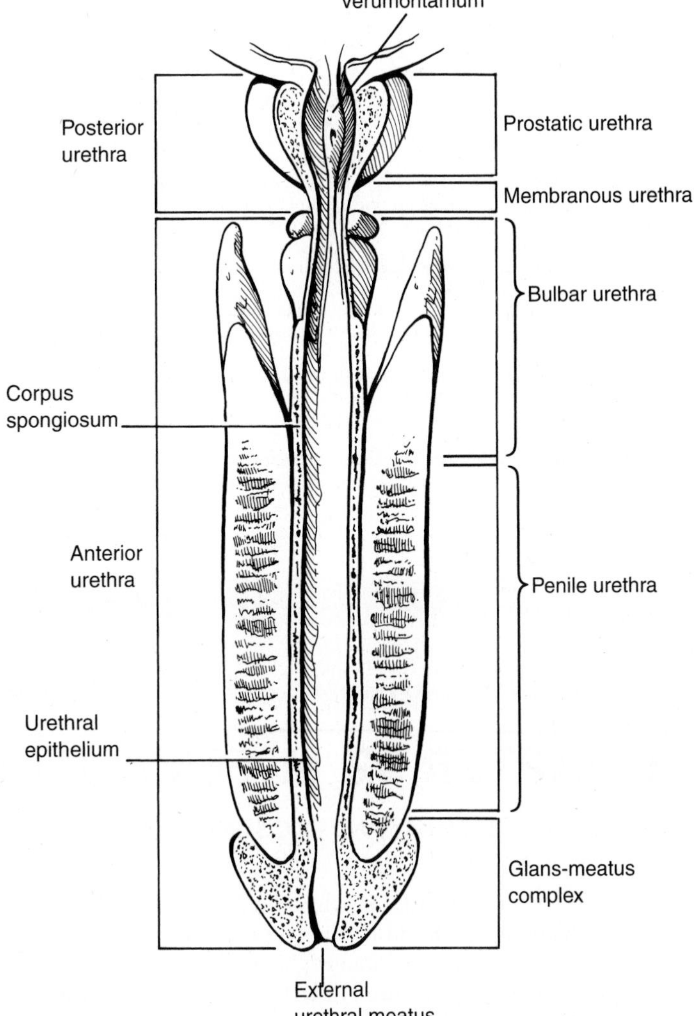


FIGURE 31.6 The male urethra and its divisions with associated histology.

## Innervation

The urethra mucosa is innervated via the urethrobulbar nerve. It is a branch of the nerve to the bulbocavernosus, which is a branch of the perineal nerve, which is derived from the pudendal nerve. A branch of the bulbocavernosus nerve at the 3 and 9 o'clock positions penetrates the striated urethral sphincter (14). The pudendal nerve, consisting of fibers from the second, third, and fourth sacral spinal nerves, is thus both motor to the urethral sphincter and sensory to the urethra and glans penis.

## Lymphatics

The lymphatic drainage of the anterior urethra is into the superficial and deep inguinal node and ultimately to the external iliac nodes. The lymphatics of the posterior (the bulbous, membranous, and prostatic) urethra can take three routes: to the external iliac nodes, to the obturator and internal iliac nodes, or to the presacral nodes.

## Contiguous Structures

The membranous urethra is covered by the fibers of the striated urethral sphincter (rhabdosphincter). Brooks et al. used computer-generated, three-dimensional reconstruction of the male pelvis from the visible human data set to show that the striated urethral sphincter is circular with abundant posterior tissue, making it more signet-ring shaped (16). Ventrally and laterally, the rhabdosphincter is separated from the membranous urethra by a thin sheath of connective tissue (15). Anteriorly the sphincter is approximately twice as long as it is posteriorly. An intrinsic smooth muscle lies between the urethral mucosa and the striated urethral sphincter. This muscle begins above the striated sphincter and then gradually thins distal to the striated sphincter (16).

The remainder of the anterior urethra lies within the corpus spongiosum lying in the ventral groove of the corpora cavernosa of the penis. The Cowper glands (bulbourethral glands) lie within the urogenital diaphragm posterior and lateral to the membranous urethra.

## *References*


1. Raz S, Caine M, Zeigler M. The vascular component in the production of intraurethral pressure. *J Urol* 1972;108:93–96.
2. Klutke JJ, Bergman A. Nonsurgical management of stress urinary incontinence. In: Ostergard DR, Bent AE, eds. *Urogynecology and urodynamics,* 4th ed. Baltimore: Williams & Wilkins, 1996:505–516.
3. Colleselli K, Stenzl A, Eder R, et al. The female urethral sphincter: a morphological and topographical study. *J Urol* 1998;160:49–54.
4. Clobes A, DeLancey JOL, Morgan DM. Urethral circular smooth muscle in young and old women. *Am J Obstet Gynecol* 2008;198:587.e1-5.
5. Oelrich TM. The striated urogenital sphincter muscle in the female. *Anat Rec* 1983;205:223–232.
6. DeLancey JOL. Functional anatomy of the female pelvis. In: Kursh ED, McGuire EJ, eds. *Female urology.* Philadelphia: JB Lippincott Co, 1994:3–16.
7. Ferner H, Staubesand J, eds, *Sobatta atlas of human anatomy,* 10th ed. Munich/Baltimore: Urban & Schwartzenberg, 1982.
8. Ek A. Innervation and receptor functions of the human urethra. *Scan J Urol Nephrol* 1997;S45:1–50.
9. Huisman AB. Aspects on the anatomy of the female urethra with special relation to urinary incontinence. *Contrib Gynecol Obstet* 1983;10:1–31.
10. Borirakchanyavat S, Aboseif SR, Carroll PR, et al. Continence mechanism of the isolated female urethra: an anatomical study of the intrapelvic somatic nerves. *J Urol* 1997;158:822.
11. Ball TP Jr, Teichman JHM, Sharkey FE, et al. Terminal nerve distribution to the urethra and bladder neck: considerations in the management of stress urinary incontinence. *J Urol* 1997;158:827.
12. DeLancey JOL. Structural support of the urethra as it relates to stress urinary incontinence: the hammock hypothesis. *Am J Obstet Gynecol* 1994;170:1713–1723.
13. Strohbehn K. Normal pelvic floor anatomy. *Obstet Gynecol Clin North Am* 1998;25:683–705.
14. Shafik A, Doss S. Surgical anatomy of the somatic terminal innervation to the anal and urethral sphincters: role in anal and urethral surgery. *J Urol* 1999;161:85–89.
15. Dalpiaz O, Mitterberger M, Kerschbaumer A, et al. Anatomical approach for surgery of the male posterior urethra. *BJU International* 2008; 102:1448–1451.
16. Brooks JD, Chao W, Kerr J. Male pelvic anatomy reconstructed from the visible human data set. *J Urol* 1998;159:868–872.


# CHAPTER 32 ■ FEMALE URETHRAL DIVERTICULUM

AHMED M. EL-ZAWAHRY AND ERIC S. ROVNER

Urethral diverticulum (UD) in women represents a challenge in both diagnosis and reconstruction for the urologist. The actual prevalence of UD is not known, but it is reported to occur in 1% to 6% of adult women (1). UD is an epithelialized cavity dissecting within the fascia of the urethropelvic ligament (Fig. 32.1) (2). This cavity forms an isolated cystlike appendage, usually with a single connection to the urethral lumen, termed the neck or ostium. Complicated UD may extend partially around the urethra to form a "saddlebag" UD, or more uncommonly anterior to the urethra (3), or circumferentially around the urethra (4).

It is generally believed that an adult UD is formed as a result of infection and obstruction of the periurethral glands. These tubuloaveolar glands are anatomically located in the

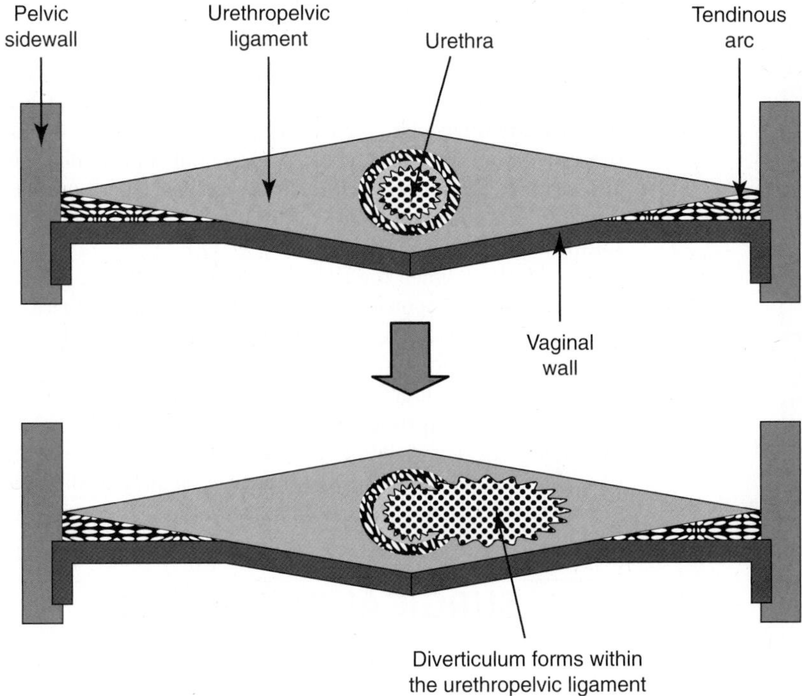


FIGURE 32.1 Diverticulum forms within the urethropelvic ligament.

distal one-third of the urethra ventral and lateral to the urethral lumen. Infection of these glands leads to abscess formation and eventual rupture of the abscess back into the urethral lumen, resulting in an epithelialized cavity in communication with the urethra.

Often, although not invariably highly symptomatic due to the location, the most common coexisting condition is probably urinary incontinence, especially stress urinary incontinence (SUI), which may coexist in up to 50% of individuals (1). Malignant and benign tumors in UD are quite rare. The most common malignant pathology in UD is adenocarcinoma, followed by transitional cell and squamous cell carcinomas. Calculi within UD may be diagnosed in 4% to 10% of cases and is most likely due to urinary stasis and/or infection.

## DIAGNOSIS

The diagnosis of UD can be made with a combination of a thorough history, physical examination, and selected imaging. The symptoms of UD are classically described as the "three Ds": dysuria, dyspareunia, and dribbling (postvoid). However, common presenting symptoms include irritative lower urinary tract symptoms, pain, and urinary tract infection (UTI), which is reported in almost one-third of patients (5). Other symptoms include a vaginal mass, hematuria, vaginal discharge, obstructive voiding symptoms, and urinary retention. Up to 20% of patients may be completely asymptomatic and are thus diagnosed incidentally on imaging or physical examination. Patients may often be misdiagnosed and treated for years for a number of unrelated conditions, such as interstitial cystitis, recurrent cystitis, vulvodynia, endometriosis, and vulvovestibulitis, before the diagnosis of UD is made.

Physical examination should include a careful inspection of the anterior vaginal wall. Masses or areas of tenderness should be noted and further examined. Suspected UD should be carefully differentiated from vaginal prolapse, including cystourethrocele. Most UD are located ventrally over the middle and proximal portions of the urethra corresponding to the area of the anterior vaginal wall 1 to 3 cm inside the introitus. During physical examination, the anterior vaginal wall may be gently "stripped" or "milked" distally in an attempt to express purulent material or urine from within the urethral lumen out through the urethral meatus, which strongly suggests the diagnosis of UD.

Endoscopic examination of the bladder and urethra is performed in an attempt to visualize the UD ostium (communication to the urethra) as well as to evaluate for other causes of the patient's presenting symptoms. A flexible cystoscope or a specially designed rigid female cystoscope with a short beak to maintain the discharge of the irrigation solution immediately adjacent to the lens is most useful in visualizing the lumen of the relatively short female urethra. During cystoscopy, simultaneous gentle compression of the bladder neck and the diverticular sac with an assistant's finger can express luminal discharge of purulent material during urethroscopy localizing the ostium.

High-quality preoperative imaging is important in the diagnosis of UD as well as in planning operative therapy. This will help to provide an accurate reflection of the relevant anatomy of the UD and its anatomical relationships. No single study can be considered the gold standard for the evaluation of UD. Furthermore, the availability and quality of individual radiological techniques is quite variable across centers. Currently available techniques for the evaluation of UD include double-balloon positive-pressure urethrography (PPU), voiding cystourethrography (VCUG), ultrasound (US), and magnetic

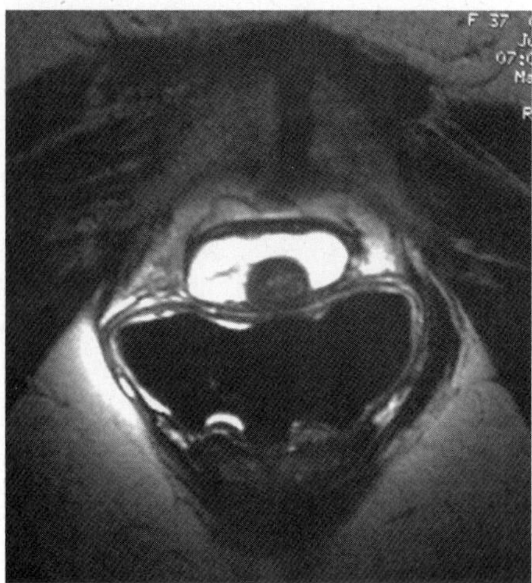

FIGURE 32.2 Axial T-2 weighted MRI of an unusual anterior urethral diverticulum.

resonance imaging (MRI) with or without an endoluminal coil (eMRI). eMRI has several distinct advantages over VCUG; however, these studies are often complementary (6). We currently utilize MRI in the evaluation of all patients with known or suspected UD as the complexity of these lesions is more readily appreciated using this technique (Fig. 32.2). Urodynamic studies, especially videourodynamics, are utilized in patients with urinary incontinence or significant voiding dysfunction in order to characterize these symptoms, especially if surgery is planned. These studies are useful in evaluating the anatomy of the UD, assessing the competence of the bladder neck, assessing bladder function, and confirming the diagnosis of SUI.

## INDICATIONS FOR SURGERY

Symptomatic patients should be offered surgical excision and reconstruction. Those with concomitant SUI can be considered for a simultaneous anti-incontinence procedure at the time of UD excision.

Asymptomatic patients may not desire surgical excision. Other patients may be unwilling or medically unable to undergo surgical excision. However, the natural history of untreated UD is unknown. In such cases, patients should be counseled that certain carcinomas or other complications such as stones or urinary incontinence may arise and that close follow-up is warranted.

## ALTERNATIVE THERAPY

Patients electing nonoperative management can be treated with daily low-dose antibacterial preparations and digital stripping of the anterior vaginal wall following micturition to prevent postvoid dribbling and reduce the risk of UTI due to stasis in the UD.

Most commonly, UD are treated with a complete excision and urethral reconstruction. However, a variety of other surgical interventions for UD have been reported. Approaches have included transurethral and open marsupialization, endoscopic unroofing, fulguration, incision and obliteration, and coagulation (1). One noteworthy alternative to excision and reconstruction is transvaginal marsupialization as described by Spence and Duckett (7). This approach may reduce operative time, blood loss, and recurrence rate but is probably only applicable to UD in very select cases involving the distal one-third of the urethra due to the risk of sphincteric injury and resulting *de novo* SUI.

In rare cases, when the UD is highly symptomatic, acutely infected, and unresponsive to antibiotic therapy, or in cases when a complete elective excision should be postponed, such as during pregnancy, a transvaginal incision (diverticulotomy) can be performed directly into the UD cavity. This will create a temporary urethrovaginal fistula from the UD ostium through the UD cavity into the vagina, thus decompressing the UD. The UD and fistula are subsequently repaired at the time of planned elective excision and reconstruction.

## SURGICAL TECHNIQUE

Excision and reconstruction is probably the most common surgical approach to UD in the modern era. The principles of the urethral diverticulectomy operation have been well described (Table 32.1). There are only a few minor differences between surgical approaches, including the type of vaginal incision (inverted "U" versus inverted "T"), whether it is necessary to remove the entire mucosalized portion of the UD, and finally, the optimal type of postoperative catheter drainage (urethra only versus urethra and suprapubic).

Preoperative preparation includes (a) antibiotic administration in patients with recurrent or persistent UTIs; (b) stripping of the anterior vaginal wall to prevent urinary stasis and recurrent UTIs; and (c) application of topical estrogen creams for several weeks prior to surgery in postmenopausal patients with atrophic vaginitis.

The patient is placed in the high lithotomy position with all pressure points well padded. We have found that the use of padded adjustable stirrups for the lower extremities greatly enhances operative access to the female perineum. A standard vaginal antiseptic preparation is applied. The use of a headlight as well as operative magnification (1.5 × to 2.0 ×) assists with the dissection and precise reconstruction. A Foley catheter (16Fr) is placed in the urethra. A suprapubic tube may

**TABLE 32.1**

**PRINCIPLES OF TRANSVAGINAL URETHRAL DIVERTICULECTOMY**

| |
|---|
| Mobilization of a well-vascularized anterior vaginal wall |
| Preservation of periurethral fascia |
| Identification and excision of the neck of the UD or ostium |
| Removal of the entire UD wall or sac (mucosa) |
| Watertight closure of the urethra |
| Multilayered, nonoverlapping closure with absorbable suture |
| Closure of dead space |
| Preservation or creation of continence |

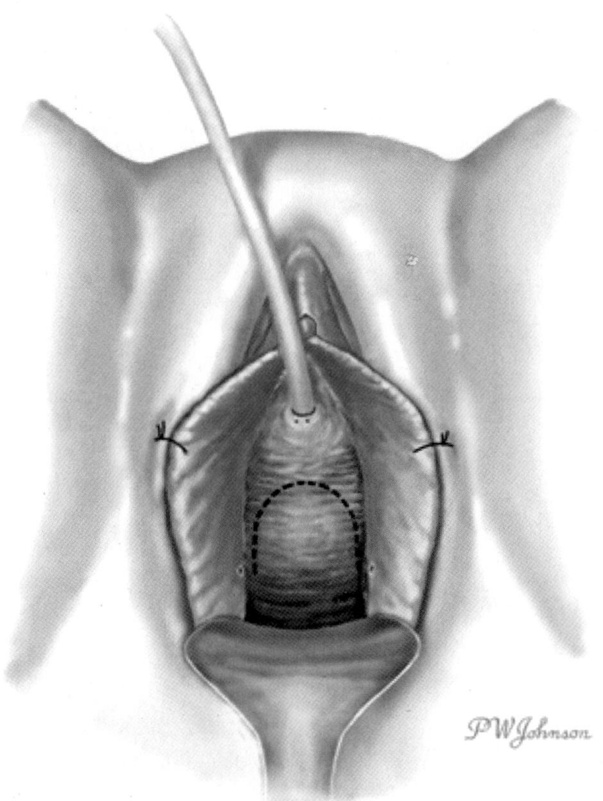

FIGURE 32.3 Incision along the anterior vaginal wall, with the base of the "U" at the level of the distal urethra, provides an excellent lateral exposure at the midvagina for transvaginal urethral diverticulectomy. (From Rovner ES. Urethral diverticula. In: Raz S, Rodriguez L, eds. *Female urology*, 3rd ed. Philadelphia: Elsevier, 2008: 825–844, with permission.)

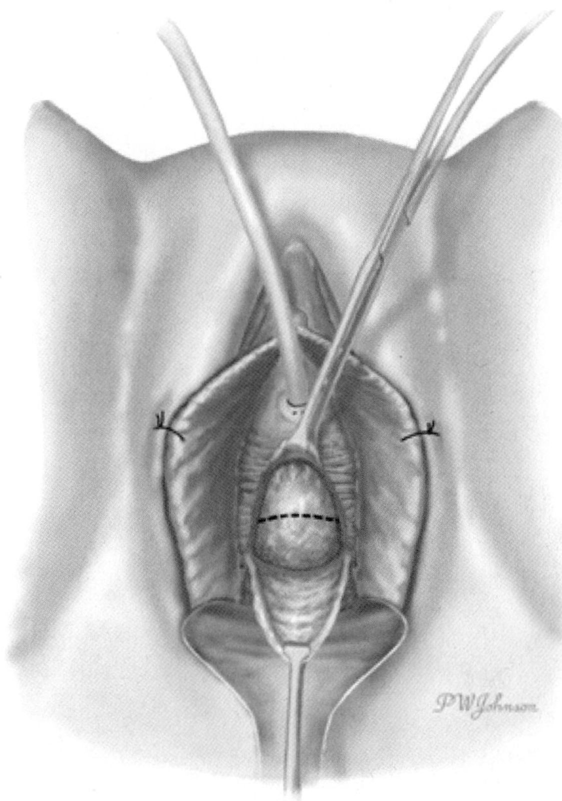

FIGURE 32.4 A transverse incision is made into the periurethral fascia. Proximal and distal layers will be carefully developed without entering the UD. (From Rovner ES. Urethral diverticula. In: Raz S, Rodriguez L, eds. *Female urology*, 3rd ed. Philadelphia: Elsevier, 2008: 825–844, with permission.)

be utilized for an additional postoperative urinary drainage if desired.

A weighted vaginal speculum and Scott retractor with hooks are placed to assist with exposure. An inverted "U" is marked out along the anterior vaginal wall proximal from the urethral meatus with the limbs extending to the bladder neck or beyond (Fig. 32.3). The inverted "U" incision provides excellent exposure laterally at the level of the midvagina and can be extended proximally as needed for lesions that extend beyond the bladder neck. Normal saline can be injected along the lines of the incision beneath the vaginal wall to facilitate dissection. A posterolateral episiotomy may be of help in some patients with a narrow introitus, especially in nulliparous women.

An anterior vaginal wall flap is created by careful dissection in the potential space between the vaginal wall and the periurethral fascia. The use of sufficient countertraction during this portion of the procedure is important in maintaining the proper plane of dissection. During the dissection it is important to preserve the periurethral fascia, maintain an adequate blood supply to the anterior vaginal wall flap, and avoid inadvertent entry into the UD. The periurethral fascia forms a distinct layer that is usually interposed between the vaginal wall and the UD; however, in some lesions it may be deficient (8). Preservation and later reconstruction of the perirurethral fascia is of paramount importance in order to prevent UD recurrence, close dead space, and avoid urethrovaginal fistula formation postoperatively. Pseudodiverticula have been described where this layer of tissue is considerably attenuated or even absent (8). In these patients, an interpositional flap, or graft such as a pubovaginal sling, may be utilized for reconstruction.

Following the completed takedown of the anterior vaginal wall flap, the periurethral fascia is incised transversely (Fig. 32.4). Proximal and distal layers of periurethral fascia are carefully developed, avoiding entrance into the UD. The UD is then grasped and sharply dissected back to its origin on the urethra within the leaves of the periurethral fascia (Fig. 32.5). In many cases it is necessary to open and enter the UD to facilitate dissection from the surrounding tissues, especially if the patient had a previous recent infection. The ostium or connection to the urethra is identified and the walls of the UD are completely excised. Every effort should be made to remove the entire mucosalized surface of the UD in order to prevent recurrence. All abnormal tissue in the area of the ostium should be removed if possible to ensure that no mucosal elements of the UD wall remain that could result in postoperative urine leakage and recurrence. Following complete excision of the UD, the urethral catheter is often seen (Fig. 32.6). The urethra can be reconstructed over a Foley catheter as small as 12Fr without long-term risk of urethral stricture and should be closed in a watertight fashion with 4-0

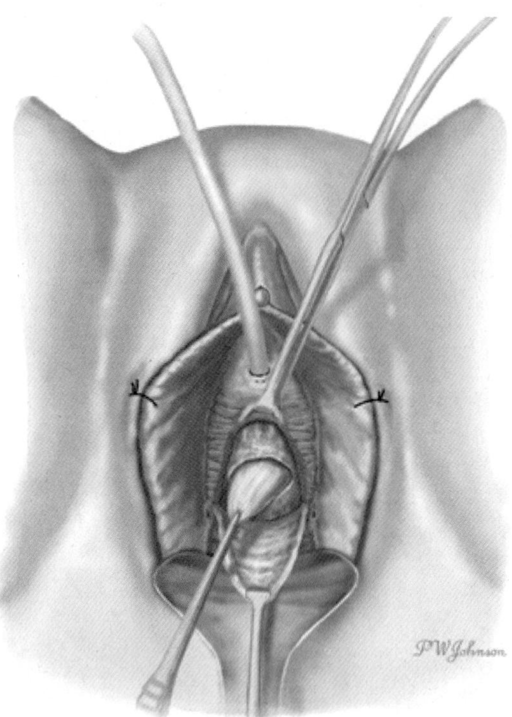


FIGURE 32.5 Following mobilization of the anterior and posterior leaves of the periurethral fascia, the urethral diverticulum is dissected back to its origin on the urethra within the leaves of the periurethral fascia. (From Rovner ES. Urethral diverticula. In: Raz S, Rodriguez L, eds. *Female urology*, 3rd ed. Philadelphia: Elsevier *[in press]*, with permission.)

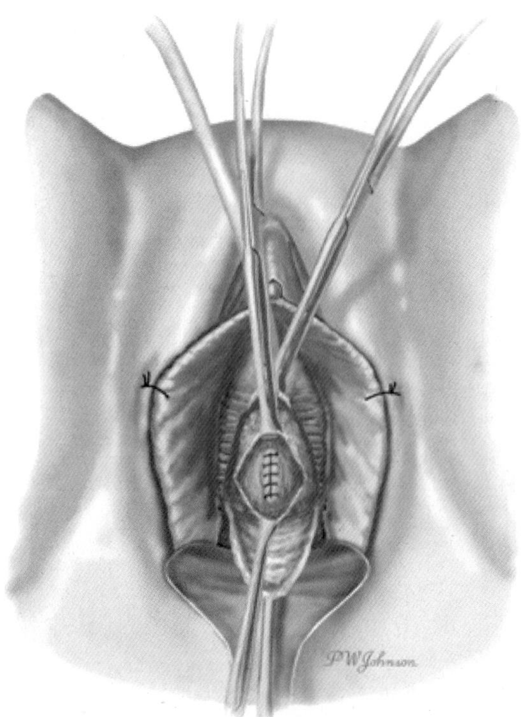


FIGURE 32.7 Closure of the urethra with absorbable suture should be watertight and tension-free. (From Rovner ES. Urethral diverticula. In: Raz S, Rodriguez L, eds. *Female urology*, 3rd ed. Philadelphia: Elsevier *[in press]*, with permission.)

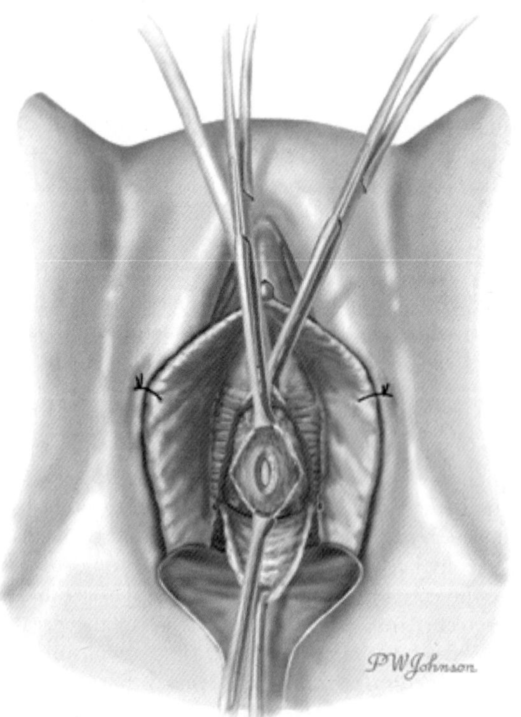


FIGURE 32.6 Following removal of the entire urethral diverticulum, the Foley catheter is often seen. (From Rovner ES. Urethral diverticula. In: Raz S, Rodriguez L, eds. *Female urology*, 3rd ed. Philadelphia: Elsevier *[in press]*, with permission.)

synthetic absorbable suture (Fig. 32.7). The closure should be tension-free and should include the full thickness of the urethral wall. The periurethral fascial flaps are reapproximated with 3-0 synthetic absorbable sutures in a perpendicular orientation to the urethral closure line in order to minimize overlap and hence the risk of postoperative urethrovaginal fistula formation (Fig. 32.8). Care is taken to secure the periurethral fascial flaps in such a way as to close all dead space.

If desired, a fibrofatty labial (Martius) flap can be harvested at this point and placed over the periurethral fascia as an additional layer of closure. Indications for such a flap are not universally agreed upon. However, in patients with poor-quality tissues or attenuated periurethral fascia, or in whom significant inflammation is encountered intraoperatively, a well-vascularized adjuvant flap such as a Martius flap may reduce the risk of wound breakdown and subsequent complications such as urethrovaginal fistula. The anterior vaginal wall flap is then repositioned and reapproximated with absorbable suture (Fig. 32.9). This completes a three-layer closure (four layers if a Martius flap is utilized). An antibiotic impregnated vaginal pack is placed postoperatively.

The vaginal packing is removed within 6 to 24 hours, and the patient is discharged home with closed urinary drainage. Antispasmodics are used liberally to reduce bladder spasms. A pericatheter VCUG is obtained at 14 to 21 days postoperatively. If there is no extravasation, the catheters are removed. If extravasation is seen, then repeat pericatheter VCUGs are performed weekly until resolution is noted. In the vast majority of cases, extravasation will resolve in several weeks with this type of conservative management.

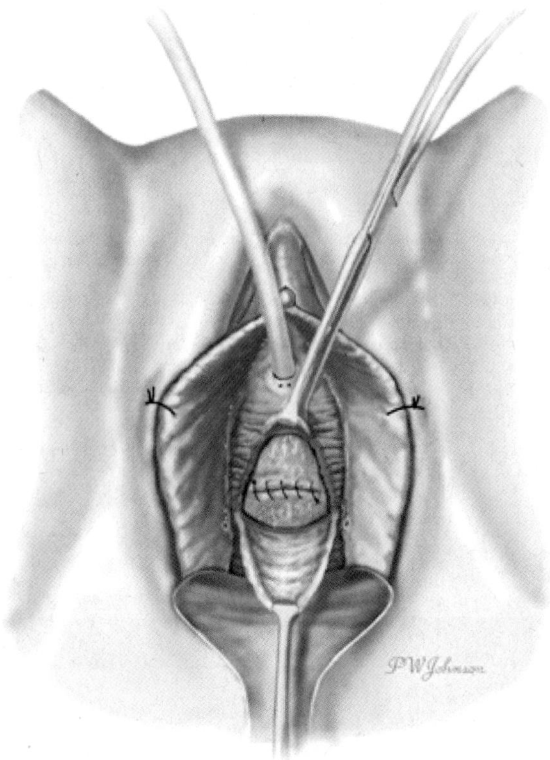


**FIGURE 32.8** Closure of the periurethral fascia should be perpendicular to the urethral closure line to minimize overlap and the risk of urethrovaginal fistula. (From Rovner ES. Urethral diverticula. In: Raz S, Rodriguez L, eds. *Female urology*, 3rd ed. Philadelphia: Elsevier *[in press]*, with permission.)

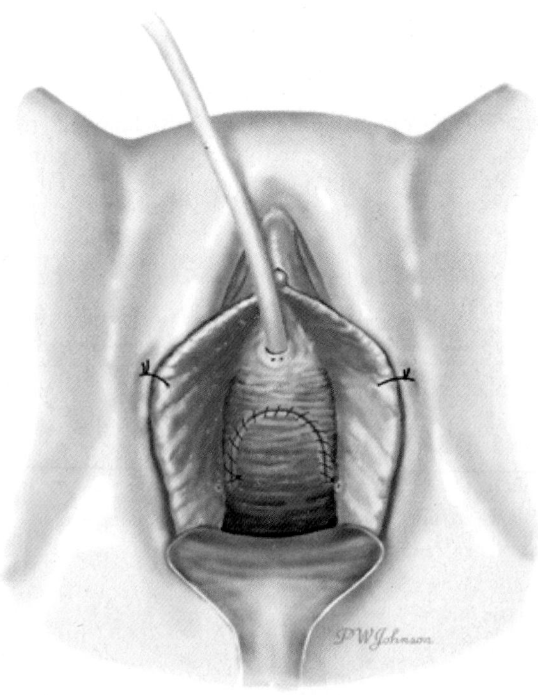


**FIGURE 32.9** Closure of the vaginal wall with reapproximation of the anterior vaginal wall flap. This completes a three-layer closure including closure of the urethra, periurethral fascia, and vaginal wall. (From Rovner ES. Urethral diverticula. In: Raz S, Rodriguez L, eds. Female urology, 3rd ed. Philadelphia: Elsevier *[in press]*, with permission.)

## COMPLICATIONS

Postoperative complications can be avoided by careful adherence to the principles of transvaginal urethral diverticulectomy. Nevertheless, complications may arise. Large diverticula (>4 cm) or those associated with a lateral or horseshoe configuration may be associated with a greater likelihood of postoperative complications (9). Complications include recurrent diverticulum (1% to 29%), stress incontinence (1.7% to 16.0%), urethral stricture (0% to 5%), and recurrent UTIs (0% to 31%) (1).

Intraoperative bleeding can be avoided by maintaining the proper plane of dissection during takedown of the anterior vaginal wall flap. If bleeding is encountered, cautery or suture ligature can be used. Excessive use of cautery should be avoided as this can lead to flap necrosis and fistula formation.

Urethrovaginal fistula is a devastating but fortunately rare complication that may result from diverticulectomy. A fistula can be located either distal or proximal to the sphincteric mechanism. A distally located fistula is usually not associated with symptoms other than perhaps a split urinary stream and/or vaginal voiding. As such a distal urethrovaginal fistula may not require repair, although some patients may request repair. Conversely, a proximal fistula located at the bladder neck or within the proximal half of the urethra in patients with an incompetent bladder neck will likely result in considerable symptomatic urinary leakage. These patients should undergo repair with or without the use of an adjuvant tissue flap such as a Martius flap to provide a well-vascularized additional tissue layer. Meticulous attention to surgical technique, good hemostasis, avoidance of infection, preservation of the periurethral fascia, a well-vascularized anterior vaginal wall flap, and a multilayered closure with nonoverlapping suture lines should minimize the potential for postoperative urethrovaginal fistula formation.

Coexisting SUI can be treated at the time of urethral diverticulectomy as noted previously. However, *de novo* SUI may occur following urethral diverticulectomy. The proximity of most urethral diverticula to the sphincter mechanism puts the patient at risk for this complication even with meticulous attention to surgical technique.

Persistence or recurrence of symptoms following diverticulectomy may occur in some patients. This may be caused by a new medical problem (e.g., UTI, etc.), a new UD, or alternatively, recurrence of the original lesion. Recurrence of a UD may be due to incomplete excision of the UD, inadequate closure of the urethra or residual dead space, or other technical factors. Ljungqvist et al. found recurrence in 11 out of 68 of their patients over 26-year follow-up with a 92% overall satisfaction (10). Repeat urethral diverticulectomy surgery can be challenging due to altered anatomy, scarring, and the difficulty of identifying the proper anatomic planes.

## OUTCOMES

The significance of appropriate preoperative patient counseling regarding surgery and postoperative expectations of cure cannot be overemphasized. Individuals with UD have a myriad of symptoms, including pain, UTIs, and urinary dysfunction. Although these are often related to the presence of the

UD, sometimes they do not resolve even with a technically successful surgery. Nevertheless, surgical outcome for the UD has generally been good. Outcome can be evaluated by resolution of the patient's symptoms or recurrence of the diverticulum. Successful excision of UD has been reported in 86% to 100% of patients.

## *References*


1. Rovner ES. Bladder and urethral diverticula. In: Wein AJ, Kavoussi L, Novick A, et al., eds. *Campbel's urology*, Vol. 9. Philadelphia: Elsevier, 2007:2361–2390.
2. Young GPH, Wahle GR, Raz S. Female urethral diverticulum. In: Raz S, ed. *Female urology*. Philadelphia: WB Saunders, 1996:477–489.
3. Vakili B, Wai C, Nihira M. Anterior urethral diverticulum in the female: diagnosis and surgical approach. *Obstet Gynecol* 2003;102:1179–1183.
4. Rovner ES, Wein AJ. Diagnosis and reconstruction of the dorsal or circumferential urethral diverticulum. *J Urol* 2003;170:82–86.
5. Ganabathi K, Leach GE, Zimmern PE, et al. Experience with the management of urethral diverticulum in 63 women. *J Urol* 1994;152:1445–1452.
6. Blander DS, Rovner ES, Schnall MD, et al. Endoluminal magnetic resonance imaging in the evaluation of urethral diverticula in women. *Urology* 2001;57:660–665.
7. Spence HM, Duckett JW Jr. Diverticulum of the female urethra: clinical aspects and presentation of a simple operative technique for cure. *J Urol* 1970;104:432–437.
8. Leng WW, McGuire EJ. Management of female urethral diverticula: a new classification. *J Urol* 1998;160:1297–1300.
9. Porpiglia F, Destefanis P, Fiori C, et al. Preoperative risk factors for surgery for urethral diverticula: our experience. *Urol Int* 2002;69:7–11.
10. Ljungqvist L, Peeker R, Fall M. Female urethral diverticulum: 26-year followup of a large series. *J Urol* 2007;177:219–224.


# CHAPTER 33 ■ RECONSTRUCTION OF THE FEMALE URETHRA

JERRY G. BLAIVAS AND RAJVEER S. PUROHIT

Reconstruction of the female urethra is technically challenging, but when done correctly can restore anatomy and function in women with a urethrovaginal fistula or urethral stricture using a single procedure. Conversely, surgical failure necessitates multiple operations with decreasing chances of success and may leave patients functionally crippled or in need of a urinary diversion. For this reason, technical proficiency and a comprehensive preoperative diagnostic examination to understand the patient's pathophysiology are mandatory. The goal of surgery should be repair of the damaged urethra in such a way as to allow the patient voluntary, unobstructed, and painless micturition.

In the developing world, the most common cause of urethral damage requiring reconstruction is urethrovaginal fistula resulting from obstetric trauma. Prolonged obstructed labor with compression of the fetal head against the symphysis pubica may cause pressure necrosis of the urethra and, consequently, the development of complicated fistulas. Cesarean section performed to relieve this condition also carries a risk of subsequent fistula formation (1). Where modern obstetric care is available, urethral damage is commonly the result of reconstructive surgery for urethral diverticulum but can also occur from bladder neck suspensions, anterior colporrhaphy, and, rarely, vaginal hysterectomy (Table 33.1). Urethrovaginal fistulas are also caused by erosion of synthetic materials placed during pelvic reconstructive surgery or anti-incontinence procedures (2), locally invasive malignancies, and long-term effects of radiation (3). Less commonly reported causes include damage from Shirodkar cerclage sutures for cervical incompetence in gravid women, complications from operative vaginal delivery, and pressure necrosis from tightly placed Kelly plication sutures over an indwelling catheter. The presence of an indwelling urethral catheter itself can cause erosive necrosis, typically in the population of paralyzed or

**TABLE 33.1**

**CAUSES OF URETHRAL DAMAGE IN A CASE SERIES OF 74 WOMEN**

| Cause | n |
|---|---|
| Urethral diverticulectomy or diverticulum | 28 |
| Urethral injury from Pereyra procedure | 18 |
| Anterior colporrhaphy | 10 |
| Fistula from other gynecologic surgery | 3 |
| Fistula or erosion associated with synthetic material | 9 |
| Urethral obstruction from previous surgery | 3 |
| Trauma | 3 |
| Obstetric injury | 2 |
| Ectopic ureter | 1 |
| Primary urethral stricture | 1 |
| Total | 74 |

From Flisser AJ, Blaivas JG. Outcome of urethral reconstructive surgery in a series of 74 women. *J Urol* 2003;169:2246–2249, with permission.

comatose patients. Finally, pelvic trauma can cause laceration of the urethra, usually when accompanied by separation or fracture of the symphysis pubica (4).

## DIAGNOSIS

A thorough history and physical examination are critical for evaluating a patient suspected of urethral injury. In our experience, pelvic examination will reveal the vast majority of injuries. If concurrent sphincteric urinary incontinence complicates the diagnosis, the urethral meatus can be occluded by the examiner's finger while the patient strains or coughs. If the anterior vaginal wall is visualized with the assistance of a speculum blade placed into the posterior fornix, urinary leakage from the fistula can usually be detected.

Cystoscopic examination is essential in the diagnostic investigation. Cystoscopy enables visualization of the extent of the pathology as well as the evaluation of both concurrent injuries or defects and the quality of the surrounding local tissue that is available for use in a reconstructive procedure. The addition of methylene blue to the cystoscopic irrigant may be useful if a fistula is suspected but has not been observed. After the surgeon occludes the urethra with a partially inflated Foley catheter, the vagina is examined for signs of urinary leakage.

It is important to recognize that urethral damage alone causes neither urinary incontinence nor detrusor instability. In patients who have coexisting urologic symptoms, the physician should be suspicious of injury to the proximal urethra and/or vesical neck. Videourodynamic examination provides vital information about the presence of involuntary bladder contractions, bladder outlet obstruction, ureteral reflex, and bladder compliance and can also identify concurrent fistulas or diverticula. A low urinary flow rate can suggest posttraumatic stricture.

Radiographic imaging is of great value in patients with urethral and urovaginal pathology. Abdominal and pelvic CT with intravenous contrast can reveal complicated fistulas that are associated with concomitant ureteral pathology. Retrograde pyelography should be performed when ureteral injury is suspected and may show ureteral injury despite a normal CT scan.

## INDICATIONS FOR SURGERY

Surgical repair is usually undertaken due to the presence of urethral obstruction, sphincteric urinary incontinence, or associated vesicovaginal fistula. We advocate the simultaneous correction of all of the coexisting anatomic and functional pathologies that led to the surgery. In patients with sphincteric incontinence, we recommend an autologous fascial pubovaginal sling with a supporting labial fat flap interposed between the vesical neck and the sling and with the vaginal mucosa closed directly over the fascial sling; however, others have alternatively proposed transvaginal bladder neck suspension in patients with favorable anatomy and incontinence due to urethral hypermobility (5).

In our experience, the majority of patients with urethral damage who also have impaired detrusor contractility, low bladder compliance, or detrusor instability improve after urethral reconstruction; however, patients with radiation damage are unique. The poor tissue quality in this subset of patients makes successful anatomic repair difficult and often results in functional problems. In this situation, supravesical diversion is often the more prudent and successful choice. In such patients, when repair of the fistula is undertaken, it may be wise to use a vascularized muscular flap as part of the initial procedure and to perform synchronous augmentation cystoplasty in patients who have low blade compliance.

Past teaching suggested that 3 to 6 months of delay was necessary to allow the quality of the local tissue to improve as inflammation and edema subsided; however, we believe that although pliable tissue must be available and free of infection and inflammation, lengthy delay is not necessary, and under the right conditions successful repair can be accomplished within days or weeks of the injury.

## ALTERNATIVE THERAPY

Alternatives to urethral reconstruction include observation, catheterization, or urinary diversion. Occasionally, women may decide against any form of surgical repair or drainage, particularly if the fistula does not result in any bothersome symptoms or if other significant medical problems preclude operative intervention. Chronic catheterization is an option if patients are too sick to undergo surgery, but this is associated with infections, stones, detrusor spasms, further urethral erosions, and the development of squamous cell cancer. In patients with radiation-induced urethral damage, a urinary diversion may be the best long-term option, although labial fat interposition and rectus or gracilis flaps combined with a buccal graft may be an alternative.

## SURGICAL TECHNIQUE

Regardless of the specific nature of the pathology and the precise procedure chosen to correct it, certain general principles should be followed: the operative site should be clearly exposed and the closure tension-free, in multiple layers, with local flaps or relaxing incisions used to mobilize the anterior vaginal wall. Appropriate postoperative bladder drainage is also essential and is accomplished through the placement of a large suprapubic catheter as well as a urethral catheter employed as a stent.

It is usually helpful to employ a well-vascularized pedicle flap to promote healing and prevent fistula formation; potential sources of this flap include the labia majora (6) and the rectus abdominis muscle (7); gracilis myocutaneous (8) or perineal artery axial fasciocutaneous (Singapore) flaps (9) may also be used. Regardless of the specific anatomic findings and the choice of vascular supply, the basic procedure is described as follows.

With the patient in the dorsal lithotomy position, cystourethroscopy is performed and the urethral orifices are visualized. Inadvertent injury to the ureter when the fistula extends close to the trigone can be avoided by placing ureteral stents and removing them at the conclusion of the case. A 14Fr percutaneous suprapubic cystotomy tube is placed under direct visualization unless concurrent abdominal incisions are planned (such as those used in autologous fascial pubovaginal

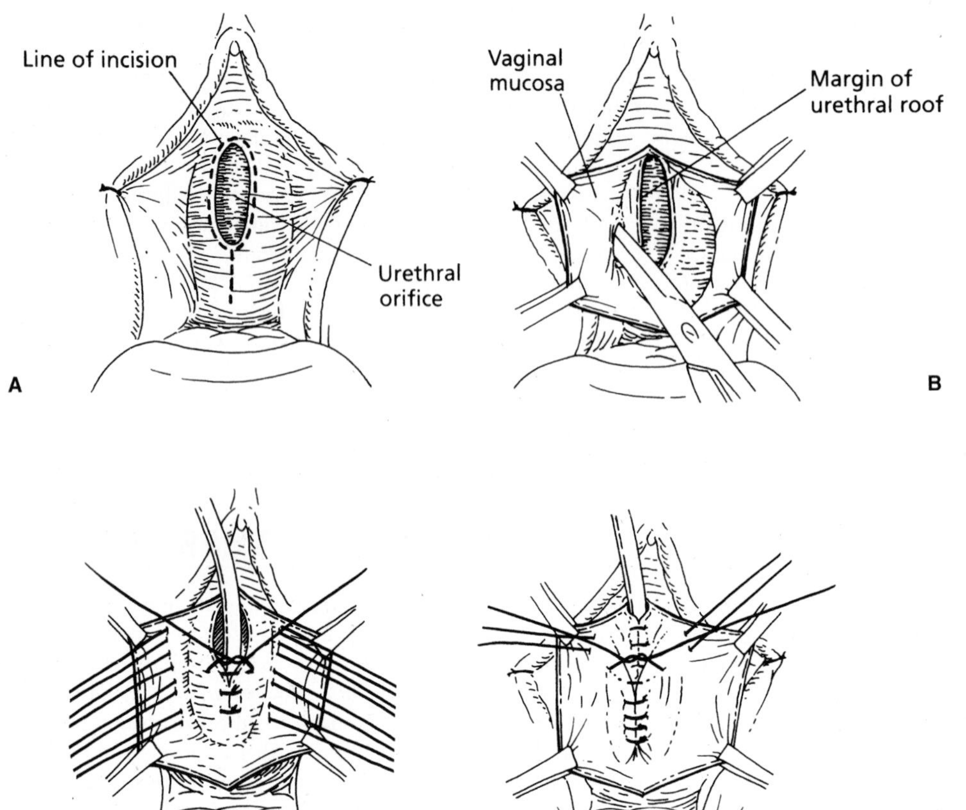


FIGURE 33.1 Bladder flap reconstruction. Tanagho anterior bladder flap reconstruction can be used in lieu of vaginal flap reconstruction. (From Tanagho EA. Bladder neck reconstruction for total urinary incontinence: 10 years of experience. *J Urol* 1981;125:321, with permission.)

sling), in which case the placement of the tube is deferred until the end of the procedure. A 16Fr urethral Foley catheter is placed and the balloon inflated to secure the catheter in place at the bladder neck.

Three basic methods are available for urethral repair, depending on the anatomic defect and the availability of local tissue for flaps: primary closure, local tissue flaps originating from the vaginal wall close to the urethra or from the bladder, or a buccal graft. Small urethral defects can be fixed with a tension-free *primary closure* (Fig. 33.1). The urethra is closed over a 16Fr catheter with interrupted 3-0 or 4-0 chromic catgut sutures, which in our experience result in less dysuria and long-term urethral pain than do longer-acting synthetic absorbable sutures. If possible, a second layer of periurethral tissue is closed over the first. The vaginal mucosa is closed using lateral flaps elevated alongside the urethral repair or, alternatively, using an inverted U incision of vaginal mucosa; chromic suture is also employed.

If insufficient urethral tissue exists for primary closure, the use of a flap is an alternative. Rotation of a U-shaped *advancement flap* of the anterior vaginal wall is one option (Fig. 33.2). The cephalad aspect of the anterior vaginal wall is mobilized

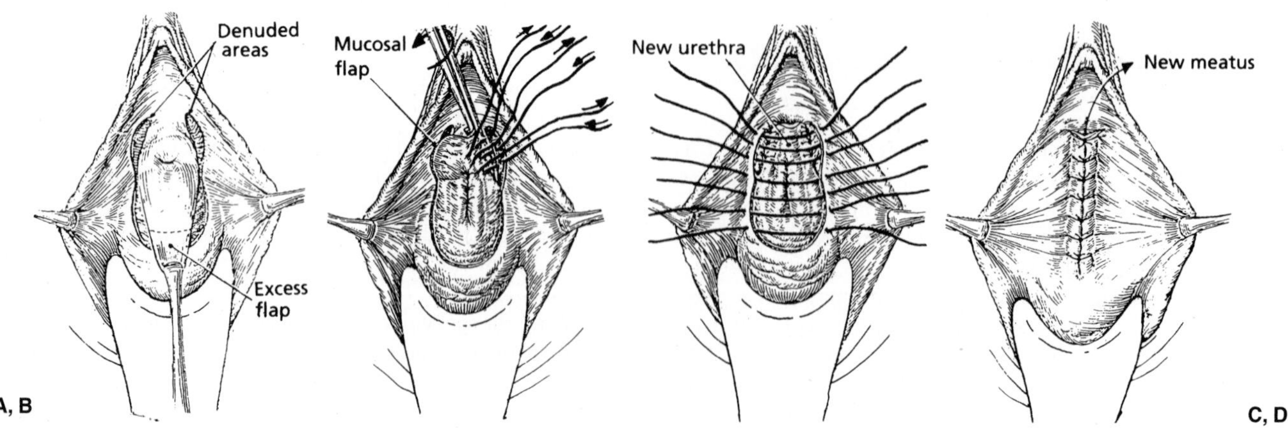


FIGURE 33.2 Primary closure. **A:** The fistula is circumscribed. **B:** The lateral vaginal wall flaps are elevated, and the lateral urethral walls are mobilized if possible. **C:** The urethra is closed primarily with interrupted sutures of 3-0 chromic catgut. The vaginal wall is closed either primarily or with a U-shaped flap, depending on the availability of local tissue. (Modified from Mattingly RF, Thompson JD. In: *Telinde's operative gynecology*, 6th ed. Philadelphia: JB Lippincott Co, 1985:662.)

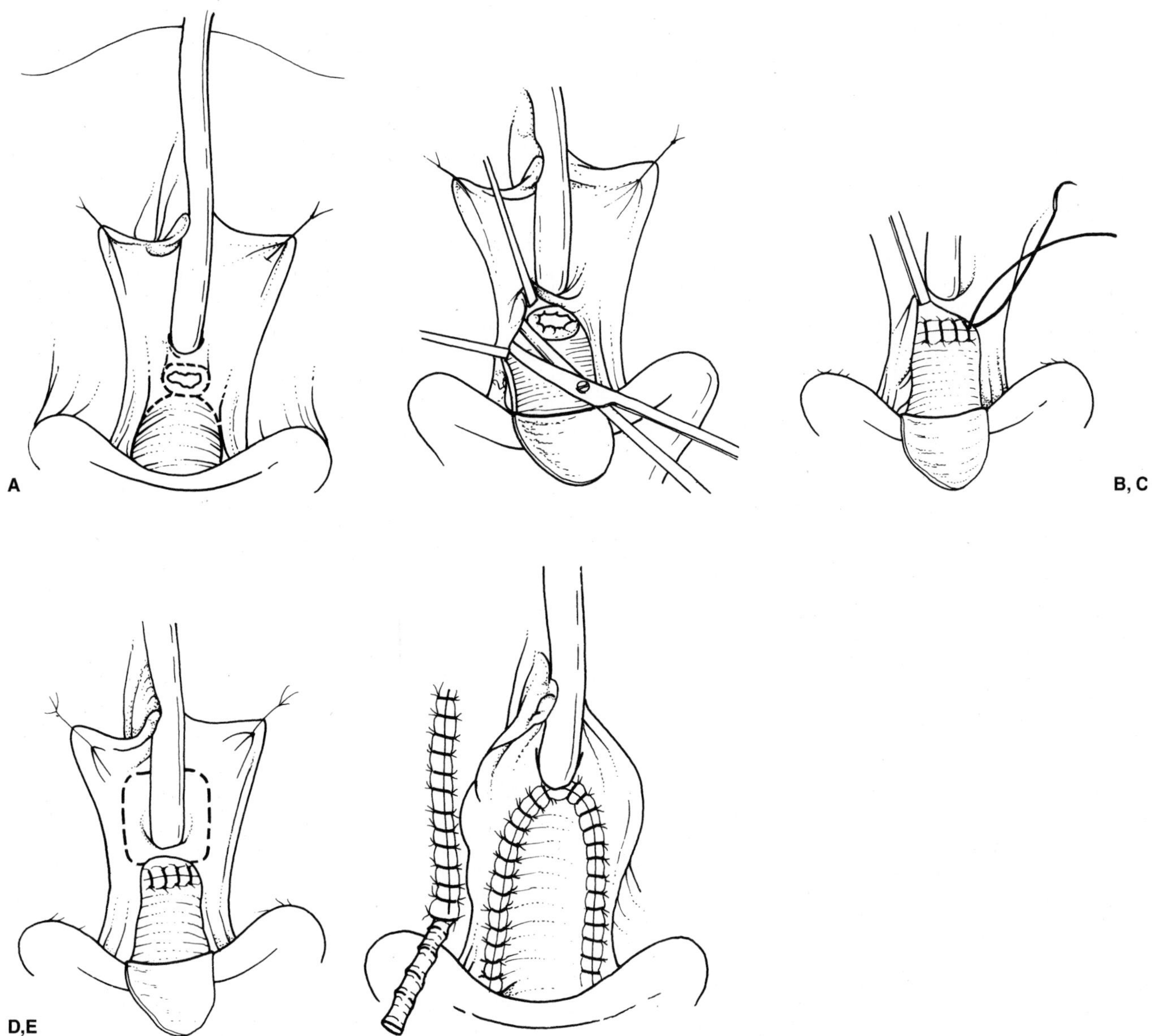


FIGURE 33.3 Advancement flap. **A:** A U-shaped incision is made with the arms of the U extending caudally as far as the planned urethral meatus. **B:** The flap is elevated and rotated 180 degrees. The flap is sutured to the edges of the parallel distal incisions over the catheter to form the new urethra. The vaginal wall is closed either primarily or with a U-shaped flap, depending on the availability of local tissue. (Modified from Mattingly RF, Thompson JD. In: *Telinde's operative gynecology*, 6th ed. Philadelphia: JB Lippincott Co, 1985:660–661.)

with Metzenbaum scissors, advanced, and rotated to form the posterior and lateral walls of the neourethra, using the urethral catheter as a guide around which the tissue is sutured. The harvested site in the vaginal wall can usually be repaired by closing the lateral and cephalad edges of the wound; however, pedicle flaps are sometimes necessary if the graft is large.

A larger vaginal wall flap can be employed as a *tube flap* (Fig. 33.3) in the case of extensive loss of urethral tissue. A rectangular incision is made with wide margins and the vaginal wall flap is rolled into a tube over the urethral catheter. It is best to provide a vascular pedicle flap for successful wound healing, and a pubovaginal sling is usually required if continence is to be achieved. As with vaginal advancement flaps, the vaginal wound may be too large for primary closure, and a secondary rotational flap of vaginal wall or labia minora can be used to close the principal defect created by the initial tube graft incisions. In our experience, gracilis myocutaneous and rectus pedicle flaps have been necessary in only 2 of over 110 patients.

In cases of extensive vaginal scarring and urethral damage, there may be insufficient vaginal wall for use in the repair. A *labia minora pedicle flap* (Fig. 33.4) is a potential solution to this problem. The labia is cut as close as possible to the site of the urethral repair and in such a manner as to allow a rotational patch graft or tube graft of labial mucosa to be employed as a neourethra that is loosely approximated over the urethral catheter. The graft with underlying vascular supply is passed beneath the vaginal wall such that the mucosal surface forms the inner wall of the reconstructed urethra.

At the conclusion of the procedure, a Penrose drain is placed in the labial harvest sites if applicable and is removed usually on postoperative day 1 or 2. The Foley catheter should

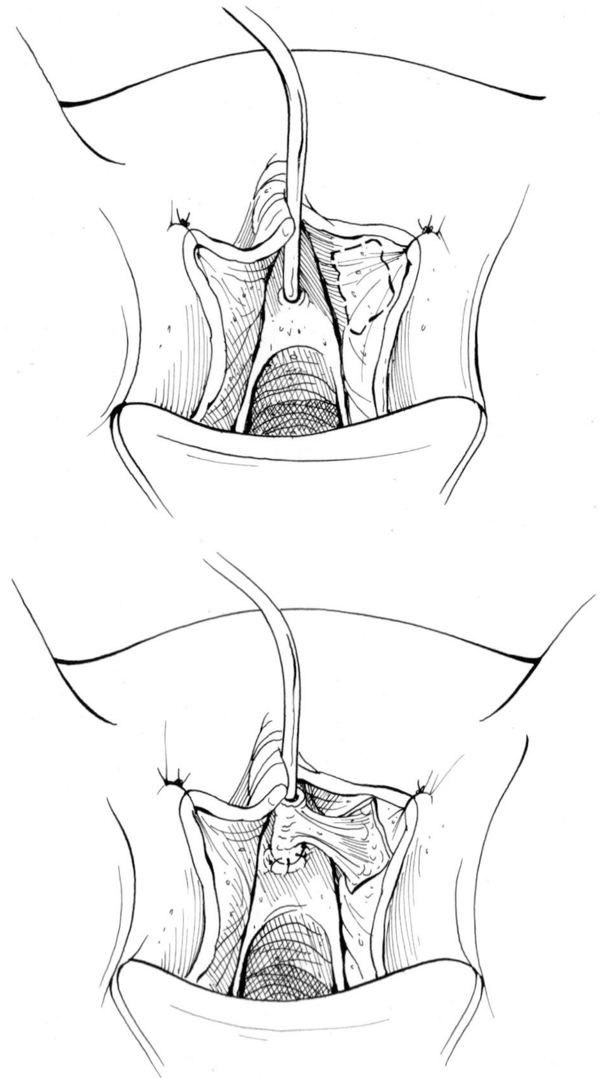

FIGURE 33.4 Tube graft. **A:** An inverted U-shaped incision is made in the anterior vaginal wall with the apex of the U at the vesical neck just proximal to the urethral fistula. The fistula is circumscribed. **B:** A plane is created in the avascular plane just underneath the vaginal epithelium, and the vaginal wall flap is reflected posteriorly. If a pubovaginal sling is to be performed, the dissection into the retropubic space is completed at this time. **C:** The urethrovaginal fistula is closed with interrupted sutures of 3-0 or 4-0 chromic catgut. **D:** Two parallel incisions are made alongside the Foley catheter, and medially based flaps are elevated. **E:** The vaginal and labial wounds are closed. (From Blavais JG. Vaginal flap urethral reconstruction. An alternative to the bladder flap neurourethra. *J Urol* 1989;41:542–545, with permission.)

be fixed in a tension-free manner to the anterior abdominal wall to prevent trauma and pressure necrosis of the repair; this catheter is usually removed within postoperative days 2 to 5, before the patient is discharged from the hospital. A voiding cystourethrogram should be performed though the suprapubic catheter about 2 weeks after the procedure. If the patient successfully voids and there is no extravasation, the suprapubic catheter can be removed; if not, the voiding trial is repeated in another 2 weeks. None of our patients has required a catheter for longer than 4 weeks.

Alternatives to vaginal wall flaps include anterior and posterior bladder flaps. Creating a neourethra using these methods is possible with a comparable degree of success to the procedures outlined previously; however, continence is not as easily achieved, with success rates of about 50% (6). Accordingly, we prefer vaginal reconstruction with anti-incontinence surgery as the preferred management of urethral injury associated with incontinence rather than employing these alternatives and their associated complications. Nonetheless, when extensive vaginal scarring in conjunction with large fistulas precludes vaginal flap reconstruction, a bladder flap procedure is an option (Fig. 33.5).

After the edges of the fistula are dissected free from the pubic rami and the anterior and inferior aspect of the bladder is separated from its attachments, a rectangular flap of anterior bladder wall is raised and rolled into a tube over a 16Fr catheter. The distal end of this tube is sutured either to the vaginal portion of the remaining urethra or at the site of the new urethral meatus. "Fixation sutures" are used to attach the neourethra/tubular bladder flap to the pubic periosteum, and a Martius fat pad is placed beneath the suture lines (6).

While skin grafts have not been widely utilized, buccal mucosal graft have been employed for repair of female urethral strictures (10,11). We generally use a two-team approach to harvesting the graft, with the oral cavity prepared and draped separately and instrument trays also kept separate. A Steinhauser mucosal retractor is used to improve visualization, and the graft harvest site is marked and lidocaine with epinephrine injected just below the mucosa. The graft is incised and removed sharply, taking care to remain in the fatty layer superficial to the buccinator muscle. Once removed, the graft is defatted and the wound closed primarily. The graft tissue has been used on the dorsal urethra, where it is quilted to the adventitia of the clitoris and the urethra anastamosed to this (10). Buccal grafts have also been sutured to the ventral (vaginal) edge of the urethra after the stricture is incised (11).

An autologous fascial pubovaginal sling can be prepared as part of the reconstructive procedure (Fig. 33.6) in cases associated with sphincteric incontinence or fistula where extensive dissection under the bladder neck puts the patient at risk for postoperative incontinence. Further, we recommend against the use of synthetic materials for concurrent incontinence surgery due to the risk of complications from erosion of the synthetic graft. It is crucial to note that if a pubovaginal sling is to be employed, it is harvested, but no vaginal dissection is performed to place the sling until after the urethra is repaired; vaginal tissue should not be compromised by additional incisions until successful repair of the urethra is complete, leaving the widest variety of possible solutions to the patient's primary problem.

A Pfannenstiel incision is made approximately two finger breadths above the symphysis pubica. The surface of the rectus fascia is freed from adherent subcutaneous tissue and two parallel horizontal incisions are made in the midline, defining the 2- to 3-cm width of the rectus fascial strip that will become the sling. These incisions are extended laterally and superiorly until approximately 10 cm of fascia is marked by the parallel incisions. The fascial strip is then freed from the underlying muscle and scar using careful sharp dissection. Each end of the sling is then secured with long 2-0 nonabsorbable monofilament sutures and a running mattress suture directed across the width of the sling. The sling is then cut free, and the security of the suspension sutures is checked by pulling each suture separately with moderate tension created by grasping each end of the fascia; it is then placed in a saline bath.

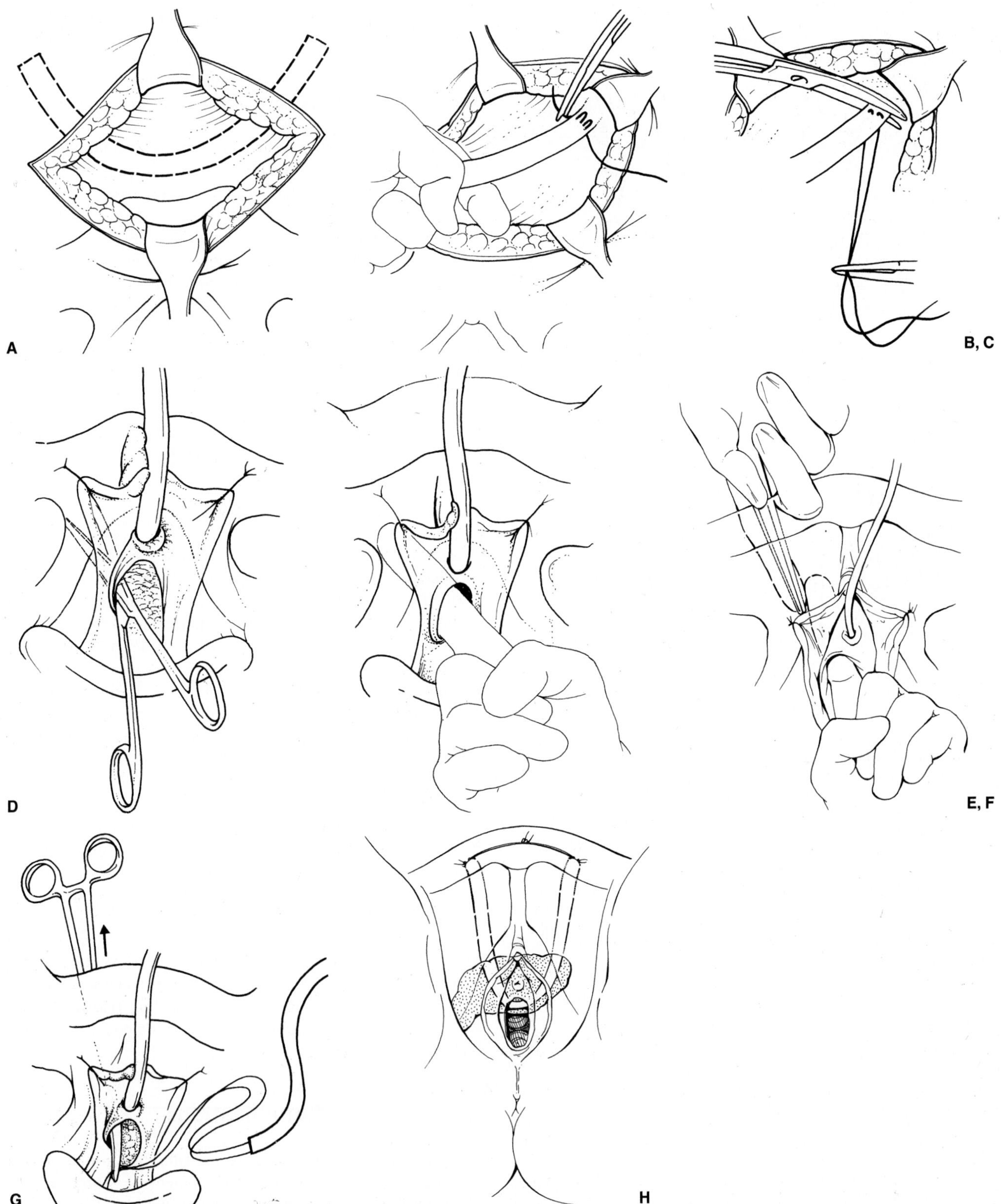


FIGURE 33.5 Labia minora pedicle graft. **A:** An oval incision in the labia minora mobilizes the labial tissue and underlying fat. **B:** The flap is passed through the wall of the labia minora and sutured into position as a neourethra with the mucosal surface of the labia becoming the interior of the neourethra.

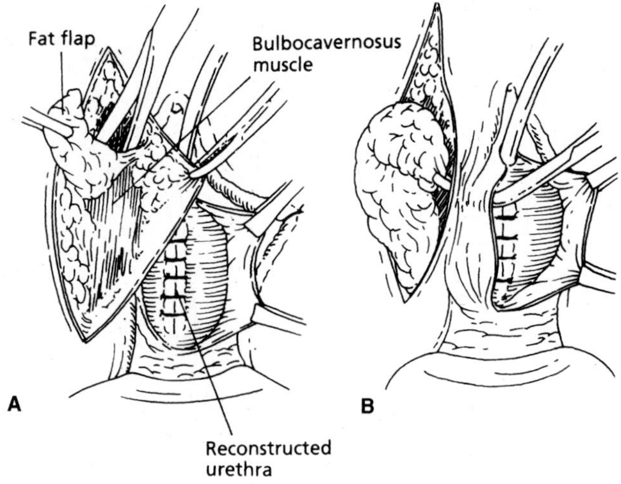


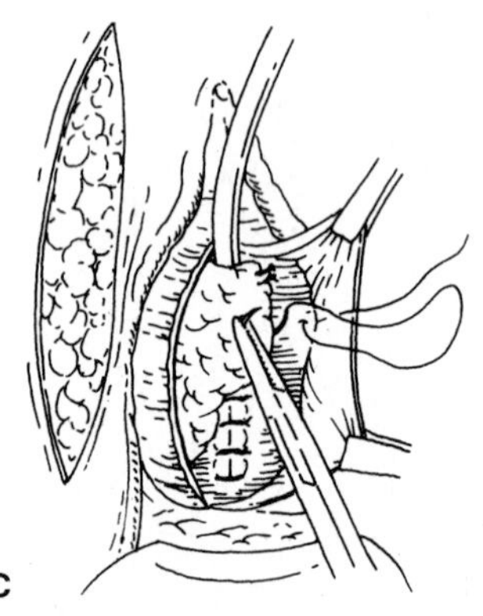


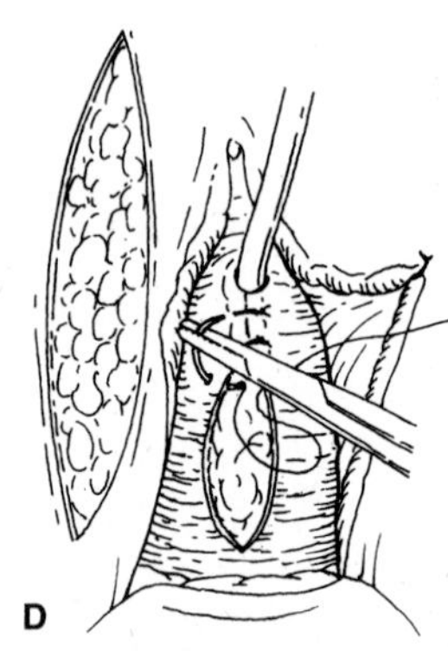


FIGURE 33.6 Pubovaginal sling. **A:** A 2- to 3-cm-wide graft is outlined with the incision kept parallel to the direction of the fascial fibers. The incision is extended laterally to the point where the fascia divides and passes to the internal and external oblique muscles. **B:** A 2-0 nonabsorbable running horizontal mattress suture is placed across the most lateral portion of the graft, and the ends are left long. **C:** Each end of the fascial graft is transected approximately 1 cm lateral to the mattress suture. **D:** Dissection is begun with Metzenbaum scissors in the avascular plane just beneath the vaginal epithelium. The tips of the scissors are directed toward the patient's ipsilateral shoulder. **E:** The endopelvic fascia is perforated with the index finger and the retropubic space is entered. **F:** A long DeBakey clamp is passed from the abdominal to the vaginal wound lateral to the urethra. **G:** The fascial graft is passed around the urethra and brought to the abdominal wound on either side. **H:** The long ends of the sling are tied together in the midline with no tension. The labial fat pad is positioned between the sling and the vesical neck. (A–G from Blavais JG. Pubovaginal sling procedure. In: Whitehead ED, ed. *Current operative urology*. Philadelphia: JB Lippincott Co, 1990: 93–101, with permission.)

The lateral edges of the vaginal incisions are retracted laterally using Allis clamps, and a closed Metzenbaum scissor is used to dissect bluntly into the retropubic space, keeping the scissor directed laterally by exerting pressure against the lateral aspect of the underside of the vaginal mucosa. There is usually a distinct and abrupt decrease in tissue resistance as the retropubic space is entered. The surgeon then places a fingertip into the dissected tract and further mobilizes the bladder neck and urethra through blunt dissection. With the surgeon's finger displacing the vesical neck medially, a long, curved (DeBakey) clamp is fed abdominally under the inferior aspect of the free rectus fascia, against the pubic periosteum, and is then guided by the surgeon's abdominal hand onto the lateral aspect of the vaginal fingertip, thus protecting the bladder from injury.

The clamp is then fed through into the vagina, where it is used to grasp and pull through one of the nonabsorbable sling sutures into the abdominal wound. The procedure is repeated on the contralateral side, and the absorbable sutures are threaded through separate small stab incisions of the inferior leaf of the rectus fascia. Following this, the rectus fascia is closed using 0 delayed absorbable monofilament suture, and the vascular pedicle graft is positioned between the pubovaginal sling and reconstructed urethra (Fig. 33.7). The vaginal mucosa is then closed, and at the conclusion of the operation the long ends of the sling are tied together in the midline over the rectus fascia without any tension at all.

## OUTCOMES

### Results

A review of published results reveals that successful anatomic reconstruction has been reported in 67% to 100% of cases, with emphasis on the need for vascular pedicle flaps to ensure viability of the repair (5,12). Continence varied from 55% to 93% in patients after a single operation, and resulting urethral obstruction varied from 2% to 41%; however, most studies did not specify the method of evaluating continence. It was clear that anti-incontinence procedures were in general successful and dramatically improved the continence rates, with postoperative incontinence in 50% to 84% of patients who underwent anatomic reconstruction only. Table 33.2 summarizes these studies.

We have performed 110 urethral reconstructive procedures in women. All but 1 underwent primary or vaginal wall repairs, and the 1 Tanagho anterior bladder flap was unsuccessful because of refractory overactive bladder. A Martius flap was used in all but 4 patients. We did not perform pubovaginal sling routinely until later in the series, and 50% of the early patients who underwent modified Pereyra procedures were incontinent; of these, all were subsequently cured or improved by a pubovaginal sling. For this reason we are strongly in favor of a pubovaginal sling for concurrent anti-incontinence surgery.

### Complications

Three patients experienced necrosis of the flap, which in one case was associated with the development of sphincteric incontinence and in one with overactive bladder. One patient had urinary obstruction from the pubovaginal sling, and one patient had an unrecognized vesicovaginal fistula that was successfully repaired transvaginally. All patients who suffered from sphincteric incontinence were cured or improved by successful reoperation at 1 year follow-up, except for one patient who declined surgery. No patients required intermittent catheterization.

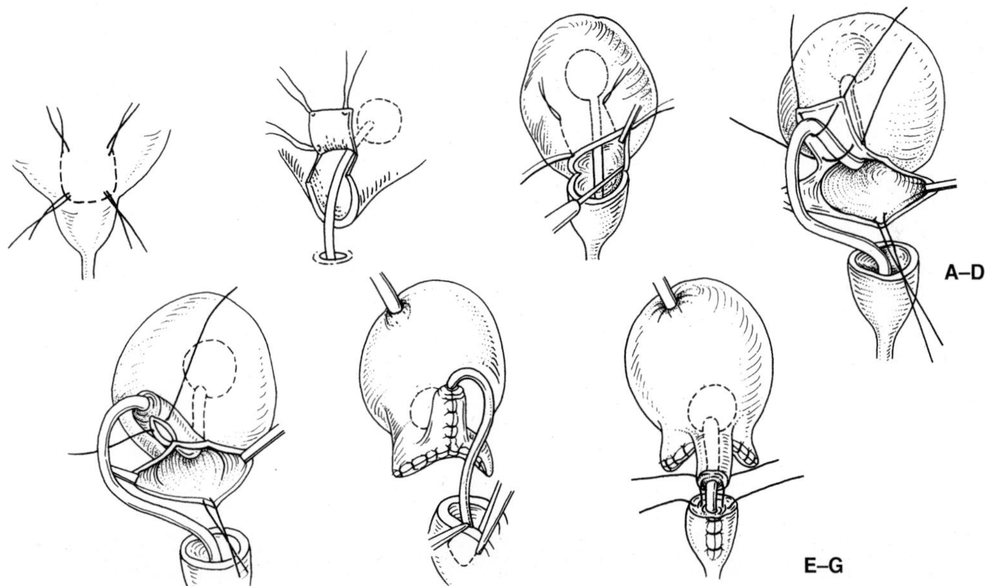


FIGURE 33.7 Vascular pedicle graft. **A:** Incisions in the labia majora expose the underlying fat pad, which is suture-ligated at its superior margin and mobilized posteriorly. **B:** The graft is drawn through a perforation in the vaginal wall. **C:** A 2-0 chromic catgut suture is used to fix the graft over the reconstruction. **D:** The vaginal wall is closed over the reconstruction. If a pubovaginal sling is performed, it is placed beneath the vaginal wall prior to the closure. (Modified from Mattingly RF, Thompson JD. In: *Telinde's operative gynecology*, 6th ed. Philadelphia: JB Lippincott Co, 1985:663.)

Urethral reconstruction in women can be highly complicated and requires considerable surgical expertise as well as a thorough diagnostic workup. In most women successful anatomic and functional repair can be achieved with a single surgical procedure employing vaginal flap reconstruction with a grafted vascular supply and a pubovaginal sling as an anti-incontinence measure. Bladder flap techniques can also be used, especially in cases of extensive vaginal scarring.

TABLE 33.2

RESULTS OF URETHRAL RECONSTRUCTION

| Reference | Number | Continence (%) | Cure/improved (%) | Anatomic repair (%) | Obstruction (%) |
|---|---|---|---|---|---|
| Xu, 2008 | 8 | 100 | 100 | — | 13 |
| Wadie, 2007 | 13 | 85[a] | 92 | — | 31 |
| Migliari, 2006 (10)[b] | 3 | 100 | 100 | 100 | 0 |
| Flisser, 2003 | 74 | 87 | 93 | — | — |
| Bruce, 2000 (7) | 6 | 83 | 100 | 100 | 0 |
| Taneer, 1993 (12) | 34 | — | 82 | 82 | — |
| Elkins, 1990 (5) | 20 | 50 | 55 | 90 | 10 |
| Mundy, 1989 | 30 | 93 | — | 93 | 41 |
| Patel, 1980 | 9 | — | 78 | 100 | 0 |
| Morgan, 1978 | 9 | 56 | 89 | 100 | 11 |
| Elkins, 1969 | 6 | 10 | 83 | 67 | 17 |
| Hamlin, 1969 | 50 | 80 | 84 | 98 | 12 |
| Gray, 1968 | 10 | 50 | 50 | — | — |
| Symmonds, 1968 | 20 | 65 | 90 | 85 | — |

[a]A second adjunctive procedure used.
[b]Buccal grafts used for repair.

## References


1. Danso KA, et al. The epidemiology of genitourinary fistulae in Kumasi, Ghana, 1977–1992. *Int Urogynecol J Pelvic Floor Dysfunct* 1996;7(3):117–120.
2. Siegel AL. Urethral necrosis and proximal urethro-vaginal fistula resulting from tension-free vaginal tape. *Int Urogynecol J Pelvic Floor Dysfunct* 2006;17(6):661–664.
3. Loran OB, Pushkar DO. Treatment of vesicovaginal fistula, simple or complicated by urethral destruction. Experience apropos of 903 cases. *J Urol (Paris)* 1991;97(6):253–259.
4. Perry MO, Husmann DA. Urethral injuries in female subjects following pelvic fractures. *J Urol* 1992;147(1):139–143.
5. Elkins TE, et al. Transvaginal mobilization and utilization of the anterior bladder wall to repair vesicovaginal fistulas involving the urethra. *Obstet Gynecol* 1992;79(3):455–460.
6. Elkins TE, DeLancey JO, McGuire EJ. The use of modified Martius graft as an adjunctive technique in vesicovaginal and rectovaginal fistula repair. *Obstet Gynecol* 1990;75(4):727–733.
7. Bruce RG, El-Galley RE, Galloway NT. Use of rectus abdominis muscle flap for the treatment of complex and refractory urethrovaginal fistulas. *J Urol* 2000;163(4):1212–1215.
8. Blaivas JG. Vaginal flap urethral reconstruction: an alternative to the bladder flap neourethra. *J Urol* 1989;141(3):542–545.
9. Zorn KC, et al. Female neo-urethral reconstruction with a modified neurovascular pudendal thigh flap (Singapore flap): initial experience. *Can J Urol* 2007;14(1):3449–3454.
10. Migliari R, et al. Dorsal buccal mucosa graft urethroplasty for female urethral strictures. *J Urol* 2006;176(4, Pt 1):1473–1476.
11. Berglund RK, et al. Buccal mucosa graft urethroplasty for recurrent stricture of female urethra. *Urology* 2006;67(5):1069–1071.
12. Blaivas JG, Heritz DM. Vaginal flap reconstruction of the urethra and vesical neck in women: a report of 49 cases. *J Urol* 1996;155(3):1014–1017.


# CHAPTER 34 ■ SURGICAL MANAGEMENT OF THE INCOMPETENT BLADDER OUTLET IN THE PATIENT WITH A NEUROGENIC BLADDER

ALIENOR S. GILCHRIST, GARY E. LEMACK, AND PHILIPPE E. ZIMMERN

Patients with a neurogenic bladder can exhibit one of two main abnormalities of the urethra and bladder neck: bladder outlet overactivity, leading to obstruction, and bladder outlet underactivity, leading to incontinence.

Detrusor contraction with involuntary contraction of the urethra and/or sphincter, known as detrusor striated sphincter dyssynergia (DSD), is a common pattern of voiding dysfunction in patients with suprasacral spinal cord lesions. Sphincterotomy is the gold standard for treatment of DSD and renders the patient completely and continuously incontinent via endoscopic incision of the external urethral sphincter at the 12 o'clock position. Sphincterotomy may also ameliorate symptoms of autonomic dysreflexia in patients suffering from this condition (7). Risks associated with the procedure include erectile dysfunction, hemorrhage, and urinary extravasation. Patients are subsequently managed with a condom catheter, which can lead to skin breakdown and ulceration. Some patients may require a concurrent bladder neck incision to treat obstruction, and in many cases a repeat incision may ultimately be required as the efficacy may diminish over time.

Incontinence in the neurogenic population can originate from sphincteric and bladder neck deficiency in addition to detrusor overactivity. Outlet insufficiency is frequently neurologic in origin but may also arise from iatrogenic destruction of tissue from long-term urethral catheter use. For patients with sphincteric incompetence, a variety of treatments exists, including injectables, slings, artificial urinary sphincters (Fig. 34.1), adjustable continence therapy, and bladder neck closure with tissue interposition.

Bladder neck closure (BNC) is an uncommon procedure that has traditionally been reserved as a final alternative for the management of the female patient with neurogenically induced intractable incontinence arising from long-term urethral catheter drainage (9,14). It has also been used in the treatment of nonneuropathic conditions such as traumatic urethral destruction or fistulas that have failed surgical repair. BNC in men is usually reserved for patients with incontinence secondary to neurogenic bladder, recalcitrant urethrocutaneous fistula, or trauma who have failed surgical correction or artificial sphincter placement. In recent years, salvage prostatectomy and BNC in the management of recurrent prostate cancer after radiation therapy and in the management of severe complications after salvage cryotherapy have been reported (5).

## DIAGNOSIS

Preoperative evaluation and patient selection are extremely important to the success of BNC. A detailed history should elicit any prior abdominal or pelvic surgeries, including previous reconstructive flaps or grafts. A thorough physical examination is important to assess for the following: (a) the presence of lower-extremity contractures that may limit vaginal access; (b) perineal skin integrity and the presence of decubitus; and (c) a body habitus that may impede successful intermittent catheterization. In patients with adequate manual dexterity or a reliable caregiver, a catheterizable efferent limb from the

TABLE 34.1

COMPARISON OF APPROACHES TO BLADDER NECK CLOSURE IN THE FEMALE PATIENT

| FACTOR | VAGINAL CLOSURE | ABDOMINAL CLOSURE |
|---|---|---|
| Multiple prior abdominal procedures | Preferred approach | Alternate approach |
| Prior radiation | No prior pelvic radiation | History of pelvic radiation |
| Postoperative drainage | Suprapubic tube drainage | Desires incontinent vesicostomy or catheterizable bladder drainage |
| Vascularized interposition | Martius flap | Omentum; rectus flap; peritoneal flap |
| Lower-extremity flexibility | Adequate | Impaired |
| Perineal skin condition | Adequate | Decubitus or infected |

bladder may be chosen for postoperative drainage. When intermittent catheterization is not feasible, postoperative bladder drainage is achieved via suprapubic tube or incontinent ileovesicostomy (8).

Evaluation of the upper urinary tract is important, and when upper-tract deterioration is noted, strong consideration must be given to supravesical diversion or bladder preservation with augmentation cystoplasty to lower intravesical pressures. A voiding cystogram may assist in detecting bladder diverticula or vesicoureteral reflux. In most cases, reflux should resolve after regularizing intravesical pressures (in the case of augment), and therefore ureteral reimplantation is typically not recommended unless severe obstruction at the level of the ureterovesical junction is noted on preoperative imaging. In the case of urethral fistula or stricture, a retrograde urethrogram or fistulogram can document the nature and extent of the patient's underlying disease.

Cystoscopy with biopsy to exclude bladder malignancy is essential for patients managed long term with indwelling catheters. The extent of urodynamic evaluation is tailored to the type of postoperative bladder management. In patients desiring continent, catheterizable access to the bladder, preoperative urodynamic or preferably video-urodynamic evaluation of bladder storage parameters such as capacity, compliance, and detrusor overactivity helps determine the need for concomitant augmentation cystoplasty.

## INDICATIONS FOR SURGERY

### Women

Patients suffering from neurogenic incontinence often have intractable leakage from urethral destruction due to the long-term effects of an indwelling urethral catheter. A common indication is the patient with advanced multiple sclerosis and detrusor overactivity resulting in leakage around the catheter or repeated catheter extrusions. Though control of incontinence has been achieved by some using a pubovaginal sling, many patients with urethral destruction and reduced urethral length are not suitable candidates for this procedure (2,10). The indications for bladder neck closure in the nonneurogenic patient are urethral destruction, severe intrinsic sphincteric deficiency that is not amenable to or has failed conventional treatment, and failed urethrovaginal fistula repair. For the woman who has failed attempts at urethrovaginal fistula closure, BNC with a continent catheterizable efferent channel, incontinent vesicostomy, or suprapubic tube may represent a viable option for management.

The vaginal approach is favored in the patient without history of prior radiation who desires suprapubic tube drainage. An abdominal approach is preferred for the patient with a history of radiation in whom vaginal tissues may be poorly vascularized and in whom omental interposition between the bladder neck and vagina is desirable. It is also the approach of choice in the patient who elects a continent efferent limb (bowel or appendix) or an incontinent ileovesicostomy, or has failed a prior attempt at vaginal closure of the bladder neck (Table 34.1) (8).

### Men

The role of BNC in men with benign disease resides in the management of refractory urethrocutaneous or urethrorectal fistula and in cases of severe neurogenic or postoperative incontinence (with low outlet resistance) when an artificial sphincter is not an option. It may also be used in the treatment of recalcitrant urethral strictures when reconstruction is impossible or undesired. BNC may be considered in conjunction with salvage prostatectomy for locally recurrent prostate adenocarcinoma after radiation therapy. Complications encountered after salvage cryotherapy, such as osteitis pubis, recurrent gross hematuria, bladder outlet obstruction, urinary incontinence, puboprostatic fistula, urethral stricture disease, and intractable perineal pain, can be managed by prostatectomy with BNC as well.

## ALTERNATIVE THERAPY

Options for local reconstruction in women with severe incontinence or fistula are limited. Though urethral reconstruction with vaginal wall or bowel is an available option, maintaining a urethral outlet that is both patent and continent can prove extremely challenging. Continence following these reconstructive procedures may be provided by autologous or synthetic sling materials, injectable bulking agents, an artificial urinary sphincter, or bladder neck reconstruction (Young–Dees) (2). In men with refractory incontinence or fistula, when previously irradiated tissue is not present, the artificial urinary sphincter and formal fistula closure are other viable alternatives.

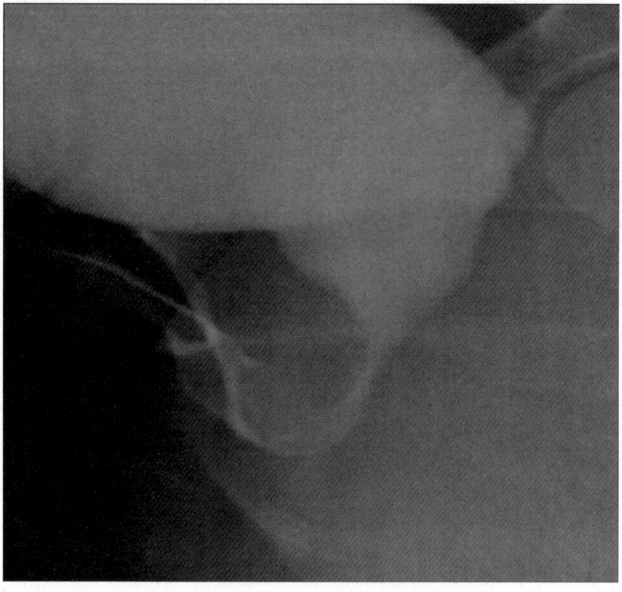

A

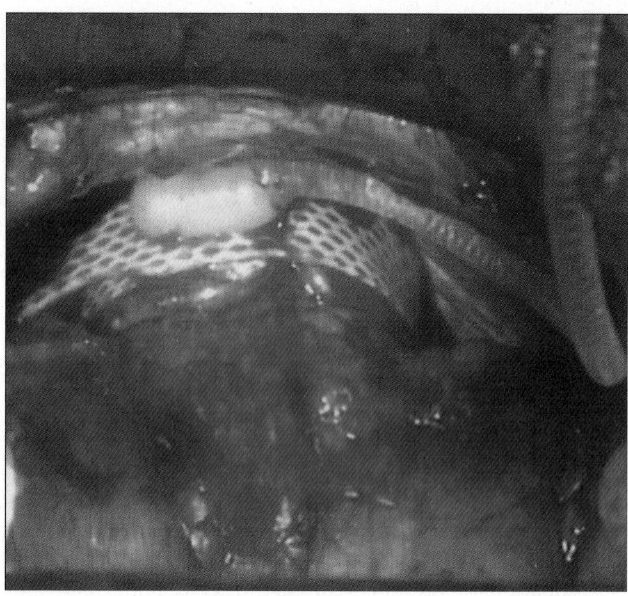

B

FIGURE 34.1 A: Lateral view cystogram in a severely incontinent woman demonstrating a wide open and incompetent bladder neck and proximal urethra. B: Intraoperative view of AUS placement at the bladder neck with a 10 cm cuff and a 61–70 cm $H_2O$ pressure reservoir in the same patient.

Historically, supravesical diversion and ureterosigmoidostomy (nonneurogenic patients) have been advocated for treatment of patients with this severity of incontinence. However, it is our opinion that BNC should be considered before embarking on these more extensive surgical options. BNC not only preserves the bladder, but it also preserves the integrity of the ureterovesical junction, thereby protecting the upper tracts. In addition, BNC is performed through either a vaginal or retropubic approach, avoiding complications associated with open abdominal surgery.

## SURGICAL TECHNIQUE

The goals of the procedure are the same for both male and female patients, regardless of the approach utilized. These goals include wide mobilization of the bladder neck to allow for tension-free closure; multilayer closure of the outlet without overlapping suture lines, thereby reducing secondary fistula formation; interposition of vascularized tissue between the vesical outlet and urethral stump or vagina; and adequate postoperative bladder drainage with a large-bore catheter.

### Vaginal Approach (Women)

The vaginal approach is preferred in the woman who will be managed with suprapubic tube drainage, has no history of prior radiation, and is not undergoing a concomitant abdominal procedure. Preoperative preparation includes antibiotics to sterilize the urine, vaginal douching, and deep venous thrombosis prophylaxis. The patient is placed in high lithotomy position with careful attention to padding of all pressure points and extremities. A Lone Star ring retractor (Houston, TX) is recommended along with a weighted vaginal speculum and headlight to provide maximal vaginal exposure. In the case of a small contracted bladder, a curved Lowsley retractor is employed to place a suprapubic tube. The patient is placed in deep Trendelenburg position to displace bowel contents, and the curved retractor is introduced through the urethra and directed to the anterior abdominal wall 1 to 2 cm above the symphysis pubica. A small suprapubic incision is made over the tip of the Lowsley, which can be palpated beneath the fascia. The tip of the retractor is then pushed out through the skin incision, and a 20Fr Foley catheter is grasped between the open jaws and delivered back into the bladder. Its intravesical position can be confirmed with cystoscopy or irrigation with normal saline.

A waterproof surgical ink pen marks the proposed inverted U-shaped vaginal wall incision. Normal saline or a dilute solution of vasopressin 60 U per 100 $cm^3$ is injected into the periurethral tissues and anterior vaginal wall to facilitate dissection of both the urethra and anterior vaginal flap. Vasopressin can reduce local bleeding (Fig. 34.1).

After a circumscribing incision has been made around the destroyed urethra, a broad-based vaginal flap is elevated (Fig. 34.2). This flap not only aids in the exposure of the remainder of the bladder neck dissection, but will also serve as an advancement flap over the closed vesical outlet and interposed labial fat pad graft. The bladder neck is freed from its lateral and anterior fascial attachments to achieve a tension-free closure (Fig. 34.3). The anterior mobilization includes detaching the bladder neck from the pubic symphysis attachments with sharp and blunt dissection and entering the retropubic space. Main concerns during this portion of the case include bleeding and injury to the bladder. Indigo carmine is given intravenously to aid in visualizing the ureteral orifices. Remnant urethral edges, when present, may be trimmed before formal closure.

The bladder neck is closed in a vertical fashion with absorbable suture (Fig. 34.4). The bladder is then filled through the suprapubic tube to ensure that the closure is

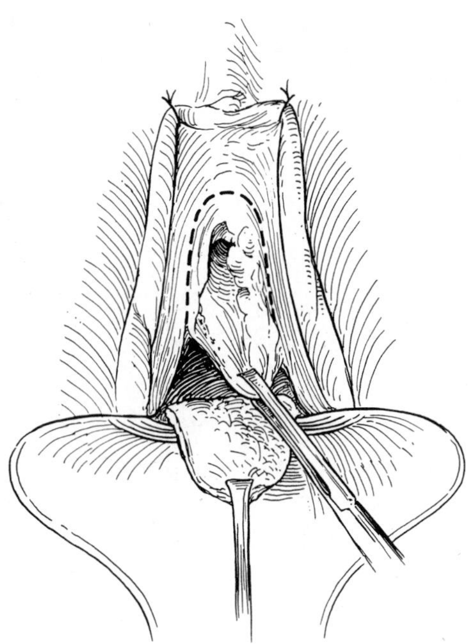

FIGURE 34.2 Elevation of the vaginal flap.

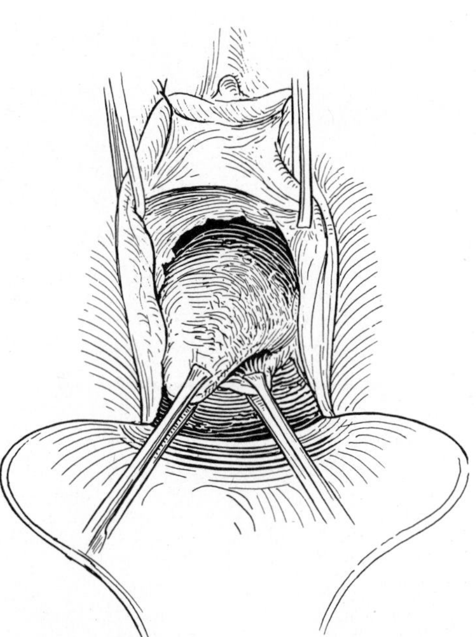

FIGURE 34.3 Detachment of the bladder neck.

watertight. To reduce the likelihood of secondary vesicovaginal fistula, a second horizontal layer of interrupted sutures imbricates the first layer in such a way that the closed bladder outlet is elevated to a position high behind the symphysis pubica (Fig. 34.5). This technique not only avoids a dependent closure but also directs the force of bladder spasms away from the vagina.

The use of a Martius flap is recommended to reinforce the bladder neck closure and reduce the risk of fistula. The technique relies on a well-vascularized fibrofatty labial pad (from the labia majora) that is based posteriorly on a labial branch

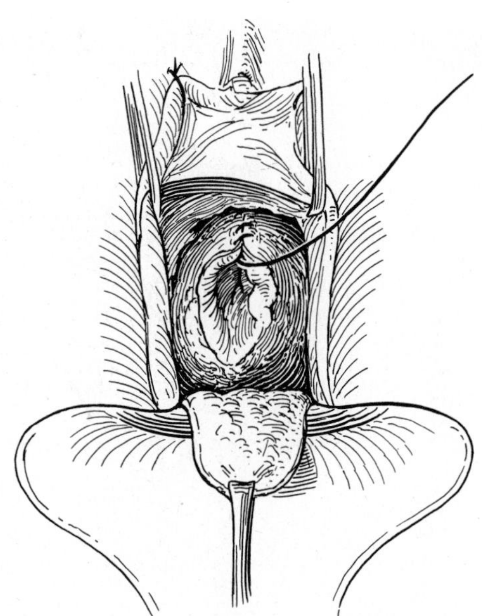

FIGURE 34.4 Primary closure with tension-free anastomosis.

of the internal pudendal artery. The Martius flap is tunneled beneath the vaginal wall and fixed in place over the bladder neck closure (Fig. 34.6). The vaginal flap is advanced to close the vagina (Fig. 34.7). The vagina is packed for 24 hours with an antibiotic-soaked pack.

## Abdominal Approach (Women)

The patient is placed in low lithotomy position with adjustable stirrups to provide continuous access to the vagina. Alternatively, if lower-extremity contractures prohibit the lithotomy position, the supine position may be used. A urethral Foley catheter is placed, and an infraumbilical midline incision is made. This incision not only provides excellent exposure but also can be extended for omental harvest or use of bowel for an efferent catheterizable limb. A Pfannenstiel incision may be considered if a chronic suprapubic tube has been chosen for long-term bladder management. The rectus muscles are retracted laterally, and the prevesical space (Retzius) is developed bluntly. The peritoneum is retracted superiorly, and a self-retaining retractor (Balfour or Bookwalter) provides exposure of the retropubic space.

By palpating the Foley catheter balloon, the bladder neck and urethra are identified. An absorbable figure-of-eight suture is placed through the distalmost aspect of the deep dorsal vein over the proximal urethra. Using electrocautery or sharp dissection, the anterior bladder neck is incised over the most distal aspect of the Foley catheter. The lip of the bladder neck is grasped with traction sutures or Allis clamps, and the Foley catheter is identified and delivered into the surgical field. After intravenous administration of indigo carmine, ureteral catheters may be placed for safe dissection of the posterior bladder neck (Fig. 34.8). Placing a hand in the vagina can help identify and maintain the appropriate plane between the posterior bladder neck and the vaginal wall. Using electrocautery or sharp dissection, the posterior bladder neck is freed from the anterior vaginal wall. This dissection

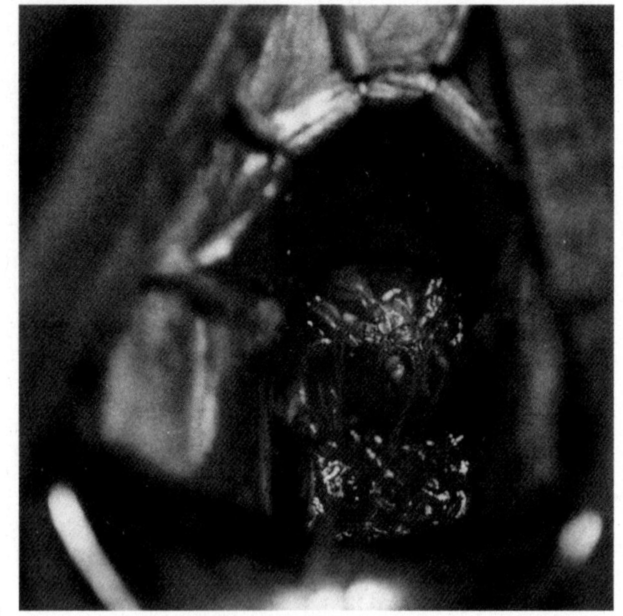


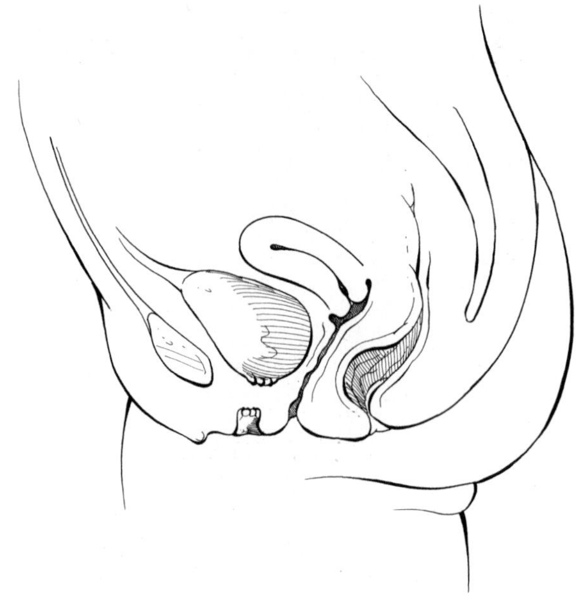


FIGURE 34.5 **A:** Photograph of closure of the bladder neck. **B:** Lateral view of bladder neck closure.

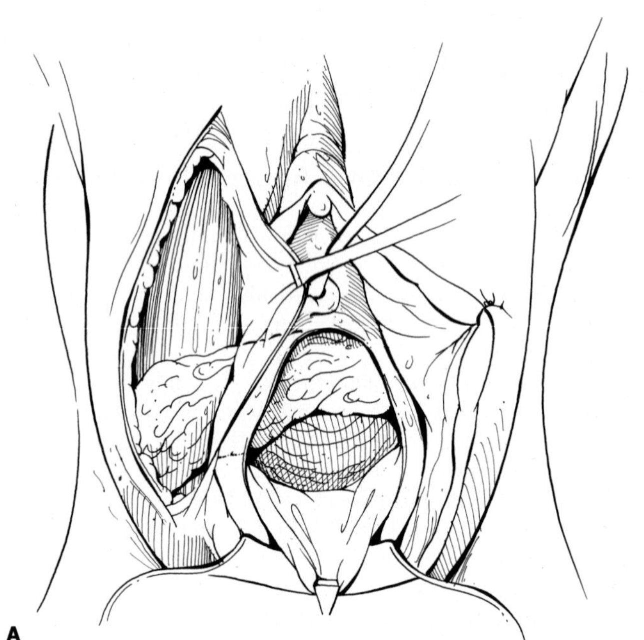


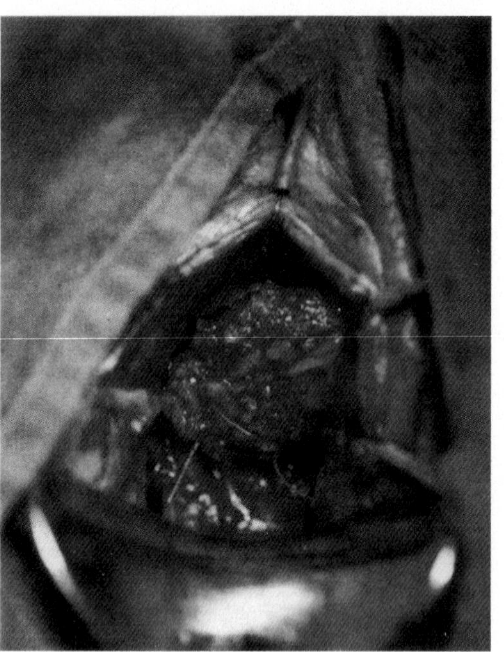


FIGURE 34.6 **A:** Martius flap tunneled beneath the labia minora. **B:** Intraoperative photograph of Martius flap to close over the bladder neck.

continues until the bladder neck is rolled up and out of its dependent position. The edges of the bladder neck are trimmed to allow approximation of healthy tissues, and the ureteral catheters are removed. If an incontinent vesicostomy or catheterizable efferent limb is selected for postoperative bladder drainage, they may be fashioned at this time. Otherwise, a large-bore (24Fr) Malecot or Foley suprapubic tube is placed at the bladder dome. The bladder neck is closed in two layers as described for vaginal closure. The bladder is then filled through the suprapubic tube to verify that the closure is watertight. A well-vascularized interposition tissue is placed over the two-layer closure to minimize the risk of fistula.

## Approach in the Man

The technique of bladder neck closure in men differs from that in women in several distinct ways: (a) lack of direct perineal access to the bladder neck; (b) limited selection of vascularized

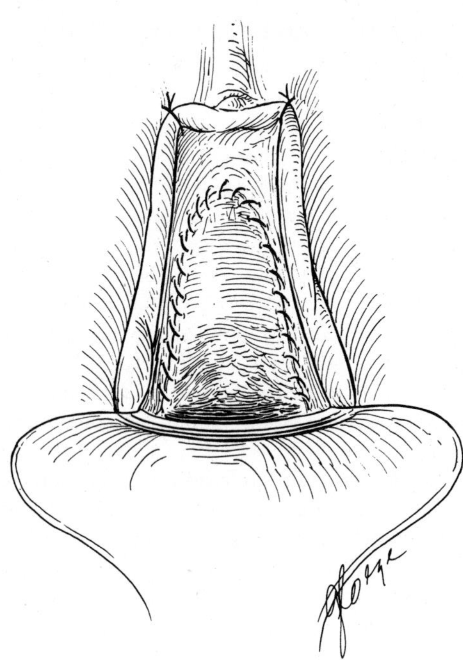

FIGURE 34.7 Closure of the vaginal flap.

interposition tissue; and (c) challenging intraoperative closure and postoperative care due to prostatic anatomy.

## Perineal Access (Men)

The perineal approach to BNC, though conceptually and technically feasible, is not considered to be the procedure of choice in the man. Perineal access to the bladder neck necessitates either a concomitant prostatectomy with its own inherent morbidity or closure of the infraprostatic urethra, a procedure associated with a high rate of spontaneous fistulization. Closure of the infraprostatic urethra, though easily performed, is not desirable for the following reasons:

1. The surgical closure continues to remain in a dependent position.
2. With the exception of a gracilis or gluteal flap, there is little opportunity for interposition of a large healthy segment of vascularized tissue.
3. Prostatic secretions can only drain in a retrograde fashion into the bladder or, in dyssynergic patients, remain trapped in the prostatic fossa, leading to high rates of fistulization.
4. Perineal closure does not preserve antegrade ejaculation and compromises future fertility.

### Abdominal Closure (Men)

The abdominal approach to bladder neck closure has two distinct advantages over perineal closure: (a) the bladder neck can be rotated anteriorly and out of a dependent position and (b) the choices for vascularized interposition are abundant (omentum, rectus flap, and peritoneal flap). Two techniques have historically been employed for abdominal closure of the bladder neck in men with benign disease: supraprostatic and infraprostatic closure. Supraprostatic bladder neck closure has been our choice as it offers several distinct advantages over infraprostatic closure. It is technically easier and does not involve deep pelvic dissection or transection of the dorsal venous complex. It also allows better mobilization of the bladder neck, resulting in a tension-free closure. Lastly, it provides opportunity for future fertility as an antegrade flow of ejaculate is preserved.

When BNC is to be performed in conjunction with salvage prostatectomy, the extirpative portion of the procedure is performed first. Description of this portion of the procedure is beyond the scope of this chapter, but those who have published reports in the care of these patients describe it as technically challenging (5). A distinct advantage of this operation, when compared to salvage prostatectomy with vesicourethral anastamosis, is that it allows for wider excision, particularly at the apex of the prostate.

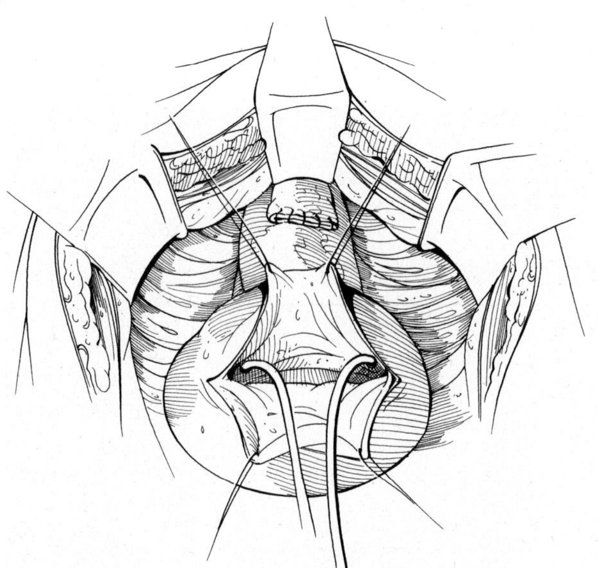



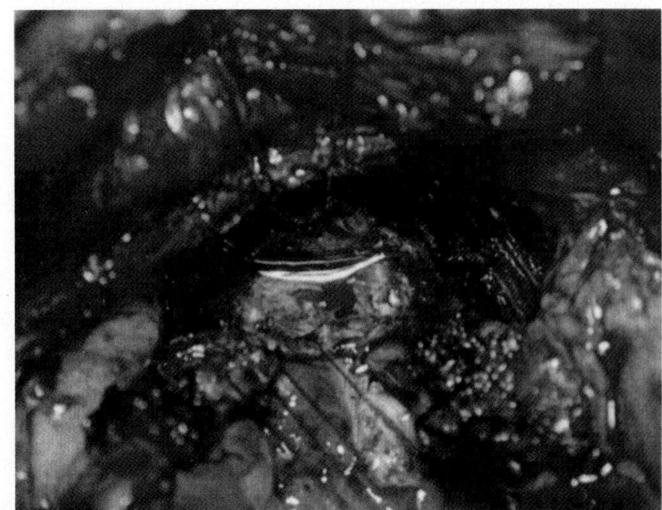



FIGURE 34.8 **A:** Opened bladder with mobilization of the bladder neck. **B:** Intraoperative photograph of divided urethral stump and mobilized open bladder neck.

After supine or low lithotomy positioning, the patient is prepared and a catheter is placed in sterile fashion. An infraumbilical vertical midline incision is performed, and the retropubic space is accessed as described earlier. The bladder neck is identified, and absorbable sutures are used to ligate the superficial dorsal venous complex at the prostatovesical junction. The prostate and vesical neck are grasped, and electrocautery or sharp dissection is then used to amputate the anterior vesical neck from the prostate. Once the bladder neck mucosa is entered, the Foley balloon may be deflated and removed to permit visualization of the posterior vesical neck. Indigo carmine and ureteral catheters are used as previously described. The posterior bladder wall is transected and the plane between the bladder and the rectum identified. Mobilization of the posterior bladder neck from the Denonvilliers fascia and rectum should continue until the vesical outlet has reached an anterior, nondependent position. Excessive mobilization should be avoided to prevent injury to the ureters or vascular pedicles of the bladder. A large-bore Malecot or Foley suprapubic tube is then placed through a separate stab incision. If an alternative bladder drainage method is desired (incontinent vesicostomy, catheterizable efferent limb), it may be constructed at this time.

Depending on its size, bladder neck closure can be performed by one of two methods. In the patient with a small bladder neck, a series of two absorbable pursestring sutures may be used to invert the outlet similar to the inversion of an appendiceal stump. For a larger bladder neck, or where closure is more difficult, the outlet may be closed in two layers as described above. Placement of a well-vascularized flap of omentum, rectus muscle, or peritoneum in the fossa between the bladder neck closure and prostate is performed to not only facilitate healing but also to help prevent fistulization (Fig. 34.9).

Concomitant prostatectomy may be planned in the case of salvage prostatectomy, or it may be indicated in the case of a strictured urethra or prostatorectal fistula that poses a problem to postoperative prostatic drainage.

### Vascularized Interposition (Men)

Following the BNC, it is highly advisable to interpose vascularized tissue between the bladder neck and the pelvic outlet to reduce the risk of secondary fistula. Choices for interposition include omentum, a flap of adjacent peritoneum, or a rectus flap. We prefer omentum because of its size, reliable blood supply, and abundant lymphatic drainage. In patients with a generous omentum, a tongue may be easily mobilized with only limited dissection. If, however, the patient is extremely thin or has had radiation or prior intra-abdominal surgery, the incision may be extended to mobilize the omentum on a pedicle supplied by the right gastroepiploic artery. The right side is preferred due to its more dependent position in the abdomen and its more generous blood supply. The omentum is positioned between the BNC and the pelvic outlet, and it is sutured in place with absorbable sutures. When a rectus flap is selected, it may be mobilized and based on an inferior epigastric vascular pedicle with careful attention to tie all lateral vascular collaterals. The mobilized rectus flap is then rotated downward and positioned as described above for omentum. Alternatively, a paravesical peritoneal flap may be interposed; however, its vascular supply may not be as reliable as that of omentum or a rectus flap. A suction drain is left in the pelvis and brought out through a separate stab wound along with the suprapubic catheter.

## Postoperative Care

Postoperative intravenous antibiotics are used for 3 to 5 days, after which patients are placed on daily oral antibiotic suppression. The suction drain is usually left for 1 to 2 days. In our experience a nasogastric tube is not usually necessary. The suprapubic tube is carefully secured to avoid kinking or dislodgement. Patients are kept on either oral or rectal anticholinergic medication (belladonna and opium suppositories) to prevent bladder spasms. A cystogram is obtained at 2 to 3 weeks to document the integrity of bladder neck closure. If

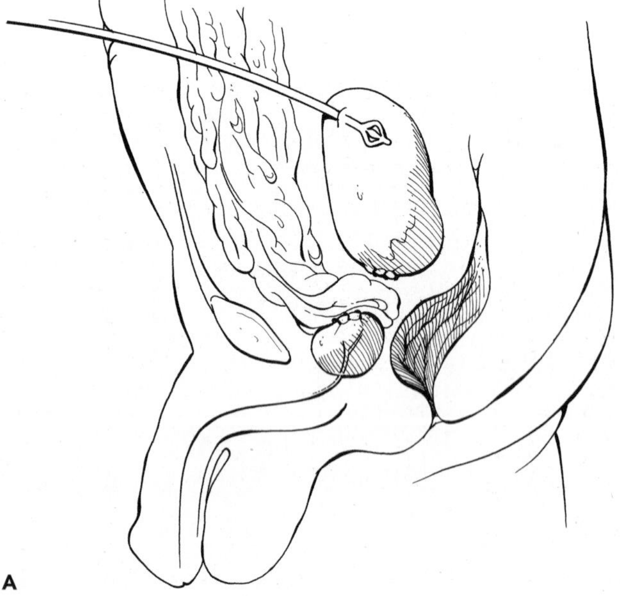


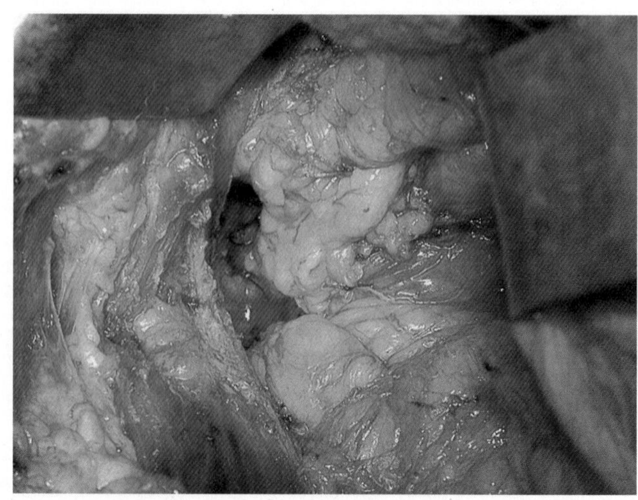


FIGURE 34.9 **A:** Omental interposition in the man. **B:** Intraoperative photograph showing omental wrap over bladder neck closure to prevent secondary vesicourethral fistula.

there is no evidence of leak or fistula, the suprapubic tube may be changed or removed if a catheterizable stoma was chosen for bladder drainage.

# OUTCOMES

## Complications

The primary complication of bladder neck closure is postoperative fistula. Such a fistula may occur as early as 1 week postoperatively or as late as 1 year. When a fistula is suspected, the patient should undergo a cystogram with a mixture of contrast and methylene blue dye. The site of leakage (vagina or perineum) should then be assessed both visually and radiographically. If a small fistula is encountered early in the postoperative period, bilateral percutaneous nephrostomies may be used to divert the urine away from the fistulous site. Reoperation is a more complex but reliable method of dealing with postoperative fistula. When the initial procedure was performed from a vaginal or perineal approach, reoperation should be performed suprapubically to allow extensive bladder mobilization and interposition of a large, well-vascularized omental flap. Supravesical diversion is reserved for patients in whom all attempts at repair have failed.

Loss of access to the bladder may also represent a source of postoperative morbidity. Loss of a suprapubic tube and closure of its tract is an underreported but not uncommon complication. Access may be re-established by using a flexible cystoscope or ureteroscope and may require fluoroscopy to negotiate the tract and pass a flexible wire down to the bladder. If this procedure fails, the patient may be given a fluid bolus and the bladder may be percutaneously accessed under sonographic guidance. Once access has been established, the tract may be dilated and a council catheter passed over the wire. Inability to catheterize a continent efferent limb may be treated similarly, and endoscopic negotiation of the conduit usually suffices to reestablish access.

## Results

Though a number of authors have reported their results with BNC, most series have been small, retrospective, and with a great deal of variability in technique (3,4,8,11). Consequently, long-term outcomes and overall success rates are difficult to judge. In series where the bladder neck is anteriorly mobilized and appropriate vascularized interposition tissue is utilized, long-term continence rates range from 83% to 100% with a 7% to 8% reoperation rate (4,6,11). In series where these principles have not been employed, fistula formation and reoperation rate range from 30% to 46% and 25% to 46%, respectively (1,3,9). In one series where female multiple sclerosis patients were treated with vaginal urethral closure and suprapubic cystostomy, approximately 80% of the patients who were continent (and available for reliable follow-up) remained continent at an average follow-up of 6.5 years (range, 2 to 17 years) (3). Upper-tract deterioration has been noted in a single series (11%) and has been causally related to the use of continent, catheterizable efferent channels in patients with persistent bladder dysfunction (1).

## *References*


1. Andrews HO, Shah PJR. Surgical management of urethral damage in neurogenically impaired female patients with chronic indwelling catheters. *Br J Urol* 1998;82:820.
2. Chancellor MB, Erhard MB, Kiilholma PJ, et al. Functional urethral closure with pubovaginal sling for destroyed female urethra after long-term catheterization. *Urology* 1994;43(4):499.
3. Eckford SB, Kohler-Ockmore J, Feneley RCL. Long-term follow up of transvaginal urethral closure and suprapubic cystostomy for urinary incontinence in women with multiple sclerosis. *Br J Urol* 1994;74:319.
4. Hensle TW, Kirsch AJ, Kennedy WA, et al. Bladder closure in association with continent urinary diversion. *J Urol* 1995;154:883.
5. Izawa JI, Ajam K, McGuire EJ, et al. Major surgery to manage definitively severe complications of salvage cryotherapy for prostate cancer. *J Urol* 2000;164:1978.
6. O'Connor RC, Stapp EC, Donnellan RM, et al. Long-term results of suprapubic bladder neck closure for treatment of the devastated outlet. *Urology* 2005;66(2):311–315.
7. Perkash I. Transurethral sphincterotomy provides significant relief in autonomic dysreflexia in spinal cord injured male patients: long-term followup results. *J Urol* 2007;177:1026.
8. Schwartz SL, Kennelly MJ, McGuire EJ, et al. Incontinent ileo-vesicostomy urinary diversion in the treatment of lower urinary tract dysfunction. *J Urol* 1994;152:99.
9. Stower MJ, Massey JA, Feneley RC. Urethral closure in management of urinary incontinence. *Urology* 1989;34(5):246.
10. Wanatabe T, Rivas DA, Smith R, et al. The effect of urinary reconstruction on neurogenically impaired women previously treated with an indwelling urethral catheter. *J Urol* 1996;156:1926.
11. Zimmern PE, Hadley HR, Leach GE, et al. Transvaginal closure of the bladder neck and placement of a suprapubic catheter for destroyed urethra after long term indwelling catheterization. *J Urol* 1985;134:554.

# CHAPTER 35 ■ SURGERY FOR URETHRAL STRICTURE DISEASE

JACK R. WALTER AND GEORGE D. WEBSTER

Urethral stricture have been described and managed since antiquity. Egyptians used reeds to dilate strictures in 1700 B.C., documenting the first nonsurgical intervention reported for the management of strictures. Urethral strictures remain a relevant disease process in present times. Their etiology remains trauma, inflammation, or ischemia, with trauma being the most common cause. Traumatic injuries may result from external violence, including blunt trauma to the perineum, pelvic fracture, or penetrating injury with knife or projectile injury. More frequently, iatrogenic injury secondary to urethral catheterization and endoscopic surgery create strictures. Inflammatory processes, including gonococcal urethritis or lichen sclerosis, can result in stricture formation. Rarely, urethral strictures can result from malignancy, typically of urethral, penile, or lymphoid origin. The central process of urethral stricture pathophysiology is progressive fibrosis of the epithelium with subsequent involvement of the underlying spongiosum. The urethral lumen narrows, leading to a weak urinary stream and difficulty voiding, culminating in complete obliteration with urinary retention. Rarely, stricture disease will lead to fistula or abscess formation.

## DIAGNOSIS

The presentation of urethral strictures ranges from insidious to obvious. Men may have stricture disease for many years and never seek evaluation or suspect they have a problem. These men are commonly diagnosed when urethral catheters are placed for surgery or when their long-standing strictures lead to bladder decompensation. Frequently, strictures present with symptoms of bladder outlet obstruction and irritative symptoms, including urgency, frequency, and dysuria. Occasionally, patients will present with microscopic or gross hematuria. Recurrent urinary tract infection can accompany these symptoms. In cases of traumatic stricture, the history will include prior urethral instrumentation or an episode of external injury.

Men with newly diagnosed strictures require a thorough history and physical examination with special attention to the genitalia. Penile length should be noted. The character, color, and laxity of penile shaft skin and preputial skin, when present, should be assessed to determine flap and graft availability. The urethra is palpated to help determine the severity of spongiofibrosis. Laboratory evaluation should include urine analysis, urine culture, and assessment of renal function. Conventional radiological studies adequately delineate urethral strictures in most men. Retrograde urethrography (RUG) provides the length, location, caliber, and multiplicity of the stricture (8). If one is unable to adequately distend the proximal uretha due to near obliteration of the lumen, voiding cystourethrography (VCUG) provides additional information. Simultaneous RUG–VCUG is indispensable in the evaluation of the obliterative urethral defect that follows pelvic fracture. Urethral ultrasonography and magnetic resonance imaging have also been used in the evaluation of urethral disease but are not as widely available. Uroflowmetry provides insight on the functional significance of the stricture. Cystourethroscopy provides little additional information in the clinic setting as visualization of the proximal urethra is limited by the stricture. Urethroscopy if performed is primarily used to rule out malignancy and complement the radiological findings.

## INDICATIONS FOR SURGERY

The presence of stricture alone does not necessitate surgical intervention as many wide-caliber strictures are of little consquence. Prior to surgery, strictures should demonstrate outlet obstruction. Stricture location and characteristics dictate initial management. In most settings dilation or optical urethrotomy is acceptable. Such intervention is rarely curative but usually temporizes the acute event for a variable duration (11). Indications for open urethroplasty include frequent urethral dilation or complications associated with dilation, including false passage, diverticulum, fistula, bacteremia, hemorrhage, and excessive pain. In addition, strictures that occur in children or long, obliterative strictures justify earlier consideration for open repair.

Numerous urethroplasty techniques have been described, and no single technique is appropriate for all strictures. Consider two broad technical groups of urethroplasty: anastomotic and substitution repairs. Anastomotic, as the name implies, involves removal of the diseased urethra and reanastomosis of the healthy ends. Substitution repairs augment or replace the urethral lumen with a pedicalized flap or graft performed in single or multiple stages. Traditionally, grafts and flaps originated from genital skin. However, buccal mucosal grafts have emerged as the preferred urethral substitute in adults due to their favorable inherent qualities and consistent availability.

The goals of any reconstructive urologic surgery are functional and anatomic success. Location, length, and etiology of the stricture as well as personal experience determine the appropriate surgical technique. Additional factors, including concominant fistulas, inflammation, and prior repairs, need to be considered. With these thoughts in mind, excellent function—urethral patency and stable sexual function—and cosmetic results are attainable.

# ALTERNATIVE THERAPY

Nonsurgical and minimally invasive alternatives exist for management of urethral stricture. Nonsurgical options include expectant management and dilation performed by the patient or physician. Minimally invasive techniques include optical urethrotomy using cold knife, electrocautery, or laser. In general, urethrotomy is contraindicated in the pendulous urethra due to the paucity of surrounding spongy tissue, which is necessary for urethral re-epithelialization. More recently transurethral placement of metallic urethral stents has been utilized. Currently, urethral stenting is discouraged in the pendulous urethra due to patient discomfort and potential compromise of erectile function. In the bulbar urethra all of the mentioned options are available. In terms of cure rates, optical urethrotomy has no advantage over urethral dilation (11). Further, if one urethrotomy or dilation fails to cure a patient, then subsequent procedures are rarely if ever successful (6). With poor success of repeat internal urethrotomy, the cost-effective strategy is to move to open surgical repair following one failed endoscopic treatment (12). Strictures that may be cured by dilation or urethrotomy are usually short (<1 cm) bulbar strictures, whereas longer strictures or those of the pendulous urethra are rarely cured by dilation or urethrotomy.

# SURGICAL TECHNIQUE

## General Surgical Principles

Prior to incision, controlled variables should be optimized. The preoperative urine culture must be negative. If the patient has an indwelling suprapubic tube, broad-spectrum oral antibiotics should be provided during the 24 hours prior to surgery. On-call parenteral antibiotics should be given. Appropriate radiological studies must be available in the operative room. The surgeon should communicate openly with anesthesia about anticipated length of surgery, expected blood loss, and type of anesthetic required. Most anterior urethral strictures can be managed with a spinal anesthetic. If one determines that a buccal mucosal graft will be needed, one should advise anesthesia that general endotracheal anesthesia is necessary. We prefer to position patients in modified lithotomy using padded Allen stirrups. Exaggerated lithotomy is rarely necessary and carries a significant risk of neuronal injury and compartment syndrome, especially with prolonged operative time (1). Staining the urethra with methylene blue assists in identifying the urethral lumen as well as differentiating urethral scar from healthy urothelium. "Table-fixed" ring retraction (Bookwalter or Omni) provides ideal exposure for bulbar or posterior urethroplasty, while nonfixed ring retraction (Lone Star) is optimal for pendulous urethroplasty. Polyglycolic acid (PGA) suture material has ideal tensile strength, absorption rate, and tissue reactivity; and 5-0 is generally used. Wound drainage when necessary is accomplished with a 7Fr closed-suction drain. Dressings should be supportive and noncompressive.

Postoperative urinary drainage should be effective and cause minimal urothelial irriation. For this purpose 12Fr silicone urethral catheters function adequately. When surgical repair in bulbar stricture disease requires a graft or flap, the catheter is fenestrated to promote drainage of the operative site (Fig. 35.1). One rarely needs suprapubic catheter drainage with anterior urethral surgery. If present, it may facilitate postoperative urethral stent management, allowing removal of the urethral catheter without requiring the patient to void. The type and location of repair determine the length of time that catheterization is required. Meatal or glanular repairs require 5 to 7 days, anastomotic repairs require 10 to 14 days, and one-stage graft repairs require 21 days of urinary drainage. Prior to catheter removal, the anastomotic lines are assessed for healing with a pericatheter RUG for all urethroplasties proximal to the fossa navicularis. If there is no extravasation at the repair site, the catheter is removed and the patient resumes normal voiding. History and examination, uroflowmetry, and RUG are performed at 3 and 12 months following repair. Subsequently, symptomatic follow-up is indicated, and some use periodic uroflow studies.

## Strictures of the Glanular Urethra

Strictures in the glanular urethra arise commonly from inflammatory conditions, instrumentation, or improper circumcision. Simple meatotomy, a glans-based Y–V advancement flap for very distal stenosis, or a ventral shaft skin onlay flap in the case of stricture involving the entire fossa navicularis may accomplish surgical repair. For Y–V advancement, a V-shaped incision is made on the dorsal aspect of the glans with the apex terminating at the urethral meatus (Fig. 35.2). A dorsal midline extension of this incision is made into the urethra to widen the lumen to accept a 22Fr sound. The glans flap can be elevated using skin hooks and sharp dissection to allow its mobilization into the most proximal limit of the dorsal urethral incision, where it is anchored with a 4-0 PGA suture. Care must be taken to leave this glans flap with a wide base to avoid vascular compromise.

More extensive strictures of the glanular and distal penile urethra should be managed according to their etiology. If one suspects lichen sclerosis (LS), biopsies may be obtained to confirm diagnosis and exclude possible malignancy. Strictures associated with LS are best repaired with nongenital skin as the penile skin is considered blighted and may eventually develop LS. In these cases, the diseased urethra is excised, the buccal mucosa is inlayed, and the urethra is left open. A second stage, during which the urethra is then tubularized, occurs 6 to 12 months later after the graft matures, and the adjacent urethra is observed for further development of LS. If extensive stricture disease is unrelated to LS, then a flap of skin obtained from the penile shaft allows repair in a single stage. The flap may be fashioned as an onlay or as a tube, depending on the extent of the disease (Fig. 35.3).

## Strictures of the Pendulous Urethra

Pendulous urethral strictures are most often repaired using an onlay flap of penile skin. Although many variations of this technique have been described, the laterally based pedicled island flap originally described by Orandi gives excellent results and is technically forgiving. It is in general suitable for repairs measuring up to 8 cm (depending on penile length), although longer repairs can be performed by harvesting a penile "J"

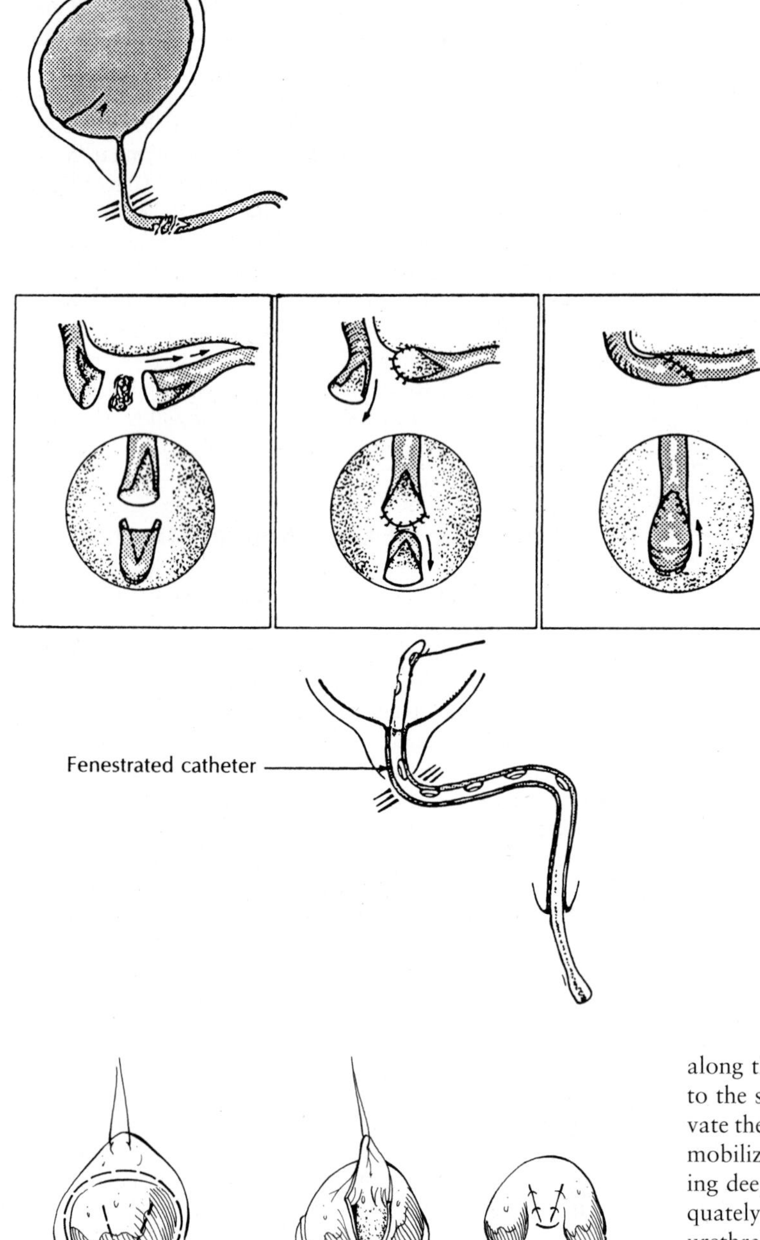


FIGURE 35.1 The fenestrated urethral catheter is optimal following urethroplasty. Either a balloon or straight catheter may be used, and fenestrations are made in the catheter shaft in the region of repair. The fenestrations allow debris and exudate to be washed away from the site of repair. Bladder irrigation cannot be performed unless the catheter is inserted all the way into the bladder so that the most distal fenestration is intravesical.

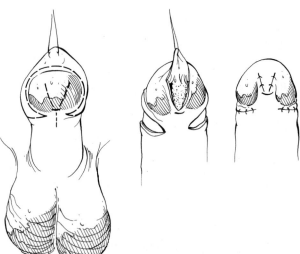

FIGURE 35.2 Glans flap meatoplasty.

flap that has a vertical and a distal circumferential component. A flap width up to 25 mm can be used without compromising penile skin closure. The patient is placed in either the lithotomy or supine frog-legged position. An incision is made along the ventral penile raphe through the Buck fascia down to the strictured segment of urethra. Using skin hooks to elevate the flap and fine scissors for dissection, one skin margin is mobilized from the corpus cavernosum for 10 to 15 mm, staying deep to the Buck fascia (Fig. 35.4). With the urethra adequately exposed, a suitable catheter or filiform is placed in the urethral lumen as a guide and the urethra incised ventrally along the stricture. This incision is then extended to expose at least 1 cm of healthy urethra proximal and distal to the stricture. An onlay flap of suitable width to achieve a 24Fr lumen (in general, 18 to 25 mm) is then outlined on the mobilized lateral penile shaft skin. The flap length corresponds to the length of the urethrotomy and is tapered at the proximal and distal ends. Care must be taken not to incorporate a significant segment of hair-bearing shaft skin in the repair.

Once the flap has been outlined, the projected new skin edges are approximated in the midline to ensure that wound closure with minimal tension is possible. The lateral aspect of the flap is then incised through the subcutaneous connective tissue, leaving the underlying dartos and deeper Buck fascia intact. With exposure of the correct tissue plane, the lateral penile shaft skin will retract with minimal additional dissection. The medial border of the island flap is then anchored to the lateral edge of the incised urethra with 5-0 PGA stay sutures. The flap is sutured to the urethra beginning at the distal margin, using a

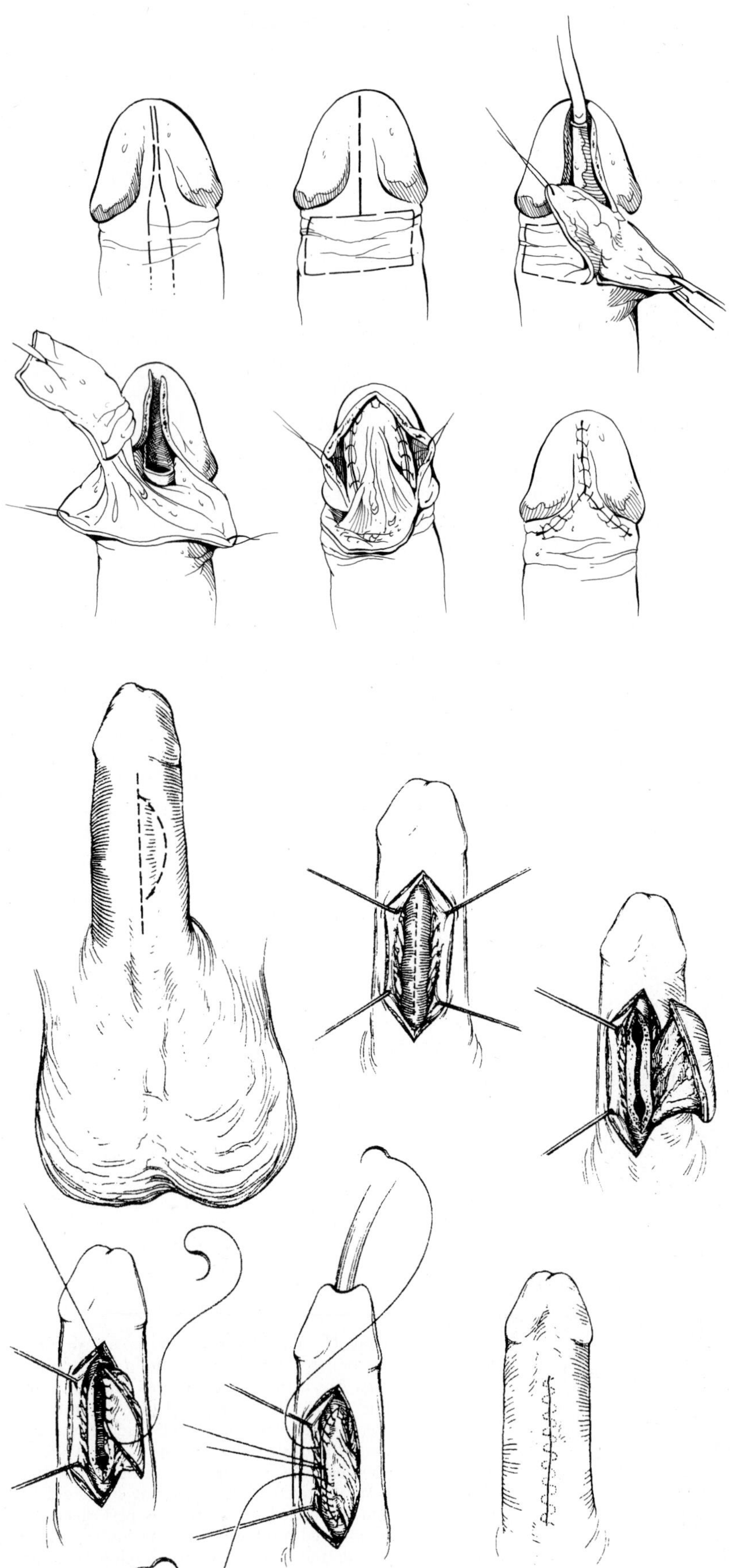

FIGURE 35.3 Repair of meatal and distal penile urethral stricture using a pedicled island of distal penile skin. This procedure allows for reapproximation of glans tissue around the neourethra, giving an excellent cosmetic and functional result.

FIGURE 35.4 Onlay urethroplasty of a pendulous urethral stricture (Orandi repair). The stricture is approached through a ventral penile incision. The outline of the skin island to be used for onlay is marked once the stricture has been opened and its length and caliber determined. The skin island is raised on a subcutaneous vascular pedicle, rotated inward, and sutured as an onlay to augment urethral caliber. Skin closure is in at least two layers to avoid fistula formation.

running 5-0 PGA suture, incorporating the urothelium in the closure. When the lateral suture line is complete, the free edge of the island flap can be rolled over and secured with 5-0 PGA stay sutures to the contralateral margin, recreating the urethral lumen. A similar running suture line is performed with 5-0 PGA to complete the onlay repair. Local wound drainage may be accomplished with a suction drain placed underneath the vascular pedicle along the length of the flap to obviate hematoma or urinoma formation, which could compromise the flap.

Wound closure is performed in two layers using 5-0 interrupted PGA sutures. Care must be taken when approximating the subdermal connective tissue of the skin margins to avoid injury to the flap pedicle. This first layer of closure covers the exposed urethral suture line and minimize the risk of fistula formation. Skin closure is performed with a running subcuticular 5-0 PGA suture. The wound is supported with adhesive strips and covered with a gauze and loosely applied Coband dressing to reduce edema formation. The urethral catheter is secured to the abdominal wall and remains in place for up to 3 weeks. If a suction drain is used, it is removed within 24 hours. The supportive dressing is taken down on postoperative day 2. The patient is allowed to ambulate on postoperative day 1, and the procedure is usually performed as an outpatient.

## Bulbar Urethral Stricture Repair

### Anastomotic Urethroplasty

Strictures of the bulbar urethra originate most commonly from straddle injuries or iatrogenic trauma during endoscopy or catheterization. Optimal management is dictated by stricture length. Strictures under 1 cm in length are best managed with excision and anastomotic urethroplasty. The patient is placed in modified lithotomy position. A midline perineal incision is made and bifurcated posteriorly 2 cm above the anus. The bulbospongiosus muscle is divided in the midline, exposing the bulbar urethra. The bulbospongiosus muscle can frequently be separated from the underlying bulbar urethra with blunt disection if the correct plane is identified. By sharply dividing the reflection of the Buck fascia lateral to the urethra as it drapes over the corporal bodies proximal to the crus, one can safely dissect the urethral circumferentially. A space deep to the Buck fascia and between the separating corporal bodies is entered on each side. This dorsal dissection, separating the urethra from the corporal bodies, is continued sharply until the entire strictured urethra has been circumferentially mobilized. One should avoid mobilization distal to the suspensory ligament of the penis if possible, as this will increase the risk of chordee and penile length shortening. Further mobility of the proximal bulbar urethra is obtained by dividing the ventral attachments to the perineal body.

Once the strictured segment is fully mobilized, the urethra is divided at the distal extent of the stricture as defined by a catheter or bougie à boule placed from the meatus. The urethra should be spatulated through the diseased segment defining the extent of disease. Complete removal of fibrotic tissue with exposure of healthy proximal and distal urethra is essential for successful repair, but no >1 cm of urethra should be excised. If the urethral ends appose in a tension-free fashion, they are spatulated sharply for 1 cm (Fig. 35.5). Using 5-0 interrupted PGA sutures, the dorsal wall of the anastomosis is

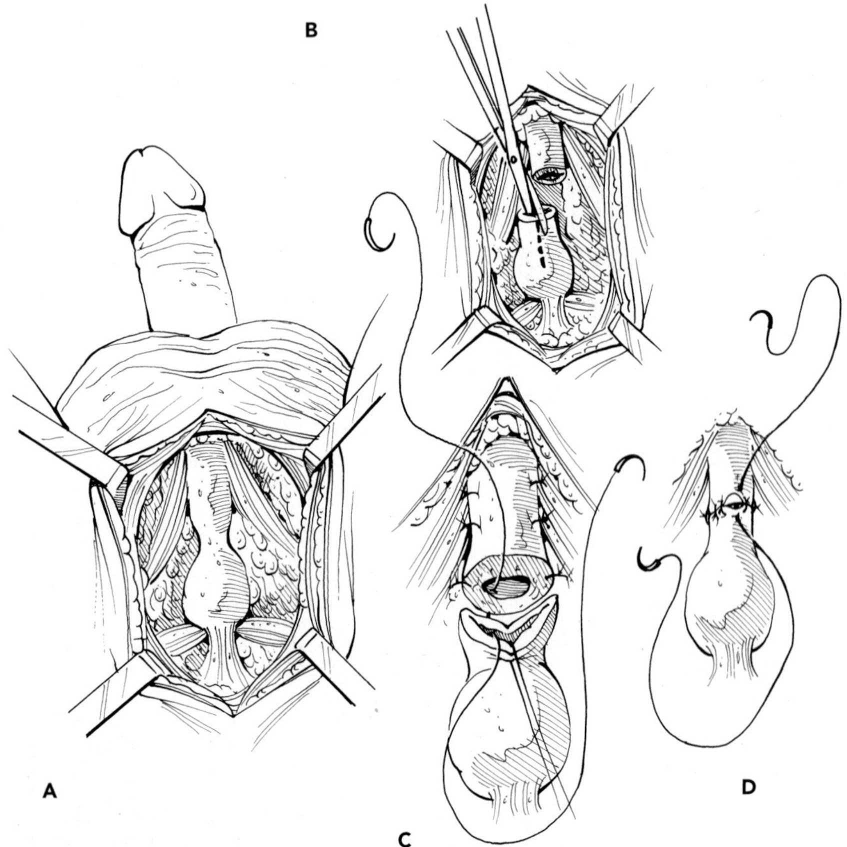


FIGURE 35.5 Anastomotic repair of bulbar urethral stricture that may follow straddle injury. **A:** The urethra is exposed through a midline perineal incision and the stricture site identified and excised. **B:** Following stricture excision, apposing spatulations of 1 cm are accomplished. **C:** The proximal urethral opening is spread-fixed to the underlying corporal body, and spatulated anastomosis is performed with interrupted sutures. **D:** The anastomosis is completed, and additional tension-relieving sutures between urethral adventitia and adjacent corporal bodies are placed to avoid anastomotic tension during erection.

completed while spread-fixing the urethra to the corporal bodies. Circumferential partial-thickness anastomotic sutures incorporating the urothelium and some of the corpora spongiosum complete the first layer of the repair on the ventral surface. A second layer of closure is accomplished using the redundant spongiosum. The bulbospongiosus muscle and the Colle fascia are approximated in the midline with interrupted 5-0 PGA sutures. Final skin closure is made with interrupted 5-0 PGA sutures. The perineum is dressed and bolstered with fluff gauze and mesh underwear. The urethral catheter is secured to the abdominal wall to minimize traction and pressure on the urethra.

### Augmented Anastomotic Urethroplasty

Excision of 1 cm of urethra and associated 1-cm spatulated repair results in a total of 2 cm of urethral shortening, an amount that can be easily accommodated by the elasticity of the mobilized bulbar urethra. As bulbar urethral strictures extend beyond 1 cm in length, the risk of chordee and shortening increases if primary anastomotic repairs are performed. A variety of alternative procedures that avoid penile shortening and chordee may be used for strictures that are >1 cm in length.

For strictures of up to 2 cm in length, stricture excision and augmented anastomotic repair is a good option (5). The 2-cm segment of stricture is excised. The urethra is then spatulated proximally and distally for 1 cm into healthy urethra on the same side. The anastomosis is then augmented with a graft (or a flap), increasing the lumen and avoiding the need for spatulation. This in effect spares an additional 1-cm loss of urethral length. In the ventral onlay, spatulation is at the 6 o'clock position (floor), and the unspatulated dorsal (roof) strips are then reapproximated end-to-end after spread-fixation, thereby securing the anastomosed urethral roof strip to the overlying corporal body. The anastomosis is not completed circumferentially, resulting in a diamond-shaped ventral urethral defect into which is laid either a graft of penile skin or buccal mucosa or, alternatively, a diamond-shaped flap of penile skin mobilized on a pedicle through the scrotum. This repair is called an augmented roof strip anastomotic procedure. It provides the advantages of an anastomosis while augmenting the repair to limit penile shortening to 2 cm, which is usually acceptable (Fig. 35.6). Alternatively, and our preference, is to perform a floor strip anastomosis, placing the augmenting graft, typically buccal mucosa, on the dorsal aspect, where it is spread-fixed to the overlying corporal body. This approach permits superior spread-fixation of the graft and therefore reduces graft shrinkage and enhances graft take because of the reliable apposition to the corporal body; it also avoids graft or flap sacculation. Consequently, since 1996, we prefer the dorsal onlay in the bulbar urethra (3).

### Onlay Bulbar Urethroplasty

As bulbar stricture length increases to >2 cm in length, it is rarely possible to complete any type of anastomotic repair without causing some penile chordee and tension on the anastomosis. In this setting we have found success using a buccal mucosal or skin graft onlay applied to the dorsal aspect of the strictured portion of the bulbar urethra (Fig. 35.7). The urethral bulb is exposed circumferentially. The distal extent of the stricture is defined with a 20Fr catheter. The urethra is rotated 180 degrees to expose its dorsal aspect. Stay sutures of 4-0 silk are placed along the exposed dorsal aspect, and the urethra is then incised along the strictured segment in the 12 o'clock (dorsal) position. The incision is extended for 1 cm into healthy urethra proximal and distal to the stricture.

Confirmation of proximal and distal patency is confirmed endoscopically and by calibration with a 24Fr bougie à boule. A suitable skin donor site, selected on the ventral penile shaft or prepuce, or a buccal mucosa graft is harvested. The graft is spread-fixed on a paraffin block and defatted. It is then fenestrated with a scalpel and sized and shaped to fit the defect created by urethral incision. The graft is then anchored in a spread-fixed fashion to the corporal bodies opposing the dorsally incised strictured urethra. The urethra is then rotated back to its normal anatomic position, and the margins of the urethral incision are sutured to the fixed graft edge and corporal body using interrupted 5-0 PGA sutures. In this fashion, the dorsal graft becomes the new urethral roof, augmenting the urethral caliber at the stricture site. This dorsal approach mitigates blood loss from a ventral bulbar incision and provides excellent graft stabilization. Of note, the residual floor of the strictured urethra functions as the foundation for the repair. If the stricture is severe, outcomes may be compromised.

## Panurethral Stricture or Failed Urethroplasty

The management of extensive stricture of the anterior urethra involving both the pendulous and bulbar portions can be extremely challenging. These are usually of inflammatory origin (often due to lichen sclerosis) and can be up to 20 cm in length. Urethral repair in these circumstances is undertaken either by combination repairs using grafts and flaps or, more conservatively, by multistaged repairs that may also use perineal inlays of full- or split-thickness skin grafts. One must consider the use of perineal urethrostomy or repeat dilations, as reconstructive results in other locations and situations are not as successful.

## One-Stage Combination Urethroplasty

One-stage combination procedures make use of both a flap repair for the pendulous portion of the urethra and a graft repair for the bulbar area, with the two procedures being performed in continuity (7). The patient is placed in the lithotomy position for access to the perineum as well as the penile shaft. In uncircumcised men the prepuce can be used as a skin graft donor site, leaving the remaining shaft skin for island pedicle flap construction. In the event there is insufficient penile skin, buccal mucosa may be used for the graft repair of the contiguous scrotal/bulbar urethra, or buccal mucosa may be preferred even in cases where penile skin is sufficient. One should avoid the use of penile skin when lichen sclerosis is present.

A ventral incision is made over the pendulous urethra, and this portion of the stricture is repaired using a ventral onlay repair in the fashion of Orandi, as described earlier. The more proximal scrotal portion of the stricture is then repaired in continuity by a dorsal or ventral onlay. This portion of the repair is approached through a separate incision in the perineum for exposure of the bulbar urethra. If a dorsal onlay is used, which is our preference, the bulbar urethra is circumferentially mobilized as far distally as the proximal limit of the penile flap

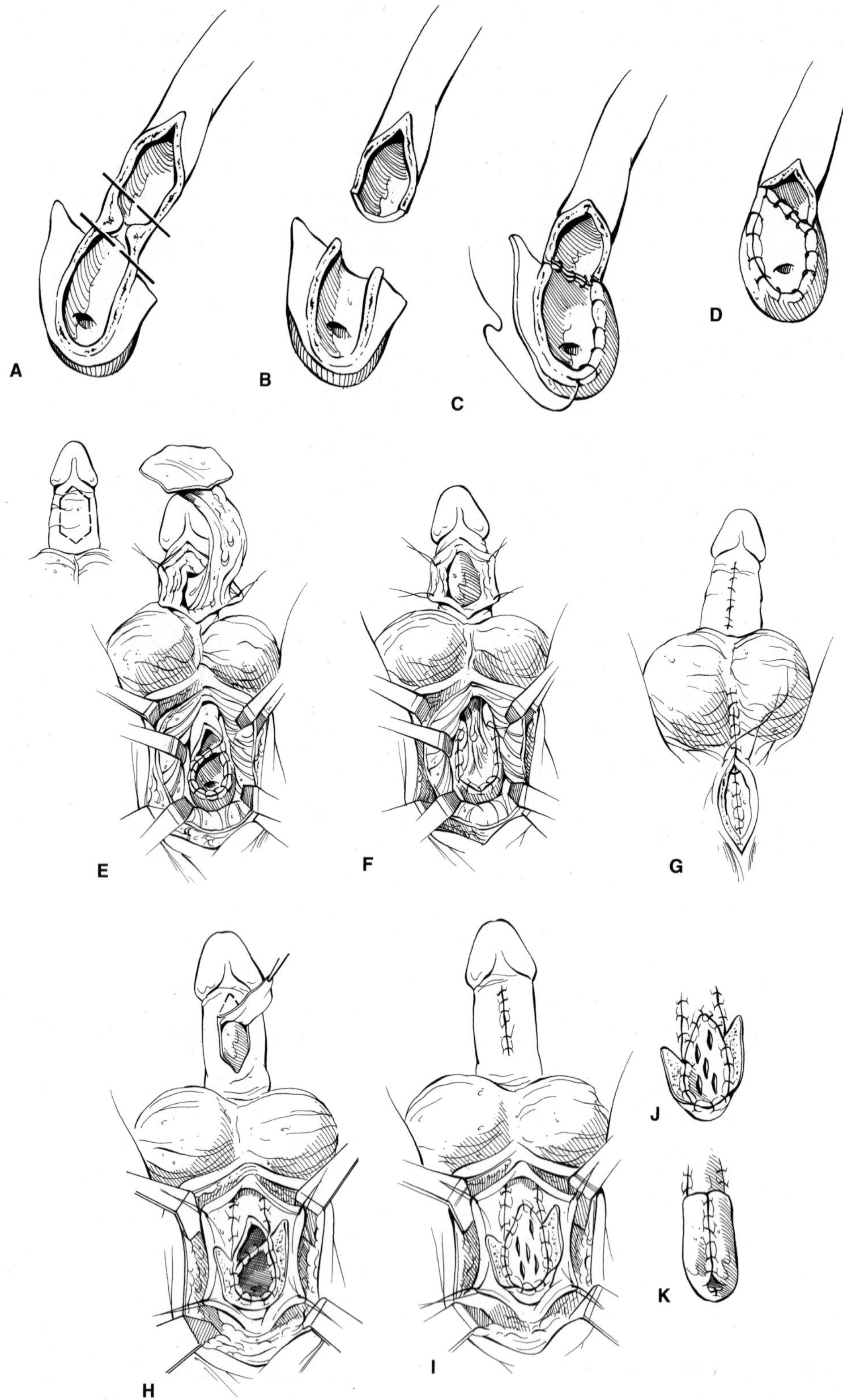


FIGURE 35.6 Augmented roof strip anastomotic repair. **A–D:** A healthy roof strip of urethra is created by stricture excision and roof strip reanastomosis. **E–G:** An appropriately sized and shaped island of ventral penile skin is mobilized on its vascular pedicle, tucked through the scrotum, and sutured over the anastomosis, augmenting its caliber (closure is in layers). **H–K:** This series illustrates the augmented roof strip anastomotic repair using a fenestrated full-thickness skin graft from the ventral penile shaft rather than a pedicled island of penile skin.

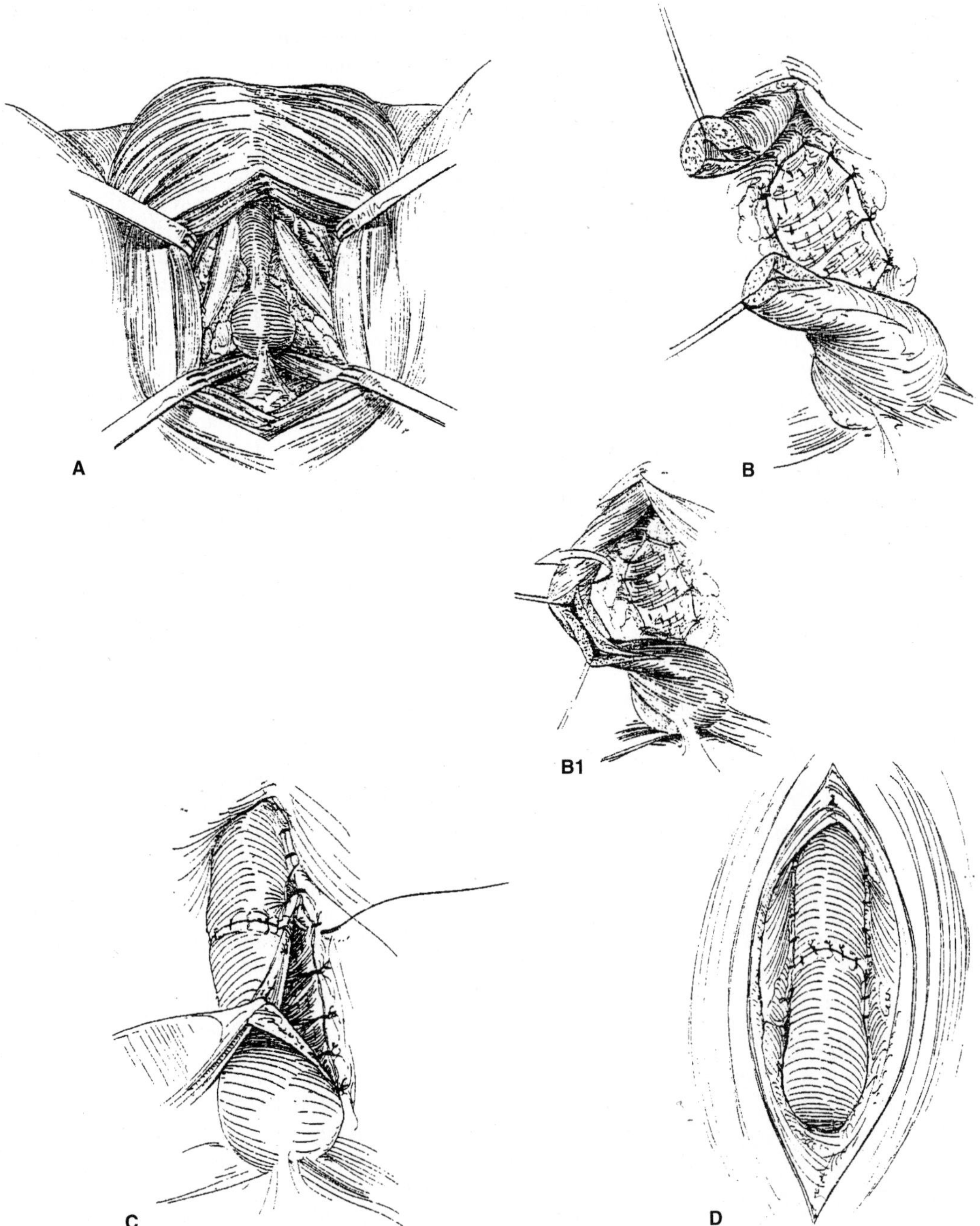


FIGURE 35.7 The dorsal onlay graft bulbar urethroplasty. **A:** Exposure of the urethra. **B, B1:** Fenestrated graft sutured to the undersurface of the corporal body. Strictured portion of the urethra either excised or rotated. **C:** Suture of the opened urethra to dorsal onlay graft. **D:** Completed repair.

repair, and the urethra is then incised dorsally through the stricture, with the distal limit being the visible ventral onlay; the dorsal onlay graft is then completed as described earlier. Hence, the long stricture is repaired by a ventral onlay flap for the pendulous portion and a dorsal onlay graft for the more proximal urethra, with the composite repair being completed nose to tail.

## Staged Repair

Extensive anterior urethral stricture disease, in particular full-length strictures, strictures complicated by fistula or inflammation, and long recurrent strictures following prior repair, is best managed by a staged repair. Historically, such repairs were performed as scrotal inlay procedures with the resultant neourethra being constructed from hair-bearing scrotal skin, which experience has proven to be a suboptimal substitute. Variations on this theme now inlay fenestrated full-thickness preputial skin, split-thickness thigh skin, or buccal mucosa alongside the marsupialized urethra in the first stage. In the second stage, the neourethra is formed by tubularization of the graft. Full-thickness skin is superior for this purpose but is not often available in communities where circumcision is common. If split-thickness skin is to be used, it is in general harvested from the thigh, which is easily accessed with a patient in the lithotomy position. The strictured anterior urethra is exposed through a ventral midline perineal incision that may bifurcate the scrotum, and the urethra is then incised along the length of the stricture to healthy urethra proximally and distally. This again is confirmed by calibrating the urethra with a 24Fr to 28Fr bougie à boule, which should pass easily through each ostium. Using a dermatome set to 20 thousandths of an inch, a split-thickness graft is harvested from the thigh and meshed to a ratio of 1.5:1.0. A strip of meshed graft measuring 3 to 5 cm is then inlayed around the marsupialized strictured urethra (Fig. 35.8). Medially it is sutured to the incised urethral margin and laterally to the incised scrotal and perineal skin edges using 5-0 PGA. This width of graft accounts for the up to 50% shrinkage that may occur with split-thickness skin, resulting in suitable graft width for a future neourethra. If buccal mucosa is inlayed (preferable but not always adequately available), a fenestrated graft of 2.5 to 3.0 cm in width is usually adequate because it undergoes less contraction. A suprapubic tube is placed for urinary diversion in the postoperative period, and the graft is dressed with an Adaptic gauze and a tie-down dressing of sterile cotton fluffs soaked in Bunnell solution. The graft is keep moist by periodic application of Bunnell solution until the dressing is removed after 5 days. Graft take is in the order of 95% or greater.

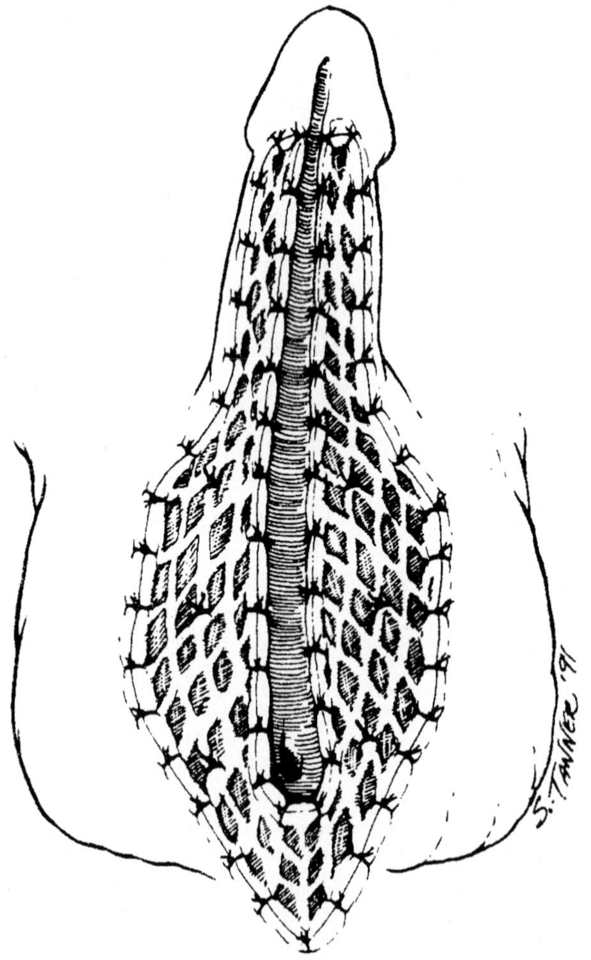


FIGURE 35.8 Staged urethroplasty for full-length stricture disease using meshed split-thickness skin graft. The meshed graft is laid alongside the marsupialized urethra so that the neourethra will be tubularized from the graft rather than from hair-bearing scrotal skin. Tubularization of the neourethra is delayed for 3 to 6 months.

The second stage is performed a minimum of 3 months later and in practice usually 6 to 12 months later to allow thorough vascularization of the graft and to allow adjacent stricture disease to declare itself. The proximal and distal urethral openings should again freely calibrate to 28Fr and 24Fr, respectively, prior to second-stage closure. If the ostia have narrowed, revision rather than dilation should be undertaken, usually using a Y–V advancement technique. Second-stage repair is begun by incising the graft circumferentially to a width that will allow neourethral tubularization to approximately 28Fr. The tubularization is performed by midline anastomosis with a running 5-0 PGA suture, interlocking every third pass, followed by a multilayer wound closure. The urethral is stented for 20 days.

# OUTCOMES

## Complications

Hematoma or hemorrhage is in general rare if meticulous attention is paid to hemostasis during the repair. Wound infection is an uncommon complication that in general presents with erythema and induration at the incision site.

Flap necrosis is uncommon in experienced hands and is most often due to technical errors in preparation of skin flaps or poor flap selection. Flap viability may also be adversely affected by prior surgery, infection, tissue ischemia, tobacco usage, and malnutrition. Contraction of 15% to 25% is anticipated for full-thickness skin grafts and must be accounted for during preparation. Removal of subcutaneous fat and fascia must be achieved for adequate exposure of the subdermal vascular plexus but should not be so excessive as to convert the graft to a split-thickness variety. Fenestration of free grafts will promote drainage of the graft bed, and a well-vascularized graft bed must be assumed, sometimes requiring redeployment of spongy tissue. Split-thickness grafts are not advocated for one-stage urethroplasty because their shrinkage is unpredictable and may be excessive (up to 50%).

Fistula is in general uncommon in adult urethral surgery but is on occasion encountered in the setting of underlying infection or vascular compromise. It most commonly occurs following repair of pendulous urethral strictures. Suprapubic urinary diversion may allow for spontaneous healing of fistulas encountered within the first few weeks following urethroplasty. Fistulas that fail to close with proximal diversion generally need reoperation after a minimum of 6 months.

With use of an oversized or poorly supported ventral onlay flap or graft, in particular in the bulbar urethra, there is on occasion formation of a redundant urethral segment in which urine may pool, leading to poor urethral emptying and recurrent infection. Urethral stones can form as a result of urinary stasis in the diverticulum or as a result of retained hair on flaps and grafts. Proper measurement of flaps and grafts to provide a 26Fr to 28Fr lumen, as well as adequate spread-fixation of the onlay, may obviate sacculation. Preoperative epilation and proper selection of donor sites can prevent the hairy urethra.

Penile curvature may result because of inappropriate procedure selection in attempting anastomotic repair or long-graft onlay repair to the pendulous urethra distal to the suspensory ligament. It may also follow excessive urethral excision (>2 cm) when performing anastomotic repair in the bulbar urethra. A downward deflection of the erect penis may also occur. Grafts of nonpenile origin frequently will not have the same elasticity as the penis, contributing to curvature.

In experienced hands erectile dysfunction as a result of anterior or posterior urethroplasty is rare. Temporary (3 months or less) impotence occurs in 53% of those who undergo anastomotic urethroplasty and in 33% of those who undergo patch repair. However, permanent impotence is unusual: 5% and 0.9%, respectively. Further, Coursey et al. reported that erectile dysfunction after anterior urethroplasty is no more common than in men who undergo circumcision (4). In a prospective evaluation of the effect of bulbar urethroplasty on erectile function using International Index of Erectile Function scores, surgery proved to have an insignificant effect (2). These results can be attributed to judicious scar excision, minimal use of electrocautery, and dissection away from the dorsally based neurovascular structures.

## Results

As understanding of urethral anatomy and tissue transfer techniques has grown, so too has the effectiveness of urethral reconstruction for stricture disease. Patency rates in excess of 90% are reported for anastomotic repairs in bulbar strictures (10). With regard to substitution repairs, tube grafts fare less well than onlay procedures, both of which are best applied to the more proximal portion of the anterior urethra. A discouraging constant annual attrition rate of 5% per year has been reported for substitution urethroplasty at follow-up of 10 years, although this is not these authors' experience (9). For repair of pendulous urethral strictures, flaps perform best in terms of patency and avoidance of penile curvature. Buccal mucosal grafts show promise and conceptually seem to be superior, but long-term data are necessary to define their emerging role in urethral reconstruction. Certainly the most common cause for stricture recurrence appears to be ongoing fibrosis in the adjacent unmanaged urethra, in particular that proximal to the repair.

## *References*


1. Anema JG, Morey AF, McAninch JW, et al. Complications related to the high lithotomy position during urethral reconstruction. *J Urol* 2000; 164:360–363.
2. Anger JT, Sherman ND, Webster GD. The effect of bulbar urethroplasty on erectile function. *J Urol* 2007;178:1009–1011.
3. Barbagli G, Selli C, Tosto A, et al. Dorsal free graft urethroplasty. *J Urol* 1996;155:123–126.
4. Coursey JW, Morey AF, McAninch JW, et al. Erectile function after anterior urethroplasty. *J Urol* 2001;166:2273–2276.
5. Guralnick ML, Webster GD. The augmented anastomotic urethroplasty: indications and outcome in 29 patients. *J Urol* 2001;165:1496–1501.
6. Heyns CF, Steenkamp JW, deDock MLS, et al. Treatment of male urethral strictures: is repeated dilation or internal urethrotomy useful? *J Urol* 1998;160:356–358.
7. Iselin CE, Webster GD. Dorsal onlay graft urethroplasty for repair of bulbar urethral stricture. *J Urol* 1999;161:815–818.
8. McCallum RW. The adult male urethra: normal anatomy, pathology and method of urethrography. *Radiol Clin North Am* 1979;17:227–244.
9. Mundy AR. The long-term results of skin inlay urethroplasty. *Br J Urol* 1995;75:59–61.
10. Santucci RA, Mario LA, McAninch JW. Anastomotic urethroplasty for bulbar urethral stricture: analysis of 168 patients. *J Urol* 2002;167: 1715–1719.
11. Steenkamp JW, Heyns CF, deKock MLS. Internal urethrotomy versus dilation as treatment for male urethral strictures: a prospective, randomized comparison. *J Urol* 1997;157:98–101.
12. Wright JL, Wessells H, Nathens AB, et al. What is the most cost-effective treatment for 1 to 2 cm bulbar urethral strictures: societal approach using decision analysis. *Urology* 2006;67(5):889–893.


# CHAPTER 36 ■ SURGERY FOR URETHRAL TRAUMA INCLUDING URETHRAL DISRUPTION

JACK MCANINCH AND BRYAN B. VOELZKE

A solid understanding of the etiology, evaluation, and management of traumatic urethral injuries is dependent upon the location of urethral trauma. The urethra is divided into anterior (pendulous and bulbar urethra) and posterior (membranous and prostatic urethra) divisions, which have specific mechanisms of injury that will influence eventual therapy and outcome. Immediate management of anterior and posterior urethral trauma predominantly involves temporizing solutions to divert urine away from the urethral injury. A small cohort of patients will be cured by these temporizing measures; however, the majority will require an invasive surgical repair 3 to 6 months after the initial injury. Early recognition and diagnosis of urethral injuries are crucial to the successful management and prevention of long-term complications. This chapter will divide the diagnosis and management of urethral trauma into anterior and posterior injuries to better enable the reader to learn how to manage their unique presentations.

# ANTERIOR URETHRAL INJURIES

The anterior urethra extends distally from the membranous urethra to the urethral meatus (Fig. 36.1). Contrary to the posterior urethra, the anterior urethra is encompassed by the corpus spongiosum, the deep (Buck) fascia, and the superficial (dartos) fascia along its entire length. The penoscrotal junction divides the shorter, proximal bulbar urethra from the longer, distal pendulous urethra. The bulbospongiosus muscle ventrally covers the bulbar urethra and terminates at the penoscrotal junction, prior to the origination of the distal pendulous urethra. The pendulous urethra closely approximates the corpora cavernosa during most of its length, with the lumen of the distal pendulous urethra dilating distally to form the fossa navicularis.

Blunt or penetrating injury can result in anterior urethral trauma; however, blunt forces predominate along the entire urethra. Etiologies include blunt compression or straddle injuries, penile fracture with concomitant urethral disruption, constriction rings, iatrogenic trauma (e.g., after Foley catheterization or endoscopic urethral surgery), and penetrating trauma (e.g., stab or gunshot wounds). Compression of the bulbar urethra against the pubic bone (straddle injury) is the most common anterior urethral injury and occurs after a direct force to the perineum compresses the relatively immobile bulbar urethra against the pubic bone. Additionally, penile constriction rings can damage the anterior urethra secondary to tissue ischemia. Foley catheterization or endoscopic urethral surgery can damage the bulbar urethra, resulting in contusion or partial urethral disruption. The true extent of iatrogenic injuries, along with trauma from constriction rings, may not become evident until many years after the original event (1). Anterior urethra injuries are rarely associated with pelvic fractures but are seen in approximately 20% of penile fractures (2). The close relation of the corpora cavernosa to the pendulous urethra contributes to this association.

## Diagnosis

Anterior urethral injuries can present in an immediate or delayed fashion. A careful history and physical examination should raise suspicion for anterior urethral injury. Straddle injuries often present in a delayed fashion with obstructive voiding symptoms and an idiopathic etiology. In a series of 78 patients with straddle injuries, 40% presented to the emergency department in an acute setting, versus 60% of patients who presented 6 months to 10 years after the original injury (3). Hematuria, difficulty voiding, penile sleeve hematoma (injury confined to the Buck fascia), and perineal "butterfly" hematoma (injury penetration to the Buck fascia) are common presenting symptoms in the acute or delayed setting. In addition to a perineal "butterfly" hematoma, penetration of the Buck fascia can allow the spread of urine and/or blood to the scrotum (dartos fascia), anterior abdominal wall (Colles fascia), and/or thighs (fascia lata).

All patients with a suspected anterior urethral injury should undergo a retrograde urethrogram prior to an attempt at urethral catheter placement. Ideally the patient should be placed obliquely at a 30- to 45-degree angle with the bottom leg flexed at 90 degrees and the top leg kept straight (Fig. 36.2). In the acute setting, associated pelvic fracture may preclude this position; therefore, a supine retrograde urethrogram should be employed to answer the simple question of whether or not the urethral lumen has been disrupted. Flexible cystoscopy has been advocated to aid the diagnosis of urethral trauma; however, we prefer radiographic imaging when possible.

The retrograde urethrogram should be performed with undiluted water-soluble contrast medium [full-strength (60%) ionic contrast medium]. A scout film provides initial information on patient position and the potential presence of a foreign body. A 12Fr Foley catheter is then placed into the fossa navicularis, and the balloon is inflated with 2 to 3 mL of sterile water to prevent

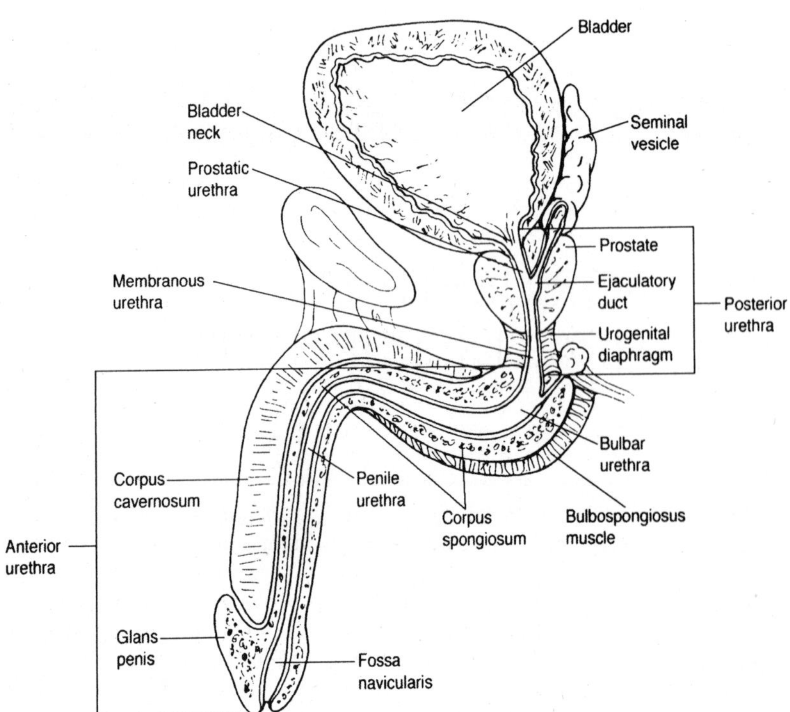


FIGURE 36.1 Anatomy of the anterior and posterior urethra.

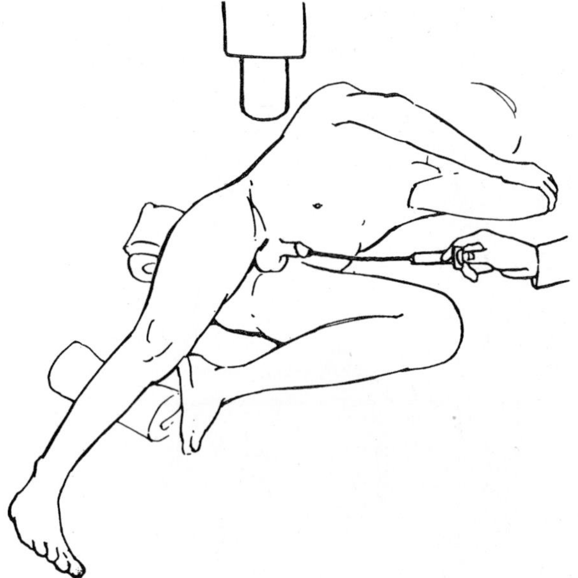

FIGURE 36.2 Proper positioning for retrograde urethrography. The patient is placed obliquely at a 45-degree angle with the bottom leg flexed and the top leg straight. Slight traction on the penis during injection of contrast helps avoid telescoping of the urethra and allows more accurate characterization of the injury.

catheter dislodgment during the urethrogram. The penis is positioned laterally on a slight stretch to provide a more descriptive study, and 20 to 30 mL of contrast is then injected in a retrograde fashion. Dynamic fluoroscopy is ideal; however, in the setting of acute trauma in the emergency department, static radiographs will suffice. The entire anterior urethra can be visualized during a retrograde urethrogram; however, the posterior urethra is typically excluded by reflex contraction of the external sphincter. If a catheter is present at the time of evaluation, then a cystogram is recommended to confirm the catheter's presence in the bladder. After documenting the correct location of the urethral catheter, a pericatheter retrograde urethrogram can delineate possible urethral injury.

Anterior urethral injuries are classified into three groups based upon radiographic, clinical, or endoscopic findings. *Contusions* appear normal on retrograde urethrogram or as urethral elongation from compression by periurethral hematoma. Contusions are best appreciated by cystoscopy in the setting of a "normal" retrograde urethrogram; however, we are not recommending cystoscopy for all "normal" urethrogram studies with a suspicious clinical history. *Partial disruptions* appear as extravasated urine on retrograde urethrogram with visualization of contrast in the urethra or bladder proximal to the injury. *Complete disruptions* appear as total extravasation without visualization of contrast in the more proximal urethra or bladder.

## Indications for Surgery

Primary surgical repair of acute anterior urethral injuries should be avoided, with the exception of a stable patient with a complete urethral disruption and an open or penetrating injury. We also recommend an attempt at anterior urethral repair in the setting of emergent surgery for penile fracture. Successful repair of all acute anterior urethra injuries is dependent upon minimal associated inflammation; therefore, surgeons should consider waiting for delayed, definitive repair when possible.

## Alternative Therapy

Alternative options to surgical repair are placement of a urethral or suprapubic catheter to divert urine from the injured area. Contusions to the anterior urethra should be managed with a urethral catheter for approximately 2 to 3 weeks followed by a retrograde urethrogram. The patient should be counseled on the possibility of delayed development of a urethral stricture at the site of contusion; however, stricture development is uncommon.

Percutaneous suprapubic catheter placement should be considered in patients with penetrating urethral trauma and hemodynamic instability, multiple associated injuries, or a long anterior urethra defect. Ultrasound guidance should be considered in the setting of a nonpalpable bladder or a history of prior abdominal surgery. If there is an associated pelvic fracture, urologists are urged to speak with orthopedic staff to ensure that future internal or external fixation hardware will not interfere with the planned suprapubic tube location. If radiographic staging was precluded by the patient's concomitant injuries, then a suprapubic cystogram and retrograde urethrogram should be done at the earliest opportunity. Broad-spectrum antibiotics are essential to maintain the sterility of extravasated urine or blood. A voiding cystogram is recommended after 3 weeks of urinary diversion. We do not advocate blind urethral catheter placement in the presence of blood at the urethral meatus, pelvic fracture, or perineal hematoma if hemodynamic instability precludes a retrograde urethrogram; however, some would argue that one attempt at urethral catheter placement by an experienced physician or urologist is acceptable.

Partial urethral disruptions diagnosed by retrograde urethrogram may be managed via various algorithms. Urinary diversion with formal repair after a minimum of 3 months to allow resolution of inflammation and maturation of scar tissue is our preference. As mentioned above, one attempt at urethral catheter placement by experienced medical personnel is acceptable; however, the possibility of creating a complete urethral disruption during this attempt should be considered. If urethral placement is unsuccessful, percutaneous suprapubic tube placement should be performed. The preservation of urethral mucosa with partial disruptions may be adequate for re-epithelialization and eventual luminal recanalization; however, if successful, we would recommend periodic evaluation with pressure-flow urine studies and counseling patients regarding the possibility of future stricture development.

Endoscopic alignment of the anterior urethra has been described in a limited series of 16 men with partial and complete bulbar straddle injuries (4). With this management, 14 out of 16 patients were successfully managed with endoscopic urethral alignment alone. The 2 failures had a history of a failed attempt at blind urethral catheter placement. The authors stressed the importance of not advancing the cystoscope past the stricture during endoscopic alignment, but rather to only pass guide wires through the urethral disruption in an attempt to prevent worsening the degree of urethral injury.

## Surgical Technique

Open surgical repair is primarily reserved for stable patients after open or penetrating injury to the anterior urethra. The patient is placed in either the supine position or lithotomy position and draped widely to allow exploration of potential concomitant injuries to the penis, testes, perineum, and rectum. Clean wounds need only minimal debridement followed by urethral closure with interrupted or running 6-0 polyglyconate monofilament (polydioxanone, Maxon) sutures over a 16Fr catheter. Contaminated wounds require thorough irrigation and debridement of devitalized tissues to ensure reapproximation of healthy tissue.

With open or penetrating bulbar urethra injuries, the patient is placed in the high lithotomy position and a vertical perineal incision is performed along the raphe. As expected, only stable patients without injury precluding the high lithotomy position should be offered acute surgical intervention. The urethra is exposed after division of Colles fascia and the bulbospongiosus muscle. As with elective bulbar urethra stricture surgery, anastomotic urethroplasty should only be considered for defects <20 mm. Surgeons should avoid acute repair of bulbar urethra defects longer than 20 mm as more complex intervention with grafts of flaps will be required. The most important tenet allowing successful outcome is a tension-free anastomosis; therefore, mobilization of the distal urethra is an important step to ensure adequate urethral length. Once adequate length is achieved, the urethral ends are spatulated (Fig. 36.3). The anastomosis is performed with interrupted 5-0 and 6-0 polyglyconate monofilament suture to create a tension-free, watertight closure. The dorsal surface is closed in one layer with 5-0 interrupted polyglyconate monofilament incorporating the urethral mucosa and spongiosal adventitia. Since the ventral bulbar urethra is vascularized by the spongy urethra, we advocate ventral closure in two layers with interrupted 6-0 polyglyconate monofilament suture (Fig. 36.4). We make no attempt to control bleeding from the spongy urethra during closure, as we theorize that the added vascularity from the spongy urethra will provide enhanced healing of the anastomosis after two-layer closure. We strongly recommend that a first-stage marsupialization of healthy proximal urethra be considered if tension-free closure cannot be achieved or if there is significant wound inflammation or contamination.

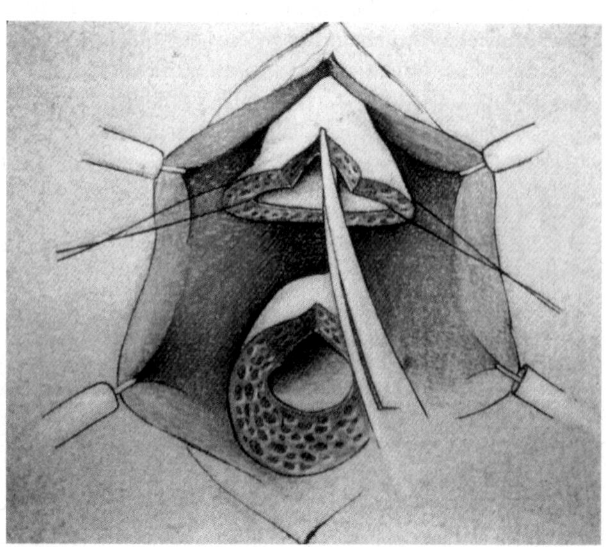

FIGURE 36.3 Repair of bulbar urethral injuries. The urethra is mobilized and spatulated in preparation for a tension-free end-to-end anastomosis.

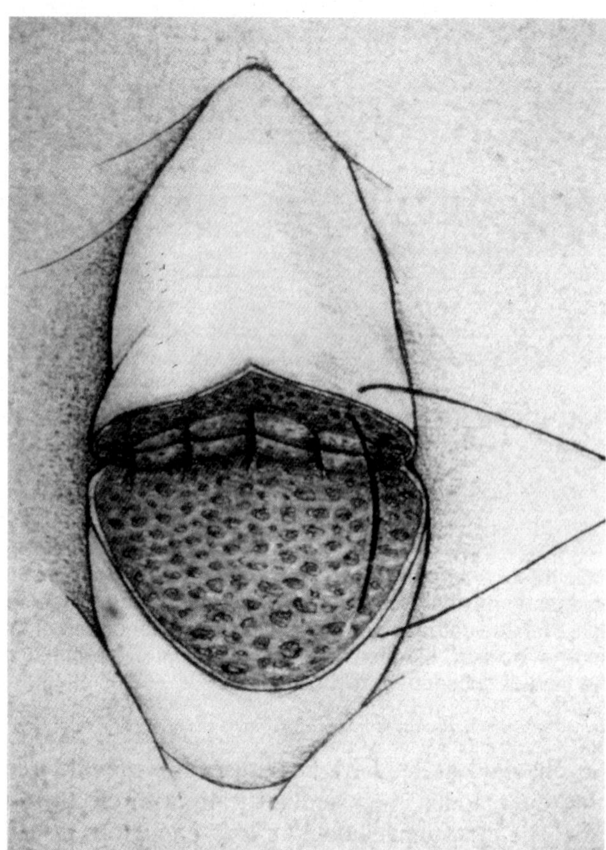

FIGURE 36.4 Repair of bulbar urethral injuries. Anastomosis is carried out with a single-layer dorsal closure and a two-layer ventral closure using interrupted 5-0 or 6-0 Maxon sutures.

Penile urethral injuries are best exposed via a subcoronal circumferential incision. Contrary to bulbar urethral injury, anastomotic repair should not be considered for defects >15 mm, as the risk of penile chordee is higher with penile anastomotic repairs. In prior editions of this textbook, we have advocated utilization of a 16Fr silicone Foley catheter; however, we now use regular latex catheters, if possible. Suppressive antibiotics are given while the catheter is in place to maintain urine sterility, with a voiding cystogram performed after 2 to 3 weeks. If extravasation is noted, we gently replace the catheter for an additional period of time with repeat imaging at the time of urethral catheter removal.

## Outcomes

### Complications

The major complications relating to anterior urethral trauma include urethral stricture formation and infection. If untreated, persistent extravasation of infected urine or blood may lead to urethral abscess, urethrocutaneous fistula, or urethral diverticula. Prolonged urine extravasation into the corpus spongiosum can also lead to added spongiofibrosis, resulting in a longer urethral stricture. Consequently, a longer anterior urethral stricture translates to more complex management with a buccal mucosa graft or fasciocutaneous flap.

With early urine diversion, a percentage of anterior urethral strictures will never progress to functional significance; however, of those that do, early diversion can limit stricture length to allow a wider array of future options. Incontinence and impotence, although common in posterior urethral injuries, are uncommon in anterior urethral injuries. Stricture recurrence after formal anastomotic urethroplasty is most common in the first 12 months. Stricture recurrence after urethroplasty is generally short and can be successfully treated in one session with internal urethrotomy.

### Results

Anastomotic urethroplasty can be successfully performed in a high percentage of patients who sustain a bulbar urethra (straddle) injury requiring surgery. The procedure has an overall success rate of approximately 95% when performed in a delayed setting (3). As mentioned previously, patients sustaining open or penetrating injuries associated with minimal inflammation are the best candidates for acute repair; otherwise, urine diversion is recommended with formal repair at a later date.

# POSTERIOR URETHRAL INJURIES

The posterior urethra is shorter than the anterior urethra and consists of the membranous and prostatic urethra (Fig. 36.1). The more proximal prostatic urethra extends from the bladder neck to the apex of the prostate and is secured to the pubic bone by the paired puboprostatic ligaments. During cystoscopy, the verumontanum marks the most distal aspect of the prostatic urethra. The proximal urethral sphincter is present within the prostatic urethra and is an extension of smooth muscle fibers of the trigone and prostatic urethra cephalad to the verumontanum. Conversely, the distal urethral sphincter encompasses smooth muscle fibers caudad to the verumontanum, including the rhabdosphincter (slow-twitch skeletal muscle fibers) (5). In the absence of a functional distal urethral sphincter, the proximal urethral sphincter can maintain urinary continence in select patients; however, the bladder must be compliant and free from periodic elevations of detrusor pressure (e.g., overactive bladder). The membranous urethra is the least supported portion of the urethra, and injury to the membranous urethra is not uncommon given its location between two relatively fixed points (prostate and bulbar urethra). Since the distal urethral sphincter is located in the membranous urethra, shear injuries leading to partial or complete membranous urethral disruption can result in distal urethral sphincter damage.

Posterior urethral trauma is almost always associated with pelvic fracture; conversely, only 10% to 15% of pelvic fractures are associated with urethral injury. Furthermore, bladder injury has also been diagnosed in 10% to 20% of patients with pelvic fracture and urethral injury (6). Since the blunt forces required to generate a pelvic fracture are significant, the associated urethral injuries are highly correlated with serious injuries (e.g., intra-abdominal and vascular injuries to the pelvic vasculature). Other sources of injury to the posterior urethra include penetrating injuries and iatrogenic injuries secondary to endoscopic or open prostate surgery.

The clinical and surgical appearance of each form of posterior urethral injury will differ. Endoscopic or open prostate surgery is associated with continuity strictures and preservation of the distal external urinary sphincter. As such, these injuries have been termed "sphincter stenoses" (bladder neck sphincters). In contradistinction, pelvic fractures are associated with urethral disruptions to the membranous urethra. These injuries have been termed "pelvic fracture urethral disruption defects" (PFUDDs). Interestingly, a recent report has found that 7 of 10 patients examined at autopsy had urethral disruption after pelvic fracture *distal* to the external urinary sphincter, disputing the historical view that these injuries occur at the interface of the fixed prostatic apex and the less supported membranous urethra (7). Additionally, urodynamic studies have demonstrated a functional rhabdosphincter at the prostatomembranous region in many patients after anastomotic posterior urethroplasty for PFUDD (5).

## Diagnosis

This section will primarily focus on PFUDD injuries, as these injuries are the most common presentations in the acute trauma setting. Given the close association of more serious concomitant injuries with PFUDD, the first goal is resuscitation of the patient. Suspicious findings after PFUDD mirror those of anterior urethral injuries, namely, hematuria, blood at the meatus, perineal hematoma, and difficulty voiding. Additionally, a high-riding prostate on digital rectal exam and specific pelvic fractures are linked with PFUDD. The prostate can appear elevated in position on digital rectal exam due to displacement from a pelvic hematoma and/or digital confirmation of the prostate may be indistinguishable from the pelvic hematoma. Regarding pelvic fractures, displacement of the inferomedial pubic bone and symphysis pubica diastasis are independently associated with urethral injury (8).

Retrograde urethrogram should be performed on all patients suspected of having PFUDD before any attempt at urethral catheter placement (Fig. 36.5). If normal, the catheter should be gently advanced into the bladder and a formal cystogram should be obtained to assess for bladder perforation. The technique for retrograde urethrogram was discussed in the section on anterior urethra injuries. A formal cystogram can be performed in the emergency department or radiology suite. Three radiographic views should be obtained, including an anterior-posterior scout film, a full-bladder anterior posterior film, and a drainage film. False-negative results are strongly correlated with inadequate filling; therefore, passive filling to discomfort or 350 mL of contrast is recommended. Other studies to further delineate posterior urethral injuries include flexible cystoscopy; however, we caution against advancing the cystoscope past the site of injury for fear of worsening the injury. Lastly, in a nonacute setting MRI can be useful to provide more descriptive analysis of complex PFUDD.

Posterior urethral injuries secondary to blunt trauma have historically been classified based upon the Colapinto and McCallum system (9). A recent modification maintains the original three classes of injury; however, this revised system also includes posterior urethral injuries that extend to the bladder neck and blunt anterior urethral injuries (Table 36.1) (10).

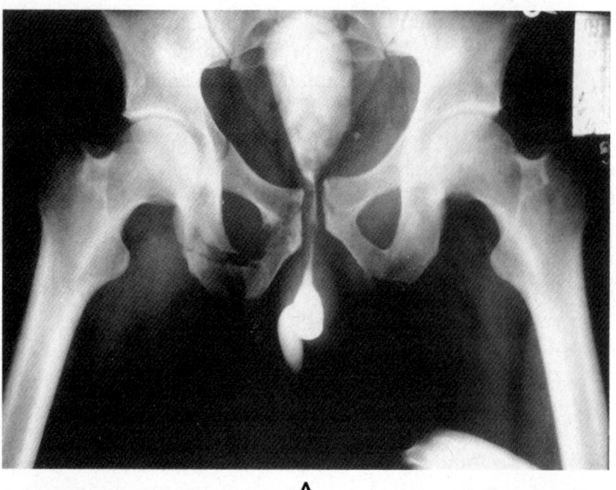
A

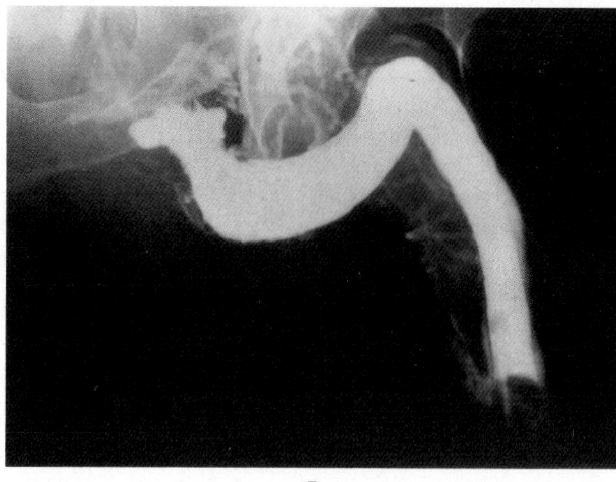
B

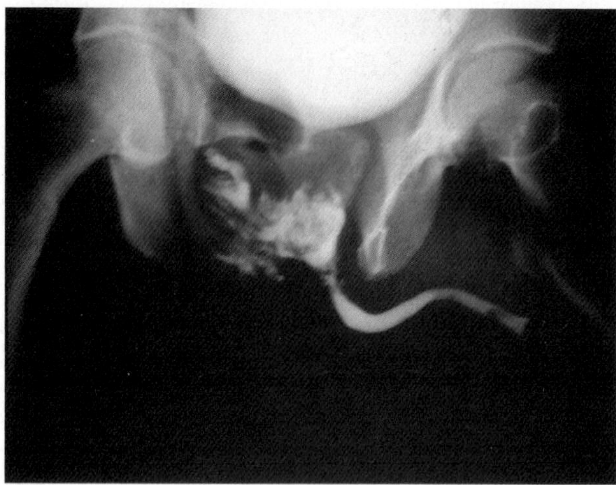
C

FIGURE 36.5 Posterior urethral injuries. **A:** Type I: stretched urethra without rupture. Note the displaced and compressed bladder and fractures of the right symphysis and superior and inferior rami. **B:** Type II: complete rupture of the membranous urethra with intact urogenital diaphragm. Note the limited extravasation and venous filling. **C:** Type III: Note the pattern of extravasation when the urogenital diaphragm is disrupted, as compared with type II. (From Dixon CM. Diagnosis and acute management of posterior urethral disruptions. In: McAninch JW, ed. *Traumatic and reconstructive urology*. Philadelphia: WB Saunders, 1996:347–355, with permission.)

**TABLE 36.1**

CLASSIFICATION OF BLUNT URETHRAL INJURIES (9)

| Class | Description |
|---|---|
| I | Posterior urethra stretched but intact |
| II | Tear of the prostatomembranous urethra above the urogenital diaphragm |
| III | Partial or complete tear of both the anterior and posterior urethra with disruption of the urogenital diaphragm |
| IV | Bladder injury extending into the urethra |
| IVa | Injury of the bladder base with periurethral extravasation simulating posterior urethral injury |
| V | Partial or complete pure anterior urethral injury |

## Indications for Surgery

Controversy and confusion exist regarding whether primary alignment or suprapubic diversion is better for acute management of PFUDD. There is no correct answer for this question, despite what has been written in the literature regarding the impact of each on eventual incontinence, impotence, and urethral stricture rates. Since each procedure is governed by different definitions for successful outcome, neither should be considered the best therapy option. The obvious benefit of primary alignment is a lower stricture rate of 56% versus the 97% stricture rate seen with suprapubic catheter placement (11). In addition, urethral strictures after endoscopic alignment can result in shorter stricture length and the possibility of a less invasive option, such as internal urethrotomy instead of formal perineal urethroplasty. Despite claims that periodic office urethral dilations are trivial to the patient, we would disagree with this assertion and counsel the patient for posterior urethroplasty to definitively treat the persistent stricture.

Impotence and incontinence outcomes in the literature can be difficult to compare, with multiple reports claiming different results after endoscopic alignment and suprapubic tube with delayed urethroplasty. In experienced centers, incontinence and impotence rates after endoscopic alignment are 4% and 36%, respectively (11). A suprapubic tube with delayed urethroplasty in the same study found minimal improvement in incontinence (2.7%) but a more significant reduction in impotence among those with erections preinjury (18% versus 36% endoscopic alignment).

Given the above findings, we would agree that endoscopic alignment and suprapubic tube placement are acceptable options for management of PFUDD; however, in the setting of a severely injured patient, we favor percutaneous suprapubic catheter placement. A review of our experience with posterior urethral disruption after pelvic trauma shows that the average stricture length was 2.08 cm during posterior urethroplasty and the delayed posterior urethroplasty was predominantly amenable to one-stage repair (12). We believe this average length of stricture is acceptable, especially given that approximately 33% of the patients in our series had a prior failed attempt at treatment (cut-to-the-light approach, urethral dilation, internal urethrotomy, and failed urethroplasty).

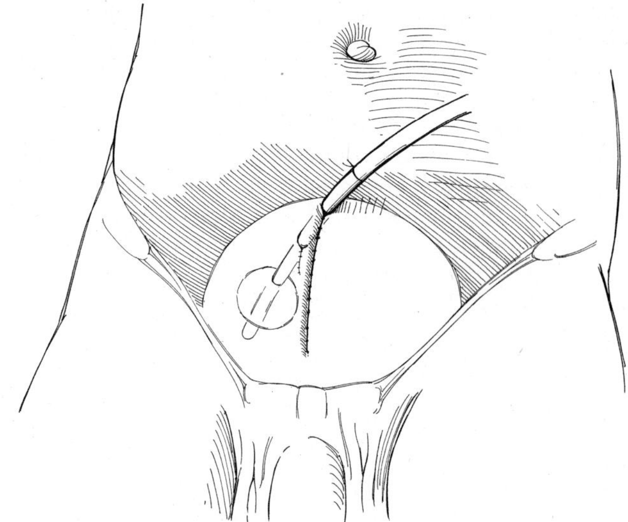

FIGURE 36.6 A large-caliber Foley catheter is placed in the bladder dome after inspection for concomitant bladder laceration. With the catheter placed through the superior end of the midline incision, bladder neck identification is facilitated at the time of subsequent reconstruction.

## Alternative Therapy

Given the association of PFUDD with bladder injury, we recommend open suprapubic cystostomy to allow repair of associated bladder injuries when present. If the patient is too unstable to allow operative exploration, then percutaneous suprapubic placement with or without ultrasound guidance is appropriate; however, percutaneous placement may be difficult if there is associated bladder injury. Therefore, we would advocate open suprapubic catheter placement after the patient is stabilized. Most bladder injuries associated with PFUDD are extraperitoneal and heal spontaneously with catheter drainage; however, if surgical management of pelvic fractures is planned, we recommend operative repair of the associated bladder injury to reduce complication rates.

Primary suture repair of PFUDD in the acute setting is associated with elevated impotence and incontinence rates. Primary suture repair of PFUDD is not recommended for this reason, and also because of the more important risk of hemorrhage and contamination associated with evacuation of the retropubic hematoma to gain access to the injury site. The only clinical scenario in which we favor acute repair of PFUDD is in the setting of a class IV injury (Table 36.1). This is because of the risk of bladder neck stenosis from urine extravasation at the bladder neck. We would also recommend repair of rectal and vaginal lacerations in this clinical scenario. Lastly, endoscopic alignment should be considered in the setting of a stable patient with a stable pelvis. Furthermore, we advocate utilization of fluoroscopy during cystoscopy to aid alignment in the safest possible manner.

## Surgical Technique

For open suprapubic catheter placement, the patient is placed in the low lithotomy position to allow simultaneous access to the rectum if needed. If orthopedic injuries preclude this positioning, a supine approach will suffice. An infraumbilical incision is made to allow access to the prevesical space anterior to the bladder dome. After placing stay sutures around the anticipated cystostomy site, the bladder is opened vertically at the bladder dome, which will provide ample exposure to examine the bladder and urethra for injury. *Strict avoidance* of dissection into the space of Retzius and lateral perivesical space is essential to prevent pelvic hemorrhage and contamination. Therefore, in the presence of an associated bladder neck or bladder base injury, intravescial repair is recommended. An additional benefit of bladder neck repair is that it prevents the laceration from extending into the external urethra sphincter complex.

Bladder lacerations, if present, should be repaired in two layers with a deeper 2-0 polyglactin (Vicyl, Dexon) suture incorporating the detrusor muscle and a superficial 4-0 chromic suture incorporating the bladder mucosa. Open suprapubic catheter placement is performed in the bladder dome, and the bladder cystostomy site is fixed in place with a pursestring suture (Fig. 36.6). We do not favor Malecot catheters, as they have a higher propensity to be accidentally dislodged. Instead, we utilize a 20Fr to 24Fr Foley catheter with an inflation balloon. The vesicostomy is closed in two layers with 2-0 polyglactin suture. Regarding associated pelvic fractures, we recommend communicating with the orthopedic service to ensure that the suprapubic tube skin site does not interfere with future operative endeavors. We do not use abdominal drains unless an associated bowel injury is present.

## Outcomes

### Complications

Complications after treatment of posterior urethral trauma are directly related to the severity of injury. Acute complications include pelvic hemorrhage and infection or abscess of the pelvic hematoma, which can occur after ill-advised retropubic exploration or attempts at pelvic hematoma evacuation.

Delayed complications include incontinence, impotence, and urethral stricture formation. Regarding impotence, recent studies have demonstrated that sexual dysfunction is commonly associated with pelvic fracture, even in the absence of urethral injury (13). Delayed return of potency has been reported after definitive urethroplasty; however, this would depend upon the severity of the initial injury (14). Nearly all patients remain continent if their bladder neck continence mechanism is undamaged; however, they should be counseled on the potential negative impact of future transurethral prostate surgery.

## Results

At our institution, delayed urethroplasty after suprapubic tube is the preferred management algorithm for PFUDD. Posterior urethroplasty has been successful for resolution of stricture in 86% of patients; however, definition of success is improved to 93% if an additional internal urethrotomy is utilized for stricture recurrence (12). Endoscopic alignment is also an appropriate management strategy in the acute setting; however, urologists should seriously consider formal urethroplasty (or referral to a tertiary care center) if internal urethrotomy or urethral dilation is unsuccessful.

## *References*

1. Hernandez J, Morey AF. Anterior urethral injury. *World J Urol* 1999; 17(2):96–100.
2. Nicolaisen GS, Melamud A, Williams RD, et al. Rupture of the corpus cavernosum: surgical management. *J Urol* 1983;130(5):917–919.
3. Park S, McAninch JW. Straddle injuries to the bulbar urethra: management and outcomes in 78 patients. *J Urol* 2004;171(2, Pt 1):722–725.
4. Ying-Hao S, Chuan-Liang X, Xu G, et al. Urethroscopic realignment of ruptured bulbar urethra. *J Urol* 2000;164(5):1543–1545.
5. Whitson JM, McAninch JW, Tanagho EA, et al. Mechanism of continence after repair of posterior urethral disruption: evidence of rhabdosphincter activity. *J Urol* 2008;179(3):1035–1039.
6. Corriere JN Jr., Sandler CM. Mechanisms of injury, patterns of extravasation and management of extraperitoneal bladder rupture due to blunt trauma. *J Urol* 1988;139(1):43–44.
7. Mouraviev VB, Santucci RA. Cadaveric anatomy of pelvic fracture urethral distraction injury: most injuries are distal to the external urinary sphincter. *J Urol* 2005;173(3):869–872.
8. Basta AM, Blackmore CC, Wessells H. Predicting urethral injury from pelvic fracture patterns in male patients with blunt trauma. *J Urol* 2007;177(2):571–575.
9. Colapinto V, McCallum RW. Injury to the male posterior urethra in fractured pelvis: a new classification. *J Urol* 1977;118(4):575–580.
10. Goldman SM, Sandler CM, Corriere JN Jr., et al. Blunt urethral trauma: a unified, anatomical mechanical classification. *J Urol* 1997;157(1):85–89.
11. Koraitim MM. Pelvic fracture urethral injuries: evaluation of various methods of management. *J Urol* 1996;156(4):1288–1291.
12. Cooperberg MR, McAninch JW, Alsikafi NF, et al. Urethral reconstruction for traumatic posterior urethral disruption: outcomes of a 25-year experience. *J Urol* 2007;178(5):2006–2010; discussion 10.
13. Metze M, Tiemann AH, Josten C. Male sexual dysfunction after pelvic fracture. *J Trauma* 2007;63(2):394–401.
14. Morey AF, McAninch JW. Reconstruction of posterior urethral disruption injuries: outcome analysis in 82 patients. *J Urol* 1997;157(2):506–510.

# CHAPTER 37 ■ CARCINOMA OF THE FEMALE URETHRA

PETER L. STEINBERG AND WILLIAM BIHRLE III

Carcinoma of the female urethra is a histologically heterogeneous disease; while most cases are squamous cell (55%) in origin, transitional cell carcinoma (TCC) and adenocarcinoma equally account for between 15% and 20% of new cases. Melanoma and clear cell carcinoma represent rare subsets of disease. Disease developing in urethral diverticuli is, most commonly, adenocarcinoma and often presents at a higher stage than the squamous carcinomas.

Disease progression occurs by way of local invasion into the muscularis of the urethra followed by extension to local structures, including the anterior vaginal wall, vulva, and bladder neck. Lymphatic spread is not uncommon; distal urethral disease migrates into the superficial and deep inguinal nodes, while more proximally based cancers spread preferentially into the pelvic lymph chain (iliac, obturator, and presacral). Metastatic disease, while uncommon at presentation, occurs via hematogenous spread to the liver, lung, bone, and brain.

Primary urethral carcinoma is extremely uncommon, accounting for <1% of adult malignancies. Urologic orthodoxy holds that urethral carcinoma is the only genitourinary malignancy with a higher incidence in women than in men. However, findings from the most recent SEER population database suggest that, with an incidence of <1 case per 100,000 women annually, urethral cancer appears to be less common in women (1,2). With the exception of adenocarcinoma in the African American population, for which the incidence in women remains elevated, there is a higher rate of all three subtypes of urethral cancer in men relative to women. Excepting adenocarcinomas, urethral carcinoma is rare in women under the ago of 60; the incidence of adenocarcinoma begins to rise about ten years earlier. Urethral cancer is distinctly uncommon in the premenopausal population. Its incidence peaks between ages 75 and 84 for TCC and squamous cancer, whereas the incidence of adenocarcinoma appears to

TABLE 37.1

STAGING OF FEMALE URETHRAL CARCINOMA

| Grabstald[a] | TNM[b] | |
|---|---|---|
| | Tx | Primary Tumor Cannot be Assessed |
| | T0 | No Evidence of Primary Tumor |
| Stage 0 | Tis | Carcinoma In Situ (CIS) |
| | Ta | Noninvasive Papillary, Polypoid, or Verrucous |
| Stage A | T1 | Invades Lamina Propria |
| Stage B | T2 | Invades Periurethral Muscularis |
| Stage C1 | T3 | Invades Anterior Vaginal Muscle or Bladder Neck |
| Stage C2 | | Invades Anterior Vaginal Mucosa |
| Stage C3 | T4 | Invades adjacent Structures Including Clitoris, Labia, or Pubis |
| Stage D1 | N1 | Regional Metastasis to Inguinal Lymph Nodes (TNM = Single Node <2 cm) |
| Stage D2 | N2 | Regional Metastasis to Pelvic Lymph Nodes (TNM = Single Node >2 cm but <5 cm or Multiple <5 cm) |
| Stage D3 | N3 | Metastasis to Lymph Nodes Above the Aortic Bifurcation (TNM = > cm Node) |
| Stage D4 | M1 | Distant Metastasis (With Any Primary Tumor) |

[a]From Grabstald H. Tumors of the urethra in men and women. *Cancer* 1973;32:1236, with permission.
[b]Modified from Beahrs OH, et al, eds. *Manual for staging of cancer*, 3rd ed. Philadelphia: JB Lippincott Co, 1988:120, with permission.

remain stable throughout. For reasons that remain conjectural, the incidence of female urethral carcinoma has dropped by 50% over the past 30 years.

Staging is based upon the tumor-nodes-metastasis (TNM) system, although many practitioners continue to use the system developed by Grabstald noted in Table 37.1.

## DIAGNOSIS

Nearly all women are symptomatic at presentation (3–5). Urinary symptoms, specifically hematuria, splayed stream, and urinary retention, indicate the presence of an obstructing lesion. Many patients have long-standing symptoms and often have been diagnosed with and treated for a myriad of benign conditions, including urethral diverticuli, caruncles, and urethral stenosis. Any process that does not respond to conservative measures should be investigated to rule out a urethral malignancy. Physical examination may reveal a palpable mass at the meatus, induration of the urethra, a mass along the anterior vaginal wall, or a mass that ball valves and protrudes from the urethral meatus. Ulceration of the meatus or the vaginal wall can also occur. The diagnosis of urethral cancer within a urethral diverticulum is a rare occurrence (5).

Endoscopy of the urethra and bladder neck and a well-performed bimanual pelvic examination are essential to tumor assessment. Examination under anesthesia, performed at the time of tumor biopsy, is essential in confirming the diagnosis and aiding in the assessment of tumor resectability. Evaluation of the proximal urethra and bladder neck for disease extension guides the recommendation for bladder-preserving techniques. Either a CT scan of the abdomen and pelvis with and without intravenous contrast or an enhanced MRI of the pelvis can help assess local extension of the tumor to the vagina or bladder, as well as the status of the pelvic lymph nodes. A chest X-ray is used to complete staging studies, and a CT of the chest may be needed in the event an equivocal lesion is noted. Liver function tests should also be assessed. Suspiciously enlarged pelvic lymph nodes may be biopsied via CT guidance or removed via laparoscopic node dissection.

## INDICATIONS FOR SURGERY

Given the rarity of this disease, there are no large-volume, randomized data to guide management. Treated disease has a 5-year survival of roughly 50% (3,4); left untreated, almost all urethral carcinomas will progress, with a mean survival of <1 year. The presence of metastatic disease or deep pelvic lymphadenopathy represents a strong contraindication to major extirpative surgery. Disease localized to the urethra may be treated in a variety of ways depending on the anatomical location and local stage. Generally, low-stage, distal cancers carry a more favorable prognosis than higher-stage and more proximally located lesions and may be amenable to less radical extirpation. There appears to be a limited role for topical ablative therapy in women presenting with superficial disease. Surgical therapy is suggested in women who are free from metastasis and will tolerate an operative intervention.

## ALTERNATIVE THERAPY

External beam radiation, brachytherapy, and local ablative therapy either alone or in combination have been reported in the treatment of both distal and proximally located tumors. Success is better with distal tumors; several small series report 5-year survival rates of 50% to 70% (5). Unfortunately, the treatment of more proximal tumors is associated with a 5-year survival rate of 30% to 50% (5). As in the case with surgery, no randomized data exist to guide treatment.

The role of chemotherapy in a neoadjuvant or adjuvant setting is also lacking in randomized data. Centers that see a larger volume of this disease often utilize chemotherapy in a neoadjuvant or adjuvant fashion, though specific management strategies cannot be suggested based on the existing literature.

There is case report evidence only that combined chemotherapy and radiation therapy can offer long-term control of female urethral cancer. Using a combination of 5-fluorouracil, mitomycin C, and/or cisplatin, as well as 30 to 60 Gy or radiation, there are reports of survival exceeding 5 years in the literature. It is emphasized, however, that these data have been accrued over a period of 20 years and consist of nine case reports (6). The failure of single-arm therapies to improve long-term outcomes has led clinicians to consider more flexible, multimodal approaches to the treatment of urethral carcinoma.

## SURGICAL TECHNIQUE

This chapter considers the operative techniques for both distal and proximal lesions of squamous and glandular origin—diseases that originate in the urethra—and bladder-sparing approaches for large distal lesions. Management using minimally invasive approaches such as neodymium or holmium: YAG lasers will not be described, as there is a paucity of data in the literature to support their use. The specific management of the female urethra in the case of TCC will not be discussed because this represents pathology of the lower urinary tract and should be considered separately.

### Distal Urethral Tumors

Tumors involving the distal third of the urethra, and especially those of the urethral meatus, are amenable to a distal urethrectomy. Preoperative preparation should include full staging studies, a detailed history and physical examination with particular attention given to a history of bleeding or anesthetic complications, and a urine culture, with any infection managed before surgery.

TED hose and sequential compression devices are mandatory for deep venous thrombosis (DVT) prophylaxis, and the use of 5,000 U of subcutaneous heparin or 40 mg of subcutaneous enoxaparin is prudent in a patient with any pelvic malignancy prior to surgery. Prophylactic antibiotics should be administered within the hour prior to the first incision, and a first-generation cephalosporin along with gram-negative coverage from an aminoglycoside should be adequate; patients allergic to penicillin can receive either vancomycin or clindamycin as an alternative gram-positive prophylactic.

The patient should be placed in the lithotomy position, with attention paid to the padding of pressure points on the legs; the patient's perineum should sit at the edge of the operating room table. After preparation and draping, a weighted vaginal speculum is placed and the labia are retracted with a 1-0 silk suture that is then secured to the drape. The use of a versatile perineal retraction system, that is, the Lone Star or Jordan-Bookwalter devices, facilitates exposure of the vaginal introitus. Placement of a Foley catheter aids in the palpation and localization of the urethra and tumor during dissection (Fig. 37.1).

Once a circumcising incision is made around the urethral meatus, it may be secured with an Allis clamp or silk tie, allowing for retraction and manipulation of the urethra during its dissection. An incision is made in the epithelium of the vagina to aid in the posterior urethral dissection. A combination of electrocautery and sharp dissection is utilized to free the urethra circumferentially, taking care not to enter the urethra and using the Foley catheter to guide the dissection. The anterior vaginal wall is also resected with a 1-cm margin of healthy tissue. A margin of 1 cm of normal tissue from the proximal margin of the tumor is desirable from an oncological standpoint. When healthy tissue has been encountered proximally, stay sutures of 3-0 Vicryl are placed into the urethra at 3 and 9 o'clock to prevent proximal migration, the specimen is amputated, and the margin is assessed with a frozen section.

Hemostasis is achieved with cautery, and the wound is copiously irrigated with normal saline. The remaining urethral stump is approximated to the edges of the vaginal incision with interrupted 3-0 Vicryl or other absorbable suture. The vaginal wall is closed with interrupted 3-0 Vicryl sutures in two layers. A vaginal pack with estrogen crème is placed, as is a new small-caliber Foley catheter. The vaginal pack is removed on postoperative day 1, and the Foley catheter is removed 7 days after surgery. The patient is placed on a general diet the night of surgery and should ambulate as soon as she has recovered from anesthesia. DVT prophylaxis is also maintained postoperatively, and antibiotics are stopped within 24 hours of surgery.

### Distal Tumors, Bladder-sparing Approach

Bladder sparing is feasible for large distal urethral tumors, including T3 disease, not involving the bladder neck. Although reports exist of bladder sparing for more aggressive tumors involving the genitalia, the high risk of local recurrence makes exenterative surgery the standard of care (4). Following resection of the diseased urethra, the bladder neck is closed and one of a variety of continent urinary diversions is performed. Currently there are no data to suggest that pelvic or inguinal lymph node sampling improves survival, though pelvic node dissection is useful for staging purposes (4).

The presurgical regimen is identical to that described for surgery of small distal disease, with the addition of a bowel preparation and clear liquids the day before surgery. Once in the operating room, the patient is placed in the low lithotomy position in Allen stirrups. Both the abdomen and the genitals are prepared into the field, and a weighted vaginal speculum is placed. Cystoscopy can be performed to place bilateral ureteral catheters if desired. To assess for tumor resectability and lymph node status, the procedure is begun through a midline or Pfannenstiel trans- or extraperitoneal incision. Surgeons with advanced laparoscopic skill may choose to perform the lymph node dissection and mobilization of the bladder neck and proximal urethra in a laparoscopic fashion. The lymph nodes are sent for frozen section analysis if it is the intent of the surgeon to alter the surgical plan in the face of lymphatic spread. There are insufficient data in the literature to either support or refute abandoning resection in the face of positive pelvic lymph nodes.

The endopelvic fascia is incised, allowing mobilization of the lateral aspects of the bladder with electrocautery. Urethral attachments to the pelvic floor are taken down with cautery and between 2-0 or 3-0 silk ties as needed. The uterus and ovaries are preserved with this approach. Once the bladder neck is mobilized, the vaginal portion of the procedure is performed. If sufficient assistance is available, this can be performed as a two-team simultaneous procedure.

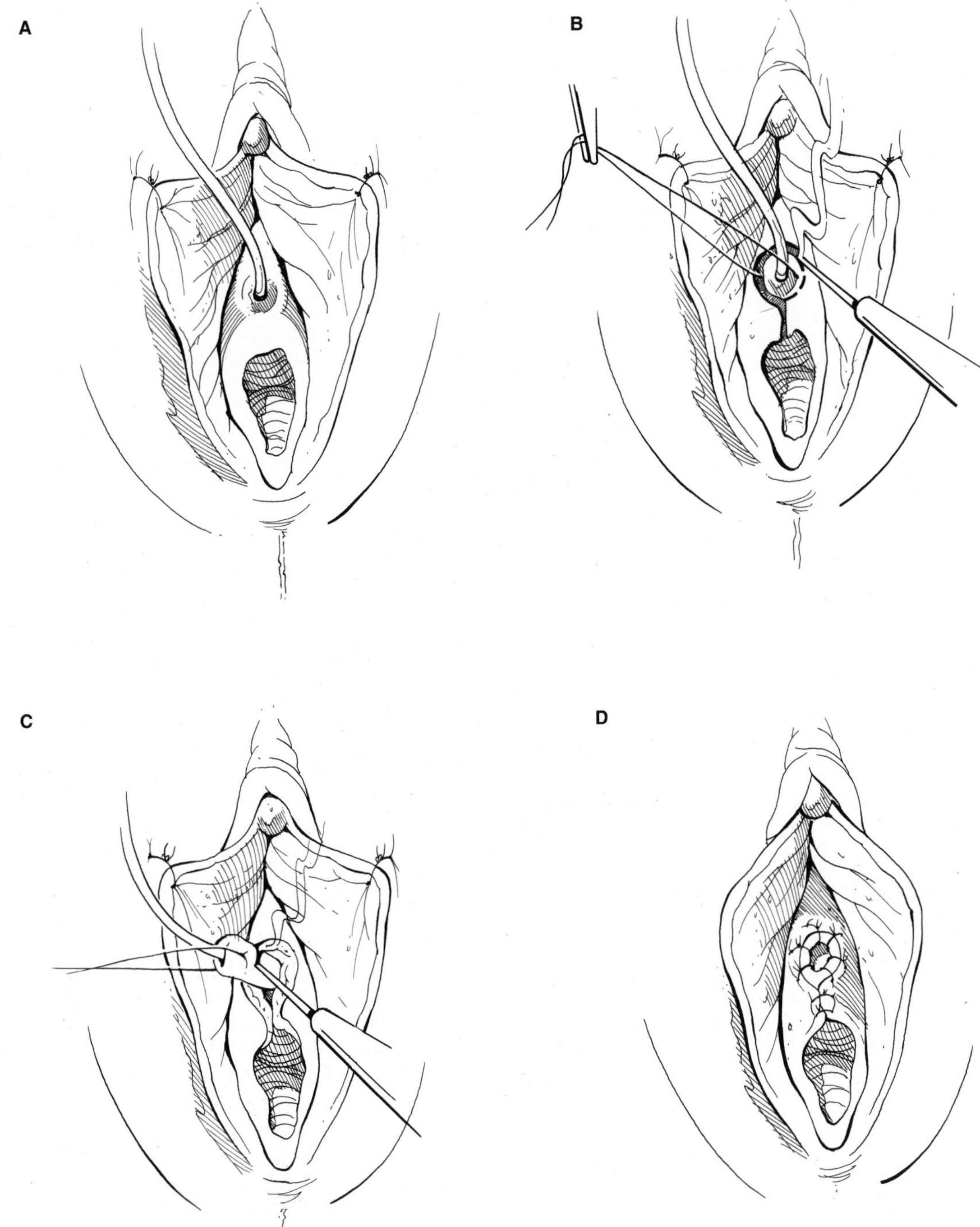


**FIGURE 37.1** Technique of distal urethrectomy.

To excise the urethra, distal bladder neck, and a margin of anterior vaginal wall, again the meatus is circumscribed with a scalpel, and then cautery and sharp dissection are used to take down the periurethral tissues proximal to the palpable tumor. The pubourethral ligaments are identified with blunt and sharp dissection and divided with cautery.

Through the abdominal incision, the bladder neck is opened anteriorly with electrocautery; the ureteral orifices are identified and cannulated with stents if these were not placed at the time of cystoscopy. With care taken to preserve the ureteral orifices, the bladder neck is divided distal to the orifices and the incision is carried through the anterior vaginal wall. The urethra, bladder neck, and vaginal wall are then removed en bloc. A frozen section is taken of the bladder neck margin, and if positive anterior exenteration is performed (Fig. 37.2).

With a negative bladder neck margin, the vaginal defect is closed in layers using a combination of 2-0 or 3-0 Vicryl or other absorbable suture on the vaginal mucosa. Large partial vaginal wall defects resulting from this resection may require coverage with a regional flap. A pudendal-based medial thigh flap or rectus flap may be necessary to close such a defect, and given the propensity toward multimodality therapy in this disease, consultation with a plastic surgeon is likely to yield the best outcome (7).

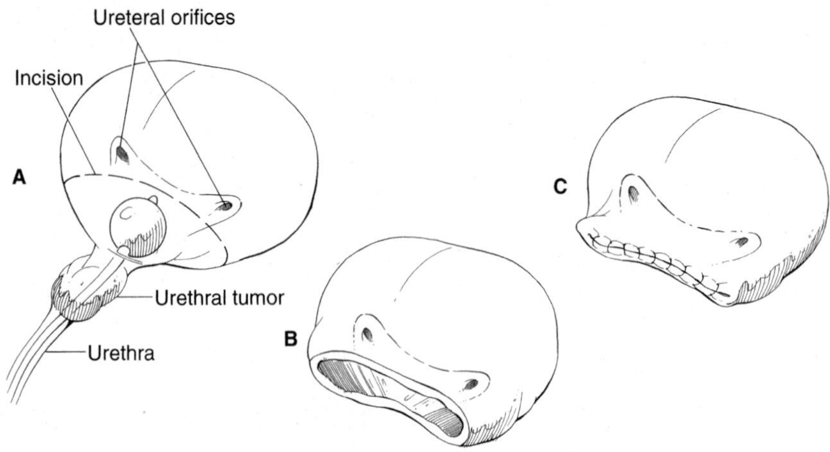


FIGURE 37.2 Technique of urethrectomy and bladder preservation by excision of the tumor at the level of the bladder neck, with subsequent bladder neck closure.

Urinary diversion is then performed, as is bladder neck closure. Postoperatively, the patient is managed with a 14Fr catheter running through the stoma, a 20Fr to 22Fr suprapubic tube, a vaginal pack, and a pelvic drain. The vaginal pack is removed 24 hours after surgery. The diversion is irrigated with normal saline every 8 hours beginning on postoperative day 1. Nasogastric suction is not needed postoperatively, and the diet can be slowly advanced, beginning with sips of clear liquids on postoperative day 1 or 2, followed by clear liquids ad lib, and finally a general diet prior to discharge (8). Return of flatus is not needed to advance the diet, though intake should be restricted if nausea or vomiting occur. The patient should ambulate as soon as she has recovered from anesthesia. DVT prophylaxis is also maintained postoperatively, and antibiotics are stopped within 24 hours of surgery.

### Proximal Urethral Tumors

For patients who have large tumors or tumors involving the bladder base, bladder-preserving approaches are not feasible and anterior pelvic exenteration is indicated. A stoma site on the abdomen is selected preoperatively for urinary diversion. Preoperative preparation is identical to that for distal tumors, and again a bowel preparation and clear liquids are utilized the day before surgery.

Radical cystourethrectomy, pelvic lymph node dissection, and urinary diversion are then performed in the standard fashion (see Chapters 19, 81, 83). For larger lesions, wide excision of the vulva, pelvic floor, and pubic rami may also be indicated. The assistance of an orthpedic and plastic surgeon is invaluable in these circumstances. Pelvic floor reconstruction with either rectus or gracilis flap will be necessary, and thus planning with a plastic surgeon is mandatory preoperatively.

## OUTCOMES

Data from multiple sources confirm that distal lesions have a better prognosis than proximal disease or panurethral disease. In a representative series, Dalbagni et al. (3) demonstrated a 71% survival in distal lesions, 48% in proximal lesions, and 24% in lesions involving the entire urethra. Local recurrence after partial urethrectomy occurs roughly 20% of the time, though this number is based on a series of 19 patients (4). Pelvic lymph node disease is associated with a poor prognosis, with only 23% disease-specific survival at 5 years (4). Disease-specific survival at 5 and 10 years is roughly 50%, with the best prognosis in low-grade, low-stage distal lesions without lymph node metastases (4). Roughly one-third of patients with stage T3 or T4 disease remain recurrence-free. The overall recurrence rate is roughly 50%, and after recurrence 71% of women are dead within 5 years (4).

## COMPLICATIONS

Distal urethrectomy is associated with urinary incontinence in nearly 40% of patients (4), a finding drawn from a number of small series. Both worsening stress and urge incontinence are reported in this series, as is a small rate of urinary retention. More proximal resections and pelvic exenteration are associated with risks of wound infection, wound dehiscence, DVT, metabolic complications from urinary diversion, and bowel-related complications. We would direct the reader to the specific chapters dealing with cystectomy and urinary diversion for a better treatment of this topic.

## *References*

1. Swartz MA, Porter MP, Lin DW, et al. Incidence of primary urethral carcinoma in the United States. *Urology* 2006;68:1164–1168.
2. http://apps.nccd.cdc.gov/uscs/Table.aspx?Group=TableAll&Year=2003&Display=n, accessed December 2, 2007.
3. Dalbagni G, Zhang ZF, Lacombe L, et al. Female urethral carcinoma: an analysis of treatment outcome and a plea for a standardized management strategy. *Br J Urol* 1998;82:835–841.
4. Zincke H, Webb MJ, Bass SE, et al. Surgical treatment for local control of female urethral carcinoma. *Urol Oncol* 2004;22:404–409.
5. Campbell MF, Wein AJ, Kavoussi LR, eds. *Campbell-Walsh urology*, 9th ed. Philadelphia: Saunders Elsevier, 2007:1018–1023.
6. Hara I, Hikosaka S, Eto H, et al. Successful treatment for squamous cell carcinoma of the female urethra with combined radio- and chemotherapy. *Int J Urol* 2004;11:678–682.
7. Pusic AL, Mehrara BJ. Vaginal reconstruction: an algorithm approach to defect classification and flap reconstruction. *J Surg Oncol* 2006;94:515–521.
8. Pruthi RS, Chun J, Richman M. Reducing time to oral diet and hospital discharge in patients undergoing radical cystectomy using a perioperative care plan. *Urology* 2003;62:661–665; discussion 665–666.

# CHAPTER 38 ■ CARCINOMA OF THE MALE URETHRA

PETER L. STEINBERG AND WILLIAM BIHRLE III

Carcinoma of the male urethra is a heterogeneous disease, encompassing transitional cell carcinoma (TCC), squamous carcinoma, adenocarcinoma, and very rare malignancies such as melanoma. This chapter focuses on management of primary malignancies of the urethra and does not discuss management of TCC of the urethra or management of urethral recurrence of TCC after cystectomy, though the operative principles are readily transferable.

Urethral cancer in men is an exceedingly rare condition, with an incidence of <1 case per 100,000 men annually (1,2). Fifty percent of male urethral cancers are of transitional cell origin, with the remainder divided principally between adenocarcinoma and squamous cell carcinoma, as well as a small number of other tumors. Recent information from the SEER database suggests that men may have a higher incidence of all three types of urethral tumor than women, indicating a major shift in the incidence ratio of this disease between the sexes (1,3). These tumors are rare in men under the age of 50; the incidence is highest between ages 75 and 84. Over the past 20 years the incidence of all urethral cancers has declined in men. Causal factors of urethral cancer may include chronic irritative processes, urethral stricture disease, and certain forms of sexually transmitted disease. Evidence of an association between human papilloma virus (HPV-16) and squamous cell carcinoma continues to mount.

Tumors of the urethra are defined by location and histology. The male urethra is divided into a number of discrete anatomical segments (Fig. 38.1). The bulbomembranous urethra is the most common site of disease (60%); the penile urethra represents another 30% of cancers, and the prostatic urethra comprises 10% of all tumors (4). The anterior portion of the urethra, penile and bulbomembranous, almost always develops squamous cell carcinomas, whereas the prostatic urethra, lined by transitional epithelium, is the site of TCC >90% of the time. Adenocarcinoma or undifferentiated tumors, which represent approximately 5% of all malignancies, usually develop in the bulbomembranous urethra.

Urethral cancers may spread through direct extension to adjacent structures or via the lymphatic system to regional lymph nodes. The anterior urethra of the male lymphatically drains into the superficial and deep inguinal nodes, and the posterior urethra drains to the pelvic lymph nodes. Palpable inguinal adenopathy is worrisome for metastatic disease, as inflammatory nodal involvement occurs infrequently. Disseminated disease is rare until late in the disease process.

## DIAGNOSIS

Nearly all men are symptomatic at presentation, though the low incidence of this disease, combined with failure on the part of the clinician to consider it, often results in a significant delay in diagnosis. In Dalbagni's series of 46 patients, 96% of men presented with some form of lower-urinary-tract symptom

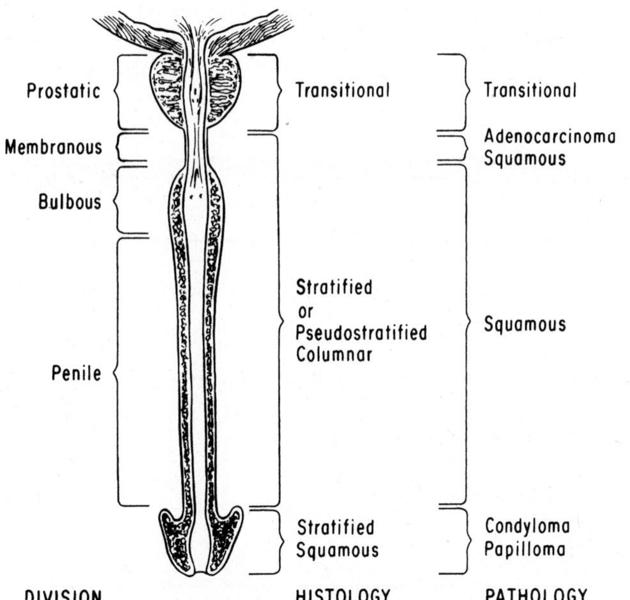


FIGURE 38.1 Changes in the histology of the epithelial lining within the divisions of the male urethra tend to dictate the pathology of the tumor most likely to occur. (From Webster GD. The urethra. In: Paulsen DF, ed. Genitourinary surgery. New York: Churchill Livingstone, 1983:567, with permission.)

or palpable mass (5). Hematuria, obstructed voiding, urethral discharge, and a palpable mass are the most common presenting symptoms and signs. Approximately 25% of men diagnosed with urethral cancer have a history of sexually transmitted infection. Fully half of these patients have been treated for urethral stricture disease; the diagnosis of cancer needs to be suspected in men with recalcitrant or nonhealing strictures (4). Urethral stricture in association with bloody discharge, penile or urethral mass, or urethrocutaneous fistula should heighten the suspicion of urethral cancer.

The diagnosis of urethral cancer is histologically confirmed by transurethral or percutaneous biopsy of the suspicious lesion. Examination under anesthesia, complete with bimanual assessment of the external genitalia, rectum, and perineum, aids in local staging of the disease. The inguinal lymph nodes are palpated, as adenopathy is usually attributable to metastatic disease rather than inflammation. Either a CT scan of the abdomen and pelvis with and without contrast or MRI of the pelvis can help assess local extension of the tumor to the rectum or bladder, as well as the status of the pelvic lymph nodes. The MRI may aid in the detection of corporal cavernosal invasion. Lung imaging with a chest radiograph, augmented by CT scanning for equivocal lesions, completes the radiological staging. Liver function tests should also be assessed.

Staging is based upon the tumor-nodes-metastasis (TNM) system.

## INDICATIONS FOR SURGERY

Given the paucity of data regarding this disorder, there are no randomized trials to support a particular treatment approach. That said, urethral cancer is a lethal disease that, if left untreated, has a median survival of <6 months. Although survival has not changed for this disease in the past 50 years, treatment still consists of extirpative surgery if the patient's condition will allow it (5). Evidence of distant metastatic disease limits treatment options to palliative measures. Local treatment is a function of the location of the disease within the urethra as well as the local stage of the malignancy. Superficial disease, especially of the penile urethra, may be managed with transurethral resection, local excision, or distal urethrectomy. Partial penectomy with a 2-cm urethral margin is the preferred treatment for disease of the distal half of the penile urethra with local invasion of the corpus spongiosum. For more proximal lesions, total penectomy is indicated. As in women, distal disease portends a better prognosis in men.

Carcinoma of the bulbomembranous urethra, often presenting at a higher stage with local extension into adjacent organs, is only occasionally amenable to local therapy, resection, or segmental excision with primary anastomosis. Radical cystoprostatectomy, complete penectomy, and pelvic lymphadenectomy represent the best option for local disease control and cure. The margins of excision may be extended into the urogenital diaphragm and pubis in an effort to extirpate locally advanced disease.

Prophylactic ilioinguinal lymphadectomy is not routinely performed.

## ALTERNATIVE THERAPY

Given the rarity of this entity, there are no randomized data to delineate the role of radiation therapy, chemotherapy, or combination therapy in this disorder. Radiation therapy and chemotherapy have been used as part of multimodality therapy or as monotherapy, but few conclusions can be inferred from most series, which are small in patient numbers and retrospective in nature. A recent series from the Lahey Clinic suggests that a combination of 5-fluorouracil, mitomycin C, and perineal, genital, and pelvic radiotherapy—an adaptation of the regimen successfully employed in the treatment of squamous carcinoma of the anus—has an 80% 5-year disease-specific survival rate, a 30% improvement over that reported in most published series (6). In this study salvage surgery was offered to patients who failed conservative therapy. General recommendations for treatment based on these data are limited due to the small cohort of patients studied. It is difficult to support or refute the role of neoadjuvant or adjuvant chemo- or radiotherapy in this disease, though the accruing data are provocative.

## SURGICAL TECHNIQUE

Given the rarity of this disease and the limited experience with management even at large referral centers, there are no randomized data to guide management. Treated disease has a 5-year survival of roughly 50%, and untreated disease has a worse prognosis (5). On the basis of these facts, surgical therapy is suggested in men who are free from metastasis and will

**TABLE 38.1**

STAGING OF MALE URETHRAL CARCINOMA

| Ray | TNM | |
|---|---|---|
| Stage 0 | Tis | Confined to Mucosa Only (In Situ) |
| Stage A | Ta | Into But Not Beyond Lamina Propria |
| Stage B | T2 | Into But Not Beyond Substance of Corpus Spongiosum or Into But Not Beyond Prostate |
| Stage C | T3, T4 | Direct Extension Into Tissues Beyond Corpus Spongiosum (Corpora Cavernosa, Muscle, Fat, Fascia, Skin, Direct Skeletal Involvement), or Beyond Prostatic Capsule |
| Stage D1 | N1, N2 | Regional Metastasis Including Inguinal and/or Pelvic Lymph Nodes (With any Primary Tumor) |
| Stage D4 | M1 | Distant Metastasis (With Any Primary Tumor) |

tolerate an operative intervention. Distal lesions have a better response to surgery than more proximal lesions, and they often are amenable to less radical curative surgery.

Tumors of the anterior urethra have a better prognosis than more proximal lesions. The surgical management of anterior lesions continues to evolve. Endoscopic ablation or local excision of the diseased urethra allows preservation of the penis in men with limited, superficial disease. Candidates for penile-sparing surgery must have well-defined disease with a negative surgical margin confirmed by frozen section analysis. Any question of the adequacy of resection or the malignant status of the proximal urethral margin should prompt the surgeon to perform a more complete extirpative procedure, including partial or total penectomy (7,8). Surgical description of partial and total penectomy is found in the chapter on surgery of the penis. Smith et al. (8) have achieved impressive results in the treatment of very distal urethral lesions by performing local excision of the involved urethra followed by penile reconstruction using skin grafts (8). The Indiana University group has recently reported a series of men with in situ carcinoma of the pendulous urethra who were treated with urethrectomy and one-stage urethroplasty with a tubularized penile fasciocutaneous pedicle flap *(personal communication)*. In men who are not candidates for immediate urethral reconstruction, creation of a penile urethrostomy maintains standing micturition.

## Urethrectomy with Penile Preservation

It must be emphasized that a penile-preserving approach is indicated for disease limited to the corpus spongiosum and urethra; any disease that extends into the corpora is best managed with partial or total penectomy. Preoperative preparation should include full staging studies, a detailed history and physical examination with particular attention to a history of bleeding or anesthetic complications, and a urine culture, with any infection managed before surgery.

TED hose and sequential compression devices provide deep venous thrombosis (DVT) prophylaxis; the use of 5,000 U of subcutaneous heparin or 40 mg of subcutaneous enoxaparin is prudent in a patient with a pelvic malignancy undergoing extirpative surgery. Prophylactic antibiotics with a first-generation cephalosporin should be administered within the hour prior to the first incision; patients allergic to penicillin can receive either vancomycin or clindamycin as an alternative. An aminoglycoside or quinolone to augment gram-negative coverage is reasonable. The patient should be placed in lithotomy, with care taken to adequately pad all pressure points on the legs and dorsum of the feet. The patient's sacrum may be elevated with a rolled towel or Gelfoam pad to facilitate exposure of the proximal bulbar urethra. The perineum, proximal thigh, genitalia, and lower abdomen are prepared into the field; the anus is excluded from the operative field by a sterile towel secured by staples to the perineum and posterior thighs. A 16Fr Foley urethral catheter is placed.

A 4- to 5-cm vertical perineal incision extending inferiorly from just below the scrotum provides exposure to the proximal portion of the anterior urethra. A Scott, Lone Star, or Jordan-Bookwalter ring retractor system facilitates exposure of the bulbar urethra. Using electrocautery, the superficial fascial and fatty tissue is dissected to the level of the bulbospongiosus muscle. The bulbospongiosus is divided sharply over the ventral aspect of the urethral bulb and dissected from the lateral aspects of the urethra. Careful, sharp dissection of the dense attachment between the dorsum of the bulb and the corpus cavernosum circumferentially liberates the urethra; a vessel loop or small Penrose drain placed around the urethra serves as a "handle" for the surgeon in mobilizing the urethra distally. Frequent palpation of the urethral catheter ensures that the plane between the spongiosum and corpora is accurately assessed (Fig. 38.2) .

As the dissection is carried distally, the penis will begin to invert into the wound. There is a tendency to overestimate the extent of distal urethral mobilization as the inverted glans is approached. Indeed, the urethral plane becomes less distinct within the spongy tissue of the glans penis. The authors find it helpful at this point to evert the penis and complete the distal urethral dissection from the meatus.

Using a no. 15 scalpel blade, the urethral meatus, including a small cuff of glanular skin, is circumscribed. A holding suture may be placed through the meatal urethra to aid in the dissection of the intraglanular portion of the urethra. Sharp and cautery dissection are used to free the urethra from its spongy glanular attachments. With the urethra liberated distally, it is maneuvered into the perineal aspect of the wound and amputated at least 2 cm proximal to the tumor. Frozen section analysis of the proximal resection margin confirms that a disease-free margin has been achieved. The wound is copiously irrigated with sterile saline, and all bleeding is arrested with cautery.

Following resection of the surgical specimen, attention is directed to the creation of a perineal urethrostomy. A site for the urethrostomy is selected ventral to the anus and, preferably, lateral to the initial skin incision. The urethra is spatulated on its ventral aspect for a distance of at least 1 cm. The urethrocutaneous anastomosis is matured with a 3-0 or 4-0 absorbable suture, such as Vicryl or Monocryl. Four 3-0 interrupted sutures are placed between the urethra and perineal skin at the apical spatulation, the distal end of the urethra, and laterally along each side of the urethra equidistant from the first two. The anastomosis is completed with 4-0 interrupted or running sutures placed between the quadrant sutures. Care is taken not to kink or twist the urethra. With the urethrostomy complete, a 16Fr Foley catheter is inserted into the bladder. The perineal incision is closed in a layered fashion; both the superficial fascia and deep dermis are approximated using a running 3-0 Vicryl or PDS suture, and the skin is closed with a running 4-0 Monocryl subcuticular stitch. The incision is covered with a layer of tissue glue, such as Dermabond or Indermil, obviating the need for a wound dressing. A generous portion of petroleum-based ointment is placed over the urethrostomy at the conclusion of the procedure. The catheter is left in place for 10 to 14 days and the urethrostomy inspected for stenotic changes on a regular basis.

## Proximal Urethral Tumors

Tumors of the posterior urethra generally present at a more advanced stage, limiting the possibility of endoscopic resection or segmental resection with end-to-end anastomosis. Bulbomembranous cancers, though responding poorly to all forms of treatment, require radical extirpative techniques to

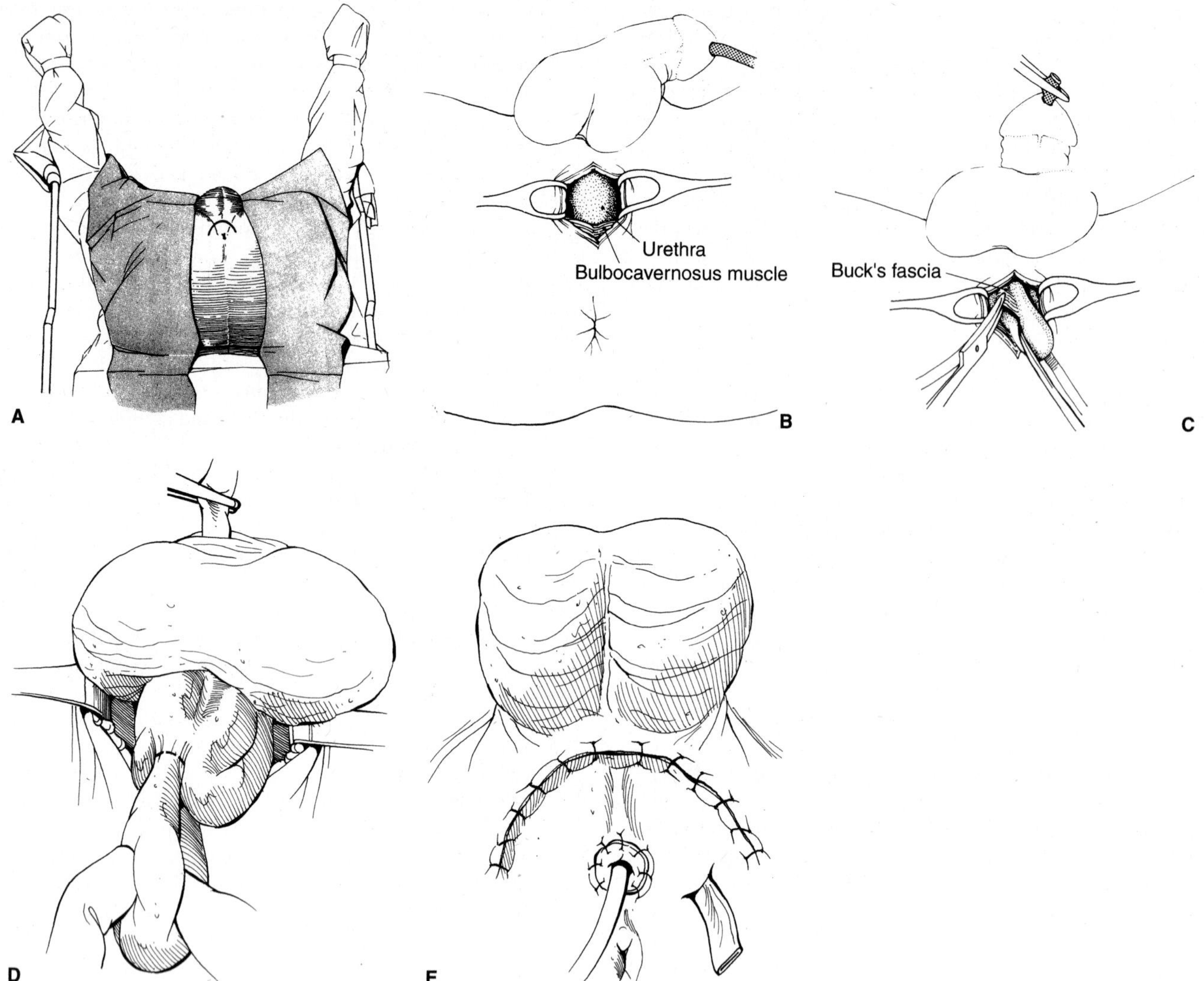


FIGURE 38.2 **A and B:** Incisions used for penile-sparing urethrectomy. **C:** The urethra is dissected off the corpora cavernosa using electrocautery. **D:** Distal dissection of the urethra results in inversion of the penis. **E:** The spatulated urethra is sewn to the skin edges with interrupted 3-0 chromic sutures, and the drain is brought out through a separate stab incision.

achieve disease control. Radical cystoprostatectomy with an en bloc total penectomy, although mutilative and disfiguring, provides the patient with his best opportunity for cure. Resection of part of the pubic arch and urogenital diaphragm may be needed to achieve an adequate surgical margin. Complete removal of the tumor may result in the creation of a large pelvic floor defect; in situations where this degree of extirpation is anticipated, consultation with a plastic surgeon will prove beneficial in planning for reconstruction and "dead space" closure. Bladder-sparing procedures may be considered when it has been confirmed, through biopsy, that the bladder neck is free of disease. The extirpative portion of the procedure is similar to what will be described herein except that the prostate and seminal vesicles are dissected, in an antegrade fashion, from the base of the bladder. Once the bladder neck has been closed, a continent or noncontinent small bowel limb (e.g., A Monti procedure) is matured to the lower abdominal wall.

A mechanical bowel preparation consisting of a clear liquid diet and oral Fleet Phospho-Soda is initiated on the day prior to surgery. Broad-spectrum antibiotics to provide coverage for gram-positive, gram-negative, and anaerobic bacteria are delivered 1 hour before the procedure. In all other respects the preparation is similar to that described for surgery of the distal urethra.

The patient is positioned in the low lithotomy position, and all pressure points are well padded. The abdominal component of the procedure is begun first; the abdominal and perineal components may be performed simultaneously by two experienced surgical teams, reducing operative time. Although an experienced laparoscopic or robotic surgeon may be capable of performing both the pelvic node dissection and the cystoprostatectomy, many urologists will feel more comfortable approaching the pelvic dissection through an open approach.

A vertical midline incision is made between the umbilicus and the pubis. The preperitoneal space is developed bluntly, and the pelvic sidewalls are cleared for the pelvic lymph node dissection. Following placement of a Bookwalter or Omni retraction device, the external iliac, obturator, and internal iliac nodes are dissected to the bifurcation of the iliac vessels and sent for frozen and permanent pathologic examination.

Next, the peritoneum is entered, the abdomen explored, and the bowel packed clear of the pelvis. The bladder is mobilized and the ureters divided as in a radical cystectomy for bladder cancer. Prostatectomy is performed in an antegrade fashion, though the puboprostatic ligaments are not divided, in the event the pubis is resected en bloc. Please see chapter on cystoprostatectomy for a complete description of this surgical technique.

With the bladder and prostate widely mobilized, a modified lambda or inverted U incision is made in the prepared perineum, extending laterally to points just medial to the ischial tuberosities. The apex of the incision is based in the midperineum. The superficial fascia is opened with cautery, and the ischiorectal fossae are bluntly developed bilaterally. After division of the perineal body, a tunnel is developed anterior to the rectum in a manner similar to the technique described for the perineal prostatectomy. The perineal contents are cleared off between the ischial tuberosities and up to the pubic arch. The suspensory ligament of the penis and the neurovascular bundles of the penis are divided between 0 silk ties (Fig. 38.3).

With mobilization of the prostate and proximal urethra complete, the penoscrotal junction is then incised circumferentially with a scalpel. The incision may be extended along the median raphe of the scrotum, joining with the previously created perineal dissection to allow for enhanced exposure of the distal bulb and pendulous urethra. Using electrocautery, the dartos fascia is divided to expose the neurovascular bundle of the penis, which is divided between silk or Vicryl ties. If the suspensory ligament has not been divided during the perineal portion of the surgery, it is done so now. With the corporal bodies and urethral spongiosum exposed, the penis may be transposed into the perineal aspect of the incision. The corpora cavernosa are then divided at the ischial tuberosities and oversewn with a running 2-0 Vicryl or PDS suture. Dissection of the spongiosum from its investing tissues is performed sharply, with care taken to avoid a positive surgical margin. Tumor invasion of the superficial periosteum of the pubic arch requires vigorous resection of the periosteum with electrocautery. Deeper involvement of the pubic bone will require removal of the inferior portion of the pubic arch with orthopedic rongeurs and surgical drills. In the face of extensive disease, consultation with an orthopedic surgeon may be necessary to achieve an adequate margin. The puboprostatic ligaments are generally divided at this time.

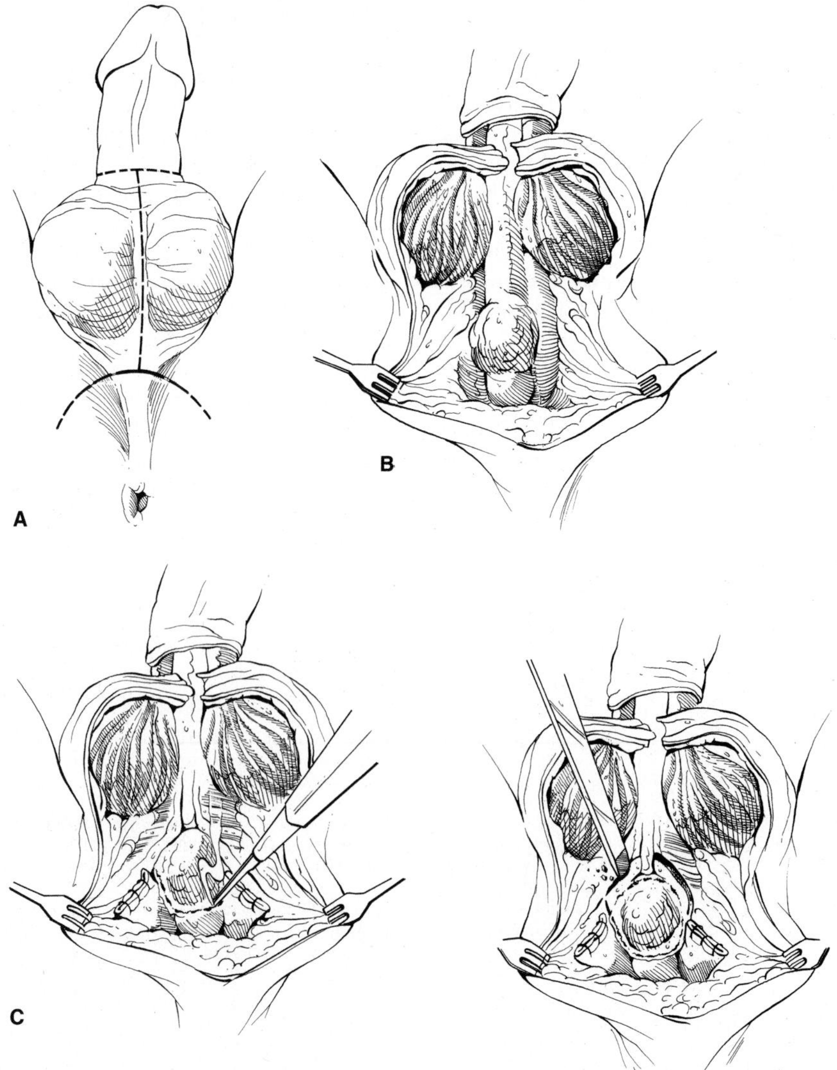


**FIGURE 38.3 A and B:** Incision used to gain access to the perineum for total penectomy, total urethrectomy, radical prostatectomy, and continent cutaneous bladder augmentation. **C:** Electrocautery and suture ligatures are used to resect the urethral mass. **D:** If pubic bone invasion is present, the pubic arch is first scored with electrocautery; then, an orthopedic hammer and chisel are used to resect the inferior pubic arch to ensure a negative margin.

With the penis free, a negative surgical margin on the pubic arch, and the cystoprostatectomy completed, the entire specimen is removed en bloc. If additional room is needed at the penile incision to remove the specimin, the scrotum can be incised along its median raphe as previously described. In patients in whom a bladder-sparing procedure is being contemplated, the bladder neck margin is assessed with frozen section. Disease found at the bladder neck should prompt the surgeon to consider complete cystectomy and urinary diversion.

The type of urinary diversion performed—conduit or continent reservoir—is a function of surgeon and patient preference and should be discussed and planned prior to surgery. We prefer a variation of the right colon detubularized continent reservoir in motivated patients capable of performing intermittent catheterization. The ileal conduit is our preferred choice of intestinal segments for patients electing an incontinent diversion; in patients with irradiated small bowel or inflammatory bowel disease, the transverse colon conduit, based on the middle or right colic arteries, provides a safe, easy-to-handle alternative to the terminal ileum.

Small pelvic defects may be filled with a pedicled flap of omentum, unhinged from the greated curvature of the stomach and based on either the right or left gastroepiploic vessels. Large perineal defects, especially those resulting from wide resection of the pubic arch, require placement of a pedicled muscle flap. Many reconstructive urologists are conversant with the gracilis muscle flap, which is relatively easy to harvest and has a reliable blood supply. Rectus abdominus or gluteal muscle flaps may be necessary to fill even larger spaces. A Jackson-Pratt drain is placed deeply in the perineal wound and brought out through a stab incision. The superficial perineal fascia is closed with a running 3-0 Vicryl suture, as is deep dermis. The skin is approximated with a running 4-0 Monocryl suture. A tissue glue such as Indermil or Dermabond is utilized to seal the skin; in such cases, no dressing is needed. A Jackson-Pratt or Penrose drain, placed abdominally in close proximity to the ureteral reconstruction, is exteriorized lateral to the midline incision.

Postoperatively patients are managed in a standard fashion (9). A nasogastric tube, placed at the time of surgery, is routinely removed on the first postoperative day. DVT prophylaxis is maintained with heparin or enoxaparin postoperatively, and antibiotics are stopped within 24 hours, unless an active infection is being treated. Patients are aggressively ambulated beginning the first night or the morning of postoperative day 1; pulmonary toilet with incentive spirometry is initiated on the day following surgery. The diet is advanced on a schedule, with sips begun on postoperative day 2 and advancing on a daily basis to a regular diet on postoperative day 5. Ketorolac is utilized to minimize opiates and help bowel function, and metoclopramide is also given to enhance motility.

## OUTCOMES

Tumors of the distal urethra enjoy the best prognosis, with a nearly 70% 5-year survival rate. In patients with superficial squamous cell carcinoma resection, laser ablation or local excision provides progression-free rates approaching 100%. More locally advanced disease requiring partial penectomy can be cured when a 2-cm urethral margin is achieved. Proximal urethral tumors, on the other hand, due to the more advanced nature of disease at presentation, respond poorly to extirpative surgery; they are associated with a 25% to 40% 5-year survival rate (5). The reported disease-specific survival rate in most series is around 50%, a figure that has changed little over the last few decades, owing, in part, to little improvement in adjuvant therapies.

## COMPLICATIONS

With penile-preserving surgery, the possibility of local recurrence dictates the need for compulsive monitoring. Endoscopic therapies and local excision may result in the development of urethral strictures. Stenotic lesions failing to respond to dilation should be evaluated for the presence of recurrent cancer. Recalcitrant benign stricture disease needs to be addressed with open urethroplasty. Stenoses of the meatus or perineal urethrostomy are common complications seen in patients undergoing partial and total penectomies, respectively, and may be managed conservatively with patient self-dilation.

Pelvic exenteration for bulbar urethral tumors carries a similar profile of complications as that seen with other exenterative procedures. Pelvic abscesses need immediate attention with open or radiological drainage. Perineal wound breakdown, especially when associated with the placement of pedicled flaps, is treated with surgical debridement and local wound care.

## *References*


1. Swartz MA, Porter MP, Lin DW, et al. Incidence of primary urethral carcinoma in the United States. *Urology* 2006;68:1164.
2. http://apps.nccd.cdc.gov/uscs/Table.aspx?Group=TableAll&Year=2003&Display=n, accessed December 2, 2007.
3. Krieg R, Hoffman R. Current management of unusual genitourinary cancers. Part 2: Urethral cancer. *Oncology (Williston Park)* 1999;13:1511–1517, 1520; discussion 1523–1524.
4. Campbell MF, Wein AJ, Kavoussi LR. *Campbell-Walsh urology*, 9th ed. Philadelphia: Saunders Elsevier, 2007.
5. Dalbagni G, Zhang ZF, Lacombe L, et al. Male urethral carcinoma: analysis of treatment outcome. *Urology* 1999;53:1126–1132.
6. Cohen MS, Triaca V, Billmeyer B, et al. Updated outcomes with coordinated chemoradiation therapy as the primary treatment for invasive carcinoma of the male urethra. Abstract presented at the 2007 NE AUA Meeting, Boston, MA.
7. Davis JW, Schellhammer PF, Schlossberg SM. Conservative surgical therapy for penile and urethral carcinoma. *Urology* 1999;53:386–392.
8. Smith Y, Hadway P, Ahmed S, et al. Penile-preserving surgery for male distal urethral carcinoma. *BJU Int* 2007;100:82–87.
9. Pruthi RS, Chun J, Richman M. Reducing time to oral diet and hospital discharge in patients undergoing radical cystectomy using a perioperative care plan. *Urology* 2003;62:661–665; discussion 665–666.

# CHAPTER 39 ■ INJECTABLE THERAPIES FOR INCONTINENCE IN WOMEN

RODNEY APPELL

The idea of increasing urethral resistance by an injectable agent is nothing new. It was first reported in 1938 (1). Twenty women had either sodium morrhuate or cod liver oil injected into the anterior vaginal wall to provoke an inflammatory response resulting in scar formation and contracture of tissue around the urethra. Seventeen patients reported being cured or improved, but pulmonary infarction and cardiopulmonary arrest were reported. In 1955 the first injections into the urethra were reported by Quackels (2). Two patients were treated successfully without complications. In 1963 Sachse (3) used Dondren, a sclerosing agent, to treat 7 women and 24 men. Four women and 12 men were reported as cured, but several patients experienced pulmonary embolism. These first bulking agents were far from ideal. Such an ideal agent would be nonimmunogenic, hypoallergenic, biocompatible, heal with minimal fibrosis, be nonmigratory, and retain its bulking effect over a long period of time (be durable) (4).

## MECHANISM

Injectable agents work by forming a "seal" through restoring mucosal coaptation. They have several advantages over surgical procedures in treating stress urinary incontinence (SUI). Compared to surgical procedures that create a functional obstruction, injectable agents restore continence by increasing urethral resistance at rest. With bulking agents, the urethra maintains its ability to funnel and open, keeping urethral resistance low during micturition. This spares a resultant increase in detrusor pressure (Pdet), which could lead to overactive bladder symptoms and/or upper-tract damage. In comparison, surgical procedures may result in increased resistance at rest and during micturition by not allowing the urethra the same physiologic movement. Most bulking agents are placed at the level of the bladder neck within the smooth muscle in the area of the continence mechanism. Since the placement is within the urethra, *intraurethral* is a more accurate term than the commonly used terms *periurethral* or *submucosal.*

## CRITERIA FOR SELECTION

Ideal patients for intraurethral bulking have SUI due to intrinsic sphincter deficiency (ISD) and a normal contractile bladder. Clues such as leaking a large amount of urine with cough or sneeze, significant leakage upon exertion, leakage while supine, bed wetting, or leakage with the sensation of urinary urgency may suggest ISD. On physical examination, the patient should have a well-supported, fixed urethra. This can be determined by placing a cotton swab through the urethra with the tip just past the urethrovesical junction. If the angle is >30 degrees from the horizontal or the change in angle is >30 degrees when the patient bears down or coughs, the patient is said to have a hypermobile rather than fixed urethra (5,6).

The use of intraurethral bulking agents in women with urethral hypermobility, type II incontinence, is an area of controversy. A comparison between pubovaginal slings and intraurethral collagen injections was performed by Kreder and Austin (7). In their study, they compared success rates in patients with ISD alone or mixed with urethral hypermobility. In the mixed group, those receiving a pubovaginal sling faired better, with a cure rate of 81% versus 25% in the collagen group. However, the collagen group only received a single injection, whereas it has been demonstrated that many patients require two to three injection sessions to affect their continence (8). In another study, despite more injections and the amount of material injected in the group with urethral hypermobility, both those with and without hypermobility had equal success (9). In a later study by Herschorn and Radomski (10), no statistically significant difference was found between those with and without urethral hypermobility. Over time, 72% remained dry at 1 year, 57% at 2 years, and 45% at 3 years, with no significant difference between the type of incontinence and time to failure. Others have documented similar findings in patients with urethral hypermobility or type II incontinence (11–14).

Urodynamics should be performed to rule out other causes of urinary incontinence, such as detrusor overactivity. Urethral function can be assessed by measuring the abdominal leak point pressure (ALPP), which is the amount of abdominal pressure (Pabd) necessary to overcome the bladder's continence mechanism. The definition of ISD by ALPP has varied from a low ALPP (60 cm $H_2O$) to an ALPP <100 cm $H_2O$. An absolute value for ALPP suggesting ISD has become unimportant due to limitations in urodynamic testing as well as different values used by different clinicians. With videourodynamics, radiographic evidence of an open bladder neck and proximal urethra without detrusor contraction during the storage phase of the bladder is felt to imply ISD.

As more is understood about the continence mechanism, it appears that most women with SUI have some component of ISD, since there are numerous women with urethral hypermobility who do not leak with significant intra-abdominal pressures. Women who do have a fixed, nonmobile urethra are, however, more likely to have a greater degree of ISD (15). Exclusion criteria for intraurethral bulking would include urinary incontinence due to abnormal detrusor contractions, active urinary tract infection, or allergy to the material used as a bulking agent.

### Key Concepts

- *Ideal patients for intraurethral bulking have SUI due to intrinsic sphincter deficiency (ISD) and a normally contractile bladder.*
- *Most women with SUI have some component of ISD.*

## INJECTION TECHNIQUES

When performing intraurethral bulking, precise placement of the bulking material into the wall of the proximal urethra near the bladder neck in the area of the continence mechanism is of the utmost importance. The plane of delivery, the tissue quality at the injection site, and the cause of incontinence are all important factors in successful therapy. If material is delivered too distally, the treatment is likely to fail and may cause irritative voiding symptoms. Prior to injection, patients are placed in lithotomy position and prepared in standard sterile fashion. A local anesthetic in the form of 20% benzocaine ointment or cream may be applied to the vestibule covering the urethra, and a topical 2% lidocaine jelly may be applied to the urethra. Approximately 4 mL of 1% lidocaine is then injected periurethrally at the 3 and 9 o'clock positions.

### Key Concept

- *Precise placement of the bulking material into the wall of the proximal urethra near the bladder neck in the area of the continence mechanism is of the utmost importance.*

## TRANSURETHRAL INJECTION

Several approaches may be taken when performing injections of bulking agents. They may be performed by placing a needle through a cystourethroscope and injecting suburothelially, also known as a "transurethral injection" (16). A 0-, 12-, or 30-degree lens is best for providing a good view of the urethra as well as the injection needle. Once the cystourethroscope is placed into the urethra and passed into the bladder, the bladder is usually drained because the patient's bladder may become distended toward the end of the procedure. The endoscope is then backed to the midurethra, at which time the needle is deployed at the 4 o'clock position. The needle is then inserted submucosally into the urethral muscle beyond the midurethra and advanced to the proximal urethra near the bladder neck. Once the desired positioning is achieved, the bulking agent is slowly delivered to allow it to spread underneath the urethral mucosa. Once the mucosa on that side has expanded to the midline, the needle is slowly withdrawn while injecting. Attention is then turned to the 8 o'clock position, where the technique is repeated again. After completion of both sides, a fair amount of coaptation should be noted.

### Key Concepts

- *Once the mucosa at the 4 o'clock position has expanded to the midline, the technique is repeated again at the 8 o'clock position.*
- *A 0-, 12-, or 30-degree lens is best for providing a good view of the urethra as well as the injection needle.*

## PERIURETHRAL INJECTION

Injections may also be performed periurethrally via a needle placed percutaneously lateral to the urethral meatus and parallel to the urethra. While the needle is placed, the urethra is visualized through a cystourethroscope (17,18). Localization of the needle tip may be facilitated by preinjecting the urethra with methylene blue during the periurethral approach (19). With the periurethral approach, there is often less bleeding, which can improve visualization. There is also less extrusion of the material injected, although this also depends upon the type of material injected. The desired amount of coaptation is the same as when performed via a transurethral technique. After the periurethral block, a 20-gauge spinal needle is placed at the 4 o'clock position into the periurethral tissue within the lamina propria. Urethroscopy is then performed as the needle is further inserted with minimal resistance up to the level of the bladder neck. The needle is then rocked in a horizontal plane to assess the location of the needle tip and ensure placement at the proper depth. The material is then injected slowly while observing for coaptation, similarly to the transurethral technique, and the process is repeated at the 8 o'clock position. If material is noted in the lumen of the urethra, the needle is removed and relocated to a more anterior position, where the injection is repeated again. Once sufficient coaptation is noted, the procedure is ended. A needle with a "bent tip" has been manufactured (Boston Scientific Inc, Natick, MA) to facilitate placement into the proper plane. With advancement of the needle, the tip is brought more medially. These needles were originally designed to ease the injection of Durasphere, since a larger bore size (18 gauge) also aids in the passage of the particles, but they certainly can be used for the periurethral injection of other bulking agents.

The differences between the transurethral and periurethral techniques were reviewed by Faerber et al. (20). They found similar outcomes with no significant differences in adverse events using collagen. Of significance, the amount of material injected was less using a transurethral approach. A prospective, randomized comparison was later performed in women with again no noted differences in efficacy, but a higher rate of urinary retention and also an increased volume of injected material were seen in the periurethral group (21). It appears that a periurethral approach tends to use larger volumes of material and has been noted to have a longer learning curve than the transurethral approach.

## ULTRASOUND GUIDANCE

Although transurethral and periurethral injections are the most commonly performed injections, injections may also be performed in women with an ultrasound probe (22). Theoretically, this technique circumvents the passage of instruments through the urethra, which may alter the placement of the bulking agent affecting coaptation. First, a transrectal ultrasound probe with a biopsy port is placed into the vagina. Once the bladder neck has been identified, a needle of the same type for transurethral injection is placed through the port. Longitudinal views by ultrasound are used to determine coaptation of the bladder neck. Studies have demonstrated that three-dimensional ultrasound views may predict long-term outcomes and may provide an objective measure for the amount of material to be placed (23). In later studies with three-dimensional ultrasound, collagen injections were shown to maintain their volume and ultrasound appearance with an associated improved continence and quality of life. It was also found that the most desirable appearance on ultrasound was either a circumferential or horseshoe configuration (24). Regardless of the technique, coaptation of the urethra is the goal.

## POSTOPERATIVE CARE

Immediate postoperative complications are rare. After completion of the procedure, the patient should demonstrate the ability to void. If the patient is in acute urinary retention, most often the patient will be able to urinate shortly after the periurethral block loses effect. Meanwhile, the patient is usually catheterized with a small 10Fr to 14Fr catheter to relieve the patient's full bladder after cystourethroscopy. An indwelling Foley catheter should be avoided since there is a theoretical risk of the bulking agent molding around the catheter and losing its effect, although there is no evidence to support that short-term catheterization decreases the efficacy of intraurethral bulking. If long-term catheterization is necessary, a suprapubic catheter until return of voiding would be best to avoid disrupting the placement of the bulking agent. Prophylactic treatment with antibiotics is recommended to avoid urinary tract infections. Many patients will require more than one treatment session to achieve maximal continence. Different waiting periods are required for each individual bulking agent. Bulking agents such as GAX-collagen can be repeated after 1 week (in the original multicenter study, a 4-week waiting period was used). With polytetrafluoroethylene, a 4-month wait is required since improved coaptation occurs with time. On repeat injection, if erosion is noted, injection into that side should be avoided until re-epithelialization occurs.

Irritative voiding symptoms may also develop after placement of bulking agents. Surprisingly, in a study by Steele et al. (13), 50% of patients were reported to have developed de novo detrusor overactivity. In a study by Cross et al. (25), 28% of patients were found to have de novo urge incontinence without ISD when undergoing urodynamics for post-treatment incontinence. Stothers et al. (26) reported a 12.6% rate of de novo urgency with urge incontinence in 337 women enrolled in a prospective trial of which 21% failed anticholinergic treatment. Commonly, minor urethral bleeding may occur. If the urethral mucosa becomes disrupted, perforation and extravasation of the bulking agent may occur. An advantage of the periurethral approach involves placement of the bulking agent without disruption of the mucosa.

### Key Concept

- *If the patient is in acute urinary retention, catheterize with a small 10Fr to 14Fr catheter to relieve the patient's full bladder.*

## INJECTABLE AGENTS

Other methods of treatment for SUI include urethropexies, slings, and artificial urinary sphincters. Often bulking agents are compared to these other methods of treatment. What has been demonstrated in some studies is that midurethral slings and Burch urethropexies tend to have higher failure rates in patients with a "fixed urethra" (27,28). These patients are better off treated with intraurethral bulking agents, bladder neck slings, or artificial urinary sphincters. Compared to injectable agents, the artificial urinary sphincter and bladder neck slings both involve undergoing a surgical procedure, which involves surgical risk as well as the risk of anesthesia, whereas the intraurethral bulking agent involves only local anesthesia and minimal complications.

Comparing the different injectable agents is a difficult task. There are few controlled, long-term studies involving commonly used bulking agents. Even within those rare studies, there are many variables that make it difficult to compare one to another. This is due to the different patients with different severities and etiologies of stress incontinence. Not all studies differentiate the results in patients with and without urethral hypermobility and/or ISD. The procedures themselves have also varied due to different technical factors such as injection technique and instrumentation. Additionally, reported results have been largely subjective rather than objective, creating a difficult situation to compare data. Variability also exists within the reported outcomes, as different criteria have been used to define *cured* or *improved*.

## AUTOLOGOUS MATERIALS

### Autologous Blood

Autologous blood is readily available and accessible. In a study of 14 women, 30 mL of blood was obtained in a heparinized syringe from the antecubital vein. Continence was achieved after two treatments. Unfortunately, all patients became incontinent again after 10 to 17 days (18).

### Autologous Fat

Although not as accessible as blood, autologous fat can be easily obtained through liposuction. In 1989 this technique was reported in 10 women (29). In a different study with 1 year follow-up, 0 of 5 men and 5 of 15 women reported improvement (30). In a study by Santarosa and Blaivas (31), 83% of 12 women with ISD were subjectively improved, although at 1 year the results were much poorer. In a randomized double-blind controlled trial of women with urethral hypermobility, fat was found to be as effective as the saline control group at 6 months (33).

These poor results are thought to be secondary to fat degradation. After injection, neovascularization never becomes adequate at the fat graft's center, leaving only a miniscule amount of viable fat, which may hinder its bulking effect. After 3 weeks, 60% of the fat injected is degraded. Once the fat is reabsorbed, inflammation occurs with resulting fibrosis, which leads to the bulking effect (31). Although this material is accessible and complications are rare, it has been reported to be associated with systemic embolization and death (33,35). Therefore, the use of autologous fat as a bulking agent is discouraged.

## BIOMATERIALS

### Glutaraldehyde Cross-Linked Bovine Collagen (GAX-Collagen)

Of all the injectables, glutaraldehyde cross-linked bovine collagen (GAX-collagen) is probably the most commonly used, with most publications describing its safety and efficacy. Before its use as a bulking agent, bovine dermal collagen was primarily used to make absorbable sutures and hemostatic agents. When used as a bulking agent, bovine collagen is cross-linked with glutaraldehyde to create a stabilized, fibrillar collagen that confers resistance to denaturation by collagenases. It consists of 35% purified bovine collagen in a phosphate buffer. The collagen itself is composed of 95% type I collagen, which is the type found predominately in ligaments and confers structural strength; however, between 1% and 5% is composed of type III collagen, which is the type abundant in vaginal tissue, giving added flexibility (36). GAX-collagen is prepared by selective hydrolysis of the collagen molecule at the nonhelicoidal amino-terminal and carboxy-terminal segments, also known as telopeptides. This serves two functions. One is to decrease the antigenicity, and the other is to increase resistance to collagenases and thus to increase the durability of the implant (37,38).

When injecting this material, the surgeon inserts the exact amount needed to achieve the desired effect, since there is no expansion or shrinking after injection. Acting as a matrix, the material promotes ingrowth of new collagen within the implant (39). Since GAX-collagen is both biocompatible and biodegradable, only minimal inflammatory changes occur (40). After 12 weeks, the collagen starts to degrade, but it persists until 19 months (41). Despite the fact that GAX-collagen is degraded, it maintains effectiveness in 80% of those who become continent, a result that is thought to be secondary to the ingrowth of new collagen (42).

One series reported that 55% of women could achieve continence after one injection session (43). In a multicenter clinical study involving 127 women with ISD, 88 patients completed 2-year follow-up. At 2 years, 46% of patients were dry and 34% were significantly improved, requiring only a single pad or tissues. Urodynamic studies also revealed a rise of 40 cm $H_2O$ in ALPP. A mean volume of 18.4 mL of GAX-collagen with a mean of 2.1 (+/− 1.5) treatment sessions was given to those who achieved continence (44). Other independent studies have supported these results (9,45,46). These reported rates have compared favorably with other treatment modalities for ISD (47). As time progresses, a noted decline in efficacy has been witnessed. Forty-five percent of elderly women were improved at 24.4 months in a report by Winters et al. (12). Of note in this group, at an average of 7.9 months, 40% required more injections; after additional material was injected, only 42% became continent again. Forty-two patients with ISD were followed at an average of 46 months by Richardson et al. (48), who reported a 40% dry rate, 43% improved rate, and 17% rate of failure. At 50 months, Corcos and Fournier (49) reported a cured rate of 30% and an improved rate of 40% in 40 women, although four women in the cured group and five women in the improved group required "maintenance" injections. In a study up to 5 years, Gorton et al. (50) reported that only 26% of 53 women reported continued improvement.

Few complications have been found with the use of GAX-collagen. In the U.S. clinical trials (51), 15% developed transient urinary retention, 5% had a UTI, and 1% experienced irritative voiding. Rates of de novo urgency and frequency have been reported to be as high as 10% (49). There has been no evidence of foreign-body response or migration (39), partly because of the small amount of glutaraldehyde in GAX-collagen, which creates minimal immunoreactivity and cytotoxicity (52). GAX-collagen is biocompatible and allows fibroblasts to deposit native collagen as well as neovascularization to occur as the implant is degraded over 12 weeks (53). After 10 to 19 months all of the implant has completely degraded (40). There have been several case reports of sterile abscesses at the injection sites, some of which required drainage (35,55).

One potential hazard of GAX-collagen involves an allergic reaction to the bovine protein, although this is reduced by cross-linking and skin testing. Approximately 4% of female patients will have a positive skin test, which precludes them from treatment (44). Despite being extraordinarily rare, delayed hypersensitivity has been reported at the skin test site. Overall, due to its complete degradation with minimal inflammatory response and lack of migration, GAX-collagen has been the most popular intraurethral bulking agent used to treat incontinence.

### Key Concepts

- *As time progresses, a noted decline in efficacy has been witnessed.*
- *Approximately 4% of female patients will have a positive skin test, which precludes them from treatment.*

## SYNTHETIC MATERIALS

### Polytetrafluoroethylene (Polytef)

Many authors have been able to demonstrate the efficacy of polytetrafluoroethylene (PTFE) as a bulking agent (58–63). Success rates have ranged from 70% to 90% with PTFE (64). This material was also studied by the Department of Technology Assessment of the American Medical Association and was found to be an easily performed, effective treatment with good short-term results (65). However, longer follow-up has proven otherwise. In one study, a 38% success rate between 21 to 72 months (mean, 49 months) was noted in women (66).

In addition to the shortcomings in long-term efficacy, rates of urinary retention have ranged from 20% to 25% (67). Transient irritative voiding symptoms may develop in approximately 20% of patients (62). Urinary tract infection has been reported to occur at a rate of 2% (61).

Of greater concern, the long-term safety profile of this agent has been brought into question. Foreign-body reaction with granuloma formation is a known risk (68). After injection, histiocytic and giant cells are responsible for this reaction. Particles have been found in blood vessels as well as lymphatics. These particles have been thought to elicit an allergic response in some patients, which is believed to be responsible for culture negative fevers in 25% of patients. Five percent of patients also complain of transient perineal discomfort with spontaneous resolution, which is also thought to be an immune-related phenomenon (67,69).

Once inside blood vessels or lymphatics, particles can migrate to distant locations. In animal models, PTFE particles have been found in pelvic lymph nodes, lungs, brain, kidneys, and spleen at 1 year (70,71). Particle migration to distant sites has been reported in humans as well. First reported by Mittleman and Marraccini in 1983 (72), a PTFE granuloma was found in the lung of a patient 2 years after injection. Claes et al. (73) reported on a patient experiencing fevers with biopsy-proven PTFE granulomas in the lung 3 years after PTFE injection. In another field, PTFE was used to inject the larynx for vocal cord paralysis. Twenty months after injection, a granuloma was found in the anterior lobe of the thyroid (74).

Despite granuloma formation, patients rarely have had any clinical consequences. It is the formation of granulomas and their association with cancer that is of more concern, although PTFE has not been linked to carcinogenesis with 30 years of use as a bulking agent for the urethra and larynx (76). In fact, there have been reported cases of cancer near PTFE injection sites, but none have demonstrated PTFE as the precipitating factor (77–79). This risk was reviewed by Dewan et al. (80). It was concluded that the available evidence did not support PTFE as a carcinogenic agent but suggested that if a risk existed, it was low. In 1995 Dewan et al. (80) reviewed the risk of both PTFE and Bioplastique in a rat model. A similar incidence of tumors was found in the PTFE, Bioplastique, and control groups. Additional late adverse events include fibrosis of the urethra and granuloma balls in the bladder at a rate of 15% (66). Currently, the U.S. Food and Drug Administration (FDA) is investigating the product.

### Key Concept

- *Particle migration with granuloma formation to distant sites has been reported, though patients rarely have had any clinical consequences.*

## Silicone Polymers (Macroplastique, Bioplastique)

Silicone polymers such as Macroplastique and Bioplastique are made of polydimethylsiloxane macroparticles suspended in a carrier hydrogel consisting of polyvinylpyrrolidone (povidone). The solid particles make up 33% of the total volume and are >100 μm in size. Silicone polymer was first used in 1992 with encouraging short-term follow-up. Like other agents as time progressed, the cure rate fell from an initial 82% to 70% at 14 months (82). In other studies with Macroplastique, 19.6% were considered cured and 41.1% significantly improved at 19 months (83). To date there has been one prospective, randomized study comparing Macroplastique to GAX-collagen in 62 women (85). The authors concluded that there was no significant objective difference between the two agents at 12 months. The only difference was that the Macroplastique group had less volume injected, although the pretreatment pad test loss was significantly less in that group.

Complications with the use of this material included urinary retention at a rate of 5.9% to 17.5%, urinary frequency at a rate of 0% to 72.4%, dysuria from 0% to 100%, and UTI from 0% to 6.25% (86). A study to determine the migratory properties of this material was performed on dogs. Small particles were found in the lungs, kidney, brain, and lymph nodes within 4 months of injection. In comparison, only one large particle was found in the lung without any associated reaction (87). In a rat model, four sarcomas with the Bioplastique group were associated with silicone particles. Given the recent controversy over silicone used in breast implants as well as the possibility of migration, it is unlikely that silicone will become a popular agent for intraurethral injections.

## Carbon-Coated Zirconium Beads (Durasphere and Durasphere EXP)

Durasphere, a new synthetic material, was approved by the FDA in 1999. It is composed of pyrolytic carbon-coated zirconium oxide beads in a 2.8% beta-glucan water-based gel. The bulking effect lasts for at least 2 years as the beads are encapsulated into the periurethral tissue. Compared to collagen, it is an inert and nonimmunogenic material, eliminating the need for skin testing. However, Durasphere can be more technically difficult to inject given its higher viscosity.

Durasphere was compared to GAX-collagen in a multicenter, randomized, controlled, double-blind study with follow-up at 1 year. The Durasphere group achieved improvement in one Stamey grade or more in 80% of patients compared to 69% of patients in the GAX-collagen group, although the difference did not reach statistical significance. Pad weights at 12 months were equivalent between the two groups. The Durasphere group had significantly less volume injected and were more successfully treated with a single injection (88). Although permanent, questions concerning longevity, similar to GAX-collagen, were brought forth. Panneck et al. (89) noted a decrease in success from 77% at 6 months to 33% at 12 months in a group of 13 women. In their study, one female patient was also noted to have asymptomatic distant particle migration into the regional and distal lymph nodes. Due to intraneedle resistance secondary to bead size, injection of Durasphere can be technically difficult. In response to this issue, Madjar et al. (90) used a periurethral approach at a single injection site. With 92% of 46 patients achieving excellent or good coaptation, 65% considered themselves cured or improved at a mean of 9.4 months. Additionally, 50% of 36 patients had a 24-hour pad test with 8 g or less of urine. Long-term data have been reported in a multicenter, comparative trial of Durasphere and GAX-collagen. Durasphere remained effective in 33% of patients at 24 months and in 21% at 36 months. Those who received GAX-collagen reported effectiveness in 19% of patients at 24 months and in 9% at 36 months. However, when controlled for differences in follow-up time, the time to failure between the two groups did not reach statistical significance. Interestingly, one third of each group felt that treatment was successful (91).

In the trials for FDA approval, the most common adverse events were acute retention ≤7 days) at 13%, dysuria at 12%, UTI at 9%, hematuria at 6%, and retention >7 days at 6%. Other adverse events occurred at ≤4% (92). There have also been case reports of sterile abscess formation.

Durasphere's beads are much larger than either PTFE or silicone polymers. In spite of their size, there have been reports of migration, although clear evidence is lacking. As determined by studies involving polytetrafluorethylene, macrophages are able to phagocytize particles smaller than 80 μm. Once phagocytized, the particles can then be carried to different parts of the body. Since Durasphere ranges from 212 to 500 μm, phagocytosis and therefore migration should not occur. Case reports involving beads found in lymphatics and other places are likely due to a high-pressure embolization effect, which may displace beads into vascular or lymphatic spaces. Delivery with large particles under low pressure should eliminate the risk of embolization. Durasphere-EXP is a modification of the original Durasphere that should allow lower-pressure injection due the smaller bead size (95 to 550 μm) yet above 80 μm to avoid migration.

## Key Concept

- *Durasphere achieved improvement in one Stamey grade or more in 80% of patients compared to 69% of patients in the GAX-collagen group, although the difference did not reach statistical significance.*

## Ethylene Vinyl Alcohol Copolymer (Tegress, Uryx)

Approved by the FDA in 2004, Tegress is composed of an 8% ethylene vinyl alcohol (EVOH) copolymer dissolved in dimethyl sulfoxide (DMSO), which is a permanent, hypoallergenic, nonimmunogenic implant. It comes prepared in 3-mL glass vials with a 3-mL DMSO-compatible syringe. The material is injected via a 25-gauge needle. Once Tegress is exposed to fluid within the tissue, the DMSO diffuses out, causing the precipitation of EVOH into a soft, spongy, hydrophilic material. The time required for the chemical reaction to occur is within 60 seconds. Care must be taken to avoid contamination of this agent with fluid prior to injection. At 1 month, an acute inflammatory response has been noted to be at its greatest. This effect lasts until 3 months, when the reaction has become more mild and localized with some resultant mineralization. There has been no evidence of EVOH affecting tissue at remote sites from the injection site. There also has been no evidence of migration.

When EVOH is used as a bulking agent, a different technique must be applied. If an excessive amount of material is injected, erosion through the urethral mucosa is likely to occur. To decrease the risk of erosion, the manufacturer suggests injecting at a more distal location in the urethra approximately 1.5 cm distal to the bladder neck. Each injection is to take place over 1 minute, with an additional minute of waiting to allow the chemical reaction to occur before removing the needle (95). When the needle is removed, a twisting motion often helps to separate the precipitated material off the needle tip and minimize the length of tail left at the injection site. Injections should not be performed until coaptation is noted, unlike with many of the other bulking agents. Urethral coaptation may suggest that too much material may have been injected.

Currently for EVOH, the only large study is from the trial for FDA approval. A multicenter, prospective, randomized trial was conducted with 177 of 253 women completing follow-up at 12 months comparing EVOH to GAX-collagen. The first 16 patients were excluded from the data since they were the first patients undergoing a new technique. At 12 months, efficacy was assessed by Stamey grade, pad weight, and quality-of-life questionnaire. Of those who received EVOH, 18.4% of patients were dry by Stamey grade compared to 16.5% of those who received collagen. The difference between the two groups regarding who had improvement by at least one Stamey grade did not reach clinical significance. In respect to pad weights, 37.8% were dry in the EVOH group compared to 32.1% undergoing collagen injection. This study resulted in FDA approval of EVOH (95,97).

In the trials for FDA approval, EVOH has been shown to have similar rates and severity of adverse events when compared to collagen. The one exception is the 16% rate of material exposure. During this study, it was noted that the exposure rate was higher with periurethral injection, and therefore this method is not recommended. Exposed material did not result in any adverse consequences and usually resolved. However, in the authors' experience, erosion rates of 37% in women and 41% in men necessitated multiple office visits for several patients with severe dysuria. Other common adverse events included UTI (29%), delayed voiding (18%), dysuria (18%), urinary urgency (14%), and frequency (13%). Interestingly, 9% of patients developed urge incontinence and 8% had worsening of incontinence. This injectable agent has been removed from utilization in the United States.

## Key Concepts

- *With EVOH, injections should not be performed until coaptation is noted, unlike with many of the other bulking agents.*

## Calcium hydroxyapatite (Coaptite)

Approved in December 2005, calcium hydroxyapatite is a synthetic agent that consists of carboxymethylcellulose in the form of an aqueous gel. Calcium hydroxyapatite is biocompatible, does not encapsulate, facilitates ingrowth of native tissues, and can be identified on radiographic studies as well as ultrasound. Another advantage includes ease of injection of material.

In a study with 1 year follow-up, 7 of 10 women reported substantial improvement in continence, a 90% decrease in mean pad weight, and an increase in mean Valsalva leak point pressure from 39 to 46 cm $H_2O$ (100). In the data for FDA approval, 158 patients received Coaptite with a mean follow-up of 11.2 months. No statistical difference was found in change in Stamey grade, pad weight, or quality of life when compared to GAX-collagen as the control. (101).

Common adverse events included urinary retention (41%), hematuria (19.6%), dysuria (15.2%), and UTI (8.3%). Changes in voiding occurred with urinary urgency at 7.6%, frequency at 7.0%, and urge incontinence at 5.7%. Two serious adverse events occurred: one erosion through the vaginal wall requiring surgery and dissection into the bladder causing tissue bridging, for which no surgical correction was needed. The overall erosion rate was 1.3% (101).

### Key Concept

- *No statistical difference was found in change in Stamey grade, pad weight, or quality of life when compared to GAX-collagen as the control.*

## FUTURE AGENTS

In patients with minimal urethrovesical junction mobility, ISD, and a stable bladder with an adequate capacity, intraurethral injections can offer treatment responses similar to that of surgical correction with minimal complications. However, most of these data are short-term; there is a scarcity of data over 5 years, with the majority of studies followed for much less time. For GAX-collagen, reinjection rates can be as high as 22% at 32 months after having achieved continence. The other injectable agents on the market have much fewer data and lack long-term follow-up. For younger patients, the cost of reinjection can become significant.

**TABLE 39.1**

| |
|---|
| Hyaluronic acid |
| Hyaluronic acid and dextranomer microspheres |
| Bioglass |
| Autologous tissue: chondrocytes (tissue engineering) in table |
| Myoblasts |
| Microballoons |

Although numerous injectable agents have entered the market over the last several years, the search for the ideal bulking agent continues. Listed in Table 39-1 are some of the current agents undergoing investigation.

## CONCLUSION

Currently, injectable agents are best used for those who are good candidates for successful treatment, those who wish to avoid a surgical procedure, or those who have problematic medical comorbidities that preclude them from undergoing surgical correction. Research continues the search for an effective, inert, nonmigratory, nonimmunogenic material that allows incorporation into native tissue, maintains its shape, and injects with ease. Currently, intraurethral bulking remains an art, as there is no exact measurement or amount of material used for each patient to achieve continence.

## *References*


1. Murless BC. The injection treatment of stress incontinence. *J Obstet Gynecol Br Emp* 1938;45:521–524.
2. Quackels R. Deux incontinences après adenectomie gueries par injection de paraffine dans la perinee. *Acta Urol Belg* 1955;23:259–262.
3. Sachse H. Treatment of urinary incontinence with sclerosing solutions: indications, results, complications. *Urol Int* 1963;15:225–244.
4. Dmochowski RR, Appell RA. Injectable agents in the treatment of stress urinary incontinence in women: where are we now? *Urology* 2000; 56[Suppl 6A]:32–40.
5. Crystle CD, Charme LS, Copeland WE. Q-tip test in stress urinary incontinence. *Obstet Gynecol* 1971;39:313–315.
6. Appell RA, Ostergard D. Practical urodynamics. *Illustrated Medicine, Female Urology Series* 1992;2:4–9.
7. Kreder KJ, Austin JC. Treatment of stress urinary incontinence in women with urethral hypermobility and intrinsic sphincter deficiency. *J Urol* 1996; 156:1995–1998.
8. Smith DN, Appell RA, Winters JC, et al. Collagen injection therapy for female intrinsic sphincter deficiency. *J Urol* 1997;152:1275–1278.
9. Herschorn S, Radomski SB, Steele DJ. Early experience with intraurethral collagen injection for urinary incontinence. *J Urol* 1992;148:1797–1800.
10. Herschorn S, Radomski SB. Collagen injections for genuine stress urinary incontinence: patient selection and durability. *Int Urogynecol J* 1997;8:18–24.
11. Faerber GJ. Endoscopic collagen injection therapy for elderly women with type I stress urinary incontinence. *J Urol* 1995;153:527A.
12. Winters J, Chiverton A, Scarpero H, et al. Collagen injection therapy in elderly women: long-term results and patient satisfaction. *Urology* 2000;55: 815–818.
13. Steele AC, Kohli N, Karram MM. Periurethral collagen injection for stress incontinence with and without urethral hypermobility. *Obstet Gynecol* 2000;95:322–331.
14. Bent AE, Foote J, Siegel S, et al. Collagen implant for treating stress urinary incontinence in women with urethral hypermobility. *J Urol* 2001;166(4): 1354–1357.
15. Winters JC. Urodynamics in the era of tension-free slings. *Curr Urol Rep* 2004;5(5):343–347.
16. O'Connell HE, McGuire EJ. Transurethral collagen therapy in women. *J Urol* 1995;154:1463–1465.
17. Appell RA. Injectables for urethral incompetence. *World J Urol* 1990;8: 208–211.
18. Appell RA. The periurethral injection of autologous blood. Presented at the American Urogynecologic Society annual meeting, Toronto, 1994.
19. Neal ED Jr, Lahaye ME, Lowe DC. Improved needle placement technique in periurethral collagen injection. *Urology* 1995;45:865–866.
20. Faerber GJ, Belville WD, Ohl DA, et al. Comparison of transurethral versus periurethral collagen injection in women with intrinsic sphincter deficiency. *Tech Urol* 1998;4(3):124–127.
21. Schulz JA, Nager CW, Stanton SL, et al. Bulking agents for stress urinary incontinence: short-term results and complications in a randomized comparison of periurethral and transurethral injection. *Int Urogynecol J Pelvic Floor Dysfunct* 2004;15:261–265.
22. Appell RA. Collagen injections. In: Raz S, ed. *Female urology*, 2nd ed. Philadelphia: WB Saunders, 1996:399–405.
23. Defreitas GA, Wilson TS, Zimmern PE, et al. Three-dimensional ultrasonography: an objective outcome to assess collagen distribution in women with stress urinary incontinence. *Urology* 2003;62:232–236.
24. Poon CI, Zimmern PE, Defreitas GA, et al. Three-dimensional ultrasonography to assess long-term durability of periurethral collagen in women with stress urinary incontinence due to intrinsic sphincteric deficiency. *Urology* 2005;65:60–64.
25. Cross CA, English SF, Cespedes RD, et al. A follow-up on transurethral collagen injection therapy for urinary incontinence. *J Urol* 1998;159:106–108.
26. Stothers L, Goldenberg SL, Leone EF. Complications of periurethral collagen injection for stress urinary incontinence. *J Urol* 1998;159(3):806–807.
27. Bergman A, Koonings PP, Ballard CA. Negative Q-tip test as a risk factor for failed incontinence surgery in women. *J Reprod Med* 1990;34(3):193–197.
28. Segal JL, Vasallo BJ, Kleeman SD, et al. The efficacy of tension-free vaginal tape in the treatment of five subtypes of stress urinary incontinence. *Int J Pelvic Floor Dysfunct* 2006;17(2):120–124.
29. Gonzalez de Garibay AS, Castro-Morrondo JM, Castro-Jimeno JM. Endoscopic injection of autologous adipose tissue in the treatment of female incontinence. *Arch Esp Urol* 1989;42:143–146.
30. Gonzalez de Garibay AS, Castillo-Jimeno JM, Villanueva-Perez PI. Treatment of urinary stress incontinence using paraurethral injection of autologous fat. *Arch Esp Urol* 1991;44:595–600.

31. Santarosa RP, Blaivas JG. Periurethral injection of autologous fat for the treatment of sphincteric incontinence. *J Urol* 1994;151:607–611.
32. Blaivas JG, Herwitz D, Santarosa RP, et al. Periurethral fat injection for sphincteric incontinence in women. *J Urol* 1994;151:419A.
33. Lee PE, Kung RC, Drutz HP. Periurethral autologous fat injection as treatment for female stress urinary incontinence: a randomized double-blind controlled trial. *J Urol* 2000;165:153–158.
34. Bartynski J, Marion MS, Wang TD. Histopathologic evaluation of adipose autografts in a rabbit ear model. *Otolaryngology* 1990;102:314.
35. Sweat SD, Lightner DJ. Complications of sterile abscess formation and pulmonary embolism following periurethral bulking agents. *J Urol* 1999;161:93–96.
36. Moalli PA, Shand SH, Zyczynski HM, et al. Remodeling of vaginal connective tissue in patients with pelvic organ prolpase. *Obstet Gynecol* 2005;106(5, Pt 1):953–963.
37. DeLustro F, Dasch J, Keefe J, et al. Immune response to allogeneic and xenogeneic implants of collagen and collagen derivatives. *Clin Orthop* 1990;260:263–279.
38. McPherson JM, Sawamura S, Armstrong R. An examination of the biologic response to injectable glutaraldehyde cross-linked collagen implants. *J Biomed Mater Res* 1986;20:93–97.
39. DeLustro F, Keefe J, Fong AT, et al. The biochemistry, biology, and immunology of injectable collagens: Contigen Bard collagen implant in treatment of urinary incontinence. *Pediatr Surg Int* 1991;6:245–251.
40. Canning DA, Peters CA, Gearhart JR, et al. Local tissue reaction to glutaraldehyde cross-linked bovine collagen in the rabbit bladder. *J Urol* 1988;139:258–259.
41. Remacle M, Marbaix E. Collagen implants in the human larynx. *Arch Otorhinolaryngol* 1988;245:203–209.
42. Appell RA. Collagen injection therapy for urinary incontinence. *Urol Clin North Am* 1994;21:177–182.
43. Appell RA. New developments: injectables for urethral incompetence in women. *Int Urogynecol J* 1990;1:117–119.
44. Appell RA, McGuire EJ, DeRidder PA, et al. Summary of effectiveness and safety in the prospective, open, multicenter investigation of Contigen implant for incontinence due to intrinsic sphincteric deficiency in females. *J Urol* 1994;151:418A.
45. Striker P, Haylen B. Injectable collagen for type 3 female stress incontinence: the first 50 Australian patients. *Med J Aust* 1993;158:89–91.
46. Swami SK, Eckford SD, Abrams P. Collagen injections for female stress incontinence: conclusions of a multistage analysis and results. *J Urol* 1994;151:479A.
47. Appell RA. Use of collagen injections for treatment of incontinence and reflux. *Adv Urol* 1992;5:145–165.
48. Richardson TD, Kennelly MJ, Faerber GJ. Endoscopic injection of glutaraldehyde cross-linked collagen for the treatment of intrinsic sphincteric deficiency in women. *Urology* 1995;46:378–381.
49. Corcos J, Fournier C. Periurethral collagen injection for the treatment of female stress urinary incontinence: 4-year follow-up results. *Urology* 1999;54:815–818.
50. Gorton E, Stanton S, Monga A, et al. Periurethral collagen injection: a long-term follow-up study. *BJU Int* 1999;84:966–971.
51. Bard CR, Inc. PMAA submission to United States Food and Drug Administration for IDE G850010, 1990.
52. Ford CN, Martin CW, Warren TF. Injectable collagen in laryngeal rehabilitation. *Laryngoscope* 1984;95:513–518.
53. Stegman S, Chu S, Bensch K, et al. A light and electron microscopic evaluation of Zyderm and Zyplast implants in aging human facial skin: a pilot study. *Arch Dermatol* 1987;123:1644–1649.
54. DeLustro F, Condell RA, Nguyen MA, et al. A comparative study of the biologic and immunologic response to medical devices derived from dermal collagen. *J Biomed Mater Res* 1986;20:109–120.
55. McLennan MT, Bent AE. Suburethral abscess: a complication of periurethral collagen injection therapy. *Obstet Gynecol* 1998;92:650–652.
56. Stothers L, Goldenberg SL. Delayed hypersensitivity and systemic arthralgia following transurethral collagen injection for stress urinary incontinence. *J Urol* 1998;159:1507–1509.
57. Berg S. Polytef augmentation urethroplasty: correction of surgically incurable urinary incontinence by injection technique. *Arch Surg* 1973;107:379–381.
58. Politano VA, Small MP, Harper JM, et al. Periurethral Teflon injection for urinary incontinence. *J Urol* 1974;111:180–183.
59. Heer H. Die Behandlung der Harnin-kontinenz mit der Teflon-paste. *Urol Int* 1977;32:295–302.
60. Lampante L, Kaesler FP, Sparwasser H. Endourethrale submukose Tefloninjektion zur Erzielung von Harninkontinenz. *Akt Urol* 1979;10:265–272.
61. Lim KB, Ball AJ, Feneley RCL. Periurethral Teflon injection: a simple treatment for urinary incontinence. *Br J Urol* 1983;55:208–210.
62. Schulman CC, Simon J, Wespes E, et al. Endoscopic injection of Teflon for female urinary incontinence. *Eur Urol* 1983;9:246–247.
63. Deane AM, English P, Hehir M, et al. Teflon injection in stress incontinence. *Br J Urol* 1985;57:78–80.
64. Appell RA. Commentary: periurethral polytetrafluoroethylene (Polytef) injection. In: Whitehead ED, ed. *Current operative urology*. Philadelphia: JB Lippincott, 1990:63–66.
65. Cole HM. Diagnostic and therapeutic technology assessment (DATTA). JAMA 1993;269:2975–2980.
66. Buckley JF, Lingham K, Meddings RN, et al. Injectable Teflon paste for female stress incontinence: long-term follow-up and results. *J Urol* 1993;149:418A.
67. Politano VA. Periurethral polytetrafluoroethylene injection for urinary incontinence. *J Urol* 1982;127:439–442.
68. Stone JW, Arnold GE. Human larynx injected with Teflon paste: histologic study of innervation and tissue reaction. *Arch Otolaryngol* 1967;86:550–562.
69. Politano VA. Periurethral Teflon injection for urinary incontinence. *Urol Clin North Am* 1978;5:415–422.
70. Malizia AA Jr, Reiman JM, Myers RP, et al. Migration and granulomatous reaction after periurethral injection of Polytef (Teflon). JAMA 1984;251:3277–3281.
71. Vandenbossche M, Delhobe O, Dumortier P, et al. Endoscopic treatment of reflux: experimental study and review of Teflon and collagen. *Eur Urol* 1994;23:386.
72. Mittleman RE, Marraccini JV. Pulmonary Teflon granulomas following periurethral Teflon injection for urinary incontinence. *Arch Pathol Lab Med* 1983;107:611–612.
73. Claes H, Stroobants D, van Meerbeek J, et al. Pulmonary migration following periurethral polytetrafluoroethylene injection for urinary incontinence. *J Urol* 1989;142:821–822.
74. Sanfilippo F, Shelburne J, Ingram P. Analysis of a Polytef granuloma mimicking a cold thyroid nodule 17 months after laryngeal injection. *Ultrastruc Pathol* 1980;1:471–475.
75. Oppenheimer BS, Oppenheimer ET, Stout AP, et al. The latent period in carcinogenesis by plastics in rats and its relation to the presarcomatous stage. *Cancer* 1958;11:204–213.
76. Hakky M, Kolbusz R, Reyes CV. Chondrosarcoma of the larynx. *Ear Nose Throat J* 1989;68:60–62.
77. Lewy RB. Experience with vocal cord injection. *Ann Otol Rhinol Laryngol* 1976;85:440–450.
78. Montgomery WW. Laryngeal paralysis-Teflon injection. *Ann Otol* 1979;88:647–657.
79. Dewan PA. Is injected polytetrafluoroethylene (Polytef) carcinogenic? *Br J Urol* 1992;69:29–33.
80. Dewan PA, Owen AJ, Byard RW. Long-term histological response to subcutaneously injected Polytef and Bioplastique in a rat model. *Br J Urol* 1995;76(2):161–164.
81. Buckley JF, Scott R, Meddings, et al. Injectable silicone microparticles: a new treatment for female stress incontinence. *J Urol* 1992;147:280A.
82. Buckley JF, Lingham K, Lloyd SN, et al. Injectable silicone macroparticles for female urinary incontinence. *J Urol* 1993;149:402A.
83. Radley SC, Chapple CR, Mitsogiannis IC, et al. Transurethral implantation of Macroplastique for the treatment of female stress urinary incontinence secondary to intrinsic sphincteric deficiency. *Eur Urol* 2001;39:383–389.
84. Tamanini JT, D'Ancona CA, Tadini V, et al. Macroplastique implantation system for female stress urinary incontinence. *J Urol* 2003;169:2229–2233.
85. Anders K, Khullar V, Cardozo L, et al. Gax-Collagen or Macroplastique: does it make a difference? *Neururol Urodynam* 1999;18:297–298.
86. Ter Meulen PH, Berghmans LC, van Kerrebroeck PE. Systematic review: efficacy of silicone microimplants (Macroplastique) therapy for stress urinary incontinence in adult women. *Eur Urol* 2003;44:573–582.
87. Henly DR, Barrett DM, Weiland TL, et al. Particulate silicone for use in periurethral injections: local tissue effects and search for migration. *J Urol* 1995;153:2039–2043.
88. Lightner D, Calvosa C, Andersen R, et al. A new injectable bulking agent for treatment of stress urinary incontinence: results of a multicenter, randomized, controlled, double-blind study of Durasphere. *Urology* 2001;58:12–15.
89. Pannek J, Brands FH, Senge T. Particle migration after transurethral injection of carbon coated beads for stress urinary incontinence. *J Urol* 2001;166:1350–1353.
90. Madjar S, Covington-Nichols C, Secrest CL. New periurethral bulking agent for stress urinary incontinence: modified technique and early results. *J Urol* 2003;170:2327–2329.
91. Chrouser KL, Fick F, Goel A, et al. Carbon coated zirconium beads in beta-glucan gel and bovine glutaraldehyde cross-linked collagen injections for intrinsic sphincteric deficiency: continence and satisfaction after extended follow-up. *J Urol* 2004;171:1152–1155.
92. United States Food and Drug Administration: Durasphere injectable bulking agent. Summary of safety and effectiveness data. www.fda.gov/cdrh/pdf/p980053.html, 1999.
93. Madjar S, Sharma AK, Waltzer WC, et al. Periurethral mass formations following bulking agent injection for the treatment of urinary incontinence. *J Urol* 2006;175:1408–1410.
94. Ritts RE. Particle migration after transurethral injection of carbon coated beads. *J Urol* 2002;167:1804–1805.
95. United States Food and Drug Administration: URYX urethral bulking agent-P030030 Part II: summary of safety and effectiveness data. http://www.fda.gov/cdrh/PDF3/p030030b, 2004.

96. Dmochowski RR, Appell RA. Advancements in minimally invasive treatments for female stress urinary incontinence: radiofrequency and bulking agents. *Curr Urol Rep* 2003;4:350–355.
97. Dmochowski RR. Tegress urethral implant phase III clinical experience and product uniqueness. *Rev Urol* 2005;7[Suppl 1]:S22–S26.
98. Hurtado EA, McCrery RJ, Appell RA. The safety and efficacy of Ethylene Vinyl Alcohol copolymer as an intra-urethral bulking agent in women with intrinsic urethral deficiency. *Int Urogynecol J* 2006 *(in press)*.
99. Hurtado EA, McCrery RJ, Appell RA. Ethylene Vinyl Alcohol copolymer as an intra-urethral bulking agent in men with stress urinary incontinence. *J Urol* 2006 *(in press)*.
100. Mayer R, Lightfoot M, Jung I. Prelimiinary evaluation of calcium hydroxylapatite as a transurethral bulking agent for stress urinary incontinence. *Urology* 2001;57:434–438.
101. United States Food and Drug Administration: Coaptite implanted device. www.fda.gov/cdrh/mda/docs/p040047.html, 2005.
102. Winters JC, Appell RA. Periurethral injection of collagen in the treatment of intrinsic sphincteric deficiency in the female patient. *Urol Clin North Am* 1995;22:673–678.
103. Biomatrix Corporation. Formal report of feasibility study of Hylagel Uro. Corporate White Paper. Ridgefield, NJ, June 2000.
104. Stenberg A, Larsson G, Johnson P, et al. DiHA Dextran Copolymer, a new biocompatible material for endoscopic treatment of stress incontinent women. *Acta Obstet Gynecol Scand* 1999;78:436–442.
105. Stenberg A, Larsson G, Johnson P. Urethral injection for stress urinary incontinence: long-term results with dextranomer/hyaluronic acid copolymer. *Int Urogynecol J Pelvic Dysfunct* 2003;14:335–338.
106. Van Kerrebroeck P, ter Meulen F, Larsson G, et al. Efficacy and safety of a novel system (NASHA/Dx copolymer using the Implacer device) for treatment of stress urinary incontinence. *Urology* 2004;64:276–281.
107. Walker RS, Wilson K, Clark AE. Injectable bioglass as a potential substitute for injectable polytetrafluorethylene. *J Urol* 1992;148:645–647.
108. Atala A, Cima LG, Kim W, et al. Injectable alginate seeded with chondrocytes as a potential treatment for vesicoureteral reflux. *J Urol* 1993;150: 745–747.
109. Bent AE, Tutrone RT, McLennan, et al. Treatment of intrinsic sphincter deficiency using autologous ear chondrocytes as a bulking agent. *Neurourol Urodynam* 2001;20:157–165.
110. Yokoyama T, Chancellor MB, Watanabe T, et al. Primary myoblast injection into urethra and bladder as a potential treatment of stress urinary incontinence and impaired detrusor contractility: long-term survival without significant cytotoxicity. *J Urol* 2000;161:307.
111. Cannon TW, Lee JY, Somogyi G, et al. Improved sphincter contractility after allogenic muscle-derived progenitor cell injection into the denervated rat urethra. *Urology* 2003;62:958–963.
112. Peyromaure M, Sebe P, Praud C, et al. Fate of implanted syngenic muscle precursor cells in striated urethral sphincter of female rats: perspectives for the treatment of urinary incontinence. *Urology* 2004;64:1037–1041.
113. Pycha A, Klinger CH, Haitel A, et al. 3 years experience with implantable microballoons for the treatment of intrinsic sphincter deficiency. *J Urol* 2000;161:307.


# CHAPTER 40 ■ PUBOVAGINAL FASCIAL SLINGS

ANNE PELLETIER CAMERON, CHRISTINA LEWICKY-GAUPP, AND EDWARD J. McGUIRE

The first urethral sling procedure was described by Giordano in 1907. This procedure was modified numerous times and employed several different sling materials, yet it never gained popularity because of the high incidence of permanent urinary retention, de novo detrusor overactivity, and urethral erosion. The pubovaginal autologous fascial sling (PVS) was repopularized by McGuire and Lytton in 1978 when they reported their modification of the technique with little morbidity and 80% success in a complicated population with urodynamic proven intrinsic sphincter deficiency (ISD)(1). In a more contemporary series with 247 patients who had either Type II or III stress urinary incontinence (SUI) and 44% patients who had concomitant urge incontinence, the authors reported a cure rate of 91% for Type II incontinence and 84% for Type III. Also in this series, of those patients with preoperative urge incontinence, 74% had resolution after surgery (2). Other authors have duplicated these results, with cure or improvement in up to 92% of women with >10 years of follow-up (3).

Female SUI is classified as being due to urethral hypermobility (Type I and Type II SUI), intrinsic sphincter deficiency (Type III SUI), or a combination of the two. In Type I and II SUI the urethral sphincter functions essentially normally, but abdominal pressure drives the sphincter into a position where its function is compromised. Therefore, procedures that correct this urethral hypermobility, such as the Burch colposuspension or synthetic midurethral slings, are effective. In contrast, ISD is characterized by a relatively immobile urethra with urethral sphincter weakness or scarring resulting in leakage with increases in abdominal pressure. This is not effectively treated by correcting only hypermobility. Splitting SUI into these two distinct categories is not quite that simple because urethral hypermobility and ISD are not mutually exclusive. It is important to note that the severities of urethral hypermobility and sphincteric incompetence are on a continuum and that both exist to some degree in all incontinent patients. Also, significant urethral hypermobility can be present in a woman, yet she can be completely continent since her sphincteric mechanism is intact (4).

Traditionally, many urologists routinely used a PVS for all types of incontinence since it effectively corrected both ISD and urethral hypermobility. In 1996 Ulmsten et al. (5) introduced an effective synthetic midurethral sling procedure that was minimally invasive and very effective for SUI secondary to urethral hypermobility [Tension-Free Vaginal Tape (TVT, Gynecare)]. In later studies, the TVT has been shown to be somewhat effective in treating ISD; however, success rates vary significantly, from 17.0% to 91.4% (6,7). The polypropylene midurethral sling and its modifications (including the transobturator route of sling placement: the TOT) have changed the landscape of stress incontinence surgery. The need to determine if a patient has a small amount of ISD versus pure hypermobility is less critical, and for many surgeons synthetic slings are their operation of choice for primary treatment of SUI. Currently, more invasive surgery like the pubovaginal sling is reserved for specific indications.

## DIAGNOSIS

Preoperative evaluation is directed toward identifying ISD, which can often be done on history, as these patients have severe leakage with minimal activity. ISD only occurs in 9% of women with SUI who have never had any incontinence surgery, but that percentage increases to 25% if they have had one prior failed incontinence surgery and to 75% after two failures (8). Concurrent urgency symptoms are not uncommon, and most patients have a history of multiple urethral or vaginal surgeries, have had radiation therapy, or are elderly. Neurologic ISD is characterized by severe incontinence with total nonfunction of the proximal sphincter and an open bladder neck on fluoroscopic urodynamics (FUDS). It is common in myelodysplasia, sacral agenesis, and T12–L1 spinal cord injuries. These injuries result in loss of the sympathetic innervation of the urethra at a central level, and the incontinence is almost always due to ISD.

## PHYSICAL EXAMINATION

The physical examination is directed toward the pelvis. A thorough vaginal examination in the supine position with a half-speculum both at rest and with straining is essential. If present, prolapse should be identified, since it can be concomitantly repaired to achieve optimal surgical success. If the patient has had previous vaginal or pelvic surgery, the mucosa should be assessed thoroughly for the possibility of a fistula or erosion of foreign material. The urethra should be palpated for lesions and then visualized at rest and with straining to assess for hypermobility. We do not routinely perform a Q-tip test, but if there is any uncertainty about the amount of hypermobility, one can be performed. A supine stress test should then be done to identify urethral incontinence. One can safely presume that a patient with an immobile urethra plus severe SUI has ISD.

## INVESTIGATIONS

One should always confirm the absence of urinary tract infection with a urinalysis. If infection is present, it must be treated preoperatively. A cystoscopy is performed if hematuria is present to rule out malignancy or if the patient has had previous incontinence surgery to rule out suture or tape erosion. Routine cystoscopy is not necessary.

Urodynamic evaluation is performed on patients with severe incontinence or mixed symptoms. A postvoid residual is measured before insertion of the urodynamic catheter. A cystometrogram is then carried out to rule out poor detrusor compliance and detrusor overactivity (DO). Poor compliance needs to be medically or surgically treated before PVS placement or the upper tracts can be at risk of deterioration after the outlet no longer leaks. Also, one needs to counsel patients that although DO may actually resolve 74% to 77% of the time (2,3), it may persist or worsen. The urodynamic abdominal leak point pressure (ALPP) is the key to diagnosing ISD. With the bladder filled to 200 mL (with children to one-half their functional bladder capacity) and the patient in an upright position, a Valsalva maneuver is performed until leakage is noted. If no leakage can be elicited with several well-performed Valsalva maneuvers, vigorous coughing can be used with the knowledge that the ALPP will be falsely elevated. If the patient has significant prolapse, it should be reduced with a vaginal pack or pessary to ensure that the prolapse is not masking the incontinence. Even if the patient has SUI without reduction of the prolapse, placement of a vaginal pack will often demonstrate a greatly reduced ALPP, which can change the contemplated procedure. The exact urodynamic definition of ISD is controversial, with some authors utilizing maximum urethral closure pressure (MUCP) $\leq$20 cm $H_2O$ (6), others valsalva leak point pressure (VLPP) $<$60 cm $H_2O$ (2), and some the combination (7). We consider an ALPP $<$60 cm $H_2O$ to be consistent with ISD. A pubovaginal sling is ideal to correct this kind of severe incontinence. Pure urethral hypermobility is an ALPP $>$90 cm $H_2O$, and a gray area exists where both hypermobility and ISD coexist between 60 and 90 cm $H_2O$. Both of these latter conditions with less severe incontinence, barring contraindications, are well suited for a midurethral sling.

## INDICATIONS FOR SURGERY

Before the era of the TVT and TOT, a pubovaginal sling could be used to treat any kind of incontinence. However, since these minimally invasive procedures carry less morbidity, they have become the primary treatment for uncomplicated stress incontinence. Pubovaginal slings are now reserved for the following specific indications:

1. **Severe ISD:** Severe ISD with an ALPP $<$60 cm $H_2O$, especially when combined with little urethral hypermobility, is poorly treated with the minimally invasive midurethral slings. Cure rates are reported to be as low as 17% if both conditions coexist (6). An autologous PVS is ideal in this instance, and success is expected to be from 84% to 92% even in the presence of DO (2,3).
2. **Neurogenic incontinence:** Children or adults with neurogenic voiding dysfunction from myelodysplasia, sacral agenesis, or T12-S1 spinal cord injury are ideal candidates for autologous PVS (Fig. 40.1). Their incontinence is invariably due to ISD, and they have both proximal sphincter dysfunction and an open bladder neck that requires a compressive sling to resolve their leakage (9). The anatomy is similar with incontinence from a pelvic nerve injury secondary to rectal surgery, a traumatic pelvic crush injury, or posthemipelvectomy incontinence. Midurethral slings are designed to be tension-free and do not compress the urethra. In addition, many of these patients have an areflexic bladder or have had augmentation cystoplasty and require lifelong clean intermittent catheterization that could cause urethral erosion in the presence of synthetic mesh. Also, the use of an autologous material for a PVS is especially important in the pediatric population since it will grow with the child and can safely allow vaginal delivery if the child has a pregnancy later in life (9).
3. **Failed midurethral sling:** If patients have persistent stress incontinence after a midurethral sling, it is possible that they had severe ISD initially. Their persistent incontinence is unlikely to be corrected by placing another midurethral sling. A prior midurethral sling does not make placement of a PVS more difficult or less successful.

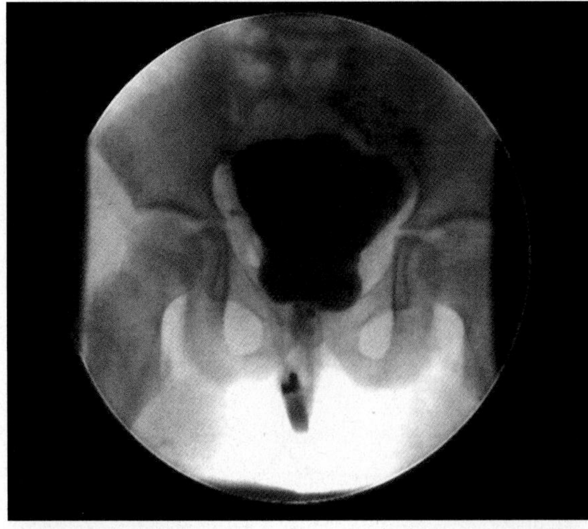

A

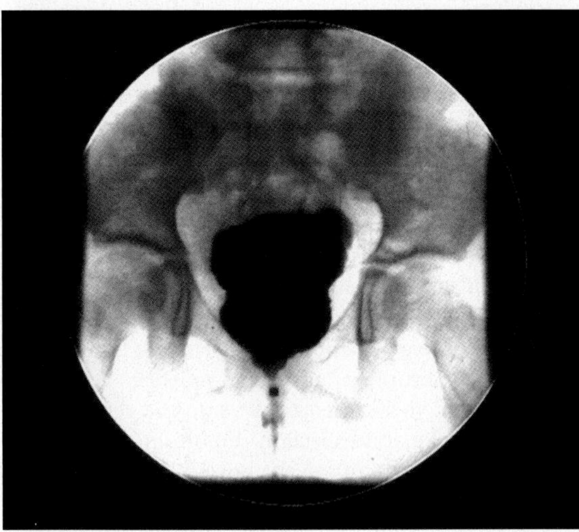

B

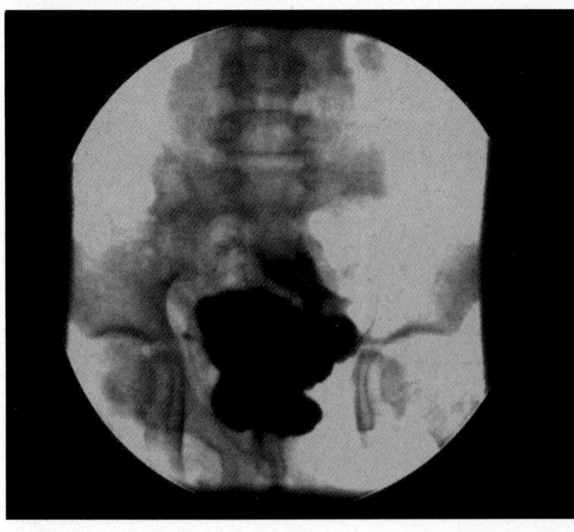

C

FIGURE 40.1 **A:** Fluoroscopic urodynamics (FUDS) image of a girl with myelomeningocele and a previous bladder augmentation with small bowel. She has an artificial sphincter in place, but it has eroded and requires removal. **B:** After removal she has severe stress incontinence from a wide-open bladder neck. **C:** A pubovaginal sling (PVS) was placed and this girl is now continent.

4. **Previous tape erosion:** Any patients with erosion of tape or mesh into the urethra are at high risk of ISD after removal and may have some urethral tissue loss. They should not have any more synthetic material placed in their vagina due to a high risk of re-erosion or urethrovaginal fistula formation. Also, any patients with persistent incontinence and a vaginal extrusion of mesh or a tape are better served with removal of the foreign body and a PVS rather than placement of more mesh.
5. **Contraindications to midurethral slings:** There are several conditions in which urethral reconstruction is necessary, such as an eroded urethra from a neglected indwelling catheter, severe urethral stricture requiring female urethroplasty, urethrovaginal fistula, or a urethral diverticulum. In these procedures, mesh cannot be left near the healing urethra because there is a significant risk of erosion and/or fistula formation. A pubovaginal sling provides another tissue layer of closure for the urethral repair that actually promotes healing. Similarly, if a patient has SUI and has had bladder or cervical radiation, the placement of synthetic material in the vagina is at high risk for complications like erosion, so only autologous tissue PVS should be used. Other specific circumstances in which the use of synthetics is contraindicated include neobladder-related SUI or any other previous bowel substitution of the urethra.
6. **Permanent clean intermittent catheterization:** In any instance where lifelong clean intermittent catheterization (CIC) will be required, an autologous material should be used, as patients are at risk for urethral erosion of their mesh.

## ALTERNATIVE THERAPY

Midurethral slings do have moderate success in cases of milder ISD, and they could be attempted with the knowledge that the success will not be equivalent to a PVS. For patients with significant comorbidities and high surgical risk, urethral calcium hydroxyapatite or collagen injections are a good option for ISD. Published results show a 74% to 71% improvement in incontinence and a 39% to 37% cure with an average of two injections (10). Urinary diversion is a last resort when a pubovaginal sling would be impossible, such as in instances of complete urethral loss or concomitant intractable vesicovaginal fistula.

## SURGICAL TECHNIQUE

A single dose of a prophylactic antimicrobial agent is administered, and the patient is given a general or spinal anesthetic. The procedure is performed in a low modified dorsal lithotomy position using Allen stirrups. A 16Fr urethral catheter is placed, and the balloon is inflated with 10 mL of water to allow palpation of the bladder neck. Preparation and draping of the patient is done in a manner to allow for the simultaneous exposure of the vagina and lower abdomen. We prefer to perform the abdominal dissection first to minimize vaginal bleeding.

In order to harvest the autologous fascial sling, an 8- to 10-cm Pfannenstiel skin incision is made 2 cm above the symphysis. This incision is carried down to the underlying fascia, and the subcutaneous fatty tissue is cleaned off the fascia. A

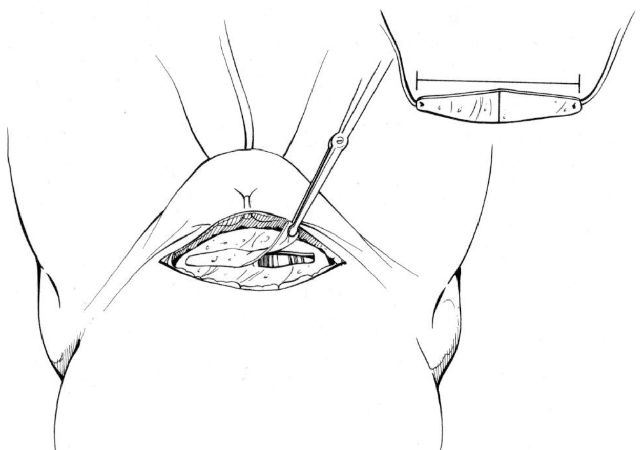

FIGURE 40.2 Harvesting of the rectus abdominis fascial sling. The sling should be at least 8 to 10 cm long and 1.5 to 2.0 cm wide in the center. The sling ends are folded and then sutured with 1-0 absorbable sutures incorporating all of the fibers.

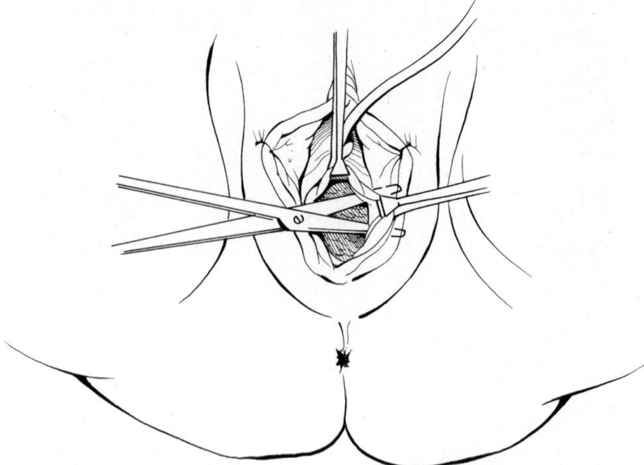

FIGURE 40.3 The vaginal dissection is performed superficially to the white periurethral fascia. With the scissors parallel to the plane of the perineum and tips pointing superiorly and laterally, the retropubic space is entered and subsequently enlarged by further advancing the scissors 1 to 2 cm and then opening them.

relatively scar-free area of fascia is selected for the sling, but even thickened and scarred fascia can be used with success. Using a scalpel, the fascia is incised 2 cm above the symphysis in the midline. With the Metzenbaum scissors, the incision is carried out laterally, parallel to the fibers. The superior leaf of the fascia is grasped with two Allis clamps and the underlying rectus muscles dissected off for a distance of 2 to 3 cm. The inferior leaf is then freed in a similar fashion. This aggressive mobilization will later allow a tension-free fascial closure. Next, the sling should be harvested from the inferior leaf. The upper leaf can alternatively be used if the tissue appears healthier or stronger. The sling should ideally be 8 to 10 cm long, 1.5 cm wide in the midline, and tapered to about 1 cm on either end (Fig. 40.2). The ends of the sling are tapered to facilitate its passage through the endopelvic fascia. Using 0-Vicryl or Prolene, both ends of the sling are then sutured 0.5 cm from the end of the sling. A figure-of-eight stitch is placed and then tied and cut, leaving 15 cm of free suture. Once the sling is harvested, it is placed in normal saline.

Attention should now be turned to the vaginal dissection. If necessary, the position of the patient's legs can be adjusted for better visualization. A weighted vaginal speculum is placed. Using the catheter as a reference, the urethrovesical junction is identified via palpation. To assist with hemostasis, the vaginal mucosa can then be injected with a dilute vasopressin solution (we prefer 10 U or 0.5 mL of vasopressin in 50 mL of normal saline). The mucosa inferolateral to the urethral meatus is grasped with two Allis clamps and traction placed superiorly for the entire vaginal part of the procedure. An inverted U incision is made in the vaginal epithelium at the level of the midurethra (1 to 2 cm proximal to the urethral meatus) using a scalpel. This flap is carefully dissected down to the level of the periurethral fascia using Church scissors and carried out laterally to the endopelvic fascia with the Metzenbaum scissors. Then, using blunt-tipped scissors, the retropubic space is entered by perforating the endopelvic fascia bilaterally using a careful "push and spread" technique (Fig. 40.3).

In the abdominal incision, the transverse fascia can be seen with medial retraction on the lateral border of the rectus muscle. It appears as a yellowish cleft where the rectus muscle inserts on the symphysis. The fascia is bluntly perforated, and a tunnel is created by hugging the posterior aspect of the pubic symphysis to avoid perforating the bladder. The blunt dissection continues distally to the level of the bladder neck (Fig. 40.4). If the patient has not had prior surgeries, this tissue plane is easily dissected. However, if the patient has had prior procedures (e.g., retropubic suspension, bone-anchored sling, or transobturator tape placement), Metzenbaum scissors may need to be used to develop the retropubic tunnels. In this instance, it is especially important to place the tips of the scissors only directly on the posterior pubis periosteum to avoid bladder or vascular injury. Also, scarring may necessitate starting the tunnel dissection between the two rectus

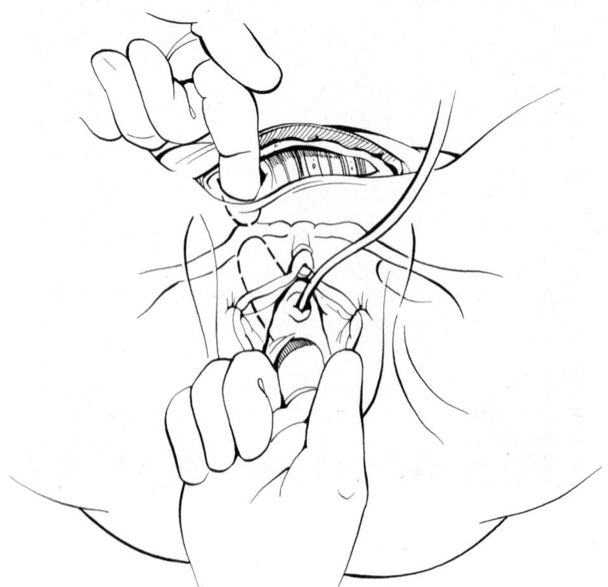

FIGURE 40.4 Blunt finger dissection creates a tunnel to the rectus muscles above. Wide dissection is unnecessary and may cause significant bleeding or bladder injury.

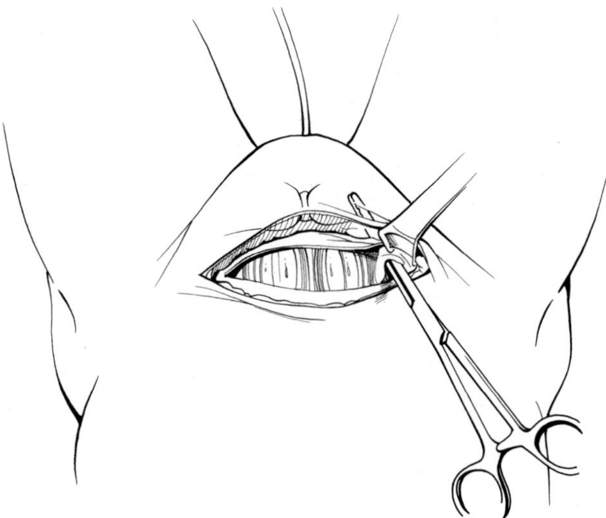

FIGURE 40.5 The approach to the retropubic space from above is located below the rectus fascia and lateral to where the rectus muscles attach to the pubic symphysis. Minimal dissection in the area allows safe and easy access to the retropubic space previously dissected by the vaginal operator.

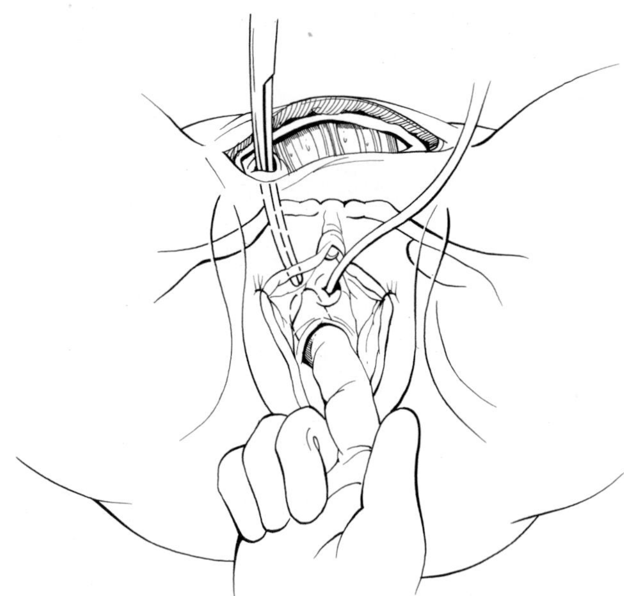

FIGURE 40.6 Using manual guidance, a Crawford clamp is passed from above toward the vaginal incision with the tip of the clamp in contact with the pubic periosteum and the vaginal operator's finger. After the passage of clamps bilaterally, cystoscopy is performed to ensure no injury to the bladder has occurred.

muscles (rather than lateral to them) before developing the retropubic space.

Ultimately, the bladder should be cleared from the created tunnels, and the tunnel should easily accommodate one finger. This step ensures that the sling will be easily advanced through the endopelvic fascia once it is placed and that the bladder will not be perforated with passage of the sling.

A long curved clamp such as the Crawford clamp or, in cases of scarring, the McGuire ligature passer, can be used to pass the sling through the created tunnels. The ligature can be passed either from "bottom to top" or "top to bottom." Generally, we prefer to pass from "top to bottom" unless there is severe vaginal scarring. In order to accomplish this, the carrier is gently advanced into the created cleft lateral to the rectus from above until its leading flat portion is in contact with the symphysis (Fig. 40.5). Now with one hand above and one below in the vagina, it is advanced along the symphysis until its tip is palpable from the vaginal incision (Fig. 40.6). Then the carrier is advanced past the bladder into the vaginal incision over one's finger. There are typically only a few millimeters of tissue that need to be perforated during this step. If more tissue is present, one has to be highly suspicious that the bladder has not been mobilized sufficiently and is at risk of perforation. The sling sutures on one end are loaded on the passer, which is then pulled back up into the abdominal incision and marked with a clamp. The same procedure is repeated on the opposite side. The sling is now in a position behind the proximal urethra with both suture ends in the suprapubic incision. After each pass of the ligature carrier, cystoscopy should be performed to ensure bladder integrity. The longevity of the sling does not depend on the sutures to hold tension (because they are absorbable); rather, it depends on the sling being well advanced into the retropubic space bilaterally. Thus, it is critical that a good portion of the sling extends into the retropubic space to allow proper fixation with healing (Fig. 40.7).

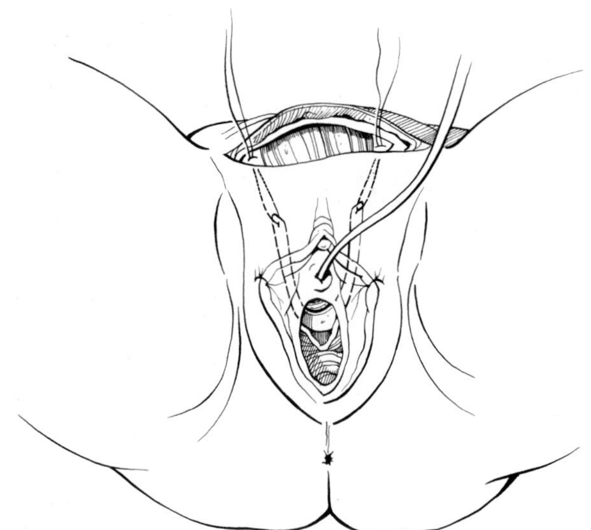

FIGURE 40.7 The sling ends are pulled well into the retropubic space to allow good fixation. The sling is seated at the proximal urethra and sutured to the periurethral fascia using 3-0 absorbable sutures.

Next, the center of the sling is anchored to the midline periurethral tissues with a fine, absorbable suture. This is to prevent malpositioning of the sling with tensioning later. The vaginal epithelium is then closed with an absorbable suture in a running fashion to maintain hemostasis.

Tensioning the sling is the final abdominal portion of the procedure. Using a pointed-tip clamp like a Tonsil, two lateral perforations are made through the inferior leaf of the rectus fascia. The sling sutures are passed through these perforations and marked with clamps. The rectus fascia is then

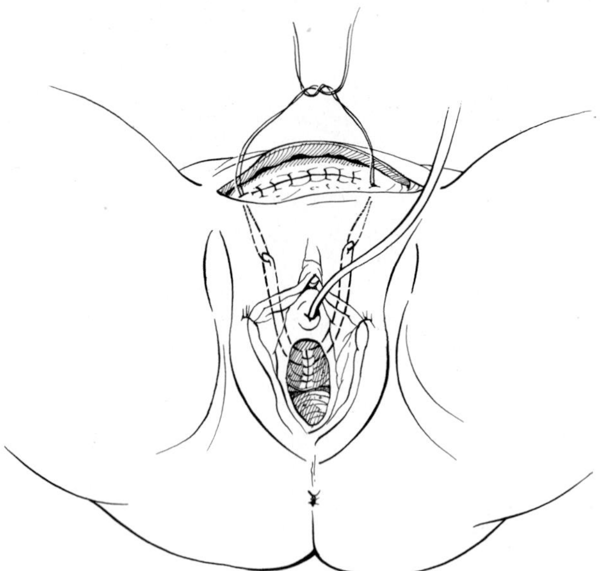

FIGURE 40.8 The sling sutures are passed through the rectus fascia before the fascia is closed. The vaginal mucosa is closed, the weighted speculum removed, and the sling sutures tied down over the rectus fascia under minimal tension.

closed using a running delayed absorbable suture (Fig. 40.8). The sling can then be tensioned. The appropriate tension is the minimum amount required to stop urethral motion. This can be judged by pulling on the transurethral catheter and ensuring that the bladder neck descends no >0.5 to 1.0 cm. A shodded clamp can be used to hold tension on the crossed sutures until this appropriate tension is obtained (Fig. 40.9). The sutures are then tied down. Two fingers should be able to be passed under the sutures in the suprapubic incision. Finally, the skin is closed with an absorbable fine suture such as 4-0 Monocryl, and a vaginal pack is placed if needed.

The urethral catheter and any vaginal packing are removed the following morning, and patients are started on CIC. Once they are adept at self-catheterization, they are discharged home. Most patients are discharged on the first postoperative day since they were given instructions on CIC preoperatively.

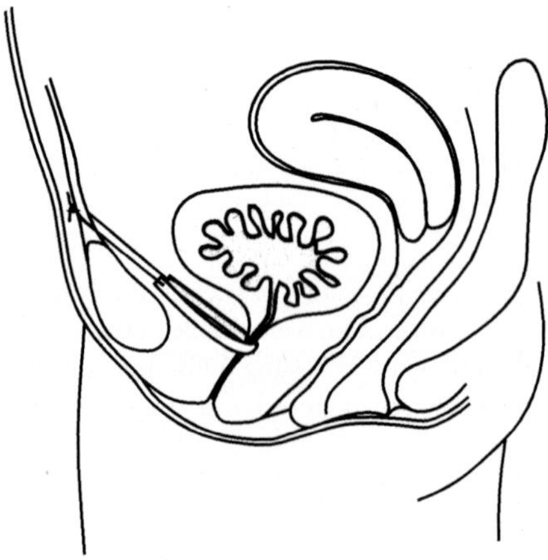

FIGURE 40.9 A lateral view of the completed pubovaginal sling procedure.

## Crossover Sling

In patients with a widely open bladder neck and proximal urethra, such as with myelomeningocele or with extremely low ALPP (<10 cm $H_2O$), more circumferential compression is required from the sling. To accomplish this, the sling can be "crossed over." The sling is harvested longer than usual (10 to 14 cm). During retropubic dissection, not only are tunnels created, but the entire retropubic space is dissected to expose the anterior bladder and proximal urethra. The sling is passed in the usual fashion and fixed on the urethra through the vaginal incision, but before passing the sling sutures through the fascial perforations, they are crossed over, allowing the sling to surround the bladder neck rather than just suspending it. The sutures are tied as usual, but tensioning is more difficult to judge since the force is compressive (Fig. 40.10).

## Alternative Graft Material

When considering choices for sling graft materials, there is much debate in the literature. Some have advocated decreasing the potential morbidity of harvesting the sling by using allografts such as cadaveric fascia (11) or other synthetic materials. However, autologous fascia has been shown to have better surgical outcomes than any of these other materials. Several synthetic materials have been used as sling material for the PVS: woven polyester injected with collagen (ProteGen, recalled from market), polytetrafluoroethylene (Gore-Tex), silicone, and polypropylene. They have all been associated with significant complications like fistulas and urethral and vaginal erosions (12), and none are in common usage for PVS.

Recently, Howden et al. (13) compared cadaveric with autologous fascial slings in 303 women. They found that the group of women who underwent placement of cadaveric fascia had a higher rate of urinary incontinence (16 versus 5 per 100 woman-years, $p = 0.0001$) and had greater reoperation rates (4 versus 1 per 100 woman-years, $p < 0.0003$) than the group with autologous fascia. Several studies have also shown

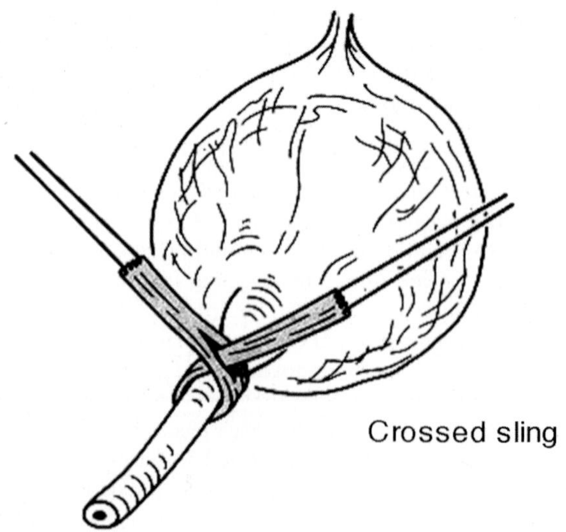


FIGURE 40.10 This crossed sling surrounds the urethra. It provides a more compressive force than a traditional sling. For ease of placement, a slit can be made in the center of the sling and the other end threaded through.

superior continence in the use of autologous fascia over the porcine xenograft Pelvichol as a PVS (14). While autologous fascia remains the sling material of choice, Pevichol is a viable alternative when native fascia cannot be harvested due to poor quality. Autologous fascia lata is a good-quality alternative to rectus fascia (11), but its use is limited because it requires another incision.

## OUTCOMES

### Complications

#### Bladder Perforation and Hematoma

Bladder perforation is very rare during PVS, since the bladder is exposed during dissection. It has been reported to occur in only 0.6% of cases in two large series (3,15). This is much lower in comparison to other surgeries for SUI like the TVT (8.6%) (7) and the Burch (3%) (15). Bladder perforation occurs during passage of the ligature from above and is detected either by cystoscopy or by observing that the urine is bloody. The clamp should be repassed and its position verified by cystoscopy. A urethral catheter should be left in place for 7 to 10 days while on antibiotic prophylaxis and a voiding trial done upon removal. Pelvic hematoma can also occur in 0.8% (2) of cases, and these patients should be followed closely for superinfection.

#### Prolonged Urinary Retention

With autologous pubovaginal slings, all women will need to initially perform CIC for a period of approximately 2 weeks, with an average of 8.4 days (2). Thus, all patients should be given preoperative instructions about CIC technique and reassured that this is a common occurrence. However, the prolonged need for CIC for >6 weeks occurs in 2.0% to 13.5% of women (2,3,14) and requires surgical intervention in 2.5% to 6.3% (2,3,15). It is our practice to surgically intervene with vaginal midline sling incision at a maximum of 4 to 6 weeks, should spontaneous voiding not return. The goal of this procedure is not to remove the sling, but to simply divide it in the middle. It is a straightforward procedure with little morbidity, and surprisingly few patients have recurrence of their SUI. Thiel et al. (16) reported a case series with 11 patients who had their PVS cut at an average of 65 days after surgery. Even after 5 years of follow-up, 7 out of 11 patients had no incontinence episodes per day, and only 1 out of 11 had more than three episodes of incontinence daily, with all 11 patients voiding spontaneously.

#### De Novo Urge Incontinence

Many patients have preexisting urge incontinence, and this should not preclude PVS placement, since as many as 74% to 77% (2,3) will actually have resolution of their urge incontinence along with their stress incontinence. De novo, or new-onset, urge incontinence will occur in 3% to 7% (2,3,15) of patients. One needs to ensure that bladder outlet obstruction is not present, since the symptoms of these two conditions often overlap. They can be differentiated with a careful history, physical examination, postvoid residual, and often urodynamic examination. For de novo urge incontinence or overactive bladder symptoms that persist in the postoperative period, anticholinergic medications are helpful and often can be discontinued after 3 months (1). If patients do have actual obstruction, they require midline sling incision.

#### Erosion

Erosion of sling material into the urethra or vagina is a difficult complication to treat, especially with synthetic materials. Although not impossible, the occurrence of autologous PVS has been reported in a few series, but the rate is estimated to be as low as 0.007% (12).

### Results

In 1998, Chaikin et al. (3) found that 92% of 251 women with Type II or Type III SUI who underwent placement of a pubovaginal sling had cure or improvement of their incontinence at a follow-up of 3 years with durable results at ten years. Similarly, Morgan et al. (2) reported continence rates of 88% at 4 years in 247 patients after sling placement. Of this cohort, 92% reported that they were "highly satisfied" with their outcomes on a quality-of-life assessment. A randomized controlled trial involving 520 women by the Urinary Incontinence Treatment Network (15) compared the PVS to the Burch colposuspension and at 2 years found the PVS to be superior in the treatment of SUI.

## CONCLUSION

The autologous pubovaginal sling is a durable and highly successful treatment for SUI. It is more invasive than the TVT or TOT, but it is the most appropriate treatment for SUI in certain specific instances like severe ISD or if the risk of erosion is high. The PVS should be included in the armamentarium of any surgeon treating SUI.

## *References*


1. McGuire EJ, Lytton B. Pubovaginal sling procedure for stress incontinence. *J Urol* 1978;119:82–84.
2. Morgan TO Jr, Westney OL, McGuire EJ. Pubovaginal sling: 4-year outcome analysis and quality of life assessment. *J Urol* 2000;163:1845–1848.
3. Chaikin DC, Rosenthal J, Blaivas JG. Pubovaginal fascial sling for all types of stress urinary incontinence: long term analysis. *J Urol* 1998;160:1312–1316.
4. Schick E, Dupont C, Bertrand PE, et al. Predictive value of maximum urethral closure pressure, urethral hypermobility and urethral incompetence in the diagnosis of clinically significant female genuine stress incontinence. *J Urol* 2004;171:1871–1876.
5. Ulmsten U, Henriksson L, Johnson P, et al. An ambulatory surgical procedure under local anesthesia for treatment of female urinary incontinence. *Int Urogynecol J Pelvic Floor Dysfunct* 1996;7:81–86.
6. Clemons J, LaSala C. The tension free vaginal tape in women with a non-hypermobile urethra and low maximum urethral closure pressure. *Int Urogynecol J* 2007;18:727–734.
7. Ghezzi F, Serati M, Cromi A, et al. Tension-free vaginal tape for the treatment of urodynamic stress incontinence with intrinsic sphincteric deficiency. *Int Urogynecol J* 2006;17:335–339.

8. McGuire E. Urodynamic findings in patients after failure of stress incontinence operations. In: Zinner NR, ed. *Female incontinence*. New York: Alan R. Liss, 1981:351–356.
9. McGuire E, Wang CC, Usilato H, et al. Modified pubovaginal sling in girls with myelodysplasia. *J Urol* 1986;135:94–96.
10. Mayer R, Dmochowski RR, Appell RA, et al. Multicentre prospective randomized 52-week trial of calcium hydroxyapatite versus bovine dermal collagen for treatment of stress urinary incontinence. *Urology* 2007;69:876–880.
11. Flynn B, Brian J, Yap W, et al. Pubovaginal sling using allograft fascia lata versus autograft fascia for all types of stress urinary incontinence: 2-year minimum followup. *J Urol* 2002;167(2, Pt 1):608–612.
12. Kobashi K, Dmochowski R, Mee SL, et al. Erosion of woven polyester pubovaginal sling. *J Urol* 1999;162:2070–2072.
13. Howden N, Zyczynski H, Moalli P, et al. Comparison of autologous rectus fascia and cadaveric fascia in pubovaginal sling continence outcomes. *Am J Obstet Gynecol* 2006;194(5):1444–1449.
14. Morgan D, Dunn R, Fenner D, et al. Comparative analysis of urinary incontinence severity after autologous fascia pubovaginal sling, pubovaginal sling and tension-free vaginal tape. *J Urol* 2007;177(2):604–608; discussion 608.
15. Albo ME, et al. Burch colposuspension versus fascial sling to reduce urinary stress incontinence. *N Engl J Med* 2007;356(21):2143–2155.
16. Thiel D, Pettit P, McClellan W, et al. Long-term urinary continence rates after simple sling incision for relief of urinary retention following fascia lata pubovaginal slings. *J Urol* 2005;174(5):1878–1881.

# CHAPTER 41 ■ SYNTHETIC MIDURETHRAL RETROPUBIC SLINGS

BHAVIN N. PATEL AND GOPAL H. BADLANI

The past decade has seen a shift from suspension procedures to sling procedures as the treatment of choice for stress urinary incontinence (SUI). The bladder neck and proximal urethra were considered zones for continence procedures in patients with SUI. Traditionally, a sling at the bladder neck, using fascia, was reserved for failed suspension or severe cases of intrinsic sphincteric deficiency (ISD).

The integral theory, proposed by Petros and Ulmsten, advanced the concept of midurethral support for a hypermobile urethra and anterior vaginal wall (1). The tension-free synthetic tape replaces and recreates the midurethral ligaments, which results in kinking or coaptation of the urethra with increase in the intra-abdominal pressure but has little or no effect on detrusor-initiated voiding or incontinence.

## DIAGNOSIS

Patients with SUI present with the complaint of involuntary urinary loss with increased intra-abdominal pressures, as in coughing, laughing, or during Valsalva. The diagnosis can be made based on history and physical examination and quantified with a pad test. Attention should be paid to any associated prolapse, symptoms of overactive bladder (OAB), urge incontinence (UI), or significant postvoid residual urine. The utility of urodynamic testing is debatable in the diagnosis of primary SUI; however, it is helpful in cases that are not as straightforward and in cases complicated by the aforementioned pathologies, and it is required in recurrent SUI after failed surgery.

In patients with associated vaginal prolapse, the SUI may be occult and become evident only with the reduction of the prolapse. Patients with OAB and/or UI with SUI should be counseled regarding the fact that their OAB or UI may not improve with a midurethral sling. Finally, patients with postvoid residual urine, depending upon its etiology, should be counseled regarding an increased risk of urinary retention after a midurethral sling.

## INDICATIONS FOR SURGERY

Those patients with SUI and a moderate to severe bother on the quality-of-life (QOL) score who fail or cannot tolerate nonsurgical modes of management should be considered for surgical correction. Patients with urethral hypermobility (indicated by >30-degree deflection on office Q-tip test), no significant prolapse, and mild to moderate intrinsic sphincteric deficiency (leak point pressures >60 cm $H_2O$) are ideal candidates for midurethral synthetic slings. Patients with ISD, lack of hypermobility, and leak point pressure (LPP) <60 cm $H_2O$ are candidates for bladder neck sling.

Prior anterior vaginal wall surgery, age over 70, obesity, and prior failed sling are not contraindications to midurethral slings but require a higher degree of skill and prior experience with vaginal surgery. Studies have demonstrated no overall difference in outcome when procedures such as vaginal hysterectomy or vault suspension are performed in conjunction with a midurethral sling (2). Severe ISD at rest with or without hypermobility, previous urethral surgery or injury, urethral diverticulum, pelvic radiation, poor vaginal epithelium, pipestem urethra, and hypersensitivity to the synthetic materials are contraindications to midurethral synthetic slings.

## ALTERNATIVE THERAPIES

Nonsurgical alternative therapies to the midurethral sling include limited fluid intake, bladder training, timed voiding, Kegel exercises, pessaries, and medical therapy, including alpha-adrenergic drugs and off-label use of imipramine and duloxetine. The use of hormone replacement therapy is controversial. The use of pads and in rare cases an indwelling catheter to deal with SUI is to be discouraged. Nonsurgical management is only efficacious in mild SUI and often does not provide adequate relief in moderate or severe SUI. Surgical alternatives include injectable bulking agents, open or laparoscopic Burch procedure, bladder neck sling, transobturator sling (TOT), and the recently introduced minisling and prepubic sling.

Injectable bulking agents work by increasing urethral resistance and are indicated in patients with ISD and a fixed (not hypermobile) urethra. There are a variety of techniques and injectable materials, each of which has a material-specific success rate that decreases as time from injection increases. They require reinjection, and complications may include sterile abscess formation, irritative voiding symptoms, pelvic pain, ectopic calcifications, and transient urinary retention.

Open Burch and midurethral sling in a randomized trial showed an equal efficacy in a short-term follow-up with decreased morbidity with the midurethral sling (3).

Bladder neck sling is indicated in patients with ISD with or without urethral hypermobility and SUI manifested by lower urethral closure pressures. The material used in the suspension varies per the surgeon's preference. To minimize the morbidity of the traditional fascial sling, synthetic and other biomaterials can be used; success with these materials has been reported (4).

Transobturator suburethral support was developed in an effort to decrease the risk of injury to adjacent structures such as large vessels, bowel, and the bladder. Its indications are the same as those for the midurethral sling described above. Compared with the midurethral sling, TOT required less operative time (5) and had similar rates of success, but it was associated with a higher rate of groin or thigh pain, vaginal injuries, and tape erosion (6).

There is limited peer-reviewed information on the use of minislings or prepubic slings.

## CHOICE OF MATERIAL

The choice of sling material is a key component of midurethral sling surgery. The materials used for the slings are divided into the following categories: autologous fascia, cadaveric allograft, xenograft, and synthetics. Rectus fascia and fascia lata have been harvested for SUI surgery. The advantages of using autologous fascia are its durability, its availability, and its nonimmunogenic quality. However, difficulty in procurement, longer operative times, increased patient morbidity, and late sling contraction limit its use today. Cadaveric allograft and xenograft tissues have also been used because they are readily available and do not require procurement from the patient. On the other hand, their costs, theoretical risk of infectious transfer, mechanical variability, and unpredictable outcome have limited their use. In our practice we reserve cadaveric allograft and xenograft to cases where synthetic mesh is contraindicated.

Synthetic meshes are readily available and highly durable, maintain their strength over time, are free of potential pathogens, and are less expensive. A variety of synthetic materials are available; the current standard is a monofilament, large-pore, soft mesh made out of polypropylene. This mesh has lower rates of erosion when compared to multifilament (Mersilene). Pore size is pivotal in allowing incorporation of host fibroblasts, macrophages, and leukocytes. Stiffness is an important factor too, as stiffer slings are more prone to erosion. Additionally, our research shows a biochemical defect in patients with SUI and prolapse resulting in a faster rate of breakdown of collagen and elastin, supporting the use of synthetic mesh (7).

## SURGICAL TECHNIQUE

An informed consent is obtained, informing the patient of expected outcomes and possible complications such as retention, de novo or persistent OAB, adjacent organ injury, recurrence of incontinence, risk of developing prolapse, erosion, and exposure of mesh, in addition to the standard surgical and anesthetic risks.

Aspirin and other anticoagulants are discontinued 5 to 7 days preoperatively. A flouroquinolone is started 48 hours prior to surgery, and the patient receives routine preanesthetic instructions for the night preceding the surgery. No food or liquid is allowed 8 to 10 hours prior to the procedure, laxatives are prescribed for patients who suffer from constipation, and preoperative labs including complete blood count, serum electrolytes, coagulation studies, urinalysis, and urine culture are obtained. The procedure should be postponed in the presence of active urinary tract infection or coagulopathy.

On the day of surgery, a parenteral antibiotic, such as a first-generation cephalosporin or a fluoroquinolone, is administered and continued for 24 hours. The choice of local anesthesia with sedation, spinal block, or general anesthesia depends on the surgeon, anesthesiologist, and patient preferences. Sequential compression devices are used on the lower extremities prior to the induction of anesthesia. The procedure is performed in the dorsal lithotomy position using Allen stirrups. The lower abdominal and pubic areas are shaved, prepared, and draped using a Lingeman Gyn surgery drape (Microtek Medical, Isolyser Healthcare, Columbus, MS).

To retract the labia, a Lone Star surgical retractor (Medical Products Inc, Houston, TX) is used. Alternatively, the labia can be sutured laterally. Weighted vaginal speculums can be used to better expose the anterior vaginal wall during dissection, but they should be removed before tensioning the sling. A 20Fr urethral catheter is placed, the bladder is drained, and the balloon is palpated at the bladder neck.

An Allis clamp is placed at the bladder neck and 1 cm proximal to the urethral meatus. Injectable Marcaine, 5 mL, is infiltrated into the anterior vaginal wall, along the midline between the two Allis clamps, to facilitate the dissection. A 2-cm midline incision is made between the urethral meatus and the bladder neck to avoid injury to the somatic and autonomic neurons that travel laterally through the anterior vaginal wall to the urethra and supply the urethral sphincter.

With Metzenbaum scissors, flaps of the anterior vaginal wall are developed bilaterally, aiming toward the ipsilateral shoulder. Traction is applied on the vaginal wall with Allis clamps to facilitate flap dissection, avoiding too much traction, which may tear the flap. Minimal bleeding is noted if the correct depth of dissection is reached.

For the suprapubic arch (SPARC) sling kit (American Medical Systems), 1% lidocaine is injected at the skin on the superior portion of the symphysis, 2.5 cm lateral to the midline. Small stab incisions are made at the areas of infiltration with a no. 15 blade knife. At this point, the bladder is once again emptied to avoid injury, and the needle is passed with

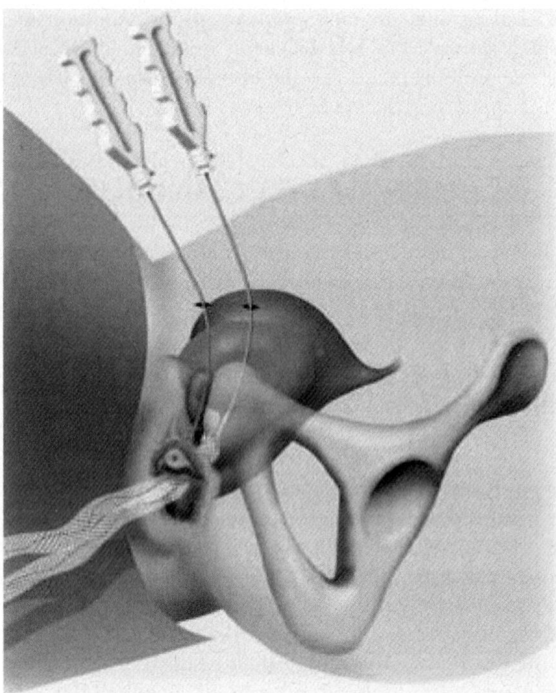

FIGURE 41.1 Placement of the suprapubic arch (SPARC) needles.

the dominant hand through the suprapubic incision behind the pubic bone. The needle is advanced toward the ipsilateral vaginal dissection, guided by contact with the posterior aspect of the bone. The needle handle is displaced posteromedially as the tip advances further through the space of Retzius.

At this point the nondominant hand should be placed along the ipsilateral vaginal dissection plane, and the needle tip should be palpated. The needle is then advanced out of the vaginal wound. This method of needle placement minimizes the risk of injuring adjacent large vessels and nerves but not the bladder or the urethra. The needle placement is then repeated on the contralateral side (Fig. 41.1). The urethral catheter is removed and cystoscopy is performed to assess for bladder injury. Injury to the bladder most commonly occurs along the superolateral aspects of the bladder. Blood seen on entering the bladder, visualization of the needle, or bladder submucosal movement with motion of the needle are all indicators of bladder injury. If bladder injury has occurred, the ipsilateral needle should be removed and repositioned once the bladder has been drained. Also, catheter drainage postoperatively for additional days is indicated. A key step here is to drain the bladder before removing the cystoscope, as the connector width is larger than the needle, resulting in possible shearing injury of the bladder wall if it is full. The sling, covered in a protective plastic sheath, is locked onto the needles with the sling indicator positioned in the midline at the midurethra. Once secured, the needles with attached sling are brought back out through the suprapubic stab incisions (Fig. 41.2).

## Tension-Free Vaginal Tape (Gynecare)

The procedure for tension-free vaginal tape (TVT) follows the same vaginal dissection as described above, for the placement of the SPARC sling. At this point, a solution of normal saline and local anesthetic is injected suprapubically at the lateral aspects of the pubic symphysis toward the ipsilateral vaginal dissection to aid in sling placement. The tip of the Foley catheter with a catheter guide is placed on contralateral traction to avoid injury to the bladder. The TVT needle is placed in the vaginal incision and aimed toward the ipsilateral scapula. The needle is advanced along the posterior aspect of the pubic bone and then brought to the skin at the lateral aspect of the symphysis, and a stab incision is made to deliver the needle through the skin. The needle placment is repeated on the contralateral side. A key step is to avoid lateral rotation of the needle and avoid proximal passage away from the bone. Cystoscopy is performed to identify bladder injury. Extra care is needed if the patient has had an open or laparoscopic procedure in the pelvis, as bowel may be adherent to the retropubic space.

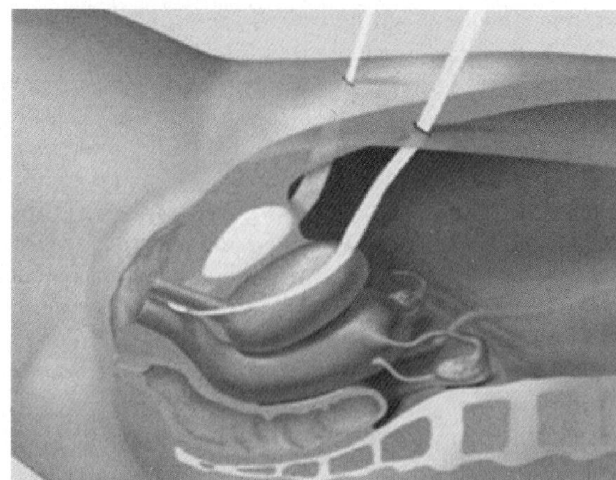

FIGURE 41.2 Anatomic lie of the midurethral sling.

The sling should be examined to ensure that no twisting has occurred. The sling is then adjusted until the appropriate tension has been achieved, avoiding too much or too little tension. This is often done by ensuring that a 22Fr cystoscopic sheath passes freely through the urethra or by placing a pair of clamps between the tape and the midurethra as the sling is adjusted. Once positioning is satisfactory, the plastic covering is cut and removed, redundant sling at the suprapubic incision is excised, and the suprapubic wounds are closed with Dermabond and the vaginal wound closed with 2-0 Vicryl suture.

At the end of the case, a Foley catheter is placed as well as a Betadine-soaked vaginal pack. Patients are then discharged with or without the Foley or kept in observation overnight, depending on surgeon preference. At discharge patients are given a 5-day course of antibiotics, pain medications, and stool softeners. They are also told to abstain from sexual activity for 4 to 6 weeks. Trial of voiding can be initiated in the recovery room if the patient has had a local anesthesia. We prefer overnight use of a Foley catheter if general or spinal anesthesia was used.

# OUTCOMES

There is good initial and durable success in treating SUI with midurethral sling compared to the standard Burch colposuspension (3). A recent prospective randomized study showed no difference in outcome between TVT (95%) and SPARC (83%) (8). These findings have been confirmed by other studies. Further comparision has shown no difference in the cure rate of SUI with TVT (95%), SPARC (90%), or TOT (94%) (8).

# COMPLICATIONS

## Perioperative Complications

Intraoperative complications are mostly related to the dissection and placement of the trocar. There have been four FDA-reported deaths due to TVTs, two associated with bowel injury, and two associated with vascular injury. During the procedure there is a risk of bleeding, infection, and injury to the bladder, urethra, ureter, bowel, vessels, and nerves. One thousand cases of TVT in Finland were reviewed (10), and the incidence of bladder injury, the most common complication during needle placement, was reported as 3.8%. The risk of postoperative bleeding was 1.9%, and that of wound infection was <1%. Mortality associated with injury to vessels has been reported but is exceedingly rare and has been mentioned previously. A key point is awareness, immediate recognition, and management of the complication.

## Postoperative Complications

Postoperative complications include outflow obstruction, de novo or persistent OAB, extrusion, and erosion. Urinary obstruction after a midurethral sling can be brief and transient or persistent. Transient postoperative obstruction is often due to edema of the urethra and the supporting structures along with pelvic pain. As the edema and pain subside, so does the obstruction. However, patients can have persistent urinary obstruction due to a combination of previously undiagnosed prolapse and/or a "tight" sling. They often present with urgency, frequency, decreased force of stream, positional voiding, and/or retention. Treatment includes anticholinergic medication with monitoring of PVR, use of CIC or consideration of sling loosening, incision, or uretholysis with or without sling revision. A recent multicenter trial of an adjustable sling is being evaluated. The cost of such a sling is considerably higher and not supported by the low rate of retention with tension-free slings.

Persistent incontinence can occur after midurethral sling. The cause, whether it is persistence of SUI, urgency- or OAB-related, urge-related, or rarely iatrogenic fistula, must be determined.

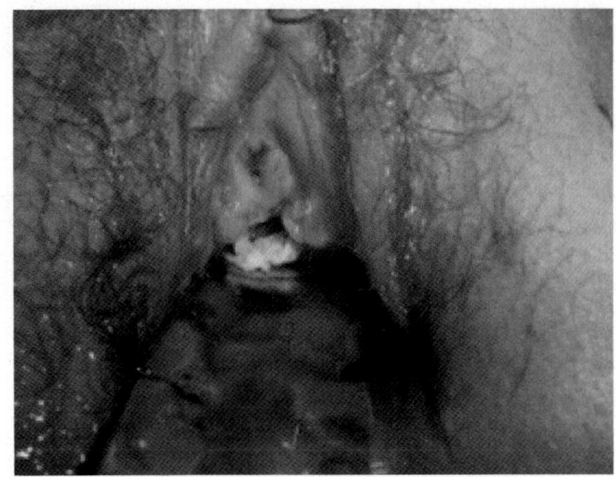

FIGURE 41.3 Vaginal extrusion of midurethral tape.

Vaginal extrusion (Fig. 41.3) of the tape usually occurs within 6 months of the initial surgery. Patients often present with vaginal discharge, dyspareunia, and feeling the tape material within the vagina. The treatment of the extrusion varies according to the degree of erosion and the patient's symptomatology, but it can include partial or complete removal of the tape and closure of the vaginal mucosa over the extrusion.

Urethral or bladder erosion can occur at any time in the postoperative course but often occurs in the first 6 months after surgery. Most patients present with recurrent SUI, hematuria, perineal pain, urinary tract infections, and/or irritative voiding symptoms. The treatment of erosion involves removal of the intraviscous sling. This can be achieved endoscopically in the urethra or laparoscopically in the bladder. A vaginal approach can result in a fistula formation and recurrence of incontinence. Thus, for a bladder erosion we prefer removing the intravesical portion with either a laparoscopic or open approach without disturbing the suburethral portion.

# CONCLUSIONS

The midurethral sling has revolutionized the approach to SUI. It allows many patients to improve their quality of life with minimal morbidity. The success depends on proper case selection and patient education.

## *References*


1. Petros PE, Ulmsten UI. An integral theory of female urinary incontinence. Experimental and Clinical considerations. *Acta Obstet Gynecol Scand Suppl* 1990;153:7–31.
2. Schraffordt Koops SE, Bisseling TM, van Brummen HJ, et al. Result of the tension-free vaginal tape in patients with concomitant prolapse surgery: a 2 year follow up study. An analysis from the Netherlands TVT Database. *Int Urogynecol J Pelvic Floor Dysfunct* 2007;18(4):437–442.
3. Ward KL, Hilton P. Tension-free vaginal tape versus colposuspension for primary urodynamic stress incontinence: 5 year follow up. *Br J Obstet Gynecol* 2008;115(2):226–233.
4. Hom D, Desautel MG, Lumerman JH, et al. Pubovaginal sling using polypropylene mesh and Vesica bone anchors. *Urology* 1998;51(5):708–713.
5. deTayrac R, Deffieux X, Droupy S, et al. A prospective randomized trial comparing tension-free vaginal tape and transobturator suburethral tape for surgical treatment of stress urinary incontinence. *Am J Obstet Gynecol* 2004;190(3):602–608.
6. Latthe PM, Foon R, Toozs-Hobson P. Transobturator and retropubic tape procedures in stress urinary incontinence: a systematic review and meta-analysis of the effectiveness and complications. *Br J Obstet Gynecol* 2007;114(5):522–531.
7. Kushner L, Mathrubutham M, Burney T, et al. Excretion of collagen derived peptides is increased in women with stress urinary incontinence. *Neurourol Urodynam* 2004;23(3):198–203.
8. Adonian S, Chen T, St-Denis B, et al. Randomized clinical trial comparing suprapubic arch sling (SPARC) and tension-free vaginal tape (TVT): one-year results. *Eur Urol* 2005;47(4):537–541.
9. Paick JS, Oh SJ, Kim SW, et al. Tension-free vaginal tape, suprapubic arc sling, and transobturator tape in the treatment of mixed urinary incontinence in women. *Int Urogynecol J Pelvic Floor Dysfunct* 2008;19(1): 123–129.
10. Kuuva N, Nilsson CG. A nationwide analysis of complications associated with the tension-free vaginal tape (TVT) procedure. *Acta Obstet Gynecol Scand* 2002;81(1):72–77.

# CHAPTER 42 ■ THE TRANSOBTURATOR APPROACH TO THE MIDURETHRAL SLING

PAUL HANISSIAN AND JAMES WHITESIDE

There has been significant innovation in the treatment of urinary incontinence over the last 15 years. In the early 1990s there was growing understanding that needle urethropexies did not have long-term efficacy compared to retropubic urethropexies and pubovaginal slings. The morbidity of these latter procedures, however, set the stage for the development of a minimally invasive approach. The tension-free vaginal tape (TVT) procedure was the first minimally invasive midurethral sling that came into use in the late 1990s. Developed by the late Ulf Ulmstem, the TVT placed a polypropylene mesh suburethrally with the use of curved needles passed transvaginally through the retropubic space and out through cutaneous abdominal incisions (1). Unlike its pubovaginal sling predecessors, the TVT mesh was not fixed to bone or fascia. The TVT mesh maintains its position through friction with the surrounding tissue and ultimately through fibroblast ingrowth into the mesh. Though clinical trials ultimately showed this procedure to have similar efficacy to more traditional approaches (e.g., Burch urethropexy [2]), rare complications such as life-threatening bowel and major vascular injury along with the requirement of cystoscopy inspired improvements in this technique.

In 2001 Delorme (3) published "Transobturator Urethral Suspension: Mini-invasive Procedure in the Treatment of Stress Urinary Incontinence in Women," introducing the transobturator approach for the placement of a midurethral sling. Using a two-dimensional Emmet needle, a polypropylene mesh was passed through thigh muscles, around the ischiopubic ramus, and into a vaginal epithelial tunnel for placement at the midurethra. This approach dramatically reduced the possibility of an intra-abdominal injury. While two approaches have evolved in the placement of the mesh (inside-out [e.g., TVT-O, Gynecare] versus outside-in [e.g., Monarc, American Medical Systems]), the transobturator procedure is relatively simple to learn and can be accomplished with minimal anesthesia in an awake patient. Controlled randomized studies have documented the safety and efficacy of the transobturator approach compared to retropubic midurethral slings (4).

## DIAGNOSIS

A thorough understanding of urinary incontinence is important before implementing therapy. Urinary incontinence as defined by the International Continence Society can be a symptom, sign, or condition. It is the condition of stress incontinence that is appropriate for surgical treatment, and a distinction needs to be drawn between stress incontinence and other types of urinary incontinence, including urge incontinence. The symptom of stress urinary leakage can alone be misleading; hence it is imperative to document the sign of stress urinary leakage before performing surgery. It is also worthwhile to understand the patient's fluid intake volume and output (i.e., bladder diary) before surgery to support the patient's perceptions of leakage and exclude other incontinence etiologies.

There is disagreement regarding the optimal preoperative testing for urinary incontinence among women. At initial evaluation, the patient should provide a urine specimen for dipstick analysis, and then urine microscopy and culture can be done as necessary. Postvoid residual volumes should be determined to assess the possibility of disordered bladder sensation or detrusor pathology leading to retention. Documentation of stress urine leakage should be done; this could include multichannel urodynamic studies or could be done with a standardized cough stress test. A cough stress test involves filling the bladder to 300 mL or to subjective fullness and then having the patient forcefully cough while in an upright position. Witness of gross urine loss from the urethral meatus during coughing is considered a positive test. The necessity of multichannel urodynamic testing is unclear, particularly in the low-risk patient, if the sign of stress urinary leakage is documented by some alternative means and the postvoid residual volumes are normal. Multichannel urodynamic testing could render insight into voiding and urethral competency issues. The reliability and value of this insight are a matter of debate. Ideally, the patient should not have urge incontinence or voiding dysfunction. Patients with mixed urinary incontinence may be appropriate candidates for a transobturator midurethral sling if their stress symptoms outweigh their urge symptoms and they recognize what the surgery could do to their incontinence problems. Urge incontinence can be exacerbated or occur de novo following surgical treatment of stress incontinence, although it is also possible that urge leakage improves following sling surgery. Information gleaned from the bladder diary can clarify ambiguous mixed urinary incontinence symptoms.

Vaginal examination and assessment for pelvic organ prolapse are essential. It has been long recognized that patients with pelvic organ prolapse (particularly anterior vaginal wall prolapse) can become newly incontinent of urine with reduction of the prolapse (occult urinary incontinence). A corollary to this recognition is that if an incontinence procedure alone is done in a woman with Stage III or IV prolapse that is not concurrently treated, postoperative urinary retention or voiding dysfunction can ensue. In addition, placement of a transobturator midurethral sling carries a higher risk of bladder injury without reduction of the prolapse at the time of insertion. The question of whether and how the prolapse should be corrected and the nuances of simultaneous continence surgery are beyond the scope of this chapter.

## INDICATIONS

Transobturator midurethral slings are indicated for urinary incontinence that by both symptom and sign is consistent with urethral incompetence and where placement of the sling could not be expected to compromise voiding (e.g., pelvic organ prolapse, diabetes, neuropathy). Stress-associated urine leakage occurs when urethral pressure is exceeded by transmitted bladder pressure. The reasons this may occur are not well understood, despite years of definitions and debate. Historically, when selecting the appropriate surgical procedure for treatment of stress incontinence, it has been considered important to distinguish between incontinence related to hypermobility of the bladder neck and incontinence related to a urethral sphincter that cannot maintain a watertight seal even at rest (e.g., intrinsic sphincter deficiency, ISD). This dichotomy, from a pathophysiologic view, could be distilled into support versus sphincter problems. In the case of a hypermobile urethra, inadequate pelvic floor support allows the urethra to escape transmitted abdominal pressure to the urethra. In the case of ISD, the urethra is fixed and theoretically does benefit from transmitted abdominal pressures, but this cannot compensate for whatever issues led to a nonfunctioning sphincteric mechanism. The dichotomy, while appealing on theoretical grounds, finds little experimental support. Although it is true that lower abdominal pressures are required to induce leakage in women whose incontinence is more subjectively severe, this relationship is fuzzy at best, and it must be accepted that the treatment outcomes among subjectively severe incontinent women will likely be less ideal than among women with subjectively less severe incontinence. This relationship is not necessarily offset by information gleaned from measurements of urethral competence (e.g., urethral pressure profilometry or leak point pressures). Indeed, the outcomes of transobturator midurethral slings appear to be independent of leak point pressures, allowing us to leave this quandary for the laboratory.

## ALTERNATIVE THERAPY

Though the most common treatments for stress incontinence are surgical, a number of nonsurgical alternatives are available for women who either do not desire surgery or who are not good surgical candidates. These approaches include behavioral techniques, medications, urethral inserts and occlusive devices, and vaginal pessaries. It would not be uncommon for more difficult cases of urinary incontinence to require more than one treatment to achieve a satisfactory outcome. Nonsurgical and nonsling surgical options (e.g., Burch urethropexy) for female urinary incontinence are beyond the scope of this chapter.

The transobturator approach to placement of a midurethral sling represents a second-generation concept based on the TVT that was popularized in the mid 1990s. Retropubic midurethral procedures continue to be popular and enjoy considerable supportive evidence. Most recently, single-incision midurethral slings (TVT-SECUR, Gynecare; MiniArc, American Medical Systems) have been introduced with claims of better safety and the possibility of office placement. These third-generation midurethral slings differ in that they are inserted through a midline suburethral vaginal incision, traverse the periurethral tissue, and are anchored in some fashion retropubically or behind the ischiopubic ramus. To date, there are no long-term efficacy and safety data for these products. Prior to 1995, traditional pubovaginal slings and retropubic procedures (e.g., Burch, Marshall-Marchetti-Krantz) were the mainstay of surgical treatment of female stress urinary incontinence. These procedures continue to be viable options; however, they are mostly reserved for patients who will otherwise need laparotomy. It is worth noting that in the SISTEr trial traditional pubovaginal slings were found to be more successful in correcting female urinary incontinence but at the price of greater morbidity relative to the Burch colposuspension (5).

## SURGICAL TECHNIQUE

In placement of a midurethral sling, the technical goal is to position the sling material through the obturator foramen and beneath the midurethra with as little trauma as possible (Fig. 42.1). Using one of the commercially available kits, a transobturator suburethral mesh is placed through three incisions: a 1- to 2-cm midline suburethral vaginal incision, and two smaller groin incisions. Device needles are passed either toward or away from the urethra, depending on the manufacturer. Table 42.1 lists various products on the market. Irrespective of the direction of passage, the needles will traverse skin; subcutaneous fat; the gracilis, adductor brevis, and obturator externus muscles; the obturator membrane; the obturator internus muscle; and the periurethral endopelvic fascia (6). Although there are differences in the type of mesh offered by the various manufacturers, there are few controlled studies comparing them. Most available mesh used in this application today are macroporous polypropylene.

Anesthesia for the procedure can be delivered by local block with sedation, by spinal block, or by general anesthesia. The patient should be administered preoperative antibiotics based on their utility in vaginal surgery; however, there is no evidence to support soaking the mesh in antibiotic solution or giving antibiotics postoperatively. Following adequate anesthesia, the

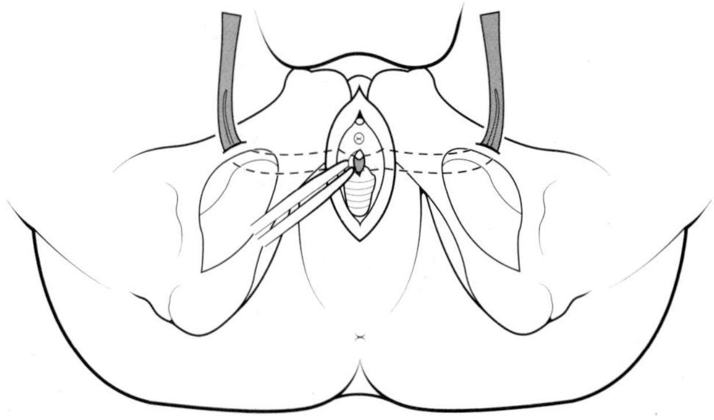

FIGURE 42.1 Transobturator tape in final anatomic position. The tape has been passed under the midurethra, through the periurethral tissues and obtuator membrane, and exits through skin incisions on the lateral thigh.

TABLE 42.1

**TRANSOBTURATOR MIDURETHRAL SLINGS**

| Name | Manufacturer | Approach |
|---|---|---|
| Aris | Coloplast[a] | Outside-in |
| Monarc | AMS[b] | Outside-in |
| ObTape | Mentor[c] | Outside-in |
| Obtyrx | Boston Scientific[d] | Outside-in |
| TVT-O | Ethicon[e] | Inside-out |
| Desara | Caldera[f] | Either |
| Uratape | Porges-Mentor[g] | Inside-out |

All of the above use a polypropylene mesh; they vary regarding pore size and weave. [a]Coloplast AVS, Copenhagen, Denmark. [b]American Medical Systems Research Corp., Minnetonka, MN. [c]Mentor Corp., Santa Barbara, CA. [d]Boston Scientific Scimed Inc., Maple Grove, MN. [e]Ethicon Inc., Somerville, NJ. [f]Caldera Medical, Inc., Agoura Hills, CA. [g]LePlessis, Robinson, France.

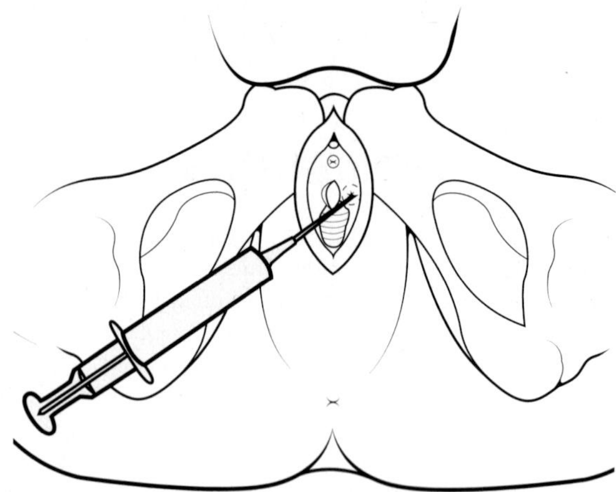

FIGURE 42.2 Blunting of the vaginal crease while injecting lidocaine helps to decrease the risk of buttonholing the vaginal mucosa as the needles are passed through the periurethral tissues.

patient is positioned in a neurologically neutral lithotomy position using padded stirrups. A Foley catheter is inserted and the position of the midurethra determined as the midpoint between the palpable Foley bulb at the bladder neck and the urethral meatus. A weighted speculum is inserted for exposure of the anterior vaginal wall. Next, 10 to 20 cc of a vasoactive solution (1% lidocaine with 1:200,000 epinephrine or vasopressin, 20 U diluted in 100 cc of sterile saline) is injected in the subepithelial vagina before making a 1.5- to 2.0-cm vertical vaginal incision at the midurethra. The injection is also carried laterally toward the vaginal sulcus medial to the ischiopubic ramus bilaterally. Ideally, the operator will see blunting of this vaginal crease as the injected epithelium expands outward (Fig. 42.2). Applying this technique may help the surgeon avoid "buttonholing" the vagina while passing the helical needles. Allis clamps are useful for grasping the vaginal epithelium for exposure.

The midurethral vaginal incision should include both the vaginal epithelium and portions of the muscularis. Too shallow of an incision may promote postoperative vaginal mesh extrusion. The operator then dissects using a fine scissors (Church, Metzenbaum, or sternotomy) in the periurethral tissues toward the ischiopubic ramus, until a tunnel is created and the tip of the surgeon's finger can touch the ischiopubic ramus. The dissection is carried out bilaterally. It is also advantageous to continue developing the plane between the vagina and urethra at the inferior aspect of the incision for approximately 0.5 cm to create a pocket for the mesh and to limit tearing the vaginal tissue with digital manipulation of the subepithelial tunnel.

The adductor longus tendon is palpated, and a marking pen is used to identify the genital crural fold below the tendon. This typically is at the level of the clitoris at the lateral edge of the labia majora (Fig. 42.3). Local anesthetic is injected along the proposed needle path followed by a small stab incision. In reference to the outside-in technique, the cut edge of the vaginal incision is grasped with an Allis clamp, and the operator's same-hand index finger is placed behind the Allis clamp into the vaginal epithelial tunnel. The needle passer is then grasped in the operator's opposite hand and positioned so that the axis of the passer is parallel to the ischiopubic ramus. The needle tip is placed perpendicular to the skin and advanced through the soft tissues around the ramus, meeting the operator's index finger that guides the needle tip out of the vaginal epithelial

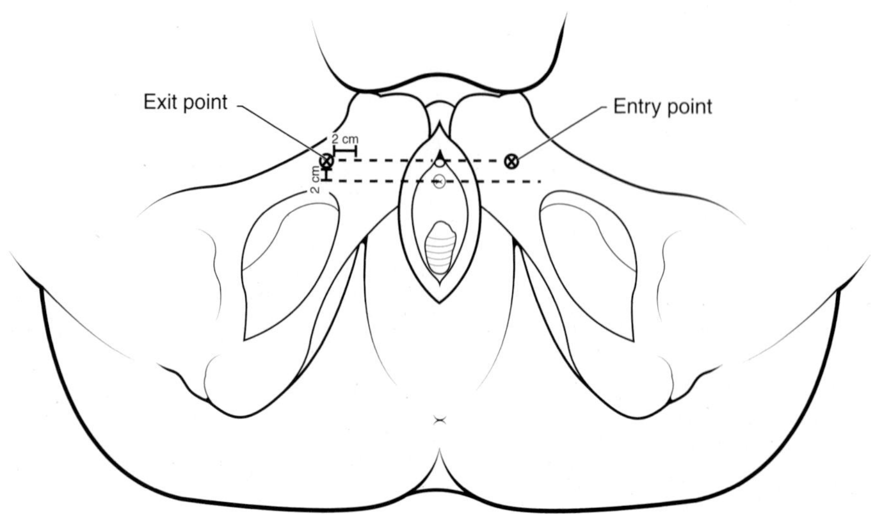


FIGURE 42.3 Demonstration of placement for the groin incisions. The patient's right side shows the exit points of the needles for the outside in technique, and the patients left side shows the entry points for the inside out technique.

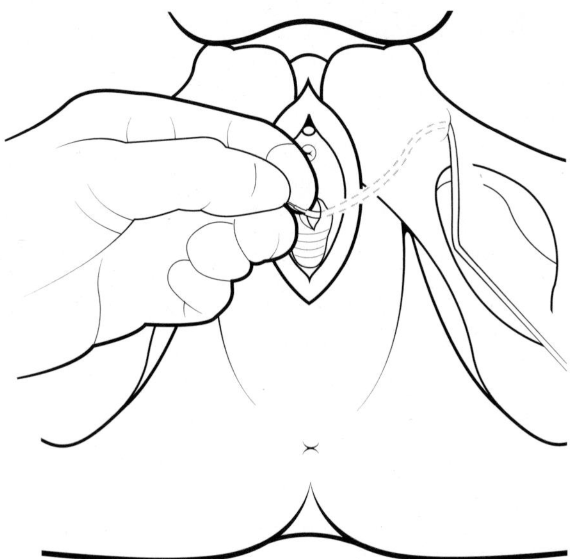

FIGURE 42.4 The needle tip is placed perpendicular to the skin and advanced through the soft tissues around the ramus meeting the operators index finger that guides the needle tip out of the vaginal epithelial tunnel lateral to the urethra.

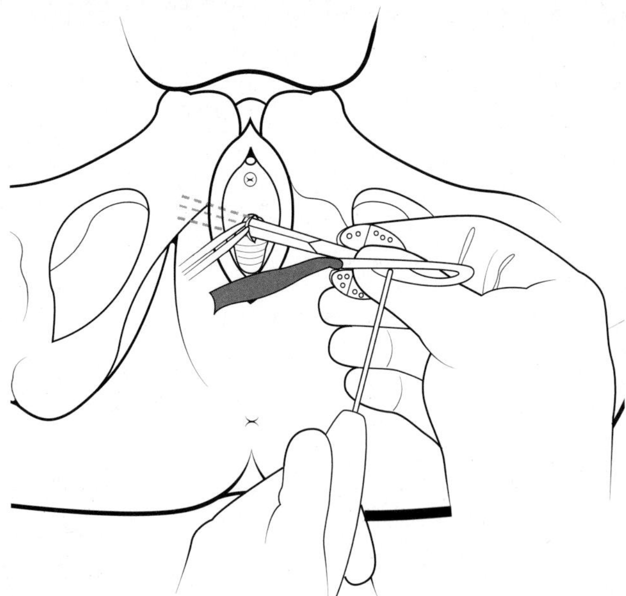

FIGURE 42.5 The winged guide is inserted into the dissected track and through the obturator membrane. The helical needle passer is then inserted through the vaginal incision following the channel of the winged guide so the tip is beyond the obturator membrane.

tunnel lateral to the urethra (Fig. 42.4). At this point, it is important to determine that the lateral sulci of the vagina are free of inadvertent mesh passage. This done, the mesh is attached to the needle and removed, reversing the path of insertion. The process is then repeated on the contralateral side. The products are marketed such that the mesh is ensheathed in plastic that overlaps in the middle. The plastic allows the mesh to slip through the tissue during placement. It is useful to place a hemostat to stabilize the overlapping plastic, ensuring that the mesh is not prematurely exposed. At this point, cystoscopy is recommended.

Although the concept for the inside-out technique is similar, the surgical steps do vary from the outside-in technique described above. Gynecare manufactures the TVT Obturator System, which includes helical passers, a plastic ensheathed polypropylene mesh, and a winged guide that facilitates introduction and passage of the helical needle passers. The groin incisions are made along a line 2 cm above the level of the urethral meatus. The exit points for the helical needle lie on this line, 2 cm lateral to the folds of the thigh (Fig. 42.3). A midline vaginal incision is then made superficial to the urethra as described above. Sharp and blunt dissection is employed to traverse the periurethral tissues to the obturator membrane, which is perforated with scissor tips. The winged guide is inserted into the dissected track and through the obturator membrane. The helical needle passer is then inserted through the vaginal incision following the channel of the winged guide so that the tip is beyond the obturator membrane (Fig. 42.5). At the starting point, the handle is 45 degrees from midline. The guide is then removed and the helical needle passer is rotated (clockwise for the patient's left side and counterclockwise for the right) while the handle is moved simultaneously toward the midline. The tip of the needle passer with an overlying plastic tube that is attached to the mesh then exits the marked groin incisions. The tubing is grasped with a clamp, and the needle passer is backed out of the plastic tubing by reverse rotation of the handle. The tubing is then pulled through the skin until the plastic-covered mesh appears. At this point, the previous steps are repeated on the contralateral side.

Once bladder and urethral integrity is confirmed by cystoscopy, the mesh is tensioned. There is considerable variability in how "proper" tension is determined. Given that a transobturator sling can be done with the patient awake, perhaps the best technique involves having the patient perform a cough stress test at a specific bladder volume (usually 300 cc). There is evidence that deeper anesthesia techniques are associated with lower treatment outcomes; however, it cannot be said that the "tailoring" of the mesh tension in the awake patient is responsible for this finding. Another technique for tensioning mesh is to place a no. 9 Hegar dilator between the mesh and the urethra before pulling back on the plastic sheaths exiting the groin incisions. Alternatively, a Babcock clamp can be used to grasp a 4-mm knuckle of mesh under the urethra before tensioning that, when released, will render "proper" tension. Care should be taken to use a similar technique on all patients. Once the appropriate tension has been determined, the mesh is stabilized, the hemostat in the middle is released, the plastic sheaths alone are grasped, and, applying equal pressure, the sheaths are removed out of the groin incisions. The vaginal epithelial incision is next closed with a running suture of delayed absorbable suture on a taper needle. The groin incisions are closed with suture or skin adhesive.

## OUTCOMES

Of equal importance to the technical issues of pelvic floor surgery is the measurement of treatment outcomes by the performing surgeon. In general, treatment outcomes can be assessed with objective or subjective measures, and these should

TABLE 42.2

INCONTINENCE SEVERITY INDEX

| How often do you experience urinary leakage? | How much urine do you lose each time? |
|---|---|
| 1. Less than once a month<br>2. A few times a month<br>3. A few times a week<br>4. Every day and/or night | 1. Drops<br>2. Small splashes<br>3. More |
| The four-level severity index is based on the following index values (1–12), which is a product of the score of each question.<br>1–2 = slight<br>3–6 = moderate<br>8–9 = severe<br>12 = very severe | |
| *Source:* Sandvik H, Seim A, Vanvik A, et al. A severity index for epidemiological surveys of female urinary incontinence: comparison with 48-hour pad-weighing tests. *Neurourol Urodynam* 2000;19(2):137–145. | |

match those used before treatment. There are several subjective survey tools to assess urinary incontinence. These tools vary in length and psychometric properties (e.g., validity, reliability, and responsiveness) and also in the degree to which they indicate the kind of incontinence. For example, the Urinary Distress Inventory (UDI) can render insight into whether the leakage is stress or urge; however, the overall score blends these issues and is less concise in assessing the overall severity of leakage. In contrast, the Incontinence Severity Index (ISI) (Table 42.2) renders a quick assessment of leakage severity but does not distinguish the kind of leakage.

Pelvic floor disorders are multidimensional issues and should be assessed with composite outcomes to capture, reasonably, as many aspects as possible. In clinical practice the burden to

TABLE 42.3

THE 3 INCONTINENCE QUESTIONS (3IQ)

1. During the last 3 months, have you leaked urine (even a small amount)?
   ☐ Yes ☐ No
   Questionnaire completed.
2. During the last 3 months, did you leak urine:
   (Check all that apply)
   ☐ a. When you were performing some physical activity, such as coughing, sneezing, lifting, or exercise?
   ☐ b. When you had the urge or the feeling that you needed to empty your bladder, but you could not get to the toilet fast enough?
   ☐ c. Without physical activity, and without a sense of urgency?
3. During the last 3 months, did you leak urine most often:
   (Check only one)
   ☐ a. When you were performing some physical activity, such as coughing, sneezing, lifting, or exercise?
   ☐ b. When you had the urge or the feeling that you needed to empty your bladder, but you could not get to the toilet fast enough?
   ☐ c. Without physical activity, and without a sense of urgency?
   ☐ d. About equally as often with physical activity as with a sense of urgency?

Definitions of type of urinary incontinence are based on responses to question 3:

| Response to Question 3 | Type of Incontinence |
|---|---|
| a. Most often with physical activity | Stress only or stress predominant |
| b. Most often with the urge to empty the bladder | Urge only or urge predominant |
| c. Without physical activity or sense of urgency | Other cause only or other cause predominant |
| d. About equally with physical activity and sense of urgency | Mixed |

*Source:* Brown JS, Bradley CS, et al. The sensitivity and specificity of a simple test to distinguish between urge and stress urinary incontinence. *Ann Intern Med* 2006;144:715–723.

patient and provider of using validated surveys to assess pelvic organ prolapse, bowel dysfunction, sexual function, and bladder function can be daunting. Subjective outcomes, as noted previously, can identify (UDI) and quantify (ISI) symptoms or assess general (SF-36) or condition-specific quality of life (Incontinence Impact Questionnaire, IIQ).

Objective outcomes include the pelvic organ prolapse quantification system (7), bladder diaries, cough stress tests, pad tests, office cystometrics with cough stress testing, and multichannel urodynamics. Although there are settings in which objective assessment would be useful in routine clinical practice (e.g., treatment failure), regular posttreatment use can be burdensome to both patient and clinician, rendering little additional information than that gathered from the subjective assessments. However, long-term outcomes data are not currently available.

## COMPLICATIONS

As with any surgical procedure, complications can arise intraoperatively or postoperatively that can have either short- or long-term sequelae. The transobturator technique was developed as a safer approach compared to the retropubic technique. The needles are unlikely to enter the peritoneal cavity, virtually eliminating the potential for bowel injury, and they do not pass near large blood vessels, making major vascular injury less likely. Regardless, brisk bleeding can ensue intraoperatively from the vaginal incision, periurethral tissues, or while passing the needles close to the obturator artery and its branches. Typically this responds to pressure applied for a short duration or vaginal packing. Vaginal mucosal damage is more likely with transobturator than retropubic midurethral slings (8). In patients with deep lateral vaginal sulci, the helical needle can "buttonhole": doubly pierce the vaginal epithelium and result in a "bridge" of mesh superficial to the epithelium. Bladder injury is less common than with retropubic techniques (9), but cystoscopy is still recommended to ensure the integrity of the bladder and urethra. Recurrent postoperative urinary tract infections should alert the physician to the possibility of mesh in the bladder. It is notable, however, that postoperative urinary tract infections can be common following any incontinence surgery.

Short-term complications of bleeding include hematomas, ecchymosis, and anemia. Vaginal erosion can present days to months postoperatively. Numerous factors may contribute to erosion, including operative technique, mesh properties (pore size, stiffness, elasticity), and tissue properties (local ischemia, infection, and tissue integrity). Depending on the extent of the erosion, it can be managed by freshening up the vaginal edges and oversewing the epithelium, or by excision of the exposed mesh followed by closure of the epithelium. Infectious complications can present in a number of ways. Cellulitis can occur in both the groin and vaginal incisions, and it can lead to mesh erosion even after the infection has cleared. Abscess formation has been reported in both the adductor muscles of the thigh and the ischiorectal fossa. Treatment of these can be challenging, as they are rare and there is minimal experience in any single institution. Based on individual cases, drainage of the abscess, debridement of the infected tissue, and removal of the mesh are options. The latter can be challenging, depending on the time course of the infection and the amount of tissue ingrowth that has occurred.

Other complications that can have either short- or long-term sequelae include new-onset detrusor instability, continued incontinence, urinary retention, nerve injuries, and pain or dyspareunia.

Rates of major complications, including abscess formation, nerve injury, and life-threatening hemorrhage, are unknown, as they are rare events and even large studies are underpowered to report them. In 2006 Boyles (10) published on complications of three commercially available transobturator slings reported to the MAUDE data base (maintained by the FDA to collect and report complications of medical devices) between January 2004 and July 2005. During this time, 173 complications were listed in 140 reports. Sixty percent of these complications were mesh erosions, and one third of those were associated with infection. One urethral erosion was reported. Two abscesses of the ischiorectal fossa presented 2 months after the surgical procedure and required drainage. Two infections involved abscesses of the adductor muscles. Four cases of neuropathy were reported, and in two of these cases the patients had difficulty with ambulation. Five cases of bleeding in excess of 300 cc were reported. There was one documented case of injury to an iliac vessel with the medial to lateral technique that required embolization in radiology. Although these data are useful for understanding the types of complications that can occur, the number of cases they are pooled from are unknown. The FDA estimates that the actual number of complications is 10 to 100 times higher than reported to the MAUDE database.

## *References*


1. Ulmsten U, Petros P. Intravaginal slingplasty (IVS): an ambulatory surgical procedure for treatment of female urinary incontinence. *Scand J Urol Nephrol* 1995;29(1):75–82.
2. Ward K, Hilton P, G. Prospective multicentre randomised trial of tension-free vaginal tape and colposuspension as primary treatment for stress incontinence [see comment]. *BMJ* 2002;325(7355):67.
3. Delorme E. Transobturator urethral suspension: mini-invasive procedure in the treatment of stress urinary incontinence in women. *Prog Urol* 2001;11(6):1306–1313.
4. Barber MD, et al. Transobturator tape compared with tension-free vaginal tape for the treatment of stress urinary incontinence: a randomized controlled trial. *Obstet Gynecol* 2008;111(3):611–621.
5. Albo ME, et al. Burch colposuspension versus fascial sling to reduce urinary stress incontinence [see comment]. *N Engl J Med* 2007;356(21):2143–2155.
6. Whiteside JL, Walters MD. Anatomy of the obturator region: relations to a trans-obturator sling. *Int Urogynecol J* 2004;15(4):223–226.
7. Bump RC, et al. The standardization of terminology of female pelvic organ prolapse and pelvic floor dysfunction. *Am J Obstet Gynecol* 1996;175(1): 10–17.
8. Latthe PM, Foon R, Toozs-Hobson P. Transobturator and retropubic tape procedures in stress urinary incontinence: a systematic review and meta-analysis of effectiveness and complications. *Br J Obstet Gynecol* 2007; 114(5):522–531.
9. Barber MD, et al. Perioperative complications and adverse events of the MONARC transobturator tape, compared with the tension-free vaginal tape. *Am J Obstet Gynecol* 2006;195(6):1820–1825.
10. Boyles SH, et al. Complications associated with transobturator sling procedures. *Int Urogynecol J Pelvic Floor Dysfunct* 2007;18(1):19–22.

# CHAPTER 43 ■ ABDOMINAL RETROPUBIC APPROACHES FOR FEMALE INCONTINENCE

LESLIE M. RICKEY

Urinary incontinence (UI) is common, with approximately 30% of women reporting any incontinence; about 25% to 50% of these cases are estimated to be stress urinary incontinence (SUI) (1–3). In addition, the number of women seeking care for UI is increasing. Office visits for UI more than doubled, from 815,832 visits in 1992 to 1,932,768 visits in 2000 (4). A recent analysis of population growth and future demand for care concluded that consults for pelvic floor disorders will increase by 45% from 2000 to 2030 (5). In terms of surgical management, one out of nine women will have surgery for a pelvic floor disorder in their lifetime, and this number represents only a subset of women who have the condition (6). About one third of the surgeries were for SUI alone, and another 20% of surgeries were performed for combined SUI and pelvic organ prolapse (POP).

Although the exact mechanism that leads to SUI is not known, proposed theories include loss of proximal urethral support, or the "hammock" theory, and intrinsic deficiency of the external urethral sphincter. Surgical procedures are directed towards correction of the deficiency, either re-establishing support of the proximal urethral or improving urethral closure. The suburethral sling procedure can be performed using autologous fascia (rectus fascia or fascia lata) or synthetic material. The sling procedures are covered in other chapters.

Urethral position depends on anterior vaginal wall support. Retropubic colposuspension, or urethropexy, aims to improve the support of the vesicourethral junction by lifting the periurethral tissue towards the pubic bone, thus restoring the proper anatomy. The procedure is believed to treat incontinence by providing improved resistance to increases in intra-abdominal pressure, resulting in more effective urethral compression. The Marshall–Marchetti–Krantz (MMK) procedure involves suturing the periurethral tissue at the level of the bladder neck directly to the periosteum of the pubic symphysis. Burch, a gynecologist, modified this technique by altering the suspension laterally to the iliopectineal line, or Cooper's ligament. The Burch technique was further modified by Tanagho, a urologist, to include a suture bridge instead of direct apposition of the anterior vaginal wall to Cooper's ligament. The Burch urethropexy has traditionally been performed via a small Pfannenstiel incision, but the laparoscopic approach has been utilized as well.

The MMK is largely a historical procedure as the Burch appears to be slightly more efficacious. In addition, the complication of osteitis pubis is specific to the MMK approach due to the placement of suture directly into the periosteum. Although the Burch urethropexy may be regarded as an outdated procedure as well, it is still a reasonable option for a woman desiring an incontinence procedure, particularly if she is undergoing a concomitant abdominal surgery. In addition, as will be discussed later in the chapter, it is indicated for an asymptomatic, stress-continent woman undergoing an abdominal sacrocolpopexy for prolapse.

## DIAGNOSIS

A thorough and detailed patient history should elicit whether the patient has stress incontinence, urge incontinence, or mixed incontinence. It is important to ascertain a history of previous incontinence or pelvic surgeries, as this may affect surgical decision making. Prolapse symptoms should also be queried, as almost two thirds of women with SUI have coexisting POP (7), and additional procedures may be necessary at the time of the incontinence surgery. Finally, it is prudent for physicians performing pelvic surgery to inquire about whether the patients Pap screening is up to date.

The physical examination should include a bimanual and speculum examination to assess the vaginal tissue and vaginal support and to rule out any pelvic masses. A positive empty supine cough stress test is highly predictive of urodynamic stress incontinence (8). Urethral hypermobility should be confirmed before considering a Burch urethropexy. Traditional teaching has utilized the cotton-tipped swab test to measure urethral hypermobility. A cotton-tipped swab is inserted transurethrally to the proximal urethra, and the patient is asked to maximally Valsalva. A deflection of >30 degrees from the resting angle during Valsalva is considered to reflect urethral hypermobility. The surgeon should inspect the lower abdominal wall for scars indicative of previous pelvic surgery and correlate with the patient's surgical history.

If the patient relates SUI symptoms and desires surgical treatment, many surgeons choose to perform urodynamics (UDS) to confirm the diagnosis. It is believed that the Burch is not as effective in women with "intrinsic sphincter deficiency," typically defined by indirect measures of urethral function, including leak point pressure <60 mm Hg or urethral closure pressure of 20 mm Hg or less. However, a randomized trial comparing Burch to sling in women with low urethral closure pressures (20 cm $H_2O$ or less) did not show a difference in subjective success between the two procedures at a mean 5 years of follow-up (84% versus 93%, respectively, $p = 0.47$) (9). Although the study was not powered to detect small differences between the treatment groups, the findings still demonstrate that the Burch procedure can be effective in women with low urethral closure pressures. Valsalva leak point pressure (VLPP) has not been shown to be a significant predictor of success after the Burch procedure (10). In addition, a retrospective review of women who underwent a Burch urethropexy with preoperative VLPPs of <60 cm $H_2O$ showed an objective success rate of 91.7%, indicating that a low VLPP is not necessarily predictive of Burch failure (11). Direct measurement of striated urethral sphincter function using electromyography suggested that women with better innervation of their urethral sphincters were more likely to be cured by the Burch urethropexy (12). In summary, there are no UDS parameters clearly predictive of Burch success or failure. Therefore, traditional urodynamic testing does not seem to aid in the surgeon's decision of which incontinence procedure to perform. However, the study can provide helpful information about the coexistence of detrusor overactivity, clarify confusing symptomatology, and confirm diagnoses in patients who have undergone previous incontinence surgeries.

## INDICATIONS FOR SURGERY

The main indication for an incontinence procedure is the presence of symptomatic SUI that adversely affects the woman's quality of life. The patient should also have the sign of transurethral loss of urine with a cough stress test or during formal urodynamic testing. Additionally, the patient must be sufficiently healthy to undergo regional or general anesthesia, be able to be placed in dorsal lithotomy position and have a habitus that allows a suprapubic incision. There appears to be a risk of worsening POP after a Burch procedure (13–15); therefore, a Burch urethropexy probably should not be performed as a solitary procedure if there is significant apical descent. Lack of urethral hypermobility and a previously failed retropubic approach would be considered indications for a suburethral sling by most pelvic surgeons.

A Burch urethropexy is also appropriate for an asymptomatic woman (without SUI) undergoing a sacrocolpopexy for POP. A randomized controlled trial showed that performing a concomitant Burch urethropexy at the time of abdominal sacrocolpopexy resulted in a decrease of new-onset postoperative SUI from 40% to 20% in stress-continent women (16).

## ALTERNATIVE THERAPY

Conservative therapies for SUI may involve use of pessaries or physical therapy for pelvic floor muscle (PFM) rehabilitation. In women successfully fitted with a pessary for UI, rates of continued use and satisfaction range from 16% to 59% at 1 year (17,18). PFM physical therapy includes both strengthening and instruction on timing of activation of PFMs to avoid leakage. A Cochrane review in 2007 supported that PFM training should be included in first-line conservative management for women with UI (19). In women with SUI who participated in a course of PFM exercise, 44% to 56% of patients were satisfied with symptom improvement and desired no further treatment (20,21).

## SURGICAL TECHNIQUE

### Open Burch Urethropexy

The patient is placed in the low dorsal lithotomy position and the vagina and abdomen are prepped and draped for combined access. A Foley catheter is placed and a Pfannenstiel incision is made. Dissection of the space of Retzius is performed (Fig. 43.1). The first and second fingers of the surgeon's nondominant hand are placed in the vagina, with one finger on each side of the urethral catheter. The bladder is retracted medially so that the perivaginal tissue lateral to the vesicourethral junction is exposed. Using the vaginal finger as a guide, a peanut sponge can be used to carefully sweep away the overlying fat until the glistening white perivaginal "fascia" is visualized. Care must be used as vaginal and pelvic veins are often encountered in this area. Palpation of the Foley balloon will help delineate the vesicourethral junction. Two figure-of-eight sutures are placed in the periurethral vaginal tissue, one at the vesicourethral junction and another more distally at the level of the midurethra. Avoid placing the sutures through any fatty tissue. Placement of the sutures into the vagina is aided by elevation of the anterior vaginal wall using the hand in the vagina (Fig. 43.2A). The vaginal finger should be used as a guide to ensure that the sutures are sufficiently lateral to the urethra. The suture bite should encompass vaginal tissue without perforating the vaginal epithelium (Fig. 43.2B). The procedure is repeated on the other side. A total of four permanent, nonabsorbable sutures such as no. 0 or no. 1 polyester (Ethibond) or polytetrafluoroethylene (Gore-Tex) sutures are placed (two on each side; Fig. 43.3A). Cooper's ligament is identified and any overlying tissue is gently swept off using a peanut sponge.

The sutures are then placed through Cooper's ligament on the respective sides (Fig. 43.3B). Note that the sutures are tied off the midline. The proximal sutures will be placed slightly

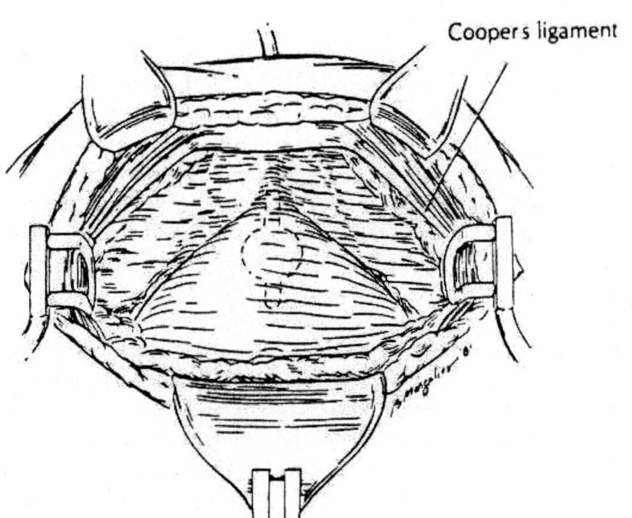


FIGURE 43.1 Retropubic space showing the bladder neck, Foley balloon, and Cooper's ligament.

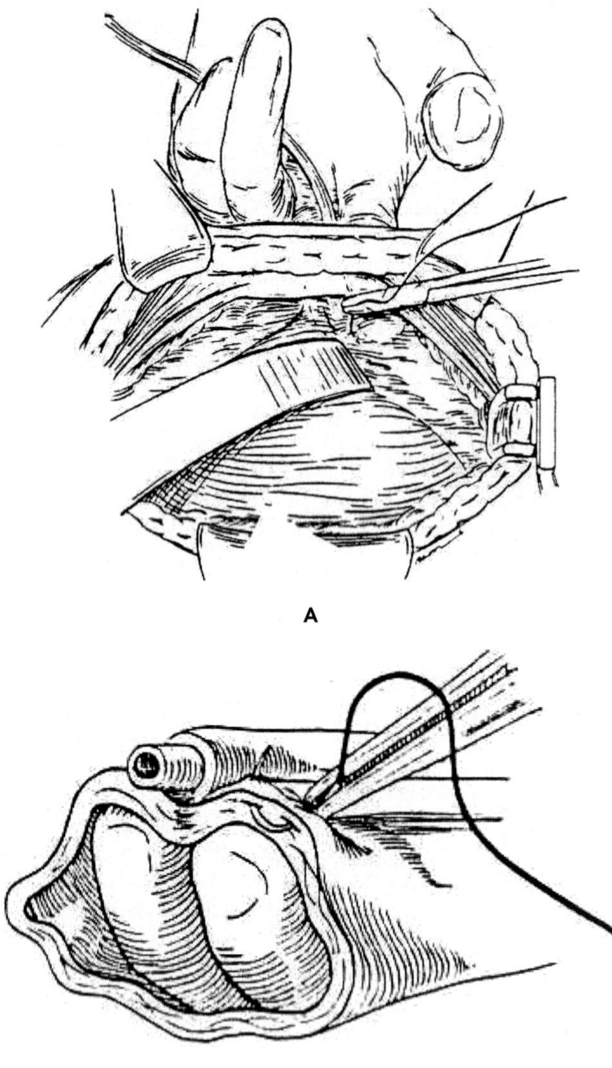

FIGURE 43.2 A: The first suture at the level of the vesicourethral junction. The surgeon's finger in the vagina helps guide the suture lateral to the urinary tract. B: The finger in the vagina also helps exclude the suture from the vaginal epithelium.

lateral to the more distal midurethral sutures. The obturator vessels and nerve pass through the obturator fascia; this obturator "notch" is the lateral limit for suture placement into Cooper's ligament and should be avoided. The assistant ties the sutures down while the operator's fingers remain in the vagina to ensure the proper degree of suspension. The operator should feel that the anterior wall is slightly lifted without overcorrection of the urethrovesical junction. It is imperative that the sutures are tied such that there is distance between Cooper's ligament and the vaginal tissue (Fig. 43.3B), seen as a suture bridge of approximately 2 cm. This prevents overcompression of the urethra, which can cause obstruction. The placement of these sutures and how tightly they are tied differ from the initial description of Burch, in which the sutures were tied down with complete approximation of the perivaginal tissue onto Cooper's ligament. After tying the sutures, cystoscopy is performed to ensure that the sutures did not perforate the bladder and that the ureters are patent. Methylene blue can be used to help identify efflux of urine from the ureteral orifices.

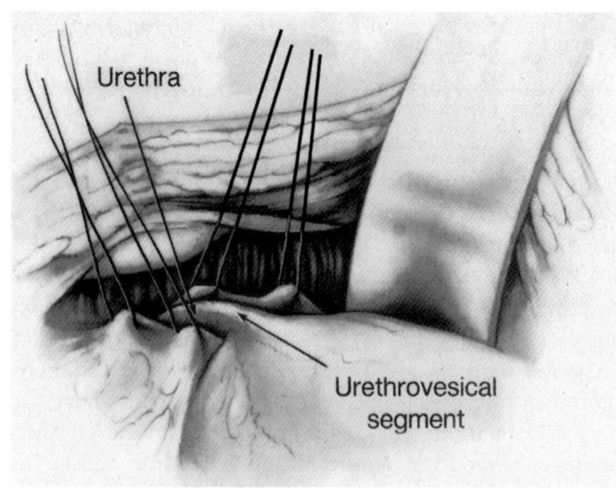


A

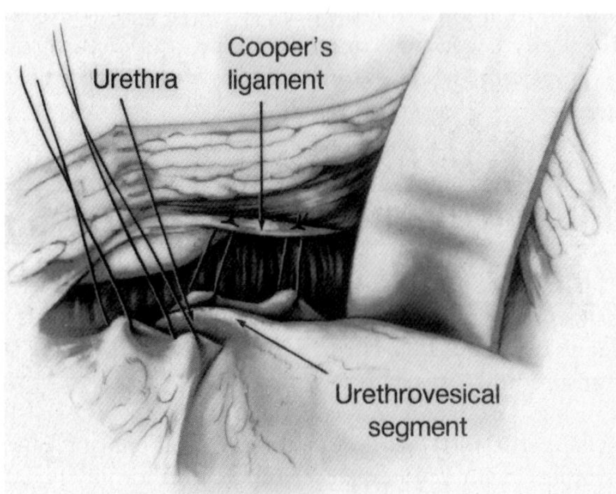


B

FIGURE 43.3 A: A total of four sutures are placed in the periurethral tissue. B: The two right-sided sutures are passed through Cooper's ligament and tied; note that there is a gap between the vaginal tissue and Cooper's ligament, creating a suture bridge.

### Laparoscopic Burch Urethropexy

Apart from the incisions, the laparoscopic Burch is performed in an identical manner to the open Burch procedure. There are a variety of port placement strategies described. A common approach is to place a 10-mm laparoscopic port at the umbilicus and two 5-mm ports in the lower lateral abdominal wall, approximately two fingerbreadths superior and medial to the anterior superior iliac spine. An additional suprapubic port is sometimes utilized. As in the open approach, cystoscopy should be performed at the end of the procedure to exclude intravesical suture and ensure ureteral patency. The laparoscopic procedure is covered in more detail in the chapter dedicated to laparoscopic surgery for urinary incontinence.

## OUTCOMES

### Results

A recent Cochrane review showed overall cure rates between 69% and 88% for open retropubic colposuspension (22). A randomized controlled trial comparing Burch to suburethral sling showed stress-specific success of 49% (compared to 66% for the sling group) at 2 years, using a very strict definition of success (23). However, there was also a lower rate of adverse events in the Burch group. The overall patient satisfaction was slightly lower in the Burch group (78% versus 86%, $p = 0.02$). Another randomized trial comparing Burch to tension-free vaginal tape (TVT) revealed 63% of women reporting cure after the Burch (versus 70% in TVT group, $p = 0.54$) at 5 years, but overall 90% of women who had undergone colposuspension were satisfied or very satisfied with the results of surgery (14). Using a negative 1-hour pad test (<1 g change in weight) for definition of cure, and using pad test data from the last available follow-up visit for missing data, the cure rates were computed as 69% for colposuspension versus 75% for TVT ($p = 0.28$).

In a randomized controlled trial comparing laparoscopic to open Burch, there were no significant differences seen at 24 months in patient-reported cure of stress incontinence (66%), although the study was not powered to detect a difference of <20% (24). There was not a significant difference in perioperative complications. Out of six cases of suture penetration into the bladder, five occurred in the laparoscopic group, but this difference did not reach statistical significance ($p = 0.11$). Mean operating time was less in the open group (87 versus 42 minutes, $p < 0.0001$), and blood loss was less in the laparoscopic group (126 versus 170 mL, $p = 0.03$). There was no difference in length of hospital stay, but the average return to normal activities was 5 days less in the laparoscopic group (24.6 versus 19.7 days, $p = 0.01$). A meta-analysis of studies comparing laparoscopic versus open Burch had similar findings of longer operating times, marginally less blood loss, decreased hospital stay, and faster return to normal activity in the laparoscopic group (25). There was not a significant difference in subjective or objective cure rates up to 2 years postoperatively.

Finally, a randomized trial comparing laparoscopic Burch to TVT with a median follow-up of 65 months concluded that the two procedures have similar long-term efficacy (26). Although only 52% of subjects in the TVT group and 43% in the Burch group reported no urine leakage under any circumstances, bothersome urine leakage was present in only 8% and 11%, respectively ($p = 0.26$), and overall patient satisfaction rates were similar as well (79% versus 88%). Operating time was less in the TVT group, but there was no difference in blood loss or hospital stay. In terms of bladder injury, there were two cystotomies in the TVT group and two patients with bladder sutures detected intraoperatively in the laparoscopic Burch group.

## Complications

Delayed bladder emptying was seen in 2% of patients after undergoing a Burch urethropexy in a large multicenter study, but no additional procedures were required for urinary retention (23). These patients may require temporary intermittent self-catheterization. Occasionally, the periurethral sutures must be released transvaginally to relieve the urethral obstruction if there is not adequate bladder emptying at 4 to 6 weeks postoperatively. New-onset urge urinary incontinence occurs in 3% to 4% of patients, and 5% report de novo urgency (14,23). In a patient with significant postoperative urgency and frequency, urinary retention and urinary tract infection should be ruled out: as many as 30% of patients may develop a urinary tract infection in the postoperative period (23).

Ureteral injuries occur in <1% of patients. Bladder injury is more common, with incidental cystotomy rates of 2% to 4%, usually due to suture passage into the bladder. A recent study showed that 2 of 329 (0.6%) patients sustained a ureteral injury and 10 of 329 (3.3%) had an incidental cystotomy when undergoing a Burch urethropexy (23). A cystoscopy at the time of surgery can aid in identifying intravesical sutures, and ureteral patency can be confirmed as well.

Approximately 8% to 13% of women are found to have vaginal vault or uterine prolapse during the follow-up period after Burch (14,15,27). The clinical significance of the prolapse has been unclear; however, a randomized controlled trial comparing Burch to TVT showed that surgery for prolapse was more common after the Burch colposuspension (7.5% versus 1.8%, $p = 0.025$) (14). Therefore, a sling may be a more appropriate choice for a woman desiring an incontinence procedure who has asymptomatic prolapse with apical descent of several centimeters or more.

## CONCLUSION

A Burch urethropexy should be considered for a woman desiring an incontinence procedure, particularly if she is undergoing a concomitant abdominal surgery, or for a stress-continent woman undergoing an abdominal sacrocolpopexy.

## *References*


1. Hunskaar S, Arnold EP, Burgio K, et al. Epidemiology and natural history of urinary incontinence. *Int Urogynecol J Pelvic Floor Dysfunct* 2000; 11(5):301–319.
2. Melville JL, Katon W, Delaney K, et al. Urinary incontinence in US women: a population-based study. *Arch Intern Med* 2005;165(5):537–542.
3. Waetjen LE, Subak LL, Shen H, et al. Stress urinary incontinence surgery in the United States. *Obstet Gynecol* 2003;101(4):671–676.
4. Thom DH, Nygaard IE, Calhoun EA. Urologic diseases in America project: urinary incontinence in women-national trends in hospitalizations, office visits, treatment and economic impact. *J Urol* 2005;173(4):1295–1301.
5. Luber KM, Boero S, Choe JY. The demographics of pelvic floor disorders: current observations and future projections. *Am J Obstet Gynecol* 2001; 184(7):1493–1501.
6. Olsen AL, Smith VJ, Bergstrom JO, et al. Epidemiology of surgically managed pelvic organ prolapse and urinary incontinence. *Obstet Gynecol* 1997;89(4):501–506.
7. Bai SW, Kang JY, Rha KH, et al. Relationship of urodynamic parameters and obesity in women with stress urinary incontinence. *J Reprod Med* 2002;47(7):559–563.
8. Lobel RW, Sand PK. The empty supine stress test as a predictor of intrinsic urethral sphincter dysfunction. *Obstet Gynecol* 1996;88(1):128–132.
9. Sand PK, Winkler H, Blackhurst DW, et al. A prospective randomized study comparing modified Burch retropubic urethropexy and suburethral sling for treatment of genuine stress incontinence with low-pressure urethra. *Am J Obstet Gynecol* 2000;182(1, Pt 1):30–34.
10. Nager CW, FitzGerald M, Kraus SR, et al. Urodynamic measures do not predict stress continence outcomes after surgery for stress urinary incontinence in selected women. *J Urol* 2008;179(4):1470–1474.
11. Bai SW, Park JH, Kim SK, et al. Analysis of the success rates of Burch colposuspension in relation to Valsalva leak-point pressure. *J Reprod Med* 2005;50(3):189–192.

12. Kenton K, FitzGerald MP, Shott S, et al. Role of urethral electromyography in predicting outcome of Burch retropubic urethropexy. *Am J Obstet Gynecol* 2001;185(1):51–55.
13. Wiskind AK, Creighton SM, Stanton SL. The incidence of genital prolapse after the Burch colposuspension. *Am J Obstet Gynecol* 1992;167(2): 395–404.
14. Ward KL, Hilton P. Tension-free vaginal tape versus colposuspension for primary urodynamic stress incontinence: 5-year follow up. *Br J Obstet Gynaecol* 2008;115(2):226–233.
15. Enzelsberger H, Helmer H, Schatten C. Comparison of Burch and lyodura sling procedures for repair of unsuccessful incontinence surgery. *Obstet Gynecol* 1996;88(2):251–256.
16. Brubaker L, Cundiff GW, Fine P, et al. Abdominal sacrocolpopexy with Burch colposuspension to reduce urinary stress incontinence. *N Engl J Med* 2006;354(15):1557–1566.
17. Robert M, Mainprize TC. Long-term assessment of the incontinence ring pessary for the treatment of stress incontinence. *Int Urogynecol J Pelvic Floor Dysfunct* 2002;13(5):326–329.
18. Farrell SA, Singh B, Aldakhil L. Continence pessaries in the management of urinary incontinence in women. *J Obstet Gynaecol Can* 2004;26(2): 113–117.
19. Hay-Smith EJ, Dumoulin C. Pelvic floor muscle training versus no treatment, or inactive control treatments, for urinary incontinence in women. *Cochrane Database Syst Rev* 2006(1):CD005654.
20. Bo K, Talseth T, Holme I. Single blind, randomised controlled trial of pelvic floor exercises, electrical stimulation, vaginal cones, and no treatment in management of genuine stress incontinence in women. *BMJ* 1999; 318(7182):487–493.
21. Nygaard IE, Kreder KJ, Lepic MM, et al. Efficacy of pelvic floor muscle exercises in women with stress, urge, and mixed urinary incontinence. *Am J Obstet Gynecol* 1996;174(1, Pt 1):120–125.
22. Lapitan MC, Cody DJ, Grant AM. Open retropubic colposuspension for urinary incontinence in women. *Cochrane Database Syst Rev* 2005(3): CD002912.
23. Albo ME, Richter HE, Brubaker L, et al. Burch colposuspension versus fascial sling to reduce urinary stress incontinence. *N Engl J Med* 2007; 356(21):2143–2155.
24. Carey MP, Goh JT, Rosamilia A, et al. Laparoscopic versus open Burch colposuspension: a randomised controlled trial. *Br J Obstet Gynaecol* 2006; 113(9):999–1006.
25. Tan E, Tekkis PP, Cornish J, et al. Laparoscopic versus open colposuspension for urodynamic stress incontinence. *Neurourol Urodyn* 2007;26(2): 158–169.
26. Jelovsek JE, Barber MD, Karram MM, et al. Randomised trial of laparoscopic Burch colposuspension versus tension-free vaginal tape: long-term follow up. *Br J Obstet Gynaecol* 2008;115(2):219–225.
27. Kwon CH, Culligan PJ, Koduri S, et al. The development of pelvic organ prolapse following isolated Burch retropubic urethropexy. *Int Urogynecol J Pelvic Floor Dysfunct* 2003;14(5):321–325.


# CHAPTER 44 ■ THE ARTIFICIAL URINARY SPHINCTER

HELEN ZAFIRAKIS AND O. LENAINE WESTNEY

The artificial urinary sphincter (AUS) is the most effective treatment for intrinsic urethral sphincter dysfunction. The three components, consisting of a cuff that is placed around the urethra, a reservoir, and a pump (Fig. 44.1), have not changed since the initial device was introduced in 1983. However, in the late 1980s several modifications were made to the device, such a narrow-backed cuff and kink-resistant tubing, that resulted in a significant reduction in the number of mechanical failures. The pump, which is placed either in the scrotum in men or the labium majorum in women, has both a mechanical pump section and a deactivation button. When activated, the cuff maintains continence by circumferential compression of the urethra. If voiding is desired, the patient uses the pump to force fluid from the cuff toward the reservoir. Fluid automatically returns into the cuff over about 2 minutes as the pressure reequilibrates in the system, allowing adequate time for bladder emptying. The deactivation button prevents the reentry of fluid in the cuff. To reactivate the device, the patient presses the pump forcefully and thus releases the poppet valve, allowing the fluid to enter the cuff and thus restore continence.

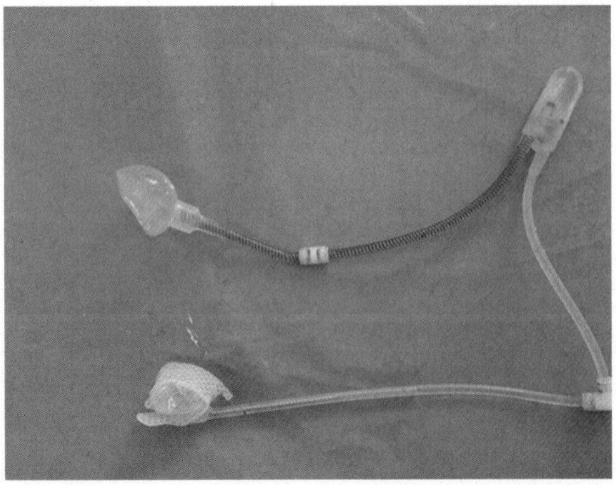

FIGURE 44.1 The AMS 800 Artificial Urinary Sphincter. The three components are the pump, the reservoir, and the cuff, connected with tubing and connectors.

## DIAGNOSIS

Physical examination should include examination of the genitalia, neurological assessment, and assessment of the integrity of the perineal skin. Investigations should include a voiding diary and cystoscopy to look at the quality of the urethral tissue, especially at the bladder neck and bulbar urethra, in order to exclude conditions that would need to be dealt with prior to placing the AUS, such as stricture disease. Fluoroscopic urodynamics are necessary to verify the cause of incontinence, assess bladder capacity and compliance, and exclude detrusor overactivity, which, in conjunction with an AUS being placed and especially in the setting of neurogenic patients, can be dangerous to kidney function over time. Urethral pressure profiles are not obligatory but may add weight to the diagnosis of intrinsic sphincter deficiency, depending on the leak point pressures.

# INDICATIONS FOR SURGERY

The most common indication for AUS insertion is postprostatectomy sphincter incompetence. Other indications include congenital or acquired neurogenic conditions of the bladder. Patients with congenital genitourinary abnormalities (such as exstrophy-epispadias complex), those with posterior trauma where the sphincter has been compromised, and female incontinence where other anti-incontinence therapies have failed may also benefit from an AUS.

The AUS is contraindicated in patients who have an intellectual or physical disability that would render them unable to utilize the device properly. Other relative contraindications include patients with progressive neuromuscular disorders who would develop such a disability in a relatively short time or patients with an untreated small-capacity or noncompliant bladder or with detrusor overactivity that is not controlled. Women with a previous history of pelvic irradiation [1] also fall into the group of relative contraindications because they may have a poor outcome with AUS due to urethral and/or vaginal device erosion.

# ALTERNATIVE THERAPIES

Alternative therapies to the artificial sphincter include closure of the bladder neck, injection of bulking agents, and urinary diversion.

# SURGICAL TECHNIQUE

## Preoperative Preparation

Urinary tract infection must be either excluded or treated if identified prior to surgery. The perineal skin must be in good condition and intact. If there is irritation of the skin due to urine contact, a catheter should be placed and then removed a week or so before implantation of the AUS. Antibiotics are given 1 hour preoperatively or at induction, and they need to cover both aerobic and anaerobic organisms. Common combinations of antibiotics include vancomycin and gentamicin or cefuroxime, and metronidazole and gentamicin (2).The patient is shaved on the operating table, not beforehand, to reduce the risk of infection. An additional measure is the use of a chlorhexidine wash to reduce the microbial load 24 hours prior to surgery. If the patient was on an intermittent catheterization program, prophylactic antibiotics should be given for 3 days leading up to surgery (3).

Spinal or general anesthesia is usually given, and the lower abdomen and genitalia are shaved carefully. A povidone-iodine or chlorhexidine wash of the skin is performed for 10 minutes, with a separate povidone-iodine or equivalent skin preparation followed by an alcohol scrub. The patient is draped to allow access to the lower abdomen, suprapubic area, and genitalia and is placed supine in a lithotomy or spreader bar position. A 16Fr Foley catheter is then placed into the bladder.

## AUS Placement in Men

### Perineal Incision

The traditional method of AUS placement involves a perineal incision. For bulbous urethra cuff placement, a midline perineal incision is made over the bulbar urethra with dissection extended to just distal to the bulbocavernosus muscle so that a 2-cm length of urethra has been dissected (Fig. 44.2). The most proximal placement of the cuff possible should be attempted. Care should be handle the corpus spongiosum gently and to avoid opening the urethral lumen. Injury to the spongiosal tissue should be repaired with a 4-0 absorbable suture rather than with cautery. Circumferential dissection of the urethra requires careful sharp removal of the midline dorsal urethra attachment to the corpora. The sound of the scissor blade when dissect in the correct plane should be a distinct snip. Once the urethral dissection is complete, the cuff size is determined using a sizer in the AUS kit. The most common

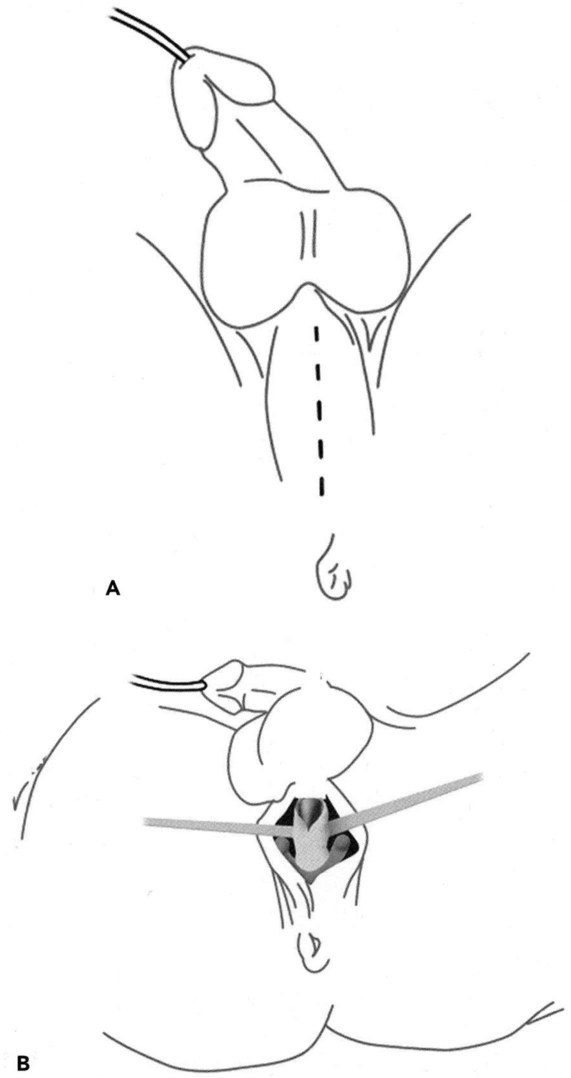


FIGURE 44.2 **A:** Diagram demonstrating the perineal incision for placement of the AUS. **B:** Dissection of the urethra. The urethra is dissected free circumferentially (demonstrated by the Penrose drain behind the urethra).

size for an adult male bulbar urethra in this position is 4.5 cm. The cuff should be snug, but not too loose or tight.

A small lateral transverse groin incision is made approximately 2 to 3 cm above the symphysis pubica to the side of the desired pump placement. A transverse 2-cm incision is made in the fascia. Closure sutures are placed in the fascia at this point prior to reservoir placement. After opening the rectus fascia, a space is developed beneath the transversalis fascia in the retropubic space for the reservoir. The reservoir is positioned and inflated to 23 to 25 mL of solution, depending on the size and number of cuffs. The most commonly selected reservoir pressure is 61 to 70 cm of water in postprostatectomy patients. The pathway for the pump tubing is developed from the suprapubic incision, beneath the Scarpa fascia, utilizing a ring clamp. The subdartos space is developed by spreading the clamp in the most dependent scrotal position. The pump should be on the lateral aspect of the scrotum with the deactivation button directed laterally. The length of tubing required to ensure continued dependent placement is facilitated by securing the tubing to the scrotal skin with a Babcock clamp until the connections are performed.

The pressure of the reservoir balloon is a balance between adequate continence and avoidance of extreme cuff pressures. Generally, in most postprostatectomy patients, a balloon with 61–70 cm of water pressure is adequate; however, where the urethra has been compromised or in cases of previous irradiation, a reduced pressure, such as 51 to 60 cm of water, is used to reduce the risk of urethral erosion and atrophy.

The cuff tubing is directed to the suprapubic incision utilizing a tubing passer. At this time, the tubing connections are completed using either the Quick Connect (American Medical Systems, Minnetonka, MN) system or tied connections. Injectable normal saline is preferred to the use of isotonic contrast solutions as these can alter the pressure dynamics in the system over time.

After inserting the AUS, the system should be cycled to ensure that it functions, then deactivated to allow healing for 4 to 6 weeks. It is important to allow the pump to partially fill prior to deactivation to decrease the difficulty of activation. This is done by waiting until there is enough fluid in the pump to create a small dimple when it is palpated as the AUS is activated, then deactivating it. Once all the components are in place and tested, the wounds are closed in layers with absorbable sutures. No urethral catheter needs to be left in situ, unless there are concerns about bladder emptying, such as in some neurogenic patients. Antibiotics are continued for 24 hours parenterally and then orally for a further 5 to 7 days. This implies that the patient can usually be discharged the following day. No drains are left. The AUS is left in the deactivated position for 6 weeks to allow healing. Patients are encouraged to gently milk the pump inferiorly to encourage maintenance of the appropriate scrotal dependency.

## Transcorporeal Cuff Placement

Patients with urethral erosion or infection of the AUS device can be difficult to manage. The cuff can be placed at a different site once the urethral tissues are ready for reimplantation; however, the urethral re-erosion rate is 11.8% (4). In some cases there is not adequate room to place a cuff in a position more proximal to the original urethral position, and using the urethra distal to the bulbar urethra can generate problems with a thin urethral wall, increasing the risk of recurrent erosion. The ability to augment in the urethra while protecting from the pressure from the cuff would theoretically decrease the risk of erosion. There are also reports of some encouraging results using a gracilis muscle transposition flap to the proximal urethra in conjunction with electrical stimulation (5).

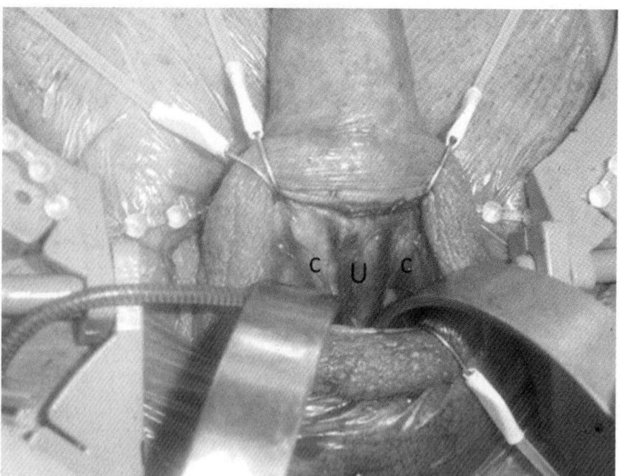


FIGURE 44.3 Initial dissection of the urethra, showing the urethra *(U)* and the corpora cavernosa *(C)* on either side.

Guralnick et al. (6) developed the technique of transcorporeal cuff placement, which utilizes a buttress of tunica albuginea from the corpora cavernosa to protect the dorsal urethral wall from erosion in cases of revision due to either erosion or atrophy. The essential principles of this technique involve utilizing a segment of urethra 2 to 3 cm distal to the bulbar urethra (where the original cuff was placed), avoiding dissection of intervening urethra. A urethral site is selected using urethroscopy, and an incision is made over the urethra at this site, exposing both the urethra and corporal bodies (Fig. 44.3). Longitudinal incisions 2.5 cm long are made in the corporal bodies bilaterally, with a tunnel being formed between the two corporotomies (Fig. 44.4A). This results in a layer of tunica albuginea attached onto the roof of the urethra, around which the new cuff is placed, giving extra protection to the urethra at this point (6) (Fig. 44.4B). The tunica left on the corpora cavernosa is reconstituted behind the cuff prior to cuff placement (Fig. 44.4C). With the supplemental tissue, the circumferential measurement is increased, allowing for larger cuff placement (6).

## Transverse Scrotal Incision for Placement of AUS

Conventional placement of the AUS is via a perineal incision and a separate suprapubic incision for the pressure-regulating balloon. In 2003, Wilson et al. (7) reported on the transverse scrotal incision, which uses a single incision to place all components of the AUS (Fig. 44.5). The patient is placed in the supine position with gentle abduction of the hips with the legs on spreader bars, rather than in the lithotomy position.

The perineum and lower abdomen are prepared and draped in the standard fashion. A 2.5- to 3.0-cm upper transverse

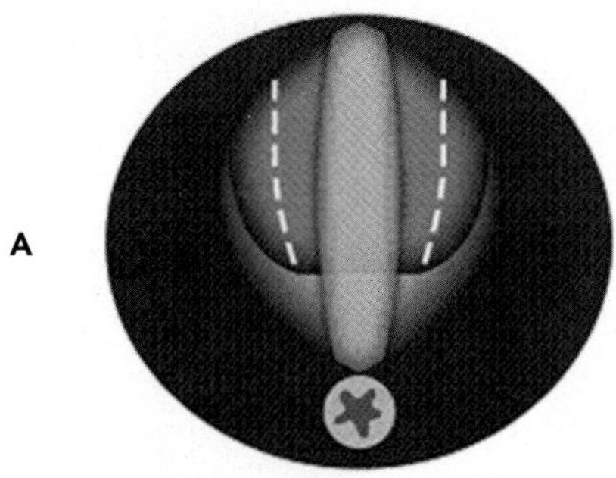


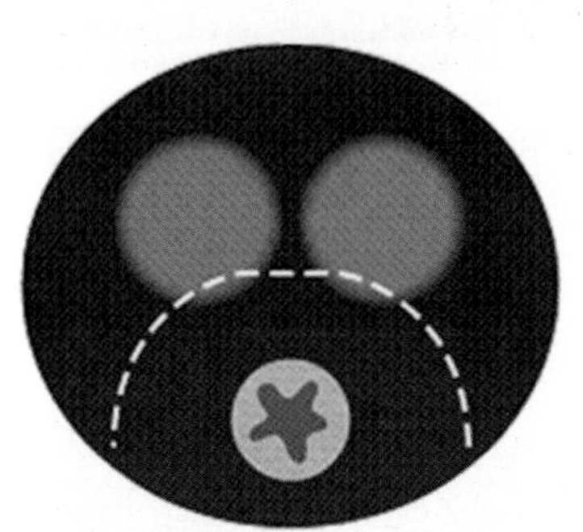


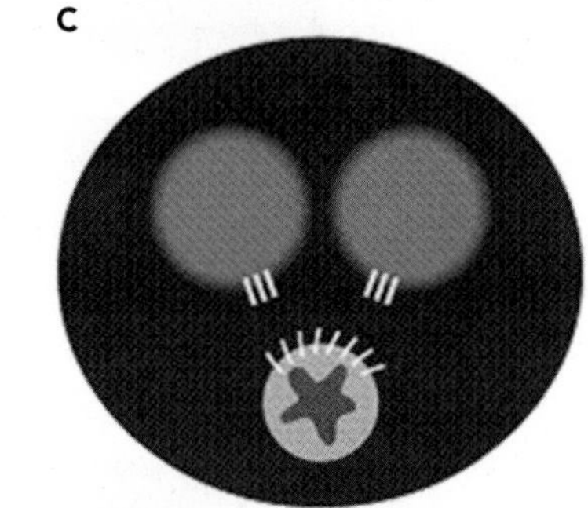


FIGURE 44.4 **A:** Transcorporeal cuff placement: Vertical corporotomies are made bilaterally. **B:** The tunica over the corpora is left attached to the urethra for extra support of urethral tissues. **C:** The remaining tunica albuginea is reconstituted behind the position of the cuff. (Adapted from Guralnick ML, et al. *J Urol* 2002;167(5):2075–2079, with permission.)

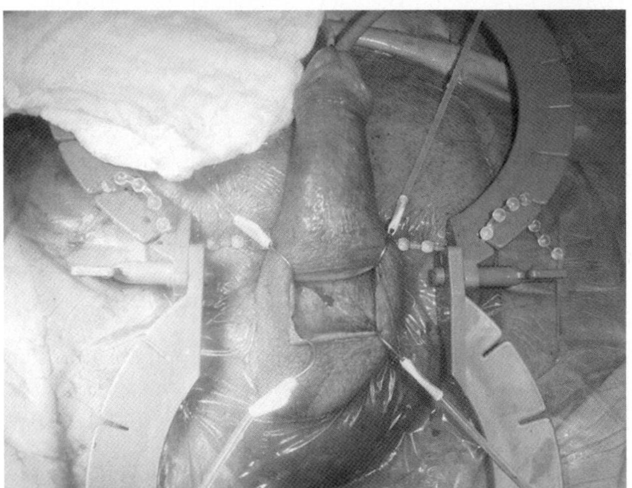

FIGURE 44.5 Transverse scrotal incision for placement of AUS with Lone Star ring retractor in place.

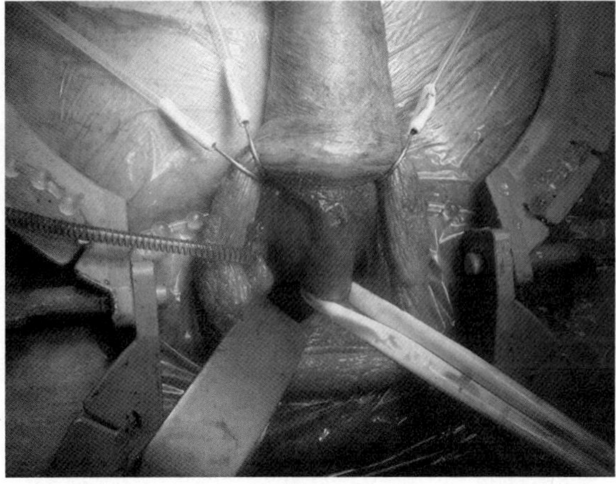


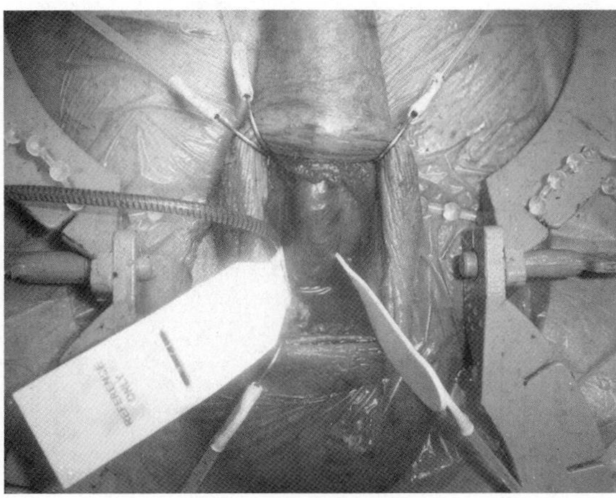


FIGURE 44.6 **A:** Transverse scrotal incision with completely dissected urethra. A Penrose drain is slung behind the urethra. **B:** Placement of the sizer to determine the size of the cuff required.

scrotal incision is made. The dissection is optimized by utilization of a self-retaining retractor combined with a dorsal meatal glans hook to stretch the penis superiorly and a penile band at the dorsal aspect of the base of the penile shaft.

The corpora are exposed proximally, and the midline attachment between the Corpora spongiosa and the scrotal septum is divided sharply (7). Pediatric Deaver retractors deavers positioned adjacent to the corpora cavernosa are utilized to retract the scrotal wall and the bulbocavernosus muscle. The dissection is carried to the level of the perineal body. The bulbar urethra is then dissected circumferentially at the desired cuff location (Fig. 44.6). Blunt dissection is used to identify the external ring, which is placed on tension by upward retraction with a Rich or Deaver retractor. Metzenbaum scissors are used to perforate the transversalis fascia just above

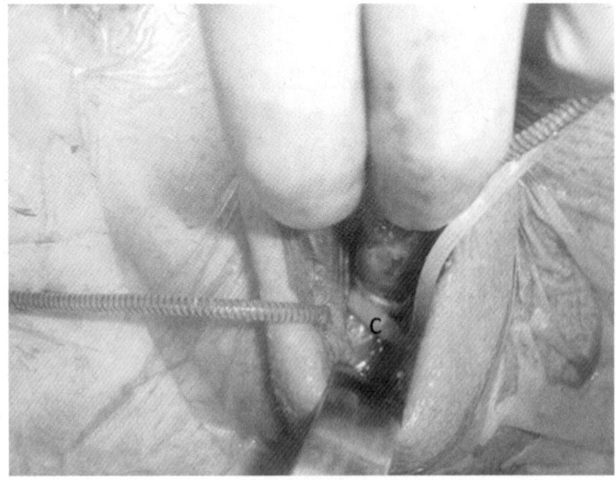


FIGURE 44.6 C: Urethral cuff *(c)* in position.

the pubic bone (7) (Fig. 44.7). The reservoir is placed and filled with either normal saline or isotonic contrast solution (Fig. 44.8). The pump is then placed in a subdartos pouch (Fig. 44.9).

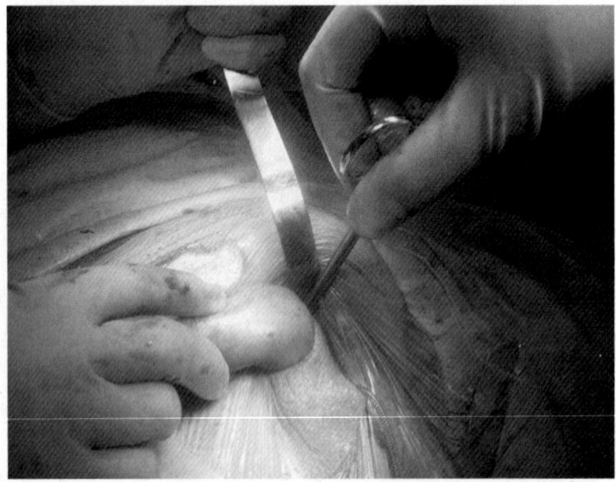

FIGURE 44.7 Through the same transverse scrotal incision, Metzenbaum scissors are used to perforate the transversalis fascia and develop the pocket for placement of the reservoir.

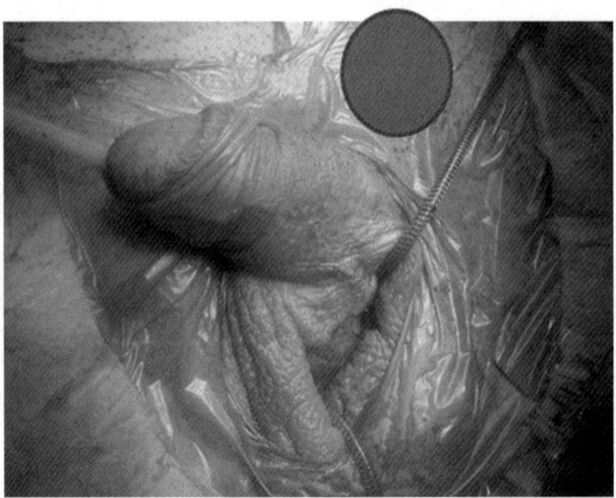

FIGURE 44.8 The reservoir is in position in the space of Retzius. The tubing connecting to the reservoir can be seen caudally. The *blue circle* represents the position of the reservoir.

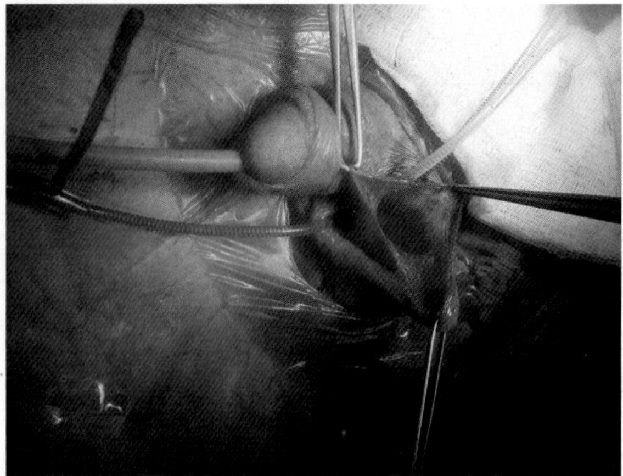

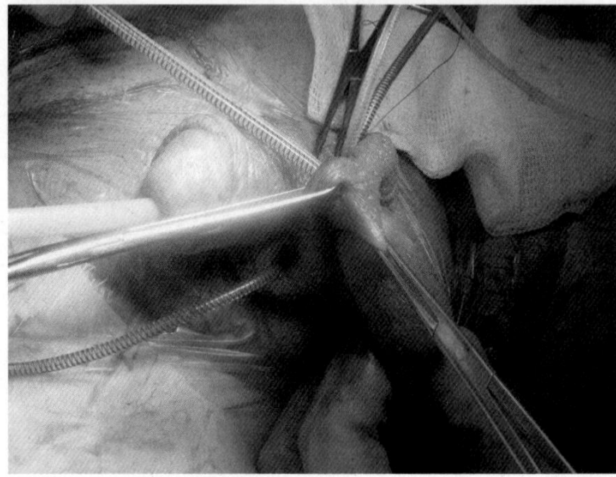

FIGURE 44.9 A: Creation of a subdartos pouch with the transverse scrotal incision for placement of the pump. B: The AUS pump is in position in the scrotum and is held by a Babcock clamp.

## Bladder Neck Cuff Placement

For bladder neck cuff placement, a suprapubic incision (either transverse or vertical) is made to allow access to the prevesical space. Blunt dissection continues to expose the endopelvic fascia, prostate, and bladder neck area. Some surgeons leave the endopelvic fascia intact while others opt to open it, but ultimately, a plane is developed between the bladder neck and the rectum posteriorly to allow room for the cuff. If additional space is required, the endopelvic fascia may be incised and the dissection can involve some of the prostate laterally and posteriorly. The bladder can also be opened to facilitate this dissection. The dorsal vein complex can usually be left undisturbed. The sizing tape is then passed around the dissected bladder neck to determine the cuff size of the AUS, and the cuff is placed. At this level, larger cuff sizes are often used 6–8 cm. The balloon is then placed in the prevesical space. The cuff tubing is passed anteriorly and the balloon tubing inferiorly and above the rectus fascia. The reservoir balloon is filled with 22 mL of fluid. The pump is placed in the ipsilateral scrotum in a subdartos space similar to the two-incision approach. The tubing is then positioned, trimmed, and connected Quick Connect connectors. At all stages of insertion of the AUS, extreme care should be taken to avoid air bubbles getting into the system by the use of rubber shods.

## AUS Placement in Women

The main indication for insertion of AUS in the female patient is in the neurogenic population, especially those with congenital neurogenic conditions, such as spina bifida. Increasingly, however, the sphincter is being placed for patients with primary, secondary, or recurrent incontinence, especially when alternative or less invasive procedures have failed. The evaluation prior to AUS insertion is the same as that previously discussed. However, the use of topical estrogens to the vaginal tissues in postmenopausal women can improve the quality and resilience of these tissues preoperatively.

There are two approaches to the female AUS: abdominal (8) and transvaginal (9). The bladder neck is the only position available for insertion of the cuff in women. There is limited urethral length, and the dissection is more difficult due to a lack of a surgical plane between the posterior urethra and vagina. This increases the risk of early erosion in this gender. The abdominal approach involves a transverse lower midline, or Pfannenstiel, incision. A 2-cm area of bladder neck is developed, carefully avoiding perforation of the urethra, bladder, and vagina (Fig. 44.10). The dissected area is measured and the cuff is placed, with the tubing away from the vaginal wall toward the desired placement for the reservoir. Next, the balloon is placed in the paravesical space, with care taken to avoid direct contact with the tubing and connections. The pump is placed in a dependent subcutaneous portion of the ipsilateral labia majora.

The transvaginal technique involves an inverted U incision in the anterior vaginal wall, centered at the level of the bladder neck. The posterior urethral and bladder neck dissection is done under direct vision; however, the anterior part of the urethra needs to be dissected bluntly and with careful sharp dissection to avoid entering the urethral lumen and bladder. If this dissection is difficult because of previous scarring, a separate supraurethral vaginal incision can be made. The cuff is then positioned once the circumferential dissection is completed. A separate small transverse suprapubic incision is used to place the reservoir balloon and the pump, which is tunneled into the labia majora. The tubing from the cuff is passed on the suprapubic incision utilizing the tubing passer. A vaginal pack is used for 24 hours, and a Foley catheter is left in place for 1 or 2 days. There have been concerns raised over an increased risk of infections and erosions using the transvaginal approach; however, in Appell's series (9), out of the 34 women studied, 56% were dry at 3 years and there were no infections or erosions reported. Others have reported conflicting opinions (10).

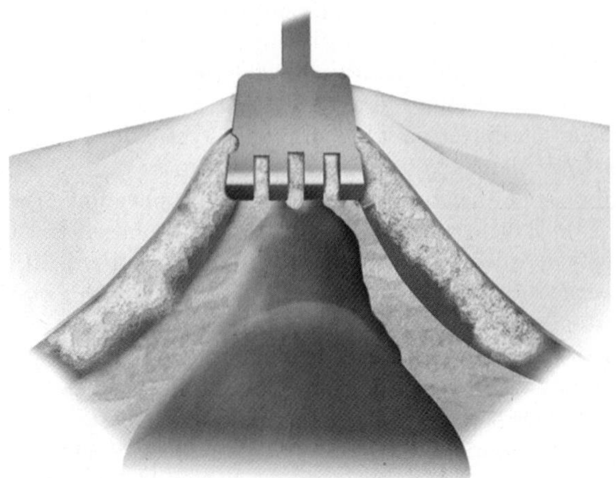

FIGURE 44.10 The abdominal approach to implantation of the AUS in women. The bladder neck region has been dissected ready for placement of the cuff.

## Synchronous AUS and Penile Implant Insertion

The transscrotal approach for insertion of the AUS has naturally led to the development of an extended procedure to place penile implants via the same incision. The upper transverse scrotal incision used to insert an AUS is also ideal for exposing the corpora for access to penile prosthesis procedures. Despite this, there have been concerns about the risk of infection and erosion with this technique. The preparation of the patient is the same as for AUS, except that the patient is supine with legs slightly abducted. After the incision is made, the septum is incised to free the corpora. The urethra is dissected enough to place a bulbar cuff, followed by corporotomy for insertion of the penile prosthesis. The reservoirs are placed in either retropubic space and the pumps in the scrotum as usual. Bhalchandra et al. (21) recommend implanting the AUS first and deactivating the device, prior to placing the penile prosthesis. They also suggest that, to reduce the rate of erosion, primary deactivation and nocturnal deactivation are used. Furthermore, they suggest the use of a low-pressure reservoir and an inflatable penile prosthesis.

## AUS in the Pediatric Population Simultaneous with Bladder Augmentation

The usual subgroup requiring AUS in the pediatric population is either those with congenital neurogenic bladder dysfunction or those with exstrophy-epispadias complex. They often have abnormal detrusor function, which can often manifest after insertion of the AUS. Studies that have looked at the medium- and long-term outcome in the pediatric group have noted excellent continence rates of 92% at 4 years (11) and 71% to 86% at 10 years (12,13). In patients with neurogenic bladder dysfunction who are inadequately controlled by antimuscarinic medication, an augmentation cystoplasty is required. Ideally, AUS placement and augmentation may be performed at the same setting. Also, post-AUS bladder dysfunction is being recognized as a potential problem. Following augmentation with AUS, the rate of needing to self-catheterize is 60% to 70% (11–14); therefore, it is important that the patient is capable of catheterizing in some way prior to operation.

Finally, the potential problem of renal failure needs to be discussed. Levesque et al. (12) reported an 11% risk of renal failure due to high bladder pressures in their population. These patients failed to attend follow-up because they were continent and otherwise well. This problem has also been seen in other studies and highlights the need to educate patients and their family about the importance of regular follow-up after insertion of an AUS, irrespective of whether they have had an augmentation.

## COMPLICATIONS

Early complications of AUS insertion are commonly urinary retention and hematoma. Urinary retention can be managed easily with either a temporary Foley catheter or intermittent catheterization. Hematomas can occur adjacent to any part of the AUS but are more commonly found around the pump.

Infection and urethral erosion are often discussed simultaneously in studies on the AUS. Although the generally quoted incidence for this serious complication is around 3%, its incidence has varied considerably and in some studies is surprisingly high. A recent review of 270 AUS patients with 36 months follow-up reports an infection rate of 5.5% and an erosion rate of 6% (15). In a long-term study with a mean follow-up of 11 years, the infection and erosion rate was 25% (13), and in Hajivassiliou's review of the literature the incidence of erosion is 12% with infection in 4% to 5% (16). Once suspected, all components of the AUS have to be removed and a period of antimicrobial treatment and recovery needs to take place before reimplantation. The standard waiting period prior to attempting replacement is usually 3 to 6 months. Erosion can occur early and is often due to an unrecognized perforation in the urethra, or it may occur late due to chronic pressure of the cuff on the urethral tissues. Previous irradiation, trauma, or urethral scarring for any reason may increase the risk of erosion. Women are also at increased risk, as discussed previously.

Mechanical failure can occur from the outset of AUS insertion or later due to wear and tear on the AUS components. The long-term incidence of revisions secondary to mechanical failure is 32% over 11 years (13); however, in one review the figure is 12% (16). This percentage has decreased to 7.6% due to developments in AUS design such as the narrow-backed cuff (17).

If incontinence recurs, one needs to consider the patient, the device, and the bladder. It may be due to the patient not using the device properly, mechanical failure of the device, urethral spongiosal atrophy, the development of detrusor overactivity, or overflow incontinence. If the device seems to be cycling correctly, one should perform urodynamics with leak point pressures and cystoscopy to investigate the cause. If urethral atrophy is the cause, the cuff can be downsized, or, if a small cuff is already in situ, another cuff can be placed in tandem or transcorporeal cuff placement can be attempted. Overactivity of the detrusor can usually be treated with antimuscarinics; however, in the neuropathic population it often requires augmentation of the bladder.

## OUTCOMES

Of the long-term follow-up studies for the AUS, Hajivassiliou (16) found that the overall continence rates are 73% with 88% improved continence. Venn et al. (13) found an overall continence rate at 10 years of 84%. The best results were in the postprostatectomy group, who had cuffs placed at the bulb (92% dry at 10 years). This group also had the least chance of infection of the AUS. The overall risk of revision was 54% (13). The continence rate in patients with postprostatectomy incontinence is excellent, with long-term continence exceeding 90% (13,17,18). The revision rate in this group is about one-third, but patient satisfaction is consistently high.

Revision rates of the AUS vary, but of the studies looking at long-term survival of grafts, the overall revision rates are between 26% and 32% (16,17). Hajivassiliou (16) found a revision rate of 32%, with 90% of revisions needing to be done within the first 3 years following insertion of the AUS. Revisions are generally due to mechanical or nonmechanical failure. Mechanical failure is usually due to leakage of the device, malfunction of the pump, or kinks in the AUS tubing. Nonmechanical failure is due to infection or erosion and urethral atrophy. The incidence of mechanical failure is between 13% and 27%, and that of nonmechanical failure is 13% to 37% (13,17,18). Problems with the pump account for the majority of mechanical failures (43.8%) (17).

In women, results of AUS are variable and population numbers often small. One recent series (19) studied the long-term follow-up of 68 female patients. They found that at 7 years, 81% were dry, with a revision rate for erosion or infection of 46%. Those with neuropathic etiologies had a continence rate of 90%, although 50% of these required revision surgery. In the Type III incontinence group, 83% were dry.

### Influence of Previous Radiotherapy on Results of AUS

Previous irradiation is known to be a risk factor for urethral erosion and the need for revision of the AUS (4). Irradiation of tissues is thought to produce a change in vascularity and fibrosis over time. It can cause hypovasculation of the urethral tissue and may affect the function of the bladder by similar mechanisms. Continence rates following insertion of the AUS in irradiated patients vary from 64% to 70% (20,22), and overall continence rates do not differ significantly between the nonirradiated and irradiated groups. Revision rates can be higher in the irradiated group, usually due to atrophy. In one study, 42% of patients had previous radiotherapy, and in this group, 51% (compared with 15% of the nonirradiated group) needed revision, mostly for urethral atrophy (22). Urethral atrophy seems to be related to intrinsic urethral hypovascularity, which has been reported in many studies looking at this group. In other studies, however, the revision rates for those with and without previous radiation treatment are similar, with rates of 25% versus 22.5% (20) and 15.4% versus 20.6% (17). The risk of infection and erosion may also be higher in irradiated patients, although evidence is inconsistent.

Cuffs are usually placed at the bulb in this group, and the cuff size is determined in the usual way by sizing the urethra. Generally, however, most authors prefer to place lower-pressure reservoir balloons to reduce the risk of pressure necrosis of the urethra and thereby reduce urethral atrophy and erosion (22,23). There is a higher reported incidence of detrusor overactivity in patients who have been previously irradiated (20,22); however, this does not seem to influence the failure rate of AUS insertion, presumably because this is treated prior to placement.

AUS insertion is currently the best long-term treatment in patients with sphincter dysfunction and previous irradiation. Despite higher revision rates, the results are good in the male population. Importantly, patient satisfaction rates are consistently high (20). In women, the results of AUS insertion in conjunction with radiotherapy are particularly poor. In one series (19), all women with a history of irradiation failed and had their AUS removed.

## *References*


1. Scott FB, Bradley WE, Timm GW. Treatment of urinary incontinence by an implantable prosthetic urinary sphincter. 1974. *J Urol* 2002;(2, Pt 2): 1125–1129.
2. Classen DC, Evans RS, Pestotnick SL, et al. Timing of prophylactic administration of antibiotics and the risk of surgical wound infection. *N Eng J Med* 1992;326:281–286.
3. Carson CC. Infections in genitourinary prostheses. *Urol Clin North Am* 1989;16:139–147.
4. Raj GV, Perterson AL, Webster GD. Outcomes following erosions of the artificial urinary sphincter. *J Urol* 2006;175(6):2186–2190.
5. Chancellor MB, Heesakkers JP, Janknergt RA. Gracilis muscle transposition with electrical stimulation for sphincteric incontinence: a new approach. *World J Urol* 1997;15(5):320–328.
6. Guralnick ML, Miller E, Toh KL, et al. Transcorporeal artificial urinary sphincter cuff placement in cases requiring revision for erosion and urethral atrophy. *J Urol* 2002;167:2075–2078.
7. Wilson SK, Delk JR, Henry GH, et al. New surgical technique for sphinter urinary control system using upper transverse scrotal incision. *J Urol* 2003; 169:261–264.
8. Scott FB. The use of the artificial sphincter in the treatment of urinary incontinence in the female patient. *Urol Clin North Am* 1985;12(2):305.
9. Appell RA. Techniques and results in the implantation of the artificial urinary sphincter in women with type III stress incontinence by a vaginal approach. *Neurourol Urodynam* 1988;7:613–619.
10. Barrett DM, Goldwasser B. The AUS: current management philosophy. 1988;5:lesson 32.
11. Singh G, Thomas DG. Artificial urinary sphincter for post-prostatectomy incontinence. *Br J Urol* 1996;77:248.
12. Levesque PE, et al. Ten-year experience with the artificial urinary sphincter in children. *J Urol* 1996;156:625–628.
13. Venn SN, Greenwell TJ, Mundy AR. The long-term outcome of artificial urinary sphincters. *J Urol* 2000;164(3, Pt 1):702–707.
14. Kryger JV, et al. The outcome of artificial urinary sphincter placement after a mean of 15 year follow up in a pediatric population. *Br J Urol* 1999;83: 1026.
15. Lai HH, Hsu EI, The Es, et al. 13 years of experience with artificial urinary sphincter implantation at Baylor College of Medicine. *J Urol* 2007;177(3): 1021–1025.
16. Hajivassiliou CA. A review of the complications and results of implantation of the AMS artificial urinary sphincter. *Eur Urol* 1999;35:36.
17. Elliot Ds, Barrett DM. Mayo clinic long term analysis of the functional durability of the AMS 800 artificial urinary sphincter: a review of 323 cases. *J Urol* 1998;159:1206–1208.
18. Singh G, Thomas DG. Artificial urinary sphincter for post-prostatectomy incontinence. *Br J Urol* 1996;77:248.
19. Thomas K, Venn SN, Mundy AR. Outcome of the artificial urinary sphincter in female patients. *J Urol* 2002;167:1720–1722.
20. Gomha MA, Boone TB. Artificial urinary sphincter for post-prostatectomy incontinence in men who had prior radiotherapy; a risk and outcome analysis. *J Urol* 2002;167(2, Pt 1):591–596.
21. Bhalchandra G, Parulkar BG, Barrett DM. Combined implantation of artificial sphincter and penile prosthesis. *J Urol* 1989;142:732–735.
22. Martins FE, Boyd SD. Artificial urinary sphincter in patients following major pelvic surgery and/or radiotherapy: are they less favorable candidates? *J Urol* 1995;153:1188–1193.
23. Perez LM, Webster GD. Successful outcome of artificial urinary sphincters in men with post prostatectomy urinary incontinence despite adverse implantation features. *J Urol* 1992;148:1166.


# CHAPTER 45 ■ THE MALE SLING FOR POSTPROSTATECTOMY INCONTINENCE: CURRENT CONCEPTS AND CONTROVERSIES

CRAIG V. COMITER

## PREVALENCE OF POSTPROSTATECTOMY INCONTINENCE

The most common cause of stress urinary incontinence (SUI) in men is iatrogenic injury during prostate surgery. The rate of incontinence following surgery for benign prostatic hyperplasia is approximately 2% (1). On the other hand, the risk of urinary incontinence is significantly higher following surgery for prostate cancer. While reports of postprostatectomy incontinence (PPI) vary, contemporary cohort studies generally agree that between 5% and 11% of patients will have enough leakage after radical prostatectomy to seek further treatment (2,3). In a recent study by Stanford et al, patients were evaluated using a self-administered questionnaire. Only 32% claimed total urinary control, 40% had occasional leakage, 7% had frequent leakage, and 2% suffered from no control at 2 years postoperatively. Regarding pad usage, 18% utilized one to two pads per day, while only 3% required 3 or more pads per day (3). Regardless of the definition of PPI, a significant minority of patients will have enough urinary leakage to require pad usage and seek further therapy.

The male sling (MS) has recently emerged as an alternative to the artificial urinary sphincter (AUS) for the surgical treatment for PPI. The modern MS is based on the early concepts described by Berry in the 1960s and Kaufman and Kishev in the early 1970s. The Kaufman and Kishev prostheses ultimately fell out of favor due to long-term failure, infectious complications, and pelvic pain, concomitant with the emergence of the modern artificial urinary sphincter (AUS). Schaeffer from Northwestern (Clemens et al., [4]) described a novel bulbourethral sling procedure in 1999. Bolsters were placed beneath the bulbar urethra to form a sling; the bolsters were suspended from the rectus fascia by sutures. However, despite excellent continence rates, 21% of patients required revision of the sling, and in 6% bolster removal was necessary secondary to infection or erosion (4). Recent alterations of the MS have been described with modification of the sling material but preservation of the concept of suburethral compression. By far, the most significant innovation affecting male sling surgery has been the use of bone screws. *This purely perineal approach transformed the surgery into a reproducible, standardized, and minimally invasive outpatient procedure.*

## DIAGNOSIS

Evaluation of a patient should begin with a detailed history of the lower-urinary-tract symptoms. However, the pathophysiology of PPI is variable, and history alone is not sufficient to distinguish between bladder causes (poor compliance, detrusor overactivity, detrusor underactivity) and outlet causes (sphincteric insufficiency or bladder outlet obstruction) of incontinence. A micturition diary is useful for quantifying frequency, incontinence episodes, and functional bladder capacity. Physical examination should focus on neurourological assessment, and urinalysis is helpful to rule out infection. Urodynamic evaluation is strongly recommended prior to consideration of invasive therapy. Filling cystometry can assess bladder storage, and outlet function may be evaluated by measurement of antegrade or retrograde leak point pressure. While the majority of men with PPI suffer from intrinsic sphincter deficiency (ISD), only 25% to 50% will have ISD alone on urodynamics. Approximately 40% of patients with ISD will demonstrate concomitant bladder dysfunction, and 15% of patients with PPI demonstrate only bladder dysfunction (5).

While patient preference and pad usage clearly dictate the implementation of surgical treatment, it is important to accurately quantify the *degree* of sphincteric incompetence, as this factor may affect the type of treatment recommended for the management of the stress incontinence. For example, patients with higher abdominal leak point pressure (ALPP) (and therefore a lower degree of ISD) tend to respond better to periurethral bulking agents than do patients with a lower ALPP. Patients with more profound sphincteric incompetence are more appropriately treated with artificial sphincter or sling surgery.

## INDICATIONS FOR SURGERY

Surgical intervention is indicated for treating bothersome SUI due to ISD that fails to adequately improve following 12 months of active conservative management. Severity, effect on quality of life, and the ability of the patient to conservatively manage incontinence must be balanced against the risks of surgery. The male sling and artificial urinary sphincter both address the underactive outlet by increasing resistance to urinary flow during storage. Resistance to leakage is created by applying pressure over a length of urethra utilizing the MS mesh or the AUS cuff. These forces are concomitantly applied to the blood supply of the compressed urethral segment, and may thereby result in urethral ischemia. Device construction, component selection, and implantation technique must therefore aim to optimize urethral compression while minimizing the risk to urethral viability.

The frequency, severity, social impact, and effect on hygiene and quality of life of the incontinence must be balanced against the ability of the patient to conservatively manage the condition. In addition, reasonable physician and patient expectations based on reproducible results of clinical efficacy, acceptable morbidity (severity, duration, and need for additional therapy), and the avoidance of serious complications are essential. The AUS and the MS should be implanted cautiously in patients with uncontrolled detrusor overactivity or decreased compliance. In addition, those conditions that may require future transurethral management are relative contraindications to outlet surgery, especially if the AUS or MS would impair transurethral access or if repeated instrumentation would put the devices at risk for infection or erosion.

## ALTERNATIVE THERAPY

### Nonoperative Management

Many patients will regain satisfactory continence within the first 12 months following prostate cancer surgery. Thus treatment within the first year is usually conservative. Unfortunately, there is currently no effective FDA-approved pharmacotherapy for intrinsic sphincter deficiency. Furthermore, blood pressure effects and a generalized lack of supportive evidence for the use of alpha-agonists have limited their utility in the management of PPI. Active conservative management therefore usually relies on fluid restriction, prompted voiding, and pelvic floor exercises. While pelvic floor exercise therapy instituted prior to radical prostatectomy aids in the earlier achievement of urinary continence, the value of the various approaches to prolonged conservative management for PPI generally remains uncertain.

Noncurative management options to control urinary leakage also include the use of an indwelling catheter, an external collection device (condom catheter or pads), or a penile clamp. However, these conservative options are not without risk. An indwelling catheter may cause recurrent urinary tract infections, stone formation, urethral injury, and even metaplastic and neoplastic changes in the bladder mucosa. A condom catheter requires a drainage bag, and with the penile shortening that commonly occurs after radical prostatectomy, it may be difficult to secure. The penile clamp may cause discomfort and skin irritation but may be particularly useful during the period of active conservative management.

Periurethral bulking agents represent another "nonoperative" treatment for PPI. Carbon-coated zirconium beads in beta-glucan gel, bovine glutaraldehyde cross-linked collagen, and polydimethylsiloxane are the most popular injectable agents for SUI in men due to ISD. "Cure" rates for transurethral (retrograde) collagen injection have generally been low for PPI, and antegrade injection does not offer any significant advantage over the retrograde technique.

### Artificial Urinary Sphincter

The AUS circumferentially occludes the urethra by exerting continuous compressive pressure. The AUS was introduced in 1973, and numerous design changes have culminated in the AMS 800 urinary prosthesis (American Medical Systems,

Minnetonka, MN; hereafter AMS). Cuff closure pressure is controlled by a balloon reservoir, generally at 61- to 70-cm $H_2O$ pressure. Normal voiding can only occur during temporary relief of urethral occlusion by activation of a scrotal pump that diverts compressive fluid from the cuff to the balloon reservoir. *Experience with the AUS for greater than three decades has demonstrated consistent and excellent results. The circumferential compression of the urethra, with an appropriately sized cuff and appropriately pressurized balloon reservoir, appears to be efficacious in treating all degrees of SUI.*

When reported by itself, the infection rate with initial AUS surgery is generally 1% to 3%, but it can be as high as 10% in patients' status after pelvic radiation and in reoperations (2). In most recent reports, with the routine practice of delayed cuff activation, erosion rates are in the range of 1% to 5% following initial surgery (2). The introduction of the narrow-backed cuff has led to substantial decreases in device failure, with nonmechanical failure decreasing from 17% to 9% and mechanical failure decreasing from 21% to 8% (2). With recurrent ISD due to urethral atrophy, revision of the AUS may be indicated. The AUS revision rate is generally 17% to 25% at 5 years since the introduction of the narrow-backed cuff (2).

## RATIONALE FOR THE MALE SLING

The impetus for the design of the modern male sling (MS) was to decrease the risk of device infection and urethral erosion, minimize the incidence of urethral atrophy that is associated with the AUS, and allow for spontaneous voiding without the need for device manipulation. The MS is a noncircumferential device that is placed with the aim of applying sufficient urethral occlusive pressure to prevent leakage yet permit normal spontaneous voiding without the need for device manipulation. Recent experience with the MS has taught several lessons regarding the management of PPI with sling surgery: (a) adequate but not excessive tension is necessary for urethral compression and continence; (b) well-designed synthetic materials have an acceptably low rate of infection and erosion; (c) adequate detrusor contractility is necessary to overcome the fixed resistance of the sling; (d) various methods of sling fixation can achieve successful urethral compression; and (e) patients with more severe or total urinary incontinence appear to have a lower success rate with the MS than do patients with more mild to moderate degrees of incontinence (6).

## SURGICAL TECHNIQUE

As the bone-anchored MS is the most commonly performed sling procedure for the treatment of PPI, the technique for this particular approach is described. The surgery is performed under general anesthesia with the patient in lithotomy position. A negative urine culture is required prior to surgery. Intravenous cephazolin (or vancomycin plus gentamycin, if allergic) is given within 1 hour of surgery. After the patient is prepared and draped in a sterile fashion, a 14Fr Foley catheter is passed per urethra to help identify the perineal portion of the urethra. A 3- to 4-cm midline incision centered over the bulbous urethra is made. The bulbospongiosa are exposed in the midline, and the medial aspects of the descending pubic rami are then exposed bilaterally. Using the InVance bone drill (AMS), three titanium bone screws, each loaded with a pair of no. 1 polypropylene or braided polyester sutures, are inserted in the medial aspect of each descending ramus: just beneath the pubic symphysis, at the level of the bulbar urethra, and midway between the proximal and distal screws (Fig. 45.1).

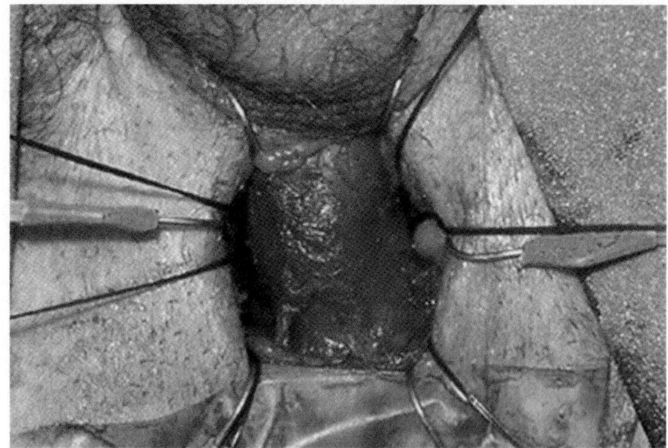

FIGURE 45.1 Three bone anchors with no. 1 polypropylene sutures are placed into each descending ramus.

Retrograde leak point pressure (RLPP) is measured via perfusion sphincterometry. With the catheter repositioned to the penile urethra and the balloon inflated with 0.5 cc saline, a 1-L saline bag is connected to the catheter via cystoscopy tubing. The RLPP is recorded in centimeters of water as the height of the fluid column above the symphysis at which fluid flow commences (6). The RLPP represents that pressure required to overcome sphincteric resistance.

A 4- by 7-cm silicone-coated polyester mesh (InteMesh, AMS) is recommended for the sling. The left-sided bone-anchored sutures are passed through the sling 0.5 cm from the left edge, equally spaced along the width of the sling, and tied down to the bone. The right-sided sutures are then passed through the sling (Fig. 45.2) and temporarily tensioned with a single throw. RLPP is again measured, and sling tension may be adjusted by moving the right sutures medially or laterally along the sling edge until an RLPP of 60 cm of water can be demonstrated. The sutures are then tied down to the pubic bone to maintain proper sling compression. The

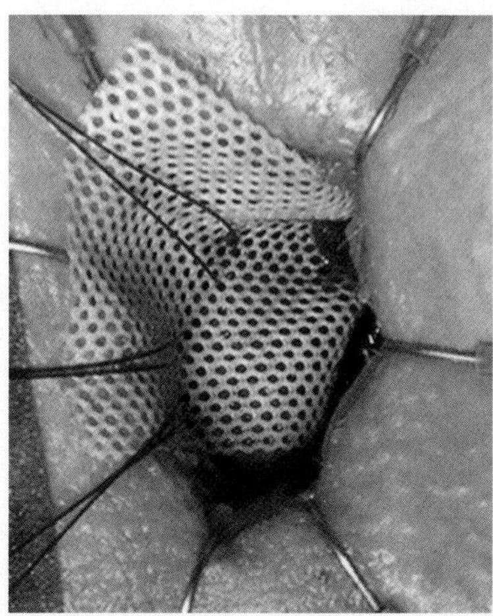

FIGURE 45.2 The left sutures have been tied and cut. The right sutures are passed through the sling. Tension is determined by how laterally or medially the right sutures are placed through the sling.

catheter is then replaced into the bladder, and the wound is irrigated with antibiotic solution and closed in multiple layers with running suture, using 2-0 polyglycolic acid suture for the deep layer, 3-0 polyglycolic acid suture for the dartos layer, and 4-0 polyglycolic acid suture for the skin. A trial of voiding is performed when the patient is able to stand comfortably to void, usually within 6 to 36 hours postoperatively. Alternatively, a 14Fr suprapubic tube may be placed intraoperatively and used to monitor residual urine volume. The suprapubic tube may be removed when residual urine volume is appropriately low (i.e., equal to the preoperative postvoid residual urine volume).

## OUTCOMES

Unlike the AUS literature, reports of the success for the MS are more difficult to interpret, as most reports come from single-institution cohorts that are hampered by small numbers and usually short follow-up.

Similar to reports of AUS surgical results, "success" depends on the definition of continence, the method of evaluation, the length of follow-up, and the experience of the surgeon. In addition, the sling material and method of tensioning may also contribute to the success or failure of the procedure. However, despite these limitations that may hinder the objective evaluation of this relatively new technique, there is relatively good consistency within the literature, with success rates for the MS generally ranging from 65% to 90% (2,6).

At the author's institution, a cohort of 48 patients with a minimum follow-up of 24 months (range, 24 to 60 months) and a median follow-up of 48 months have been followed since they underwent MS surgery between 1999 and 2003. Twenty patients had follow-up of at least 48 months, and 35 patients had follow-up of at least 36 months. The average age was 67.6 ± 9.7 years. Six patients had a previous artificial urinary sphincter, 8 had adjuvant radiation treatment (XRT), 2 had primary XRT, and 9 had a previous collagen injection. All patients rated their incontinence as a "big problem" on the UCLA Prostate Cancer Index (PCI) incontinence score, and all used three or more pads daily. Preoperative mean RLPP was 27.3 ± 8.0 cm of water, and patients used an average of 4.6 ± 2.1 pads per day. The median preoperative UCLA PCI incontinence score was 63 (scale of 0 to 500) (6).

At a mean follow-up of 48 months (range, 24 to 60 months), the median UCLA PCI incontinence score improved to 343, and postoperative pad usage decreased to a mean of 1.0 ± 1.7 pads per day. Overall, 31 out of 48 patients (65%) were cured of their leakage (no problem, no pads), 7 out of 48 (15%) were much improved (small problem, 1 pad), 3 out of 48 (6%) were mildly improved (moderate problem, 2 pads daily), and 7 out of 48 (15%) failed (big problem, 3 or more pads). Thirty-eight out of 48 patients (79%) were cured or much improved and were "socially continent," using 0 to 1 pad per day (6).

Previous collagen injection and previous *adjuvant* XRT did not affect outcome, but both patients with primary XRT failed, and 5 out of 6 patients (83%) who had previously had AUS implantation failed. In the group of 7 patients who failed to improve, 2 had primary XRT, 5 had previous AUS, and 1 had pelvic trauma.

**TABLE 45.1**

**URODYNAMIC EFFECT OF MALE SLING ON VOIDING**

| | $Q_{max}$ (mL/s) | $P_{det}Q_{max}$ (cm water) |
|---|---|---|
| Preoperative | 19.2 ± 9.7 | 40.3 ± 9.2 |
| Postoperative | 17.7 ± 6.5 | 45.8 ± 14.7 |

Urodynamic evaluation of a subgroup of 22 volunteer patients at an average of 25 months follow-up revealed an increase in RLPP from a mean of 30.4 ± 15.7 to 59.9 ± 9.7 cm water following sling surgery ($p < 0.001$). There was no significant change between intraoperative RLPP and RLPP on postoperative urodynamics (59.9 ± 9.7 versus 56.7 ± 10.4 cm water). No patient demonstrated BOO on urodynamics preoperatively, and none developed iatrogenic bladder outlet obstruction (BOO) following sling surgery. The average maximum flow rate ($Q_{max}$) following surgery (17.7 ± 6.5 mL per second) did not significantly differ from preoperative $Q_{max}$ (19.2 ± 9.7 mL per second) Nor was there a significant change in detrusor pressure at $Q_{max}$ ($P_{det}Q_{max}$), averaging 40.3 ± 9.2 cm water preoperatively and 45.8 ± 14.7 cm water postoperatively (Table 45.1). Average postvoid residual urine was 17 ± 26 mL (range, 0 to 94 mL). While 4 patients demonstrated detrusor overactivity (DO) postoperatively, none developed symptomatic de novo urgency or urge urinary incontinence postoperatively.

## COMPLICATIONS

The infection or erosion rate for the MS is quite low (2.1%), and the rate for the need for revision (secondary to bone-anchor dislodgement) is 4.2% (6). In addition, there have been no reported instances of urethral atrophy resulting in recurrent incontinence. Bothersome scrotal pain or numbness affects 5% to 16% of patients, which typically resolves within 3 months (6).

## CONTROVERSIES IN MALE SLING SURGERY

### Tensioning Sling

Unlike the woman with urethral hypermobility and preserved intrinsic sphincter function, the male with SUI suffers mostly from ISD. And just as one measures the circumference of the urethra to determine appropriate AUS cuff size, one should measure sling tension to provide sufficient urethral compression when placing the MS as a surgical treatment for ISD. Various successful tensioning techniques have been described, including measurement of leak point pressure, tensioning based on "cough leakage," and tensioning based on visual estimation. The author recommends perfusion sphincterometry, with a goal of 60 to 70 cm water compression pressure based on the well-known success of the 61- to 70-cm water balloon pressure of the AUS. Ullrich and Comiter (7) demonstrated that patients who achieve a RLPP of 60 cm have a better outcome than those who demonstrated a lower compression pressure. Furthermore, in patients who have undergone surgery with targeted tensioning based on measurement of RLPP, there have been no instances of prolonged urinary retention (6).

## Sling Material

It is vital that synthetic material be utilized so that the tension can be maintained adequately over time. The rate of infection with synthetic material is acceptably low.

## Contraindications

Similar to AUS surgery, MS surgery is contraindicated in patients who may require future transurethral surgery (e.g., recurrent urolithiasis, transitional cell carcinoma, or unstable anastomotic or urethral stricture disease). Not only might the MS impair transurethral access, but also repeated instrumentation may put the devices at risk for infection or erosion. In addition, sling surgery should be carefully considered in patients with uncontrolled detrusor overactivity or decreased compliance, as increasing outlet resistance will not help either of these conditions and could theoretically put the upper urinary tract at risk.

## Detrusor Hypocontractility

Bladder contractility can be measured preoperatively via pressure flow study. In patients with normal detrusor contractility, there have been no reported instances of prolonged postoperative urinary retention when using 60 cm water RLPP as an intraoperative guide to sling tensioning (6). Whereas the AUS can be deflated to allow voiding with abdominal straining, the fixed resistance of the sling will interfere with Valsalva voiding. *Therefore, in patients with detrusor hypocontractility, AUS implantation is recommended rather than MS surgery.*

## Radiation

Full-course external beam radiotherapy appears to be a contraindication to sling surgery. In fact, radiation was the only factor that predisposed to failure of the Northwestern sling (success rate was only 29% for irradiated patients, versus 68% for nonirradiated patients) (4). Interestingly, the success rate for bone-anchored MS surgery is not adversely affected by *adjuvant* radiation following prostatectomy (6).

## Severe Incontinence

Two recent reports demonstrated that patients with more severe incontinence preoperatively are at higher risk for postoperative incontinence following sling surgery (8). Experience with the AUS for greater than three decades has demonstrated consistent and excellent continence results for all levels of urinary incontinence (7). The circumferential compression of the urethra, with an appropriately sized cuff and appropriately pressurized balloon reservoir, appears to be efficacious in treating most cases of male SUI. *Thus, in men with severe incontinence (>450 g per 24 hours urinary leakage), AUS may be more appropriate than MS surgery.*

## Sling Failure

In the case of suboptimal continence following sling surgery, it is preferential to leave the previously placed sling in situ and to place the AUS cuff distal to the sling, via a transscrotal approach. This approach has two advantages: (a) it avoids the previous operative field, minimizing dissection through potentially scarred tissue; and (b) it leaves the proximally placed sling as a partially effective compressive device, similar to a tandem-cuff AUS. In cases where the surgeon elects to place the AUS cuff transperineally, the previous sling neither renders the operation more difficult nor decreases AUS efficacy (2,6). The silicone-coated polyester sling is only partially incorporated into the subcutaneous or periurethral tissue, and it is relatively straightforward to remove. The bulbospongiosus may then be split and dissected off the underlying spongy urethra without difficulty, and the AUS may be placed in routine fashion.

## Previous AUS Surgery or Previous MS Surgery

In patients who have failed previous AUS surgery or previous MS surgery, AUS is preferred over the MS, as previous AUS implantation and explantation may contribute to urethral fibrosis, thereby preventing adequate urethral coaptation with the ventrally placed sling (2,6) In cases of severe urethral atrophy, double-cuff AUS placement or transcorporal AUS cuff placement may be indicated.

## Transobturator Male Sling

The advent of bone screws has simplified the sling procedure and obviated the need for an abdominal incision, and subsequently the bone-anchored perineal sling has become the most common sling surgery for PPI. However, despite the small size of the perineal incision, bothersome, albeit temporary, scrotal pain or numbness affects 5% to 16% of patients and can last for up to 3 months (2,6). Such pain is likely due to irritation of pudendal nerve branches along the medial pubic rami in the area of the bone screws and/or to the sling "pulling" the pubic rami toward each other. Other limitations include the theoretical risk of osteitis and osteomyelitis, and the high cost of the disposable drill and bone screws. Hence there is a quest for a suburethral sling independent of bone-anchor fixation, which at the same time does not rely on retropubic suture placement and the associated risk of bladder injury.

This has led to a recent interest in an MS placed via a transobturator approach. However, a recent report comparing transobturator sling and retropubic sling demonstrated that the tension-free transobturator sling has been shown to be six times more likely to fail than a retropubic sling in women with significant ISD, due to the fact that the transobturator placement of the sling results in lower upward tension on the urethra than with retropubic slings (9). *Since PPI is due to ISD rather than urethral hypermobility, it is unlikely that a transobturator sling alone can provide enough urethral resistance for adequate continence in men with PPI.*

A recent series of 20 patients who underwent transobturator sling placement (AdVance, AMS) for PPI had disappointing results, with a continence rate of only 40% at 6 weeks postoperatively (10). Klingler and Marberger (11) observed in their series of removal of unsuccessful transobturator slings that there was significant narrowing and kinking of the urethra, which led to voiding symptoms and elevated residual urine without providing significant continence. They hypothesized that the narrow transobturator sling could not adequately stabilize the posterior urethra and bladder neck, but rather produced a narrow and suboptimal urethral compression.

It appears, based on these early reports, that the transobturator approach, by ventral elevation and compression of the bulbous urethra, may not be an adequate substitute for the more distal urethral compression against the perineal membrane and pubis provided by a perineal sling. On the other hand, the transobturator ventral urethral elevation and compression may be more successful as an *adjunct* to the perineal sling, rather than a *substitute* for it, by adding a component of ventral urethral elevation to the urethral compression provided by the perineal sling. Comiter and Rhee (12) have recently described a combination transobturator-plus-suprapubic sling utilizing a 5.5- by 7-cm woven polypropylene sling with two 1.5- by 22.5-cm inferior extensions and two 1.5- by 25-cm superior extensions (Fig. 45.3A). The inferior extensions are passed via a transobturator approach, providing ventral urethral elevation and compression, and the superior extensions are passed via a suprapubic approach, providing broad perineal urethral compression, similar to the bone-anchored sling (Fig. 45.3B). This combination sling, using the VIRTUE sling system (Coloplast, Minneapolis, MN), was initially evaluated in a cadaveric study, with each of the two sling components mediating increased urethral resistance (as demonstrated by urethral pressure profilometry). Two patients with severe ISD who had failed previous artificial sphincter placement, each requiring six pads per day, have realized total resolution of their SUI at >1 year follow-up (12).

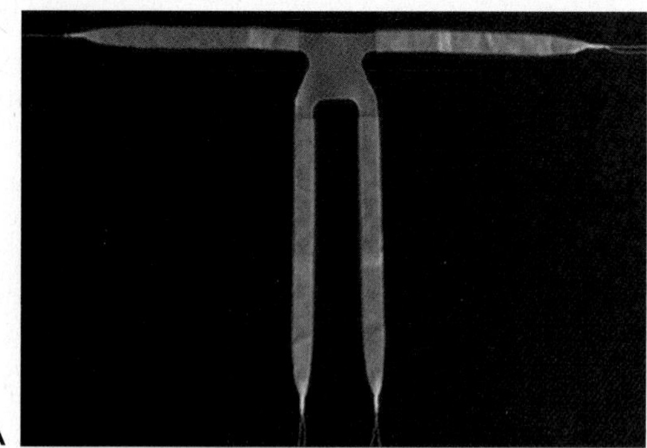

A

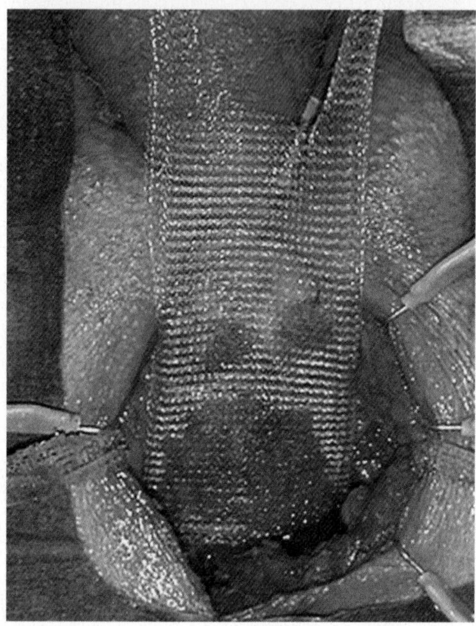

B

**FIGURE 45.3 A:** The combined transobturator-prepubic VIRTUE (Coloplast, Minneapolis, MN) sling. **B:** The inferior extensions are passed in a transobturator fashion, and the superior extensions are passed suprapubically.

## SUMMARY

Male SUI is usually iatrogenic and can be a bothersome complication of prostate cancer surgery, causing approximately 10% of patients to seek further treatment. After 12 months of active conservative management, surgical intervention is often indicated. Transurethral injection of bulking agents, while minimally invasive, has not proven successful in either the short or long term. The AUS and suburethral sling are both safe and efficacious treatments for PPI secondary to ISD.

For severe incontinence, including total urinary incontinence due to profound sphincteric insufficiency, the AUS appears to have higher efficacy than does the MS. For more mild to moderate SUI, where the patient has sufficient intrinsic sphincteric function to store urine but leaks during strenuous activity, the success rates for the two procedures appear more or less equivalent. While the AUS has a longer track record of success than the more recently described MS, the complication rate and revision rate for the latter appear lower, at least in the short term. And while spontaneous voiding without the need for device manipulation is a relative advantage of the MS, the patient must have adequate detrusor contractility to realize this benefit. Both techniques represent efficacious and acceptably safe methods for the treatment of PPI, yet each has its specific role in managing patients with various degrees of leakage.

## *References*


1. McConnell JD, Barry MJ, Bruskewitz RC. Benign prostatic hyperplasia: diagnosis and treatment. Agency for Health Care Policy and Research. *Clin Pract Guidelines Quick Ref Guide Clin* 1994;8:1–17.
2. Staskin DR, Comiter CV. Surgical treatment of male sphincteric urinary incontinence. The male perineal sling and artificial urinary sphincter. In: Wein AJ, Kavoussi LR, Novick AC, et al., eds. *Campbell-Walsh urology*, 9th ed. Philadelphia: WB Saunders, 2006:2391–2404.
3. Stanford JL, Feng Z, Hamilton AS, et al. Urinary and sexual function after radical prostatectomy for clinically localized prostate cancer: The Prostate Cancer Outcomes Study. *JAMA* 2000;283:354–360.

4. Clemens JQ, Bushman W, Schaeffer AJ. Questionnaire based results of the bulbourethral sling procedure. *J Urol* 1999;162:1972–1976.
5. Foote J, Yun S, Leach GE. Postprostatectomy incontinence. Pathophysiology, evaluation, and management. *Urol Clin North Am* 1991;18:229–241.
6. Comiter CV. The male perineal sling: intermediate-term results. *Neurourol Urodynam* 2005;24:648–653.
7. Ullrich NF, Comiter CV. The male sling for stress urinary incontinence: urodynamic and subjective assessment. *J Urol* 2004;172:204–206.
8. Fischer MC, Huckabay C, Nitti VW. The male perineal sling: assessment and predication of outcome. *J Urol* 2007;177:1414–1418.
9. Miller JJ, Botros SM, Akl MN, et al. Is transobturator tape as effective as tension-free vaginal tape in patients with borderline maximum urethral closure pressure? *Am J Obstet Gynecol* 2006;195:1799–1804.
10. Rehder P, Gozzi C. Transobturator sling suspension for male urinary incontinence including post-radical prostatectomy. *Eur Urol* 2007;52:860–867.
11. Klingler HC, Marberger M. Incontinence after radical prostatectomy: surgical treatment options. *Curr Opin Urol* 2006;16:60–64.
12. Comiter CV, Rhee EY. The ventral urethral elevation plus sling: a novel approach for the treatment of stress urinary incontinence. *BJU Int* 2008;101:187–191

# CHAPTER 46 ■ SACRAL NEUROMODULATION

SARAH E. MCACHRAN, RAYMOND R. RACKLEY, AND SANDIP VASAVADA

The refractory overactive bladder represents one of the most challenging problems in urology as well as a clinical problem that significantly erodes patient quality of life. Symptoms include urinary frequency, urgency, urge incontinence, and nocturia. Initial treatment for patients with overactive bladder without any remediable anatomic cause is anticholinergic therapy. For patients who are not candidates for, refractory to, or cannot tolerate anticholinergic pharmacotherapy, options are limited. Augmentation cystoplasty, in which a piece of small or large intestine is used to enlarge the bladder, has traditionally been offered as a last resort. However, this is a major operation with significant potential short-term and long-term complications. Even without complications, most patients are troubled by the need for lifelong intermittent bladder catheterization after such reconstructive procedures. Sacral neuromodulation (SNM) offers an alternative to patients who have failed more conservative treatments and may be considering irreversible surgical options.

The neuromodulation that we practice today has its roots in the 1960s work of Boyce, Dees, Caldwell, and Nashold, who experimented with various modes of bladder stimulation including a transurethral approach, direct detrusor stimulation, pelvic nerve and pelvic floor stimulation, and finally spinal cord stimulation. The pioneering work of Tanagho and Schmidt in the 1980s demonstrated that the stimulation of the sacral nerve root S3 generally induces detrusor and sphincter action (11). The U.S. Food and Drug Administration (FDA) approved SNM for intractable urge incontinence in 1997 and for urgency-frequency and nonobstructive urinary retention in 1999. Later labeling was changed to include "overactive bladder" as an appropriate diagnostic category. Since its inception, >40,000 InterStim neurostimulators (Medtronic, Inc., Minneapolis, MN) have been implanted for the three approved indications for SNM of the lower urinary tract (LUT).

## MECHANISMS OF ACTION OF SACRAL NERVE STIMULATION

### Overactive Bladder

The ability to volitionally store and evacuate urine is modulated by several centers in the brain. It is thought that patients with overactive bladder may have suffered an insult that effectively unmasks involuntary bladder contractions (Fig. 46.1) (6). SNM of these primitive reflexes may restore normal micturition by suppressing or inhibiting interneuronal transmission in the bladder reflex pathway (6). This inhibition may, in part, modulate the sensory outflow from the bladder through the ascending pathways to the pontine micturition center (PMC), thereby preventing involuntary contractions by modulating the micturition

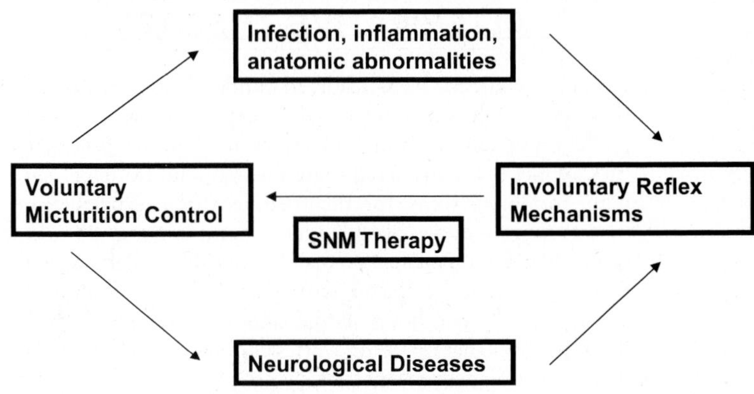


FIGURE 46.1 The concept of SNM is to modulate the abnormal involuntary reflexes of the lower urinary tract and restore voluntary control. (Adapted from Leng WW, Chancellor MB. How sacral nerve stimulation neuromodulation works. *Urol Clin North Am* 2005;32:11–18.)

reflex circuit. In clinical practice, SNM improves abnormal bladder sensations, involuntary voids, and detrusor contractions. Interestingly, voluntary voiding is preserved.

### Urinary Retention

To allow for complete bladder emptying, detrusor contractions must be coordinated with urethral sphincteric relaxation. When the suprasacral pathways that coordinate sphincteric activity are altered, the guarding and urethral reflexes that allow for urine storage without leakage still exist and cannot be turned off. This may result in urinary retention and is seen in certain patients with spinal cord injury and detrusor sphincter dyssynergia. These patients have functional detrusor contractions but are unable to coordinate this with a relaxed urethral sphincter, resulting in urinary retention. Inhibition of the guarding reflexes may improve urinary retention. SNM is postulated to turn off excitatory flow to the urethral outlet and facilitate bladder emptying.

## DIAGNOSIS

A thorough history will help delineate the nature (acute vs. chronic) and help classify the causes (neurogenic, anatomic, postsurgical, functional, inflammatory, and/or idiopathic) of a patient's LUT symptoms. Physical examination should focus on ruling out treatable causes of incontinence such as stress urinary incontinence and pelvic organ prolapse. Levator tone and function are assessed with rectal and vaginal examination; evidence of high-tone pelvic floor muscle dysfunction is often seen in patients who suffer from both overactive bladder and idiopathic urinary retention. A neurourologic examination should be performed to check for saddle sensation, sphincter tone, and intact bulbocavernosus reflex. Postvoid residual urine volume is determined. Urinalysis and urine culture are routinely performed. Urine cytology should be considered to screen for bladder cancer and bladder carcinoma in situ in those patients who present with refractory symptoms of dysuria and urgency or frequency, especially with coexistent hematuria.

Voiding diaries are invaluable. They provide an objective assessment of symptoms for both initial evaluation and for assessing response to treatment. For patients with overactive bladder, the number of voids and incontinence episodes per 24-hour period, voided volumes, and degree of urgency should be assessed. For patients with idiopathic retention, the amount spontaneously voided versus the catheterized volume per 24-hour period is useful information. Urodynamic studies (UDS) including cystometrogram, pressure-flow studies, and electromyography (EMG) of sphincters and pelvic floor muscles are performed on a selected basis. Many patients without known neurologic disorders can be thoroughly evaluated with the use of a voiding diary and a focused history and physical examination of the pelvis. However, EMG is recommended in suspected cases of neurogenic bladder dysfunction, detrusor sphincter dyssynergia, or Fowler syndrome and may be considered for evaluation of inappropriate pelvic floor muscle behavior. Additionally, urodynamics may be used to rule out treatable causes of urinary incontinence or obstruction.

Cystourethroscopy may be helpful. Urethral strictures and bladder neck contractures or fibrosis can be diagnosed. Bladder wall trabeculation may help to confirm a clinical suspicion of bladder outlet obstruction or neurogenic pathology.

## INDICATIONS FOR SURGERY

As yet, there are still no clear predictive factors suggesting who will and will not be helped with SNM. Therefore, all patients with voiding dysfunction, both overactive bladder and idiopathic urinary retention, who are not helped by other measures may be considered candidates. A therapy trial, whether a peripheral nerve evaluation (PNE) or Stage 1 of a two-stage implant, is a minimal-risk, reversible procedure, making it the ultimate predictive test for patient selection (8).

There are several important contraindications to SNM. In patients with anatomic changes such as bony abnormalities of the sacrum, access to the sacral neural foramina may be difficult or impossible. Patients with cognitive impairment rendering them incapable of operating the device or giving appropriate feedback regarding the level and comfort of stimulation are poor candidates. Because of the unknown teratogenic potential of electrical stimulation, it has been considered contraindicated in pregnant women with various voiding dysfunctions. However, women with electrical stimulation devices for pelvic health conditions who become pregnant may simply turn off their devices when considering, and during, pregnancy.

SNM is relatively contraindicated for those patients who have an anticipated need for future magnetic resonance imaging (MRI). The potential hazards of MRI include motion, dislocation, or torquing of the implanted pulse generator (IPG), heating of the leads, and damage to the IPG, resulting in painful stimulation. A recent pilot study from Toronto evaluated eight patients with sacral nerve stimulator devices as they underwent MRI examinations at 1.5 T to study areas outside the pelvis (3). Patients were monitored continuously during and after the procedure. Voiding diaries were collected after the procedure and compared with previous records. No patient experienced painful stimulation during or after the MRI, and there were no changes in perception of stimulation. Furthermore, there were no changes in voiding diaries after the MRI. Until further evidence is collected proving the safety of MRI for this population, we advocate removal of the neuroelectrode lead without removal of the pulse generator prior to elective MRI. Following the MRI procedure, a new neuroelectrode may be placed and connected to the previously implanted and preserved pulse generator.

## ALTERNATIVE THERAPY

Generally, patients are considered candidates for SNM once they have failed other forms of therapy. For the overactive bladder population, anticholinergics tend to be prescribed first. While still considered experimental, clinical experience with botulinum toxin for the treatment of neurogenic and nonneurogenic overactive bladder is accumulating. As a last resort, bladder augmentation may be considered. Patients with idiopathic urinary retention, particularly when attributable to a hypertonic pelvic floor, should undergo a course of pelvic floor physical therapy with a physical therapist who specializes in treating pelvic floor disorders.

## SURGICAL TECHNIQUE

The procedure consists of two stages: a testing stage or first stage and an implantation stage or second stage. Since its introduction, several modifications have been made in the technology, with resultant changes in the surgical technique.

The most significant of these changes was the shift from peripheral nerve evaluation to the anchored lead staged procedure, and finally to the current tined lead staged procedure. The tined lead was introduced in 2002 and offers the advantage of simplified placement of the stimulation lead through a percutaneous approach without the need for lead anchoring to the fascia, significantly minimizing the invasiveness of the procedure (10). The lead is secured through the action of the tines (Fig. 46.2). Another surgical modification was the movement of the location of the IPG unit from the lower anterior abdominal wall to the posterior gluteal region.

The peripheral nerve evaluation was originally developed to evaluate whether or not patients would respond to SNM before implanting the IPG. Before the inception of the tined lead, implantation required a significant sacral incision and dissection to anchor the lead to the sacral fascia. A less invasive screening test was therefore desirable before committing the patient to permanent implantation. Unfortunately, the PNE lead is precarious, and it is often difficult to replicate placement with the permanent lead and therefore to replicate patient responses. Several reports have confirmed lower response rates and a higher rate of lead migration with the PNE (5). Therefore, after the introduction of the significantly less invasive tined lead, the two-stage implantation approach gained favor. However, the PNE still has proponents because it can be performed in the office setting with local anesthesia, thereby eliminating one trip to the operating room.

### PNE Test Stimulation

The patient is placed prone with slight flexion at the hips to position the sacrum horizontally. A jelly roll or other buttress

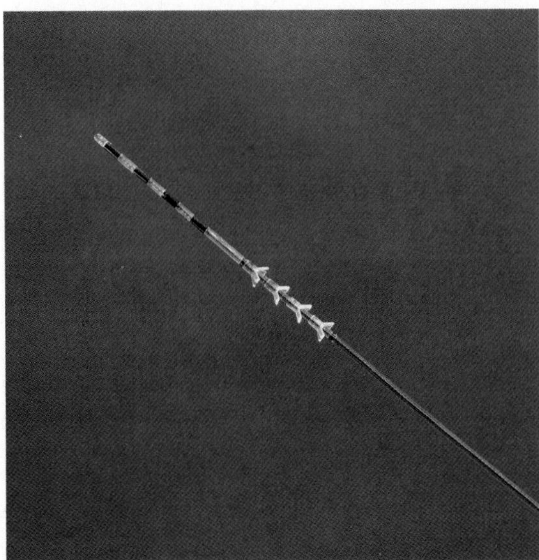

FIGURE 46.2 The tined lead allows for suture-free anchoring to the fascia. (From Medtronic, Inc. © 2006, with permission.)

TABLE 46.1

PATIENT TEST BOX SETTINGS

| | | |
|---|---|---|
| Rate | | 15 Hz |
| Amplitude | | Off |
| Rate and pulse width selection switch | | Position A |
| Pulse width | | 210 microseconds |
| Amp limit | | 10 V |
| Electrode select switches: | 0 | Minus |
| | 1 | Off |
| | 2 | Off |
| | 3 | Plus |

can be used. The sacrum and buttocks are prepared and the patient is draped so that the sacrum, buttocks, and feet are exposed, allowing observation of the bellows and great toe response. The ground pad is placed on the patient's heel or calf. The red plug of the long test stimulation cable is connected to the grounding pad. The black plug is connected to the test stimulation cable and the other end to the test stimulator. The initial settings for the test stimulator can be seen in Table 46.1.

### Locating Sacral Landmarks

There are several methods to locate the S3 neural foramen, the desired location for tined lead placement (Fig. 46.3). Using surface landmarks, the S3 foramen is generally located 2 to 3 cm off the midline on either side approximately 9 to 11 cm cephalad to the tip of the coccyx. If the sciatic notch can be

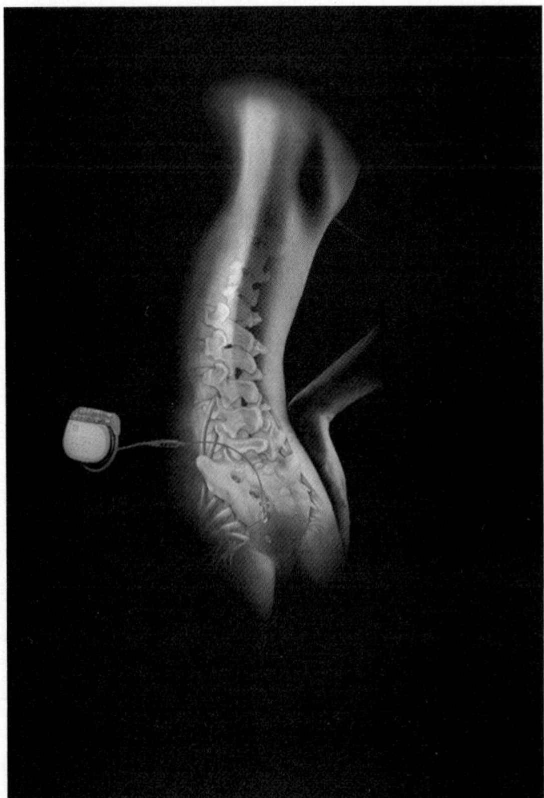

FIGURE 46.3 The S3 foramen is the desired location for the lead. (From Medtronic, Inc. © 2006, with permission.)

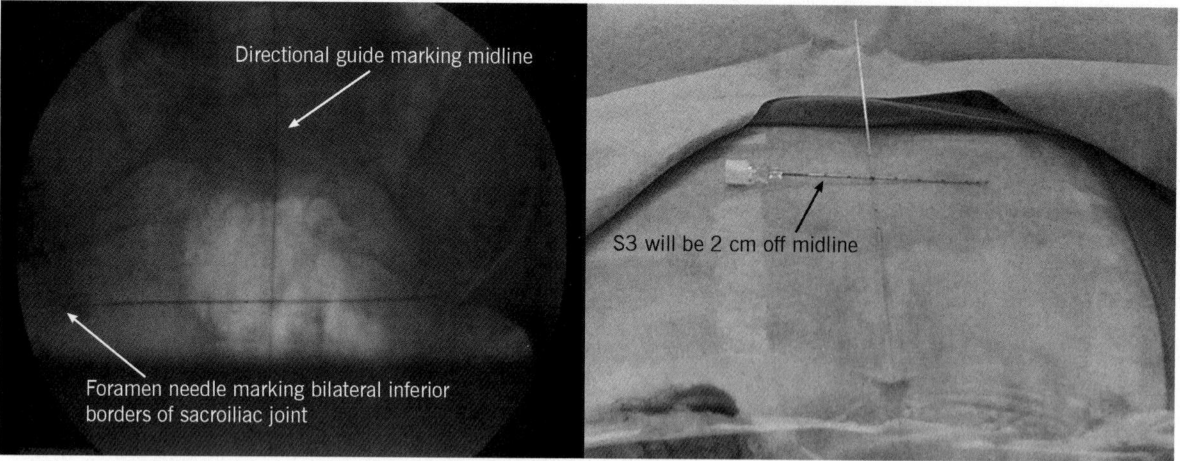


FIGURE 46.4 Chai and Mamo's "cross-hair" technique for S3 localization. Fluoroscopic image and surface image of the same patient. The midline is marked by the directional guide, which is placed over the spinous processes of the lower lumbar vertebrae. The foramen needle is placed so that it connects the most inferior border of the sacroiliac joints. The S3 foramina are located approximately 2 cm lateral to the junction of the two lines.

palpated, this provides a useful landmark as well. A line is drawn connecting the sciatic notches bilaterally, and an intersecting line is drawn at the midline of the sacrum. The S3 foramen can be located approximately 1 fingerbreadth, or 2 cm, lateral to the midline of the sacrum along the line connecting the sciatic notches. Less reliably, one can look for the least curved portion of the sacrum by balancing a pen on the sacral crest. This marks the level of the S4 foramen; S3 will be located about 2 cm cephalad to S4.

In 2001, Chai and Mamo (1) introduced the use of the "cross-hair" fluoroscopic technique for S3 localization (Fig. 46.4). An anterior and posterior fluoroscopic image is used to locate the inferior borders of the sacroiliac joints. This is marked with a foramen needle. The directional guide can be used to identify the spinous processes in the midline. A sterile marker is used to trace a line along the path of both needles, creating a "cross-hair." The S3 foramen can be found approximately 2 cm lateral to the cross-hairs on either side.

## Inserting the Foramen Needle

After injecting a buffered lidocaine solution into the skin, the subcutaneous layers and bony surface of the sacrum in the vicinity of the selected foramen are anesthetized. Care is taken not to inject anesthetic into the foramen itself as this can anesthetize the nerve intended for test stimulation. The foramen needle comes in two lengths, 3.5 and 5.0 in. After the appropriate needle is selected, it is inserted at the desired site at an angle perpendicular to the bony surface of the sacrum, thus causing it to pierce the skin at approximately a 60-degree angle (Fig. 46.5).

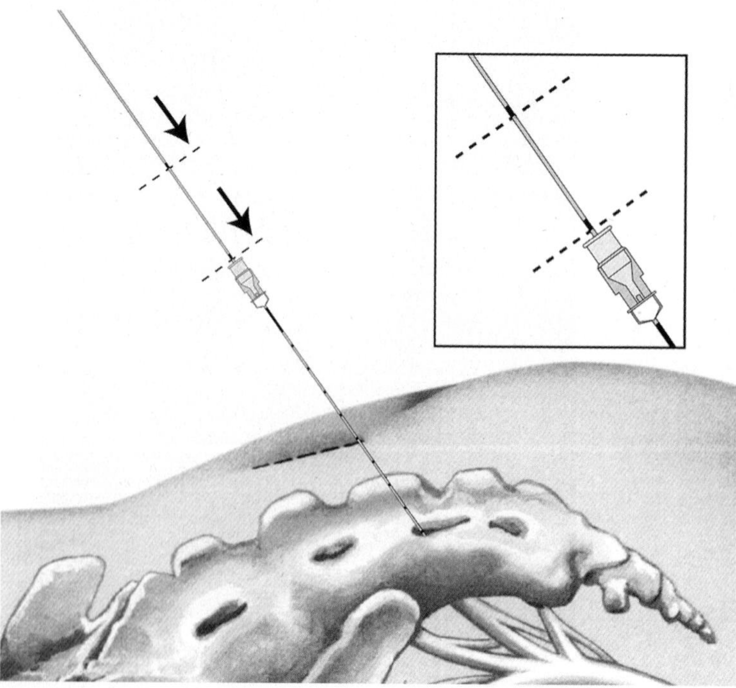

FIGURE 46.5 A wire is passed through the foramen needle so that the foramen needle can be exchanged for the introducer sheath. Note that the foramen needle is inserted at a 60-degree angle to the skin. (From Medtronic, Inc. © 2006, with permission.)

**TABLE 46.2**

SACRAL NERVE RESPONSES

| SACRAL NERVE | MOTOR AND SENSORY RESPONSE |
|---|---|
| S2 | Motor: Plantar flexion of the entire foot with lateral rotation and clamp movement of the anal sphincter<br>Sensory: Sensations in the leg and buttock |
| S3 | Motor: Dorsiflexion of the great toe and a Bellows reflex (anal wink)<br>Sensory: Parasthesias or sensation of pulling in the rectum, scrotum, or vagina |
| S4 | Motor: Bellows reflex only<br>Sensory: Sensation of pulling in the rectum only |

The operator should walk off the bone by feeling the needle as it drops through the foramen. The J hook of the patient cable is then attached to the black, uninsulated portion of the needle, just below the hub. Beginning at zero, the amplitude of the test stimulator is then slowly increased until the desired response is seen. The nerve is tested for the appropriate motor response: dorsiflexion of the great toe and bellows contraction of the perineal area (Table 46.2). The so-called bellows reflex represents contraction of the levator muscles. A fluttering or tugging sensation in the rectum, vagina, or labia is considered the ideal sensory response.

When the desired response is confirmed, the stimulation lead is placed. After the stylet is removed from the foramen needle, the test lead is threaded through the foramen needle until the depth indicator on the lead is properly aligned with the needle. The distal indicator aligns with the hub of the 3.5-in. needle, and the proximal indicator aligns with the hub of the 5-in. needle. Care must be taken as the lead is delicate and easily damaged. The lead is stimulated once again. After the appropriate response is confirmed, the foramen needle and lead stylet are removed, leaving the lead in place. Once the lead stylet is removed, the lead cannot be repositioned. The lead is taped to the patient's skin to secure it, leaving the proximal end exposed. The ground pad is relocated to the patient's lower back. The lead is connected to the test stimulation cable and the test stimulator. It should not be left in place for >7 days.

## Stage 1 Tined Lead Placement

For Stage 1, preoperative intravenous antibiotics are given and standard aseptic techniques for the implantation of foreign bodies are implemented. An intravenous dose of either a cephalosporin, vancomycin, or a fluoroquinolone is preferred. Either general anesthesia or monitored anesthesia care (MAC) is used. MAC is preferable as it allows the patient to communicate sensory responses during the procedure. If a general anesthetic is used, no long-acting muscle relaxants should be administered as they can inhibit motor responses. The patient is prone and the buttocks are held apart using wide tape retraction so that the anus is visible during test stimulation. The anus and tape are prepared into the sterile field and then covered with a separate plastic drape until visualization of the anus is required. The patient's feet will also need to be visible during the procedure.

The foramen needle is inserted at a 60-degree angle to the skin, approximately 1 to 2 cm cephalad to the marked location of the S3 foramen. If the patient is obese, the 5-in. needle should be used and the insertion point may need to be even more cephalad. Because the pelvic plexus and pudendal nerve run alongside the pelvis, the needle should be placed just inside the ventral foramen. Fluoroscopy is used to confirm needle position. The nerve is tested for the appropriate motor response. The foramen needle is exchanged for the introducer sheath over the directional guide, and the lead is passed so that the electrodes, numbered 0 (distal) through 3 (proximal), are positioned with electrodes 2 and 3 straddling the ventral surface of the sacrum (Fig. 46.6). Test stimulation is repeated on each electrode and the responses are observed. An S3 response should be noted at a minimum of two of the four electrodes. Once the operator is satisfied with the position, the sheath is removed, releasing the tines that anchor the lead (Fig. 46.6). Confirmation of an S3 sensory response, a sensation of stimulation in the perineum, is not required to confirm proper placement if the correct S3 motor response is observed

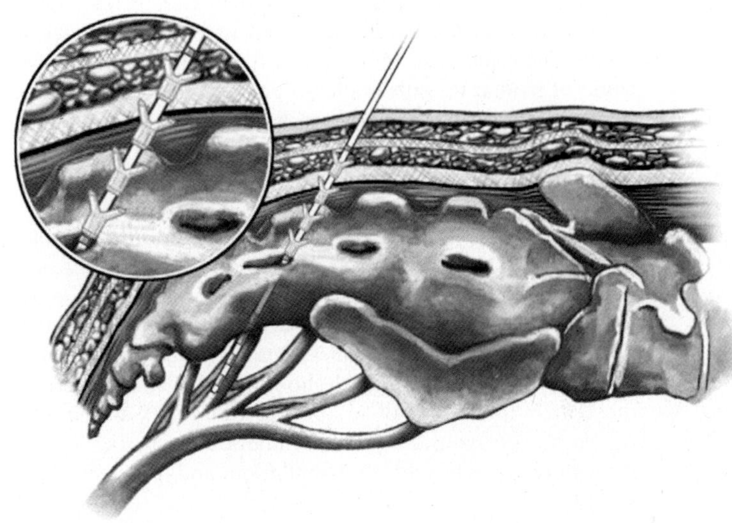

FIGURE 46.6 The foramen needle is exchanged for the introducer sheath over the directional guide, and the lead is passed so that the electrodes, numbered 0 (distal) through 3 (proximal), are positioned with electrodes 2 and 3 straddling the ventral surface of the sacrum. (From Medtronic, Inc. © 2006, with permission.)

(2). However, if a motor response is absent despite what appears to be fluoroscopically appropriate placement, the patient's sedation is lightened and sensory responses are elicited. Patient verification of the correct sensory response can then confirm proper localization. Fluoroscopically appropriate lead placement demonstrates the lead curving cephalad to caudad on the lateral image and with electrodes 2 and 3 straddling the interior portion of the sacrum. The lead should lie medial to lateral on the anteroposterior image.

A 2- to 4-cm incision into the subcutaneous tissues in the upper lateral buttock is made below the beltline, 3 to 5 cm below the superior iliac crest with the outer edge of the incision meeting the posterior axillary line. This will be the site for connecting the permanent lead to the percutaneous extension lead wire. If the screening trial is successful, this connection site will be the site of implantation for the IPG. The permanent lead is transferred to the medial aspect of the lateral buttock incision using the tunneling device. The lead is then connected to the extension wire and the tunneling device is used again to transfer the extension wire from the medial aspect of the incision to an exit point on the contralateral side of the back. The long tunnel created by this transfer reduces the occurrence of infection from the percutaneous exit site of the wire. The extension wire is connected to the test stimulator. The pocket is closed in two layers with a deep, interrupted 2-0 absorbable suture layer and a superficial, running 4-0 absorbable suture layer to close the skin. Patients are able to resume their normal activities immediately but are advised to limit excessive movement, such as during high-impact exercises, for the duration of the trial period.

The external generator can be flexibly programmed for the duration of the intended trial while patients record their symptoms and bladder function in a voiding diary. If there is >50% improvement in the symptoms or voiding function, a Stage 2 procedure is performed.

### Stage II

At the Stage 2 procedure, the IPG is placed. Fluoroscopy is not required during Stage 2 when a permanent neuroelectrode has been placed for the Stage 1 procedure; however, if a PNE was performed for Stage 1, then fluoroscopic confirmation of the neuroelectrode placement is advised. The buttock incision overlying the lead connections is opened, the percutaneous extension wire is removed, and the extension lead is secured to the permanent lead and subsequently to the IPG. The newer-generation IPG, the InterStim II, is connected directly to the permanent lead without the need for an extension lead (Fig. 46.7). It is smaller than the original IPG but also has a shorter battery life. The IPG pocket should be large enough to accommodate the IPG without tension and deep enough to prevent erosion and provide cosmetic results. The etched side of the IPG faces up when it is inserted into the pocket. The lead should be wrapped around the IPG, not placed on top of the IPG. This protects the lead if the pocket needs to be reopened for revision or IPG replacement. Prior to closing the incision in two layers, impedances should be checked.

Patients are discharged after patient education regarding the test stimulator and with prescriptions for oral pain medication and 1 week of oral antibiotics, either cephalosporins or fluoroquinolones.

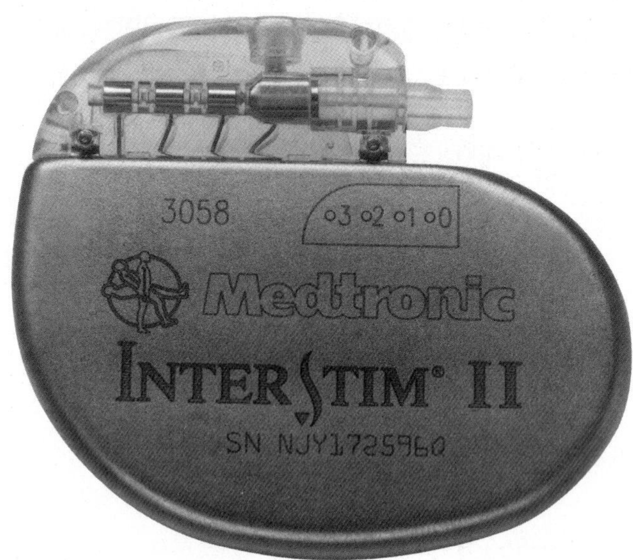


FIGURE 46.7 The InterStim II. (From Medtronic, Inc. © 2006, with permission.)

## COMPLICATIONS

The sacral nerve stimulation study group has published several reports on the efficacy and safety of the procedure for individual indications (9). The complications were pooled from the different studies based on the fact that the protocols, devices, efficacy results, and safety profiles were identical. A total of 581 patients were recruited, 219 of whom underwent implantation of the InterStim system. The complications were divided into problems related to percutaneous test stimulation and postimplant-related problems. Of the 914 test stimulation procedures done on the 581 patients, 181 adverse events occurred in 166 of these procedures (18.2% of the 914 procedures). The vast majority of complications were related to lead migration (108 events, 11.8% of procedures). Technical problems and pain represented 2.6% and 2.1% of the adverse events. For the 219 patients who underwent implantation of the InterStim system (lead and generator), pain at the neurostimulator site was the most commonly observed adverse effect at 12 months (15.3%). Surgical revisions of the implanted neurostimulator or lead system were performed in 33.3% of cases (73 of 219 patients) to resolve an adverse event. These included relocation of the neurostimulator because of pain at the subcutaneous pocket site and revision of the lead for suspected migration. Explantation of the system was performed in 10.5% for lack of efficacy. One should consider the fact that at the time, the generator was implanted in the lower abdomen.

Hijaz et al. (5) have presented algorithms for the troubleshooting of SNM problems. Generator site infection is best treated with explanation of the whole system. Despite attempts to salvage some of these patients, follow-up revealed that the infection persisted in all and eventual explantation was inevitable. The troubleshooting algorithm includes the search for causes of (a) pocket (IPG site) discomfort; (b) recurrent symptoms; (c) stimulation occurring in the wrong area of pelvis; (d) no stimulation; and (e) intermittent stimulation.

## OUTCOMES

The original reported outcomes of SNM for the indications of idiopathic urgency-frequency and urge incontinence were derived from two studies that randomized patients to active or delayed therapy, as well as reports from numerous prospective and retrospective reviews of case series and registry databases.

Schmidt et al. (7) reported on SNM therapy in 76 patients with refractory urge incontinence. During the 6-month study period, at 16 different centers, patients were randomized to active or delayed therapy (control group). Of the 34 patients receiving active SNM therapy, 16 (47%) were completely dry, and an additional 10 (29%) demonstrated a >50% reduction in incontinence episodes.

In a similar study design, Hassouna et al. (4) reported the outcomes of SNM for refractory urgency-frequency conditions in 51 randomized patients. At 6 months patients in the active SNM group showed improvement in the number of daily voids (16.9 ± 9.7 to 9.3 ± 5.1), volume voided (118 ± 74 to 226 ± 124 mL), degree of urgency (rank score of 2.2 ± 0.6 to 1.6 ± 0.9), and quality-of-life measures. At 6 months post implant, stimulators in the active group were turned off and urinary symptoms returned to baseline values. After reactivation of SNM, sustained efficacy was documented at 12 and 24 months.

In 2007, the results of a 5-year, prospective, multicenter trial confirmed the long-term efficacy of SNM in patients with refractory urge incontinence, urgency-frequency, and retention (12). Seventeen centers enrolled 163 patients, and 152 patients underwent permanent implantation. Voiding diaries were collected annually for 5 years. Study patient retention was fairly good: at 5 years a total of 105 patients completed follow-up and 87 completed the voiding diary. At 5 years after implantation, 68% of patients with urge incontinence, 56% with urgency-frequency, and 71% with retention had successful outcomes, confirming the durability of this therapy.

## *References*


1. Chai TC, Mamo GJ. Modified techniques of S3 foramen localization and lead implantation in S3 neuromodulation. *Urology* 2001;58(5):786–790.
2. Cohen BL, Tunuguntla HS, et al. Predictors of success for first stage neuromodulation: motor versus sensory response. *J Urol* 2006;175(6): 2178–2180; discussion 2180–2181.
3. Elkelini MS, Hassouna MM. Safety of MRI at 1.5 tesla in patients with implanted sacral nerve neurostimulator. *Eur Urol* 2006;50(2):311–316.
4. Hassouna MM, Siegel SW, et al. Sacral neuromodulation in the treatment of urgency-frequency symptoms: a multicenter study on efficacy and safety. *J Urol* 2000;163(6):1849–1854.
5. Hijaz A, Vasavada SP, et al. Complications and troubleshooting of two-stage sacral neuromodulation therapy: a single-institution experience. *Urology* 2006;68(3):533–537.
6. Leng WW, Chancellor MB. How sacral nerve stimulation neuromodulation works. *Urol Clin North Am* 2005;32(1):11–18.
7. Schmidt RA, Jonas U, et al. Sacral nerve stimulation for treatment of refractory urinary urge incontinence. Sacral Nerve Stimulation Study Group. *J Urol* 1999;162(2):352–357.
8. Siegel SW. Selecting patients for sacral nerve stimulation. *Urol Clin North Am* 2005;32(1):19–26.
9. Siegel SW, Catanzaro F, et al. Long-term results of a multicenter study on sacral nerve stimulation for treatment of urinary urge incontinence, urgency-frequency, and retention. *Urology* 2000;56(6)[Suppl 1]:87–91.
10. Spinelli M, Giardiello G, et al. New sacral neuromodulation lead for percutaneous implantation using local anesthesia: description and first experience. *J Urol* 2003;170(5):1905–1907.
11. Tanagho EA, Schmidt RA, et al. Neural stimulation for control of voiding dysfunction: a preliminary report in 22 patients with serious neuropathic voiding disorders. *J Urol* 1989;142(2, Pt 1):340–345.
12. van Kerrebroeck PE, van Voskuilen AC, et al. Results of sacral neuromodulation therapy for urinary voiding dysfunction: outcomes of a prospective, worldwide clinical study. *J Urol* 2007;178(5):2029–2034.


# CHAPTER 47 ■ SURGICAL TREATMENT OF PELVIC ORGAN PROLAPSE: ANATOMY OF THE PELVIC FLOOR

ARIANA L. SMITH, JA-HONG KIM, AND SHLOMO RAZ

The etiology of pelvic organ prolapse (POP) is multifactorial, with at most 40% of cases being attributable to genetics (1). Other factors that contribute to the development of prolapse include aging, hormonal status, birth and surgical trauma, pudendal neuropathy, elongation or detachment of support, and myopathy. While genetic and environmental effects are being investigated and preventive measures sought, there remain millions of women who have developed or will develop POP in their lifetime.

Understanding pelvic floor anatomy is critical for any pelvic surgeon before undertaking reconstructive surgery. Not only restoring pelvic floor anatomy but also maintaining and restoring appropriate function is essential for successful patient outcomes. Therefore, it is crucial to understand the complex combination of muscles, ligaments, and fascia that act dynamically to provide support to the female pelvic anatomy, including the urethra, bladder, uterus, and rectum. When normal mechanisms of support fail, pelvic floor relaxation and organ descent occurs. Depending on the compartment affected, symptoms may vary from voiding dysfunction and urinary incontinence to bowel dysfunction and stool incontinence.

Numerous techniques are available for surgical repair of POP, and many of these will be described in upcoming chapters. This chapter will review female pelvic anatomy and musculofascial support, emphasizing the supporting structures that allow normal voiding and defecatory function, as well as the pathophysiology of pelvic floor relaxation, with a description of the various components of POP.

# ANATOMY OF PELVIC SUPPORT

Conceptually, the vaginal canal can be divided into three compartments that have distinct anatomic structures: (i) the anterior compartment, which includes the urethra, bladder neck, and bladder, (ii) the superior compartment, which includes the uterus and cul-de-sac after hysterectomy, and (iii) the posterior compartment, which includes the rectum, anal canal, and perineum. These compartments have functional and anatomic interactions such that the function and support of one compartment depend on intact support of the others. Structurally, the vaginal and pelvic anatomy starts with a framework of bones and ligaments that are lined with fascia and muscles. These structures are intimately related and in some cases are continuations of each other, especially in the case of ligaments and fascia.

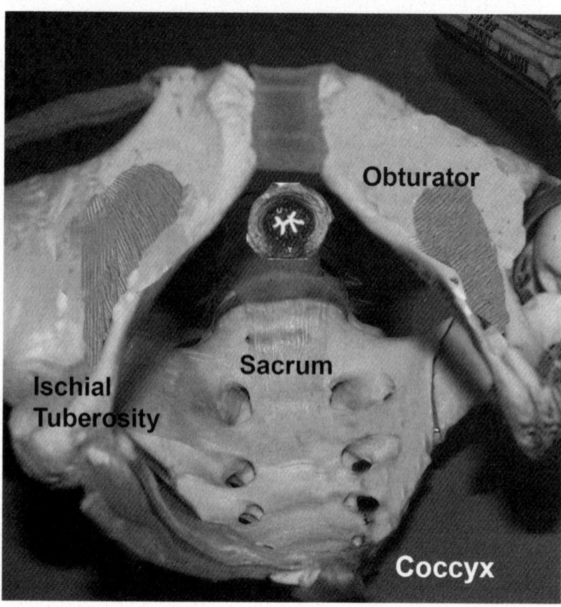


FIGURE 47.1 The framework of the pelvic floor is formed by the pubic symphysis, pubic rami, and sacrum. The ischial tuberosities divide the pelvic floor into the anterior and posterior compartments. The urethra is shown in the anterior compartment behind the pubic symphysis. The obturator fascia is an important area of anchoring for pelvic support.

## The Pelvic Diaphragm

### Bones

The framework of the pelvic floor is provided by the bony structures, including the pubis, ilium, ischium, sacrum, and coccyx. The pelvic bones create a diamond shape, with the pubic symphysis and coccyx at the apices and the ischial tuberosities dividing the diamond into anterior and posterior compartments (Fig. 47.1). The anterior or urogenital triangle contains the clitoris, urethra, and vaginal vestibule. The posterior or anal triangle contains the anal canal and anal sphincter. The pubic rami, ischial spines, and sacrum are important anchoring points of muscular and fascial structures in the pelvis (2).

### Ligaments

The name *ligament* has been given to what are truly dense condensations of connective tissue in the pelvis.

**Pubourethral Ligaments.** The pubourethral ligaments anchor the urethra anteriorly to the inferior ramus of the pubic symphysis (Fig. 47.2). They also divide the urethra into proximal and distal halves, with the proximal, intra-abdominal portion responsible for passive, involuntary continence. The midportion, or the striated external sphincter, is responsible for active, voluntary continence. The distal third of the urethra is simply a conduit for urine passage and does not significantly change function when damaged or removed.

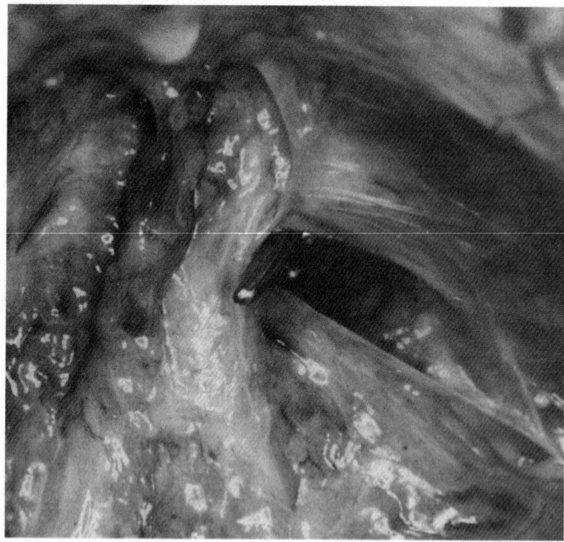

FIGURE 47.2 Abdominal view of the pelvis in a cadaver. The retropubic space has been entered from the vaginal side, detaching the urethropelvic ligaments from the lateral pelvic wall and exposing the pubourethral ligament.

**Urethropelvic Ligaments.** The urethropelvic ligaments are a condensation of periurethral fascia that provides anatomic support of the bladder neck and proximal urethra to the lateral pelvic wall (Fig. 47.3). They do so by anchoring the urethra laterally to the arcus tendineus fasciae pelvis (ATFP, see below). The urethropelvic ligaments provide elastic, musculofascial support to the bladder outlet, thereby maintaining passive continence. Voluntary or reflex contractions of the pelvic floor increase the tensile force across these ligaments, enhancing outlet resistance and preventing incontinence. Thus, restoration of these ligamentous structures is critically important in the surgical correction of stress incontinence.

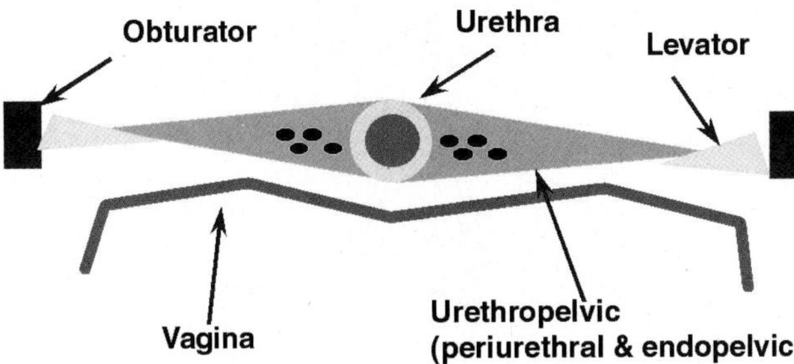


FIGURE 47.3 Urethropelvic ligaments supporting the urethra to the levator musculature of the lateral pelvic sidewall. In patients with multiple deliveries, the levator musculature is weakened and the ligament is thin, elongated, or detached from the lateral pelvic wall.

**Vesicopelvic Ligaments.** The vesicopelvic ligaments anchor the bladder to the pelvic sidewall. During voluntary or reactive pelvic floor contraction (i.e., contraction of the levator muscles), the ligamentous structures tighten and elevate the bladder, preventing mobility and descent into the vagina. Restoration of these ligaments is important in the correction of anterior wall prolapse, or cystocele.

**Cardinal–Sacrouterine Ligament Complex.** The cardinal ligaments, or ligaments of Mackenrodt, are thick, triangular condensations of pelvic fascia that originate from the greater sciatic foramen and insert into the cervix and vaginal wall. They also extend to the perivesical fascia, providing support to the bladder base (Figs. 47.4 and 47.5). These ligaments contain numerous blood vessels branching from the hypogastrics that supply the uterus and upper vagina (2). The cardinal ligaments fuse posteriorly with the sacrouterine ligaments, which stabilize the uterus, cervix, and upper vagina

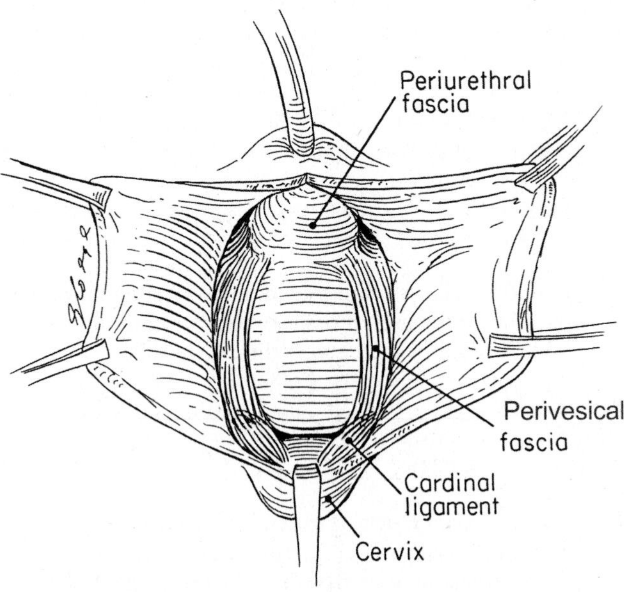


FIGURE 47.4 The vaginal wall has been dissected free to expose the anterior support of the bladder and urethra. The periurethral fascia covers and supports the urethra distally. The perivesical fascia covers the bladder wall from the bladder neck to the cervix. The cardinal ligaments are attached to the cervix in the midline with proximal extensions to the bladder. They provide important support to the bladder base.

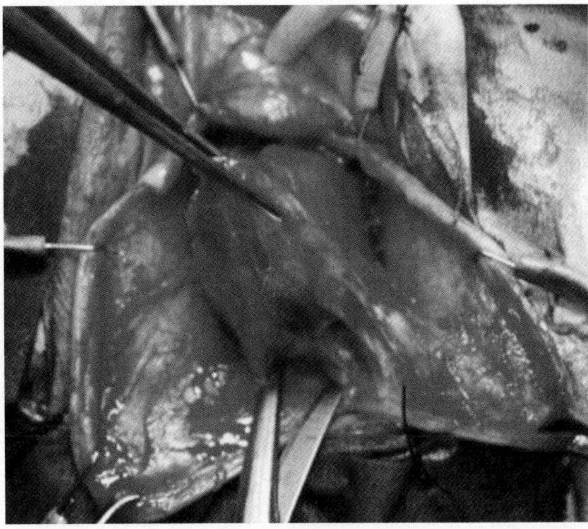

FIGURE 47.5 Dissection of the bladder wall during repair of grade IV cystocele exposes the cardinal ligaments as they attach to the bladder base.

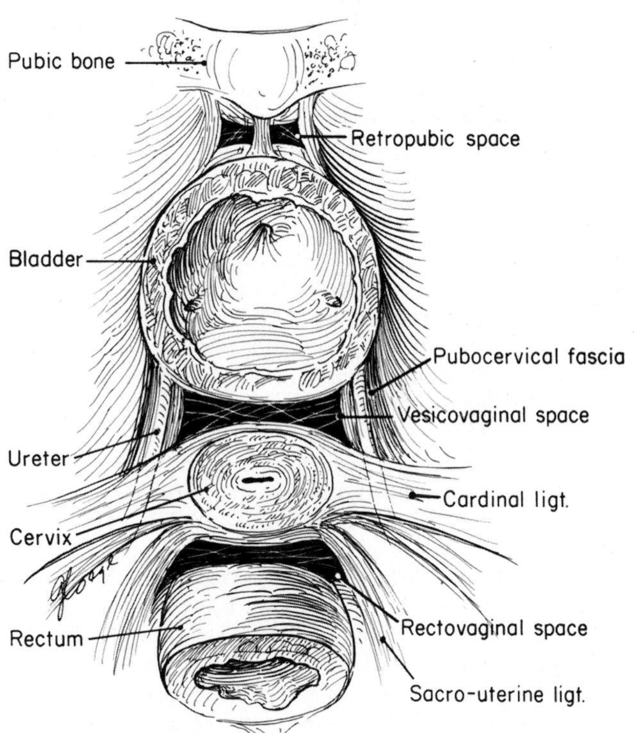


FIGURE 47.6 Uterine support and its relations to the bladder and rectum. The cardinal ligaments provide support of the cervix to the lateral pelvic wall.

posteriorly toward the sacrum (3) (Fig. 47.6). The sacrouterine ligaments originate from the second, third, and fourth sacral vertebrae and insert posterolaterally into the cervix and vaginal fornices (4). The trauma of vaginal delivery can cause relaxation of the cardinal-sacrouterine complex and allow descent of the cervix and uterus. Poor surgical technique at the time of hysterectomy may not restore the ligaments to the midline position, thus allowing a wide gap for the bladder to herniate. It is very important to reapproximate the cardinal ligaments in the midline when repairing anterior or posterior wall prolapse.

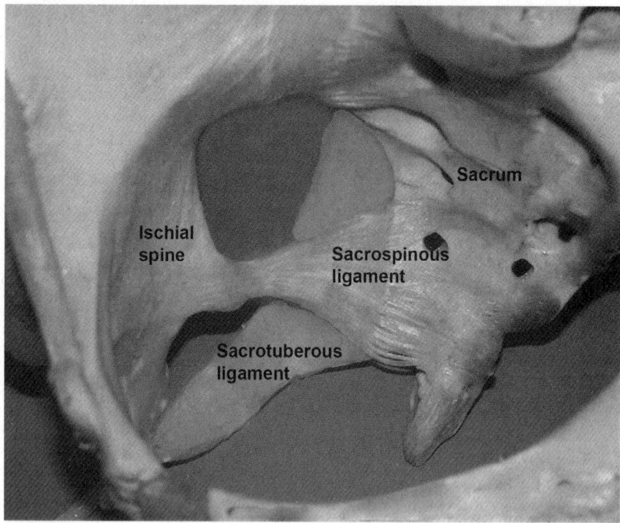


FIGURE 47.7 The sacrospinous ligament is an important area of anchoring for vaginal vault suspension.

**Broad Ligaments.** The broad ligaments provide additional uterine support superior to the previously named structures. They attach the lateral walls of the uterine body to the pelvic sidewall and contain the fallopian tubes, the round and ovarian ligaments, and the uterine and ovarian vessels. The broad ligaments are covered by an anterior and posterior sheet of peritoneum.

**Sacrospinous Ligaments.** The sacrospinous ligaments span the posterior portion of the pelvic floor, from the ischial spines to the sacrum and coccyx (Fig. 47.7). The coccygeus muscle lies over the top of the sacrospinous ligament and is a very important landmark in vaginal surgery. Cephalad to the coccygeus muscle, the lumbosacral plexus spreads its fibers, which if injured can cause chronic debilitating pain. Lateral to the coccygeus muscle the pudendal nerves and vessels traverse in the canal of Alcock. Also in this area is the ureter, which can be occluded with a suture placed too laterally (5).

**Perineal Body.** The perineal body is a tendinous structure located in the midline of the perineum between the anus and vaginal introitus. It provides a central point of fixation for the transverse perineal muscles, which extend from the ischial tuberosities laterally (6) (Fig. 47.8). The perineal body provides an additional level of support to the posterior vaginal wall and rectum, incorporating the levator ani, bulbocavernosus muscle, and transverse perineal musculature as well as the external anal sphincter. This level of support is elastic in nature, allowing distortion and recoil during childbirth and intercourse.

## Fascia

Like vaginal ligaments, there are no true vaginal fascias. The structures commonly called fascia are condensations of connective tissue separating the vagina from the urethra, bladder, cervix, or rectum (7). The fascia overlying the pelvic floor musculature plays a critical role in pelvic support. Both sides of the muscle, the abdominal side and the vaginal side, are covered with fascia, and therefore the fascia comprises two components. On the abdominal side it is called endopelvic fascia and represents a continuation of the transversalis fascia.

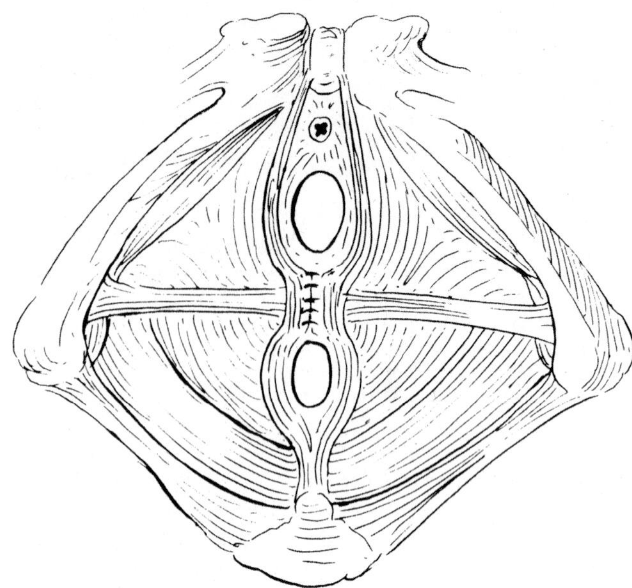

FIGURE 47.8 Repair of the perineal body. The bulbocavernosus muscle, the transverse perineal muscles, and the anal sphincter fibers are approximated to recreate the central tendon of the perineum.

**Pubocervical Fascia.** On the vaginal side is it often referred to as the pubocervical fascia, but can be divided into discrete areas of specialization depending on the associated organ it supports (periurethral and perivesical fascia). As a whole, the pubocervical fascia is a trapezoid-shaped continuous sheet of connective tissue support that extends from the pubic symphysis to the cervix and laterally to the ATFP (8). The fascia is fused to the bony scaffold by the cardinal ligaments laterally and the sacrouterine ligaments posteriorly.

**Arcus Tendineus Fasciae Pelvis.** ATFP is a curvilinear condensation of pelvic fascia that arises from the obturator internus muscle and runs from the pubic symphysis to the ischial spines (Fig. 47.9). This tendinous arc of the obturator is the line of insertion of the levator muscles on the obturator fascia. This crucial structure provides musculofascial attachment for the anterior and posterior pelvic organs. It also provides an anchoring point during reconstructive surgery of organs that have descended.

**Periurethral Fascia.** Around the urethra, the periurethral fascia represents two wings of tissue extending from the urethra to the ATFP, fused by the pubourethral ligaments.

**Perivesical Fascia.** Around the bladder, the perivesical fascia extends as wings from the bladder to the ATFP, fused by the vesicopelvic ligaments.

**Prerectal/Pararectal Fascia.** Prerectal and pararectal fascia extends from the cardinal-sacrouterine complex to the perineal body and is sometimes referred to as the rectovaginal septum.

## Musculature

The striated musculature supporting the pelvic floor is composed of the levator ani muscles and the coccygeus muscles. Together they cradle the visceral contents of the pelvis, providing dynamic support.

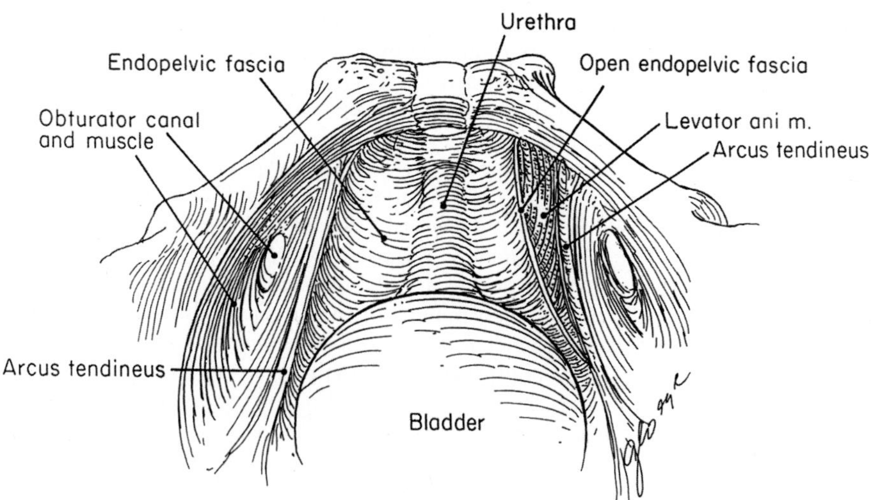


FIGURE 47.9 View of the anterior pelvis. The endopelvic fascia covers the bladder and urethra. The levator musculature is attached to the arcus tendineus fasciae pelvis.

**Levator Ani.** The levator ani has two main components, the pubococcygeus and the iliococcygeus, which are named according to their origin from the pelvic sidewall (9). This broad sheet of muscle extends from the pubic symphysis to the ischial spines and coccyx, taking origin from the ATFP laterally. These muscle groups have overlying endopelvic fascia that allows direct attachment to the bladder, urethra, vagina, uterus, and rectum to permit active visceral control (Fig. 47.10). These muscles supply support during increases in intra-abdominal pressure, preventing organ descent and more importantly preventing the release of urine and stool (2). The medial fibers of the pubococcygeus muscles are also referred to as the puborectalis muscle or "pullator" because of its role in pulling forward the anal canal and distal vagina, closing the levator hiatus.

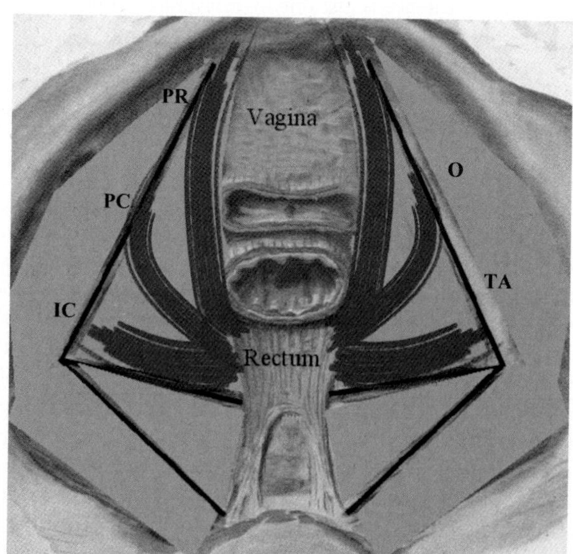


FIGURE 47.10 Pelvic support provided by the levator ani muscles. The levator ani is divided into two main segments: the pubococcygeus and the iliococcygeus. These muscles take origin in the arcus tendineus fasciae pelvis, a thickening of the obturator fascia. The medial portion of the pubococcygeus, the puborectalis, forms a sling around the distal rectum. PR, puborectalis; PC, pubococcygeus; IC, iliococcygeus; O, obturator musculature; TA, tendinous arc.

**Coccygeus.** The posterior portions of the levator ani, together with the coccygeus muscle, provide a horizontal plate from the rectal hiatus to the coccyx. This plate maintains a normal vaginal and uterine axis. The uterus and proximal vagina, as well as the bladder and rectum, lie horizontally on this plate, preventing their descent. Resting tone of the levator ani and coccygeus, as well as reflex and voluntary contraction, acts to pull the vagina and rectum forward, closing the lumens of these structures. Re-establishing this axis is important for re-establishing normal anatomy and sexual function as well as long-term success in prolapse surgery.

**Levator Hiatus.** The levator hiatus is a U-shaped midline aperture in the levator ani that allows passage of the urethra, vagina, and rectum (Fig. 47.11). These structures are supported by a fascial hammock, the urogenital diaphragm, as they exit the pelvis (10). Fibers from the pubococcygeus enter

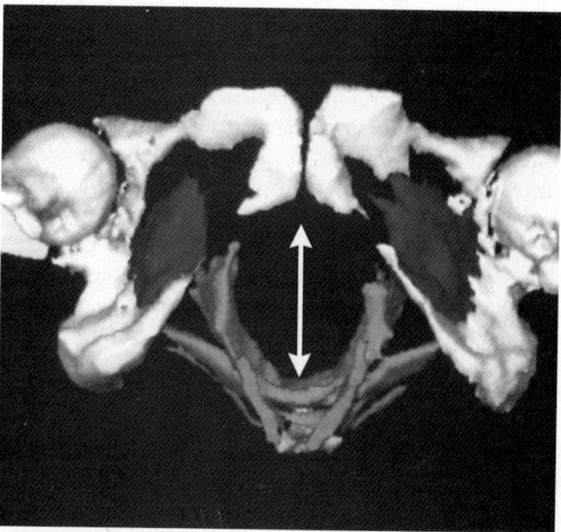

FIGURE 47.11 Three-dimensional MRI reconstruction of the levator musculature, bony pelvis, and obturator musculature in a patient with multiple deliveries. The levator hiatus is widened (*arrow*); this represents the distance between the rectal canal and the pubic bone, called the puborectal line.

into the hiatus and surround the urethra and anus, forming the sphincter musculatures.

### Areas of Special Interest: Obturator Anatomy

Prior to the introduction of the transobturator tape, the obturator anatomy was rarely studied. With the dramatic increase in the number of procedures performed in this area and the arising complications, it is important for all urologists to understand the anatomic landmarks. The adductor longus tendon is a major landmark for trocar passage and protects the patient from injury to the neurovascular bundle. Safe entry and exit zones exist when the patient is properly positioned and landmarks are obeyed. When a sling is placed using this technique, it is important to understand that the mesh sling is placed through the obturator internus muscle via passage of the trocar (Fig. 47.1). Complications are possible as a result of this placement; these include walking difficulty and pain with contraction of the obturator internus muscle.

## PATHOPHYSIOLOGY OF PELVIC FLOOR DYSFUNCTION

### Mechanisms of Urethral Continence

Bladder outlet resistance in women is attained by several factors working together to provide continence at rest and during stress maneuvers. Urethral anatomy, including functional length and elastic closure, is an important determinant of continence. In addition, activity of the muscular pelvic floor with its associated connective tissue elements helps maintain outlet resistance during times of increased intra-abdominal pressure. The anatomic position of the urethra is another factor contributing to continence. Each of these entities will be discussed separately to provide a basis for understanding the pathophysiology of pelvic floor relaxation.

Structural support of the urethra alone is not enough for the maintenance of urinary continence; there are also integral features of the urethra that contribute. The urethra is made up of three functional anatomic components that result in an elastic, dynamic conduit with mucosal coaptation. The urethral mucosa is transitional epithelium with numerous infoldings that allow distensibility and closure with excellent coaptation. Beneath the mucosa is a spongy tissue made up of vascular networks, analogous to the corpus spongiosum in men. Surrounding the spongy tissue is a thin musculofascial envelope, the periurethral fascia, which appears as a glistening, white membrane during surgery. These three components contribute to form a coaptive seal. Surrounding the mucosa are layers of smooth and striated muscle that are part of the sphincter mechanism. These muscles are under both voluntary and involuntary control. When functioning properly, they maintain enough compression, or resistance, of the urethra to prevent leakage of urine.

Both the bladder neck and urethra are normally maintained in a high retropubic position relative to the more dependent bladder base, creating a valvular effect. The bladder neck and urethra are supported by a musculofascial layer that suspends these structures from the pubic bone and pelvic sidewalls, thereby preventing their descent during increases in intra-abdominal pressure (11). Further, direct transmission of intra-abdominal forces to a well-supported proximal urethra increases its resistance and promotes coaptation (12). Relaxation of the pelvic floor as well as weakening of the urethropelvic ligaments and midurethral complex produces significant posterior and downward rotation of the urethra and bladder neck. This anatomic repositioning of the urethra and bladder neck to a more dependent pelvic position eliminates the valvular effect. Thus, a poorly supported urethra will tend to funnel and open during increases in intra-abdominal pressure. Interestingly, the same mechanism of restoring continence by repositioning the urethra higher than the bladder base and trigone (classic Burch procedure) can produce outlet obstruction in patients who develop a secondary cystocele. This occurs due to a kinking effect when the prolapsing bladder drops further below the suspended urethra.

Essentially, three mechanisms of support maintain continence during increases in intra-abdominal pressure: (i) the backboard effect of urethral support maintained by the periurethral fascia and urethropelvic ligaments, (ii) the valvular effect at the bladder neck, and (iii) the voluntary and reflex contraction of the pelvic floor.

With aging there is a decrease in skeletal and smooth muscle density as a result of atrophy. This can affect the urethral sphincter mechanism as well as the contributing pelvic floor. Continence should therefore be perceived as a dynamic function that changes with age. As a result, surgery for repair should not be viewed as a cure that will last forever, but rather as a treatment. Current methods are not actually curing the defect in urethral function but rather temporizing or treating the symptoms. Therapies aimed at cure are being employed using stem cells to regenerate smooth and striated muscle.

Stress incontinence is just one manifestation of pelvic relaxation. Often other pelvic defects coexist and should be addressed simultaneously.

### Cystocele

When defects in pubocervical fascia exist, a cystocele develops (Fig. 47.12). Usually the defect is in both the lateral fascia and the midline of the fascia, with also a notable defect in cuff support (13). The defect can be treated by using a trapezoid-shaped piece of mesh and anchoring it to the obturator fascia laterally (via the ATFP), the sacrouterine complex apically, and the bladder neck distally, thus reapproximating the trapezoid-shaped pubocervical fascia. This is usually performed in combination with anterior colporrhaphy, or plication of the pubocervical fascia in the midline. Because of the risk of de novo stress incontinence after cystocele repair, many authors recommend performing a concomitant sling at the time of bladder repair. We agree with this. In fact, there is evidence to support not only a decrease in incontinence, but also a decrease in recurrence of prolapse when a sling is added to the repair (14). It is also important to reapproximate the cardinal ligament complex in the midline to support the bladder base and prevent recurrence.

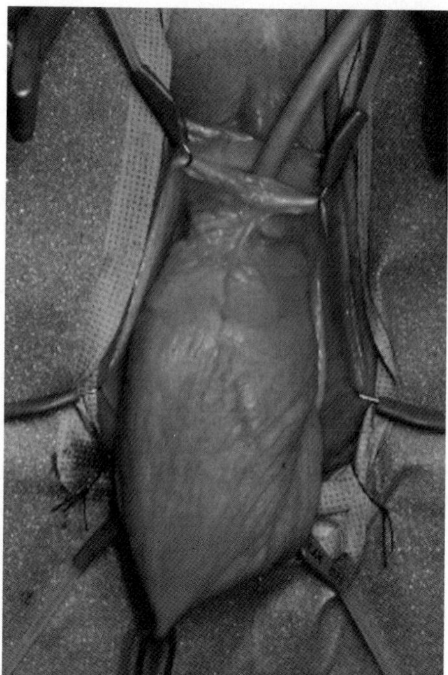

FIGURE 47.12 Severe prolapse of the anterior vaginal wall with central and lateral defect. The normal H-shape of the vagina is lost. The lateral walls of the vagina are detached from supporting structures, allowing downward displacement and disappearance of the lateral sulci.

### Rectocele

The posterior vaginal wall has a complex fascial and muscular arrangement that provides support not only to the vagina but also to the rectum, perineum, and anal sphincter. There are four components that contribute to failing posterior support: prerectal/pararectal fascia attenuation, perineal membrane widening, levator hiatus widening, and descent of the levator plate. Rectocele is a poor name to encompass all of these defects. It is important to address and repair all of these potential weaknesses and avoid segmental repairs—in particular, reinforcing attenuated prerectal and pararectal fascia by plication or with mesh, reapproximating the levator musculature to close the levator hiatus, and rebuilding the perineal body to provide normal introital size and improved support. These measures prevent descent of the organs and the need for secondary surgery.

## RESTORATION OF SUPPORT

The normal vaginal length is approximately 8 to 9 cm, with the ischial spines as a good landmark. The caliber should approximate two fingerbreadths. The axis should be such that the vagina rests on the levator plate in a banana shape, much like its natural position (Fig. 47.13). The proximal half of the vagina is practically horizontal resting over the levator plate. We can see that the axis of the vagina points down to S4–S5 (Fig. 47.14), not to the promontory where sacrocolpopexy is often performed. Suspending the vaginal cuff to this location can allow the formation of other defects, specifically enteroceles and rectoceles. Simply placing the cuff to the sacrospinous ligament restores proper anatomy, allows approximation of the perivesical and perirectal fasciae, and prevents recurrent prolapse. Lateral, anterior, and posterior dissection allows one to obtain good strong tissue for plication of the anterior and posterior vaginal walls. Anteriorly the surgeon must extend dissection to the inferior pubic ramus at the level of the obturator muscle, and posteriorly dissection must be taken to the rectal gutter, the groove between the rectum and the iliococcygeus muscle. The distal vagina is elevated with closure of the perineal defect, allowing achievement of normal introital caliber and shape.

Placement of the vault suspension sutures can be daunting. It is important to understand where it is safe and where it is dangerous to place these sutures. These sutures should be

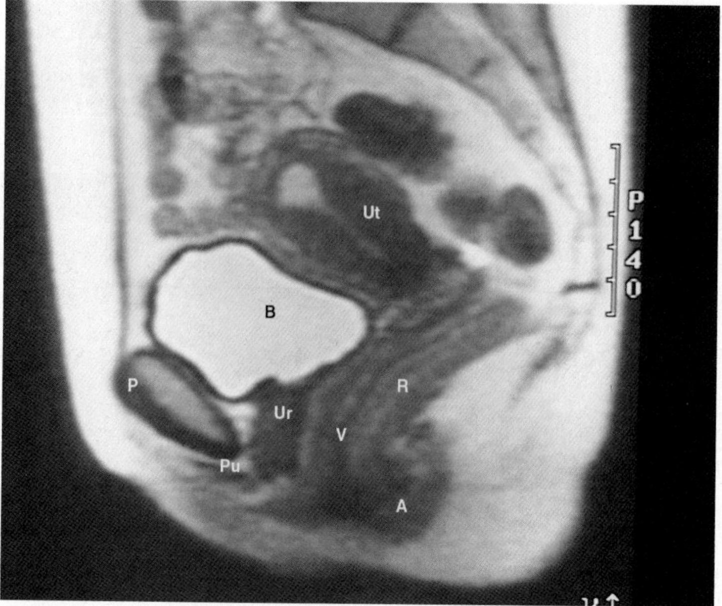


FIGURE 47.13 Dynamic MRI in a patient with normal vaginal support. The banana-shaped vaginal curvature is seen. The angulation between proximal and distal vagina (located at the level of the proximal anal canal) points to the insertion of the puborectalis musculature. P, pubic bone; Ur, urethra; PU, pubourethral ligaments; R, rectum; A, anal canal; B, bladder; U, uterus.

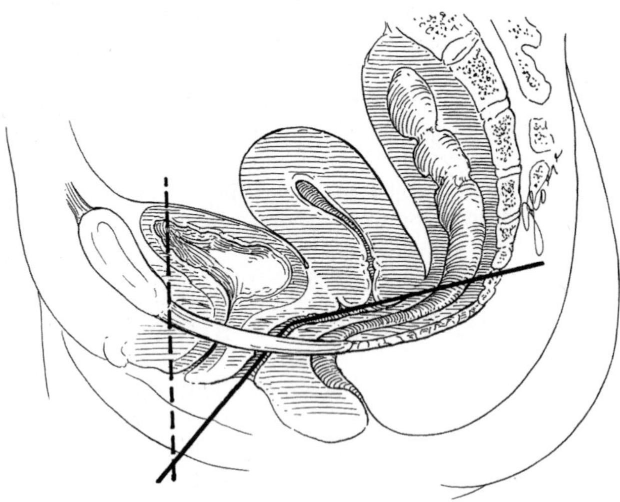

FIGURE 47.14 Vaginal support. The distal vagina is approximately 45 degrees from the vertical axis and the proximal vagina is approximately 10 degrees from the horizontal axis. The angulation between the two areas marks the insertion of the puborectalis muscle, which pulls the vagina anteriorly.

placed in the sacrospinous ligament with the needle pointing downward rather than laterally or superiorly in the direction of other important structures (Fig. 47.7). It is imperative to avoid going cephalad to the sacrospinous ligament, as the lumbosacral plexus can be injured or trapped with a suture. The ureter can be damaged, as can the pudendal nerve, if the needle is placed laterally. T-shaped soft polypropylene mesh is used to replicate cardinal–sacrouterine support by anchoring the cuff to the sacrospinous ligament.

The importance of a thorough evaluation and complete repair of the whole pelvic floor cannot be overemphasized. Segmental repairs allow exaggeration of pre-existing defects due to functional and anatomic changes. Repair of concomitant prolapse also has an important impact on the outcome of stress incontinence surgery (10). The reverse has also been found to be true: the addition of a sling procedure to anterior colporrhaphy reduces the cystocele recurrence rate by 50% (14). These findings are likely due to the dissipation of intra-abdominal pressure in the setting of POP. With restoration of strong support to the pelvic organs, there is more efficient transmission of abdominal pressure to the urethra and therefore better continence (10). The need to augment support with mesh or biologic fascia is debated. Most experts in the field believe that supporting the patient's weakened fascia can achieve a more durable response.

Regardless of technique, three basic tenets must be obeyed in pelvic reconstruction: (i) restoration of normal vaginal depth, caliber, and axis, (ii) prevention of further POP, and (iii) restoration and maintenance of normal bladder, bowel, and sexual function (7).

## *References*


1. Altman D, Forsman M, Falconer C, et al. Genetic influence on stress urinary incontinence and pelvic organ prolapse. *Eur Urol* 2008;54(5):918–922.
2. Klutke CG, Siegel CL. Functional female pelvic anatomy. *Urol Clin North Am* 1995;22:487–498.
3. Baden WF, Walker T. The anatomy of uterovaginal support. In: Baden WF, Walker T, eds. *Vaginal Defects*. Philadelphia: Lippincott, 1992:25–50.
4. DeLancey JO, Richardson AC. Anatomy of genital support. In: Hurt WG, ed. *Urogynecologic Surgery*. Gaithersburg, IL: Aspen Publishers, 1992: 19–33.
5. DeLancey JO. Surgical anatomy of the female pelvis. In: Rock JA, ed. *Te Linde's Operative Gynecology*. Philadelphia: Lippincott-Raven, 1997: 63–93.
6. Brooks JD. Anatomy of the lower urinary tract and male genitalia. In: Wein AJ, Kavoussi LR, Novick AC, et al., eds. *Campbell-Walsh Urology*. 9th ed. Philadelphia: Saunders-Elsevier, 2007:43–46.
7. Twiss CO, Triaca V, Konijeti R, et al. Reconstructive surgery for pelvic floor relaxation. In: Montague D, Angermeier KW, Ross J, Gill I, eds. *Textbook of Reconstructive Urologic Surgery*. Informa Healthcare Press, London , 2008: 532–552.
8. DeLancey JO. Fascial and muscular abnormalities in women with urethral hypermobility and anterior vaginal wall prolapse. *Am J Obstet Gynecol* 2002;187:93–98.
9. Redman JF. Surgical anatomy of the female genitorurinary system. In: Buchsbaum HJ, Schmidt JD, eds. *Gynecologic and Obstetric Urology*. Philadelphia: WB Saunders, 1993:25–60.
10. Raz S. *Atlas of Transvaginal Surgery*. 2nd ed. Philadelphia: WB Saunders, 2002.
11. Nitti V, Blaivas JG. Urinary incontinence: epidemiology, pathophysiology, evaluation, and management overview. In: Wein AJ, Kavoussi LR, Novick AC, et al., eds. *Campbell-Walsh Urology*. 9th ed. Philadelphia: Saunders-Elsevier, 2007:2046–2077.
12. Enhorning G. Simultaneous recording of intravesical and intra-urethral pressure. A study on urethral closure in normal and stress incontinent women. *Acta Chir Scand Suppl* 1961(276):1–68.
13. Scarpero HM, Nitti VW. Anterior vaginal wall prolapse: mild/moderate cystoceles. In: Vasavada SP, Appell RA, Sand PK, et al., eds. *Female Urology, Urogynecology, and Voiding Dysfunction*. New York: Marcel Dekker, 2005:575–594.
14. Goldberg RP, Koduri S, Lobel RW, et al. Protective effect of suburethral slings on postoperative cystocele recurrence after reconstructive pelvic operation. *Am J Obstet Gynecol* 2001;185:1307–1313.


# CHAPTER 48 ■ VAGINAL HYSTERECTOMY FOR UTERINE PROLAPSE

JA-HONG KIM, ARIANA L. SMITH, AND SHLOMO RAZ

Hysterectomy is the second most commonly performed surgical procedure in the United States, with 66% of the cases done through the abdominal approach, followed by the vaginal route in 22% and the laparoscopic route in 12% (1). The most common indications for hysterectomy are uterine fibroids (33%) and menstrual disorders (17%), followed by prolapse (13%) and endometriosis (9%). There is a growing body of evidence has shown that vaginal hysterectomy is the preferred surgical route due to shorter operative time, fewer postoperative complications, and a shorter hospital stay (2,3). More importantly, it avoids the morbidity of an abdominal incision and offers optimal opportunity to correct and prevent pelvic organ prolapse. Relative contraindications for vaginal hysterectomy include a large uterus in proportion to a narrow introitus, ovarian pathology, previous cesarean delivery, endometriosis, and a history of pelvic inflammatory disease, which may result in extensive scarring in the pelvis, making dissection difficult. The ultimate decision regarding the surgical approach to hysterectomy, however, rests on the surgeon's experience and preference. As a genitourinary surgeon, one should be familiar with the surgical principles and technique of vaginal hysterectomy, as it is a crucial component of female pelvic reconstruction.

This chapter will focus on four major concepts that are important to performing a successful vaginal hysterectomy for uterine prolapse: (i) pertinent female pelvic anatomy as it relates to the pathophysiology of uterine prolapse, (ii) standard evaluation, including a focused history and imaging, (iii) surgical technique, highlighting the principles for vascular control and restoring vaginal support, and (iv) review of potential complications and outcomes.

## SURGICAL ANATOMY

The female pelvic organs are supported by the dynamic interaction between their connective tissue attachments (ligaments and fascia) and the pelvic floor muscles (levator ani muscle group and coccygeus), which provide a firm yet elastic base on which they rest. Histologically, the term *endopelvic fascia* is used to describe this continuous network of connective tissue that envelops all of the pelvic organs and connects them to supportive musculature and pelvic bones, which is located on the peritoneal side. On the vaginal side, the fasciae acquire different nomenclature and are distinctively named according to their anatomic location and the organ that they support. The thick condensations of the connective tissue are further organized to a trilevel support system that was described by De Lancey as they relate to the pathophysiology of uterovaginal prolapse (4). Level I refers to the fused ligamentous complex in the most cephalad portion (cervix and upper vagina) that maintains vaginal length and horizontal axis. Level II support is provided by the paravaginal attachments along the length of the vagina to the arcus tendineus fasciae pelvis. Level III support describes the most inferior or distal portions of the vagina, including the perineum.

The pear-shaped uterus consists of the corpus and the cervix and lies in the medial axial position, anteverted with the vertical axis of the uterus perpendicular to the axis of the vagina. The corpus or body of the uterus is enclosed between the double-layered broad ligaments, which contain the fallopian tubes, the round and ovarian ligaments, and the uterine and ovarian vessels. No fixed uterine support is provided by the broad ligaments, as demonstrated by its ability to enlarge without restriction during pregnancy. Thus, the main uterine support is provided by the uterosacral and cardinal (Mackenrodt) ligaments, which attach to the cervix from the posterior and lateral sides, respectively. Together, the fused uterosacral–cardinal ligament complex represents level I support and attaches the upper vagina, cervix, and lower uterine segment to the sacrum and lateral pelvic sidewalls at the piriformis, coccygeus, levator ani, and arcus tendineus. During hysterectomy, these ligaments must be carefully identified and controlled, as they will be incorporated into the vaginal cuff to successfully re-establish proper vault support.

The natural vaginal axis is a banana shape, with the upper third of the vagina lying in a horizontal position and the apex directed towards the lower sacrum (S3–S5). This axis is normally maintained partly by the support of the levator ani and coccygeus muscle group, especially during increased intra-abdominal pressure. Therefore, complete correction of uterovaginal prolapse at the time of hysterectomy should include not only reattachment of the cardinal and uterosacral ligaments to the vaginal vault, but also vault or apical suspension to the area of the coccygeus to re-establish the banana-shaped axis. In the substance of the coccygeus lies a cordlike structure called the sacrospinous ligament, which extends from the ischial spines on each side to the lower portion of the sacrum and coccyx. This sacrospinous ligament provides a consistently strong site for apical fixation that can restore vaginal depth and axis. It is crucial to accurately identify this important structure when placing vault suspension sutures, as the pudendal neurovascular bundle, lumbosacral plexus, and ureters live in close proximity and can be injured during suture placement. Various techniques for vault suspension at the time of hysterectomy have been described in the literature, and a thorough comparison of these procedures is beyond the scope of this chapter. There is no randomized control study that has shown long-term superiority of one technique over the other. In our experience, bilateral fixation of the vaginal cuff to the origin of the uterosacral–cardinal ligament at the coccygeus–sacrospinous ligament complex provides the optimal restoration of vaginal depth and vault support with minimal morbidity. We routinely utilize a piece of soft polypropylene mesh to add strength to the uterosacral–cardinal ligament complex, which is often attenuated in patients undergoing vaginal hysterectomy for prolapse repair.

## PATHOPHYSIOLOGY OF UTERINE PROLAPSE

Although the exact etiology of pelvic prolapse has yet to be clearly defined, many risk factors have been proposed in the development of prolapse. Bump and Norton (5) categorized these risk factors into four categories: (i) **predisposing** factors are genetics, race, and gender; (ii) **inciting** factors are pregnancy and delivery, surgery, myopathy, and neuropathy; (iii) **promoting** factors are obesity, smoking, pulmonary disease, constipation, and recreational or occupational activities that cause chronic increases in intra-abdominal pressure; and (iv) **decompensating** factors are aging, menopause, debilitation, and medications. Any of the above risk factors can result in attenuation of the uterosacral–cardinal ligament complex or breaks along the endopelvic fascia. Furthermore, muscle atrophy of the levator ani and coccygeus can lead to a wider levator hiatus and a compromise in the excretory function of the bladder and rectum. The loss of uterine support causes the cervix to move anteriorly, and the uterus then begins to shift posteriorly such that the intra-abdominal pressure is then directed on the anterior surface of the uterus. The uterus becomes progressively more retroverted until the axis of the uterus is essentially vertical. This position allows uterine prolapse to occur (6).

## DIAGNOSIS

Standard evaluation of the patient with uterine prolapse includes a comprehensive history and physical examination, focusing on urinary and defecatory symptoms, sexual function, reproductive status, and other pelvic pathology. Urinary or bowel symptoms may be present if there is prolapse of other organs. Less commonly, a patient presents because uterine prolapse was incidentally found on routine physical examination. Validated questionnaires measuring symptom severity, impact on quality of life, voiding log, and sexual function can be premailed to allow the patient time to consider her symptoms. An important piece of information in the patient's surgical history is whether the patient had a partial hysterectomy. Often, what is assumed to be uterine descent is only cervical descent resulting from a supracervical hysterectomy. It is also important to ask about any uterine pathology, such as endometriosis, fibroids, and pelvic inflammatory disease, which can influence surgical planning.

Postvoid residual urine volume and urinalysis are obtained for all patients. Urodynamic evaluation is not routinely performed for prolapse patients unless there is a history of stress or urge incontinence, incomplete emptying, obstructive voiding complaints, or bothersome overactive bladder symptoms. For these patients with urinary symptoms, we recommend assessment of the lower urinary tract with a videourodynamic evaluation and office cystoscopy. It is important to recognize that stress incontinence may be masked by the prolapse, which can cause kinking of the urethra. As many patients with prolapse are elderly, detrusor instability secondary to obstruction versus hyperreflexia secondary to an occult neurologic condition must be ruled out in this patient population. Cystoscopy is useful to rule out any intrinsic urethral or bladder lesions that may be contributing to lower urinary tract symptoms.

General, gynecologic, and basic lower neurologic examination should be performed on every woman with prolapse. Occasionally, surgical scars detected on the abdominal examination can provide an important piece of surgical history that was previously unmentioned. The pelvic examination begins with external genitalia inspection for atrophy, discharge, episiotomy scars, and integrity of the perineum. The uterus and cervix is assessed for size, mobility, and any abnormal gross pathology. The anterior, posterior, and apical vaginal walls are examined separately with the aid of a half speculum to assess the presence of other prolapse such as cystocele or rectocele. The size of the introitus and evidence of vaginal stenosis should be noted, as a size disproportion between the uterus and vaginal opening may limit transvaginal delivery of the uterus. Physical examination should be performed both in the supine and standing positions. The severity of prolapse may not be appreciated in the supine position. In both positions the patient needs to perform a Valsalva maneuver to fully elicit the prolapse. The physical examination should be repeated at the time of surgery with the patient under anesthesia. Often, with anesthesia-induced relaxation of the pelvic floor, the degree of uterine descent and other prolapse becomes more pronounced. The screening neurologic examination should evaluate gross sensory and motor function of both lower extremities, and lumbosacral function. This can be quickly achieved by assessing pelvic floor muscle strength, anal sphincter resting tone, voluntary anal contraction, and perineal sensation.

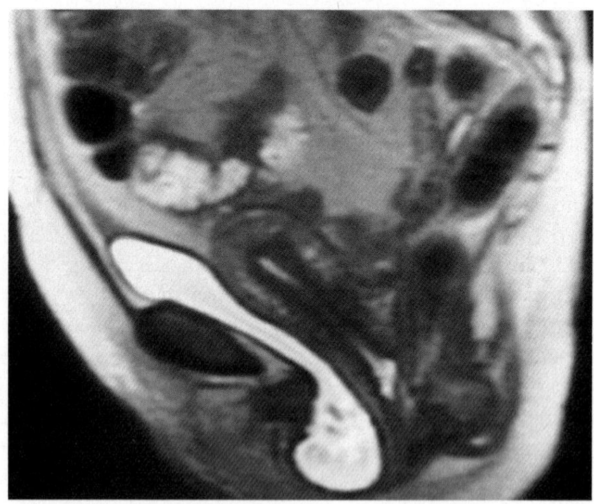

FIGURE 48.1 Magnetic resonance imaging (MRI) of the pelvis. Dynamic MRI of the pelvis demonstrating uterine and bladder prolapse.

Imaging of the upper urinary tracts is recommended since patients with uterine prolapse may have associated hydronephrosis. Our preferred imaging modality to assess the presence of hydronephrosis as well as other pelvic pathology is dynamic magnetic resonance imaging (MRI). Dynamic MRI is unrivaled in its ability to characterize pelvic soft tissue, and thereby it can accurately diagnose other uterine and ovarian pathology. It is a relatively simple, noninvasive test that takes only minutes to complete. No contrast is used as the bladder is distinct on T-2 weighted images. Sagittal images are taken of the pelvis with the patient at rest and then performing the Valsalva maneuvers. Uterine or other pelvic organ prolapse is readily identified with this imaging modality (Fig. 48.1).

The Pelvic Organ Prolapse Quantification System (POP-Q) is a commonly used staging system for describing vaginal prolapse and is based on physical examination (7). We classify uterine prolapse based on the dynamic MRI findings. Prolapse is classified in reference to the puborectalis hiatus. The puborectalis hiatus is formed by the puborectalis muscle (the most inferior part of the levator ani) and includes the urethra, vagina, and rectum. The degree of prolapse is measured by 2-cm increments. Mild uterine prolapse is 0 to 2 cm distal to the hiatus, moderate prolapse is 2 to 4 cm, and severe prolapse is >4 cm distal to the hiatus (8).

## ALTERNATIVE THERAPY

Nonsurgical alternative therapy to hysterectomy and vault suspension for uterine prolapse is no treatment, pelvic floor muscle training, or pessary. These options are reserved for those patients who are deemed poor candidates for surgery. Uterine-sparing procedures can be offered to patients who wish to maintain fertility or have strong opinions regarding sexual and personal identity related to the uterus and cervix. Obliterative procedures, such as colpocleisis, are also viable options for the appropriate patient population.

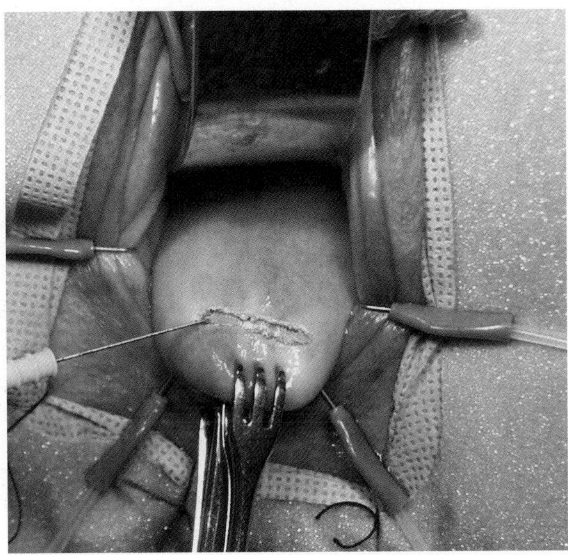

FIGURE 48.2 Incision: A circumferential incision is made approximately 1 cm from the cervical os with electrocautery.

## SURGICAL TECHNIQUE

As previously mentioned, vaginal hysterectomy alone is not sufficient to relieve symptoms of uterine prolapse or restore functional anatomy. Thus, every effort must be made to recreate normal pelvic anatomy with adequate support of the vaginal vault and functional depth. These measures include reapproximating the bladder and rectum to close the cul-de-sac and fixing the vaginal apex to the origin of the uterosacral–cardinal ligament at the coccygeus-sacrospinous ligament complex for vault support.

Broad-spectrum prophylactic antibiotics are administered preoperatively. Compression stockings are placed prior to incision to prevent venous thromboembolic events. Following successful induction of anesthesia, the patient is placed in the high lithotomy position. Care should be taken to avoid hyperflexion of the hips, which can result in femoral neuropathy. An iodine-based solution is used to cleanse the skin from the suprapubic area to the posterior perineum. Sutures are used to retract the labia laterally and a weighted speculum is inserted for vault exposure. A Lowsley retractor is used to place a suprapubic tube in every patient undergoing hysterectomy, and the bladder is drained by both urethral and suprapubic catheters. A ring retractor with skin hooks is used to maintain exposure. The cervix is grasped at the 12 o'clock and 6 o'clock positions using Lahey clamps to maintain the axis. A circumferential incision is made at the cervicovaginal junction using electrocautery (Fig. 48.2). The vagina and bladder base is dissected off the cervix for several centimeters. The anterior cul-de-sac is carefully entered using sharp dissection (Fig. 48.3A). Gentle downward traction, visualization of the glistening surface of the uterus, and limiting the dissection to the midline of the uterus help to minimize risk of cystotomy. Once the anterior cul-de-sac is entered, we use electrocautery to extend the incision laterally to allow placement of a Heaney retractor (Fig. 48.3B).

The posterior cul-de-sac is entered similarly, and the peritoneum is opened sharply using curved Mayo scissors (Fig. 48.4). Any adhesions encountered should be lysed with limited sharp dissection to allow placement of another Heaney retractor. If

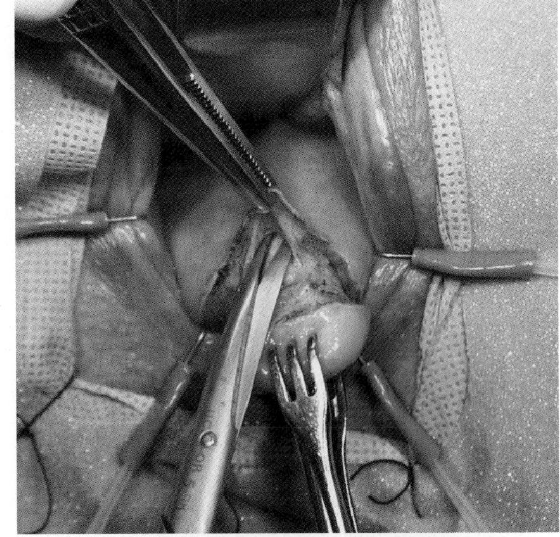

A

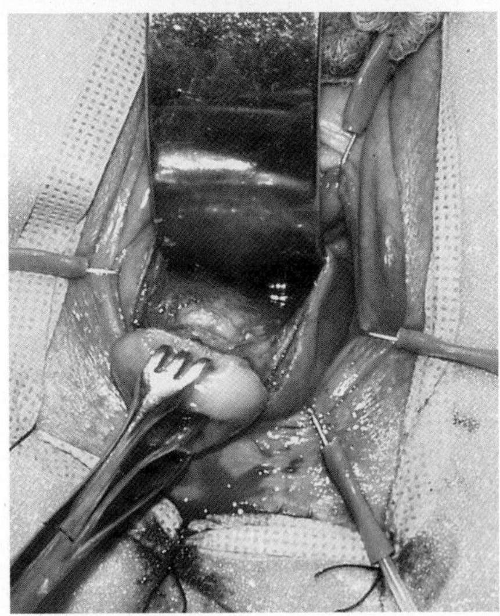

B

FIGURE 48.3 Exposure of the anterior uterus: Sharp dissection is used to (A) expose the anterior cul-de-sac and (B) place a Heaney retractor.

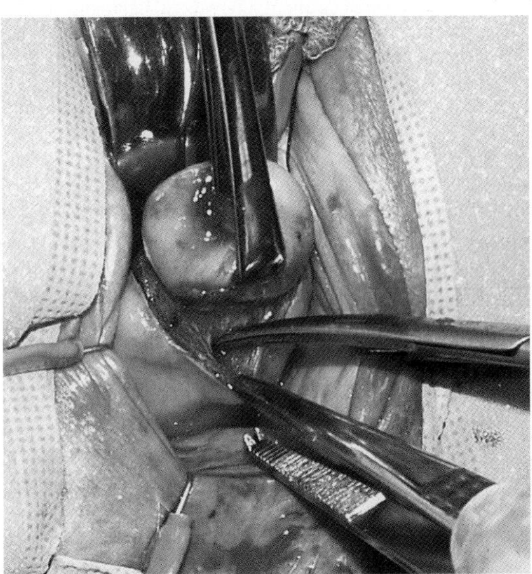

FIGURE 48.4 Exposure of posterior cul-de-sac and sharp entry into the peritoneum.

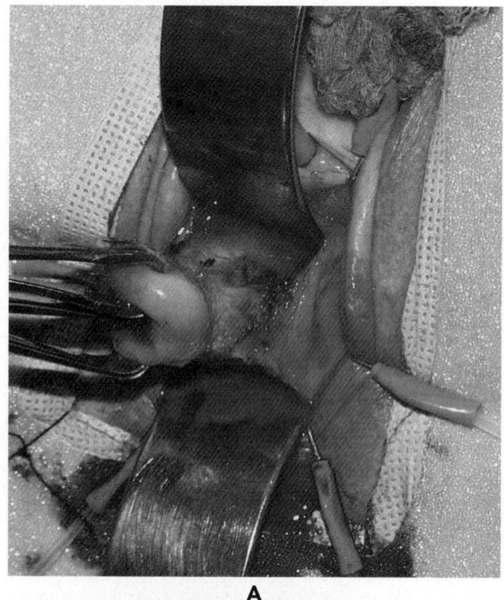

A

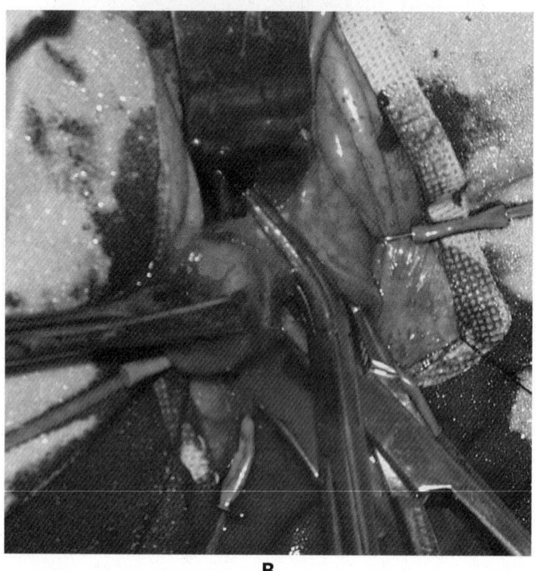

B

FIGURE 48.5 Isolation of cardinal–uterosacral ligaments. Right-angle and Phaneuf clamps are used in succession to (**A**) better delineate the cardinal–uterosacral complex before (**B**) transection.

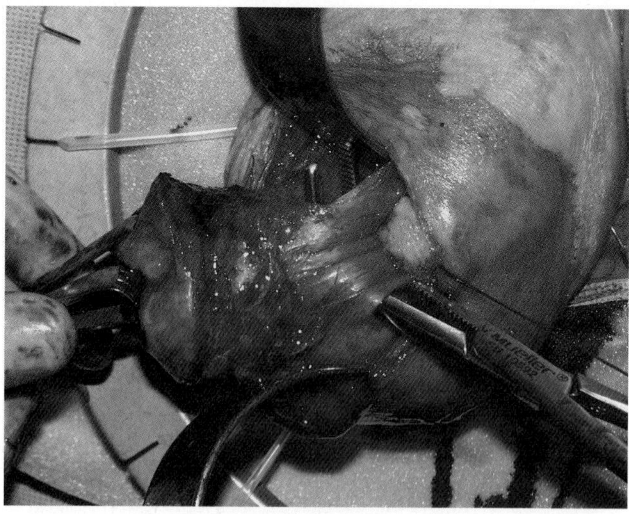

A

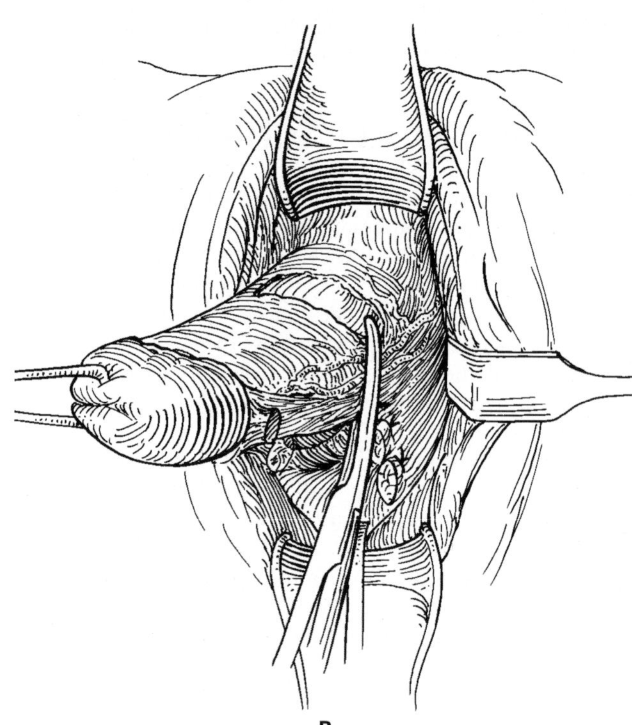

B

FIGURE 48.6 The uterine pedicles are carefully identified (**A**), isolated, and divided (**B**).

difficulty is encountered when attempting to enter the peritoneum, the hysterectomy can be initiated in an extraperitoneal fashion by severing the uterosacral ligament and caudal portions of the cardinal ligament close to the cervix. This maneuver mobilizes the uterus to provide better visualization.

Next, the uterosacral and cardinal ligament complex is divided by placing the cervix on careful traction and passing a large right-angle clamp from the posterior cul-de-sac parallel to the cervix. The right-angle clamp is used to expose the ligament, which is then grasped with a Phaneuf clamp and ligated with electrocautery (Fig. 48.5). The stumps are oversewn with figure-of-eight 0 Vicryl sutures. The ends of the sutures are clamped and secured on the ring retractor. Then the uterine pedicles are carefully identified, isolated, and divided in similar fashion (Fig. 48.6). After the contralateral ligament and pedicles are likewise controlled, the uterus can then be manually everted and brought outside the introitus (Fig. 48.7). Safe entry into the anterior peritoneum can be made by placing a finger anteriorly over the uterine fundus to elevate the peritoneum. Electrocautery can then be used to incise the peritoneum overlying the surgeon's finger. The broad ligaments are now ligated as above (Fig. 48.8). If an oophorectomy is not planned, the ovarian attachments are also now divided. The uterus is finally removed. A circular arrangement of the six ligated pedicles and their attached sutures remain (Fig. 48.9).

After hysterectomy, the vault support and vaginal depth must be restored. This is accomplished by obliterating the cul-de-sac to prevent enterocele recurrence and by sacrospinous fixation of the apex to recreate the natural banana shape. To perform this procedure correctly and safely, the surgeon must be familiar with the pararectal anatomy and obtain adequate

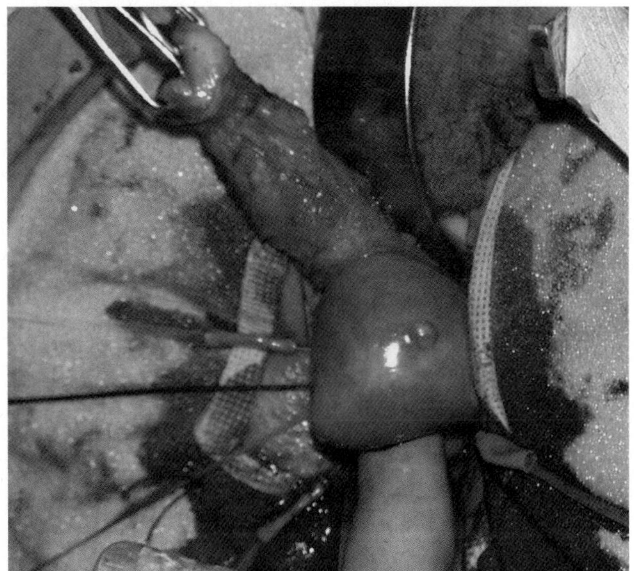

FIGURE 48.7 Eversion of the uterus. After the bilateral cardinal–uterosacral ligaments have been ligated, the uterus is manually everted.

exposure. First, the patient is placed in Trendelenburg position, and two Betadine-soaked laparotomy pads are placed intraperitoneally to pack away the peritoneal contents. Next, the coccygeus–sacrospinous ligament complex is identified by palpating the ischial spine and tracing the taut triangular band of fascia medially and posteriorly as it attaches to the edges of the sacrum. Next, we use two Allis clamps to grasp the area of the future vaginal cuff and apply downward traction toward the coccygeus–sacrospinous ligament complex to determine the extent of the apical prolapse and associated pelvic support defects. If concomitant cystocele still exists after reducing the apical prolapse, we will perform a formal cystocele repair. Otherwise, we will incise an oval shaped soft polypropylene mesh with two arms, which is designed so that the horizontal arms are attached to the corresponding sides of the vaginal cuff (at the uterosacral–cardinal ligament complex). The middle circular portion of the mesh is incorporated extraperitoneally to reinforce the pursestring closure of the cul-de-sac (Fig. 48.10).

The technique of bilateral sacrospinous ligament fixation is challenging due to the difficulty in maintaining good visualization in the deep pelvis through the vagina and the risk of injuring the pudendal vessels, the lumbosacral plexus, and the ureters, which are in close proximity. To optimize this exposure, three retractors are employed: (i) a long-handled Breisky is placed anteriorly to retract the peritoneal contents from descending; (ii) another Breisky or Heaney is used to displace the rectum laterally; and (iii) a Heaney retractor is then carefully placed posteriorly just distal to the tight cordlike coccygeus-sacrospinous ligament complex. We begin by placing a 1-0 Vicryl suture brought from outside the vaginal wall into the peritoneal cavity (in the area of the ligated uterosacral–cardinal ligament complex) (Fig. 48.11). Instruments are switched to a long-handled needle driver and long gastroplasty forceps to place that same suture in figure-of-eight fashion in the coccygeus–sacrospinous ligament complex on the corresponding side (Fig. 48.12). The direction of the needle must be horizontal, since one can easily damage the nearby neurovascular structures and ureters. It helps to

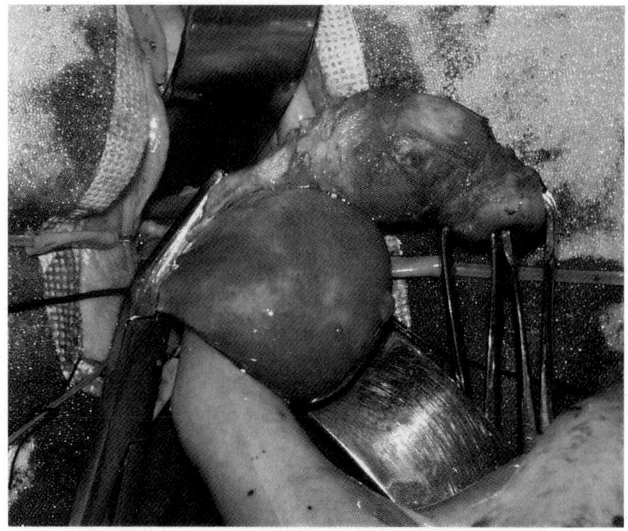

A

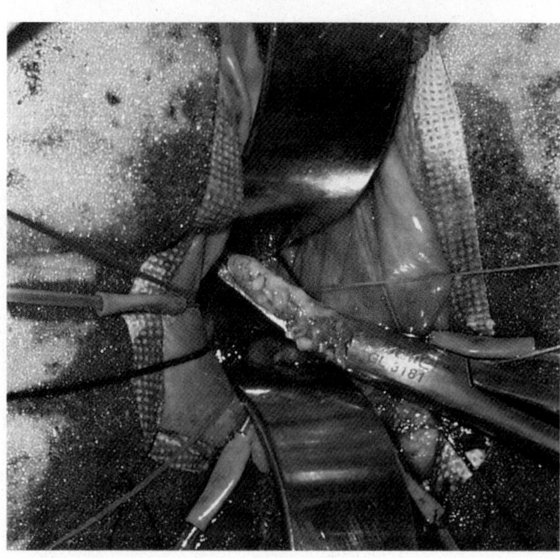

B

FIGURE 48.8 Division of the broad ligament. The surgeon's index finger is (**A**) inserted into the peritoneal cavity and hooked around the broad ligament, which is (**B**) then ligated in the same fashion as the cardinal–uterosacral ligaments.

carefully palpate and identify the tight cordlike sacrospinous ligament structure in the substance of the coccygeus prior to suture placement. The same suture is then brought through one end of the mesh, then exited through the vaginal wall just above the area of the uterosacral–cardinal ligament complex, and tagged separately. The adjunctive use of mesh is necessary because we cannot rely on the native attenuated connective tissues to suspend the vaginal vault. A second 1 Vicryl suture is placed on the contralateral side in the exact same fashion.

Two pursestring sutures of 1 Vicryl are now placed to close the cul-de-sac. These sutures incorporate the prerectal fascia, the uterosacral–cardinal ligament complex, the broad ligaments, segment of the circular mesh, segment of the circular mesh, and the perivesical fascia (Fig. 48.13). It is important to stay in the midline when incorporating the perivesical fascia to avoid ureteral injury. The pursestring sutures are tagged at this time. The sutures of the previously ligated pedicles of the broad ligaments and the uterosacral–cardinal ligament

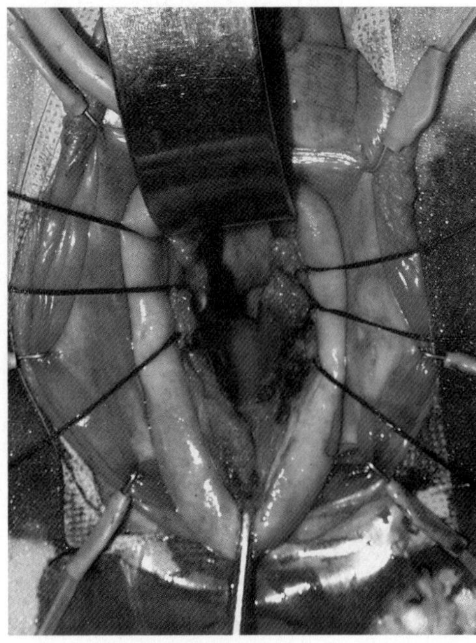

FIGURE 48.9 A circular arrangement of the six ligated pedicles and their attached sutures remain.

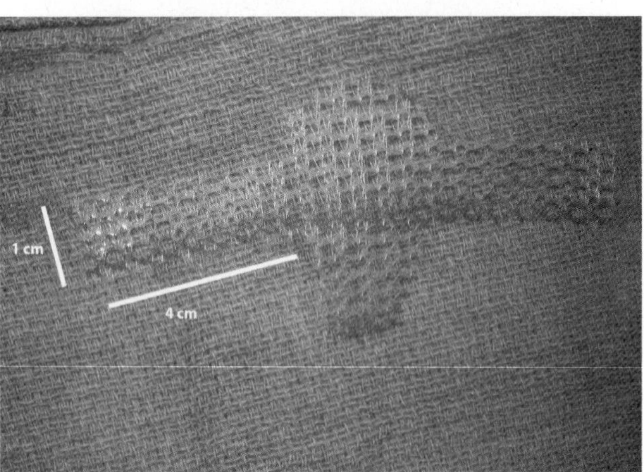


FIGURE 48.10 The oval shaped soft polypropylene mesh with horizontal arms is used to add strength to vault support. The horizontal arms are attached to the corresponding sides of the vaginal cuff (at the uterosacral–cardinal ligament complex). The middle circular segment of mesh is used to reinforce the pursestring closure of the cul-de-sac.

complex are identified on each side and tied in the midline. The pursestring culdoplasty sutures are now cinched and tied. If simultaneous repair of other prolapse is planned, it is now performed. The sacrospinous ligament vault suspension sutures are tied last after any cystocele repair and vaginal cuff closure. It is important to use Allis clamps to grasp and push down the vault to the sacrum while tying down the vault suspension sutures to achieve optimal depth.

Cystoscopy is performed routinely after giving indigo carmine and a bolus of 500 mL normal saline to assess for a healthy jet stream of urine from the ureteric orifices prior to tying down the vault suspension sutures. If there is any question of ureteric injury, the repair is taken down systematically starting with the vault suspension sutures to correct the problem. Vaginal depth is restored when the vault suspension sutures are tied down. Excess vaginal wall is excised before closure with an absorbable suture. Finally, if rectocele is planned, it is performed at this time. A detailed description of rectocele and cystocele repair will not be addressed in this chapter.

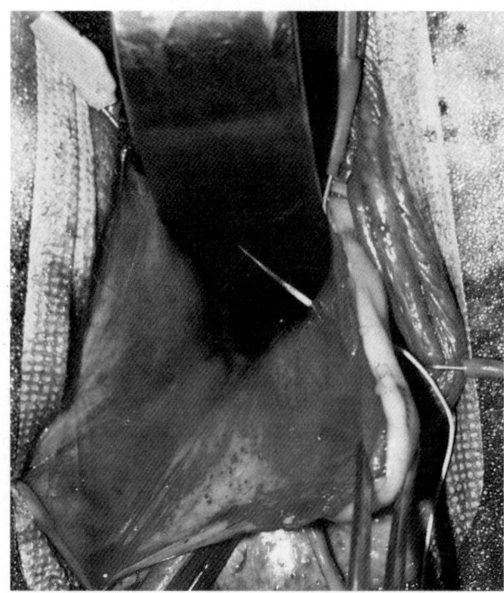

FIGURE 48.11 A 1 Vicryl suture brought from outside the vaginal wall into the peritoneal cavity in the area of the ligated cardinal–uterosacral complex.

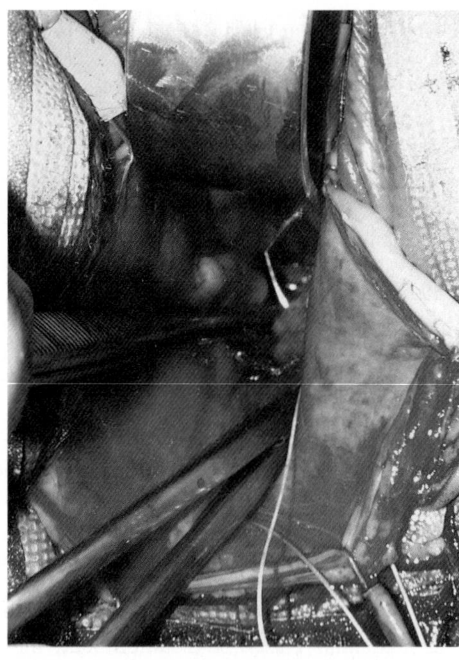

FIGURE 48.12 The same suture is placed in figure-of-eight fashion in the coccygeus–sacrospinous ligament complex.

## OUTCOMES

### Complications

Hysterectomy is a relatively safe procedure. Intraoperative complications include cystotomy (especially in patients with history of cesarean delivery), ureteral injury, hemorrhage, and gastrointestinal injury, although these complications occur less frequently compared to when the abdominal approach is used (9–11). Interestingly, bladder and ureteral injury occurs less

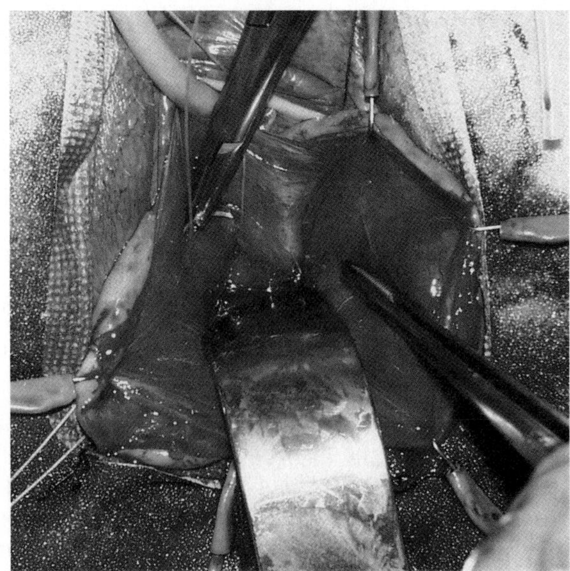

FIGURE 48.13 Placement of pursestring culdoplasty sutures. Inside the peritoneal cavity, two 1 Vicryl pursestring sutures are placed to obliterate the cul-de-sacs and approximate the prevesical and prerectal fascia.

commonly with the vaginal approach. By performing routine cystoscopy, we are able to diagnose and address any ureteral injury in a systematic fashion by taking down any offending suture and/or placing a ureteral stent if needed (12).

Complications during and after surgery include infection (cuff cellulitis or abscess), bleeding, urinary retention, rectal injury, bladder injury, mesh erosion, bowel obstruction, fistulas, and ileus. Our patients are discharged on postoperative day 2 with a capped suprapubic tube and instructed to check postvoid residuals. The suprapubic tube is removed when the residuals are <50 mL. Ileus may also occur but usually responds to conservative treatment. Delay in bowel function >3 days should be taken seriously, with appropriate assessment to rule out bowel injury or colonic obstruction (from misplaced vault suspension sutures). Avoiding abdominal incision facilitates early ambulation and fewer respiratory complications. Apical cure rate of uterine prolapse following vaginal hysterectomy range from 88–100% (13). The majority of cases of recurrent prolapse involve only the upper vagina and are asymptomatic. Prolapse that develops following hysterectomy may be an enterocele that was missed at the time of surgery or, more commonly, that occurred because of insufficient closure and/or support of the cuff. An enterocele may also develop postoperatively if other affected compartments are not repaired. Absence of the normal vaginal axis promotes prolapse of the cuff.

Ureterovaginal and vesicovaginal fistulas occur in 0.09% to 0.5% and 0.6%, respectively, of cases (6). Adequate anterior retraction of the bladder, ligation of the pedicles close to the cervix, and avoidance of lateral placement of the pursestring sutures in the perivesical fascia aid in the prevention of bladder and ureteral injury.

### Results

In regard to overall postoperative genitourinary function, Roovers et al used validated questionnaires to assess urogenital symptoms and quality of life after prolapse surgery and found improvement in all domains and quality of life following vaginal hysterectomy (14). Sexual function has always been a concern following hysterectomy. Recent data indicate that hysterectomy actually improves sexual functioning and overall quality of life. Rhodes et al. found that following hysterectomy, the occurrence of sexual relations and orgasm increased, while the rates of dyspareunia and low libido decreased (15). Similarly, researchers from the Maine Medical Assessment Foundation concluded that hysterectomy relieved pelvic pain, fatigue, depression, and sexual dysfunction and improved the overall quality of life 1 year after surgery (16).

## CONCLUSION

All genitourinary and pelvic reconstructive surgeons should be familiar with the relevant female pelvic anatomy and surgical technique of vaginal hysterectomy, which is being performed in increasing numbers in this country. Vaginal hysterectomy is considered the preferred surgical approach for treatment of benign uterine pathology, especially uterine prolapse, since it avoids the morbidities associated with an abdominal incision and has lower rates of bladder and ureteral injury. Successful vault suspension is an integral part of vaginal hysterectomy to restore normal vaginal axis and functional depth.

## *References*


1. Nationwide Inpatient Sample (NIS) of the Healthcare Cost and Utilization Project (HCUP). April 19. www.hcupnet.ahrq.gov.
2. Johnson N, Barlow D, Lethaby A, et al. Surgical approach to hysterectomy for benign gynecological disease. *Cochrane Datahse Syst Rev* 2006, Issue 2. Art. No.:CD003677.
3. Montefiore ED, Rouzier R, Chapron C, et al. Surgical routes and complications of hysterectomy for benign disorders: a prospective observational study in French university hospitals. *Hum Reprod* 2006;22:260–265.
4. De Lancey JOL. Anatomic aspects of vaginal eversion after hysterectomy. *Am J Obstet Gynecol* 1992;166:1717–1724.
5. Bump RC, Norton PA. Epidemiology and natural history of pelvic floor dysfunction. *Obstet Gynecol Clin North Am* 1998;25:723.
6. Chopra A, Stothers L, Raz S. Uterine prolapse. In: Raz S, ed. *Female Urology*, 2nd ed. Philadelphia: WB Saunders, 1996:457–464.
7. Bump RC, Mattiasson A, Bo K, et al. The standardization of terminology of female pelvic organ prolapse and pelvic floor dysfunction. *Am J Obstet Gynecol* 1996;175:10–17.
8. Barbaric ZL, Marumoto AK, Raz S. Magnetic resonance imaging of the perineum and pelvic floor. *Top Magn Reson Imag* 2001;12:83–92.
9. Dicker RC, Greenspan JR, Strauss LT, et al. Complications of abdominal and vaginal hysterectomy among women of reproductive age in the United States. The collaborative review of sterilization. *Am J Obstet Gynecol* 1982;144:841–848.
10. Gitsch G, Berger E, Tatra G. Trends in thirty years of vaginal hysterectomy. *Surg Gynecol Obstet* 1991;172:207–210.
11. Scott JR, Sharp HT, Dodson MK, et al. Subtotal hysterectomy in modern gynecology; a decision analysis. *Am J Obstet Gynecol* 1997;176:1186–1191.
12. Kim JH, Moore C, Jones JS, et al. Management of ureteral injuries associated with vaginal surgery for pelvic organ prolapse. *Int Urogynecol J Pelvic Floor Dysfunct* 2006;17:531–535.
13. Dietz V, Koops S, van der Vaart C. Vaginal surgery for uterine descent; which options do we have? A review of the literature. *Int Urogynecol J* 2009;20:349–356.
14. Roovers JP, van der Vaart CH, van der Bom JG, et al. A randomized controlled trial comparing abdominal and vaginal prolapse surgery: effects on urogenital function. *BJOG* 2004;111:50–56
15. Rhodes JC, Kjerulff KH, Langenberg PW, et al. Hysterectomy and sexual functioning. *JAMA* 1999;282:1934–1941.
16. Carlson KJ, Miller BA, Fowler FJ Jr. The Maine Women's Health Study I: Outcomes of hysterectomy. *Obstet Gynecol* 1994;83:556–572.

# CHAPTER 49 ■ CYSTOCELE AND ANTERIOR VAGINAL PROLAPSE

MELISSA R. KAUFMAN, HARRIETTE M. SCARPERO, AND ROGER R. DMOCHOWSKI

Anterior compartment vaginal prolapse, commonly referred to as cystocele (1), is the most common category of pelvic floor relaxation. Anterior defects arise from weakening of the endopelvic fascia and herniation of pelvic viscera into the potential space of the vagina. Compromise of the levator fascia and laxity of pelvic floor musculature both result in structural defects causing loss of pelvic floor support and subsequent formation of anterior compartment prolapse.

The fascia of the levator floor has a primary supportive function for not only the anterior vaginal wall but also the bladder and urethra in composite. DeLancey (2) elegantly described three levels of vaginal support to elucidate the proximal and distal structures involved in pelvic organ biomechanics. The abdominal aspect of this fascia is referred to as the endopelvic fascia, while the vaginal side is termed perivesical fascia at the level of the bladder base and periurethral fascia at the level of the bladder neck. The term *pubocervical* often refers to the combined periurethral and perivesical fascia complex. The vaginal and abdominal components of these fascial sheets fuse laterally at their insertion into the tendinous arch of the obturator internus, formally termed the arcus tendineus fasciae pelvis (ATFP), which forms a pelvic sidewall anchor for these structures.

When viewing vaginal support from cephalad to caudad, the uterosacral–cardinal ligament complex supports the upper vagina and cervix and anchors them to the pelvic sidewall (Fig. 49.1). In the midvagina, the vesicopelvic ligament, composed of endopelvic and perivesical fascia, extends from the ATFP of the pelvic sidewall to the bladder base and anterior vaginal wall. Distally, the urethropelvic ligaments provide support from the urethral meatus to the bladder neck. The ATFP, which is actually a thickened condensation of the obturator internus fascia and endopelvic fascia, provides a lateral insertion for all these structures. Indeed, the sturdy shelf of the ATFP provides a stabilization point for the entire pelvic floor hammock (3,4). Cystocele defects are commonly associated with other forms of pelvic relaxation, namely loss of support of the uterus and vaginal apex resulting in uterine or enterocele vault prolapse and/or loss of posterior compartment support with ensuing perineal relaxation and rectocele as well as functional deficits such as incontinence.

Defects of the anterior compartment may produce either isolated urethral or bladder support defects or a combination of deficiencies of both structures. Loss of structural integrity surrounding the urethra can result in urethral hypermobility without a concomitant cystocele defect being identified. Cystocele defects tend to be more complex and may involve isolated central, lateral, or combination defects (Fig. 49.2). Lateral, or paravaginal, cystoceles result from disruption or separation of the condensation of the vesical pelvic ligament to the arcus tendineus on either side of the vagina. Central defect cystoceles result from attenuation of the pubocervical fascia without compromise of the urethropelvic and vesicopelvic ligaments. Central defect cystoceles are often associated with

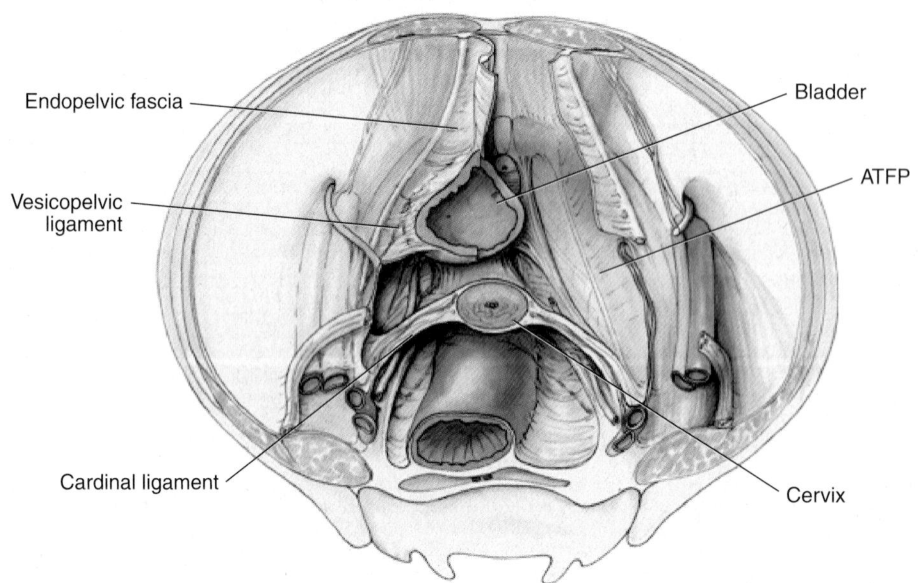


FIGURE 49.1 The vesicopelvic ligament supporting the bladder is composed of endopelvic and perivesical fascia. The cardinal ligaments support the upper vagina and cervix and anchor them to the pelvic sidewall.

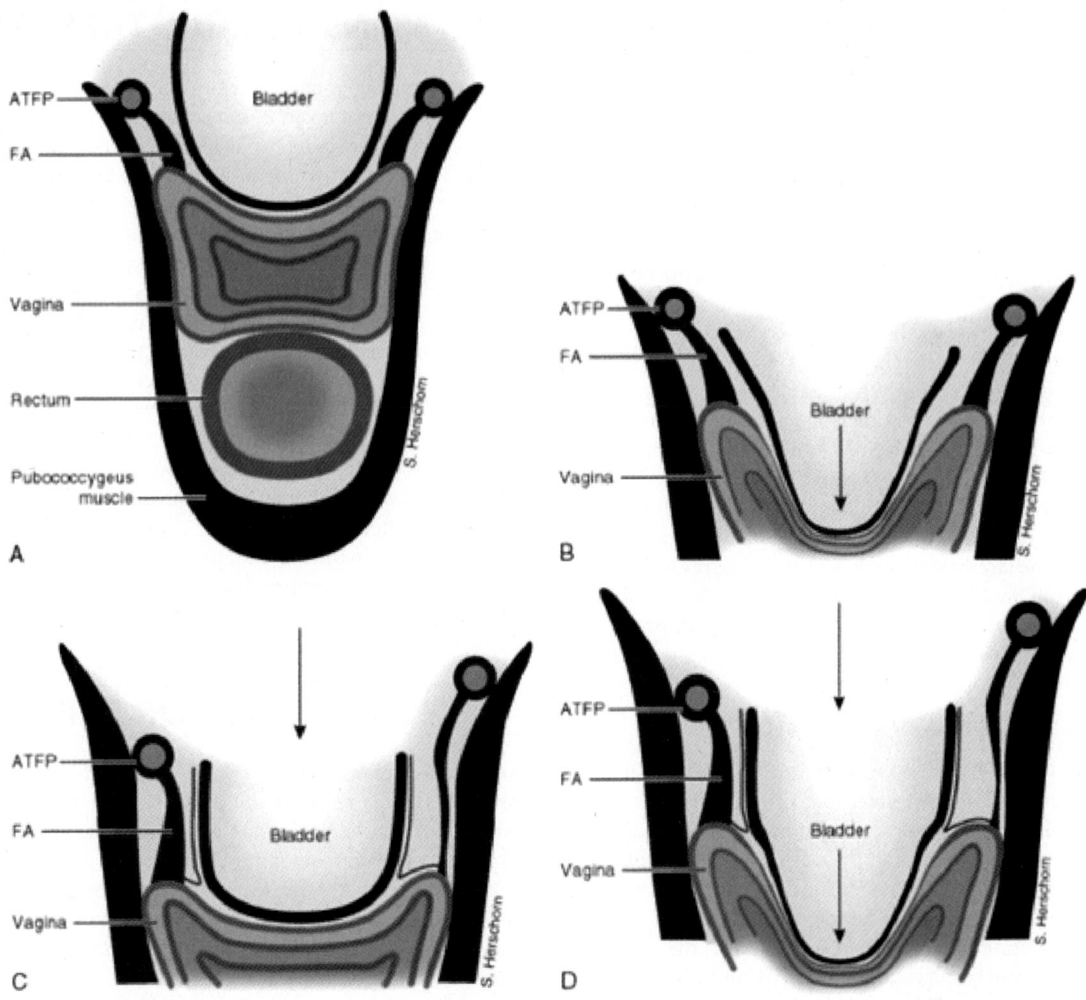


FIGURE 49.2 Defects of the anterior compartment may result in either isolated urethral or bladder support defects or a combination of support defects of both structures. **A:** Cross section demonstrating bladder support to fascial attachments (FA) and the arcus tendineus fasciae pelvis (ATFP). **B:** Central cystocele. **C:** Lateral support defect. D: Combined central and lateral anterior prolapse. (Reprinted with permission from Herschorn S. Vaginal reconstructive surgery for sphincteric incontinence and prolapse. In: Walsh PC, ed. *Campbell-Walsh Urology*, 9th ed. Philadelphia: Saunders, 2007.)

attenuation of upper vaginal support as well, including loss of cardinal ligament support, which on occasion will manifest as a concomitant enterocele. Isolated central defects actually represent the minority of diagnosed anterior prolapse cases, with the most frequent presentation being a combination cystocele (5). Lateral defects are more numerous and are often associated with urethral hypermobility (6). When combined central and lateral defects are present, more severe degrees of prolapse regularly result.

## DIAGNOSIS

Anterior compartment prolapse produces a diversity of symptoms, including "mass effect" discomfort such as perineal or intravaginal bulge or sensation of a mass in the vagina, stress or urge urinary incontinence, dyspareunia, low back pain, vaginal irritation or bleeding due to excoriation of exposed vaginal mucosa, recurrent urinary tract infections, voiding dysfunction, and in exceptional cases defecatory symptoms. Women may be required to manually reduce the anterior prolapse for successful voiding. Surprisingly, even large cystoceles can be totally asymptomatic. Profound cystocele defects may be associated with angulation of the proximal urethra by the bladder base, resulting in concomitant incomplete emptying, obstructive voiding symptoms and urinary retention. Severe cystoceles might also precipitate upper urinary tract changes, including hydronephrosis and, rarely, renal failure due to urethral or ureteral obstruction. Smaller cystoceles could be responsible for dyspareunia or incontinence only during sexual activity and, in select individuals, provoke early presentation prior to the onset of pelvic descensus symptoms.

Physical examination of the vagina will demonstrate a mass occupying the anterior vaginal wall from the vaginal apex or cervix, if hysterectomy has not been performed, extending to the bladder neck and/or urethra. If significant pelvic relaxation is present, this anterior prolapse may actually protrude from the vaginal introitus with activity or may present exteriorized at rest. Vaginal examination with the patient in dorsal lithotomy position with a full bladder is aided by the lower blade of a Graves speculum. The examination should include anatomy at rest and with straining maneuvers to evaluate for stress incontinence, urethral hypermobility, and the degree of anterior prolapse. Examination should also focus on the integrity of the bladder base and presence or absence of defects in the lateral vaginal fornices. Isolated central defect cystoceles will present with a large anterior vaginal wall bulge that blunts the vaginal rugae with preservation of the lateral fornices. However, central cystoceles are often associated with lateral defects with little preservation of the paravaginal support. Unfortunately, physical examination is not particularly reliable or accurate for diagnosis of paravaginal defects (7). With isolated central defects, urethral hypermobility is often not noted; however, this finding is not universal. Lateral cystoceles are usually associated with combined anterior vaginal wall defects and urethral hypermobility. Bimanual examination or placement of an instrument such as a curved ring forceps in the lateral sulci may help reveal paravaginal defects. Evaluation should be repeated in the standing position to discover more subtle defects, to recapitulate the prolapse experienced during daily activity, and to identify concomitant apical or posterior prolapse.

Cystocele grading uses several different taxonomies, with the Baden-Walker being the simplest and most reproducible and the Pelvic Organ Prolapse Quantification System (POP-Q) providing the most descriptive method, often reserved for research protocols (8,9). Vaginal apical examination is crucial to locate the vaginal cuff and identify other forms of prolapse that may be present posteriorly or behind the cuff, such as enterocele and/or high rectocele. The location of the cuff establishes the usual limit of surgical dissection for the vaginal cystocele repair, and recognition of cuff position facilitates evaluation of a concomitant enterocele.

During the pelvic examination, it is imperative to ascertain the presence or absence of urinary incontinence. With significant anterior compartment defects, urinary urgency and urge incontinence from detrusor instability may be identified. The possibility of bladder outlet obstruction should be considered in patients who have undergone a prior incontinence procedure and developed de novo anterior prolapse. In those patients, a hyperangulated or nonmobile urethra with increased urinary residuals and symptoms compatible with outlet obstruction should warrant consideration of urethrolysis prior to or at the time of cystocele correction. Reduction of the prolapse during the vaginal examination with a speculum, packing, or pessary will on occasion unmask occult stress urinary incontinence. Video urodynamic evaluation may be indicated for these patients to best discover any contributing obstructive voiding component, as this patient may experience persistent outlet obstruction postoperatively and should be alerted to the risk of long-term catheterization. Some reconstructive surgeons advocate preoperative videourodynamics for all prolapse patients to assess for bladder dysfunction and provide a baseline for comparison (10). If the prolapse patient possesses additional lower urinary tract symptoms, office cystoscopy may be useful to illuminate concomitant bladder or urethral pathology. In complicated scenarios, dynamic magnetic resonance imaging (MRI) of the pelvis can provide dramatic anatomic information on the type and degree of pelvic organ prolapse and aid in operative planning.

## NONSURGICAL THERAPY

Optional management strategies for pelvic floor descensus include pelvic floor exercises, physical therapy combined with biofeedback, and behavioral modifications, although efficacy is usually confined to incontinence and not prolapse. The utilization of topical estrogens may augment the symptomatic response to this intervention in those patients who demonstrate vaginal mucosal atrophy and have a component of associated urinary irritative symptoms. Estrogens may also bolster vaginal tissues for improved tolerance of pessaries. A patient with an asymptomatic small cystocele, adequate vesical emptying, and no incontinence does not require surgical intervention.

Large prolapse defects can often be managed effectively with pessary placement. This option should be discussed with all women who experience symptoms of anterior compartment mass effect, as substantive clinical improvement may result. In some women, the use of a pessary may actually unmask occult incontinence and nullify any symptomatic benefit that the device has conveyed.

## INDICATIONS FOR SURGERY

Surgical intervention is predicated on several factors. Symptoms arising from the anterior prolapse, including incomplete emptying, vaginal mass, perineal prolapse, or the presence of urinary incontinence are the cornerstone indications for repair. The presence of dyspareunia should be carefully considered, as this symptom often coexists with cystocele mass effect complaints. Dyspareunia as an isolated indication for surgery, however, must be judiciously evaluated as the complaint may or may not respond to anatomic correction.

The choice of appropriate technique for operative management of anterior prolapse is based upon the degree and severity of the patient's incontinence, the magnitude of the cystocele, the underlying nature of the fascial defect, and the presence of concurrent voiding dysfunction. Comprehensive surgical planning also includes identification of associated prolapse elements, including enterocele, rectocele, and apical prolapse defects, as well as possible indications for concurrent hysterectomy.

The type of anterior compartment repair is suggested by the preoperatively defined fascial defect, although patients should always be counseled that intraoperative findings may alter the prescribed course of therapy (Table 49.1). Central fascial defects may be managed with a plication type of repair and/or an interposition graft repair with or without concomitant sling, dependent upon the presence of incontinence. Indeed, an isolated central defect repair is rare in the absence of a concomitant stress incontinence procedure.

Lateral defect repairs may be performed with a variety of techniques, including multiple-point suspensions as well as vaginal paravaginal repairs or abdominal paravaginal repairs combined with an incontinence intervention. Severe cystoceles with attendant central and lateral defects require simultaneous stress procedures as well as interpositional graft placement to compensate for complete disruption of the supportive pelvic floor structures.

Lower-grade cystoceles may be effectively repaired by outlet procedures performed at the level of the bladder neck,

**TABLE 49.1**

**OPTIONS FOR ANTERIOR PROLAPSE REPAIR SUMMARIZED BY CLASSIFICATION OF DEFECT**

| *Anterior prolapse repair options* | | |
|---|---|---|
| Central Defect | Lateral Defect | Combination Defect |
| anterior colporrhaphy<br>interposition graft<br>± incontinence procedure | suspensions<br>vaginal paravaginal<br>abdominal paravaginal<br>+ incontinence procedure | interposition graft<br>+ incontinence procedure |

including pubovaginal slings and earlier forms of suspensions such as needle suspensions.

Recent innovative approaches to be discussed below include transobturator techniques for tension-free placement of polypropylene mesh that will accommodate both central and paravaginal fascial deficits and are often accomplished in conjunction with placement of a polypropylene midurethral sling. However, the surgeon must always consider to risks of transvaginal mesh placement and carefully select patients for such procedures.

## SURGICAL TECHNIQUE

### Repair of Combination Defects with Interposition Graft

Simultaneous lateral and central defects with associated urethral hypermobility may be addressed by a combined mesh inlay and pubovaginal sling procedure (Fig. 49.3). The choices for mesh interposition include synthetic, xenograft, autograft of free full-thickness vaginal wall, as well as allograft materials. Long-term data are not yet available to support one material as preferred; however, some evidence exists from experience with alternative slings that may be extrapolated to these inlays (11–13). When considering synthetic materials, polypropylene, polyglactin 910, and polyglycolic acid meshes are all viable choices. Polyglactin 910 and polyglycolic acid materials are conformal, modestly rigid, and, most importantly, eventually degraded and replaced by host fibrosis. Newer knitted filament polypropylene meshes, although permanent, elicit minimal inflammatory response and have pore sizes that allow excellent tissue ingrowth. Allografts that are fresh frozen appear to have poor durability, whereas those that are solvent deactivated or radiated maintain structural integrity, which has translated to increased durability. Dermis xenografts are the most conformal to underlying tissues and are less rigid and relatively less expensive, but some iterations tend to encapsulate as opposed to integrate into the tissue (14).

Defect repair may be approached either with a single-component interposition that serves as both bladder base and urethral support (14) or with a two-component interposition with separate strips of material providing the sling and the anterior compartment repair. The authors favor the two-component method, particularly considering the advent of midurethral tapes for use in cases of urethral hypermobility.

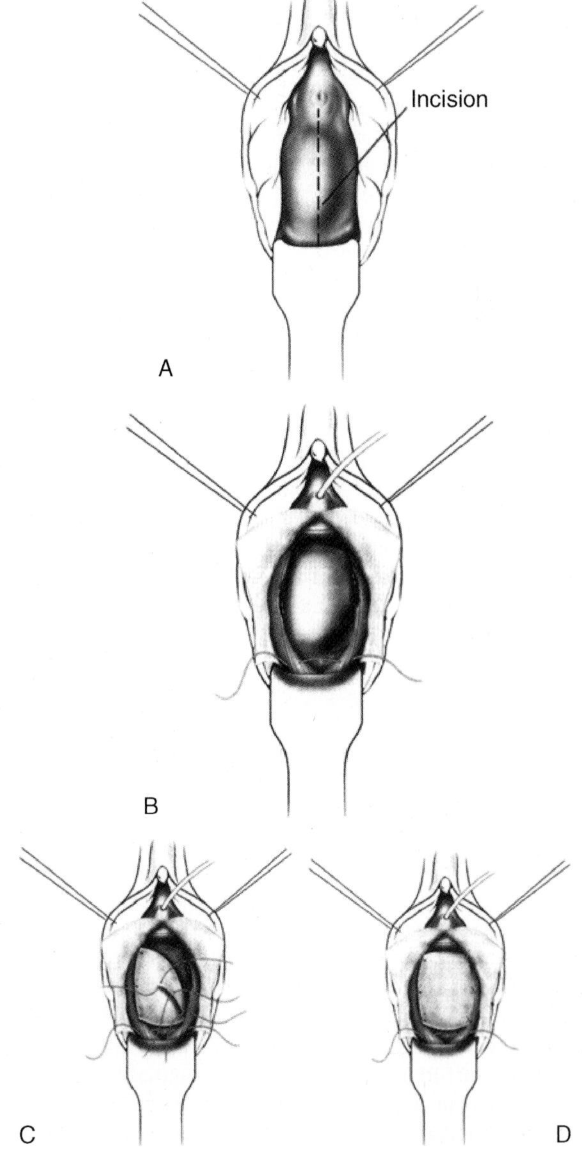


FIGURE 49.3 **A:** The incision for the interposition graph is made in the midline from the midurethra to vaginal apex. **B:** After completion of dissection and entry into the retropubic space, identification of the cardinal ligament complex and the obturator internus is completed. The area of the cardinal ligament complex on either side is identified and the ligaments are reapproximated to reconstruct the vaginal apex. **C:** The interposition graft is inlaid in the defect. Sutures are placed sequentially in the obturator internus fascia and through the inlay material. **D:** Final repair demonstrating placement of the free graft from the bladder neck to vaginal apex.

Consideration should be given to concurrent stabilization of the vaginal apex with cardinal ligament plication sutures and/or apical suspension to the iliococcygeus muscle fascia or the sacrospinalis ligament. Inlay repairs tackle both central and lateral defects. Further paravaginal defect correction may also be fashioned by suture placement through the vesicopelvic ligaments and subsequent suspension to the anterior rectus fascia.

After appropriate administration of perioperative antibiotics (16) and placement of graded compression stockings and pneumatic compression devices, the patient is placed in hydraulic stirrups in the dorsal lithotomy position. After preparation of the abdomen, perineum, and vagina, the posterior compartment is draped away from the surgical field. However, if the surgeon is concerned that access to the rectum may be required, an adherent drape may be placed for an isolation barrier that will still permit entrance. A weighted speculum and a ring retractor are used for vaginal exposure. A 16Fr indwelling catheter is inserted and the incision delineated on the anterior vaginal wall in the midline extending from the midurethra to the vaginal apex (Fig. 49.3). The anterior vaginal wall overlying the cystocele is infiltrated with 20 to 50 cc of either normal saline or dilute vasoconstrictor for hydrodissection prior to incision with a scalpel. Lateral vaginal flaps are then developed by sharp dissection of the vaginal wall away from the underlying attenuated pubocervical fascia. The appropriate plane is recognized by the glistening white pubocervical fascia, with the vaginal wall itself often noted to be very thin in this plane. Dissection in the incorrect plane is usually associated with significant bleeding and inability to identify the underlying fascia. When placing mesh in the anterior compartment, some authors advocate developing a thicker vaginal flap that preserves some muscularis on the vaginal epithelium to decrease the risk of mesh extrusion. Placement of an Allis clamp on the lateral aspect and supporting the vaginal wall inferior to the clamp with the index finger can facilitate proprioception of the proper plane and substantially aid dissection. Once the dissection of the vaginal wall has been completed to the fornix on either side of the bladder neck, sharp dissection is utilized to enter the retropubic space immediately under the arch of the pubis. This plane is in general avascular and should separate well from the underlying fascial components. In previously operated cases, this space may be difficult to identify and it is important to utilize sharp, shallow dissection in immediate tactile proximity to the arch of the symphysis pubis to avoid inadvertent entry into pelvic viscera such as the bladder and urethra.

After sharp entry into the retropubic space, blunt lateral and anterior dissection is carried out to extend the space, palpate the arcus tendineus and ischial spine, and mobilize the bladder and urethra. Subsequently, dissection is performed to the vaginal cuff in a line parallel to the vaginal vault. During this dissection in posthysterectomy patients, the stump of the uterine arterial complex is commonly encountered, and bleeding may occur due to disruption of remaining vessels. Suture ligature with 4-0 polydioxanone should be contemplated to avoid persistent blood loss during the reconstructive segment of the operation. Cautery should be minimized to avoid devascularization of the underlying tissues. The authors prefer bipolar diathermy for vessel coagulation.

Apical dissection should be meticulous so as to identify any enterocele component; if found, the defect is excised and closed. Apical enteroceles may be small and somewhat obscured by the bladder base descensus. The uterosacral ligaments can often be identified at this level of the dissection, and when found, plication with a 0 or 2-0 synthetic absorbable suture (SAS) can be performed. For high-grade cystocele, placement of sutures posteriorly in the iliococcygeus muscle fascia will provide further support and stability to the anterior compartment repair. These sutures are then brought through the vaginal apex to be tied at the completion of the procedure, after the vaginal wall has been closed. Once dissection of the retropubic space is completed and it is freely mobile, a pubovaginal sling is placed. The sling may be autologous tissue harvested through a separate abdominal incision, or if a midurethral transvaginal tape is selected, it should be placed through a separate incision following final closure of the anterior repair. For autologous fascial slings, ligature passage needles are directed from suprapubic to vaginal incisions on either side of the proximal urethra and bladder neck with digital guidance. Once placed, cystoscopy is performed to exclude needle entry into the bladder or urethra. Suspending sutures of 0 or 1 polydioxanone are placed through either end of the sling material and the suspending suture is then transposed from vaginal to suprapubic incisions using the ligature carrier. The sling is then affixed to the underlying periurethral fascia with 4-0 SAS. Following these steps, absorbable 1 polydioxanone sutures are placed in the obturator internus fascia at the level of the ATFP in an interrupted manner from the bladder neck to vaginal apex. This step usually requires two to four sutures in sequence. A sheet of graft material is tailored to the dimensions of the defect and affixed to the preplaced sutures in the arcuate internus fascia. The material should be placed loosely under the bladder base from the bladder neck to vaginal apex. Apical relocation sutures are then delivered through the vaginal wall, utilizing a free needle to pass the blunt end of the suture. Next, the vaginal wall is closed with running 2-0 SAS, and in our experience, it is rarely necessary to trim excess vaginal mucosa. If previously brought through the vaginal wall, apical relocation sutures are tied at this juncture.

After completion of the above steps, cystoscopy is again performed to ensure no penetration of graft or sutures into the bladder has occurred, as well as confirming bilateral efflux from the ureteral orifices and assessing the degree of reduction of the prolapse at the bladder base with the inlay material. Sling tension is then set by loosely tying the suspension sutures over two fingers, followed by closure of the suprapubic incision. Vaginal packing impregnated with estrogen cream is placed at the conclusion of the procedure. The vaginal pack is removed 12 to 24 hours postoperatively and the urinary catheter is removed for a voiding trial. If this is not successful, an indwelling catheter is reinserted or clean intermittent catheterization may be instituted. Alternatively, if a suprapubic tube has been placed at the time of surgery, the patient cycles the suprapubic tube during at-home convalescence. Patients are counseled to refrain from lifting over 5 lbs or engaging in intercourse for 6 weeks postoperatively.

## Repair of Isolated Central Defect Cystoceles

Primary colporrhaphy of isolated central defects with a well-supported, nonobstructive urethra may be performed with plication of the pubocervical fascia (Fig. 49.4). Urethral sphincteric function should be evaluated to determine if a concurrent sling is indicated. Patient preparation and positioning are similar to the previously described procedure utilizing mesh. The anterior vaginal wall is infiltrated with injectable saline and a single midline incision is formed from the bladder neck to vaginal apex. The anterior vaginal wall is then dissected off the underlying attenuated pubocervical fascia utilizing countertraction with Allis clamps facilitated by the operative finger of the nondominant hand. This technique splays and flattens the tissue, easing dissection and identification of the correct surgical plane. The dissection is continued to the level of perivesical fascia. Once this is reached, the retropubic space is entered and the defect is defined from the introitus to vaginal apex.

Repair commences with reapproximation of the pubocervical fascia with 2-0 interrupted SAS along the base of the bladder from the bladder neck to vaginal apex. The fascial plication effectively relocates the cystocele behind the reconstituted pelvic floor. This repair may be bolstered with absorbable mesh to reduce the cystocele during plication and further strengthen the fascial reapproximation. The cardinal ligaments should also be reapproximated in the midline to secure the apex of the repair. The cardinal ligaments are then corrected with interrupted 2-0 absorbable sutures.

Cystoscopy is performed to ensure that the bladder is intact and ureteral efflux is present. Vaginal closure is then carried out utilizing a running 2-0 absorbable suture.

## Vaginal Paravaginal Repair

The paravaginal procedure performed through a vaginal incision does not use inlay material, instead exploiting the ATFP as an anchoring point for sutures placed through the anterior vaginal wall on either side of the bladder base (17). The surgical field is prepared as above with dissection of the retropubic space, which frees the base of the bladder from the pelvic floor. Once the dissection is complete, the bladder base is retracted medially with curved retractors and the ischial spine is palpated. A 1-0 permanent suture is placed into the white line of the ATFP just distal to the spine. A series of four to six 1-0 sutures are then placed in sequence to the urethrovesical junction. These sutures are then passed through the pubocervical fascia and vaginal wall beneath the bladder base from the bladder neck to the apex of the vagina. These steps are repeated on the contralateral side and then all are tied to reduce the cystocele. Subsequent sutures of 1-0 delayed absorbable material may be used to plicate the vaginal muscularis prior to closure.

## Needle Suspension

These procedures rely on a sequence of sutures placed through the pubocervical fascia that are then secured to the anterior rectus muscle (18). The authors find these types of procedures are of minimal utility for most patients. Preparation is similar to the previously described inlay repair. Two parallel anterior vaginal wall incisions that extend from the bladder neck to the vaginal apex are created. These incisions are made on either side of the midline in an oblique fashion so as to be able to reflect the lateral wall off the underlying anterior vaginal wall. Once the incisions are completed, sharp dissection is carried out laterally to enter the retropubic space and identify the attenuated edge of the pubocervical fascia. In addition, the location of the cardinal ligament complex at the apex of the vagina is identified on either side.

After vaginal dissection has been completed, four or six suspending sutures of 1 polypropylene are placed in the pubocervical fascia in pairs—two proximal at the vaginal apex, two midvaginal, and two distal at the level of the bladder neck. Sutures are placed to incorporate the pubocervical fascia and, at the vaginal apex, the cardinal ligaments. The most distal sutures are placed in the midurethral complex. These sutures are then transferred from the vaginal to the suprapubic incision using specially designed needle carriers. This repair may be augmented with SAS mesh or other inlay materials affixed to the pubocervical fascia with 0 or 2-0 SAS or PDS sutures. The vaginal wall is closed with a 2-0 absorbable suture, and finally the suprapubic incision is irrigated and closed.

## Abdominal Repairs

The abdominal approach for cystocele repairs is exclusively for lateral defects (5) (Fig. 49.5). This approach yields superb visualization of the lateral defect and surrounding structures. Also, retropubic incontinence procedures or slings may both be performed with this approach (19). Preparation includes positioning the patient in the low lithotomy or frog-leg position so as to have sterile access to the vagina. A lower-abdominal incision is made, either horizontal or transverse.

The retropubic space is entered and developed on either side of the bladder and urethra to identify the obturator internus fascia. This is best performed bluntly, with the suction tip or a sponge stick, so as to sweep the overlying adipose tissue from the underlying structures. The ischial spine is identified and the white line of the ATFP traced from its origin at the ischial spine to the urethrovesical angle. The fascial defect will often be easily identifiable once this dissection is complete. The surgeon may also place a sponge stick or the nondominant hand in the vagina to displace the vaginal wall superiorly and better demonstrate the edges of the fascial defect.

Once dissection is complete, four to six interrupted sutures are placed in the disrupted edges of the defect to reappose the obturator internus fascia and the medially displaced pubocervical fascia. After all sutures are placed, they are tied sequentially. Prior to closure of the abdomen, cystoscopy is performed to exclude suture entry into the bladder and confirm ureteral efflux.

## Innovative Transobturator Approaches

Several comprehensive pelvic organ prolapse systems have recently been released and are gaining substantial acceptance from urologists and urogynecologists for the treatment of cystocele. These mesh-based systems utilize the minimally invasive approach of a vaginal incision with a reproducible, standardized kit allowing simultaneous repair of multiple fascial defects (Perigee, American Medical Systems, Minnetonka, MN; and Anterior Prolift, Gynecare, Somerville, NJ). Current systems allow anchoring of allograft, xenograft, or polypropylene mesh through the obturator foramen and into the ATFP with specially designed passage devices (Figs. 49.6 and 49.7). The appropriate placement of these supporting materials allows simultaneous repair of both central and lateral defects. Patient

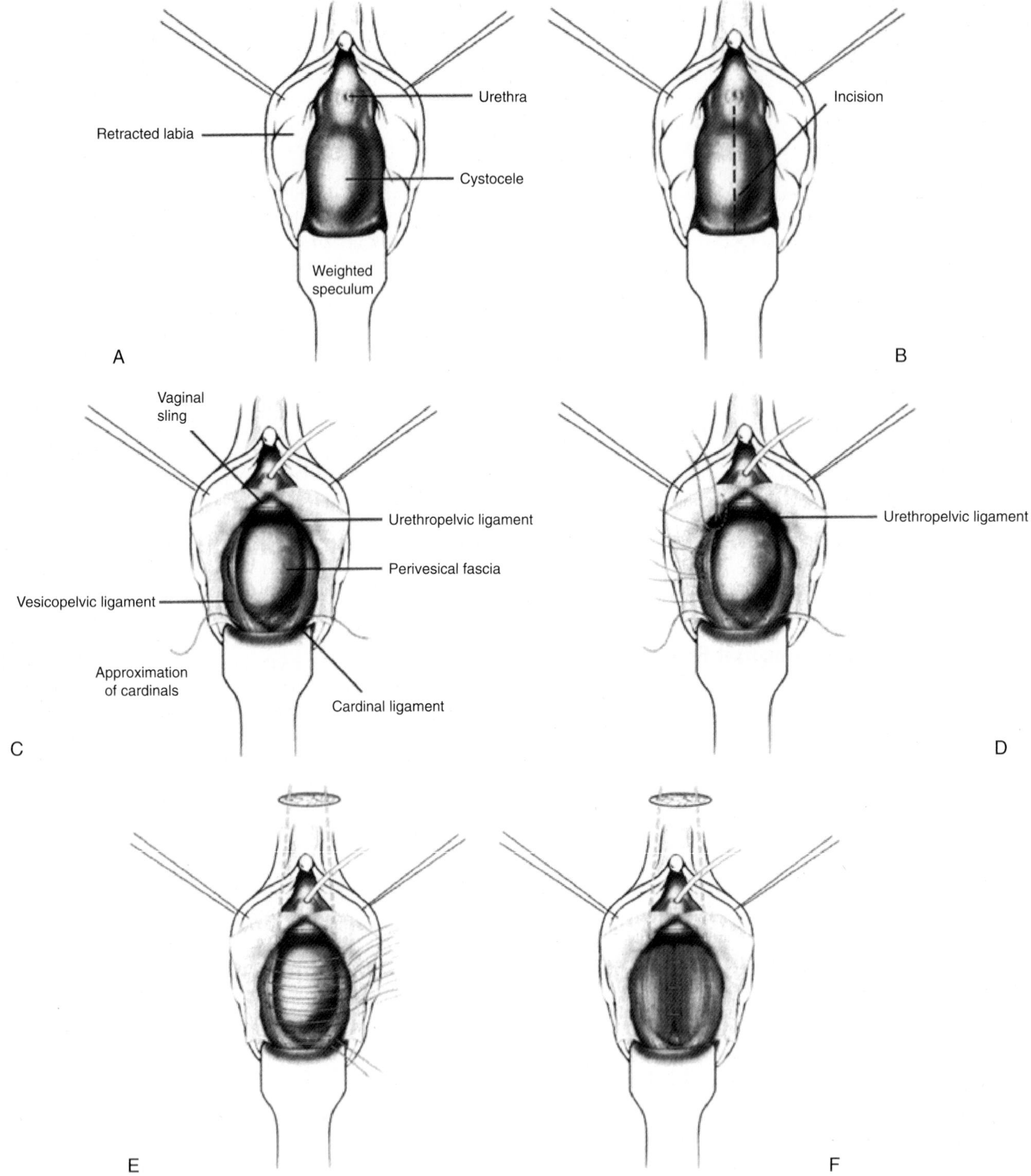


FIGURE 49.4 **A:** Demonstration of the central cystocele defect with preservation of the lateral vaginal sulci. **B:** A midline incision is created from the midurethra to vaginal apex in the vaginal wall. The retropubic space is developed on either side of the urethra and bladder. **C:** The vesicopelvic ligaments are identified, as are the cardinal ligaments. The cardinal ligament complex is reconstituted in the midline with sutures so as to provide apical support for the repair. **D:** For those repairs involving suture suspension techniques, sutures may be placed throughout the vesical pelvic ligament and transposed from the vaginal to suprapubic area for subsequent stabilization. These steps are repeated on the contralateral side. **E:** In those circumstances where plication alone is performed, sutures are placed across the base of the bladder from the vesicopelvic ligament on one side to the vesicopelvic ligament on the contralateral side and the two structures are reapproximated. **F:** Completion of combined plication repair with needle suspension of the proximal urethra and bladder neck.

preparation and positioning are similar to anterior colporrhaphy, except draping of the operative field must include the medial thigh overlying the obturator foramen. A urethral catheter is placed and hydrodissection of the anterior vaginal wall performed with saline or a dilute vasoconstrictor prior to creating a midline incision from the bladder neck to the vaginal apex.

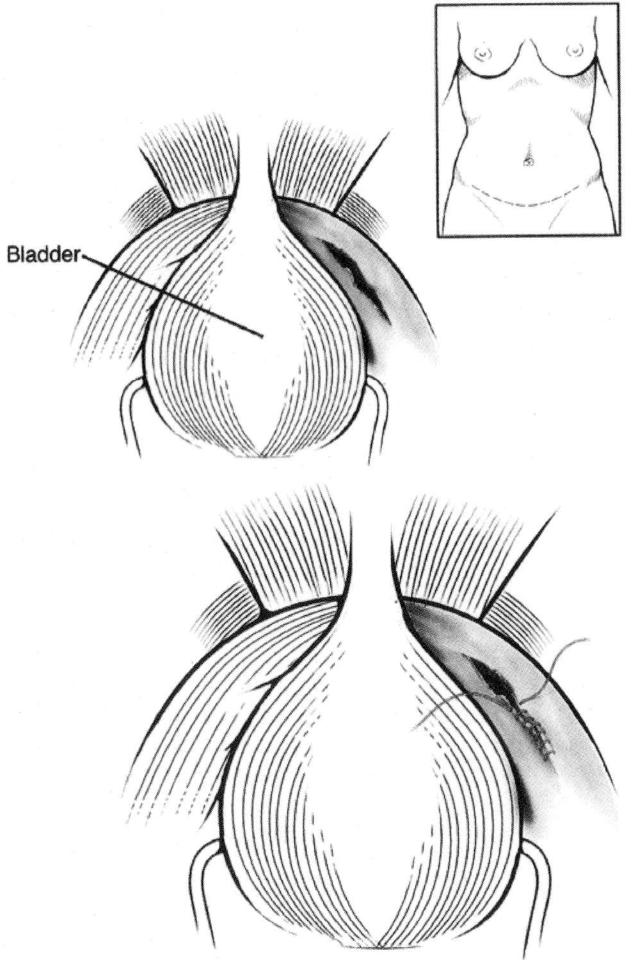


FIGURE 49.5 Positioning and incision for retropubic repair of lateral cystocele defects. A Pfannenstiel incision is made in the lower abdomen to expose the retropubic space. The dissection exposes the obturator internus fascia, and the fascial defect is identified as seen in the right aspect of the diagram. Using interrupted delayed absorbable or permanent sutures, the disrupted fascial edges are reapproximated. The sutures are placed from the ischial spine to the level of urethrovesical angle as noted.

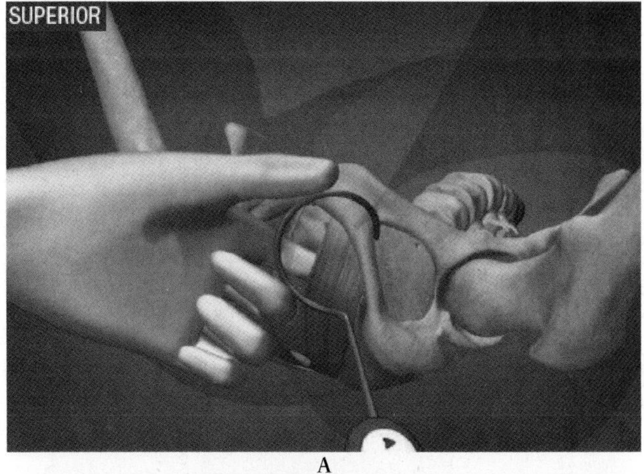


A

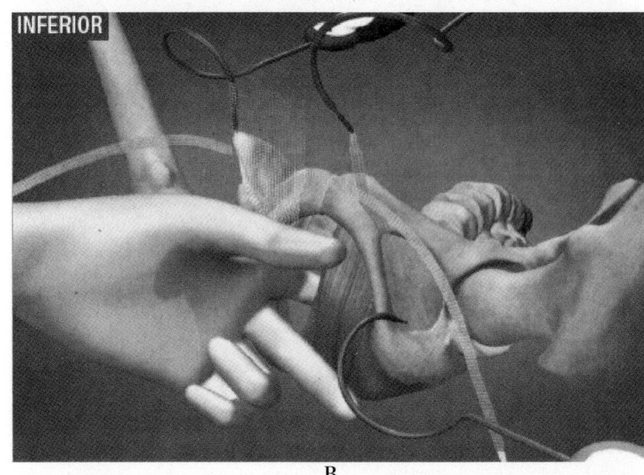


B

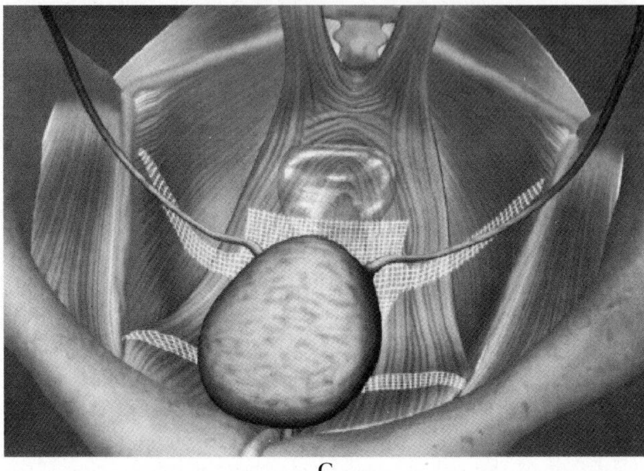

C

FIGURE 49.6 Perigee mesh placement. **A and B:** Helical needles are passed through the superior and inferior medial aspects of the obturator foramen to secure the graft arms. **C:** Final placement of the graft demonstrating fixation points in the arcus tendineus fasciae pelvis. (Reproduced with permission from American Medical Systems, Inc.)

Vaginal epithelial flaps are intentionally created so as to be thicker for purposes of graft coverage. Lateral dissection proceeds to the endopelvic fascia, but entry into the retropubic space is not performed. The surgeon must be able to palpate the ischial spine for appropriate placement of the proximal graft arm. External skin incisions are made over the medial border of the obturator foramen and the passage devices are delivered from the outside to the inside of the vaginal dissection with guidance of the surgeon's finger. The distal incision is at the level of the clitoris, and the proximal incision is 2 cm inferior and 1 cm lateral to the clitoral incision. The distal trocar is placed in the ATFP at the level of the bladder neck and the proximal trocar is placed approximately 2 cm distal to the ischial spine. Cystoscopy is performed at this juncture to ensure no violation of the bladder has occurred during dissection or trocar passage. The graft is attached to the passage devices and guided back out of the skin incisions. Tension is set by manipulation of the graft arms and cystoscopy is again performed to ensure bilateral ureteral reflux. The graft is secured proximally with 2-0 absorbable suture and the vaginal incision closed with 2-0 SAS. Tailoring of redundant anterior vaginal wall skin is not recommended, as redundant mucosa will contract and may provide an additional barrier for prevention of mesh extrusion. Skin incisions may be closed with 4-0 SAS subcuticular sutures or secured with a biologic tissue adhesive. Using a separate

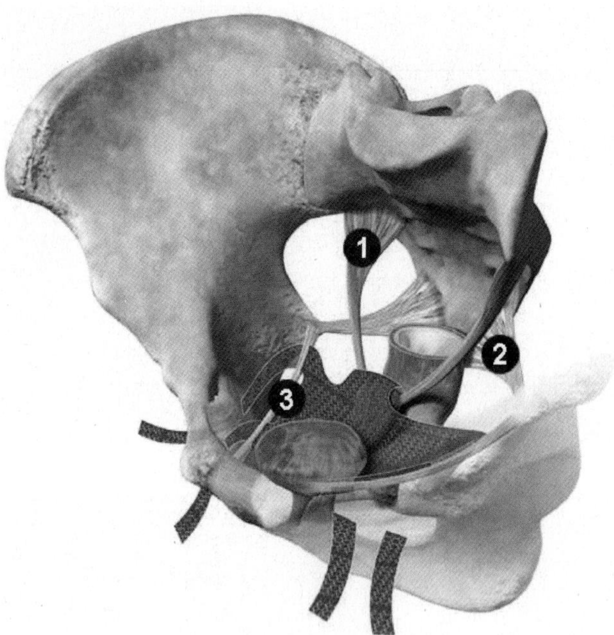


FIGURE 49.7 Prolift mesh placement with critical landmarks—1 denotes uterosacral ligament, 2 indicates sacrospinous ligament, and 3 overlies the arcus tendineus fasciae pelvis, demonstrating the position of graft anchoring through this fascial condensation. (Reproduced with permission from Gynecare, Inc.)

midline incision, a midurethral sling can now be placed for treatment of concomitant incontinence.

# OUTCOMES

## Complications

Significant intraoperative complications occur relatively infrequently with anterior vaginal prolapse repairs. In addition to the general risks of hemorrhage and urinary or soft tissue infections, the most common complication seen with cystocele repair is injury to underlying structures such as the urethra, bladder, and rarely, other pelvic viscera, including bowel. Incidental cystostomy may be repaired with a layered closure with absorbable suture, nonopposing suture lines, and maximization of urinary drainage. Although reported to occur at an incidence of <2%, the prolapse surgeon must always be cognizant of the risk of ureteral damage or obstruction (20). Cystoscopic evaluation intraoperatively should indicate the possibility of ureteral obstruction with nonreflux from one side. Sutures may be removed at this time prior to completion of the procedure. Stenting should be considered only in the case of significant disruption or trauma to the ureteric orifice. Failure to recognize ureteral injury intraoperatively sets the stage for one of the most devastating complications of anterior prolapse repair, namely ureterovaginal or vesicovaginal fistula.

Increasing use of permanent mesh materials for prolapse repair may increase the risk for erosions, infections, sinuses, fistulas, and development of robust vaginal granulation tissue (13,21). Nonabsorbable suture present in the bladder can result in stone formation or recurrent infections and should be removed and relocated. The use of the transobturator approach has added the variable of leg pain due to inexact placement of trocars during graft insertion. When encountered, this pain may be persistent and quite troublesome.

Postoperative voiding dysfunction may be caused by detrusor instability, urethral obstruction, or recurrence of the cystocele. Resolution of preoperative urgency will occur in up to 63% of patients (22); however, de novo detrusor instability will occur in approximately 5%. Although degrees of urinary retention may occur in patients on a transient basis, prolonged obstruction manifests in <1% of women. Poor or inadequate detrusor contractility may be a reason for incomplete emptying and should be predictable on the basis of preoperative urodynamic evaluation. Clean intermittent catheterization or long-term indwelling catheterization may be indicated in these patients.

Persistent dyspareunia, pelvic pain, or vaginal stenosis may ensue from aggressive plication and/or excision of vaginal mucosa. However, the majority of women appear to have improved dyspareunia after surgery, largely due to resolution or improvement of stress urinary incontinence (23). In those women who had deterioration of sexual function, the majority of cases appear to be associated with simultaneous posterior colporrhaphy (24). Vaginal shortening from inadequate apical reconstruction also may contribute to dyspareunia. Finally, late-onset apical prolapse and enterocele formation may occur due to alterations of the vaginal axis and insufficient repair of the apex. Meticulous attention to apical reconstruction should avert this consequence.

## Results

Long-term results for these procedures are still undergoing evaluation, and as evidenced by recent meta-analysis, most published studies reflect uncontrolled case series (25). Results should reveal cure of prolapse and remediation of incontinence. Risk factors for operative failure may include advanced age, hormonal depletion, inadequate preoperative identification of all anatomic defects, incomplete surgical reconstruction, or technical failure (26). In addition, obesity, chronic pulmonary disease, bowel dysmotility, and genetic predisposition have also been implicated in surgical failure. Some studies have reported that interpositional grafts convey a significant reduction in prolapse recurrence, with plication repairs demonstrating only a moderate success rates (25,27); however, other authors have found similar objective anatomic outcomes (28).

Vaginal paravaginal repairs have reported failure rates of 3% to 14% at 1 year (29). The six-corner bladder suspension has shown reasonable results at 2 years. Combined repairs have a small associated risk of cystocele and enterocele formation but have been reported to have a 94% success rate for cure of incontinence.

Little data have yet to be published on the transobturator mesh kits, but short-term results appear promising, with up to 95.3% anatomic correction of the anterior compartment, with an acceptable complication profile (30–32). Enthusiasm for these early results must be tempered by emerging reports of exceptional complications possible with extensive transvaginal mesh procedures (33).

## References

1. Abrams P, Cardozo L, Fall M, et al. The standardisation of terminology of lower urinary tract function: report from the Standardisation Sub-committee of the International Continence Society. *Am J Obstet Gynecol* 2002;187:116–126.
2. DeLancey JO. Anatomy and biomechanics of genital prolapse. *Clin Obstet Gynecol* 1993;36:897–909.
3. DeLancey JO. Anatomic aspects of vaginal eversion after hysterectomy. *Am J Obstet Gynecol* 1992;166:1717–1724.
4. DeLancey JO. Structural support of the urethra as it relates to stress urinary incontinence: the hammock hypothesis. *Am J Obstet Gynecol* 1994;170:1713–1720.
5. Richardson AC, Edmonds PB, Williams NL. Treatment of stress urinary incontinence due to paravaginal fascial defect. *Obstet Gynecol* 1981;57:357–362.
6. Delancey JO. Fascial and muscular abnormalities in women with urethral hypermobility and anterior vaginal wall prolapse. *Am J Obstet Gynecol* 2002;187:93–98.
7. Barber MD, Cundiff GW, Weidner AC, et al. Accuracy of clinical assessment of paravaginal defects in women with anterior vaginal wall prolapse. *Am J Obstet Gynecol* 1999;181:87–90.
8. Baden WF, Walker T. Evolution of the defect approach. In: *Surgical Repair of Vaginal Defects*. Philadelphia: J.B. Lippincott, 1992:13–17.
9. Bump RC, Mattiasson A, Bo K, et al. The standardization of terminology of female pelvic organ prolapse and pelvic floor dysfunction. *Am J Obstet Gynecol* 1996;175:10–17.
10. Scarpero HM, Nitti VW. Anterior vaginal wall prolapse: mild/moderate cystoceles. In Vasavada SP, Appell RA, Sand P, et al., eds. *Female Urology, Urogynecology, and Voiding Dysfunction*. Boca Raton, FL: Taylor and Francis, 2005:575–594.
11. Gomelsky A, Dmochowski RR. Biocompatibility assessment of synthetic sling materials for female stress urinary incontinence. *J Urol* 2007;178:1171–1181.
12. Herschorn S. The use of biological and synthetic materials in vaginal surgery for prolapse. *Curr Opin Urol* 2007;17:408–414.
13. Ridgeway B, Chen CC, Paraiso MF. The use of synthetic mesh in pelvic reconstructive surgery. *Clin Obstet Gynecol* 2008;51:136–152.
14. Kobashi KC, Mee SL, Leach GE. A new technique for cystocele repair and transvaginal sling: the cadaveric prolapse repair and sling (CAPS). *Urology* 2000;56:9–14.
15. Cole E, Gomelsky A, Dmochowski RR. Encapsulation of a porcine dermis pubovaginal sling. *J Urol* 2003;170:1950.
16. Wolf JS, Bennett CJ, Dmochowski RR, et al. Best Practice Policy Statement on Urologic Surgery Antimicrobial Prophylaxis. *J Urol* 2008;179(4):1379–1390.
17. Shull BL, Benn SJ, Kuehl TJ. Surgical management of prolapse of the anterior vaginal segment: an analysis of support defects, operative morbidity, and anatomic outcome. *Am J Obstet Gynecol* 1994;171:1429–1436.
18. Raz S, Stothers L, Young GP, et al. Vaginal wall sling for anatomical incontinence and intrinsic sphincter dysfunction: efficacy and outcome analysis. *J Urol* 1996;156:166–170.
19. Burch JC. Urethrovaginal fixation to Cooper's ligament for correction of stress incontinence, cystocele, and prolapse. *Am J Obstet Gynecol* 1961;81:281–290.
20. Kwon CH, Goldberg RP, Koduri S, et al. The use of intraoperative cystoscopy in major vaginal and urogynecologic surgeries. *Am J Obstet Gynecol* 2002;187:1462–1471.
21. Altman D, Falconer C. Perioperative morbidity using transvaginal mesh in pelvic organ prolapse repair. *Obstet Gynecol* 2007;109:303–308.
22. Nguyen JK, Bhatia NN. Resolution of motor urge incontinence after surgical repair of pelvic organ prolapse. *J Urol* 2001;166:2263–2266.
23. Azar M, Noohi S, Radfar S, et al. Sexual function in women after surgery for pelvic organ prolapse. *Int Urogynecol J Pelvic Floor Dysfunct* 2008;19:53–57.
24. Weber AM, Walters MD, Piedmonte MR. Sexual function and vaginal anatomy in women before and after surgery for pelvic organ prolapse and urinary incontinence. *Am J Obstet Gynecol* 2000;182:1610–1615.
25. Maher C, Baessler K, Glazener CM, et al. Surgical management of pelvic organ prolapse in women. *Cochrane Database Syst Rev* 2007;CD004014.
26. Whiteside JL, Weber AM, Meyn LA, et al. Risk factors for prolapse recurrence after vaginal repair. *Am J Obstet Gynecol* 2004;191:1533–1538.
27. Sand PK, Koduri S, Lobel RW, et al. Prospective randomized trial of polyglactin 910 mesh to prevent recurrence of cystoceles and rectoceles. *Am J Obstet Gynecol* 2001;184:1354–1362.
28. Weber AM, Walters MD, Piedmonte MR, et al. Anterior colporrhaphy: a randomized trial of three surgical techniques. *Am J Obstet Gynecol* 2001;185:1296–1304.
29. Weber AM, Walters MD. Anterior vaginal prolapse: review of anatomy and techniques of surgical repair. *Obstet Gynecol* 1997;89:311–318.
30. Altman D, Vayrynen T, Engh ME, et al. Short-term outcome after transvaginal mesh repair of pelvic organ prolapse. *Int Urogynecol J Pelvic Floor Dysfunct* 2008;19(6):787–793.
31. Fatton B, Amblard J, Debodinance P, et al. Transvaginal repair of genital prolapse: preliminary results of a new tension-free vaginal mesh (Prolift technique)—a case series multicentric study. *Int Urogynecol J Pelvic Floor Dysfunct* 2007;18:743–752.
32. Gauruder-Burmester A, Koutouzidou P, Rohne J, et al. Follow-up after polypropylene mesh repair of anterior and posterior compartments in patients with recurrent prolapse. *Int Urogynecol J Pelvic Floor Dysfunct* 2007;18:1059–1064.
33. Yamada BS, Govier FE, Stefanovic KB, et al. Vesicovaginal fistula and mesh erosion after Perigee (transobturator polypropylene mesh anterior repair). *Urology* 2006;68:1121–1127.

# CHAPTER 50 ■ TRANSVAGINAL REPAIR OF APICAL PROLAPSE

KATIE N. BALLERT AND VICTOR W. NITTI

Most women who present with pelvic organ prolapse (POP) have a combination of pelvic floor support defects affecting multiple compartments (anterior, apical, and posterior). In our opinion, the majority of anterior prolapse cases significant enough to require repair have an apical component. In addition, we believe that the high recurrence rate after POP repair may in part be due to failure to adequately address the apical component. For example, Shull et al. (1) demonstrated a reduced rate of recurrence (by 7%) after vaginal repair of large POP by routine performance of a transverse defect repair.

After hysterectomy, the apical portion of the vagina is supported by sheet-like extensions of the endopelvic fascia that attach it to the pelvic sidewall and levator ani fascia, referred to as the paracolpium (Fig. 50.1) (2). The paracolpium provides two levels of support. Level I, or upper support, "suspends" the vagina, attaching it to the pelvic sidewall. Level II,

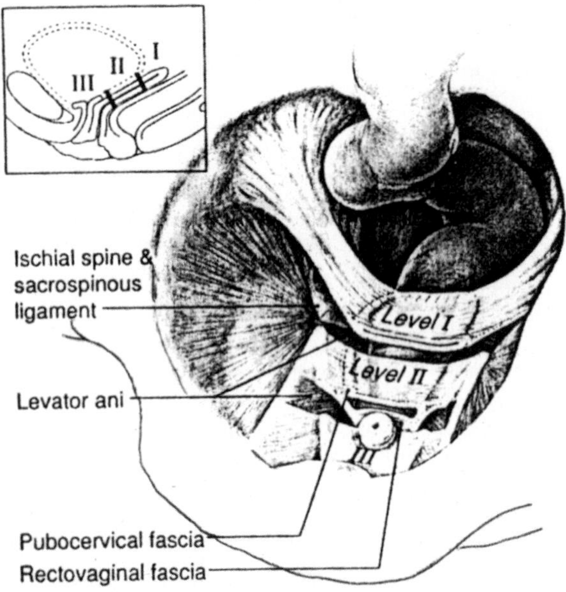


FIGURE 50.1 Level I (suspension) and level II (attachment). In level I the paracolpium suspends the vagina from the lateral pelvic walls. Fibers of level I extend both vertically and also posteriorly toward the sacrum. In level II the vagina is attached to the arcus tendineus fasciae pelvis and superior fascia of levator ani. (From DeLancey JOL. Anatomic aspects of vaginal eversion after hysterectomy. *Am J Obstet Gynecol.* 1992;166:1717–1728, with permission.)

or midvaginal support, which includes the pubocervical fascia, "attaches" the midvagina more directly to the pelvic walls, including the levator fascia and arcus tendineus. Damage to mid-level support usually results in anterior and posterior defects, while damage to upper-level support results in apical prolapse, including enterocele and/or vault or uterine prolapse.

## DIAGNOSIS

Prolapse is described in terms of anterior, apical, and posterior as opposed to "cystocele, enterocele, and rectocele." This is because most cases of prolapse are multicompartmental, and the support of one pelvic structure is dependent on the support of other structures. Second, it is sometimes difficult to tell on physical examination exactly what organs are prolapsed. An enterocele may present as anterior prolapse (usually in conjunction with a cystocele), apical prolapse, posterior prolapse, or a combination, depending on where the break in support is located. It is also important to ascertain if the vaginal vault is prolapsed, as this will affect the type of repair performed.

The extent of prolapse is first evaluated with the patient in the lithotomy position. The presence of urethral mobility, stress incontinence, and anterior, apical, and posterior prolapse should be assessed. The patient should be instructed to cough and perform a Valsalva maneuver to assess the effect of increased abdominal pressure on the prolapse. With the prolapse reduced (manually or with a ring forceps, packing, or pessary), the patient should be asked to cough and perform a Valsalva maneuver to evaluate for occult stress incontinence. To ascertain the full extent of the prolapse, the patient should also be examined in the standing position with one foot elevated on a stool. The degree of prolapse of each compartment may be quantified using a variety of systems. Currently, the Pelvic Organ Prolapse Quantification System (POP-Q) is the most comprehensive (3). Imaging studies, including cystography, defecography, ultrasound, computerized tomography scan, and magnetic resonance imaging, may also be used to help define pelvic anatomy if necessary.

## INDICATIONS FOR SURGERY

In general, the degree of pelvic prolapse and the severity of the symptoms it causes are the main indications for treatment. Low-stage prolapse is often asymptomatic and does not require treatment. Treatment is typically driven by the patient's symptoms, which may include an uncomfortable feeling of prolapse that may limit activity, obstructive voiding symptoms, and/or constipation. POP may be associated with stress incontinence, which may ultimately drive the patient toward treatment. The patient's age, general health, performance status, degree of sexual activity, and expectations from treatment will play a role in the type of treatment or surgical procedure performed. Finally, some patients may suffer serious sequelae of prolapse, such as hydronephrosis from ureteral obstruction or urinary retention from urethral obstruction.

## ALTERNATIVE THERAPY

Nonsurgical treatment involves supporting the pelvic floor with a device such as a pessary. Pessaries come in a variety of shapes and sizes and are fit depending on the patient's size and anatomy and the components of the prolapse. Many women find pessaries a satisfying alternative to surgery that can comfortably control the symptoms of pelvic prolapse, while others are unable to maintain a pessary due to their specific anatomy or cannot use one due to symptoms such as discomfort, bothersome discharge, or bleeding. For those women who do not remove the pessary, regular follow-up (every 1 to 3 months) is necessary so the pessary can be removed, cleaned, and replaced and the patient examined.

## SURGICAL TECHNIQUE

There are several options for surgical management of apical prolapse. Prolapse can be approached vaginally or abdominally depending on its degree, patient characteristics, and desired outcomes. While the focus of this chapter is on transvaginal repair, there are situations where the abdominal approach (either open or laparoscopic) is preferred, such as in young women with vaginal vault prolapse or those with failed transvaginal procedures (4). In the frail elderly population, colpocleisis, in which the entire vagina is closed, may also be considered.

### Transvaginal Enterocele Repair

Transvaginal enterocele repair may be performed either intraperitoneally or extraperitoneally. In cases of large enterocele, we prefer the intraperitoneal approach; however, in cases where the enterocele is small or difficult to find, an extraperitoneal approach may be appropriate. There are several variations of the repair, depending on the degree of prolapse and

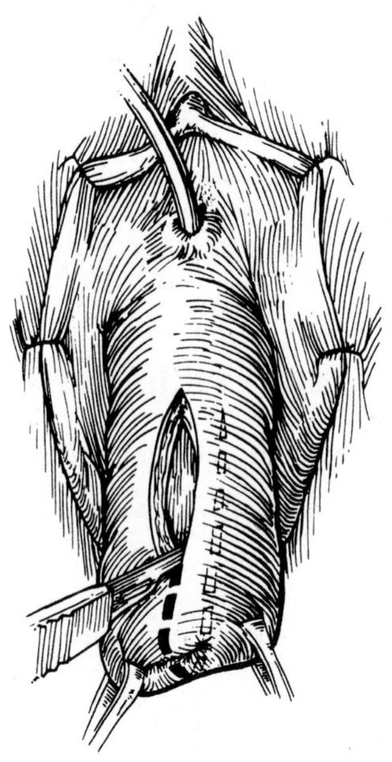

FIGURE 50.2 The vaginal wall is grasped with two Allis clamps and brought outside the vaginal introitus. A midline incision is made. (From Nitti VW. Transvaginal enterocele repair with variations. *Contemp Urol* 1994;6:50–64, with permission.)

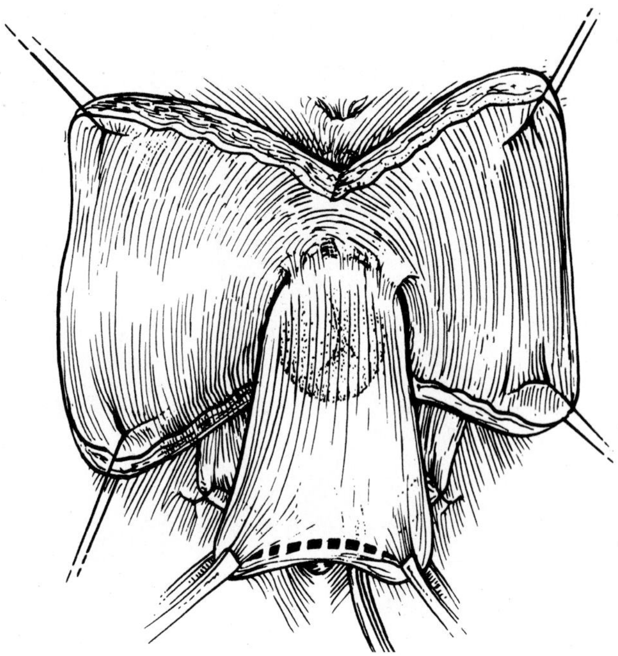

FIGURE 50.3 Enterocele sac completely dissected to its neck. (From Nitti VW. Transvaginal enterocele repair with variations. *Contemp Urol* 1994;6:50–64, with permission.)

whether or not a vault suspension is necessary, yet most variations start with the basic intraperitoneal repair.

The patient is placed in the dorsal lithotomy position. She is prepped, with attention placed on adequately scrubbing the inside of the vagina. If necessary, the labia are retracted with silk sutures. A Scott ring retractor (Lone Star Medical Corp.) is useful in exposing the operative field.

The first step in intraperitoneal repair is to isolate the enterocele sac. This is begun by grasping the prolapsed vaginal wall with two Allis clamps and bringing it outside of the vaginal introitus. A longitudinal incision is made in the vaginal wall along the entire length of the enterocele (Fig. 50.2). The vaginal wall is then carefully dissected away from the underlying pubocervical fascia and enterocele sac. In the initial dissection, care must be taken to stay very superficial and develop the proper plane. This is best accomplished by placing the curve of the Metzenbaum scissors against the vaginal wall. A finger can be placed on the outside of the vaginal wall to stabilize the initial dissection. Once the proper plane is entered, it is usually easy to dissect the vaginal wall away from the underlying enterocele sac. Care taken here will prevent early entry into the peritoneal cavity. The dissection of the enterocele is continued all the way to the neck of the enterocele sac (Fig. 50.3). After the enterocele has been completely isolated, the sac is opened and the peritoneal cavity is entered. At this time, one may see small bowel, omentum, or ovary and fallopian tube in cases where previous hysterectomy without oophorectomy has been performed (Fig. 50.4).

The next step is closure of the enterocele defect or pouch of Douglas. Retraction of the peritoneal contents is best performed using a moist pediatric laparotomy pad and a narrow Deaver or Heaney retractor. Placing the patient in the Trendelenburg position so that abdominal organs fall slightly cephalad assists with this. The enterocele repair begins posteriorly while the abdominal contents are retracted anteriorly

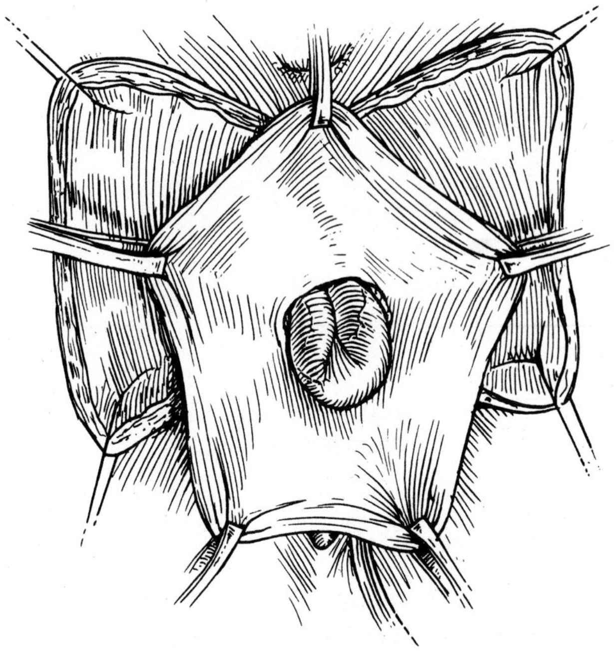

FIGURE 50.4 The enterocele sac is opened, exposing intra-abdominal contents. (From Nitti VW. Transvaginal enterocele repair with variations. *Contemp Urol* 1994;6:50–64, with permission.)

using the retractor. A no. 1 polyglactic acid (PGA) suture is first placed through the peritoneum and into the prerectal fascia that overlies the rectum (Fig. 50.5). A circumferential closure of the defect is then performed by placing the purse-string suture laterally in the right uterosacral–cardinal ligament complex, anteriorly in the peritoneum overlying the base of the bladder, laterally on the left in the uterosacral–cardinal

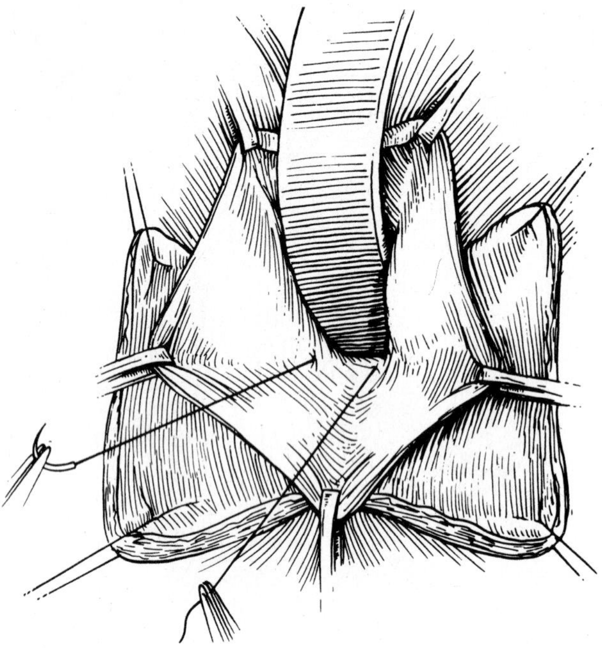

FIGURE 50.5 A Deaver retractor is used to retract abdominal contents so that pursestring sutures can be placed. (From Nitti VW. Transvaginal enterocele repair with variations. *Contemp Urol* 1994;6:50–64, with permission.)

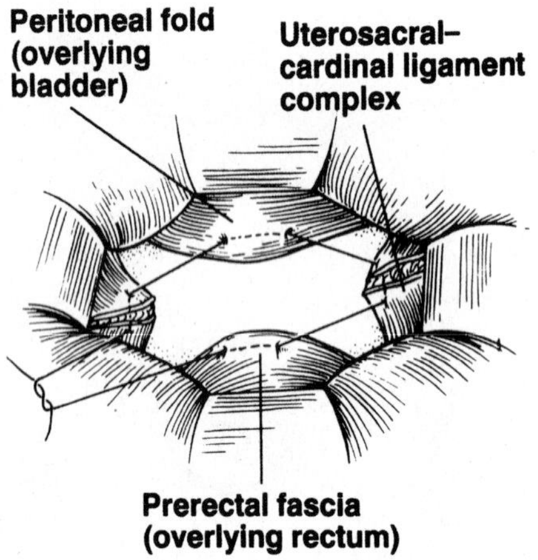


FIGURE 50.6 Placement of pursestring sutures. (From Nitti VW. Transvaginal enterocele repair with variations. *Contemp Urol* 1994;6:50–64, with permission.)

ligament complex, and finally again posteriorly in the prerectal fascia (Fig. 50.6). After this pursestring suture has been placed, a second one may be placed in the identical structures in close proximity to the first. If one is not going to perform a further vault suspension, it is especially important to incorporate the uterosacral–cardinal ligament complex into the closure, as this will be the main support of the vaginal apex. In addition, care should be taken to place these sutures deep enough to ensure that adequate vaginal depth can be achieved. When an additional apical support procedure is preformed, the main purpose of the pursestring suture is simply to close the peritoneum. After all sutures are placed, the assistant cinches down and places tension on one of the pursestrings while the surgeon ties the other. After this has been tied, the second pursestring (if placed) is tied in a similar manner. The excess enterocele sac may be excised and the ends oversewn with a 2-0 PGA suture.

Cystoscopy is performed to document that there has been no injury to the bladder. Ureteral injury is ruled out by intravenous indigo carmine. Excess vaginal wall is then excised, and the vaginal wall is closed with a 2-0 PGA suture incorporating deep tissue to obliterate any dead space. Antibiotic-impregnated vaginal packing is placed for 24 hours.

## Enterocele Repair with Vault Suspension

In most cases of enterocele, the vaginal apex is also prolapsed and requires new support. It is also common to have concomitant anterior and posterior defects, and therefore repair of more than one compartment is typically necessary. There are several techniques commonly used to accomplish a transvaginal vault suspension, and the best technique is still debated. We will review nonaugmented repairs, including the McCall culdoplasty, the uterosacral ligament suspension, the sacrospinous ligament fixation, and the iliococcygeus fixation, as well as augmented repairs, including sacrospinous ligament fixation with mesh. Lastly, we will briefly discuss uterine-sparing procedures and the mesh kits that have recently emerged as treatment options for POP.

## Nonaugmented Repairs

### McCall Culdoplasty

In 1957 McCall (5) originally described a technique of posterior culdoplasty used to correct enterocele at the time of vaginal hysterectomy. Several modifications of the procedure have been reported, but the concept remains the same. As described above, retraction of the peritoneal contents is best performed using a moist pediatric laparotomy pad and a narrow Deaver retractor with the patient in the Trendelenburg position. Permanent or delayed absorbable suture can be used for the internal McCall sutures. The suture is passed through one uterosacral ligament approximately 2 cm above its cut edge. Successive passes are then made through the posterior peritoneum, and lastly the suture is placed through the contralateral uterosacral ligament. The suture is not tied, and additional sutures are placed in a similar fashion as needed (Fig. 50.7). After all of the internal McCall sutures have been placed, one or two external McCall sutures are placed using delayed absorbable suture. External McCall sutures are placed through the vaginal epithelium (from outside to inside), through the peritoneum and the ipsilateral uterosacral ligament. Similar to the internal McCall sutures, successive passes are again made through the posterior peritoneum until the contralateral uterosacral ligament is reached. The suture is then passed through the peritoneum and the vaginal epithelium close to the entry point. The internal sutures are each tied, followed by the external sutures, which suspend the vaginal wall at the level of the uterosacral ligaments.

### Uterosacral Ligament Fixation

Suspension of the vaginal vault to the uterosacral ligaments, as described by Shull et al. (1), provides a more natural vaginal axis than the sacrospinous ligament fixation. Without the posterior deflection of the vagina caused by fixation to the

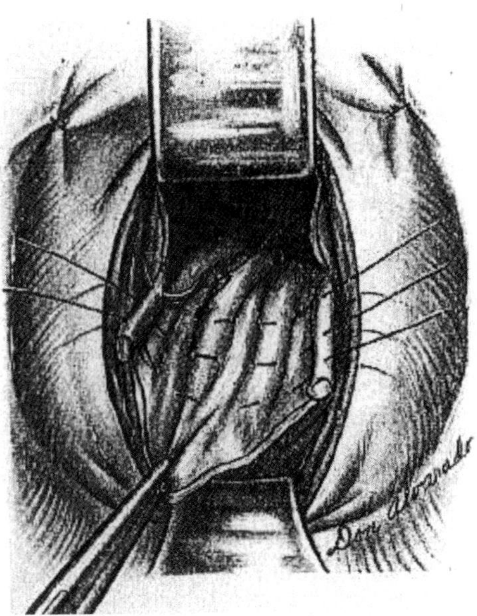

FIGURE 50.7 Placement of internal McCall sutures. (From McCall ML. Posterior culdoplasty: surgical correction of enterocele during vaginal hysterectomy: a preliminary report. *Am J Obstet Gynecol* 1957;10:595–602, with permission.)

sacrospinous ligament, the risk of prolapse of the anterior vaginal compartment is reduced. Identification of the uterosacral ligaments posthysterectomy can be difficult. Their origin is at the sacrum, and they reflect anteromedially toward insertion at the cervix. After the uterus and cervix are removed, these ligaments meld into the surrounding connective tissue. The optimal site of fixation to the uterosacral ligament is in the intermediate portion of the ligament, which has fewer vital adjacent structures and is a strong fixation site, and tension on this area has little effect on the nearby ureter. The ischial spine can be used to reliably identify the intermediate portion of the uterosacral ligament. Sutures should be placed at the level of the ischial spine, 1 cm posterior to the anteriormost palpable margin of the uterosacral ligament. The uterosacral ligament is very close to the intrapelvic ureter and the ureter can be injured if incorporated by one of the sutures or kinked by traction from a suture. The intraperitoneal approach, however, allows for better visualization and thus better suture placement compared to the visualization in the narrow, deep pararectal space.

A vertical midline incision is made in the vaginal epithelium. The vaginal wall is then carefully dissected away from the underlying pubocervical fascia and enterocele sac and the enterocele sac is entered and the bowel is packed away as described above for transvaginal enterocele repair. The following technique is as described by Shull et al. (1) in 2000, with minor modifications. The remnants of the uterosacral ligaments are identified posterior and medial to the ischial spines at approximately the 4 o'clock and 8 o'clock positions. An Allis clamp can be used to apply traction to the tissue and the uterosacral ligament can be palpated towards the sacrum. Two or three delayed absorbable or permanent (Ethibond) sutures (double-armed) are placed through the uterosacral ligaments on each side. In an effort to minimize ureteral injury, it is recommended that sutures be passed in a lateral-to-medial fashion as the surgeon has better control over the entry point of the needle than its exit point. Central defects in the pubocervical

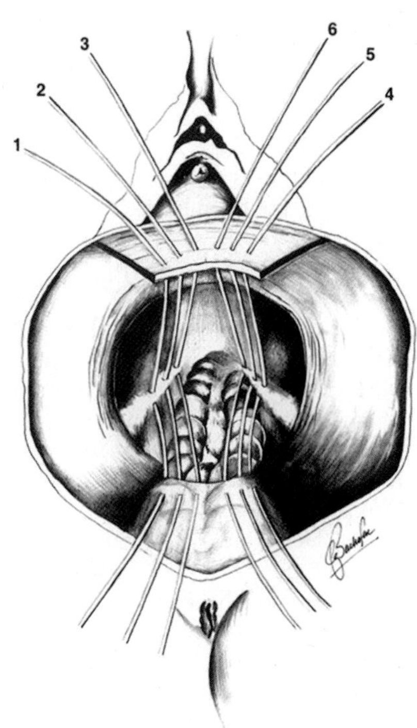


FIGURE 50.8 Sutures are placed in uterosacral ligaments bilaterally. One arm of each suture is placed in the pubocervical fascia and the other in the rectovaginal fascia. (From Shull BL, Bachofen C, Coates KW, et al. A transvaginal approach to repair of apical and other associated sites of pelvic organ prolapse with uterosacral ligaments. *Am J Obstet Gynecol* 2000;183:1365–1373, with permission.)

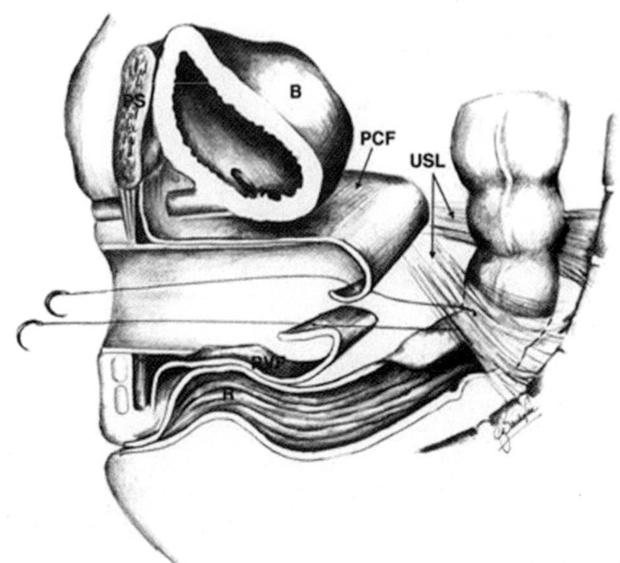


FIGURE 50.9 Sagittal view of suspensory suture in uterosacral ligament (USL), pubocervical fascia (PCF), and rectovaginal fascia (RVF). (From Shull BL, Bachofen C, Coates KW, et al. A transvaginal approach to repair of apical and other associated sites of pelvic organ prolapse with uterosacral ligaments. *Am J Obstet Gynecol* 2000;183:1365–1373, with permission.)

and rectovaginal fascia are repaired by plication. The double-armed sutures are placed through the pubocervical and rectovaginal fascia (Figs. 50.8 and 50.9). The distal remnants of the uterosacral ligaments are then plicated across the midline. The previously placed absorbable suspension sutures may be placed through the posterior vaginal wall. If one prefers, two permanent sutures and one absorbable suture (to be brought through the vaginal wall) can be used. Intravenous indigo carmine is administered. The vaginal epithelium is then closed as described previously, and the suspension sutures are tied, but left long and tagged. Cystoscopy is performed with indigo carmine as described above, and once ureteral patency is ensured the suspension sutures are trimmed.

### Sacrospinous Ligament Fixation

Sacrospinous ligament fixation is used to correct vault prolapse when the anterior vaginal wall is well supported, or it can be used with simultaneous anterior repair. Vaginal depth and axis are restored by posterior fixation of the vaginal vault to the sacrospinous ligaments. The sacrospinous ligament stretches from the ischial spine to the sacrum and is covered by the coccygeus muscle.

Once the enterocele repair is complete, the posterior vaginal wall must be opened far enough distally to facilitate dissection to the sacrospinous ligament. When a simultaneous rectocele repair is to be performed, the entire posterior vaginal wall is opened through the perineum. After the posterior vaginal wall is incised in the midline, it is gently dissected laterally from the underlying prerectal fascia for a short distance. Next, the sacrospinous ligament must be identified. This is done by penetrating the right or left rectal pillar (pararectal fascia) sharply and entering the pararectal space (Fig. 50.10). Blunt dissection of the pararectal space can be performed with a combination of finger dissection and the use of deep Breisky-Navratil retractors. This dissection is performed until the sacrospinous ligament is palpated and the overlying coccygeus muscle is seen. The Breisky-Navratil retractors will help expose the ligament. Once the ligament is identified, a no. 1 permanent braided suture is placed through the ligament and coccygeus muscle complex 2 cm medial to the ischial spine, which is also identified by palpation. It is important to place the suture in this position to avoid injury to the pudendal nerve and vessels, which run just below the ischial spine. It is also important to include the strong ligament in addition to the overlying coccygeus muscle. These tasks can be made easier by carefully dissecting over the ligament with a spreading motion of the Metzenbaum scissors and with the aid of a Kittner dissector. Visualization of the ligament itself helps avoid incorrect placement of the sutures. Another helpful tool is the Capio transvaginal suture-capturing device (Boston Scientific). This tool allows for placement of the suture and retrieval of the needle in this deep and narrow space with just the depression of a lever on the instrument's end. It has greatly simplified suture placement in our procedures. Tension should be placed on the suture to make certain that it is in the strong ligament. A second suture should be placed adjacent to the first. Each of these sutures is then placed through the vaginal wall, excluding the epithelial layer at the level of the apex, approximately 1 cm apart, and left untied. If a rectocele is present, it is repaired at this time. The apex of the vagina can be directed under finger guidance to the deepest possible portion, where it will be fixed. The vaginal wall is then closed with a running interlocking 2-0 PGA suture, and then the previously placed sacrospinous ligament fixation sutures are individually tied. Antibiotic-impregnated vaginal packing is then placed.

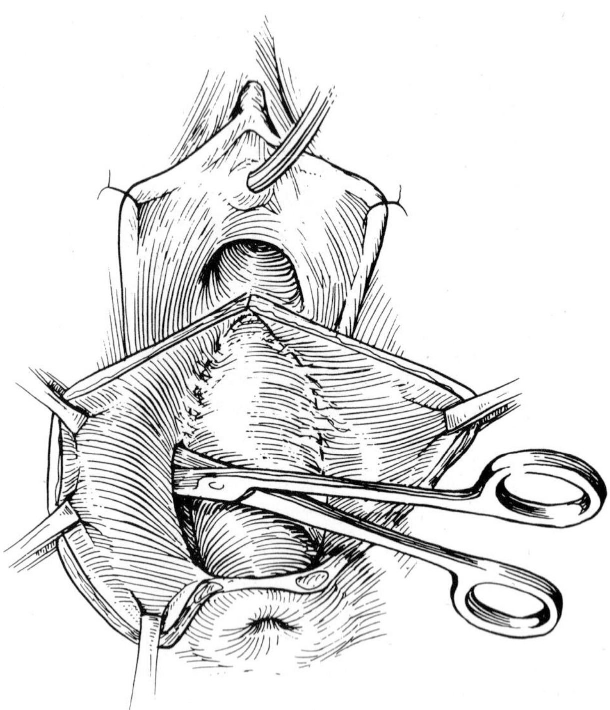

FIGURE 50.10 Dissection for sacrospinous ligament fixation. The rectal pillars are sharply penetrated and the pararectal space is entered. The space is widened with blunt dissection to expose the superior surface of the pelvic diaphragm. The sacrospinous ligament can then be palpated and the coccygeus muscle overlying it can be seen. (From Nitti VW. Transvaginal enterocele repair with variations. *Contemp Urol.* 1994;6:50–64, with permission.)

After sacrospinous ligament fixation, recurrences usually occur in the anterior vaginal compartment. This observation has led some investigators to try a modification of the sacrospinous ligament fixation meant to reduce recurrences in the anterior compartment by avoiding the downward deflection of the vagina. The anterior approach to sacrospinous ligament fixation approaches the ligament from the retropubic space and dissection of the ipsilateral paravaginal space from the level of the bladder neck to the ischial spine. Theoretically this approach should reduce postoperative vaginal narrowing and posterolateral deviation of the upper vagina, resulting in improved functional outcome. An additional modification is the bilateral anterior sacrospinous ligament fixation. Bilateral fixation should provide additional support and longevity over a single fixation point and may also increase the area of the vagina over the pelvic floor, improving its ability to withstand increases in intra-abdominal pressure. A limitation of this technique is that not all women have vaginal anatomy that is able to stretch to bilateral ligaments.

### Iliococcygeus Fixation

Iliococcygeus or prespinous fixation for vaginal vault prolapse is yet another method to suspend the vaginal vault, created to address what was considered to be a high rate of anterior compartment prolapse after sacrospinous ligament fixation and damage to the pudendal neurovascular bundle. In an iliococcygeus fixation the vaginal apex is fixed bilaterally to the iliococcygeus fascia using one no. 1 polydioxanone suture. The incision and dissection are carried out posteriorly. The rectovaginal fascia is dissected off the posterior vaginal wall laterally all the way to the pelvic sidewall. The ischial spine and sacrospinous ligament are identified as a landmark for the iliococcygeus fascia, which will be found anterior to them.

Cystoscopy with indigo carmine is recommended with each of the previous procedures to evaluate for bladder injury and ureteral patency.

## Mesh-Augmented Repairs

The use of mesh at the time of POP repair is becoming increasingly popular. This is in part due to the high incidence of recurrence following primary repair. However, there are minimal long-term safety and efficacy data on graft utilization in pelvic reconstruction.

There are various mesh-augmented repairs described in the literature. In 2004, Shah et al. (6) described a procedure using polypropylene mesh for total pelvic reconstruction. Subsequently, Amrute et al. (7) described their modification, in which a tension-free method is used for the anterior arms of the mesh. A horizontal incision is made at the most dependent portion of prolapsed vagina. Sharp and blunt dissection is performed extraperitoneally towards the ischial spine and sacrospinous ligament bilaterally. Two delayed absorbable sutures are placed bilaterally in the sacrospinous ligament (1 cm medial to the ischial spine) using the Capio needle driver. The vaginal epithelium is dissected off the bladder sharply, and if necessary the endopelvic fascia is imbricated with absorbable suture. Sharp dissection of the periurethral space is performed superiorly toward the retropubic space. An approximately 6 × 8-cm piece of polypropylene mesh is configured in an H and the anterior arms are sutured to the arms of a BioArc device (American Medical Systems). Using the BioArc needle passers, the anterior arms are passed retropubically through the anterior abdominal wall. The distal edge of the mesh is positioned at the level of the midurethra. Cystoscopy is performed to place a suprapubic tube, the bladder is evaluated to identify injury, and indigo carmine is administered to assess ureteral patency. The sacrospinous ligament sutures are passed through the lateral arms of the mesh and tied down. The sutures are then brought through the posterolateral aspect of the vaginal mucosa. Absorbable sutures are placed as needed to prevent folding and kinking of the mesh. The vagina is then closed in a running fashion.

Our current mesh-augmented repair for patients with severe apical and anterior prolapse includes a simultaneous paravaginal and apical repair using soft polypropylene mesh and involves sacrospinous ligament fixation through an anterior approach. It is a modification of the technique described by Shah et al. (6). The prolapsed anterior vaginal wall is grasped with Allis clamps and infiltrated with 1% lidocaine with epinephrine. A vertical midline incision is made from the area of the bladder neck to the vaginal apex. The vaginal wall is dissected off the bladder and the enterocele sac to the level of the endopelvic fascia. The enterocele sac may be opened and repaired as described above for transvaginal enterocele repair or simply reduced, depending on its size. After repair of the enterocele, the endopelvic fascia is perforated and the space of Retzius entered bilaterally. A Capio needle driver is then used to place a 2-0 Vicryl suture into the arcus tendineus at the level of the bladder neck and 1 cm above the ischial spine, as well as a PDS suture into the sacrospinous ligament. These sutures are placed bilaterally (Figs. 50.11 and 50.12). A piece of soft

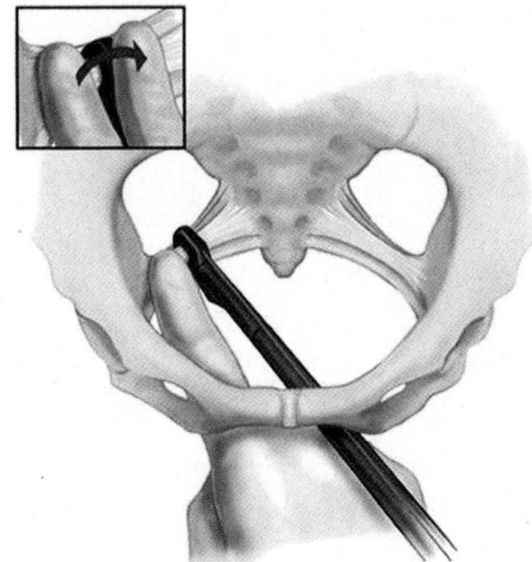

FIGURE 50.11 Placement of 2-0 PDS suture into sacrospinous ligament using a Capio needle driver. (From Boston Scientific Corporation, with permission.)

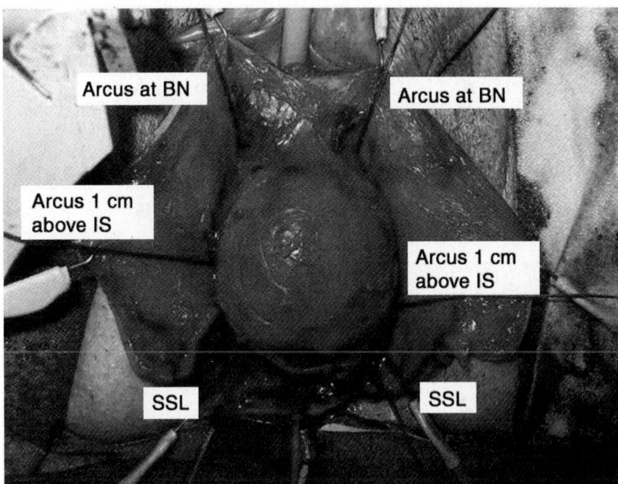


FIGURE 50.12 Sutures are placed in the arcus tendineus at the level of the bladder neck and 1 cm above the ischial spine as well as into the sacrospinous ligament bilaterally.

polypropylene mesh is then configured in the shape of a trapezoid approximately 5 cm wide at the top, 10 cm wide at the bottom, and 10 cm long (Fig. 50.13). The previously placed Vicryl sutures are then placed in the mesh with the narrow portion corresponding to the level of the bladder neck, the middle portion corresponding to the level of the ischial spines, and the widest portion of the mesh at the level of the sacrospinous ligament. The sacrospinous ligament sutures are tied down first and left long. The sutures 1 cm above the ischial spine and the sutures at the bladder neck are then tied down and cut. The wound is irrigated with antibiotic solution. Cystoscopy after intravenous indigo carmine is then performed to ensure ureteral patency. The sacrospinous ligament sutures are passed through the vaginal wall bilaterally at the vaginal apex, about 2 cm from the midline. The proximal two thirds of the vaginal wall is closed, and then the sacrospinous ligament sutures are tied down. The remainder of the anterior vaginal wall is closed. Sometimes a small amount of vaginal wall is excised prior to completing the closure. We have recently modified our procedure

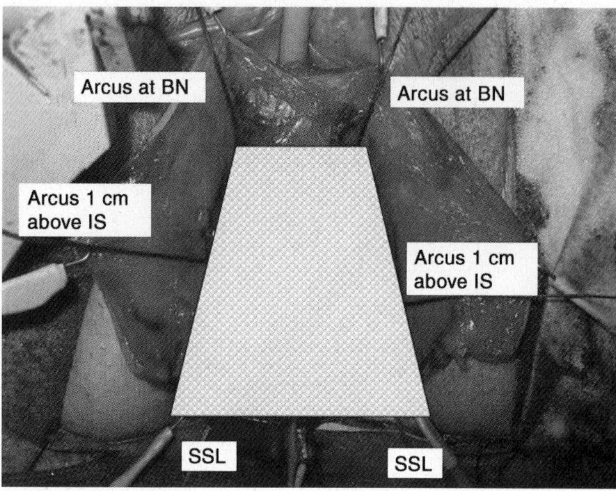


FIGURE 50.13 Soft polypropylene mesh configured in the shape of a trapezoid (approximately 5 × 5 × 10 cm).

to include an anterior colporrhaphy with plication of the pubocervical fascia across midline prior to placement of sutures into the arcus tendineus and sacrospinous ligament. Unfortunately this is not demonstrated in the figures.

## Transvaginal Procedures for Preservation of the Prolapsed Uterus

There has been a recent trend towards uterine-sparing procedures despite limited long-term data. Various vaginal, abdominal, and laparoscopic techniques have been described.

### Manchester Procedure

The Manchester procedure was originally described in 1888 by Archibald Donald of Manchester, England, and subsequently modified by W.E. Fothergill (8). It is an alternative to vaginal hysterectomy for patients with uterine prolapse, cervical elongation, and nonattenuated uterosacral–cardinal ligaments. A circumferential incision is made around the cervix (similar to the incision for a vaginal hysterectomy). The vaginal epithelium is dissected off the cervix. The cardinal ligament, including the cervical branch of the uterine artery, is clamped, divided, and suture-ligated bilaterally. A portion of the cervix is then amputated with a scalpel. Sturmdorf sutures are placed to invaginate the vaginal epithelium into the cervical os. The previously ligated cardinal ligaments are sewn to the anterior cervical stump. Anterior and posterior colporrhaphy procedures are performed as needed, and the vaginal epithelium is closed.

On occasion, we have performed a uterine-preserving transvaginal mesh-augmented sacrospinous ligament fixation repair. We typically prefer the abdominal approach when preserving the uterus. However, in patients in whom an abdominal approach is not ideal and mild (grade II or less) uterine prolapse exists in the setting of more severe anterior prolapse (a rare situation), this approach may be considered. It is performed in a similar fashion as the above-described sacrospinous ligament fixation. A midline incision is made in the anterior vaginal wall from the level of the bladder neck to the cervix. The dissection is then performed as described previously. An anterior colporrhaphy is performed, suturing the pubocervical fascia across midline and securing it to the cervix at the most proximal extent. The Capio needle driver is used as described previously to place Vicryl sutures in the arcus tendineus at the level of the bladder neck and just above the ischial spine. It is also used to place a PDS suture in the sacrospinous ligament bilaterally. A 5 × 5 × 10-cm trapezoidal piece of polypropylene mesh (same as previously) is fashioned and secured using the previously placed sutures. The mesh is also secured to the paracervical fascia in the midline using Vicryl suture. Cystoscopy is performed prior to passing the previously placed PDS sutures through the vaginal wall just lateral to the cervix. Anecdotally, we have had some success with this procedure, but no long-term data are available.

## Mesh Prolapse Repair Devices

Recently a number of prepackaged mesh kits have been marketed for prolapse repair. These kits include polypropylene meshes with various arms that are anchored by passage through support tissues (including the sacrospinous ligament, iliococcygeus muscle, and arcus tendineus) using insertion trocars. We have very limited experience with these procedures, and there are currently no long-term data regarding their use. Further discussion is beyond the scope of this text.

# OUTCOMES

The results of apical prolapse repair are difficult to evaluate because the definition of success varies between studies and few studies report long-term follow-up. Colombo and Milani (9) found no statistical difference in recurrence of vault prolapse in a retrospective study comparing sacrospinous ligament fixation and McCall culdoplasty (8% versus 3%, respectively). Shull et al. (1) reported "optimal anatomic outcomes" in 87% of patients undergoing uterosacral fixation, while Karram et al. (10) reported that 89% of women expressed satisfaction following the procedure. Success rates ranging from 8% to 97% have been reported for traditional sacrospinous ligament fixation (11,12). Shull et al. (13) and Meeks et al. (14) reported 95% and 96% cure rates following iliococcygeus fixation, while more recently Maher et al. (15) reported equal efficacy when comparing the iliococcygeus fixation to sacrospinous ligament fixation.

There are even fewer data regarding outcomes of mesh-augmented repairs. Amrute et al. (7) reported a 5.2% recurrence rate and a 2.1% rate of vaginal erosion with a mean follow-up time of 31 months.

## Complications

In all the previous procedures, the major risks are bleeding due to vascular injury, nerve entrapment, ureteral injury or kinking, bowel injury, wound infection, and persistent or recurrent prolapse. During placement of the pursestring sutures of an enterocele repair, one must take care not to disturb the ovarian vessels, which lie near the uterosacral–cardinal complexes. The pudendal vessels and nerve, which lie beneath the sacrospinous ligament, are at high risk of injury during sacrospinous ligament fixation. Pudendal entrapment may occur if sutures are placed too laterally, whereas the sciatic nerve is at risk if the sutures are placed too cephalad. Pelvic and gluteal pain, although usually transient, can occur as a result of injury to the pudendal and sciatic nerves. The intrapelvic ureter is intimately associated with the uterosacral ligaments but can be injured or kinked by any of the transvaginal vault suspensions. Ureteral injury or kinking in cases of vault suspension has a reported rate of 1% to 11% (10). The anterior vaginal compartment is at highest risk for persistent or recurrent prolapse, but in many cases this prolapse is asymptomatic and does not require reoperation.

## *References*


1. Shull BL, Bachofen C, Coates KW, et al. A transvaginal approach to repair of apical and other associated sites of pelvic organ prolapse with uterosacral ligaments. *Am J Obstet Gynecol* 2000;183:1365–1373.
2. Delancey JOL. Anatomic aspects of vaginal eversion after hysterectomy. *Am J Obstet Gynecol* 1992;166:1717–1728.
3. Bump RC, Mattiasson A, Bo K, et al. The standardization of terminology of female pelvic organ prolapse and pelvic floor dysfunction. *Am J Obstet Gynecol* 1996;175:10–17.
4. Sze EH, Kohli N, Miklos JR, et al. A retrospective comparison of abdominal sacrocolpopexy with Burch colposuspension versus sacrospinous fixation with transvaginal needle suspension for the management of vaginal vault prolapse and coexisting stress incontinence. *Int Urogynecol J Pelvic Floor Dysfunct* 1999;10:390–393.
5. McCall ML. Posterior culdoplasty: surgical correction of enterocele during vaginal hysterectomy: a preliminary report. *Am J Obstet Gynecol.* 1957;10:595–602.
6. Shah DK, Paul EM, Rastinehad AR, et al. Short-term outcome analysis of total pelvic reconstruction with mesh: The vaginal approach. *J Urol* 2004;171:261–263.
7. Amrute KV, Eisenberg ER, Ardeshir RR, et al. Analysis of outcomes of single polypropylene mesh in total pelvic floor reconstruction. *Neurourol Urodynam* 2007;26:53–58.
8. Fothergill W. Anterior colporrhaphy and amputation of the cervix combined as a single operation for the use in the treatment of genital prolapse. *Am J Surg* 1915;29:161.
9. Colombo M, Milani R. Sacrospinous ligament fixation and modified McCall culdoplasty during vaginal hysterectomy for advanced uterovaginal prolapse. *Am J Obstet Gynecol* 1998;179:13–20.
10. Karram M, Goldwasser S, Kleeman S, et al. High uterosacral vaginal vault suspension with fascial reconstruction for vaginal repair of enterocele and vaginal vault prolapse. *Am J Obstet Gynecol* 2001;185:1339–1342.
11. Holly RJ, Varner RE, Gleason BP, et al. Recurrent pelvic support defects after sacrospinous ligament fixation for vaginal vault prolapse. *J Am Coll Surg* 1995;180:444–448.
12. Nichols DH. Sacrospinous fixation for massive eversion of the vagina. *Am J Obstet Gynecol* 1982;142:901–904.
13. Shull BL, Capen CV, Riggs MW, et al. Bilateral attachment of the vaginal cuff to iliococcygeus fascia: an effective method of cuff suspension. *Am J Obstet Gynecol* 1993;168:1669–1674.
14. Meeks GR, Washburne JF, McGehee PR, et al. Repair of vaginal vault prolapse by suspension of the vaginal to iliococcygeus (prespinous) fascia. *Am J Obstet Gynecol* 1994;171:1444–1454.
15. Maher CF, Murray CJ, Carey MP, et al. Iliococcygeus or sacrospinous fixation for vaginal vault prolapse. *Obstet Gynecol* 2001;98:40–44.


# **CHAPTER 51** ■ POSTERIOR VAGINAL PROLAPSE REPAIR

LIOR LOWENSTEIN AND ELIZABETH R. MUELLER

Pelvic organ prolapse (POP) is prevalent in the United States, with approximately 200,000 surgeries in women annually (1). An epidemiologic study of a large U.S. northwest health care population suggests that a woman has an 11.1% risk of undergoing POP surgery by the age of 80. Over the next 30 years it is predicted that the number of women seeking care for pelvic floor disorders will increase by 45% (2).

One of the confounding factors in diagnosing and treating POP is that "less than perfect" support of the anterior and posterior vaginal walls is a normal finding in the majority of vaginally parous women. Swift (3) reported on vaginal examination findings of 497 women who presented for their annual Pap and pelvic examination. All women were >18 years of age, with a median parity of two. The incidence of cases in which the leading edge of the most prolapsed segment was 1 cm distal to the hymen or beyond was 52%, with only 6% of women demonstrating no prolapse or perfect support. Likewise, the Women's Health Initiative hormone replacement clinical trial performed baseline pelvic examinations on 16,616 women with a uterus (4). They found that 41% of women aged 50 to 79 years had POP on physical examination. The vaginal compartment most frequently associated with the prolapse was the anterior vaginal wall (also known as cystocele) at 34%, followed by the posterior compartment (rectocele, 19%) and uterine prolapse (14%). Parity and obesity were strongly associated with an increased risk for prolapse.

Posterior vaginal wall prolapse is thought to be herniation of the posterior vaginal wall or anterior rectal wall into the lumen of the vagina. Vaginal childbirth is one of the most frequent risk factors associated with prolapse. Labor and vaginal delivery results in damage to the pudendal nerve and disruption of connective tissue and muscular attachments. Denonvilliers fascia, which is fused to the inner layer of the posterior vaginal wall, may be torn during vaginal delivery at its caudal and lateral attachments to the perineal body. Nonobstetric risk factors associated with POP include pelvic surgery, conditions leading to elevated intra-abdominal pressure (e.g., obesity and chronic constipation with excessive straining), inherited connective tissue disorders (e.g., Ehlers-Danlos and Marfan syndromes), and genetic predisposition. Though menopause is often cited as a risk factor for POP, several researchers have failed to find an association with estrogen status. Suspension of the anterior vaginal wall for incontinence procedures such as the Burch urethropexy is also a risk factor for apical prolapse. This is most likely due to the change in the vaginal axis following the surgical procedure, resulting in abdominal forces being directed over the genital hiatus instead of the posterior levator ani.

The symptoms attributed to POP are numerous and include colorectal and urinary symptoms, dyspareunia, pelvic heaviness, and the protrusion of the vaginal wall beyond the introitus. Bowel symptoms such as constipation, incomplete bowel emptying, straining, splinting to defecate, and anal incontinence are common in women and are often attributed to posterior vaginal prolapse (5). Of all of these symptoms, the most reliable predictor of POP appears to be simply the self-reported presence of a palpable bulge at the introitus. Numerous studies have demonstrated that bowel symptoms do not correlate with the degree of POP or objective measures of anorectal function (6); however, these symptoms may improve following surgical intervention, as we will discuss later.

## DIAGNOSIS

At our institution, the physical examination of a patient with suspected POP is initially done with the patient in the standing, straining position and the physician seated or kneeling. If a bulge is palpable past the introitus on straining, then we place our fingers in the vagina and determine the extent of the prolapse.

Following the standing examination, the woman undergoes a complete gynecologic examination including bimanual examination in the dorsolithotomy position. The pelvic examination of the vagina (especially the apical segment) can be facilitated by using the lower blade of a Graves speculum. The single blade is placed against the anterior wall and then the posterior wall of the vagina during Valsalva, for the evaluation of the opposing wall and apex. Isolated distal protrusion of the posterior vaginal wall with lack of descent of the vaginal apex represents an isolated rectocele. Often the viscera behind the vaginal wall cannot be accurately determined. For example, prolapse of the posterior vaginal wall and apex in a woman who has had a hysterectomy may be due to small bowel herniation (enterocele) or a defect in the rectovaginal fascia (rectocele). A bimanual straining rectovaginal examination with a finger simultaneously in the rectum and the thumb in the vagina can help distinguish rectocele from an enterocele. An enterocele will often fill the space between the two viscera, while a rectocele will result in no change in the plane.

The two most commonly used systems to document the degree of prolapse are the Pelvic Organ Prolapse Quantification (POP-Q) and the Baden-Walker. The POP-Q consists of nine measurements and describes the topography of the vagina, genital hiatus, and perineal body. The anterior, posterior, and apical compartments are described and the prolapse stage is based on the compartment that is most prolapsed relative to the hymenal remnant. The Baden-Walker grading system is based on the position of the most protruding part of the vagina relative to the hymen and is usually reported as the prolapse grade.

One of the possible explanations for the high recurrence rate in prolapse repairs (~30%) is that concomitant vaginal defects are not recognized at the time of surgery. Apical prolapse may go unrecognized during the supine examination. We evaluated the relationship between the anterior, posterior, and apical compartment in 325 consecutive new patients (7). Thirty-nine percent had a previous hysterectomy and only 3% had a previous anterior, posterior, or apical repair. The vaginal apex (POP-Q point C) strongly correlated with the most prolapsed portion of the anterior vaginal wall, Ba (Spearman $\rho = 0.835, p < 0.001$), and moderately correlated with the most prolapsed portion of the posterior vaginal wall, Bp (Spearman $\rho = 0.556, p < 0.001$). Of 113 women who had the leading edge of the posterior vaginal wall at the introitus or beyond, a significant amount of concurrent apical prolapse was present (Fig. 51.1).

Radiologic imaging may be indicated more for understanding the cause of defecatory dysfunction than for diagnosing POP. Defecography involves dynamic evaluation of the pelvic floor, providing both structural and functional information. Standardization of the testing and interpretation of defecography is not established, however, and therefore it is not recommended for routine clinical use, although it can be helpful in "high" rectoceles when an enterocele is suspected. Magnetic resonance imaging (MRI) has been used to describe the location of the defects during POP, but we do not routinely use it in our practice.

## ALTERNATIVE THERAPIES

Asymptomatic patients or women with minor symptoms may report little or no bother as a result of the disorder, and observation or watchful waiting is appropriate. Pelvic floor muscle rehabilitation may be offered despite the lack of data supporting its use to prevent progression.

Mechanical support, such as a pessary, can be used to reduce the POP. Support pessaries are made of silicon or soft plastic and can be offered to women with symptomatic POP who prefer a nonsurgical approach. Other indications include women who are poor surgical candidates because of medical comorbidities, or patients needing temporary relief of pregnancy-related POP or incontinence. In most patients, the pessary can be fitted successfully in one or two office visits. Women with symptomatic improvement are taught to place and remove the pessary at least twice weekly and prior to intercourse and should return every 6 to 12 months. Women who cannot remove the pessary will leave it in continuously and return every 3 months for pessary care. They may benefit from vaginal estrogen cream, unless contraindicated, to reduce the risk of erosion. If vaginal erosion develops, the pessary should be removed and vaginal estrogen cream applied until the erosion is healed. The pessary can then be replaced, although a reduction in pessary size is advisable. Pessaries generally are less effective in supporting the posterior vaginal wall than in apical and anterior vaginal wall prolapse.

## INDICATIONS FOR SURGERY

Due to the possibility of postoperative dyspareunia, it is believed that an isolated rectocele should not be repaired unless the patient is bothered by symptoms. Our practice is to refer

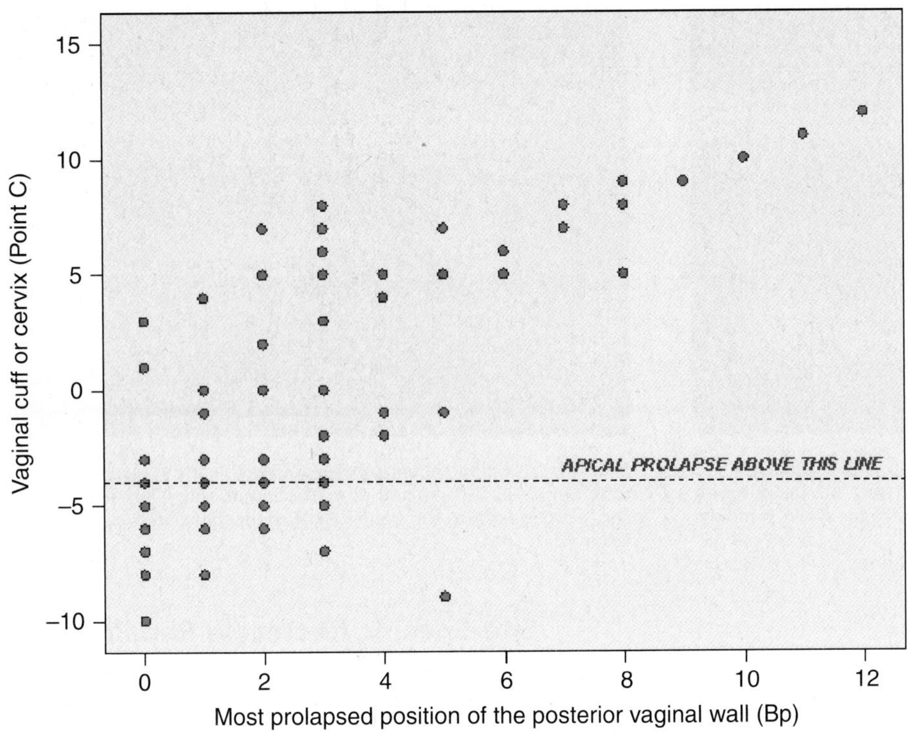


FIGURE 51.1 A scatter plot of the leading edge of the posterior vaginal wall and the vaginal apex in 122 women who had the leading edge of the posterior vaginal wall at the introitus or beyond in a standing straining exam.

the patient to colorectal surgery or occupational therapy for defecation disorders prior to undergoing a procedure for posterior vaginal wall prolapse.

Numerous factors must be considered when counseling patients about the best surgical treatment:

- Surgical route
- Durability
- Recovery time
- Immediate and delayed postoperative complications

# SURGICAL TECHNIQUES

There are three surgical routes that may be used for rectocele repair: abdominal, transanal, and transvaginal. Among the different surgical routes, the transvaginal approach is the most commonly practiced route for the "noncolorectal" surgeon. The abdominal approach is indicated for rare cases when rectocele is associated and repaired with the rectal prolapse. The transanal route was thought to be indicated for cases of small distal rectocele. Today, this is less commonly practiced because of the possible impairment of the anal sphincter as a result of its dilatation during the surgery. Although rectocele repair has been practiced for >100 years, the most effective surgical treatment remains undetermined.

As stated earlier, the position of the vaginal apex or cervix is well correlated to the most prolapsed part of the posterior and anterior vaginal walls in women with POP. When performing sacrocolpopexy, the apical segment is resuspended and the vaginal axis is adequately restored; the anterior and posterior vaginal walls are also restored to a nonprolapsed position without additional anterior or posterior repairs (8).

The following procedures are indicated for women who have a distal defect of the posterior vaginal wall or who are having a concomitant apical suspension.

## Posterior Colporrhaphy

Posterior colporrhaphy is still commonly practiced today by general gynecologists and urologists. Our protocol includes giving 2 g of cefoxitin intravenously at the start of the procedure. Though we find that bowel preparation is often recommended before surgery by our colleagues, this has not been our practice.

Following the administration of general or spinal anesthesia, the patient is positioned in the dorsal lithotomy position with her legs in Yellofin stirrups (Allen Medical Systems). Care is taken to ensure the neural safety and positioning of all four extremities. She is prepped and draped in a sterile fashion and a Foley catheter is inserted.

A bimanual examination is performed to reassess the POP and ensure that the surgical procedures chosen are adequate (Fig. 51.2). A self-retaining vaginal wall retractor such as the Lone Star (Lone Star Medical Products) is placed. Twenty milliliters of 1/200,000 epinephrine/saline solution is injected into the submucosal tissue to aid in the dissection and help with hemostasis. The posterior commissure of the vagina is clamped approximately 2 to 3 cm from the midline on the right and left with Allis clamps. A transverse incision is made in between the two Allis forceps. In cases where perinorrhaphy is performed concomitantly, an additional incision is made in the perineum to remove a triangular piece of skin, allowing exposure of the perineal body, as will be discussed in a later section. A vertical incision is made in the posterior vaginal mucosa from the middle of the transverse incision reaching the apex of the rectocele, which is held by an Allis clamp in the midline (Fig. 51.3). Using a Metzenbaum scissors the vaginal mucosa is dissected from the underlying perirectal fascia using a "snip and push" technique. Once an avascular plane is established, an index finger wrapped with a moist vaginal laparotomy sponge can be used for further dissection, although this technique should be abandoned if significant tissue resistance is met. It is also

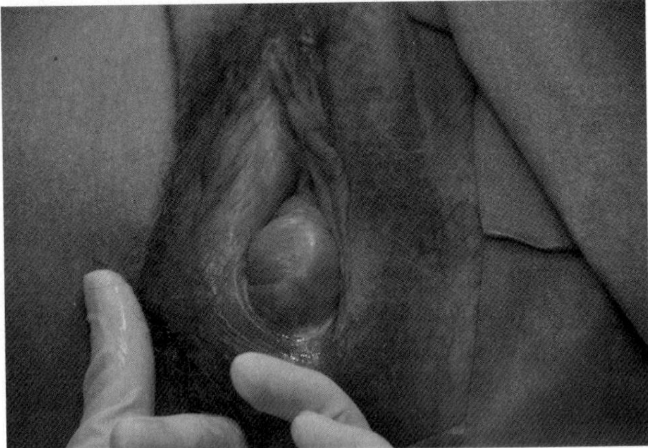

FIGURE 51.2 Rectal examination of a woman with a rectocele. The vaginal apex is 6 centimeters proximal to the hymen but the posterior vaginal wall distal edge protrudes past the introitus when standing. Notice how by placing the nondominant hand's third digit in the rectum, the thumb and index finger can still be utilized by the operating surgeon.

important to do the dissection close to the vaginal wall side to avoid incising the rectum. The dissection is extended upward in the midline to well above the bulge of the rectocele (Fig. 51.4). At this point it is necessary to obtain sufficient hemostasis to identify the anatomic structures.

The surgeon then should insert the nondominant middle finger into the rectum, which allows the thumb and index finger to be available to the surgeon. The bulge is reduced to aid in the identification of the lateral rectovaginal fascia. Care is taken not to incorporate the levator ani (levator plication), since this can result in vaginal distortion, constriction, postoperative pain, and dyspareunia. The rectovaginal fascia is plicated to the midline using a series of interrupted size 0 polyglactin sutures (Fig. 51.5) that are initially tagged and then tied in succession. The distal end of the rectovaginal septum (imbricated rectovaginal fascia) is then attached to the reconstructed perineal body (perineorrhaphy) if this is performed. Any redundant vaginal epithelium that crosses the midline is excised, and the vaginal epithelium is closed with 3-0 poliglecaprone 25 (Monocryl) absorbable sutures (Fig. 51.6).

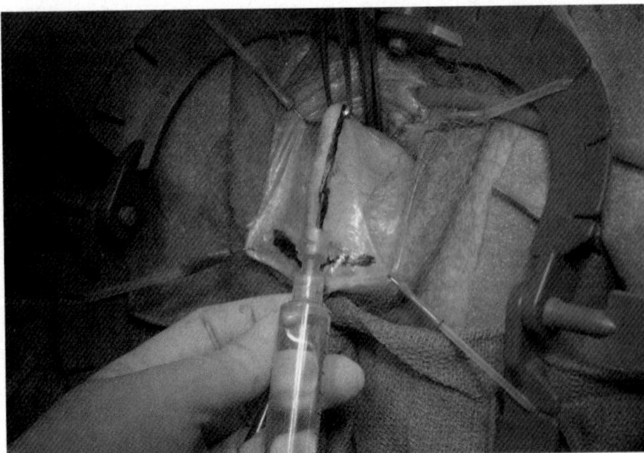

FIGURE 51.3 The proximal end of the rectocele is grasped with an Allis clamp and the midline and transverse incisions are marked. Injection of local anesthetic with epinephrine can help with developing a plane.

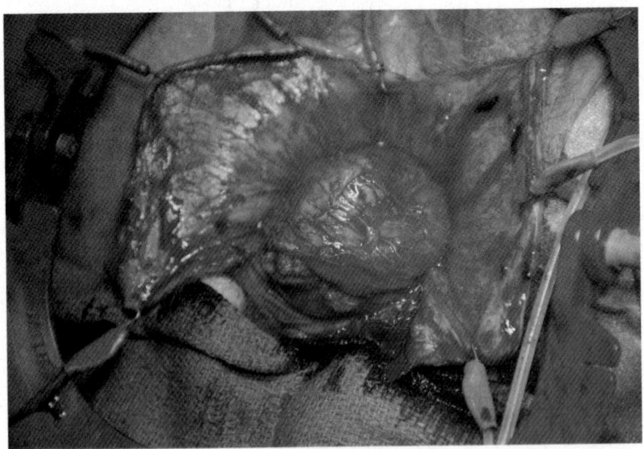

FIGURE 51.4 The vaginal epithelium overlying the rectocele is dissected off using a "snip and push" technique with Metzenbaum scissors held at a 90° to the vaginal epithelium. The excess epithelium is removed.

## Site-Specific Rectocele Repair

The site-specific repair of rectocele was proposed by Richardson et al. (9) in 1976. This technique is based on Richardson's observations during cadaveric dissection that rectoceles are the result of a specific defect in the rectovaginal fascia.

The initial steps of this procedure are similar to the classic posterior colporrhaphy. The vaginal epithelium is opened and dissected from the underlying rectovaginal fascia. A rectal examination assists in the identification of the edges of the defect, which are grasped with forceps. The defect is repaired with interrupted 0 polyglactin sutures (Vicryl); they are usually placed cranial to caudal, as opposed to the side-to-side placement in a posterior repair. Again, care is taken to avoid

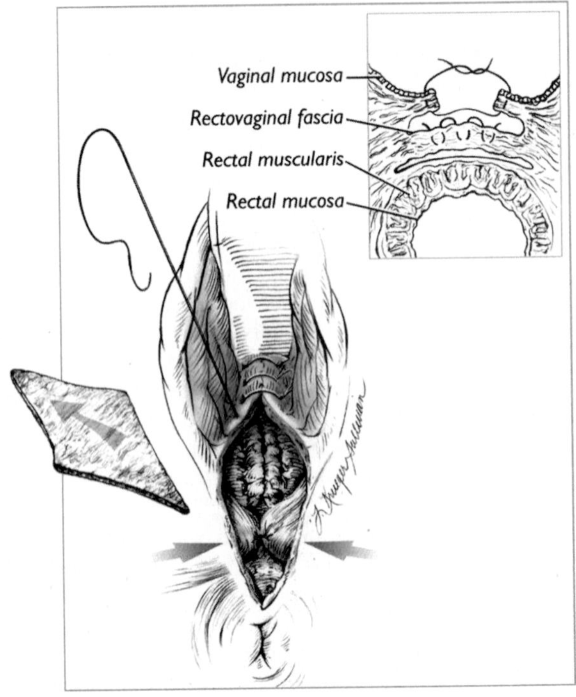


FIGURE 51.5 The rectovaginal fascia is identified lateral to the rectocele. Absorbable interrupted sutures are placed in the rectovaginal fascia bilateral. The sutures are tagged and then tied down in succession.

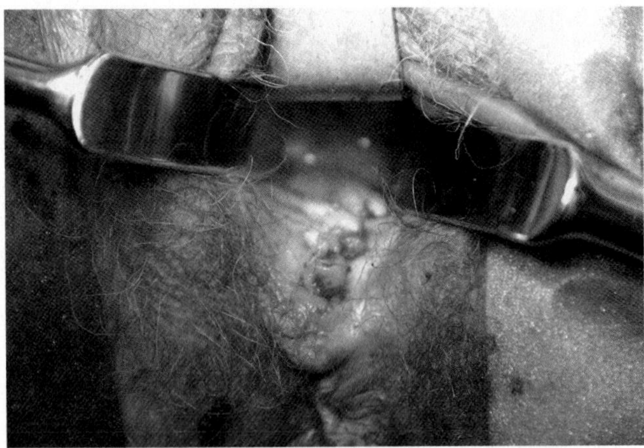

FIGURE 51.6 Examination of the posterior vaginal wall following the posterior repair.

the incorporation of any healthy muscle that could result in dyspareunia. If indicated, the perineal body is reconstructed. The vaginal epithelium is closed as previously described.

## Reconstruction of the Perineal Body

The perineal body is located between the vaginal introitus and the anus, and attached to it are the following structures: bulbocavernosus muscles, superficial transverse perineal muscles, levator ani muscles, the external anal sphincter, and the rectovaginal fascia (Fig. 51.7). Due to its lateral and superior support there is limited downward movement of the perineal body. Rectoceles that recur or are symptomatic with defecatory disorders may actually be disorders of exaggerated perineal descent due to the detachment of the perineal body to the rectovaginal septum.

Reconstruction of the perineal body starts with placement of Allis clamps on the lateral edges of the posterior commissure of the vagina that also grasp the underlying bulbocavernosus muscles. When brought together in the midline, they represent the lower edges of the reconstructed introitus. Care must be taken not to overly narrow the introitus especially because the relaxation of the pelvic floor during anesthesia can often lead to miscalculations in the resulting introitus. A triangular piece of vaginal epithelium is removed so as not to damage the underlying superficial transverse perineal muscles (Fig. 51.8). The bulbocavernosus muscles are plicated with midline interrupted size 0 polyglactin sutures (Fig. 51.9) and the epithelium is closed with a running absorbable suture. Preservation of the size of the genital hiatus is important for women who wish to remain sexually active.

## Posterior Repair with Biologic and Synthetic Materials

In an attempt to improve the anatomic cure rates, several variations have been used for correcting the posterior prolapse. The use of synthetic or biologic material as reinforcement or replacement of weak fascia was derived originally from general surgery and has been advocated in gynecologic surgery. The most widely used biologic materials are human freeze-dried cadaveric fascia lata, solvent-dehydrated fascia lata (Tutoplast), porcine dermal graft (Pelvicol), and decellularized human cadaveric dermis (Alloderm, Repliform).

Synthetic materials can be classified as absorbable or permanent. Their use has increased since they were first described in 1995 for the management of stress urinary incontinence and POP. The most commonly used absorbable synthetic graft is polyglactin 910, while polypropylene is commonly used as a nonabsorbable material. Most published data on graft materials are related to incontinence surgery and abdominal colpopexy. There is no standardized method to place the graft. The graft is placed through the vaginal incision as another layer of support after plication of the rectovaginal fascia. Transverse and anteroposterior dimensions of the prolapsed segment are measured. A graft of similar size is placed and secured by delayed absorbable or nonabsorbable 0 sutures. The redundant vaginal mucosa is then excised and the mucosa is closed using an absorbable continuous suture with no tension.

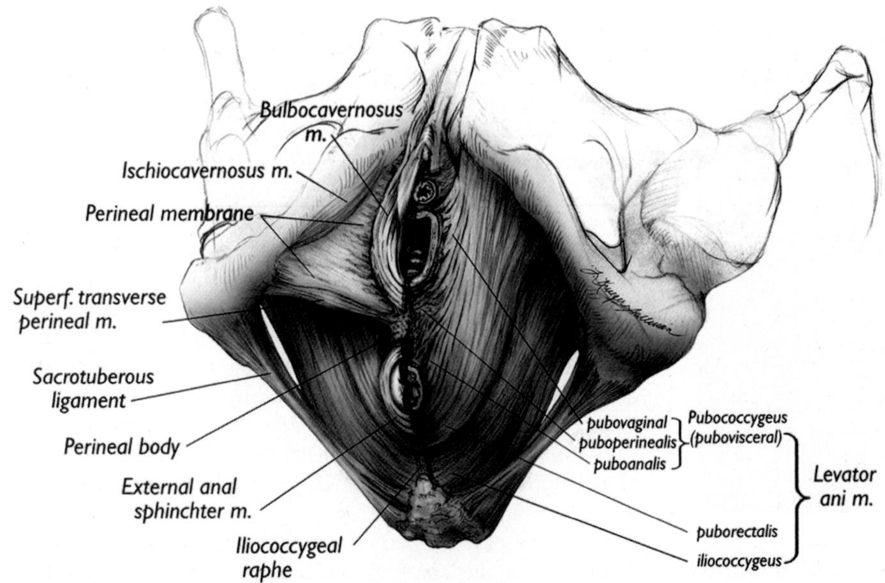


FIGURE 51.7 Inferior view of the pelvic floor. Superficial perineal muscles and perineal membrane have been removed on the left to show attachments of the levator ani (LA) muscles to the distal vagina, anus, and perineal body.

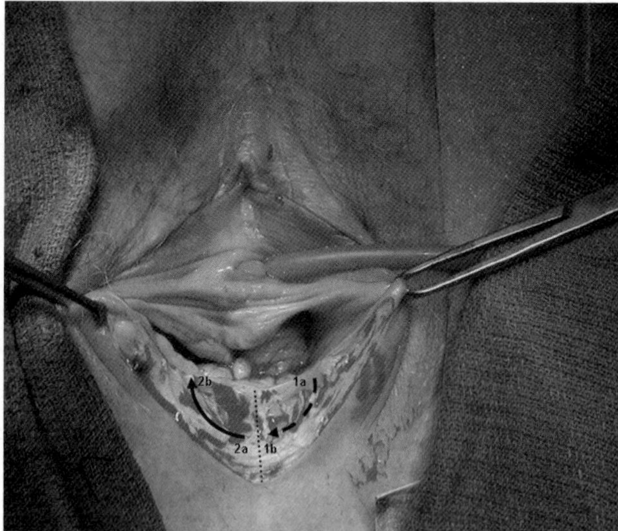


FIGURE 51.8 Perineorrhapy incision. The perineorrhapy incision is diamond-shaped and only the epithelium is removed. With a finger in the rectum, interrupted sutures are placed lateral to medial (1) with the first pass and then medial to lateral (2) and then tied down.

## Postoperative Care

In our practice, women who have undergone a repair of a posterior vaginal wall defect are admitted to the hospital overnight for pain management and observation. An ice pack to the perineum every couple hours can reduce postoperative edema and pain in women who have had a perineorrhaphy. A voiding trial is typically performed the day of discharge (most often postoperative day 1). A repeat voiding trial is performed by a visiting nurse 3 or 4 days later in the patient's home for those who fail initially. Women are discharged home, to return in 2 weeks, with a bowel regimen consisting of fiber, stool softeners, and a "plan" if they have not had a bowel movement for a couple of days. Oral pain medications, including anti-inflammatory agents and narcotics, may be prescribed. We instruct all women that they are limited to no lifting over 10 pounds and "nothing in the vagina" for 6 weeks.

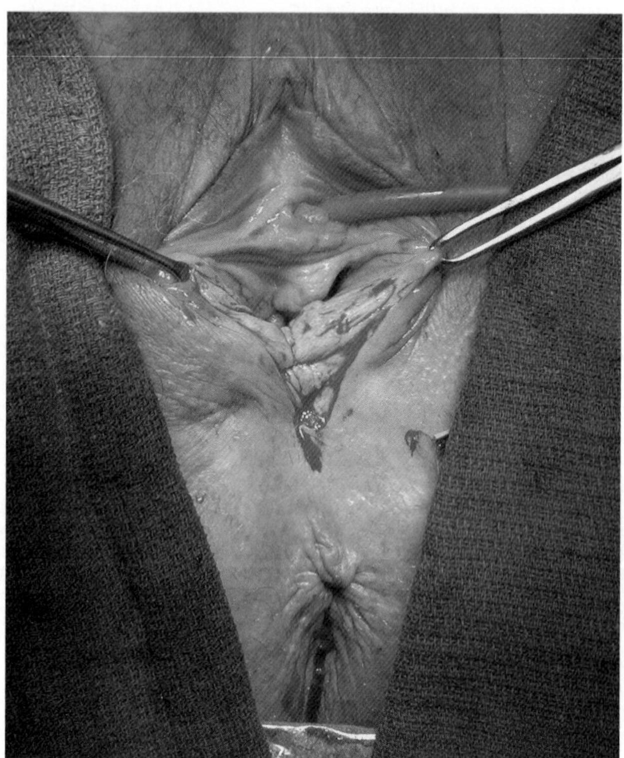

FIGURE 51.9 The perineum after three sutures are placed. The genital hiatus has decreased in size and the perineal body is reconstructed.

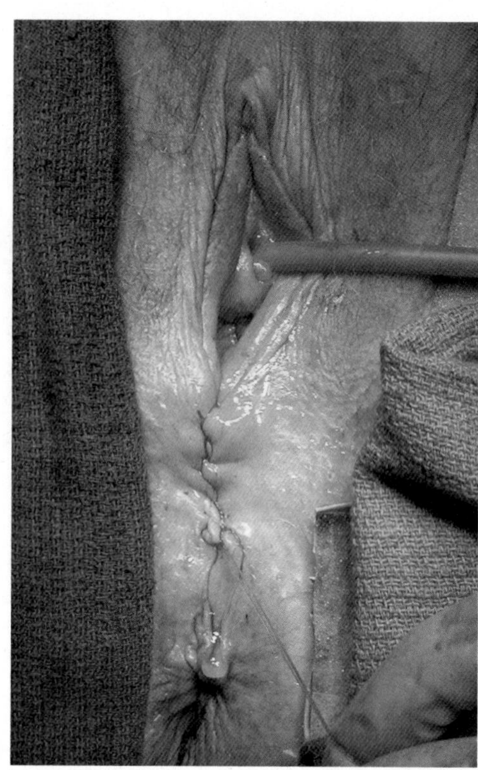

FIGURE 51.10 Following the reconstruction of the perineal body, the epithelium is closed using a running absorbable suture. The genital hiatus demonstrated has been constructed for a non-sexually active woman.

# OUTCOMES

## Results

Despite the fact that transvaginal colporrhaphies have been the preferred surgical procedure for rectocele repair among gynecologic surgeons for over 100 years, there are few data regarding the long-term anatomic success. In different case series, the anatomic cure rate ranges from 76% to 96% for posterior and from 56% to 100% for site-specific defects (10). A recent Cochrane review of surgical management for prolapse reported that transvaginal repair is superior to a transanal approach for posterior vaginal wall prolapse, with a lower recurrence rate (RR 0.28; 95% CI, 0.009–0.64) (11).

Posterior colporrhaphy was found to be effective in alleviating symptoms of vaginal bulge (4–64%), constipation (22–100%), and fecal incontinence (4–36%). Thus, the functional improvement is not always correlated with anatomic success.

Over the past 20 years there have been several case series reporting on the anatomic success of posterior repair with graft material, with cure rates ranging from 89% to 100% for a follow-up period of 3 to 60 months. Variability of the cure rate can be partially explained by the different definitions and tools used to assess anatomic cure.

## Complications

The most common immediate complications associated with repair of rectocele are injury to the rectum, constipation, infection, perirectal hematoma, and inclusion cyst. When the rectal lumen is inadvertently opened during dissection of the rectum from the vaginal mucosa, the defect must be closed during surgery. The most important factor is recognition at the time of the injury, as neglected cases may result eventually in rectovaginal fistula. The risk of passing suture through the rectal mucosa is diminished by placing a finger in the rectum at the time of suturing. If a stitch is felt on rectal examination it should be removed transvaginally, not through the rectum.

Constipation should be avoided and is one of the major threats to the success of the surgery; therefore, the problem is best addressed prior to undergoing surgical repair.

Dyspareunia rates of 21% to 27% have been reported following posterior repair (12) and are linked to the levator ani plication that is commonly done. Weber et al. (5) reported similar rates without a plication. Rectocele repairs using synthetic mesh may result in both dyspareunia and *hispareunia. Hispareunia* or *partner dyspareunia* is a term we use to describe the pain resulting from penile exposure to the eroded mesh during intercourse. The extent of this phenomenon is unknown.

According to the literature, the rate of erosion via the vaginal route varies from 12% to 30% (13). The true rates of erosion may be higher than reported due to the short follow-up in most studies. The type of mesh used affects erosion rates; however, no synthetic mesh seems to be completely spared from this phenomenon.

Typically, women with mesh erosion present with persistent vaginal discharge or bleeding and possible dyspareunia and require transvaginal trimming of the exposed portion of the mesh. Successful treatment of vaginal mesh erosion with estrogen cream has been reported (13), but in our experience estrogen has not been effective.

## *References*

1. Olsen AL, Smith VJ, Bergstrom JO, et al. Epidemiology of surgically managed pelvic organ prolapse and urinary incontinence. *Obstet Gynecol* 1997;89:501–506.
2. Luber KM, Boero S, Choe JY. The demographics of pelvic floor disorders: current observations and future projections. *Am J Obstet Gynecol* 2001; 184:1493–1501.
3. Swift SE. The distribution of pelvic organ support in a population of female subjects seen for routine gynecologic health care. *Am J Obstet Gynecol* 2000;183:277–285.
4. Hendrix SL, Clark A, Nygaard I, et al. Pelvic organ prolapse in the Women's Health Initiative. *Am J Obstet Gynecol* 2002;186:1160–1166.
5. Weber AM, Walters MD, Ballard LA, et al. Posterior vaginal prolapse and bowel function. *Am J Obstet Gynecol* 1998;179:1446–1450.
6. Bradley CS, Brown MB, Cundiff GW, et al. Bowel symptoms in women planning surgery for pelvic organ prolapse. *Am J Obstet Gynecol* 2006; 195:1814–1819.
7. Rooney K, Mueller E, Kenton K, et al. Isolated anterior vaginal wall repairs is highly correlated with apical prolapse. *Am J Obstet Gynecol* 2006; 195:1837–1840.
8. Guiahi M, Kenton K, Brubaker L. Sacrocolpopexy without concomitant posterior repair improves posterior compartment defects. *Int Urogynecol J Pelvic Floor Dysfunct* 2008;19(9):1267–1270.
9. Richardson AC, Lyon JB, Williams NL. A new look at pelvic relaxation. *Am J Obstet Gynecol* 1976;126:568–573.
10. Cundiff GW, Fenner D. Evaluation and treatment of women with rectocele: focus on associated defecatory and sexual dysfunction. *Obstet Gynecol* 2004;104:1403–1421.
11. Maher C, Baessler K, Glazener CM, et al. Surgical management of pelvic organ prolapse in women. *Cochrane Database Syst Rev* 2007:CD004014.
12. Haase P, Skibsted L. Influence of operations for stress incontinence and/or genital descensus on sexual life. *Acta Obstet Gynecol Scand* 1988;67: 659–661.
13. Dwyer PL, O'Reilly BA. Transvaginal repair of anterior and posterior compartment prolapse with ATrium polypropylene mesh. *Br J Obstet Gynecol* 2004;111:831–836.

# CHAPTER 52 ■ ABDOMINAL SACRAL COLPOPEXY

J. CHRISTIAN WINTERS AND SCOTT DELACROIX, JR.

Pelvic organ prolapse (POP) is a common yet complex medical condition that can significantly impair a woman's quality of life. POP can occur at multiple sites, and therefore the effect of these defects on a woman's symptoms may vary. One of the more complex types of POP is vaginal vault prolapse (VVP), and its incidence is reported to be 18.2% of all women with prolapse (1). In fact, many would suggest that any descensus of the anterior compartment near the hymenal ring or beyond is associated with VVP. VVP usually occurs as a result of multifactorial muscular and connective tissue disorders that result in weakening of the supporting structures of the vaginal apex—the cardinal and uterosacral ligaments. In most cases this is accompanied by defects elsewhere on the pelvic floor, such as central or lateral cystocele, high or low rectocele, enterocele, or perineal body laxity. Up to 72% of patients with VVP have been shown to have other pelvic floor defects in some combination (2). For any patient undergoing surgical correction for prolapse, it is paramount to recognize all potential defects prior to surgery. Undiagnosed and untreated vault prolapse will almost always ensure recurrence of a surgically corrected cystocele (1). It has also been demonstrated that an isolated abdominal repair of VVP without addressing concomitant pelvic floor defects may lead to decreased patient satisfaction and the need for secondary vaginal repair.

Finally, there are numerous reports of occult stress urinary incontinence manifesting after vaginal vault prolapse repair (3). There is evidence to support the use of prophylactic anti-incontinence procedures at the time of VVP repair in women with occult stress urinary incontinence (3).

This chapter will discuss the abdominal sacral colpopexy (ASC) for the correction of VVP. One must consider incorporating ancillary vaginal or anti-incontinence procedures with ASC because an untreated symptomatic secondary defect or undiagnosed occult stress urinary incontinence (3) will significantly impair overall patient satisfaction.

## DIAGNOSIS

Patients with VVP will often complain of pelvic pressure, vaginal protrusion, dyspareunia, difficulty walking, and back pain. Bowel and genitourinary symptoms vary from urinary and fecal incontinence to difficult elimination or sexual dysfunction. Patients with severe prolapse may need to manually reduce the prolapse to evacuate the rectum or void. Women with severe prolapse or uterine procidentia may develop recurrent urinary tract infections or hydronephrosis due to angulation of the ureters.

A thorough physical examination is needed to establish the diagnosis of VVP and to demonstrate other pelvic floor defects and/or occult stress urinary incontinence. During the examination every segment of the pelvic floor should be evaluated in a systematic manner—the anterior vaginal wall, the vaginal apex (or cervix), the posterior vaginal wall, and the perineum (Table 52.1).

**TABLE 52.1**

**COMPARTMENT-SPECIFIC DEFECTS AND FEMALE PELVIC ORGANS COMMONLY AFFECTED**

| LOCATION | DEFECT |
|---|---|
| Urethra | Occult stress incontinence<br>Hypermobility |
| Anterior vaginal wall | Lateral cystocele<br>and/or<br>central cystocele |
| Vaginal apex | Vaginal vault prolapse |
| Posterior superior vaginal wall | Enterocele<br>and/or<br>high rectocele |
| Posterior inferior vaginal wall | Rectocele |
| Perineum | Incompetent perineal body |

The pelvic examination begins with the patient in the lithotomy position, utilizing a Valsalva maneuver. If all areas of the pelvic floor can be assessed in this position, the examination is completed. Urethral mobility can almost always be assessed visually, but in rare equivocal cases, a cotton-tipped applicator test can be performed. In many cases, it will be difficult to assess low-grade or moderate VVP, especially in posthysterectomy patients without the cervix as an anatomic landmark. "Dimples" at the lateral apex of the vagina can sometimes be used to locate the cuff. These dimples usually represent the point of attachment of the uterosacral ligaments. The examiner's fingers are placed at the vaginal apex. If the fingers descend halfway to the hymeneal ring or further on Valsalva, significant vault prolapse is present. Once again in the supine position, the anterior and posterior compartments are assessed independently. Half of a vaginal speculum is initially used to compress the posterior compartment while the examiner assesses the anterior compartment for abnormal descent. The posterior compartment can then be assessed by replacing the speculum to support the anterior vaginal wall. It is important to distinguish prolapse high along the posterior vaginal wall as either a high rectocele or an enterocele. This can be accomplished by bimanual rectovaginal examination in the supine or standing position to detect enterocele. In an enterocele, there is a defect between the pubocervical fascia and rectovaginal fascia that allows predominantly small intestine to press against the vaginal epithelium. If no enterocele sac is palpated between the rectum and vagina (examiner's fingers), the defect is most likely a high rectocele. The perineal body should provide definition between the anterior and posterior perineal triangles. Prior episiotomy scars and defects in this area should be noted. In equivocal or difficult examinations where the full extent of the prolapse may not be appreciated, the patient can be evaluated while standing. The Pelvic Organ Prolapse Quantification (POP-Q) can be used as an adjunct to the examination, particularly when performing serial examinations or exchanging data (4).

Lower urinary tract function should be assessed in all patients, whether symptomatic or not. As previously noted, stress urinary incontinence can be unmasked by correction of POP of any type. After reduction of the POP by vaginal packing or pessary, a Valsalva stress test with a full bladder is performed in the standing position. Care should be taken not to falsely support and occlude a hypermobile urethra and thus obtain a false-negative result.

Urodynamic testing is strongly advised to delineate bladder and urethral function. With the prolapse reduced, the examiner assesses for the presence of stress urinary incontinence. If present, the degree of sphincteric deficiency is quantified using abdominal leak point pressures. In addition, urodynamic testing allows the examiner to assess the quality of bladder storage and quantify the contractility of the bladder during emptying. Women with impaired contractility or those who void by abdominal straining may have more difficulty voiding after surgery. These women may need counseling regarding this issue, particularly if an anti-incontinence procedure is performed. These voiding dynamics are easily diagnosed with urodynamic evaluation. Patients with fecal dysfunction, particularly incontinence, may be evaluated with additional studies such as anorectal manometry, transrectal ultrasonography, and an electromyographic latency study. An assessment of sexual function should be performed; one may consider the use of a validated questionnaire such as the Prolapse and Incontinence Sexual Questionnaire (PISQ-12) (5).

## INDICATIONS

An individualized approach to patients with advanced POP should be undertaken after consideration of multiple factors. The surgeon must consider all site-specific defects present as well as the patient's urinary, bowel, and sexual function. It is of paramount importance to determine the most bothersome symptoms for the patient and to highlight the patient's goals and expectations of treatment. Following this, the patient's general medical condition and other factors are considered when deciding on a management plan.

There is no panacea for POP, as each procedure has advantages, disadvantages, and risks. ASC should be considered an excellent treatment option in the following cases: failed previous vaginal repair; recurrent enterocele and/or VVP; isolated high-grade apical prolapse and/or enterocele; and a younger woman with an active lifestyle who desires to continue sexual intercourse.

In these patients ASC is an excellent choice because it maximizes functional vaginal length and provides a near-normal vaginal axis. As discussed above, other pelvic floor defects and occult stress urinary incontinence can be addressed at the same time.

## ALTERNATIVE THERAPY

Pessary placement is a nonsurgical option that is often unsatisfactory in severe cases of prolapse. In cases of total vaginal prolapse, pessary placement can be impossible. The need for daily cleansing, replacement, discomfort, and vaginal erosion are some of the disadvantages to long-term pessary placement.

A colpocleisis is a safe and effective alternative treatment of POP, especially in elderly patients. It does not preserve normal anatomy and is an option only in a patient not desiring future sexual activity.

Vaginal methods of prolapse repair, including unilateral or bilateral sacrospinous ligament fixation, plication of the uterosacral ligament (McCall) with culdoplasty, or iliococcygeus fascial fixation, are also alternatives to abdominal sacral colpopexy. Sacrospinous ligament fixation will result in significant changes in the vaginal axis and has a higher incidence of anterior compartment defect recurrence and rectal, vascular, or neural complications. Plication of the uterosacral ligament with culdoplasty is difficult in posthysterectomy patients, with a higher potential for ureteral injury. In addition, there is concern regarding the functional integrity of the uterosacral remnant (6). Iliococcygeus fascial fixation will result in vaginal shortening.

## SURGICAL TECHNIQUE

All patients are administered a mechanical bowel preparation preoperatively. Thromboembolic elimination stockings and sequential compression devices are used. Open, robotic-assisted laparoscopic and pure laparoscopic approaches have all been described. The principles of the operation remain the same regardless of approach, and we will describe the open technique of ASC. The critical elements of the operation include:

- Permanent mesh (type I macroporous, monofilament) as graft material
- Secure suture fixation of the graft to the sacral promontory and vaginal cuff
- Complete enterocele reduction and culdoplasty
- Anti-incontinence procedure as indicated

The patient is positioned in the low lithotomy position, providing both transvaginal and transabdominal access. A low midline abdominal incision is preferred by the authors to allow exposure of the sacral promontory. A Pfannenstiel incision may also be chosen in younger patients, although exposure may be slightly more difficult. The following is a description of the operative technique of ASC and abdominal enterocele repair.

Once the incision is made and the peritoneal cavity entered, it is essential to achieve excellent exposure by freeing all adhesions in the pelvis and packing the bowel out of the pelvis above the level of the sacral promontory. Next, an incision is made in the posterior peritoneum over the sacral promontory, extending inferiorly along the right lateral aspect of the rectum (Fig. 52.1). Electrocautery is used when dividing the fatty tissue over the promontory. Diathermy cautery forceps are useful in this dissection. Excessive blunt dissection is avoided in this area as shearing of presacral veins with severe bleeding may occur. Care is taken to avoid the middle sacral vein traversing over the promontory. As the fatty tissue is dissected free, the anterior surface of the sacral promontory is visualized, usually by identification of the anterior longitudinal ligament.

Two or three sutures of no. 0 Ethibond (Ethibond Excel polyester suture; Ethicon Inc., Johnson & Johnson, Somerville, NJ), using a MO-7 needle, or no. 0 Prolene (polypropylene suture material; Ethicon Inc.), using a MO-6 needle, are placed into the periosteum over the sacral promontory (Fig. 52.1).

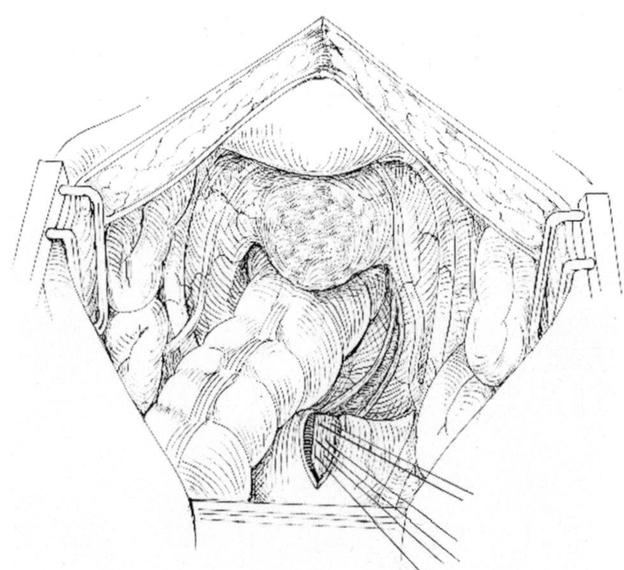

FIGURE 52.1 Incision of posterior peritoneum extending into pelvis lateral to rectum. Note secure suture placement into the sacral promontory.

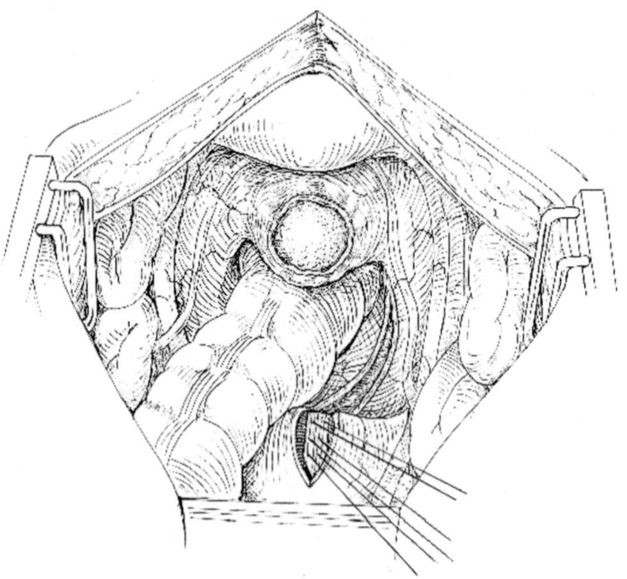

FIGURE 52.2 Peritoneum over vaginal cuff incised. Note: Dissection is made easier by use of EEA sizer.

These sutures are safely secured for later placement into the graft. Alternatively, commercially available tacking devices may be used for securing the graft to the sacral promontory.

The peritoneum over the vaginal cuff is excised, and the peritoneum is dissected off the cuff of the vagina (Fig. 52.2). A 2.0-cm-wide segment of graft is sutured to the exposed vaginal cuff using six sutures of 2-0 Ethibond (Fig. 52.3). Monofilament nonabsorbable mesh is recommended (see Outcomes later). The graft is secured to the vagina by folding over the cuff of the vagina and allowing the long end of the graft to exit posteriorly and extend to the sacrum. Alternatively, a T-shaped configuration of the graft may be created. The short arm of the T is placed on the top of the vagina, and the long arm of the T is secured to the lower end of the vagina. The enterocele sutures (Fig. 52.4) are placed into the long arm of the T on the lower side of the vagina.

After placing an obturator in the vagina (large end-to-end anastomosis sizers are useful), the enterocele sac is identified and secured with an Allis clamp. If the enterocele is large, several pursestring sutures or linear 2-0 Ethibond sutures are

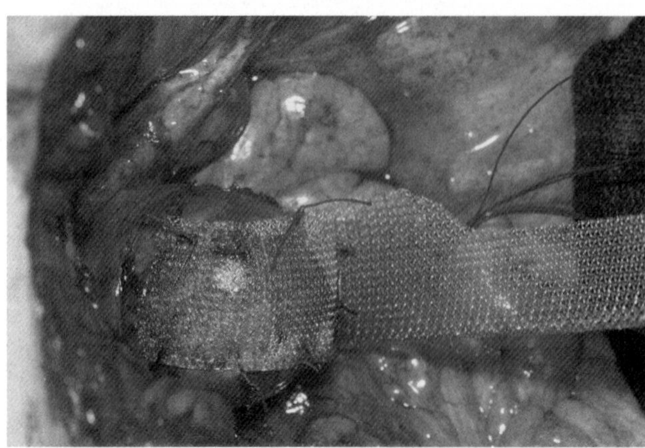

FIGURE 52.3 Intraoperative view: Permanent graft secured to vaginal apex.

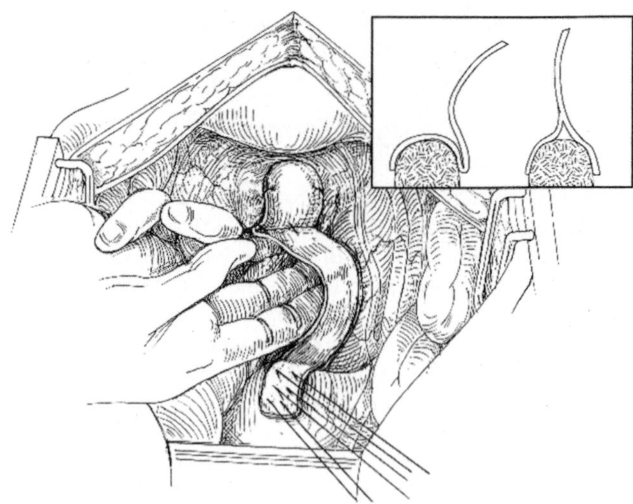

FIGURE 52.4 Final graft position. Inset shows different methods of graft attachment. Long extension of graft secured posteriorly.

placed into the enterocele sac to obliterate it (Fig. 52.5). This will reduce the cul-de-sac and facilitate the culdeplasty.

A Halban culdoplasty is performed by placing linear sutures (2-0 Ethibond) through the posterior peritoneum and on the outer surface of rectum up to the vaginal cuff (Fig. 52.6). The central sutures are placed through the obliterated enterocele sac to prevent recurrence of enterocele. Upward retraction of the graft will assist in exposing the cul-de-sac. Usually four to six sutures are used to complete adequate cul-de-sac closure. (At this step, the central sutures from the culdoplasty are placed through the long arm of the T, if used.)

Using the preplaced sutures on the sacral promontory, the graft is secured to the promontory. Care must be taken to avoid excessive tension. Placing the obturator all the way into the vagina but not pushing the vagina upward establishes the proper length of the graft. The graft is placed around the right lateral aspect of the rectum. A space of two fingerbreadths between the graft and the rectum prevents compression of the rectum over the graft (Fig. 52.7). The excessive length of the graft is trimmed after fixation to the sacrum.

The graft is positioned in the retroperitoneal space by closing the presacral peritoneum over the graft and covering the

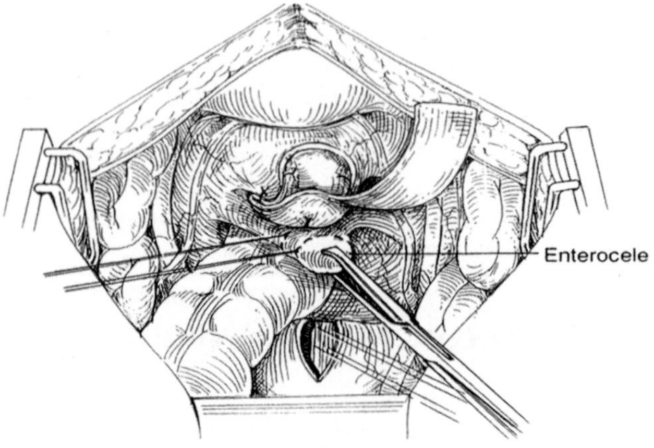


FIGURE 52.5 Isolation of enterocele from above. If enterocele is large, it may be reduced by plicating with pursestring sutures prior to cul-de-sac closure.

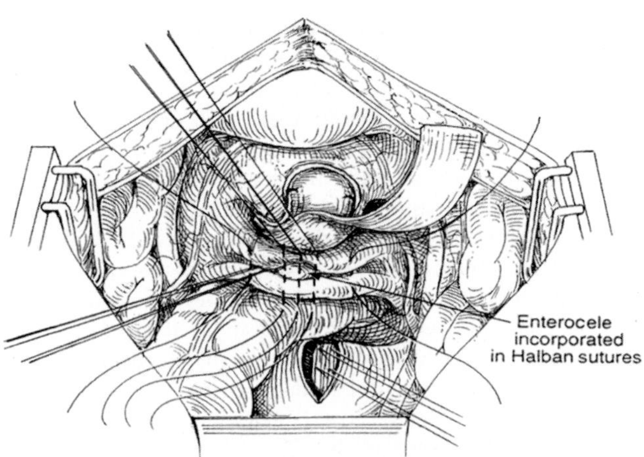


FIGURE 52.6 Halban cul-de-plasty: longitudinal sutures placed to close cul-de-sac.

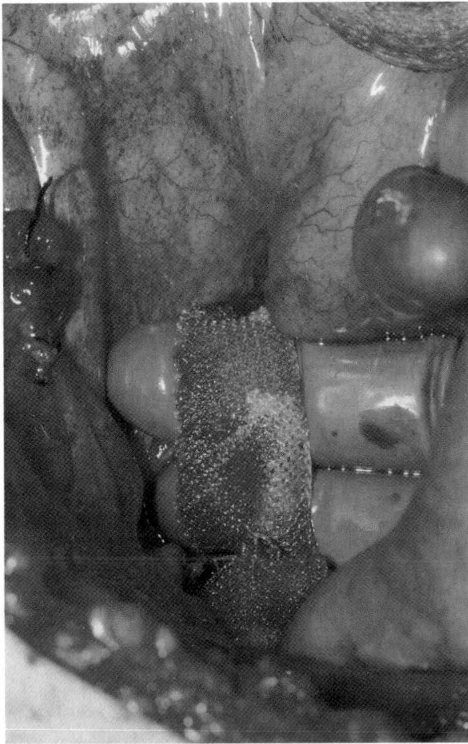

FIGURE 52.7 Intraoperative view: graft in final position. Note minimal tension placed on graft material. Incised peritoneum will be closed over graft after securing graft.

graft on the vagina with the superior edge of the peritoneum over the vagina (Fig. 52.8). Stress incontinence procedures (if indicated) are then performed. The patient is then examined to determine if any ancillary prolapse repairs are needed.

## OUTCOMES

### Results

In the indicated patient, the goal of pelvic reconstruction is to preserve vaginal depth and normal vaginal axis while repairing POP. This should be done through a procedure with a low

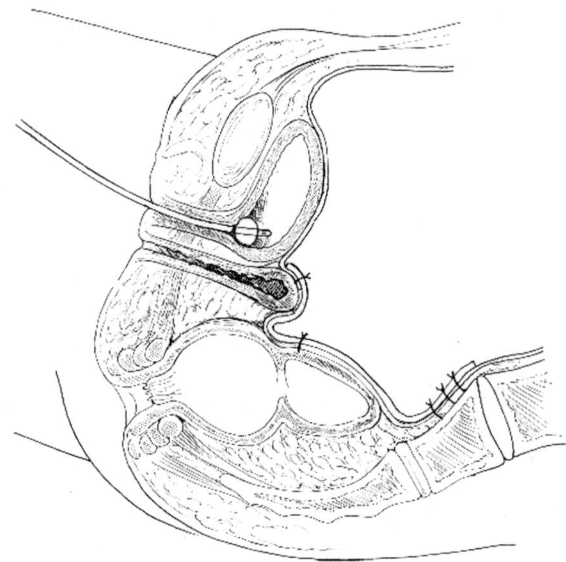

FIGURE 52.8 Final result. Graft positioned below posterior peritoneum by closing the previously incised peritoneum over the mesh.

complication rate, minimal morbidity, and a low recurrence rate. ASC maintains a functional vagina and restores maximal vaginal length and support by securing the vaginal apex to the periosteum of the sacrum (7). In a comparative study, the vaginal length was longer after ASC compared to sacrospinous fixation (7). The abdominal approach allows excellent exposure to the pelvis and allows complete obliteration of the pouch of Douglass (Halban culdoplasty).

A nonabsorbable monofilament synthetic mesh should be used for fixation during the ASC. In a study by Culligan et al. (8), patients undergoing ASC using either absorbable cadaveric fascia lata graft (Tutoplast) or nonabsorbable monofilament polypropylene were randomized. The objective failure rate for recurrence at any other vaginal site was 14 out of 44 in the fascial group and 4 out of 45 in the mesh group (RR 3.58, 95% CI 1.28–10.03) (9).

There are numerous reports by multiple authors that confirm the success of ASC. Success rates >90% have been reported and the durability of this procedure has also been documented (10–12). There are several randomized, prospective trials comparing sacrospinous ligament fixation (SSLF) with abdominal sacral colpopexy (13). In a comparative study between ASC versus vaginal repair, Benson et al. (11) reported a lower success rate with vaginal repair and an equivalent hospital stay between the two groups. Lo and Wang (12) reported on their results of ASC versus SSLF at a duration of 2.1 years: 94.2% success with ASC compared to 80% with SSLF. Maher et al. (10) reported on a comparative study between ASC and SSLF. At 2 years of follow-up, symptoms and anatomic success were equivalent, but asymptomatic failures to introitus and recurrent cystoceles were less after ASC. Overall, vaginal procedures have a higher rate of recurrent anterior defects even when performed in the setting of a concomitant anterior repair (colporrhaphy).

The assessment, determination, and treatment (if present) of occult stress urinary incontinence should be the standard by which patients with significant POP warranting surgical correction are addressed. Brubaker et al. (3) reported the importance of performing simultaneous Burch culposuspension in women undergoing ASC. In a prospective, controlled trial, 23.8% of women who underwent Burch procedures at the time of ASC reported bothersome stress urinary incontinence compared to 44.1% of women who underwent ASC alone. These findings occurred in women regardless of the presence or absence of occult stress urinary incontinence. This study clearly demonstrates that women undergoing ASC are at significant risk for developing stress urinary incontinence postoperatively, even in the absence of preoperative symptoms. The implications of these findings should be discussed with patients in advance of surgery. However, some patients may have significant obstructive voiding symptoms and no evidence of stress urinary incontinence on preoperative evaluation. A selective approach may be warranted in these patients, with the caveat that a midurethral sling can be placed at a later date with minimal difficulty. In patients who have symptomatic or occult stress urinary incontinence, the authors prefer midurethral sling placement at the time of ASC, due to the common coexistence of intrinsic sphincter deficiency.

Other advantages of ASC include consistent anatomy that is less reliant on deficient pelvic connective tissue, the ability to perform the most definitive enterocele repair via abdominal culdoplasty, and the fact that urologists are comfortable with pelvic surgery. The ASC is a procedure that should be easily incorporated into the surgical repertoire of urologists, providing excellent correction of VVP.

## Complications

Complications can be divided into intraoperative complications and postoperative complications. In a comprehensive review by Nygaard et al. (13), intraoperative complications included hemorrhage or transfusion (4.4%), cystotomy (3.1%), enterotomy (1.6%), and ureteral injury (1.0%). Postoperative complications included urinary tract infection (10.9%), wound infection (4.6%), ileus (3.6%), deep venous thrombosis or pulmonary embolism (3.3%), and small bowel obstruction (1.1%). The risk of significant bleeding has been reported from 1.6% to 4.4% and may be controlled with the use of stainless steel thumbtacks (14). Significant hemorrhage can occur from disruption of the presacral vessels. This complication may be reduced when fixation of the graft is performed high on the sacral promontory. Mesh erosion into the sigmoid colon has been reported (15) and is avoided by meticulous placement of the mesh while ensuring an adequate space between it and the sigmoid colon. Erosions are heralded by persistent pain, discharge, irritative voiding symptoms, or infections, and clinicians must be vigilant in follow-up (16). In a recently reported meta-analysis, the rate of mesh erosion into the vagina was reported at 3.4% to 5.4%; the rate may vary depending on the type of mesh used (13,17). Erosions are more prevalent with Teflon or Gore-Tex type of materials and are rare with macroporous, monofilament meshes. The incidence of mesh erosion is increased when performing a sacral colpoperineopexy (15). Concurrent hysterectomy has a theoretical risk of increasing infection or erosion of the graft, given the chance of contamination from vaginal microbes; however, current evidence is contradictory, and no randomized trials have addressed this issue (13). In 60 patients undergoing concomitant hysterectomy using a two-layer closure of the vaginal cuff followed by ASC with synthetic nonabsorbable monofilament mesh, the erosion rate was 0.8% compared to 0% in the 64 patients with a prior hysterectomy (18). In patients undergoing a combined operation, supracervical hysterectomy or a meticulous two-layer imbricated closure of the vaginal cuff can be performed to reduce the risk of mesh erosion at the vaginal cuff.

## *References*


1. Winters J, Cespedes R, Vanlangendonk R. Abdominal sacral colpopexy and abdominal enterocele repair in the management of vaginal vault prolapse. *Urology* 2000;56:55–63.
2. Richter K. Massive eversion of the vagina: pathogenesis, diagnosis and therapy of the true prolapse of the vaginal stump. *Clin Obstet Gynecol* 1982;25:897–912.
3. Brubaker L, Cundiff G, Weber A, et al. Abdominal sacral colpopexy with Burch colposuspension to reduce stress urinary incontinence. *N Engl J Med* 2006;354:1557–1566.
4. Bump RC, Mattiasson A, Bo K, et al. The standardization of terminology of female pelvic organ prolapse and pelvic floor dysfunction. *Am J Obstet Gynecol* 1996;175:10–17.
5. Rogers RG, Coates KW, Kammerer-Doak D, et al. A short form of the Pelvic Organ Prolapse/Urinary Incontinence Sexual Questionnaire (PISQ-12). *Int Urogynecol J* 2003;14(3):164–168.
6. Cole EE, Leu PB, Gomelsky A, et al. Histopathological evaluation of the uterosacral ligament: is this a dependable structure for pelvic reconstruction? *BJU Int* 2006;97(2):345–348.
7. Given FT. Vaginal length and sexual function after colpopexy for complete uterovaginal eversion. *Am J Obstet Gynecol* 1993;169:284–287.
8. Culligan PJ, Murphy M, Blackwell L, et al. Long-term success of abdominal sacral colpopexy using synthetic mesh. *Am J Obstet Gynecol* 2002; 187(6):1473–1482.
9. Maher C, Baessler K, Glazener CM, et al. Surgical management of pelvic organ prolapse in women. *Cochrane Database of Systematic Reviews (Online)* 2007;3:CD004014.
10. Maher CF, Qatawneh AM, Dwyer PL, et al. Abdominal sacrocolpopexy or vaginal sacrospinous colpopexy for vaginal vault prolapse: a prospective randomized study. *Am J Obstet Gynecol* 2004;190:20–26.
11. Benson JT, Lucente V, McClellan E. Vaginal versus abdominal reconstructive surgery for the treatment of pelvic support defects: a prospective randomized study with long-term outcome evaluation. *Am J Obstet Gynecol* 1996;175:1418–1422.
12. Lo T-S, Wang AC. Abdominal colposacropexy and sacrospinous ligament suspension for severe uterovaginal prolapse: a comparison. *J Gynecol Surg* 1998;14:59–64.
13. Nygaard I, McCreery R, Brubaker L, et al. Abdominal sacral colpopexy: a comprehensive review. *Obstet Gynecol* 2004;104:805–823.
14. Timmons MC, Kohler MF, Addison WA. Thumbtack use for control of presacral bleeding with description of an instrument for thumbtack application. *Obstet Gynecol* 1991;78:313–315.
15. Rose S, Bunten CE, Geisler JP, et al. Polypropylene mesh erosion into the bowel and vagina after abdominal sacral colpopexy. *J Pelvic Med Surg* 2006;12(1):45–47.
16. Karlovsky M, Thakre A, Badlani G, et al. Biomaterial for pelvic floor reconstruction. *Urology* 2005;66:469–475.
17. Wu JM, Wells EC, Hundley AF, et al. Mesh erosion in abdominal sacral colpopexy with and without concomitant hysterectomy. *Am J Obstet Gynecol* 2006;194(5):1418–1422.
18. Brizzolara S, Pillai-Allen A. Risk of mesh erosion with sacral colpopexy and concurrent hysterectomy. *Obstet Gynecol* 2003;102(2):306–310.

# SECTION V ■ VAS DEFERENS, SEMINAL VESICLE, TESTIS

MARC GOLDSTEIN

# CHAPTER 53 ■ ANATOMY OF THE EPIDIDYMIS, VAS DEFERENS, AND SEMINAL VESICLE

HOWARD H. KIM AND MARC GOLDSTEIN

The formation of a spermatozoan from precursor cells does not signify its readiness to fertilize an oocyte. It must travel a vast distance and learn fundamentals such as swimming before debuting in the world and laying claim to its female counterpart. Fortunately, the excurrent ductal system of the male reproductive tract provides specialized facilities for this journey, as a nursery, dormitory, finishing school, and test track. The anatomic features that make this system so exquisitely suited for nurturing and educating sperm also make it vulnerable to injury and malfunction; imagine how easily the elongated single duct of the epididymis is injured or blocked. The components of the excurrent ductal system (Fig. 53.1) can be organized into a logical order, the epic journey of a spermatozoan from its origin at the germinal epithelium to its dramatic exit at the ejaculatory duct with assorted encounters in between.

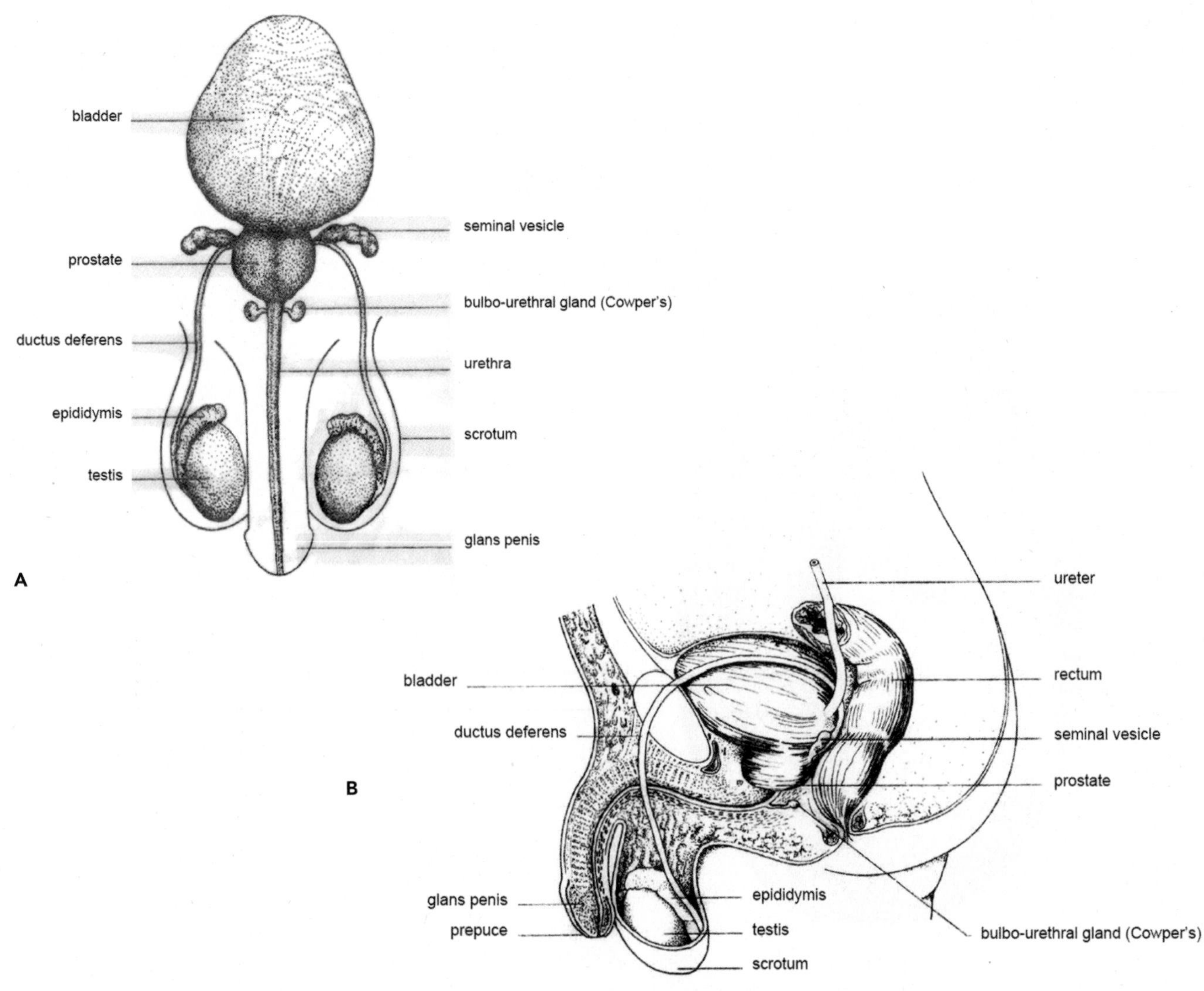


FIGURE 53.1 **A:** Front overview of the male excurrent ductal system. **B:** Side overview.

# EPIDIDYMIS

## Physical Examination

Careful assessment of the epididymides during the physical examination of an infertile patient is as important as the testicular evaluation. The consistency of the epididymis can help differentiate obstructive from nonobstructive causes of azoospermia. A large and turgid feel to the epididymis implies obstruction of sperm outflow, whereas a small and flaccid epididymis indicates a likely problem of spermatogenesis. Tenderness to palpation can indicate the presence of inflammation or infection. Palpation of a cystic structure originating from the epididymis indicates the presence of a spermatocele; aspiration of the cyst fluid revealing sperm confirms the diagnosis. In patients presenting with acute scrotal pain, the presence of a paratesticular or epididymal nodule or "blue dot" and absence of testicular pain help to distinguish testicular torsion from torsion of the testicular appendages.

## Development

The epididymis develops from the portion of the mesonephric duct that was directly associated with the mesonephros; all mesonephric tubules degenerate along with the mesonephros, except the vasa efferentia, which become highly convoluted tubules (11). In humans, the epididymis is well developed by 16 weeks of gestation, and secretory activity of the epididymal cells has been observed by 25 weeks of gestation (12).

## Anatomy

The epididymis is a single tubule 6 to 7 m in length with the cauda forming half of the length (Fig. 53.2); the long distance provides gametes both time and resources to mature during their travel down the tract (32,34). The rete testis gives rise to 8 to 12 ductuli efferentes that penetrate the tunica albuginea and form the lobules that comprise the caput of the epididymis (34). Anatomically, the epididymis is divided in three parts, the caput (head), the corpus (body), and the cauda (tail). More specifically, the epididymis is composed of the terminal part of the ductuli efferentes, the ductus epididymis, and the initial portion of the vas deferens (34). Each segment of the epididymis features the characteristic size and shape of the ducts, epithelial lining, contractile elements, innervation, and vascularization (34).

The luminal shape on transverse section of the epididymis varies from the irregular stellate shape in the ductuli efferentes to the regular, round, or oval shape in the ductus epididymis to

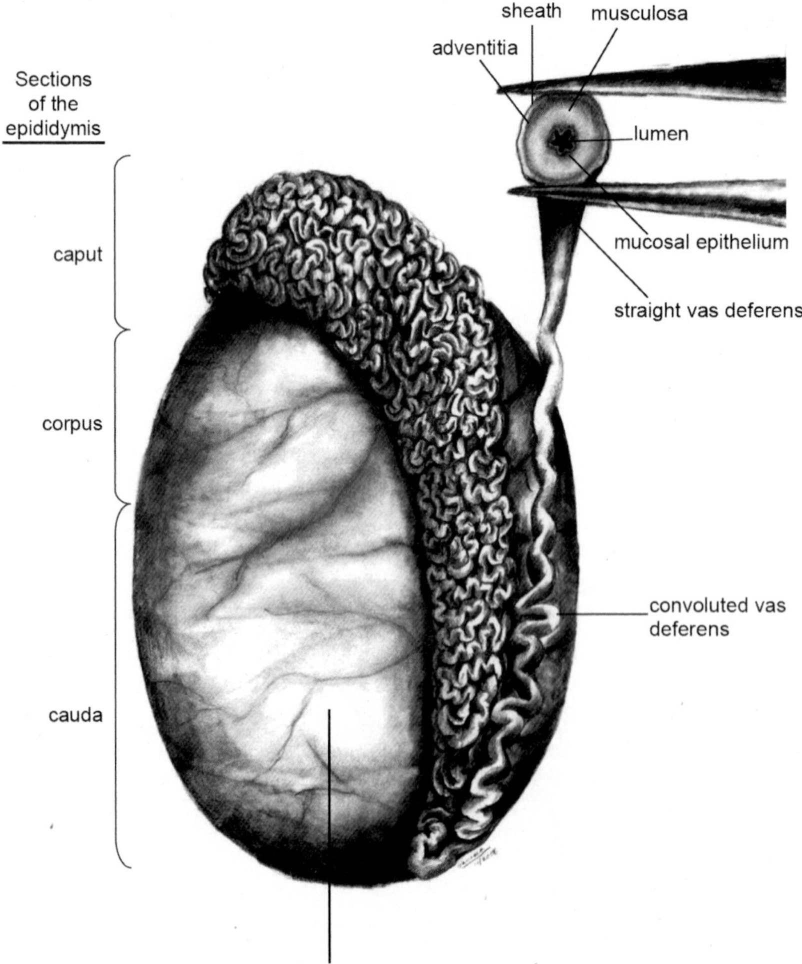


FIGURE 53.2 Epididymis and vas deferens.

the wide irregularity of the cauda epididymis (34). The duct constricts at the caudal section before it widens considerably (34). The luminal shape and size reflect the different function of each segment as well as the different cellular components contained within. The epithelium of the ductuli efferentes is prismatic; at least two cell types, some with cilia and others with microvilli, are gathered according to size in a single layer with their apical poles joined by junctional complexes (34). As variant cell morphologies may reflect adaptations of the same cell, different investigators report different numbers of cell types. The epithelium of the ductus epididymis is a prismatic pseudostratified type with basal and chief cells, among other cell types (34). The epithelial transition from the cauda to the initial portion of the vas deferens is progressive, without striking changes in the cellular organization (34). The sheath enclosing the entire epididymis contains a continuous layer of contractile cells, organized circularly or in a light spiral, with rare longitudinal bundles outside the circular layers (34). In the cauda, the contractile cells are replaced by smooth muscle cells forming three layers, inner and outer longitudinal and intermediate circular, that thicken and continue into the vas deferens (34).

The delicate structure of the epididymis makes it vulnerable to iatrogenic injury. The epididymis may be violated during procedures such as hydrocelectomy, spermatocelectomy, and orchiopexy, especially if the epididymis is adherent to the tunica vaginalis. Furthermore, unlike vascular injuries, which declare themselves immediately with hematoma or ecchymosis formation, epididymal injury may not be evident until the patient later presents for fertility evaluation. Hopps and Goldstein (16) reported the restoration of spermatozoa in the ejaculate in five of six patients following microsurgical repair of iatrogenic epididymal injury from hydrocelectomy. Blockage of the epididymis is not limited to iatrogenic injuries; trauma, infection, inflammation, and even blockage of the vas deferens (i.e., vasectomy) and subsequent increase in intraluminal pressure can result in epididymal obstruction.

### Blood Supply

The epididymis is supplied by the spermatic and funicular vascular pedicles (7). An intra-abdominal branch of the spermatic artery divides to feed the corpus, and an inguinal branch divides to feed the caput (7). The funicular pedicle consists of the deferential artery, which is a branch of the internal iliac artery or from a branch of the internal iliac artery, usually the superior vesical artery, and runs along the vas deferens onto the cauda; and the funicular artery, which starts at the vesicular artery and supplies the vas deferens and the cauda; the funicular artery is thought to be the most important contribution to the main muscular epithelium of the cauda (7). Just as the hypogastric artery is now referred to as the internal iliac artery, the funicular vessel has fallen out of favor and is rarely referenced outside of historical anatomy texts. A more recent description of epididymal blood supply attributes the testicular (internal spermatic) artery as the source of the superior epididymal artery of the globus major of the epididymis and the cremasteric artery as the origin of the inferior epididymal artery of the globus minor of the epididymis (17).

In humans, the testicular vascular and epididymal vascular systems form anastomoses (7); this redundancy is helpful to microsurgeons performing vasectomy reversals and other scrotal procedures that can potentially interrupt blood supply to the testis or epididymis. Despite this contact with the testicular blood supply, the epididymis is generally independent of the testicular vascular network, and there is little direct hormonal exchange by this route, although the direct linkage of the lymphatic drainage of the testis and epididymis allows for passage of testicular hormones into the epididymis (7). The capillary network of the epididymis is much more extensive than that of the testis, with the density of microvessels reflecting the concentration and demands of the specialized epithelial cells (7).

### Innervation

Sympathetic nerve endings are concentrated in the corpus and cauda of the epididymis with progressive density approaching the vas deferens, consistent with their contractile role during ejaculation (34). In the ductuli efferentes and proximal epididymis, the sympathetic nerves form a loose peritubular plexus without penetrating between the cells (34). The distal portion of the epididymis demonstrates intermittent contractions during ejaculation, in contrast to the peristaltic activity of the proximal epididymis (34). Mean transit time of sperm in the epididymis of humans is 12 days (26).

## Function

In addition to the transport of spermatozoa with smooth muscle contractions, the epididymis stores and facilitates maturation of the spermatozoa. Fluid resorption at the caput epididymis concentrates sperm by 20-fold (9). Turner et al. (33) hypothesized that the dilution of epididymal fluid on ejaculation along with the addition of electrolytes promote sperm motility. Acott et al. (1,4) presented evidence that sperm motility may depend on changes in intrasperm cyclic adenosine monophosphate (cAMP) levels and the binding of a forward motility protein of epididymal origin. The epididymis also synthesizes and secretes proteins thought to be involved in the development of motility and fertilizing capacity (18). Studies in rats have demonstrated reconstruction of membrane glycoproteins of spermatozoa resulting from interactions with epididymal secretory proteins as part of the maturation process (5). The maturation process within the epididymis is dependent on androgens. In a study of the rat epididymis, castration resulted in changes in the ultrastructural organization of the epididymal epithelium and inhibition of secretory function (22). Fertilization with spermatozoa from the caput epididymis is possible, however. Silber (30) performed vasoepididymostomy in 51 patients with blockage at the caput epididymis; pregnancy rates with spermatozoa from the proximal and distal caput were 33% and 50%, respectively.

# VAS DEFERENS

## Physical Examination

The most important aspect of the physical examination of the vasa deferentia is to simply confirm their presence (Fig. 53.3). About 95% of men with cystic fibrosis have congenital bilateral absence of the vasa deferentia (CBAVD) (6). As over 70% of men with CBAVD have mutations in at least one allele of the cystic fibrosis transmembrane conductance regulator (CFTR) gene detectable by routine testing methods, couples with CBAVD wanting to conceive should undergo genetic testing (6).

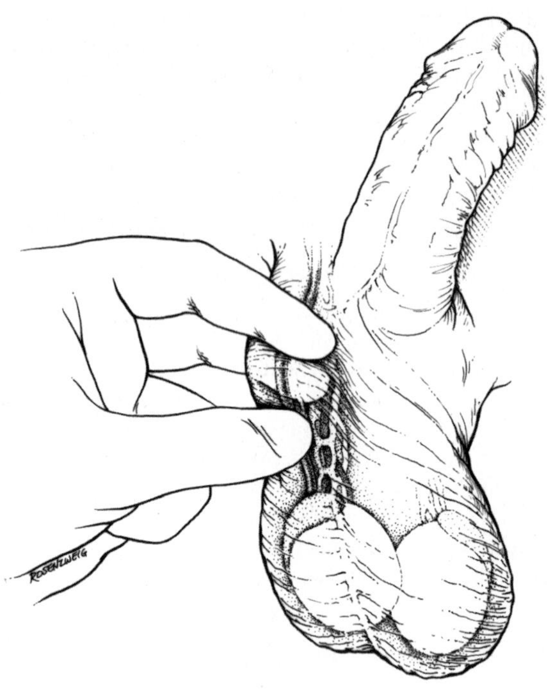

FIGURE 53.3 Palpation of the vas deferens on physical examination. (From Goldstein M. Surgical management of male infertility and other scrotal disorders. In: *Campbell's urology*, 8th ed. Philadelphia: WB Saunders, 2002:1532–1587, with permission.)

In addition, abdominal ultrasonography should be performed to assess the man for associated renal anomalies. Schlegel et al. (27) reported 26% of men with unilateral congenital absence of the vas deferens and 11% of men with CBAVD to have renal agenesis. Scrotal ultrasonography is helpful in detecting other urogenital anomalies, such as contralateral ejaculatory duct and epididymal or vasal obstruction in men with unilateral congenital absence of the vas deferens (13).

## Development

The vas deferens is formed by the portion of the mesonephric duct from the mesonephros to the urogenital sinus (11). The vas deferens is taken along with the testis during its descent and inguinal passage; the vas deferens is progressively stretched during this process (11).

## Anatomy

The vas deferens stretches about 45 cm in length as it travels from the cauda epididymis through the inguinal canal to join the seminal vesicle behind the bladder and form the ejaculatory duct that empties into the prostatic urethra (35). The lumen of the scrotal portion averages about 330 $\mu$m in diameter. Two distinct histologies divide the vas deferens into the vasal portion, comprising the proximal 40 cm of length, and the ampullary portion, comprising the distal 5 cm (35). The cylindrical vasal portion is 2 to 4 mm in diameter and resembles the cauda epididymis (35). In contrast, the ampulla is dilated and fusiform and resembles the seminal vesicle (35).

The thick, muscular wall (>1 mm thickness) of the vas deferens contrasts with its narrow lumen (0.5 mm) (35). It is composed of three layers: mucosa, musculosa, and adventitia. The mucosa (60 $\mu$m thickness) is lined by a tall columnar epithelium containing chief cells, dark or pencil cells, mitochondrion-rich cells, and basal cells (35). The muscular layer forms >80% of the wall thickness, and the component large smooth muscle cells are arranged in an outer and inner longitudinal orientation with a thick middle circular or spiral layer (35). The adventitia contains blood vessels and nerves (35).

The vas deferens is vulnerable to injury, especially in its course through the inguinal canal. Inguinal hernia repair in both adults and children is an important cause of vasal obstruction. In adults, the vas deferens can become entangled in the synthetic mesh of the hernia repair. In children, the vas deferens can be ligated inadvertently with the hernia sac. The vas is only 1 mm in external diameter before puberty and 2 mm after midpuberty (24). In a report by Sheynkin et al. (29), 7.2% of 472 men surgically explored for obstructive azoospermia had an iatrogenic injury to the vas deferens. Twenty patients had undergone pediatric inguinal hernia repair, and 10 patients had undergone adult inguinal hernia repair, the two most common etiologies of vasal injury. Overall, vasal injury was secondary to bilateral inguinal hernia repair in 19 patients, to unilateral inguinal hernia repair in 11, to renal transplantation in 2, to appendectomy in 1, and to spermatocelectomy in 1 (29).

### Blood Supply

The blood supply to the vas deferens is derived from the deferential artery, which originates from the internal iliac artery (28). The vas deferens features two distinct vascular networks: the larger vessels of the adventitia provide branches that penetrate the musculosa centripetally to the lamina propria, where a dense capillary network resides in the subepithelium (28). In rat studies, a distinct subepithelial sinusoidal network is seen, and the sinusoidal network is thought to function during ejaculation in increasing intraluminal pressure (14,23,28,31). The deferential artery is surrounded by a dense adrenergic network, and it contracts and relaxes in response to different agonists, demonstrating that it plays an active role in regulating the vasal blood supply (21). Venous drainage occurs via the deferential vein, which travels along the vas deferens to empty into the hypogastric vein (28).

### Innervation

The high density of the adrenergic nerve endings of the distal epididymis continues into the three layers of the vas deferens (28), although it has been noted that adrenergic innervation in humans is less extensive than in other species (2). Cholinergic neurons have also been demonstrated in the vas deferens (28).

# SEMINAL VESICLE

## Physical Examination

Palpation of the seminal vesicles provides important information for urologic specialists in oncology or fertility. Ideally, the former group uses the digital rectal examination of the seminal vesicles to feel for their involvement in prostate cancer and the latter group to collect evidence for ejaculatory duct obstruction in men with azoospermia and low-volume ejaculate. In reality, unless the examiner is blessed with long, slender digits, the seminal vesicles are difficult to reach for adequate palpation. Although transrectal ultrasonography cannot substitute for the tactile assessment of cancer, infertility specialists fortunately can use this noninvasive test to help diagnose ejaculatory duct obstruction when the seminal vesicles elude the reach of their index fingers. Seminal vesicle dilatation >1.5 cm and other signs, including dilatation of the ejaculatory duct, calcifications within the duct, and the presence of midline cysts on transrectal ultrasonography, suggest the diagnosis of ejaculatory duct obstruction. However, transrectal ultrasonography is less accurate than the traditional diagnostic combination of testicular biopsy and vasography (Fig. 53.4).

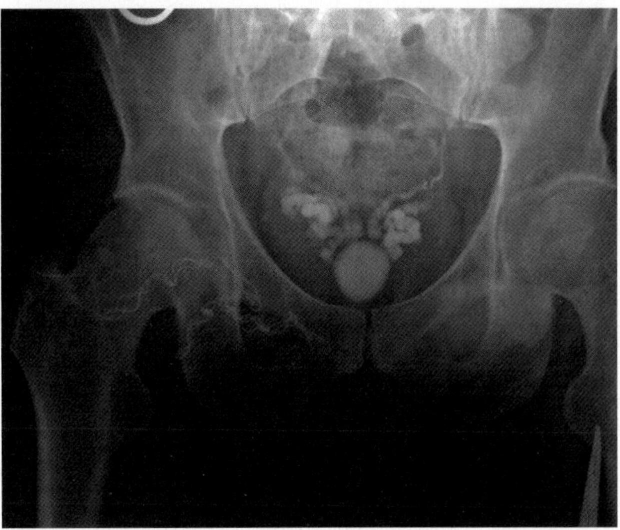

FIGURE 53.4 Left vasogram demonstrating contrast in the vas deferens, seminal vesicle, and bladder, indicating patency of the left excurrent ductal system. Residual contrast seen in right seminal vesicle from previously performed right vasogram.

## Development

The caudal end of the Wolffian duct develops into the seminal vesicle, first as a dilatation, then as an evagination (15). This simple tube branches into a lobular structure during its development, organizing into ducts draining into a principal excretory duct (15). The few differentiated cuboidal cells that line the Wolffian duct during fetal life undergo several modifications with the production of androgens by the fetal testis and are eventually replaced at puberty by a glandular epithelium (15). In humans, the seminal vesicles are relatively undifferentiated during infancy and adolescence and develop their secretory activity between 16 and 18 years of age (3,15).

## Anatomy

The seminal vesicles (Fig. 53.5) are exocrine glands that empty into the ejaculatory ducts (Fig. 53.6). They enrich the sperm with proteins, enzymes, fructose, and other substances, contributing 46% to 80% of the total ejaculate volume (20). As such, the seminal vesicles are designed to optimize their secretory function. The three layers of the seminal vesicle wall include villous mucosa, smooth muscle, and external sheath (10). The mucosa consists of a pseudo-stratified epithelium containing granular columnar cells and ovoid basal cells resting on a basement membrane surrounded by loose connective tissue replete with elastic fibers (10). The histology of the seminal vesicle is identical to that of the ampulla of the vas deferens (10). The epithelium is composed of principal secretory cells, basal cells, and duct cells, which are considered variants of principal cells (3,10). The principal cells metabolize the secretory components of seminal vesicle plasma and are dependent on androgens and other hormones such as prolactin for growth and activation (10).

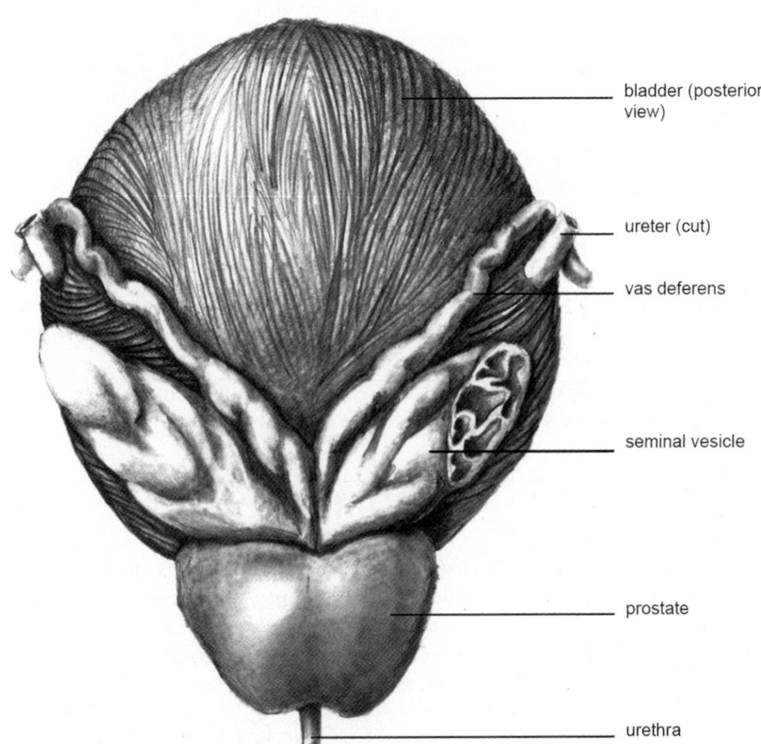


FIGURE 53.5 Seminal vesicles, posterior view.

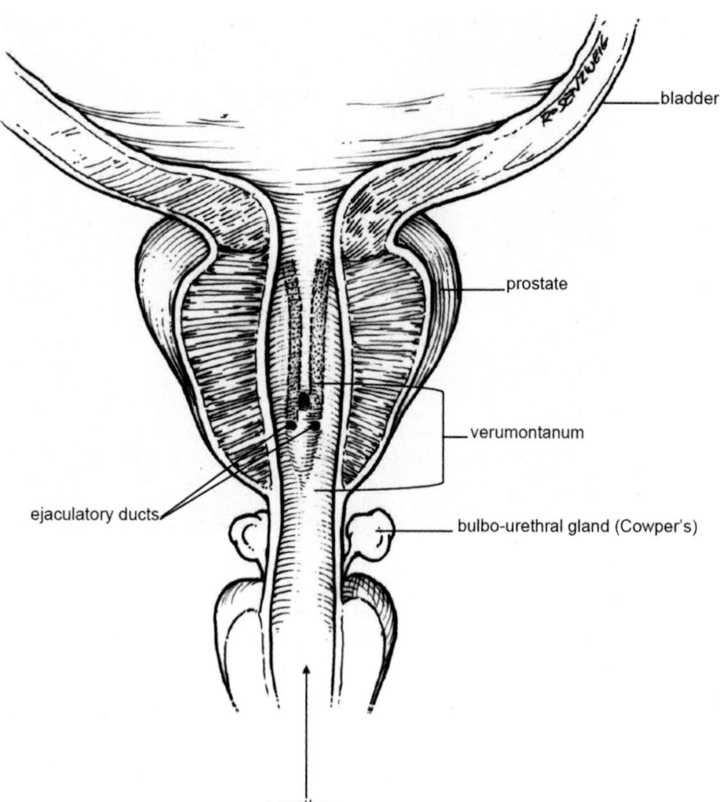


FIGURE 53.6 Ejaculatory ducts. (Adapted from Goldstein M. Surgical management of male infertility and other scrotal disorders. In: *Campbell's urology*, 8th ed. Philadelphia: WB Saunders, 2002:1532–1587.)

### Blood Supply

The seminal vesicle receives its blood supply from the internal iliac artery via the vesiculodeferential artery (28). Venous outflow is provided by the prostatic plexus and the inferior vesical plexus, which in turn drain into the internal iliac vein (28).

### Function

The seminal plasma, composed of fluid from the seminal vesicles, prostate, and accessory glands, contains a wide range of substances, including inorganic ions, low-molecular-weight organic molecules such as citrate, reducing sugars, amino acids, and prostaglandins (28). Using a rat model system, Clavert et al. (8) examined the role of the seminal vesicle fluid on fertility. They concluded that seminal plasma prevents agglutination of sperm, stabilizes the sperm cytoplasmic membrane, coats antigens on the sperm surface, forms a coagulum to prevent loss of deposited sperm, and in the female genital tract stimulates smooth muscle activity and inhibits lymphocytic reactions (8).

## ACCESSORY GLANDS

### Prostate

Although an important organ of the male reproductive tract, the prostate is featured in its own chapters and will not be reviewed here.

### Bulbourethral (Cowper) Glands and Urethral Glands

Bulbourethral glands are paired multilobular glands that are located at the penile bulb and empty into the urethra (28). A fibroelastic capsule and a thick striated compressor muscle surround a network of elastic and muscle fibers separated by connective tissue septa (28). A single layer of cuboidal or squamous cells lines the ducts, while mucuslike cells line the glandular alveoli (25,28). The bulbourethral glands receive their blood supply from the artery to the bulb of the penis as well as the internal pudendal artery, the urethral artery, the perineal artery, and the anastomosis of the cystic inferior and internal pudendal arteries (19,28). Motor nerves control the smooth muscle contraction, vascular tone, and secretory activity of the accessory glands (28). Primary innervation of the smooth muscle of the accessory glands is provided by adrenergic fibers arising from the ipsilateral pelvic plexus (28). The vasculature is innervated by a separate system of nerves traveling with the blood vessels (28). Urethral glands or the glands of Littre open into the urethra and, similar to bulbourethral glands, secrete mucus during intercourse.

## SUMMARY

The anatomic features of the epididymis, vas deferens, and seminal vesicle reflect their function. An understanding of the anatomy of the excurrent ductal system facilitates the diagnostic workup and physical examination as well as the surgical management of male fertility disorders.

## *References*


1. Acott TS, Johnson DJ, Brandt H, et al. Sperm forward motility protein: tissue distribution and species cross reactivity. *Biol Reprod* 1979;20: 247–252.
2. Alm P. On the autonomic innervation of the human vas deferens. *Brain Res Bull* 1982;9:673–677.
3. Aumüller G. *Prostate gland and seminal vesicles*. Berlin: Springer, 1979.
4. Brandt H, Acott TS, Johnson DJ, et al. Evidence for an epididymal origin of bovine sperm forward motility protein. *Biol Reprod* 1978;19:830–835.
5. Brown CR, von Glos KI, Jones R. Changes in plasma membrane glycoproteins of rat spermatozoa during maturation in the epididymis. *J Cell Biol* 1983;96:256–264.
6. Chillon M, Casals T, Mercier B, et al. Mutations in the cystic fibrosis gene in patients with congenital absence of the vas deferens. *N Engl J Med* 1995;332:1475–1480.
7. Clavert A, Cranz C, Brun B. Epididymal vascularization and microvascularization. In: Bollack C, Clavert A, eds. *Progress in reproductive biology*, Vol. 8. Basel: S. Karger, 1981:48–57.
8. Clavert A, Gabriel-Robez O, Montagnon D. Physiological role of the seminal vesicle. In: Bollack C, Clavert A, eds. *Progress in reproductive biology and medicine*, Vol. 12: *Seminal vesicles and fertility*. Basel: S. Karger, 1985:80–94.
9. Courot M. Transport and maturation of spermatozoa in the epididymis of mammals. In: Bollack C, Clavert A, eds. *Progress in reproductive biology*, Vol. 8: *Epididymis and fertility: biology and pathology*. Basel: S. Karger, 1981:67–79.
10. Dadoune JP. Functional morphology of the seminal vesicle epithelium. In: Bollack C, Clavert A, eds. *Progress in reproductive biology and medicine*, Vol. 12: *Seminal vesicles and fertility*. Basel: S. Karger, 1985:18–35.
11. Gier HT, Marion GB. *Development of the mammalian testis*, Vol. 1: *Development, anatomy, and physiology*. New York: Academic Press, 1970.
12. Grignon G, Hatier R, Malaprade D. Histogenesis of the epididymis. In: Bollack C, Clavert A, eds. *Progress in reproductive biology*, Vol. 8. Basel: S. Karger, 1981:12–20.
13. Hall S, Oates RD. Unilateral absence of the scrotal vas deferens associated with contralateral mesonephric duct anomalies resulting in infertility: laboratory, physical and radiographic findings, and therapeutic alternatives. *J Urol* 1993;150:1161–1164.
14. Hamilton DW, Cooper TG. Gross and histological variations along the length of the rat vas deferens. *Anat Rec* 1978;190:795–809.
15. Hatier R, Grignon G, Guedenet JC. Development of the seminal vesicles. In: Bollack C, Clavert A, eds. *Progress in reproductive biology and medicine*, Vol. 12: *Seminal vesicles and fertility*. Basel: S. Karger, 1985:4–7.
16. Hopps CV, Goldstein M. Microsurgical reconstruction of iatrogenic injuries to the epididymis from hydrocelectomy. *J Urol* 2006;176: 2077–2079; discussion 2080.
17. Jabren GW, Hellstrom WJG. Trauma to the external genitalia. In: Wessells H, McAninch JW, eds. *Urological emergencies: a practical guide*, 1st ed. Totowa, N.J.: Humana Press, 2005;71–93.
18. Jones R, Brown CR, Von Glos KI, et al. Hormonal regulation of protein synthesis in the rat epididymis. Characterization of androgen-dependent and testicular fluid-dependent proteins. *Biochem J* 1980;188:667–676.
19. Lasinski W, Sikorski A. Arterial vascularization of the human bulbourethral glands [in French]. *Bull Assoc Anat (Nancy)* 1975;59:911–918.
20. Lundquist F. Studies on the biochemistry of human semen; the viscosimetric determination of hyaluronidase. *Acta Physiol Scand* 1949;17:44–54.
21. Medina P, Chuan P, Noguera R, et al. Reactivity of human deferential artery to constrictor and dilator substances. *J Androl* 1996;17:733–739.
22. Moore HD, Bedford JM. Short-term effects of androgen withdrawal on the structure of different epithelial cells in the rat epididymis. *Anat Rec* 1979;193:293–311.
23. Ohtani O, Gannon BJ. The microvasculature of the rat vas deferens: a scanning electron and light microscopic study. *J Anat* 1982;135:521–529.
24. Pryor JL, Fusia T, Mercer M, et al. Injury to the pre-pubertal vas deferens. II. Experimental repair. *J Urol* 1991;146:477–480.
25. Riva A, Usai E, Cossu M, et al. The human bulbo-urethral glands. A transmission electron microscopy and scanning electron microscopy study. *J Androl* 1988;9:133–141.
26. Rowley MJ, Teshima F, Heller CG. Duration of transit of spermatozoa through the human male ductular system. *Fertil Steril* 1970;21:390–396.
27. Schlegel PN, Shin D, Goldstein M. Urogenital anomalies in men with congenital absence of the vas deferens. *J Urol* 1996;155:1644–1648.
28. Setchell BP, Maddocks S, Brooks DE. *Anatomy, vasculature, innervation, and fluids of the male reproductive tract*, 2nd ed., Vol. 1. New York: Raven Press, 1994.
29. Sheynkin YR, Hendin BN, Schlegel PN, et al. Microsurgical repair of iatrogenic injury to the vas deferens. *J Urol* 1998;159:139–141.
30. Silber SJ. Apparent fertility of human spermatozoa from the caput epididymidis. *J Androl* 1989;10:263–269.
31. Suzuki F. Microvasculature of the mouse testis and excurrent duct system. *Am J Anat* 1982;163:309–325.
32. Turner TT. De Graaf's thread: the human epididymis. *J Androl* 2008;29:237–250.
33. Turner TT, D'Addario D, Howards SS. Further observations on the initiation of sperm motility. *Biol Reprod* 1978;19:1095–1101.
34. Vendrely E. Histology of the epididymis in the human adult. In: Bollack C, Clavert A, eds. *Progress in reproductive biology*, Vol. 8. Basel: S. Karger, 1981:21–33.
35. Vendrely E. Structure and histophysiology of the human vas deferens. In: Bollack C, Clavert A, eds. *Progress in reproductive biology and medicine*, Vol. 12: *Seminal vesicles and fertility*. Basel: S. Karger, 1985:8–17.


# CHAPTER 54 ■ SEMINAL VESICLE AND EJACULATORY DUCT SURGERY

JAY I. SANDLOW

## SEMINAL VESICLE SURGERY

The seminal vesicles are paired male organs with no female homologue. They develop as a dorsolateral bulbous swelling of the distal mesonephric duct at approximately 12 fetal weeks. The blood supply to the seminal vesicle is from the vesiculodeferential artery, a branch of the umbilical artery. Venous drainage is from the vesiculodeferential veins and the inferior vesical plexus. The seminal vesicles are innervated by the pelvic nerve and the hypogastric nerve. The hypogastric nerve sends both adrenergic and cholinergic fibers to the seminal vesicles. Lymphatic drainage is via the internal iliac nodes (1).

Primary pathology within the seminal vesicles is rare; secondary lesions are more common. In the past, insufficient imaging methods led to infrequent definition of either primary or secondary seminal vesicle pathology. The use of transrectal ultrasonography (TRUS), computerized tomography (CT), and magnetic resonance imaging (MRI) has improved diagnostic visibility and facilitated the diagnosis and treatment of seminal vesicle pathology. The necessity of surgical intervention is rare, but indications include congenital cysts with infection and/or obstruction causing infertility, ureteral ectopy into a seminal vesicle with resultant obstruction or dysplasia of the ipsilateral kidney, and primary tumors, either benign or malignant. Surgical access to the seminal vesicles is mostly via routes familiar to the urologic surgeon, but surgery on the seminal vesicles alone (without adjacent organ removal) is a unique challenge.

## Diagnosis

The normal seminal vesicle on TRUS is an elongated, flat, paired structure between the rectum and the bladder just superior to the prostate and is typically not palpable on digital rectal examination. The diagnosis of seminal vesicle neoplasms can be difficult because they often do not cause symptoms until late in their course. General symptoms that may occur include urinary retention, dysuria, hematuria, or hematospermia. A mass is often palpable above the prostate and is usually not tender. TRUS is usually the next step in diagnosis and may be accompanied by needle aspiration or biopsy for diagnosis. CT or MRI would then be appropriate to stage the patient and may also be used to stage solid lesions within the pelvis, as well as to confirm the hemorrhagic nature of suspicious masses. Because prostate cancer may be mistaken for primary seminal vesicle cancer, serum prostate-specific antigen (PSA), as well as tissue immunohistochemical stains for PSA, should, if positive, help define the prostate as the site of primary malignancy. In infertile patients who present with azoospermia, or in patients with hematospermia or coital pain, TRUS is the initial imaging study. Contrast vasography accurately images the vas deferens and ampullary–seminal vesicle junction but is less reliable than TRUS for seminal vesicle pathology.

## Alternative Therapy

There are relatively few alternatives to treatment of seminal vesicle masses, unless they are infected. Antibiotics may be utilized in this case. Many of the benign masses are asymptomatic and may be observed. Ejaculatory duct obstruction can also be observed if fertility is not an issue or if the couple desires sperm acquisition with in vitro fertilization.

## Indications for Surgery

Treatments of conditions of the seminal vesicles alone are limited to (i) transperineal/transvesical aspiration of seminal vesicle cysts or abscesses, (ii) transurethral unroofing of seminal vesicle cysts or abscesses, (iii) laparoscopic or robotic dissection, and (iv) open resection of one or both seminal vesicles.

Most procedures performed on the seminal vesicles are related to radical surgery for the treatment of urethral, prostate, bladder, or rectal cancer. Treatments specific to the seminal vesicle include transrectal aspiration of cysts or abscesses, transurethral unroofing of abscesses and obstructing cysts, and open resection for refractory infections, to excise an ectopic ureter, or to remove benign or malignant masses.

If a solid lesion identified in the seminal vesicle shows no evidence of local spread and is benign on biopsy, treatment is dependent on symptoms. If the patient is asymptomatic, close follow-up consisting of repeat rectal examination and TRUS to determine subsequent growth of the tumor is reasonable. If the mass enlarges or if the patient has symptoms referable to the mass, simple seminal vesiculectomy is advisable. This may be accomplished through one of several routes described below. If the mass is quite large and solid and demonstrates questionable margins, or if the biopsy shows malignant cells, the treatment of choice is quite different. Because fewer than 10 cases of primary tumors of the seminal vesicles have been treated at any one institution, it is difficult to define optimal treatment with any degree of certainty. Radical excision, which usually includes a cystoprostatectomy with pelvic lymphadenectomy, is the treatment of choice unless the tumor is extremely small. This recommendation is based on the extensive nature of the majority of the cancers when detected. The excision may include the rectum (total pelvic exenteration) if it is thought to be invading the surrounding structures. Adjuvant therapy has no proven efficacy, although the only long-term survivors in the literature received radical surgery with subsequent pelvic radiation therapy or androgen deprivation therapy. No chemotherapeutic regimen is known to be efficacious.

## Surgery

The most useful open surgical methods include transperineal, similar to radical perineal prostatectomy; transvesical, achieved by incising through the posterior bladder wall; paravesical; retrovesical; or transcoccygeal. Over the past decade, the laparoscopic or robotically assisted approaches to benign seminal vesicle lesions have been found to be remarkably direct and associated with much less postoperative morbidity than the open surgical approach (2). The choice of surgical approach, of course, depends partly on the characteristics of the lesion to be treated but probably more on the experience and expertise of the surgeon. For the most part, congenital lesions require an abdominal approach so that the ipsilateral kidney can be dealt with concomitantly, if necessary. Such lesions may be dealt with by laparoscopic or open surgical intervention. Benign lesions may be approached perineally; however, the risk of impotence is high even if a nerve-sparing approach is attempted. Larger benign tumors or cysts are best handled by an anterior abdominal approach, although a transcoccygeal method may be as useful. Again, the transperitoneal or retroperitoneal laparoscopic approach has great merit for such lesions. Patients with malignancy require radical extirpation, which commonly includes cystoprostatoseminal vesiculectomy and pelvic lymphadenectomy. This operation is no different from a routine procedure for bladder cancer and, thus, is not described here.

### Preoperative Preparation

Preoperative preparation for laparoscopic, robotic, or open seminal vesicle surgery depends on the extent of the pathology and the planned incision. Transperineal, transcoccygeal, and transvesical approaches should be prefaced by a complete bowel preparation. Most surgeons use a mechanical preparation with GoLytely orally the evening before surgery, followed by the standard antibiotic bowel regimen. Some method to prevent phlebothrombosis in the legs, such as use of intermittent compression stockings during and immediately after surgery, is advisable.

## Surgical Technique

A variety of open surgical approaches to the seminal vesicles have been described, of which the most useful are the transvesical, transperineal, and laparoscopic.

### Transvesical Approach

The transvesical approach to the seminal vesicle has been described by numerous authors (3). A midline extraperitoneal suprapubic incision is made up to the umbilicus, and the rectus muscles are separated on the midline. The space of Retzius is opened by downward displacement of the transverse fascia on the pubis, and an Omni retractor is placed to expose the anterior bladder wall. Care is taken during this dissection not to injure the epigastric vessels on either side of the pubis. The bladder is opened longitudinally approximately 7 to 10 cm, ending 2 to 3 cm away from the bladder neck. Moist 4 × 8 sponges are placed on the bladder wall laterally and at the dome of the bladder, and specialized blades are placed to put the open bladder on stretch. Although it is not necessary, it is preferable to place long 8Fr feeding tubes in the ureters at this point to define the orifices and to help with identification of the subtrigonal ureters to prevent their injury later in the dissection. Using a Bovie cutting stylet, a vertical incision is made through the trigone on the posterior midline approximately 5 cm in length (Fig. 54.1A). Alternatively, a transverse incision just above the bladder neck can be used, but it is not preferred. The vertical incision is deepened through the bladder muscle, and the ampullae of the vas should be recognized directly beneath the bladder neck. They can be dissected by scissors down to their entrance into the prostate and then either ligated and divided or left intact, depending on the pathology, as described in the perineal approach. Just lateral to the ampullae on the prostate base, the seminal vesicles should be identified and the plane surrounding them entered easily unless there has been prior inflammatory disease (Fig 54.1B). The seminal vesicles should be encircled and dissected completely free. Metal clips should be placed on the vascular pedicle and a 2-0 chromic tie on the distal end at the prostate. A clip is placed across the proximal end of the vas to prevent seminal vesicle contents from obscuring the field, and then the vesicle is transected and removed. If there is a moderate-sized cyst, the dissection is more involved but is usually made simple because the perivesical plane is usually more pronounced. The plane may be very difficult to establish if there was prior vesiculitis, and in this instance the ureteral catheters are a welcome safeguard—care must be taken not to dissect completely through Denonvilliers fascia posteriorly and into the rectum. The posterior bladder incision is then closed with a running 2-0 absorbable suture in the muscle layer, followed by a running 4-0 absorbable suture in the mucosal layer. The ureteral stents and 4 × 8 sponges are removed, a 20Fr urethral catheter is placed, and the anterior bladder wall is closed as the posterior wall was. Suprapubic tube placement is an option but is not necessary. A suction drain is placed through a separate stab incision and positioned in the prevesical space away from the suture line. The urethral catheter is typically removed in 5 to 7 days. This approach is more prone to blood loss and ureteral injury than the perineal approach, but a rectal laceration is much less likely.

### Transperineal Approach

The transperineal approach to seminal vesiculectomy is virtually identical to radical perineal prostatectomy, described in

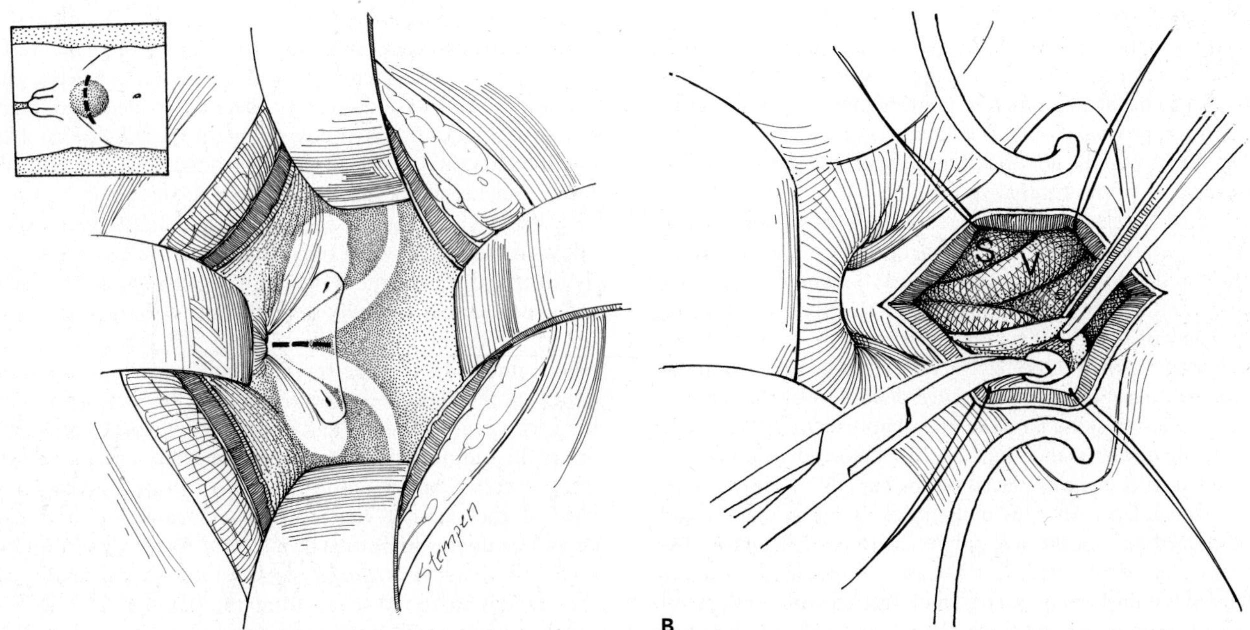


FIGURE 54.1 The transvesical approach to the seminal vesicle. **A:** Vertical incision in the trigone to expose the retrovesical seminal vesicle. **B:** Dissection of the vas ampullae and seminal vesicles.

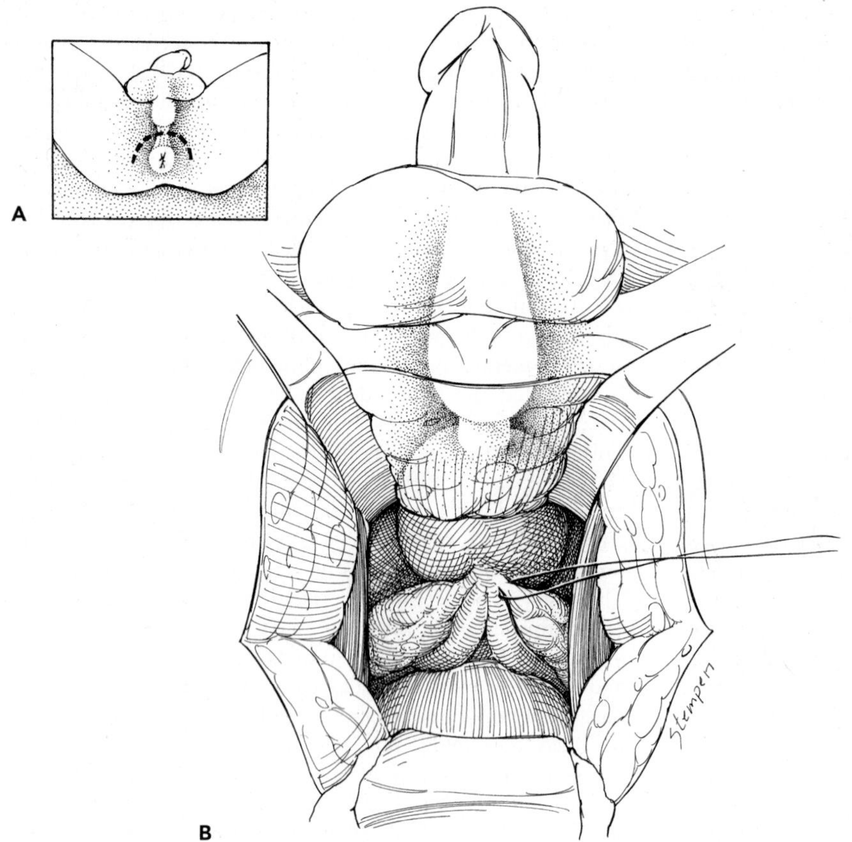


**FIGURE 54.2** The transperineal approach. **A:** U-shaped incision in the perineum with takedown of the central tendon. **B:** Exposure and ligation of the seminal vesicles after incising Denonvilliers fascia.

Chapter 29. An exaggerated dorsal lithotomy position is used to elevate the perineum so that it is parallel to the floor. An inverted-U incision is made in the perineum and the central tendon is divided (Fig. 54.2A). An anterior retractor stretches the rectal sphincter superiorly, allowing visualization of the glistening anterior rectal fascia fibers. The rectourethralis is divided near the prostatic apex and a weighted speculum is placed, dropping the tented rectum. To adequately expose the seminal vesicle, the rectum should be dissected off the posterior surface of the prostate to a point higher than that needed for perineal prostatectomy. Denonvilliers fascia is then incised transversely or in the midline (if nerve-sparing) on the prostate near the base of the seminal vesicles.

Seminal vesicle dissection is facilitated by posterior traction on the prostate provided by placement of a Lowsley retractor in the bladder. Medially, the ampullae and seminal vesicles are apparent after Denonvilliers fascia is incised (Fig. 54.2B). The ampullae can be spared for the excision of a simple seminal vesicle cyst or small tumor but may need to be resected in the setting of cancer or infection. After dissection of the seminal vesicle at the prostatic base, an absorbable tie of 2-0 suture is used to ligate the gland (Fig. 54.2B). Before division of the seminal vesicle, a clip is placed on the cut end of the organ to minimize spillage. An Allis or Babcock clamp is then placed on the freed base of the seminal vesicle to ease the apical dissection. The vascular pedicle at the apex of the gland is usually observed within 1 cm of the tip and is ligated with small metal clips, allowing gland removal. The wound is closed in layers as outlined for perineal prostatectomy. A Penrose drain is left in the area of dissection for 24 hours or until no drainage is noted. This approach is well tolerated, and patients are usually discharged within 24 to 48 hours of surgery.

## Paravesical and Retrovesical Approaches

The paravesical incision is used in children, when there is a large unilateral cyst that lies lateral to and above the bladder, and when nephroureterectomy is required. A midline or Pfannenstiel extraperitoneal suprapubic incision is made. The bladder is finger-dissected away from the lateral pelvic sidewall on the affected side. The vas deferens is identified, placed on tension, and dissected down toward the base of the bladder. If the seminal vesicle mass is distended, it should be visible rather quickly as the vas comes close to the bladder posteriorly. Placing a catheter in the bladder and emptying it usually allows the plane between the bladder and the cyst to be readily identified. The plane is incised with scissors, and the seminal vesicle cyst is carefully dissected away sharply. When the tip of the cyst is clearly identified, a 1-0 chromic suture is placed into it to provide traction, making further dissection easier. As the dissection proceeds, it must be remembered that the ureter crosses the vas and must be identified to prevent its injury. In addition, the superior vesicle artery and perhaps the inferior vesicle artery may be sacrificed to gain access to the base of the seminal vesicle. This will cause no harm and should be done without major concern. As the dissection proceeds, the bladder is progressively rolled over medially, and the mass is dissected away from the bladder laterally. The plane is easily maintained with sharp dissection. Any vessels feeding the seminal vesicles should be suture-ligated or metal-clipped. As the prostate is approached, caution must be used

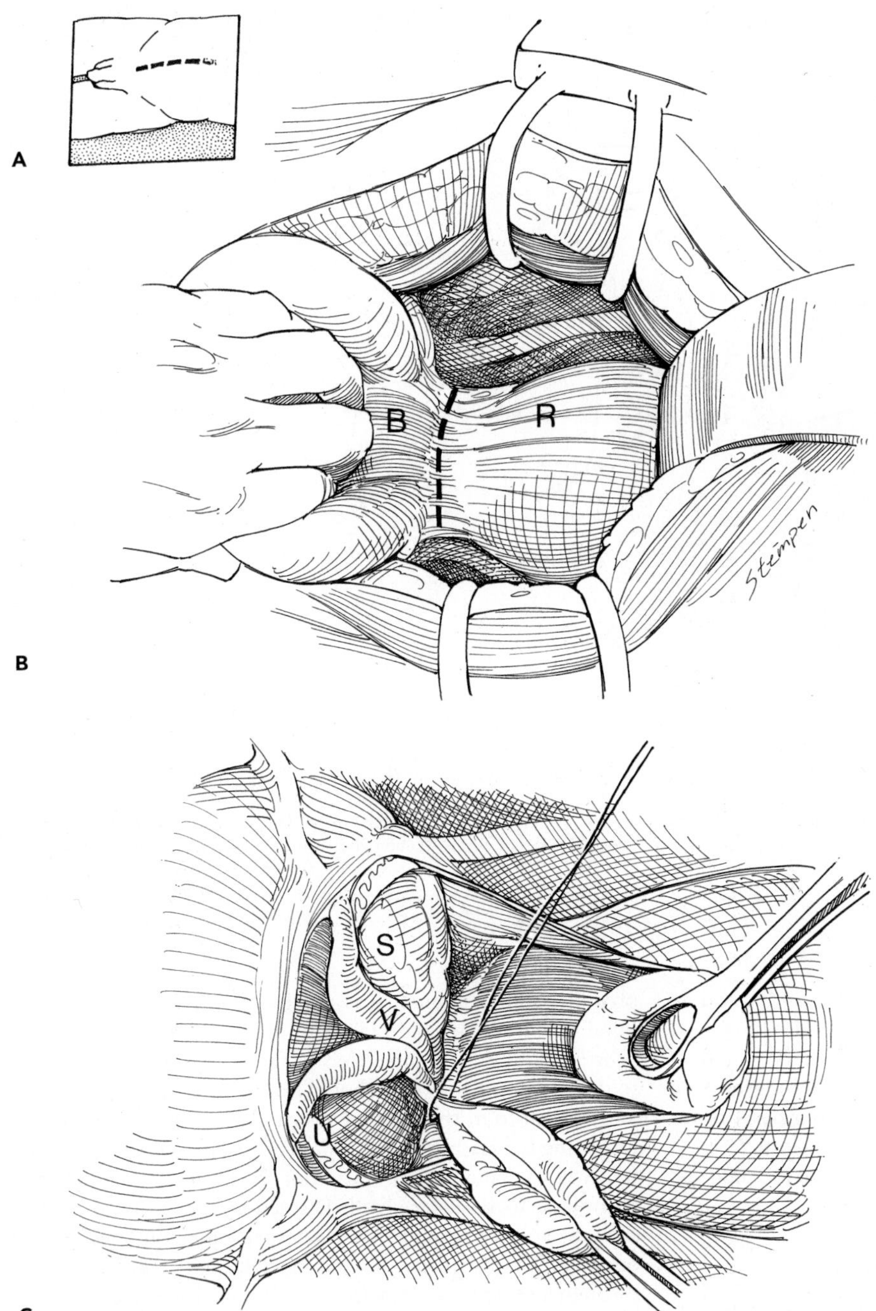


FIGURE 54.3 The retrovesical approach. **A:** Midline infraumbilical incision. **B:** Incision of the posterior peritoneum over the rectum in the cul-de-sac. **C:** Exposure of the vas ampulla and seminal vesicle behind the bladder.

to stay directly on the mass so as not to injure the neurovascular bundle lying just lateral to the seminal vesicle. At the prostate base, the neck of the seminal vesicle is encircled and ligated with a 2-0 absorbable suture. A clamp is placed across just distal to the tie, and the seminal vesicle is severed. There may be no need to clip the vas. A suction drain is placed in the bed of the seminal vesicle and brought out through a separate stab incision. The wound is then closed in layers. Postoperative care is as previously described, except with this approach, the drain can be removed within 24 hours if there is no drainage, and the urethral catheter can be removed within 24 hours. The patient may be discharged within 2 to 3 days. Complications include ureteral injury and excessive blood loss. If the principles outlined earlier are followed, these are unlikely events.

The retrovesical approach should be considered in patients requiring bilateral excision of small seminal vesicle cysts or benign masses (4). A midline suprapubic incision is made into the peritoneal space (Fig. 54.3A). A catheter is placed, and the urine is evacuated. The reflection of the peritoneum over the rectum at the posterior bladder wall is incised transversely, with care taken not to incise into the rectum (Fig. 54.3B). The bladder is peeled back from the rectum progressively with sharp dissection until the ampullae of the vasa and the tips of the seminal vesicles come into view (Fig. 54.3C). The seminal vesicles are dissected down to the base of the prostate, much as described in the transvesical approach, and the neck of the seminal vesicle is ligated and divided bilaterally. The ampullae are usually not taken unless necessary. A suction drain is left in the area posterior to the bladder and brought out as before.

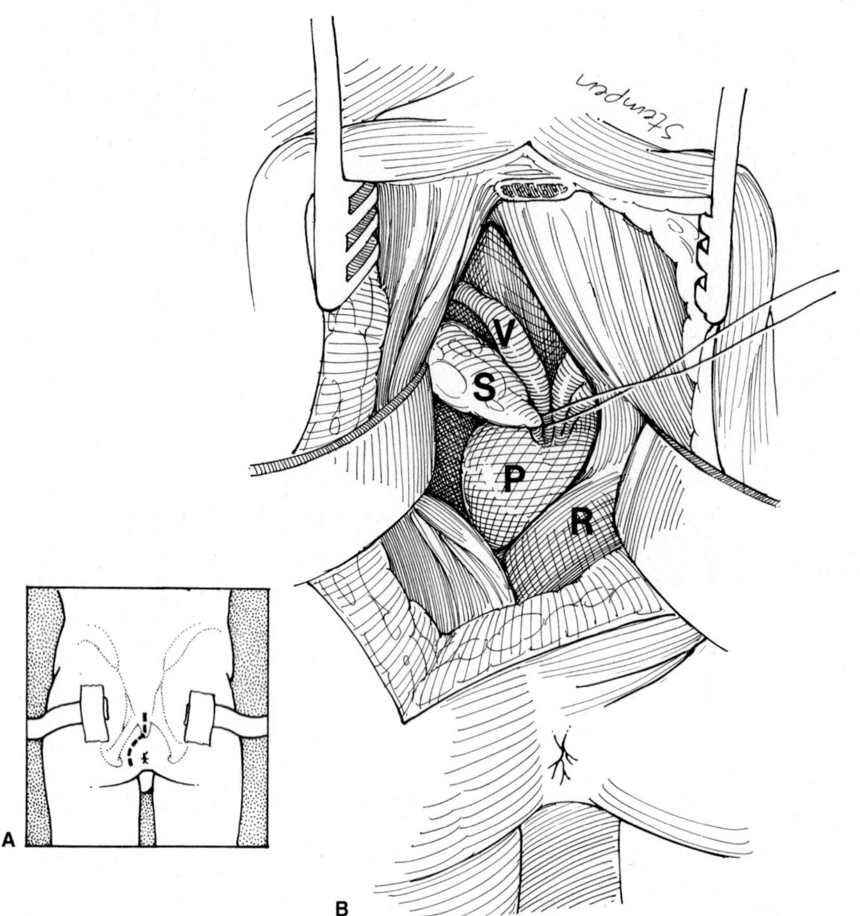


FIGURE 54.4 The transcoccygeal approach. **A:** The incision is made over the coccyx and curved along the gluteal cleft. **B:** Denonvilliers fascia is incised deep to the rectum to expose the prostate and seminal vesicles.

Postoperative care is as per the description for a paravesical resection. Complications include rectal injury, bladder laceration, and hemorrhage. In this situation, a rectal injury would be within the peritoneum well above the levator ani muscles. After a two-layer closure as before, strong consideration should be given to placement of omentum over the closure between the bladder base and the rectum, as well as to a temporary colostomy.

## Transcoccygeal Approach

The transcoccygeal approach may not be familiar to most urologic surgeons and is unlikely to be a common choice owing to fear of rectal injury and impotence. In individuals for whom the perineal or supine position may be difficult to maintain, or who have had multiple suprapubic or perineal surgeries, the transcoccygeal approach may be very useful. The patient is placed on the table, ventral side down (prone) and in a relative jackknife position (5). The incision is made in an L shape from midway on the sacrum (10 cm from the tip of the coccyx) and angled at the tip of the coccyx down the gluteal cleft within 3 cm of the anus (Fig. 54.4A). The incision is carried down to the lateral side of the coccyx, which is dissected free from the underlying rectum and eventually totally removed. The gluteus maximus muscle layers are moved aside, and the rectosigmoid is encountered and dissected carefully from the underside of the sacrum. With careful dissection, the lateral wall of the rectum on the side of the lesion is dissected medially from the levator ani muscle and surrounding tissue until the prostate is encountered. It is possible that the neurovascular bundle will be recognized from this approach. Once the prostate is palpated, dissection of the tissue directly superior to the base on the midline should reveal the ampulla of the vas and, lateral to it, the seminal vesicle (Fig. 54.4B). If difficulty dissecting the rectum away from the prostate is encountered, a finger in the anus via an O'Connor sheath will allow the correct plane to be determined. Dissection and removal of the seminal vesicles should follow the principles outlined previously. A Penrose drain should be left in the area, exiting through a separate stab incision at closure. The rectum should be carefully scrutinized for injury; if any injury is found, it is closed in two layers. The wound is closed in layers as well. Postoperative care does not differ from that previously described; similar to the perineal approach, the patient should have a rapid and easy recovery. The drain should be removed within 2 to 3 days if there is no drainage.

## Laparoscopic Technique

Most laparoscopic surgery performed on the seminal vesicles has been in conjunction with radical prostatectomy. It is known that dissection of the ampulla of the vas and seminal vesicles is a challenging part of a perineal prostatectomy, and thus prior mobilization of these structures made this easier. Its application for benign seminal vesicle pathology is limited to case reports or small series (2).

Patients are placed supine with the arms carefully padded and tucked in by the sides. Access to the perineum is usually

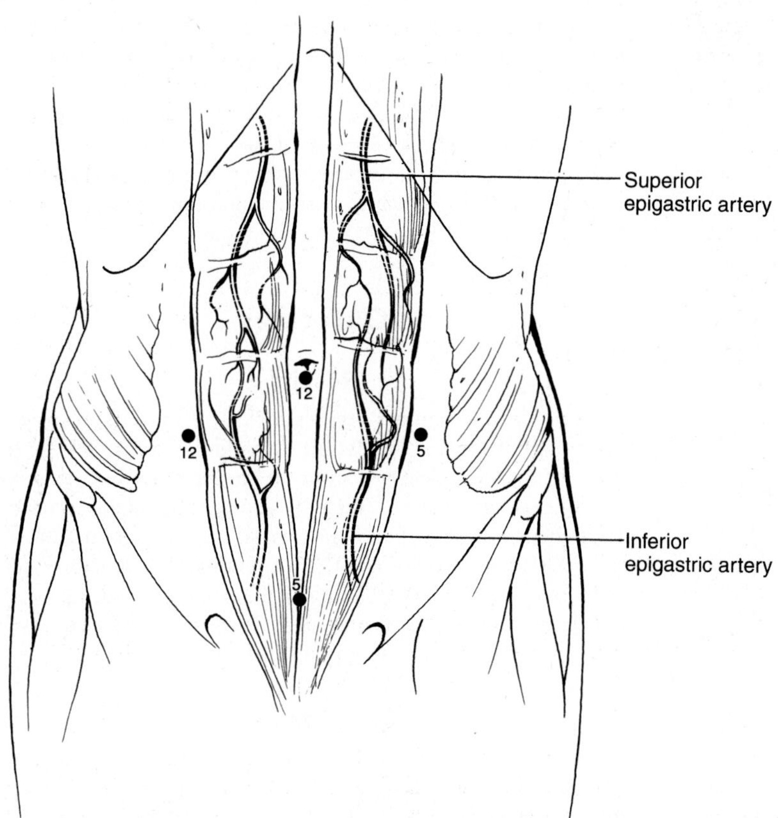


FIGURE 54.5 Optimal sites (*black spots*) of access for transabdominal laparoscopic seminal vesicle excision. Numbers represent trocar size in millimeters.

not necessary for benign seminal vesicle pathology, whereas if a laparoscopic or robotic prostatectomy will be performed in addition, the legs are abducted but left straight with the use of an operating table that allows a split-leg arrangement. If possible the low lithotomy position is avoided so as to minimize the risk of lower extremity thrombosis or neuromuscular injury. Patients are carefully strapped to the operating table with wide cloth tape across the chest and thighs as steep Trendelenburg (approximately 20 degrees) is required for deep pelvic laparoscopic visualization. After the patient is prepared and draped, a Foley catheter is inserted into the bladder under sterile conditions. An orogastric tube placed in the stomach is optional.

A transperitoneal approach is preferred for benign seminal vesicle lesions. After establishing a suitable pneumoperitoneum up to 15 mm Hg with the Veress needle placed at the inferior or superior umbilical crease, four laparoscopic ports are usually adequate for seminal vesicle benign pathology excision. These ports, varying from 5 to 12 mm in size, may be placed in a diamond shape (Fig. 54.5) or a horseshoe shape. With the patient in steep Trendelenburg, the peritoneum just anterior to the rectum in the rectovesical pouch (pouch of Douglas) is incised transversely between the two obliterated umbilical ligaments. Large seminal vesicle cysts are usually easily visualized and the dissection is carried close to the seminal vesicles so as to avoid injury to surrounding viscera and the neurovascular bundle. Use of bipolar coagulation is highly recommended over monopolar energy so as to minimize injury to these surrounding structures. The dissection can be completed using laparoscopic scissors and curved graspers using blunt and sharp dissection. The main arterial branch to the tip of the seminal vesicle is easily handled with bipolar coagulation, but a laparoscopic clip is also a good choice. The seminal vesicle should be dissected caudally down to its juncture with the ampulla of vas and then clipped en bloc. With completion of the dissection, the specimen is placed in an entrapment device (LapSac, Cook Urological Inc., Spencer, IN) or an Endocatch bag (US Surgical, Tyco Healthcare, Norwalk, CT) and extracted through one of the larger laparoscopic ports. Large cysts may be aspirated prior to extraction so as to minimize the specimen size and obviate the need for enlarging the incision. Hemostasis and surrounding visceral integrity are assured and then the laparoscopic ports are closed in the usual fashion.

In select cases, a concomitant ipsilateral nephroureterectomy may be required should an atrophic kidney have an ectopic ureter draining into the seminal vesicle. It is recommended that the laparoscopic nephroureterectomy be performed prior to the seminal vesicle dissection. Thus, the patient would begin the procedure in a modified lateral decubitus position and then the operating table would be rotated so as to bring the patient into a relative supine and Trendelenburg direction. The operative details of laparoscopic nephrectomy for benign disease are described in Chapter 124.

Laparoscopic robotic assistance for surgery of the seminal vesicles has usually been performed in conjunction with radical prostatectomy. The technique, with respect to port placement and approach, is almost identical to the standard laparoscopic route described (6).

Although the transperitoneal laparoscopic/robotic approach to the seminal vesicles offers improved visualization to the seminal vesicles, the latter's close proximity to bladder, rectum, ureter, and neurovascular bundle must be appreciated by the surgeon. Transperitoneal incision in the pouch of Douglas, which is too anterior, may lead to perforation of the posterior bladder wall. Subtle hints that the surgeon may be dissecting too anterior would be the appearance of the detrusor musculature, which is quite vascular and tends to bleed easily. Should a hole be made in the bladder, it can be repaired laparoscopically or robotically without undue difficulty.

Similarly, the rectal wall may be incised at any point in the seminal vesicle mobilization. Assuming the patient has received a satisfactory bowel preparation, such rectal lacerations may be laparoscopically or robotically repaired in two layers. The anal sphincter is dilated at the termination of the procedure and the patient's diet is advanced slowly. Electrocautery must be used judiciously when in close proximity to the rectum. Use of precise bipolar coagulation is recommended.

The distal ureter runs close to the tip of the seminal vesicle. Any tubular structure that is lateral to the seminal vesicle may be the vas arching upwards towards the internal ring, but it also could be the ureter. The surgeon may easily become disoriented to which ampulla of the vas is being dissected, leading to the dissection shifting too far lateral and possibly injuring or transecting the ureter. Injection of intravenous methylene blue quickly confirms the ureteral injury. Should this unfortunate complication occur, the ureter could possibly be repaired by laparoscopic or robotic suturing. However, a ureterovesical reimplantation may be required and necessitate open surgical conversion. Placement of a double-J ureteral stent following repair is wise, and a pelvic drain is strongly advised in the presence of any bladder, rectal, or ureteral injury that may have occurred during the course of laparoscopic or robotic seminal vesicle dissection.

Finally, the neurovascular bundle is just lateral to the tips of the seminal vesicles. Injury to this structure will impair erectile function and create a serious problem, especially to the potent patient who may be undergoing seminal vesicle excision for benign disease.

Although data are limited for laparoscopic and robotic excision of benign seminal vesicle pathology alone, this approach appears to afford superb visualization with minimal postoperative morbidity and shorter hospitalization compared to the open surgical alternatives (2). In most cases, the seminal vesicle is excised laparoscopically or robotically in conjunction with radical prostatectomy or cystoprostatectomy.

### Endoscopic Treatment

**Transurethral Resection.** If the cyst or abscess is adjacent to the prostate (not in the middle or distal end of the seminal vesicle), it may be possible to unroof the cavity with a deep transurethral resection into the prostatic substance, just distal to the bladder neck at the 5 or 7 o'clock position. However, urinary reflux, with resultant postvoid dribbling, and infection are potential complications (7). Previous reports have detailed endoscopic treatment of seminal vesicle abscesses using semirigid ureteroscopes, as well as drainage of a seminal vesicle cyst cystoscopically with an incision using a Collins knife (1).

## Outcomes

### Results

Resection of the seminal vesicles for cystic and inflammatory diseases is in general successful, although large case series are rare. Seminal vesicle extirpation for cancer has also been successful, but the rarity of this indication prohibits an accurate assessment of survival and cure rates. Strict categorization of the 100 reported cases of primary seminal vesicle cancer reveals that fewer than 50% are truly primary to the seminal vesicle (8). In general, reconstructive surgery in children using these approaches has resulted in satisfactory outcomes.

### Complications

Each approach to seminal vesicle surgery is associated with unique complications. The relative complication rates with these approaches are outlined in Table 54.1. Limited extraperitoneal rectal injuries can be handled with formal two-layer closure. Rectal injury with the retrovesical approach is intra-abdominal, however, and may require the placement of omentum over the repair or even temporary colostomy. Most bladder injuries can be closed primarily. The most important point about ureteral injuries is their recognition. Most ureteral injuries can be treated adequately with stents for 7 to 10 days.

# EJACULATORY DUCT SURGERY

The ejaculatory ducts are paired, collagenous, tubular structures that commence at the junction of the vas deferens and seminal vesicle, course through the prostate, and empty into the prostatic urethra at the verumontanum. There are three distinct anatomic regions to the ejaculatory duct: the proximal and largely extraprostatic portion, the middle intraprostatic segment, and a distal segment that is incorporated into the lateral aspect of the verumontanum in the prostatic urethra (9).

**TABLE 54.1**

RELATIVE COMPLICATION RATES OF THE DIFFERENT SURGICAL APPROACHES TO THE SEMINAL VESICLE

| Approach | Rectal Injury | Impotence | Bladder or Ureteral Injury | Risk for Blood Transfusion | Other Risks |
|---|---|---|---|---|---|
| Other | Moderate | High | Moderate | Moderate | Thromboembolic |
| Transvesical | Low | Low | High | Low | Fistula |
| Transperineal | High | High | Moderate | Moderate | Thromboembolic |
| Para/Retrovesical | Moderate | Low | Moderate | Low | Low |
| Transcoccygeal | High | High | Low | Low | Low |
| Laparoscopic | Low | Low | Unclear | Low | Air Embolism |

The duct consists of three histologic layers: an outer muscular layer, a collagenous middle layer, and an inner mucosal layer (10). The muscular layer is absent in the distal segment.

## Indications for Surgery

Patients with ejaculatory duct obstruction sufficient to cause coital discomfort, recurrent hematospermia, or infertility should be considered candidates for transurethral treatment. Infertility with duct obstruction can present with low ejaculate volume and azoospermia or low ejaculate volume with decreased sperm density ($<20 \times 10^6$ sperm per mL) or impaired sperm motility (<30% motility). Anatomic findings suggestive of obstruction and lesions located within approximately 1 to 1.5 cm of the verumontanum are usually amenable to transurethral management.

## Diagnosis

Ejaculatory duct obstruction causes infertility in 5% of azoospermia cases. Duct obstruction can result from seminal vesicle calculi, mullerian duct (utricular) or wolffian duct (diverticular) cysts, postsurgical or postinflammatory scar tissue, calcification near the verumontanum, or congenital atresia (7). Classically, this condition presents as hematospermia, painful ejaculation, or infertility with azoospermia. Associated risk factors include evidence of prior urinary tract infection or trauma and perineal pain or discomfort. It is important to discontinue medications that may impair ejaculation. An abbreviated list of these medications is found in Table 54.2. Ejaculatory duct obstruction is suggested by finding enlarged, palpable seminal vesicles on rectal examination. The diagnosis is confirmed by a combination of findings:

1. An ejaculate volume <1.0 mL and a pH <7.0 that contains no sperm or fructose
2. A TRUS demonstration of dilated seminal vesicles (>1.5 cm in width) or dilated ejaculatory ducts (>2.3 mm) in association with a cyst, calcification, or stones along the duct

Recently, high-resolution TRUS has virtually replaced the more invasive vasography for this diagnosis. MRI with endorectal coil is recommended in suspicious cases without TRUS findings as it is excellent for the detection of small cysts. To complete the evaluation for infertility, it is important that the serum follicle-stimulating hormone (FSH) and testosterone levels be normal. Testicular volume should also be normal. A testis biopsy confirming ongoing sperm production may be helpful but is not always necessary.

**TABLE 54.2**

**MEDICATIONS ASSOCIATED WITH IMPAIRED EJACULATION**

| |
|---|
| Antihypertensive agents |
| α-Adrenergic blockers (prazosin, phentolamine) |
| Thiazides |
| Antipsychotic agents |

Not all patients with ejaculatory duct obstruction have dilated seminal vesicles, and not all patients with dilated seminal vesicles have ejaculatory duct obstruction. This has led to refinements in diagnostic techniques. Jarow (9) found that seminal vesicle sperm aspiration with TRUS more accurately defined affected patients. With a 30-cm, 21-gauge needle (Williams, Chiba, or oocyte retrieval needle), the seminal vesicles are aspirated transrectally or transperineally during TRUS (Fig. 54.6A). The aspirate is then examined under 400 × phase microscopy for sperm. The finding of more than three sperm per high-power field is considered positive and suggestive of obstruction. Importantly, the duration of sexual abstinence prior to aspiration can influence the findings. Seminal vesicle aspiration should be performed with <24 hours of sexual abstinence. Despite the fact that aspiration does not anatomically localize the site of blockage or differentiate between physical blockage and functional obstruction, it confirms that spermatogenesis is ongoing and that epididymal obstruction is unlikely.

Injection of nonionic contrast (50% Renografin) into the seminal vesicles after seminal vesicle aspiration, followed by formal radiographic imaging, can be a useful retrograde study of seminal vesicle and vasal anatomy in suspected obstruction (Fig. 54.6B). Also, a good-quality pelvic and inguinal vasogram can be obtained in most patients (Fig. 54.6B). Fluoroscopy or a kidney-ureter-bladder (KUB) plain film is taken after the injection of 5, 10, and 20 mL of contrast to delineate excurrent duct anatomy. Helpful maneuvers include (i) having the patient in the 15- to 30-degree reverse Trendelenburg position for radiographs to "open up" the pelvic outlet and minimize overlying pelvic bone density and (ii) placing a Foley catheter with 5 mL of water in the balloon on slight traction during contrast injection to reduce the spillage of contrast into the bladder that "clouds" the radiograph. As seminal vesiculography is more invasive than simple aspiration, it may require mild intravenous sedation and is best performed at the time of transurethral surgery.

Injection of diluted indigo carmine or methylene blue (1:5 dilution with saline) into the seminal vesicle with TRUS instead of contrast is termed seminal vesicle chromotubation. When performed with cystoscopy it can assess whether or not there is antegrade flow of dye from the seminal vesicle into the prostatic urethra (Fig. 54.6C). In fact, "patency," with chromotubation, defined by the presence of dye egressing from the ejaculatory duct orifices after seminal vesicle injection, may be the most accurate way to diagnose complete ejaculatory duct obstruction, unilateral or bilateral (11).

## Surgical Technique

Transurethral resection of the ejaculatory ducts (TURED) is performed in the outpatient setting. Following the administration of light general or regional anesthesia and a single dose of a broad-spectrum antibiotic, the patient is placed in the dorsal lithotomy position with a rectal drape (O'Connor). Formal cystourethroscopy is performed. Careful examination is made of the areas lateral to the verumontanum within the prostatic urethra to visualize either ejaculatory duct orifice. A small resectoscope (24Fr) and electrocautery loop are inserted and the verumontanum is resected in the midline (Fig. 54.7). The resection is performed with pure cutting current to minimize cauterization of the delicate ejaculatory ducts. Often several

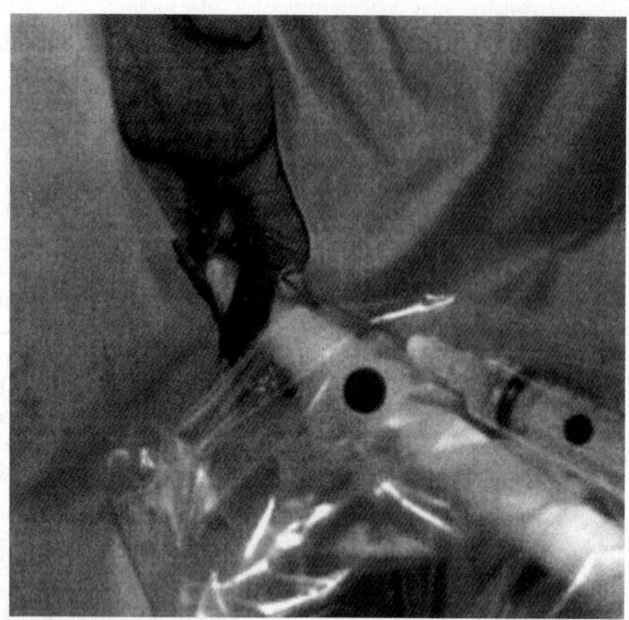
A

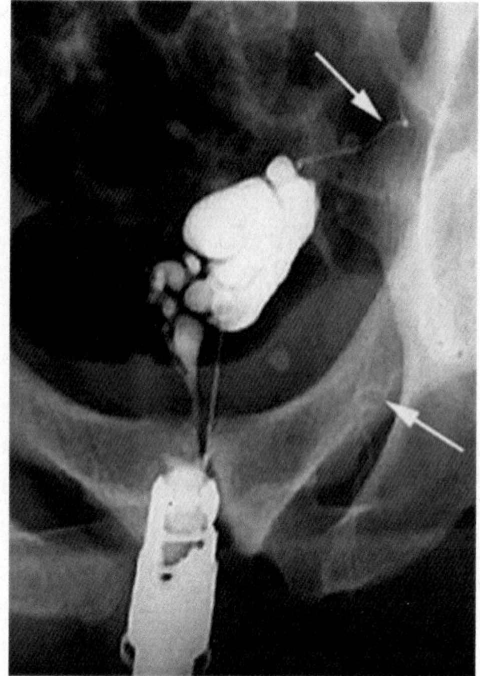
B

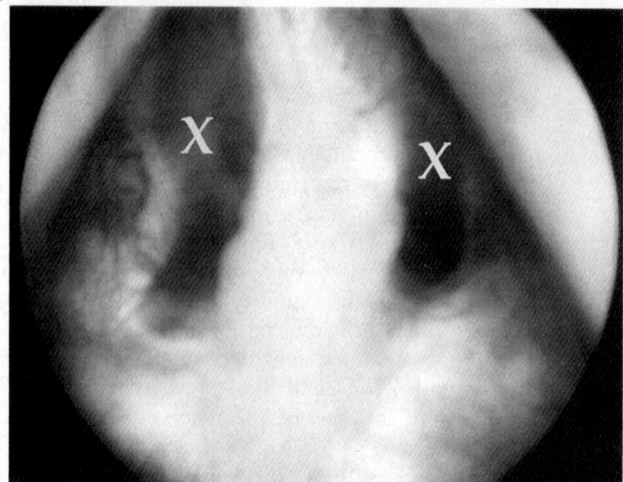

C

FIGURE 54.6 A: Working setup for transrectal ultrasound (TRUS) aspiration of seminal vesicles. *Large black dot* points out the TRUS probe inserted into the rectum and *small gray dot* is placed on the syringe and needle used for aspiration. B: Normal TRUS seminovesiculogram showing seminal vesicle and ejaculatory ducts with contrast. *Arrows* show the pelvic and inguinal vas deferens. C: Normal TRUS chromotubation. Cytoscopic view of methylene blue egressing from both ejaculatory duct orifices (*white Xs*) after injecting the seminal vesicles.

passes of the cutting loop are required to visualize the ejaculatory duct openings within the prostate. This can mean relatively deep dissection in a small prostate gland, a situation that can make even an experienced transurethral surgeon feel uneasy. At the correct level of resection, cloudy, milky fluid can usually be seen effluxing from the opened ducts. After resection, large bleeding blood vessels are lightly cauterized, with care taken to avoid fulguration of the duct openings. Because the area of resection is at the prostatic apex, near both the external urethral sphincter and the rectum, careful and constant positioning of the resectoscope is essential. A finger placed in the rectum can help avoid rectal injuries and assist in keeping the resectoscope tip proximal to the external sphincter. A small Foley catheter is placed for 24 to 48 hours and removed on an outpatient basis. Oral antibiotics are given while the catheter is in place. After such treatment for infertility, intercourse is resumed after 7 days, and a formal semen analysis is checked as early as 2 weeks and then at regular intervals thereafter, until semen quality stabilizes.

Several useful aids can ensure that the resection is performed safely and completely. With an endoscopic needle, the milky ejaculatory duct fluid can be sampled transurethrally during the procedure and inspected with microscopy for sperm. The use of simultaneous, real-time TRUS during the resection is a valuable addition to this procedure. The exact location of the lesion to be resected can be determined by TRUS and the depth of resection continuously assessed during the resection. Similarly, TRUS can be used to guide the instillation of indigo carmine or methylene blue into the seminal vesicles with a long, 20-gauge Chiba needle before the resection. The dye is subsequently visualized on relief of obstruction.

## Outcomes

### Results

Long-term relief of postcoital and perineal pain after TURED can be expected in 60% of patients (12). Hematospermia has

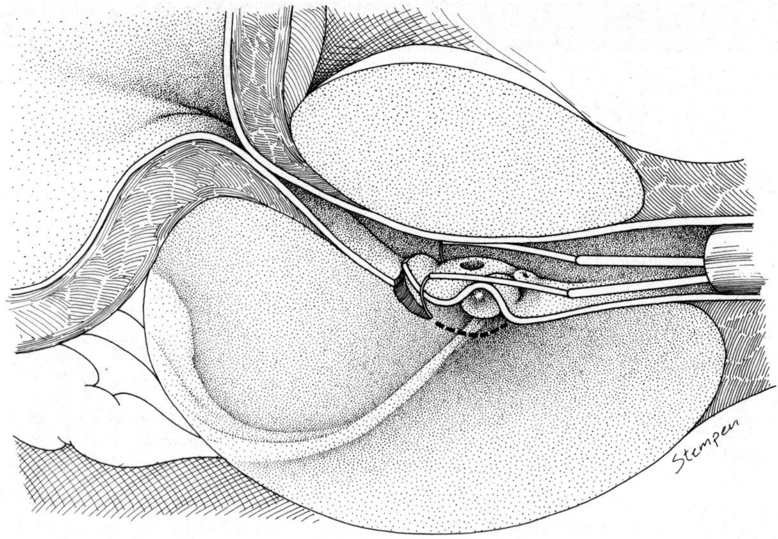


FIGURE 54.7 Transurethral resection for ejaculatory duct obstruction. Midline resection of the verumontanum is shown. Lateral and deeper resection may be necessary depending on the site and reason for duct obstruction. (Conceptualized by Paul Stempen)

also been effectively treated with TURED, but the literature on this indication remains anecdotal. There is convincing evidence from several large series of patients treated for infertility that a 20% to 30% pregnancy rate can be expected from TURED (13,14). In one series, men treated for either low-volume azoospermia or low-volume oligoasthenospermia were equally likely (65% to 70%) to show improvements in semen quality after TURED (14). From a recent series, it appears that obstruction due to cysts responds better to TURED than that due to calcification (15).

Several caveats of TURED surgery should be emphasized to the patient preoperatively. Roughly 13% of men treated by TURED for low-volume azoospermia will convert to normal-volume azoospermia. Among these patients, some have evidence of secondary obstruction at the level of the epididymis that requires epididymovasostomy. Epididymal obstruction may reflect the effects of time and blockage on other portions of the delicate male ductal system. Notably, 4% of patients treated for low-volume oligoasthenospermia may become azoospermic after TURED, presumably from scar tissue formation. We now recommend preoperative sperm cryopreservation if TURED is planned for this indication.

## Complications

The expected complication rate from TURED surgery is approximately 20% (7). The most common complications are self-limited hematospermia, hematuria requiring recatheterization, and urinary tract infection. More concerning, but less frequent, are epididymitis and a "watery" ejaculate. High-volume watery ejaculate is presumed secondary to the reflux of urine retrograde through the ejaculatory ducts into the seminal vesicles or into opened cysts, as suggested by the finding of creatinine in the ejaculates of TURED patients. In addition to the social implications of this, the exposure of sperm to urine may impair fertility potential. Several potentially major but rarely reported complications include retrograde ejaculation, rectal perforation, urinary incontinence, and recurrent seminal vesicle infection.

## ACKNOWLEDGMENTS

The author would like to thank Drs. Paul Turek and Howard Winfield for their previous works that contributed to this chapter.

## *References*

1. Sandlow JI, Winfield HN, Goldstein M. Surgery of the scrotum and seminal vesicles. In: *Campbell-Walsh Urology*, 9th ed. Philadelphia: WB Saunders, 2007;1098–1127.
2. McDougall EM, Afane JS, Dunn MD, et al. Laparoscopic management of retrovesical cystic disease: Washington University experience and review of the literature. *J Endourol* 2001;15:815–819.
3. Politano VA, Lankford RW, Susaeta R. A transvesical approach to total seminal vesiculectomy: a case report. *J Urol* 1975;113:385–388.
4. Silva DeAssis J. Seminal vesiculectomy. *J Urol* 1952;68:747–753.
5. Kreager JA, Jordan WP. Transcoccygeal approach to the seminal vesicles. *Am Surg* 1965;31:126–127.
6. Menon M, Tewari A, Peabody J. The VIP Team. Vattikuti Institute prostatectomy: technique. *J Urol* 2003;169:2289–2292.
7. Fisch H, Lambert SM, Goluboff ET. Management of ejaculatory duct obstruction: etiology, diagnosis, and treatment. *World J Urol* 2006;24(6): 604–610.
8. Benson RC Jr, Clark WR, Farrow GM. Carcinoma of the seminal vesicle. *J Urol* 1984;132:483–485.
9. Jarow JP. Seminal vesicle aspiration in the management of patients with ejaculatory duct obstruction. *J Urol* 1994;152:899–901.
10. Nguyen HT, Etzell J, Turek PJ. Normal human ejaculatory duct anatomy: a study of cadaveric and surgical specimens. *J Urol* 1996;155:1639–1642.
11. Wu DS, Shinohara K, Turek PJ. Ejaculatory duct chromotubation as a functional diagnostic test in ejaculatory duct obstruction. *J Urol* 1999; 161:1357A.
12. Farley S, Barnes R. Stenosis of ejaculatory ducts treated by endoscopic resection. *J Urol* 1973;109:664–666.
13. Pryor JP, Hendry WF. Ejaculatory duct obstruction in subfertile males: analysis of 87 patients. *Fertil Steril* 1991;56:725–730.
14. Turek PJ, Magana JO, Lipshultz LI. Semen parameters before and after transurethral surgery for ejaculatory duct obstruction. *J Urol* 1996; 155:1291–1293.
15. Kadioglu A, Cayan S, Tefekli A, et al. Does response to treatment of ejaculatory duct obstruction in infertile men vary with pathology? *Fertil Steril* 2001;76:138–142.

# CHAPTER 55 ■ VASECTOMY

DOUGLAS G. STEIN

As the most dependable method of contraception and one that requires virtually no compliance, vasectomy is an ideal choice for those men who have made a mature, informed decision to have no more children, and especially for men who have difficulty with compliance. As a result, 11% of the U.S. population relies on vasectomy as their primary method of birth control, and the incidence of vasectomy is approximately 500,000 per year in the United States. While it has been noted that vasectomy is the "most common procedure involved in malpractice claims against urologists" (1), vasectomy accounted for only 8 of 469 (1.7%) urology malpractice claims closed with indemnity payment between 1985 and 2004 for one liability carrier in New York (2). So, while urologists need not avoid vasectomy to decrease perceived high liability, they need to be thoroughly versed in the management of men seeking vasectomy.

## DIAGNOSIS

In most practices, a "consultation visit" includes counseling about vasectomy and a brief physical examination to help determine whether the surgeon and the patient feel comfortable with office vasectomy under local anesthesia or whether, in rare circumstances, general anesthesia in an operating room is indicated for reasons of patient anxiety or features on physical examination that could make vasectomy more difficult in an office setting. Such features include incomplete testicular descent (either untreated or status post orchiopexy); scarring due to prior scrotal surgery; a small tight scrotum; obesity with thick spermatic cords; very thin vasa; large hydrocele, spermatocele, or varicocele; or extreme scrotal hypersensitivity. In this practice of about 2,000 vasectomies per year, general anesthesia is never utilized. Counseling is accomplished online by a personal counseling video, a very informative web page, and a written consent that includes alternatives, potential complications, and pre- and postprocedure instructions. Medical and surgical (prior scrotal conditions and surgeries) histories are reviewed by the physician. Sedatives are not routinely used.

## INDICATIONS FOR SURGERY

While no strict criteria exist for determining which patient should be offered vasectomy, the Electronic Code of Federal Regulations for sterilization of persons in federally assisted family planning projects (Title 42 CFR, Part 50, subpart B) specifies that the individual be at least 21 years of age and mentally competent when consent is obtained, that consent be obtained with certain procedures, and that 30 days pass between the date of consent and the date of vasectomy.

## ALTERNATIVE THERAPY

Especially because vasectomy should always be presented as a permanent form of contraception, a full disclosure of alternative contraceptive methods must be a part of informed consent. While condoms are the only other alternative available to men, men should have a thorough understanding of the options available to women, even though these provide less control for the male. When features of the male anatomy (obesity, tight scrotum, thin vasa, or scarring from prior scrotal surgery) would make vasectomy difficult for the vasectomist at his or her skill level, couples considering permanent contraception should be asked to consider tubal ligation for the woman or the opinion of a vasectomist with more experience, as complication rates are lower for vasectomies performed by more experienced vasectomists. While not guaranteed successful, sperm storage should also be considered by vasectomy candidates as an insurance policy that may enable paternity after vasectomy, if vasectomy reversal fails to restore fertility.

## SURGICAL TECHNIQUE

Nearly all surgical procedures involve three steps: (i) anesthesia, to allow the procedure to proceed without pain, (ii) access, or how the surgeon gets to the target organ, and (iii) technique, how one manages the target organ, the actual vasectomy.

### Anesthesia

For vasectomy, general anesthesia or heavy intravenous sedation in an operating room setting may be preferred by anxious patients and by surgeons who simply find it easier than using local anesthesia for anxious or technically challenging patients. For young healthy men, the risks are minimal, but the costs may make it prohibitive for men without health insurance coverage.

Most vasectomies are performed in an office setting under local anesthesia. Administration with a needle is the most common and traditional technique, but since 2002, no-needle anesthesia has made vasectomy much more acceptable, especially for men who "just hate needles."

Needle local anesthesia is accomplished after the scrotum is prepped and draped. A 27-gauge 1.5-inch needle is commonly used to create a skin wheal over the point at which the vas is held beneath the skin (Fig. 55.1). Then the needle is advanced proximally its full length adjacent to the vas in the direction of the external ring. Two mL of anesthetic is injected into the vas sheath as the needle is withdrawn. (A 30-gauge 1-inch needle causes less of a poke but requires more time and strength for injection. The anesthetic can be lidocaine without epinephrine

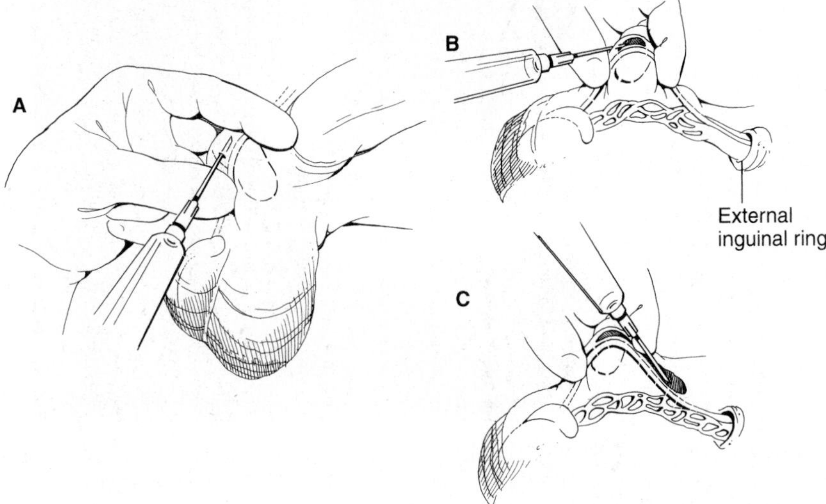


FIGURE 55.1 The right vas deferens is manipulated to the midline raphe and anesthetized.

[1% burns a bit <2%] or a mixture of lidocaine and bupivacaine to delay the onset of the mild discomfort that usually occurs on the day of the procedure.) The surgeon then either lifts and injects the other vas or proceeds with the vasectomy on this side, employing the traditional incisional technique or the no-scalpel technique (see below). The contralateral vas sheath is injected similarly, either through the same skin wheal if the vasectomy is to be performed through a single midline opening (preferred) or through a second skin wheal if the surgeon is more comfortable with accessing the vas through separate lateral wall openings.

No-needle local anesthesia for vasectomy involves the use of a jet injector, the most popular of which is the MadaJet (MADA, Inc., Carlstadt, NJ). Use of no-needle local anesthesia has become more widespread, popularized by Weiss and Li (3). The MadaJet (Fig. 55.2) emits an extremely thin 0.1- to 0.2 mL stream of anesthetic (a 50:50 mixture of 2% lidocaine and 0.5% bupivacaine is preferred) strong enough to penetrate the skin and underlying tissue to a depth of 2 to 5 mm, depending on the factory setting of the particular MadaJet. No-needle anesthesia is administered after the scrotal wall is shaved but before the formal scrotal preparation with povidone-iodine. The vas is lifted into position beneath the skin at the preferred access site (anterior midline or lateral scrotal wall), the overlying skin is prepared with alcohol, the fluted tip of the MadaJet is positioned over the vas (Fig. 55.3), and the release button is pressed to discharge the anesthetic through the skin and around the vas. The procedure is repeated one or two times along the path of the vas at 4- to 5-mm intervals. Medication entry sites are barely visible as minute dots, surrounding which are 2- to 3-mm areas of anesthetized skin. If the right vas is lifted to the midline and injected 2 mm to the left of the median raphe, and if the left vas is then lifted to the midline and injected 2 mm to the right of the median raphe, the patient develops a square of anesthetized skin about 4 to 5 mm on each side centered on the midline and the scrotal septum receives four to six doses of the anesthetic. Through the anesthetized square, the no-scalpel vasectomy (NSV) is performed.

For the occasional vasectomy, needle anesthesia is more convenient unless the surgeon wishes to appeal to those men who "just hate needles."

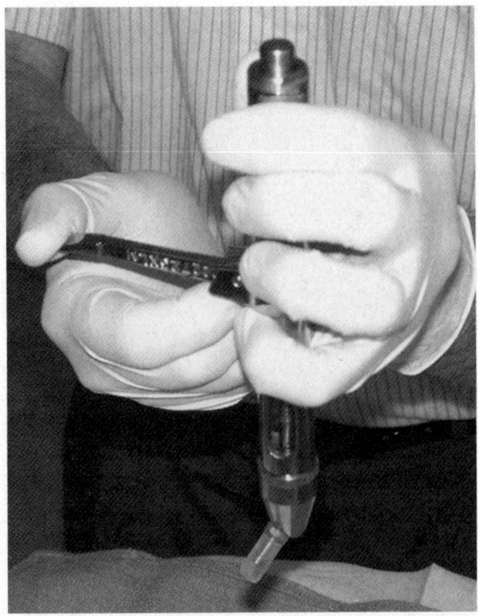

FIGURE 55.2 Cocking a MadaJet with an angled head. The release button is at the top.

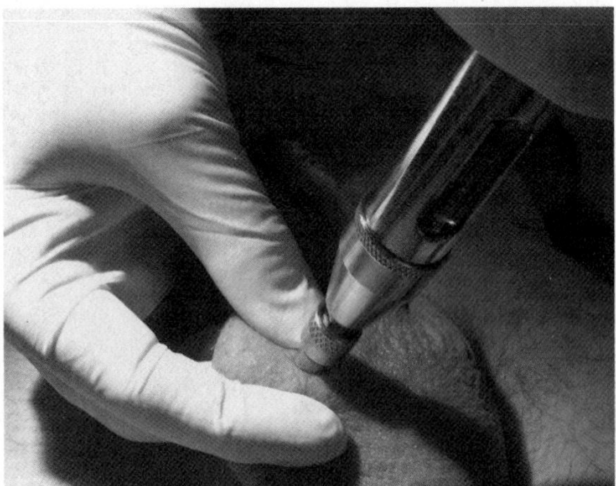

FIGURE 55.3 Positioning a MadaJet with a straight head over the right vas, while it is held beneath the median raphe using a three-finger technique.

## Access

Using the traditional approach, access to the vas is accomplished through a 1- to 1.5-cm horizontal or vertical incision in each lateral scrotal wall or through a single incision in the midline, wherever the vas was previously anesthetized using needle or MadaJet. The vas, held beneath the incision and still within its sheath, is grasped with an Allis or small towel clamp. Then the fibrous tissue around the vas is incised longitudinally with the scalpel, exposing the vas itself, which is then grasped with an Adson forceps, and a section is lifted through the sheath. Surgeons familiar with NSV instruments but more comfortable with an incisional approach often prefer to use the NSV ringed forceps to both secure the vas and lift it from its sheath.

The no-scalpel approach utilizes two special instruments and a three-finger technique (Fig. 55.4). Access to both vasa is via a single small opening in the anterior midline of the scrotal wall (anesthetized with needle- or MadaJet-applied lidocaine), but there is no reason why the same instruments could not be used with lateral wall incisions for surgeons more comfortable with that approach. After the scrotum is prepared with povidone-iodine and draped, needle anesthesia is utilized (see above) or the pinpoint marks in the skin made by the MadaJet are located and the site marked by inserting and gently spreading the tips of the pointy NSV hemostat. Locating the pinpoint MadaJet injection application sites can be difficult, especially in dark-skinned men, so this step and the remainder of the vasectomy may be much easier with the magnification provided by 2× optical loupes. The vas, most commonly located on the posterior aspect of the spermatic cord, is swept medially and lifted into position beneath the anesthetized site using a three-finger technique. While the vas is draped over the middle finger and stabilized with the thumb of the nondominant hand, the skin is drawn tightly over it with the index finger of the same hand. The vas is grasped with the NSV ringed forceps (Fig. 55.5). When the overlying skin is thin, the initial grasp incorporates the skin. When the overlying skin is very thick, some surgeons will find it easier to spread the skin and underlying fascia enough to introduce the NSV ringed forceps through this opening and grasp the vas within its sheath. One tip of the pointy NSV hemostat is then introduced into the lumen of the vas and removed. The NSV hemostat is then closed and both tips are introduced into the lumen of the vas at the same spot. The tips are spread to a width twice that of the vas, splitting the vas open longitudinally and spreading all overlying layers. One tip of the NSV hemostat is then used to "hook" the vas (Fig. 55.6) and lift it from its sheath as the ringed forceps is removed. The ringed forceps is then used to grasp one wall of the vas and deliver a 1- to 3-cm loop of it from its sheath (Fig. 55.7).

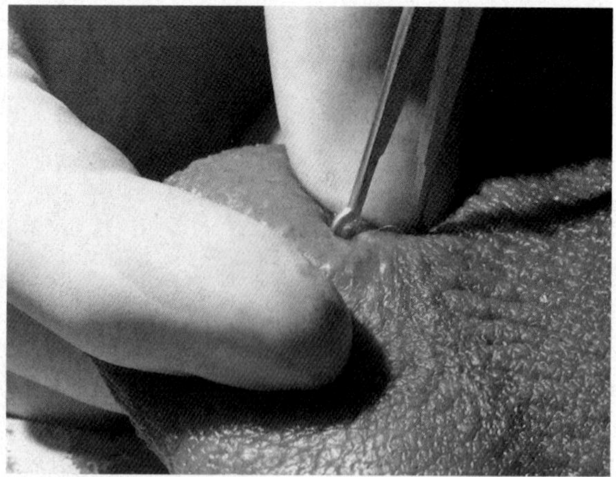

FIGURE 55.5 Held using the three-finger technique, the right vas is grasped with the no-scalpel vasectomy (NSV) ringed forceps.

## Occlusion

Numerous methods for establishing vasal obstruction have been described, and most surgeons employ a combination of luminal cauterization, ligation, division, excision, and fascial interposition with either a suture ligature or hemoclip (4) (Figs. 55.8, 55.9, 55.10, and 55.11). The objective should be very low failure and low complication rates, without removing so much vas, especially in young patients, that vasectomy reversal is rendered extremely difficult. "Early" failure is said to occur when the postvasectomy patient has motile sperm or

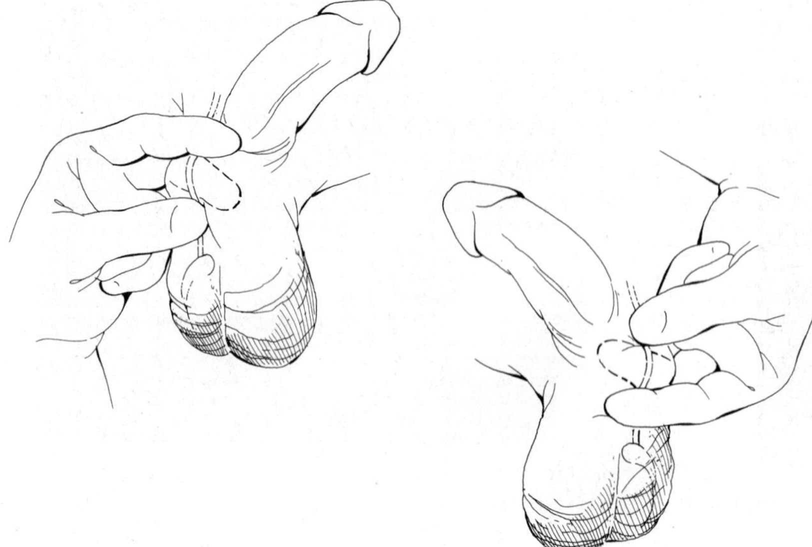

FIGURE 55.4 The three-finger technique for isolating the (A) right and (B) left vas deferens.

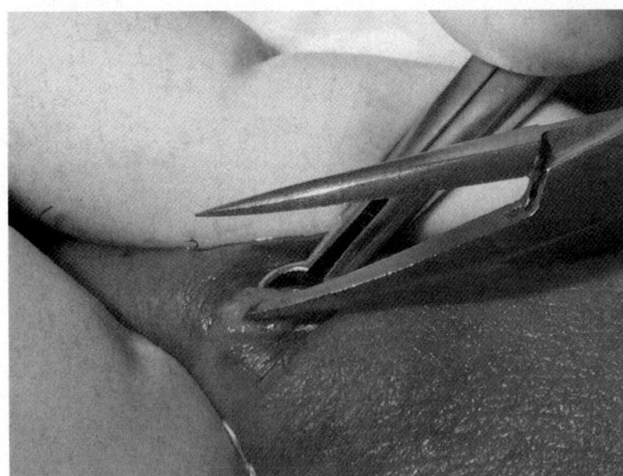

FIGURE 55.6 After the vas and overlying layers are split by spreading with the pointy hemostat, the pointy hemostat is used to hook the vas as the no-scalpel vasectomy (NSV) ringed clamp is released.

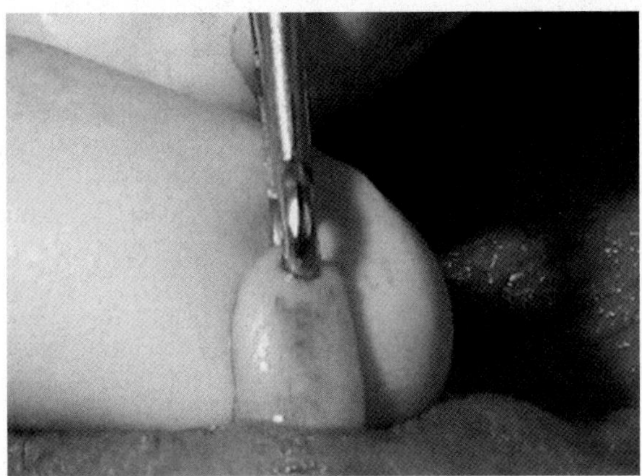

FIGURE 55.7 A loop of vas is delivered.

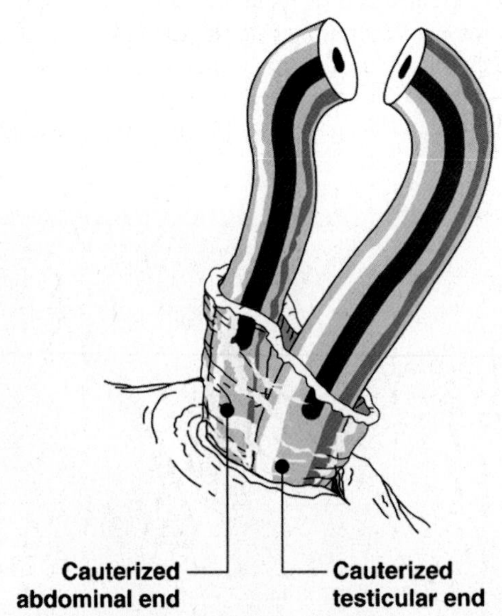


FIGURE 55.8 Cauterization of both ends without excision of a segment or fascial interposition. (Copyright and courtesy of Barone MA, Irsula B, Chen-Mok M, et al., and the Investigator Study Group. Effectiveness of vasectomy using cautery. *BMC Urol* 2004;4:10, http://www.biomedcentral.com/1471-2490/4/10)

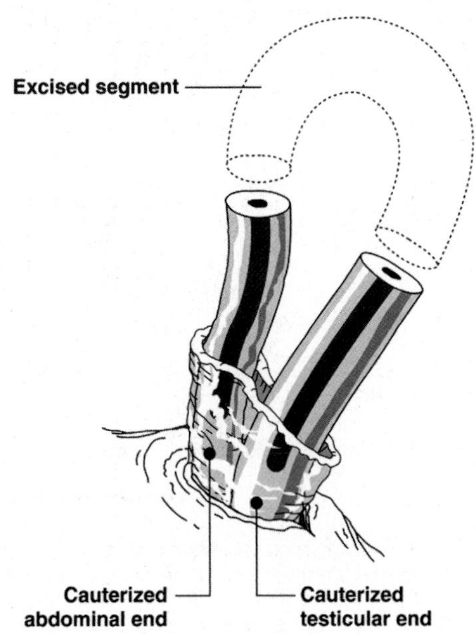


FIGURE 55.9 Cauterization of both ends with excision of a segment but no fascial interposition. (Copyright and courtesy of Barone MA, Irsula B, Chen-Mok M, et al., and the Investigator Study Group. Effectiveness of vasectomy using cautery. *BMC Urol.* 2004;4:10, http://www.biomedcentral.com/1471-2490/4/10)

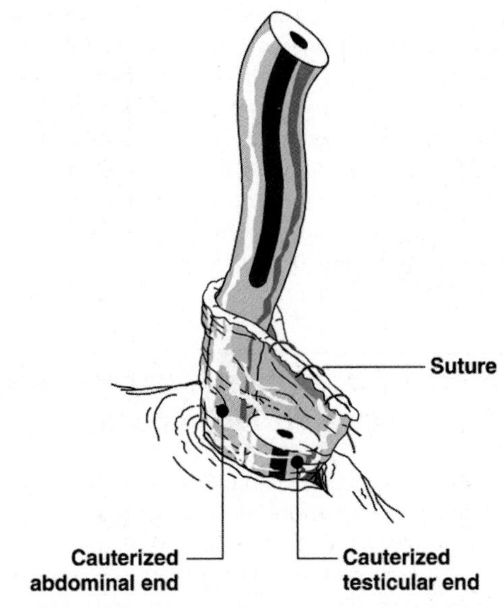


FIGURE 55.10 Cauterization of both ends with fascial interposition over the testicular end (abdominal end left outside sheath) using suture. (Copyright and courtesy of Barone MA, Irsula B, Chen-Mok M, et al., and the Investigator Study Group. Effectiveness of vasectomy using cautery. *BMC Urol* 2004;4:10., http://www.biomedcentral.com/1471-2490/4/10)

significant numbers (>100,000/mL) of nonmotile sperm in the semen 6 months after vasectomy. Recanalization within the tissue between the two severed ends occurs frequently during the 1 to 2 months following vasectomy but usually scars off. Early failure occurs when recanalization does not scar off but rather persists. "Late" failure is the return of motile sperm to the semen of a patient previously diagnosed as azoospermic, an event caused by delayed recanalization and usually discovered as a result of a surprise pregnancy.

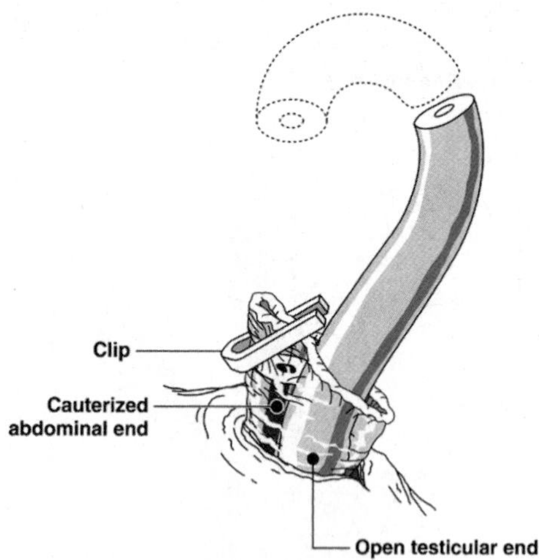


FIGURE 55.11 Cauterization of the abdominal end only (open-ended technique) with fascial interposition over the abdominal end (testicular end left outside sheath) using a hemoclips. (Copyright and courtesy of Barone MA, Irsula B, Chen-Mok M, et al., and the Investigator Study Group. Effectiveness of vasectomy using cautery. *BMC Urol* 2004;4:10, http://www.biomedcentral.com/1471-2490/4/10)

There are numerous reviews of surgical techniques (5,6). Ligation without division has a high early failure rate, even when employing a specially designed clip rather than a suture ligature or hemoclip (7). Cauterization without division might be expected to create adequate obstruction by scarring in some patients but is not routinely used because of an anticipated high failure rate, given that cautery and division (without excision of a segment or fascial interposition) resulted in the only failures in a study of the effectiveness of various cautery techniques (4). Early recanalization and failure rates are highest for ligation and excision without fascial interposition and lowest for thermal cautery with fascial interposition (4,8). This is the rationale for the following technique.

## Preferred Anesthesia, Access, and Occlusion Techniques

The no-needle, no-scalpel vasectomy with thermal cauterization and hemoclip fascial interposition is performed as follows. An elastic lasso is applied at the coronal sulcus and an attached hemostat is snapped onto the shirt to keep the penis elevated. Most patients, coached by online instructions and telephone staff, shave the night before so that the skin is not so sensitive to the alcohol used to prepare it for application of the no-needle anesthesia. If needed, the anterior scrotal wall is shaved with a single-edge shaver. No-needle local anesthesia is applied to each vas in turn at a midline location as described previously. The scrotum is then formally prepped with povidone-iodine and draped with a fenestrated 18 × 24-inch drape. If no-needle anesthesia is not used, needle anesthesia is applied as described previously.

After local anesthesia, the no-scalpel technique described previously is utilized to deliver a loop of vas from its sheath (see Fig. 55.7). It is very important that the vas be opened a few millimeters lengthwise to confirm complete penetration of the sheath and to allow grasping of the vas wall with the ringed forceps. The NSV pointy hemostat is passed along theundersurface of the vas at the apex of the loop and gently spread to push the vasal vessels away from a 1- to 2-cm segment of vas

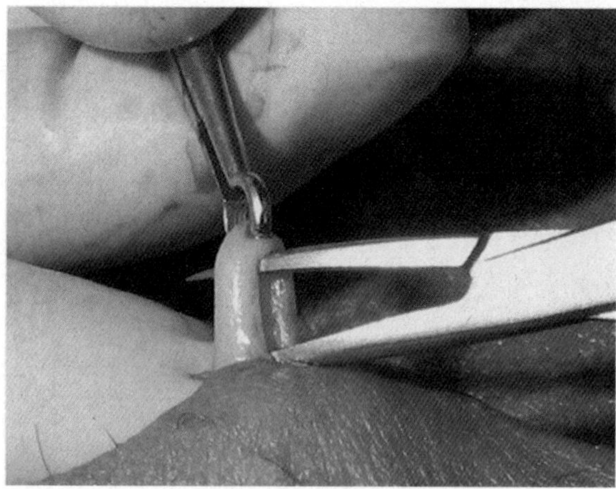

FIGURE 55.12 The no-scalpel vasectomy (NSV) pointy hemostat is used to spread vessels away from a 1- to 2-cm length of vas.

(Fig. 55.12). At the prostatic end of the segment, a small vasotomy opening is made with one tip of the pointy NSV hemostat (Fig. 55.13). A battery-powered wire loop thermocautery tip is introduced into the upper end and advanced 5 to 10 mm toward the prostate (Fig. 55.14). It is activated just long enough to sear the mucosal lining of the vas so that it will seal off by scarring. If applied too long, causing the full thickness of the wall to blanch, the cauterized segment may slough, negating the effectiveness of cautery in contributing to obstruction of the vas. Then the thermocautery unit or a scissors is used to divide the vas where the vasotomy was made. The prostatic end slips up into the vas sheath and the margins of the sheath are brought together and tented over the buried end with a conventional Halsted hemostat (Fig. 55.15). If there are any bleeding vessels near the sheath margins, these can be included in the hemostat to provide hemostasis. At this point, the testicular end is still secured with the ringed clamp. The hemostat is now brought down to a position below the ringed clamp (toward the foot of the table) and transferred to the nondominant hand. A medium hemoclip is applied to the tissue in the hemostat alongside the testicular end of the vas, drawing the sheath around the testicular end so that it cannot slip back inside. When the hemostat is removed, the clip rotates back cephalad and sits parallel to the testicular end (Fig. 55.16)

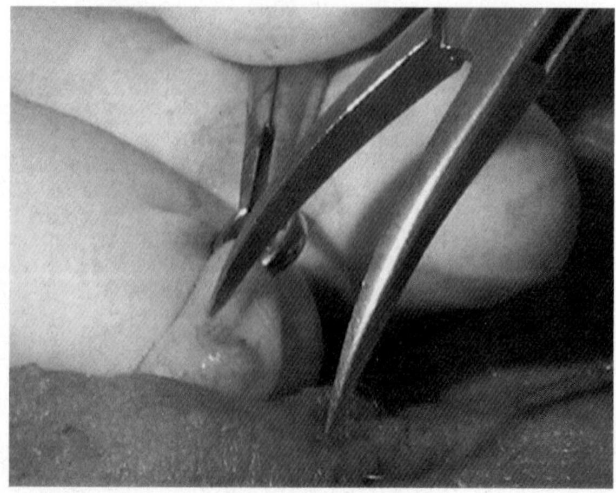

FIGURE 55.13 The no-scalpel vasectomy (NSV) pointy hemostat is used to make a small vasotomy opening in the abdominal end.

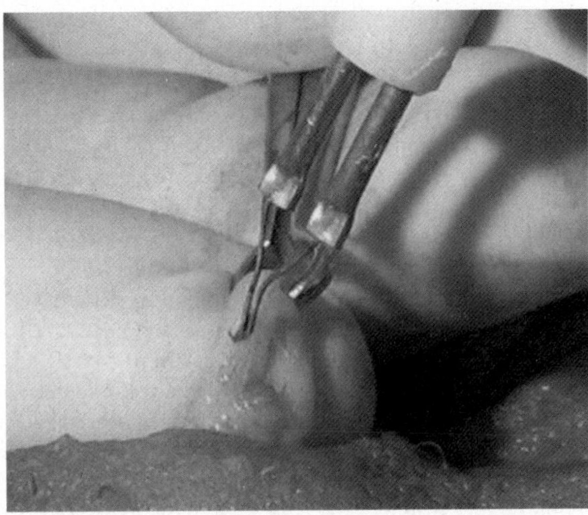

FIGURE 55.14 The tip of a thermocautery unit is introduced into the abdominal end.

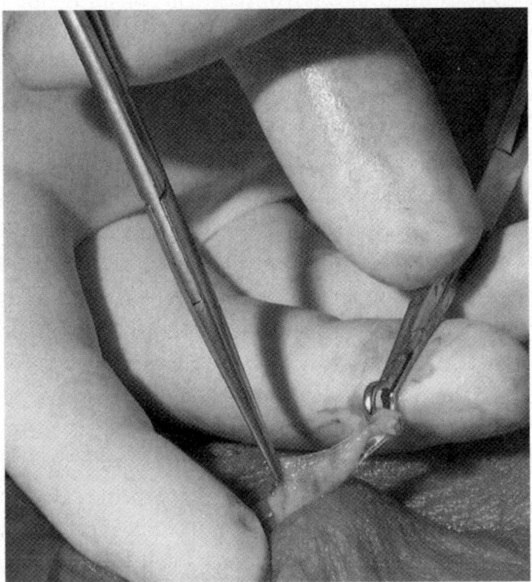

FIGURE 55.15 After the abdominal end is divided, it slips up into the vas sheath and a Halsted hemostat is used to close the sheath margins over the now-buried abdominal end.

so that it will not hang up on scrotal wall fascia as it released back into the scrotum. Be careful that the sheath is not drawn so tightly around the lower end that it indents the surface, compromising blood flow to the segment outside the sheath. Should that end slough, the remaining stump would be inside the sheath, defeating the intent of fascial interposition. An additional hemoclip can be applied for hemostasis if necessary. The ringed clamp on the testicular end is opened and the divided vas ends fall back into the scrotum. The testicular end is not ligated or cauterized, making this an open-ended technique. The same procedure is repeated on the other side.

The patient is instructed to recline on the day of the surgery. Ice packs are recommended by many surgeons to decrease the risk of hematoma formation. On the day after surgery, patients may walk and drive ad lib but should avoid yard work, sports, and heavy lifting. They may shower, then continue use of scrotal supports for 2 more days. Two days after the vasectomy, patients may return to normal activities and sex but should limit aggressive athletic workouts to half of the normal routine to see if they are ready for normal routines thereafter.

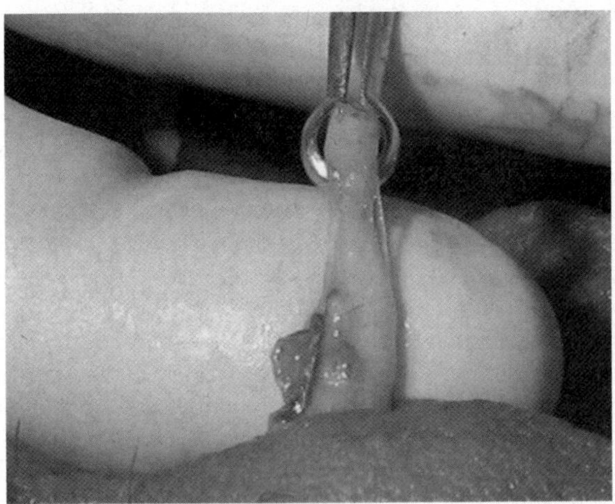

FIGURE 55.16 When the hemostat is removed, the hemoclipped sheath over the buried abdominal end rotates back to its original position.

## Follow-Up Semen Analysis

If a fresh specimen contains fewer than 100,000 nonmotile sperm per milliliter (1 sperm per 400× high-power field with many light microscopes), as will be the case for 95% at 12 weeks, no further testing is necessary, as 99.7% of these cases will achieve azoospermia or rare nonmotile sperm by 24 weeks (4) and the risk of pregnancy with fewer than 100,000 nonmotile sperm per milliliter is extremely low (9,10). If a sample older than 2 hours (motility evaluation not reliable) shows no sperm in 10 high-power fields, which would be fewer than 10,000 sperm per milliliter, no further testing is necessary. If any sperm are seen in 10 high-power fields at 8 weeks, another container or mailer is provided. If sperm are seen at 12 weeks in a second unfresh specimen, evaluation of a fresh specimen is required. Labrecque et al. (8,10) propose a nomogram suggesting that testing be repeated every 4 to 6 weeks and that failure due to "persistent" recanalization (some cases will scar closed) be considered probable only if motile sperm persist over 6 months. When 100,000 or more non-motile sperm per milliliter persist for over 6 months, failure should be considered, but even this is considered overly cautious by some (11,12).

# OUTCOMES

## Results

Using fascial interposition with a hemoclip to bury the testicular end, over the past 16 years and approximately 10,800 vasectomies, four patients (0.04%) experienced early failure (motile sperm at 4 months) and required repeat vasectomies, and four patients (of whom we are aware), again 0.04%, experienced late failure (pregnancy and confirmation of motile seminal sperm or paternity >1 year after azoospermia). Since February 2007, the author has buried the prostatic end of the vas, hoping for an even lower failure rate. As of May 2008 and 2,465 vasectomies with burial of the prostatic end, there has been one early failure (again 0.04%) and no late failures. It is still too early to present a rate of late failures and to determine whether abdominal-end fascial interposition is superior to testicular-end fascial interposition.

## Complications

### Early

Three levels of hematoma are possible: small (2–3 cm) incidental hematomas following needle or no-needle anesthesia will usually resolve within a few days; medium (3–5 cm) hematomas due to delayed bleeding of a weakened small vessel may take 2–3 weeks to resolve; for large (>5 cm) hematomas, surgical drainage should be considered to decrease the duration of morbidity. Reported rates average about 2% but are higher (4.6%) for surgeons who perform few vasectomies (1 to 10 per year) and lower (1.6%) for surgeons who perform many vasectomies (>50 per year). The incidence is lower with NSV (0.3% versus 1.4%), during which tissue is spread for exposure of the vas, than with traditional vasectomy.

Postvasectomy inflammation can occur anywhere from 3 days to years following vasectomy. Patients who have had little discomfort following vasectomy may "out of the blue" develop swelling and tenderness at the vasectomy site or within the epididymis and convoluted vas "upstream" from the vasectomy site. Most cases are unilateral and respond quickly to nonsteroidal anti-inflammatories.

Infection with conventional incisional vasectomy has been reported to occur in 1.4% of cases compared with a rate of 0.1% with NSV (13). The most severe and obvious cases develop into scrotal abscesses that require surgical drainage. There is one published report of lethal gangrene due to beta-hemolytic strep with onset 2 days after vasectomy in a previously healthy young man.

### Late

Sperm granulomas form at the vasectomy site to varying degrees in up to 60% of patients. A granuloma probably forms when sperm leak from the testicular end of the divided vas and cause the inflammation needed for their absorption, typically in the second or third week following vasectomy. This actually vents the congestion and inflammation that often occurs upstream in the proximal vas and epididymis and may enhance the prognosis for success with a future vasovasostomy. Open-ended vasectomy expectedly reduces the risk of pain due to congestive epididymitis, but paradoxically does not increase the risk of tender sperm granuloma (14) and actually reduces it. For granulomas that are exquisitely tender, most patients will respond to nonsteroidal anti-inflammatories. Some may also respond to an injection of a steroid near the granuloma, but some will require surgical excision.

Chronic pain of the scrotal contents after vasectomy is a syndrome with various names: postvasectomy pain syndrome (PVPS), congestive epididymitis, postvasectomy orchalgia, and chronic testicular pain (15). In two studies conducted 7 to 12 months following vasectomy, 14.7% of men described some degree of chronic discomfort of the scrotal contents; approximately 1% described the pain as "quite severe and noticeably affecting quality of life" (16), and 1% to 2% expressed regret over having had the vasectomy because of pain. Rates were about the same at 10 years following vasectomy, indicating that the incidence does not increase or decrease with time. PVPS is thus defined as intermittent or constant unilateral or bilateral testicular pain for >3 months following vasectomy, severe enough to interfere with daily activities and cause the patient to seek medical attention. There are no predictors as to which patients will develop it, there is no clear-cut etiology, and there is no best treatment. The syndrome is not due to infection, so antibiotics are not helpful. Medical treatment options include nonsteroidal anti-inflammatories, scrotal support, nerve blocks, and tricyclic antidepressants. Surgical treatments include conversion to open-ended vasectomy, vasectomy reversal, epididymectomy, and orchiectomy (15).

Prolonged sexual dysfunction following vasectomy is rare.

Through the years questions have been raised about an association between vasectomy and a variety of subsequently diagnosed disease states, including atherosclerosis, prostate cancer, glomerulonephritis, and primary progressive aphasia. So far, reviews of the initial studies point out methodologic factors, and subsequent studies have not been able to support any association between vasectomy and any disease states (17).

## *References*


1. Pryor JL. Vasectomy. Chapter 54 in Graham SD, Gleen JF, Keane TE, eds. *Glenn's Urologic Surgery*, 6th ed. Philadelphia: Lippincott Williams & Wilkins, 2004.
2. Perrotti M, Badger W, Prader S, et al. Medical malpractice in urology, 1985 to 2004: 469 consecutive cases closed with indemnity payment. *J Urol* 2006;176:2154–2157.
3. Weiss RS, Li PS. No-needle jet anesthetic technique for no-scalpel vasectomy. *J Urol* 2005;175:1677–1680.
4. Barone MA, Irsula B, Chen-Mok M, et al., and the Investigator Study Group. Effectiveness of vasectomy using cautery. *BMC Urol* 2004;4:10.
5. Clenney TL, Higgins JC. Vasectomy techniques. *Am Fam Physician* 1999; 60:137–152.
6. Labrecque M, Dufresne JA, Barone MA, et al. Vasectomy surgical techniques: a systematic review. *BMC Med* 2004;2:21.
7. Levine LA, Abern MR, Lux MM. Persistent motile sperm after ligation band vasectomy. *J Urol* 2006;176:2146–2148.
8. Labrecque M, Hays M, Chen-Mok M, et al. Frequency and patterns of early recanalization after vasectomy. *BMC Urol* 2006;6:25.
9. Haldar N, Cranston D, Turner E, et al. How reliable is a vasectomy? Long-term follow-up of vasectomised men. *Lancet* 2000;356:43–44.
10. Labrecque M, Barone MA, et al. Letter to the editor. *J Urol* 2005;174:791.
11. Edwards IS. Earlier testing after vasectomy, based on the absence of motile sperm. *Fertil Steril* 1993;59:431–436.
12. DeKnijff DW, Vrijhof HJ, Arends J, et al. Persistence or reappearance of nonmotile sperm after vasectomy: does it have clinical consequences? *Fertil Steril* 1997;67:332–335.
13. Nirathpongporn A, Huber D, Krieger JN. No-scalpel vasectomy at the King's Birthday Vasectomy Festival. *Lancet* 1990:335:894–895.
14. Denniston GC, Kuehl L. Open-ended vasectomy: approaching the ideal technique. *J Am Board Fam Pract* 1994;7:285–287.
15. Christiansen CG, Sandlow JI. Testicular pain following vasectomy: a review of post-vasectomy pain syndrome. *J Androl* 2003;24:293–298.
16. Leslie TA, Illing RO, Cranston DW, et al. The incidence of chronic scrotal pain after vasectomy: a prospective audit. *BJU Int* 2007;100(6):1330–1333.
17. Brannigan RE. *Any Associated Diseases with Vasectomy?* Lecture Summaries, Society for the Study of Male Reproduction Annual Meeting, 2008:15.

Barone MA, Nazarali H, Cortes M, et al. A prospective study of time and number of ejaculations to azospermia after vasectomy by ligation and excision. *J Urol* 2003;170:892.

Benger JR, Swami SK, Gingell JC. Persistent spermatozoa after vasectomy: a survey of British urologists. *Br J Urol* 1995;76:376.

Dhar NB, Bhatt A, Jones JS. Determining the success of vasectomy. *BJU Int* 2006;97:773.

Li PS, Li S, Schlegel PN, et al. External spermatic sheath injection for vasal nerve block. *Urology* 1992;39:173.

Sokal D, Irsula B, Hays M, et al., and the Investigator Study Group. Vasectomy by ligation and excision, with or without fascial interposition: a randomized controlled trial. *BMC Medicine* 2004;2:6.

Hartanto VH, Chenven ES, DiPiazza DJ, et al. Fournier gangrene following vasectomy. *Infect Urol* 2001;14(3):80–82.

Viddeleer AC, Lycklama A, Nijeholt GA. Lethal Fournier's gangrene following vasectomy. *J Urol* 1992;147:1613–1614.

# CHAPTER 56 ■ VASOEPIDIDYMOSTOMY

PETER T. K. CHAN

Azoospermia may be due to bilateral obstruction at any point of the male excurrent ductal system, which comprises the efferent ductules, epididymis, vas deferens, and the ejaculatory ducts. Primary obstructive azoospermia is most commonly due to bilateral obstruction of the epididymides, if the iatrogenic cause of vasal obstruction postvasectomy is excluded. Obstructive azoospermia due to epididymal obstruction can be corrected by microsurgical reconstruction with vasoepididymostomy.

Vasoepididymostomy is considered the most technically challenging operation in male reproductive microsurgery. With the introduction of optical enhancement, microsurgical end-to-end single-tubule anastomosis was introduced by Silber (9) in 1978, and end-to-side anastomosis by Wagenknecht et al. (10) Berger (1) described a tubular intussusception using three double-armed microsutures placed to an epididymal tubule in a triangular fashion (Fig. 56.1). Subsequently, Marmar (7) modified this technique, using only two microsutures placed perpendicularly to the epididymal tubule for the anastomosis (Fig. 56.2). Chan et al. (2,3) reported placing the two microsutures longitudinally to the epididymal tubules, allowing the incision on the tubules to be made longitudinally (longitudinal intussusception vasoepididymostomy [LIVE]) and resulting in a larger lumen of epididymal inflow to the anastomosis.

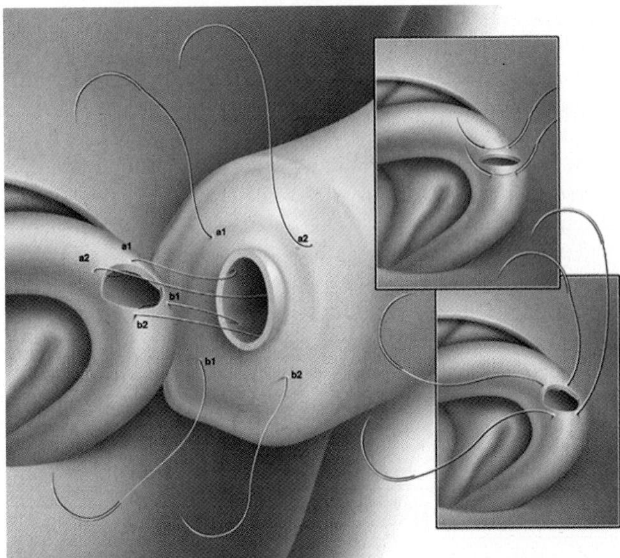


FIGURE 56.2 Two-needle intussusception vasoepididymostomy. This technique allows the use of two double-armed sutures to provide a four-point fixation on the vasal end for the anastomosis.

## DIAGNOSIS

A thorough history and physical examination often provide important clues that can lead to the diagnosis of epididymal obstruction. In North America, by far the most common cause of epididymal obstruction is prolonged vasal obstruction after vasectomy. Besides a vasectomy, other history that may suggest an obstruction include previous surgeries, instrumentation, or trauma in the groin, pelvis, scrotum, prostate, or urethra or prior epididymoorchitis. A family history of cystic fibrosis suggests that the patient may be a carrier of mutations in the cystic fibrosis transmembrane conductance regulator gene (congenital bilateral absence of vas deferens with epididymal obstruction).

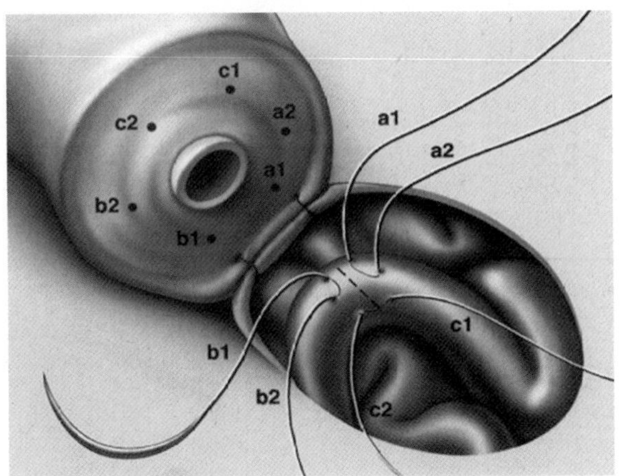


FIGURE 56.1 Triangulation intussusception end-to-side vasoepididymostomy. Three double-armed microsutures are placed in a triangulation fashion on the epididymal tubule, which is opened in the center of the triangle formed. The ends of the sutures are placed on the vasal end to complete the anastomosis.

The physical examination should include a complete examination of the scrotum, vas deferens, testes, and epididymides. Findings suggestive of epididymal obstruction include a vasectomy performed in the proximal convoluted vas, a full epididymis or epididymal cysts with normal testicular volume and texture, and the time since the vasectomy. The presence of a vasal sperm granuloma reduces the risk of epididymal obstruction. Congenital bilateral absence of the vas deferens on scrotal examination represents another finding consistent with obstruction of the excurrent ductal system. Semen analyses demonstrating azoospermia with normal ejaculation volume, pH, and fructose level are consistent with isolated bilateral epididymal obstruction.

The diagnoses of unilateral obstruction and partial epididymal obstruction are difficult to make or confirm, as these patients generally do not present with azoospermia, but rather with infertility with a combination of oligo-, astheno-, and teratospermia. If unilateral or partial epididymal obstruction is suspected clinically and vasoepididymostomy or other surgical reconstruction of the excurrent ductal system is contemplated, cryopreservation of sperm preoperatively should be considered as it is possible that the semen profile may decline significantly postoperatively if the reconstructive surgery fails.

Epididymal obstruction is generally an intraoperative diagnosis, as suggested by the presence of active spermatogenesis within the testis and the absence of sperm in a patent vas deferens. Although additional evaluations, including cystoscopy and various imaging studies, including scrotal and transrectal ultrasound, computerized tomography, and magnetic resonance imaging, may provide information that is consistent with epididymal obstruction, they are neither sensitive nor specific enough to diagnose epididymal obstruction and are generally not required prior to vasoepididymostomy.

Active spermatogenesis must be confirmed prior to attempting reconstruction of the excurrent ductal system. Confirmation of active spermatogenesis can be obtained through bilateral testicular biopsy performed as an isolated procedure ahead of time. Histologically, the cross section of each seminiferous tubule should have over 20 mature spermatids. Alternatively, cytologic examination of testicular aspiration for spermatozoa intraoperatively prior to vasoepididymostomy may confirm the presence of active spermatogenesis.

## INDICATIONS

Vasoepididymostomy is indicated in cases of obstructive azoospermia due to epididymal obstruction. Vasoepididymostomy should be performed in epididymal tubules that contain abundant sperm (motile or immotile) or sperm parts (heads and tails). Absence of abundant sperm or sperm parts indicates that the level of epididymal obstruction is located more proximally, where the anastomosis should be performed. Vasoepididymostomy should not be attempted in the absence of vasa, when the vasal gap is too big to be bridged despite appropriate surgical maneuvers for tissue mobilization, or in case of azoospermia due to testicular failure (nonobstructive azoospermia).

## ALTERNATIVE THERAPY

Besides microsurgical reconstruction with vasoepididymostomy, men with azoospermia due to epididymal obstruction may have sperm retrieved surgically from the epididymides (microscopic [MESA] or percutaneous [PESA] epididymal sperm aspiration) or from the testes (testicular sperm aspiration [TESA] or testicular sperm extraction [TESE]) for intracytoplasmic sperm injection (ICSI) to achieve pregnancy with their partners. With the increasing popularity and availability of assisted reproductive technologies such as in vitro fertilization and ICSI, the safety and efficacy of these technologies have improved significantly in recent years. Particularly for couples in whom the female partners are of advanced reproductive age or have significant female-factor infertility, sperm retrieval combined with ICSI can be an effective alternative to allow them to conceive as early as possible.

## SURGICAL TECHNIQUE

A light general anesthesia is preferred. Slight movements are greatly magnified by the operating microscope and may disturb performance of the anastomosis. In the absence of any clinical evidence of complicated obstruction (e.g., multiple previous failure of reconstruction attempts, large vasal gap, significant fibrosis in scrotal structure on physical examination), regional anesthesia with sedation can be employed in cooperative and motivated patients. Appropriate intraoperative intravenous antibiotics should be considered, particularly in cases with a significant past history of infection in the genitourinary tract.

### Preparation of the Vas

A high scrotal incision (Fig. 56.3) is preferred to allow adequate mobilization of the inguinal portion of the vas to anastomose to the epididymis without any tension. When isolating the vas, its periadventitial sheath should not be stripped off to preserve its blood supply. As the epididymis lies laterally in the posterior aspect of the testis, the vas should be mobilized and isolated lateral to the rest of the spermatic cord to allow a more direct contact with the epididymis for the anastomosis. In patients who had a previous vasectomy, the vas should be transected at the vasectomy site to evaluate whether the testicular vas contains sperm and whether a vasoepididymostomy is indicated. The cut surface of the testicular end of the vas deferens is inspected with the operating microscope under 15× to 25× magnification. A healthy, white mucosal ring should be seen that springs back immediately after gentle dilation with a 2- to 3-mm microvessel dilator. The muscularis should appear smooth and soft. A gritty-looking muscularis layer indicates the presence of scar/fibrotic tissues. Healthy bleeding should be noted from both the cut edge of the mucosa as well as the surface of the muscularis. If the blood supply is poor or the

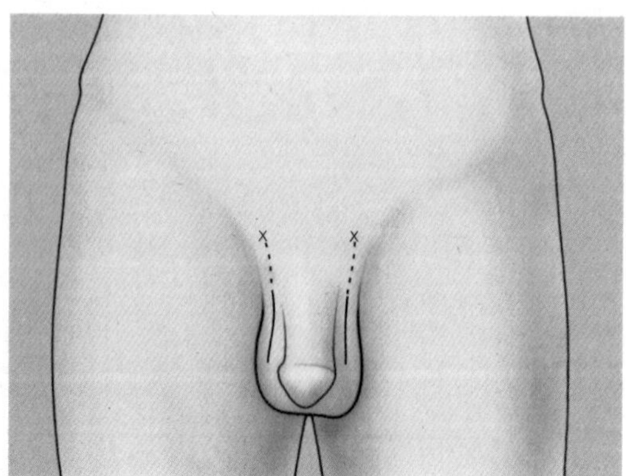

FIGURE 56.3 A high scrotal incision (*solid lines*) for vasoepididymostomy allows to option to extend the incision (*dotted lines*) towards the external inguinal ring (marked by X) for mobilization of the abdominal vas to bridge a larger gap for the anastomosis.

muscularis is gritty, the vas should be recut until healthy tissue is found.

In patients with primary epididymal obstruction with no previous vasectomy, the vas is isolated at the junction of the straight and convoluted vas, where it is hemitransected with a 15-degree ophthalmic knife. Transection of the vas at this area will allow the maximal length of straight vas to be preserved to allow a tension-free vasoepididymostomy to be performed. The vasal fluid is sampled and evaluated under light microscopy. The absence of sperm and sperm parts in the vasal fluid indicates epididymal obstruction. On the other hand, the presence of abundant motile sperm indicates the absence of epididymal obstruction, and evaluation of vasal patency distally is essential to identify the location of the obstruction. In this case, the hemitransected vas can be reapproximated with interrupted 10-0 and 9-0 microsutures in two layers.

Patency of the abdominal end of the vas should be confirmed by saline vasogram in which a 24G soft angiocatheter connecting to a syringe containing 1 to 3 cc of saline is used to cannulate the vas. Easy injection of saline towards the abdominal vas confirms patency. If patency is not certain, a dye vasogram using 1 to 3 cc of 1:10 diluted indigo carmine should be performed. After injection of dye, bladder catheterization should review blue or green dye in the urine to confirm patency. If patency is not confirmed, formal vasography with diluted water-soluble radiographic contrast medium can be used to locate the obstruction.

## Identification of the Appropriate Epididymal Tubule

After confirming that a vasoepididymostomy is necessary and that the abdominal vas is patent and of adequate length, the testis within the tunica vaginalis is delivered outside the wound. A longitudinal incision is made on the anterior aspect of the tunica vaginalis. In long-term epididymal obstruction, a small hydrocele is often noted when opening the tunica vaginalis. The epididymis is then inspected under the operating microscope at 16× to 25× magnification to select an anastomotic site above the area of suspected obstruction. Often, a discrete yellow sperm granuloma is noted, above which there is indurated epididymis and dilated tubules, and below which the epididymis is soft and the tubules are collapsed.

Selection of the correct level of the epididymal tubule for anastomosis should not be a random event. The diameter of the epididymal tubule increases gradually from caput to cauda. Anastomosing to the larger tubule may result in a higher patency rate. Once a potential epididymal tubule for the anastomosis is identified, a relatively avascular area of the epididymal tunica is grasped with sharp jeweler's forceps and tented upward. A 3- to 4-mm buttonhole is made in the tunica with microscissors to create a round opening that matches the outer diameter of the prepared vas deferens.

If the level of obstruction in the epididymis is not clearly demarcated, choose a tubule distally and puncture it with a 10-0 needle to aspirate epididymal fluid and examine it microscopically. If sperm are not found, proceed in an identical fashion proximally. Once sperm are identified, seal the puncture with a bipolar cautery and begin the anastomosis a few millimeters proximally along the epididymal tubule. Since the microsutures are to be placed longitudinally, a straight segment of the tubule is more preferable than one that is curved. This would allow the needle bites to run further along the tubule and a longer incision to be made longitudinally between the two needles.

## Preparation of the Epididymal Tubule

The epididymal tunic covering the tubule is thick and tough. On the other hand, the bare epididymal tubule underneath is thin and delicate, and extra care should be taken to avoid accidentally puncturing it, resulting in leakage of epididymal fluid and collapse of the tubule. After the initial cut on the epididymal tunic, there is often still a thin layer of residual tunic covering the epididymal tubule. Use of indigo carmine on the tissue may enhance visualization of the residual overlying tunic. The residual tunica should be dissected off fully with a combination of sharp and blunt dissection to expose the bare epididymal tubule underneath and to facilitate its intussusception into the vasal lumen when completing the anastomosis.

The vas deferens is drawn up through an opening in the tunica vaginalis and secured in proximity to the anastomotic site with two to four interrupted sutures of 6-0 polypropylene placed through the vasal adventitia and the tunica vaginalis. Care should be taken to avoid taking too deep a bite with the suture; this may result in accidental closure of the vasal lumen, rendering failure of the surgery. The vasal lumen should reach the opening in the epididymal tunica easily, with length to spare. To avoid tension or kinking of the vas, the surgeon should inspect the position and orientation of the vas not only when the testicle is delivered outside, but also when the testicle is placed back into the scrotum. The posterior edge of the epididymal tunica is then approximated to the posterior edge of the vas muscularis and adventitia with two or three interrupted sutures of 9-0 nylon (Fig. 56.4). This is done in such a way as to bring the vasal lumen in close approximation to the epididymal tubule selected for anastomosis. Adequate hemostasis of the vas and the epididymal tunic is essential, as the fluid in the epididymis cannot dissolve blood clot, which may obstruct the anastomosis.

## Longitudinal Intussusception Vasoepididymostomy

The LIVE procedure is our preferred method of microsurgical vasoepididymostomy as it greatly simplifies the procedure while yielding the highest patency rate among the various alternative techniques that we have employed (4–6). To allow even distribution of the suture points, four microdots are placed with a micro marking pen on the vasal ends to demarcate the exit points of the suture needles to be placed on the vas (Fig. 56.4A). For the anastomosis, we prefer to use 1-inch monofilament 10-0 nylon sutures, double-armed with 70-micron-diameter taper-point needles. Double-armed sutures

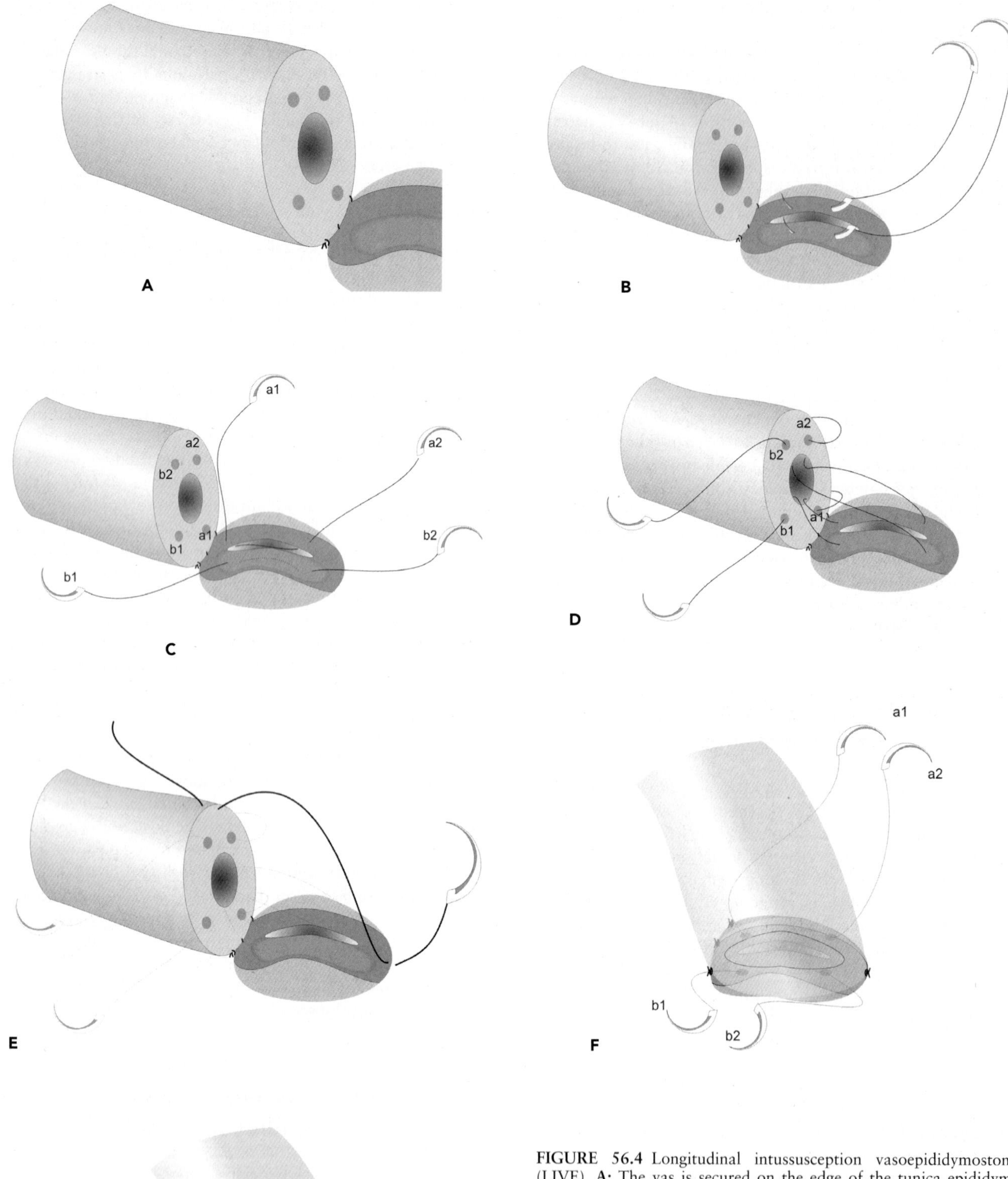


FIGURE 56.4 Longitudinal intussusception vasoepididymostomy (LIVE). **A:** The vas is secured on the edge of the tunica epididymis with two or three 9-0 sutures with its lumen opposing the midportion of the isolated epididymal tubule. **B:** Placement of the two double-armed 10-0 mucosal sutures in a longitudinal fashion on the tubule that is opening with a longitudinal incision between the needles. **C and D:** The sutures are pulled through and placed in an inside-out fashion on the vasal ends. **E and F:** A 9-0 tension-reducing suture is placed to position the vasal lumen in direct opposition with the epididymal lumen prior to tying the mucosal sutures. **G:** When the epididymal tubule is aligned in parallel with the vasal lumen, both mucosal sutures can be tied to their own ends to complete the anastomosis.

allow inside-out placement of the needles on the mucosa, eliminating the need for manipulation of the mucosa and the possibility of back walling. Modification of the LIVE technique for the use of longer double-armed needles or single-armed needles will be described later.

The vas is secured with 9-0 nylon sutures on the edge of the tunica epididymis opening, with the vasal lumen positioned at the center of the selected epididymal tubule. Under the highest magnification of the operating microscope (25× to 40×), the needles of two double-armed 10-0 microsutures are placed longitudinally on the epididymal tubule (Fig. 56.4B). Leave the microneedles in the epididymal tubule until it is ready to be incised longitudinally. Since the diameter of the needle (70 microns) is significantly larger than the suture diameter (17 microns), pulling through the needle will result in leakage of the epididymal fluid. The collapse of the epididymal tubule, along with the impaired visibility from the cloudy epididymal fluid, makes it difficult to place an additional suture or to make a precise opening in the tubule for the anastomosis.

Using a 15-degree ophthalmic knife, the tubule is incised longitudinally between the two needles of the 10-0 sutures (Fig. 54.4B). The epididymal fluid is then aspirated with a 5-microliter micropipette or with a 24G angiocatheter connected to a syringe for aspiration. The fluid is examined for sperm under light microscopy. We generally recommend that the surgeon evaluate the epididymal fluid himself or herself with a bench-top light microscope intraoperatively. This allows a quicker and more accurate answer to be obtained and avoids drying of the slide during transit to a pathologist/cytologist outside the operating room, which may compromise the interpretation.

If motile sperm are found, cryopreservation of the sample should be considered for future use with ICSI should the anastomosis fail. Generally, if the level of the epididymal tubule is carefully selected, the fluid inside is likely to contain sperm or sperm parts. Absence of abundant sperm or sperm parts in the fluid indicates that obstruction is still proximal to the selected segment of tubule and anastomosis should not be performed there.

The needles of the two double-armed 10-0 sutures are then pulled through and placed to the mucosa in the vasal ends in an inside-out fashion through the four microdots (Figs. 56.4C, 56.4D). Depending on whether the selected epididymal tubule for the anastomosis lies parallel (Fig. 56.4) or perpendicular (Fig. 56.5) to the vas, the placement of the needles on the vas may vary.

## Completing the Anastomosis

To avoid tearing the 10-0 sutures out of the epididymal tubule during tying, it is necessary to position the vas to allow the vasal and epididymal lumina to be in direct opposition to each other. This is achieved by placing a 9-0 tension-reducing suture approximating the epididymal tunic to the vasal sheath prior to tying the 10-0 microsutures (Figs. 56.4E, 56.4F). This 9-0 suture is tied loosely to allow visualization of the anastomosis during tying of the 10-0 sutures. Just prior to tying, the ends of each of the 10-0 sutures should be gently pulled until the opposite end just begins to move. This prevents having a loose loop of suture in the anastomosis and ensures that the epididymal mucosa is plastered against the vasal mucosa prior to tying. When setting up the anastomosis, in order to achieve the lowest tension possible without kinking the vas, the vasal lumen usually may end up lying parallel (Fig. 56.4) or perpendicular (Fig. 56.5) to the direction of the epididymal tubule. The ends of sutures for tying should be chosen carefully according to the orientation of the vas with respect to the direction of the epididymal tubule. In the setting when the vas and the epididymal tubules are parallel to each other, the two sutures are tied with their own ends on either side of the stay suture (Figs. 56.4F, 56.4G). In the setting when the vas and the epididymal tubules are perpendicular to each other, it is not necessary to push the ends of the 10-0 sutures on the same side of the 9-0 tension-reducing suture to tie. Instead, the two 10-0 sutures can simply be cross-tied to each other (Figs. 56.5B, 56.5C).

The advantages of LIVE include providing a four-point fixation at the mucosal anastomosis using two double-armed microsutures and allowing a larger epididymal lumen to be created with a longitudinal incision on the tubule. A watertight outer-layer anastomosis between the vasal sheath and the epididymal tunic is crucial to avoid leakage of fluid, which can lead to formation of sperm granuloma. We recommend placing 10 to 12 interrupted sutures of 9-0 nylon for the outer layer closure (Fig. 56.5D). Care should be taken to avoid injury to the peripheral epididymal tubules during the placement of needles on the epididymal tunic.

LIVE is a delicate procedure. Errors can occur at several crucial points of the surgery, requiring the anastomosis to be performed more proximally. Examples may include absence of sperm or sperm parts in the epididymal fluid, tearing of the epididymal tubule, or breakage of a mucosal suture. In any of these cases, a new spot more proximally in the epididymis should be identified to redo the anastomosis. The surgeon should not feel frustrated when it is necessary to take down the setup and redo the procedure at a more proximal site. Although it is time-consuming to redo an anastomosis, the extra time is well worth it. Vasoepididymostomy is a delicate operation where the outcome is highly dependant on technical perfection.

## Closure

After careful hemostasis and copious irrigation of the tissue, the tunica vaginalis should be closed with absorbable sutures and the testis returned intrascrotally in the correct orientation. Care should be taken to avoid any tension when manipulating the testis and spermatic cord after a delicate anastomosis is completed. With careful control of hemostasis, the risk of scrotal edema or hematoma can be minimized and drainage is generally not necessary.

## Maneuvers to Gain Extra Length to Bridge a Larger Gap

The simplest maneuver that should be attempted first to gain length to bridge a larger gap for the anastomosis is to mobilize the abdominal vas superiorly towards the external inguinal ring. The skin incision may be extended towards the external

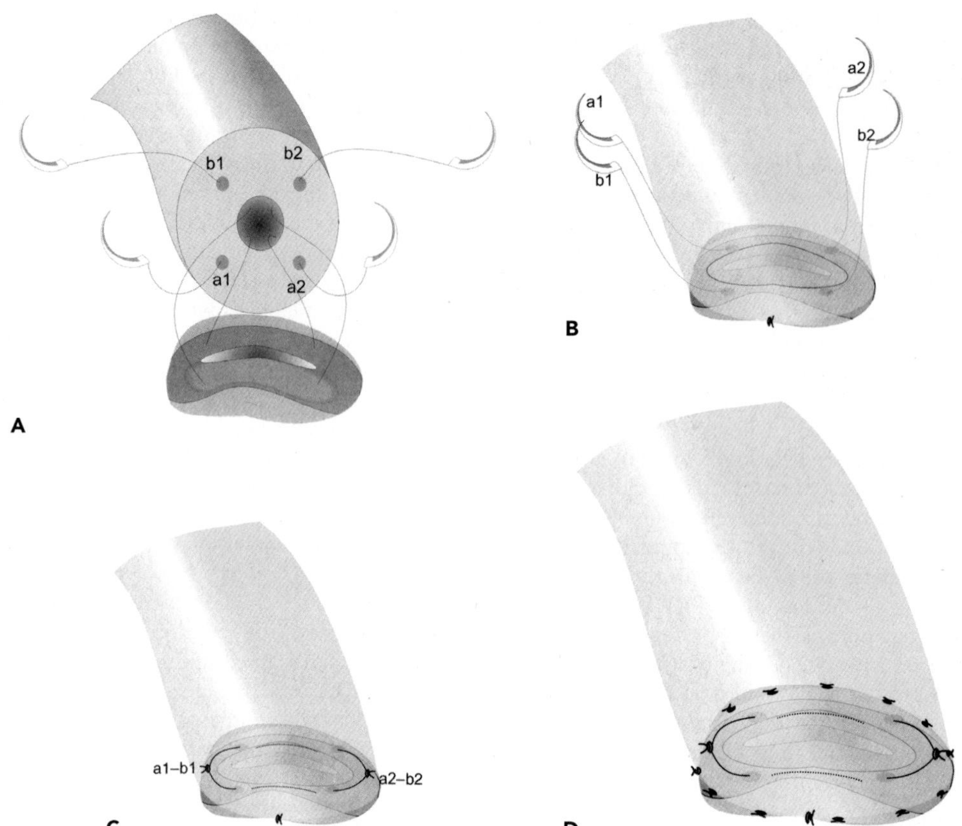


FIGURE 56.5 Longitudinal intussusception vasoepididymostomy (LIVE) when the epididymal tubule lies perpendicular to the vasal lumen. **A:** After pulling through the 10-0 mucosal sutures from the epididymal tubules, they are placed on the vasal end according to the plan for tying. **B:** A 9-0 tension-reducing suture is placed to position the vasal lumen in direct opposition with the epididymal lumen prior to tying the mucosal sutures. **C:** In this scenario, the mucosal sutures can be cross-tied with the end of the other mucosal suture to complete the anastomosis. **D:** Ten to 12 9-0 sutures are placed on the vasal sheath and the tunica epididymis to complete the outer layer of the anastomosis.

inguinal ring to facilitate this maneuver. Care should be taken to avoid stripping the periadventitial sheath to compromise the vasal blood supply. When there is still inadequate length of the vas deferens to reach the dilated epididymal tubule without tension, the cauda and corpus epididymis can be dissected off the testis and flipped up to obtain additional length (Fig. 56.6). To do this, the full depth of the epididymis is encircled with a small Penrose drain at the level of obstruction and, under 8× to 16× magnification, it is dissected distally off the testis, yielding sufficient length to perform the anastomosis (4). Usually, a surgical plane can be developed between the epididymis and testis, and injury to the epididymal blood supply can be minimized by staying right on the tunica albuginea of the testis. The inferior and if necessary the middle epididymal branches of the testicular artery are doubly ligated and divided to free an adequate length of epididymis. The superior epididymal branches entering the epididymis at the caput are always preserved and can provide adequate blood supply to the entire epididymis. The tunica vaginalis in then closed over the testis with absorbable suture, which prevents drying of the testis and thrombosis of the surface testicular vessels during the anastomosis. The dissected epididymis can remain outside the tunica vaginalis for the anastomosis.

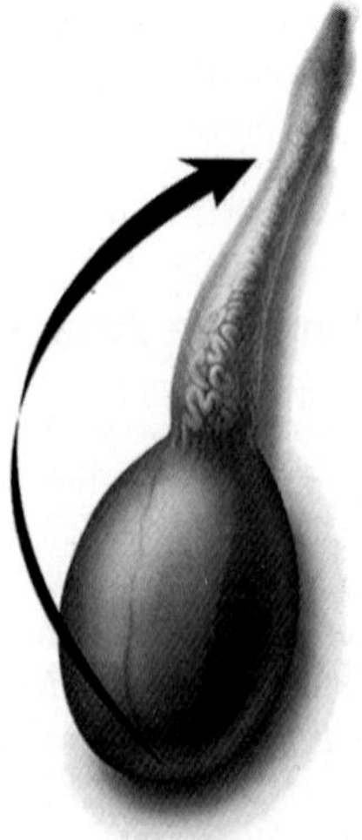

FIGURE 56.6 The corpus and caudal epididymis can be dissected off from the testis tunica albuginea and brought superiorly to bridge a massive vasal gap.

## Use of Single-Armed Microsutures for Longitudinal Intussusception Vasoepididymostomy

LIVE can be performed using 10-0 single-armed sutures, which are less costly than the double-armed ones (8). The disadvantage is that two of the four needle placements on the vasal end have to be done in an outside-in fashion. Two 10-0 sutures are first placed on the vas in an outside-in fashion. If the selected epididymal tubule lies perpendicularly to the vasal lumen, it is recommended to place the two needles on the two dots on the same side as the dominant hand of the surgeon (Fig. 56.7A). If the selected tubule lies in parallel to the vas, the sutures can be first placed on the two upper microdots and then pulled through the vasal lumen (Fig. 56.7B). Insertion of a 2- to 3-mm microvessel dilated during the outside-in placement of the needle may further decrease the risks of back walling of the vasal lumen mucosa. The LIVE procedure can then be performed in a similar fashion, with the two needles placed on the epididymal tubules where a longitudinal incision is made between the needles. The sutures are then pulled through and placed to the remaining two microdots marked on the vasal end in an inside-out fashion to complete the anastomosis. Tying of the two single-armed sutures can follow the same principle as described previously.

## Use of Long Double-Armed Microsutures for Longitudinal Intussusception Vasoepididymostomy

LIVE can be performed using a single long (6-inch) double-armed microsuture. Similar to the use of single-armed microsutures, the disadvantage is that two of the four needle placements on the vasal end have to be done in an outside-in fashion. The two needles at each end are first placed in the vas in an outside-in fashion. If the selected epididymal tubule lies perpendicularly to the vasal lumen, it is recommended to place the two needles on the two dots on the same side as the dominant hand of the surgeon (Fig. 56.8A). If the selected tubule lies in parallel to the vas, the sutures can be first placed on the two upper microdots and then pulled through the vasal lumen (Fig. 56.8B). Insertion of a 2- to 3-mm microvessel dilated during the outside-in placement of the needle may further decrease the risks of back walling of the vasal lumen mucosa.

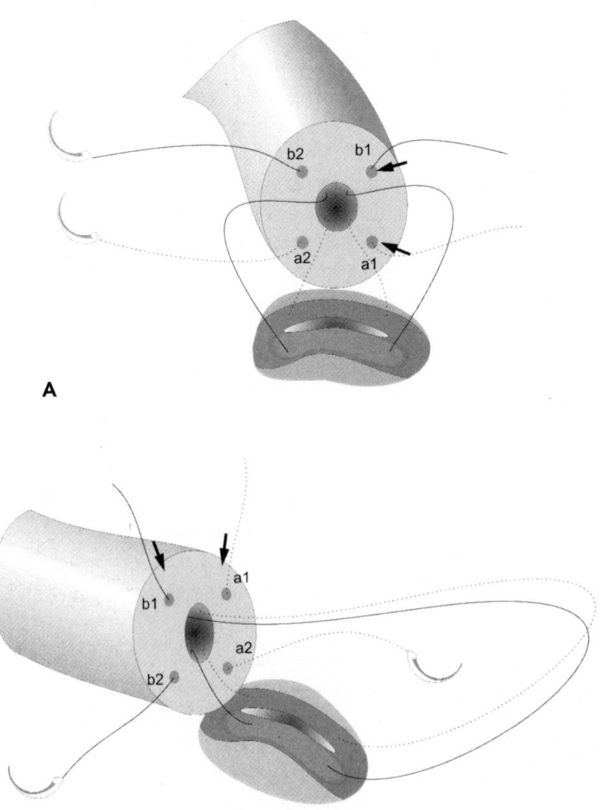


FIGURE 56.7. **A:** Placement of single-armed microsutures for longitudinal intussusception vasoepididymostomy (LIVE) when the epididymal tubule is in parallel to the vasal lumen. The *arrows* indicate the placement of the first bites of the two sutures. **B:** Same technique when the epididymal tubule is perpendicular to the vasal lumen. The *arrows* indicate the placement of the first bites of the two sutures when the surgeon is right-handed.

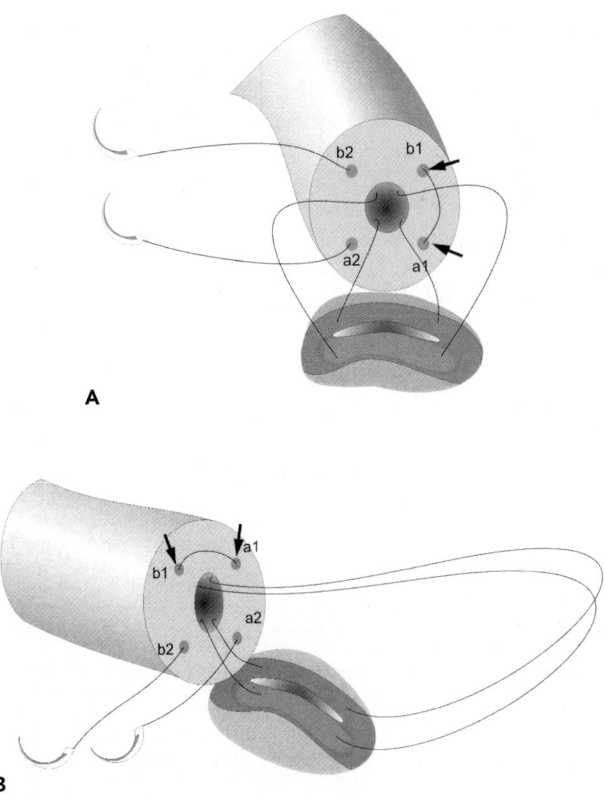


FIGURE 56.8. **A:** Placement of a long double-armed microsuture for longitudinal intussusception vasoepididymostomy (LIVE) when the epididymal tubule is in parallel to the vasal lumen. The *arrows* indicate the placement of the first bites of the two needles. **B:** Same technique when the epididymal tubule is perpendicular to the vasal lumen. The *arrows* indicate the placement of the first bites of the two needles of the suture when the surgeon is right-handed.

The LIVE procedure can then be performed in a similar fashion, with the two needles first placed on the epididymal tubules where a longitudinal incision is made between the needles. The sutures are then pulled through and placed to the remaining two microdots marked on the vasal end in an inside-out fashion to complete the anastomosis. Since a single double-armed suture is used in this case, suture tying needs to be done only once. Care must be taken to ensure there is no loose loop of suture before tying; otherwise, leakage of epididymal fluid may occur.

# OUTCOMES

## Results

We recently reported our clinical experience of microsurgical LIVE in a series of 72 men with azoospermia due to epididymal obstruction (3). The mean age of the subjects was 39.3 years. The etiologies of obstruction were postvasectomy (69%), infection (22%), iatrogenic (5%), trauma (1%), and idiopathic (3%). The median duration of obstruction was 18.7 years. Previous failed attempts at reconstruction were noted in 38% of patients. Mean follow-up period was 16.3 months.

The patency rate, defined as >10,000 sperm per milliliter of semen at any time postoperatively, was 92%. Early patency was achieved in 73% of subjects at 4 to 6 weeks postoperatively. The median best sperm count was 12.9 × $10^6$/mL, with a 23% rate of forward motility. The late "shut-down" rate, defined as the percentage of subjects who had sperm postoperatively but later became persistently azoospermic, was 4% at 1 year postoperatively. The median duration of the procedure was 55 minutes per anastomosis.

Among patients with follow-up over 1 year, the natural pregnancy rate was 31%. Median time to achieve natural pregnancy was 15.3 months. An additional 39% of patients achieved pregnancy with assisted reproduction, all using fresh ejaculated sperm.

## Complications

Potential surgical complications associated with vasoepididymostomy include wound infection, scrotal edema, hematoma, orchalgia, and persistent epididymal obstruction (surgical failure). Most of these complications are self-limiting and can be managed conservatively. More devastating complications such as ischemic epididymal fibrosis and testicular atrophy may be encountered rarely. The risk of complications increases in patients who have multiple previous unsuccessful reconstruction attempts with a significant extent of tissue fibrosis in the scrotal contents, or in cases where additional dissection is required to mobilize the vas or the epididymis to bridge a larger gap for the anastomosis.

Patients should also be instructed on the various preventive measures, such as avoidance of strenuous physical activities immediately postoperatively, use of an ice pack for wound or scrotal compression to prevent the development of hematoma or edema, and avoidance of ejaculation for up to 4 weeks to minimize the risks of disruption of the anastomosis due to the force of propulsion of the excurrent ductal system from orgasm.

Postoperatively, semen analyses may be performed at 1 month and subsequently every 2 to 3 months. Patients who have motile sperm return to the ejaculate should consider cryopreserving sperm, as initially patent anastomoses may eventually shut down. From our experience with LIVE, the great majority of patients who have a patent anastomosis will have sperm in the ejaculate in the first 6 months. It is rare for patients who have been persistently azoospermic in the first 6 months postoperatively to have the anastomoses open up. Persistently azoospermic men without cryopreserved sperm can opt for a redo vasoepididymostomy or surgical sperm retrieval by various techniques combined with ICSI to achieve pregnancy with their partner.

## *References*

1. Berger RE. Triangulation end-to-side vasoepididymostomy. *Journal of Urology,* 1998;159:1951–1953.
2. Chan PT, Li PS, Goldstein M. Microsurgical vasoepididymostomy: a prospective randomized study of 3 intussusception techniques in rats. *J Urol* 2003;169:1924–1929.
3. Chan PT, Lee R, Li PS, et al. *Six Years of Experience with Microsurgical Longitudinal Intussusception Vasoepididymostomy (LIVE): A Prospective Analysis.* Abstract presented at the 2008 Annual Meeting of the American Urological Association.
4. Chan PTK, Goldstein M. Vasectomy and vasectomy reversal. In: Kandeel FR, ed. *Male Reproductive Dysfunction.* New York: Informa Healthcare, 2007:385–405.
5. Chan PTK, Goldstein M. Reproductive tract reconstruction and vasectomy reversal. In: Chan PTK, Goldstein M, Rosenwaks Z, eds. *Reproductive Medicine Secrets.* Philadelphia: Hanley & Belfus, 2004:112–135.
6. Chan PT, Brandell RA, Goldstein M. Prospective analysis of outcomes after microsurgical intussusception vasoepididymostomy. *BJU Int* 2005; 96(4): 598–601.
7. Marmar JL. Modified vasoepididymostomy with simultaneous double needle placement, tubulotomy and tubular invagination. *Journal of Urology* 2000;163:483–486.
8. Monoski MA, Schiff J, Li PS, et al. Innovative single-armed suture technique for microsurgical vasoepididymostomy. *Urology* 2007;69(4): 800–804.
9. Silber SJ. Microscopic vasoepididymostomy: specific microanastomosis to the epididymal tubule. *Fertility and Sterility* 1978;30:565–571.
10. Wagenknecht LV, Klosterhalfen H, Schirren C. Microsurgery in andrologic urology. I. Refertilization. *Journal of Microsurgery* 1980;1:370–376.

# CHAPTER 57 ■ VASOVASOSTOMY

MARC GOLDSTEIN AND HOWARD H. KIM

Of the 500,000 men undergoing vasectomy each year in the United States, an estimated 2% to 6% will ultimately seek reversal (1). Despite the proven safety and efficacy of reversal surgery, vasovasostomy is not universally accepted. A significant drawback to vasovasostomy is the variable time interval to recovery of fertile sperm from the ejaculate, which is especially problematic for patients with partners of advanced maternal age. The lack of access to a microsurgeon trained in the vasovasostomy and vasoepididymostomy procedures is another potential limitation. With the widespread availability of assisted reproductive techniques (ART), some have questioned the need for complex reconstructive procedures for postvasectomy infertility.

Microsurgical vasovasostomy was first described in the 1970s by Earl Owen and Sherman Silber. Owen reported a patency rate of 98% in his series of 50 patients (2). Silber noted that normal sperm counts can be achieved in up to 95% of patients (3). This technique has been refined even further since its introduction, and similar, if not better, success rates have been reported recently by dedicated urologic microsurgeons (4). Most cost-benefit analyses have found that reversal procedures are the most efficacious and economical management of postvasectomy infertility (5), even in men with previous failed vasectomy reversal (6), demonstrating that microsurgical reconstruction is an important treatment option in appropriately selected patients.

## DIAGNOSIS

The preoperative workup for men requesting vasectomy reversal is straightforward. Confirmation of previous natural fertility is often sufficient documentation of spermatogenesis. However, if the patient has never fathered children in the past or if he has obstructive azoospermia without a history of prior vasectomy, further workup is necessary. The workup includes a full history, physical examination, and basic laboratory tests, including a semen analysis, and should be performed in conjunction with evaluation of the female partner. An obstructive etiology such as complications from a previous hernia repair may be revealed in the medical history.

### Physical Exam

The physical examination provides important clues about the likelihood for successful reversal surgery. Testicular volume and consistency mirror the spermatogenesis status; soft, small testes suggest impaired spermatogenesis, and a testicular biopsy may be necessary prior to reconstruction. An indurated epididymis or an ipsilateral hydrocele may predict the presence of a secondary epididymal obstruction, which would necessitate a vasoepididymostomy.

Physical findings specific to the vasectomy site include the presence of a sperm granuloma and the length of the vasal gap. Sperm granulomas are found in 10% to 30% of men undergoing reversal surgery (7). The presence of a sperm granuloma can serve as a pop-off valve for the efferent ductile system, protecting the epididymis from the detrimental effects of increased intratubular pressure, and increases the likelihood of vasovasostomy being required instead of vasoepididymostomy. A large gap between the obstructed vasal ends may require inguinal extension of the scrotal incision and additional dissection to ensure a tension-free anastomosis.

### Laboratory Evaluation

A semen analysis with examination of the centrifuged pellet is the primary laboratory test obtained prior to reversal surgery. Up to 10% of patients will have sperm with tails in the centrifuged pellet at a mean of 10 years after vasectomy (8), a finding indicative of likely sperm in at least one has deferens, meaning a vasovasostomy will almost certainly be possible on at least one side with a good overall prognosis for return of sperm to the ejaculate. An elevated level of serum follicle-stimulating hormone (FSH) suggests poor spermatogenesis in men with small, soft testes, which may precipitate further diagnostic workup. In men with elevated serum FSH levels or in men without prior fertility, the serum antisperm antibody assay helps to make a case for obstructive azoospermia with active spermatogenesis (9).

## INDICATIONS FOR SURGERY

Although an overwhelming majority of vasovasostomies are performed in men with postvasectomy infertility, a significant number of men undergo repair for iatrogenic injury to the vas deferens. In a series of 472 patients surgically explored for obstructive azoospermia, 7.2% had an iatrogenic injury (10). Mode of injury included inguinal hernia repair (more frequently pediatric hernia surgery), renal transplantation, appendectomy, and spermatocelectomy (10). Because these patients often have longer vasal defects, impaired blood supply, and longer obstructive intervals, surgery is usually more challenging technically and outcomes are worse.

### Prognostic Factors

Several patient and partner factors influence the outcome of reversal surgery and should be considered during the preoperative evaluation. These factors include prior fertility, age at vasectomy, medical and surgical history subsequent to vasectomy, obstruction interval, and partner's age and fertility status. The chance for successful pregnancy following vasectomy reversal decreases from 56% in patients whose partners are 20 to 39 years of age to 14% in those whose partners are age 40 or older (11). Men with the same partners from before the vasectomy procedure also fare better, perhaps due to proven previous fecundity together and shorter time interval since vasectomy (12). Regarding time interval between the initial vasectomy and subsequent reversal surgery, we found patency and pregnancy rates of 91% and 89%, respectively, for obstruction interval of <5 years and 89% and 44%, respectively, for obstruction interval of >15 years (13). The Vasovasostomy Study Group had similar results: they reported patency and pregnancy rates of 97% and 76%, respectively, for obstruction interval of <3 years, which fell to 71% and 30% for obstruction interval of 15 years or more (14). Finally, as a significant number of reversals actually require vasoepididymostomy on one or both sides, the surgeon must be comfortable with performing both surgeries.

## ALTERNATIVE THERAPY

Alternatives to vasovasostomy include in vitro fertilization (IVF) with intracytoplasmic sperm injection (ICSI) using retrieved sperm, donor sperm insemination, and adoption. Selecting between vasovasostomy and vasoepididymostomy based on intraoperative vasal fluid findings will be discussed later in this chapter. With the availability of IVF/ICSI, the use of donor sperm or adoption for postvasectomy infertility is rare.

## SURGICAL TECHNIQUE

### Operating Room Set-up

A two-headed operating microscope with 6× to 32× power magnification is used (Fig. 57.1). Foot pedal controls allow the surgeon to zoom and focus the field of view without interrupting the surgery. The microscope is used for most of the procedure, with the exception of the opening incision and closure. Although the operation can be performed in the standing position, the use of specially designed microsurgical chairs increases the stability of the surgeon's chest and arms (Fig. 57.2). By standing or sitting on the patient's right side, the right-handed surgeon is in position to place the more difficult abdominal end vasal sutures with the forehand.

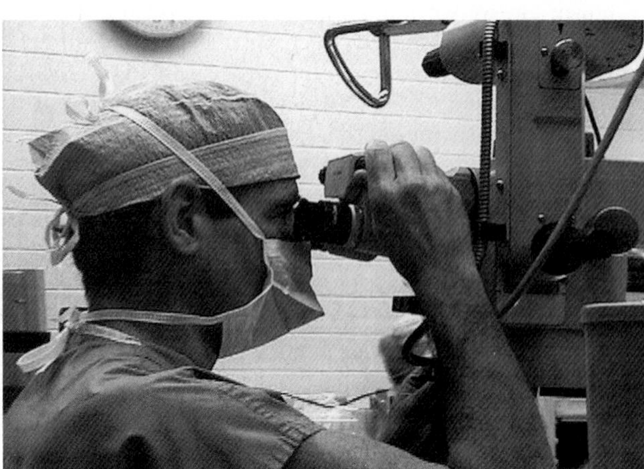

FIGURE 57.1 The operating microscope has two heads for the surgeon and the assistant. Microscope settings are checked before starting the procedure. (All photos courtesy of Marc Goldstein, MD and Philip S. Li, MD)

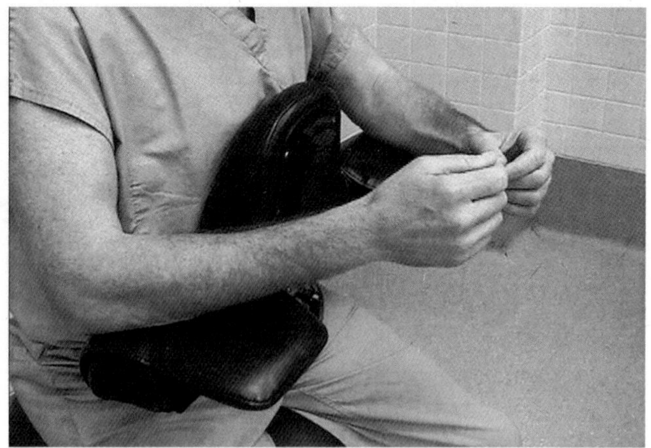

FIGURE 57.2 The specially designed microsurgical chair adjusts for optimal support of the chest and arms.

### Anesthesia

Although regional anesthesia can be used for uncomplicated vasovasostomies, general anesthesia is preferred to minimize disruptive motion when placing the delicate anastomotic sutures, especially during complex or prolonged reconstructive procedures. The patient's ability to remain still and the surgeon's experience and comfort level should be considered in selecting the type of anesthesia.

### Incision

After a dose of intravenous cefazolin and standard surgical preparation of the groin and genitalia in the supine position, the external inguinal ring is marked on both sides (Fig. 57.3). Careful palpation of the vasectomy site helps to determine the level of the incisions, usually high vertical scrotal incisions at

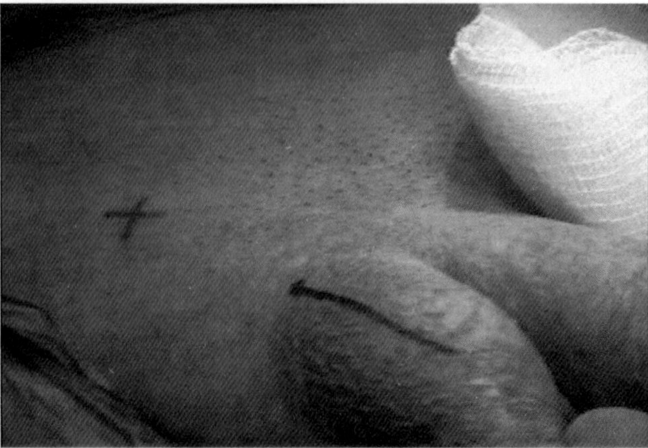

FIGURE 57.3 **A:** The right surgical incision is marked over the scrotal skin. The external inguinal ring is marked with an *X*. The incision is at least 1 cm away from the penis.

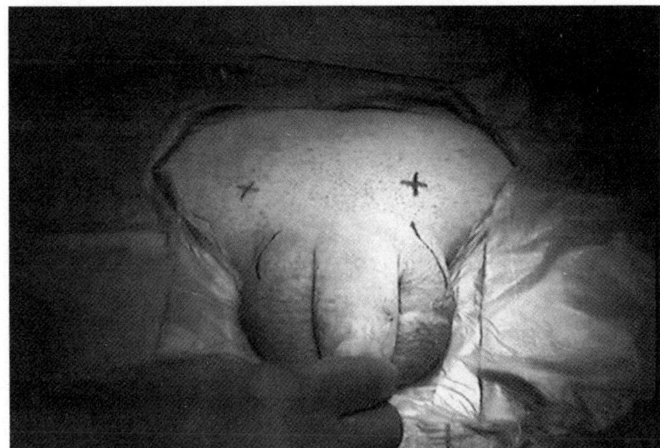

FIGURE 57.3 B: The skin incisions for both sides are marked.

least 1 cm lateral to the base of the penis for optimal cosmetic results. The incision should be long enough to allow delivery of the testis; the tunica vaginalis should be kept intact to optimize exposure of the vas deferens (Figs. 57.4–6). The incision may be extended toward the external ring if a high vasectomy or large vasal gap is encountered. Alternatively, if the site of vasal disruption is even higher, such as in the case of inguinal obstruction secondary to herniorrhaphy, an inguinal incision is

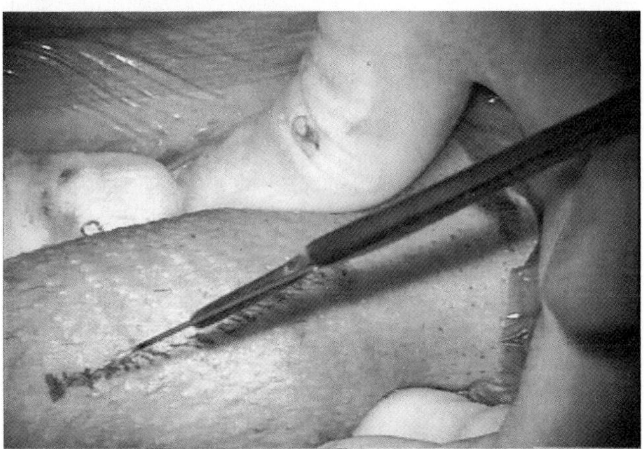

FIGURE 57.4 The skin incision is made with a #15 blade.

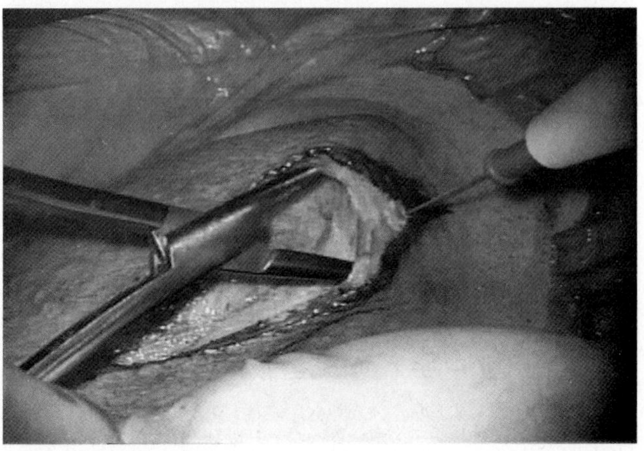

FIGURE 57.5 Electrocautery is used for the underlying dartos layer.

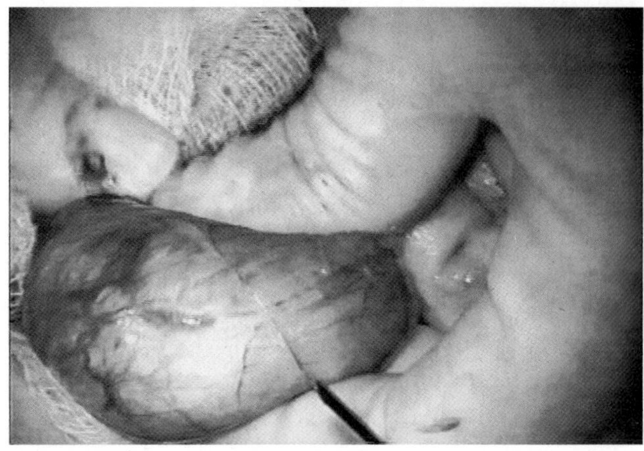

FIGURE 57.6 The testis is delivered into the field, with the tunica vaginalis intact.

preferred. Incision through the scar from the previous surgery usually leads directly to the obstruction. Even if the epididymis needs to be exposed, the testis can be delivered through the inguinal incision or through a separate scrotal incision.

## Exposure of the Vasa Deferentia

Adequate exposure of the vas deferens is critical for achieving a tension-free anastomosis (Fig. 57.7). To preserve the blood supply of the vas deferens, the correct dissection plane must be achieved along the vasal sheath; venturing too close to the sheath endangers the periadventitial vasal blood supply, whereas straying too far away from the sheath jeopardizes the testicular artery. Injury to the testicular artery can result in testicular atrophy, as the deferential artery likely has been disrupted during the previous vasectomy. The operating microscope should be used for this dissection with at least 10× power magnification to provide adequate visualization and to minimize risk of injury to the vessels. After gentle blunt dissection of the vas deferens, two Babcock clamps are placed above and below the obstructed segment (Fig. 57.8). Finding the proper dissection plane can be facilitated by transilluminating the sheath with the operating light (Fig. 57.9). A curved mosquito clamp is used to puncture this space at two points on either side of the vasectomy site (Fig. 57.10), and two quarter-inch Penrose

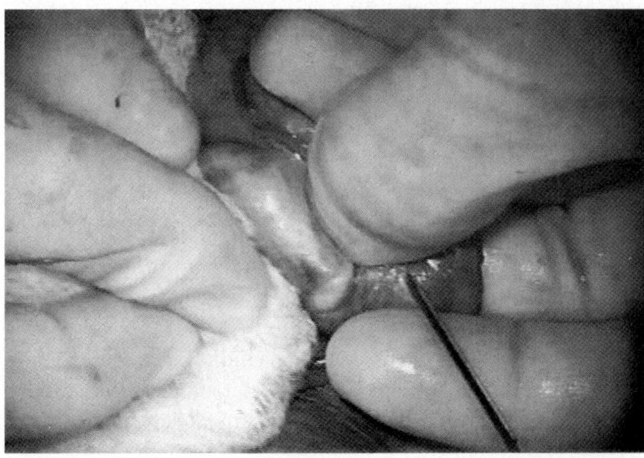

FIGURE 57.7 Blunt dissection with a gauze-covered finger releases the vas deferens from the surrounding tissue.

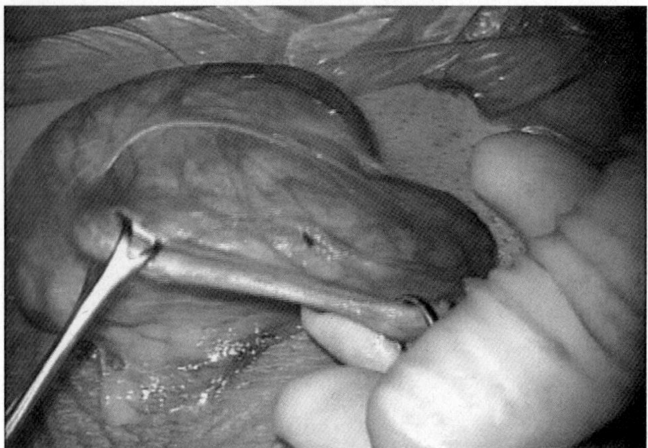

FIGURE 57.8 Two Babcock clamps are placed along the length of the vas deferens.

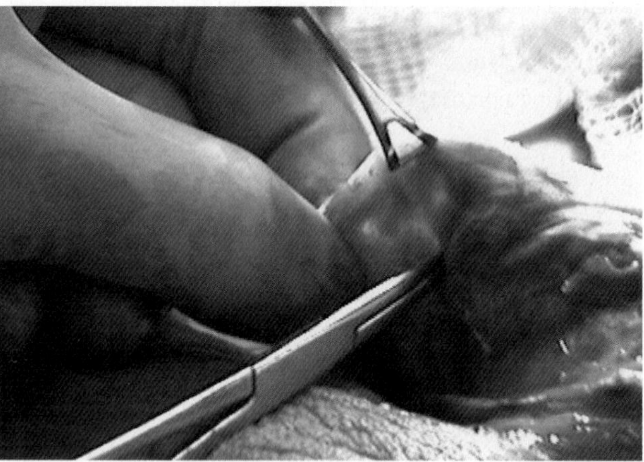

FIGURE 57.9 Transilluminating the tissue surrounding the vas deferens by bringing the operating light low helps to identify the correct dissection plane.

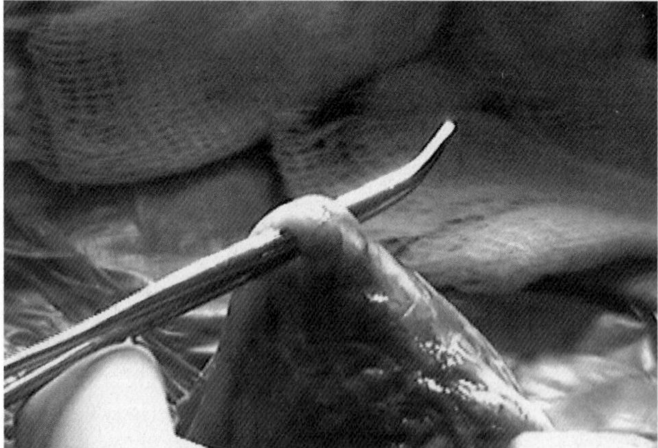

FIGURE 57.10 The plane between the vas deferens and the surrounding tissue is pierced with a Crile clamp.

drains are pulled through to serve as handles to traction the vas deferens while gently separating the surrounding tissue with both blunt and sharp dissection with small fine Metzenbaum scissors (Fig. 57.11).

Length is more difficult to achieve on the abdominal portion of the vas deferens. Several maneuvers can be used to achieve

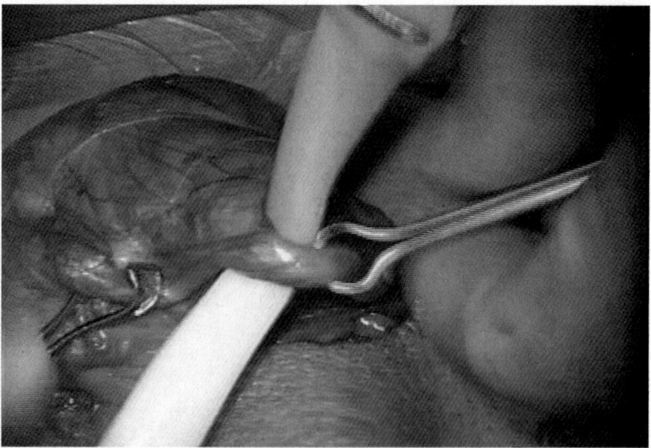

**A**

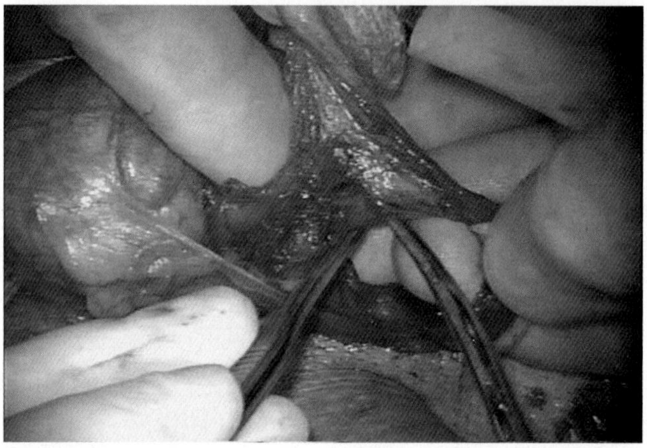

**B**

FIGURE 57.11 **A:** Quarter-inch Penrose drains are brought through the two openings made by transillumination. **B:** Using traction on the Penrose drains, the vas deferens is released using both blunt and sharp dissection.

additional length when a long vasal gap is encountered. Blunt dissection with the index finger through the external inguinal ring can release the abdominal vas deferens almost to the level of the internal inguinal ring without opening the external oblique aponeurosis. Distally, the convoluted vas deferens can be dissected from the epididymal tunica (Figs. 57.12 and 57.13). Up to 6 cm of additional length can be achieved with

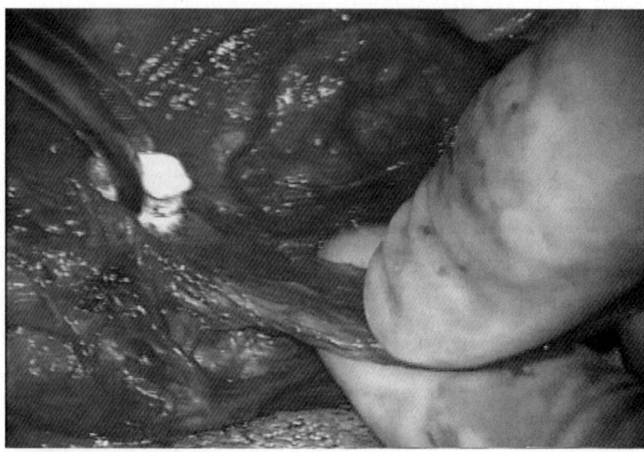

FIGURE 57.12 The vas deferens is freed distally to the level of the convolutions.

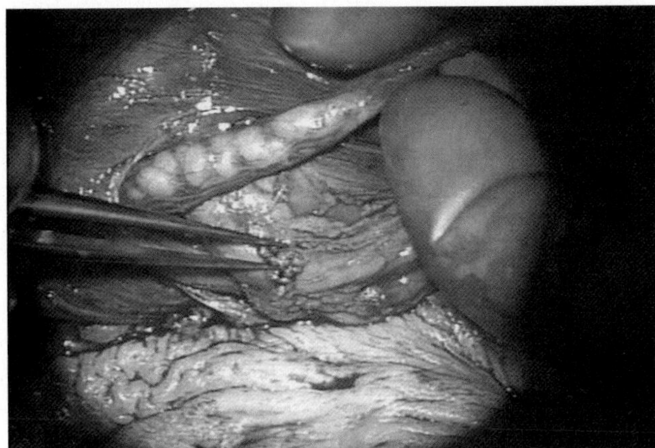

FIGURE 57.13 The convoluted vas deferens is fully exposed.

these techniques. Another 4 to 6 cm can be released by further dissection of the epididymis from the testis, up to the level of the caput epididymis. Again, the blood supply must be carefully preserved. Finally, the Prentiss maneuver can provide up to 10 cm of vasal length when used in combination with the other techniques.

## Preparation of the Vasa Deferentia

The obstructed segment, along with any associated vasectomy clips or sperm granuloma, is excised, first on the testicular side using an ultrasharp knife and a slotted 2-mm, 2.5-mm, or 3-mm-diameter nerve-holding clamp (Accurate Surgical & Scientific Instruments Corp., Westbury, NY). The slotted nerve-holding clamp allows for a perfect 90-degree transection (Figs. 57.14 and 57.15). Under 15× to 25× magnification, three distinct layers—the mucosa, muscularis, and adventitia—can be visualized. The mucosa should be white and elastic and the muscularis smooth and supple. Evidence of bleeding at each layer demonstrates a healthy blood supply. If the blood supply is in question, or if the muscularis appears gritty and fibrotic, additional transections should be made until the appearance of healthy tissue (Fig. 57.16). The deferential artery and vein are ligated with 6-0 Vicryl. The micro-bipolar coagulation forceps, set at 2.5 to 3.5 watts, help control the smaller bleeders, but care should be taken to avoid thermal injury to the mucosa.

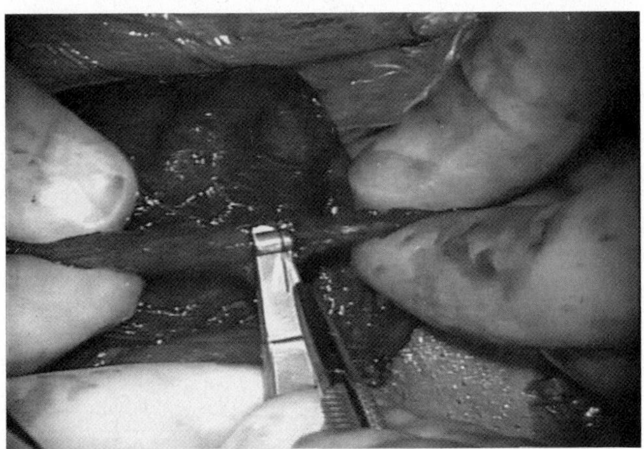

FIGURE 57.14 The slotted nerve-holding clamp and the ultrasharp knife help to make perfect 90-degree transections of the vas deferens.

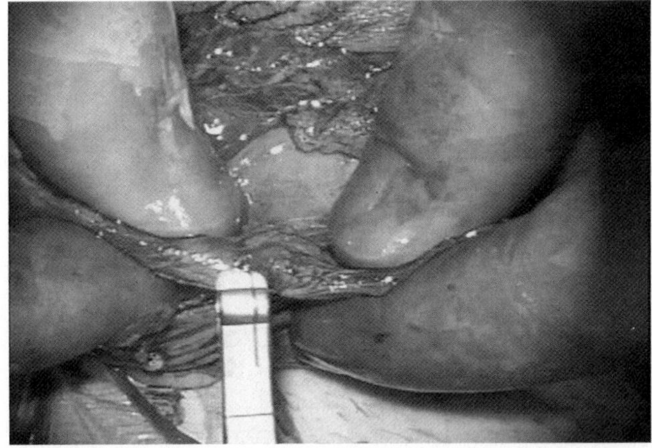

A

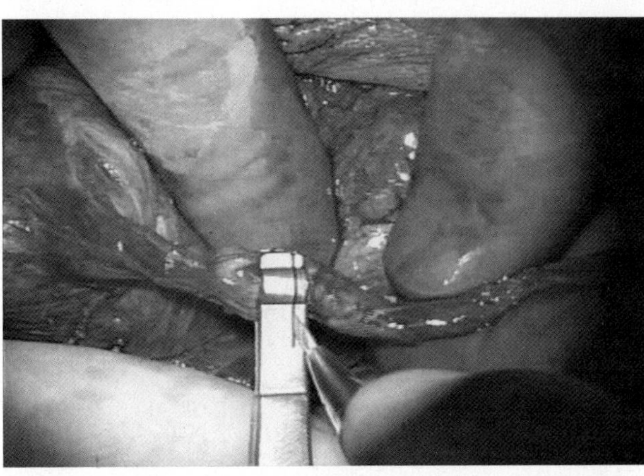

B

FIGURE 57.15 **A:** Sperm granulomas are found in 10% to 30% of men undergoing vasovasostomy. **B:** The initial cut is made on the testicular side of the obstructed segment or sperm granuloma.

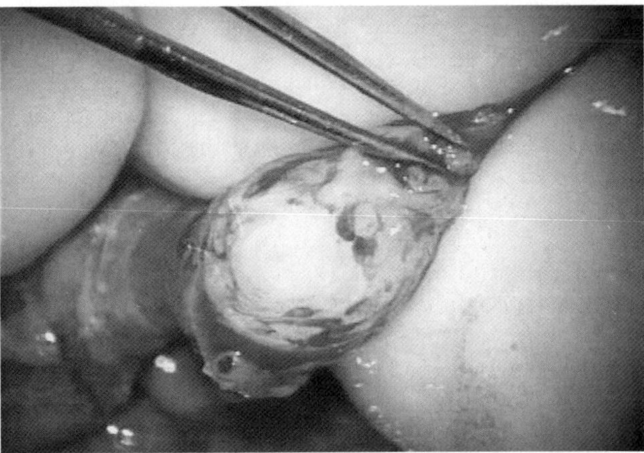

FIGURE 57.16 An unhealthy segment of vas deferens demonstrates white, avascular vasal layers surrounded by fibrotic scar tissue.

## Examination of Vasal Fluid

The testicular end of the vas deferens is milked and a touch-prep is made using a glass slide (Fig. 57.17). The fluid is mixed with a drop of lactated Ringer's solution and a cover slip is placed. The slide is immediately examined under 40× power magnification using a separate microscope setup (Fig. 57.18).

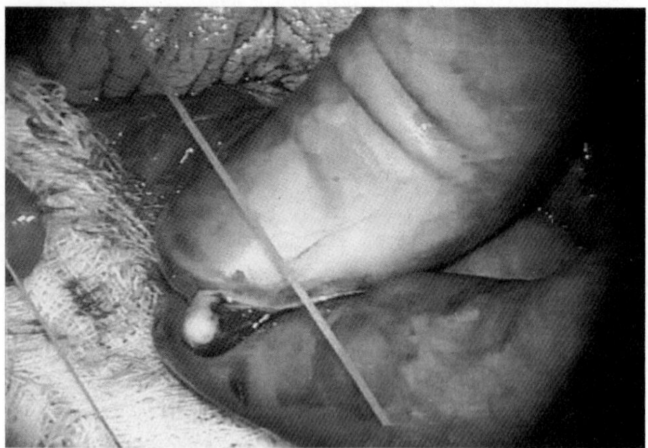

FIGURE 57.17 A touch-prep of the vasal fluid is made by blotting the freshly cut testicular portion of the vas deferens onto a glass slide.

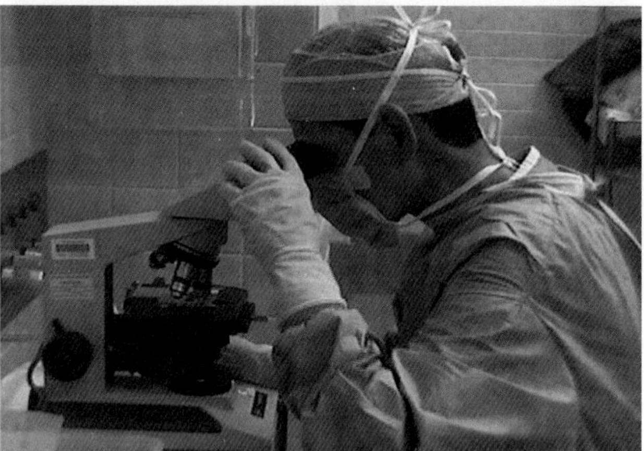

FIGURE 57.18 A separate microscope setup should be used to examine the vasal fluid under 40× magnification.

In its review of vasectomy reversal, the Practice Committee of the American Society for Reproductive Medicine (ASRM Guidelines) graded the sperm quality of vasal fluid as follows: grade 1, mainly normal motile sperm; grade 2, mainly normal nonmotile sperm; grade 3, mainly sperm heads; grade 4, only sperm heads; and grade 5, no sperm (15). Vasovasostomy is a good option for grades 1 through 4. If no sperm are found in the vasal fluid (grade 5), the gross appearance of the vasal fluid can help in deciding between vasovasostomy and vasoepididymostomy (Table 57.1). Cloudy, water-soluble fluid indicates the best chance for the eventual return of sperm to the semen, and thick, white, greasy toothpaste-like material indicates the worst prognosis (Fig. 57.19). Although a standard algorithm has not been established, the general recommendation is to proceed with vasovasostomy if sperm are identified in the vasal fluid or if the quantity of the fluid is copious and watery. Vasoepididymostomy should be considered if the vasal fluid is absent or if the quality of the fluid is thick, white, and creamy. If no fluid can be expressed for evaluation, the testicular end of the vas deferens is barbitaged with 0.1 mL of saline using a 24-gauge angiocatheter sheath, and the resultant fluid is examined (Fig. 57.20). In the presence of large sperm granulomas, the testicular end of the vas is minimally dilated with very little or no luminal fluid; barbitage with milking often expresses a small amount of fluid with sperm.

The abdominal end of the vas deferens is similarly transected and inspected. The lumen is gently dilated with a microvessel dilator and about 1 mL of saline is injected with a 24-gauge angiocatheter sheath to confirm patency. In assessing patency of the testicular and abdominal ends of the vasa deferentia, the surgeon must consider the left and right sides

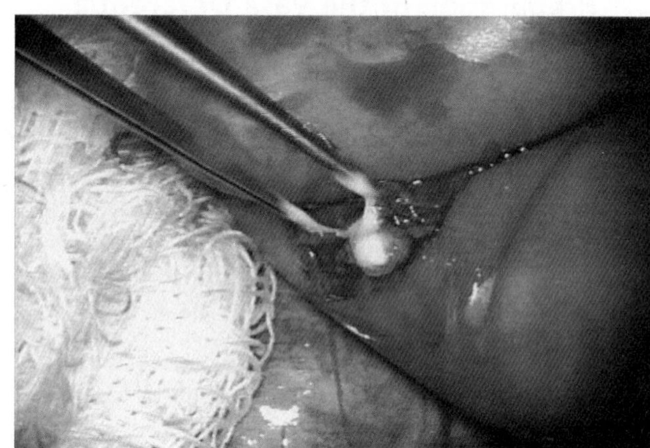

FIGURE 57.19 A thick, greasy, "toothpaste" consistency indicates a poor prognosis for sperm in the vasal fluid.

TABLE 57.1

EVALUATION OF VASAL FLUID

| Gross appearance | Microscopic appearance | Grade | Indicated surgery |
|---|---|---|---|
| Copious, cloudy, thin, water soluble | Sperm with tails | 1, 2 | Vasovasostomy |
| Copious, creamy yellow, water-soluble | Many sperm heads, occasional sperm with short tails | 3, 4 | Vasovasostomy |
| Scant fluid, sperm granuloma present | Barbitage fluid with sperm | 1–5 | Vasovasostomy |
| Copious, crystal clear, watery | No sperm | 5 | Vasovasostomy |
| Scant, white, thin fluid | No sperm | 5 | Vasoepididymostomy |
| Copious, thick, white, toothpaste-like, water-insoluble | No sperm | 5 | Vasoepididymostomy |
| Dry | No sperm | 5 | Vasoepididymostomy |

Typical intraoperative findings on vasal fluid evaluation and the recommended procedure for each finding are listed.

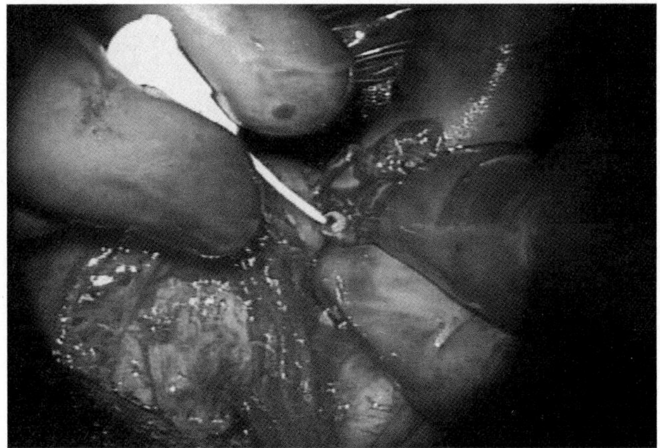

FIGURE 57.20 If the vas deferens is "dry," a 24-gauge angiocatheter sheath is used to barbitage the lumen with saline.

together, with the fundamental principle that one good anastomosis is superior to two tenuous connections. For example, if a right epididymal obstruction and a left abdominal vas blockage are encountered, a single crossed vasovasostomy should be performed. Specifically, crossed vasovasostomy should be considered in the following circumstances: (i) unilateral inguinal obstruction of the vas deferens with an atrophic contralateral testis, or (ii) obstruction or aplasia of the inguinal vas or ejaculatory duct with a contralateral epididymal obstruction. Although this technique requires opening of the scrotal septum, it is much easier than an inguinal vasovasostomy.

## Anastomosis of the Vasa Deferentia

In preparation for the anastomosis, the two ends of the vas deferens are stabilized without tension using a microspike approximating clamp (Fig. 57.21) (16). A tongue blade encased in a 1-inch Penrose drain serves as a platform for suturing (Fig. 57.22). The entire setup is brought up through a slit in a rubber dam (Fig. 57.23); the rubber dam provides a contrasting field for the black sutures and prevents the sutures from adhering to tissue.

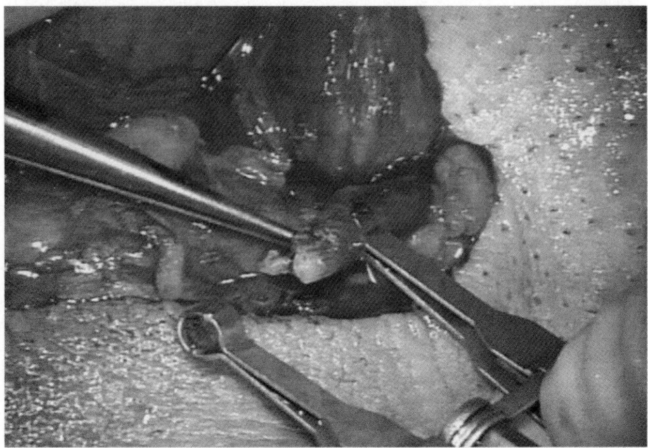

FIGURE 57.21 The microspike approximating clamp stabilizes the two ends of the vas deferens for suturing.

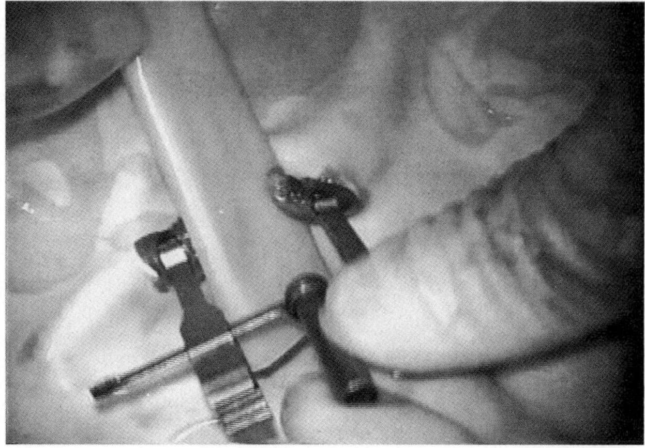

FIGURE 57.22 A tongue blade wrapped with 1-inch Penrose drain provides a platform for suture placement.

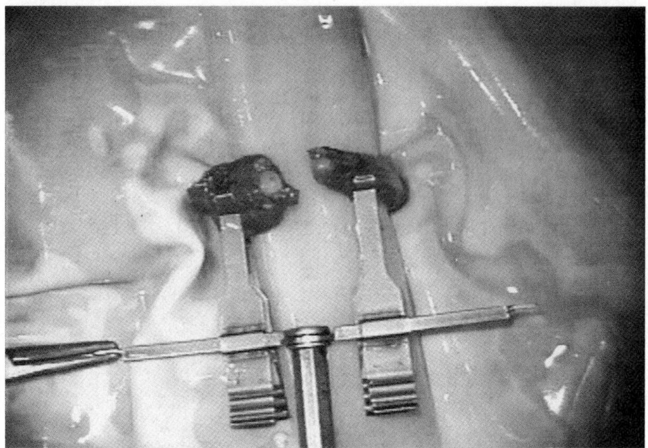

FIGURE 57.23 A rubber dam prevents sutures from sticking and getting lost in the surrounding tissue.

## The Microdot Technique for Multilayer Microsurgical Vasovasostomy

A microtip marking pen (Devon Skinmarker Extra Fine #151, Devon Industries, Buffalo, NY) is used to make six equidistant dots on the face of each transected vas deferens; the dots of one vasal end should mirror those of the other end to prevent twisting or distortion of the anastomosis (Fig. 57.24). The dots are made at the 1, 3, 5, 7, 9, and 11 o'clock positions on the muscularis, roughly halfway between the adventitia and the mucosa. This blueprint ensures precise suture placement and a watertight closure even with markedly discrepant luminal diameters.

Six monofilament 10-0 nylon double-armed sutures with 70-micron-diameter taper-point needles (Sharpoint, Surgical Specialties Corp., Reading, PA, or Ethicon, Inc., Somerville, NJ) are placed, starting with the three anterior positions (Figs. 57.25 and 57.26). Each suture begins within the lumen and exits at the dot; this inside-out placement of the sutures minimizes mucosal manipulation and reduces the risk of backwalling. The mucosal lumen can be stained with indigo carmine and gently dilated with the microvessel dilator as needed to facilitate suture placement (Fig. 57.27). Although methylene blue causes an immediate reduction in sperm motility and

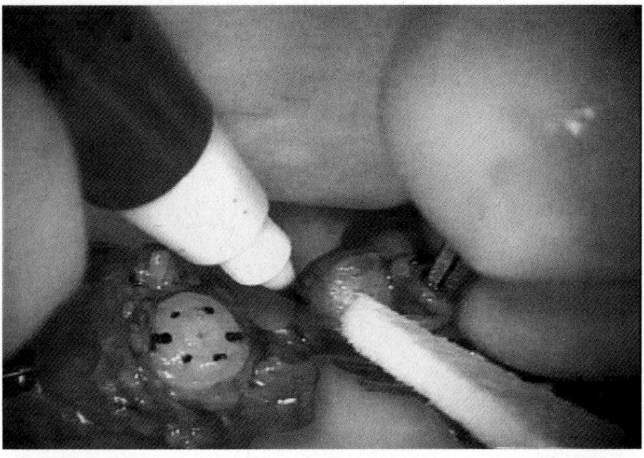

A

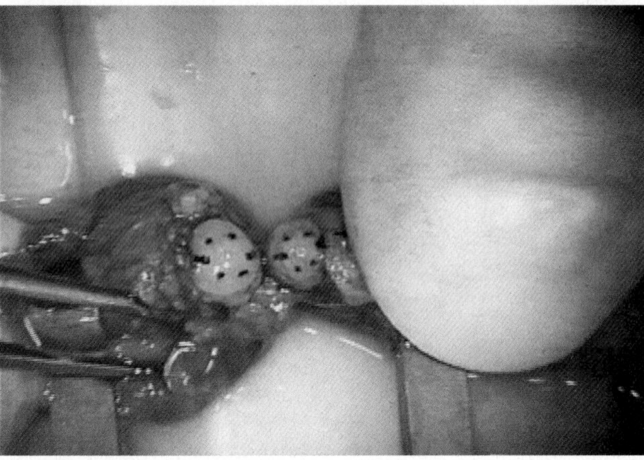

B

FIGURE 57.24 **A:** The microdots are made on the clock face of each cut vasal end using a microtip marking pen. **B:** The microdots should be symmetrical and mirror the corresponding side. Note the size discrepancy of the two vasal ends, with the larger dilated testicular end resulting from occlusive pressure.

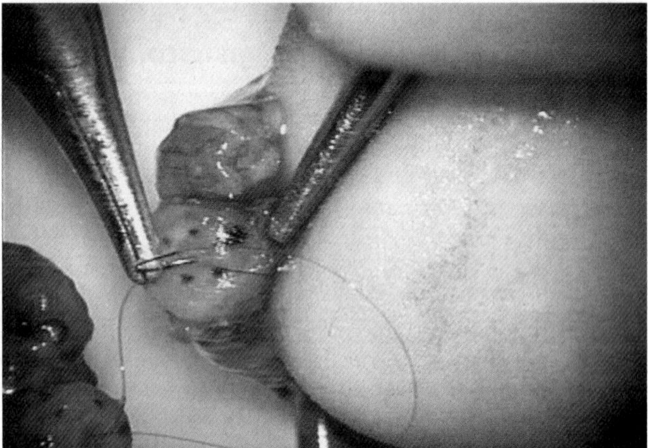

FIGURE 57.25 The placement of the 10-0 nylon mucosal sutures is guided by the microdots. Additional fine-tuning of the suture placements can be made at the surgeon's discretion.

should be avoided in reversal surgery, indigo carmine may be used (17). Each suture should include a small amount of mucosa and one third to one half of the muscularis, and the same amount of tissue should be included on each side. After the three anterior mucosal sutures are tied, two monofilament 9-0

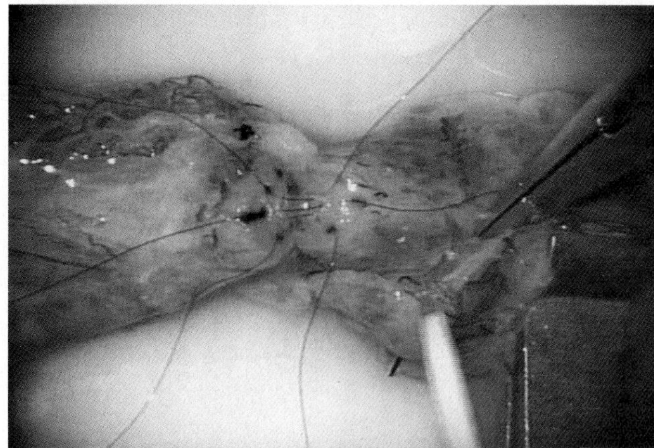

FIGURE 57.26 Three anterior mucosal sutures are placed and tied.

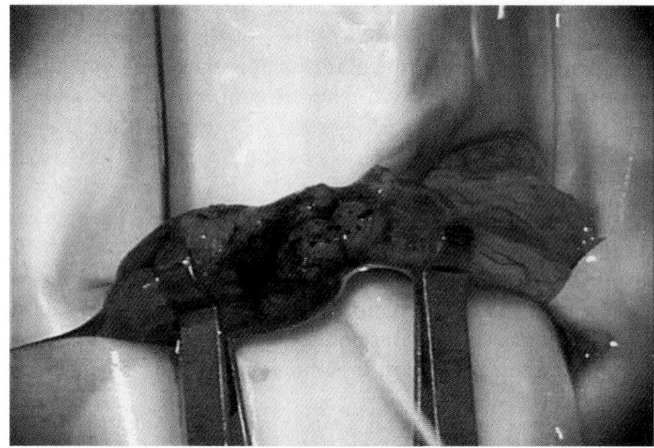

FIGURE 57.27 Visualization of the mucosal edge is improved with the application of indigo carmine.

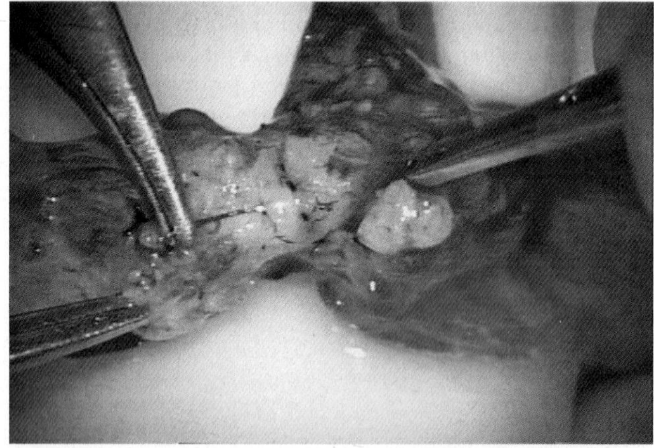

FIGURE 57.28 Monofilament 9-0 nylon deep muscularis sutures are placed in between the three anterior mucosal sutures.

nylon deep muscularis sutures are placed in between these three, without including the mucosa, and tied (Fig. 57.28).

The vas deferens is rotated 180 degrees and the remaining three mucosal sutures are placed in a similar fashion (Fig. 57.29). Before the final mucosal suture is tied, the vasal lumen is irrigated with heparinized lactated Ringer's solution to discourage clot formation. Four deep muscularis sutures are placed between the recently placed mucosal sutures for a circumferential two-layer closure. Four to six monofilament 9-0

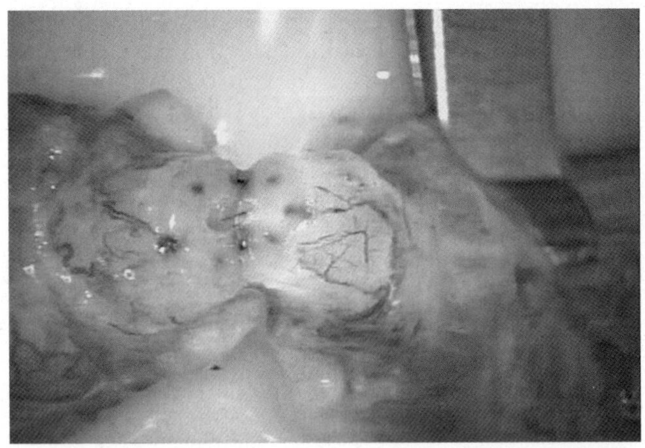

A

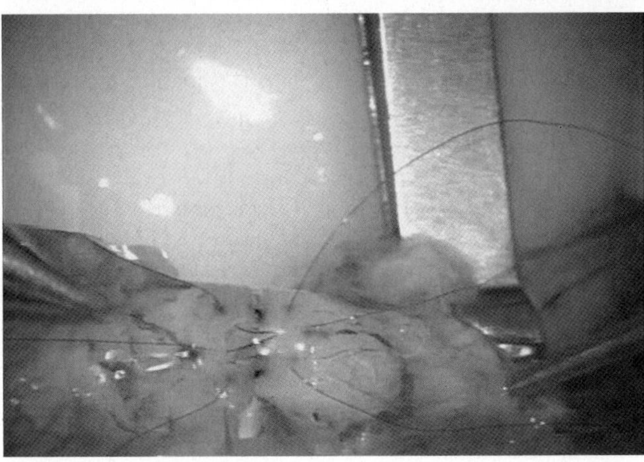

B

FIGURE 57.29 **A:** The vas deferens is rotated 180 degrees for placement of the remaining sutures. **B:** The sutures are placed in the same sequence as on the other side.

nylon sutures placed between the deep muscularis sutures within the adventitia constitute the third closure layer. Finally, the vasal sheath is reapproximated with six interrupted 8-0 nylon sutures, which protects the anastomosis from tension and enhances vascularization across the anastomosis (Fig. 57.30).

Chances for a successful operation are optimized by following the basic principles of anastomotic surgery, including mucosa-to-mucosa approximation of healthy well-vascularized tissue with minimal handling using atraumatic technique. The anastomosis should be leak-proof and tension-free. As sperm are highly antigenic, leakage at the anastomosis can develop into a sperm granuloma and provoke an inflammatory reaction, potentially leading to failure of the vasovasostomy (18). Tension on the anastomosis may result in late stricture and failure after an initial period of sperm in the ejaculate.

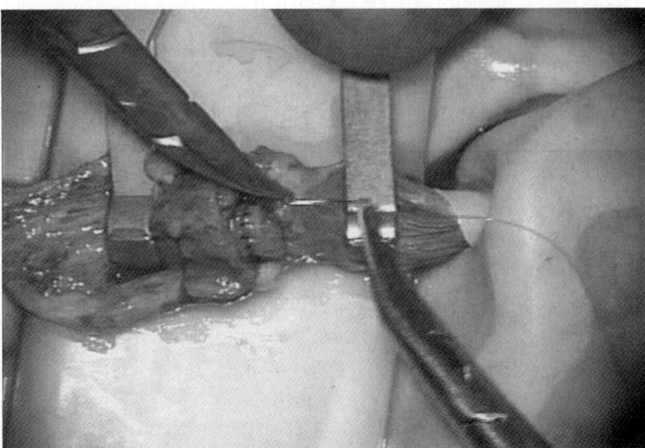

FIGURE 57.30 The vasal sheath is reapproximated with 8-0 nylon sutures, covering and protecting the anastomotic sutures.

## Special Circumstances

If unhealthy tissue or blood supply results in cutback of the testicular portion of the vas deferens to the convoluted segment (Fig. 57.31), anastomosis to the convoluted portion of the vas deferens follows the same principles as for the standard anastomosis, with a few additional considerations. A perfect 90-degree transection must be achieved; the convoluted segment is even more vulnerable to an oblique cut, resulting in insufficient mucosa and muscularis on one side. The surgeon must resist the temptation to unravel the convoluted segment lest the maneuver compromise the blood supply. Instead, additional length can be achieved with careful dissection of the vas deferens away from the epididymal tunica. During the suturing, taking too-large bites of the convoluted segment increases the risk for perforation of adjacent convolutions. In a series of 48 patients undergoing vasectomy reversal

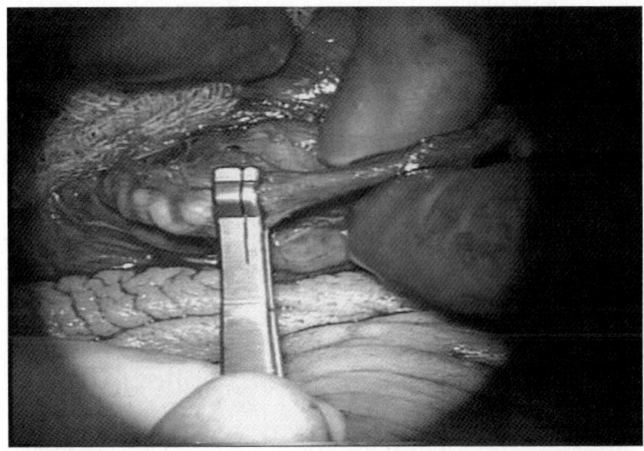

A

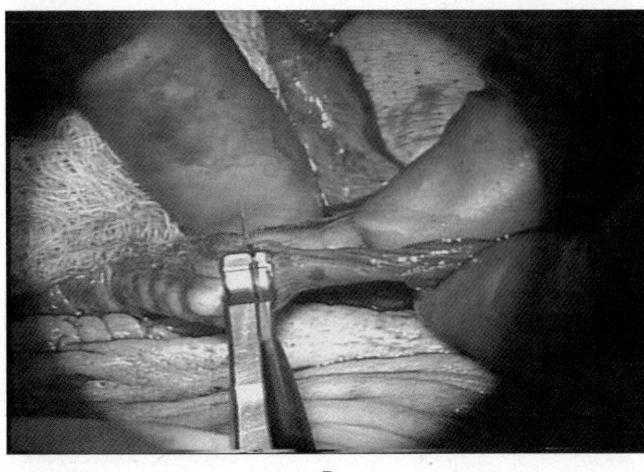

B

FIGURE 57.31 **A:** If additional length is necessary, the convoluted segment is carefully dissected free. **B:** The vasal cut is made at the juncture of the straight and convoluted portions.

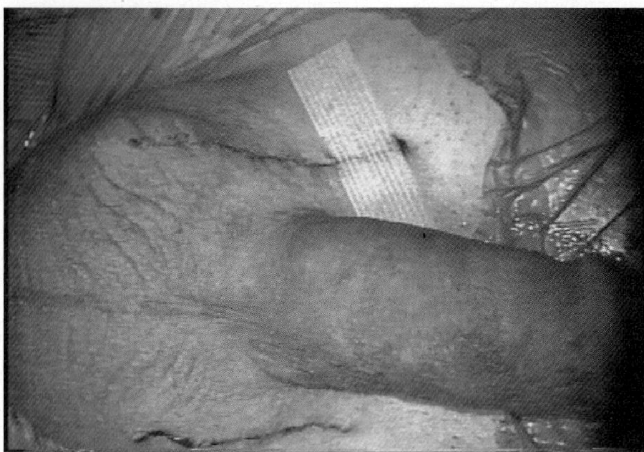

FIGURE 57.32 After closure, the nonscrotal portion of the incision is reinforced with adhesive skin-closure strips.

involving the convoluted vas deferens, the patency and natural pregnancy rates were 88% and 48%, respectively, comparable to outcomes with the standard technique (19).

In a less frequently encountered scenario, significant shortage of vasal length during a crossed vasovasostomy may warrant a testicular transposition. This maneuver takes advantage of the superior length of the spermatic cord to the vas deferens. Tension on the vas deferens is relieved by simply moving the testes to the contralateral hemiscrotum through an opening in the septum.

### Closure

After the four-layer anastomosis, the dartos layer is approximated with interrupted 4-0 Monocryl followed by a subcuticular skin closure with 5-0 Monocryl (Fig. 57.32). Penrose drains may be necessary with extensive dissection (Fig. 57.33); as reversal surgery is performed on an ambulatory basis, explicit instructions are given to the patient for self-removal the following day.

### Postoperative Care and Follow-Up

Bacitracin ointment and sterile gauze dressing are applied to the closure, followed with fluff-type gauze and a snug-fitting athletic supporter. The supporter should be worn at all times, even at nighttime, for 6 weeks. Thereafter, the supporter is worn during athletic activity until pregnancy is achieved. Light activity may be resumed in 3 days and heavy activity in 3 weeks. The patient is instructed to avoid sexual activity and ejaculation for 4 weeks. Hydrocodone with acetaminophen and a nonsteroidal anti-inflammatory drug are used for postoperative pain management. Semen analyses are obtained at 1, 3, and 6 months after surgery and every 6 months thereafter.

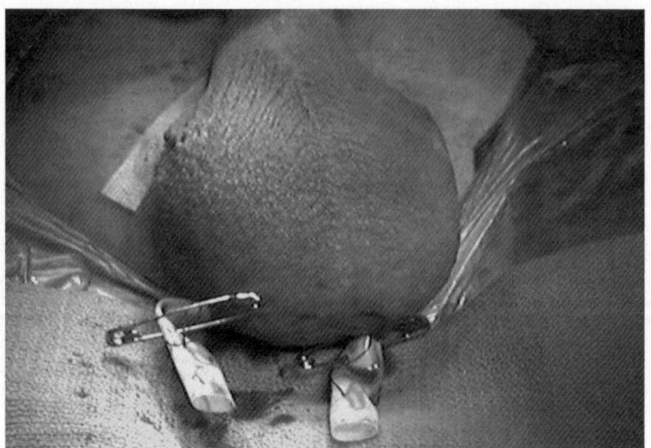

FIGURE 57.33 Penrose drains exiting the dependent portion of the scrotum provide wound drainage for cases involving extensive dissection.

## OUTCOMES

### Results

In our published series of 194 consecutive cases, patency was achieved in 99.5% of cases when sperm were found in the vasal fluid on at least one side at the time of surgery (4). The pregnancy rate in the first 100 cases was 54%, which increased to 64% when female factor infertility was excluded (4). Pregnancy rates were 82% to 89% for obstructive intervals of 0 to 15 years but significantly lower, 44%, with obstructive intervals >15 years (13). Persistent azoospermia beyond 6 months after surgery is an indication of likely immediate surgical failure. Late failure after initial patency were observed in 12% of men by 14 months after surgery, an event usually preceded by progressive loss of motility on semen analyses, followed by decreasing sperm counts (20). Because of the possibility for late stricture formation, we recommend cryopreservation of semen specimens when motile sperm are found in the ejaculate.

Failure of vasectomy reversal may be due to unrecognized epididymal obstruction and compromised anastomosis, among other causes. With patency and pregnancy rates of 67% and 30%, respectively, repeat vasectomy reversal surgery remains a viable option (21). Prognostic factors for successful initial vasectomy reversal also apply to repeat procedures.

### Complications

Vasovasostomy is a safe procedure with a low risk for significant complications. Although hematoma formation is the most common acute complication of vasectomy reversal surgery, only seven small hematomas occurred in our series of 2,100 cases (unpublished data). All resolved in 6 to 12 weeks without intervention. No wound infections occurred. Sperm granulomas, which often precede eventual obstruction, formed in about 5% of our patients (unpublished data). In an animal study, sperm granulomas were present in 99% of failed anastomoses in rats undergoing vasovasostomy (18).

### Cost-Benefit Analyses

To address the comparative utility of reversal surgery and ART, several cost-benefit analyses have been performed. Pavlovich and Schlegel (5) reported a cost per delivery after vasectomy reversal of $25,475 with a delivery rate of 47%, whereas the cost per delivery after sperm retrieval and ICSI was $72,521 with a delivery rate after one cycle of ART with sperm retrieval of 33%. Furthermore, a systematic review of four cost-benefit analyses comparing these two approaches also reported results favoring vasectomy reversal surgery (22). Another study found the cost of microsurgical epididymal sperm aspiration with ICSI/IVF to be 2.4 times higher than vasectomy reversal, even in men with previous failed vasectomy reversal (6).

Vasovasostomy is a safe and cost-effective management option for postvasectomy infertility. Although the average interval until pregnancy after successful microsurgical reconstruction is 12 months, reversal surgery has significant advantages over ART: the normal partner avoids treatment and subsequent children are possible without the need for further intervention. The ASRM Guidelines recommend the use of microsurgical reconstruction if the obstructive interval following a vasectomy is <15 years and no female fertility risk factors are present (15). The use of ICSI with sperm retrieval is recommended if advanced female age (>37 years of age) or fertility factors requiring IVF (e.g., tubal disease) are present, if the chance for success is greater with this technique, or if the couple prefers this method for financial or other reasons (15).

## *References*


1. Goldstein M. Vasectomy reversal. *Compr Ther* 1993;19:37–41.
2. Owen ER. Microsurgical vasovasostomy: a reliable vasectomy reversal. *J Urol* 2002;167:1205.
3. Silber SJ. Perfect anatomical reconstruction of vas deferens with a new microscopic surgical technique. *Fertil Steril* 1977;28:72–77.
4. Goldstein M, Li PS, Matthews GJ. Microsurgical vasovasostomy: the microdot technique of precision suture placement. *J Urol* 1998;159:188–190.
5. Pavlovich CP, Schlegel PN. Fertility options after vasectomy: a cost-effectiveness analysis. *Fertil Steril* 1997;67:133–141.
6. Donovan JF Jr, DiBaise M, Sparks AE, et al. Comparison of microscopic epididymal sperm aspiration and intracytoplasmic sperm injection/in-vitro fertilization with repeat microscopic reconstruction following vasectomy: is second attempt vas reversal worth the effort? *Hum Reprod* 1998;13: 387–393.
7. Goldstein M. Surgical management of male infertility and other scrotal disorders. In Walsh PC, Retik AB, Vaughan DE, et al., eds. *Campbell's Urology*, Vol. 2. Philadelphia: WB Saunders, 1997:1331–1377.
8. Lemack GE, Goldstein M. Presence of sperm in the pre-vasectomy reversal semen analysis: incidence and implications. *J Urol* 1996;155:167–169.
9. Lee R, Ullery BW, Ehrlich JR, et al. Value of serum antisperm antibodies in diagnosing obstructive azoospermia. *J Urol* 2007;639(suppl. 177): abstract 1927.
10. Sheynkin YR, Hendin BN, Schlegel PN, et al. Microsurgical repair of iatrogenic injury to the vas deferens. *J Urol* 1998;159:139–141.
11. Gerrard ER Jr, Sandlow JI, Oster RA, et al. Effect of female partner age on pregnancy rates after vasectomy reversal. *Fertil Steril* 2007;87:1340–1344.
12. Chan PT, Goldstein M. Superior outcomes of microsurgical vasectomy reversal in men with the same female partners. *Fertil Steril* 2004;81: 1371–1374.
13. Boorjian S, Lipkin M, Goldstein M. The impact of obstructive interval and sperm granuloma on outcome of vasectomy reversal. *J Urol* 2004; 171:304–306.
14. Belker AM, Thomas AJ Jr, Fuchs EF, et al. Results of 1,469 microsurgical vasectomy reversals by the Vasovasostomy Study Group. *J Urol* 1991; 145:505–511.
15. Practice Committee of the American Society for Reproductive Medicine. Vasectomy reversal. *Fertil Steril* 2006;86:S268–271.
16. Goldstein M. Microspike approximator for vasovasostomy. *J Urol* 1985; 134:74.
17. Sheynkin YR, Starr C, Li PS, et al. Effect of methylene blue, indigo carmine, and Renografin on human sperm motility. *Urology* 1999;53: 214–217.
18. Hagan KF, Coffey DS. The adverse effects of sperm during vasovasostomy. *J Urol* 1977;118:269–273.
19. Sandlow JI, Kolettis PN. Vasovasostomy in the convoluted vas deferens: indications and outcomes. *J Urol* 2005;173:540–542.
20. Matthews GJ, Schlegel PN, Goldstein M. Patency following microsurgical vasoepididymostomy and vasovasostomy: temporal considerations. *J Urol* 1995;154:2070–2073.
21. Matthews GJ, McGee KE, Goldstein M. Microsurgical reconstruction following failed vasectomy reversal. *J Urol* 1997;157:844–846.
22. Garceau L, Henderson J, Davis LJ, et al. Economic implications of assisted reproductive techniques: a systematic review. *Hum Reprod* 2002;17: 3090–3109.


# CHAPTER 58 ■ MICROSURGICAL VARICOCELECTOMY

ARMAND ZINI AND ZIV MAIANSKI

A varicocele is an abnormal dilation of the pampiniform plexus of the testis. It is reported that 35% to 40% of infertile men have a palpable varicocele (dilated testicular veins), whereas the prevalence of a varicocele in the general male population is about 15% (1,2). Despite extensive study, the exact mechanism by which varicocele influences fertility remains unclear. Various theories continue to be discussed, such as abnormal testicular temperature regulation with elevated scrotal temperature, reduced perfusion of the affected testicle due to venous stasis and backflow of toxic substances of either adrenal or renal origin, and changes in the testicular endocrine milieu (2). The effect of varicocelectomy on male fertility is also controversial (3,4). Uncontrolled studies have generally shown improved semen quality and pregnancy outcome after surgery (3). On the other hand, the results of randomized, controlled studies of varicocelectomy for clinical varicocele are equivocal (4,5). Nonetheless, varicocelectomy remains a commonly treated condition in men with infertility in North America (6). The benefit of varicocele repair must be balanced by the risk associated with the procedure itself. Therefore, it is important to select the procedure with the highest success and lowest complication rate.

## DIAGNOSIS

Varicoceles develop during early adolescence, at which time they usually produce no symptoms. Therefore, in the adolescent, the detection of a varicocele is by routine physical examination of healthy individuals. In contrast, in the majority of adult cases, the patient is referred to the urologist following a poor semen analysis. On occasion the patient may provide a history of dull scrotal ache or heaviness upon prolonged standing or exertion.

The physical examination should be performed in a warm room. The patient should be examined in the standing and supine positions, before and after a Valsalva maneuver. Careful palpation of the pampiniform plexus and measurement of testicular size (preferably by a standard orchidometer) are essential. The Valsalva maneuver can provoke engorgement of the plexus. Long-standing varicocele can induce a reduction in volume of the affected testis, usually the left one.

Varicoceles can be classified into one of three grades based on physical examination:

1. Grade I: small, palpable, following Valsalva maneuver only
2. Grade II: moderate, clearly palpable but not visible
3. Grade III: large, visible enlargement of the pampiniform plexus

Scrotal ultrasound including Doppler is a valuable tool to confirm the physical findings when the clinical exam is difficult (e.g., in obese men, when there has been prior scrotal surgery, or when the testicle has a high scrotal position) and for objective measurement of testicular size.

Abnormalities in semen analysis include a decrease in sperm concentration and motility and an increase in abnormal morphologic forms classically described as "stress pattern." However, none of these seminal findings are specific to varicocele.

## INDICATIONS

The indications for repairing varicoceles in adolescents include the following:

1. Palpable left varicocele with associated ipsilateral testicular atrophy (with the volume of the left testis being at least 20% less than that of the right)
2. Palpable varicocele with abnormal semen analysis results
3. Large symptomatic (painful) varicocele
4. Bilaterally palpable varicocele with testicular atrophy

Although prophylactic treatment of adolescent varicocele (for prevention of future infertility) is not recommended, it is important to follow untreated patients, since no test can predict whether an adolescent will be fertile or infertile.

Based on the Best Practice Policies for Male Infertility of the American Urological Society (5), varicocele treatment should be offered to the male partner of a couple attempting to conceive when all of the following are present:

1. A varicocele is palpable.
2. The male partner has one or more abnormal semen parameters or sperm function test results.
3. The couple has documented infertility.
4. The female partner has normal fertility or potentially correctable infertility.

In addition, testicular pain associated with varicocele (in the absence of other pathology), psychological concern regarding future fertility, and cosmetic reasons are all relative indications. Varicocele repair is not indicated in men with normal semen analyses or a subclinical (nonpalpable) varicocele.

## ALTERNATIVE THERAPY

Several approaches exist for varicocelectomy, including retroperitoneal and inguinal open techniques, microsurgical inguinal and subinguinal approaches, laparoscopic repairs, and radiographic embolization. The microsurgical varicocelectomy, low inguinal or subinguinal, as first described by Marmar et al. (7), is preferred by many urologist and male infertility experts because it is associated with a higher success rate and lower morbidity than nonmicrosurgical techniques (8,9).

The subinguinal approach is associated with less operative and postoperative pain than the inguinal approach because, with the former technique, the external oblique aponeurosis is not opened. However, the subinguinal approach is more challenging owing to the greater number of vessels (arteries and veins) encountered at the subinguinal level compared to the inguinal canal.

## SURGICAL TECHNIQUE

For the subinguinal approach, optical magnification is mandatory to avoid injury to the testicular artery and lymphatic vessels. For a better cosmetic result in the case of bilateral varicocelectomy, we recommend marking the incision sites (Fig. 58.1). The inguinal area is prepared and draped in the standard sterile way.

We start with a 2- to 3-cm oblique skin incision centered over the external inguinal ring, as previously described (Fig. 58.2) (8). The incision is deepened through the Camper and Scarpa fasciae by lifting these layers with a mosquito clamp and dividing the tissue with monopolar electrocautery. The spermatic cord is exposed by placing two small Richardson retractors at the extremities of the incision and by sliding a finger along the course of the spermatic cord, starting at the

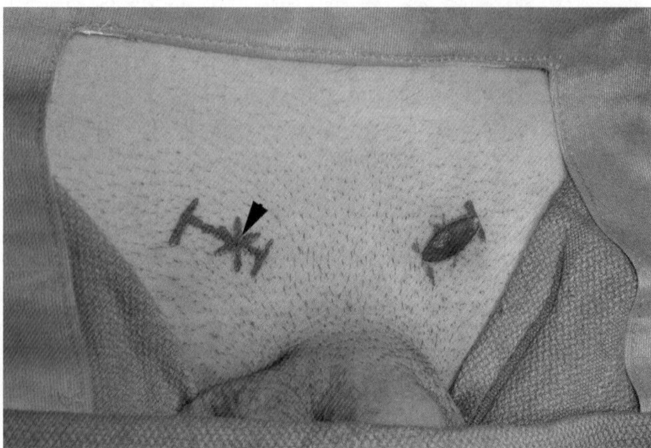

**FIGURE 58.1** The position of the right and left subinguinal incisions (approximately 2.5 cm long) for microsurgical varicocelectomy. The *arrowhead* points to the location of the right external inguinal ring.

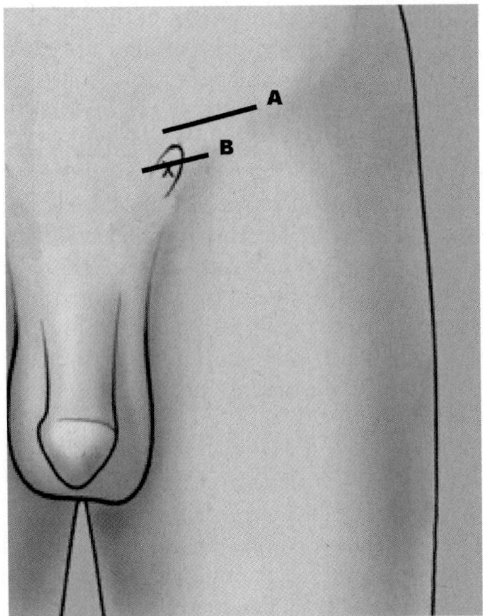


FIGURE 58.2 Illustration demonstrating the location of the inguinal *(A)* and subinguinal *(B)* incisions for microsurgical varicocelectomy (the position of the external inguinal ring is shown).

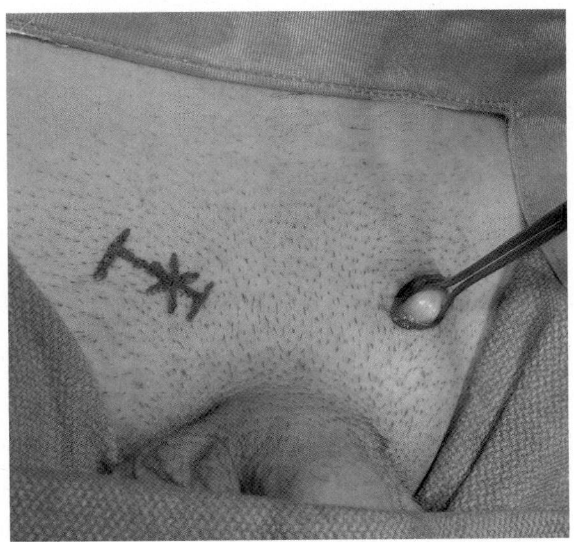

FIGURE 58.3 The spermatic cord is grasped with the Babcock clamp and delivered through the incision.

external ring and ending at the upper scrotum. The cord is then grasped with a Babcock clamp (Fig. 58.3), delivered, and placed over a large (1-in.) Penrose drain. During this maneuver, care is taken to spare the ilioinguinal nerve and the genital branches of the genitofemoral nerve. The testicle is then delivered through the wound by gently pulling on the cord and pushing the testicle cephalad. Once the testicle is delivered, the gubernacular veins and external spermatic perforators are exposed, clipped, and divided (Fig. 58.4).

The testicle is returned to the scrotum, and the spermatic cord is elevated on a large Penrose drain. The microscope is then brought into the operating field and the cord examined under 8× to 15× magnification. The external and internal spermatic fasciae are gently lifted (Fig. 58.5) and incised in the direction of the fibers using the monopolar electrocautery.

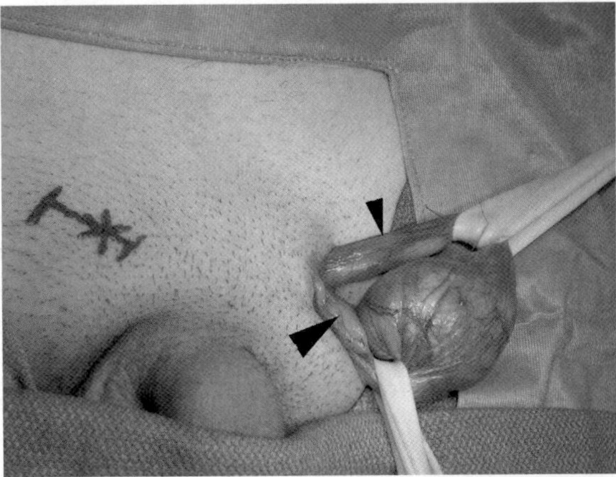

FIGURE 58.4 The testicle is delivered through the subinguinal incision. The spermatic cord *(small arrowhead)* and the gubernaculum *(large arrowhead)* are depicted.

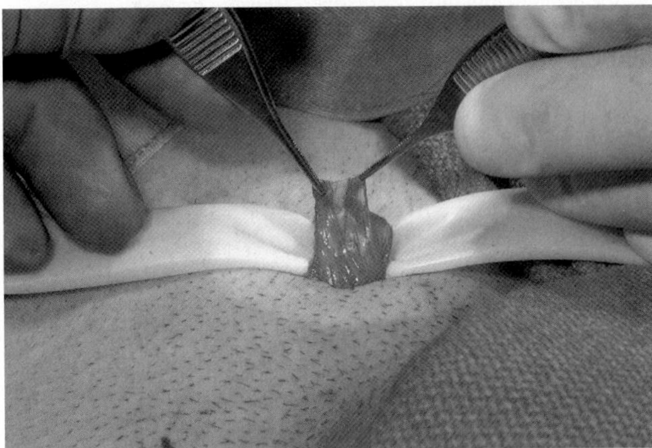

FIGURE 58.5 The external spermatic fascia is lifted with two smooth forceps in preparation for longitudinal incision of this fascia.

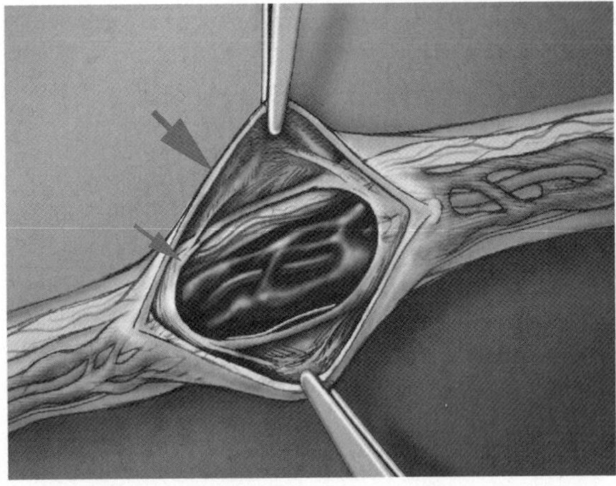

FIGURE 58.6 Illustration demonstrating the spermatic cord after longitudinal incision of the external *(large arrow)* and internal spermatic fasciae *(small arrow)*.

The internal spermatic vessels are exposed and examined (Fig. 58.6).

To simplify the procedure and protect the vas deferens and its vessels from potential injury during subsequent cord dissection, we first create a window between the internal spermatic vessels and the external spermatic fascia such that the internal

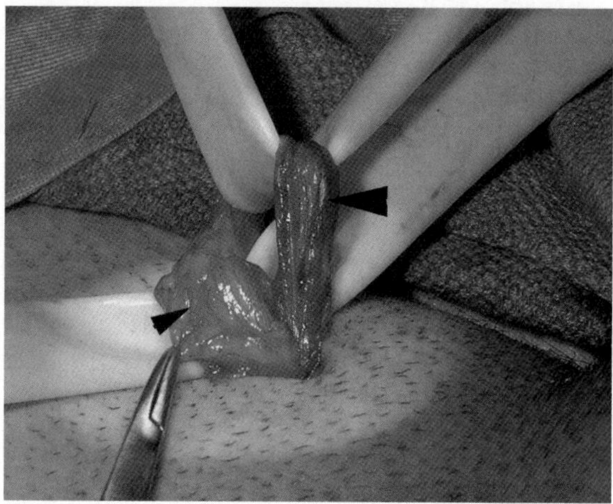

FIGURE 58.7 The spermatic cord is divided into two packages with a 1-in. Penrose drain between (a) the contents of the internal spermatic fascia *(large arrowhead)* and (b) the remainder of the cord, including the vas deferens and cremasteric fibers *(small arrowhead)*.

spermatic vessels are separate from the external spermatic fascia and its associated structures (cremasteric fibers, external spermatic vessels, vas deferens and its vessels) (10). A second Penrose drain is then introduced between the internal spermatic vessels and the external spermatic fascia and its associated structures (Fig. 58.7).

We first dissect the contents of the internal spermatic fascia (lying on top of the most superficial Penrose drain). Subtle pulsations will usually reveal the location of the underlying internal spermatic artery(ies). Once identified, the artery is dissected free of all surrounding veins by blunt dissection using a microsurgical needle driver and is then encircled with a 2-0 silk ligature for identification. Care is taken to also identify and isolate a number of lymphatics (usually three to six channels), and these are also encircled with a 2-0 silk ligature. All internal spermatic veins are clipped or ligated (with 4-0 silk) and divided. At the end of the first dissection, the cord is skeletonized such that only the identified artery(ies) and lymphatics are preserved.

We then elevate and dissect the contents of the external spermatic fascia (lying between the two Penrose drains). The vas deferens and its associated vessels are readily identified and preserved. Any cremasteric artery is also preserved. The remaining cremasteric fibers and veins are ligated and cut, thus skeletonizing the cord. At the completion of varicocelectomy, the cord should contain only the testicular artery or arteries, vas deferens and associated vessels, and spermatic cord lymphatics. The wound is irrigated with 1% Neomycin irrigation, and the Scarpa and Camper fasciae are closed with a single 3-0 chromic catgut suture. The incision is infiltrated with 0.5% Marcaine solution with epinephrine, and the skin is closed with a running 4-0 Vicryl subcuticular closure reinforced with Steri-Strips. A dry sterile dressing is applied.

## OUTCOME

Several publications have addressed the efficacy of varicocelectomy as a treatment for male infertility. In general, varicocelectomy is associated with an improvement in several sperm parameters and with pregnancy rates in the range of 40% to 60% (3). However, most of these studies are retrospective, nonrandomized, and heterogeneous (3). Several recent reviews have critically examined the results of randomized, controlled trials of varicocelectomy. When all randomized trials are evaluated (including studies of subclinical varicocele and those of men with normal semen parameters), the data do not support the practice of varicocelectomy for male infertility (4). However, in North America, it is not common practice to treat subclinical varicoceles and/or men with normal semen parameters (6). In a recent analysis including only randomized studies of clinical varicoceles with abnormal semen parameters, the data support the practice of varicocelectomy for male infertility (5).

Most studies of adolescents with varicocele indicate that varicocelectomy has a beneficial effect on testicular function. In general, surgery is indicated in boys with testicular atrophy and/or abnormal semen parameters. Controlled studies indicate that at follow-up evaluation (1 to 15 years), varicocelectomy is associated with higher sperm parameters and higher testicular volumes than no treatment (11,12).

## COMPLICATIONS

There are three complications specific to varicocelectomy:

1. Hydrocele formation. This complication is believed to be due to ligation of lymphatic channels. The postoperative incidence of hydrocele is significantly lower with microscopic surgery (0% to 0.69%) than it is with the retroperitoneal approach (7% to 9%), laparoscopic ligation (12%), or conventional inguinal varicocelectomy (3% to 30%) (8,9). Hydrocele repair (hydrocelectomy) is indicated for the management of a large, symptomatic (painful) hydrocele.
2. Recurrence. This generally results from incomplete ligation of collateral venous channels. The recurrence rate associated with microsurgery (<2%) is significantly lower than that with the retroperitoneal (15% to 25%), inguinal (5% to 15%), and laparoscopic approaches (5% to 15%) (8,9). This complication can be corrected by a repeat surgical procedure or by radiographic embolization. However, a redo varicocelectomy is often technically challenging and may pose a greater risk of complications (e.g., testicular atrophy, hydrocele).
3. Testicular ischemia and atrophy. These are a result of injury to the testicular artery. The incidence is likely very low owing to the collateral vasculature (vasal and external spermatic arteries) supplying the testicle.

## SUMMARY

The use of the operating microscope during varicocelectomy allows for better identification (and preservation) of the testicular artery and lymphatic channels and for complete ligation of small collateral venous branches. Therefore, microsurgical varicocelectomy reduces the potential for complications to a minimum and, as such, is considered superior to nonmicrosurgical varicocelectomy (inguinal or subinguinal). However, microsurgical varicocelectomy, particularly the subinguinal approach, remains a technically challenging procedure that requires microsurgical expertise.

## *References*


1. Nagler HM, Luntz RK, Martinis FG. Varicocele. In: Lipshultz LI, Howard SS, eds. *Infertility in the male*, 3rd ed. St. Louis, MO: Mosby–Year Book, 1997:336–359.
2. Fretz PC, Sandlow JI. Varicocele: current concepts in pathophysiology, diagnosis, and treatment. *Urol Clin North Am* 2002;29:921–937.
3. Schlesinger MH, Wilets IF, Nagler HM. Treatment outcome after varicocelectomy: a critical analysis. *Urol Clin North Am* 1994;21:517–529.
4. Evers JL, Collins JA. Assessment of efficacy of varicocele repair for male subfertility: a systematic review. *Lancet* 2003;361:1849–1852.
5. Ficarra V, Cerruto MA, Liguori G, et al. Treatment of varicocele in subfertile men: the Cochrane Review—a contrary opinion. *Eur Urol* 2006; 49:258–263.
6. Sharlip ID, Jarow JP, Belker AM, et al. Best Practice policies for male infertility. *J Urol* 2002;167:2138–2144.
7. Marmar JL, DeBenedictis TJ, Praiss D. The management of varicoceles by microdissection of the spermatic cord at the external inguinal ring. *Fertil Steril* 1985;43:583–588.
8. Goldstein M, Gilbert BR, Dicker AP. Microsurgical inguinal varicocelectomy with delivery of the testis: an artery and lymphatic sparing technique. *J Urol* 1992;148:1808–1811.
9. Cayan S, Kadioglu TC, Tefekli A, et al. Comparison of results and complications of high ligation surgery and microsurgical high inguinal varicocelectomy in the treatment of varicocele. *Urology* 2000;55(5):750–754.
10. Zini A, Fischer MA, Bellack D, et al. Technical modification of microsurgical varicocelectomy can reduce operating time. *Urology* 2006;67:803–806.
11. Sayfan J, Siplovich L, Koltun L, et al. Varicocele treatment in pubertal boys prevents testicular growth arrest. *J Urol* 1997;157:1456–1457.
12. Paduch DA, Niedzielski J. Repair versus observation in adolescent varicocele: a prospective study. *J Urol* 1997;158:1128–1132.


# CHAPTER 59 ■ TESTIS BIOPSY AND TESTICULAR SPERM EXTRACTION (TESE)

PETER N. SCHLEGEL

Testicular biopsy may serve as a diagnostic or therapeutic procedure, or both. Testicular biopsy is indicated for the classification of azoospermia as obstructive (where normal sperm production is documented on biopsy) or nonobstructive (where sperm production is markedly abnormal). For azoospermic men, testicular sperm extraction (TESE), a surgical procedure involving retrieval of one or more samples of testicular tissue, may procure spermatozoa that can be used for successful treatment with assisted reproduction. Whereas testicular biopsy was previously used only to document normal sperm production prior to possible reconstruction of reproductive tract obstruction, men with impaired sperm production (serum follicle stimulating hormone [FSH] more than three times normal levels) may be candidates for testis biopsy or TESE.

## TESTIS BIOPSY

A testis biopsy is performed to document the level of sperm production. It is used to determine whether obstruction is present for an azoospermic man with palpable vasa deferentia. Testis biopsy can also provide some diagnostic information for men with nonobstructive azoospermia. Since a single biopsy samples very little of the testis, it may not definitively determine if sperm are present in any area of the testis for men with nonobstructive azoospermia. Only men with a serum FSH less than three times the upper limit of normal levels will have normal sperm production. Azoospermic men with small or soft testes are highly unlikely to have sperm production, but some of these men have limited foci of spermatogenesis that can provide sperm for assisted reproduction. All men (that we have evaluated) with congenital absence of the vas deferens, normal serum FSH levels, and normal-volume (>15-cc) testes had sperm production, obviating the need for biopsy. If performed for diagnostic purposes, biopsy should be performed on both testes, since substantial differences in sperm production may be present without a palpable difference in the testes. Up to 10% to 15% of men will have a substantial difference in sperm production in the two different testes.

A second relative indication for testis biopsy is for the evaluation of azoospermic men with presumed abnormal production. These men with nonobstructive azoospermia (NOA) will typically have soft or small testes and an elevated FSH level. Although these patients are not expected to have completely normal production and reproductive tract obstruction, in selected cases sperm may be retrieved from the testis and used with assisted reproduction (intracytoplasmic sperm injection; ICSI). A biopsy may be of value in providing some prognostic information on which patients are candidates for ICSI. Unfortunately, a diagnostic biopsy is performed randomly and evaluates only a limited number of the hundreds of highly coiled seminiferous tubules within the testis. Subsequent attempts at sperm retrieval are dependent on finding the most advanced spermatogenic pattern of production in the 600 to 800 tubules present within each entire testis. An initial, random diagnostic biopsy that demonstrates at least one spermatozoon predicts the subsequent finding of sperm on attempted TESE in 80% to 95% of patients. The observation of at least germ cells (spermatogonia or spermatocytes) on diagnostic biopsy predicts subsequent sperm retrieval with TESE for about 50% of patients. In all cases, the chance of sperm retrieval is determined by the most advanced pattern of sperm production on diagnostic biopsy, not the predominant pattern. For men who have only tubules with Sertoli cells in their lumen, the chance of sperm retrieval from another area of the testis is at least 35% to 40%. Therefore, the prognostic value of a diagnostic biopsy in NOA is limited.

Diagnostic information on the status of spermatogenesis is most reliably determined on evaluation of a thin-sectioned stained fixed tissue specimen. Specimens for tissue evaluation can be obtained by open biopsy, needle biopsy, or, occasionally, fine needle aspiration. Given the potential inadequacy of needle biopsy or fine needle aspiration, with its attendant risks to the vasculature of the testis, the open biopsy technique is preferable. The biopsy should be performed prior to reconstruction (rather than simultaneous to vasoepididymostomy) in most cases, so that a definitive analysis of sperm production is possible on fixed sections prior to further exploration. In addition, vasography is superfluous at the time of biopsy and should be avoided because of the risk of vasal injury or stricture.

## Technique

For open biopsy, the procedure may be done under local or general anesthesia. The testis must be accurately positioned with the scrotal skin tightly stretched over the testis, and the epididymis must be secured in a posterior position. A 1-cm incision is made transversely over the midportion of the testis (Fig. 59.1). The incision is carried out down to the tunica vaginalis. Cutting through this tunic is confirmed intraoperatively by the release of a small amount of clear fluid, expressed from within the space of the tunica vaginalis. A stay suture is placed through a nonvascularized region of the testis, preferably in a superior, medial, or lateral position. Nonreactive suture such as nylon or polypropylene is preferred. Optical loupes or an operating microscope may help identify vessels under the tunica albuginea, limiting the risk of injury to the testicular blood supply. A 0.5-cm incision is made through the tunica albuginea with a sharp no. 11 blade or a fine ophthalmic knife. A small sample of seminiferous tubules should extrude easily through this incision. If a sample is not easily delivered, the incision may not be long or deep enough. Excessive pressure to extrude tubules may adversely affect the architecture of the specimen. The sample should be cut off sharply and placed directly into Bouin solution or buffered glutaraldehyde. The use of formalin is avoided because of the deleterious effects that it has on tubular architecture. A "wet prep" of the cut seminiferous tubular surface or a "squash prep" of a separate piece of tubules on a glass slide, bathed with lactated Ringer solution and compressed with a cover slip, can be immediately examined under the microscope. The presence of sperm alone does not guarantee obstruction; however, only men with motile sperm are highly likely to have distal obstruction.

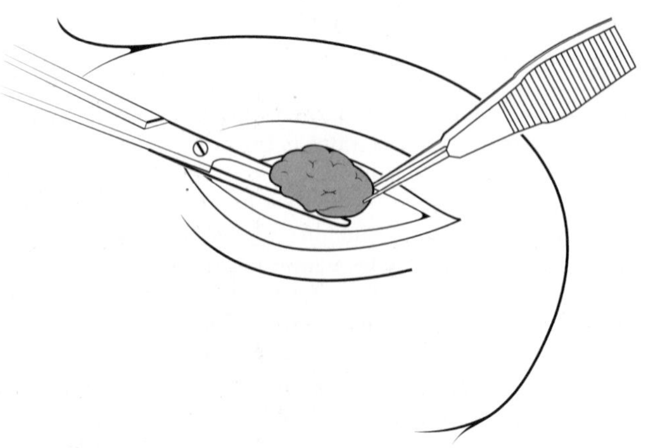

FIGURE 59.1 Technique for open testicular biopsy.

The tunical levels and the skin should both be closed to encourage hemostasis. Generous injection of 0.25% bupivacaine into the tunica vaginalis space and the subcutaneous areas provides excellent local anesthesia postoperatively.

## "Quick Prep" Cytologic Evaluations for Men with Presumed Obstruction

Since introduction of the testis biopsy as a diagnostic tool by Hotchkiss (3) and Charney (4), a variety of refinements in technique have been proposed to improve its usefulness. The role of a testis biopsy is to evaluate spermatozoal production and, indirectly, the presence or absence of reproductive tract obstruction. Since formal testis biopsy requires fixation, embedding, and staining of specimens for interpretation, biopsy and reproductive tract reconstruction must occur at different times. Quantitative analysis of testicular sperm production is possible by counting the number of mature spermatids per round tubule, as described by Silber and Rodriguez-Rigau (5). Several techniques have attempted to provide additional information or "quick analysis" from testis biopsy specimens.

### Technique: Touch Prep

The touch prep (testicular touch imprint) is a cytologic smear of fluid from the cut surface of testicular parenchyma. The touch prep is performed during testis biopsy by taking a clean glass slide and placing it on the cut surface of seminiferous tubules after obtaining a specimen for permanent section. The slide is applied to the cut surface in several areas and immediately cytofixed with a commercial spray or 95% ethyl alcohol. The smear is subsequently stained via the Papanicolaou technique. Identification of individual spermatogenic cells as well as mature spermatozoa is possible. The most important role of the touch prep is to differentiate between late maturation arrest and complete spermatogenesis. Late maturation arrest may be difficult to assess on biopsy, since mature sperm with tails are uncommonly seen on the thin slice of a histologic slide, and quantitation of spermatozoal production is usually inferred from the number of mature spermatids present on fixed testis biopsy specimens. Quantitation of spermatozoa on touch prep allows direct evaluation of whether late maturation arrest may be present. Detection of fully formed testicular sperm morphology is also possible. A diagnosis of late maturation arrest spares the patient unnecessary scrotal exploration and even possible partial epididymectomy in a futile attempt at reconstruction.

Little published data exist regarding the frequency of late maturation arrest or the sensitivity (or specificity) of the touch prep technique. If late maturation arrest is very uncommon and false-positive results occur with the touch prep, then it is possible that more patients may be denied reconstructive microsurgery than are benefited by diagnosis of late maturation arrest. Certainly, the touch prep can be of great value when late maturation arrest is suspected.

### Technique: Wet Prep

A wet prep is performed after the standard biopsy specimen has been atraumatically transferred into Bouin solution. For the wet prep, a small additional piece of testis is placed on a clean glass side with Ringer lactate, and the tissue is compressed under a glass cover slip. Analysis of this specimen can be performed immediately in the operating room. The presence or absence of sperm is documented, and the motility of sperm can also be evaluated.

The presence or absence of sperm is not very predictive of the findings on fixed permanent sections, but the presence of sperm motility may be of importance. A review of 100 consecutive testis biopsy and wet prep evaluations at Cornell indicated that histology (complete spermatogenesis) and cytology (presence of sperm on wet prep) were concordant in only 81% of biopsies. However, the presence of motile sperm had a 100% positive predictive value for the presence of reproductive tract obstruction. For the 18 cases where motile sperm were present, it would have been safe to proceed with microsurgical reconstruction of the reproductive tract. The converse is not applicable; the absence of motile sperm did not predict the absence of obstruction. In fact, 47 out of 65 men (72%) with obstruction did not have motile sperm present on wet prep.

Further data collection will be helpful to fully evaluate the relevance of sperm motility on wet prep examination during testis biopsy. Based on the data available, the presence of motile testicular sperm is highly suggestive of the presence of distal obstruction.

## Summary: Testis Biopsy

Testis biopsy is a diagnostic technique to assess spermatogenesis. It is most useful to determine whether obstruction is the cause of azoospermia. It is possible to take additional tissue during this diagnostic procedure that can be frozen for subsequent therapeutic trials of assisted reproduction. Cytologic evaluation, performed concurrently with standard testicular biopsy, may provide important adjunctive information. Touch prep techniques allow for the detection of late maturation arrest, not evaluable on fixed permanent sections. Touch prep techniques allow for evaluation of the presence of sperm within the seminiferous tubule, without removing an additional piece of testicular parenchyma. The wet prep technique allows an evaluation of sperm motility. The presence of sperm motility appears to be highly indicative of the presence of obstruction. Further information regarding the frequency of late maturation arrest and the endurance of the predictive value of wet prep sperm motility is needed. At present, cytologic techniques should best be considered adjuncts to, not a replacement for, careful evaluation of fixed permanent testicular biopsy specimens.

# SPERM RETRIEVAL FOR ASSISTED REPRODUCTION

It had long been thought that sperm exiting the testis lack maturity, motility, and fertilizing capability and that transit through the epididymis is essential to the acquisition of these features. ICSI has changed our view of the functional capacity of testicular spermatozoa; these sperm are now routinely used to effect pregnancies using in vitro fertilization (IVF) with ICSI. In the unobstructed setting, sperm quality improves as the spermatozoa travel from caput to cauda epididymis; however, this is not true in the obstructed setting. In reproductive tract obstruction, improved motility is seen in sperm retrieved from the areas of the epididymis closer to the testis (caput) compared to the distal end of the epididymis (cauda). In contrast, sperm from the cauda region of an obstructed epididymis are in advanced stages of degeneration and necrosis. Normal sperm are absent or rare, whereas macrophages filled with phagocytized sperm remnants or sperm with blunt or coiled tails are seen in abundance. This finding is often referred to as "inverted motility." Therefore, in some cases, it is possible that better sperm quality can be found in the testis.

Although it has long been thought that sperm exiting the testis are immature and incapable of fertilization, this holds true only in the unobstructed system. In obstruction, better-quality sperm can be found proximally, in the rete testis, vasa efferentia, or caput epididymis, and the more distal (cauda) epididymis is the site of sperm degeneration. These factors should be taken into account during any attempt at sperm retrieval.

## Nonobstructive Azoospermia: Heterogeneity of Sperm Production

It has previously been shown that human testicular histology is heterogeneous; that is, there can be small foci of abnormal spermatogenesis adjacent to normal seminiferous tubules. The converse of this previously casual observation is now the cornerstone of treatment for men with nonobstructive azoospermia. Successful sperm retrieval is possible in most TESE attempts in men with nonobstructive azoospermia, despite diagnostic testis biopsy specimens showing predominantly maturation arrest or Sertoli cell-only. The ability to retrieve sperm from the testes of men with nonobstructive azoospermia is independent of testicular size and FSH level but dependent on the most advanced level of spermatogenesis identified. All standard parameters of testicular evaluation (testicular volume, FSH, inhibin B levels) evaluate overall function of the testis. Since sperm retrieval and pregnancy are dependent on finding sperm in just one small focu of the testis, the only predictor of successful treatment is the most developed region of the testis, not the predominant pattern of testicular histology, overall testicular volume, or FSH. These observations suggest that nearly all cases of male factor infertility can potentially be treated.

## Intracytoplasmic Sperm Injection

Without question the most significant advance in the treatment of male infertility has been the technique of intracytoplasmic sperm injection or ICSI. The procedure involves the deposition of a single sperm directly into the oocyte cytoplasm with a micropipette. The advantages of this technique are that it bypasses all oocyte barriers so that even severely abnormal spermatozoa can successfully fertilize as long as the spermatozoon is viable. At this point, ICSI has been applied successfully to obstructive and nonobstructive azoospermia with fresh and thawed spermatozoa obtained from the epididymis and testis.

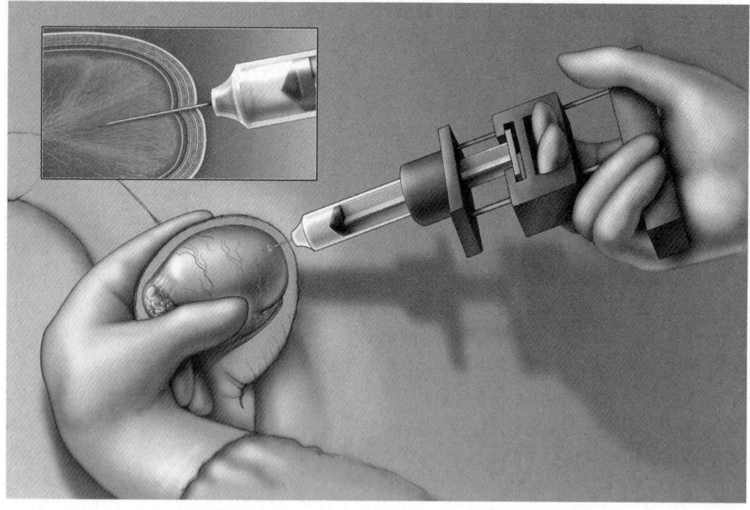

FIGURE 59.2 Technique of fine needle aspiration of testis.

As ICSI has been more widely applied, it has become evident that female factors, not male, present the primary limitations to ICSI success in couples unable to achieve a pregnancy.

## Percutaneous Testicular Sperm Aspiration

As mentioned above, it was previously thought that sperm retrieved from the testis were incapable of fertilization. However, it is now well established that testicular sperm can be used effectively with ICSI, although the cytogenetic abnormality rate is higher in testicular than in epididymal or ejaculated sperm. Although testicular sperm retrieval has been reported in cases of obstructive azoospermia after epididymal aspiration attempts failed, the primary indication for open testicular sperm retrieval today should be for sperm acquisition in nonobstructive azoospermia.

Testicular sperm can be recovered using fine needle aspiration (FNA), percutaneous biopsy, or an open technique. The technique of percutaneous fine needle aspiration of the testis was initially described as a diagnostic procedure in azoospermic men. In this procedure, the testis is stabilized between the surgeon's thumb and forefinger and a needle is inserted along the long axis of the testis. The needle is withdrawn slightly and redirected in order to disrupt the testicular architecture. The procedure is repeated until adequate testicular material has been aspirated. A Franzen needle holder can be used to provide negative pressure for needle aspiration (Fig. 59.2).

## Percutaneous Testicular Biopsy (PercBiopsy)

A technique of percutaneous biopsy of the testis has also been described. A 15-gauge biopsy gun with a short (1-cm) excursion is used to retrieve testicular tissue (Fig. 59.3). Anesthesia is achieved with a spermatic cord block, and multiple biopsies can be obtained through a single entry site. The patient may be prepared for this procedure by the topical application of local anesthetic as EMLA cream (Astra-Zeneca Pharmaceuticals, Worcester, MA). The core needle provides better sperm yield than fine needle aspiration and is relatively simple to use.

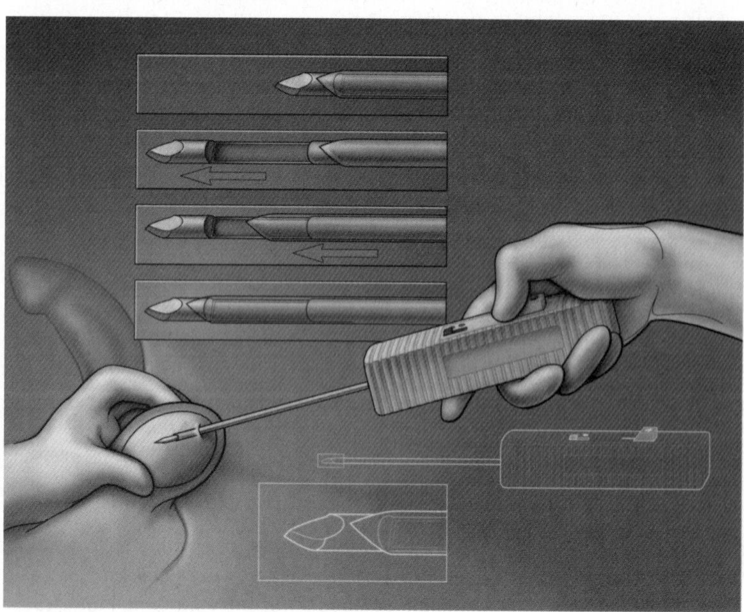

FIGURE 59.3 Technique of percutaneous testicular biopsy (PercBiopsy).

## Testicular Sperm Extraction

Testicular sperm retrieval using an open biopsy technique (TESE) is rarely, if ever, indicated for men with obstructive azoospermia. The procedure is more invasive and is not needed in obstructive azoospermia to allow sperm retrieval. If an open procedure is performed, then our experience is that over 99% of men (184 out of 185) with obstructive azoospermia will have approximately 100 × $10^6$ or more sperm retrieved from the epididymis with microsurgical epididymal sperm aspiration (MESA). Sperm retrieval from the epididymis is far more efficient than testicular biopsy extraction in that it provides better sperm yield and motility when compared to that obtained with TESE in obstructive azoospermia. This provides sperm quantities sufficient for a virtually unlimited number of ICSI attempts. If testicular sperm retrieval is planned because of patient preference or if microsurgical expertise is not available, then PercBiopsy is the recommended approach.

## Nonobstructive Azoospermia

Testicular access is required for sperm retrieval in nonobstructive azoospermia since pockets of sperm production are limited and evaluation of large areas of the testis or multiple biopsies are usually needed to retrieve sperm. Although testicular fine needle aspiration has been used to retrieve spermatozoa in azoospermic men, documentation of its effectiveness is lacking for men with nonobstructive azoospermia. Two controlled studies have shown that open biopsy has a substantially higher yield of sperm for men with nonobstructive azoospermia (1,2). An alternative approach is to perform testis biopsies with intentional cryopreservation. However, this approach may lead to unnecessary biopsies, since up to 35% of "azoospermic" men will have sperm found with careful examination of the ejaculate on the day of planned simultaneous TESE-ICSI. In addition, sperm "retrieved" from the testis and frozen may not survive the freeze-thaw process in nonobstructive azoospermia. Moreover, multiple biopsies may be needed to retrieve sperm in men with nonobstructive azoospermia, and a simultaneous biopsy-by-biopsy analysis is required with careful analysis by an experienced embryologist. A microsurgical approach to TESE is presented herein.

## Microdissection Testicular Sperm Extraction (MicroTESE)

Microsurgical TESE offers the advantages of improved yield of spermatozoa per biopsy, less tissue removal (and less risk of testicle loss), and improved identification of blood vessels within the testicle, minimizing the risk of vascular injury and loss of remaining functional areas of the testis.

On the day of, or preferably on the day before, oocyte retrieval, scrotal exploration is performed through a median raphe incision under local or general anesthesia, and sperm are retrieved using an open technique. In order to confirm accurate identification of the testis, observe all testicular vessels, and avoid any injury to the epididymis, delivery of the testis is routinely performed.

Testicular blood vessels under the tunica albuginea are identified with 6× to 8× optical magnification. An avascular region near the midportion of the medial, lateral, or anterior surface of the testis is chosen, and a generous incision in the tunica albuginea is created with a 15-degree ultrasharp knife, avoiding any capsular testicular vessels. With this approach, direct visualization of large areas of the testis can be achieved, which allows for either large sample biopsies or microdissection. Since the incision is directed at an avascular region, the sperm retrieval procedure is less traumatic than multiple "blind" biopsies. The testis is opened widely to allow direct examination of all areas of testicular parenchyma. Dissection between the tubules is also needed to view tubules that are not exposed with the initial approach (Fig. 59.4). The microdissection technique that we have applied allows the removal of tiny (2 to 3 mm; 3- to 5-mg volumes) of testicular tissue with improved sperm yield (1). The tubules containing sperm can often be identified visually under an operating microscope after opening the testis, when approximately 10× to 15× magnification is used to assist the biopsies. The tubules containing sperm production are directly identified based on their large size and white color. If all tubules appear uniform at high power magnification, then dissection is performed to allow access to other regions of the testis. Finally, if no sperm have been seen in microdissected samples, additional searching throughout testicular tissue is done, avoiding the centrifugal testicular vessels that course parallel to and between the septae that separate seminiferous tubules.

The excised testicular tubular segments are placed in buffered human tubal fluid or a similar culture medium supplemented with 6% Plasmanate. Isolation of individual tubules from the mass of coiled testicular tissue is achieved by initial dispersal of the testis biopsy specimen using scissors, preferably in a small Petri dish. Additional dispersion of tubules is achieved by passing the suspension of testicular tissue through a 24-gauge angiocatheter. Individual tubules may also be evaluated directly in the embryology laboratory immediately prior to ICSI, but the evaluation of sperm in the operating room during TESE provides critical information to the surgeon to determine how much dissection and/or removal of tissue is necessary.

Intraoperatively, a "wet prep" of the suspension is preferably examined under phase-contrast microscopy at 200× power in the operating room. If no spermatozoa are seen, then (a) additional samples of tissue are obtained through the same tunical incision, (b) the remainder of the testis is examined by evaluating the exposed regions of testicular tissue and (c) exposure of deeper tubules is effected by dissecting between the septae and everting the testicular tissue, and then (d) examination of the contralateral testis is performed if no sperm have been found. The sperm extraction process is complete when sperm are reliably identified in the wet preparation of a biopsy specimen. Otherwise sperm extraction attempts are stopped when all areas of the testis have been examined. Care must be taken to preserve vessels between and within the septae of the testis that contain the tubules. Additional incisions beyond the initial wide incision should be avoided, as they could adversely affect the blood supply to the testis. Operating through a limited incision may not allow the surgeon to adequately control bleeding within the testis. Not only does this potentially obscure the testicular tissue, but the scar tissue that develops within the testis postoperatively is primarily caused by postoperative bleeding within the testicle. Therefore, meticulous hemostasis with bipolar cautery during the procedure is important.

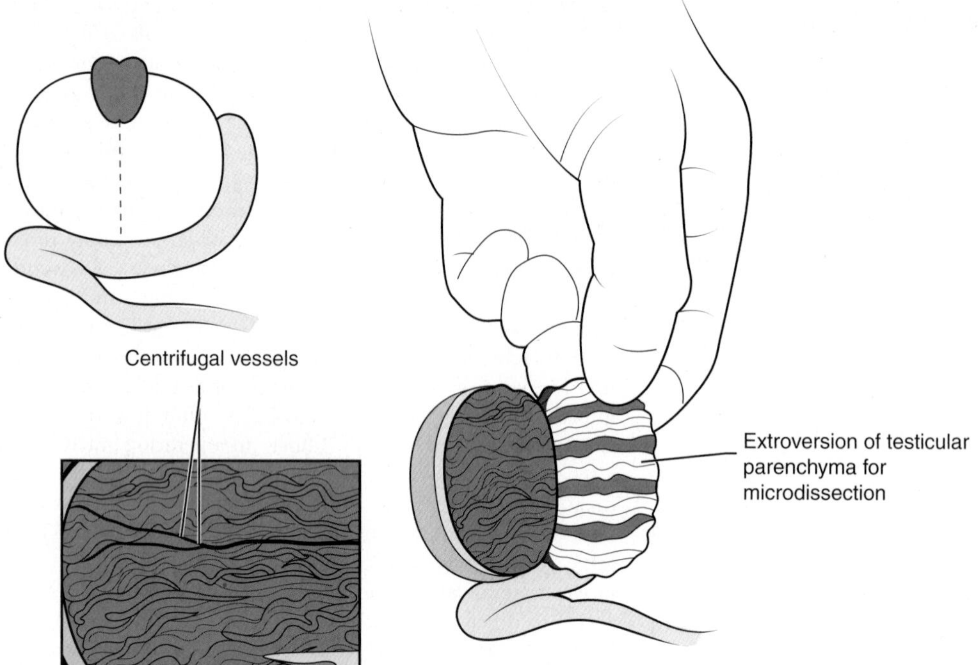


FIGURE 59.4 Exposure during microdissection testicular sperm extraction (TESE).

Subsequent processing of the testicular tissue suspension, including mechanical disruption and/or additional enzymatic digestion of the specimens, is performed in the IVF laboratory. Aliquots of tissue can also be processed for cryopreservation.

## Results of TESE for Nonobstructive Azoospermia

We have done microdissection TESE on over 865 men with nonobstructive azoospermia. Sperm retrieval rates for azoospermic men are 63%. Once sperm are obtained, the testicular sperm will fertilize 55% of oocytes injected using the ICSI technique. Clinical pregnancies (fetal heartbeat seen on ultrasound) are obtained during 48% of successful sperm retrieval attempts for couples with nonobstructive azoospermia. Ongoing or delivered pregnancies occurred for 43% of successful attempts at sperm retrieval.

No etiology of azoospermia provided an absolute predictor for the presence or absence of sperm within the testes, except for the presence of complete deletions of the AZFa or AZFb regions of the Y chromosome. (Testicular volume and serum FSH levels did not predict sperm retrieval.) Sixty-four attempts at sperm retrieval-ICSI have been made where the man had testicular failure because of prior chemotherapy treatment. Sperm were obtained in 53% of attempts, slightly more commonly in men previously treated with platinum-based regimens for germ cell tumor (73%) than in men treated for lymphoma with cytoxan-based regimens (48%). Of 91 attempts at sperm retrieval for men who have Klinefelter syndrome (47, XXY; nonmosaic), sperm were found for 68% of men, and clinical pregnancy (fetal heartbeat on ultrasound) was achieved in 43% of cases once sperm were retrieved.

## Summary: Sperm Retrieval

Sperm retrieval for use with the advanced form of assisted reproduction, ICSI, is now possible for many men with nonobstructive azoospermia. Men with azoospermia may have unique genetic defects, such as Y chromosome microdeletions, that should be evaluated prior to an attempt at conception. In obstructive azoospermia, several options exist to allow for sperm retrieval rates approaching 100%. In nonobstructive azoospermia, TESE is required and sperm retrieval is less certain. At the Weill Cornell Medical Center, 63% of couples with nonobstructive azoospermia have sperm retrieved from the testis with TESE, and 48% of couples achieved a clinical pregnancy using testicular sperm in nonobstructive azoospermia. Since some couples will not have sperm retrieved with TESE, the use of frozen donor spermatozoa as backup should be discussed with couples prior to simultaneous TESE-ICSI attempts.

## *References*

1. Schlegel PN. Testicular sperm extraction: microdissection improves sperm yield with minimal tissue excision. *Hum Reprod* 1999;14:131–135.
2. Amer M, Ateyah A, Hany R, et al. Prospective comparative study between microsurgical and conventional testicular sperm extraction in non-obstructive azoospermia: follow-up by serial ultrasound examinations. *Hum Reprod* 2000;15(3):653–656.
3. Hotchkiss RS. Testicular biopsy in the diagnosis and treatment of sterility in the male. *Bull NY Acad Med* 1942;18:600–605.
4. Charney CW. Testicular biopsy: its value in male infertility. *J Am Med Assoc* 1940;115:1429–1432.
5. Silber SJ, Rodriguez-Rigau LJ. Quantitative analysis of testicle biopsy: determination of partial obstruction and prediction of sperm count after surgery for obstruction. *Fertil Steril* 1981;36(4):480–485

# CHAPTER 60A ■ EPIDIDYMAL SPERM ASPIRATION

CIGDEM TANRIKUT AND MARC GOLDSTEIN

Obstructive azoospermia is the blockage of the male reproductive tract resulting in complete absence of sperm in the ejaculate. Up to 40% of azoospermic patients undergoing fertility evaluation will have an obstructive etiology (4). Fortunately, cases of obstructive azoospermia now comprise the most treatable of male factor problems owing to the development of advanced reproductive techniques: in vitro fertilization (IVF) and intracytoplasmic sperm injection (ICSI).

Obstruction may be either congenital or acquired, occurring along any point of the male excurrent ductal system: epididymis, vas deferens, or ejaculatory duct. Congenital causes of obstructive azoospermia include congenital absence of the vasa deferentia and idiopathic epididymal obstruction. Acquired reasons for reproductive tract obstruction include prior vasectomy, previous genitourinary tract infection, iatrogenic injury related to prior surgery, and a history of pelvic or scrotal trauma. This chapter focuses on common techniques used in the setting of obstructive azoospermia to surgically extract sperm from the epididymis for use with a concurrent IVF-ICSI cycle or for purposes of cryopreservation for future IVF-ICSI cycles.

## DIAGNOSIS

Azoospermia in a man with normal-volume testes (≥20 cc) and normal serum follicle stimulating hormone (FSH <8.0 U per L) suggests an obstructive etiology. If neither vas deferens is palpable on physical examination, obstructive azoospermia is due to congenital bilateral absence of the vasa deferentia (CBAVD), a reproductive tract anomaly associated with cystic fibrosis. Men with genetic mutations of the cystic fibrosis transmembrane conductance regulator (CFTR) gene may lack segments anywhere from the epididymis to the seminal vesicle, with resultant obstructive azoospermia (2,11). Screening for the CFTR gene mutation should be performed in the patient as well as in his partner, and genetic counseling should be provided.

Patients with obstructive azoospermia due to vasectomy will be apparent upon obtaining patient history. If physical examination reveals normal testicular volume and FSH is in the normal range, no further evaluation is warranted prior to proceeding with sperm extraction.

In patients with suspected or known obstructive azoospermia presenting with testis atrophy and/or elevated FSH, a testis biopsy may be considered to confirm normal spermatogenesis, proceeding with concurrent epididymal or testicular sperm extraction if sperm are identified.

## INDICATIONS FOR SURGERY

Although many postvasectomy patients are candidates for microsurgical reconstruction via vasovasostomy or vasoepididymostomy (see Chapters 56 and 57), not all such patients are willing or able to undergo reconstruction. Obstructive azoospermia related to blockages of the epididymides or vasa deferentia, regardless of etiology, may be addressed via surgical sperm retrieval followed by IVF-ICSI.

## ALTERNATIVE THERAPY

Surgical alternatives to epididymal sperm extraction in men with obstructive azoospermia include testicular sperm extraction via a variety of methods (see Chapter 59). Sperm obtained from men with chronically obstructed reproductive tracts usually have poorer motility and decreased fertilizing capability as compared with ejaculated sperm. The use of ICSI is essential to achieve optimal results with either epididymal or testicular sperm; thus the female partner must be willing and able to go through with an IVF cycle if surgically extracted sperm are to be used. Other alternatives about which the couple should be counseled include the use of donor sperm or adoption.

## SURGICAL TECHNIQUE

Sperm may be retrieved from the epididymis using either microsurgical or percutaneous techniques (Table 60A.1). Microsurgical epididymal sperm aspiration (MESA) can be performed on the same day as the partner's oocyte retrieval or at a separate time interval prior to oocyte retrieval with cryopreservation of procured sperm. Percutaneous epididymal sperm aspiration (PESA) does not often yield numbers of sperm sufficient to allow for cryopreservation and, therefore, should be performed synchronously with egg retrieval. Regardless of when sperm aspiration is performed relative to oocyte retrieval, it is imperative that an intraoperative sample be assessed under phase-contrast microscopy by a qualified embryologist to assess the quality of the sample.

In patients with obstructive azoospermia, sufficient quantities of sperm are generally obtained from aspiration on one side; however, the patient should be counseled that a bilateral procedure may be necessary.

TABLE 60A.1

COMPARISON OF MESA AND PESA

| | ADVANTAGES | DISADVANTAGES |
|---|---|---|
| Microsurgical epididymal sperm aspiration (MESA) | • Lower risk for complications, less risk for spermatic cord or epididymal damage<br>• Large numbers of sperm may be obtained and cryopreserved in multiple aliquots during single procedure | • General anesthesia preferred<br>• Requires microsurgical skills<br>• More expensive<br>• Longer recovery |
| Percutaneous epididymal sperm aspiration (PESA) | • No microsurgical skill required<br>• Local anesthesia ± sedation<br>• Can be done in office | • Higher risk of complications, including hematoma, pain, and vascular injury to testes and epididymis<br>• Variable success in obtaining sperm<br>• Smaller quantity of sperm obtained than with MESA |

## Microsurgical Epididymal Sperm Aspiration (MESA)

MESA is most easily performed with the patient under general anesthesia, although spinal or local anesthesia may be used. The patient is supine on the operating table and anesthesia is induced. The scrotum is shaved and sterilely prepared and draped. A longitudinal median raphe or transverse hemiscrotal incision is made. The testis is delivered through the incision to gain direct access to the epididymis. The operating microscope is brought into the field at this time. The surgeon's nondominant hand is used to hold the testicle while stabilizing the epididymis between the thumb and index finger. Under the operating microscope at 10× to 15× magnification, the microtipped bipolar forceps are used along the longitudinal plane of the epididymal tunic to create an avascular plane. The tunic is incised gently using a 15-degree ophthalmic microknife, taking care not to violate the underlying epididymal tubules. Hemostasis is attained using the bipolar cautery. A dilated epididymal tubule is selected and isolated, then incised with the microknife (Fig. 60A.1A). In an obstructed epididymis, sperm within the more caudal aspect tend to be of poorer quality, and better-quality sperm are usually found within the body or head of the epididymis, so the tubule should be selected accordingly. The epididymal fluid is touched to a sterile glass slide, a drop of saline is added, a cover slip is placed, and then the fluid is immediately examined under a bench microscope. When motile sperm are identified, a dry micropipette (5 μL; Drummond Scientific Co., Broomall, PA) or a standard hematocrit pipette is placed adjacent to the effluxing epididymal tubule (Fig. 60A.1B). Using an in-line syringe for aspiration is not recommended, as the negative pressure generated may disrupt the delicate epididymal mucosa. Sperm-containing fluid will be drawn into the pipette by simple capillary action (5). Two pipettes may be used simultaneously in order to expedite sperm recovery. The highest rate of flow is observed immediately after incising the tubule. Sperm quality progressively improves after the initial washout. Gentle compression of the testis and epididymis using the thumb and index finger or a smooth-tipped microforceps enhances flow from the incised tubule. With patience, 25 to 50 μL of highly concentrated epididymal fluid can be recovered, containing approximately 75 million sperm. This is diluted in multiple aliquots of 2 to 3 mL of human tubal fluid medium, such that there are approximately 5 million sperm per milliliter. Those specimens not used immediately for IVF-ICSI are cryopreserved for possible future use. If no sperm or immotile sperm are obtained at the initial incision site or the quantities acquired are inadequate, additional incisions are made more proximally along the epididymis or even at the level of the efferent ductules until motile sperm are obtained.

Once adequate quality and quantity of sperm are attained, the tubular incisions may be closed using 10-0 Prolene or bipolar cautery. After ensuring meticulous hemostasis, the edges of the epididymal tunic are reapproximated using a 6-0 or 8-0 nonabsorbing monofilament suture in a running fashion. The testis is reduced into the hemiscrotum, and the scrotal incision

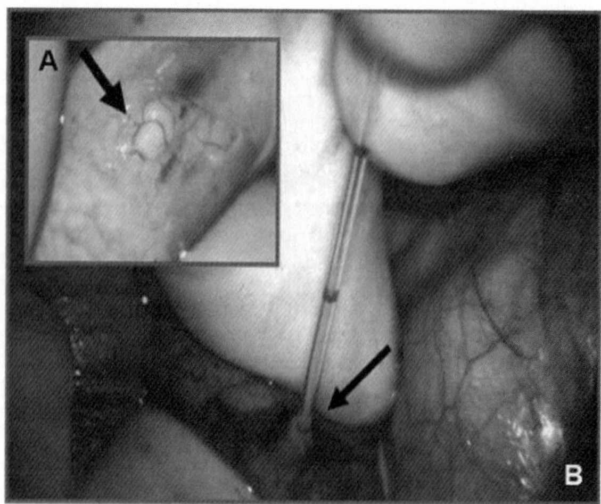


FIGURE 60A.1 Microsurgical epididymal sperm aspiration. **A:** Selection and isolation of dilated tubule (10× magnification). **B:** Aspiration of sperm into micropipette by capillary action (15× magnification).

is closed in layers in standard fashion. Fluffed gauze and an athletic supporter are placed on the patient prior to waking from anesthesia.

## Percutaneous Epididymal Sperm Aspiration

Percutaneous epididymal sperm aspiration (PESA) is a simpler method of obtaining epididymal sperm that does not require microsurgical experience (1). It may be performed under local anesthesia via spermatic cord block, with or without the use of intravenous sedation. After initiation of anesthesia and sterile preparation and draping of the scrotum, the testis is stabilized manually with the nondominant hand or by the assistant. The surgeon grasps the epididymis between thumb and index finger. A small (21- or 22-gauge) needle is percutaneously inserted into the epididymis, and an attached syringe containing a small amount (approximately 0.1 cc) of human tubal fluid is used to gently aspirate fluid from the epididymis. A small amount of this fluid is assessed under a bench microscope to confirm the presence of sperm and ascertain motility. Multiple punctures may be required to obtain sufficient sperm-containing fluid. If no sperm are retrieved, as occurs in at least 20% of sperm retrieval attempts (6), then one must proceed with MESA, testis biopsy, or testicular aspiration.

Given that the numbers of sperm retrieved with PESA are often not sufficient to allow for cryopreservation, repeat procedures may be warranted for multiple IVF cycles. In addition, there is a risk for the development of scrotal hematoma or injury to the epididymal or testicular vessels given the blind nature of this procedure.

# OUTCOMES

## Complications

Complications after either procedure are infrequent and include wound infection, scrotal hematoma, epididymal scarring, and injury to the spermatic cord vasculature, possibly leading to testis atrophy and impaired testis function. Scrotal exploration is rarely indicated for management of any of these complications. Given the blind nature of PESA, the risks of hematoma, scarring, and spermatic cord injury are higher than those associated with MESA.

## Results

An experienced microsurgeon can retrieve sperm from the epididymis via MESA in over 99% of patients with obstructive azoospermia (7,10). Similar success rates are possible even if previous scrotal procedures have been performed or if extensive scarring is present. If the entire epididymis is obliterated from prior surgery or infection, the efferent ductules of the testis can still be exposed by reflection of the caput epididymis; one should be able to aspirate sperm from at least one of these tubules.

Reported sperm extraction rates via PESA are somewhat lower than those reported for MESA, averaging about 80% (3). The ability to cryopreserve sperm obtained from men with obstructive azoospermia can help alleviate concerns regarding coordination of sperm extraction with oocyte retrieval, as well as offer the possibility of avoiding repeat sperm extraction if good quantities of motile sperm are obtained at the initial extraction. No clearly identified differences in outcomes between the use of fresh or cryopreserved and thawed sperm have been demonstrated (9).

Using surgically extracted epididymal sperm warrants IVF with ICSI to accomplish oocyte fertilization. Successful fertilization rates using ICSI in conjunction with surgically retrieved epididymal sperm are approximately 72% (8). Fertilization and pregnancy rates for both MESA and PESA are comparable. Of critical importance for successful outcomes, however, is the collaborative effort of the urologist along with the embryology team and reproductive endocrinologist.

## *References*


1. Craft IL, Khalifa Y, Boulos A, et al. Factors influencing the outcome of in-vitro fertilization with percutaneous aspirated epididymal spermatozoa and intracytoplasmic sperm injection in azoospermic men. *Hum Reprod* 1995;10:1791–1794.
2. Daudin M, Bieth E, Bujan L, et al. Congenital bilateral absence of the vas deferens: clinical characteristics, biological parameters, cystic fibrosis transmembrane conductance regulator gene mutations, and implications for genetic counseling. *Fertil Steril* 2000;74:1164–1174.
3. Glina S, Fragoso JB, Martins FG, et al. Percutaneous epididymal sperm aspiration (PESA) in men with obstructive azoospermia. *Int Braz J Urol* 2003;29:141–145.
4. Jarow JP, Espeland MA, Lipshultz LI. Evaluation of the azoospermic patient. *J Urol* 1989;142:162–165.
5. Matthews GJ, Goldstein M. A simplified technique of epididymal sperm aspiration. *Urology* 1996;47:123–125.
6. Meniru GI, Gorgy A, Batha S, et al. Studies of percutaneous epididymal sperm aspiration (PESA) and intracytoplasmic sperm injection. *Hum Reprod Update* 1998;4:57–71.
7. Nudell DM, Conaghan J, Pedersen RA, et al. The mini-micro-epididymal sperm aspiration for sperm retrieval: a study of urological outcomes. *Hum Reprod* 1998;13:1260–1265.
8. Palermo GD, Schlegel PN, Hariprashad JJ, et al. Fertilization and pregnancy outcome with intracytoplasmic sperm injection for azoospermic men. *Hum Reprod* 1999;14:741–748.
9. Prabakaran SA, Agarwal A, Sundaram A, et al. Cryosurvival of testicular spermatozoa from obstructive azoospermic patients: the Cleveland Clinic Experience. *Fertil Steril* 2006;86:1789–1791.
10. Schlegel PN, Palermo GD, Alikani M, et al. Micropuncture retrieval of epididymal sperm with in vitro fertilization: importance of in vitro micromanipulation techniques. *Urology* 1995;46:238–241.
11. Stuhrmann M, Dörk T. CFTR gene mutations and male infertility. *Andrologia* 2000;32:71–83.

# CHAPTER 60B ■ EPIDIDYMECTOMY

DAVID M. NUDELL AND LARRY I. LIPSHULTZ

The epididymis is a complex tubular network that connects the testicular efferent ducts to the vas deferens. In total, the single epididymal tubule measures 3 or 4 m. In its coiled form, the epididymal tubule is contained within the tunica vaginalis of the epididymis, creating a crescent-shaped organ intimately attached to the posterolateral aspect of the testis. The epididymis is anatomically divided into caput, corpus, and cauda regions (head, body, and tail, respectively) (Fig. 60B.1). While there are histologic differences in the delicate epididymal tubule between these regions, there are no gross and discrete dividing lines between the regions. The blood supply to the caput and body of the epididymis arises from a division of the testicular artery. The cauda epididymis is usually supplied by a branch of the vasal artery, but rich anastomotic connections usually exist. The epididymis functions primarily in sperm transport and maturation.

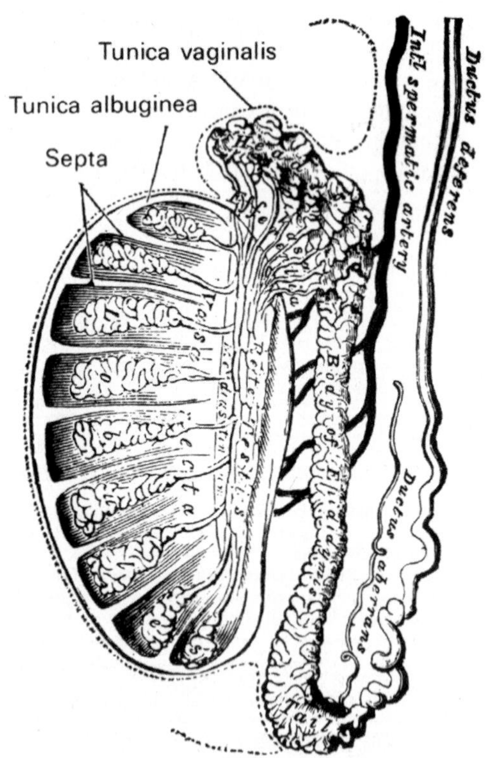


**FIGURE 60B.1.** Sagittal section of the testis and epididymis. The epididymis is seen attached to the posterolateral aspect of the testis. The efferent ducts (vasa efferentia) of the testis consist of 10 to 20 channels draining individual lobes of the testis into the globus major of the epididymis. The epididymal tubule gradually gains more smooth muscle components as it progresses toward the vas deferens, which is seen exiting the inferior, most distal aspects of the epididymis.

## DIAGNOSIS

This procedure is performed rarely, and the diagnostic steps are individualized to each patient.

## INDICATIONS FOR SURGERY

Currently, epididymectomy is done more commonly for complex epididymal cystic disease, chronic scrotal pain, or postvasectomy pain syndromes. Other indications are for abscess or chronic infections of the epididymis.

## ALTERNATIVE THERAPY

Surgical removal of all or part of the epididymis is done uncommonly, especially with the availability of broad-spectrum antibiotics. In the past, most cases were performed for abscess, chronic infection, or tuberculosis of the epididymis. In cases of scrotal abscess, the epididymis may be removed in an attempt to save the testis from overwhelming orchitis (1). If tuberculosis is suspected, it is critical to obtain appropriate cultures at the time of surgery.

## SURGICAL TECHNIQUE

After administration of appropriate antibiotics if necessary, either general or local anesthesia is induced. If local anesthesia is used, a generous cord block and infiltration of the skin overlying the incision will be adequate. A transverse scrotal incision is made that is just large enough to deliver the testis, epididymis, and distal vas deferens. The initial incision may be carried down through the tunica vaginalis without extensive dissection of the plane between the tunica vaginalis and dartos muscle layer. This will allow delivery of the intravaginal contents. Often, the distal vas deferens can be accessed in this way as well. If extensive scarring or infection has occurred, it may be necessary to dissect the tunica vaginalis free of the dartos muscle layer due to dense adhesions. In these cases, sharp dissection of the testis and epididymis from the undersurface of the tunica vaginalis will usually be necessary as well. In cases performed for postvasectomy pain, it is important to remove the epididymis and vas all the way up to and including the vasectomy site or sperm granuloma (2). If performed for other reasons, the vas may be divided and ligated at the junction of the convoluted and straight vas with an absorbable suture. In

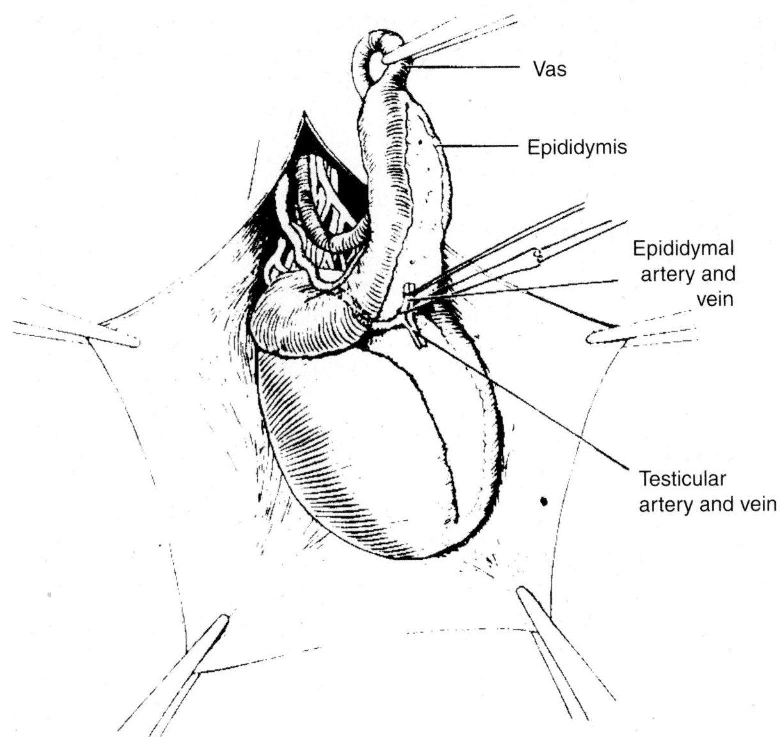


FIGURE 60B.2. Drawing demonstrating the correct plane of dissection during epididymectomy. The main spermatic cord structures are seen posterior and medial as they enter the testis. Injury to these structures can be avoided by dissecting only the plane between the epididymis and testis, which will usually contain only epididymal blood supply. The vascular pedicle to the epididymis may be encountered in the dissection plane between the testis and epididymis. The exact location of this blood supply can be variable.

patients with complex cystic disease, it is critical to ascertain the desire for future fertility. If fertility is still desired, epididymectomy should be avoided. If surgery is necessary in this situation, the larger cysts should be removed from the epididymis individually with the use of an operating microscope to avoid epididymal tubular obstruction.

After the vas is divided, it is dissected back to the vasoepididymal junction and dissection begun in the plane between the epididymis and the testis (Fig. 60B.2). Optical loupe magnification can be helpful in maintaining the correct plane and avoiding injury to the testis or spermatic cord vessels. The dissection is done sharply with fine Iris-type scissors and Bovie cauterization. The epididymis is grasped between the thumb and index finger of the nondominant hand and elevated off the testis as the dissection progresses from inferior to superior. The epididymal artery may be encountered midway up the dissection of the epididymis, but its exact location may be variable. If encountered, the artery should be ligated. The main spermatic cord blood supply containing the testicular artery will usually be found medial and posterior to the dissection in the region of the head or proximal body of the epididymis (Fig. 60B.2). In cases where the normal anatomy is distorted, it is important to avoid dissection into the spermatic cord, as this will lead to testicular infarction and subsequent atrophy. The most superior attachment of the epididymis to the testis consists of the testicular efferent ducts. These can be ligated with a single absorbable suture or cauterized. At this point, the specimen can usually be removed intact.

After the area is irrigated, the epididymal bed is inspected closely for bleeding. Vessels can be cauterized or ligated with small, absorbable sutures. The edges of the tunica along the bed of the epididymis should be approximated with several absorbable sutures for further hemostasis and to prevent leakage of testicular sperm from the efferent ducts. If extensive dissection has been performed or purulent material was encountered, a drain should be left in place that exits in a dependent fashion. Otherwise, the tunica vaginalis is closed with a running absorbable suture followed by closing the dartos layer and skin with interrupted or running absorbable sutures.

# OUTCOMES

## Complications

Complications of epididymectomy include hematoma formation, orchitis, skin infection, chronic pain, and infertility. Inadvertent injury to the spermatic cord during a difficult dissection may lead to testis atrophy.

## Results

The results of epididymectomy vary with the indications for surgery. In patients with complex, symptomatic cystic disease, patient satisfaction is usually high following surgical removal (3). In patients with chronic orchalgia, epididymectomy has produced poor results, with around 50% improvement rates in several series (3–5). This may not be surprising given the high incidence of perineural fibrosis found in the pathology specimens from patients undergoing epididymectomy for pain syndromes (2). However, in well-selected patients, satisfaction as high as 90% has been obtained (5). Poor predictors of success include pain extending into the groin region, failure to alleviate pain following a well-placed spermatic cord block, and normal appearance of the epididymis on preoperative ultrasound (5). Selective denervation of the spermatic cord may be another alternative to epididymectomy for chronic pain syndromes (6). This technique involves skeletonizing the spermatic cord surgically, leaving only the vas deferens, a few lymphatic channels, and the testicular artery intact. This procedure is best accomplished through a subinguinal incision with the use of an operating microscope. The long-term results of this relatively new approach remain to be determined.

For patients with postvasectomy pain syndromes, epididymectomy results have been mixed. In general, about 50% of patients report long-term satisfaction and prevention of ongoing pain following epididymectomy (2). As mentioned, it is important in these cases to include the vas deferens up to and including the vasectomy site in the surgical specimen.

Epididymectomy is performed most commonly for complex cystic disease, chronic pain syndromes, postvasectomy pain syndromes, and nonhealing infections. There are slight but important differences in the technique used for each of these indications. For example, during epididymectomy performed for postvasectomy pain syndromes, excision of the proximal vas up to and including the vasectomy site is necessary. This is not necessary in patients with cystic disease or with idiopathic orchalgia. In patients with cystic disease who desire fertility, epididymectomy should be avoided and the larger cysts, if necessary, should be removed microsurgically. In patients with infection, it is important to obtain appropriate intraoperative cultures and insert a dependently directed drain.

## *References*


1. Chen TF, Ball RY. Epididymectomy for post-vasectomy pain: histological review. *Br J Urol* 1991;6:407–413.
2. Heidenreich A, Olbert P, Engelmann UH. Management of chronic testalgia by microsurgical testicular denervation. *Eur Urol* 2002;41:392–397.
3. Padmore DE, Norman RW, Millard OH. Analyses of indications for and outcomes of epididymectomy. *J Urol* 1996;156:95–96.
4. Sweeney P, Tan J, Butler MR, et al. Epididymectomy in the management of intrascrotal disease: a critical reappraisal. *Br J Urol* 1998;81:753–755.
5. West AF, Leung HY, Powell PH. Epididymectomy is an effective treatment for scrotal pain after vasectomy. *BJU Int* 2000;85:1097–1099.
6. Witherington R, Harper WM IV. The surgical management of acute bacterial epididymitis with emphasis on epididymotomy. *J Urol* 1982;128:722–725.


# CHAPTER 61 ■ EJACULATION INDUCTION PROCEDURES: PENILE VIBRATORY STIMULATION AND ELECTROEJACULATION

DANA A. OHL, SUSANNE A. QUALLICH, JENS SØNKSEN, NANCY L. BRACKETT, AND CHARLES M. LYNNE

Anejaculatory infertility is a relatively uncommon etiology of failure to conceive, but in certain patient populations, this condition may be the most common cause of infertility. Men with anejaculatory infertility have dysfunction of some portion of the normal ejaculatory reflex system, preventing the emission of semen during normal sexual activity. These neuroanatomic components of the ejaculatory response include (a) penile dorsal nerves carrying efferent sensory stimuli to the spinal cord at S2–4; (b) descending pathways from the brain to carry cerebral input down to the ejaculatory center at T10–L2; (c) ascending pathways from S2–4 to coordinate sensory input at T10–L2; (d) sympathetic outflow at T10–L2, carried via the sympathetic chain, the inferior mesenteric plexus, and pelvic sympathetics, ending in the walls of the ejaculatory organs, the seminal vesicles, vas deferens, prostate, and bladder neck, to effect seminal emission and bladder neck closure; and (e) pudendal nerves to stimulate the periurethral skeletal muscle, to create the projectile phase of the reflex. Stimulation of the brain and genitalia results in a coordinated response culminating in emission of sperm and seminal plasma into the urethra, followed shortly by rhythmic contractions of the periurethral muscle against a tightly closed bladder neck, resulting in projectile expulsion of semen from the urethra.

There are several types of ejaculatory dysfunction, including premature ejaculation, retrograde ejaculation, and anejaculation. Men with premature ejaculation and retrograde ejaculation are not appropriate for penile vibratory stimulation (PVS) and electroejaculation (EEJ), favoring other treatment algorithms. Candidates for ejaculation induction procedures are those men who are unable to initiate a normal ejaculatory reflex due to neurologic conditions. The most common cause seen in practice is spinal cord injury (SCI), due to the fact that SCI men are able to ejaculate only 10% to 20% with normal coitus (8). Other etiologies include surgical sympathectomy from retroperitoneal lymph node dissection, aortic surgery, or perirectal dissection, diabetic neuropathy, transverse myelitis, multiple sclerosis, and spinal bifida. In these neurologic conditions, segments of the normal neuroanatomic structures are nonfunctioning, leading to absence of seminal emission. In uncommon cases, anorgasmia from a psychogenic source may be a reason to utilize ejaculation induction procedures.

## DIAGNOSIS

The diagnosis of anejaculation is made primarily by history. Certainly in individuals with the profound neurologic conditions mentioned previously, such as spinal cord injury, there is little mystery as to the source of their infertility. The history needs to capture other risk factors, such as prior surgery, a diagnosis of diabetes, and any neurologic symptoms that may indicate an occult condition. In individuals who are relatively neurologically intact, such as a diabetic neuropath, a history of normal orgasm sensation, without seminal fluid emitted per urethra, is key. One needs to inquire for signs of retrograde ejaculation, such as cloudiness in the urine immediately after ejaculation. In men with psychogenic anorgasmia, which tends to be lifelong, the history may be more problematic, as these men may have never experienced a normal orgasm. The clinician may need to have the man describe in detail the events that occur during sexual activity to determine if the man is experiencing orgasm or not.

There are few diagnostic tests necessary in most men prior to a trial of an ejaculation induction procedure. Information about spermatogenesis can be indirectly obtained with a serum follicle stimulating hormone (FSH) level and by finding a normal testicular volume on physical examination. If the FSH is elevated, a testis biopsy might be indicated. If there is a question of retrograde ejaculation, postorgasm urine is examined to look for sperm. In men with retrograde ejaculation, or those with peripheral neuropathy (diabetic neuropathy or surgical sympathectomy), a trial of sympathomimetic agents may induce antegrade ejaculation, thus preventing the need for ejaculation induction. Finally, prior to performing procedures on men with anejaculation, a fertility evaluation of the female partner ensures that a suitable recipient for assisted reproductive techniques (ARTs) is available.

## INDICATIONS FOR EJACULATION INDUCTION PROCEDURES

Men with anejaculation who wish to induce a pregnancy in their female partners are candidates for PVS or EEJ. These procedures are not aimed at restoring sexual function, but merely serve as a method to retrieve sperm that might be used for ARTs. Indeed, many men find these procedures uncomfortable. Therefore, the goal of using PVS and EEJ is procreation.

Penile vibratory stimulation is useful in men who are anejaculatory from SCI. Since this procedure requires an intact ejaculatory reflex arc, men with peripheral neuropathies and those with incomplete lesions are suboptimal candidates. PVS has a higher success rate in SCI men with complete lesions, lesions above T8, upper motor neuron characteristics (spastic), and intact bulbocavernosus and hip flexion reflexes. The success rate markedly drops off with the lower levels of injury associated with lower motor neuron injury characteristics. However, because of the relative noninvasiveness of PVS compared to EEJ, it is reasonable to attempt PVS in all SCI men prior to attempting EEJ.

EEJ is utilized for SCI men who fail PVS and in all other etiologies of anejaculation. However, cost analysis of the results of EEJ with ARTs has led to the recommendation that non-SCI men rarely should undergo EEJ (7). In men with normal sensation, a general anesthetic is needed to perform EEJ, and the added cost of the anesthetic changes the cost-effectiveness calculations. Although it may still be reasonable to utilize EEJ in the non-SCI population, the clinician needs to strongly consider the alternative procedures noted below.

## ALTERNATIVE THERAPIES

The goal in ejaculation induction procedures is to obtain sperm to be used in ARTs. Therefore, the choice of ART is dependent on the sperm quality delivered by the ejaculation induction procedure. For instance, if a procedure delivers sperm with >10 million total motile sperm (TMS), then a simple ART procedure, such as intrauterine insemination (IUI), will have a reasonable chance of a pregnancy. However, if the TMS is between 1 and 10 million, then standard in vitro fertilization (IVF) will be necessary to give reasonable pregnancy rates. If the TMS drops below 1 million sperm, intracytoplasmic sperm injection (ICSI) in conjunction with IVF is necessary to give reasonable pregnancy rates. Finally, in an SCI man who exhibits exceptional semen quality with PVS, patient-directed PVS procedures in the home setting, followed by patient-directed vaginal insemination, may result in pregnancy.

In general, ejaculation induction procedures are aimed at utilizing IUI in an attempt to optimize cost-effectiveness. If IUI is determined not to be cost-effective as compared to IVF, the advantage of ejaculation induction is lost. In fact, when analyzing the effectiveness of EEJ when coupled with IUI in men without SCI, the increased cost of the required anesthetic changes the analysis to favor proceeding directly to the more costly IVF procedure, based on pregnancy rates and the cost of the procedures (7). Since there are methods other than EEJ to deliver adequate numbers of sperm for IVF, these procedures merit discussion.

In men who require an anesthetic to perform EEJ, it is cost-effective to bypass the EEJ procedure and go directly to sperm aspiration procedures (described elsewhere in this book), in conjunction with IVF, and ICSI of the partner's oocytes (7). However, some IVF clinics proceed directly to sperm aspiration procedures in all men, without consideration of PVS or IUI, even for SCI subjects. The authors disagree with this algorithm, based on cost-effectiveness analysis (5).

Finally, a discussion of options in the anejaculatory patient would not be complete without mentioning the possibility of donor artificial insemination and adoption. This information is discussed with the couple, but the subjects themselves need to decide whether to forego attempts at conception with the male partner's sperm and use these techniques.

## TECHNIQUES

### Penile Vibratory Stimulation

Penile vibratory stimulation depends on an intact reflex arc to be successful. The general idea is that the penis is overstimulated with a carefully designed vibrator, overcoming the ejaculatory reflex threshold. Sensory input is carried via the dorsal nerves into the sacral cord. These impulses then ascend into the ejaculatory center at the thoracolumbar cord, where sympathetic fibers carry a signal to the ejaculatory organs, causing them to contract. Since a complete ejaculatory reflex is elicited, there is also coordination of bladder neck closure during emission to prevent retrograde ejaculation, as well as pulsatile rhythmic contraction of the periurethral muscles, causing, in turn, pulsatile projectile ejaculation. The neurophysiologic events that occur during PVS are indistinguishable from a normal ejaculatory reflex, other than the fact that it is not associated with sexual activity, as well as the lack of sensation and control of the SCI subject.

The choice of the vibrator directly impacts ejaculation success rates. A study performed by Sønksen et al. (9) found that ejaculation rates when utilizing a vibrator with amplitude of 1.0 mm was only 32% in a cohort of SCI men. When challenging the same group of men with a vibrator with peak-to-peak amplitude of 2.5 mm, the ejaculation rate was 91%. In this study, amplitudes of commercially available vibrators were measured, and it was found that manufacturers' specifications were highly inaccurate and were not dependable enough to make choices in the types of devices to be used for patients. These observations led to development of a commercially available device produced with medical indication standards and FDA approval for use in ejaculation induction procedures in SCI men (Fig. 61.1). The authors recommend that this FDA-approved device be used in clinical PVS.

The initial PVS should be done in the clinic setting to ensure that there are no complications. PVS can be performed on a treatment table or with the patient remaining in his wheelchair. Although retrograde ejaculation is very uncommon with PVS, it is prudent to catheterize the bladder prior to the first procedure and again immediately after the procedure to check for sperm in the bladder. Catheterization must be done with a plastic catheter with nonspermicidal lubricant. If after the first procedure it is determined that no retrograde ejaculation is present, subjects will characteristically not develop this over time, and the catheterization may be omitted from future procedures.

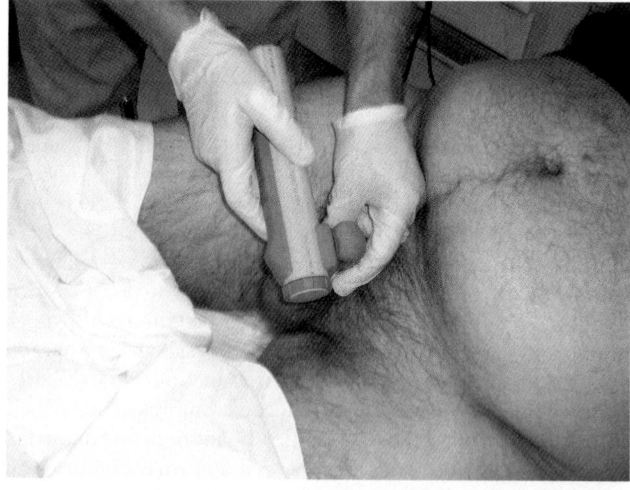

A

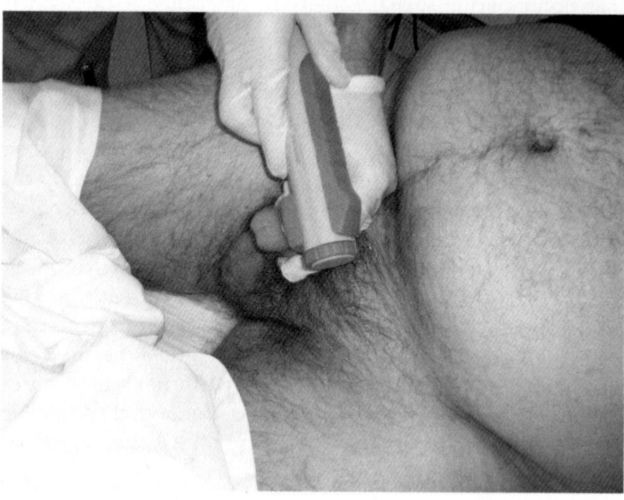

B

FIGURE 61.2 Different SCI patients will respond to different stimulation positions. **A:** Placement of the vibrator head at the frenulum. **B:** Placement of the vibrator head on the dorsum of the glans penis.

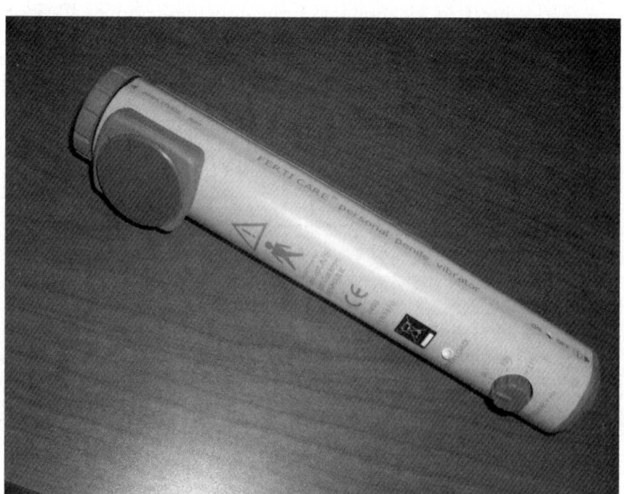


FIGURE 61.1 The FertiCare vibrator (Multicept APS, Copenhagen, Denmark) is the only device approved by the FDA for the purpose of penile vibratory ejaculation.

An automated blood pressure cuff is used to monitor blood pressure during the procedure, in case autonomic dysreflexia with extreme blood pressure increase occurs in response to the stimulation. SCI men with lesions above T6 are prone to dysreflexia. In such patients, consideration must be given to prophylactic administration of sublingual nifedipine 10 to 20 mg. Autonomic dysreflexia is discussed in more detail in the "Complications" section of this chapter.

The vibrator is placed on the patient's penis to deliver the stimulation. In most subjects, the stimulation area most likely to result in a positive response is the frenulum, although there is individual variation that can be sorted out with trial and error (Fig. 61.2).

The vibrator is placed on the penis with an initial amplitude of 2.5 mm and a frequency of 100 Hz. Enough pressure to get the device close to dampening is used to ensure delivery of an adequate power of vibration. The stimulation is applied until ejaculation occurs, or for a total of 3 minutes. If no ejaculation is reached within 3 minutes, there may be sensory fatigue and a rest period is indicated. One can resume stimulation again after a rest period of 1 minute, with consideration given to increasing the amplitude in half-centimeter increments up to 4.0 mm at maximum.

During stimulation, characteristic muscular responses can be seen and can give clues to the operator that ejaculation may be imminent. With application of the vibrator, abdominal and periurethral muscle contractions are typical. Piloerection is also common. When ejaculation is near, there is tonic contraction of leg and abdominal muscles, followed by rapid release and spastic, sometimes jerking, contractions of the muscles, coincident with the actual ejaculation process. If the vibration is discontinued just prior to ejaculation when such premonitory signs are seen, the complete reflex will continue without interruption. Discontinuation at this time may limit blood pressure rise in those prone to dysreflexia and may also prevent overstimulation and sensory fatigue, allowing multiple stimulations to be successful. If multiple attempts are made, one can continue with another stimulation period after a rest period of 1 minute (2).

An assistant is responsible for ensuring that the ejaculate is collected in a sterile specimen container. The assistant can also be very helpful in ensuring the comfort of the patient and watching for complications. Such assistance in monitoring for complications ensures having another set of eyes on the blood pressure monitor and checking verbally with the patient for any symptoms of dysreflexia, such as headache.

After the procedure, most patients feel quite well. There may be a general reduction in reflex activity that may lead to limitation of spasticity and bladder activity. The blood pressure of those who have received prophylactic nifedipine should be measured after assuming the sitting position.

## Electroejaculation

Rectal probe EEJ has been used in animal husbandry quite regularly for some time. The first use in men with spinal cord injury was reported in 1948 (4), but no pregnancies from electroejaculated sperm were reported until the 1970s. Further isolated reports ensued for many years until Bennett refined the procedure and presented a series of United States pregnancies from EEJ of SCI men (1).

Historically, it was assumed that EEJ worked via direct stimulation and contraction of the ejaculatory organs. However, recent research has shown that the electrical stimulation appears to initially cause high-pressure contraction of the pelvic floor and periurethral muscles, leading to a partially coordinated reflex with seminal emission and contraction of the bladder neck and rhythmic, although somewhat disorganized, contractions of the periurethral muscles, leading to expulsion of semen (11). Although there are many components of the reflex that are similar to PVS, the less organized reflex response leads to incomplete coordination and the likely possibility that some of the ejaculate will be emitted in a retrograde fashion.

Since retrograde ejaculation is a distinct probability, it is important to prepare the patient to limit toxicity of the sperm-urine contact. The authors favor limitation of fluid intake in order to limit urine production during the procedure. Subjects are instructed to take ½ teaspoon of sodium bicarbonate 12 hours and 2 hours prior to the procedure to alkalinize the urine. In SCI men with recurrent urinary tract infections, consideration is given for a short course of prophylactic antibiotics. To clear the rectum of feces, SCI men are instructed to perform their normal bowel evacuation the night before the procedure. Non-SCI men are instructed to empty the rectum with the assistance of an enema.

Although most non-SCI men should not undergo EEJ, there may be compelling reasons to proceed. These may include evidence of very high sperm production, increasing the chance of an IUI success; or religious objections to IVF, necessitating the use of IUI. In non-SCI men, EEJ is a very painful procedure and must be performed under anesthesia. General anesthesia has been the most common modality in practice. The discussion of the procedure that ensues will assume that the subject is an SCI man, who does not require anesthesia.

There is only one device that is FDA-approved for EEJ of SCI men. This is the Seager unit. Virtually all modern experience with EEJ has been with this machine. The unit consists of a central power generator and cords that may be attached to a variety of rectal probes. The central unit has a stimulation counter and a read-out of probe temperature so that overheating may be monitored. There is a heat sensor fail-safe that cuts power to the unit if temperature rises to unsafe levels. The EEJ equipment setup and additional supplies are shown in Fig. 61.3.

EEJ is performed on the treatment table. The patient begins supine, and an automated blood pressure cuff is applied to monitor for dysreflexia. In those prone to dysreflexia, consideration is given for prophylactic sublingual nifedipine, 10 to 30 mg. Since EEJ is capable of providing a very noxious stimulus that can create a dysreflexia situation in prone individuals, subjects are instructed to inform the staff if a headache or palpitations arise.

The bladder is catheterized in all EEJ cases, due to the propensity for retrograde ejaculate (Fig. 61.4). Five to 20 mL of a sperm-friendly medium from the assisted reproduction lab is instilled into the bladder (Fig. 61.5). A plastic catheter with nonspermicidal lubricant is used for the pre- and post-procedure catheterizations to limit sperm toxicity.

The subject is then turned into the lateral decubitus position (Fig. 61.6), and rectoscopy is performed to ensure that no lesions are seen (Fig. 61.7). If significant inflammation is seen due to bowel program activity or colitis, the procedure should be canceled for the day and rescheduled. Any inflammatory condition of the colon will only be made worse by running electrical energy into the area.

The probe is inserted far enough into the rectum such that the limit of the plastic is located just at the anal sphincter (Fig. 61.8). The electrodes should be completely internalized inside the rectum. The conductive characteristic of the rectal mucosa allows efficient flow without much heat generation. However, if the electrodes are applied externally to the skin, the very high resistance of the skin will cause significant heat release and put the patient at risk for perineal burn. The electrodes are positioned anteriorly, facing the ejaculatory organs.

Electricity is delivered in waves of increasing voltage. The first stimulation is 2.5 to 5.0 V and is increased by 2.5 to 5.0 V per stimulation. The degree of rectal contact and individual characteristics lead to differences in resistance, such that with the same voltage, differences in electrical flow (milliamperes) may be seen. In general, a guideline of a maximum delivery of 1,000 mA at peak stimulation should be used, and that is usually seen with a voltage delivery of 30 to 35 V (Fig. 61.9).

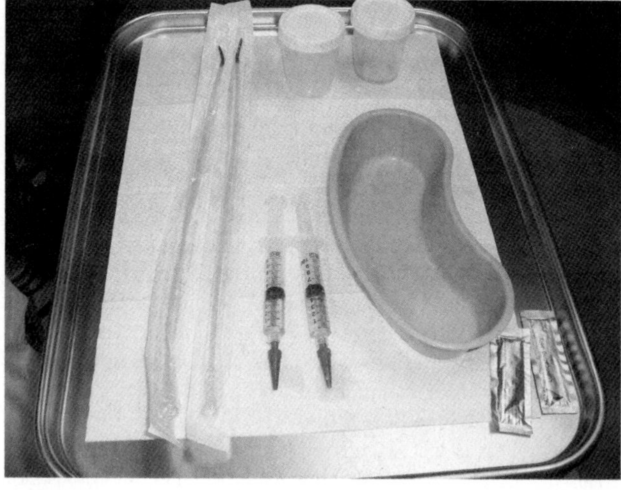

A

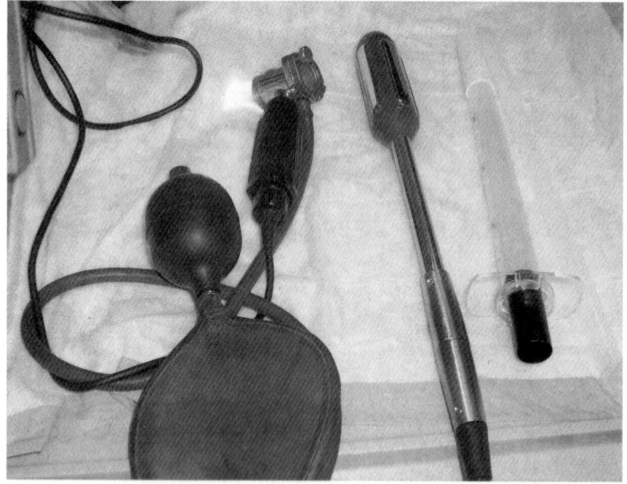

B

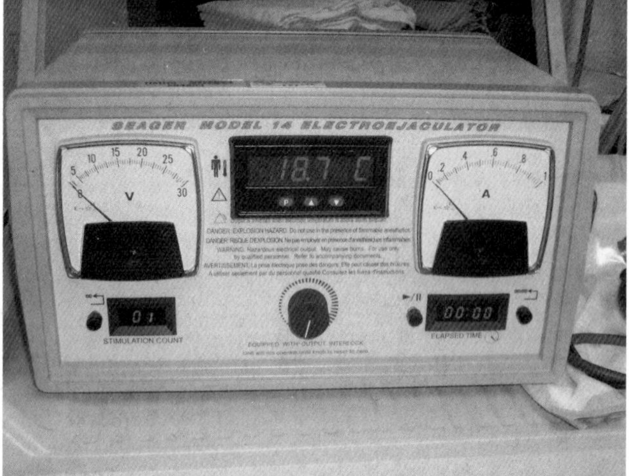


C

FIGURE 61.3 Electroejaculation equipment. **A:** Sigmoidoscope and rectal probe. **B:** Additional equipment, including plastic catheters, non-spermicidal lubricant packets, media for instillation into the bladder, basin for draining the urine, and specimen containers for the antegrade and retrograde specimens. **C:** Seager Model 14 Electroejaculator. Meters give voltage and current delivery, stimulation count and time, and probe temperature. The central rheostat is turned by the operator to alter voltage.

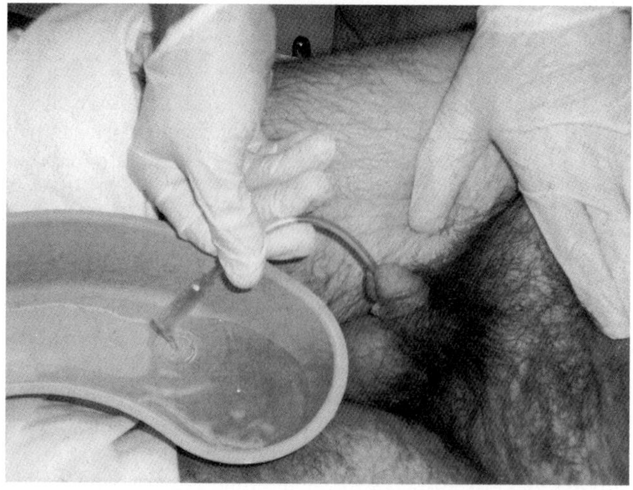

FIGURE 61.4 The bladder is emptied prior to electroejaculation.

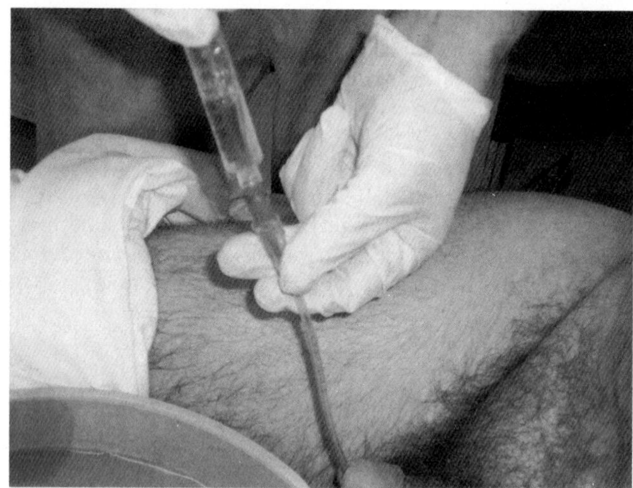

FIGURE 61.5 Sperm-friendly medium is instilled into the bladder in anticipation of retrograde ejaculation.

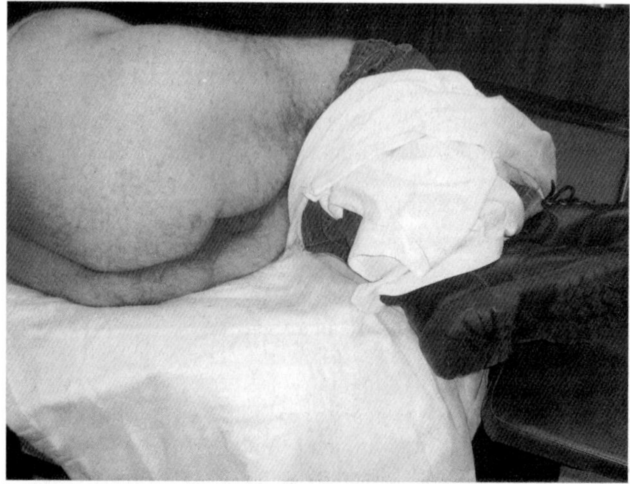

FIGURE 61.6 The lateral decubitus position allows access for insertion of the rectal probe and access to the penis for retrieving antegrade ejaculate.

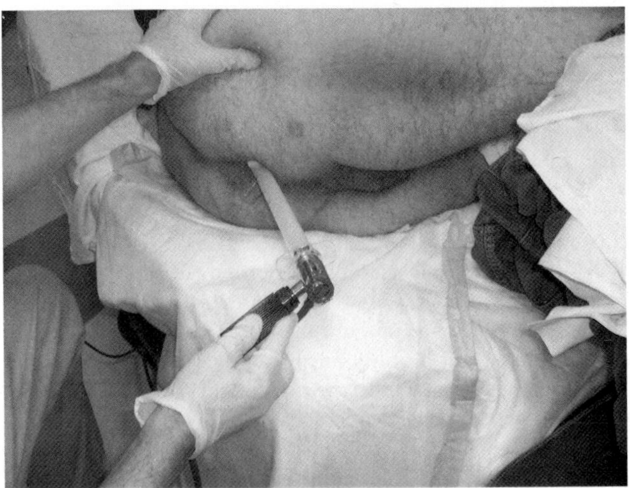

FIGURE 61.7 Rectoscopy is performed before and after the electrical stimulation.

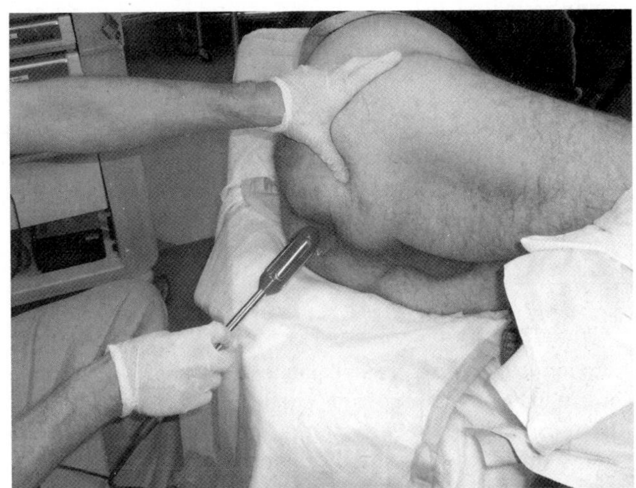

A

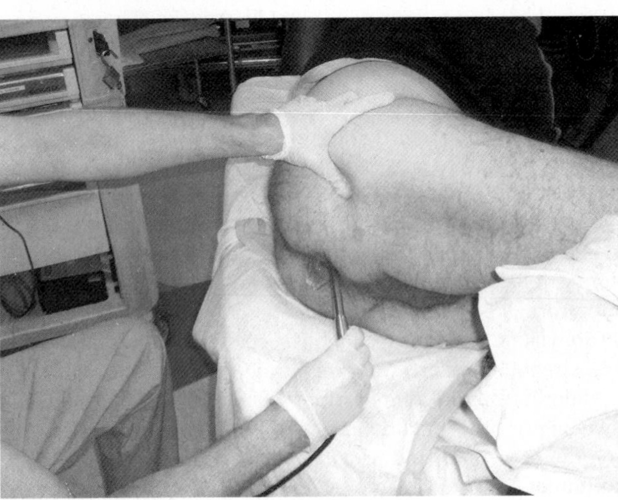

B

FIGURE 61.8 Rectal probe insertion. **A:** The well-lubricated probe is placed into the rectum. **B:** Final probe position with the electrodes completely inside the sphincter. The electrodes are positioned facing anteriorly.

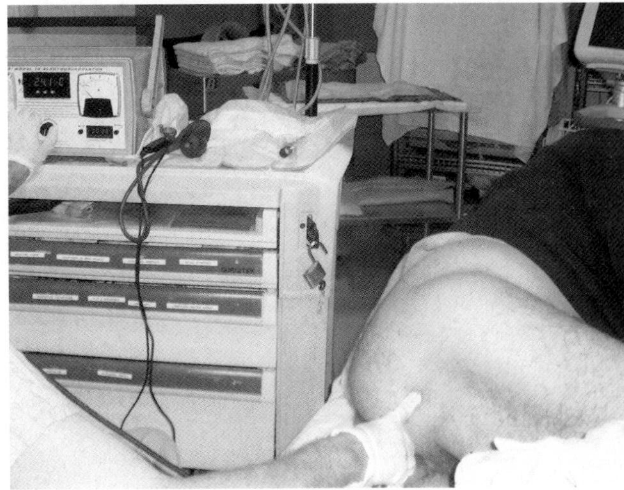

FIGURE 61.9 The operator is maintaining probe position with the right hand, while moving the rheostat on the machine to alter voltage delivery.

Waves are delivered with a relatively rapid rise to the chosen voltage for that stimulation, held for 5 seconds, and then abruptly cut off. During the time of electrical silence, the ejaculatory response develops over a few seconds, and ejaculation actually occurs during the silent phase. In the past the standard thinking was to leave an electrical baseline of 100 mA, never reaching zero again. However, the change from the older technique to the one described above has led to a significant reduction in the percentage of retrograde ejaculate (3,6).

During stimulation, there can be significant abdominal and leg muscle contractions. Piloerection can be seen also, and this also may indicate an adequate level of stimulation. In the electrically silent period between contractions, and during ejaculation, visible contraction of the perineal and periurethral muscles may be seen, again attesting that adequate stimulation is being given.

An assistant holds a cup over the penis to ensure that any antegrade ejaculate is collected (Fig. 61.10). Since ejaculate

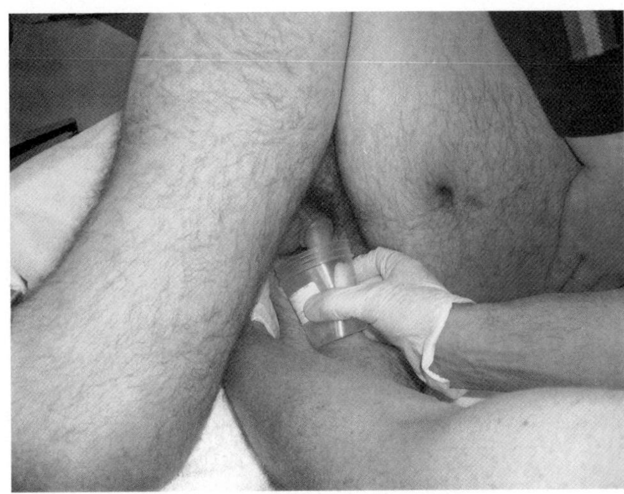

FIGURE 61.10 The assistant is maintaining the position of the urethral meatus inside the specimen container to collect the antegrade ejaculate.

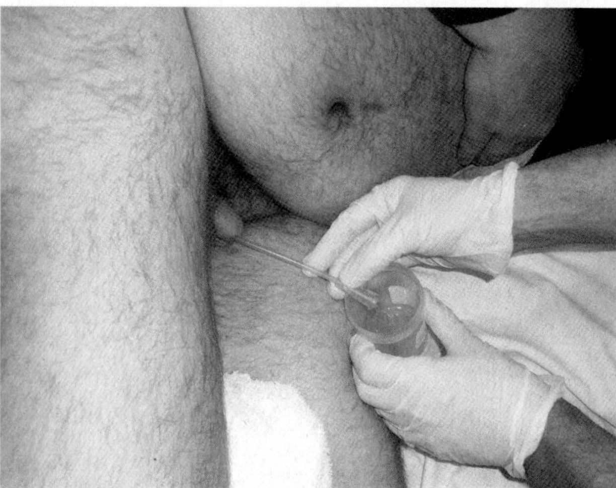

FIGURE 61.11 Following electrical stimulation, the subject is once again catheterized to retrieve the retrograde fraction of the ejaculate.

may be retained in the urethra, gentle milking on the underside of the urethra in an antegrade fashion may help in the expulsion. The assistant can also aid in monitoring the blood pressure and any patient complaints of dysreflexia.

When no more fluid is expelled following a stimulation cycle, or if probe temperature reaches 39.5°C, the procedure is terminated. The probe is removed and rectoscopy performed again to ensure that no burn, bleeding, or perforation is seen. The subject is then catheterized again to extract the postejaculation urine (Fig. 61.11). A plastic catheter is used to avoid sperm adhering to it, and nonspermicidal lubricant is used, for obvious reasons. After extraction of bladder contents, the bladder is irrigated with the sperm-friendly medium for complete removal of retrograde ejaculate. Both specimens are submitted to the laboratory for analysis and processing (Fig. 61.12).

Similar to PVS, patients feel quite well after EEJ, and they may also feel a reduction in skeletal muscle and bladder spasticity for 12 to 24 hours after the procedure.

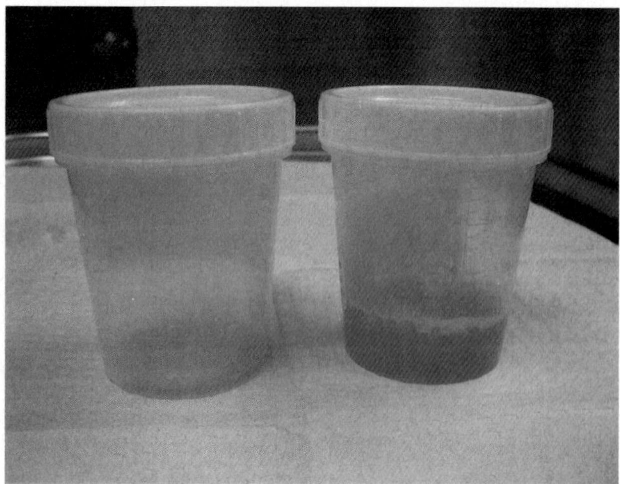

FIGURE 61.12 The specimens from a typical EEJ procedure include a small-volume antegrade ejaculate and a larger-volume retrograde fraction.

## OUTCOMES

In SCI men, PVS is approximately 60% successful in inducing an ejaculatory response. The best results are seen in men with spasticity, in those with lesions above T8, and in those with intact bulbocavernosus and hip flexion reflexes, where ejaculation rates can be as high as 90%. EEJ, however, is nearly universally successful in causing seminal emission.

Unfortunately, the sperm quality from PVS and EEJ in SCI men is poor. This includes abnormalities of gross semen parameters and abnormal sperm function. Typically, sperm numbers are high, but motility and viability are very low. Other abnormalities seen include poor overnight survival, decreased ability to penetrate cervical mucus, and lower fertilizing capability, as compared to control sperm. This limits the success rates in series of men attempting conception.

Sperm obtained from ejaculation induction procedures are sent to the assisted reproductive laboratory for processing by standard preparation techniques. The specimens can be utilized for IUI or IVF, depending on the couple's situation and the sperm quality. The largest series of EEJ coupled with ARTs demonstrated an IUI cycle fecundity of 11% per cycle and 35% per couple. A single attempt of EEJ coupled with IVF gave a 43% pregnancy rate (7).

In men with exceptional semen quality, couples may be taught to perform PVS at home and do vaginal insemination. In a series of men in Germany, Denmark, and the United States, 73 of 169 couples had a pregnancy (43%). Ninety-nine pregnancies in these 169 couples were achieved (10).

## COMPLICATIONS

Autonomic dysreflexia is a phenomenon seen in higher spinal cord lesions. When a noxious stimulus is delivered, such as EEJ, the initial response is for the sympathetic nervous system to raise the blood pressure. Regulatory mechanisms including vascular baroreceptors give rise to modulation of the response from brainstem centers. The sympathetic outflow responsible for the blood pressure rise is located below T6. Therefore, in a man with a spinal cord injury above T6, the brainstem centers cannot communicate with the sympathetic outflow, leading to an autonomous, and unchecked, response. Therefore, the periphery is responding to the noxious stimulus with extreme rises in blood pressure, without normal control mechanisms stopping this reflex response.

EEJ and PVS are efficient stimuli that can induce dysreflexia. In susceptible subjects, dangerous rises in blood pressure can be seen, resulting in a risk for stroke. Blood pressure monitoring is essential in men with T6 or above lesions. Prophylactic nifedipine is highly successful in limiting the risk of extreme blood pressure rise during the procedures (12).

Specific minor complications from PVS may include skin swelling or bruising, discomfort from muscle contraction during the procedure, and urinary retention in reflex voiders due to limitation of reflex activity following the procedure.

There have been very rare reports of rectal injury or burn from EEJ, which is obviously a major complication, but the incidence is extremely low. Patients may also experience some discomfort during the procedure and temporary urinary retention, as in PVS.

## *References*


1. Bennett CJ, Ayers JW, Randolph JF Jr, et al. Electroejaculation of paraplegic males followed by pregnancies. *Fertil Steril* 1987;48:1070–1072.
2. Bird VG, Brackett NL, Lynne CM, et al. Reflexes and somatic responses as predictors of ejaculation by penile vibratory stimulation in men with spinal cord injury. *Spinal Cord* 2001;39:514–519.
3. Brackett NL, Ead DN, Aballa TC, et al. Semen retrieval in men with spinal cord injury is improved by interrupting current delivery during electroejaculation. *J Urol* 2002;167:201–203.
4. Horne HW, Paull DP, Munro D. Fertility studies in the human male with traumatic injuries of the spinal cord and cauda equina. *N Engl J Med* 1948;239:959–961.
5. Kafetsoulis A, Brackett NL, Ibrahim E, et al. Current trends in the treatment of infertility in men with spinal cord injury. *Fertil Steril* 2006;86:781–789.
6. Ohl DA, Sønksen J, Bolling R. New stimulation pattern for electroejaculation based on physiological studies. *J Urol* 2000;163[Suppl]:1522.
7. Ohl DA, Wolf LJ, Menge AC, et al. Electroejaculation and assisted reproductive technologies in the treatment of anejaculatory infertility. *Fertil Steril* 2001;76:1249–1255.
8. Sønksen J, Biering-Sørensen F. Fertility in men with spinal cord or cauda equina lesions. *Semin Neurol* 1992;12:106–114.
9. Sønksen J, Biering-Sørensen F, Kristensen JK. Ejaculation induced by penile vibratory stimulation in men with spinal cord injuries. The importance of the vibratory amplitude. *Paraplegia* 1994;32:651–660.
10. Sønksen J, Lochner-Ernst D, Brackett NL, et al. Vibratory ejaculation in 169 spinal cord injured men and home insemination of their partners. *J Urol* 2008;175[Suppl]:656.
11. Sønksen J, Ohl DA, Wedemeyer G. Sphincteric events during penile vibratory ejaculation and electroejaculation in men with spinal cord injuries. *J Urol* 2001;165:426–429.
12. Steinberger RE, Ohl DA, Bennett CJ, et al. Nifedipine pretreatment for autonomic dysreflexia during electroejaculation. *Urology* 1990;36:228–231.


# CHAPTER 62 ■ ANATOMY OF THE TESTIS

HOWARD H. KIM AND MARC GOLDSTEIN

A working knowledge of anatomy is vital for all surgeons, but it is perhaps especially critical for male reproductive urologists. In addition to knowing which nerves and lymphatics to avoid injuring during surgery and which collateral blood supply to depend on when a particular blood vessel is transected, the infertility specialist must understand the surgical anatomy in the context of spermatogenesis and reproductive physiology. Fortunately, the male reproductive anatomy has clinically relevant physical examination findings that facilitate the commitment of major principles to memory.

## INTRODUCTION TO MALE REPRODUCTIVE SYSTEM

### Physical Examination

Although representing only a minor subset of infertile men, endocrine disorders are often associated with characteristic findings on physical examination and are generally treatable with hormonal manipulation. Physical assessment of the hypothalamic-pituitary-gonadal (HPG) axis begins as soon as the infertile patient disrobes for the examination. Body habitus and secondary sex characteristics such as body hair distribution provide clues to disruption of the HPG axis and its potential role in the fertility status of the patient. For example, men with Kallmann syndrome or hypogonadotropic hypogonadism (HH) can present with delayed pubertal development or midline defects such as anosmia and cleft palate. In Kallmann syndrome, the olfactory axons fail to establish connections with the developing olfactory bulb during development, resulting in problems with gonadotropin-releasing hormone (GnRH) secretion. GnRH neurons use olfactory nerve migration for their own travel to the forebrain (12). Other disorders, such as androgen-insensitivity syndromes, can present with impaired secondary sex development or infertility.

### Hypothalamic-Pituitary-Gonadal Axis

Reproductive hormones are controlled by the hypothalamus, which releases GnRH in a pulsatile fashion, on average every 90 to 120 minutes from its preoptic and arcuate nuclei (Fig. 62.1). GnRH stimulates the anterior pituitary to release luteinizing hormone (LH) and follicle stimulating hormone (FSH). LH in turn stimulates the production of testosterone by Leydig cells, while FSH supports spermatogenesis in Sertoli cells. Both androgens and estrogens feed back to inhibit LH release, and inhibin, produced by the Sertoli cells, decreases FSH release.

## TESTIS

### Physical Examination

The physical examination of an infertile man reveals a wealth of information. Body habitus is assessed. Late closure of the epiphyses due to lack of adequate testosterone results in an arm span that exceeds height, or a pubis-to-foot distance that exceeds pubis-to-crown distance by >5 cm. Gynecomastia, feminized body habitus, and sparse male hair distribution complete the picture characteristic of either HH or Klinefelter syndrome. Evaluation of the scrotal contents is the centerpiece of the examination. A scrotum warmed with a heating pad to relax the dartos muscle and a securely private room optimize patient comfort and subsequently yield

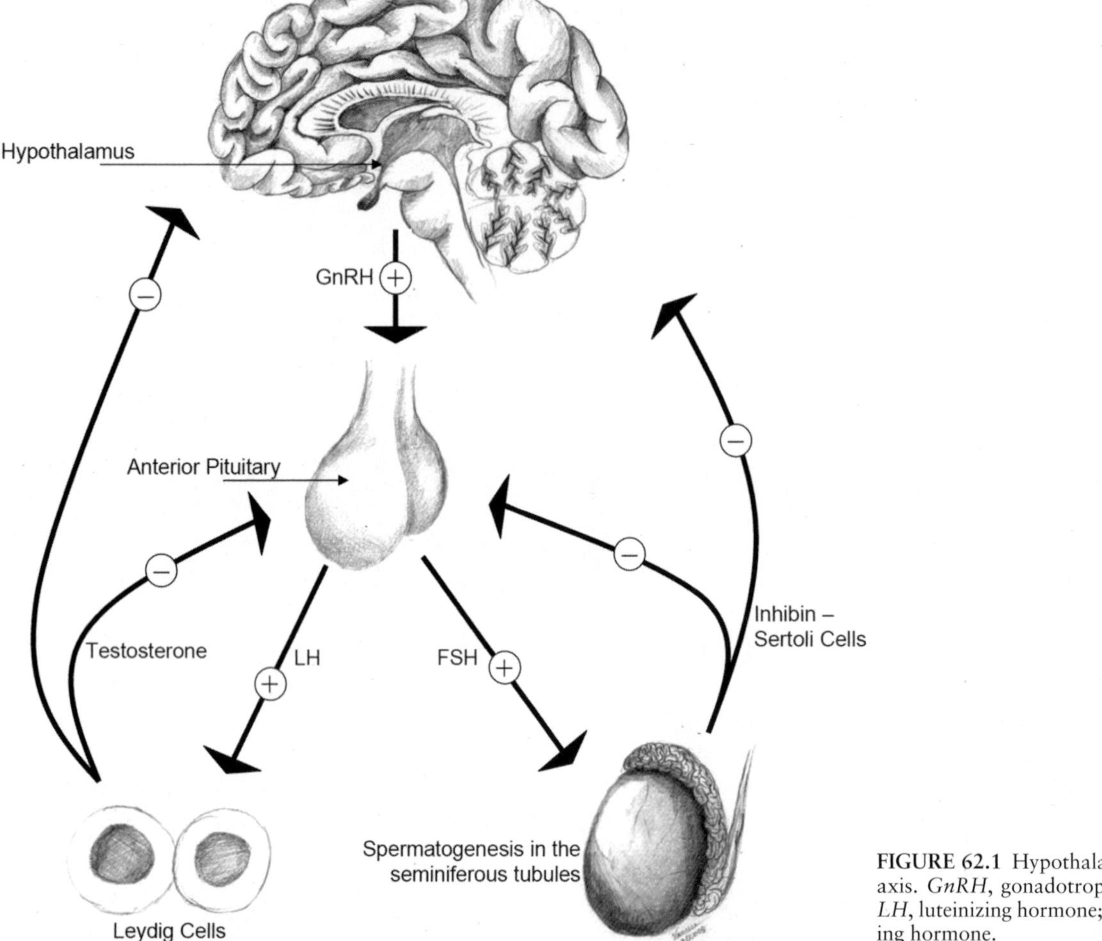


FIGURE 62.1 Hypothalamic-pituitary-gonadal axis. *GnRH*, gonadotropin-releasing hormone; *LH*, luteinizing hormone; *FSH*, follicle stimulating hormone.

a superior examination. The testes should be checked for size and consistency. Testes measure 15 to 25 cu cm in volume (45) and 4.5 to 5.1 cm in longitudinal length (60) in young healthy men. Testes decrease in size with age (27). Size directly correlates to spermatogenesis, as seminiferous tubules comprises 80% of testicular volume (5). Although a variety of devices are available for testis size measurement, including calipers, punched-out orchidometers, and scrotal ultrasonography, we prefer the standard Prader orchidometer for quick and easy assessment of testis volume. Assessment of testis consistency is equally important. A soft, mushy feel to the testis implies diminished spermatogenic capacity. Taken together, size and consistency help differentiate nonobstructive from obstructive causes of azoospermia.

## Development

Primordial germ cells migrate from the yolk sac to the genital ridge of the mesonephros, where they join somatic cells to form the primary epithelial or medullary cords (55). The testes arise from the primordial germ cells at 7 to 8 weeks of development (25) under the direction of the SRY gene of the Y chromosome (58). The component cells of the testis, Leydig and Sertoli cells, begin production of testosterone and müllerian inhibiting substance/antimüllerian hormone (MIS/AMH), respectively (65). AMH transcription is regulated by many transcription factors, including steroidogenic factor 1 (SF-1), SRY HMG box related gene 9 (SOX9), Wilms tumor 1 (WT1), and a zinc finger transcription factor (GATA-4) (11). Testosterone preserves the wolffian duct, and MIS/AMH induces degeneration of the adjacent müllerian duct (23). The wolffian duct of the regressing mesonephros combines with the developing gonad to form the epididymis, ductus deferens, ampulla, and seminal vesicles (55).

## Descent

The developing testis is anchored by two ligaments, the cranial suspensory ligament and the caudal genitoinguinal ligament or gubernaculum (23). Although we have an incomplete understanding of the mechanism of testicular descent, the process can be conceptualized as occurring in three simplified steps: nephric displacement, transabdominal movement, and inguinal passage. In the first stage, occurring about gestation day 55, the gubernaculum and the wolffian and müllerian ducts pull the gonad posteriorly as the metanephros moves anteriorly into the space recently vacated by the mesonephros (15). As the abdominal cavity of the fetus enlarges, the gonad maintains its proximity to the inguinal canal by dynamic changes to the suspensory ligaments. Under hormonal control, the gubernaculum enlarges and the cranial suspensory ligament regresses, facilitating descent (24) at 8 to 15 weeks of gestation (23). Testosterone induces regression of the cranial suspension ligament (61), whereas gubernacular development depends on insulinlike hormone 3 (Insl3) produced by the Leydig cell (13,43). At 25 to 35 weeks of gestation (23), the gubernaculum pushes through the inguinal canal, leading the testis outward into its final position (55). Calcitonin gene-related peptide (CGRP), found in the sensory branches of the genitofemoral nerve, appears to control gubernacular growth and direction of migration (23,68). The process ends with the regression of the gubernaculum (66).

## Capsule

Medical students are all too familiar with the seven layers of the scrotal wall: skin, dartos muscle, superficial perineal fascia, external spermatic fascia, cremasteric fascia, internal spermatic fascia, and the parietal layer of the tunica vaginalis (Fig. 62.2). But not many know that the testicular capsule consists of more than just the tunica albuginea. The testicular capsule is distinctly separate from the scrotal layers and is composed of its own three layers: the visceral layer of the tunica vaginalis (an outer thin serous layer composed of attenuated mesothelial cells), the tunica albuginea (a fibrous membrane, composed of collagen fibers and fibroblasts, that forms the bulk of the capsule), and the tunica vasculosa (a thin, delicate areolar layer with occasional networks of tiny blood vessels) (9). The tunica albuginea forms septations that separate the testis into lobules; the blood supply travels along these septations (9). Along the posterior border of the testis, the tunica albuginea thickens to form the mediastinum testis, which houses the channels of the rete testis and the initial portions of the vasa efferentia (Fig. 62.3) (9). Contractility of the testicular capsule (49) may be involved in the regulation of blood flow into the testis (53).

## Blood Supply

The internal spermatic or testicular, deferential, and external spermatic or cremasteric arteries are the major blood supply

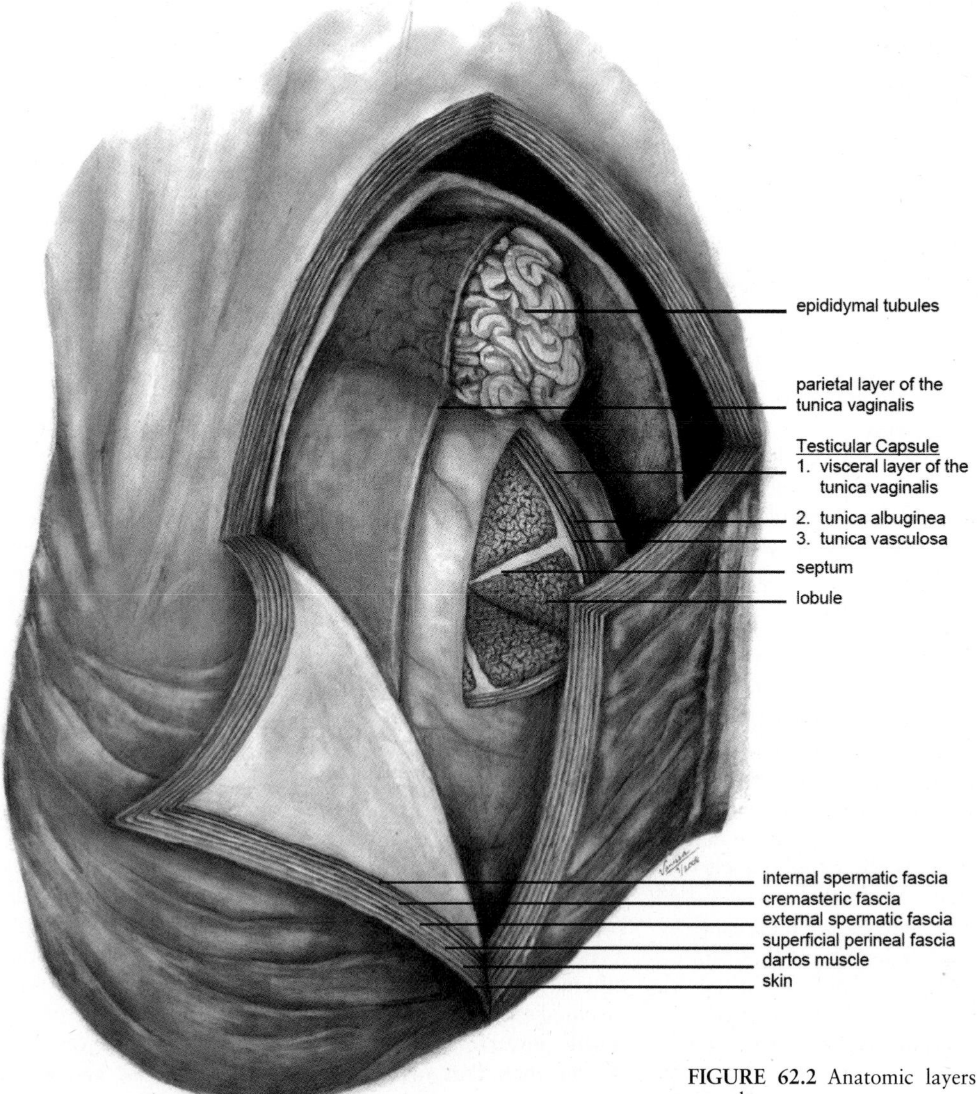


FIGURE 62.2 Anatomic layers of the scrotal wall and testicular capsule.

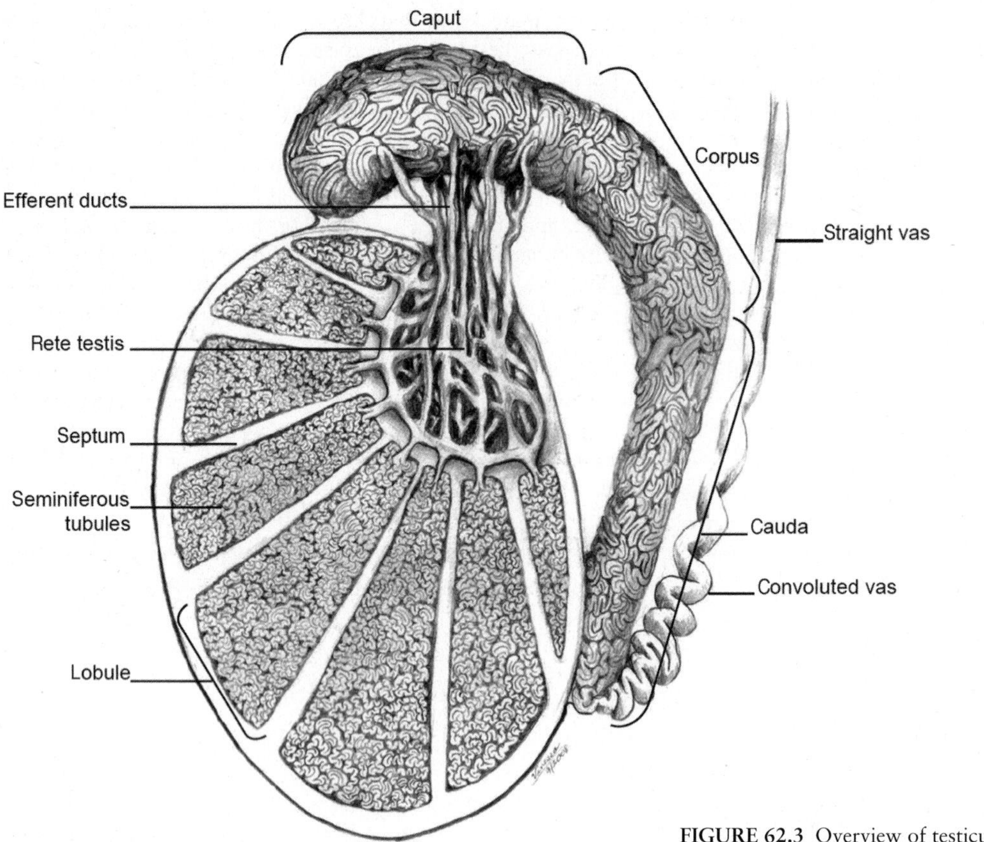


FIGURE 62.3 Overview of testicular anatomy.

to the testis (Fig. 62.4) (18). The internal spermatic artery arises from the aorta at L2-3, just below the origin of the renal arteries, and travels over the psoas major muscle, the ureter, and the genitofemoral nerve (41). The right testicular artery also lies anterior to the inferior vena cava and posterior to the third part of the duodenum, the right colic artery, the ileocolic artery, the root of the mesentery, and the terminal ileum; the left testicular artery lies posterior to the inferior mesenteric vein, the left colic artery, and the lower descending colon (41). The artery enters the spermatic cord as a single vessel before branching several times, sometimes as high as the internal inguinal ring (34). Studies have noted that the testicular artery often has one to three branches supplying the upper and lower poles of the testis (41).

Despite variant views on testicular blood supply, the predominant understanding is that the arteries supplying the parenchyma arise on the free border and run up toward the mediastinum before turning and branching out into the parenchyma (54). The testicular arteries penetrate the posterior aspect of the tunica albuginea and send parenchymal branches anteriorly as they travel inferiorly. Large branches also cover the inferior pole of the testis. The medial and lateral aspects of the midtestis have relatively fewer arterial branches compared to the anterior and inferior aspects (53). Color Doppler ultrasonography with point spectral analysis has demonstrated the low vascular resistance of the testis, in contrast to the high vascular resistance of the epididymis and peritesticular tissues (39).

The deferential artery branches from the inferior vesical artery and travels along the vas deferens in the spermatic cord to the convoluted portion of the epididymis at the cauda (34). The cremasteric artery forms off the inferior epigastric artery and travels superficially in the cremasteric fascia and tunica vaginalis to widely cover the surface of the testis and spermatic cord (34). Large-caliber anastomotic channels between the testicular and deferential arteries have been demonstrated in 87% of human testes specimens (34). The deferential artery forms its anastomosis at the cauda epididymis, whereas the testicular artery forms its anastomosis by a branch anywhere from near the internal inguinal ring to the tunica albuginea (34). The cremasteric artery has contributed to the anastomosis in 50% of the specimens studied (34). The relative contributions of each artery to the overall blood supply can be estimated by noting their diameters; Harrison and Barclay (18) and Harrison (17) reported that the sum of the cremasteric and deferential diameters was equal to the diameter of the testicular artery in one third of the cases. The diameter of the testicular artery is equal to or greater than the sum of the deferential and cremasteric artery diameters in 57.5% of cases (47). Raman and Goldstein (47) point to the Poiseuille law ($Q = \pi\alpha^4 P8\eta L$), in which the rate of blood flow through a vessel ($Q$) is related to the fourth power of the radius ($\alpha$), the difference in blood pressure at the two ends ($P$), the viscosity of blood ($\eta$), and the length of the vessel ($L$); because of the fourth power of the radius, blood flow of a large vessel is greater than that of two smaller vessels whose combined

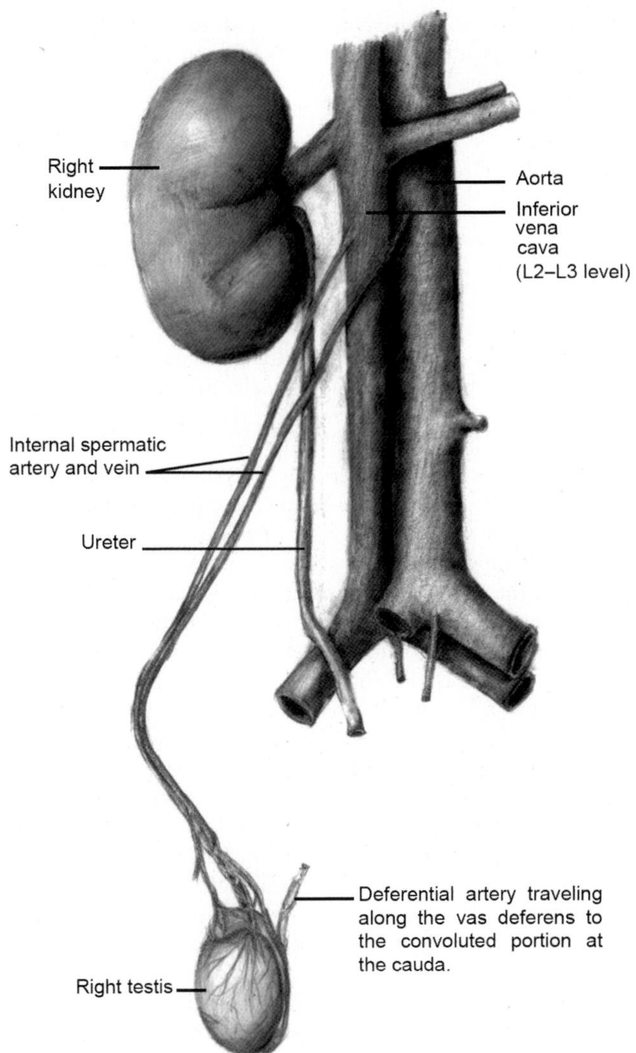


**FIGURE 62.4** Testicular blood supply. Not pictured: cremasteric artery.

diameter equals that of the larger vessel. Raman and Goldstein (47) concluded that the testicular artery contributes significantly more to the testicular blood supply than the combined flow of the deferential and cremasteric arteries. This fact may be relevant in procedures involving ligation of the testicular artery with dependence on collateral blood flow, such as non–artery-sparing laparoscopic varicocelectomy. Although several studies have reported no testicular atrophy in adults and adolescents who had their testicular arteries ligated during varicocelectomy (29,38,59), other studies have demonstrated significant sequelae of testicular artery ligation (30,44,57).

The layout of the testicular blood supply has important implications for several urologic procedures. In the surgical management of cryptorchidism with intentional ligation of the testicular artery, manipulation of the vas deferens should be minimized to preserve the deferential artery (34). Also, the testicular artery must be ligated above the origin of its anastomotic branch to take advantage of collateral circulation from the other arteries (34). Even venous drainage plays a significant role in the surgical anatomy of the testis. Deferential veins provide the only outlet for venous drainage following

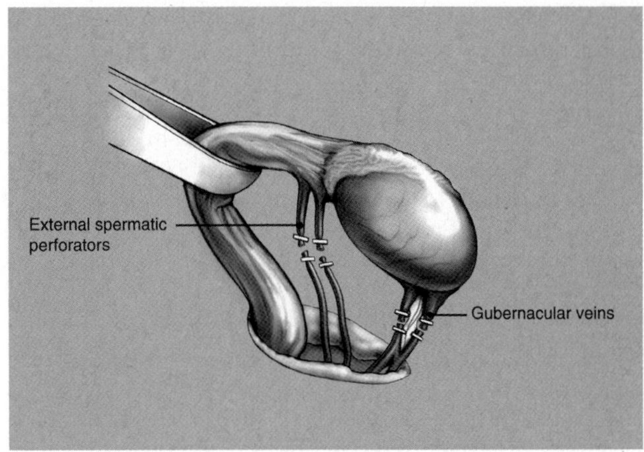


**FIGURE 62.5** Varicocelectomy. In addition to ligation of the internal spermatic veins, external spermatic and gubernacular veins must be identified and clipped to prevent varicocele recurrence. (From Goldstein M. Surgical management of male infertility and other scrotal disorders. In: *Campbell's urology*, 8th ed. Philadelphia: WB Saunders, 2002:1532–1587, with permission.)

varicocelectomy (Fig. 62.5). If the patient simultaneously or subsequently undergoes vasectomy, the deferential venous drainage may be compromised. Lee et al. (35) advocate microsurgical technique to avoid this outcome of insufficient venous drainage when performing both vasectomy and varicocelectomy in the same patient. In another example of relevant surgical venous anatomy, the importance of gubernacular veins and their contribution to varicocele has been debated. Although Ramasamy and Schlegel (48) reported no benefit of testicular delivery and ligation of gubernacular veins when performing varicocelectomy, Murray et al. (42) found presumed scrotal collaterals in 7% of recurrent varicoceles.

Knowledge of the layout of the testicular blood supply minimizes the risk for significant bleeding and compromise of the arterial supply during surgical sperm retrieval (51). The branches of the testicular artery are vulnerable to injury with their superficial course beneath the tunica albuginea. In one study, significant arterial blockage resulted from placement of a traction suture through the lower pole of the testis (26). Each septal compartment created by the tunica albuginea encapsulates at least one centrifugal artery with surrounding seminiferous tubules (53). Mostafa et al. (41) divided the testis into three vascular zones: the rich vascular areas comprising the upper pole, mediastinum testis, and posterolateral segments; the moderate vascular area of the middle third of the lateral surfaces; and the poor vascular areas of the anterior border and anterolateral surfaces.

The location of the testes outside the main body cavity makes them vulnerable to traumatic injury and torsion. Within the body, the long distance of travel across several anatomic planes by the internal spermatic artery and the other structures of the spermatic cord, as well as their delicate nature, exposes them to iatrogenic injury. Spermatic cord structures, including the testicular artery, may be injured during an inguinal hernia repair. In adults, the use of mesh for hernia repair can involve the spermatic cord with inflammation or direct obstruction. In children, the fine structures of the spermatic cord can be ligated inadvertently along with the hernia sac. The testicular artery and lymphatics may be compromised during varicocelectomy. Even with microsurgical technique, accidental artery ligation has occurred in approximately 1% of 2,102 cases (4). Of these, 5% resulted in testicular atrophy; the low incidence of morbidity was attributed to the preservation of the cremasteric and/or secondary testicular arteries (4).

Venous channels run independent of arteries, draining into surface veins of the tunica albuginea or into a central vein near the mediastinum; these veins feed the pampiniform plexus (54). Lymph fluid of the testis and epididymis travels in the spermatic cord to the lumbar or para-aortic lymph nodes (40,55).

## Countercurrent Heat Exchange

The control of blood flow to the testis is a complex collaboration of many factors, including nervous and hormonal control, temperature, and posture (54). As for all organ systems, blood flow is critical for testicular function and its effects on the system as a whole. Beyond the importance of flow rate to the inflow of oxygen and nutrients, the delivery of androgens to the body relies on testicular blood flow (54). Furthermore, the countercurrent heat exchange system of the testicular vasculature has been widely discussed in the context of varicocele pathophysiology. The arteries are intimately intermingled with the veins along the spermatic cord with the surrounding pampiniform plexus (64), allowing for efficient heat exchange and cooling of the testis. As a result of this mechanism, the blood entering the testis is 2°C to 4°C lower than rectal temperature (1), and intratesticular temperatures are 3°C to 4°C lower than rectal temperature (32).

## Blood–Testis Barrier

The relative isolation of the testis fluid is attributed to the blood–testis barrier formed by inter–Sertoli cell tight junctions (63). Lipid solubility, not molecular size, is the main determinant of substance entry into the testis fluid, although glucose and testosterone are two substances that enter more rapidly than expected (55). The barrier is established at puberty, and once formed is resistant to disruption (55). Efferent duct ligation and subsequent distention of the seminiferous tubules is one way to disrupt the barrier (55). The blood–testis barrier may serve to optimize tubular conditions for meiosis, and the immunological isolation of the testis fluid may be a secondary benefit (55). Men with failure of the barrier (i.e., men having undergone vasectomy) can form antibodies against their own spermatozoa (55). Holash et al. (21) hypothesized that testicular microvessels form part of the blood–testis barrier. They reported several markers of barrier properties, such as glucose transporter and P-glycoprotein, in testicular microvessels analogous to brain microvessels. They also found intertubular Leydig cells adjacent to microvessels to express the astrocyte markers glial fibrillary acidic protein, glutamine synthetase, and S-100 protein; astrocytes help to maintain barrier features in brain microvessels (21).

Sperm cells must travel from the basal compartment to the adluminal and luminal compartments. Two theories exist to explain how spermatocytes cross the blood–testis barrier during the course of spermatogenesis. In the "zipper" theory, tight junctions at the basal domain of Sertoli cells break down to allow passage of spermatocytes as new tight junctions are formed behind them (37). In the "repetitive removal of membrane segments" theory, stress created by spermatocytes alters tight junction fibrils (37).

## Innervation

No somatic nerves supply the testis. Scrotal and spermatic branches of the genitofemoral and ilioinguinal nerves as well as sympathetic fibers along the testicular artery mediate testicular pain (19). The genital branch of the genitofemoral nerve innervates the cremaster muscle and scrotal skin, and a branch of the ilioinguinal nerve innervates the skin of the upper scrotum and base of the penis. Spermatic cord traction during scrotal surgery may even activate peritoneal stimulation (62). Autonomic innervation is provided by the superior spermatic nerve and the inferior spermatic nerve (14). The superior spermatic nerve originates from the celiac and aortic plexuses and travels along the testicular vessels to form the major nerve supply of the testis (14). Sympathetic fibers originate in thoracic segments 10 and 11, whereas the parasympathetic fibers come from the vagus nerve (14). The inferior spermatic nerve travels with the ductus deferens and through the epididymis to innervate the lower pole of the testis (14). Sympathetic fibers originate in the inferior mesenteric and hypogastric plexuses, and parasympathetic fibers branch from the pelvic nerve (14). Evidence from animal models indicates that the nerve supply to the testis helps regulate its endocrine function. However, the precise function of testicular innervation in humans remains unclear.

Testicular pain is a common referral for urologists and can be secondary to infection, inflammation, trauma, varicoceles, hydroceles, and other causes. Orchialgia can be acute or chronic, and it is best treated by addressing the underlying disorder, such as varicoceles. As another example, vasectomy reversal can alleviate postvasectomy pain syndrome. However, the etiology of chronic testicular pain remains unknown in up to 25% of patients even after extensive workup (8). For these men, treatment ranges from psychological support to medication, from regional nerve blocks to surgery (36). Inguinal orchiectomy is one option, providing complete pain relief in 75% of patients in one study (8). In another study, however, orchiectomy failed in 80% of patients (6). Understanding the innervation of the testes and scrotum can help to target surgical management. Levine and Matkov (36) reported microsurgical denervation of the spermatic cord, including branches of the ilioinguinal and genitofemoral nerves and autonomic fibers, to provide complete pain relief in 76% and partial relief in 9%. Heidenreich et al. (19) reported a 96% complete response rate.

## Seminiferous Tubules

The seminiferous tubules contain the germinal epithelium. They form the bulk of the testis, with 15 to 25 m of length per gram of tissue in humans (3,55). As the testis declines in size with age, there is a corresponding shortening of the

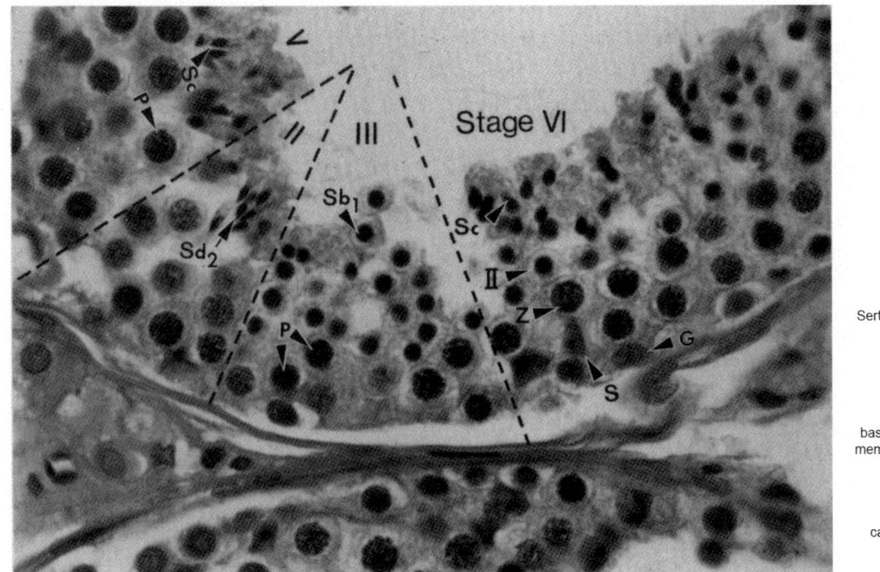


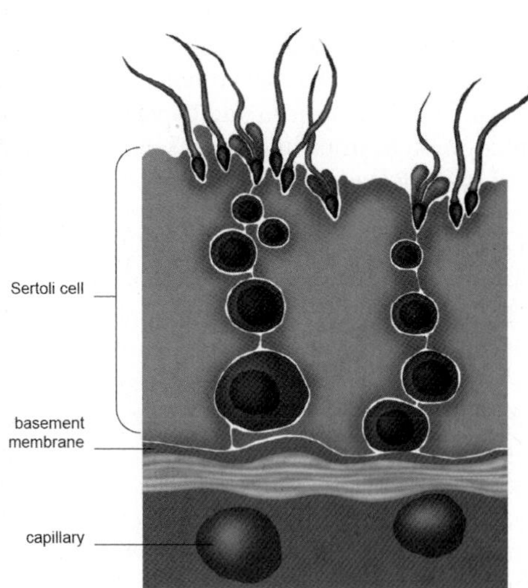


FIGURE 62.6 Normal spermatogenesis showing several cellular associations (stages) in a seminiferous tubular cross section. *Sb1*, round spermatid; *Sc* and *Sd2*, elongated spermatids; *II*, secondary spermatocyte; *P*, pachytene spermatocyte; *Z*, zygotene spermatocyte; *G*, spermatogonia; *S*, Sertoli cells (hematoxylin and eosin, magnification 1,000×). (From Jow WW. Testis biopsy. In: Goldstein M, ed. *Surgery of male infertility.* Philadelphia: WB Saunders, 1995:15, with permission.) Inset: Exaggerated, schematic illustration of the blood–testis barrier formed by tight junctions of Sertoli cells.

seminiferous tubules (33,55). The tubules are a series of convoluted loops with their two ends opening into the rete testis; they are further organized into about 300 lobules, with one to four tubules per lobule (55). The tubular wall has four layers: an internal noncellular layer or basement membrane, an internal cellular or intralamellar layer containing smooth muscle cells, an external noncellular layer similar to the internal noncellular layer, and an external cellular layer organized from cells of the intertubular mesenchyme (7). This flexible wall regulates the entry of fluid and substances and may contribute to the transport of spermatozoa with rhythmic peristaltic contractions (7).

## Germinal Epithelium

### Germ Cells and Spermatogenesis

A cross-sectional view of a seminiferous tubule demonstrates the wall with basement membrane enclosing Sertoli cells and sperm cells at various stages of development. Spermatogenesis involves three distinct processes: mitotic renewal of constituent stem cells, called spermatogonia; meiotic halving of the chromosomal number of the sperm product; and structural development of the mature spermatozoan (10). Spermatogenesis begins near the basement membrane, and the cells migrate toward the lumen as they develop, a process facilitated by the Sertoli cells (10).

Spermatogonia (2N) have significant contact with the basement membrane of the seminiferous tubule. They are classified as type A dark, type A pale, and type B based on their appearance on electron microscopy (10). Cells undergoing meiosis are identified as spermatocytes. In meiosis I, the diploid primary spermatocyte (2N becomes 4N with DNA replication), which has duplicated its DNA, forms two haploid secondary spermatocytes (2N). In meiosis II, the chromatids of each chromosome of the secondary spermatocyte divide to form spermatids (1N). In transforming the spermatid into a spermatozoan, spermiogenesis involves multiple steps, including acrosome formation, nuclear changes, neck and tail formation, and reorganization of the cytoplasm (10).

### Supporting Cells

In addition to the germ cells, supporting cells, also called folliculous cells, small epithelial cells, or indifferent cells, reside in the seminiferous tubules (7). These somatic elements originate from the coelomic cells of the gonadic crests and organize into sex cords shortly after sexual differentiation (7). The supporting cells increase their numbers by mitosis prior to spermatogenesis, and they gradually convert to Sertoli cells with the onset of spermatogenesis (7).

### Sertoli Cells

Sertoli cells are polymorphous and highly cohesive (7). The size and shape of Sertoli cells vary over the course of the seminiferous epithelial cycle (7). The shape has been described as a short body adjacent to the basement membrane with multiple sheetlike cytoplasmic projections extending toward the lumen, the form of these projections altered by surrounding germ cells (10). Each Sertoli cell spans the basement membrane to the tubular lumen and encloses clusters of germ cells (Fig. 62.6).

The seminiferous epithelial cycle refers to the simultaneous development of several germ cell generations within the seminiferous tubule, in which the cycles of different generations are coordinated (7). In humans, the duration of the seminiferous epithelial cycle is 64 days (20), and the duration of spermatogenesis is 74 to 76 days (56).

The Sertoli cell has many functions. The Sertoli-Sertoli tight junctional complexes effectively separate the exterior and interior compartments of the seminiferous epithelium (2). The Sertoli cell also secretes numerous products, including inhibin, androgen-binding protein (ABP), testicular transferrin and ceruloplasmin (iron and copper transport proteins), plasminogen activators, and growth factors (2). It even produces and metabolizes steroid hormones, although on a much smaller scale than Leydig cells (2). The secretory capacity of the Sertoli cell is bidirectional, which means it can secrete into both the tubular lumen and the interstitium and systemic circulation (67). In addition to supplying nutrition, adhesion, and transport functions to cells undergoing spermatogenesis, Sertoli cells may regulate apoptosis of germ cells (46). Sertoli cell function is regulated primarily by FSH and testosterone, although other substances, such as insulin, glucagon, calcitonin, estrogens, other steroid hormones, and vitamins, play a supporting role (2). Surrounding cells such as germ cells, Leydig cells, and myoid cells interact with the Sertoli cell by cell-cell contacts and paracrine factors (2). The Sertoli cell population is a major determinant of testicular size along with germ cells (2). The ratio of germ cells to Sertoli cells is estimated at 16:1 (2,67).

## Interstitial Tissue

The interstitium surrounding the seminiferous tubules is composed of loose fibrous connective tissue and a network of blood vessels, nerves, and lymphatics. The interstitial tissue also contains cells including fibroblasts, reticular cells, macrophages, plasma cells, lymphocytes, mast cells, and epithelioid cells called Leydig cells (22).

### Leydig Cells

Organization of the Leydig cell within the interstitium varies by species, but in humans Leydig cells form small aggregations near blood and lymphatic vessels (10). LH stimulates the production of androgens by the Leydig cell through several mechanisms, including acceleration of synthesis of the proteins involved in steroidogenesis and augmentation of cholesterol transport to and within the mitochondria (16). Leydig cells communicate extensively with Sertoli cells and germ cells via paracrine regulation of testicular function (50). There are two generations of Leydig cells in humans: fetal and adult. Fetal Leydig cells originate from undifferentiated mesenchymal cells at 8 weeks of gestation and regress starting at 14 weeks (5). Adult Leydig cells are evident at puberty (5). The gradual decline in plasma testosterone with advancing age correlates with age-related attrition of Leydig cells (28) or may possibly be due to alterations in LH function and oxidative damage to proteins involved in steroidogenesis (69).

### Rete Testis and Efferent Ducts

The rete testis is a network of anastomosing channels located at the testicular hilum along the epididymal edge of the testis (55). Cells lining the rete testis vary from squamous to columnar and are joined near the lumen by specialized junctions (55). The rete testis is closely associated with the testicular artery at the surface of the testis (55). Sperm and fluid flow from the rete testis and travel through efferent ducts to reach the epididymis (55). These ducts are lined with principal and ciliated cells (55). Although these cells have minimal secretory capacity, the ciliated cells may be involved with fluid resorption (55). In contrast to the rete testis, the efferent ducts are bathed by a dense subepithelial capillary bed (31).

## SUMMARY

Our current knowledge of male reproductive anatomy and physiology is a culmination of research spanning more than a century. Recent advances in molecular techniques have revealed some of the underlying mechanisms, such as cell signaling, involved in spermatogenesis and development of the reproductive tract. This chapter reviewed the basic anatomy of the testis, a simplified framework that can be filled in with future developments in the field.

## *References*

1. Agger P. Scrotal and testicular temperature: its relation to sperm count before and after operation for varicocele. *Fertil Steril* 1971;22:286–297.
2. Bardin CW, Cheng CY, Mustow NA, et al. *The Sertoli cell*, 2nd ed., Vol. 1. New York: Raven Press, 1994.
3. Bascom KF, Osterud HL. Quantitative studies of the testicle. II. Pattern and total tubule length in the testicles of certain common mammals. *Anat Rec* 1925;31:159–169.
4. Chan PT, Wright EJ, Goldstein M. Incidence and postoperative outcomes of accidental ligation of the testicular artery during microsurgical varicocelectomy. *J Urol* 2005;173:482–484.
5. Codesal J, Regadera J, Nistal M, et al. Involution of human fetal Leydig cells. An immunohistochemical, ultrastructural and quantitative study. *J Anat* 1990;172:103–114.
6. Costabile RA, Hahn M, McLeod DG. Chronic orchialgia in the pain prone patient: the clinical perspective. *J Urol* 1991;146:1571–1574.
7. Courot M, Hochereau-de Reviers MT, Ortavant R. Spermatogenesis. In: Johnson AD, Gomes WR, Vandemark NL, eds. *The testis*, Vol. 1: *Development, anatomy, and physiology*. New York: Academic Press, 1970: 339–432.
8. Davis BE, Noble MJ, Weigel JW, et al. Analysis and management of chronic testicular pain. *J Urol* 1990;143:936–939.
9. Davis JR, Langford GA, Kirby PJ. *The testicular capsule*, Vol. 1: *Development, anatomy, and physiology*. New York: Academic Press, 1970.
10. de Kretser DM, Kerr JB. *The cytology of the testis*, 2nd ed., Vol. 1. New York: Raven Press, 1994.
11. de Santa Barbara P, Moniot B, Poulat F, et al. Expression and subcellular localization of SF-1, SOX9, WT1, and AMH proteins during early human testicular development. *Dev Dyn* 2000;217:293–298.
12. Duke VM, Winyard PJ, Thorogood P, et al. KAL, a gene mutated in Kallmann's syndrome, is expressed in the first trimester of human development. *Mol Cell Endocrinol* 1995;110:73–79.
13. Emmen JM, McLuskey A, Adham IM, et al. Hormonal control of gubernaculum development during testis descent: gubernaculum outgrowth in vitro requires both insulin-like factor and androgen. *Endocrinology* 2000; 141:4720–4727.
14. Gerendai I, Banczerowski P, Halasz B. Functional significance of the innervation of the gonads. Endocrine 2005;28:309–318.

15. Gier HT, Marion GB. *Development of the mammalian testis*, Vol. 1: *Development, anatomy, and physiology*. New York: Academic Press, 1970.
16. Hall PF. *Testicular steroid synthesis: organization and regulation*, 2nd ed., Vol. 1. New York: Raven Press, 1994.
17. Harrison RG. The distribution of the vasal and cremasteric arteries to the testis and their functional importance. *J Anat* 1949;83:267–282.
18. Harrison RG, Barclay AE. The distribution of the testicular artery (internal spermatic artery) to the human testis. *Br J Urol* 1948;20:57–66.
19. Heidenreich A, Olbert P, Engelmann UH. Management of chronic testalgia by microsurgical testicular denervation. *Eur Urol* 2002;41:392–397.
20. Heller CG, Clermont Y. Kinetics of the germinal epithelium in man. *Recent Prog Horm Res* 1964;20:545–575.
21. Holash JA, Harik SI, Perry G, et al. Barrier properties of testis microvessels. *Proc Natl Acad Sci U S A* 1993;90:11069–11073.
22. Hooker CW. The intertubular tissue of the testis. In: Johnson AD, Gomes WR, Vandemark NL, eds. *The testis*, Vol. 1: *Development, anatomy, and physiology*. New York: Academic Press, 1970:483–550.
23. Hutson JM, Hasthorpe S. Abnormalities of testicular descent. *Cell Tissue Res* 2005;322:155–158.
24. Hutson JM, Hasthorpe S. Testicular descent and cryptorchidism: the state of the art in 2004. *J Pediatr Surg* 2005;40:297–302.
25. Hutson JM, Hasthorpe S, Heyns CF. Anatomical and functional aspects of testicular descent and cryptorchidism. *Endocr Rev* 1997;18:259–280.
26. Jarow JP. Clinical significance of intratesticular arterial anatomy. *J Urol* 1991;145:777–779.
27. Johnson L, Petty CS, Neaves WB. Age-related variation in seminiferous tubules in men. A stereologic evaluation. *J Androl* 1986;7:316–322.
28. Kaler LW, Neaves WB. Attrition of the human Leydig cell population with advancing age. *Anat Rec* 1978;192:513–518.
29. Kass EJ, Marcol B. Results of varicocele surgery in adolescents: a comparison of techniques. *J Urol* 1992;148:694–696.
30. Koontz AR. Atrophy of the testicle as a surgical risk. *Surg Gynecol Obstet* 1965;120:511–513.
31. Kormano M, Reijonen K. Microvascular structure of the human epididymis. *Am J Anat* 1976;145:23–27.
32. Kurz KR, Goldstein M. Scrotal temperature reflects intratesticular temperature and is lowered by shaving. *J Urol* 1986;135:290–292.
33. Langford GA, Silver A. Proceedings: Histochemical localization of acetylcholinesterase-containing nerve fibres in the testis. *J Physiol* 1974; 242: 9P–10P.
34. Lee LM, Johnson HW, McLoughlin MG. Microdissection and radiographic studies of the arterial vasculature of the human testes. *J Pediatr Surg* 1984;19:297–301.
35. Lee RK, Li PS, Goldstein M. Simultaneous vasectomy and varicocelectomy: indications and technique. *Urology* 2007;70:362–365.
36. Levine LA, Matkov TG. Microsurgical denervation of the spermatic cord as primary surgical treatment of chronic orchialgia. *J Urol* 2001;165: 1927–1929.
37. Lui WY, Mruk D, Lee WM, et al. Sertoli cell tight junction dynamics: their regulation during spermatogenesis. *Biol Reprod* 2003;68:1087–1097.
38. Matsuda T, Horii Y, Yoshida O. Should the testicular artery be preserved at varicocelectomy? *J Urol* 1993;149:1357–1360.
39. Middleton WD, Thorne DA, Melson GL. Color Doppler ultrasound of the normal testis. *AJR Am J Roentgenol* 1989;152:293–297.
40. Moller R. Arrangement and fine structure of lymphatic vessels in the human spermatic cord. *Andrologia* 1980;12:564–576.
41. Mostafa T, Labib I, El-Khayat Y, et al. Human testicular arterial supply: gross anatomy, corrosion cast, and radiologic study. *Fertil Steril* 2008; 90(6):2226–2230.
42. Murray RR Jr, Mitchell SE, Kadir S, et al. Comparison of recurrent varicocele anatomy following surgery and percutaneous balloon occlusion. *J Urol* 1986;135:286–289.
43. Nef S, Parada LF. Cryptorchidism in mice mutant for Insl3. *Nat Genet* 1999;22:295–299.
44. Penn I, Mackie G, Halgrimson CG, et al. Testicular complications following renal transplantation. *Ann Surg* 1972;176:697–699.
45. Prader A. Testicular size: assessment and clinical importance. *Triangle* 1966;7:240–243.
46. Print CG, Loveland KL. Germ cell suicide: new insights into apoptosis during spermatogenesis. *Bioessays* 2000;22:423–430.
47. Raman JD, Goldstein M. Intraoperative characterization of arterial vasculature in spermatic cord. *Urology* 2004;64:561–564.
48. Ramasamy R, Schlegel PN. Microsurgical inguinal varicocelectomy with and without testicular delivery. *Urology* 2006;68:1323–1326.
49. Rikimaru A, Shirai M. Responses of the human testicular capsule to electrical stimulation and to autonomic drugs. *Tohoku J Exp Med* 1972;108: 303–304.
50. Saez JM, Perrard-Sapori MH, Chatelain PG, et al. Paracrine regulation of testicular function. *J Steroid Biochem* 1987;27:317–329.
51. Schlegel PN. Microsurgical techniques of epididymal and testicular sperm retrieval. In: Goldstein M, ed. *Atlas of the Urologic Clinics of North America: Surgery for male infertility*, Vol. 7. Philadelphia: WB Saunders, 1999:109–129.
52. Schlegel PN. Surgical anatomy and diagnostic procedures. In: Goldstein M, ed. *Surgery of male infertility*, 1st ed. Philadelphia: WB Saunders, 1995: 3–7.
53. Schlegel PN, Hardy MP, Goldstein M. Male reproductive physiology. In: Wein AJ, Kavoussi LR, Novick AC, et al., eds. *Campbell-Walsh urology*, Vol. 1. Philadelphia: Saunders Elsevier, 2006.
54. Setchell BP. *Testicular blood supply, lymphatic drainage, and secretion of fluid*, Vol. 1: *Development, anatomy, and physiology*. New York: Academic Press, 1970.
55. Setchell BP, Maddocks S, Brooks DE. *Anatomy, vasculature, innervation, and fluids of the male reproductive tract*, 2nd ed., Vol. 1. New York: Raven Press, 1994.
56. Sharpe RM. *Regulation of spermatogenesis*, 2nd ed., Vol. 1. New York: Raven Press, 1994.
57. Silber SJ. Microsurgical aspects of varicocele. *Fertil Steril* 1979;31:230–232.
58. Sinclair AH. New genes for boys. *Am J Hum Genet* 1995;57:998–1001.
59. Student V, Zatura F, Scheinar J, et al. Testicle hemodynamics in patients after laparoscopic varicocelectomy evaluated using color Doppler sonography. *Eur Urol* 1998;33:91–93.
60. Tishler PV. Diameter of testicles. *N Engl J Med* 1971;285:1489.
61. van der Schoot P. The name cranial ovarian suspensory ligaments in mammalian anatomy should be used only to indicate the structures derived from the foetal cranial mesonephric and gonadal ligaments. *Anat Rec* 1993;237:434–438.
62. Verghese ST, Hannallah RS, Rice LJ, et al. Caudal anesthesia in children: effect of volume versus concentration of bupivacaine on blocking spermatic cord traction response during orchidopexy. *Anesth Analg* 2002;95: 1219–1223, table of contents.
63. Waites GM, Gladwell RT. Physiological significance of fluid secretion in the testis and blood-testis barrier. *Physiol Rev* 1982;62:624–671.
64. Waites GMH. *Temperature regulation and the testis*, Vol. 1: *Development, anatomy, and physiology*. New York: Academic Press, 1970.
65. Warne GL. Advances and challenges with intersex disorders. *Reprod Fertil Dev* 1998;10:79–85.
66. Wensing CJ, Colenbrander B. Normal and abnormal testicular descent. *Oxf Rev Reprod Biol* 1986;8:130–164.
67. Wing TY, Christensen AK. Morphometric studies on rat seminiferous tubules. *Am J Anat* 1982;165:13–25.
68. Yong EX, Huynh J, Farmer P, et al. Calcitonin gene-related peptide stimulates mitosis in the tip of the rat gubernaculum in vitro and provides the chemotactic signals to control gubernacular migration during testicular descent. *J Pediatr Surg* 2008;43:1533–1539.
69. Zirkin BR, Chen H, Luo L. Leydig cell steroidogenesis in aging rats. *Exp Gerontol* 1997;32:529–537.

# CHAPTER 63 ■ SIMPLE ORCHIECTOMY

BRETT S. CARVER AND SHERRI M. DONAT

Simple orchiectomy involves the removal of one or both testes at the distal spermatic cord, usually through an anterior transscrotal approach, although it has also been described through a suprapubic approach (9). It is used in the treatment of benign intrascrotal processes and as a method of androgen ablative therapy in patients with advanced prostate cancer.

Among men in the United States, prostate cancer is the most commonly diagnosed malignancy, with 186,320 new cases projected to be diagnosed in 2008 and approximately 28,660 deaths attributed to it (1). Since Huggins and Hodges (7) first demonstrated the therapeutic benefit of hormonal ablation in the treatment of advanced prostate cancer, bilateral scrotal orchiectomy has been commonly utilized as a means of removing the testosterone-producing tissue, thereby bringing serum levels to castrate levels. Although it has been by tradition used only for treatment in patients with advanced or metastatic disease, it is currently being evaluated for patients with presumed localized disease in both neoadjuvant and adjuvant settings to determine if it has any benefit in decreasing the chance of local or systemic recurrence and improving survival when used in combination with the traditional monotherapies of surgery or radiation (4).

## DIAGNOSIS

The initial diagnosis of prostate cancer is usually made through a combination of digital rectal exam, prostate-specific antigen level, patient symptoms, and transrectal ultrasound-directed biopsy, although it is on occasion found incidentally on transurethral resection for obstructive benign disease. Advanced disease may involve lymph nodes, bone, or, less commonly, visceral or soft tissue lesions and may be documented by physical examination, elevated prostatic acid phosphatase levels, abnormal bone scan, computerized tomography scan, magnetic resonance imaging, plain film bone survey, or chest X-ray. Lymph node involvement may be determined by biopsy of enlarged nodes seen on imaging studies or unexpectedly during the pelvic lymph node dissection for a radical prostatectomy.

Benign intrascrotal processes such as epididymal orchitis or devitalization of testicular tissue by trauma or torsion are diagnosed by physical examination, patient symptoms, nuclear testicular examinations, color Doppler ultrasonic examinations, and/or surgical exploration. In general, inflammatory processes show increased flow on both nuclear scans and Doppler flow studies and processes causing devascularization show decreased or no flow on nuclear and Doppler flow studies. However, if there is any question as to whether an acute scrotum represents a testicular torsion versus an epididymal orchitis, it should be surgically explored immediately to answer the question and render the appropriate treatment.

## INDICATIONS FOR SURGERY

The primary indication for bilateral scrotal orchiectomy is advanced prostate cancer requiring hormonal ablation as treatment. Other indications for simple orchiectomy include benign intrascrotal disorders such as a traumatic injury to the testis requiring partial or complete removal of the devitalized tissue, testicular necrosis following prolonged torsion, and severe epididymal orchitis that is refractory to antimicrobial therapy.

Malignant diseases of the testes, such as suspected germ cell tumor, should never be managed with a simple orchiectomy through a transcrotal approach. Suboptimal approaches to testicular neoplasms, including scrotal orchiectomy and transscrotal biopsy, can alter the normal lymphatic drainage of the testis and increase the burden of therapy for the patient (3). A meta-analysis of 206 cases of scrotal violation reported a local recurrence rate of 2.9%, compared to 0.4% for patients treated with inguinal orchiectomy, but no difference in systemic relapse or survival were appreciated (3). Therefore, if there is any suspicion of testicular cancer, a radical orchiectomy through an inguinal incision should be performed.

## ALTERNATIVE THERAPY

There are now several agonist analogues of gonadotropin-releasing hormone that inhibit the pituitary gonadal axis, resulting in the downregulation of luteinizing hormone–releasing hormone receptors and subsequent decrease in gonadotropin secretion. These are equally effective in achieving hormonal ablation and provide an alternative to orchiectomy in patients for whom the psychological implications of the surgery are too great (4); however, the cost effectiveness of surgery is certainly superior to that of chemical castration. While the use of bilateral orchiectomy for the management of metastatic prostate cancer has declined with the implementation of gonadotropin-relasing hormone agonists or antagonists, a recent study demonstrated that, with changes in Medicare reimbursement, the rates of surgical castration have increased over recent years (14).

Alternatives to the total removal of the testis and epididymis have been explored and include subcapsular orchiectomy and subepididymal orchiectomy (2,6,8,12). These give the cosmetic effect of a testis being present but also achieve the therapeutic goal of androgen ablation. There has been some controversy (10) over the efficacy of subcapsular orchiectomy since it was first described in 1942 by Riba (12); however, multiple modern studies have demonstrated its efficacy and suggest that any residual testosterone production is most likely a result of incomplete removal of the intratesticular contents (2). Testicular prostheses are also available for use in patients who desire a better cosmetic result, and these may be placed in either the tunica vaginalis or within the tunica albuginea (13). Kihara and Oshima (8) have also described an epididymal-sparing orchiectomy with insertion of a pedicled fibrofatty tissue graft to preserve scrotal cosmesis after bilateral orchiectomy. This type of procedure may be complicated by epididymitis, which can be minimized by performing a vasectomy at the time of the procedure (6). Advantages of a fibrofatty tissue graft over implants or prostheses are that there are no risks of developing autoimmune disorders and rupture or migration complications.

## SURGICAL TECHNIQUE

### Simple Orchiectomy

This procedure may be performed with local, regional, or general anesthesia. Local anesthetic sensory blockade is obtained by infiltrating the spermatic cord in the region of the vas deferens in the high scrotum just below the pubic tubercle with a 0.5% bupivacaine solution. Care must be taken to ensure that the block is not injected intravascularly by drawing back on the syringe prior to injecting the medication. The same solution is then injected subcutaneously at the site of the anterior scrotal incision. Sensory blockade should then be tested by pinprick before the beginning of the procedure.

### Scrotal Approach

The anterior scrotal wall is shaved to remove existing hair, and the scrotum and genitalia are prepared in a sterile manner. A 2.5- to 3.0-cm midline incision is made just through the skin along the median raphe in the anterior scrotal wall using a no. 15 blade scalpel while the assistant pushes a testicle toward the incision between his or her thumb and index finger so that the testicle lies directly under the incision (Fig. 63.1). By electrocautery, the incision is then carried down through

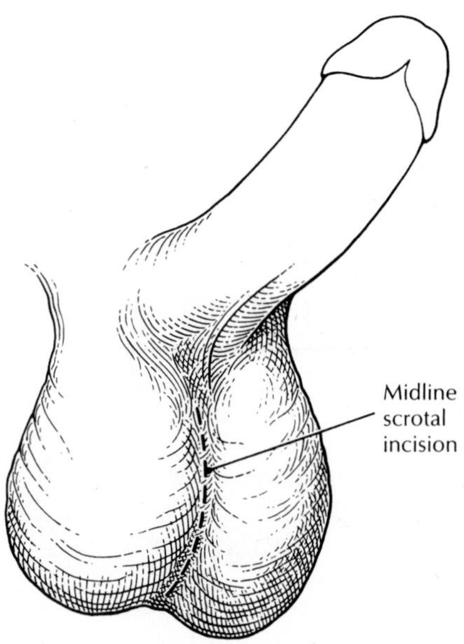


FIGURE 63.1 A midline scrotal incision over the median raphe allows access to both testes.

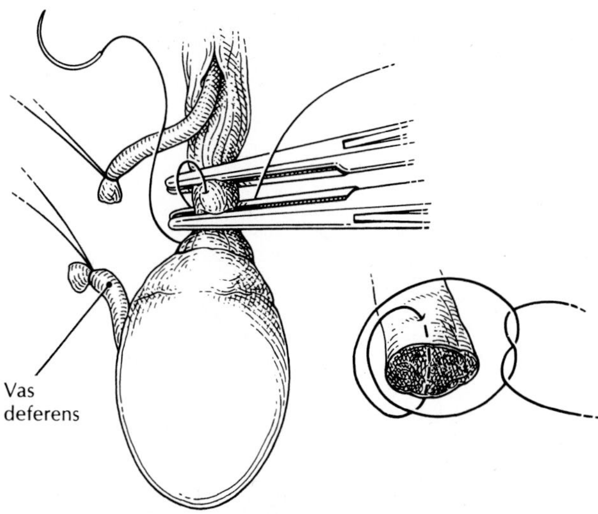


FIGURE 63.2 The vas deferens is ligated separately from the vascular structures of the cord. The vascular structures are double ligated with both a free tie proximally and a suture ligature distally using 0 Vicryl.

the dartos and cremasteric layers until the parietal portion of the tunica vaginalis is incised directly over the testis. This is usually evidence by a gush of fluid from the peritesticular space. The incision in the tunica vaginalis is lengthened in both directions far enough to allow exposure of the entire testicle through the wound. The surrounding tunics are freed from the spermatic cord by a combination of blunt and sharp dissection. Meticulous hemostasis may be obtained in each layer as it is entered with electrocautery. Once the spermatic cord is isolated, the vas deferens is separated, doubly clamped, divided, and ligated with 2-0 Vicryl ties (Fig. 63.2). The remainder of the cord structures may be divided into one or more bundles and are doubly clamped on the proximal side and singly clamped on the distal side. Once divided, the proximal portion of the cord is ligated with a 0 Vicryl free tie behind the most proximal clamp, which is then removed, and a 0 Vicryl suture ligature is placed just distal to the free tie (Fig. 63.2). Before the cord is released to retract proximally, the tunics, dartos, and subcutaneous areas are again inspected for hemostasis. Once this is felt to be adequate, the cord is allowed to retract and attention is turned to the opposite testicle. It is then removed through the same midline incision in the same manner. This leaves two openings in the tunica vaginalis and dartos layers, which are separated by a median septum. These deep layers are then closed in one layer using a 3-0 Vicryl running suture. Allis clamps are placed at either end of the median septum to facilitate the exposure (Fig. 63.3). The skin is then closed with interrupted 3-0 chromic sutures and a gauze dressing is applied. Drains are not required but can be considered if there is doubt about hemostasis. Compression or turban dressings may also be used if there is concern over postoperative hemostasis or edema.

### Suprapubic Approach

This approach is advantageous in patients in whom one wants to avoid a scrotal incision and/or place testicular prostheses at the time of the orchiectomy. The patient again is placed in the supine position and the suprapubic area is shaved. A

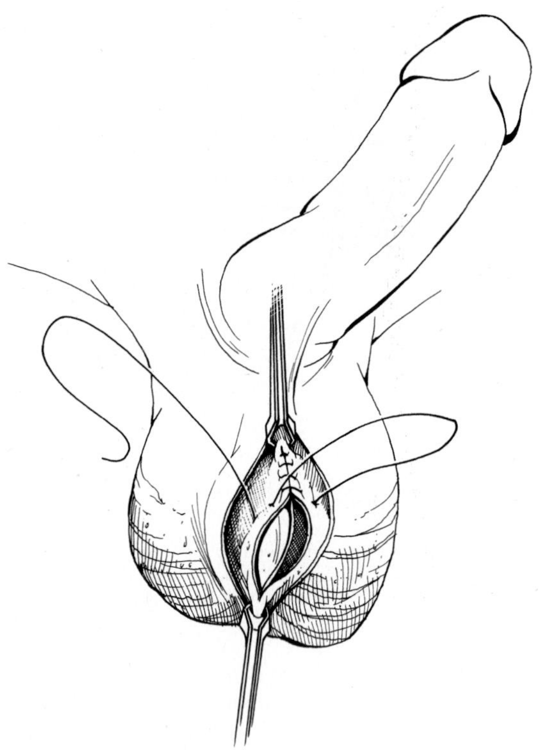

FIGURE 63.3 Closure of the deep layers of the scrotum, including the dartos musculature and testicular tunics laterally and the midline septum in one running layer.

4- to 5-cm transverse incision is made in the midline approximately 2 to 3 cm above the pubic symphysis (Fig. 63.4). This is extended down through the subcutaneous tissues to the level of the rectus fascia using electrocautery. The subcutaneous tissue is then swept bluntly toward the external inguinal ring, exposing the distal spermatic cord, which is then isolated just distal to the ring in the upper scrotum (Fig. 63.5). Right-angle retractors are helpful to obtain exposure during this dissection by moving the incision toward the side being worked on. The spermatic cord is looped with a Penrose drain and the testicle is delivered into the wound by placing upward pressure on the scrotum and testicle, with simultaneous upward traction on the cord with the Penrose drain. The gubernaculum is then divided, which mobilizes the testicle (Fig. 63.5). The vas deferens and spermatic cord are then divided as previously described. If testicular prostheses are desired, they are then placed into the empty scrotum after adequate hemostasis is ensured, and a pursestring suture of 3-0 silk is used to close the neck of each hemiscrotum (Fig. 63.6). The Scarpa fascia is closed with 3-0 Vicryl suture, and the skin is closed with a 4-0 Vicryl subcuticular suture reinforced with benzoin and Steri-Strips.

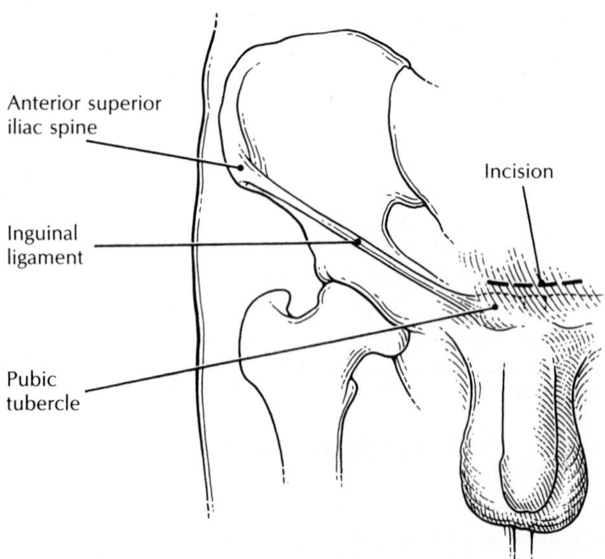


FIGURE 63.4 A midline suprapubic incision 2 to 3 cm above the pubis allows access to both testes at a level just below the external ring.

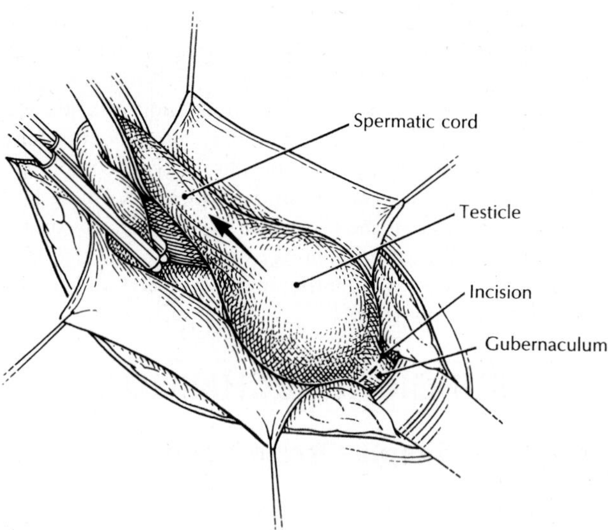


FIGURE 63.5 Isolation of the cord with a Penrose drain. Division of the gubernaculum allows complete mobilization of the testis from the scrotum.

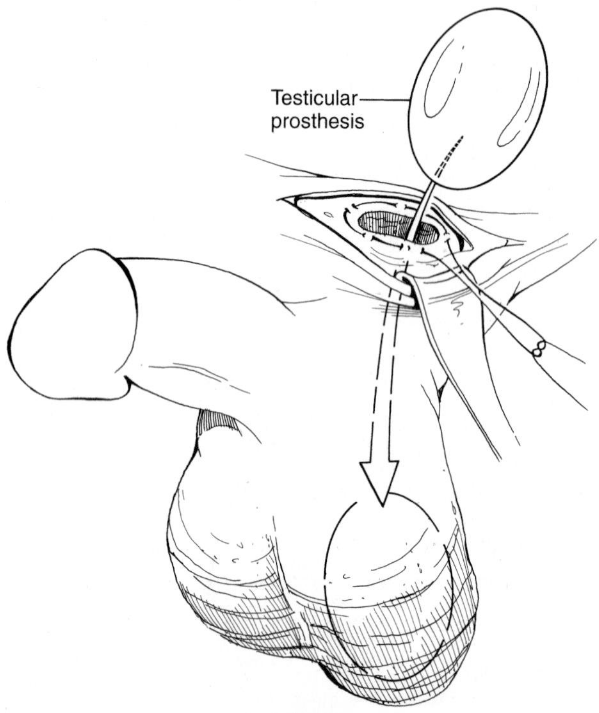


FIGURE 63.6 If a prosthesis is desired, it is placed into the empty hemiscrotum. To prevent migration, a pursestring suture is used to close the neck of the hemiscrotum, eliminating the need for an anchoring suture.

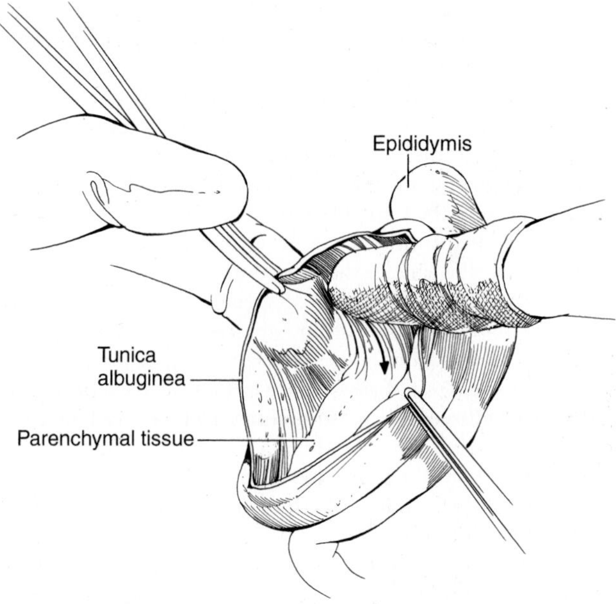


FIGURE 63.7 The tunica albuginea is opened in midline opposite the epididymis and the contents are swept bluntly to the midline attachment.

## Subcapsular Orchiectomy

This approach is used in patients who desire the cosmetic effect of testicles being present without the use of testicular prostheses. The operation is approached through the anterior scrotum as previously described (Fig. 63.1). Once the testicle is delivered to the wound, the tunica albuginea is opened in midline in a cephalad-to-caudad fashion. Hemostats are placed on the edges of the capsule to provide traction, and an index finger is placed behind the capsule to invert it (Fig. 63.7). This maneuver facilitates the removal of the parenchymal contents, which are swept to the midline using a gauze sponge. The midline attachment of the parenchyma is divided using electrocautery, and the remainder of the interior capsule is cauterized to ensure hemostasis and complete destruction of all testicular parenchyma (Fig. 63.8). This technique has also been described using a $CO_2$ laser (15). The tunica albuginea is then closed using a running 3-0 Vicryl suture (Fig. 63.9) and the residual testicular tunics, adnexa, and cord are returned to the scrotum. The deep layers of the scrotum are closed in one layer as previously described, as is the skin (Fig. 63.3).

## Subepididymal Orchiectomy

This is another procedure offered as an alternative to simple scrotal orchiectomy for a more acceptable cosmetic result. Again, the initial exposure to the testicles is the same as previously described for the anterior scrotal approach (Fig. 63.1). Once the testicle is delivered to the wound, a vasectomy is performed including double ligation and division to minimize the possibility of postoperative epididymitis (6). A line of dissection between the cleavage plane of the testis and the epididymis is utilized (Fig. 63.10). Dissection is started at the head of the epididymis, and the epididymal tissue is clamped for hemostasis. Care must be taken to secure the spermatic artery entering the testis at a point between the midportion and the tail of the epididymis. The clamped epididymal tissue is ligated using a

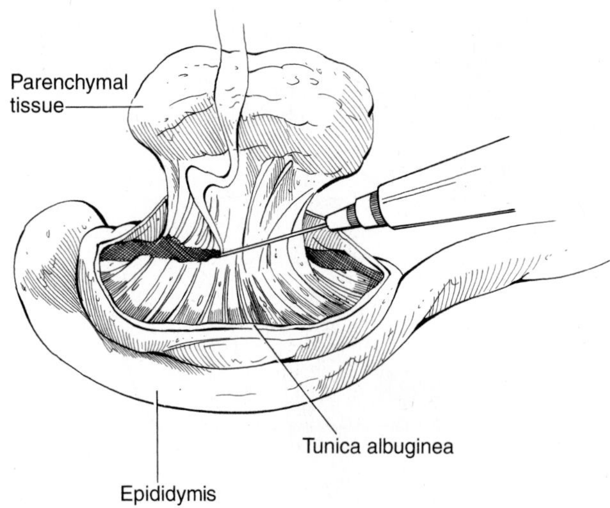


FIGURE 63.8 The parenchymal tissue is then removed at its midline attachment with electrocautery and the internal surface of the capsule is cauterized.

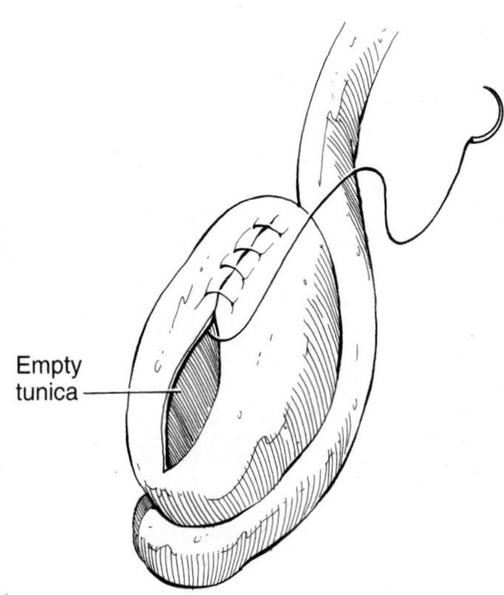


FIGURE 63.9 The tunica albuginea is reapproximated with a running 3-0 Vicryl suture.

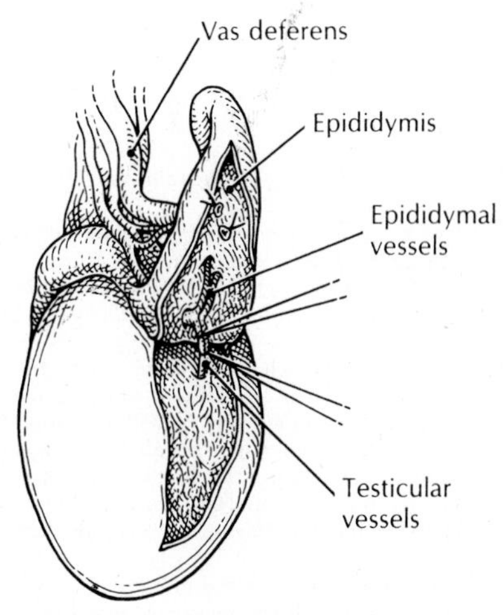


FIGURE 63.10 Dissection of the testis from the epididymis, ligating the epididymal side over clamps with Vicryl suture.

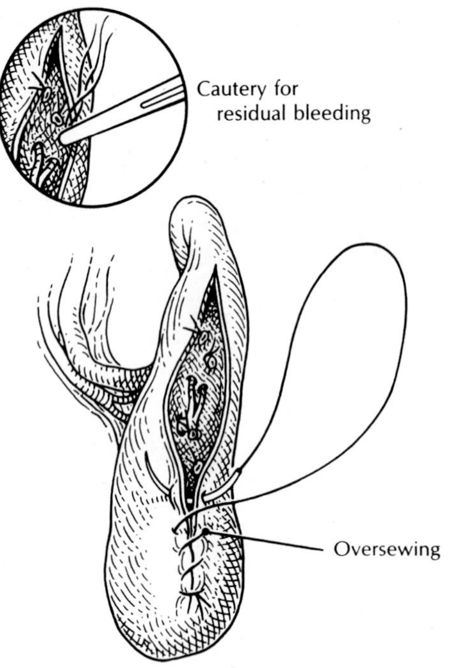


FIGURE 63.11 After removal of the testis and further hemostasis with electrocautery, the tunica of the epididymis is closed over the raw surface using a running suture.

3-0 Vicryl suture. Meticulous hemostasis is then obtained using electrocautery, and a running 3-0 Vicryl suture on a tapered needle is used to approximate the edges of the tunica albuginea over the raw surface of the epididymis (Fig. 63.11). The remaining spermatic cord and epididymis are replaced into the scrotum, which is closed as previously described.

# OUTCOMES

## Complications

Complications can include infection, hematoma, edema, and the inadvertent removal of a testicular neoplasm through the scrotal approach. Of these, hematoma can be a significant problem because of the distensible nature of the scrotum, which prevents any tamponade effect. Re-exploration with evacuation of the hematoma and placement of a drain may be required but can be ineffective when the bleeding dissects subcutaneously in the dartos layer. This has led to the development of several preventative measures to achieve adequate compression of the area postoperatively, including turban-type dressings or compression of the scrotal wall over a gauze bolster as described by Oesterling (11). These techniques should not be substituted for being meticulous in obtaining hemostasis at the time of the procedure.

Infection, depending on the degree of severity, is managed by incision and drainage of any abscess pockets. This is followed by local wound care, which may include wet-to-dry dressing changes, sitz baths, and whirlpool with debridement of any devitalized tissue. Antibiotics can be used in cases where there is induration only and no abscess to drain or in combination with the incision and drainage procedure if needed. If antibiotics are used, they should be directed by the results of wound cultures.

If a testicular neoplasm has been inadvertently removed through a scrotal approach, the remaining inguinal spermatic cord should be removed, as well as a wide excision of the scrotal scar. The hemiscrotum should also be removed if there was any known tumor spillage during the transscrotal procedure. This usually results in cure rates similar to those for conventional initial radical inguinal orchiectomy (5).

## Results

The effectiveness of scrotal orchiectomy in terms of achieving adequate hormonal ablation in patients with prostate cancer can be easily determined by measuring serum testosterone levels postcastration, which are reduced by approximately 90%. Castrate levels of testosterone have reportedly been achieved by 2 and 15 hours after surgery (2,4). Prostate-specific antigen levels, patient symptoms, and patient survival may be followed to determine the procedure's effectiveness in terms of disease control. Side-effects may include loss of libido, impotence, and hot flashes.

**For benign intrascrotal processes such as epididymal orchitis unresponsive to antibiotics, or devitalized tissues secondary to torsion or trauma, simple orchiectomy is curative.**

## *References*

1. Jemal A, Siegel R, Ward E, et al. Cancer statistics 2008. *CA Cancer J Clin* 2008;58(2):71–96. Epub 2008 Feb 20.
2. Arcadi JA. Rapid drop in serum testosterone after bilateral subcapsular orchiectomy. *J Surg Oncol* 1992;49:35.
3. Capelouto C, Clark P, Ransil B, et al. A review of scrotal violation in testicular cancer: is adjuvant local therapy necessary? *J Urol* 1995;153: 1397–1401.
4. Cassady JR, Hutter JJ, Whitesell LJ. Prostate cancer. In: Vogelzang NJ, Scardino PT, Shipley WU, et al., eds. *Comprehensive textbook of genitourinary oncology*. Baltimore: Williams & Wilkins, 1996:557–828.
5. Giguere JK, Stablein DM, Spaulding JT, et al. The clinical significance of unconventional orchiectomy approaches in testicular cancer. A report from the Testicular Cancer Intergroup Study. *J Urol* 1988;139:1225.
6. Glenn JF. Subepididymal orchidectomy: the acceptable alternative. *J Urol* 1990;144:942.
7. Huggins C, Hodges CV. Studies on prostatic cancer: the effect of castration, of estrogen, and of androgen injection on serum phosphatases in metastatic carcinoma of the prostate. *Cancer Res* 1941;1:293.
8. Kihara K, Oshima H. Cosmetic orchiectomy using pedicled fibrofatty tissue graft for prostate cancer: a new approach. *Eur Urol* 1998;34:210.
9. Klein EA, Herr HW. Suprapubic approach for bilateral orchiectomy and placement of testicular prosthesis. *J Urol* 1990;143:765.
10. O'Conor VJ, Chaing SP, Grayhack JT. Is subcapsular orchiectomy a definitive procedure? *J Urol* 1963;89:236.
11. Oesterling JE. Scrotal surgery: a reliable method for the prevention of postoperative hematoma and edema. *J Urol* 1990;143:1201.
12. Riba LW. Subcapsular castration for carcinoma of the prostate. *J Urol* 1942;48:384.
13. Solomon AA. Testicular prosthesis: a new insertion operation. *J Urol* 1972; 108:436.
14. Weight CJ, Klein EA, Jones JS. Androgen deprivation falls as orchiectomy rates rise after changes in reimbursement in the US Medicare population. *Cancer* 2008;112:2195.
15. Wishnow KI, Johnson DE. Subcapsular orchiectomy using the $CO_2$ laser: a new technique. *Lasers Surg Med* 1988;8:604.

# CHAPTER 64 ■ INGUINAL ORCHIECTOMY

DAVID A. SWANSON

Testicular tumors are relatively rare (only 2 to 3 cases per 100,000 men; an estimated 8,090 new cases in the United States in 2008) (8). When they occur, 94% are germ cell tumors and the rest are tumors of the gonadal stroma and secondary tumors of the testis. In black men throughout the world, germ cell tumors occur infrequently, but because they do occur, this diagnosis cannot be excluded on the basis of race alone. Although the etiology of testicular tumors is not known, there is a relatively high association (reported in up to 12% of tumors) with a history of cryptorchidism; in 20% of such cases, the tumor is in the normally descended testis. Orchidopexy does not prevent the subsequent development of tumor; it simply makes the diagnosis easier to establish. Carcinoma in situ (CIS) is also known to be associated with cryptorchidism, and data support the hypothesis that at least some, if not all, germ cell tumors originate as CIS (7).

## DIAGNOSIS

Most testicular tumors present as a palpable nodule or painless swelling of the testis, often discovered incidentally by the patient or his sex partner. The differential diagnosis of a testicular mass includes tumor, epididymitis, and epididymoorchitis (the two most common diagnoses other than cancer), torsion (the diagnosis of which also requires surgery), and, less commonly, hernia, hydrocele, spermatocele, varicocele, hematoma, and hematocele. The patient with cancer may complain of a dull ache or sense of heaviness. Acute onset of pain is relatively rare and usually indicates bleeding within the tumor or associated epididymitis. Signs and symptoms may be secondary to metastatic spread.

When careful bimanual examination of the testis reveals an intratesticular mass, with or without an associated epididymal mass or tenderness, testicular tumor must be suspected. A transscrotal ultrasound is a widely available, rapid, sensitive, noninvasive, and inexpensive way to determine whether there is a solid mass within the tunica albuginea (12). Color Doppler ultrasound might on occasion help differentiate testicular torsion. Magnetic resonance imaging can also demonstrate the presence of an intratesticular mass but has no established advantage over a careful physical examination plus ultrasound exam. With rare exceptions, all solid masses within the testis should be considered malignant until proven otherwise, and all require surgical intervention.

Patients with testicular tumors commonly have elevated tumor markers, in particular β-human chorionic gonadotropin and α-fetoprotein. However, the presence of normal marker levels does not exclude malignancy, and there is in general no advantage to waiting for the marker results before operating, although blood should always be drawn for these tests before orchiectomy (12).

## INDICATIONS FOR SURGERY

The presence of an intrascrotal mass that cannot be clearly localized to outside the tunica albuginea is sufficient indication for surgical exploration through an inguinal approach. Although a sense of urgency is appropriate, it is not necessary to consider inguinal orchiectomy an emergency procedure; it can be scheduled during regular operating hours.

## ALTERNATIVE THERAPY

For the patient who has equivocal findings on physical examination and ultrasound that make the diagnosis of epididymitis tenable, a short course of antibiotics may be tried. If there is no prompt improvement (<10 to 14 days), or if the serum tumor markers are elevated, inguinal exploration should be performed. Although radical (inguinal) orchiectomy is standard therapy for a solid lesion within the tunica albuginea, partial orchiectomy might be appropriate in the patient with a solitary testis or bilateral testicular masses or in the patient whose preoperative evaluation makes the diagnosis of an epidermoid cyst of the testis highly likely (3,5,6,11). The selection criteria, technique, and results of organ-sparing surgery of the testis are presented in Chapter 65.

## SURGICAL TECHNIQUE

Although regional anesthesia is acceptable, general anesthesia is preferred because of the short duration of the surgery and the possible reflex response to traction on the testicle and cord. With the patient in the supine position, and after adequate anesthesia, the lower abdominal wall, penis, and scrotum are cleaned with a surgical scrub and draped in a sterile fashion so that the palpable testicular mass and ipsilateral hemiscrotum are accessible in the surgical field. By tradition, an oblique skin incision is made approximately 2 cm superior to the inguinal ligament and parallel to that ligament, extending approximately 8–10 cm laterally from just above the pubic tubercle to a point overlying the external inguinal ring. I prefer a more horizontal incision, extending approximately 5 to 8 cm from one fingerbreadth above the superior aspect of the external inguinal ring laterally toward the internal inguinal ring, which might be slightly more cosmetic (Fig. 64.1).

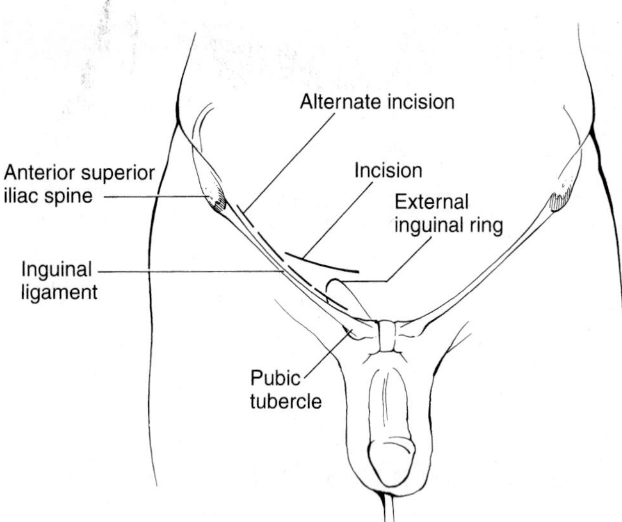


FIGURE 64.1 An almost horizontal incision from just cephalad to the external inguinal ring laterally almost to the internal ring provides adequate exposure and an excellent cosmetic result. Alternatively, the incision may be made parallel to the inguinal ligament.

The incision with the knife or electrocautery should be deepened through the subcutaneous tissue until the external oblique aponeurosis is reached. There are usually one or two significant veins that traverse this incision. They should be isolated and secured with hemoclips or 3-0 plain or chromic catgut sutures before being cut. When the external oblique aponeurosis is cleaned sufficiently to be well visualized, it is helpful to place one or two small self-retaining Gelpi (or similar) retractors in the wound to improve exposure. Next, the scalpel is used to make a small incision in the external oblique aponeurosis midway between the internal and external inguinal rings, in the direction of its fibers. Metzenbaum scissors are inserted through this opening, and the closed scissors are pushed with slight upward pressure underneath the aponeurosis to the external inguinal ring and then laterally toward the internal ring (Fig. 64.2A). This helps ensure that the ilioinguinal nerve will not be cut during the next step, which is to push the partially opened Metzenbaum scissors from the point of incision into the external inguinal ring and then laterally toward the internal ring as required, thus splitting the aponeurosis and opening the roof of the inguinal canal (Fig. 64.2B). Careful inspection will usually reveal the ilioinguinal nerve, which should be freed up carefully by blunt and sharp dissection for the length of the incision. It can then be retracted out of the surgical field by passing two small hemostats underneath the nerve, grasping the superior edge of the aponeurosis, and retracting it in a cephalad direction. It may also help to grasp the inferior edge of the aponeurosis and retract it as well to fully expose the inguinal canal.

This will expose the spermatic cord, although it may not appear distinct because of the cremasteric muscle fibers surrounding the cord, which merge into the internal oblique muscle. Using a gauze sponge wrapped around the fingertip (Fig. 64.3A) or a peanut (Kittner) sponge (Fig. 64.3B), the plane between the spermatic cord and the floor of the inguinal canal is bluntly developed until it can be encircled with a thumb and forefinger. It is usually easiest to both initiate the dissection and completely encircle the cord at the level of the pubic tubercle. Once it is ascertained that all components of the cord are included, the operator should pass a 0.5-in. Penrose drain around the cord (Fig. 64.3C), elevate it with gentle traction, and free up the cord laterally to the internal

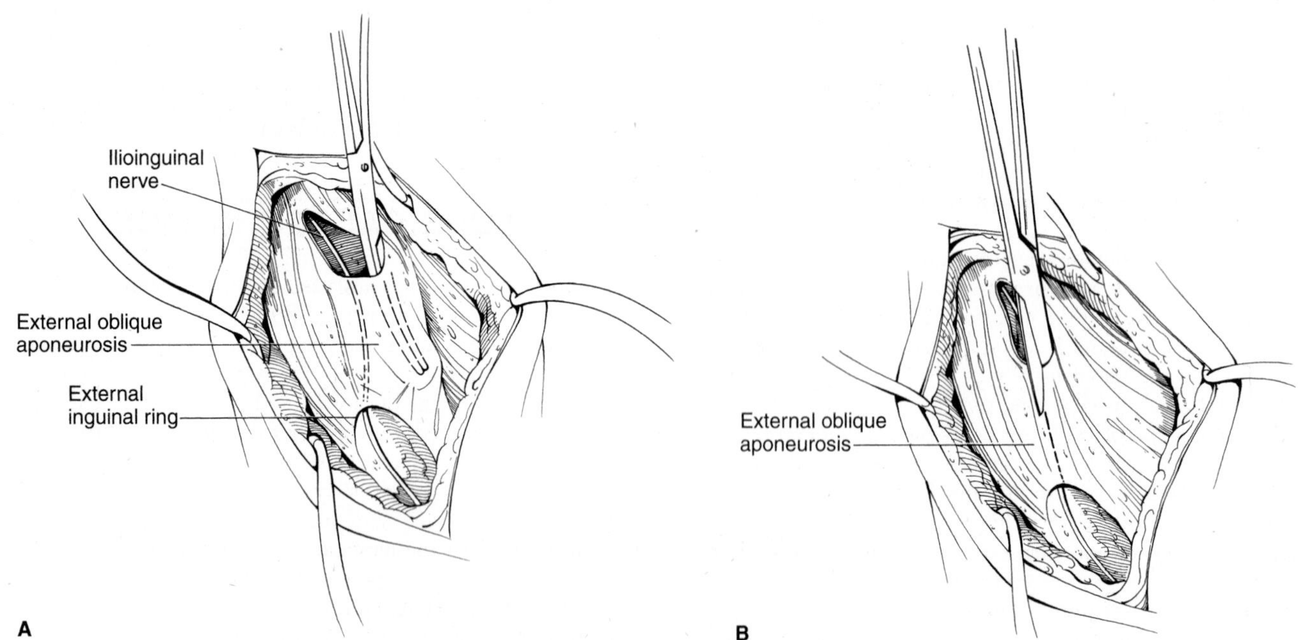


FIGURE 64.2 **A:** The external oblique fascia is entered and tented up over the length of the inguinal canal before cutting to help ensure that the ilioinguinal nerve is not injured. **B:** The external oblique fascia is incised over the spermatic cord, and the incision is extended into the external ring.

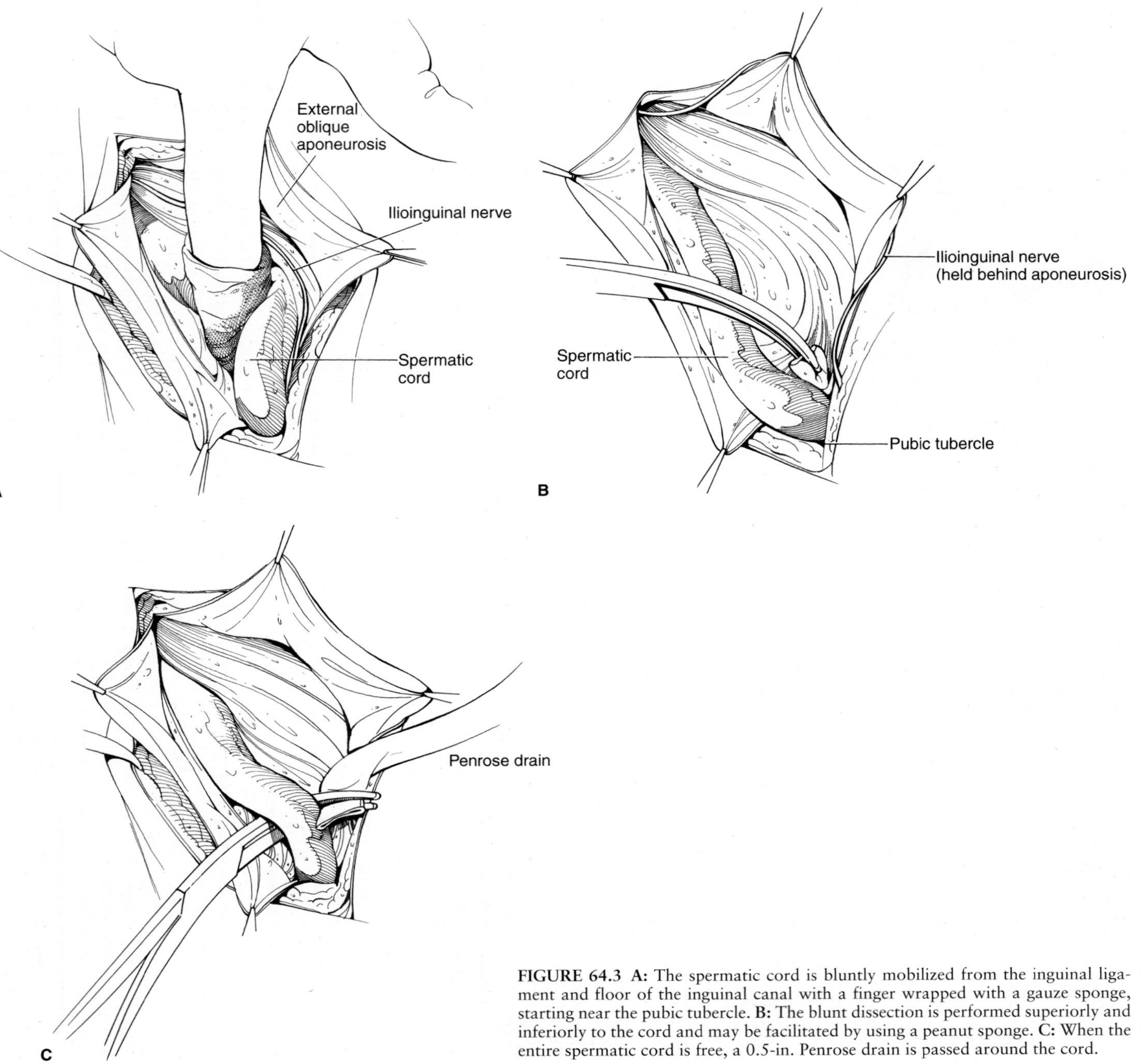


FIGURE 64.3 **A:** The spermatic cord is bluntly mobilized from the inguinal ligament and floor of the inguinal canal with a finger wrapped with a gauze sponge, starting near the pubic tubercle. **B:** The blunt dissection is performed superiorly and inferiorly to the cord and may be facilitated by using a peanut sponge. **C:** When the entire spermatic cord is free, a 0.5-in. Penrose drain is passed around the cord.

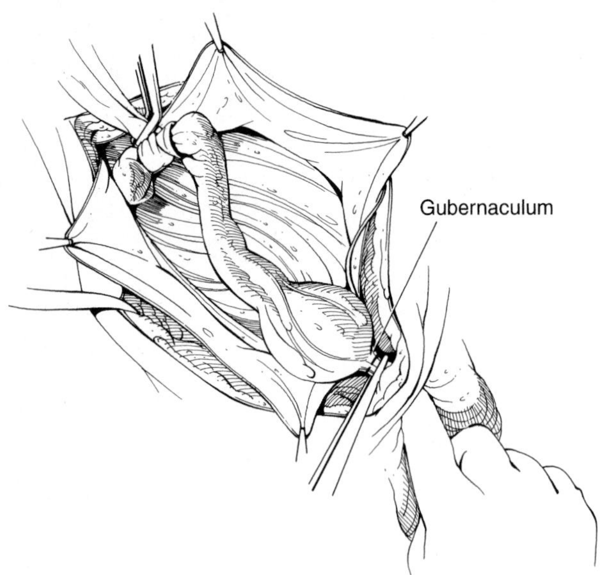


FIGURE 64.4 The Penrose drain is encircled twice around the cord just distal to the internal ring and clamped to act as a tourniquet. A finger outside the scrotum helps push the testis into the surgical field. The gubernaculum is clamped and cut, and the scrotal side of the gubernaculum is tied.

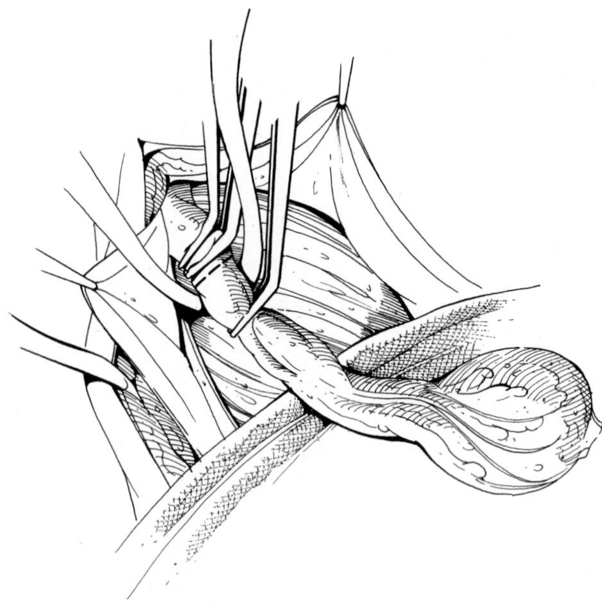

FIGURE 64.5 The spermatic cord is triple-clamped just distal to the internal ring (two clamps proximal and one distal to the Penrose tourniquet) and cut after careful inspection of the testis, which has been isolated from the surgical field on a sterile towel.

ring using predominantly blunt dissection, although some sharp dissection may be required. Care should be taken in approaching the internal ring that the inferior epigastric vessels are not injured, and the spermatic cord should be inspected carefully to ensure that an indirect inguinal hernia, which could contain bowel or bladder, is not present. At this point, the spermatic cord should be occluded firmly with either a soft rubber-shod clamp or, as I prefer, a 0.5-in. Penrose drain encircled twice around the cord, tightened in a tourniquet fashion, and secured with a Kelly or right-angle clamp (Fig. 64.4). The operator should be sure to leave enough spermatic cord distal to the internal ring to permit it to be double-clamped later without first removing the tourniquet.

It is now possible to mobilize the testis from the scrotum and through the opened external inguinal ring into the inguinal canal and surgical field. Upward pressure on the external skin of the hemiscrotum and testis, coupled with gentle traction on the spermatic cord, will in general define the circumferential fibromuscular attachments that need to be cut or, better, electrocoagulated to completely free up the testis (Fig. 64.4). Great care should be taken not to rupture the mass and spill tumor contents. At the most inferior aspect of the testis, there may be a well-defined gubernaculum that needs to be clamped and cut, being careful to exclude scrotal skin, and tied with 2-0 or 3-0 chromic catgut.

At this point, the surgeon should isolate the testis and spermatic cord, now free to the level of the internal ring, with sterile towels and carefully inspect the testis. If the diagnosis is still in doubt, the surgeon may open the tunica vaginalis and expose the tunica albuginea of the testis. If doubt still persists, which should happen only rarely, a small incision may be made in the tunica albuginea to permit insertion of a finger for palpation of the testicular parenchyma. If all of these maneuvers fail to exclude tumor, the surgeon should proceed with radical orchiectomy rather than risk returning a testis with tumor to the scrotum. I want to emphasize that it is only rarely necessary to open even the tunica vaginalis and far more rare to open the tunica albuginea or perform a biopsy.

To complete the orchiectomy, the spermatic cord should be double-clamped at the level of the internal ring and proximal to the Penrose tourniquet with two Kelly or heavy right-angle clamps; a third clamp is added to occlude the cord just distal to the Penrose tourniquet (Fig. 64.5). The surgeon then transects the cord and removes the testicle, with attached spermatic cord, from the surgical field. The cord is tied behind the most proximal clamp with a 0 silk tie, and a suture ligature of 0 silk is placed behind the most distal clamp. One of the two sutures should be left long for later identification of the stump of the cord if a retroperitoneal lymph node dissection is performed. Some surgeons prefer to tie the cord in two portions, separating the spermatic vessels and the vas deferens, and double-tying both portions of the cord. In either case, after the cord is securely tied, it should be allowed to retract through the internal ring into the retroperitoneum.

Next, the surgeon should carefully inspect the entire floor of the inguinal canal as well as the scrotal compartment by everting the scrotal wall into the surgical field with upward external pressure on the most dependent portion of the hemiscrotum. All sites of bleeding, even tiny ones, should be controlled with electrocautery and then irrigated with sterile water. It is prudent to perform a final inspection for complete hemostasis at this point before closure. Closure begins with careful inspection of the inguinal floor. If it seems weak, it can be reinforced with several interrupted sutures in a standard hernia repair. If not, the ilioinguinal nerve should be released and the external oblique aponeurosis closed with interrupted 2-0 silk or 2-0 Prolene sutures, placing the sutures at varying

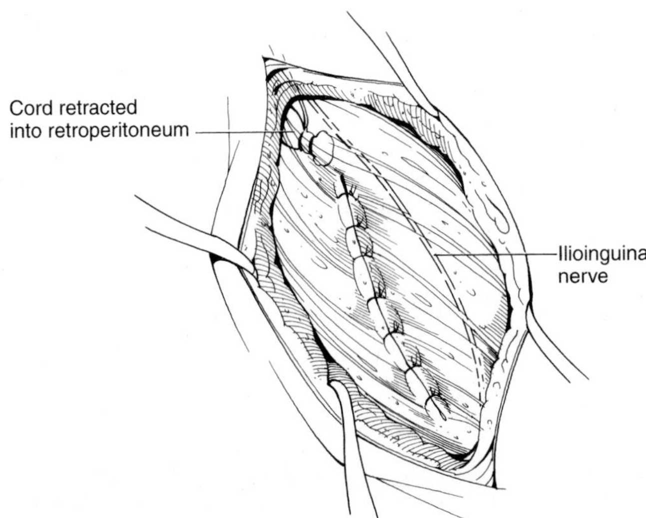


FIGURE 64.6 The stump of the cord retracts back through the internal ring into the retroperitoneum; one suture is left long. The external oblique fascia is closed with interrupted sutures placed at varying distances from the cut edge and completely closing the external ring.

distances from the aponeurotic edge to prevent a linear tear and taking care to exclude the ilioinguinal nerve (Fig. 64.6). The closure should begin at the level of the internal ring and extend medially as close to the pubic tubercle as possible because there is no longer any reason to have an external inguinal ring. A drain is not necessary or advisable. The wound should be irrigated once again and the skin incision closed with clips or with a running subcuticular suture of 4-0 Vicryl or Monocryl. The wound is covered with a dry sterile dressing and the scrotum is gently compressed with either fluffed gauze sponges held in place with an athletic supporter or by gently wrapping the scrotum with a loosely applied turban dressing of Kling, Kerlix, or Coban. An ice pack should be avoided because it has little impact on swelling and is a source of considerable discomfort.

Patients may resume a regular diet and ambulation when completely awake and may be discharged. Most patients require oral narcotic analgesics for pain control for several days.

# OUTCOMES

## Complications

Many would consider the most serious complication to be scrotal violation, which in the past required hemiscrotectomy and now requires irradiation to the scrotum (for seminoma). In truth, little data demonstrate reduced survival following scrotal contamination (9,10). Nonetheless, there is virtually no reason why the testis should be approached transscrotally if the diagnosis of possible testicular tumor has been even considered. At the least, a transscrotal approach prevents early control of venous outflow in the cord before manipulation of the tumor, leaves spermatic cord behind, potentially alters lymphatic drainage of the testis, risks tumor contamination of the scrotum (10), and may preclude consideration of surveillance as a treatment option, although this has been challenged (1).

The most common actual complication is probably an intrascrotal hematoma. Because the scrotum is such an expansile organ with loose areolar tissue beneath the dermis, bleeding may continue because of a lack of tamponade, and the resulting hematoma may grow quite large. These scrotal hematomas usually become organized and quite firm and may even raise the question of residual or recurrent tumor. Nonetheless, if the hematoma does not become infected (which would require surgical drainage), it can almost always be followed expectantly and will eventually regress. Ideally, this complication should be prevented. The depths of the inguinal canal and entire inner surface of the scrotal wall should be thoroughly and compulsively inspected and electrocoagulated to ensure hemostasis. The surgeon can facilitate this, as described earlier, by everting the scrotal wall with a finger positioned on the most dependent portion of the external scrotal wall. After hemostasis appears adequate, the surgeon should irrigate with sterile water and inspect again. Although the turban dressing used in bilateral orchiectomy, which completely collapses the scrotum, is not possible, it is possible to use a modified turban dressing that is wrapped firmly enough to collapse the hemiscrotum ipsilateral to the orchiectomy but not so tight as to cause pain because of pressure on the remaining testis.

It is also possible to get a retroperitoneal hematoma if the ligature(s) on the spermatic cord pull off or if there is an injury to one of the inferior epigastric vessels. Although rare, retroperitoneal hematoma and other potential complications have prompted one team of clinicians to advocate orchidectomy at the external ring (low cord) instead of at the internal ring (high cord) (2). Nonetheless, despite an absence of apparent increase in relapse rate with this alternate surgical approach, they present no data to show fewer complications and no proven advantage to a quicker operation or to leaving the inguinal flooor intact. In the absence of such data, this approach is not recommended (4). Retroperitoneal hematoma can be prevented virtually always by a properly tied ligature with adequate length of spermatic cord distal to it so it cannot slip off. A suture ligature on the spermatic cord offers an additional measure of security. Injury to the epigastric vessels can be avoided by careful dissection of the proximal spermatic cord at the level of the internal inguinal ring. This complication is usually discovered incidentally at the time of further staging evaluation with a computed tomography scan, although an unexplained and occult blood loss may prompt investigation. If bleeding has stopped when the problem is discovered, it does not require specific treatment; the hematoma should ultimately be reabsorbed.

## Results

Properly performed inguinal orchiectomy with the spermatic cord taken at the level of the inguinal ring is potentially curative if the tumor is still confined to the testis. Except for treatment of a complication, reoperation is virtually never required, although additional surgical procedures may be performed later to remove regional lymph nodes.

## References


1. Aki FT, Bilen CY, Tekin MI, et al. Is scrotal violation per se a risk factor for local relapse and metastases in stage I nonseminomatous testicular cancer? *Urology* 2000;56:459–462.
2. Ashdown DA, Bodiwala D, Liu S. Is high cord radical orchiectomy always necessary for testicular cancer? *Ann R Coll Surg Engl* 2004; 86;289–291.
3. Atchley JT, Dewbury KC. Ultrasound appearances of testicular epidermoid cysts. *Clin Radiol* 2000;55:453–512.
4. Hayes M, Smart CJ, Mead GM. Inguinal orchidectomy [Comment]. *Ann R Coll Surg Engl* 2005;87:488–492.
5. Heidenreich A, Engelmann UH, Vietsch HV, et al. Organ preserving surgery in testicular epidermoid cysts. *J Urol* 1995;153:1147–1150.
6. Heidenreich A, Weissbach L, Höltl W, et al., for the German Testicular Cancer Study Group. Organ sparing surgery for malignant germ cell tumor of the testis. *J Urol* 2001;166:2161–2165.
7. Hoei-Hansen CE, Rajpert-De Meyts E, Daugaard G, et al. Carcinoma in situ testis, the progenitor of testicular germ cell tumours: a clinical review. *Ann Oncol* 2005;16: 863–869.
8. Jemal A, Thomas A, Siegel R, et al. Cancer statistics, 2008. *CA Cancer J Clin* 2008;58:71–96.
9. Leibovitch I, Baniel J, Foster RS, et al. The clinical implications of procedural deviations during orchiectomy for nonseminomatous testis cancer. *J Urol* 1995;154:935–939.
10. Pizzocaro G. Editorial comment. *J Urol* 1995;154:939.
11. Sloan JC, Beck SDW, Bihrle R, et al. Bilateral testicular epidermoid cysts managed by partial orchiectomy. *J Urol* 2002;167:255–256.
12. Steele GS, Kantoff PW, Richie JP. Staging and imaging of testis cancer. In: Vogelzang NJ, Scardino PT, Shipley WU, et al., eds. *Comprehensive textbook of genitourinary oncology*, 3rd ed. Baltimore: Lippincott Williams & Wilkins, 2005:587–595.


# CHAPTER 65 ■ ORGAN-PRESERVING SURGERY IN TESTICULAR TUMORS

AXEL HEIDENREICH

Testicular germ cell tumors (TGCTs) are the most common neoplasms in young men, with bilateral simultaneous and sequential tumors arising in 2% to 3% of patients. Bilateral orchiectomy is still recommended as the gold standard treatment; it results in infertility, lifelong dependency on androgen substitution, and psychological distress due to castration at a young age. Because most testicular cancer patients are going to be longtime survivors with modern therapeutic approaches, long-term morbidity should be omitted whenever possible; cure of cancer might only be achieved if quality of life following therapy can be restored to pretreatment levels. Considering these quality-of-life issues, organ-sparing surgical approaches have been developed in patients with bilateral testicular cancer or in selected patients with a germ cell tumor arising in a solitary testicle.

## DIAGNOSIS

The diagnosis of testicular cancer is usually made by the appearance of a mass in the testicle that on ultrasonography appears solid or appears to have some cystic components (2). Serum markers, including β-human chorionic gonadotropin and α-fetoprotein, are routinely drawn prior to surgery.

## INDICATIONS FOR SURGERY

Patients in whom preservation surgery is contemplated should have enough testicular parenchyma for maintaining physiological testosterone synthesis, which requires that the diameter of the tumor should not exceed 2 cm (3,7). Preoperative serum testosterone and serum luteinizing hormone (LH) levels should be in the normal range. Elevated LH levels in the presence of normal testosterone levels indicate compensated Leydig cell insufficiency. These patients bear a high risk to develop hypogonadism with the need for androgen substitution following surgery. In addition, a semen analysis should be obtained to assess fertility and to discuss the option of cryopreservation (3,5). Also, testicular ultrasonography must be performed preoperatively because this usually represents the imaging modality of choice to assess the intratesticular location and diameter of the tumor. Scrotal magnetic resonance imaging appears only to be necessary if there is more than tumor suspected or if there is a very high suspicion for a benign testicular lesion (6).

## ALTERNATIVE THERAPY

The alternative to testicular-sparing surgery is bilateral orchiectomy, which will require lifelong hormonal replacement. Other problems associated with bilateral orchiectomy include infertility and the psychological impact of the procedure on the patient, who is usually a young male.

## SURGICAL TECHNIQUE

An inguinal approach is chosen with the skin incision being made about two fingerbreadths above and parallel to the inguinal ligament (Fig. 65.1). The incision extends from the external inguinal ring cephalad for about 5 cm and is carried down to the external oblique fascia (Fig. 65.2). Care is taken not to injure the ilioinguinal nerve, which runs laterally just underneath the fascia.

The spermatic cord is identified and isolated at the level of the pubic tubercle (Fig. 65.3), secured with a half-inch Penrose

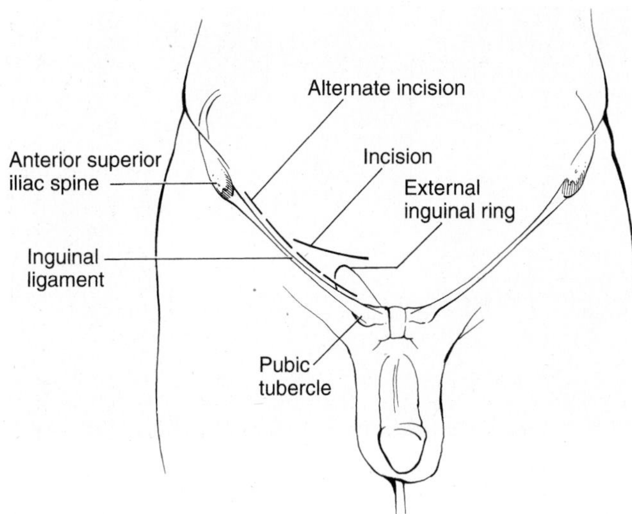


FIGURE 65.1 Inguinal incision for exploration of the testicle in relation to anatomic landmarks of the groin.

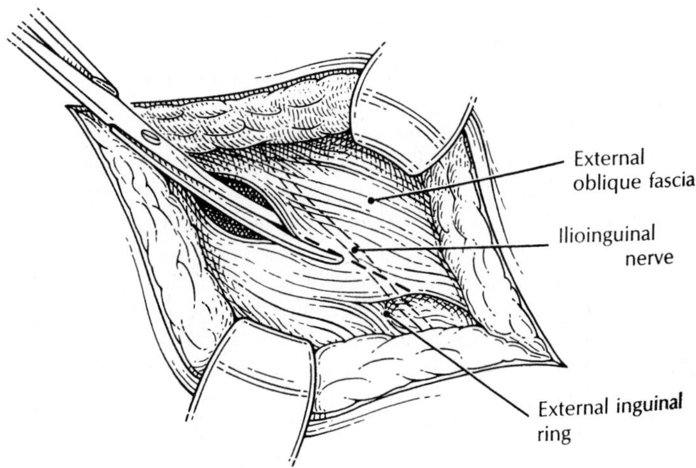


FIGURE 65.2 Incision of the external oblique fascia and its close relationship to the ilioinguinal nerve.

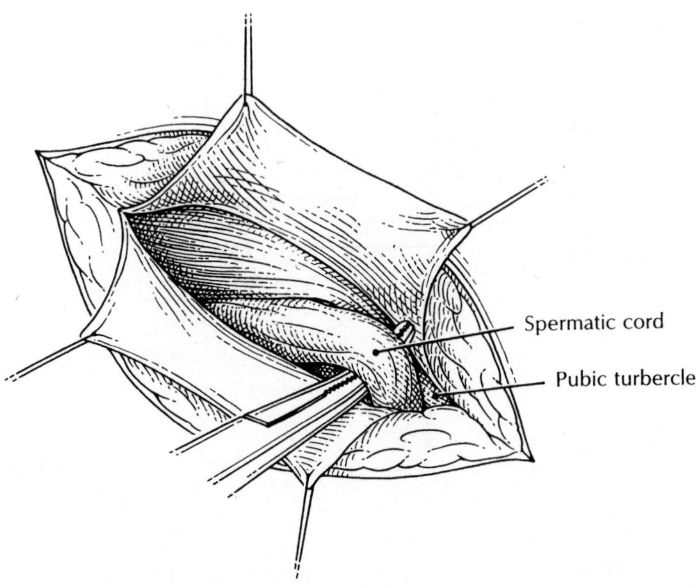


FIGURE 65.3 Delivery of the spermatic cord after the external oblique fascia has been opened.

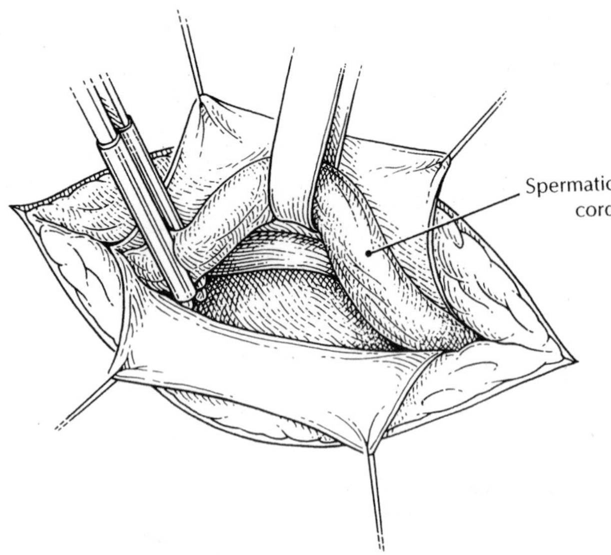


FIGURE 65.4 Mobilization of the spermatic cord up to the internal inguinal ring; the cord may be cross-clamped if desired.

drain, and mobilized back to the internal inguinal ring (Fig. 65.4). As in the case of radical orchiectomy, the spermatic cord might be cross-clamped with a rubber-shod clamp prior to delivering the testicle in the operating field. In this scenario, all following manipulations should be performed under cold ischemia by placing the testicle in crushed ice.

On the other hand, it is also possible to deliver the testicle into the operating field without cross-clamping the spermatic cord; we know that simple tumor cell shedding will not result in an increased frequency of distant metastases unless the tumor cells harbor molecular characteristics enabling them to adhere to the vascular endothelium, invade adjacent organs, and induce neovascularization. The testicle is delivered by slight traction on the spermatic cord and inversion of the scrotum; the gubernaculum is divided between two clamps and suture-ligated with 3-0 silk ties (Fig. 65.5).

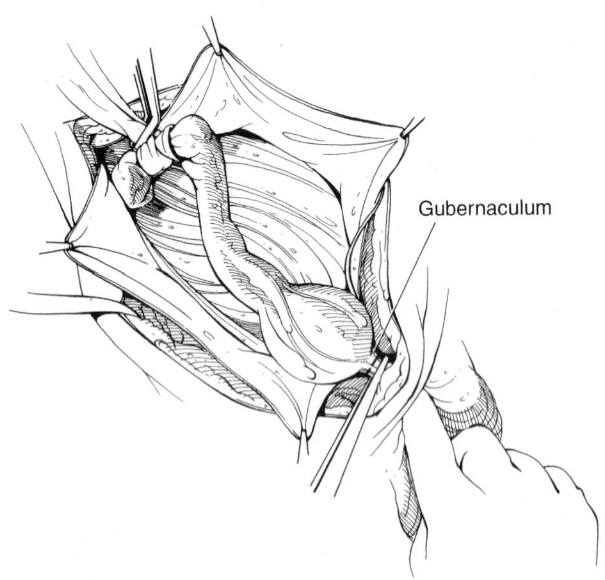


FIGURE 65.5 The testicle is delivered, and the gubernaculum may be divided and suture-ligated.

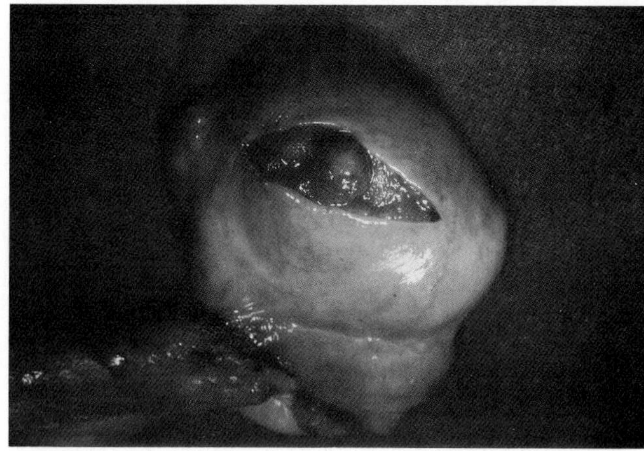

FIGURE 65.6 Incision of the tunica albuginea just above the testicular tumor.

The operating field is draped with laparotomy pads, and the tunica vaginalis is opened anteriorly; depending on the size and the intratesticular location of the tumor, it might be located underneath the tunica albuginea by simple palpation. In the presence of small testicular lesions, intraoperative ultrasonography with a 7.5-MHz scanner might be used for visualization and detection (1).

The tunica albuginea is incised just above the tumor (Fig. 65.6); because small testicular lesions usually present with a pseudocapsule, the surrounding testicular parenchyma can be scraped away with the blade of a scalpel (Fig. 65.7). Following the enucleation procedure, four additional biopsies are taken from the tumor bed to exclude tumor infiltration (Fig. 65.8), and all specimens are sent for frozen section examination (FSE). At least in our hands, FSE has turned out to represent a reliable technique to differentiate between benign and malignant tumors. Another biopsy is taken from the peripheral testicular parenchyma, fixed in Bouin or Stieve solution, and sent for pathohistologic analysis to exclude associated testicular intraepithelial neoplasia. After careful bipolar coagulation of small intratesticular blood vessels, the tunica albuginea is closed with a 4-0 Vicryl running suture

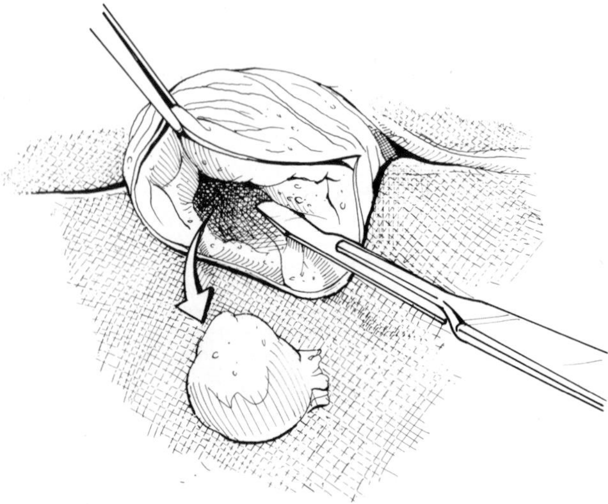

FIGURE 65.7 The tumor is surrounded by a firm pseudocapsule.

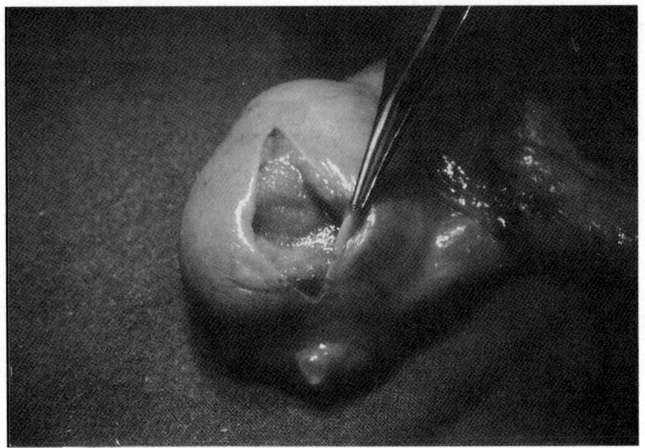

FIGURE 65.8 Additional quadrant biopsies following the enucleation procedure.

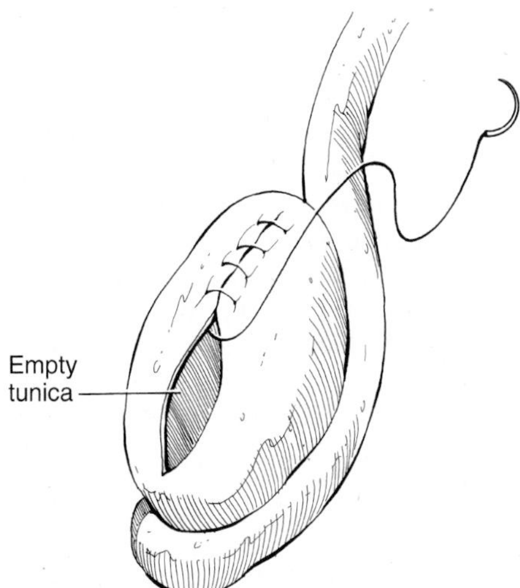


FIGURE 65.9 Running suture of the tunica albuginea.

(Fig. 65.9), the tunica vaginalis is closed with a Vicryl 3-0 running suture, and the testicle is replaced in the scrotum, taking care not to twist the spermatic cord. A formal orchidopexy for the testicle is not necessary. The skin is closed with an absorbable, intracutaneous running suture; usually, no drains are placed. Postoperatively, the patient should receive potent analgesics and antiphlogistics to reduce uncomfortable testicular pain.

# OUTCOMES

## Complications

Potential complications include hemorrhage and loss of the testicle. Eight-five percent to 92% of patients have maintained adequate androgen levels (5).

## Results

The initial study with a limited number of patients showed a 5-year survival rate of 92% and the maintenance of physiological testosterone serum levels in 92% without the need for androgen substitution (5). These findings resulted in the German Testicular Cancer Study Group criteria for proper patient selection, surgical technique, and follow-up based on the review of a large patient cohort with a median follow-up of >8 years. The disease-free survival rate was 99%, local recurrences developed in 5.5%, and normal testosterone serum levels were maintained in 85% of the patients.

The use of testicular-sparing surgery in testicular cancer requires that there be close follow-up for possible recurrence. The best modality for local follow-up is transscrotal ultrasonography. We recommend the first ultrasound to be done 4 to 6 weeks postoperatively, a time when scar tissue has replaced the intraparenchymatous traumatic edema; thereafter, scrotal imaging should be performed at 2-month intervals for the first year to adequately document the developing scar tissue for further follow-up studies (5). In patients who have undergone local radiation therapy postoperatively, periodic ultrasonography can be safely omitted and the patients should be educated to self-palpate the testicle. In patients who have not undergone adjuvant local radiation, periodic ultrasonography should be performed twice annually due to the high risk of local recurrence. In patients who develop a local recurrence, secondary orchiectomy has to be performed and androgen substitution has to be initiated (3–5).

In summary, organ-preserving surgery in patients with testicular germ cell tumors is feasible in patients with bilateral testis cancer or germ cell tumor in a solitary testicle. The procedure should be performed in conjunction with biopsies of the tumor bed and the resection rim and frozen section analysis, as well as a biopsy of the peripheral parenchyma. Follow-up in these patients should be either postoperative radiation of the remaining testicle with 18 Gy or very close follow-up. As this is still a controversial procedure, it may be best performed in a center experienced in the management of testicular cancer.

## *References*


1. Buckspan MB, Klotz PG, Goldfinger M, et al. Intraoperative ultrasound in the conservative resection of testicular neoplasms. *J Urol* 1989;141: 326–327.
2. Fuse H, Shimazaki J, Katayama T. Ultrasonography of testicular tumors. *Eur Urol* 1990;17:273–275.
3. Heidenreich A, Bonfi R, Derschum W, et al. A conservative approach to bilateral testicular germ cell tumors. *J Urol* 1995;153:10–13.
4. Heidenreich A, Höllt W, Albrecht W, et al. Testis-preserving surgery in bilateral testicular germ cell tumors. *Br J Urol* 1997;79:253–257.
5. Heidenreich A, Weissbach L, Höltl W, et al., for the German Testicular Cancer Study Group. Organ sparing surgery in malignant germ cell tumors of the testis. *J Urol* 2001;166:2161–2165.
6. Menzner A, Kujat C, König J, et al. MRI in testicular diagnosis: differentiation of seminoma, teratoma and inflammation using a statistical score. *Rofo Fortschr Geb Rontgenstr Neuen Bilgeb Verfahr* 1997;166:514.
7. Weissbach L. Organ preserving surgery of malignant germ cell tumors. *J Urol* 1995;153:90–93.

# CHAPTER 66 ■ RETROPERITONEAL LYMPHADENECTOMY

MICHAEL LEVERIDGE AND MICHAEL A. S. JEWETT

Carcinoma of the testis is the most common malignancy occurring in men aged 20 to 35. Most testicular malignancies are germ cell in origin and are classified as seminoma or nonseminomatous germ cell tumors (NSGCT), with the latter including embryonal carcinoma, teratoma and teratocarcinoma, choriocarcinoma, and yolk sac tumors. Treatment usually begins with radical inguinal orchiectomy to remove the primary tumor and to make a tissue diagnosis. Lymphovascular invasion (LVI) and embryonal carcinoma (EC) are the principal risk factors for metastasis. A staging workup follows. This chapter discusses the indications for retroperitoneal lymphadenectomy in testis cancer and describes the technique in primary and postchemotherapy settings.

## DIAGNOSIS

The majority of testis cancers are diagnosed following radical inguinal orchiectomy for a painless testicular mass. Less frequently, patients present with a symptomatic testis mass, or signs or symptoms of metastatic disease that lead to a presumptive or pathologically confirmed diagnosis.

The propensity for and the patterns of metastasis in germ cell tumors form the basis of the staging workup and the staging system used to describe the extent of disease. This information will dictate treatment. As the testes originate in utero as intra-abdominal structures, their primary lymphatic drainage, and therefore first metastatic tumor landing site, is to the retroperitoneum. The primary landing zones differ for each testis. Right-sided testis tumors metastasize first to interaortocaval nodes along the route of the supplying vessels, then with decreasing frequency to the precaval, para-aortic, and paracaval nodes (crossover may occur from right to left in the retroperitoneum). Left-sided masses metastasize to the para-aortic nodes, and with decreasing frequency to the precaval and interaortocaval nodal regions (1). Further lymphatic metastasis occurs via the thoracic duct, which may lead to mediastinal or supraclavicular adenopathy. Hematogenous metastatic disease is less common than lymphatic and can originate from the testis or can gain entry to the systemic circulation via the thoracic duct. The lungs are the most common hematogenously seeded sites.

Retroperitoneal nodal staging is based on the number and size of metastatic nodal deposits (2). N0 disease is when the retroperitoneal computerized tomography (CT) imaging is clinically negative with no nodes ≥10 mm, although normal-sized nodes along the gonadal drainage may be considered suspicious. N1 disease is when there are fewer than five enlarged nodes, none >2 cm. N2 disease involves more than five nodal deposits, or disease between 2 and 5 cm, while N3 disease has a greatest diameter >5 cm.

The retroperitoneum in patients with germ cell tumors is best examined using CT. Coronal views can be particularly helpful in examining the presence of and extent of disease. Plain films or CT of the chest should be used to assess for metastatic disease to the lungs or mediastinum.

Serum tumor markers are important in the assessment of the patient before and after orchiectomy, as well as in disease monitoring after retroperitoneal or systemic treatment. The serum alpha-fetoprotein (AFP) and beta-human chorionic gonadotropin (HCG) are elevated in up to 80% of patients before orchiectomy, and their persistence after removal of the primary tumor may be considered an indicator of metastatic disease, even in the setting of a negative imaging workup. The serum half-lives of AFP and HCG are 5 to 7 days and 24 to 36 hours, respectively, and so serial measurements may be needed until a nadir is reached before determining that markers are persistently elevated.

## INDICATIONS FOR SURGERY

Primary retroperitoneal lymphadenectomy or lymph node dissection (RPLND) is less widely practiced than it once was but is considered for patients with stage I NSGCT, especially in the setting of adverse pathologic risk factors (presence of LVI and predominant or pure EC) in the primary tumor, as an alternative to surveillance (3). Those without adverse risk factors have a low risk of progression and are generally managed by initial active surveillance. Persistently elevated markers after orchiectomy, with or without nodal metastases, are generally managed with chemotherapy due to a 50% or more risk of systemic metastatic disease beyond the retroperitoneum.

Patients with N1 low-volume disease may also be managed with primary RPLND if markers are very low or normal. If the nodal diameter is >5 cm in any dimension, or if there are numerous small nodes, these patients have a high likelihood of systemic disease and are managed with primary chemotherapy. The management of nodal disease 2 to 5 cm in axial dimension is controversial, and many centers recommend initial primary chemotherapy as although RPLND provides 50+% control if markers are low or normal.

The most common indication for retroperitoneal lymphadenectomy is in the postchemotherapy setting (pcRPLND). Patients with a residual retroperitoneal mass(es) after primary chemotherapy for NSGCT are candidates for surgery because of a 50% incidence of viable germ cell tumor or teratoma (which may expand) (4). Histology of the residual mass can determine future treatment, as residual carcinoma is usually an indication for further chemotherapy (5). Residual retroperitoneal disease occurs infrequently after radiation and/or chemotherapy for seminoma, but these patients should be considered for RPLND if resolution does not occur, particularly if a PET scan is positive. These masses tend to disappear slowly after radiation therapy, and so a retroperitoneal mass may be initially closely observed.

## ALTERNATIVE THERAPY

Surveillance remains a very reasonable alternative for testis cancer patients with a negative staging workup. A recent systematic review of surveillance in stage I germ cell cancer revealed a 28% relapse rate in patients with NSGCT (3), with the implication that RPLND would represent overtreatment in approximately 70% of cases. One percent of the patients in these studies died of testis cancer during follow-up. Recurrence outside of the retroperitoneum will not be prevented by RPLND. These studies of early-stage germ cell tumors have uncovered several prognostic factors relating to the primary tumor that have predictive value regarding risk of relapse. Vascular or lymphovascular invasion is consistently related to increased risk of relapse, as are an increased proportion of embryonal histology, the absence of yolk sac elements, higher local stage (particularly involvement of spermatic cord tissue), and the presence of mature teratoma (3). In patients without adverse risk factors, a stringent surveillance protocol can be followed with 10% to 15% risk of progression, sometimes treatable by RPLND alone. High-risk patients, in our experience, have about a 50% chance of progression, so any treatment will be unnecessary in about 50%. Nonrisk adapted surveillance can be practiced, reserving treatment for those who clearly need it. Surveillance requires frequent assessments with history, physical examination, serum marker measurement, and chest and abdominal imaging. As the majority of relapses occur in the first year of surveillance, visits are undertaken at 2-month intervals for the first 2 years (CT of the abdomen can be done every 4 months), with increasing intervals between assessments afterwards.

There is also evidence for primary chemotherapy for clinical stage I NSGCT, with a relapse rate of 1.5% to 7.0% in the retroperitoneum (6). Indeed, a recent German clinical trial of 382 men randomized to RPLND versus a single cycle of bleomycin, etoposide, and cisplatin suggested an increase in relapse-free survival in the chemotherapy cohort at a median follow-up of 4.7 years (7). The incidence of late relapse and long-term toxicity has not been described.

Chemotherapy and RPLND each have a role in low-volume retroperitoneal adenopathy. False-positive imaging can occur in up to 30% of patients, but with increased size of the retroperitoneal mass there is an increased likelihood that adenopathy represents active tumor. Our practice is to advise primary chemotherapy in those patients with a retroperitoneal mass >5 cm in any dimension, or with elevated markers.

Subfertility affects an increased proportion of testis cancer patients primarily, and it can be further compromised with any treatment of advanced disease. Consideration of sperm banking should be encouraged.

## SURGICAL TECHNIQUE

### Primary Procedure (No Previous Treatment)

The patient is positioned supine, with central venous and epidural lines placed at the discretion of the attendant anesthesiologist. A midline incision is made from the xiphisternum to approximately midway between the umbilicus and pubis, and subcutaneous tissue and fascia are divided (Fig. 66.1A). The fascia adjacent to the xiphisternum is undermined and incised. The falciform ligament may be ligated and divided. A thoracoabdominal incision can also be used, particularly in early-stage left-sided tumors whose primary dissection will be in the para-aortic and interaortocaval areas, but this is rarely done today. The peritoneum is entered and thoroughly explored.

The right colon is reflected medially following the plane anterior to the perinephric fascia (Fig. 66.1B). This dissection can be carried up to the hepatic flexure as needed. The right ureter is identified and protected during the mobilization of the right colon, and it will later constitute the lateral limit of the node dissection. The incision is carried around the cecum, and the posterior peritoneum is incised medially along the root of the small bowel mesentery, ending at the ligament of Treitz (Fig. 66.1C). The right colon and small bowel are then dissected off the retroperitoneum until the left renal vein is visualized and accessible superiorly and the perinephric fascia is evident laterally. The small intestine and right colon are placed in a bowel bag and rotated onto the patient's chest. The inferior mesenteric vein may be ligated and divided to facilitate outward rotation of the pancreas for optimal retroperitoneal exposure, although the left colon can also be taken down. The left renal vein is mobilized and the tissue overlying it is divided, with care to identify and ligate or clip larger lymphatic channels as they may be encountered. The superior margin must be carefully controlled to avoid chylous ascites, as with all superior borders of dissection around the hilum and behind the crura of the diaphragm. The retroperitoneum is now fully exposed to begin the dissection with a clear field of view.

### Templates for Dissection

Dissection templates in the retroperitoneum are based on the lymphatic drainage patterns of the involved testis. Many surgeons do a full bilateral dissection for all cases, but the initial efforts to achieve nerve sparing without necessarily identifying the nerves intraoperatively lead to defining templates to include the most likely nodes to be involved. For right-sided testis tumors, the upper border of the renal veins marks the superior extent of dissection (Fig. 66.2A). Suprahilar dissections are no longer performed unless there is gross adenopathy in the renal hilum, but in fact, much of the suprahilar tissue is pulled down and removed during a thorough dissection.

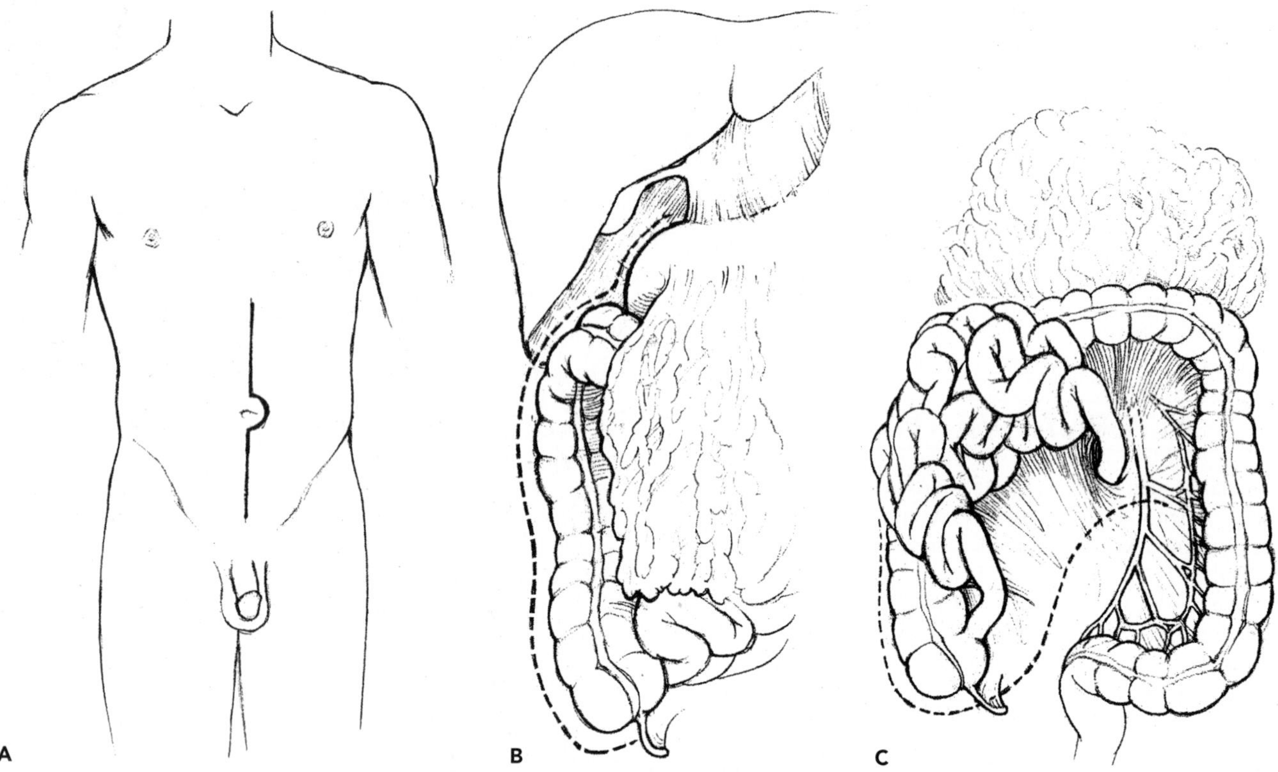


FIGURE 66.1 **A:** Midline incision from xiphoid to symphysis. **B:** Incision of the line of Toldt to allow reflection of the right colon and exposure of the retroperitoneum. **C:** Continuation of line of peritoneal incision around the root of the bowel mesentery.

Paracaval and interaortocaval nodes are removed, as are para-aortic nodes to the level of the takeoff of the inferior mesenteric artery. The nodes along the right common iliac artery are removed to the bifurcation of the common iliac artery. The dissection extends laterally to the right ureter. The upper border of the renal veins is the superior limit of dissection in the left-sided template as well (Fig. 66.2B). Para-aortic nodes are removed with the left ureter as the lateral limit and the bifurcation of the left common iliac artery as the inferior limit of dissection. Interaortocaval nodes are removed above the takeoff of the inferior mesenteric artery. In either case, suspicious or enlarged nodes are indications for a full bilateral dissection (Fig. 66.2C).

In the presence of clinically positive nodes that number less than five, with none larger than 2 cm, similar templates as outlined above may be used. Caveats include the potential for left para-aortic (17%) and left iliac (7%) nodal disease in right-sided tumors, which would not be included in a strict template dissection (8). Two percent of patients will have suprahilar nodal disease in the interaortocaval region. These may be recognized and removed if grossly abnormal, but routine dissection here is not necessary given the low incidence of disease. This additional dissection does not contribute to additional patient morbidity, unless more lumbar vessels are ligated, which may incur a greater incidence of postoperative back pain.

In the setting of more extensive nodal disease, a full bilateral template is indicated (Fig. 66.2C). In this case the superior extent of dissection lies at the origin of the superior mesenteric artery, 1 to 2 cm superior to the renal arteries. The lymphadenectomy extends laterally to the ureters, posteriorly to the psoas muscle and the anterior spinal ligament, and inferiorly to the ipsilateral midexternal iliac artery and contralateral common iliac artery bifurcation.

## Nerve-Sparing Retroperitoneal Lymph Node Dissection

The postganglionic sympathetic nerves arising from the lumbar sympathetic chains are responsible for seminal emission. Until 1988, they were routinely sacrificed, and many patients lost antegrade ejaculation and therefore fertility. The modification of RPLND allows identification and preservation of these nerves (9). The sympathetic fibers innervating the seminal vesicles and vasa deferentia arise as postganglionic fibers from T12-L3. The sympathetic trunks lie on the medial borders of the psoas muscles bilaterally, lateral to the lumbar vertebral bodies. The right trunk lies posterior to the middle of the inferior vena cava (IVC), and the lateral border of the aorta conceals the left trunk (Fig. 66.3). Their ganglia are rounded or fusiform and of variable size (up to 10 mm). The postganglionic nerves course anteromedially over the aorta, whereupon they form a network of fibers (Fig. 66.4). These nerve fibers condense to form the inferior mesenteric and hypogastric plexuses, which can exhibit variable location despite names approximating adjacent aortic branches. The nerves that connect these plexuses are termed intermesenteric nerves. One rationale for limiting the inferior dissection in a unilateral template to the inferior mesenteric artery origin is to

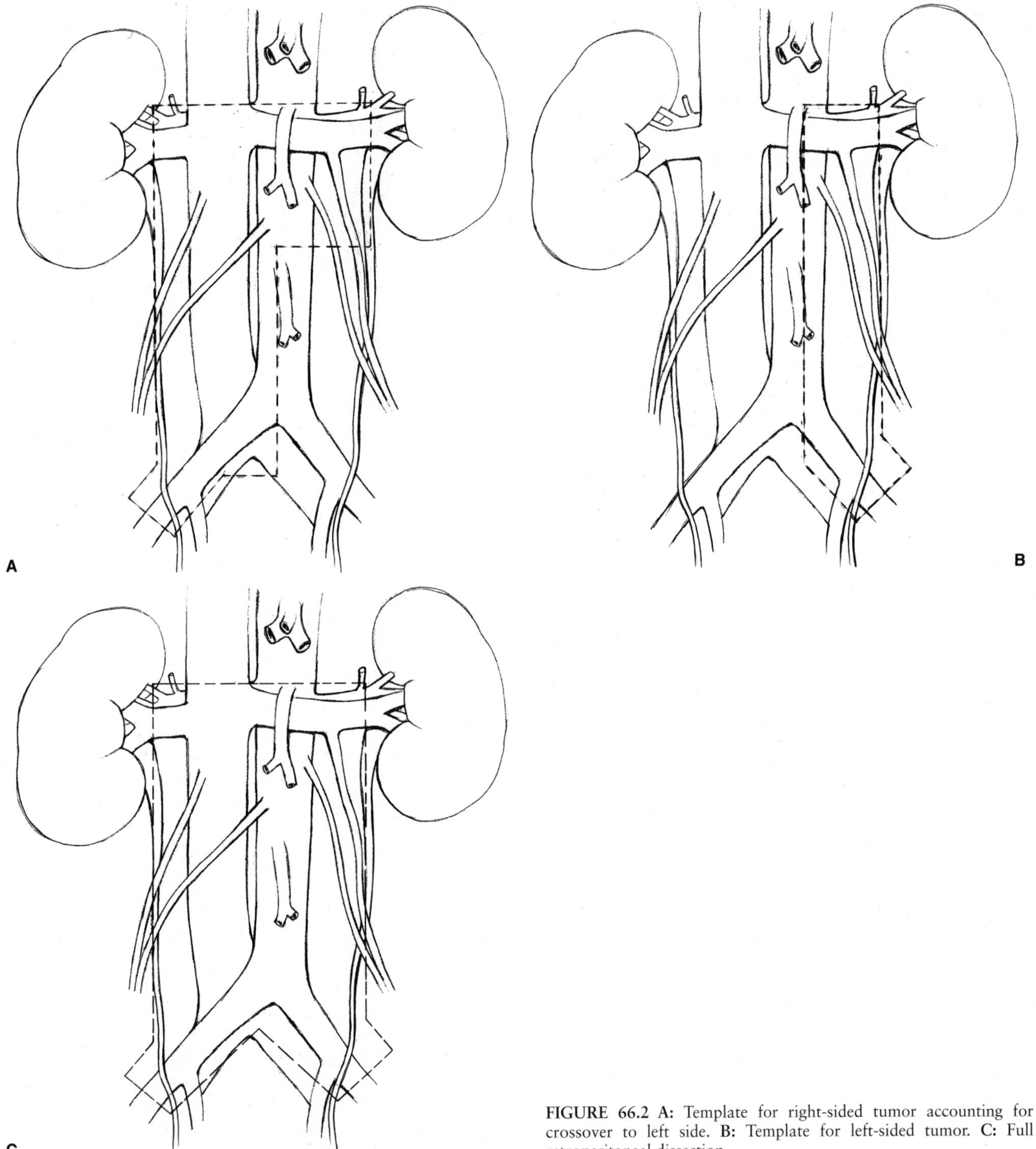


FIGURE 66.2 **A:** Template for right-sided tumor accounting for crossover to left side. **B:** Template for left-sided tumor. **C:** Full retroperitoneal dissection.

avoid the ipsilateral hypogastric plexus, which commonly overlies the aortic bifurcation and interiliac angle. The hypogastric and pelvic nerves emanate from these ganglia to course inferiorly and supply the prostate, bladder, urethra, periurethral glands, seminal vesicles, and vasa deferentia.

Dissection begins by incising the tissue on the anterior surface of the IVC in its midline, avoiding transection of obvious nodes. The adipose tissue is dissected medially to expose the left side of the IVC from the left renal vein to the common iliac vein, with care taken to ligate or cauterize small vessels as they are encountered (Fig. 66.5A). Careful lateral mobilization of the cava is performed, with ligation of lumbar veins as needed (Fig. 66.5B). The right sympathetic chain is encountered posterior to the midline of the IVC (Fig. 66.3). The lumbar veins tend to run medial to the sympathetic chain but may be found lateral to it, or occasionally branching around it. The individual nerves running anteromedially from the ganglia of the chain pass above and medial to the lumbar

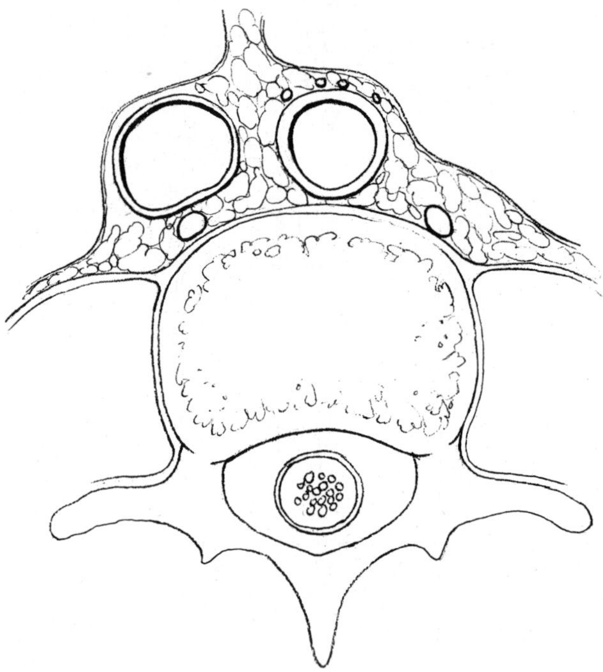

FIGURE 66.3 Relationship between the great vessels and sympathetic trunks.

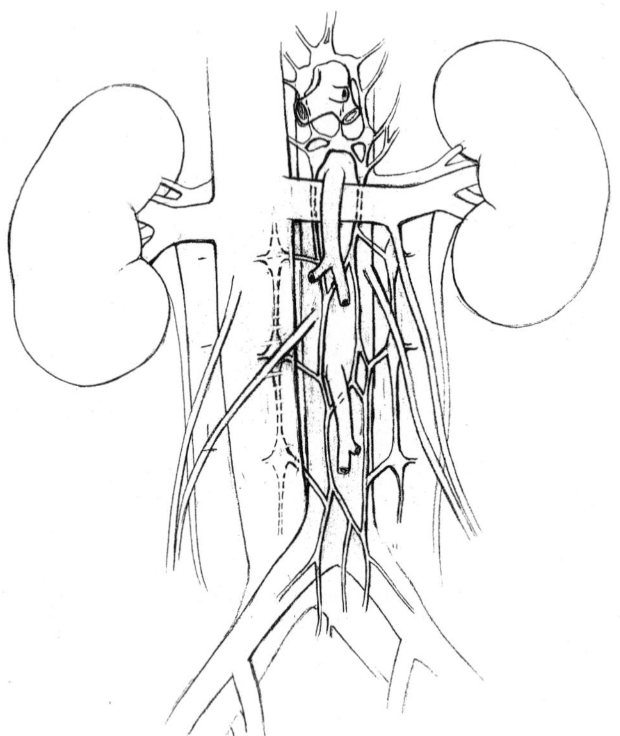

FIGURE 66.4 Anatomy of the lumbar sympathetic nerves.

veins, which serve as good landmarks. They can be individually skeletonized from the underlying tissue, which is ultimately mobilized posteriorly and removed superiorly or inferiorly. Dissection may be helped with the use of the Hydro-Jet dissector.

The left ureter is identified across the midline under the inferior mesenteric vessels posterior to the mesocolon. A plane is developed between the inferior mesenteric vessels anteriorly and the retroperitoneal lymphatic and adipose tissue posteriorly. The inferior mesenteric artery occasionally must be sacrificed, and if done should be ligated and cut several centimeters from its origin at the aorta. This allows direct access to the left side. The left ureter is identified in this plane and is mobilized to the perinephric tissue, which can be reflected laterally to identify the psoas muscle. The tissue medial to the ureters and perinephric tissue represents the para-aortic nodal bed (Fig. 66.6). It can be seen above at the level of the left renal vein as well as from below. For right-sided tumors, the left gonadal vein is a marker of the lateral limit of dissection at the renal hilum, but some surgeons sacrifice it and go more laterally to be sure that retrograde tumor cell spread to nodes in this area is removed if present. This tissue is carefully reflected medially to identify the ganglia of the left sympathetic chain, and the postganglionic nerves can be seen coming off to run anteromedially (Fig. 66.3). Fibers from a higher ganglion may be encountered anterior to either renal artery, and they can be difficult to preserve. It is not clear that they are necessary to preserve antegrade ejaculation. Similarly, nerves running along the inferior mesenteric artery are clearly seen but not always preserved with no obvious detriment.

At this point the patient's sympathetic anatomy has been elucidated, and anteromedially coursing fibers from the sympathetic chains are preserved lateral to the aorta. The aorta can now be exposed. Careful dissection along the aorta is then undertaken. The previously identified sympathetic nerves are followed from the side and preserved as they cross in front of the aorta and coalesce into plexuses. The plexuses that condense at and below the inferior mesenteric artery origin form the hypogastric nerves that provide sympathetic innervation to pelvic structures. Careful skeletonization and preservation of these structures allow the complete removal of para-aortic and interaortocaval nodal tissue, as well as tissue overlying the aortic bifurcation, common iliac veins, and sacral promontory, with maintenance of emission and ejaculation. It is our practice to limit inferior dissection to the common iliac artery bifurcation, taking care to preserve the genitofemoral nerves. The remnant ipsilateral spermatic cord is removed, along with as much vas deferens as possible and the spermatic vessels in their attachments to the retroperitoneum.

It is not always possible to preserve all postganglionic nerves, as nodal metastases or tumor masses may involve or lie immediately adjacent to them. Ejaculation does not rely on the preservation of all nerves, and so there should be no hesitation to sacrifice ipsilateral (or even in a limited manner bilateral) nerves to ensure complete removal of disease. The right-sided nerves are generally more prominent and easier to preserve.

At this point the retroperitoneum as defined by the limits of dissection should be clear of all lymphatic and adipose tissue surrounding the aorta and IVC, and postganglionic nerves should be intact beside and overlying the aorta. The contents of the bowel bag are returned to the abdomen. The peritoneum can be reapproximated with absorbable suture. The fascial incision is closed with a running no. 1 suture, with occasional interrupted figure-of-eight sutures. The skin is closed as per the surgeon's preference. Drains and nasogastric

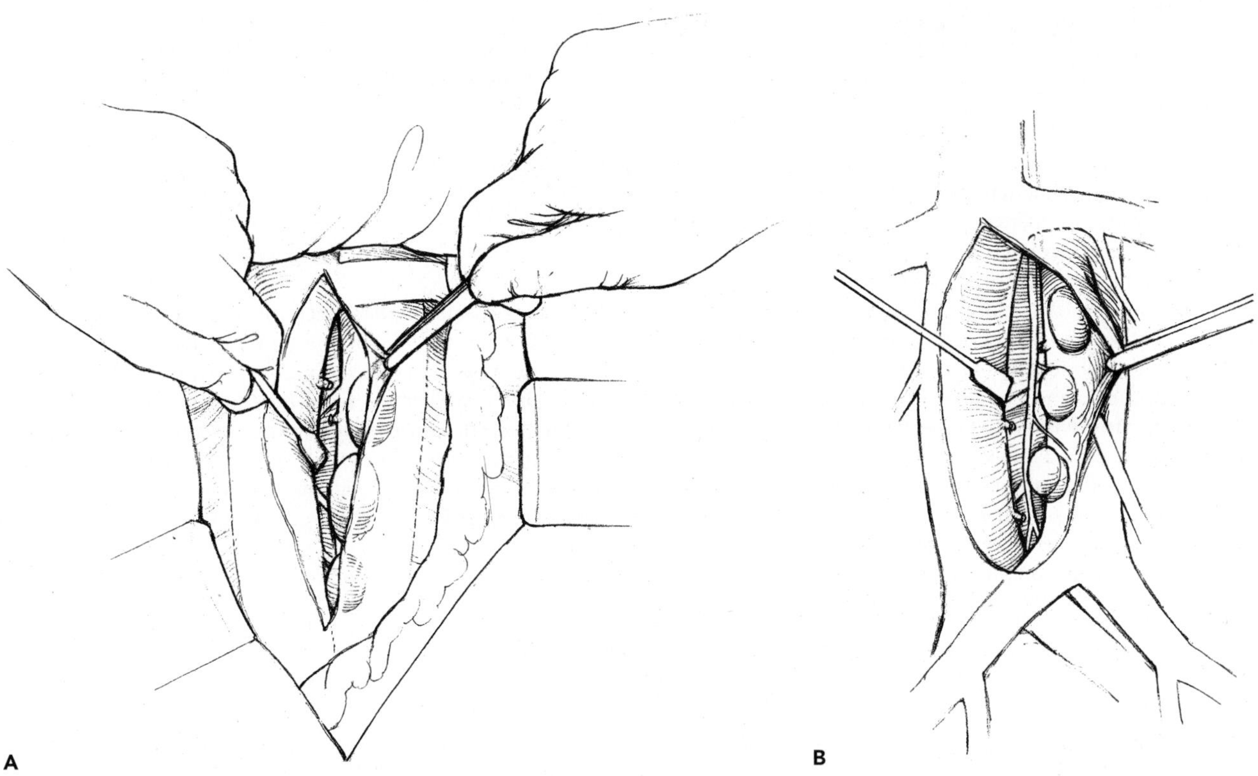


FIGURE 66.5 **A:** Dissection between the vena cava and aorta. **B:** Retraction of the great vessels allows exposure of the lumbar vessels, which may be ligated.

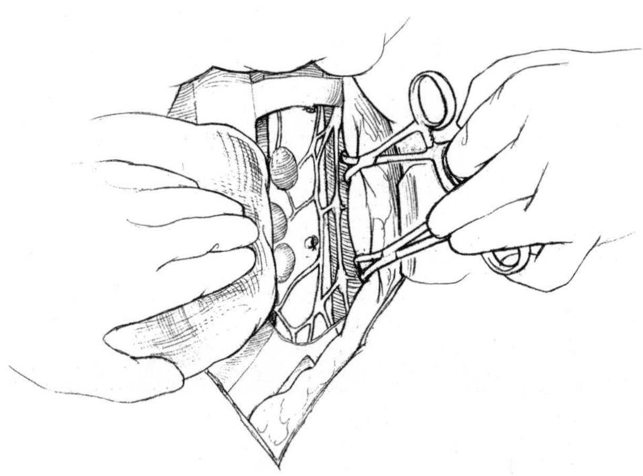

FIGURE 66.6 Reflection of the left ureter and adipose tissue.

suction are not routinely used. A urethral catheter is left in if there is an epidural.

## Postchemotherapy Retroperitoneal Lymphadenectomy

There is debate regarding whether patients with a postchemotherapy mass warranting resection should undergo a full bilateral template dissection or if oncologic control with fewer adverse outcomes can be obtained through excision of the mass and the template as above. Removing the mass alone is not recommended due to the frequent micrometastases in adjacent nodes (10). Recent case series, however, have demonstrated a low retroperitoneal recurrence rate in patients treated with unilateral template postchemotherapy procedures, with excellent maintenance of antegrade ejaculation (11). The postchemotherapy procedure can be complicated by large tumor masses outside of typical templates, which may mandate en bloc nephrectomy, or occasionally resection of significant portions of the aorta or IVC. This has become less common with the reduction in the proportion of cases with active cancer to <10% in current series. Vascular surgery expertise may be required. Small lacerations of great vessels can be repaired with monofilament 5-0 or 6-0 sutures.

It is important to clear the nodal and lymphatic tissue at the upper limits of dissection in particular. The lymphatics are often prominent anterior and behind the right crus of the diaphragm. Nodal tissue may be present behind the right crus and can be removed from below if not overly bulky, sparing the patient a thoracotomy. Similarly, nodal tissue may be present along the course of the ipsilateral gonadal vessels and vas; these structures should be carefully inspected and removed along with any nodal tissue along their lengths.

If the mass is confined and permits, nerve-sparing dissection can be performed in up to 50% of patients. This is particularly difficult where the tumor is adherent to the great vessels, when skeletonization of the nerves is difficult and dissection can appear to be subadventitial. Normal vascular and retroperitoneal anatomy can be distorted, and blood loss can be sudden; therefore, the surgeon and the anesthetist must be experienced.

# OUTCOMES

## Complications

Intraoperative complications in primary RPLND are generally confined to damage of the renal vasculature and great vessels. Complication rates are increased in postchemotherapy procedures. If an appropriate plane cannot be developed between the mass and the aorta or IVC, it may be more prudent to resect part of the vessel and primarily close it or employ a vascular graft.

Chylous ascites and lymphocele represent infrequent but potentially serious complications that stress the importance of careful identification and obliteration of lymphatic vessels intraoperatively. Most lymphoceles resolve spontaneously, while some will require percutaneous drainage. They may occasionally exert a mass effect and cause gastrointestinal symptoms, flank pain, or ureteric obstruction.

Pulmonary physiotherapy and early mobilization will limit the incidence of lung complications such as atelectasis and pneumonia. Patients who have received bleomycin as part of their chemotherapy regimen are at particular risk of pulmonary complications.

Careful and successful sympathetic nerve preservation is effective in preserving antegrade ejaculation and seminal emission.

## Results

Retroperitoneal lymphadenectomy provides pathologic staging. Patients with low-volume germ cell metastasis in the specimen progress in approximately 30% of cases without adjuvant chemotherapy. Chemotherapy in these patients may be avoided and can be given in the salvage setting in the case of relapse. Alternatively, all patients with pathologically proven retroperitoneal carcinoma may be given adjuvant chemotherapy with excellent cure rates, but 50% or more are treated unnecessarily.

## *References*


1. Donohue JP, Zachary JM, Maynard BR. Distribution of nodal metastases in nonseminomatous testis cancer. *J Urol* 1982;128:315–320.
2. Greene FL, Page DL, Fleming ID, eds. *AJCC cancer staging manual*, 6th ed. Lippincott-Raven Publishers, 2002.
3. Groll RJ, Warde P, Jewett MA. A comprehensive systematic review of testicular germ cell tumor surveillance. *Crit Rev Oncol Hematol* 2007;64(3): 182–197.
4. Sim HG, Lange P, Lin DW. Role of post-chemotherapy surgery in germ cell tumors. *Urol Clin North Am* 2007;34:199–217.
5. Steyerberg EW, Gerl A, Fossa SD, et al. Validity of predictions of residual retroperitoneal mass histology in nonseminomatous testicular cancer. *J Clin Oncol* 1998;16(1):269–274.
6. Stephenson AJ, Sheinfeld J. Management of patients with low-stage nonseminomatous germ cell testicular cancer. *Curr Treat Options Oncol* 2005; 6:367–377.
7. Albers P, Siener R, Krege S, et al. and the German Testicular Cancer Study Group. Randomized phase III trial comparing retroperitoneal lymph node dissection with one course of bleomycin and etoposide plus cisplatin chemotherapy in the adjuvant treatment of clinical stage I nonseminomatous testicular germ cell tumors: AUO Trial AH 01/94 by the German Testicular Cancer Study Group. *J Clin Oncol* 2008;26(18):2966–2972.
8. Donohue JP, Thornhill JA, Foster RS, et al. The role of retroperitoneal lymphadenectomy in clinical stage B testis cancer: the Indiana University experience (1965 to 1989). *J Urol* 1995;153:85–89.
9. Jewett MA, Kong YS, Goldberg SD, et al. Retroperitoneal lymphadenectomy for testis tumor with nerve sparing for ejaculation. *J Urol* 1988; 139(6):1220–1224.
10. Carver BS, Shayegan B, Eggener S, et al. Incidence of metastatic nonseminomatous germ cell tumor outside the boundaries of a modified postchemotherapy retroperitoneal lymph node dissection. *J Clin Oncol* 2007;25(28):4365–4369.
11. Steiner H, Peschel R, Bartsch G. Retroperitoneal lymph node dissection after chemotherapy for germ cell tumors: is a full bilateral template always necessary? *BJU Int* 2008;102(3):310–314.


# CHAPTER 67 ■ TORSION OF THE TESTICLE

BLAKE W. MOORE AND HARRY P. KOO

Testicular torsion is a surgical emergency that demands prompt recognition and treatment to preserve testicular function. This condition occurs when the spermatic cord twists upon itself, leading to vascular compromise and a possible testicular loss from prolonged ischemia. The need for timely assessment and intervention is heightened by the fact that hours often elapse between the onset of symptoms and the urologist's evaluation. Despite the continuing advancements in radiologic imaging of the acute scrotum, history and physical examination consistent with acute testicular torsion are often sufficient to warrant immediate surgical exploration.

Torsion of the spermatic cord has been recognized in all age groups, with the majority of patients presenting during adolescence. The annual incidence of testicular torsion in men under the age of 25 years is estimated to be 1 in 4,000 (1). The peak incidence has uniformly been seen in the 12- to 18-year-old age range (accounting for 65% of all torsions), with a second, much smaller peak in the perinatal period (1,2). A large

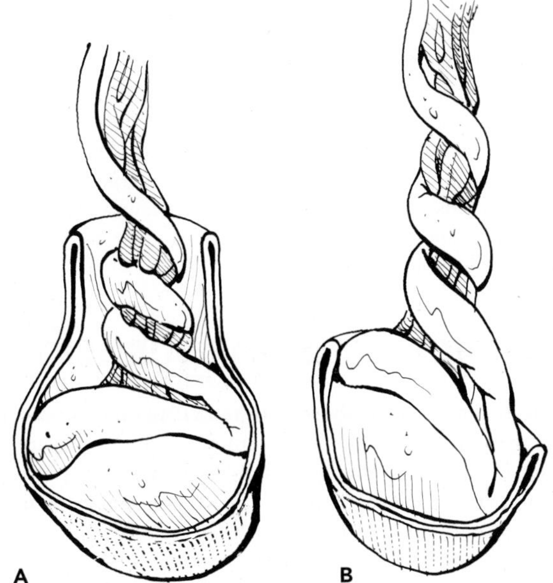


FIGURE 67.1 **A:** Extravaginal torsion, typical of a neonatal testicular torsion. The tunica vaginalis is involved with the twist of the spermatic cord. **B:** Intravaginal torsion, usually seen after the neonatal period, involves the spermatic cord below the reflection of the tunica vaginalis onto the spermatic cord.

study found that 7% of the cases involved an undescended testicle, and it was speculated that testicular torsion was 10 times more common in patients with undescended testes (3). Curiously, a number of investigations have demonstrated unequal laterality, with the left testicle being affected more frequently. Bilateral torsion is said to account for fewer than 5% of all cases (3,4).

Testicular torsion can be classified as extravaginal or intravaginal based on whether the twisting is above or below the reflection of the tunica vaginalis onto the spermatic cord (Fig. 67.1). Extravaginal torsion occurs when the tunica vaginalis is not securely attached to the scrotum, allowing the testicle and the tunica vaginalis to rotate as a unit along the longitudinal axis. This variant is virtually always limited to the perinatal population and may take place antenally or postnatally, a distinction that has important prognostic and therapeutic implications. A review by Das and Singer (5) found that 72% of perinatal torsions occur in utero. With *intravaginal* torsion, twisting of the spermatic cord occurs entirely within, but does not involve, the tunica vaginalis. This type of torsion affects patients outside of the perinatal age group, although it has been reported on rare occasion in newborns.

Several anatomic factors contribute to intravaginal torsion. The tunica vaginalis normally covers the anterior surface of the testis and extends varying distances over the epididymis and the spermatic cord. In the "bell clapper" variant, the tunica vaginalis inserts at an abnormally high location on the spermatic cord, causing the testis to be suspended freely within the tunical cavity. The "bell clapper" variant has been seen in 12% of testes at postmortem (6). In addition, the mesorchium may have a narrow attachment onto the testicle, allowing the testis to assume a more horizontal position within the scrotum. These factors contribute to increased testicular motility within the tunica vaginalis and facilitate rotation of the testis about the spermatic cord.

# DIAGNOSIS

## Perinatal Torsion

In the newborn, local and systemic symptoms of torsion may be scarce, delaying presentation and diagnosis. The patient with antenatal torsion may present with a large, firm, painless scrotal mass. Parents may report a swollen scrotum with discolored skin. In postnatal torsion, similar symptoms develop in a newborn with a previously normal scrotal examination. However, torsion that occurs after birth is more likely to cause systemic symptoms such as irritability or lack of appetite. Parents may also note an acute onset of redness and swelling of the scrotum.

In newborns, the physical exam may be the only indicator of testicular torsion. The neonate is usually in no acute distress, though a postnatal onset is more likely to cause general discomfort. An abdominal or inguinal mass may be found in the case of an undescended testis. The scrotal skin may be discolored, ranging from erythematous to blue-black, depending on the degree and duration of torsion. Chronic changes are more frequently seen with antenatal torsion.

## Torsion of the Testicle in Children, Adolescents, and Adults

Torsion outside of the perinatal population is usually associated with a more acute symptomatology. The classical presentation is described as a sudden onset of severe, unilateral testicular pain, with swelling of the testicle. With time, the patient may complain of swelling and redness of the scrotum.

The most common etiologies of scrotal pain are testicular torsion, torsion of testicular appendage, and epididymitis. Differentiating these disease processes can sometimes be problematic. In general, historical features (fever, nausea/vomiting, dysuria, sexual activity, history of trauma) were not helpful in differentiating testicular torsion from other conditions. In a retrospective review of 90 patients presenting with acute scrotum, the only statistically significant finding from history was that patients with testicular torsion or torsion of testicular appendage had a shorter duration of symptoms (<12 hours) when compared with patients with epididymitis (7).

Older patients typically have more acute findings on physical exam. Almost invariably, the testicle will be swollen and exquisitely tender. Scrotal edema and erythema are usually present. In many cases the affected testicle assumes a retracted, horizontal lie. A detectable secondary hydrocele could be found in up to 50% of patients. Loss of the cremasteric reflex is suggestive of testicular torsion, and in several series it was universally absent (6,7). These characteristic findings all point toward an etiology of testicular torsion, but it must be remembered that no single finding is pathognomonic.

## Torsion of Testicular Appendages

Four testicular appendages have been identified: the appendix testis (hydatid of Morgagni), the appendix epididymis, the paradidymis (organ of Giraldés), and the vas aberrans of Haller. Each of these is susceptible to torsion, but the overwhelming

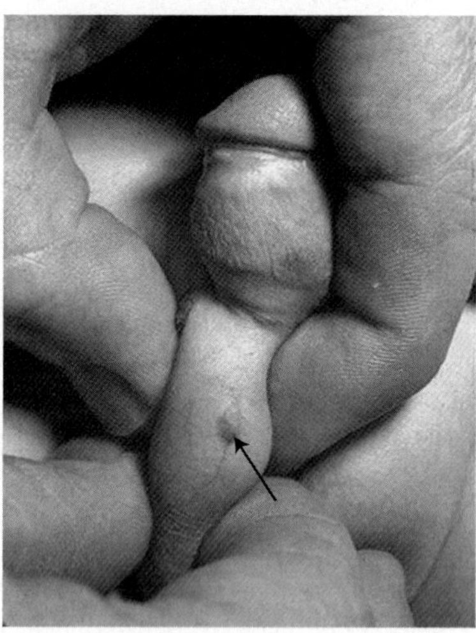

FIGURE 67.2 Torsion of appendix testis showing the "blue dot sign" *(arrow)*.

majority of twisted appendages involve the appendix testis. In the pediatric age group, appendiceal torsion is nearly as common as testicular torsion and accounts for 20% to 40% of acute scrotum cases (8). Torsion of a testicular appendage is often characterized by a gradual onset and few systemic symptoms. Early in the course of torsion of the appendix testis, physical examination may reveal a tender mass located at the upper pole of the testicle, sometimes adherent to the overlying skin. In our experience, it has been quite rare to see a small area of ecchymotic skin at the upper pole ("blue dot sign"), which is pathognomonic for torsion of the appendix testis (Fig. 67.2). In almost all cases the testicle has a normal orientation and the cremasteric reflex is intact (4). With time, torsion of the testicle and torsion of an appendage can become clinically indistinguishable. Imaging with Doppler ultrasound frequently shows a hyperechoic mass at the upper pole of a normal-appearing testicle. If the clinician is completely confident in the diagnosis of appendage torsion, the condition can be treated symptomatically. Therapy consists of bedrest, scrotal elevation, and nonsteroidal anti-inflammatory agents as needed. Symptoms should begin to resolve within 1 to 2 weeks as the infarcted appendage is gradually resorbed. If testicular torsion cannot be ruled out with certainty, urgent surgical exploration is needed.

Testicular torsion is a clinical diagnosis and is proven at the time of surgery. Radiologic studies may support the diagnosis, but negative imaging should not preclude exploration when clinical suspicion is high. Nonetheless, diagnostic examinations should be performed when testicular torsion is considered unlikely and the clinician has concluded that the patient has a nonsurgical condition.

Color Doppler ultrasound is widely utilized in the evaluation of scrotal abnormalities and has been studied in patients with testicular torsion. The capacity to view both blood flow and anatomic detail is particularly useful in assessing the scrotal contents and can provide valuable information about other pathologic conditions. Because of the prompt availability, low costs, short duration, and convenience of this examining method when compared with alternative diagnostic tools such as magnetic resonance imaging (MRI) or scintigraphy, sonography has become the primary diagnostic modality in evaluating the acute scrotum (9). Color Doppler ultrasound has been reported to have a sensitivity of 89% to 100% and a specificity of 97% to 100% in diagnosing testicular torsion (7,9). Lack of intratesticular blood flow and testicular enlargement are characteristic findings. Gunther et al. (9) have noted that central arterial perfusion was a reliable diagnostic parameter to exclude testicular torsion. However, arterial blood flow ceases only after venous obstruction and edema develop, which can lead to a false-negative result early in the torsion. Intermittent torsion may also go undiagnosed. As with many radiographic technologies, interpretation is highly dependent on the experience of the technician or radiologist.

## INDICATIONS FOR SURGERY

Management of the newborn with testicular torsion is an area of controversy. To understand treatment in this age group, it is important to define the condition as prenatal or postnatal. Torsion that presents acutely *after* birth requires emergent surgical exploration. The nonviable testicle should undergo orchiectomy while evidence of viability should prompt detorsion with orchidopexy. We recommend fixation of the contralateral testis, regardless of the condition of the affected testicle. In the case of bilateral torsion (both prenatal and postnatal), the threshold for performing bilateral orchidopexy should be lower in an effort to preserve testicular function. The most common scenario in the perinatal period is the case of prenatal torsion, in which the baby is found to have chronic changes and a nonviable testicle. These neonates should undergo elective orchiectomy with contralateral testis fixation once anesthesia risk assessment has been stabilized (within 1 to 2 days of diagnosis). Operative risk is a concern, but in a series of 27 patients with perinatal torsion who underwent exploration 2 hours to 2 months after birth, there were no surgery- or anesthesia-related complications (10). Regular follow-up is needed to assess testicular size and pubertal development, and the services of an endocrinologist should be considered when hormonal dysfunction is expected (e.g., bilateral torsion). The option for testicular prosthesis placement in childhood should be discussed with the parents of orchiectomy patients.

The principles of management for patients beyond infancy are similar to those for newborns, though the more acute presentation in the older group provides greater opportunity for testicular salvage. To reiterate, a history and physical exam consistent with testicular torsion demand immediate surgical exploration. Orchiectomy is needed for the nonviable testicle, while a viable testis should be untwisted and fixed to the scrotum. Orchidopexy should be performed to protect the contralateral testicle. Testicular prostheses are available for adults and can be placed during the initial operation or at a later date. Evidence of testicular atrophy should be noted during follow-up visits. Furthermore, it is important to discuss with patients the increased risk of subfertility.

## ALTERNATIVE THERAPY

Some clinicians recommend that manual detorsion should be attempted. Studies evaluating the success rate for manual detorsion have produced conflicting evidence. Clinicians who adopt this strategy must do so on the premise that it does not substitute for or delay surgery. Because the majority of testes twist inward (right testicle clockwise and left counterclockwise as viewed from the foot of the bed), manual detorsion should occur in the opposite direction. Nerve block of the spermatic cord can facilitate this maneuver, but it may also conceal the relief of detorsion or the pain of manipulation in the wrong direction. Successful manual detorsion should be followed by immediate surgical exploration.

While currently limited to animal models, medical adjuncts may one day be implemented, along with surgical management, to minimize the sequelae associated with testicular torsion. Pentoxifylline, a methyl xanthine derivative that decreases blood viscosity and platelet aggregation, appears to improve blood flow to both testes and unilateral torsion (11). Nitric oxide has been shown to have a protective effect against histopathologic change in the contralateral testicle, presumably through the regulation of blood flow (12).

## SURGICAL TECHNIQUE

Aside from the choice of incision, the surgical treatment for perinatal and childhood/adult (intravaginal) testicular torsions is essentially the same. For perinatal torsion, we use an inguinal approach on the affected side. The reason for doing so is that with extravaginal torsion (Fig. 67.3), there is a rare chance that another problem may exist, such as a hernia or tumor, that is best treated superior to the scrotum.

For intravaginal torsion, a vertical midline incision is our preferred approach to explore both testes. Two separate hemiscrotal incisions may also be used with excellent cosmetic results. Following incision to the level of the dartos muscles, the affected testis is moved under the midline incision. The layers of tunicae can be gently separated using a hemostat to minimize bleeding. The final few layers of tunicae are opened in a vertical fashion to expose the testis. A torsed testis usually appears dark blue or black (Fig. 67.4). Following manual detorsion, the testis is inspected for viability. If the viability of the testis is in question, the detorsed testis is wrapped in a warm moist sponge to recover while the contralateral testis is being pexed. If there still remains concern about the viability, a small nick can be made in the tunica albuginea to expose the seminiferous tubules, which should appear dusky to pink.

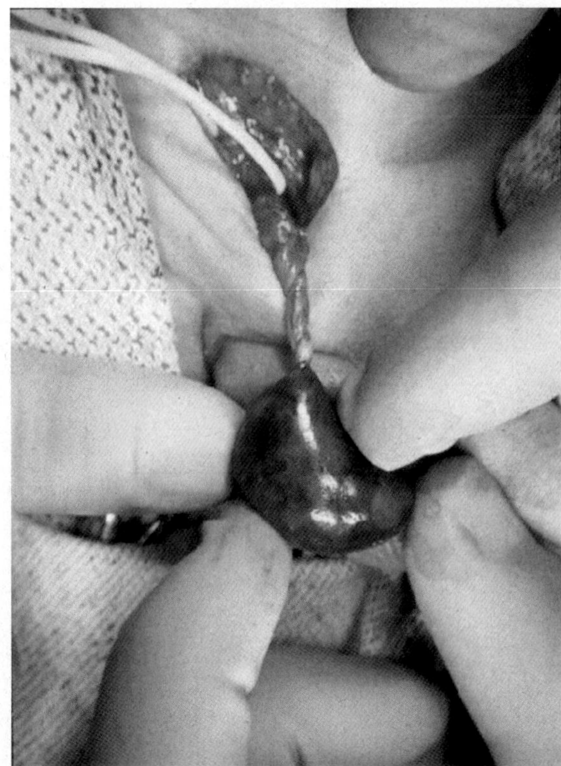

FIGURE 67.3 Exposure of the right spermatic cord and testicle through an inguinal incision reveals a case of extravaginal torsion.

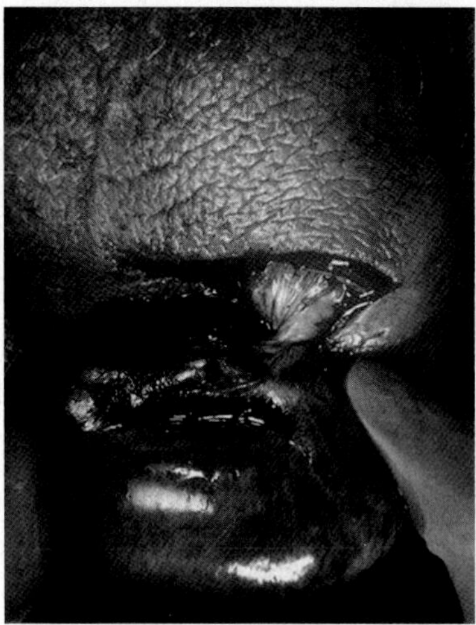

FIGURE 67.4 Intravaginal testicular torsion in an adolescent.

A nonviable testis should be removed to avoid possible continued symptoms and possible infection and to reduce the possibility of contralateral testicular damage from antisperm antibodies. We routinely do not place a testicular prosthesis at the time of orchiectomy. For the individuals who request a testicular prosthesis, we have performed delayed placement of solid silicone prostheses through a low inguinal incision.

The techniques for fixation of the viable detorsed testis and the contralateral testis still remain debated. Some of the controversy includes fixation with or without eversion of the tunica vaginalis, the use of absorbable or nonabsorbable suture, and fixation at two or three sites on the testis (13–15). We believe that the most important step in the fixation is the eversion of the tunica vaginalis (Fig. 67.5). This step produces two effects: (a) the testis is in an extravaginal position, and thus would not be at risk for intravaginal torsion; (b) everting the tunica vaginalis allows for contact between the tunica albuginea and the dartos. As an additional step, we perform two-point fixation of superior and inferior peritesticular tissue using absorbable (Vicryl) or nonabsorbable (Prolene) sutures.

## OUTCOMES

### Complications

The most significant complication of testicular torsion is infarction of the gonad. This event depends on the duration and degree of torsion and is managed by orchiectomy. A testicle that is viable at the time of surgery may later become atrophic despite orchidopexy, and it must be monitored closely by physical exam. Abnormal semen analysis and contralateral testicular apoptosis are also recognized sequelae following testicular torsion (16,17). Therefore, the risk of subfertility should be discussed with the patient. Although rare, torsion of a previously pexed testicle may occur.

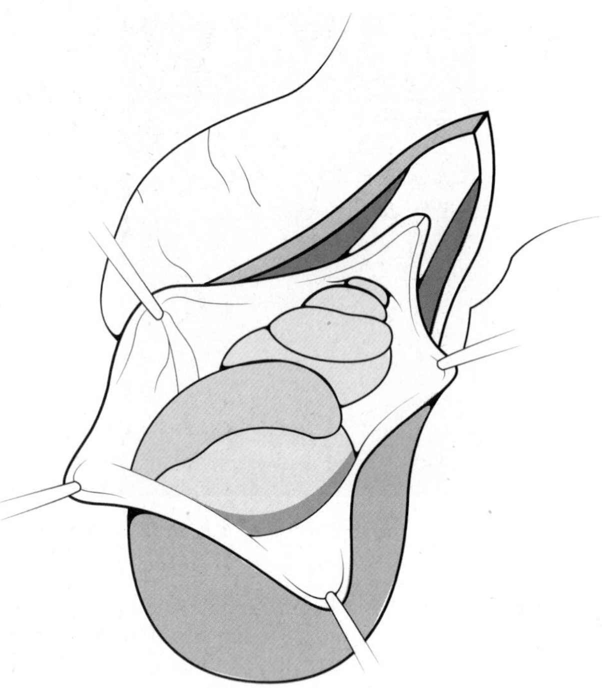

FIGURE 67.5 Scrotal incision with open tunica vaginalis reveals an intravaginal torsion.

## Results

The primary determinants of testicular viability are the degree to which the spermatic cord twists and the duration of torsion. The literature reports dismal salvage rates in newborns (as low as 5%); however, these accounts do not always distinguish between prenatal and postnatal torsion. Very few cases of testicular salvage have been reported with an antenatal event. An aggressive approach to postnatal torsion is likely to improve the rate of testicular salvage for this subset of patients, which was 20% in a recent study (10). Long-term assessment of fertility in patients with perinatal torsion is lacking.

Determining the duration of symptoms is easier in patients outside of the newborn age group, for obvious reasons. Workman and Kogan (18) found that patients who underwent surgery within 6 hours of onset had testicular salvage rates of 83% to 97%. This figure dropped to 55% to 85% between 6 and 12 hours of onset, and after 24 hours the salvage rate fell to <10%. These statistics are consistent throughout the literature. Notably, testicular salvage does not necessarily imply normal testicular function. A number of studies have demonstrated that men with testicular torsion are prone to subfertility and abnormalities of the contralateral testicle.

In summary, testicular torsion is a urologic emergency that is diagnosed clinically and treated by immediate surgical exploration. The decision to perform orchiectomy versus orchidopexy of the affected testicle is based on the viability of the testis at the time of exploration. In either case, contralateral orchidopexy should be performed. The anatomic abnormalities that predispose the patient to testicular torsion are well established; however, the mechanisms responsible for long-term testicular dysfunction and contralateral testicular damage are under investigation. Rates of testicular salvage have improved dramatically since the first recorded case of testicular torsion in 1840. With heightened awareness of the signs and symptoms on the part of patients and physicians, along with a better understanding of the pathophysiologic mechanisms, immediate and long-term outcomes of testicular torsion will continue to improve.

## *References*


1. Anderson J, Williamson R. Testicular torsion in Bristol: a 25 year review. *Br J Surg* 1988;75:988–992.
2. Melekos M, Asbach HW, Markou SA. Etiology of the acute scrotum with regard to age distribution. *J Urol* 1988;139:1023–1025.
3. Williamson RCN. Torsion of the testis and allied conditions. *Br J Surg* 1976;63:465–476.
4. Van Glabeke E, Khairouni A, Larroquet M, et al. Acute scrotal pain in children: results of 543 surgical explorations. *Pediatr Surg Int* 1999;15: 353–357.
5. Das S, Singer A. Controversies of perinatal torsion of the spermatic cord: a review, survey and recommendations. *J Urol* 1990;143:231–233.
6. Cuckow PM, Frank JD. Torsion of the testis. *BJU Int* 2000;86:349–353.
7. Kadish HA, Bolte RG. A retrospective review of pediatric patients with epididymitis, testicular torsion, and torsion of testicular appendages. *Pediatrics* 1998;102:73–76.
8. Turgut AT, et al. Acute painful scrotum. *Ultrasound Clin* 2008;3:93–107.
9. Gunther P, Schenk JP, Wunsch R, et al. Acute testicular torsion in children: the role of sonography in the diagnostic workup. *Eur Radiol* 2006;16: 2527–2532.
10. Pinto KJ, et al. Management of neonatal testicular torsion. *J Urol* 1997; 158:1196–1197.
11. Savas C, Dindar H, Aras T, et al. Pentoxifylline improves blood flow to both testes in testicular torsion. *Int Urol Nephrol* 2002;33:81–85.
12. Dokucu AI, Oztürk H, Ozdemir E, et al. The protective effects of nitric oxide on the contralateral testis in prepubertal rats with unilateral testicular torsion. *BJU Int* 2000; 85:767–771.
13. Bellinger MF, et al. Testicular torsion: late results with special regard to fertility and endocrine function. *J Urol* 1980;124:375–378.
14. Lent V, Stephani A. Eversion of the tunica vaginalis for prophylaxis of testicular torsion recurrences. *J Urol* 1993;150:1419–1421.
15. Rodriguez LE, Kaplan GW. An experimental study of methods to produce intrascrotal testicular fixation. *J Urol* 1988;139:565–567.
16. Bartsch G, Frank S, Marberger H, et al. Testicular torsion: late results with special regard to fertility and endocrine function. *J Urol* 1980;124: 375–378.
17. Hadziselimovic F, Geneto R, Emmons LR. Increased apoptosis in the contralateral testes of patients with testicular torsion as a factor for infertility. *J Urol* 1998;160: 1158–1160.
18. Workman SJ, Kogan BA. Old and new aspects of testicular torsion. *Semin Urol* 1988;6:146–157.

# CHAPTER 68 ■ SCROTAL TRAUMA AND RECONSTRUCTION

TIMOTHY O. DAVIES AND GERALD H. JORDAN

The anatomy of the male genitalia is quite complex. In the scrotum, there are multiple fascial layers (Fig. 68.1 and 68.2). From the standpoint of trauma, however, most of the fascial layers are relatively unimportant. The Buck's fascia is related to the deep penile structures and is important in the containment of periurethral processes or the occasional hematoma associated with injury to the corpora cavernosa and/or corpus spongiosum. In the scrotum, the analogous fascia to the Buck's fascia—the external spermatic fascia—is usually uninvolved with scrotal trauma (Fig. 68.2).

Culp (3) has classified injuries to the external male genitalia into five categories: nonpenetrating, penetrating, avulsions, burns, and radiation injuries (both direct and indirect). Nonpenetrating injuries result from either a crushing or sudden deforming force to the scrotum. These forces can cause severe damage to the internal structures without disrupting the skin. With any nonpenetrating trauma to the scrotum or perineum, one must suspect and rule out injury to the corpus spongiosum and urethra.

## DIAGNOSIS

Penetrating injuries to the genitalia frequently involve the urethra. Most of these injuries require exploration, irrigation, and removal of foreign-body material, if any, with anatomic repair and drainage (Level of Evidence, LOE 4) (4). If there is any suspicion of urethral injury, a retrograde urethrogram

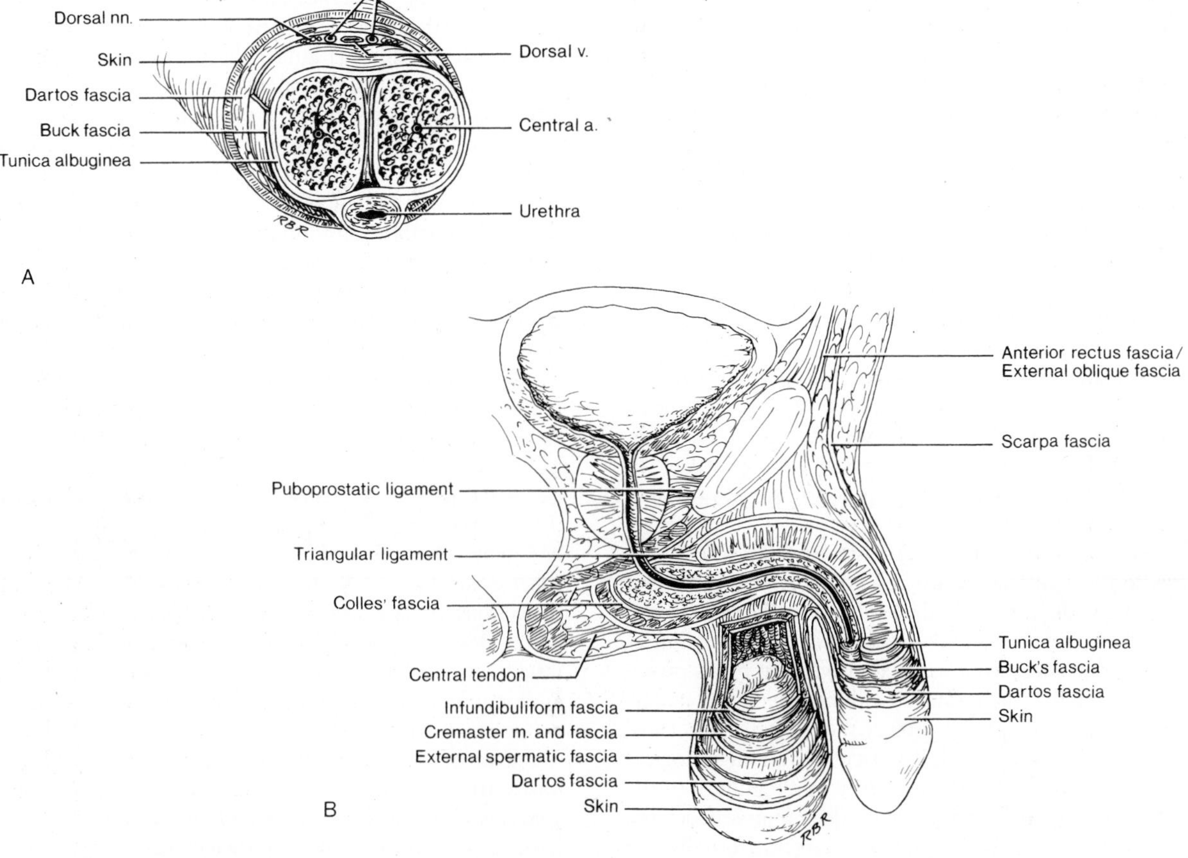


FIGURE 68.1 **A:** Cross section of the penis illustrating the fascial and structural components of the shaft of the penis. **B:** Sagittal section of the pelvis demonstrating the fascial layers and structural component.

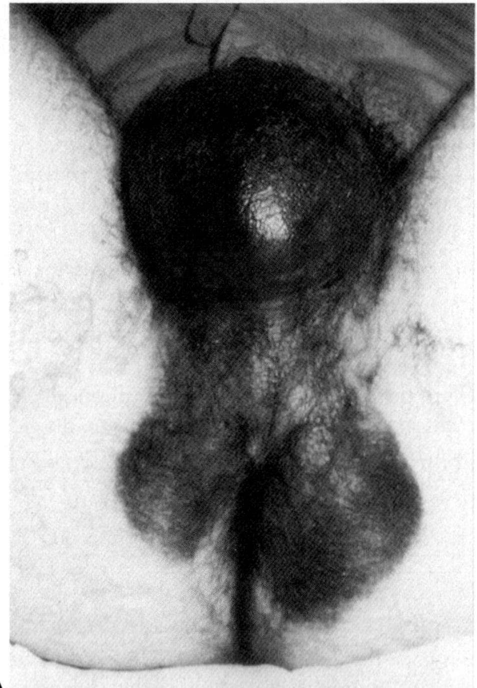


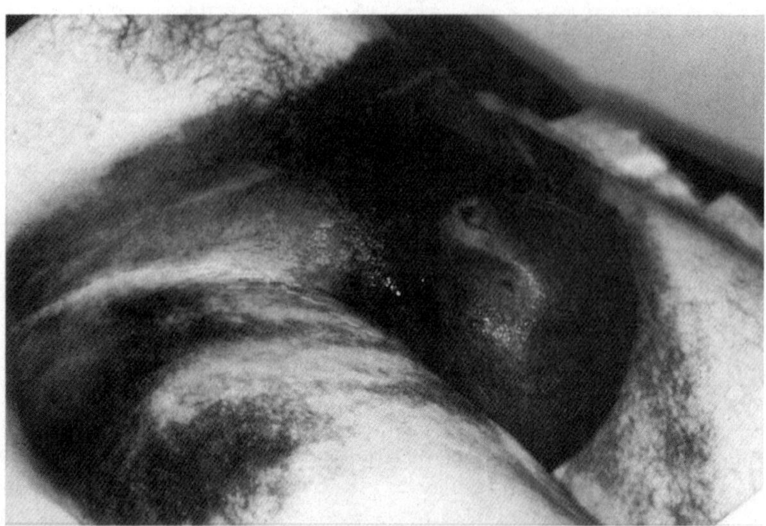


FIGURE 68.2 **A:** Perineal view of a trauma patient illustrating a hematoma contained by Colles fascia (classic butterfly hematoma). **B:** Same trauma patient illustrating the containment of the hematoma by the extended Colles layer, that is, the fascia lata of the thigh and extending onto the abdomen beneath the Scarpa fascia.

should be performed, and cystoscopy should be performed if further clarification of the injury is required. Saline should be used for irrigation in these cases. Because of the position of the urethra beneath the scrotum and perineum, significant penetrating injuries to the scrotum can also often miss the urethra.

Avulsion injuries of the genital skin most frequently involve the scrotal skin and occur when the patient's clothing becomes entangled in machinery. The loose scrotal tissues ensnare, and as the clothing is ripped off, so is the loose genital skin. These avulsion injuries vary from minimal injuries, which are essentially nothing more than lacerations, to emasculating injuries, which take not only the skin but also the deep structures. Usually, the deep penile structures are not avulsed, as the injury, fortunately, takes only the skin and the dartos fascia/tunica dartos, leaving the underlying Buck's fascia of the penis and the fascial layers surrounding the testicle intact. Occasionally, the testicle ensnares in the skin and is avulsed. In most cases of avulsion, bleeding is not a problem, as the skin and fascia are avulsed in a plane between the fascial structures related to the deep structures and the superficial fascia.

Burns to the genitalia are usually not isolated injuries but reflective of a wider area of body burn. Chemical burns are in general only superficial and involve the skin. Thermal injuries can be deep, but often, even with extensive deep burns proximate to the genitalia, the multiple clothing layers (i.e., underwear and other clothing) can protect the genitalia. Electrical burns disseminate via the deep vascular and neurological structures, and what may appear to be a minimal burn to the skin and scrotum may have significant deep injury associated with it, and this can be devastating. However, usually the deepest burns associated with electrical contact occur at the site of the current inflow and the ground site. These sites are usually not the genitalia. However, it is not uncommon to have thermal burns in concert with electrical burns, as frequently the clothing is ignited by the electrical spark. Thus, with electrical burns, fortunately, if the genitalia are involved it is usually a more superficial process.

Radiation injuries to the genitalia can occur either from direct exposure to the genitalia or from the effects of radiation on the venous and lymphatic drainage. Now, by and large, we do not see complications of direct radiation to the genitalia, as radiation for penile lesions is rarely undertaken. The secondary effects of radiation, as seen in the scrotum, are usually manifested by chronic lymphedema, lymphangiectasia, and, in some cases, chronic recurring cellulitis.

To this list of traumas must be added the patient who has required significant debridement because of rapidly progressive, multiorganism fasciitis (Fournier's gangrene). Fournier's gangrene is often seen with processes of the anus or rectum, such as missed perianal abscess. Likewise, processes involving the urethra, such as periurethral abscess, can accompany Fournier's gangrene. Many times Fournier's gangrene is associated with other comorbidities, such as diabetes mellitus. Many of these patients present late, and aggressive surgical debridement (LOE 2), while lifesaving, usually leaves a significant defect (4). If the fasciitis is associated with pathophysiology of the urethra and/or anus, then these situations must be managed and resolved before reconstruction (5). Recently there have been descriptions of the use of unprocessed honey to augment or provide an alternative treatment to wide surgical excision. Honey apparently contains antimicrobial agents and enzymes to digest necrotic tissue as well as to promote epithelial growth (6).

Also, in recent years we have seen several patients who have attempted to enhance the size and bulk of their genitalia

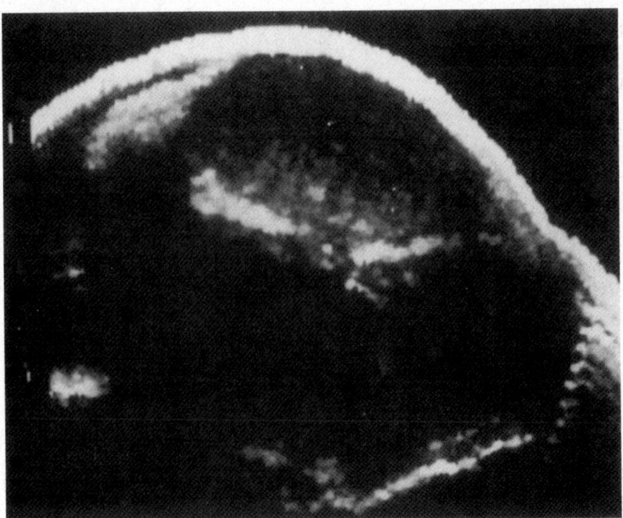

FIGURE 68.3 B-scan ultrasound demonstrating the classic distribution of a scrotal contusion (scrotal wall hematoma). Note the testis displaced anteriorly, with the hematoma contained in the multiple fascial layers of the scrotum.

with the injection of lipid-containing substances such as paraffin or petroleum jelly or inert substances such as silicone. In these cases, one is often confronted with a fulminant cellulitis that must be treated with broad-spectrum antibiotics. Later, one sees a sclerosing granulomatous process that can be troubling to the patients. In some cases, the skin must be excised along with the deeper involved structures, but it is not unusual to be able to excise the deep process and leave the skin that survives either on its random dermal blood supply or, in some cases, on the tunica dartos fasciocutaneous blood supply.

A contusion of the scrotum, that is, scrotal hematoma, can be confused with a fracture of the testicle. The latter injury implies disruption of the tunica albuginea and visceral tunica vaginalis of the testicle. With a scrotal contusion the hematoma usually is noted to be posterior and lateral to the testicle (Fig. 68.3), whereas with fracture of the testicle the parenchyma of the testis is not normal and is often associated with a hematocele (Fig. 68.4). Physical examination remains the cornerstone in the diagnosis of blunt testicular trauma. However, the

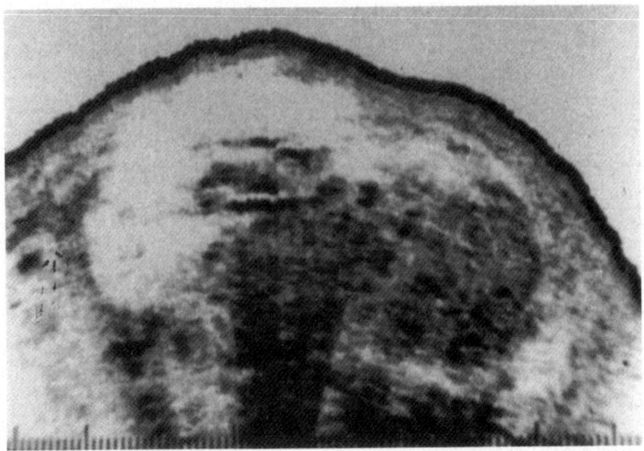

FIGURE 68.4 B-scan ultrasound of a patient with a fracture of the testicle. Note the disrupted parenchymal pattern of the testicle, the hematocele, and the demonstration of extruded seminiferous tubules within the hematocele.

use of ultrasonography in the diagnosis of testicular trauma can be helpful in situations when the physical examination is difficult to perform or interpret. Ultrasonography is the most sensitive and specific imaging technique, with heterogeneity of the parenchyma of the testicle suggestive of testicular rupture (LOE 2) (4). In the presence of penetrating trauma to the genitalia, a retrograde urethrogram is always indicated because of the close proximity to the urethra. In all cases of genital avulsion, other than a simple scrotal avulsion, a complete evaluation of the urethra must be done, along with a rectal examination and possibly flexible sigmoidoscopy.

## INDICATIONS FOR SURGERY

Exploration of the scrotum is indicated if the patient has sustained either blunt or penetrating injury to the testicle (LOE 3) (4). Scrotal reconstruction is required following complex lacerations and avulsion injuries. If a patient has required excision for chronic cellulitis, lymphangiectasia, and lymphedema, split-thickness skin graft reconstruction of the scrotum is very effective and provides cosmetically very acceptable results. If the lymphedematous process is due to a local process, then often the lateral scrotum and the posterior scrotum are free of the process because the lymphatic drainage is lateral and often uninvolved. In these cases lateral scrotal flap reconstruction is often very effectively employed.

If, however, the process causing the scrotal lymphedema is "systemic" (i.e., Charles's disease, secondary to pelvic irradiation, etc.), then Split-thickness Skin Graft (STSG) reconstruction is always the best approach. The lymphatics of the skin are carried in the reticular dermis (the deep layer of the dermis). If a thick STSG is used to reconstruct the genitalia, in cases of lymphedema, thelymphedema can significantly recur in the graft. One must be careful of the patient with scrotal lymphedema without "involvement of the penile skin"; following scrotal reconstruction, often the penile skin becomes edematous. Following burn injury to the genitalia, almost always graft reconstruction can be undertaken, and it offers extremely good functional and cosmetic results.

## ALTERNATIVE THERAPY

Contusions of the scrotum are usually treated with bedrest, analgesia, and scrotal elevation. Scrotal elevation can be accomplished very efficiently with a Bellevue-style (a taped suspensory dressing to elevate the scrotum) bridge or with scrotal support.

## SURGICAL TECHNIQUE

### Scrotal Hematomas and Blunt Testicular Injury

There is little to be accomplished in exploring the scrotal hematoma secondary to external blunt trauma, as the hematoma is usually disseminated throughout the highly elastic layers of the scrotum and does not form a drainable hematoma per se (3). On the other hand, if there is a testicular

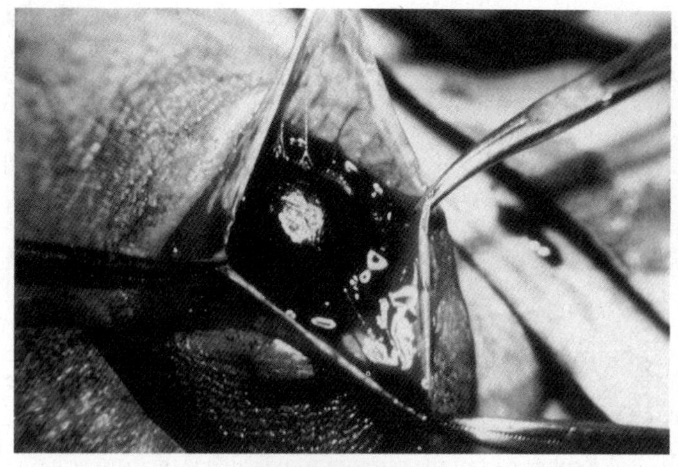

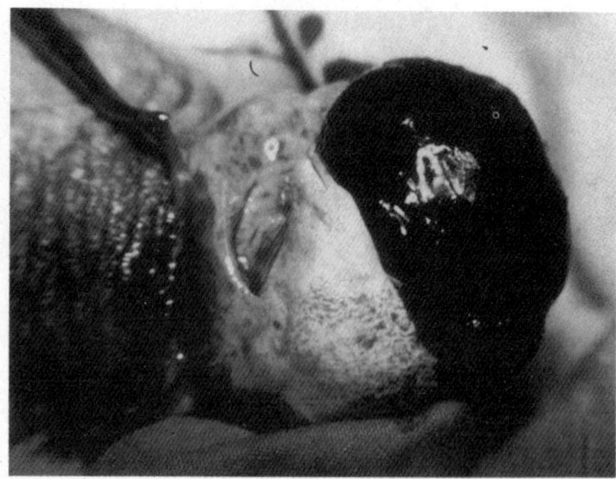

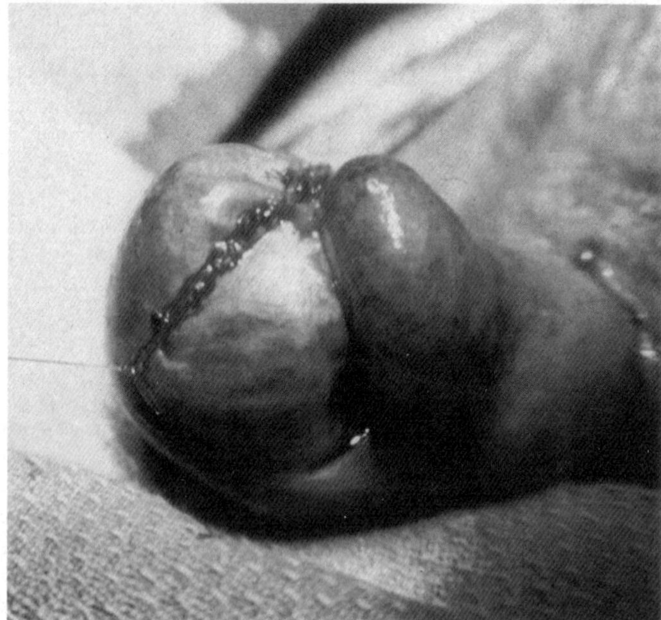

FIGURE 68.5 **A:** Patient with fractured testicle; the skin has been opened, as has the vaginal space. Note the draining hematocele fluid with clots affixed to the seminiferous tubules. **B:** The testicle has been delivered. Note the clot attached to the extruded tubules. **C:** Appearance of the testicle following repair.

injury, exploration and repair of the testicle are indicated (Fig. 68.5). Exploration consists of exposure of the testicle. The space of the tunica vaginalis is opened, the hematocele is drained, seminiferous tubules are debrided, and the tunica albuginea is closed. The remaining viable testicular tissue should be salvaged for endocrine function and psychological impact (LOE 2) (4). In the past, polyglycolic (PGA) suture was used; however, now we use polydioxanone suture, although Monocryl is also an option. The parietal tunica vaginalis is left open and is reflected as would have been done for a hydrocele. The scrotum is drained and closed with 3-0 PGA suture, chromic suture, or Monocryl. Alternatively, in cases of testicular fracture secondary to either blunt or penetrating injury, rather than using aggressive debridement and primary closure of the tunica albuginea, one can close the testis with a tunica vaginalis graft or island.

## Penetrating Injuries to the Genitalia

Penetrating injuries have been subclassified as either simple or complicated. By and large, complicated injuries imply urethral involvement, amputation, or near-total amputation; and with regard to the scrotum they imply amputation of or injury to the testicle, with or without amputation of the overlying scrotal skin (Fig. 68.6). Simple lacerations are managed with primary closure and drainage, if indicated. In the case of amputation of the testicles, testicular microreplantation has been performed, including vasovasostomy, along with reapproximation of the vasculature of the spermatic cord (Fig. 68.7). The testicle is placed, as quickly as possible, in a sterile bag in saline-soaked gauze, and that bag is placed in a second bag filled with saline slush for cold preservation. Unlike amputation of the penis, where successful replantation has been done as long as 18 to 24 hours from the injury, the testicle must be replanted by 6 to 8 hours due to the very high metabolic rate of the testicular tissue.

There can be some difficulty in identifying the vessels in the spermatic cord, although they are somewhat compartmentalized. Identifying the artery proximally is not difficult, and identification of the distal artery in the severed organ can be aided by examining the relationship of the compartments to the vas deferens. Coaptation of the artery and a number of veins is optimal using 9-0 or 10-0 Prolene, depending on the

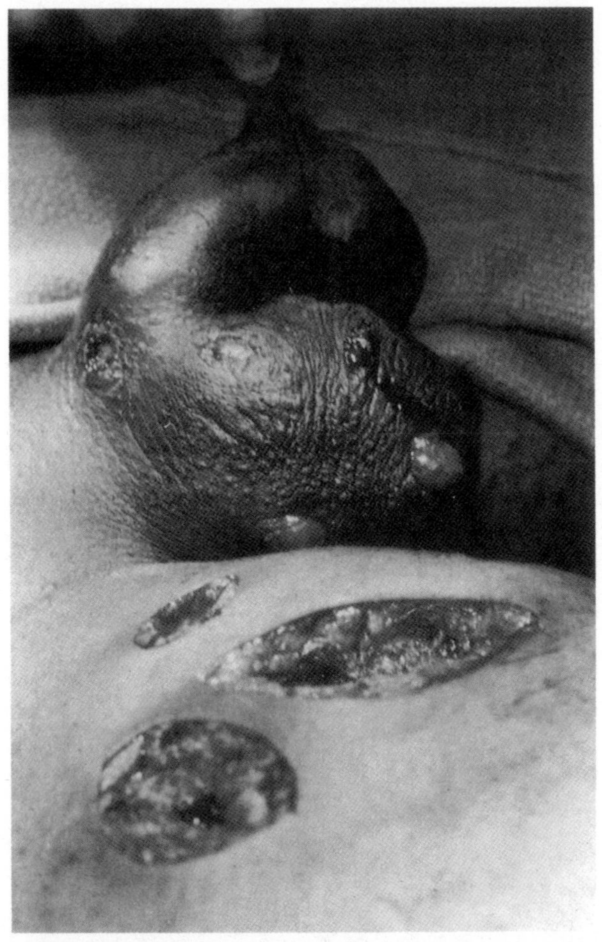

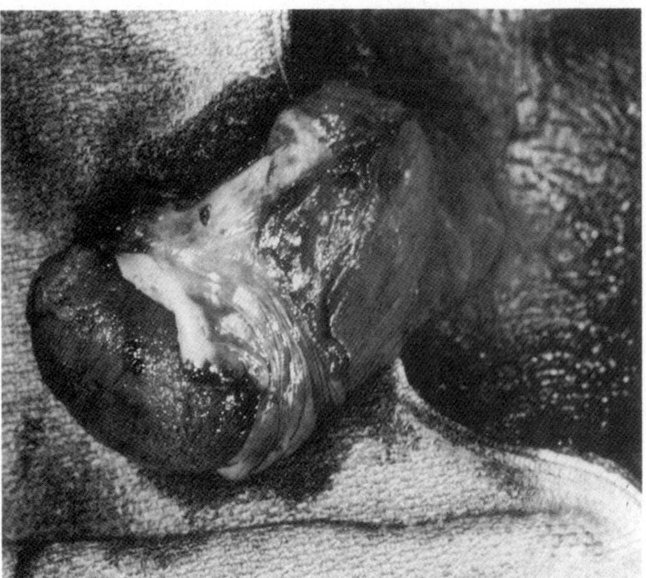

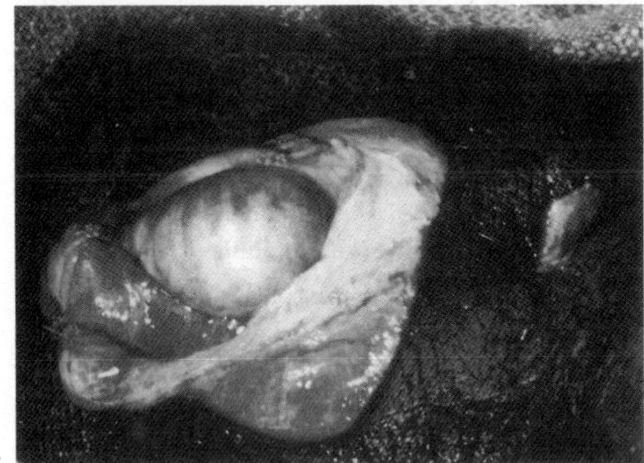

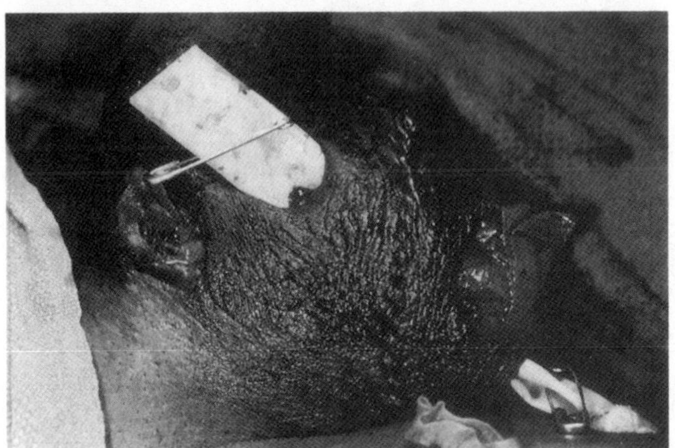

FIGURE 68.6 **A:** Young patient with complex penetrating trauma to the thigh and genitalia. Retrograde urethrogram, rectal examination, and flexible sigmoidoscopy were normal. The patient's scrotum was explored. **B:** The patient's right testicle is delivered; note the intact seminiferous tubule pattern with virtual complete disruption of the tunica albuginea. **C:** Appearance of the same testicle *(B)* following reconstruction of the tunica albuginea with primary closure. **D:** Appearance of the genitalia with the gunshot wounds debrided and the right hemiscrotum drained. Dr. Michael Coburn, Baylor University, Department of Urology, Personal Communication, (January 16, 2009, Norfolk, Virginia) has assembled a series of patients with similar injuries to that illustrated. In those cases, the testicle was closed with a parietal tunica vaginalis patch. He reports good results with this technique.

size of the respective vessels. Vasovasostomy can be done using 9-0 or 10-0 Prolene or nylon sutures, either with a classic microscopic two-layer technique or a single-layer "tricorner" technique, depending on the surgeon's preference.

If possible, the testicle should not be covered with a graft but either placed in a thigh pouch and later liberated or, if there is some remaining redundancy of the scrotum, covered primarily with reapproximation of the remaining scrotal tissues.

Obviously, if the patient arrives without his amputated testicle, then hemostasis must be ensured. Usually the vessels are in spasm, but they clearly can come out of spasm later. The wound should be irrigated and, if contaminated, packed to be closed by secondary intention. If the wound is clean, then primary closure or primary grafting can be performed.

## Avulsion Injuries

Small scrotal avulsions are managed as simple lacerations with either primary or delayed closure and drainage, as would be indicated for any laceration (LOE 3; Fig. 68.8) (4). For larger injuries, the emergency management consists of allowing the

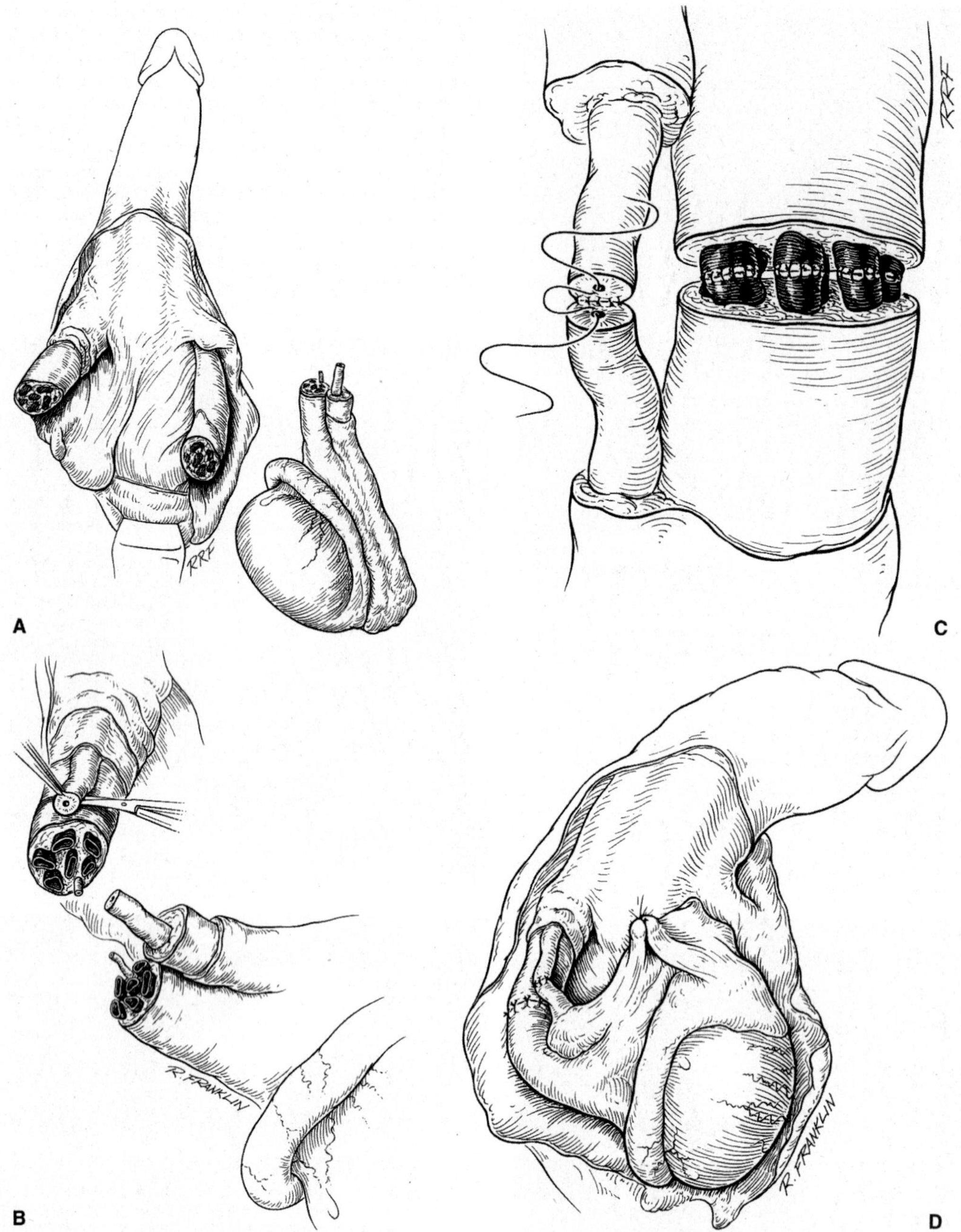


**FIGURE 68.7** **A:** Appearance of a patient following bilateral testicular amputation and scrotal amputation. The patient presented with only his right testicle. The left testicle could not be found at the trauma scene. **B:** The right testicle is reanastomosed to the left (longer) spermatic cord. **C:** Note the appearance of the debrided spermatic cord and the debrided distal spermatic cord going to the testicle. Vasovasostomy was performed with a two-layer microscopic technique. Microscopic coaptation of the spermatic artery and multiple spermatic veins was performed. **D:** Appearance of the replanted testicle before closure of the scrotum.

injury to completely demarcate (Fig. 68.9). The area of the avulsed scrotum should be managed with cold saline packs and observed over 12 to 24 hours. Clear demarcation will occur and allow the surgeon to debride only the tissue that is nonviable. Debridement with closure is then performed (LOE 3) (4).

If a primary closure cannot be accomplished with the remaining scrotal tissue, then the surgeon has several options. One option is to place the testicles in thigh pouches to be later liberated and later replaced to the area of the scrotum. The preferable option is to perform a primary reconstruction of the scrotum using a mesh split-thickness skin graft. The graft should be harvested 0.016 to 0.018 in. thick and then meshed on a 1.5- to 1.0- meshing template. The testicles must be fixed in position using permanent suture or absorbable suture that is slowly absorbed so that they do not migrate beneath the

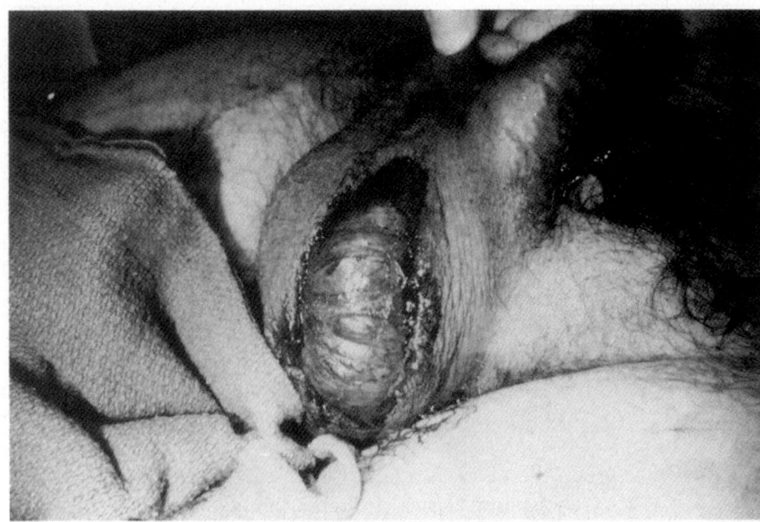
A

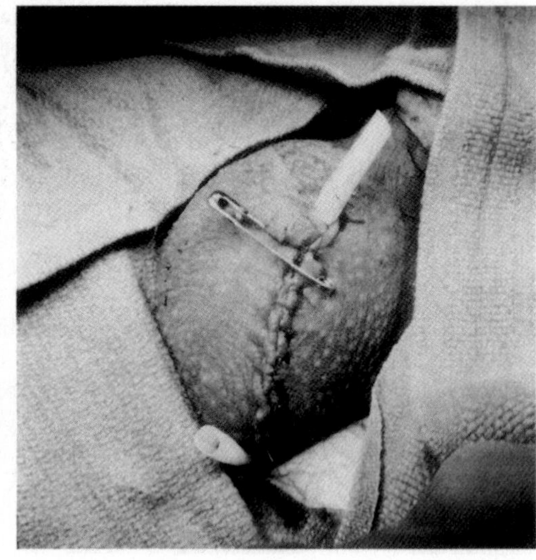
B

FIGURE 68.8 **A:** Appearance of a left scrotal avulsion injury. The patient was injured in a motorcycle accident in which his trousers were ripped off as he departed the motorcycle. **B:** Appearance after closure. Primary closure is performed with drainage.

graft. The meshing of the graft allows for escape of serum and blood products from beneath the graft, but it also allows the graft to configure to the complex contours of the underlying testicles. The vaginal space is left open, and the parietal tunica vaginalis is reflected to fix the testicle in place. The graft is then applied immediately to the testicles, suturing it to the surrounding skin. It is the opinion of some authors that grafting directly on the visceral tunica vaginalis or tunica albuginea can lead to a situation where there is chronic testicular pain. This has not been the author's (GHJ) experience. Unless the wound is markedly contaminated, cases so managed have yielded very successful results.

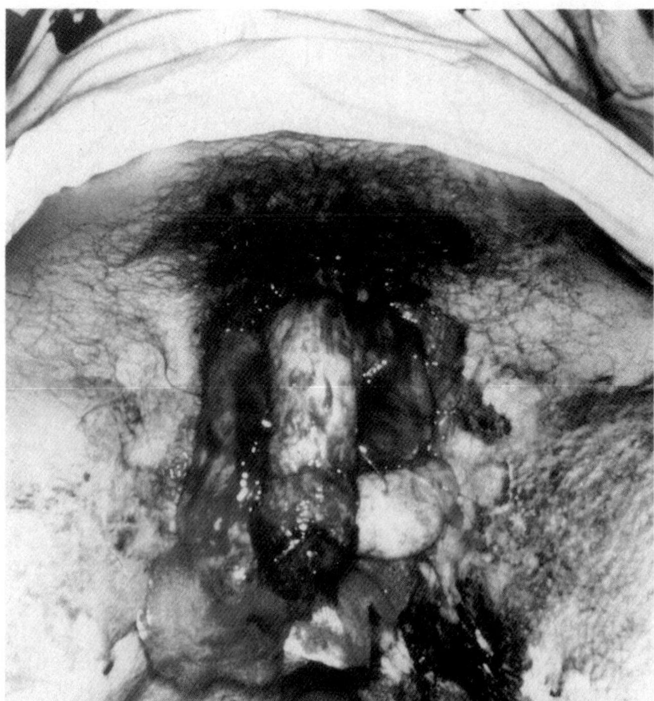
A

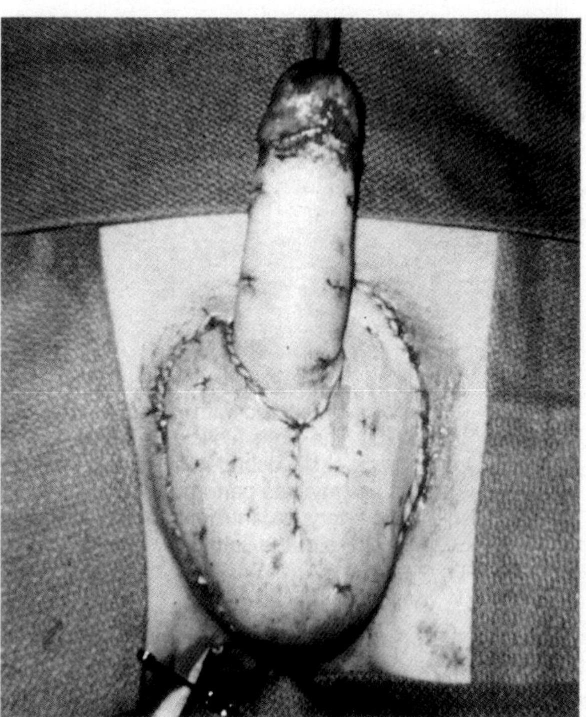
B

FIGURE 68.9 **A:** Large avulsion injury of the genitalia. The patient was injured when his clothing was ensnared in the power takeoff mechanism of a tractor. Note the exposed shaft of the penis and the exposed testicles bilaterally. **B:** The appearance after reconstruction with a split-thickness skin graft. The patient was observed for 24 hours, allowing the wounds to demarcate. In this case, both the shaft of the penis and the scrotum were reconstructed with a sheet split-thickness skin graft.

The grafts should be bolstered using Xeroform gauze or one of the other commercially available fine meshed gauzes applied directly to the graft, with Dacron batting soaked in saline and mineral oil placed over the finely meshed gauze. Lately we have favored the use of the high-density polyethylene sheeting (N-Terface, Richardson, TX 75083–2297, Winfield Laboratories, Inc.) to prevent adherence and subsequent graft displacement with bolster removal. The bolster is held in place with 4-0 chromic sutures. Unless there is an associated urethral injury, the patient can be "diverted" with a soft Foley catheter. In patients in whom the avulsion injury extends near to the anus, colostomy may be required. It must be emphasized that local skin flaps are not recommended for primary closure in these cases.

Should the testicles be avulsed, replantation is not an option. During the avulsion injury, the vasculature is stretched before giving way to the force, and the endothelial damage can be significant and unpredictable.

In patients in whom the avulsion injury is tantamount to emasculation, these injuries are often associated with significant injuries to the adjacent tissue. Reconstruction assumes a very secondary position, as these patients require lifesaving steps. The vast majority of these patients will require colostomy, suprapubic cystostomy, and multiple dressing changes over the posttrauma course, and they often present with significant bleeding.

In general, the scrotal skin is highly distensible, and even a small fragment can be expanded to cover a large defect with a good functional result. There has been concern regarding the effect of implantation of the testes in thigh pockets on spermatogenesis, although there are few clinical data to support this concern.

## Genital Burns

The emergency therapy of genital burns is similar to that for any burn. The scrotum can be dressed, open, with topical antibiotic ointments such as Silvadene, or a closed antibiotic dressing regimen can be used. The integrity of the urethra must be determined when the patient presents. A Foley catheter can be placed in the patient who has burns to his genitalia. If there is evidence of urethral burn, then most would suggest diversion with suprapubic cystostomy. If the burns to the genital and perineal area are extensive, then an occasional patient will require colostomy. If the subscrotal urethra is involved in the burn, no attempt at initial reconstruction should be made. In the case of the infant or young male, the move to a suprapubic tube should be made quickly if the need for a urethral catheter is at all prolonged.

The genital tissues are remarkably vascular. Debridement of the genitalia, in general, should be accomplished carefully. Aggressive debridement should be avoided, as many of the tissues will recover and are nonreproducible. Whirlpools and tank soaks are useful for gentle debridement and cleansing, and they may be done early on, two to three times per day.

Chemical burns rarely involve the structures deep to the skin and are managed with copious irrigation and then as with a thermal burn (LOE 4). If a patient has evidence of an electrical burn to the area of the genitalia, the patient must be observed for 12 to 24 hours and then explored. In electrical burns, the initial management is aimed at debridement, and reconstruction can be offered later as the situation dictates (Fig. 68.10).

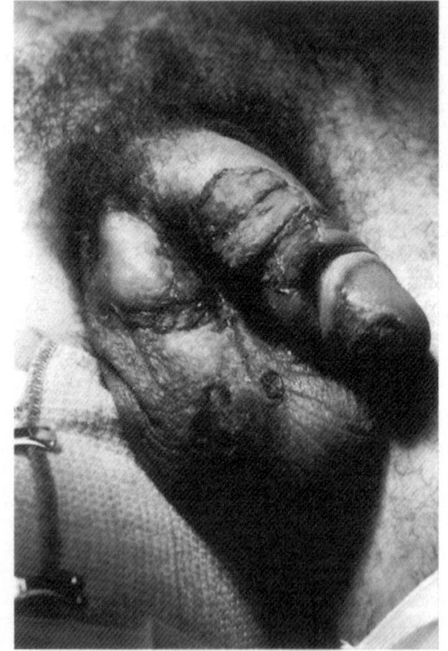
A

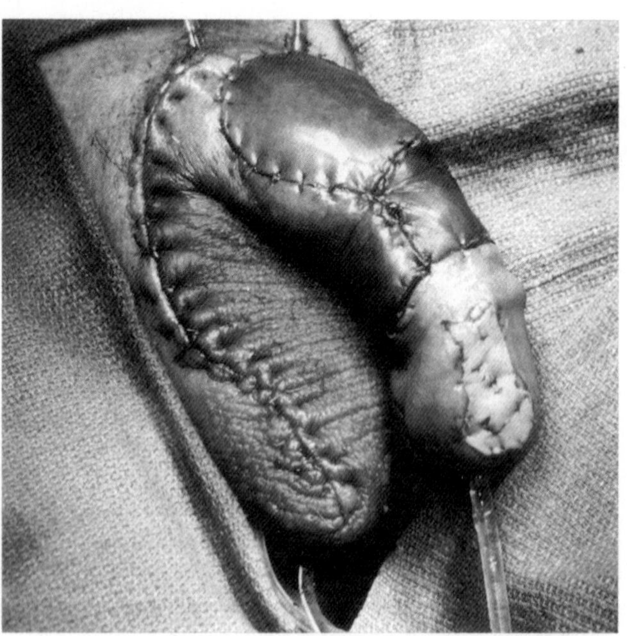
B

FIGURE 68.10 **A:** The appearance of the genitalia in a patient who was burned in a steam-line accident. Note the burns to the glans, the dorsum of the shaft of the penis, and the right hemiscrotum. **B:** In this particular case, reconstruction of the glans was accomplished with a small split-thickness skin graft. Reconstruction of the shaft of the penis was accomplished with a penile skin island flap; the patient was uncircumcised, and the ventral skin was mobilized to the dorsum. The scrotal burn was completely excised, and primary reconstruction of the right hemiscrotum was accomplished. This particular patient demonstrates all of the possibilities for reconstruction following burn debridement.

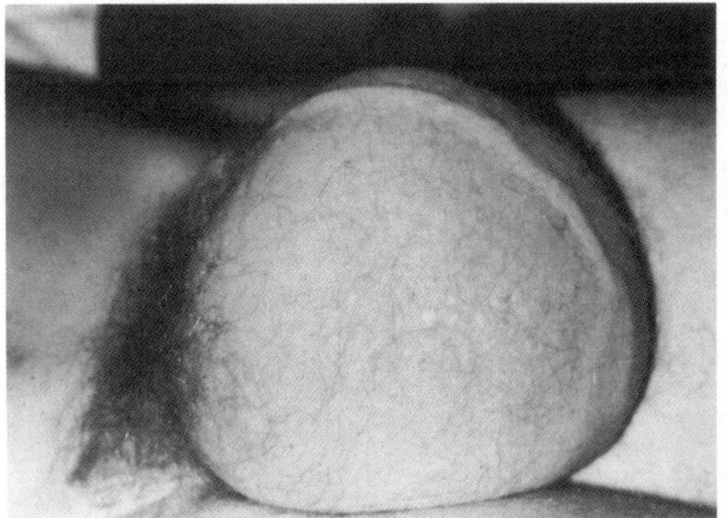

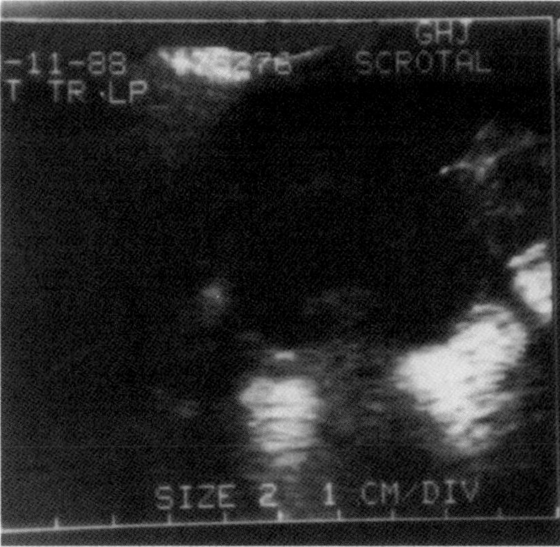


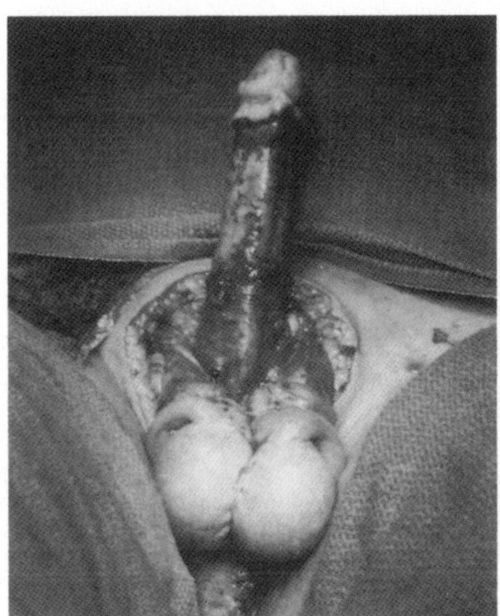

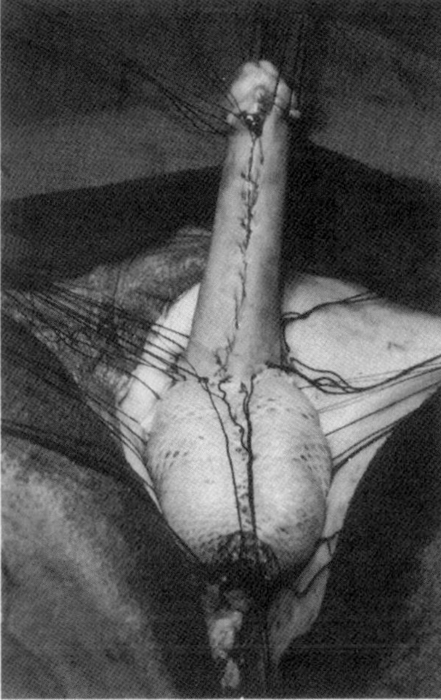

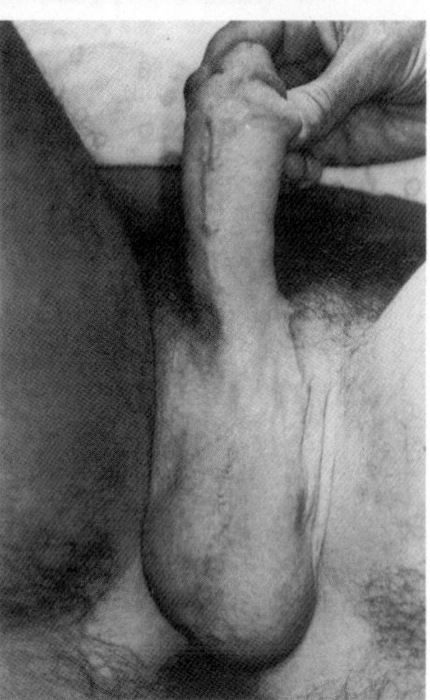

FIGURE 68.11 Appearance of a young man with chronic genital lymphedema following irradiation therapy for Hodgkin lymphoma. **A:** Appearance of the massively lymphedematous scrotum. **B:** B-scan ultrasound demonstrating the large hydrocele. Note the normal testis posteriorly. **C:** Appearance of the genitalia after debridement of the lymphedematous tissue. Note that orchidopexy has been performed. **D:** Immediate appearance following reconstruction of the shaft of the penis with a split-thickness skin graft and reconstruction of the scrotum with a meshed split-thickness skin graft. **E:** Appearance of that same patient 6 months postoperatively. Note the small amount of residual lymphedema of the preputial cuff. Further note the redundant appearance of the scrotal graft.

## Radiation Injuries

In the case of scrotal lymphedema and recurrent cellulitis, all layers of the scrotum should be excised, to the level of the external spermatic fascia (Fig. 68.11). It is not uncommon for the patient also to have large hydroceles (2).

The vaginal space should be opened and the parietal tunica vaginalis then reflected and incorporated in the orchidopexy. Reconstruction can be accomplished, using split-thickness skin grafts, as already discussed, and on the scrotum these grafts can be meshed as discussed earlier. In addition, the meshing seems to improve the cosmetic result by giving the appearance of the normal scrotal rugations (1). Full-thickness skin grafts should not be used. The cosmetic results achieved in these patients, so reconstructed, are excellent. The use of lateral scrotal flaps as mentioned previously is worthy of consideration in properly selected patients (Fig. 68.12). Radiated patients in general are not candidates, as the problem is with the "systemic" lymphatic drainage and not just the lymphatics of the skin per se.

## Fournier's Gangrene

If the primary process has resulted in extensive debridement of the scrotum, the testicles can be placed in thigh pouches with the intention of later replacing the testicles in their normal

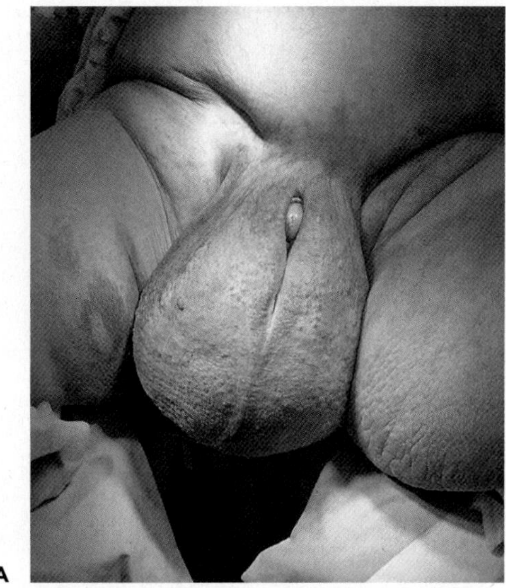


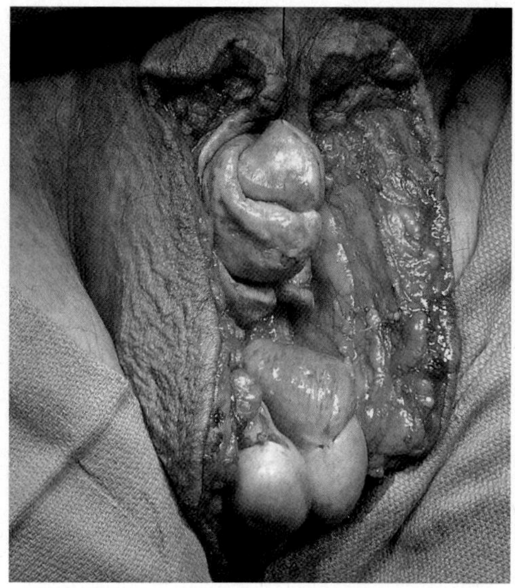


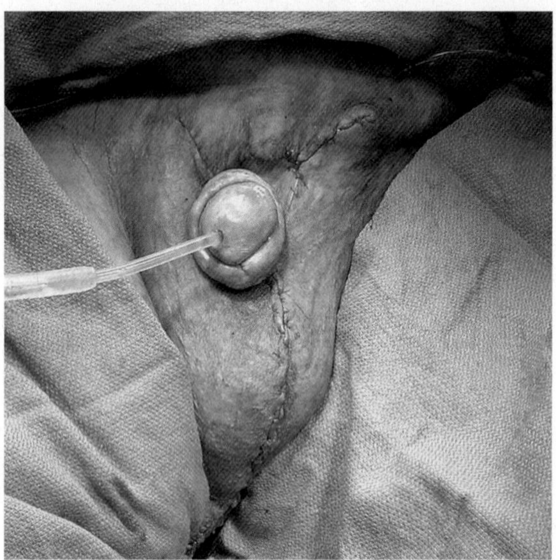

FIGURE 68.12 **A:** Preoperative appearance of a chronically lymphedematous scrotum. **B:** Intraoperative appearance following the resection of the lymphademateous scrotum, exposed testicles, and lateral scrotal flaps. **C:** Immediate postoperative appearance of the closure of the scrotum in the midline using lateral scrotal flaps.

anatomic area and for scrotal reconstruction. The author's (GHJ) preferred approach was described by McDougal and is illustrated in Fig. 68.13. The lateral defects on the thigh can often be closed *per primam* or can be grafted.

For most patients, however, the scrotal excisions do not necessitate placing the testicles in thigh pouches, but instead they can be dressed in the wound (7). These patients often require multiple dressing changes and wet-to-dry debridements. These techniques can be used in combination with negative pressure dressings or vacuum-assisted closure (VAC) devices to reduce the defect size more quickly. When reconstruction is undertaken, the testicles must be fixed in their normal anatomic position. It is my custom to open the parietal tunica vaginalis and reflect it, and, as already described, graft techniques can be utilized to restore the scrotum. Although local flaps can be used, the cosmetic results achieved with local flaps are usually less than optimal in most of these circumstances when compared to reconstruction techniques utilizing split-thickness skin grafts. Interestingly, these mesh split-thickness skin grafts not only remain supple, but in many cases (as has been shown), will actually become redundant.

## OUTCOMES

### Complications

Complications of scrotal trauma and reconstruction are primarily related to inadequate appreciation of the degree of injury with subsequent necrosis of additional skin. It is important for the surgeon to adequately debride the devitalized skin, which may require more than one trip to the operating room. The failure of a skin graft to take is usually a result of technical errors such as accumulation of fluid under the graft, inadequately prepared graft bed, or continual slippage of the graft over the bed, which does not allow capillary ingrowth.

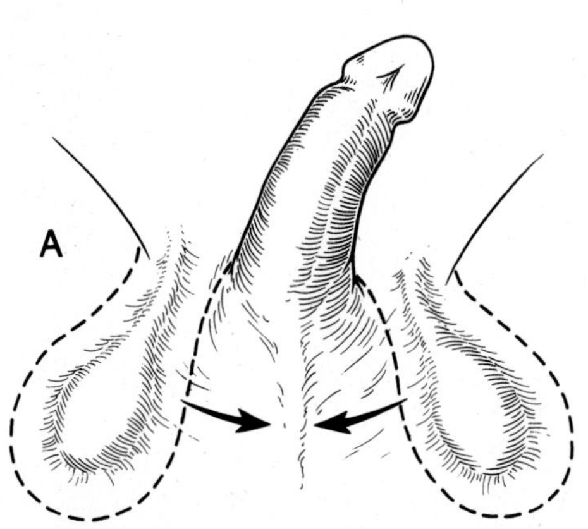


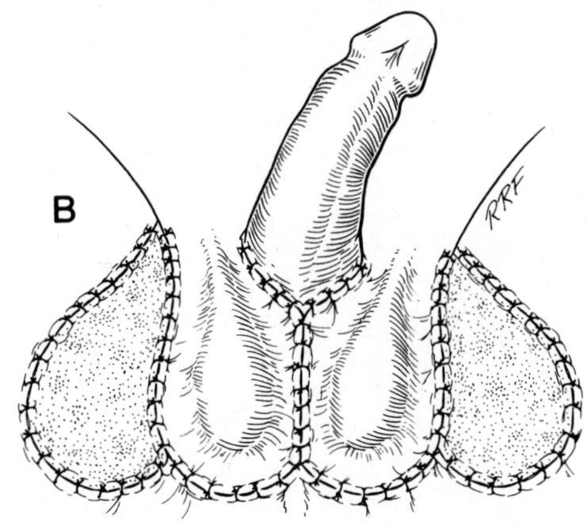


FIGURE 68.13 Technique after McDougal for liberation of testicles that have been placed in thigh pouches. Note that the testicles are mobilized with random thigh skin flaps and transposed to the midline to reconstruct the scrotum. The lateral defects can be closed *per primam* or can be grafted.

## Results

As with most surgical conditions, prompt diagnosis and management of acute testicular injuries is paramount to maintaining testicular function. Burns, avulsion, and radiation injuries require aggressive debridement of devitalized tissue to minimize infection and to prepare a healthy graft bed. Reconstruction of the scrotal skin, most often performed with meshed STSG, offers excellent graft take and survival with acceptable cosmetic results in closing the resultant defect.

## *References*


1. Arneri V. Reconstruction of the male genitalia. In: Converse J, ed. *Reconstructive plastic surgery*, 2nd ed. Philadelphia: WB Saunders, 1977: 3902–3921.
2. Charles RH. The surgical technique and operative treatment of elephantiasis of the generative organs based on a series of 140 consecutive successful cases. *Ind Med Gaz* 1901;36:84.
3. Culp D, Genital Injuries: Etiology and Initial Management. *Urol Clinics* NA 1977; 4 (1): 143–156.
4. Jordan GH, Gilbert DA. Male genital trauma. *Clin Plast Surg* 1988; 15:431.
5. Morey AF, Metro MJ, Carney KJ, et al. Consensus on genitourinary trauma: external genitalia. *BJU Int* 2004;94(4):507–515.
6. Jordan GH, Gilbert DA. Management of amputation injuries of the male genitalia. *Urol Clin North Am* 1989;16:359–367.
7. Tahmaz L, Erdemir F, Kibar Y, et al. Fournier's gangrene: Report of thirty-three cases and a review of the literature. *Int J Urol* 2006;13:960–967.
8. Jordan GH, Schlossberg SM, Devine CJ. Surgery of the penis and urethra. In: Walsh PC, et al., eds. *Campbell's urology*, 7th ed., Vol. 3. Philadelphia: WB Saunders, 1997:3316–3394.
9. McDougal WS, Persley L. Traumatic Injuries of the Genitourinary System. *International Perspective in Urology*, Vol. 1. Baltimore/London, 1981:43.

# CHAPTER 69 ■ ANATOMY OF THE PENIS AND SCROTUM

SAM D. GRAHAM, JR.

The penis is composed of three columnar bodies, a pair of which are larger, dorsally located, and extend the length of the penis (Fig. 69.1). These two columnar bodies contain cavernosal vascular tissue and are called the corpora cavernosa.

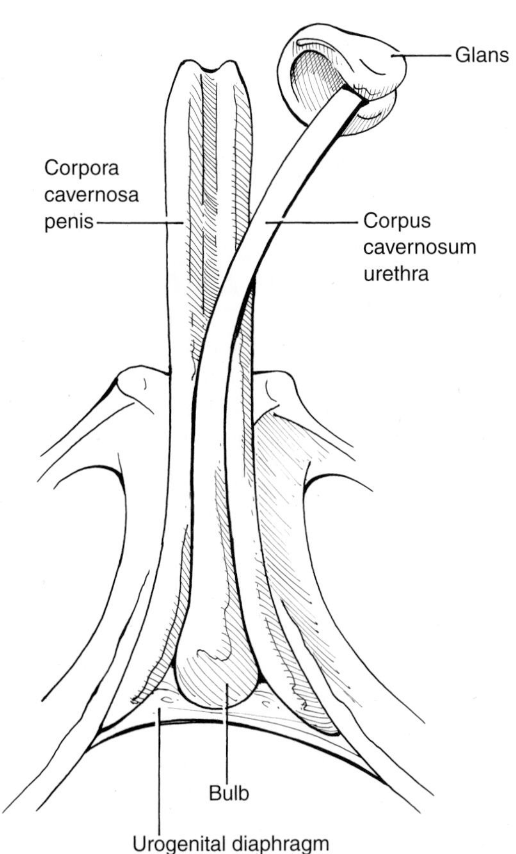


FIGURE 69.1 Anatomy of the three corporal bodies comprising the penis.

Proximally the corpora cavernosa taper to form the crus and are attached to the pubic arch. Each corpus is closely applied to the other, separated only by a septum, for most of the distal penis. The corpora cavernosus is supported at its base by the ischiocavernosus muscles, which arise from the inner surface of the ischial tuberosity and are innervated by the perineal nerves.

The third columnar body, the corpus spongiosum, contains the urethra, and the distal end is bulbous, forming the glans penis. The corpus spongiosum is attached proximally to the perineal membrane and at the most proximal portion is larger, forming the bulb.

Each of the corporal bodies is encased in its own tunica albuginea, and the three corporal bodies are surrounded by the Buck fascia, which is a continuation of the Colles fascia (Fig. 69.2). The Buck fascia is attached posteriorly to the urogenital diaphragm and anteriorly forms the suspensory ligament. There is little vascular communication between the corpora cavernosa and the corpus spongiosum. There is, however, vascular communication between the two corpora cavernosa via pectiniform septa in the distal corpora.

## VASCULAR ANATOMY

The superficial penile artery lies between the superficial and Buck fascia and originates from the external pudendal artery, which in turn is a branch of the femoral artery. This artery, along with a corresponding vein, supplies the penile skin and is located between the superficial penile fascia and the Buck fascia. The deep arterial supply arises from the internal iliac artery, which initially branches into the internal pudendal artery and then into the penile artery. As the penile artery exits the urogenital diaphragm, it branches into the bulbourethral, cavernosus, and urethral arteries. The cavernosus artery is the direct supply of the corpora cavernosa. The penile artery continues along the corpora cavernosa as the dorsal artery.

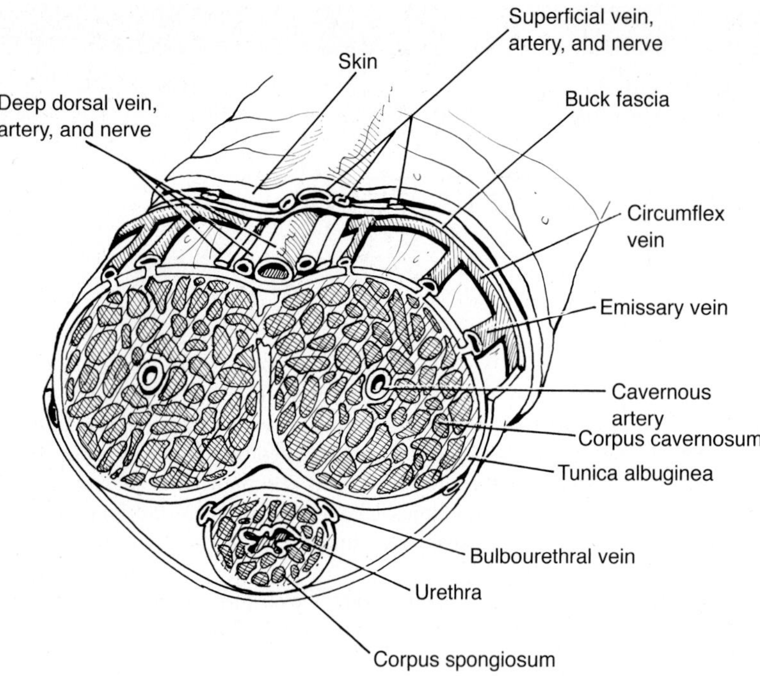


FIGURE 69.2 Cross section of the penis demonstrating fascial layers as well as vascular and neural anatomy.

The corpus spongiosum is supplied by the bulbourethral artery proximally, circumflex arteries from the dorsal artery along its shaft. The glans is supplied by the dorsal artery. The dorsal artery, the deep dorsal vein, and the dorsal nerve are enclosed within the Buck fascia.

The superficial penile vein drains into the external pudendal vein. The circumflex and deep dorsal veins drain into the plexus of Santorini, as do the crural and cavernosal veins (Fig. 69.3).

## LYMPHATIC ANATOMY

The lymphatics of the penile skin drain into the superficial inguinal and subinguinal lymph nodes. The lymphatics of the glans penis empty into the subinguinal and external iliac nodes. The deep lymphatics drain into the hypogastric and common iliac nodes.

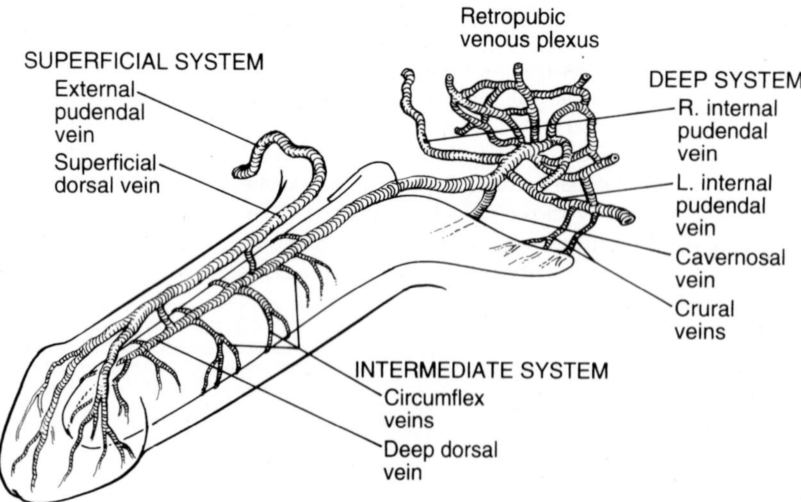


FIGURE 69.3 Venous drainage of the penis.

# CHAPTER 70 ■ PARTIAL AND TOTAL PENECTOMY IN THE MANAGEMENT OF INVASIVE SQUAMOUS CELL CARCINOMA OF THE PENIS

ANTONIO PURAS BAEZ AND ALEX M. ACOSTA MIRANDA

Squamous cell carcinoma of the penis is an epidermoid tumor arising in the glans or mucosal lining of the prepuce. Its incidence follows a distinct geographic, racial, and socioeconomic distribution. The tumor is age-related, showing an age-specific rate of increase with each decade and having its peak incidence at the fifth and sixth decades (9). An earlier age of onset and a high proportion of younger patients have been reported in areas of high incidence, such as Africa, India, and South America (8). In Puerto Rico the age-adjusted incidence is around 5 per 100,000 men (7), whereas in the United States and Europe it accounts for only 0.4% to 0.6% of all malignancies in men (8).

Although the precise etiology of penile carcinoma remains undetermined, numerous factors have been associated with the risk of developing squamous cell carcinoma of the penis, such as chronic irritation, poor genital hygiene, the presence of an intact foreskin, phimosis, smegma, and viruses.

There is increasing evidence for a sexually transmitted viral etiology in penile cancer. Human papilloma viruses (HPV), especially types 16, 18, 31, and 33, are the most frequently detected types in penile cancer. Other investigators have shown an association between the use of tobacco products and penile tumors. It appears that an enclosed preputial environment associated with poor genital hygiene of the foreskin, chronic irritation, and exposure to certain etiologic agents, such as viruses, smegma, and hydrocarbons, may also play a causative role in the development of this tumor.

## DIAGNOSIS

Patients with penile carcinoma may present with lesions that are a subtle induration or erythema of the glans or foreskin, a papule, a warty growth, or a large exophytic lesion with purulent discharge and cellulitis. These lesions are usually nonpainful, and there is a delay in patient presentation due to self-denial, ignorance, fear, and personal neglect (12).

Penile lesions such as erythroplasia of Queyrat, leukoplakia, cutaneous horn, balanitis xerotica obliterans, condyloma acuminatum, advanced melanoma, and giant condyloma may resemble squamous cell carcinoma of the penis and must be considered in the differential diagnosis.

Penile lesions should be examined thoroughly and assessed in regard to location, tumor growth, size, and infiltration of the corporal bodies and urethra. Careful examination of the inguinal area and pelvis is of extreme importance for staging and assessment of lymph node status. The lesion should be cultured and the patient started on appropriate antibiotic therapy. Any suspicious growth or ulceration should be biopsied, and meticulous pathologic analysis should be done for the depth and type of invasion, the presence of microvascular permeation, and the histologic grade of the tumor prior to initiation of any therapeutic modality.

The definite diagnosis is made by biopsy of the lesion (Fig. 70.1) following appropriate antibiotic therapy. Adequate anesthesia is obtained with 1% local lidocaine, and a 1.5-cm elliptical wedge of tumor tissue is removed (Fig. 70.2). The biopsy should include tumor growth and adjacent neighboring normal tissue to be examined for tumor infiltration. The incision is closed with interrupted 3-0 chromic catgut. We prefer to perform a wedge biopsy as a separate procedure and discuss with the pathologist the tumor grading, type of growth, and presence of microvascular permeation prior to initiation of any definite therapeutic modalities. Patients with tight phimosis who have purulent discharge and a palpable mass or induration concealed underneath the foreskin should be

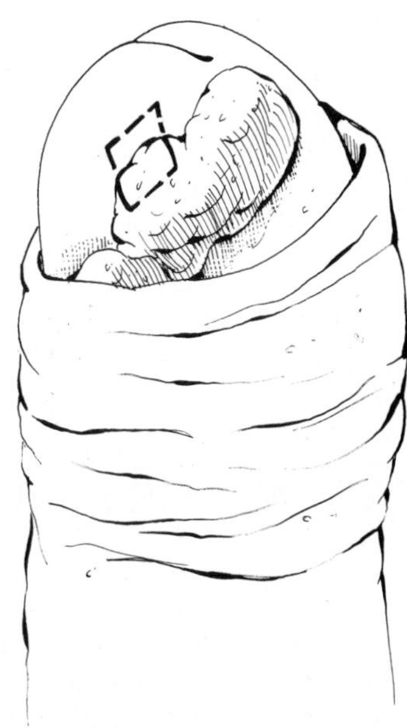

FIGURE 70.1 Wedge biopsy of the penile lesion. Biopsy should include tumor growth and adjacent neighboring normal tissue to be examined for tumor infiltration.

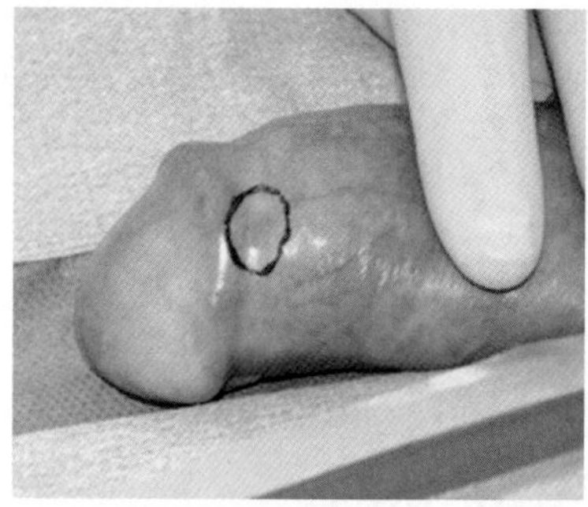
A

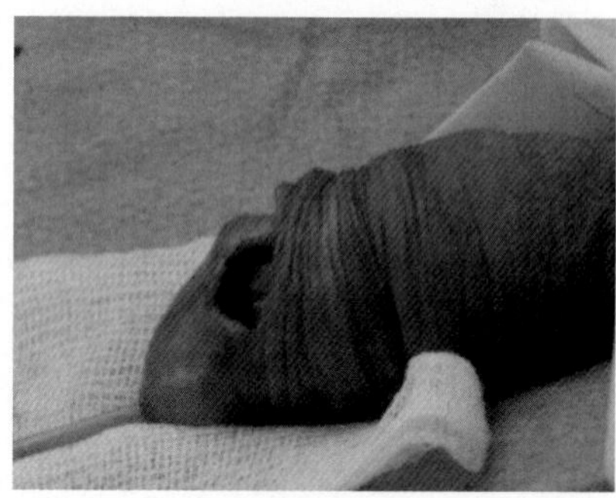
B

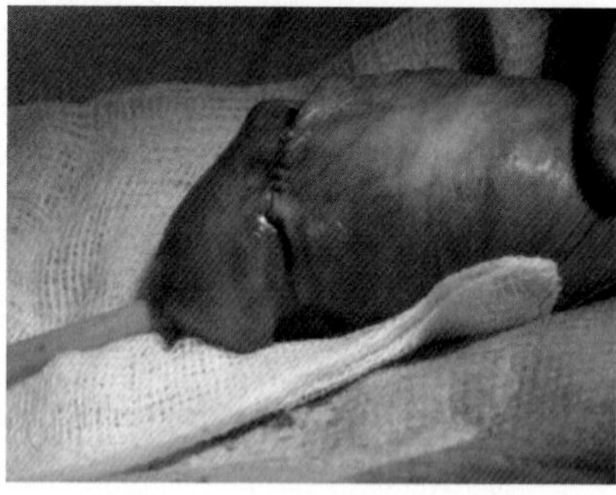
C

FIGURE 70.2 Wedge biopsy with wide excision at coronal sulcus. A: Tumor growth and adjacent normal tissue margins are marked. B: Wedge biopsy. C: Repaired defect with advancement of penile shaft skin.

managed with a dorsal slit incision, long enough to retract the prepuce and adequately examine and biopsy any suspicious lesion or growth.

Further assessment of local invasion to the corpora and spongiosum can be done with MRI. This radiologic cross-sectional modality has been shown to be highly accurate in the local staging of penile cancer and in surgical planning for the possible institution of conservative surgical treatments over more extensive procedures (5).

## INDICATIONS FOR SURGERY

Survival of patients with carcinoma of the penis depends primarily on the tumor grade, the depth of invasion, and the status of the regional nodes. The primary therapeutic goal in the management of penile carcinoma should be complete tumor excision, regional lymphatic control, and a functional, cosmetic penis. Surgery plays a prominent role in the management and control of the primary lesion. If adequately performed, it will assess the histologic grade, depth, and type of tumor invasion and in many cases can be curative.

## ALTERNATIVE THERAPY

Various nonsurgical therapeutic modalities, including radiation therapy, chemotherapy, and a combination of these, have been used in the treatment of the primary lesion. Penile-sparing procedures such as micrographic excision (Mohs micrographic surgery) and laser procedures have been utilized in other cutaneous malignancies and have been investigated in penile cancer.

Mohs micrographic surgery is a technique of excision of the lesion in thin horizontal layers using microscopic examination of the entire undersurface of each layer and systematic use of frozen sections. Two techniques by which microscopic control of the tumor is achieved have been described. The first technique is a fixed tissue technique in which the tissues are subjected to in situ chemical fixation with zinc chloride paste before excision of successive layers. In the fresh tissue technique, a local anesthetic is injected and the tissues excised in a fresh, unfixed state and examined by frozen section. The fresh tissue technique is recommended for small tumors, whereas for larger infiltrative lesions the fixed technique will provide control of bleeding from the relatively noncontractile vessels of the erectile tissues of the glans and corpora cavernosa. Cure rates for low-stage lesions that are <1 cm in diameter are close to 100%, while cure rates for lesions >3 cm drop to around 50%. It appears that microscopically controlled tumor excision provides an effective treatment alternative for managing some types of penile cancer with good cosmetic results. Complications related to most micrographic surgical techniques are meatal stenosis and disfigurement of the glans.

Laser therapy has been used in the treatment of penile carcinoma with highly satisfactory cosmetic results as well as good local tumor control. The major advantage of laser therapy for carcinoma of the penis is the destruction of the tumor with penile preservation and function; it also gives the advantages of destroying tissue, sealing small vessels and nerve endings, and reducing the incidence of postoperative bleeding and pain. The main disadvantage of laser surgery is the difficulty of obtaining histologic documentation and determining the depth of penetration by the tumor; it appears that the site and depth of penetration of the primary lesion correlate with its curability. Bandieramonte et al. (1) were able to resect T1 tumors at the glans penis by using a very short pulse and high peak power at the base of the lesion and at the meatus, providing precise excision of the specimen for histologic examination; however, a 15% recurrence rate was reported.

In a select group of patients with morphologically and anatomically suitable penile cancer with low-grade, low-stage disease, conservative surgical techniques are safe and can provide similar tumor control when compared to conventional, more radical resections. The tumor size, location, and pathologic characteristics should dictate the treatment of the primary penile lesion (2).

## SURGICAL TECHNIQUE

### Circumcision and Glans-Sparing Surgery

Patients presenting with small lesions involving the prepuce may be adequately managed by wide excision with a 1.5-cm margin. Microscopic examination by frozen section should be

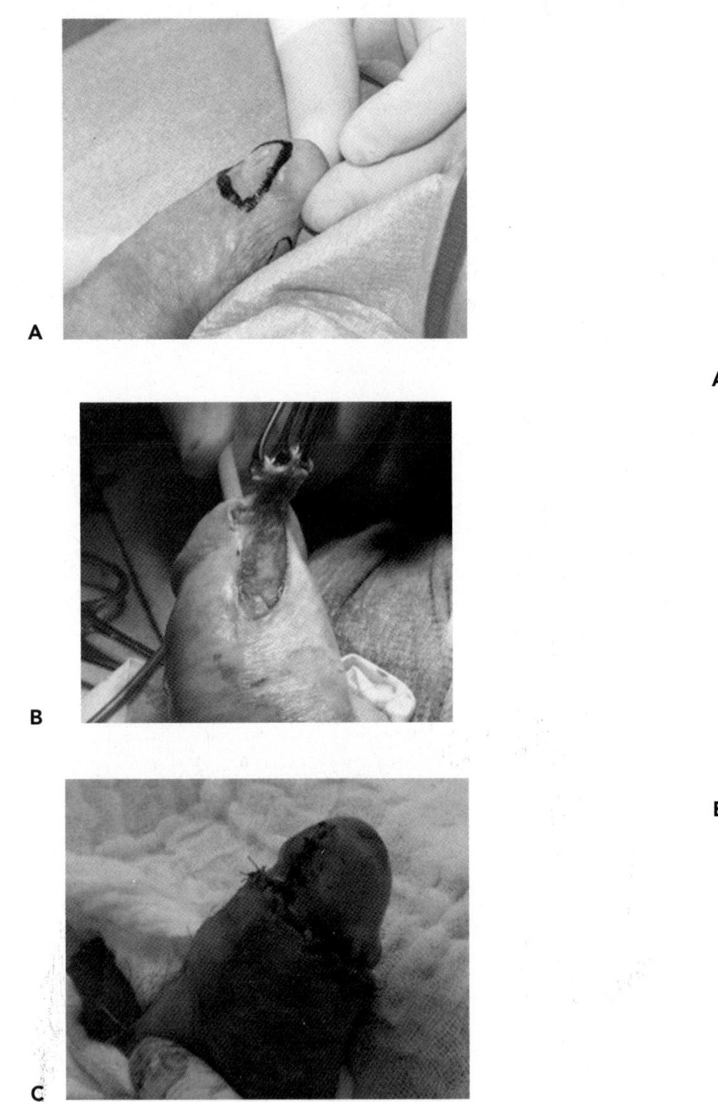

FIGURE 70.3 Excision of recurrent penile carcinoma at the frenular aspect of glans. **A:** Tumor growth with margins. **B:** Wedge excision with care to avoid damage to urethra. **C:** Repaired defect.

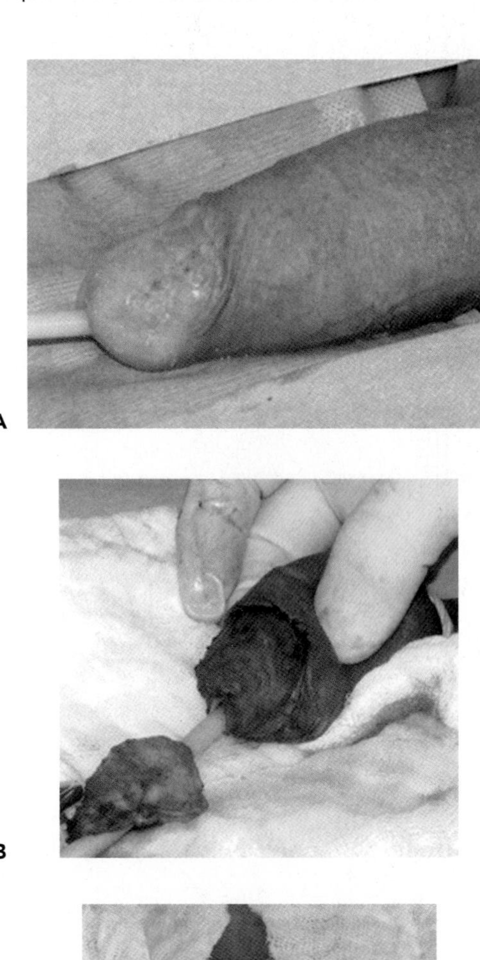

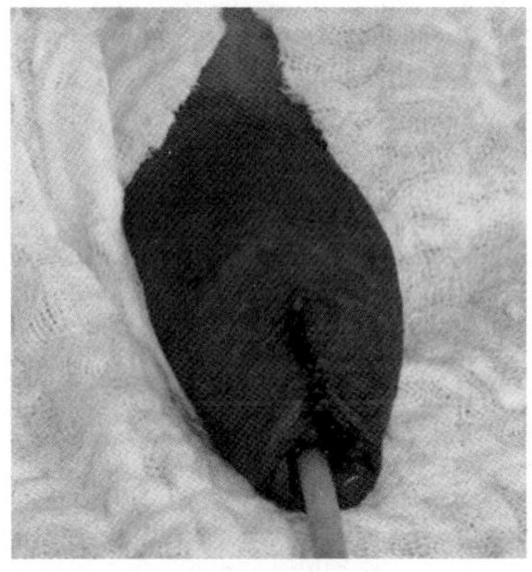

FIGURE 70.4 Glansectomy. **A:** Patient with recurrent carcinoma of the glans penis following radiation therapy. **B:** Glans is excised with preservation of a 1-cm urethral stump. **C:** Skin is closed longitudinally.

performed to obtain a tumor-free margin due to the high risk of recurrence.

The histopathologic slides should be reviewed with the pathologist with special attention to the patterns of tumor growth, grading, depth of invasion, and microvessel infiltration. Suspicious lesions at the glans or coronal sulcus should be biopsied and proved to be free of tumor. Selected patients with superficial tumors of the shaft can be managed with a wide excision by excising around 2 cm of normal skin. The skin defect can be covered by a full-thickness skin graft, which results in a functional and cosmetically appealing phallus without jeopardizing the cancer control surgical aspects. Small lesions at the glans may be treated with local excision and primary closure of the surgical defect (Fig. 70.3). Glansectomy can result in a very satisfactory cosmetic penile appearance after reconstruction, preserving penile length and function while offering an oncologically safe and effective procedure for patients with glans-confined low-grade squamous cell tumors (Fig. 70.4). In some rare cases large exophytic, low-grade, well-differentiated noninvasive lesions can be managed with organ-sparing surgery with complete disease-free status on long-term follow-up, but each case must be individualized accordingly.

The incidence of local recurrence may be increased with penile-preserving strategies. This carries a poor prognosis and may represent regional lymphatic spread. With careful patient selection and meticulous follow-up, some patients with invasive penile carcinoma can benefit from penile-preserving surgery.

## Partial Penectomy

Partial penectomy for squamous cell carcinoma of the penis provides excellent local control with a low recurrence rate and acceptable maintenance of urinary and sexual function. Invasive tumors involving the glans and coronal sulcus can be adequately managed by a partial penile amputation excising

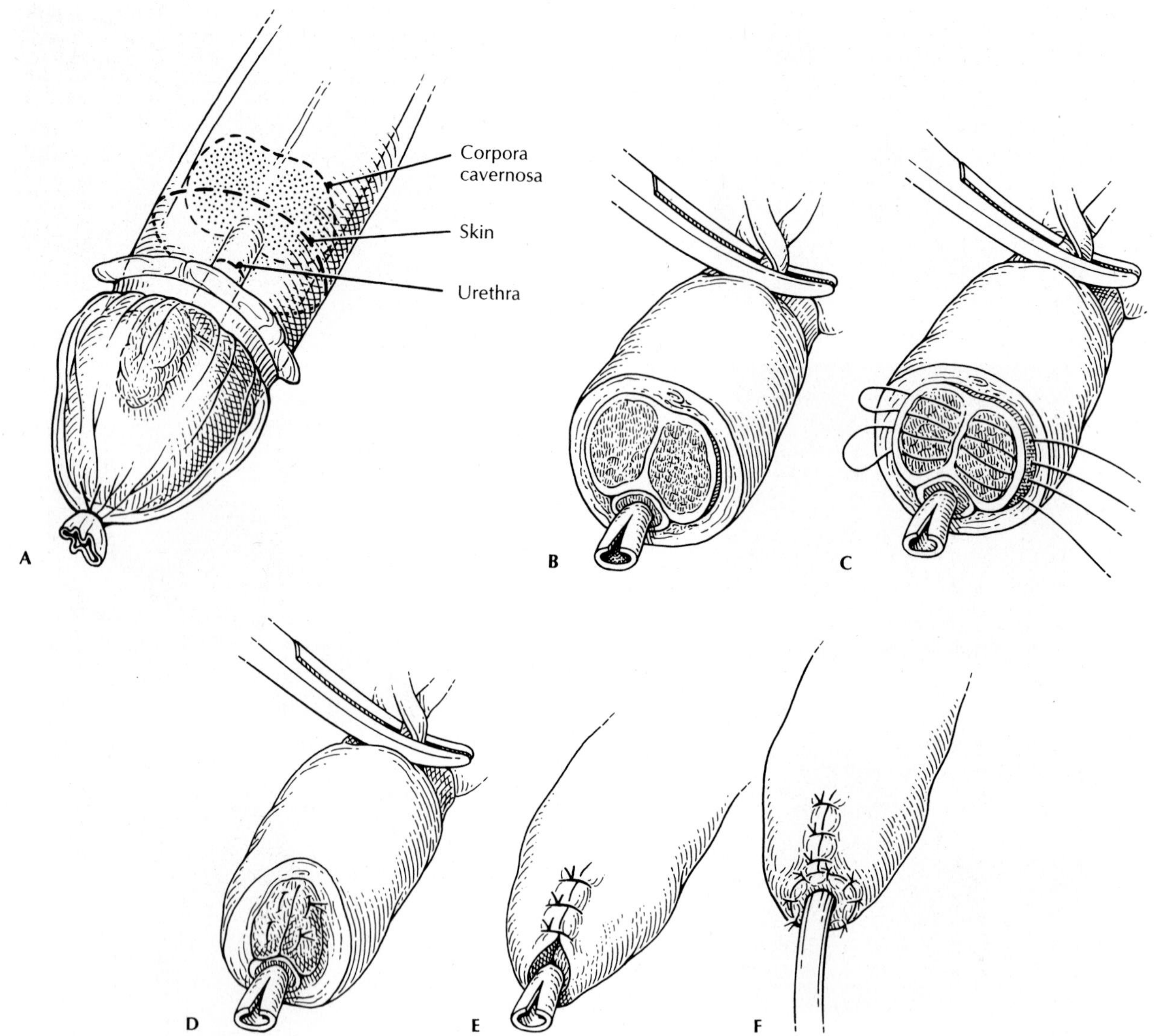


FIGURE 70.5 Partial penile amputation. A: A condom catheter is placed over the tumor and a circumferential incision is marked on the skin 2 cm proximal to the lesion. B: A 14Fr catheter or 0.25-in. Penrose drain is placed as a tourniquet at the base of the penis. The skin and Buck fascia are incised onto the tunica albuginea. Corpora cavernosa are sharply divided down to the urethra. The urethra is dissected free from the corpus spongiosum, and a 1-cm stump projects distally to the corpora cavernosa. C: The urethra is spatulated on its dorsal surface, and the corporal ends are closed with horizontal mattress sutures incorporating the Buck fascia, tunica albuginea, and intracavernosal septum. D: The tourniquet is released and adequate hemostasis is obtained. E: The dorsal skin is closed longitudinally. F: Ventral approximation of the penile skin to the urethra is begun and continued dorsally. The remaining dorsal skin is closed longitudinally.

around 1.5 to 2.0 cm of normal tissue proximal to the margin of tumor infiltration (Fig. 70.5). In most instances, this should leave a functional penis of >4 cm in length, which allows standing micturition and enough rigidity and length for vaginal penetration. Frozen sections of the proximal margins are necessary to confirm tumor-free resection and a recurrence rate of 10% or less. Partial penectomy has consistently been shown to give better oncological results than conservative treatment in the local management of the T1-stage tumor.

The procedure can be performed under local, regional, or general anesthesia. The patient is placed in the supine position. The lesion and urine should be cultured preoperatively and appropriate parenteral antibiotics started prior to the surgical procedure. The penis is prepared with a povidone-iodine solution and the tumor isolated using a sterile condom or glove that is sutured in place using 3-0 silk sutures. A 0.25-in. Penrose drain or 14Fr Red Robinson catheter is applied as a tourniquet at the base of the penis. A circumferential incision is marked on the skin 1.5 to 2.0 cm proximal to the lesion. The skin is incised circumferentially, and the superficial and deep dorsal veins are divided and ligated using 3-0 silk sutures. The Buck fascia is incised onto the tunica albuginea of the corpora. The corpora cavernosa are sharply divided down to the urethra and the central cavernosal arteries ligated on each side.

The urethra is dissected free from the corpus spongiosum in such a manner that an approximately 1-cm stump projects distally to the transected corpora cavernosa. The urethral stump and transected corpora are then washed with gentamycin solution. The corporal ends are closed with horizontal mattress sutures of 2-0 Vicryl incorporating the Buck fascia, tunica albuginea, and intercavernosal septum. The penile base tourniquet is then released, and all minor vessels are fulgurated or ligated until adequate hemostasis is obtained. Skin closure can be performed either in the classic longitudinal fashion or using a buttonhole technique in which a flap of dorsal penile skin is left, a crescentic buttonhole incision in the skin flap is made, and this flap is then rotated ventrally toward the urethra. In both techniques the urethra is spatulated dorsally and sutured to the skin using 4-0 Vicryl. The remaining skin is closed using 3-0 Vicryl sutures. A 16Fr Foley catheter is left indwelling to closed straight drainage for 48 hours, and the wound is dressed with triple antibiotic and Vaseline gauze.

### Total Penectomy

Patients with large, extensive, and infiltrating lesions involving the glans and midshaft of the penis, in which the location precludes adequate excision with a functional residual penile remnant, are managed by total penectomy (Fig. 70.6). The patient is placed on lithotomy position and the lesion is prepared with povidone-iodine solution. Appropriate antibiotic therapy should be started before the procedure according to penile and urine culture results. A condom catheter or sterile glove is secured to the base of the penis with interrupted 3-0 silk sutures. An elliptical incision is made around the base of the penis and extended through the subcutaneous tissues until the surface of the pubis is reached. All vessels and lymphatics are either fulgurated or ligated. The suspensory ligaments of the penis are isolated with a right-angle clamp and divided. The dorsal vein and penile arteries are identified, clamped, ligated, and divided. The penis is then reflected cephalad, the Buck fascia is opened ventrally, and the urethra is dissected free from the corpora cavernosa with sharp and blunt dissection. At the distal bulbar region, the urethra is divided, leaving enough length to reach the perineum. The corpora cavernosa are dissected up to the ischiopubic rami, sutured, and ligated with 2-0 Dexon sutures and then transected. The specimen should be removed with a 2-cm tumor-free margin.

The urethra is dissected to the area of the urogenital diaphragm to obtain an unangulated straight course to the perineal urethrostomy site. The urethra is tagged with 3-0 catgut sutures. A 1-cm ellipse of skin and subcutaneous tissues is removed from the midperineum just midway between the anus and scrotum. A tunnel is developed in the perineal subcutaneous tissue using a curved clamp, and the urethra is drawn into the perineal incision, with care taken to avoid angulations in the urethra. The urethra is then spatulated dorsally, and a V-inlay of skin can be created and anastomosed to the urethra using 3-0 or 4-0 Vicryl. A watertight technique should be used to prevent urinary leakage under the flap. An 18Fr Foley catheter is inserted, and 0.25–in. Penrose drains are left to drain each side of the scrotum. The scrotal incision is closed transversally to allow elevation of the scrotum away from the perineal urethrostomy using a two-layered closure with Vicryl 3-0. Triple antibiotic is placed over the wound incision and around the perineal urethrostomy. A Vaseline gauze, pressure dressing, and scrotal support are applied for 24 hours. The Penrose drains are usually removed in 48 hours, and the Foley catheter should be removed when the urethrostomy is well healed.

Lesions involving the perineum and anterior abdominal wall may need adjuvant preoperative chemotherapy in an attempt to downsize the tumor. If no adequate response is observed, the patient will need complete removal of the neoplasm, which may result in total emasculation and may require a musculocutaneous flap closure. In some rare instances cystoprostatectomy with urinary diversion will be necessary.

## OUTCOMES

### Complications

The most common complication of partial and total penectomy is meatal stenosis. The V-inlay technique has been used to decrease the stenosis at the urethral opening. Some institutions also advocate the use of a "loop" cutaneous urethrostomy, instead of the classic end cutaneous urethrostomy, during total penectomy, which may better preserve the distal urethral blood supply and thus minimize the tendency for the urethral meatus to develop stenosis. Patients should be aware of this complication and instructed to start self-dilation as soon as they notice a decrease in the urine stream.

Patients with partial and total penectomy suffer serious psychological and physical trauma with major changes in their quality of life. They should undergo psychiatric evaluation and counseling and receive emotional support in which the family and a team of social workers, psychologists, and physicians should take an active role. Some authors have proposed that the classic 2-cm excision margin is not necessary and a more conservative approach might still offer adequate cancer control while providing a more cosmetic and functional penile remnant.

Various techniques for penile reconstruction have been described and include the radial forearm flap and the use of innervated forearm osteocutaneous flaps combined with big toe pulp for reconstruction of the glans. These complex reconstructive procedures require a multidisciplinary approach and are usually performed at specialized referral centers.

### Results

Surgery plays a prominent role in the treatment and control of the primary lesion in squamous cell carcinoma of the penis. The presence and extent of metastasis to the inguinal nodes are the most important prognostic factors for survival in patients with penile cancer (6). Patients who are at risk or have persistent adenopathy following treatment to the primary lesion should undergo early regional inguinal lymphadenectomy. It has been shown that early resection of lymph node metastases in patients with penile carcinoma improves survival. Histologic grade, stage, and lymphovascular involvement are important parameters for selecting patients for "early" lymphadenectomy. Patients with microscopic disease to the inguinal nodes and well-differentiated tumor are at low risk for developing pelvic lymph node involvement and thus have a good 5-year cancer-specific survival. Survival drops

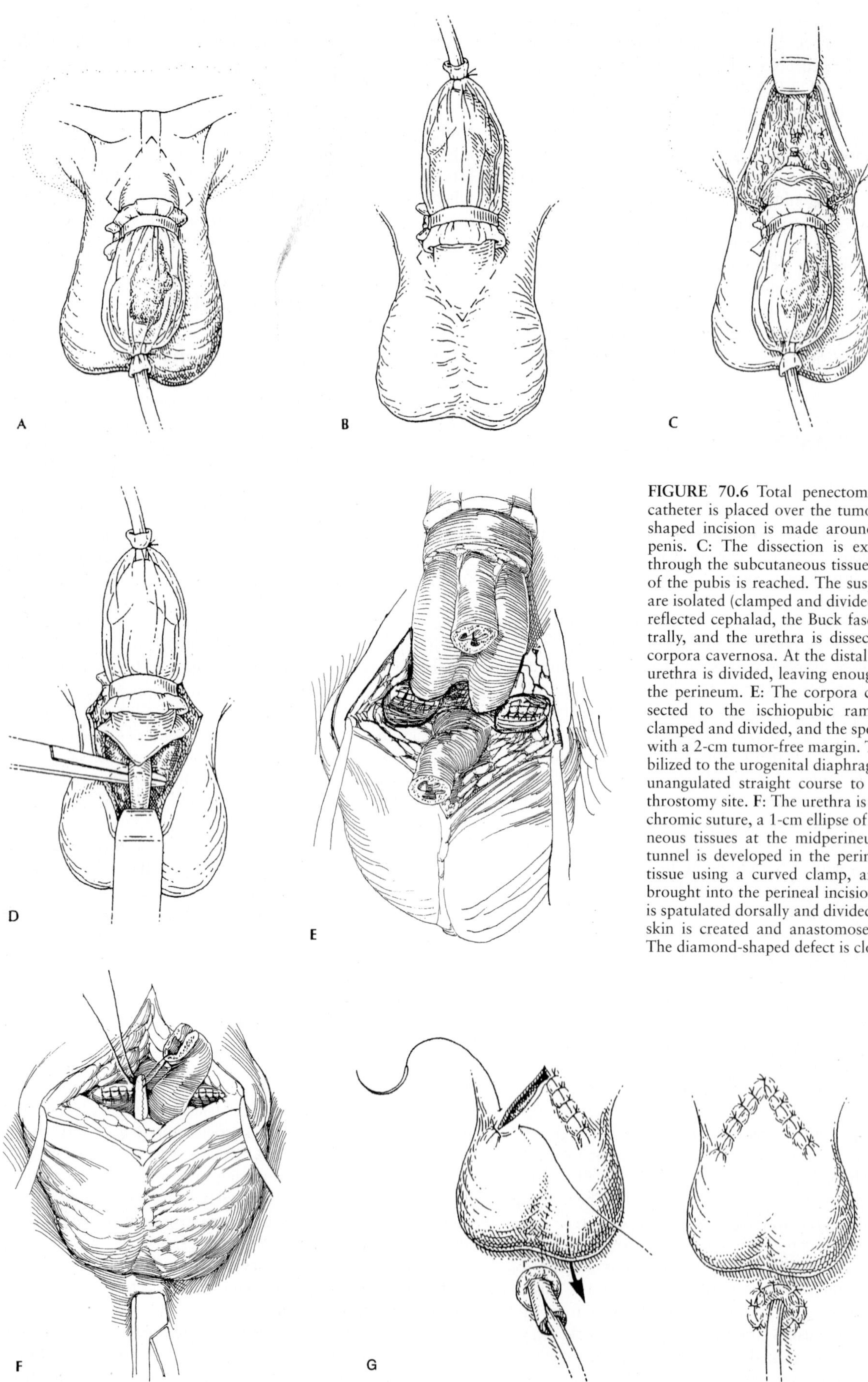


FIGURE 70.6 Total penectomy. A: A condom catheter is placed over the tumor. B: A diamond-shaped incision is made around the base of the penis. C: The dissection is extended superiorly through the subcutaneous tissues until the surface of the pubis is reached. The suspensory ligaments are isolated (clamped and divided). D: The penis is reflected cephalad, the Buck fascia is opened ventrally, and the urethra is dissected free from the corpora cavernosa. At the distal bulbar region the urethra is divided, leaving enough length to reach the perineum. E: The corpora cavernosa are dissected to the ischiopubic rami, the crura are clamped and divided, and the specimen is removed with a 2-cm tumor-free margin. The urethra is mobilized to the urogenital diaphragm to maintain an unangulated straight course to the perineal urethrostomy site. F: The urethra is tagged with a 3-0 chromic suture, a 1-cm ellipse of skin and subcutaneous tissues at the midperineum is removed, a tunnel is developed in the perineal subcutaneous tissue using a curved clamp, and the urethra is brought into the perineal incision. G: The urethra is spatulated dorsally and divided, and a V-inlay of skin is created and anastomosed to the urethra. The diamond-shaped defect is closed.

significantly in the presence of multiple nodal involvement, pelvic metastasis, and extranodal extension of cancer.

Several investigators have noted a correlation between tumor grade, regional metastasis, and survival. Well-differentiated tumors seldom demonstrate nodal involvement and have a high disease-specific survival. Tumors that exhibit a compact, vertical growth are usually high-grade neoplasms, associated with regional nodal metastasis (3). Slaton et al. (11) evaluated 48 patients with invasive squamous carcinoma of the penis and examined the prognostic factors for lymph node metastasis using univariate and multivariate analysis. These authors concluded that the pathologic stage of the penile tumor, vascular invasion, and >50% poorly differentiated cancer were independent prognostic factors for inguinal lymph node metastasis. These data clearly establish the significance of histologic grade, patterns of tumor growth, depth of invasion, and vascular permeation in predicting regional spread and survival.

Several new techniques are being applied to achieve local and regional lymph node control in patients with penile cancer. Dynamic sentinel lymph node biopsy is a promising technique in evolution that may become an alternative to superficial or modified inguinal dissection techniques with intraoperative frozen section, which remain the "gold standard" for defining the presence of microscopic lymph node metastases (4).

Sánchez-Ortiz and Pettaway (10) reviewed the M. D. Anderson Cancer Center series and proposed that follow-up regimens should be tailored according to high-risk recurrence stratification factors that include men treated with phallus-sparing strategies such as laser ablation, topical therapies, or radiotherapy; patients with clinically negative inguinal lymph nodes who are managed without lymphadenectomy despite high-risk primary tumors (pT2–3, grade 3, vascular invasion); and those with lymph node metastases after lymphadenectomy. Less rigorous surveillance protocols should be instituted in patients with low-risk primary tumors (pTis, pTa, pT1, grades 1–2) and those with negative inguinal nodes after lymphadenectomy whose primary tumors were managed with partial or total penectomy (10).

Squamous cell carcinoma of the penis, although a rare entity, represents a formidable challenge for the practicing urologist. Every therapeutic modality should be individualized to achieve the ultimate goals of complete tumor excision of the primary lesion, provision of a cosmetic functional penis, and early regional lymph node control.

## *References*


1. Bandieramonte G, Santoro O, Boracchi P, et al. Total resection of glans penis surface by $CO_2$: laser microsurgery. *Acta Oncol* 1988;27:575.
2. Bissada NK, Yakout HH, Fahmy WE, et al. Multi-institutional long-term experience with conservative surgery for invasive penile carcinoma. *J Urol* 2003;169(2):500–502.
3. Cubilla AL, Barreto J, Vaballero C, et al. Pathologic features of epidermoid carcinoma of the penis: a prospective study of 66 cases. *Am J Surg Pathol* 1993;17:753–763.
4. Izawa J, Kedar D, Wong F, et al. Sentinel lymph node biopsy in penile cancer: evolution and insights. *Can J Urol* 2005;12[Suppl 1]:24–29.
5. Kayes O, Minhas S, Allen C, et al. The role of MRI in the local staging of penile cancer. *Eur Urol* 2007;51(5):1313–1318.
6. Korets R, Kopie TM, Snyder ME, et al. Partial penectomy for patients with squamous cell carcinoma of the penis: The Memorial Sloan Kettering experience. *Ann Surg Oncol* 2007;14(12):3614–3619.
7. Marcial V, Puras A, Marcial VA. Neoplasms of the penis. In: Holland JF, Frei E, Bast R Jr, et al., eds. *Cancer medicine*, 4th ed. Baltimore: Williams & Wilkins, 1996:2165–2175.
8. Muir C, Waterhouse J, Mack T, et al., eds. *Cancer incidence in five continents.* Lyon, France: International Agency for Research on Cancer, 1987; Publication 88.
9. Puras A, Rivera J. Invasive carcinoma of the penis: management and prognosis. In: Oesterling JE, Richie JP, eds. *Urologic oncology,* 1st ed. Philadelphia: WB Saunders, 1997:604–617.
10. Sánchez-Ortiz RF, Pettaway CA. Natural history, management, and surveillance of recurrent squamous cell penile carcinoma: a risk-based approach. *Urol Clin North Am* 2003;30(4):853–867.
11. Slaton JW, Morgenstern N, Levy DA, et al. Tumor stage, vascular invasion and percentage of poorly differentiated cancer: dependent prognosticators for inguinal lymph node metastasis in penile squamous cancer. *J Urol* 2001;165:1138–1142.
12. Sufrin G, Huben R. Benign and malignant lesions of the penis. In: Gillenwater JY, Grayhack JT, Howards SS, et al., eds. *Adult and pediatric urology*, 2nd ed. St. Louis, MO: Mosby–Year Book, 1991:1643–1678.


# CHAPTER 71 ■ INGUINAL LYMPHADENECTOMY FOR PENILE CARCINOMA

SHAHIN TABATABAEI AND W. SCOTT McDOUGAL

Squamous cell carcinoma of the penis tends to spread locally to regional lymph nodes long before distant metastases occur. Approximately 50% of patients have lymph node involvement at presentation. Metastatic spread to the locoregional lymph nodes occurs in a stepwise fashion along the normal route of penile lymphatic drainage. The disease first spreads to the superficial and deep inguinal nodes, followed by the pelvic nodes (i.e., external iliac and obturator lymph nodes). Although tumor metastasis to the contralateral inguinal nodes is common, pelvic cross-drainage has not been reported.

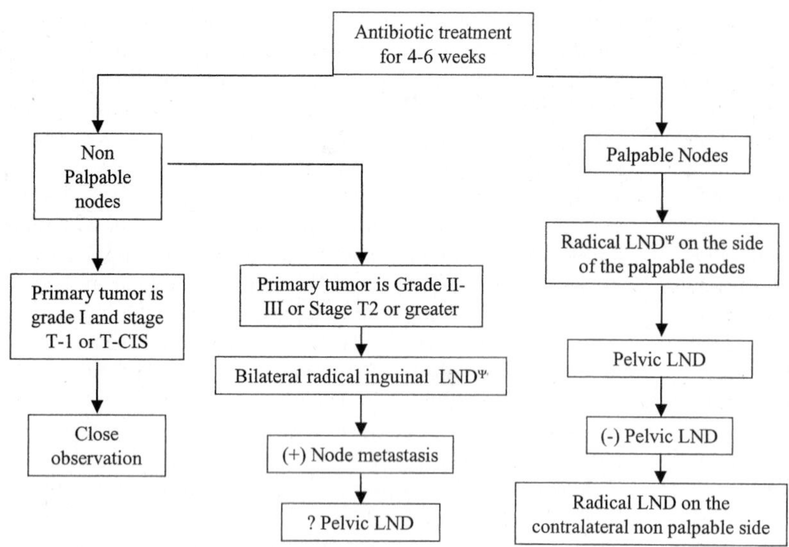


FIGURE 71.1 Management of inguinal lymph nodes following primary surgery for carcinoma of the penis. *LND*, lymph node dissection.

The most important prognostic factors for survival in men with invasive squamous cell carcinoma of the penis are the presence and extent of inguinal lymph node metastasis (1). Although penile carcinoma metastatic to the lymph nodes portends a poorer prognosis, aggressive surgical excision of the involved nodes is associated with increased long-term survival with a possible cure in 30% to 60% of patients with inguinal lymph node metastasis (1,2). This is not true if the tumor has spread to the pelvic lymph nodes, however, in which case there is a <10% survival rate. There is currently no effective chemotherapy for patients with disease beyond the inguinal nodes. Without treatment, patients with metastatic disease die within 2 years.

Until recently, inguinal lymphadenectomy had been associated with significant morbidity (30% to 90%) and up to 3% mortality. Further, previous studies reported up to a 50% false-positive rate in patients with clinically enlarged lymph nodes. These reports have generated considerable controversy regarding the indications for a lymphadenectomy in patients with penile carcinoma.

## DIAGNOSIS

The diagnosis is secured at the time of biopsy and definitive treatment of the primary lesion (Chapter 66). A computerized tomography (CT) scan of the abdomen and pelvis is important for staging the pelvic nodes.

## INDICATIONS FOR SURGERY

In the last two decades, improvements in surgical and perioperative techniques have considerably decreased the complication rates of inguinal lymphadenectomy. In addition, accurate prognostic factors to predict lymph node involvement have been better defined. Therefore, a more proactive approach to treating penile cancer may be taken. Tumor grade and depth of invasion help predict the lymph node involvement (1–3). In patients with grade 1 squamous cell carcinoma (SCC) of the penis, 24% to 37% may have inguinal lymph node involvement, while almost 82% of patients with grade 3 tumors have positive inguinal lymph nodes (3,4). Patients with carcinoma in situ and verrucous carcinoma of the penis are considered low risk as there is no evidence that these lesions metastasize. Patients with tumor stage T2 or greater (invasion into the corpora) have a 30% to 66% incidence of positive nodes. When stage and grade are combined, those with grade 3 and/or those with stage T2 or greater have an 80% incidence of positive nodes (3).

We advocate early lymphadenectomy in high-risk patients with nonpalpable groin adenopathy (5). Figure 71.1 summarizes our current approach to managing inguinal lymph nodes in these patients. As shown in the algorithm, all patients with penile cancer undergo 4 to 6 weeks of antibiotic therapy before the inguinal lymphadenectomy. It has been shown that most patients with ulcerative, penile SCC have infectious lymphangitis. Inguinal lymphadenectomy in the absence of appropriate antibiotic treatment may significantly increase the risk of complications after the surgery.

Controversies regarding unilateral versus bilateral groin dissection have been resolved by recent data and studies indicating that lymphatic cross-drainage to the contralateral side does occur. Therefore, we strongly recommend bilateral inguinal lymphadenectomy.

The role of pelvic lymphadenectomy and whether the lymphadenectomy should start in the groin or pelvis are also controversial issues. Many studies indicate that involvement of pelvic lymph nodes is an ominous sign, and almost all of these patients succumb to the disease in <2 years. Indeed, the knowledge of pelvic lymph node status has prognostic significance and may change the surgical approach. If the pelvic lymph nodes are positive, the surgical intention will be focused on palliation. In these situations, we still perform inguinal lymphadenectomy, but only on clinically palpable inguinal nodes, to prevent lesions from penetrating through the skin and/or invading into the femoral vessels, which may result in fatal femoral artery bleeding. In these cases, we do not proceed to contralateral inguinal lymphadenectomy for nonpalpable contralateral nodes. Pelvic lymphadenectomy could also serve as a tool for accurate staging in patients who are candidates for adjuvant or neoadjuvant chemotherapy protocols.

In patients with negative palpable inguinal lymph nodes who are at high risk for inguinal node involvement, several approaches have been proposed to minimize morbidity. These include (a) modified inguinal lymphadenectomy, (b) sentinel lymph node biopsy (SLNB), and (c) intraoperative lymph node mapping (IOLM). Some investigators suggest a modified inguinal lymphadenectomy for the side with nonpalpable inguinal lymph nodes and then radical lymphadenectomy only if the superficial lymph nodes are positive for cancer on the frozen section. This approach differs from radical dissection in four respects: (a) The skin incision is smaller, (b) the lymph nodes lateral to the femoral artery or dorsal to the fossa ovalis are spared, (c) the saphenous vein is preserved, and (d) the sartorius muscle is not transposed. Proponents of this approach point to evidence that there is decreased morbidity without any increase in mortality (6). The main argument against this approach is that it relies heavily on intraoperative frozen section diagnosis of lymph node involvement, which may be inaccurate (7).

Another approach is sentinel node biopsy. Lymphangiograms performed via the dorsal penile lymphatics demonstrate drainage into a specific lymph node center, which is most often located between the superficial epigastric and superficial external pudendal veins. Studies have suggested that the sentinel lymph node is the first site of metastasis and is often the only lymph node involved. Although the concept is intriguing, the location of the sentinel node varies, and therefore clinicians have not found it particularly useful (8).

Based on the experience with breast and melanoma cancers, IOLM of the inguinal nodes has been proposed to address the shortcomings of SLNB. The technique involves injecting a vital blue dye and/or technetium-labeled colloid adjacent to the primary lesion and following its drainage to a specific node in the inguinal region. This node is designated the sentinel node. The goal is to eliminate the anatomic variability of the sentinel node location. Although preliminary results with IOLM are promising, lack of long-term follow-up, as well as the associated learning curve and technical difficulties of the procedure, limits its current use (9). We do not recommend IOLM as a standard approach at this time.

At the present time it seems that because of the unreliabiliy of SLNB and the technical aspects of IOLM and its associated learning curve, superficial lymphadenopathy and modified inguinal lymphadenopathy are considered more informative and accurate for staging and carry minimal morbidity.

## ALTERNATIVE THERAPY

The value of radiation therapy and chemotherapy is still uncertain. These treatments are currently considered palliative. In patients with positive inguinal lymph nodes, the survival rate is significantly less when treated with radiation therapy than when treated with surgery. Based on the encouraging results of adjuvant radiation therapy in squamous cell carcinoma of the head and neck, some investigators advocate the use of preoperative radiation therapy in patients with large, fixed regional nodes (>4 cm in size and/or extracapsular extension). In the absence of surgical contraindications (medical comorbidities, patient's refusal, bulky, infected lymphadenopathy with distant metastasis), we are not in favor of inguinal area radiation, as flap viability may be compromised and there is no proven survival benefit in penile cancer. At the present time inguinal radiotherapy is reserved only for inoperable nodes and palliative purposes.

Experience with chemotherapy in penile carcinoma is hampered by a limited number of cases and lack of prospective trials. Cisplatin, iphosphamide, taxol, bleomycin, vincristine, 5-fluorouracil, and methotrexate, as single agents or as combinations, have all been shown to provide a partial response in selected cases. The use of chemotherapy as adjuvant or neoadjuvant therapy may be beneficial, although the optimum chemotherapy regimen remains to be determined.

## SURGICAL TECHNIQUE

All patients undergo a thorough metastatic workup including abdominal and pelvic CT scan, chest X-ray, and liver function tests. All patients complete 4 to 6 weeks of appropriate antibiotic therapy following excision of the primary lesion and wound closure, to treat any associated infection and decrease the risk of postoperative wound infection. Intravenous antibiotics with appropriate skin flora coverage are administered 1 hour prior to the skin incision. Adequate hydration should be ensured before surgery. Antiembolism stockings and pneumatic compression boots are applied to the lower extremities prior to induction of anesthesia.

## SURGICAL ANATOMY

The lymphatics of the skin of the penis, scrotum, and perineum drain into the superficial and deep inguinal nodes. The superficial fascia of the thigh (fascia lata) separates the superficial inguinal nodes from the deep nodes. Extensive work by Daseler et al. (10) on inguinal lymph node dissection suggests that five node groups exist in the superficial inguinal area (Fig. 71.2A) (10):

1. Central nodes at saphenofemoral junction
2. Superolateral nodes around the superficial circumflex vein
3. Inferolateral nodes around the lateral (femoral) cutaneous and superficial circumflex veins
4. Superomedial nodes around the superficial external pudendal and superficial epigastric veins
5. Inferomedial nodes around the greater saphenous vein

Overall, 4 to 25 lymph nodes are present in the superficial groups. All of these nodes are situated below the globular fat of the superficial fascia called the Camper fascia.

The deep inguinal nodes are located medial to the femoral vein in the femoral canal (Fig. 71.2B). The most cephalad deep inguinal node, known as the node of Cloquet, is located between the femoral vein and the lacunar ligament. Deep inguinal nodes drain to obturator, hypogastric, and external iliac lymph nodes, which in turn drain to the common iliac and para-aortic nodes.

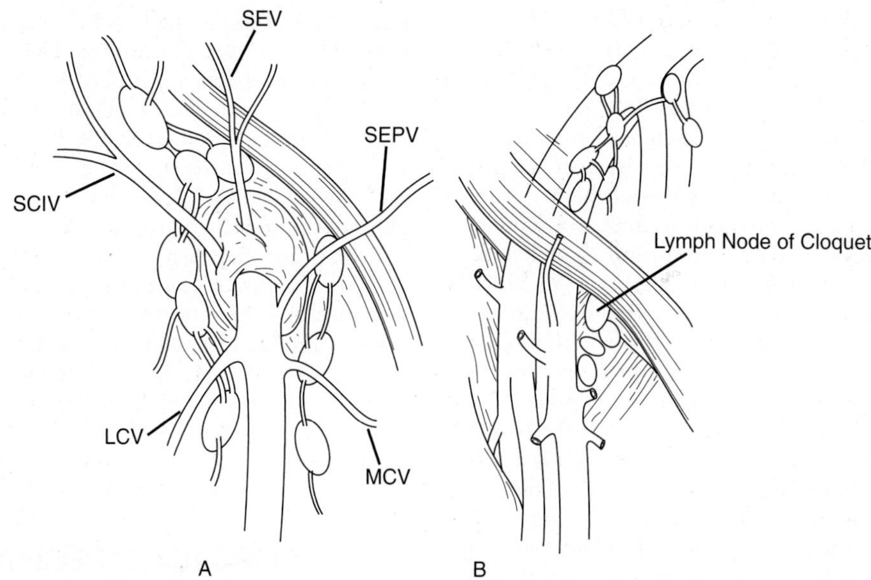


**FIGURE 71.2 A:** Superficial lymph nodes and the five tributaries of the saphenous vein: medial *(MCV)* and lateral *(LCV)* cutaneous, superficial external pudendal *(EPV)*, superficial circumflex iliac *(SCIV)*, and superficial epigastric *(SEV)*. These veins should be ligated and the surrounding package removed with preservation of the saphenous vein. **B:** Deep inguinal lymph nodes, which in general number two to four. The most cephalad lymph node is the node of Cloquet.

Blood supply to the inguinal skin derives from superficial branches of the femoral artery (i.e., superficial external pudendal, superficial circumflex iliac, and superficial epigastric arteries). Corresponding veins parallel the arteries that join into the greater saphenous vein as it joins the femoral vein at the fossa ovalis. These arteries are ligated in the inguinal lymphadenectomy. Skin flap viability depends on anastomosing vessels within the superficial globular fat of the Camper fascia that track from lateral to medial along the skin lines, parallel to the inguinal ligament. In theory, the transverse skin incision is least likely to compromise blood supply.

## Radical Inguinal Lymphadenectomy

The patient is placed in the supine position with the ipsilateral hip abducted and the ipsilateral knee flexed (Fig. 71.3). The dissection margins for the classic radical inguinal lymphadenectomy cover the area outlined superiorly by a line drawn from the superior margin of the external inguinal ring to the anterosuperior iliac spine (ASIS), medially by a line drawn from the pubic tubercle 15 cm down the medial thigh, and laterally by a line drawn from the ASIS extending 20 cm inferiorly (Figs. 71.3 and 71.4). A line drawn between the inferior end of the lateral and medial margins marks the inferior limit of the dissection. An incision is made 3 to 4 cm inferior and parallel to the inguinal crease over the medial thigh from the lateral to medial limits of the dissection. The femoral vessels should be palpable in the medial aspect of the incision. We have modified this approach to include more tissue above the inguinal ligament—see section entitled "Suprainguinal Dissection in Inguinal Lymphadenectomy" following.

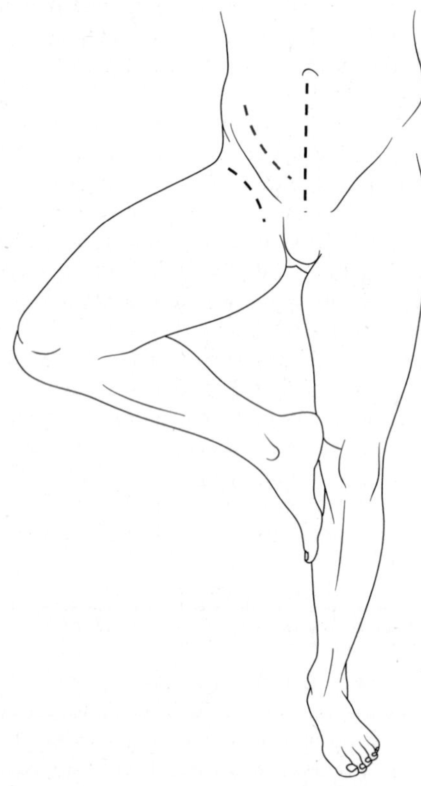

**FIGURE 71.3** The patient is positioned with the hip abducted and knee flexed. The skin incision is demarcated by the line drawn two fingerbreadths below the inguinal crease (classic dissection) or two fingerbreadths above the groin crease.

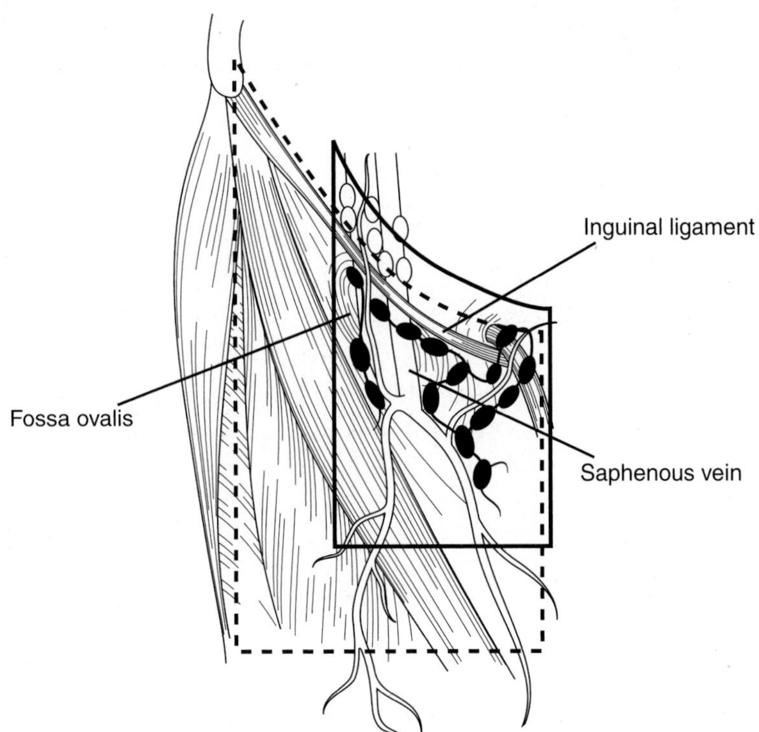


FIGURE 71.4 Comparison of limits of dissection of modified inguinal lymphadenectomy *(solid line)* with classic groin dissection *(dotted line)*. Note that with the modified groin dissection the dissection is medial to the midpoint of the femoral artery. *Black*, superficial inguinal nodes; *white*, deep inguinal nodes; *gray*, external iliac nodes.

Skin flaps are developed superiorly and inferiorly as the first step of the dissection. Elevation of the skin edges with skin hooks allows dissection within the superficial fatty fascia of the thigh. At the junction of the superficial globular fat and the deeper membranous fat, the tissues are separated. The skin and globular fat are elevated off of the deep membranous fascia and the Scarpa fascia cephalad to a point 4 cm above the inguinal ligament. The skin flaps are protected by gentle elevation with Deaver retractors placed over moist sponges. Inferior traction on the lymphatic package with a small sponge under the left hand provides countertraction to facilitate dissection in the proper plane.

Dissection is carried down through the Scarpa fascia onto the external oblique aponeurosis. The external inguinal ring and emerging spermatic cord are identified medially and retracted as dissection extends to the pubic tubercle. The fat and lymphatics are separated from the spermatic cord and base of the penis medially. Vascular and lymphatic channels are meticulously ligated to prevent postoperative fluid accumulation under the skin flaps. The fatty lymph packet is elevated off of the external oblique fascia to the inferior border of the inguinal ligament (Poupart ligament), where the femoral vessels are identified within the femoral sheath (Fig. 71.5A).

The medial (adductor longus muscle) and lateral (sartorius muscle) borders of the dissection are identified next, and the fascia lata is incised over the muscles. The muscles are traced to their confluence at the apex of the femoral triangle, representing the inferior limit of dissection. The resulting triangular packet of lymphatics and fat needs only to be elevated off its deep margin to complete the dissection. Care must be taken not to retract the adductor longus medially or the sartorius muscle laterally as the dissection will extend too far caudally (i.e., confluence of the two muscles will be displaced caudally).

The saphenous vein is identified medially and preserved if possible. Although this vessel is by tradition sacrificed during radical lymphadenectomy, this achieves no therapeutic benefit and may increase morbidity. If massive lymphadenopathy exists, however, the saphenous vein should be removed. The femoral sheath is incised over the femoral artery and vein. Medial dissection isolates the lymph node of Cloquet between the Cooper and Poupart ligaments, lateral to the lacunar ligament. The femoral sheath is stripped inferiorly to the apex of the femoral triangle, as the fascia overlying the sartorius and adductor longus is stripped distally. The deep lymph nodes are removed from their location between the femoral artery and vein. The superficial cutaneous perforating arteries and veins are ligated as they are encountered on the surface of the femoral artery and saphenous vein, leaving the intact saphenous to join the femoral vein, in the area of the now absent fossa ovalis. It is important to limit the lateral aspect of dissection along the femoral sheath to the anterior surface of the femoral artery. Dissection laterally on the femoral sheath can injure the femoral nerve beneath the iliaca fascia (deep to the fascia lata), and posterolateral dissection can injure the profunda femoris artery.

When this dissection is complete, the superficial and deep lymphatics are removed together en bloc. The wound is irrigated liberally. The exposed femoral vessels are covered by mobilizing the sartorius from its insertion on the anterior superior iliac spine, transposing it over the vessels, and securing its cephalad margin to the inguinal ligament with 2-0 silk suture (Fig. 71.5B). Blood supply to the sartorius arises from its medial and inferior aspects, and care must be taken to protect

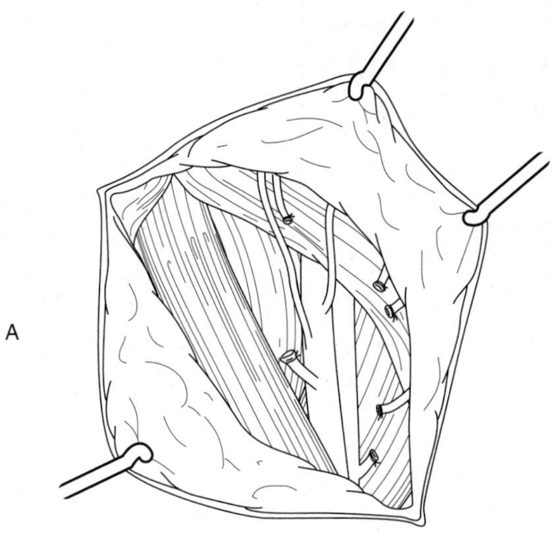


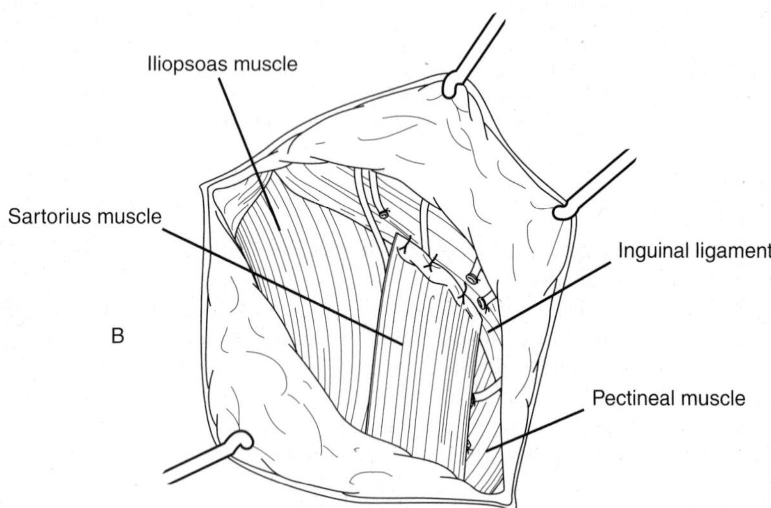


FIGURE 71.5 **A:** Raised groin flaps and the completed groin dissection. **B:** The sartorius muscle is detached at the anterior superior iliac spine and moved medially, thus providing for coverage of the vessels. **B:** The transferred sartorius muscle is sutured to the inguinal ligament.

these vessels during mobilization. The medial edge of the muscle can be tacked to the adductor longus to ensure coverage of the femoral vein. If pelvic lymphadenectomy has been performed simultaneously, this dissection should join with the distal limit of the pelvic dissection and allow free communication with the pelvis. To prevent herniation, the Cooper ligament should be secured to the shelving edge of the Poupart ligament with permanent suture (2-0 Proline) without compromising the lumen of the femoral vein.

At this point the wound edges will be inspected for nonviable tissue. Any suspicious area with doubtful vascularization should be excised. Some have suggested giving an ampule of fluorescein intravenously and inspecting the skin edges with a Wood lamp for viability. We have not found this technique to be particularly useful.

A Jackson-Pratt drain is placed beneath the subcutaneous tissue and brought out inferiorly. The skin flaps are tacked to the surface of the exposed muscles with 3-0 chromic sutures and the wound closed with nylon sutures or staples. A light-pressure dressing is applied for the first 12 hours. Care is taken not to apply excessive pressure, which might further compromise blood supply in the skin flaps.

Parenteral antibiotics are continued for 48 hours and then converted to oral agents. The patient is maintained on bedrest for 1 day and ambulated on the second postoperative day. Deep vein thrombosis (DVT) prophylaxis, that is, thromboembolic stockings or pneumatic compression boots, is crucial. The drain is removed when the patient is ambulatory and drainage is <30 cc per day. Patients are instructed to use thromboembolic stockings for at least 6 months after the surgery. Hospital stockings are converted to fitted compression stockings 1 month postoperatively.

## Modified Inguinal Lymphadenectomy

The skin is incised transversely 2 cm below the groin crease for a distance of 10 cm. Skin flaps are raised in the same manner as described previously for a distance of approximately 8 cm cephalad and 6 cm caudally. Cephalad dissection onto the external oblique is performed as in radical lymphadenectomy, and the medial extent of dissection is identical. The lateral dissection is more limited, however. After opening the femoral sheath, dissection lateral to the femoral artery is not performed. The sartorius is not exposed, and dissection inferiorly on the fascia lata and femoral sheath extends only to the caudal edge of the fossa ovalis (Fig. 71.4). The saphenous vein is preserved in the superficial nodal package, and the deep lymphatics below the fascia lata between the femoral vessels and medial to the femoral vein along the adductor longus fascia up to the Cooper ligament are removed. Postoperative management is similar to that for radical lymphadenectomy.

### Suprainguinal Dissection in Inguinal Lymphadenectomy

As mentioned previously, the primary lymphatic drainage of carcinoma of the penis is to the superficial inguinal region, which is mostly inferior to the inguinal ligament. This is the basis for the surgical approach, and hence for placing the incision inferior to the inguinal ligament.

In a number of cases we have noted that the metastasis from penile carcinoma occurs in lymph nodes above the inguinal ligament. Indeed, in some cases the only involved nodes have been superior to the inguinal ligament. For this reason, we have begun to place the incision above the groin crease (2 cm above the inguinal ligament) with the dissection extending at least to the level of the symphysis pubica, skeletonizing the cord structures and the external oblique medially and extending the incision laterally to the anterior superior iliac spine. The standard groin lymph node dissection is performed caudally.

It is important to encompass the soft tissue above the inguinal ligament as lymphatic drainage from the penis may extend directly to nodes above the inguinal ligament and superficial to the external oblique fascia. There is little additional morbidity in extending the groin dissection to this level, and we have found that skin flap viability is better preserved when compared to incisions placed several centimeters below the groin crase. Although this is slightly more difficult for the most caudal portion of the groin dissection, the decreased need to retract flaps for the dissection of the groin around the femoral vessels at the level of the inguinal ligament likely reduces trauma to the skin. We have found that this extended incision encompasses an area of nodal drainage that may be missed with the standard groin dissection; indeed, in some patients positive nodes would have been missed with a standard groin dissection. Furthermore, we believe that the incision for this extended dissection improves skin flap survival.

### Inguinal Reconstruction after Inguinal Lymphadenectomy

Large groin defects may be created after inguinal lymphadenectomy for bulky metastatic penile cancer. Many types of flaps have been described and advocated to cover large defects in the groin, when extensive dissections are required. The goal is to provide muscle bulk to protect the femoral vessels and full-thickness skin for wound coverage. This will allow for the least morbidity postoperatively and the least likelihood of femoral vessel rupture should adjuvant radiotherapy be required. Flaps described to accomplish this purpose have included a tensor fascia lata myocutaneous flap, a gracilis myocutaneous flap, an abdominal rotation flap, a rectus abdominis myocutaneous flap, a deep inferior epigastric artery myocutaneous flap, a thigh rotational skin flap, and a scrotal advancement flap. Most of these reconstructive procedures are performed in collaboration with a plastic or reconstructive surgeon.

Recently, we proposed the use of an abdominal cutaneous advancement flap as an alternative for primary skin closure of large groin defects (11). The procedure involves sartorius muscle transfer for vascular coverage followed by elevation of the ipsilateral abdominal wall, immediately anterior to the underlying rectus and external oblique fascia, cephalad to the level of the umbilicus. This provides enough mobility for closing a gap of up to 12 cm (Fig. 71.6A and B). For patients with larger (up to 20 cm) gaps, a midline incision is made to the xiphoid process and the entire overlying skin and subcutaneous tissue immediately superficial to the rectus abdominus and external oblique muscle are raised on the ipsilateral side of the defect. The flap is then moved caudad to cover the defect (Fig. 71.6C). Jackson-Pratt drains are employed beneath the flap. Postoperative management is similar to that for the standard inguinal lymphadenectomy described previously. The simplicity, lower morbidity, and excellent cosmetic results are the main advantages of this procedure. The technique may be utilized for bilateral groin defects as well. Abdominal scars (paramedian, appendectomy, Gibson, or flank incision) may compromise the blood supply to the flap and are considered relative contraindications to this approach.

## OUTCOMES

### Complications

Skin necrosis, wound infection, vascular injuries, lower-extremity lymphedema, DVT, and death are some of the potential complications. Skin necrosis and wound infection are probably the most feared complications. Older series report up to 30% flap necrosis. Improved understanding of the cutaneous blood supply, avoidance of the vertical skin incision, improved surgical technique, and appropriate use of perioperative antibiotics have resulted in significant reduction in mortality, skin necrosis, and wound infection—to negligible levels—in several recent reports (12).

### Results

Currently, surgical intervention is the most effective approach to treat SCC of the penis. Early inguinal lymphadenectomy can improve survival in the high-risk patient. Expectant follow-up may be offered to low-risk patients with clinically negative groin nodes who comply with comprehensive, close observation.

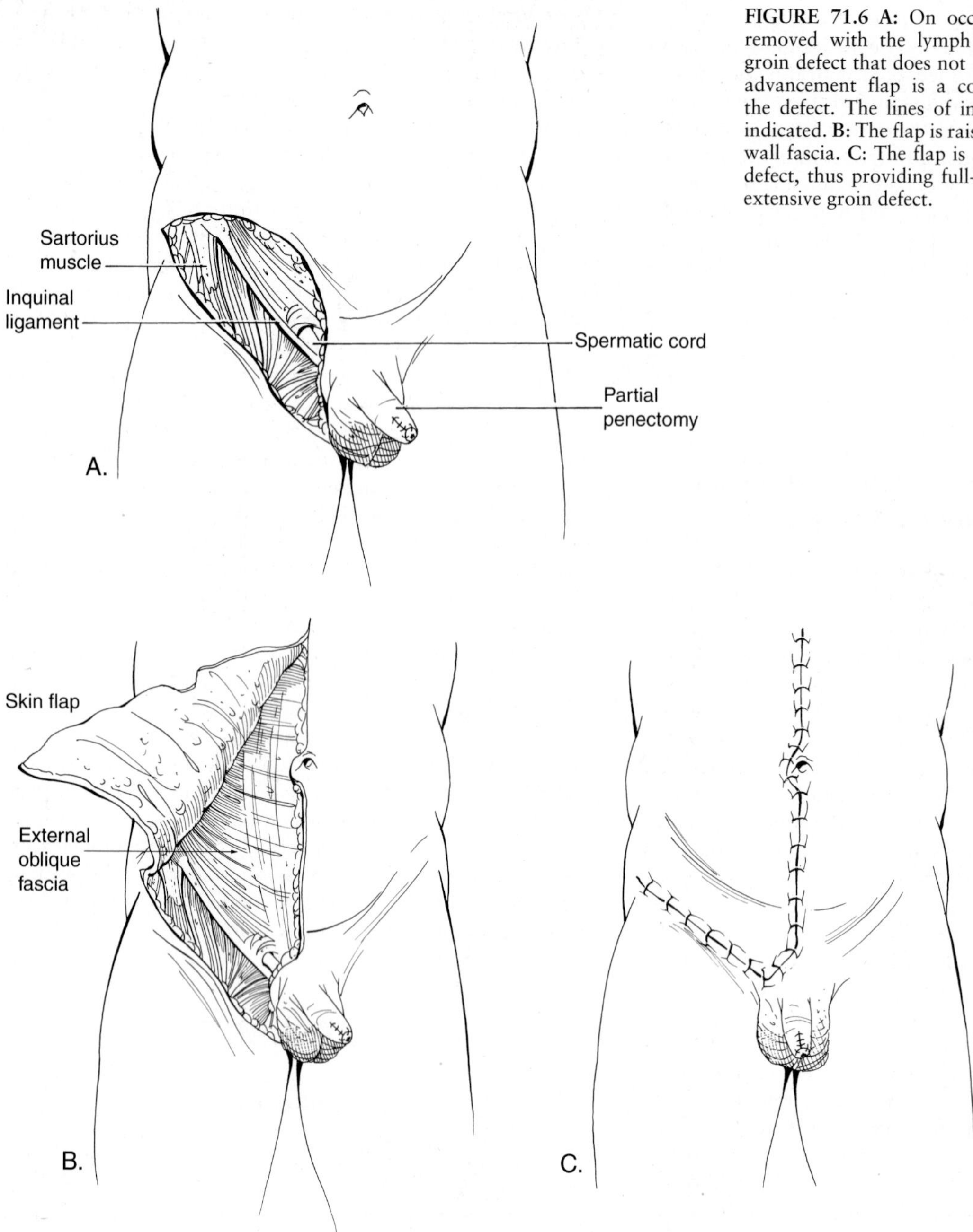


**FIGURE 71.6 A:** On occasion overlying skin must be removed with the lymph nodes, thus creating a large groin defect that does not allow primary skin closure. An advancement flap is a convenient method of covering the defect. The lines of incision for raising the flap are indicated. **B:** The flap is raised superficial to the abdominal wall fascia. **C:** The flap is advanced and sutured over the defect, thus providing full-thickness skin coverage to the extensive groin defect.

## *References*


1. McDougal WS, Kirchner FK Jr, Edwards RH, et al. Treatment of carcinoma of the penis: the case for primary lymphadenectomy. *J Urol* 1986;136(1): 38–41.
2. Horenblas S, van Tinteren H. Squamous cell carcinoma of the penis. IV. Prognostic factors of survival: analysis of tumor, nodes and metastasis classification system. *J Urol* 1994;151(5):1239–1243.
3. McDougal WS. Carcinoma of the penis: improved survival by early regional lymphadenectomy based on the histological grade and depth of invasion of the primary lesion. *J Urol* 1995;154(4):1364–1366.
4. Horenblas S, van Tinteren H, Delemarre JF, et al. Squamous cell carcinoma of the penis. III. Treatment of regional lymph nodes. *J Urol* 1993;149(3): 492–497.
5. McDougal WS. Preemptive lymphadenectomy markedly improves survival in patients with cancer of the penis who harbor occult metastases. *J Urol* 2005;173(3):681.
6. Catalona WJ. Modified inguinal lymphadenectomy for carcinoma of the penis with preservation of saphenous veins: technique and preliminary results. *J Urol* 1988;140(2):306–310.
7. Lopes A, Rossi BM, Fonseca FP, et al. Unreliability of modified inguinal lymphadenectomy for clinical staging of penile carcinoma. *Cancer* 1996; 77(10):2099–2102.
8. Pettaway CA, Pisters LL, Dinney CP, et al. Sentinel lymph node dissection for penile carcinoma: the M. D. Anderson Cancer Center experience. *J Urol* 1995;154(6):1999–2003.
9. Izawa J, Kedar D, Wong F, et al. Sentinel lymph node biopsy in penile cancer: evolution and insights. *Can J Urol* 2005;12[Suppl 1]:24–29.
10. Daseler E, Hanson BJ, Reimann AF. Radical excision of the inguinal and iliac lymph glands. *Surg Gynecol Obstet* 1948;87:679–694.
11. Tabatabaei S, McDougal WS. Primary skin closure of large groin defects after inguinal lymphadenectomy for penile cancer using an abdominal cutaneous advancement flap. *J Urol* 2003;169:118–120.
12. Milathianakis C, Bogdanos J, Karamanolakis D. Morbidity of prophylactic inguinal lymphadenectomy with saphenous vein preservation for squamous cell penile carcinoma. *Int J Urol* 2005;12(8):776–778.

# CHAPTER 72 ■ SURGICAL TREATMENT OF PEYRONIE DISEASE

URI GUR AND GERALD H. JORDAN

Peyronie's disease is characterized by the formation of a fibrous lesion within the tunica albuginea of the corpora cavernosa (Fig. 72.1). This lesion or "plaque" is believed to be caused by repetitive microvascular trauma (3). It is proposed that trauma, either acute or chronic, is sustained during intercourse, with subsequent scar formation in susceptible individuals. The plaque's inelasticity results in a functional shortening of the corporal body on the most affected side, resulting in deformity during erection. The incidence of Peyronie's disease has recently been estimated at up to 3% or as high as 7% to 9% of the general male population (9,10).

Patients most commonly present with dorsal curvature. Fortunately, only a small proportion of patients with Peyronie's disease have deformity requiring surgical intervention. Surgical intervention should be regarded as palliation of the deformity only and not as cure.

## DIAGNOSIS

The diagnosis of Peyronie's disease can usually be made with a focused history and physical examination. On history, it is imperative to elicit the duration of symptoms, the progression of the penile deformity, and the degree of sexual dysfunction. Erectile dysfunction, to some degree, is felt by many surgeons to be almost uniformly present. This may represent the psychological impact incurred from living with a genital deformity but may also be due to several organic causes.

The physical examination should be focused on delineating plaque location, size, and opposing plaque formation (if present). An attempt to elicit known disease associations such as Dupuytren's contracture or other elastic tissue fibromatosis should be made. Objective evaluation of penile curvature with home-taken photographs of the erect penis, we find, is extremely helpful. Plain radiographs are effective in demonstrating plaque calcification, believed to be a sign of plaque maturity. Plaque calcification is also easily demonstrated with ultrasonography (1). The plaque can be imaged by both CT and MRI, both being unnecessary except for the possibility of using MRI to "stage" the phase of disease for research or study protocol purposes (5), or in a rare patient where the diagnosis is not certain and a concern for a possible malignancy arises.

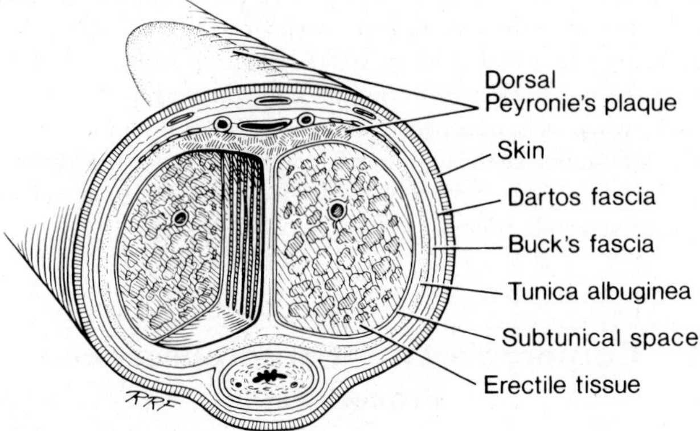


FIGURE 72.1 Cross-sectional penile anatomy with dorsal Peyronie's plaque.

It is important to evaluate and define the surgical candidate's preoperative erectile function. Prospective surgical patients, at our center, are evaluated with color duplex ultrasound (CDU) in the presence of pharmacologically induced erection. Abnormalities in the resistive index and end-diastolic velocity, at our institution, prompt further testing with dynamic infusion cavernosometry/cavernosography (DICC). In addition, one must determine if acceptable intercourse can be accomplished by enhancement of erectile rigidity alone. In this scenario, patients may be best served with a pharmacologic erection program as an alternative to surgery.

A frank discussion of treatment goals with the couple is imperative. The patient should be assured that the process is not malignant or life-threatening. The goal of surgery is to straighten the penis and maintain erectile function so that satisfactory intercourse can be achieved.

Couples must be aware that pre-existing penile shortening and erectile dysfunction will not be improved by straightening procedures. Rigidity may be improved by straightening the penis, but truly improved erectile function does not occur. Evaluation with a sex therapist can help patients and partners adjust to these new sexual expectations.

## INDICATIONS FOR SURGERY

Although medical treatments targeting the evolution of scar tissue have largely been unsuccessful, an attempt at treating Peyronie's disease medically may be beneficial for patients prior to surgical intervention, provided the patient is in the immature or active phase of the disease. A surgical candidate must meet certain criteria. First, the disease process must be stable and the "plaque" mature and quiescent. In review, the signs of disease quiescence include unchanged penile deformity for a minimum of 6 months, with the resolution of pain associated with erection. Moreover, before surgical intervention most investigators recommend a minimum 12-month waiting period from disease onset. The experienced examiner may recognize the clinical findings of a mature or calcified plaque and could elect to intervene earlier than this arbitrary time period. Once disease stability exists, indications for surgical intervention are penile deformity and/or erectile dysfunction that precludes intercourse.

Three general techniques exist for the surgical management of Peyronie's disease: (a) corporoplasty or plication procedures, (b) plaque incision or excision with grafting, and (c) penile prosthesis insertion with plaque modeling or incision with or without grafting. Many protocols have been published describing the treatment of Peyronie's disease, but the best outcome depends on an individualized approach. Straightening techniques are appropriate for patients with adequate erectile function in whom penile straightening alone will achieve satisfactory intercourse.

Plication procedures involve shortening the tunica albuginea on the side opposite the plaque; this may eventually shorten the penis, but it carries the advantages of being less technically demanding, of involving a more rapid convalescence, and in most series of having a smaller risk of postoperative erectile dysfunction.

Plication or corporoplasty procedures may be the preferred option for ventral curvatures, as historically this subset of patients has demonstrated poor outcomes with grafting procedures. Incision or excision of the Peyronie's plaque with grafting of the corporotomy defect is a more technically complex procedure and may incur a higher risk of postoperative erectile dysfunction. Patients with severe curvature, hourglass deformity, or inadequate penile length are more amenable to incision or excision with grafting over corporoplasty or plication techniques that can further shorten or deform the erect penis. At our institution we prefer the technique of plaque incision with grafting and use this even for severely calcified plaques. However, there are cases where large, extensively calcified plaques may require plaque excision with grafting.

Last, insertion of penile prostheses for Peyronie's disease was once considered a panacea but for most patients is now reserved for those with severe erectile dysfunction. In patients with severe curvature, prosthetic implantation can be done in conjunction with an incision and grafting procedure. Modeling the plaque intraoperatively after prosthesis placement is remarkably successful and often avoids the need for incision. The technique of penile prosthesis insertion is covered in Chapter 74.

## ALTERNATIVE THERAPY

Medical management includes oral agents, topical agents, with or without delivery modalities, and intralesional injection protocols. Several surgeons are also examining the efficacy of plaque expansion using devices that put traction on the penis. As mentioned, the surgical management of Peyronie disease should be viewed as a palliation of the mechanical effects of the disease rather than a cure. In a patient with erectile dysfunction, with or without curvature, penile prosthesis insertion should be contemplated. Many patients will refuse prosthetic implantation based on personal bias.

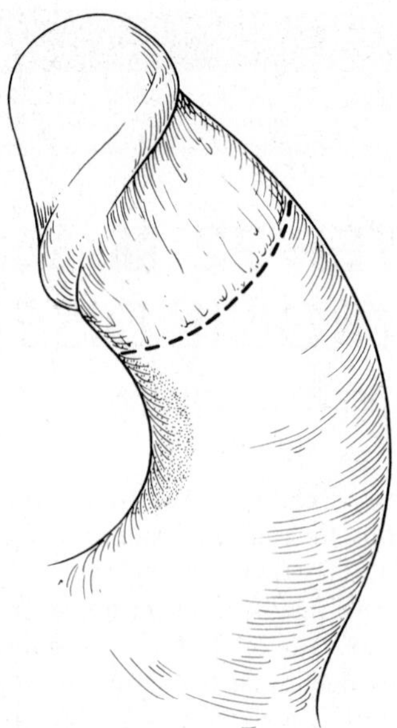

FIGURE 72.2 Dorsal penile curvature with incision marked at the circumcision scar.

## SURGICAL TECHNIQUE

### Skin Incision

The initial skin incision is dependent on plaque location and the procedure to be performed. As previously mentioned, corporoplasty or plication procedures address the aspect of the corpora cavernosa opposite the plaque (most involved aspect), whereas plaque incision or excision techniques approach the plaque directly. The dorsum of the corpora cavernosa is best exposed by a circumferential degloving incision. If the patient has been previously circumcised, then the incision should be performed through the circumcision scar (Fig. 72.2). Approaching the penis through the previous circumcision scar has not been problematic, even when the scar is displaced proximally. The penile shaft is degloved to its base by sharply dissecting the dartos fascia from the underlying Buck's fascia. This maneuver gives good exposure for midshaft and distal lesions. For very proximal plaques or patients with a redundant prepuce, a second peripenile or periscrotal incision may be helpful. After degloving the shaft of the penis, the surgeon delivers it into the counterincision, laying the shaft skin aside and covering it with a warm soaked gauze dressing. This protects the penile skin from trauma until the end of the procedure, when it is returned to the shaft. Ventral exposure can also be achieved through a midline incision on the ventral aspect of the penis, which we prefer, as this results in less postoperative penile edema.

### Corporoplasty or Corporoplication Procedures

Several techniques have been described to "plicate" the curvature associated with Peyronie's disease. At our institution, procedures are performed with the patient in the supine position, via a degloving incision for dorsal "plication," and a midline ventral incision for ventral "plication."

An artificial erection is created to accurately define the point of maximal curvature using a pressure infuser with 0.9% saline. The use of a tourniquet for control of bleeding or induction of an artificial erection is not favored as proximal curvatures can be concealed. The Buck's fascia opposite the site of maximal curvature is sharply incised and elevated from the underlying tunica albuginea. Correction of dorsal curvature requires identification of the corpus spongiosum ventrally. For ventral curvature, care must be taken to avoid injury to the dorsal neurovascular structures. Once the tunica albuginea is exposed, "plication" of the corpora can be performed in several ways. Creation of an ellipse corporotomy defect with reapproximation of the corporal edges using 4-0 polydioxanone sutures effectively counteracts the opposing lesion (11). The tunica albuginea may be excised or tucked underneath the corporotomy closure. Correction of curvature can also be achieved by plicating the tunica albuginea by a number of techniques that use nonabsorbable sutures without incising the tunica albuginea (4). One technique of corporoplasty uses the Heineke-Mikulicz technique, which horizontally closes a vertical incision of the tunica (12). Once acceptable straightening is achieved, the penis is closed anatomically in layers, and we place a small-caliber, closed-suction drain superficial to the Buck fascia.

## Plaque Incision and Grafting

After incision and degloving, exposure for the incision of a dorsal plaque requires elevation of the dorsal neurovascular bundle concurrently with the Buck's fascia. This can be approached by several techniques. One technique involves making bilateral incisions lateral to the corpus spongiosum and then dissecting the Buck's fascia and the dorsal neurovascular bundle off the lateral and dorsal aspects of the corpora cavernosa. Alternately, a dorsal plaque can be approached through the bed of the deep dorsal vein with a modified vein dissection and excision.

This is done by sharply opening the Buck's fascia over the path of the deep dorsal vein to the level of the penopubic ligaments (Fig. 72.3). The dorsal vein is elevated and ligated as proximally as possible without detaching the penopubic attachments and then distally to the "trifurcation" of the vein (Fig. 72.4). The circumferential veins are ligated at their junction with the deep dorsal vein. The dorsolateral neurovascular structures are reflected off the tunica albuginea in concert

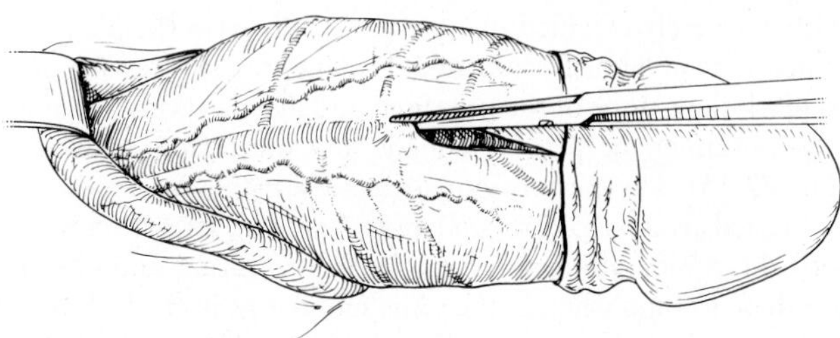

FIGURE 72.3 Incision of the Buck's fascia overlying the dorsal vein after penile degloving.

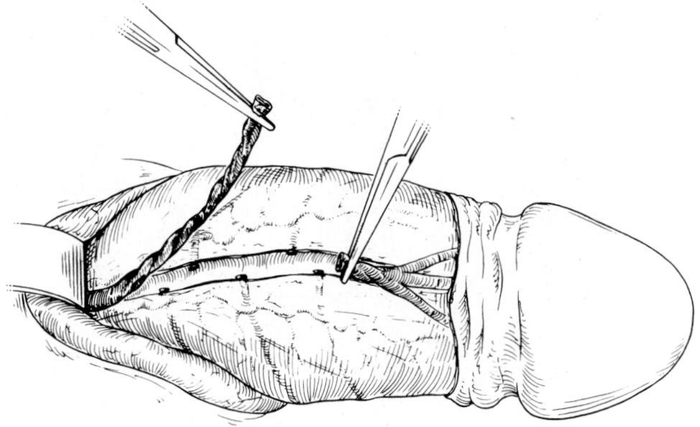

FIGURE 72.4 Deep dorsal vein dissection and ligation.

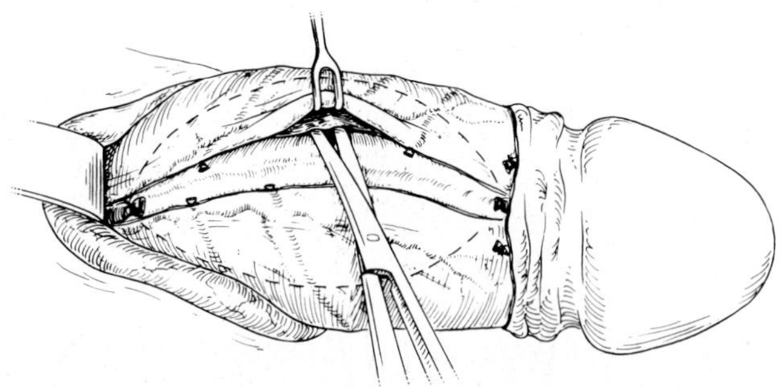

FIGURE 72.5 Elevation of the Buck's fascia concurrently with the dorsal neurovascular structures.

with the inner lamina of the Buck's fascia. The Buck's fascia is widely mobilized from the base of the penis to the coronal margin and to the lateral aspect of the penis (Fig. 72.5). If necessary, the glans can be partially detached from the tips of the corporal bodies in order to expose distal dorsal plaques. Austoni E and Perovic S, Personal Communication, Peyronie's Meeting, Washington, DC attended by Dr. Charles J. Devine, Jr., have both advocated penile disassembly for certain patients with Peyronie's disease; however, the complication rate can be significantly higher. Approaching the dorsal plaque through the bed of the dorsal vein is our favored approach.

Once appropriately exposed, the extent of the plaque can be determined by palpating the surface of the tunica albuginea. After creation of an artificial erection, an H-shaped incision is marked at the point of maximal curvature (Fig. 72.6).

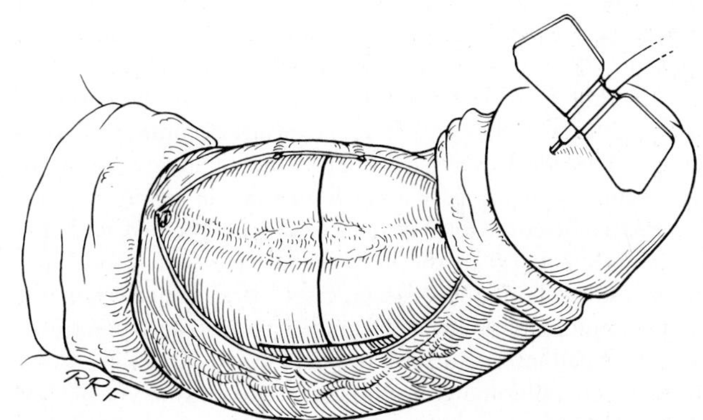

FIGURE 72.6 An H-shaped incision marked at the point of maximal deformity.

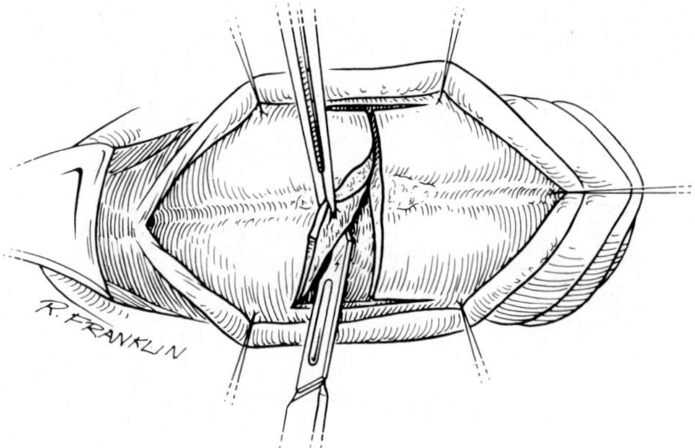


FIGURE 72.7 Incision of the tunica albuginea.

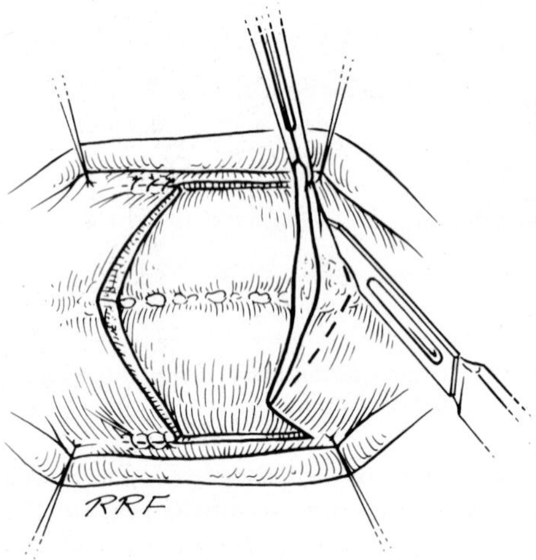


FIGURE 72.8 Creation of a square defect in the tunica albuginea. Darting incisions are performed if indentation persists.

Once the incision is created, the "flaps" of the H are elevated and allowed to "slide" (Fig. 72.7). During this maneuver the thickened septal fibers are divided from their attachment to the tunica albuginea. Complete release of all of the thickened fibers appears integral to achieving good straightening. It is not necessary to remove thickened septal fibers, and it is unnecessary and potentially harmful to remove any spongy erectile tissue. A square defect is then created by suturing the flap corners into place with interrupted 4-0 polydioxanone sutures. If an indentation exists after corporotomy, darting incisions are made to allow for expansion of the defect (Fig. 72.8).

After the incision is completed, we measure the corporotomy defect with the penis flexed to ensure accurate graft coverage. The ideal graft material is not known. We have preferentially in the past used dermis at our institution (2). Alternatively, corporotomy defects can be patched with the saphenous vein (8) or the deep dorsal vein with good long-term results. Temporalis fascia, fascia lata, tunica vaginalis, and nonautologous pericardial grafts have also been described, as have small intestinal submucosa (Surgisis Biodesign, Cook Medical Inc., Bloomington, IN) grafts. Recently we have used the Surgisis Biodesign graft at our institution with good outcomes. A recent comparative report (7) was shown to be at least equivalent to the dermal graft. Tunica vaginalis lacks tensile strength and is best applied to small defects. Prosthetic (e.g., Gore-Tex, silastic) grafts, historically, have tended to fibrose and contract. The authors feel that caution should be used when applying these "grafts" in the absence of concurrent prosthetic implantation.

The dermal graft is obtained from the nonhirsute area of abdominal skin located superior and lateral to the iliac crest (Fig. 72.9). The Surgisis Biodesign graft requires soaking when removed from the package. There is a "fuzzy side" and a smooth side. For no good reason, we have always placed the "fuzzy side" inward. By hyperflexing the penis, the graft is placed approximately 30% larger than the corporotomy defect in all dimensions.

Once tailored, the dermal graft or the Surgisis Biodesign graft is sewn into the corporotomy defect using interrupted 4-0 polydioxanone sutures followed by a running locked 4-0 polydioxanone suture (Fig. 72.10). An artificial erection is performed after graft placement to ensure a watertight suture line and an acceptably straight penis. Any leaks, if present, are oversewn. An obvious disadvantage, as opposed to "off-the-shelf grafts," is the time necessary for graft harvest as well as donor site morbidity.

We have found that curvature can be corrected with a single incision and grafting in the majority of instances. Some patients will require an additional "touch-up" plication or in the rare case a second incision of the plaque. Incision as opposed to excision limits the size of the applied graft and may be more reliable in preserving erectile function (Dr. Friedhelm Schreiter, International Reconstructive Live-Surgery Congress, Genitourinary Reconstructive Surgeons Meeting, Hamburg, Germany, February 28-March 2, 1999). The penis is closed as described previously for surgical plication. We have also noted that in patients where erect penile length is not equivalent to stretched length, the Surgisis Biodesign graft may be more likely to inadequately correct the curvature as opposed to autografts.

Recently, we have modified our technique of "H incision" in an effort to more efficiently correct the curvature without the need for touch-up plications. The site of maximal curvature is identified and marked. However, a strip of tunica albuginea, a thick cross member of the H, is marked (Fig. 72.11). The H is incised with the flaps elevated and detached from the septal fibers as already described (Fig. 72.12). The strip of the H is excised and the flap sutured as already described (Fig. 72.13). The resulting corporotomy defect is grafted (Fig. 72.14).

## Plaque Excision and Grafting

Plaque excision (vs. incision) may be required in the patient with a severely calcified plaque. In this scenario the plaque is exposed as previously discussed. Prolene stay sutures are used to mark the plaque at the proximal and distal aspects. An incision outlining the plaque is made and the plaque is excised (Fig. 72.15). The corporotomy defect left by plaque excision is converted from ovoid to stellate by creating lateral incisions into the tunica albuginea (Fig. 72.16). Grafting and closure are then accomplished in the same manner as in the technique of plaque incision and grafting. In most cases the calcified plaque can be removed without excising the entire thickness of the tunica, and that is our favored approach.

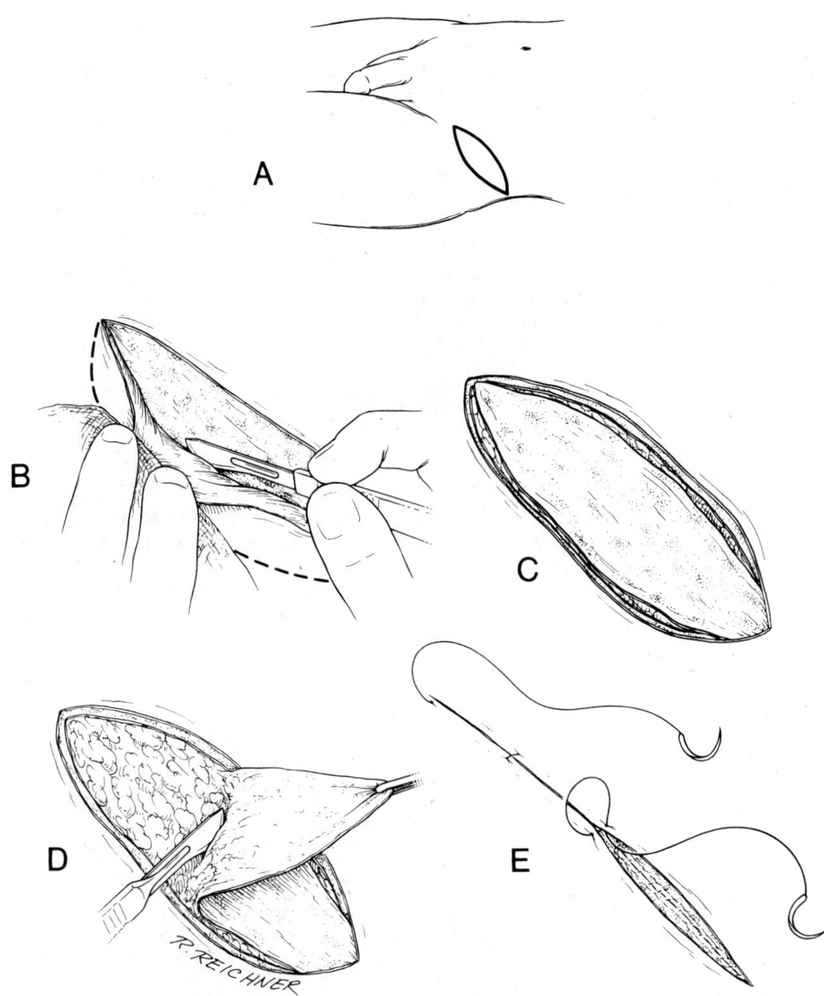


FIGURE 72.9 Dermal harvest from the nonhirsute skin above the iliac crest.

## POSTOPERATIVE CARE

A loosely applied Bioclusive (Johnson&Johnson Medical Limited, Gargave, Skipton, UK) dressing is used to dress the penis. Mildly compressing Conform gauze dressing (Tyco Healthcare Group LP, Mansfield, MA) is wrapped around the Bioclusive to reduce edema and keep the surgical spaces collapsed around the suction drains. The compressing dressing is removed in 4 hours and the glans is checked every 30 minutes during this interval. A 14Fr Foley catheter is placed intraoperatively and left for 24 hours. The drains are, in general, removed on postoperative day 1 and the patient is discharged the same day. Erections are suppressed with diazepam and amyl nitrite for a short period postoperatively.

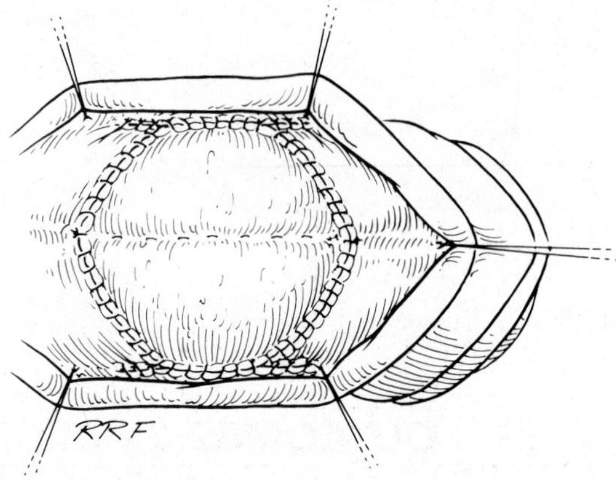


FIGURE 72.10 Watertight closure of the corporotomy after dermal graft.

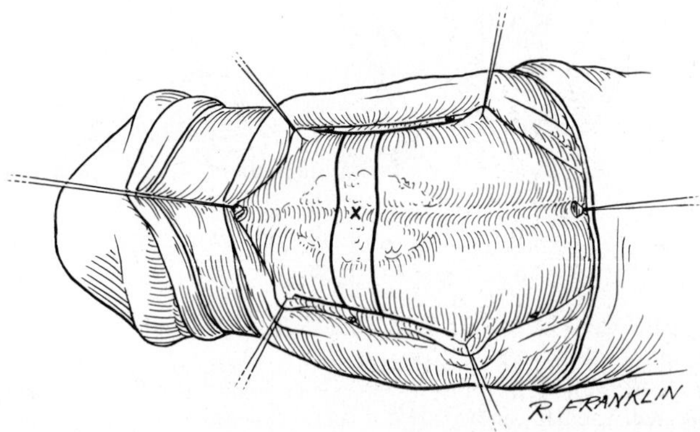


FIGURE 72.11 Modification of the sliding H technique, in which a small strip is excised at the point of maximal curvature. The stitch marks that point. (From Jordan GH. Peyronie's disease. In: Wein AJ, Kavoussi LR, Novick AC, et al., eds. *Campbell-Walsh urology*, 9th ed. Philadelphia: Saunders Elsevier, 2007:818–838, with permission.)

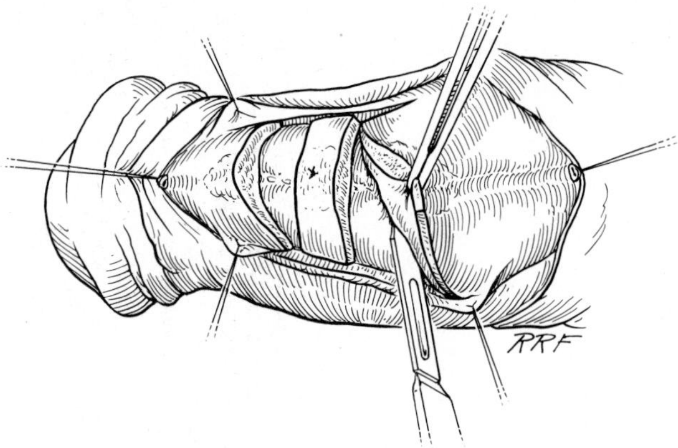


FIGURE 72.12 The incisions are made; the H flaps are incised and elevated from the underlying erectile tissue. The septal fibers are divided. The septal fibers are detached back to the point of normal tunica albuginea both proximally and distally. This maneuver is extremely important in achieving straightening with this technique. Note the expansion of the corporotomy defect. (From Jordan GH. Peyronie's disease. In: Wein AJ, Kavoussi LR, Novick AC, et al., eds. *Campbell-Walsh urology*, 9th ed. Philadelphia: Saunders Elsevier, 2007:818–838, with permission.)

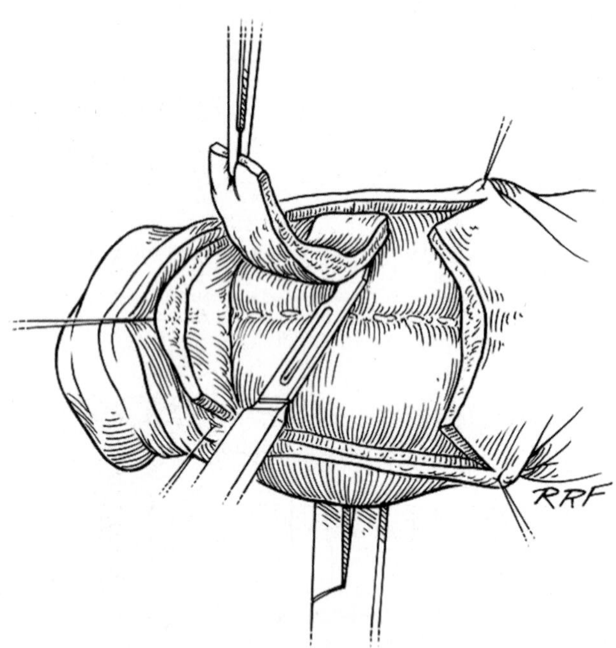


FIGURE 72.13 The transverse strip is excised; the H flaps are then sutured. The flap can be darted if lateral expansion is needed. (From Jordan GH. Peyronie's disease. In: Wein AJ, Kavoussi LR, Novick AC, et al., eds. *Campbell-Walsh urology*, 9th ed. Philadelphia: Saunders Elsevier, 2007:818–838, with permission.)

After that, erections are felt to be beneficial and integral to good graft healing. Levine (13) and Moncado, Personal Communication at Experts in Urology Conference, London, England, June 12–16, 2007, are using a mechanical stretching device to distend the penis and graft postoperatively and are encouraged that the results seem better.

After 2 weeks, patients are encouraged to have erections but refrain from intercourse. At about 10 to 12 weeks postoperatively, patients may resume sexual intercourse.

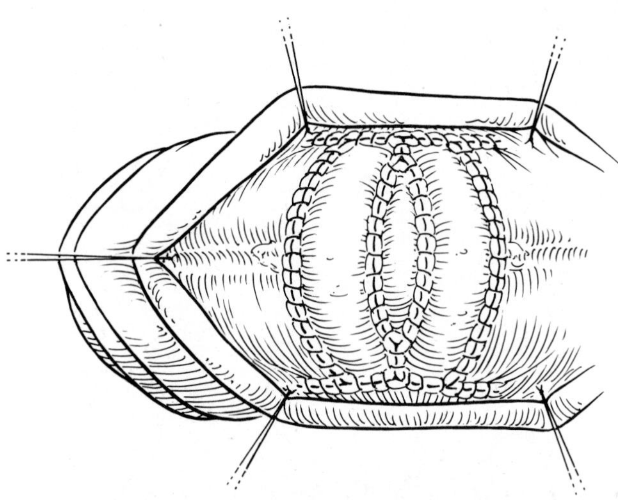

FIGURE 72.14 Alternatively, the corporotomy defect can be replaced with a vein graft. Notice that the vein graft is oriented so that the circumferential distensibility allows long axial lengthening. (From Jordan GH. Peyronie's disease. In: Wein AJ, Kavoussi LR, Novick AC, et al., eds. *Campbell-Walsh urology*, 9th ed. Philadelphia: Saunders Elsevier, 2007:818–838, with permission.)

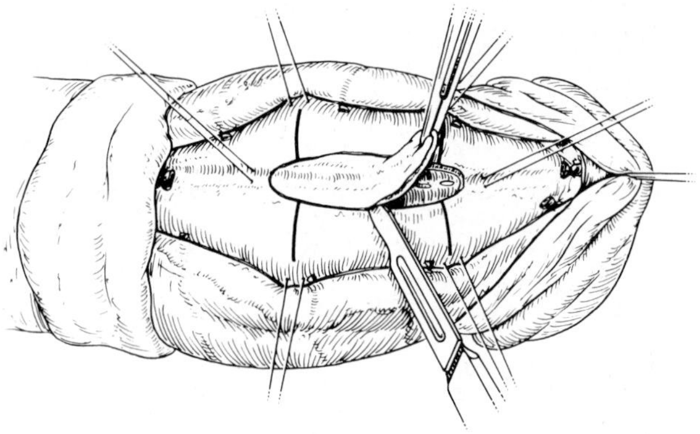

FIGURE 72.15 Excision of Peyronie plaque.

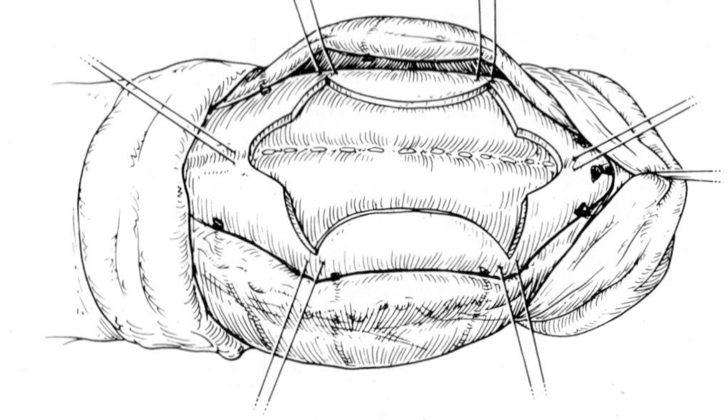

FIGURE 72.16 Creation of stellate defect after plaque excision.

## OUTCOMES

A successful reconstructive procedure for Peyronie disease results in a satisfactory straightening of the penis such that any residual deformity does not interfere with sexual intercourse.

A second component of success is preservation of adequate erectile function. In our experience surgical success correlates linearly with preoperative erectile function (6). Patients with good erectile function have a surgical success rate in the range of 85%. Poor preoperative erectile function correlates strongly with a poor surgical outcome, and these patients may be best managed with prosthesis placement. The demonstration of corporal veno-occlusive dysfunction preoperatively seems to correlate strongly with diminished success (i.e., poor preservation of erectile function), particularly with grafting operations.

The ultimate goal of surgery is to resume satisfactory sexual intercourse by correcting penile curvature without further diminishing erectile function. With proper patient selection, surgical correction for Peyronie disease yields reliable results.

## COMPLICATIONS

Early postoperative complications include hematoma formation, wound infection, and persistent penile edema. Meticulous hemostasis with bipolar cautery, the use of small closed-suction drains, and careful tissue handling can minimize the risk of these complications.

Patients should be informed of the risk of experiencing a change in glanular sensation. This applies predominantly to those patients requiring dissection of the Buck's fascia dorsally. The vast majority of patients recover adequate glanular sensation, and it is unusual for persistent bothersome neuropathies of the glans to occur.

Late and chronic complications may include the risk of a bothersome granuloma ("lump") formation after the use of permanent sutures during a plication procedure. Recurrent disabling curvature is uncommon but may occur. Patients requiring grafting with dermis should be counseled that during the late phase of maturation the graft tends to contract and may be inelastic enough to recreate some of the curvature. Patients can be reassured that this is transient and that straightening will occur when the graft softens.

The most frequently encountered "complication" is that of diminished penile rigidity postoperatively. With plication procedures this occurs in approximately 5% to 6% of patients and with grafting procedures in approximately 12% to 15% of cases. Erectile dysfunction can occur as a consequence of surgery but may also represent the natural history of the patient. Many of these patients benefit from the addition of pharmacologic therapy to enhance their erectile function.

## *References*


1. Altaffer LF III, Jordan GH. Sonographic demonstration of Peyronie plaques. *Urology* 1981;17(3):292–295.
2. Devine CJ Jr, Horton CE. Surgical treatment of Peyronie's disease with a dermal graft. *J Urol* 1974;111:44.
3. Devine CJ Jr, Somers KD, Jordan GH, et al. Proposal: trauma as the cause of the Peyronie's lesion. *J Urol* 1997;157:285.
4. Gholami SS, Lue TF. Correction of penile curvature using the 16-dot plication technique: a review of 132 patients. *J Urol* 2002;167:2066.
5. Hauck EW, Hackstein N, Vosshenrich R, et al. Diagnostic value of magnetic resonance imaging in Peyronie's disease—a comparison both with palpation and ultrasound in the evaluation of plaque formation. *Eur Urol* 2003;43:293–300.
6. Jordan GH, Angermeier KW. Preoperative evaluation of erectile function with dynamic infusion cavernosometry/cavernosography in patients undergoing surgery for Peyronie's disease: correlation with postoperative results. *J Urol* 1993;150:1138.
7. Kovac JR, Brock GB. Surgical outcomes and patient satisfaction after dermal, pericardial, and small intestinal submucosal grafting for Peyronie's disease. *J Sex Med* 2007;4(5):1500–1508.
8. Lue TF, El-Sakka AI. Venous patch graft for Peyronie's disease. Part I: Technique. *J Urol* 1998;160:2047.
9. Mulhall JP, Creech SD, Boorjian SA, et al. Subjective and objective analysis of the prevalence of Peyronie's disease in a population of men presenting for prostate cancer screening. *J Urol* 2004; 171(6, Pt 1):2350–2353.
10. Mulhall JP, Schiff J, Guhring P. An analysis of the natural history of Peyronie's disease. *J Urol* 2006;175(6):2115–2118; discussion 2118.
11. Pryor JP, Fitzpatrick JM. A new approach to the correction of the penile deformity in Peyronie's disease. *J Urol* 1979;122:622.
12. Yachia D. Modified corporoplasty for the treatment of penile curvature. *J Urol* 1990;143(1):80–82.
13. Levine LA, Newell M, Taylor FL. "Penile traction therapy for treatment of Peyronie's disease" a single-center pilot study. *J Sex Med* 2008 June; 5(6): 1468–73.


# CHAPTER 73 ■ PRIAPISM

TRINITY J. BIVALACQUA AND ARTHUR L. BURNETT

Priapism is defined as an erectile disorder in which erection persists uncontrollably without sexual purpose. This disorder is likely a result of disturbances in the mechanisms governing erection physiology as it relates to regulatory control of penile detumescence and initiation and maintenance of penile flaccidity. Priapism represents one of the greatest challenges in therapeutic management among erectile disorders. During a single episode of ischemic priapism, blood fails to drain from the corporal sinusoids, resulting in prolonged painful erection. The pain associated with priapism is perceived to be a consequence of tissue ischemia and increased pressure generated within the corporal bodies. This condition frequently results in erectile dysfunction (ED), and therefore prompt management is indicated. The natural sequelae of untreated ischemic priapism or recurrent stuttering priapism is global penile fibrosis with significant impairments in erectile mechanisms, resulting in an overall rate of ED as high as 59% (1–3).

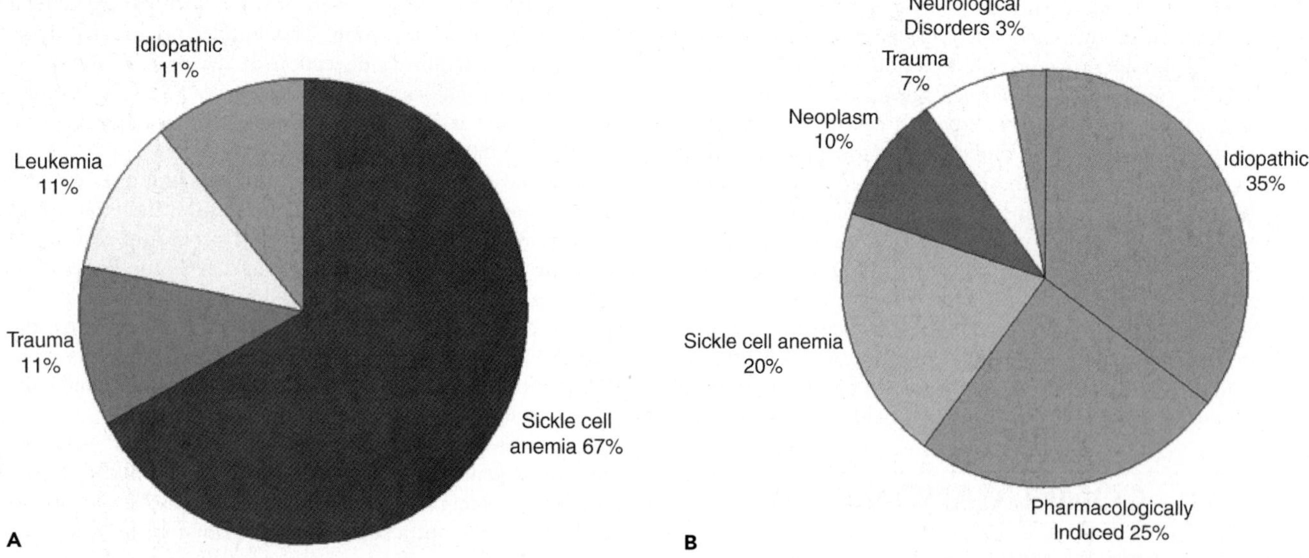


**FIGURE 73.1** Pie graphs demonstrating the percentage of (**A**) pediatric (<18 years) and (**B**) adult (>18 years) patients suffering from priapism.

Ischemic (venous, low-flow) priapism is more prevalent than nonischemic (arterial, high-flow) priapism. Ischemic priapism due to pharmacologic, hematologic, or neurogenic causes is a condition whereby there is a persistent, painful erection characterized clinically by absent cavernous blood flow. Failure to recognize this as an emergency and instigate immediate treatment may lead to corporal tissue ischemia or anoxia, fibrosis, and long-term ED. After 24 hours there is evidence of irreversible smooth muscle cell necrosis, destruction of the vascular endothelium, and exposure of the basement membrane with adherence of thrombocytes (4). Nonischemic priapism commonly follows an episode of trauma to the perineum or genitalia resulting in increased flow through cavernosal arteries, which leads to the formation of arteriocavernous shunts with increased well-oxygenated arterial flow into the cavernous tissue and may not need urgent surgical attention.

Priapism is associated with a number of diverse disease states, and a number of clinical contexts have risk associations for developing the disorder (1,5,6). Etiologic categories include trauma, neurological conditions (multiple sclerosis, spinal cord tumor with compression), hematologic dyscrasias (sickle cell anemia, thrombophilia, and thalassemia), malignancies, intracavernous injection therapy (prostaglandin $E_1$, papaverine, and combination therapy), pharmacologic and drug exposure (psychotropic and antidepressant medications, and illicit drugs), and idiopathic circumstances (Fig. 73.1) (1). Urogenital carcinomas can cause priapism either by local invasion and growth into the adjacent tissue or by the hematogenous, lymphatic, or retrograde venous routes. Priapism associated with malignancy may be ischemic secondary to veno-occlusion or nonischemic secondary to high arterial blood flow.

In principle, ischemic priapism consists of an imbalance of vasoconstrictive and vasorelaxatory mechanisms, thus predisposing the penis to hypoxia and acidosis. In vitro studies have demonstrated that when corporal smooth muscle strips are exposed to hypoxic conditions, significant apoptosis results, and alpha-adrenergic stimulation fails to induce corporal smooth muscle contraction (7). Additional pathophysiologic mechanisms involved in the progression of ischemia-induced fibrosis are the upregulation of hypoxia-induced growth factors such as transforming growth factor-β (8). Recently, we have shown that recurrent priapism is a manifestation of defective phosphodiesterase type 5 (PDE5) regulatory function in the penis, resulting from altered endothelial nitric oxide and cyclic guanosine monophosphate (cGMP) signaling in the organ and recurrent priapism (9,10).

## DIAGNOSIS

The diagnosis and classification of priapism are based on clinical evaluation, including laboratory tests and corporal blood gas evaluation via aspirated blood directly from the corpora cavernosa. On initial evaluation, patients should have a detailed history and physical examination, with emphasis on possible causative factors (Fig. 73.2). Historical features should include the duration and previous episodes of priapism, a detailed medical and social history to evaluate for hematologic or neurologic conditions, and illicit drug use (cocaine). Physical examination should assess the penis and perineum, inspecting for any neurologic defects and pelvic or penile masses, and checking the perineum for evidence of recent trauma. Laboratory tests should include a complete blood count, reticulocyte count, and sickle cell anemia screen when appropriate, as well as urinalysis and urine toxicology.

Patients with significant sustained penile pain with a rigid penis and soft glans are more likely to have ischemic priapism, whereas patients with nonischemic priapism will have a semierect penis without pain. Corporal blood gas analysis will help delineate the type of priapism. Acidotic (pH $<7.25$, $pO_2 <30$ mm Hg, $pCO_2 >60$ mm Hg) penile blood gas indicates ischemic priapism, whereas a blood gas consistent with arterial blood gas (pH $> 7.4$, $pO_2 >90$ mm Hg, $pCO_2 <40$ mm Hg) is suggestive of nonischemic priapism. To further determine the type of priapism, color duplex Doppler ultrasound may be

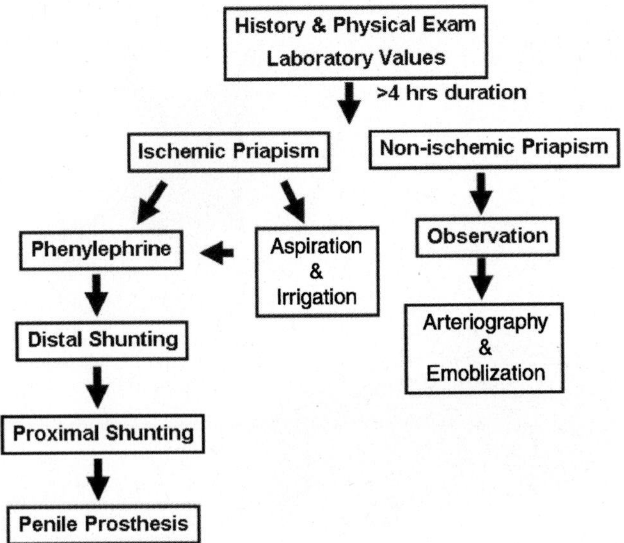


FIGURE 73.2 Algorithm for the management of priapism. (Adapted from Montague DK, Jarow J, Broderick GA, et al. Members of the Erectile Dysfunction Guideline Update Panel; American Urological Association. American Urological Association guideline on the management of priapism. *J Urol* 2003;170:1318–1324.)

performed to evaluate cavernosal arterial inflow (1,11). No cavernosal artery flow is pathognomonic for ischemic priapism, whereas a ruptured cavernosal artery with unregulated arterial flow and blood pooling may be seen in the nonischemic form of priapism. After the correct form of priapism is determined, then rapid medical and/or surgical intervention is a necessity. In ischemic priapism, definitive first-line treatment consists of evacuation of blood and irrigation of the corpora cavernosa along with intracavernous injection of an alpha-adrenergic sympathomimetic agent before initiating any surgical treatment (Fig. 73.2). If the diagnosis of nonischemic priapism is confirmed by ultrasound imaging, then embolization of the ruptured cavernous artery angiographically may be indicated after initial observation and supportive therapy (Fig. 73.2).

## INDICATIONS FOR SURGERY

The goal of therapy is to relieve pain and decompress the corporal bodies, thus reducing anoxia and the risk of tissue necrosis or injury. Ischemic priapism of >4 hours warrants decompression of the corpora cavernosa. One can proceed earlier if a patient is in severe pain, but action *must* be taken if 4 hours have elapsed (Fig. 73.2). Typically, if treatment is delayed, tissue injury and risk for development of ED may occur. A dorsal nerve block or local penile shaft block with lidocaine is usually performed. Then, a scalp vein needle (19- or 21-gauge) is inserted directly in the penile shaft for therapeutic aspiration of old blood and injection of alpha-adrenergic agonists (sympathomimetics) (5,6). Hemodynamic monitoring is recommended to monitor potential side-effects, such as hypertension, headache, reflex bradycardia, tachycardia, and cardiac arrhythmia, which may result from medication entry into the systemic circulation. The alpha-1 selective agonist phenylephrine is preferred for this application since it minimizes the risk of cardiovascular side-effects. Phenylephrine in a dose of 100 to 200 μg is injected via the same needle into the corpora cavernosa and observed for 5 minutes.

If the penis is still rigid, then aspiration of blood and injection of phenylephrine (100 to 200 μg) is performed until detumescence occurs. If the penis remains tumescent after a reasonable duration and dose escalation of phenylephrine (1 mg of diluted phenylephrine >1 hour), then another Doppler ultrasound can be performed to evaluate the status of cavernosal arterial flow in the penis. Re-evaluation may be warranted at this time because the penis may simply be edematous with restored corporal arterial flow and not in a persistent ischemic state. It is recognized that ischemic priapism of extended durations, that is, >48 hours, is unlikely to resolve with intracavernous injection or irrigation therapy; therefore, surgical shunting should be performed in a timely manner.

## ALTERNATIVE THERAPY

Aspiration or irrigation in combination with intracavernous injection therapy represents first-line therapy in patients with underlying etiologic disorders such as sickle cell anemia and other hematologic disorders, metastatic neoplasia, or other causes having standard treatments. For priapism related to sickle cell disease, medical therapies such as intravenous hydration, oxygenation, alkalinization, and exchange transfusion may be performed. However, these interventions should not lead to delays in intracavernous therapies directed at the end organ. The use of antiandrogens or gonadotropin-releasing hormone agonists is successful for the treatment of recurrent stuttering priapism. The use of sympathomimetic intracavernous injection therapy with phenylephrine is also successful in patients with stuttering priapism. The use of other agents such as baclofen and digoxin is less efficacious.

## SURGICAL TECHNIQUE

Surgical management of ischemic priapism represents a surgically created fistula that allows blood to drain from the corpora cavernosa until the penile compartment syndrome has subsided. Ideally, the surgically created fistula will spontaneously close after the priapic event has resolved. Before proceeding to distal corporoglanular surgical shunt procedures, the placement of needles into the corpora cavernosa distally and proximally at the penile crura with the patient in lithotomy position offers an approach for maximally irrigating the corporal bodies. Distal corporoglandular shunts represent the first-line surgical therapy because they are easy to perform and have fewer complications (Fig. 73.2) (1,11,12).

### Corporoglanular (Winter) Shunt

Under local or general anesthesia, a penile-glans block is performed to ensure adequate local anesthesia. The tips of the rigid corpora cavernosa are palpated, and a large biopsy needle

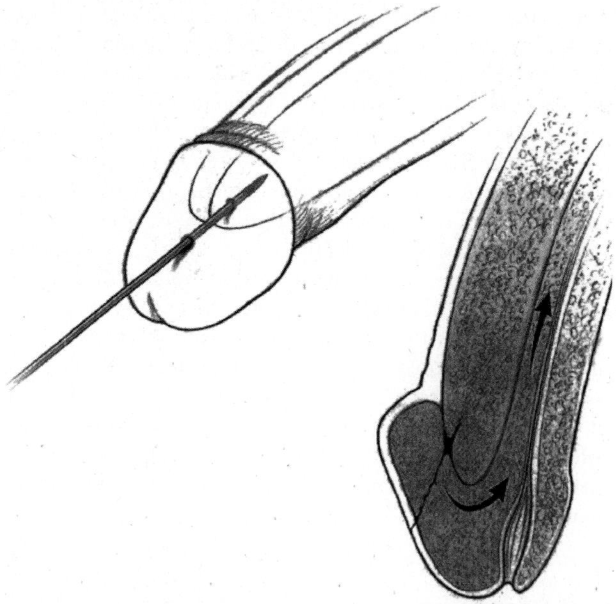

FIGURE 73.3 Corporoglanular (Winter) shunt. A needle is placed through the glans penis into the corpora cavernosa in order to make multiple core biopsy windows or fistulas between the glans and each corporal body. (Adapted from Burnett AL. Priapism. In: Wein AJ, Kavoussi LR, Novick AC, et al., eds. *Campbell-Walsh urology*, 9th ed. Philadelphia: Saunders Elsevier, 2007:839–849.)

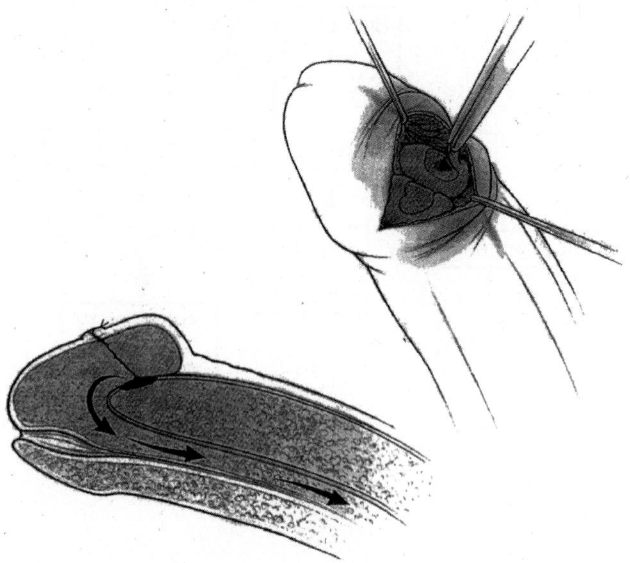

FIGURE 73.4 Corporoglanular (Al-Ghorab) shunt. An incision is made dorsally into the glans penis, and portions of the distal corpus cavernosum are excised as a vent for blood drainage. (Adapted from Burnett AL. Priapism. In: Wein AJ, Kavoussi LR, Novick AC, et al., eds. *Campbell-Walsh urology*, 9th ed. Philadelphia: Saunders Elsevier, 2007:839–849.)

is inserted through the glans into the corpus cavernosum several times (1,11,12). This results in multiple core biopsy windows or fistulas between the glans and each corporal body (Fig. 73.3). Several biopsy core fistulas are necessary to create enough communicating channels to cause detumescence. The puncture site is closed with a figure-of-eight 3-0 chromic suture. The patient is instructed to squeeze the penis every few minutes for the next 12 hours to lessen blood pooling in the penis. If partial (>50%) erection persists, the procedure is repeated or an alternative shunt is used. An adequate result is evidenced by swelling of the glans and detumescence.

## Corporoglanular (Ebbehoj and T-) Shunt

The Ebbehoj shunt procedure involves the use of a no. 11 blade scalpel passed percutaneously several times through the glans into the corpus cavernosum (1,11,12). This results in several larger fistulas between the glans and each tip of the corpus cavernosum. The scalpel blade is inserted into the corpora away from the urethral meatus and pulled back to create an opening in the tunica albuginea between the glans and corporal bodies. A modification of the Ebbehoj shunt is the T-shunt procedure (1,11,12). A no. 10 blade scalpel is placed vertically through the glans penis into the corpus cavernosum. The scalpel is then turned 90 degrees away from the urethra and pulled out. This maneuver creates a T-shaped opening in the tunica albugenia. Both of these shunts can be performed unilaterally or bilaterally if necessary. In theory, this T-shunt should provide a large enough fistula between the corpora cavernosa and spongiosal tissue of the glans for detumescence. Closure of the defects in the glans is performed using 3-0 chromic sutures, especially for the T-shunt.

## Corporoglanular (Al-Ghorab) Shunt

If the previous percutaneous distal shunts are unsuccessful, then an Al-Ghorab shunt is performed (1). Typically, distal shunts fail because a large enough window between the priapic corpora cavernosa and corpus spongiosum does not exist (Fig. 73.4). This shunt is usually done under general anesthesia in combination with a penile-glans block. A tourniquet is placed around the penis. A 2-cm transverse incision is made on the dorsum of the glans 1 cm distal to the coronal sulcus. A transverse incision is not recommended in the distal penile shaft proximal to the corona because this incision may cut sensory nerves to the dorsal aspect of the glans and possibly cause distal atrophy. The tips of the corpora cavernosa should be separated from the glans and transfixed with 2-0 sutures or grasped with a Kocher clamp so that they will not withdraw during detumescence, and a circular cone segment of tunica albuginea approximately 5 by 5 mm should be sharply excised from each corporal body. Dark blood will drain from the corporal bodies, and once detumescence occurs, then reapproximation of the skin with 3-0 chromic sutures is performed. Care is taken not to obliterate the spongy vascular space of the glans penis.

## Corporospongiosal Shunts

A proximal corporospongiosal shunt is performed in rare circumstances (1,11,12). When distal shunts are unsuccessful or technically unachievable, then a proximal shunt may be performed to re-establish blood drainage and thus produce penile detumescence. However, these surgical maneuvers are often ineffective, lead to significant ED, and have a number of potential complications. For the Quackel or Sacher shunt, the

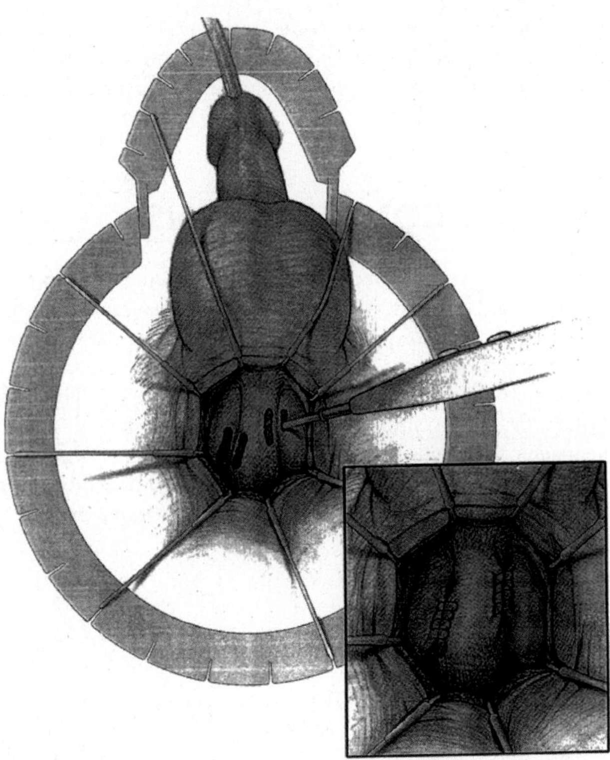

FIGURE 73.5 Quackel or Sacher shunt, a proximal cavernospongiosal (corporospongiosal) shunt procedure. Openings are placed in a staggered fashion connecting a cavernosum and spongiosum bilaterally for blood drainage.

patient is placed in lithotomy position and the bulbocavernosus muscle is dissected off the corpus spongiosum. A longitudinal incision or excision of 1-cm-long ellipses of tissue is made in the spongiosal and corporal bodies (Fig. 73.5). Care is taken to avoid incising the urethra, which would result in a fistula. The incisions or excisions are made in close proximity to each other in order to suture the defects together. The walls of the two openings in the spongiosum and corpora are sewn together in a running fashion using 5-0 polydioxanone suture. It may be necessary to perform bilateral shunting procedures if detumescence is not satisfactory. This technique involves staggering positions of the proximal shunts on the spongiosal and corporal bodies to avoid urethral fistulas.

## Corporo–Saphenous Vein Shunt

The Grayhack shunt is rarely performed due to the technical difficulties of the surgical approach and lack of efficacy and complication rate (1,11,12). For this shunt, an incision is made at the penile base and the tunica albuginea of the corpus cavernosum is exposed. Next, the femoral artery is palpated and an incision is made at the saphenofemoral junction, which is approximately 3 to 4 cm below the inguinal ligament. The saphenous vein is identified and mobilized for a distance of approximately 10 cm distal to the fossa ovalis. The surgeon ligates the vein distally and burrows beneath the skin with the index finger to join the two incisions. An ellipse of tunica albuginea 1.5 by 0.5 cm is excised, and the vein is drawn without tension or torsion into the penile wound; then the vein is spatulated and anastomosed to the tunica albuginea using a continuous 5-0 polydioxanone suture. A dry dressing is applied, and a standard protocol of intermittent squeezing is recommended.

## Corporo–Deep Dorsal Vein Shunt

As with the previous two shunts, the Barry shunt is a last resort for a patient with severe priapism refractory to distal shunt maneuvers (1,11,12). With this shunt, a 4-cm skin incision is made at the base of the penis. The superficial or deep dorsal vein is identified, taking care not to injure the dorsal artery or sensory nerves. The vein is ligated distally and divided. The proximal limb is spatulated on its ventral surface and anastomosed to the corpora cavernosa end-to-side in a tension-free manner. The penile skin is replaced and sutured at the base.

## Nonischemic Priapism

The initial management of nonischemic priapism is observation. The diagnosis is confirmed by detecting high flow or the site of rupture with color duplex Doppler imaging in combination with normal arterial blood gas analysis. Spontaneous resolution of untreated nonischemic priapism occurs in >50% of patients. Therefore, the patient is advised about chances for spontaneous resolution, complication risks after treatment (ED, abscess, neurological sequelae), and lack of significant adverse consequences resulting from delayed therapy for many months. Early presentation of nonischemic priapism can be managed with ice or pressure packing to cause vasospasm and thrombosis of the ruptured artery to efficiently close the fistula. If the fistula does not close, selective angiographic arterial embolization may be needed. This should be performed in concert with interventional radiology. Use of nonpermanent materials is associated with less ED rates postprocedure (5% vs. 39% with permanent substances); therefore, these biomaterials are preferred. If angiographic embolization fails, then penile exploration and direct surgical ligation of sinusoidal fistulas or pseudoaneurysms may be performed with the assistance of intraoperative color duplex ultrasonography.

# OUTCOMES

## Postoperative Management

After shunt procedures the patient should receive perioperative and postoperative antibiotics. It is important to avoid circular pressure dressings that may compromise the shunt and decrease venous drainage. Intermittent manual squeezing and milking of the penis will help keep the shunt open and prevent recurrence of priapism. The penis often still appears partially erect after shunting procedures due to postischemic hyperemia. Color duplex Doppler imaging may be performed to document penile vascular arterial blood flow status if desired after corporoglanular and proximal shunts. Additionally, intracavernosal pressure monitoring may help evaluate the effectiveness of the shunt procedures.

### Perspective

The most common complication of priapism is complete ED, which has been reported as high as 59% (2,3). The most critical factor in maintaining potency is immediate treatment of men presenting with priapism. Patients treated within 12 to 24 hours will more likely have a favorable response than those with delayed treatment. Patients with prolonged priapism (>36 hours) and recurrent episodes are more likely to suffer ED as a result of impaired smooth muscle function and fibrosis. This group of patients will ultimately proceed to a penile prosthesis because pharmacologic erectogenic therapy will fail. Nonischemic priapism has the best prognosis in the preservation of erectile function.

The Grayhack and Barry shunts are less efficacious in reducing priapism, perhaps due to the small-caliber size of the veins, especially regarding the Barry shunt. These are historical procedures proposed to alleviate severe priapic events and in practice have not been as successful as expected. Therefore, corporoglanular and corporospongiosal shunt procedures are preferred.

## COMPLICATIONS

Complications associated with shunt procedures are urethral damage and fistulas, bleeding, purulent cavernositis, skin necrosis, abscess, and pulmonary embolus after the Grayhack procedure. Since most shunts appear to close in time, it is believed that shunting does not cause permanent ED. However, failure of venous shunts to close spontaneously will lead to venogenic ED. Penile vascular dysfunction after shunt procedures may be a direct result of the repeated and prolonged priapism itself with significant fibrosis of the erectile compartments.

## *References*


1. Burnett AL. Priapism. In: Wein AJ, Kavoussi LR, Novick AC, et al., eds. *Campbell-Walsh urology*, 9th ed. Philadelphia: Saunders Elsevier, 2007: 839–849.
2. Earle CM, Stuckey BGA, Ching HL, et al. The incidence and management of priapism in western Australia: a 16 year audit. *Int J Impot Res* 2003;15: 272–276.
3. Adeyoju AB, Olujohungbe ABK, Morris J, et al. Priapism in sickle cell disease; incidence, risk factors and complications—an international multicentre study. *BJU Int* 2002;90:898–902.
4. Spycher MA, Hauri D. The ultrastructure of the erectile tissue in priapism. *J Urol* 1986;135:142–147.
5. Montague DK, Jarow J, Broderick GA, et al. Members of the Erectile Dysfunction Guideline Update Panel; American Urological Association. American Urological Association guideline on the management of priapism. *J Urol* 2003;170:1318–1324.
6. Berger R, Billups K, Brock G, et al. AFUD Thought Leader Panel on Evaluation and Treatment of Priapism. Report of the American Foundation for Urologic Disease (AFUD) Thought Leader Panel on evaluation and treatment of priapism. *Int J Impot Res* 2001;13[Suppl 5]: S39–S43.
7. Broderick GA, Gordon D, Hypolite J, et al. Anoxia and corporal smooth muscle dysfunction: mechanism for ischemic priapism. *J Urol* 1994;151: 259–262.
8. Ul-Hasan M, El-Sakka AI, Lee C, et al. Expression of TGF-beta-1 mRNA and ultrastructural alterations in pharmacologically induced prolonged penile erection in a canine model. *J Urol* 1998;160:2263–2266.
9. Bivalacqua TJ, Burnett AL. Priapism: new concepts in the pathophysiology and new treatment strategies. *Curr Urol Rep* 2006;7:497–502.
10. Burnett AL, Bivalacqua TJ, Champion HC, et al. Long-term oral phosphodiesterase 5 inhibitor therapy alleviates recurrent priapism. *Urology* 2006; 67:1043–1048.
11. Lue TF, Pescatori ES. Distal cavernosum-glans shunts for ischemic priapism. *J Sex Med* 2006;3:749–752.
12. Bochinski DJ, Deng DY, Lue TF. The treatment of priapism—when and how? *Int J Impot Res* 2003;15[Suppl 5]:S86–S90.


# CHAPTER 74 ■ PENILE PROSTHESIS IMPLANTATION

CULLEY C. CARSON

While erectile dysfunction has been described since ancient times, adequate treatment has only been available for the last four decades. The era of implantable devices began with the development of silicone-based prosthetic materials in the late 1960s as a result of the U.S. space program (4). Modern penile prosthetic devices were first developed in the early 1970s when Small et al. (6) along with Scott et al. (5) reported the implantation of penile prosthetic devices into the corpora cavernosa to fill the corpora cavernosa and provide a physiologically functional erection with good cosmetic results. These devices have undergone multiple revisions and redesigns between the early prosthetic devices and the currently implanted inflatable penile prostheses. Mechanical malfunction rates in these early devices, however, were reported in excess of 60% of cases. Current inflatable prosthetic devices have a far more improved mechanical reliability. These current devices can be divided into semirigid, mechanical, and multiple-component inflatable penile prostheses, of which there are two- and three-piece models available.

The semirigid rod and mechanical prostheses available today are the successors of the devices designed in the 1970s (Table 74.1). These devices, while easier to implant, have few

**TABLE 74.1**

**AVAILABLE PENILE PROSTHESES**

| Semirigid rods | Inflatable |
|---|---|
| AMS 600 (AMS) | 700 CX (AMS) |
| Malleable (Coloplast) | 700 LGX(AMS) |
| Dura II (AMS) | Alpha 1 (Coloplast) |
| | Ambicor (AMS) |

advantages over the newer inflatable devices because infection and mechanical malfunction rates are similar. The semirigid devices consist of a central metal core and a silicone elastomer rod, whereas the mechanical Duraphase implant is a series of disks held in position by a central cable. The latter design facilitates positioning of the implant between uses.

The three-piece inflatable penile prostheses vary in construction from three-layer silicon, Dacron, Lycra, or silicone to a single layer of silicon or Bioflex (Fig. 74.1). Options include girth expansion and/or length elongation. Aneurismal dilatation is rare with both of these cylinder designs, but it has been reported. Similarly, other design changes—including replacement of stainless steel connectors with plastic connectors, addition of nonkinked tubing, single design construction, Teflon cylinder input sleeves, and multiple-layer cylinders—have improved the longevity of these devices. These modifications have decreased mechanical malfunction rates from >30% to <5%. The most significant recent advance is the coating of three-piece implants to reduce infection risk.

The three-piece inflatable penile prostheses continue to be the most satisfactory prostheses once they are implanted and while they remain functional. These prosthetic devices produce the most natural-appearing erection in girth and length,

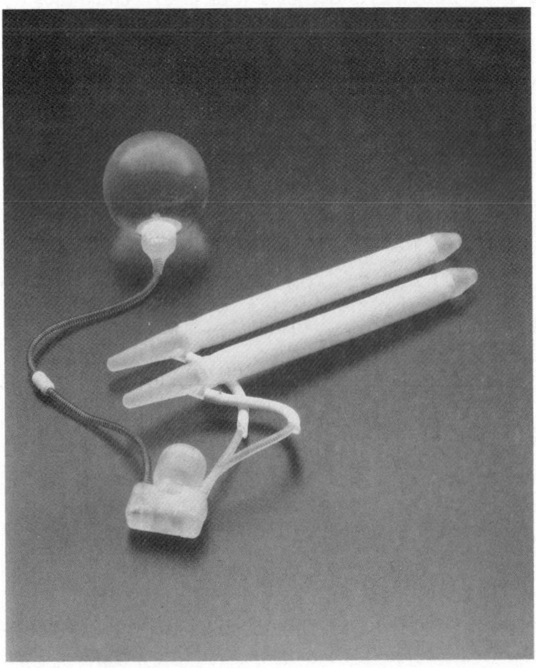

FIGURE 74.1 American Medical Systems' AMS 740CX three-piece inflatable penile prosthesis.

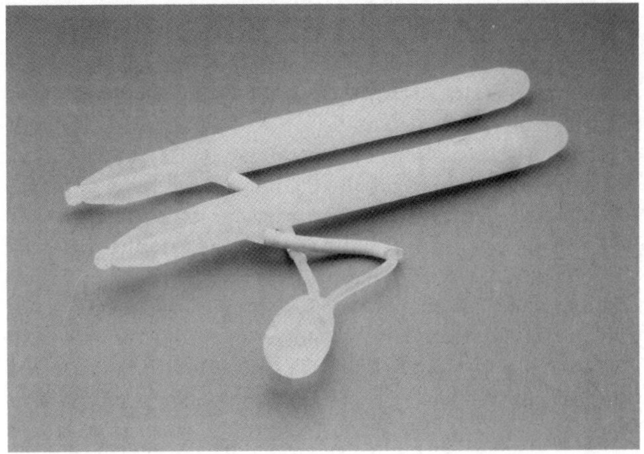

FIGURE 74.2 American Medical Systems' Ambicor two-piece inflatable penile prosthesis.

with satisfactory rigidity and excellent flaccidity for optimal concealment. They also have advantages for many patients with complex penile implantations because the flaccid position removes pressure from the corporal cavernosa and decreases the possibility of erosion in these highly difficult implantations.

To improve the ease of surgical implantation by removing a portion of the prosthesis placed within the abdominal region, two-piece prostheses were designed (Fig. 74.2). Because these two-piece inflatable prostheses remove the separate reservoir, additional fluid is available either by a larger scrotal pump or a combination of a proximal cylinder and pump reservoir. Although these devices provide adequate erection in many patients, the limited reservoir capacity decreases flaccidity and may, in some patients, diminish rigidity. These prostheses are especially difficult to deflate in patients with small penises and frequently provide inadequate rigidity in patients with longer penises. While less optimal than three-piece devices, these two-piece implants may be ideal for patients in whom reservoir placement is difficult or contraindicated. Such patients as renal transplant recipients and patients who have undergone significant radical pelvic exenteration procedures may benefit from two-piece devices.

## DIAGNOSIS

The diagnosis of erectile dysfunction can be obtained by history. The clinician should determine whether the erectile dysfunction is situational or constant, whether the degree of dysfunction is partial or total, and also include the details of the relationship with the partner. Any coexisting conditions such as diabetes, vascular disease, smoking, medications (especially steroids, hormones, antihypertensives, or antidepressants), and use of alcohol or drugs should be identified. Physical examination should include the genitalia, including the testes, hair distribution, femoral and distal lower-extremity pulses, and the penis for Peyronie plaques or other abnormalities. Nocturnal tumescence studies, cavernosometry, cavernosography, and penile Doppler are useful in some patients in securing the diagnosis.

## INDICATIONS FOR SURGERY

Although there are a variety of penile prosthesis designs currently available for implantation, not all patients with erectile dysfunction are candidates for penile prosthesis implantation. Penile prostheses are generally the procedure of last resort for those men failing more conservative measures such as oral PDE5 inhibitors, vacuum erection device, urethral alprostadil, and cavernosal injection therapy. For those men in whom penile prostheses are suggested, careful counseling before penile implant procedures will limit many of the problems with postoperative dissatisfaction. Once the discussion and demonstration of penile implant varieties have been carried out, patients can be counseled about the most appropriate penile prosthesis for their individual use. Patients may choose a specific prosthetic type based on their needs and preferences (1). Younger patients with normal manual dexterity and patients who wear stylish, form-fitting, athletic clothing or who shower in public at a health club or other athletic facility often choose a three-piece inflatable penile prosthesis because appearance in the flaccid position is better than with other designs. For these patients, implantation of a semirigid rod penile prosthesis requires a significant lifestyle change, and they are better served with an inflatable-type prosthesis. Similarly, patients with Peyronie disease, secondary implantation, or significant peripheral neuropathy such as occurs in severe diabetes are best served with an inflatable penile prosthesis because interior tissue pressures are diminished between uses and the possibility of extrusion is diminished.

For patients in whom the convenience of inflation and deflation is not important, the risks and mechanical malfunctions may outweigh the disadvantage of a malleable penile prosthesis (Fig. 74.3). Such patients as paraplegics who require an external urinary collection device, those with inadequate manual dexterity, or those with significant obesity may be better served with a malleable penile prosthesis.

## ALTERNATIVE THERAPY

Alternative therapy includes sexual counseling, vacuum erection devices, intracavernosal injection therapy, intraurethral medication, or oral PDE5 inhibitor medications. Less commonly used therapies include penile vascular (arterial or venous) surgery.

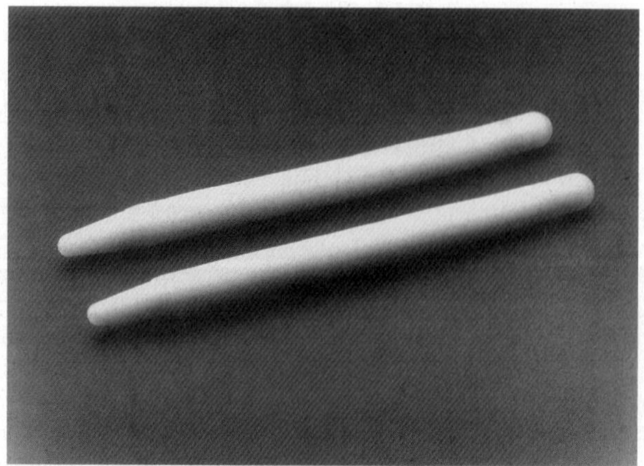

FIGURE 74.3 American Medical Systems' AMS 600 malleable penile prosthesis.

## SURGICAL TECHNIQUE

Surgical implantation of penile prostheses can be carried out using a variety of surgical approaches and incisions. Semirigid and malleable prostheses can be implanted through a distal penile approach. Multiple-piece prostheses, however, can be implanted by the infrapubic or penoscrotal approach. While individual surgeons have a variety of rationales for each of these approaches, there does not appear to be any clear advantage in patient satisfaction or outcome between the two approaches. Patient anatomy may dictate appropriate choice. Patients with previous abdominal surgical procedures where reservoir placement is difficult may be better served with an infrapubic approach, whereas patients with massive obesity may be better approached through a penoscrotal incision. Two-piece devices, because there is no separate reservoir, are best implanted through a penoscrotal incision.

### Distal Penile Approach

A distal penile approach is usually the best approach for insertion of a semirigid or mechanical penile prosthesis. This incision heals well, allows complete corporeal dilation, and facilitates rod placement. After placement of a Foley urethral catheter, a circumcoronal incision is carried out >180 degrees of the subcoronal region of the penis. Dissection is carried down to the layer of the Buck fascia, taking care to avoid the dorsal penile nerves, which course within the Buck fascia. After the Buck fascia is identified, stay sutures are applied to the two corpora through the tunica albuginea lateral to the penile nerves. These longitudinal incisions can be extended as much as is necessary for dilation and cylinder insertion. The corporal dilation is begun with Metzenbaum scissors to establish a track in the corporal tissue. Dilation then follows with Hegar, Brooks, or Dilamezinsert dilators to 9 to 11 cm, depending upon the required cylinder girth (Fig. 74.4). Once the corpora are sized using a Furlow or other dilator, the cylinders can be placed (Figs. 74.5 and 74.6). A small vein retractor can be used to facilitate placement of the distal end of the cylinder. The corporotomy is closed with 2-0 absorbable, synthetic sutures. With noninflatable cylinders, a penile block can be performed and a noncompression dressing is applied.

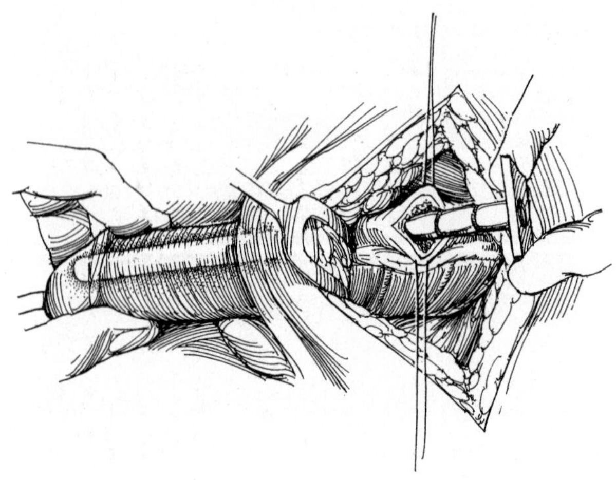

FIGURE 74.4 Corporal dilation using Brooks dilators.

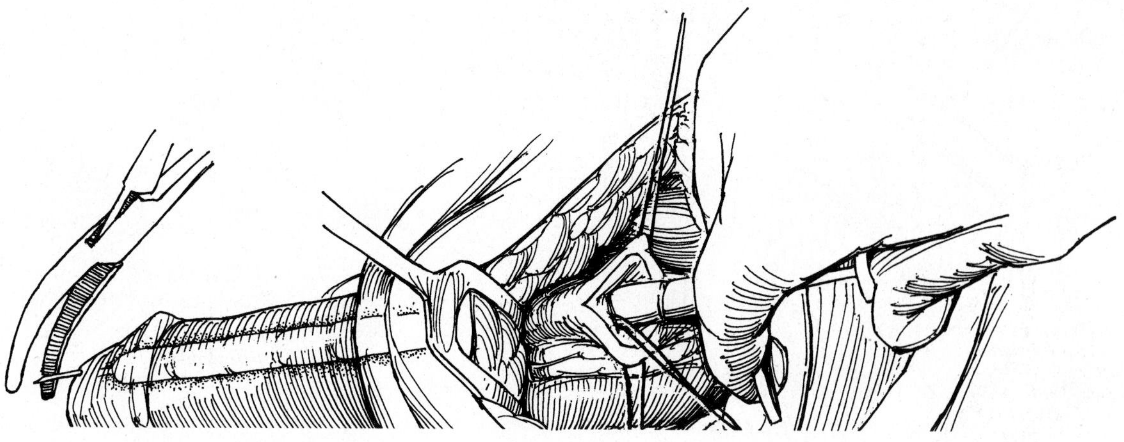

FIGURE 74.5 Prosthesis cylinder loaded onto Furlow inserter and placed into the corporal tunnel.

## Infrapubic Approach

The infrapubic approach allows better visualization of the reservoir placement than the penoscrotal approach. However, because of the proximity of the dorsal neurovascular bundle in the infrapubic approach, injury is possible, resulting in decreased distal penile sensation in some patients. The infrapubic approach is usually carried out with a horizontal incision approximately one fingerbreadth below the symphysis pubica, allowing implantation with an easily concealed incision once the pubic hair regrows (Fig. 74.7). In patients with significant obesity or a previous midline incision, however, a midline incision carried out just to the base of the penis facilitates exposure of the corpus cavernosum and improves ability for corpus cavernosum dilation. After incision of the subcutaneous tissue, the dissection is continued to the rectus fascia. The rectus fascia is incised horizontally and dissected cephalad for approximately 2 to 3 cm. A midline separation of the rectus muscles is carried out using sharp and blunt dissection. A pouch is created bluntly beneath the rectus muscles to comfortably insert the inflatable reservoir without compression (Fig. 74.8).

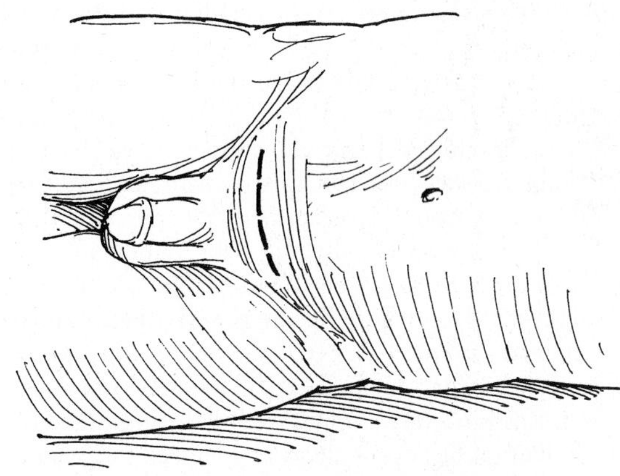

FIGURE 74.7 Infrapubic incision for prosthesis implantation.

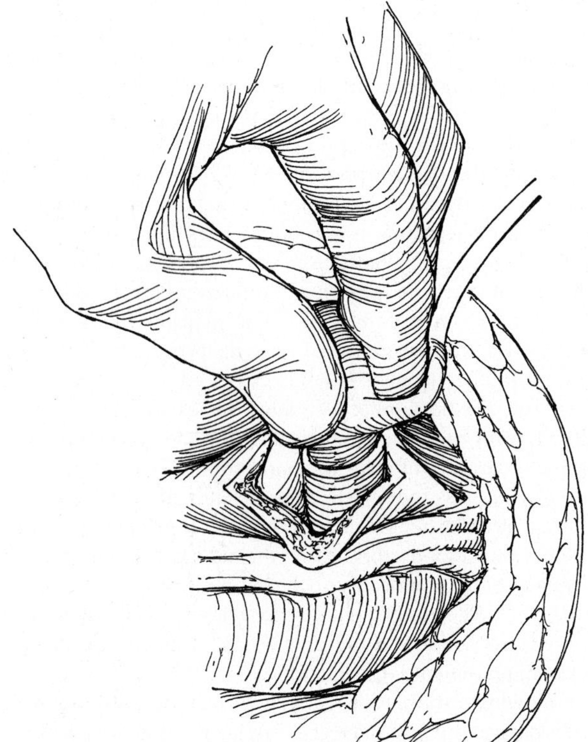

FIGURE 74.6 Placement of proximal cylinder base.

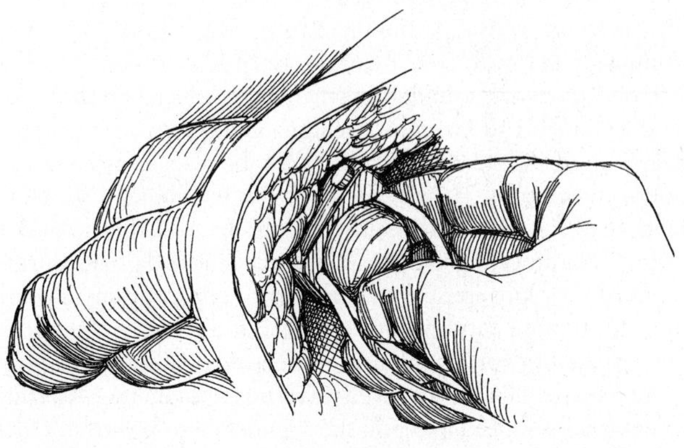

FIGURE 74.8 Blunt dissection establishes a location for the pump device.

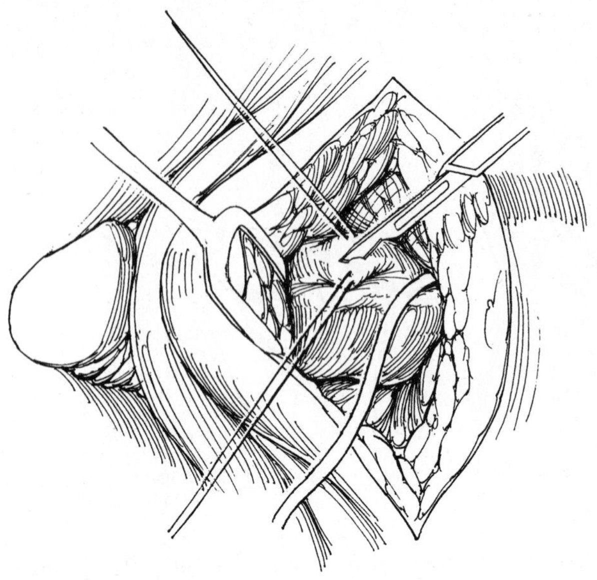

FIGURE 74.9 Corporotomy incision between two stay sutures, avoiding the dorsal neurovascular bundles.

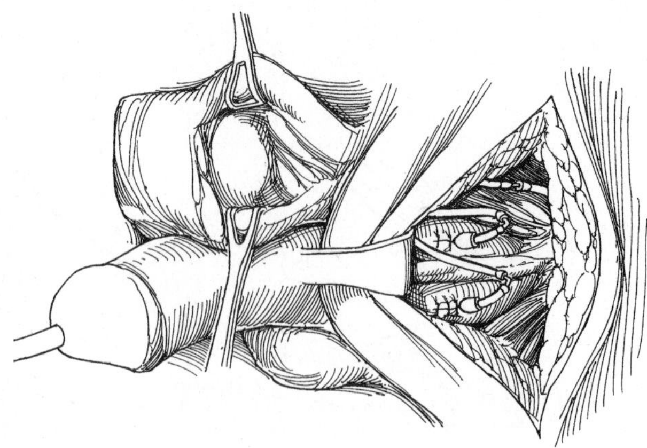

FIGURE 74.10 Device in place with connections complete.

Dissection is then carried out over the corpora cavernosa. Sharp and blunt dissection is begun on either side of the fundiform ligament identifying the dorsal neurovascular bundle. Note that the dorsal nerves of the penis lie approximately 2 to 3 mm lateral to the deep dorsal vein. Once the Buck fascia has been dissected free from the tunica albuginea, the shiny white tunica albuginea is fixed with traction sutures. A corporotomy incision is then carried out between the traction sutures and the corpora cavernosa entered (Fig. 74.9). The corporotomy incision can be carried out with scalpel or electrocautery. Metzenbaum scissors are then used to carefully initiate the tunneling of the corpora cavernosa, gently spreading the cavernosal tissue both proximally, until the ischial tuberosities and crura of the corpora are encountered, and distally, palpating the glans penis to identify the distalmost aspect of dilation. Hegar dilators from size 9 to 12 or Brooks, Pratt, or Dilamezinsert dilators can be used. If corporeal fibrosis is encountered, Rosillio cavernatomes can be used to dilate to size 12. Once dilation has been adequately carried out bilaterally, the Furlow introducer or Dilamezinsert is used to measure the corpora cavernosal length using a traction suture as a central point of reference. The proximal and distal measurements are added to identify total corporal length and obtain appropriately sized inflatable cylinders. A length slightly less than measurement is usually obtained to permit comfortable positioning of the cylinders. Rear tip extenders of size 0.5, 1.0, 2.0, or 3.0 cm or combinations thereof are placed on the proximal cylinder end to adjust length. Once measurement has been obtained, interrupted sutures can be placed for later corporotomy closure. The advantage to this technique is the elimination of suture needles close to the area of the inflatable cylinder, diminishing the possibility of cylinder damage during corporotomy closure. Other methods of corporotomy closure include running sutures with or without a locking technique. Once the corporotomy sutures are placed, cylinders are positioned in the dilated corpora cavernosa using the inserting tool with distal needle to pull the cylinders into position. Once positioned, it is essential to visualize the cylinder in the corpus cavernosum to ensure that there is no kinking and that complete proximal and distal seating has taken place (Fig. 74.10). The corporal incision should be placed proximal enough to allow easy exit of the input tube and minimize contact between the cylinder and input tube. Closure of the corpora cavernosum is carried out with traction on the cylinder placement suture to maintain it in a flat, nonkinking position and ensure adequate seating. Following placement of cylinders and closure of the corporotomy incision, cylinder inflation can be tested by placing fluid in each of the cylinders through the input tubes, gently inflating the prosthesis to identify any abnormalities in position, curvature, or other problems.

A finger is then placed in the most dependent portion of the scrotum lateral to the testicle on the right or left side. The finger is then pushed to the area of the external inguinal ring, and any adipose tissue in this area is dissected free to expose the dartos fascia. The dartos fascia is thoroughly cleaned to allow pump placement. Following development of this subcutaneous pouch for the pump, the pump is positioned in the most dependent portion of the scrotum and temporarily fixed into position using a Babcock clamp. The inflatable reservoir is then placed in the previously constructed subrectus pocket and filled with an appropriate volume of normal saline or water/radiographic contrast media. Before connection, it is important to release pressure on the filling syringe and determine if any backfilling is seen. This backfilling or backpressure may predict autoinflation in the postoperative period. Tubing connection is then carried out using quick connectors or suture tie plastic connectors. The snap-on connectors are used for Mentor prostheses. In a redo prosthesis in which a residual tubing segment is connected to a new device piece, suture tie plastic connectors must be used. The tubing is tailored prior to connection to allow for adequate pump positioning is carried out prior to connection. Shodded clamps are used to compress the tubing, and the ends of the tubing, once tailored, are flushed with inflation fluid to eliminate small particles and blood clots. After the tubing is connected, the adequacy of the connection is tested by gently pulling on the connectors. All shodded clamps are removed and the device is inflated and deflated on multiple occasions to ensure adequate location, placement, and erection.

Following testing, thorough irrigation with antibiotic solution is carried out and the rectus fascia closed with interrupted sutures. The wound is then closed in the standard fashion with two layers of subcutaneous tissue and a subcuticular skin suture. A dry sterile dressing is applied, a Foley catheter placed if necessary, and an ice pack applied. Suction drains could be used at the surgeon's discretion.

Postoperatively patients are instructed to maintain their penis in a Sutherland position for 4 to 6 weeks. Tight underwear and athletic supporters are not used in an effort to maintain the pump in its most dependent position.

## Penoscrotal Approach

Three-piece inflatable penile prostheses, as well as semirigid and two-piece prostheses, can be implanted by a transverse or vertical penoscrotal incision. This approach has distinct advantages in obese patients and is the most common approach for routine penile prosthesis implantation. Because the penoscrotal approach requires differentiation of the corpora cavernosa from the corpus spongiosum during resection, initial placement of a Foley catheter is necessary for this approach. The incision is placed in the upper portion of the scrotum and is usually horizontal, one fingerbreadth below the penoscrotal junction.. The Scott/Lone Star retractor (Lone Star Medical Products, Stafford, TX) facilitates exposure with this incision. Once the skin incision has been carried out, dissection is continued lateral to the corpus spongiosum and urethra to expose the corpora cavernosa. Incision, dilation, and closure of the corpora cavernosa are similar to those described previously for the infrapubic incision, but synthetic absorbable sutures must be used with this approach because the suture line may be palpable postoperatively (Fig. 74.11). Cylinder sizing and placement are as described above. Pump placement is likewise in the most dependent portion of the scrotum just above the dartos fascia, with positioning using a Babcock clamp.

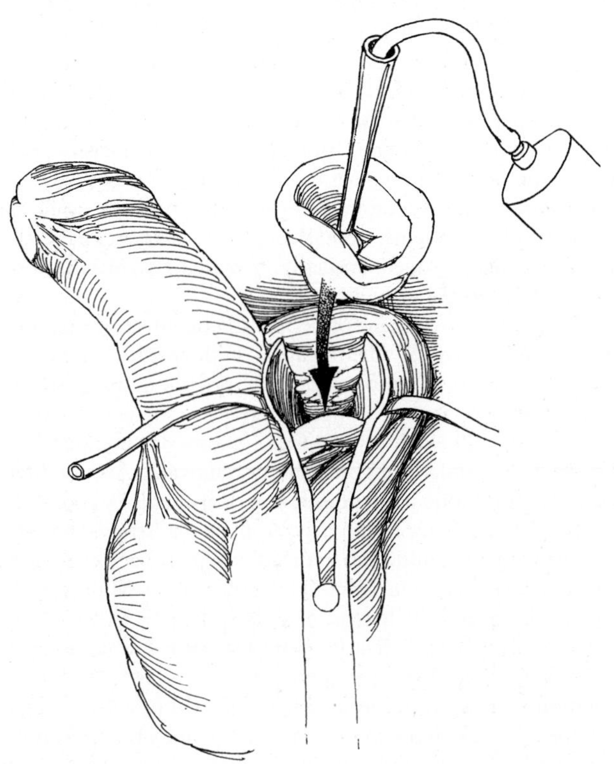

**FIGURE 74.11** Penoscrotal incision with exposure of corpora cavernosa.

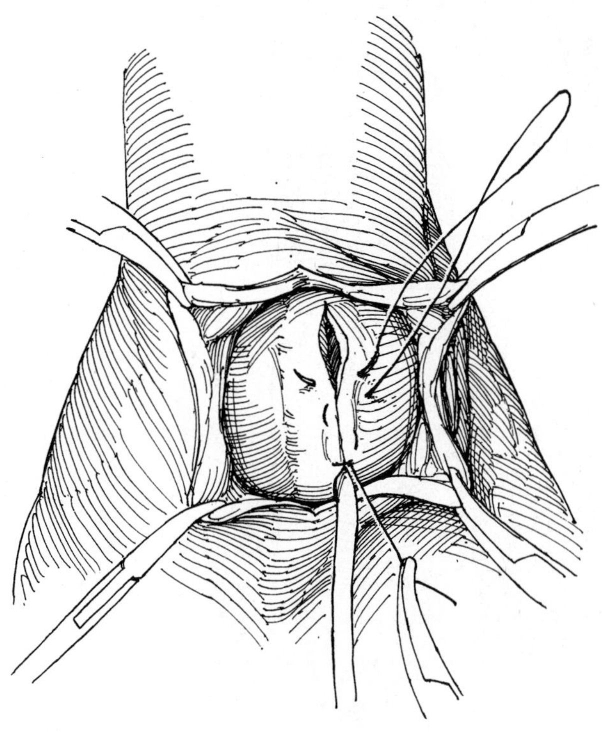

**FIGURE 74.12** Reservoir placement with penoscrotal approach.

Dissection for reservoir placements can be carried out with a second separate infrapubic incision but is more commonly performed through the penoscrotal incision (Fig. 74.12). The scrotal skin incision is retracted to the area of the external inguinal ring, and dissection is carried out medial to the spermatic cord. The transversalis fascia is identified and incised sharply using Metzenbaum scissors placed firmly against the pubic tubercle. Dissection is carried out using a combination of sharp and blunt dissection. Dilation is carried out with the index finger after incision of the transversalis fascia and with gentle blunt dissection using a large Kelly clamp. The reservoir balloon is then positioned over the index finger and placed in the perivesical space. Inflation of the reservoir is carried out with care that no backpressure is observed. If refilling of the syringe occurs, the reservoir is removed and reservoir pocket enlargement must be carried out. Once the reservoir is placed and inflated and the tubing is connected as previously described, the device is tested in inflation and deflation (Fig. 74.13). Closure is carried out with a subcuticular suture in the standard fashion. In men with a penoscrotal skin web, the horizontal skin incision can be closed in a midline fashion to enhance functional penile length.

Perioperative antibiotic treatment is critical in diminishing the incidence of perioperative infection and prosthetic removal. The Inhibizone (American Medical Systems, Minnetonka, MN) coating consisting of rifampin and minocycline or the lubricious coating of the Titan implant (Coloplast Inc, Minneapolis, MN), which allows antibiotics to adhere to the Bioflex, has reduced infection risk by threefold. An initial perioperative dosage of an antibiotic agent effective against the most common infectious pathogens should be administered 1 to 2 hours prior to surgery and continued for 24 hours postoperatively. The choice of an aminoglycoside with a first-generation cephalosporin, ampicillin/sulbactam, a cephalosporin alone, vancomycin, or a fluoroquinolone is appropriate for prophylaxis of the most common

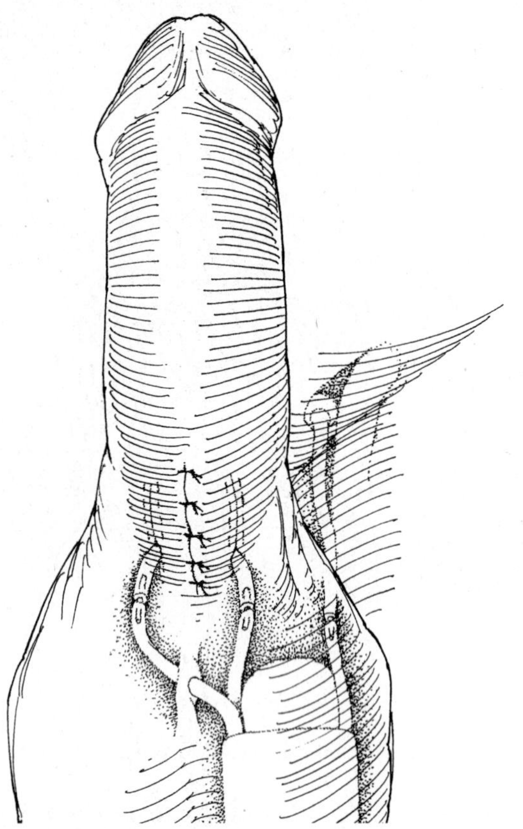

FIGURE 74.13 Pump placed for penoscrotal approach.

infections from *Staphylococcus epidermidis*. Patients may be discharged for 7 days of continued antibiotic therapy. The use of antibiotic-coated penile implants, while reducing the incidence of postoperative infection, does not preclude the need for systemic, perioperative antibiotics. The penile prosthesis remains deflated for 4 weeks while healing occurs. Prior to activation, the patient is advised to retract the pump into his scrotum on a daily basis, and tight underwear and athletic supports are avoided to maintain pump position. A return office visit for activation of the device is carried out once discomfort has resolved. Patients are advised to inflate and deflate the device on a daily basis for 4 weeks to allow tissue expansion around the prosthesis. Most patients can then begin use of their device 4 to 6 weeks after implantation.

# OUTCOMES

## Complications

Despite careful counseling, many patients enter penile prosthesis procedures with expectations that cannot be met by penile prosthesis surgery. Decreased penile length compared with the preimplant state, decreased penile sensation, "coolness" of the penis and glans penis, and chronic pain, as well as partner dissatisfaction, are among the complaints patients may voice despite adequate surgical implantation and satisfactory mechanical functioning. Fortunately, these complaints are unusual, and >90% of patients report satisfaction with their prostheses. Many patients who are dissatisfied with their penile prostheses will benefit from sexual counseling or continued counseling assistance from the implanting surgeon to be sure that they are able to operate the device satisfactorily and understand its use.

Most patients' dissatisfaction results from difficulty with operation of the device and unrealistic expectations. Preoperative discussions with patients should include the concept that penile prostheses do not create normal erections but only support the penis for sexual activity. Penile prosthesis surgery brings about the ability to resume sexual functioning and vaginal penetration, but decreased penile sensation, length, and engorgement may result. Patients should also be advised that a penile prosthesis will not improve libido or ejaculation. Patients frequently report delayed or difficult ejaculation initially following penile prosthesis surgery. This delay is primarily a result of inadequate preparation, stimulation, and psychological adjustment to the prosthesis. Most patients require 3 to 6 months of prosthesis use with careful attention to presexual stimulation before ejaculation routinely returns to preoperative levels. Because the prosthesis neither improves nor detracts from preoperative ejaculatory ability, patients must be counseled regarding their preoperative ejaculatory ability before prosthesis placement.

The most worrisome postoperative complication is infection, which occurs in fewer than 10% of all patients. Perioperative prosthetic infections can, however, occur at any time in the postoperative period in patients with penile or other prosthetic devices. Patients continue to be at risk for hematogenously seeded infections from gastrointestinal, dental, or urologic manipulations as well as remote infections. Patients must be counseled to request antibiotic coverage if remote infections occur. Most periprosthetic infections are caused by gram-positive organisms such as *S. epidermidis*, but fungi or gram-negative organisms such as *Escherichia coli* and *Pseudomonas* are also common culprits. Severe gangrenous infections with a combination of gram-negative and anaerobic organisms have also been identified and frequently result in significant disability and tissue loss. Patients at increased risk for perioperative infections include diabetics, patients undergoing penile straightening procedures or circumcision with prosthetic implantation, patients with urinary tract bacterial colonization, and immunocompromised patients, such as posttransplant patients. Spinal cord injury patients have also been reported to have a specially increased risk of infections, with rates reported as high as 15%.

Appropriate treatment of periprosthetic infections requires early and immediate identification with institution of parenteral antibiotic therapy and early prosthesis removal (2). Conservative treatment would dictate a healing period of 3 to 6 months followed by repeat prosthesis implantation. Satisfactory results with prosthesis removal, a 5- to 7-day course of antibiotic irrigation, followed by additional replacement has been reported for selected patients. Better long-term results with no additional morbidity can be achieved with the prosthesis salvage technique reported by Mulcahy (4). This technique—which requires removal of the infected implant and vigorous irrigation using solutions of antibiotics, povidone-iodine, hydrogen peroxide, and a repeat of these solutions—is successful in >75% of infected prostheses (2).

The most common complication of penile prosthesis function is mechanical malfunction. Mechanical malfunction has declined from rates as high as 61% to levels below 5% since the 1970s (3,7). Aneurismal dilation of inflatable cylinders, both American Medical Systems and Mentor, kinks in tubing, reservoir leakage, and pump malfunction have been limited by device modifications. Fluid leak, however, continues to be a problem for many inflatable penile prostheses. These mechanical malfunctions require replacement of the leaking portion of the inflatable portion of the prosthesis. If a nonfunctioning prosthesis has been in place >4 years, however, it is usual practice to replace the entire device to reduce further mechanical malfunction (1).

Semirigid rod penile prostheses are associated with fewer mechanical problems; the most common complication associated with these prostheses is cylinder erosion through skin or urethra. Prosthesis fracture or breakage has been reported, and patients may return 6 to 8 years postimplantation with complaints of decreased rigidity of their semirigid rod, indicating fracture of the central prosthetic cylinder wires. These wire fractures usually cannot be appreciated radiographically unless the prosthesis is put on stretch once it has been explanted. Replacement of these devices is indicated when patients note decreased rigidity. Prosthesis extrusion or erosion is most common in diabetics and spinal cord injury patients, especially those requiring urinary management with catheter placement or with condom catheter collection devices.

Extrusion can also occur beneath the penile skin distally from vigorous dilation or remotely from trauma or repeated use. These extrusions are characterized by distal penile pain with use. Correction can be carried out with the use of a patch graft, but a better approach is rerouting with no grafting material. Rerouting is associated with less infection and pain and a reduced recurrence rate.

## Results

Long-term function and use have been confirmed in studies of patients who have had implants as long as 10 years (3). While partner satisfaction notes are few, patients have a >90% satisfaction, and those with functioning devices for >5 years use them 27 times monthly (3). Other studies have confirmed that patient satisfaction is greater than with any other erectile dysfunction treatment modality (1).

## *References*


1. Carson CC. Penile prosthesis implantation: surgical implants in the era of oral medication. *Urol Clin North Am* 2005;32(4):503–509.
2. Carson CC. Diagnosis, treatment and prevention of penile prosthesis infection. *Int J Impot Res* 2003;15[Suppl 5]:S139–S146.
3. Carson CC, Mulcahy JJ, Govier FE. Efficacy, safety and patient satisfaction outcomes of the AMS 700CX inflatable penile prosthesis: results of a long-term multicenter study. AMS 700CX Study Group. *J Urol* 2000;164: 376–380.
4. Mulcahy JJ. Long-term experience with salvage of infected penile implants. *J Urol* 2000;163:481–482.
5. Scott FB, Bradley WE, Timm GW. Management of erectile impotence. Use of implantable inflatable prosthesis. *Urology* 1973;2:80–82.
6. Small MP, Carrion HM, Gordon JA. Small-Carrion penile prosthesis. New implant for management of impotence. *Urology* 1975;5:479–486.
7. Mulcahy JJ, Austoni E, Barada JH, et al. The penile implant for erectile dysfunction. *J Sex Med* 2004;1(1):98–109.


# CHAPTER 75 ■ PENILE VENOUS SURGERY

AUDREY C. RHEE, MARK R. LICHT, AND RONALD W. LEWIS

Although the exact incidence of vasculogenic erectile dysfunction (ED) is not known, arterial insufficiency and/or venous leakage of varying etiology probably account for the majority of cases of ED. Sustaining a rigid erection depends on both adequate perfusion pressure of the erectile bodies via arterial inflow and maintenance of intracavernosal pressure by increased venous outflow resistance. The trapping of blood within the expanding corporal bodies during erection by direct compression of subtunical venules as they exit through the tunica albuginea is known as the corporal veno-occlusion mechanism. Venous leak ED refers to the inability of an individual to maintain a rigid erection because of abnormal venous outflow from the corpora cavernosa secondary to failure of the corporal veno-occlusive mechanism. Failure of full expansion of the sinus spaces due to sinus smooth muscle malfunction or replacement with fibrous tissue probably accounts for the majority of veno-occlusive dysfunction. Focal defects in the integrity of the tunica albuginea or congenital or arteriogenic abnormal venous channels may be a less frequent source of veno-occlusive disorders. In this chapter, we discuss the diagnosis of venogenic ED and detail the surgical correction of this form of ED by penile venous dissection and ligation.

## DIAGNOSIS

A history and physical examination help identify patients who may have venous leak ED. Patients present with complete loss of erection, decreased penile rigidity, or rapid loss of erection during intercourse. Medication side-effects, significant cardiovascular disease, psychologic disorders, and tobacco use should be excluded as contributing causes of ED. Penile trauma, surgery for priapism or Peyronie disease, and previous endoscopic incision of urethral strictures can all lead to focal defects in the corporal veno-occlusive mechanism (7).

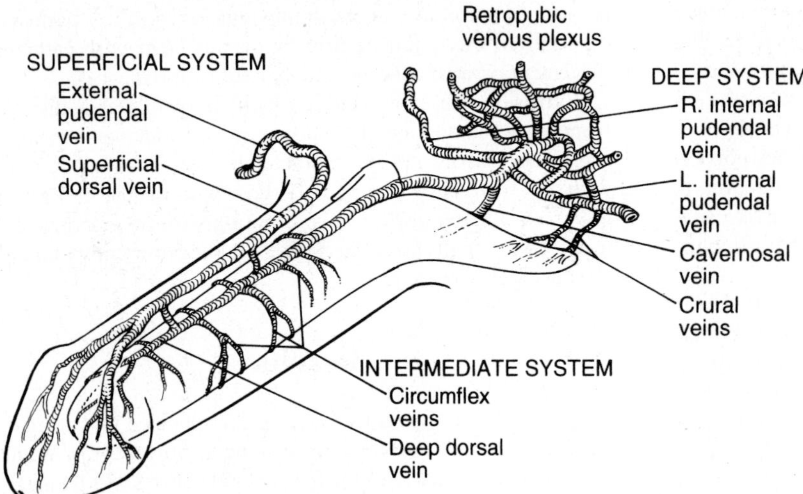


**FIGURE 75.1** Penile venous anatomy.

The first diagnostic test that we employ in the diagnosis of venogenic ED is color penile duplex Doppler ultrasonography. This test allows for the evaluation of both penile arterial inflow (peak systolic velocity) and veno-occlusion (end-diastolic velocity), as well as for observing the erectile response to the intracavernosal injection of a vasodilating agent. Our preferred injection agent is 0.25 mL of a Tri-Mix agent (containing 6 mg of papaverine, 0.2 mg of phentolamine, and 2 $\mu$g of prostaglandin $E_1$). Patients with measured end-diastolic velocities >3 cm per second for up to 20 minutes (measured at 5-minute intervals) after the administration of the vasodilating agent despite normal arterial inflow, a peak systolic velocity >30 cm per second, are likely to have venogenic ED (4). Patients who obtain a full rigid erection within 10 minutes of injection that lasts for 30 minutes probably have no clinically significant vascular disease. Our practice is to reinject and to measure values every 5 minutes for 20 minutes if after the first injection the response is not a full erection or not equal to the best attained erection at home. Patients who achieve only tumescence or who rapidly obtain a rigid erection that dissipates within 15 to 20 minutes are suspected of having a venous leak.

Infusion pharmacocavernosometry and pharmacocavernosography are the definitive tests for diagnosing venous leak ED and visualizing the sites of leakage. Knowledge of the anatomy of the venous drainage of the penis is critical in interpreting this study (Fig. 75.1). Two 19-gauge needles are placed into each of the corpora cavernosa. One is connected to a pressure transducer, and the other is connected to an infusion pump with metered delivery rates of heparinized saline. After injection of a vasodilating agent, the need for a flow rate of >20 mL per minute of saline to maintain a rigid erection at an intracorporeal pressure of at least 90 mm Hg is indicative of corporal veno-occlusive dysfunction. A maintenance flow rate between 10 and 20 mL per minute is considered borderline for venous leakage. Others have used lower flows to maintain as diagnostic cutoff. Excessively high maintenance flows (>50 mL per minute) usually indicate massive venous runoff, and these patients do not do well with veno-occlusive surgery (12). Isosmotic contrast material is infused into the corpora at the previously defined maintenance flow rate from cavernosometry, and then Anterior Posterior (AP) and oblique radiographs of the penis are taken (cavernosography). The most common sites of venous leakage seen in patients with veno-occlusive dysfunction are the deep dorsal vein, the cavernosal veins, and the circumflex veins at the base of the penis. A large amount of drainage into all of these systems is a contraindication to surgery, since these patients do not do well.

## INDICATIONS FOR SURGERY

Patients must meet strict criteria to be selected for venous surgery. Candidates must first have a history that is consistent with venous leak ED, corroborated by color duplex Doppler ultrasonography or intracavernosal test injection findings. Other causes of ED should be ruled out. Normal penile arterial inflow must also be documented in response to an intracavernosal injection agent because patients with concomitant arterial disease often have a poor outcome after venous surgery. Pharmacocavernosometry and pharmacocavernosography must confirm veno-occlusive dysfunction and outline the sites of leakage. Patients should have no medical contraindications to surgery. There is no strict age limit, but we prefer to perform venous surgery on patients <65 years old. Sasso et al. (12) advise veno-occlusive dysfunction for patients <50 years of age.

Patients need to eliminate all tobacco use at least 6 months before surgery. Finally, patients must select venous surgery only after presentation of alternative forms of therapy and discussion of the <50% long-term expected success rates (>2 years). We also perform venous surgery in conjunction with penile arterial revascularization in select patients with both focal arterial disease and veno-occlusive dysfunction (8).

## ALTERNATIVE THERAPY

Patients with venous leak ED have other effective surgical and nonsurgical options to consider instead of penile venous dissection and ligation. Some patients with mild to moderate veno-occlusive disorders will respond to oral phosphodiesterase inhibition therapy for ED. Vacuum erection devices create an adequate erection by drawing blood into the penis with negative pressure in the vacuum cylinder tube. An occlusion band placed at the base of the penis prevents outflow of blood and substitutes for a faulty veno-occlusive mechanism. Self-injection of intracavernosal vasodilating agents at higher doses can often produce a functional erection in patients with mild to moderate venous leak. Patients with severe leakage, however, will most often not respond to injection therapy. Combining self-injection with an occlusion band is also helpful in maintaining an erection in some patients. Implantation of a penile prosthesis effectively replaces the natural veno-occlusive mechanism with a mechanical device capable of producing a sufficiently rigid erection. A short-time high success rate (68.7%) with an embolization of the deep dorsal vein technique was reported in 2000 by Peskircioglu et al. (10). A goal-directed approach is used to help the patient select an appropriate form of therapy.

## SURGICAL TECHNIQUE

Patients receive a dose of intravenous cephalosporin or a fluoroquinolone within an hour before surgery. Surgery is performed under either general intubated or spinal anesthesia. The patient is positioned supine with legs abducted to allow easy access to the perineum. If crural ligation and banding are planned as part of the operative procedure, then a dorsal lithotomy position is preferred. A lighted suction device can facilitate illumination of the deep infrapubic dissection. An intraoperative Doppler probe can be helpful in localizing small arteries in this region. Optical magnification can be used for the dissection, although we do not routinely use it. The operative field is prepared and draped in a sterile fashion from the umbilicus to the perineum, and an 18Fr Foley catheter is placed for the purpose of bladder drainage and facilitating urethral identification during the dissection.

An infrapubic curvilinear anterior peripenile scrotal incision is made with a no. 15 blade (Fig. 75.2). The superior extent of the incision is the inferior border of the pubis, and the inferior extent is the median raphe of the scrotum below the penile shaft. Superficial tissue is dissected free of the corporal bodies with sharp and blunt dissection. Communicating veins joining the deep and superficial drainage systems are isolated, ligated with 3-0 plain gut sutures, and divided. The penile skin is then inverted into the wound to gain exposure to the superficial and deep venous systems (Fig. 75.3). Any other venous trunks of the superficial system that receive tributaries from the corpora are ligated with absorbable suture material and divided at this time (Fig. 75.4).

A 19- or 21-gauge butterfly needle is placed into the base of the corpus cavernosum and fixed in place to the tunica albuginea with a 3-0 chromic pursestring suture (Fig. 75.5). The cavernosal tissue receives an injection of 30 mg of papaverine (or similar vasodilating agent[s]), followed 10 minutes later by indigo-carmine colored saline (12 mL in 250 mL of saline) to help visualize abnormally effluxing veins. The butterfly needle tubing is clamped for the duration of the procedure and is

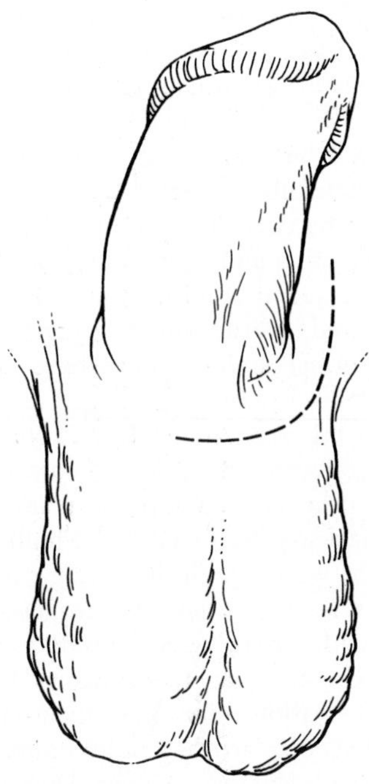

FIGURE 75.2 Peripenile scrotal incision for penile venous surgery.

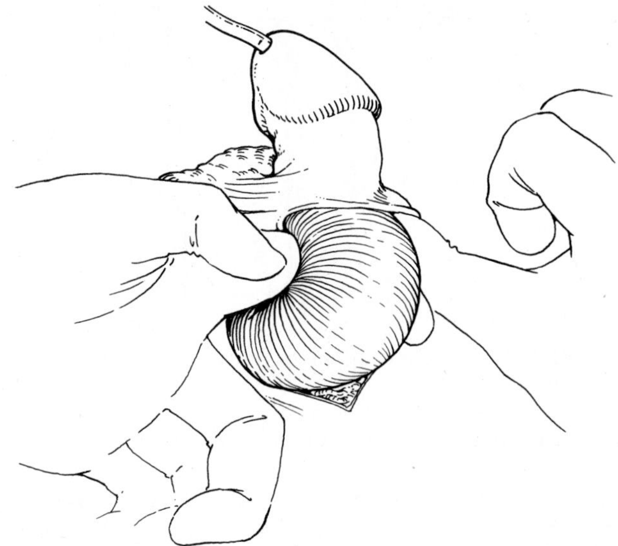

FIGURE 75.3 Inversion of the penile shaft into the wound.

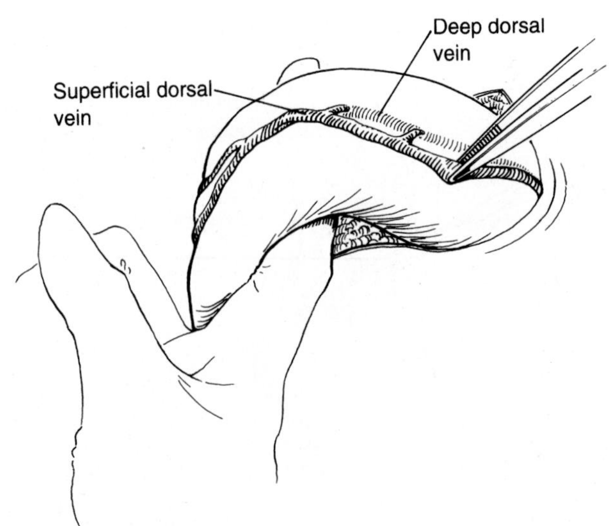


FIGURE 75.4 Ligation of superficial veins with connections to the corpora.

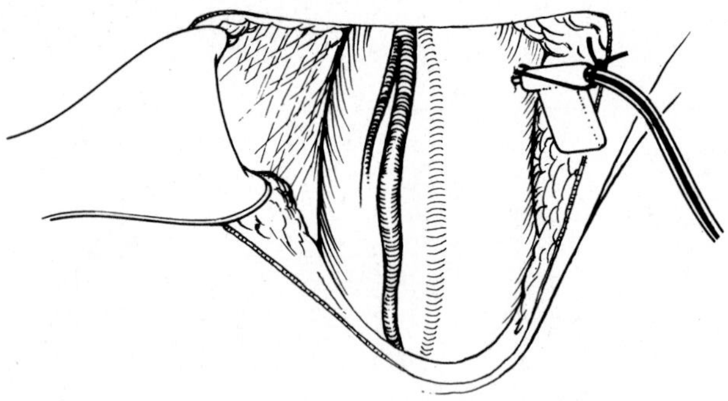

FIGURE 75.5 Placement of a butterfly needle for intraoperative cavernosometry.

used again after the dissection to perform intraoperative cavernosometry. A 3/8–in. Penrose drain is looped around the penile shaft between the corpora. This allows retraction of the penile skin, allows elongation and stabilization of the penile shaft, and affords exposure for the proximal vein dissection.

The superficial fundiform ligament is identified at the base of the penis and is divided to expose the underlying suspensory ligament. The suspensory ligament is then sharply divided close to the underside of the pubic symphysis (Fig. 75.6). The suspensory ligament must be completely taken down to expose the deep infrapubic region. Care is taken to identify and divide small veins emanating from the underside of the pubis and joining the superficial drainage system as well as veins perforating the Buck fascia to connect the deep and superficial systems at this level. Failure to ligate these vessels can lead to significant bleeding, which can be difficult to control and obscure exposure for the proximal portion of the venous dissection.

Deep in the infrapubic region, the Buck fascia is opened in the midline over the deep dorsal vein. The vein usually has a single large main trunk at this level. The deep dorsal vein is dissected free of the tunica albuginea, ligated with 0 silk ties, and divided (Fig. 75.7). Inferior to the deep dorsal vein, the cavernosal veins can be identified in the penile hilum at this time. They may be divided if they are a major source of leakage. Great care is taken to preserve the cavernosal arteries and nerve trunks that lie lateral to these veins.

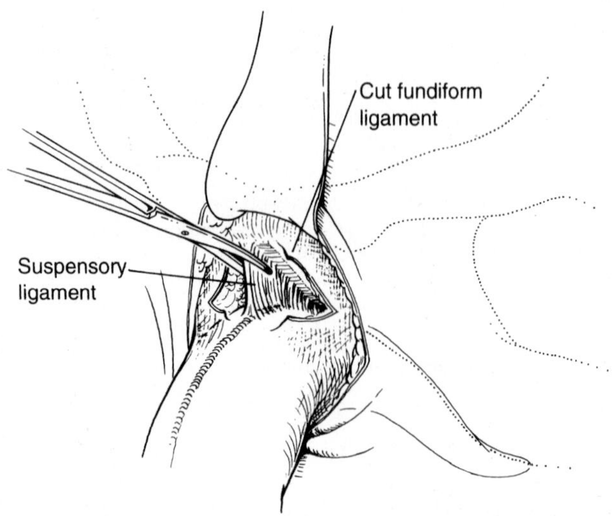


FIGURE 75.6 The suspensory ligament is divided to expose the base of the penis.

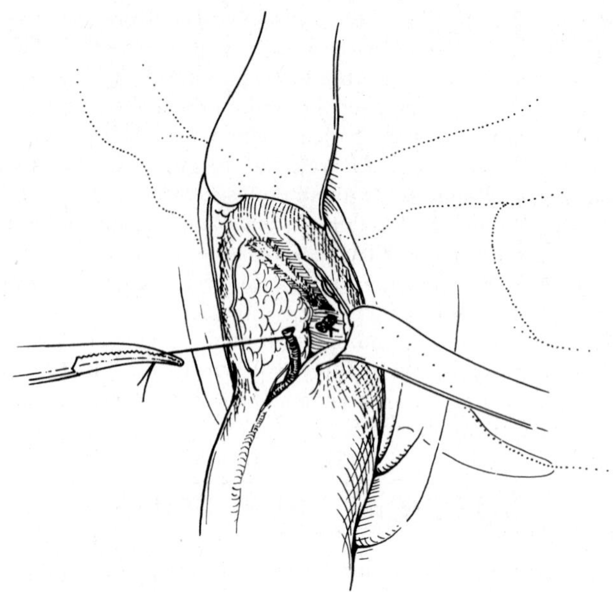

FIGURE 75.7 Division of the deep dorsal vein in the infrapubic region.

If the deep dorsal vein is a significant source of abnormal penile drainage, then it is dissected from the infrapubic region along the penile dorsal midline under the Buck fascia distally toward the glans. It is important to stay in the midline during the dissection to avoid the laterally located dorsal arteries and nerves. Circumflex and emissary veins encountered on either side of the deep dorsal vein are ligated with 3-0 plain gut sutures and divided (Fig. 75.8). Bipolar electrocoagulation on low setting can be used to cauterize some small vessels along the shaft.

Sometimes the deep dorsal vein is composed of two trunks along the penile shaft, and each must be dissected separately. Dissection continues until several fanning tributaries constitute the deep dorsal vein approximately 1 cm from the glans. Rarely, a large vein arises from the tunica albuginea and penetrates the Buck fascia to join the deep dorsal vein. Ligation of this vein may create a sinusoidal defect in the tunica, which must be closed with a 3-0 chromic figure-of-eight suture ligature. The junction between the corpora cavernosa and the spongiosum is carefully inspected as well, and circumflex veins connecting the two structures are ligated and divided.

After vein dissection and ligation are completed, 30 mg of papaverine or equivalent is injected into the corpora via the butterfly needle, and cavernosometry is performed 10 minutes later. If the abnormal draining veins have been eliminated, then a rigid erection is easily maintained at a flow of saline considerably $<5$ mL per minute (Fig. 75.9). Following this, the suspensory ligament is reapproximated with a 0 silk suture ligature between the infrapubic periosteum and the penile shaft. A no. 10 Jackson-Pratt fenestrated bulb suction drain is then placed in the wound with the tubing exiting via a separate stab incision lateral to the surgical incision. The Scarpa fascia is closed with a running 3-0 chromic suture, with care taken to approximate equal tissue planes to minimize the chance of scar formation resulting in fixation of the base of the penis. The skin edges are then reapproximated with a running subcuticular 3-0 Monocryl suture. The wound is covered with a standard sterile dressing, and the penis is snugly

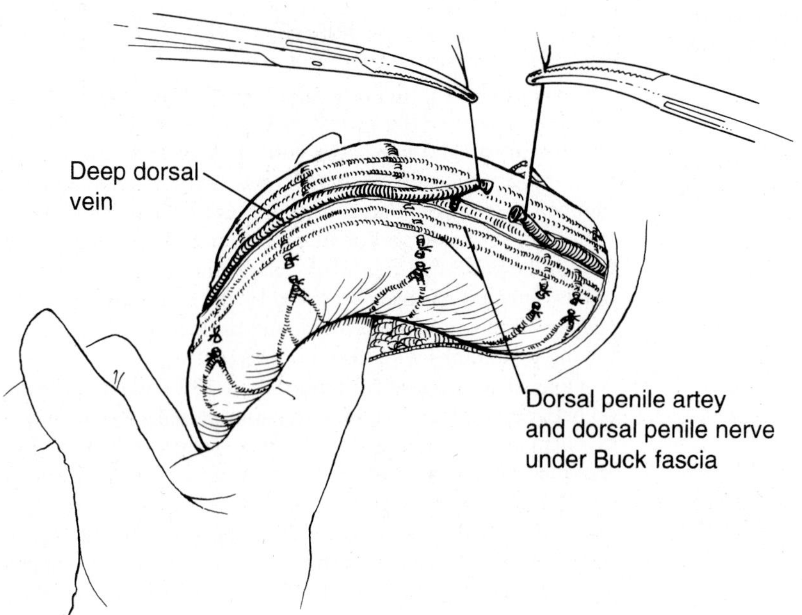


FIGURE 75.8 Division of circumflex and emissary veins on both sides of the deep dorsal vein.

wrapped with a self-adherent Coban wrap. Care is taken to avoid glanular edema from a dressing that is too tight. The Foley catheter and the dressing are removed the day after surgery. The drain is removed as soon as drainage is negligible, usually in 24 to 48 hours. Patients are discharged from the hospital on postoperative day 2 or 3. They are advised against engaging in intercourse for 6 weeks.

## Crural Banding and Other Procedures

If the crural veins are found to be the only source of major venous leakage by cavernosography, we perform a crural banding procedure. The crura are exposed near the bulb of the urethra via a perineal incision, and a 1/4-in. Mersilene ribbon (Ethicon, Inc.) is used to band the crura (Fig. 75.10). Veins

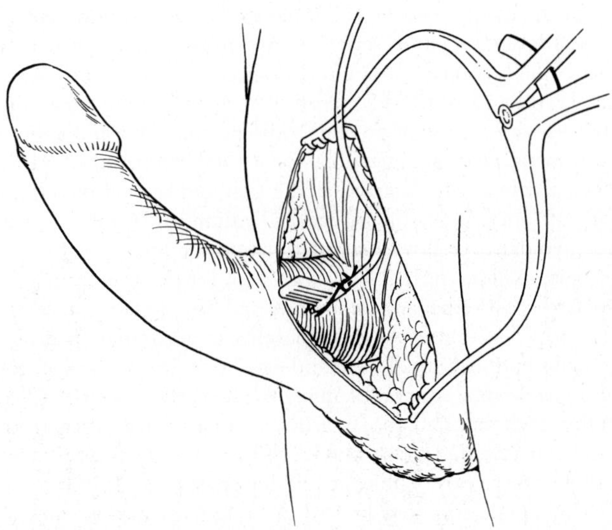

FIGURE 75.9 Cavernosometry after completion of the dissection confirms correction of the venous leak.

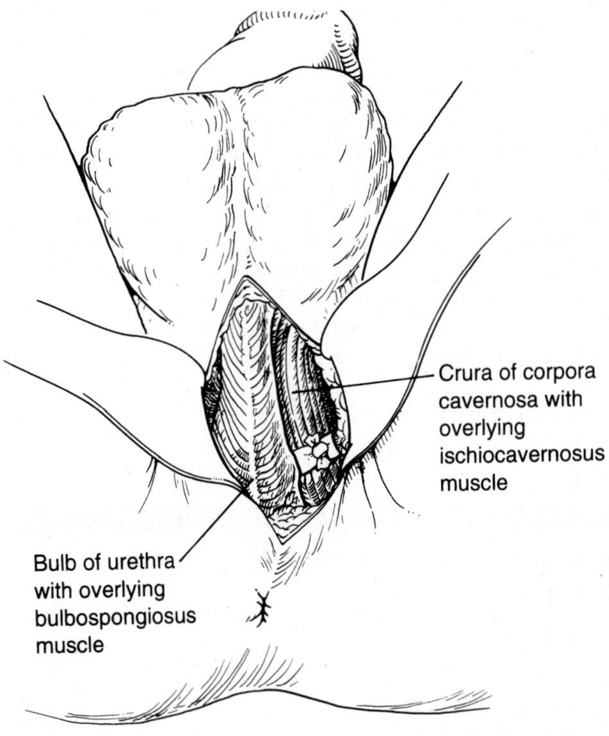


FIGURE 75.10 Crural banding to correct venous leakage from crural veins.

draining from the edge of the crura are ligated as well. Crural banding is not routinely performed at the time of deep dorsal vein ligation and is usually a secondary procedure. Lue's group described (11) recently published their case series on crural ligation in 11 patients. Cavernosometry and cavernosography were utilized to diagnose these patients with crural leakage. At mean follow-up of 34 months, 9 of 11 patients noted marked improvement in their erectile function.

Another secondary procedure that is rarely employed is spongiolysis. Via a penile scrotal incision, the corpus spongiosum is exposed and stripped away from the ventral surface of the corpora cavernosa. All communications between the two structures are ligated or coagulated.

More direct approaches to site-specific areas may be used to treat focal venous outflow abnormalities. These can be due to trauma, previous patent shunts for priapism, Peyronie disease primary or secondary venous outflow sites, or venous leaks secondary to previous stricture repair.

# OUTCOMES

## Complications

Table 75.1 lists the complications that have been encountered after penile venous surgery. Complications can be divided into immediate and long-term. Most patients experience some superficial bruising of the shaft and scrotum. Penile edema is usually moderate and resolves within 2 to 3 weeks. The incidence of penile edema has decreased since our use of a compression dressing and a closed wound drainage system. Painful nocturnal erections often occur for the first 24 to 48 hours after surgery. Infrequently, this may last for longer than 1 week. Wound infection and true hematoma rarely occur. Care taken during the infrapubic portion of the dissection can eliminate the risk of postoperative hematoma.

Despite careful reapproximation of the suspensory ligament after the vein dissection is complete, approximately 20% of patients complain of penile shortening. The amount of perceived loss of length, however, is rarely clinically or functionally significant. Hypoesthesia or numbness of the glans or shaft of the penis is a common occurrence after surgery. Patients who report a loss of sensation often experience a diminished ability to achieve orgasm as well. In most cases, though, penile sensation returns completely within 7 to 9 months. Infrequently, wound scar contractures occur that lead to true penile tethering. In these cases, revision surgery is necessary, consisting of release of scar tissue and skin Z-plasty.

**TABLE 75.1**

**COMPLICATIONS OF PENILE VENOUS SURGERY**

| |
|---|
| Immediate |
| Common |
| Penile and scrotal bruising |
| Penile edema |
| Painful nocturnal erections |
| Rare |
| Wound infection |
| Hematoma |
| Long-term |
| Common |
| Penile shortening |
| Decreased penile sensation |
| Decreased ability for orgasm |
| Rare |
| Wound scar contractures and penile tethering |

## Results

Although individual reports of successful vein ligation procedures date back to the early 1900s, the modern era of penile venous surgery did not begin until the development of accurate and appropriate diagnostic and surgical techniques. A number of surgeons have since reported on the initial and long-term success rates for this procedure. A detailed tabulation of the published results of veno-occlusive surgery for sexual dysfunction has been prepared by the senior author of this chaper (9). Some of these outcomes are discussed in the following paragraphs with also more recent data.

Donatucci and Lue (2) reported on 100 patients operated on between 1986 and 1988. Forty-four patients (44%) had an excellent result, defined as a complete return of spontaneous erections rigid enough for penetration, and 24 patients (24%) noted some improvement in rigidity. All patients were followed for longer than 1 year after surgery. Knoll et al. (5) reported a 46% excellent response to surgery in 41 patients followed for an average of 28 months. Claes and Baert (1) similarly reported a return of normal erectile function in 30 of 72 patients (42%) and a partial response in 23 others (32%). Patients were all followed for >1 year.

Lewis (8) reported on 60 patients, of whom 16 (27%) initially had return of normal erections. Seventeen other patients (28%) experienced improved rigidity and were able to have intercourse with the aid of intracavernosal pharmacologic injections for a combined success rate of 55%. All patients were followed for at least 2 years. Over time, 13 of the 33 patients (39%) who initially experienced a successful result later reported failure of the procedure. Kropman et al. (6) also reported a 40% late failure rate at a mean follow-up of 28 months in 10 of 20 patients who initially experienced a successful result from surgery.

The best long-term results were reported by Sasso et al. (12) in 1999. Seventeen of 23 patients (74%) had normal erections within 1 year of venous ligation surgery, and 12 of 17 maintained normal spontaneous erectile function long-term. The authors describe strict operative selection criteria, including the need to determine a crucial percentage of smooth muscle (>30%) in the corporeal tissue found on preoperative biopsy.

Most recently Hsu et al. (3) have reported a repeat venous dissection and ligation series in 45 men who failed their first meticulous surgery. Long-term successful erections were achieved in 35 of the 45 men (78%), with 4 more obtaining success with the use of prostaglandin $E_5$ inhibitors and 3 more with intracavernous injection, for a total improved of 91%. They attribute their success in the first and second operation series to meticulous microsurgery ligation of 76 to 125 sites and avoidance of Bovie coagulation and suction.

Several different factors can account for the approximately 40% to 50% immediate failure rate and 75% long-term failure rate of penile venous surgery. Inability to accurately diagnose concomitant arterial disease and less extensive venous dissection probably accounts for many of the early patient failures in the series reported above. With the use of stricter diagnostic inclusion criteria and a more aggressive surgical approach, many of these early failures could have been avoided (3).

Collateralization has limited the long-term success rates of other types of venous surgery as well. Hsu et al. (3) describe most failures as due to residual veins, not recurrent veins. A final reason for failure is that the ligation of penile veins may not address the true underlying pathologic disorder in many patients. Sinus smooth muscle disease that prohibits the expansion of the tunica albuginea and the subsequent compression of subtunical venules has been postulated as a major cause of veno-occlusive dysfunction (13). To date, though, no practical test is available to accurately diagnose this entity. Penile venous surgery remains a reasonable surgical option for highly selected patients with venous leak impotence, particularly those with focal or iatrogenic etiology.

## *References*


1. Claes H, Baert L. Cavernosometry and penile vein resection in corporeal incompetence: an evaluation of short-term and long-term results. *Int J Impot Res* 1991;3:129.
2. Donatucci CF, Lue TF. Venous surgery: are we kidding ourselves? In: Lue TF, ed. *World book of impotence*. London: Smith-Gorthdon and Co, 1992: 221–227.
3. Hsu GL, Chen HS, Hsieh CH, et al. Insufficient response to venous stripping surgery: is the penile vein recurrent or residual? *J Androl* 2006; 27:700.
4. King BF, Lewis RW, McKusick MA. Radiologic evaluation of impotence. In: Bennett AH, ed. *Impotence. Diagnosis and management of erectile dysfunction*. Philadelphia: WB Saunders, 1994:52–91.
5. Knoll LD, Furlow WL, Benson RC. Penile venous ligation surgery for the management of cavernosal venous leakage. *Urol Int* 1992;49:33.
6. Kropman RF, Nijeholt AABL, Giespers AGM, et al. Results of deep penile vein resection in impotence caused by venous leakage. *Int J Impot Res* 1990;2:29.
7. Lewis RW. Venogenic impotence. Diagnosis, management, and results. *Probl Urol* 1991;5:567.
8. Lewis RW. Venous surgery in the patient with erectile dysfunction. *Atlas Urol Clin North Am* 1993;1:21.
9. Lewis RW. Munarriz R. Vascular surgery for erectile dysfunction. In: Wein AJ, et al., eds. *Campbell-Walsh urology*, 9th ed. Philadelphia: Saunders Elsevier, 2007:802–817.
10. Peskircioglu L, Tekin I, Boyvat F, et al. Embolization of the deep dorsal vein for the treatment of erectile impotence due to veno-occlusive dysfunction. *J Urol* 2000;163:472.
11. Rahman N, Dean R, Carrion R, et al. Crural ligation for primary erectile dysfunction: a case series. *J Urol* 2005;173:2064.
12. Sasso F, Gulino G, Weir J, et al. Patient selection criteria in the surgical treatment of veno-occlusive dysfunction. *J Urol* 1999;161:1145.
13. Wespes E, Moreira De Goes P, Sattar AA, et al. Objective criteria in the long-term evaluation of penile venous surgery. *J Urol* 1994;152:888.


# CHAPTER 76 ■ MICROVASCULAR ARTERIAL BYPASS SURGERY FOR ERECTILE DYSFUNCTION

IRWIN GOLDSTEIN AND MARTIN BASTUBA

When a middle-aged or elderly man (age 50 or more years) presents to a physician with complaints of consistent or persistent inability to obtain and/or maintain a penile erection for satisfactory sexual activity, the "new" thinking is that the diagnosis is likely organically based erectile dysfunction. This is especially true if the patient also has a history of diabetes, hypertension, high cholesterol, cigarette smoking, or myocardial infarction (1). This contemporary knowledge represents a shift in understanding; 40 years ago, at the time of Masters and Johnson, most of erectile dysfunction was thought to be psychogenic in origin and sex therapy and cognitive behavior therapy were the primary treatment options. There are widespread data to support an organic vascular pathophysiologic basis of erectile dysfunction in strong association with endothelial dysfunction in older men with vascular risk factors (2).

However, when a young man (age teens to 40 years) presents to a physician with complaints of erectile dysfunction, the "old" thinking still prevails and the diagnosis most likely to be considered is psychogenically based erectile dysfunction. Why do practitioners have such great difficulty accepting the existence of vasculogenic erectile dysfunction in younger men? Unfortunately, many physicians who evaluate younger men do not seek a history of blunt perineal trauma. Endothelial dysfunction resulting in focal arterial occlusive disease can be associated with a history of blunt trauma (3). Evidence for trauma-associated focal arterial obstructive pathology is well established in the medical literature for several other arterial beds (4). Such arterial beds include the radial artery (construction workers), the axillary artery (crutch-related injuries), and the popliteal artery (football players). The distal internal pudendal, common penile, and proximal cavernosal arteries are susceptible to blunt trauma by virtue of the anatomic relationship to the ischiopubic rami within the Alcock canal. They can be injured during bicycle riding (5) and other sources of straddle injuries such as blows to the perineum during martial arts.

The aim of this chapter is to expand the knowledge concerning microvascular arterial bypass surgery as a therapeutic option for young patients with erectile dysfunction secondary to focal arterial obstructive pathology. Data supporting the existence of traumatic-associated vasculogenic erectile dysfunction and the associated diagnostic and therapeutic paradigm in young men will be reviewed. The overall goal is to stimulate basic science and clinical research in the management of young men with erectile dysfunction.

## ERECTILE FUNCTION PHYSIOLOGY

Penile erectile function results following autonomic cavernosal nerve stimulation (6). Nitric oxide synthase (NOS), an enzyme in lacunar space vascular endothelial cells and autonomic cavernosal nerve endings, facilitates the synthesis of nitric oxide (NO) from molecular oxygen and L-arginine. During sexual stimulation, nitric oxide (NO) activates guanylyl cyclase, an enzyme that facilitates the synthesis of the second messenger, cyclic guanosine monophosphate (cGMP) from guanosine triphosphate (GTP). The elevated concentrations of cGMP result in lowered intracellular calcium, thus promoting penile smooth muscle relaxation. Biologic consequences of NO-cGMP relaxation include increased arterial blood inflow, engorgement of the lacunar spaces, lengthening and enlargement of the corporal erectile tissue within the constrained tunica albuginea, and eventual subtunical venule occlusion with increased penile venous outflow resistance and corporal veno-occlusive function (7).

## ERECTILE DYSFUNCTION PATHOPHYSIOLOGY

The NOS-NO-cGMP pathway is, in part, interfered with by multiple organic pathophysiologies, including hypogonadism, hypothyroidism, and metabolic conditions such as diabetes and reduced insulin sensitivity, metabolic syndrome, low testosterone, elevated body mass index, elevated waist circumference, abnormal lipids, elevated blood pressure, sedentary lifestyle, cigarette smoking, and increased age. Endothelial dysfunction ultimately leads to reduced arterial blood inflow and arterial systolic perfusion pressures during erection (8).

### Focal Endothelial Dysfunction Secondary to Trauma-Associated Erectile Dysfunction

There is a puzzling resistance to acknowledge that focal endothelial dysfunction may also occur following blunt trauma to the distal internal pudendal, common penile, and proximal arteries. These critical arteries to erectile function lie in close proximity to the hard bony surface, the lateral aspect of the Alcock canal, the ischiopubic rami. Endothelial injuries induced by blunt trauma may be classified as either nondenuded or denuded. While some nondenuded endothelial injuries may spontaneously heal, some progress to frank endothelial dysfunction, increased permeability, and thrombogenicity to eventually, over a variable time period, focal atherosclerosis, focal arterial lumen stenosis, and reduced systolic arterial perfusion pressures. Denuded endothelial injuries that result following blunt trauma to the arterial wall often result in medial smooth muscle cell proliferation, smooth muscle cell migration, myointimal thickening, extracellular matrix production, and progressive occlusive arterial pathology over time, leading to diminished systolic arterial perfusion pressures and diminished erectile hardness during sexual stimulation.

### Bicycle Riding and Erectile Dysfunction

Data in the peer review medical literature of an appropriate level of scientific evidence show an association of erectile dysfunction with those who ride bicycles.

Marceau et al. (9) studied a community-based population exceeding 1,700 men 40 to 70 years of age. The odds ratio for men developing moderate to severe erectile dysfunction who acknowledged riding >3 hours per week was 1:72. This analysis was performed where covariates were factored, such as age, energy expenditure, body mass index, cigarette smoking, depression, cancer, high blood pressure, and diabetes.

Schrader et al. (10) published a unique National Institute for Occupational Safety and Health study of bicyclists involving the determination of nocturnal penile tumescence activity as recorded by RigiScan and perineal or nose pressure recorded by specialized pressure-sensitive sheets placed over the rider's saddle. They reported a significant inverse correlation between the magnitude of nose pressure values and the percentage of sleep time in erection. Control subjects exhibited >30% sleep time in erection, whereas those who rode with nose pressures exceeding 1,000 and 2,000 U revealed <20% sleep time in erection.

Dettori et al. (11) reported on the erectile dysfunction characteristics of several hundred men who performed long-distance bicycle rides. In those men who exceeded 328 kilometers, who complained of current perineal numbness, and who used a saddle with a cutout (which acted to lower surface area contact and increase perineal compressure pressures), a surprising 18% were found at risk for developing erectile dysfunction.

Cohen and Gross (12) studied >30 male cyclists and examined transcutaneous penile oxygen pressures. Compared to values obtained during standing, cyclists who straddled on commercially available saddles with nose extensions such as the Vetta Lite, Terry, and Specialized exhibited significant reductions in transcutaneous penile oxygen pressures.

Leibovitch and Mor (13) performed a literature search of 62 articles in the peer review medical literature on bicycling and genitourinary disorders. They reported that 13% to 24% of bicyclists in the literature claimed erectile dysfunction. They concluded that although bicycling is associated with established cardiovascular benefits, it was a not infrequent cause of injury to the genitourinary system.

Bacon et al. (14) reported that the risk of developing erectile dysfunction among the >20,000 men in the Health Professional Follow-up Study who were healthy and had good or very good erectile function before the study decreased as the subjects reported increasing metabolic energy transfer units (METS) during various exercise forms, including bicycling. The authors also performed a unique multivariate and total physical activity subanalysis of the data by the various exercise forms. The risk of developing erectile dysfunction among healthy participants who had good or very good erectile function before the study (and no prostate cancer) was reduced at the highest tertile of physical activity such as jogging, running, swimming, tennis, rowing, and squash or raquetball. Curiously, there was no risk lowering for bicycle riding.

Goldstein et al. (19) reported in the *Journal of Sexual Medicine* a prospective study recording cavernosal artery peak systolic velocity values using duplex Doppler ultrasound in men who lay supine, sat on the examination table, straddled a saddle, sat on a two-cheek noseless seat, and then lay supine. In all subjects who straddled a saddle, peak systolic velocity values approached zero. All remaining interventions were associated with mean peak systolic velocity values that were not significantly different from each other and that ranged from 20 to 26 cm per second. It was estimated that the compression pressure on the perineum while bearing body weight on a bicycle saddle exceeded 300 mm Hg (15).

Another study published in the *Journal of Sexual Medicine* was performed, for the first time with women bicyclists. This study is being reported because it is likely that blunt perineal trauma causes similar injuries to perineal contents in women. Other than the pudendal artery, critical structures in the Alcock canal in both genders include the pudendal nerve. In this study, female bicyclists were compared to female runners for the value of vibration quantitative sensory testing by biothesiometry. Female bicyclists had significantly lowered sensation in the clitoris, labia, and vaginal introitus compared to runners (16).

An additional study in the *Journal of Sexual Medicine* examined whether noseless bicycle saddles would be an effective intervention for alleviating deleterious health effects, erectile dysfunction, and groin numbness caused by bicycling on the traditional saddle with a protruding nose extension. Ninety bicycling police officers from five metropolitan regions in the United States (Northwest, Southern, Desert West, Midwest, and Southeast) using traditional saddles were evaluated prior to changing saddles and then again after 6 months of using the noseless bicycle saddle. The findings showed that use of the noseless saddle resulted in a reduction in saddle contact pressure in the perineal region. There was a significant improvement in penile tactile sensation, and the number of men who used no-nose saddles and who indicated they had not experienced genital numbness while cycling for the preceding 6 months rose from 27% to 82%. Use of the noseless saddle also resulted in significant increases in erectile function as assessed by the initial evaluation. With few exceptions, bicycle police officers were able to effectively use no-nose saddles in their police work, and 97% of officers completing the study continued to use the no-nose saddle afterward. In summary, for the first time, a prospective study of healthy policemen riding bikes using wider no-nose bike saddles for 6 months revealed improved perineal sensation and improved erectile function. Changing saddles changed physiology (17).

## DIAGNOSTIC TESTING

The overall goal of microvascular arterial bypass surgery is to create an alternative arterial inflow route around obstructive arterial lesions in the hypogastric-cavernous arterial bed. The specific objective of the surgery is to increase the cavernosal arterial perfusion pressure and arterial blood inflow in patients with vasculogenic erectile dysfunction secondary to pure arterial insufficiency. Young men, without other vascular risk factors, who have erectile dysfunction of a pure arteriogenic nature represent the ideal patient population for this procedure.

The diagnostic algorithm is aimed at ensuring that this operation is performed on the ideal candidate, that is, one in whom there is erectile dysfunction purely on the basis of arterial insufficiency. All young patients with a history suggestive of trauma-associated impotence (pelvic fractures and perineal trauma) should undergo a comprehensive history, physical examination, and psychologic interview. They should have a routine endocrinologic evaluation to ensure adequate circulating levels of unbound, free testosterone. Duplex Doppler ultrasonography should be performed to provide diagnostic hemodynamic data (cavernosal peak systolic and end-diastolic velocities) and preoperative information such as the presence of communicating branches from the dorsal to the cavernosal artery. Finally, vascular assessment by dynamic infusion cavernosometry should be considered to document the degree of arterial pressure gradients between the brachial artery and the cavernosal arteries and to further evaluate the veno-occlusive function. Following hemodynamic diagnosis, if the patient has pure arterial insufficiency, a selective internal pudendal arteriogram should be performed to confirm the location of the obstructive lesion, most often in the common penile or cavernosal artery(ies), and to select the best inferior epigastric artery (18).

## SURGICAL CRITERIA

The success of this operation is based on the selection of the correct operative candidate and the microsurgical capabilities of the surgeon. To this end, the following represents a list of criteria to ensure optimum results. The criteria are as follows:

1. The patient's history is characterized by (a) intact libido, (b) a consistent reduction in erectile rigidity during sexual activity, (c) variable sustaining capability with the best maintenance of the rigidity during early morning erections, and (d) poor spontaneity of erections, taking much effort and excessive time to achieve the poorly rigid erectile response.
2. Normal hormonal and neurologic evaluation.
3. Suspicion of arterial insufficiency as evidenced by reduced peak systolic velocity values during duplex Doppler ultrasonography and increased arterial gradients during cavernosal artery occlusion pressure determination using dynamic infusion cavernosometry.
4. Normal veno-occlusive parameters during both duplex Doppler ultrasonography and dynamic infusion cavernosometry.
5. The presence of a distal occlusive lesion in one or both hypogastric-cavernous arterial beds, usually within the common penile artery or cavernosal artery, that is amenable to distal bypass (Fig. 76.1).
6. The presence of an inferior epigastric artery of sufficient length to allow anastomosis to the dorsal artery (Fig. 76.2).
7. The presence of a communication branch(es) between the dorsal artery and the cavernosal artery distal to the occlusion that will allow the inflow of new blood and the development of increased intracorporal pressure.

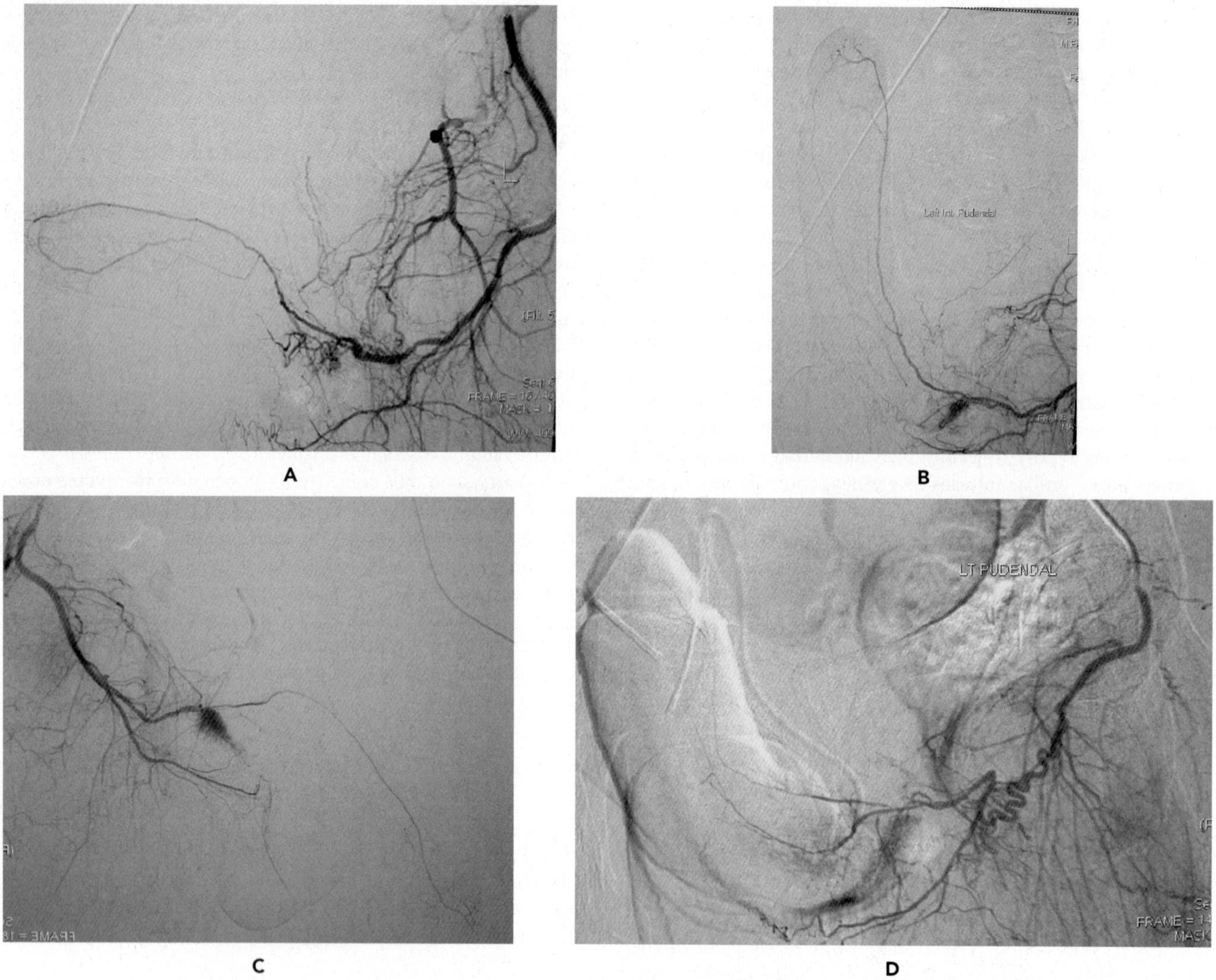

A B C D

FIGURE 76.1 The presence of a distal occlusive lesion on selective internal pudenal arteriography in one or both hypogastric-cavernous arterial beds, usually within the common penile artery or cavernosal artery that is amenable to distal bypass, is an inclusion criterion for microvascular arterial bypass surgery.

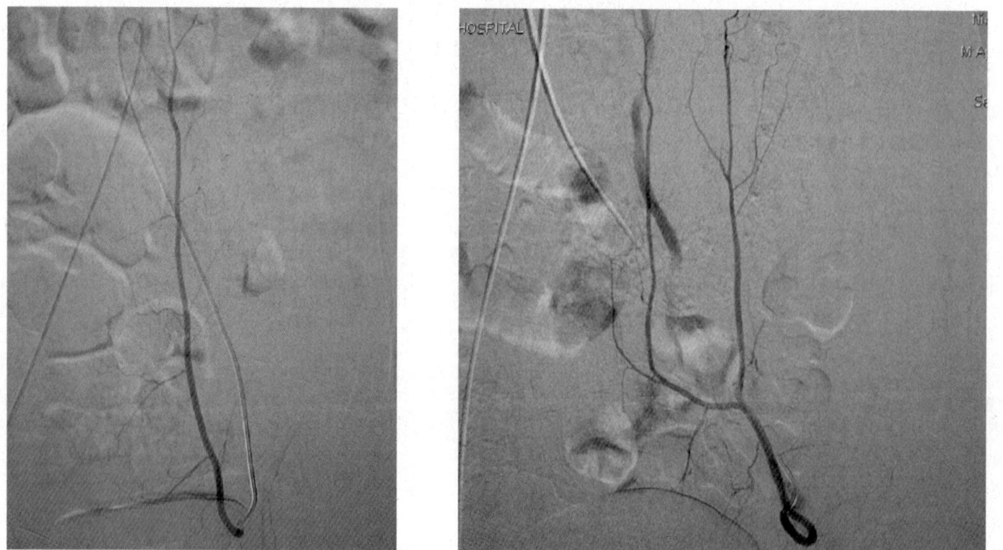


A B

FIGURE 76.2 **A:** An inferior epigastric artery of sufficient length to allow anastomosis to the dorsal artery. **B:** The inferior epigastric artery bifurcates too early to provide sufficient donor artery length. This will place the anastomosis under risk for excessive tension.

## ALTERNATIVE THERAPY

Nonsurgical treatment options for young men with erectile dysfunction include psychotherapeutic, hormonal, pharmacologic, and external device interventions. Surgical treatment options consist primarily of penile prosthesis insertion.

## SURGICAL TECHNIQUE

The patient is placed supine on the operating table and his arms secured next to his body to minimize upper-extremity nerve injuries. As this operation may last in excess of 5 hours, great care must be taken in the positioning and padding of the limbs, in particular the neurovascular points on the upper limbs. Sequential compressive devices are placed aouund each calf. General endotracheal anesthesia with complete muscle relaxation provides complete skeletal muscle (especially the rectus muscle) relaxation and facilitates harvesting the donor inferior epigastric artery vessel. The patient's abdomen and genitalia are carefully shaved, prepared, and draped, following which a 16Fr Foley catheter is placed using sterile technique. The patient is given one dose of preoperative antibiotics (cefazolin or vancomycin if penicillin allergic). From a technical standpoint, the operation can be divided into three stages: dorsal artery dissection, inferior epigastric artery harvesting, and microsurgical anastomosis (19).

### Dorsal Artery Dissection

A curvilinear incision is made, in general on the side opposite the planned abdominal incision for the donor inferior epigastric artery harvesting (Fig. 76.3A). The advantages of this incision are that it offers (a) excellent proximal and distal exposure of the penile neurovascular bundle, (b) the ability to preserve the fundiform ligament preventing penile shortening,

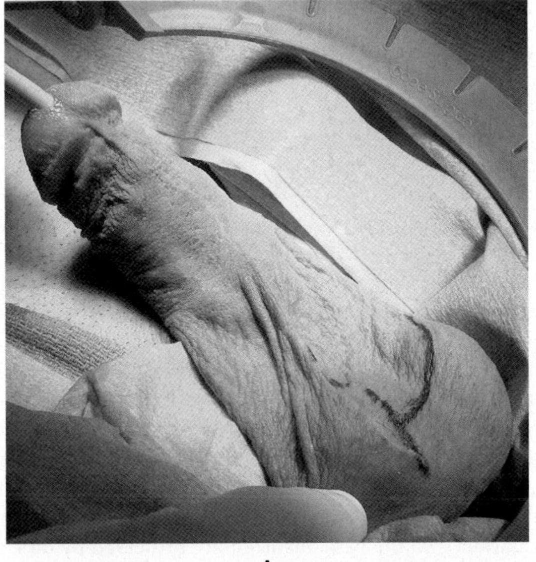

A

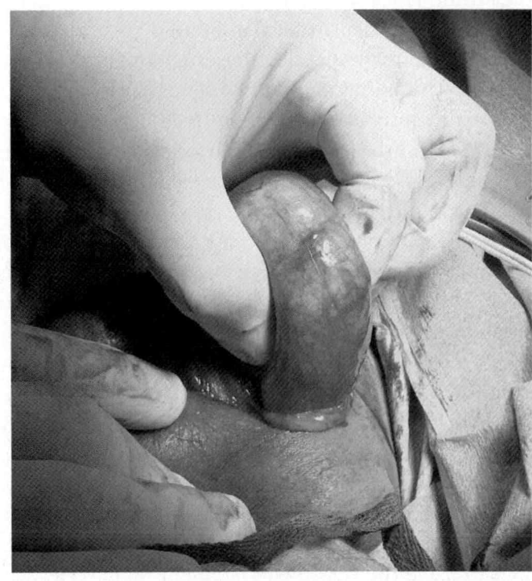

B

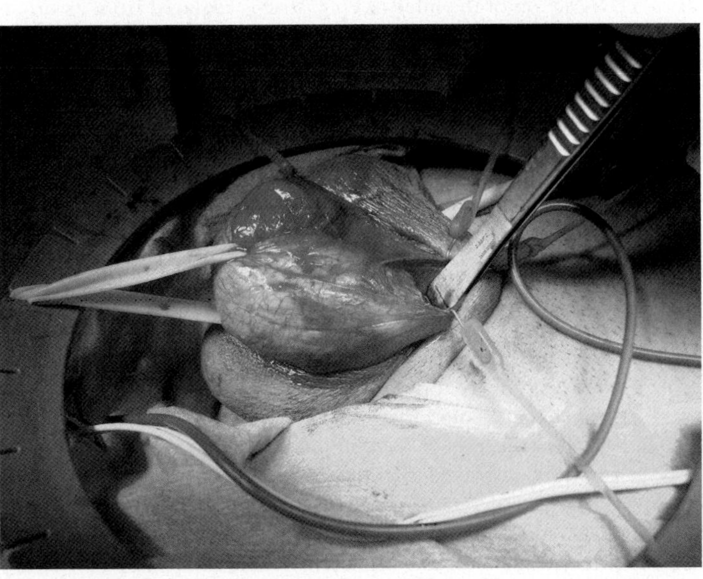

C

FIGURE 76.3 **A:** A curvilinear incision is made, in general on the side opposite to the planned abdominal incision for the donor inferior epigastric artery harvesting. The advantages of this incision are that it offers (a) excellent proximal and distal exposure of the penile neurovascular bundle, (b) the ability to preserve the fundiform ligament, preventing penile shortening, and (c) the absence of unsightly postoperative scars on the penile shaft or at the base of the penis. Use of a Scott ring retractor with its elastic hooks maximizes operative exposure of the penis with a minimum of assistance. **B:** The penis is inverted through the skin incision, with care taken to push the glans in fully. **C:** The preselected right or left dorsal penile artery is identified. The course of the appropriate dorsal artery is followed proximally underneath the fundiform ligament, with care being taken to leave the fundiform ligament intact. Blunt dissection is performed under the proximal aspect of the fundiform ligament above the pubic bone toward the external ring.

and (c) the absence of unsightly postoperative scars on the penile shaft or at the base of the penis. Use of a Scott ring retractor with its elastic hooks maximizes operative exposure of the penis with a minimum of assistance.

The incision is made 2 fingerbreadths from the base of the penis, from a point opposite the ventral root of the penis, to the scrotal median raphe. This incision is carried down through the dartos layer using blunt dissection. The ipsilateral tunica albuginea is subsequently identified at the midpenile shaft. With the penis stretched, blunt finger dissection along the tunica albuginea is performed in a distal direction deep and inferior to the spermatic cord structures along the lateral aspect of the penile shaft, avoiding injury to the fundiform ligament.

The penis is then inverted through the skin incision, with care taken to push the glans in fully (Fig. 76.3B). The penis must not be tumesced during this maneuver. If a partial erection is present, an intracavernosal alpha-adrenergic agonist (100 μg phenylephrine) should be administered. Blunt finger dissection around the distal penile shaft enables a plane to be established between the Buck fascia and the Colles fascia, and a Penrose drain is secured in this plane.

Exposure of the neurovascular bundle and, in particular, the right and left dorsal penile arteries is now performed. The arteries are usually obvious, located on either side of the deep dorsal vein and surrounded by the dorsal nerves. Isolation of the dorsal penile arteries for such arterial bypass surgery requires limited dissection at this time in the procedure; thus, ischemic, mechanical, and thermal trauma to the dorsal penile arteries may be minimized. To avoid injurious vasospasm, topical papaverine hydrochloride irrigation is applied frequently. In this way, preservation of endothelial and smooth muscle cell morphology during dorsal artery preparation is ensured. This is very critical as the room temperature of the operating room, the use of room temperature irrigating solution, and even the skin incision can induce vasoconstriction, spasm, and possible endothelial cell damage.

The preselected right or left dorsal penile artery is identified. The course of the appropriate dorsal artery is followed proximally underneath the fundiform ligament, with care being taken to leave the fundiform ligament intact (Fig. 76.3C). Blunt dissection is performed under the proximal aspect of the fundiform ligament above the pubic bone toward the external ring. This dissection enables the inferior epigastric artery to pass from its abdominal location to the appropriate location in the penis while simultaneously preserving the fundiform ligament. The penis is placed back in its normal anatomic position and the inguinoscrotal incision is temporarily closed with staples.

## Harvesting of the Inferior Epigastric Artery

A transverse semilunar abdominal incision following Langer lines is the preferred incision. The transverse incision provides excellent operative exposure of the inferior epigastric artery and heals with a more cosmetic scar compared to those observed with paramedian skin incisions. The starting point of the transverse incision is approximately three-fourths of the total distance from the pubic bone to the umbilicus in the midline (Fig. 76.4). It extends laterally along Langer lines for approximately 5 cm. The rectus fascia is incised vertically. The junction between the rectus muscle and underlying preperitoneal fat is identified and the preperitoneal space is entered. The rectus muscle is reflected medially.

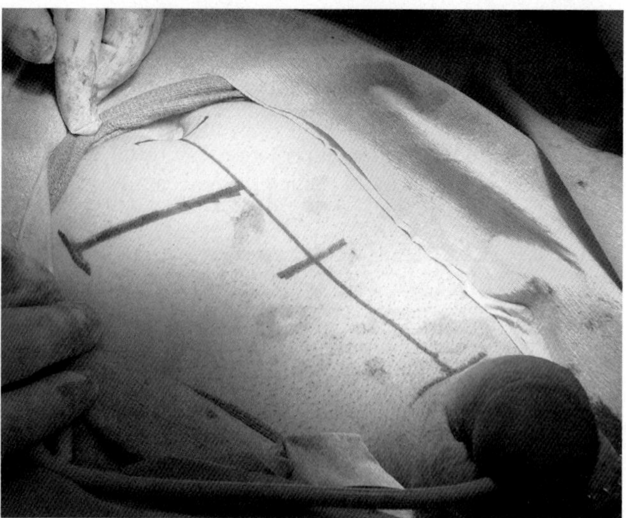

FIGURE 76.4 A transverse semilunar abdominal incision following Langer lines is the preferred incision. The transverse incision provides excellent operative exposure of the inferior epigastric artery and heals with a more cosmetic scar compared to those observed with paramedian skin incisions. The starting point of the transverse incision is approximately three-fourths of the total distance from the pubic bone to the umbilicus in the midline. It extends laterally along Langer lines for approximately 5 cm.

The inferior epigastric artery and its two accompanying veins are located beneath the rectus muscle in the preperitoneal plane. The ring retractor is again utilized to optimize operative exposure. It is critical to harvest an inferior epigastric artery of sufficient length to prevent tension on the microvascular anastomosis. Application of topical papaverine is utilized on the inferior epigastric artery throughout the dissection. Thermal injury is avoided using low-current microbipolar cautery set at the minimum level necessary for adequate coagulation, and the vasa vasorum are preserved by dissecting the artery en bloc with its surrounding veins and fat. Dissection of the inferior epigastric is required from its origin at the level of the external iliac artery to a point at the level of the umbilicus.

The transfer route of the neoarterial inflow source is prepared from the abdominal perspective prior to transecting the vessel distally (the penile transfer route has previously been dissected). The temporary scrotal staples are removed and the penis is reinverted. The internal ring on the side of the harvested artery is identified lateral to the origin of the inferior epigastric artery. Using blunt finger dissection through the inguinal canal, a long fine vascular clamp is passed through the fenestration in the fundiform ligament and the external and internal inguinal rings, and a Penrose drain is placed to protect this transfer route.

The donor inferior epigastric artery vascular bundle is transected at the level of the umbilicus between two LigaClips and carefully inspected for any proximal bleeding points. This donor artery should pulsate briskly (Fig. 76.5A). All attachments to the retroperitoneal fat are carefully removed prior to artery transfer as any attachments will diminish donor artery length and place the subsequent anastomosis with the dorsal

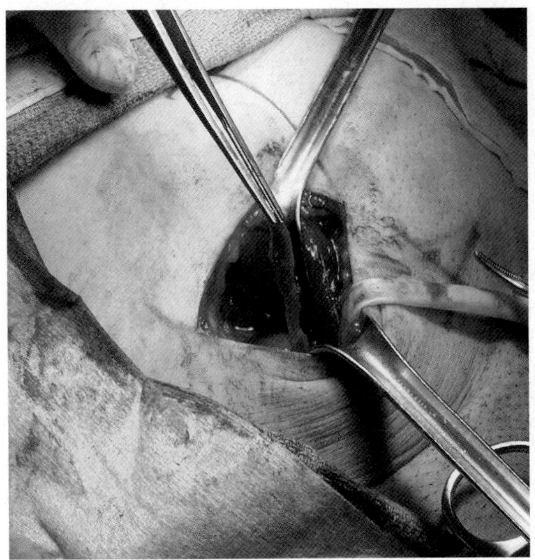
A

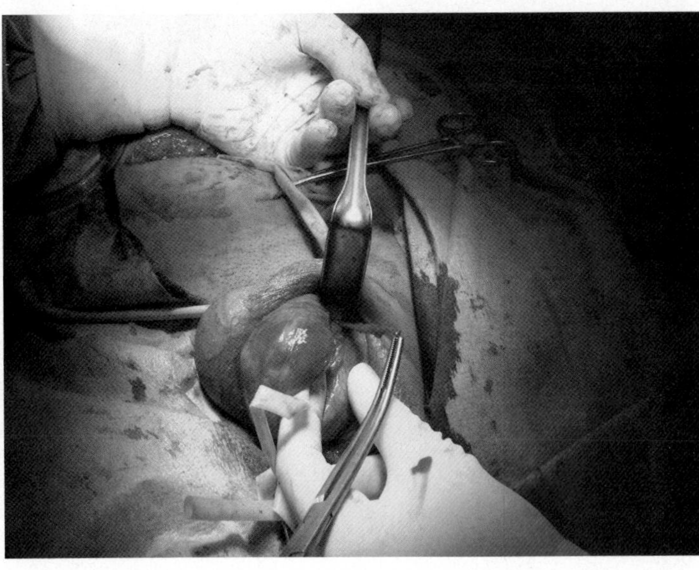
B

FIGURE 76.5 **A:** The donor inferior epigastric artery vascular bundle is transected at the level of the umbilicus between two LigaClips and carefully inspected for any proximal bleeding points. This donor artery should pulsate briskly. All attachments to the retroperitoneal fat are carefully removed prior to artery transfer as any attachments will diminish donor artery length and place the subsequent anastomosis with the dorsal artery at risk due to excessive tension. **B:** Using blunt finger dissection through the inguinal canal, a long fine vascular clamp is passed through the fenestration in the fundiform ligament and the external and internal inguinal rings, and a Penrose drain is placed to protect this transfer route. The inferior epigastric vascular bundle is transferred to the base of the penis. It should be briskly pulsating and of adequate length.

artery at risk for being made under undue tension. The long fine vascular clamp is brought through the internal inguinal ring again, this time to grasp the end of the transected inferior epigastric artery. The inferior epigastric vascular bundle is transferred to the base of the penis (Fig. 76.5B). It should be briskly pulsating and of adequate length. The origin of the inferior epigastric artery should be inspected for kinking or twisting. Following the achievement of complete hemostasis, closure of the abdominal wound is performed in two layers. The rectus fascia is closed utilizing a running 0 polyglycolic acid suture, one suture started at either end of the incision. On-Q SilverSoaker catheters, which will stay in place postoperatively for 48 to 72 hours, are placed below and above the rectus fascia, and 0.5% Marcaine is delivered at 2 mL per hour through each catheter (Fig. 76.6A). The skin edges are opposed using 4-0 Monocryl, and Dermabond is applied over the skin incision. On-Q SilverSoaker catheters are secured to the skin temporarily using Steri-Strips (Fig. 76.6B).

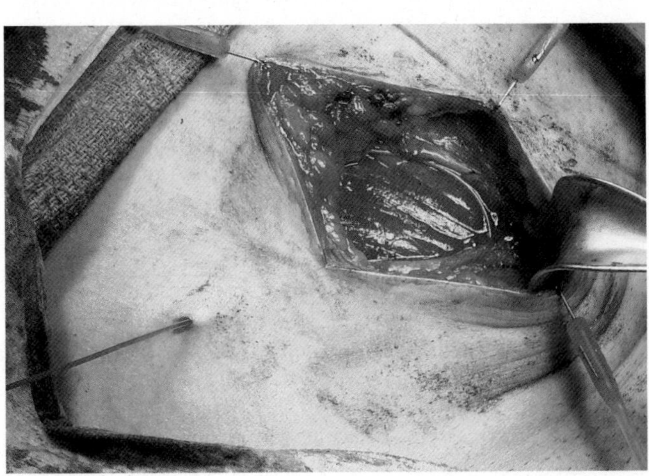
A

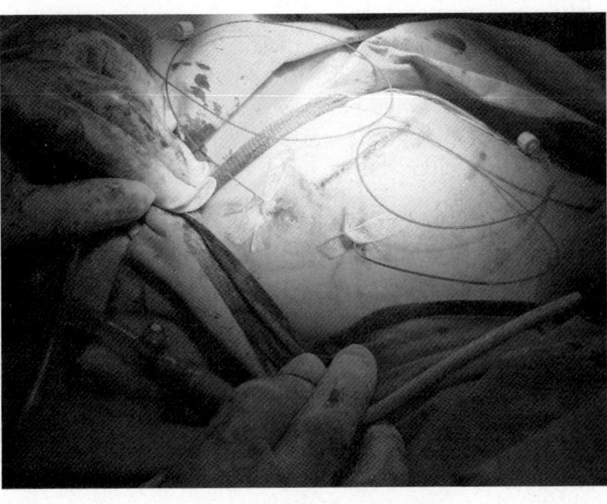
B

FIGURE 76.6 **A:** On-Q SilverSoaker catheters, which will stay in place postoperatively for 48 to 72 hours, are placed one each below and above the rectus fascia, and 0.5% Marcaine (plain) is delivered at 2 mL per hour through each catheter. **B:** The skin edges are opposed using 4-0 Monocryl, and Dermabond is applied over the skin incision. The On-Q SilverSoaker catheters are secured to the skin temporarily using Steri-Strips.

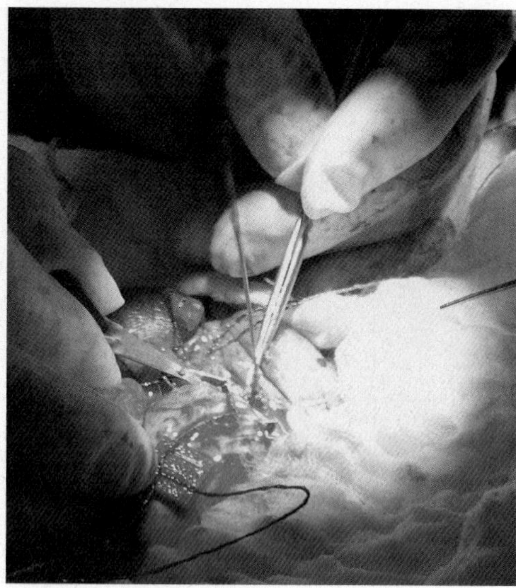

A

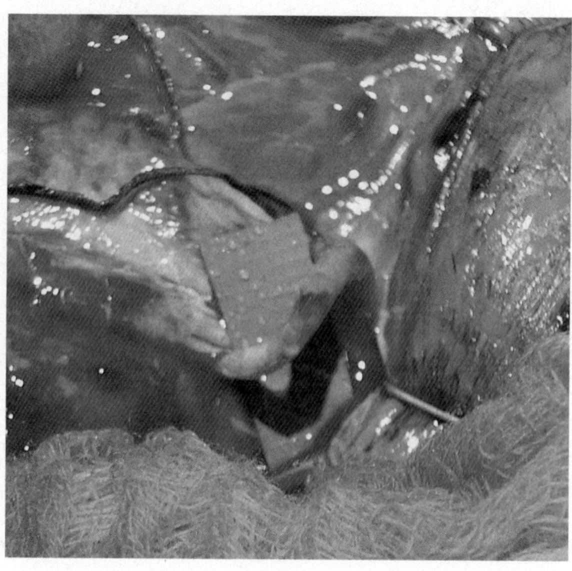

B

FIGURE 76.7 A: Prior to the anastomosis, it is appropriate to assess the integrity of the donor inferior epigastric perfusion pressure. Grossly this is assessed by temporarily removing pressure on the gold-plated (low-pressure) aneurysm vascular clamps under minimal tension. The donor artery should exhibit brisk arterial inflow. B: Following release of the temporary occluding vascular clamps on the dorsal penile artery, the anastomosed segment should reveal arterial pulsations along its length and retrograde into the inferior epigastric artery. Such an observation implies a patent anastomosis. At this time, the inferior epigastric artery gold-plated aneurysm clamp may be removed. The intensity of the arterial pulsations in the anastomosis usually increases.

## Microvascular Anastomosis

A ring retractor and the associated elastic hooks are utilized once again on the inguinoscrotal incision and the fenestration of the fundiform ligament to gain exposure of the proximal dorsal neurovascular bundle. The pulsating inferior epigastric artery is placed against the recipient dorsal penile arteries, and a convenient location is selected for the vascular anastomosis. The anastomosis is created based on the arteriographic and duplex Doppler ultrasound findings. An end-to-end anastomosis is best under conditions whereby dorsal penile artery communications exist to the cavernous artery. In addition, an end-to-end anastomosis transfers perfusion pressure more effectively than an end-to-side anastomosis with less turbulence.

For intraluminal arterial irrigation, we utilize a dilute papaverine, heparin, and electrolytic solution believed to be capable of inhibiting the early development of myointimal proliferative lesions during surgical preparation.

The appropriate dorsal penile artery segment is freed from its attachments to the tunica albuginea, with care being taken to avoid injury to any communicating branches to the cavernosal artery. Vascular hemostasis of this segment of the dorsal penile artery may be achieved with or gold-plated (low-pressure) aneurysm vascular clamps under minimal tension for the minimal of operating time. The only location where the adventitia must be carefully removed is at the site of the vascular anastomosis, that is, the distal end of the inferior epigastric artery and the free end of the dorsal artery, to avoid causing subsequent thrombosis. If segments of adventitia enter the anastomosis, the patency of the anastomosis is in jeopardy as adventitia activates clotting factors from the extrinsic clotting system. The remaining adventitia should be preserved in the vessels as the vasa vasorum provide a nutritional role to the vessel wall. The preservation of the adventitia is also important in terms of vessel innervation.

Prior to the anastomosis, it is appropriate to assess the integrity of the donor inferior epigastric perfusion pressure. This is assessed grossly by temporarily removing pressure on the gold-plated (low-pressure) aneurysm vascular clamps under minimal tension (Fig. 76.7A). The donor artery should exhibit brisk arterial inflow. A plastic colored background material is used to aid in vessel visualization under the microscope. An end-to-end anastomosis is performed between the inferior epigastric artery and the dorsal artery using interrupted 10-0 Nylon sutures (single-armed, 100-mm, 149-degree curved needle) under 10× magnification. Sutures are usually passed from the outside of the inferior epigastric artery (1 mm from the cut edge) to the inside lumen and then from the inside of the dorsal artery lumen to the outside wall of the dorsal artery (1 mm from the cut edge) and then tied. Usually 15 or more interrupted sutures are used. All sutures used to complete the anastomosis are inserted equidistant from each other to avoid an uneven anastomosis.

Following release of the temporary occluding vascular clamps on the dorsal penile artery, the anastomosed segment should reveal arterial pulsations along its length and retrograde into the inferior epigastric artery. Such an observation implies a patent anastomosis. At this time, the inferior epigastric artery gold-plated aneurysm clamp may be removed. The intensity of the arterial pulsations in the anastomosis usually increases (Fig. 76.7B). On occasion, the application of a small amount of hemostatic material may be needed to aid in promoting hemostasis from suture needle holes in the vessel walls.

After complete hemostasis has been achieved and correct instrument and sponge counts are ensured, closure of the inguinoscrotal incision may begin. The dartos layer is reapprox-

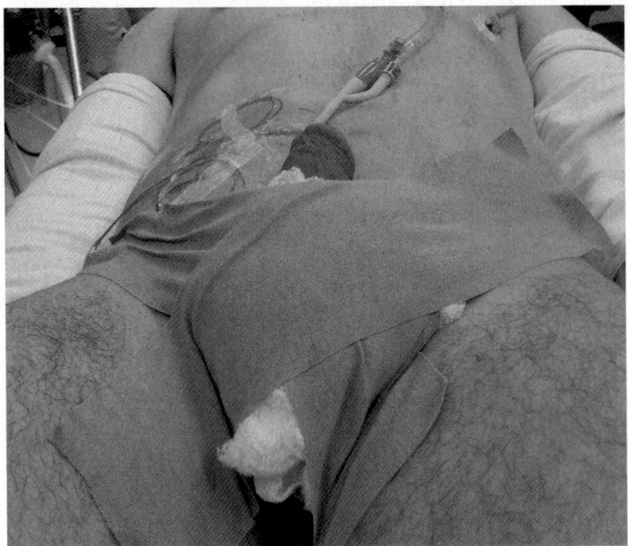

FIGURE 76.8 After complete hemostasis has been achieved and correct instrument and sponge counts are ensured, closure of the inguinoscrotal incision may begin. The dartos layer is reapproximated using 3-0 polyglycolic acid sutures in a running fashion. The skin edges are opposed using 4-0 Monocryl, and Dermabond is applied over the skin incision. The On-Q SilverSoaker catheters are coiled and secured to the skin with Tegaderm. A compressive scrotal dressing is placed using fluffs and Elastoplast. The Foley catheter is left to closed-system gravity drainage overnight.

imated using 3-0 polyglycolic acid sutures in a running fashion. The skin edges are opposed using 4-0 Monocryl, and Dermabond is applied over the skin incision. The On-Q SilverSoaker catheters are resecured to the skin with Tegaderm. A compressive scrotal dressing is placed using fluffs and Elastoplast. The Foley catheter is left to closed-system gravity drainage overnight (Fig. 76.8).

## COMPLICATIONS

Mechanical disruption of the microvascular anastomosis and subsequent uncontrolled arterial hemorrhage may occur from blunt trauma in the first few postoperative weeks following coitus or masturbation, or from accidents. Abstention from sexual activities involving the erect penis is recommended until 6 weeks postoperatively. Other complications include penile pain and diminished penile sensation from injury to the nearby dorsal nerve. Loss of compliance of the suspensory and fundiform ligaments postoperatively may lead to diminished penile length. Preserving the two ligaments has markedly minimized those complications in our series. Glans hyperemia, once a complication seen when anatomoses between the inferior epigastric artery and the deep dorsal vein (dorsal vein arterialization) were performed, is no longer seen because we no longer perform this kind of anastomosis.

## RESULTS

Microvascular arteral bypass surgery has been performed in this above fashion since 1981. An estimated 1,500 procedures have been performed over >25 years. It is estimated that the success rate (clinically relevant improvement in erectile function) is approximately 65% to 70%. Since relocating to San Diego, a review has been made of the latest 30 microvascular arterial bypass procedures using postoperative validated outcome scales, ultrasonography, and arteriography. The scores of the International Index of Erectile Function have improved significantly in the total score, the erectile function domain, the desire domain, the orgasm domain, the intercourse satisfaction domain, and the overall satisfaction domain. There has been marked and significant lowering of the sexual distress scale. Postoperative duplex Doppler ultrasonography has confirmed marked increases in cavernosal artery peak systolic velocity. Postoperative selective inferior epigastric arteriograms have been performed that have documented intact arterial anastomoses between the inferior epigastric artery and the dorsal penile artery with subsequent visualization of contrast in the cavernosal artery (Fig. 76.9). Finally, use of On-Q pump delivery of Marcaine for 48 to 72 hours has resulted in significant lowering of postoperative morphine and Percocet while the patients have simultaneously experienced excellent pain relief.

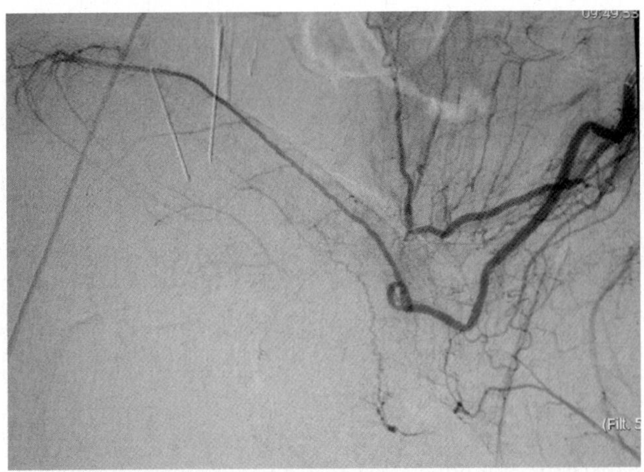

A

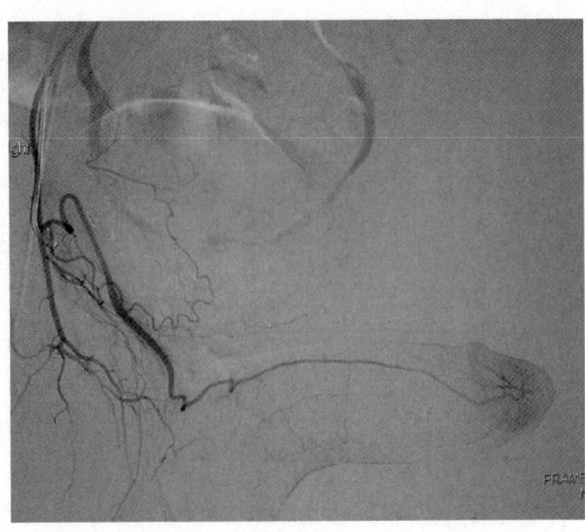

B

FIGURE 76.9 Postoperative selective inferior epigastric arteriograms document intact arterial anastomoses between the inferior epigastric artery and the dorsal penile artery with subsequent visualization of contrast in the cavernosal artery.

## *References*

1. Mulhall J, Teloken P, Barnas J. Vasculogenic erectile dysfunction is a predictor of abnormal stress echocardiography. *J Sex Med* 2009 (epub ahead of print).
2. Miner M, Billups KL. Erectile dysfunction and dyslipidemia: relevance and role of phosphodiesterase type-5 inhibitors and statins. *J Sex Med* 2008; 5(5):1066–1078; epub 2008 Mar 5.
3. Zimmerman P, d'Audiffret A, Pillai L. Endovascular repair of blunt extremity arterial injury: case report. *Vasc Endovasc Surg* 2008 (epub ahead of print).
4. Shakeri AB, Tubbs RS, Shoja MM. The most common anatomical sites of arterial injury in the extremities: a review of 75 angiographically-proven cases. *Folia Morphol (Warsz)* 2006;65(2):116–120.
5. Levine FJ, Greenfield AJ, Goldstein I. Arteriographically determined occlusive disease within the hypogastric-cavernous bed in impotent patients following blunt perineal and pelvic trauma. *J Urol* 1990;144(5):1147–1153.
6. Saenz de Tejada I, Angulo J, Cellek S, et al. Physiology of erectile function. *J Sex Med* 2004;1(3):254–265.
7. Burnett AL. Nitric oxide in the penis-science and therapeutic implications from erectile dysfunction to priapism. *J Sex Med* 2006;3(4):578–582.
8. Sáenz de Tejada I, Angulo J, Cellek S, et al. Pathophysiology of erectile dysfunction. *J Sex Med* 2005;2(1):26–39.
9. Marceau L, Kleinman K, Goldstein I, et al. Does bicycling contribute to the risk of erectile dysfunction? Results from the Massachusetts Male Aging Study (MMAS). *Int J Impot Res* 2001;13(5):298–302.
10. Schrader SM, Breitenstein MJ, Clark JC, et al. Nocturnal penile tumescence and rigidity testing in bicycling patrol officers. *J Androl* 2002;23(6): 927–934.
11. Dettori JR, Koepsell TD, Cummings P, et al. Erectile dysfunction after a long-distance cycling event: associations with bicycle characteristics. *J Urol* 2004;172(2):637–641.
12. Cohen JD, Gross MT. Effect of bicycle racing saddle design on transcutaneous penile oxygen pressure. *J Sports Med Phys Fitness* 2005;45(3): 409–418.
13. Leibovitch I, Mor Y. The vicious cycling: bicycling related urogenital disorders. *Eur Urol* 2005;47(3):277–286.
14. Bacon CG, Mittleman MA, Kawachi I, et al. A prospective study of risk factors for erectile dysfunction. *J Urol* 2006;176(1):217–221.
15. Munarriz R, Huang V, Uberoi J, et al. Only the nose knows: penile hemodynamic study of the perineum-saddle interface in men with erectile dysfunction utilizing bicycle saddles and seats with and without nose extensions. *J Sex Med* 2005;2(5):612–619.
16. Guess MK, Connell K, Schrader S, et al. Genital sensation and sexual function in women bicyclists and runners: are your feet safer than your seat? *J Sex Med* 2006;3(6):1018–1027.
17. Schrader SM, Breitenstein MJ, Lowe BD. Cutting off the nose to save the penis. *J Sex Med* 2008;5(8):1932–1940.
18. Goldstein I, Lurie AL, Lubisich JP. Bicycle riding, perineal trauma, and erectile dysfunction: data and solutions. *Curr Urol Rep* 2007;8(6): 491–497.
19. Goldstein I, Bastuba M, Lurie A, et al. Penile revascularization. *J Sex Med* 2008;5(9):2018–2021.

# CHAPTER 77 ■ PENILE TRAUMA

DANIEL I. ROSENSTEIN, ALLEN F. MOREY, AND JACK W. MCANINCH

Trauma to the penis is an uncommon event. Because of the relatively protected position of the penis between the thighs and pubic bone, it is usually able to avoid direct injury from external forces. Nonetheless, penile trauma may arise from both blunt and penetrating injuries. Such injuries present unique and difficult management problems to the urologic surgeon, in particular regarding long-term cosmesis, voiding function, and future potency. Major blunt penile injuries include penile rupture and skin loss from strangulation or degloving injuries. Penetrating penile trauma is usually secondary to stab or gunshot wounds and thus seldom occurs in the absence of associated genital, urethral, or major organ injury, except in the event of bites and self-inflicted wounds. Due to the wide disparity in the causes, diagnosis, and treatment, this chapter is divided into three parts: penile rupture, penile skin loss, and penetrating penile trauma.

## PENILE RUPTURE

The most common blunt injury involving the penis is rupture of the corpora cavernosa, or penile fracture. This almost invariably occurs when the erect penis is forced to bend in an irregular fashion, such as when it accidentally impinges on the pubis or perineum after slipping out of the vagina during sexual intercourse (11). The remainder of cases are caused by falls out of bed with an erect penis, masturbation, or manipulation of the erect penis. The patient often reports a cracking or popping noise at the time of injury, leading to immediate detumescence and rapid onset of discoloration and swelling over the site of injury. There is frequently a delay in presentation to the hospital—presumably secondary to patient embarrassment.

### Diagnosis

The diagnosis of penile rupture is easily made by physical examination along with the appropriate history. Swelling and discoloration may or may not be limited to the penis, depending on the integrity of the Buck fascia. If the Buck fascia is intact, the hematoma will be contained and will not usually spread below the base of the penis, resulting in the typical "eggplant" deformity (Fig. 77.1). However, if the laceration in the tunica albuginea involves the Buck fascia, extravasation will be contained by the Colles fascia and ecchymosis will extend in a "butterfly" distribution over the perineum, scrotum, and lower abdomen. Examination may reveal angulation of the penis away from the side of rupture because of the mass effect of the hematoma. In addition, focal tenderness and a palpable defect in the tunica albuginea may help localize the fracture site. There is often a clot lying over or near the fracture site that corresponds to the site of cavernosal rupture.

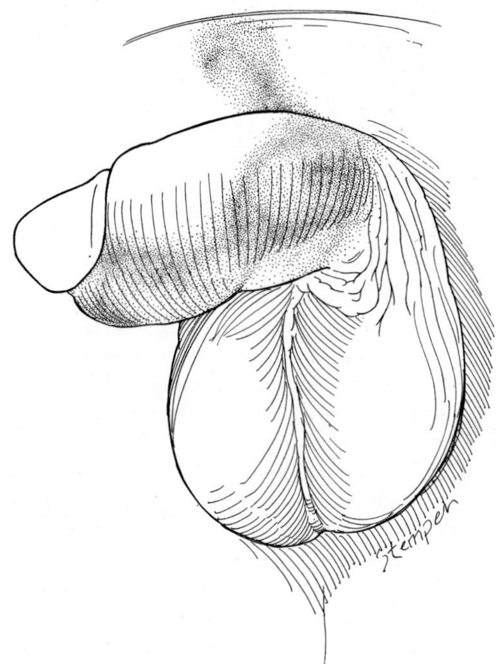

FIGURE 77.1 Fractured penis displaying the pathognomonic "eggplant deformity" with swelling and discoloration extending to the base of the shaft. The penis usually bends away from the side of injury because of the hematoma.

Penile rupture can occur anywhere along the shaft, including the base of the penis, where the corpora are fixed by the penile suspensory ligament. The fracture is typically located at the base of the penis, just proximal to the penoscrotal junction. In general only one corporal body is injured, although both corpora and the corpus spongiosum can be affected depending on the severity of the injury. Most patients are able to urinate normally, but the urologist must maintain a high index of suspicion for urethral injury. Failure to void spontaneously may signify compression of the urethra by hematoma but should lead to evaluation of urethral injury by retrograde urethrography (RUG). Urethral injury occurs in up to one third of cases and usually consists of partial disruption, although complete transection can result (10). RUG is mandatory in all patients with blood at the urethral meatus, hematuria of any extent, or inability to void (11). However, because RUG is easy to perform and provides reliable results, we perform it routinely in all cases of suspected penile rupture. Adjunctive imaging studies in penile fracture (including ultrasound, magnetic resonance imaging, and cavernosography) are usually unnecessary as the clinical picture is frequently adequate to initiate therapy.

## Indications for Surgery

Although penile fractures can be managed nonoperatively, the literature shows a clear advantage to early operative repair (10,11). This approach results in faster recovery, shorter hospital stay, less morbidity, and less long-term penile curvature. The goals of acute exploration are evacuation of the hematoma and primary repair of the laceration.

## Alternative Therapy

Conservative treatment consists of cool compression dressings, anti-inflammatory agents, and sedatives to reduce erections. This results in eventual resorption of the hematoma and scar formation at the site of the tunical rupture.

## Surgical Technique

The patient is placed in a supine position and a Foley catheter is placed to facilitate identification of the urethra and urinary drainage. Exposure is usually obtained through a subcoronal circumferential incision, and the penile skin is degloved down to the base. The distal circumferential incision is favored because it allows both exposure of the ruptured corpus and adequate assessment of the contralateral corpus and corpus spongiosum. Alternatively, an incision may be made on the shaft directly over the fracture site. This approach is only useful if the fracture is palpable preoperatively as the corporal bodies may not be easily explored through this incision. Further, the corpus spongiosum cannot be directly inspected via this approach.

Following the circumcising incision, the corpus spongiosum is carefully inspected to evaluate for potential urethral injury. Inspection of the fracture site usually reveals a transverse laceration, between 0.5 and 2.0 cm long, in the tunica albuginea of the proximal penile shaft (4). After evacuation of the hematoma and irrigation, minimal debridement of nonviable wound edges may be necessary before closure with interrupted 4-0 Maxon sutures (Fig. 77.2). The surgeon should not probe the exposed cavernous tissue unnecessarily as this may elicit troublesome bleeding. A tourniquet may be used intraoperatively to control hemorrhage. Lacerations may run directly under the dorsal neurovascular bundle located on the dorsal

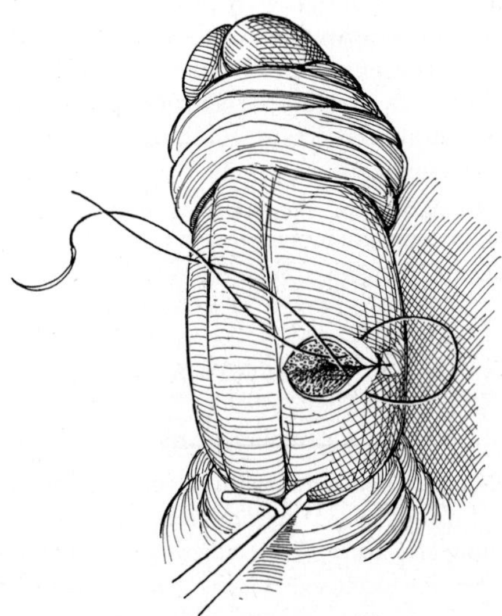

FIGURE 77.2 Identification and repair of penile fracture. A distal circumferential subcoronal incision is made and skin and soft tissue are mobilized off the underlying corporal bodies down to the base of the penis. This maneuver exposes the transverse laceration in the tunica albuginea. The laceration is repaired using interrupted 4-0 Maxon with the knots buried. Exposed corporal erectile tissue should not be probed or explored as this may cause troublesome bleeding.

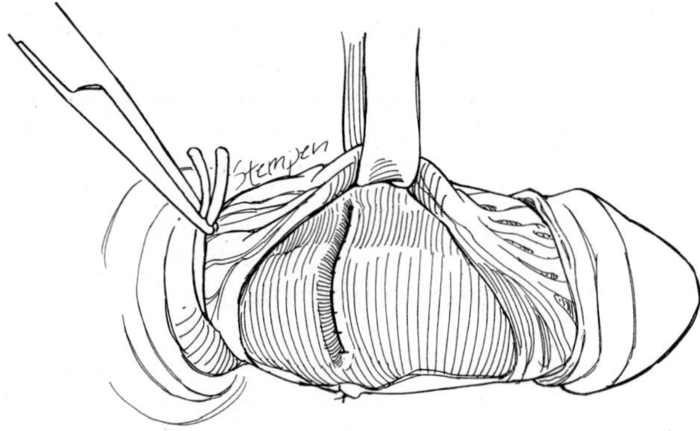


FIGURE 77.3 Penile fracture extending beneath dorsal neurovascular bundles. Elevation of the ipsilateral dorsal neurovascular bundle facilitates repair of lacerations and protects these structures from inadvertent injury. Division of the deep dorsal vein in the midline provides access to the correct surgical plane beneath the ipsilateral neurovascular bundle.

surface of the corpora at approximately the 10 and 2 o'clock positions (Fig. 77.3). This necessitates careful dissection of these structures off the corpora to allow a safe, watertight closure. Division of the deep dorsal vein facilitates unilateral dissection of the neurovascular bundle off the underlying corpus cavernosum. The penile skin is then replaced and the subcoronal incision is closed with interrupted 4-0 chromic sutures. If the patient is uncircumcised, the prepuce must be closely monitored for development of subcoronal edema. Postoperatively, a loose compression dressing (Coban) is gently placed, and the urethral catheter may be removed on postoperative day 1. Systemic antibiotics, anti-inflammatory agents, and fibrinolytics are unnecessary. Most patients can be discharged home within 1 to 2 days of surgery. Sexual activity can be resumed at about 4 to 6 weeks. Painful erections may be present in the early postoperative period. Suppression of erections with benzodiazepines or amyl nitrate may provide symptomatic relief.

When urethral transection occurs in the context of penile rupture, we advocate primary repair with interrupted 5-0 or 6-0 Maxon sutures over a 16Fr silicone catheter. In cases of complete urethral transection, additional urinary diversion through a percutaneous suprapubic cystostomy tube may be prudent (11). A voiding cystourethrogram (VCUG) should be carried out at approximately 14 days postrepair to document adequate healing before catheter removal.

## Outcomes

### Complications

Many patients treated conservatively or with delayed repair have some form of sexual dysfunction, such as painful erection, disabling curvature, or erectile dysfunction secondary to cavernous-venous occlusive disease (1,14). Patients with a missed urethral injury associated with penile fracture are also at risk of periurethral abscess, stricture, and fistula formation.

### Results

Patients who have operative repair within 48 hours of the injury have excellent functional results. In two relatively large studies, none of the patients with early operative repair experienced impotence, penile curvature on erection, or painful intercourse (4,11).

# PENILE SKIN LOSS

## Diagnosis

Penile skin loss can occur from necrotizing infection, burns, constrictive bands, or degloving injuries from blunt or penetrating trauma. Dog and human bites may also result in considerable penile skin loss. When the skin loss is secondary to infection (e.g., Fournier gangrene), repeated debridement with antibiotics and moist dressing changes must be instituted to prepare the underlying tissue for delayed reconstruction. If the wounds are grossly contaminated, the testes may be placed in subcutaneous thigh pouches with a view toward delayed scrotal reconstruction. Avulsions are most often caused by power tool injuries or motor vehicle accidents, although this injury may rarely be self-inflicted secondary to insertion of the penis into vacuum cleaners and other suction devices (1). Because of the laxity of penile skin, the avulsion usually extends just to the subcutaneous dartos layer, leaving the corporal bodies uninvolved. Immediate repair is frequently possible in cases of traumatic skin loss. If immediate closure is to be attempted, the wound edges must be clean and viable and hemostasis must be excellent to avoid delayed skin necrosis and sloughing.

## Indications for Surgery

Partial penile skin loss, especially in the distal shaft, is best managed by rotational mobilization of a local skin flap. Primary closure may be appropriate if the defect is short and there is abundant remaining shaft skin. Extensive skin loss, whether from the injury itself or surgical debridement, usually requires tissue transfer for repair. In impotent patients, the penis can be buried under a scrotal flap with the glans left exposed to allow micturition (Fig. 77.4) (5). The penis may be liberated at a later date using the scrotal skin as a graft to cover the previously denuded area. In sexually active patients, a thick (0.016- to 0.018-in.), nonmeshed split-thickness skin graft is used. Thick split-thickness grafts are preferred because they are non–hair-bearing, have minimal contraction, and offer excellent cosmesis and viability. If sexual function is not a concern, a thinner skin graft may be harvested and meshed. The avulsed skin that is still attached on a viable pedicle can be gently washed and reapplied with the knowledge that it may need to be debrided at a later time. Completely avulsed penile skin will usually not survive as a free graft if reapplied to the denuded penile shaft.

## Alternative Therapy

There are no alternatives to surgery.

## Surgical Technique

The patient is placed supine and both the genitals and a carefully chosen donor site are prepared into the field. The anterolateral thigh provides thickness, texture, and color resembling

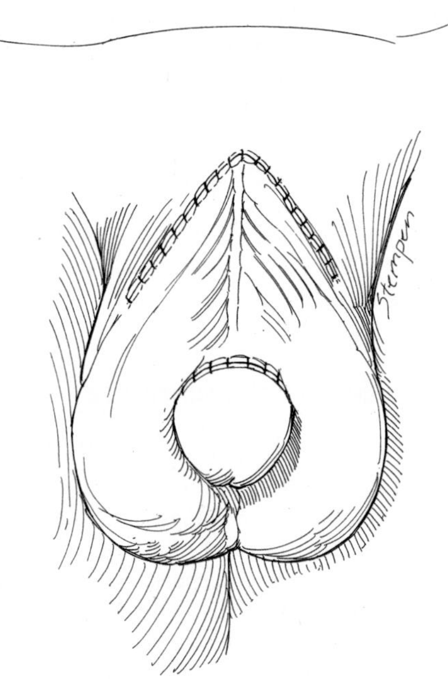

FIGURE 77.4 Scrotal tunnel maneuver for penile skin coverage. The penis shaft may be buried beneath a flap of scrotal skin to provide skin coverage, leaving the glans exposed. This is a viable option in older patients who either were impotent before their injury or who have sustained severe associated injuries.

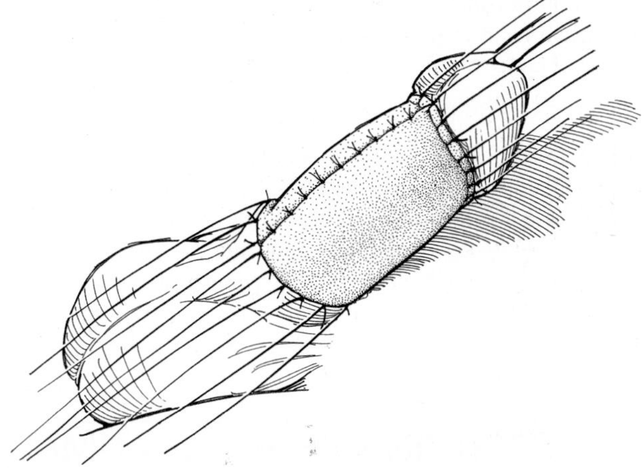

FIGURE 77.5 Penile split-thickness skin graft. A thick (0.016- to 0.018-in.) split-thickness skin graft is applied to the denuded penile shaft. The distal skin is discarded to just beneath the corona when a circumferential graft is indicated. The graft is placed with the seam in the midline ventrally and secured with 5-0 chromic sutures to itself and along the shaft, while 4-0 silk sutures placed proximally and distally are left long to secure a bolster dressing.

penile skin and is therefore the preferred donor site. Alternatively, the medial or posterior thigh or buttock may be used as a skin donor site. A Foley catheter is placed to prevent postoperative urinary contamination. The shaved donor site is coated with sterile mineral oil, and a Brown or Padgett dermatome (10-cm-wide strip) is used to harvest the graft in an approximately 0.018-in. thickness. The graft is then tailored to fit the defect on the shaft. The donor site may be dressed with fine mesh gauze under slight pressure to ensure adequate hemostasis. Placement of a semipermeable plastic or silicone membrane (e.g., Biobrane) directly against the donor site helps reduce contamination. After about 24 hours, the Biobrane is adherent to the donor site and the redundant edges may be trimmed. This dressing usually falls off spontaneously after 2 weeks.

To prepare the penile shaft for grafting, it must be sharply debrided of all devitalized tissue and any chronic granulation tissue. It is imperative to prepare the recipient site so that the graft will have adequate blood supply. Debridement of the glans should be avoided, but all nonviable skin, including the distal prepuce, should be excised up to the coronal sulcus. Native penile skin distal to the graft will become edematous because of disruption of native lymphatic and venous drainage along the shaft. Hemostasis in the graft bed is essential to prevent hematoma formation under the graft.

Once prepared, the penis is stretched and the graft applied circumferentially around the shaft. The graft seam is placed at the ventral aspect to simulate the appearance of the median raphe (Fig. 77.5). The graft is sutured in place using interrupted 5-0 chromic sutures. Chordee formation has in general not been a problem because the graft will have minimal longitudinal contraction. The graft is secured to itself and along the shaft with interrupted 5-0 chromic sutures. Several 4-0 Vicryl sutures are placed at the proximal and distal graft edges and left long to use as bolster tieover sutures. A Xeroform dressing is placed directly on the graft. A bolster dressing is then fashioned using mineral oil–soaked cotton and fluffs. The whole dressing is secured in place using the bolster sutures, leaving the glans visible for inspection. To keep the penis in a vertical position, a padded plastic splint is placed around the bolster dressing. This housing may be fashioned out of a 500-cc sterile water container.

Postoperatively, the patient is kept at strict bedrest until the dressing is removed, usually after 5 days, when the Foley catheter is also removed. Immobilization of the penis in the extended position maintained by the bolster is critical for graft survival. Broad-spectrum antibiotics and administration of subcutaneous heparin for deep venous thrombosis prophylaxis are useful adjuncts. We do not routinely administer medications to reduce frequency of erections unless they are painful for the patient. Erections may provide natural tissue expansion, and the grafts usually slide easily along the loose areolar tissue superficial to the Buck fascia. Once the penile dressing is removed, twice-daily sitz baths can be started to enhance epithelialization and reduce bacterial contamination.

## Outcomes

### Complications

The common causes of early failure of penile skin grafting are infection, shearing forces causing graft separation, and underlying hematoma. It is imperative that the graft bed be free of infected granulation tissue and any necrotic tissue. Shearing forces disrupt the blood supply to the new graft and are prevented by the penile splint and bolster dressing, provided the patient is cooperative with strict bedrest for 5 days. It is critical that the penis be maintained in the extended position within the bolster dressing as this will prevent folding or telescoping of the fresh graft on the penile surface. Hematoma causes failure by creating poor contact between the graft and the recipient bed. It is prevented by ensuring meticulous hemostasis of the graft bed prior to laying the graft in place.

Meshed grafts allow better dissipation of hematoma fluid but are discouraged in potent patients because of their increased degree of contraction.

#### Results

Long-term results of reconstruction have been excellent, with successful graft take exceeding 90%. Sensation remains absent in the grafted skin but is retained in the glans and in deeper structures. Potency is unaffected by this type of reconstruction. Most patients have satisfactory intercourse after reconstruction. Cosmetic and functional results of nonmeshed, thick split-thickness penile grafts are superior to either meshed grafts or scrotal flaps.

## PENETRATING PENILE TRAUMA

Penetrating trauma to the penis is most often caused by firearms but can also result from stab wounds, industrial accidents, self-mutilation attempts, and bites. In all cases, general principles of management include judicious debridement and hemostasis within the wound as well as careful exploration and repair of corporal and urethral injuries. Most civilian penile gunshot wounds are caused by low-velocity missiles, which cause damage only in the path of the bullet. Penetrating penile injuries are a more common genitourinary injury during wartime, possibly because of inadequate genital coverage by protective body armor (12). Associated wounds of the thigh and pelvis are common and may require urgent exploration and repair. Successful treatment of penetrating penile injuries must address and preserve normal voiding, potency, and penile cosmesis.

### Diagnosis

Genital injury is determined by careful physical examination, with special attention paid to the trajectory of the bullet and initial hemostasis. The finding of a palpable corporeal defect in combination with an expanding penile hematoma or significant bleeding from the entry/exit wound is highly predictive of corporeal injury and should prompt expedient exploration (7). The exam should include a vascular (glanular capillary refill) and penile sensory assessment (9). Urethral injury, which occurs in 25% to 40% of penetrating injuries to the penis, should be excluded with RUG in all cases (6). The triad of no blood at the meatus, absence of hematuria, and normal voiding suggests that there is no urethral injury; however, penetrating trauma can cause urethral injury without clinical signs of damage. Cystography, intravenous pyelography, and scrotal ultrasonography may be necessary to evaluate associated urologic injuries. Cavernosography is rarely indicated in this setting (9).

### Indications for Surgery

Penetrating injury to the penis most often requires surgical exploration. In addition, patients with unstable major organ injury will be unable to undergo immediate exploration. In these cases, initial treatment consists of hemostasis and packing of major wounds. Penetrating injury causing major skin loss will require tissue transfer for satisfactory coverage, but associated corporal and urethral injuries must be repaired before the skin grafting. Immediate primary closure or reconstruction should take place only with a clean wound that is in general <8 hours old.

### Alternative Therapy

Single pellet wounds with small entrance sites and superficial stab wounds in which there is no active bleeding or hematoma may not require surgical exploration (3).

### Surgical Technique

The operation consists of judicious debridement of devitalized tissue and hemostasis. The wound must be copiously irrigated to remove all foreign bodies, including powder from shotgun pellets and pieces of clothing. Bleeding almost always occurs from a lacerated corporal body but may also be from disrupted superficial veins. The primary objective of surgical exploration is control of corporal bleeding and repair of corporal defects. The corpora are well vascularized, and extensive debridement is usually unnecessary and will hinder future potency. We thus do not recommend extensive exploration of erectile or glanular tissue. Hemostasis is obtained by gentle compression and watertight closure of the tunica albuginea alone, usually with interrupted 4-0 Maxon sutures. Urethral injuries are repaired with 5-0 Vicryl sutures over a silicone catheter. A devitalized urethra must be carefully debrided, and primary repair with a tension-free anastomosis can usually be accomplished. Associated scrotal and spermatic cord injuries are treated with debridement and, if necessary, orchiectomy or ligation of the vas deferens. The skin can be closed primarily unless viable skin edges cannot be approximated. In contaminated wounds or those encountered after 8 hours, immediate skin closure or grafting is not recommended and the wound is packed instead. Once the wound is clean, delayed primary closure, staged reconstruction, or healing by secondary intention may be selected. An important contraindication to debridement and primary closure is the case of massive tissue destruction often associated with close-range shotgun blasts. These should be debrided and allowed to declare themselves in terms of the extent of injury. They may then be repaired in a staged fashion. It appears that longer-range injuries due to shotgun blasts may create multiple low-velocity wounds with less significant blast effect. Carefully selected longer-range shotgun injuries have been successfully managed with immediate debridement and primary repair (13).

Penile bites deserve special mention as they can rapidly progress to severe infection. Wounds should be copiously irrigated and all devitalized tissue debrided. All wounds should be left open and prophylactic antibiotics administered. Antibiotic treatment should cover gram-positive and gram-negative organisms as well as anaerobic gram-negative rods. The most common colonizing organisms in the mouth of a dog include *Pasteurella*, *Streptococcus*, and *Staphylococcus* species (2). Hospitalization with frequent wound inspection and intravenous antibiotics is necessary in those with delayed presentation or with increased risk factors such as steroid use, diabetes, or immunodeficiency syndromes. Close follow-up is mandatory in all outpatients.

## Outcomes

### Complications

Early complications of penetrating penile trauma include rebleeding and infection. Because the corpora are heavily vascularized, breakdown of repair in the tunica albuginea is rare. A small minority will report superficial sensory loss, pain with erection, and rapid detumescence. Complications attributable to the urethral injury include urethral stricture, periurethral abscess, and urethrocutaneous fistula.

### Results

Excellent functional results can be expected except in those cases of high-velocity injuries where massive tissue destruction has occurred. Most patients report retained potency without penile curvature and with satisfactory cosmetic results (5,8). Patients who develop late penile curvature in the absence of palpable corporeal defects or plaques may have scarring and contraction of the underlying cavernosal tissues and the intercavernous septum (7).

## *References*


1. Armenakas NA, McAninch JW. Use of skin grafts in external genital reconstruction. In: McAninch JW, ed. *New techniques in reconstructive urology*. New York: Igaku-Shoin, 1996:127–141.
2. Cummings JM, Boullier JA. Scrotal dog bites. *J Urology* 2000;164:57.
3. Goldman HB, Dmochowski RR, Cox CE. Penetrating trauma to the penis: functional results. *J Urol* 1996;155:551.
4. Gomez RG. Genital injuries: presentation and management. In: McAninch JW, ed. *Problems in urology*. Philadelphia: JB Lippincott Co, 1994:279–289.
5. Gomez RG. Genital skin loss: reconstructive techniques. In: McAninch JW, ed. *Problems in urology*. Philadelphia: JB Lippincott Co, 1994:290–301.
6. Gomez RG, Castanheira AC, McAninch JW. Gunshot wounds to the male external genitalia. *J Urol* 1993;150:1147.
7. Hall SJ, Wagner JR, Edelstein RA, et al. Management of gunshot injuries to the penis and anterior urethra. *J Trauma* 1995;38:439.
8. McAninch JW. Management of genital skin loss. *Urol Clin North Am* 1989;16:387.
9. Miller KS, McAninch JW. Penile fracture and soft tissue injury. In: McAninch JW, ed. *Traumatic and reconstructive urology*. Philadelphia: WB Saunders, 1996:693–698.
10. Nicolaisen GS, Melamud A, Williams RD, et al. Rupture of the corpus cavernosum: surgical management. *J Urol* 1983;130:917.
11. Orvis BR, McAninch JW. Penile rupture. *Urol Clin North Am* 1989;16:369.
12. Salvatierra O, Rigdon WO, Norris DM, et al. Vietnam experience with 252 urological war injuries. *J Urol* 1969;101:615.
13. Tigert R, Harb JJ, Hurley PM, et al. Management of shotgun injuries to the pelvis and lower genitourinary system. *Urology* 2000;55:193.
14. Volz LR, Broderick GA. Conservative management of penile fracture may cause cavernous–venous occlusive disease and permanent erectile dysfunction. *J Urol* 1994;151:358A.


The opinions expressed herein are those of the authors and are not to be construed as reflecting the views of the US Armed Forces or the Department of Defense.

# CHAPTER 78 ■ PENILE REPLANTATION

URI GUR AND GERALD H. JORDAN

Penile amputation is a rare injury in the Western world, arising largely from attempts at self-emasculation or as the result of violent assault. It may also arise secondary to industrial work accidents or as a war injury. Injuries amounting to penile amputation have also been reported as a rare complication of circumcision (5). The largest single series of penile amputation injuries comes from Thailand, where in the 1970s an epidemic of approximately 100 cases was reported (1). In these cases, adulterous husbands had their penises amputated by their humiliated wives while they slept. Unfortunately, only 18 of 100 cases in this series were successfully replanted using microsurgical techniques, as the amputated penis was often rapidly disposed of by the wife. Thus, experience with penile replantation is largely based upon case reports and smaller series. Despite the rarity of this injury, good functional and cosmetic results are routinely attainable using the microsurgical approach to penile replantation.

Psychotic patients who carry out self-emasculation may be broadly divided into two categories. The more common subgroup includes schizophrenic patients in a decompensated (actively psychotic) state. One study found that 87% of self-emasculating patients were psychotic at the time of injury (3). These patients are usually victims of command hallucinations that coerce the patient to mutilate his genitals.

Because these patients respond well to psychiatric rehabilitation, they are unlikely to repeat an attempt at self-mutilation, provided they remain under chronic pharmacotherapy and surveillance (3,9). Penises should therefore be replanted in a timely manner following amputation, with psychiatric support throughout the patient's admission and probably lifetime. Nonpsychotic patients who self-emasculate are often diagnosed with severe personality disorders. These patients are more difficult to rehabilitate.

While early attempts at penile replantation were frequently fraught with complications including skin and glans slough, the majority of these attempts were successful at salvaging the penis with corporal reapproximation alone. This field was revolutionized in 1976, when two independent groups described the first successful penile replantations using microvascular techniques (2,11). Since that time, microneurovascular repair has been considered the standard of care in penile replantation and has provided superior results with regard to postoperative sensation, erectile function, and overall graft viability, with durable results in the long term (1).

The remarkable ability of an amputated penile tip to survive even in the absence of penile arterial and venous reanastomosis attests to the unique vascular supply of the penis. It seems that the sinusoidal blood within the corporal bodies sufficiently approximates arterialized parameters, thus adequately nourishing the distal bodies and skin early on without having to depend upon collateral vessel development. Microvascular reanastomosis has further decreased skin and glans slough because the skin may be perfused directly rather than via corporal perforators.

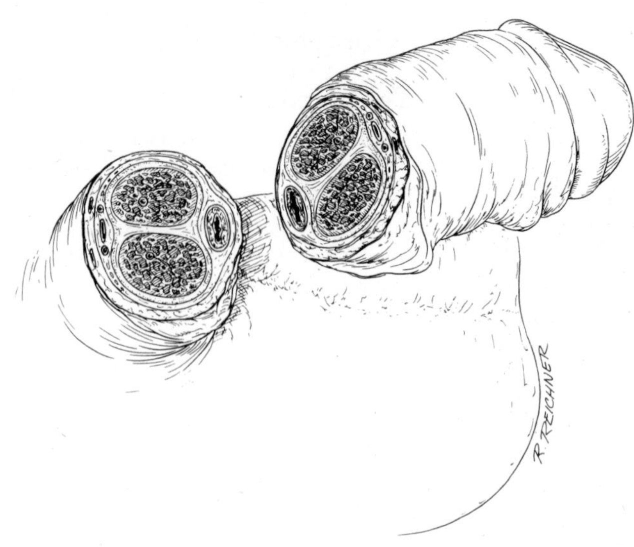


FIGURE 78.1 The typical appearance of a penile amputation injury. (From Jordan GH, Gilbert DA. Management of amputation injuries of the male genitalia. *Urol Clin North Am* 1989;16:359–367, with permission.)

## DIAGNOSIS

The physical diagnosis is obvious with complete loss of the distal penis. As already mentioned, most patients who have self-inflicted wounds will have responded to a command psychosis. Others have severe personality disorders. Thus, the surgery staff must work closely with a psychiatrist for these patients, as the emasculation is only a symptom of the underlying disease. Traumatic amputations either from an assault or industrial equipment will also likely have a postsurgical need for psychiatric evaluation.

All of these patients should be aware of the potential for loss of the penis if replantation is not successful, as well as the potential for erectile dysfunction.

## INDICATIONS FOR SURGERY

Because penile tissue has a remarkable resistance to prolonged ischemia (10), all attempts to replant the penile remnant should be carried out unless the penis has been extremely mutilated. Replantation has been successful despite cold ischemic times of 24 hours or longer. Most patients have sharply lacerated their penises, with clear anatomic structures and vessels often visible both in the stump and the distal portion (Fig. 78.1). The penis should be preserved with the "bag-within-a-bag" technique (Fig. 78.2). This serves to increase ischemic tolerance. The amputated penis is wrapped in saline-soaked gauze in a sterile plastic bag. This bag is then immersed in ice slush. The patient should be kept warm and peripherally vasodilated throughout the procedure as well as in the postoperative period.

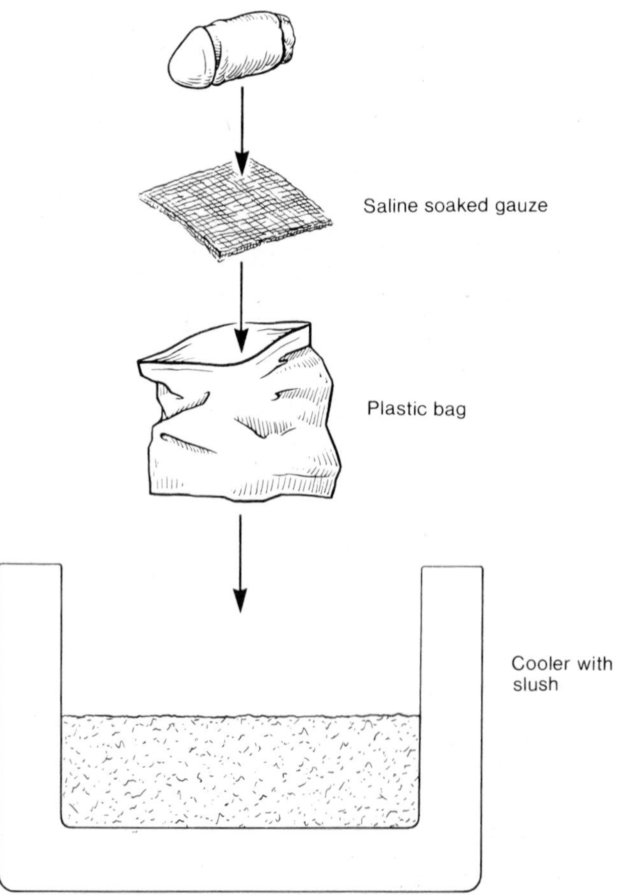


FIGURE 78.2 Illustration of the bag-within-a-bag technique of organ emergent cold storage. The amputated part of the penis is placed on a saline-soaked gauze sponge, within a sterile (if possible) plastic bag. The plastic bag is then immersed in a second container of iced slush. (From Jordan GH. Initial management and reconstruction of male genital amputation injuries. *Trauma Reconstr Urol* 1996;57:673–681, with permission.)

## ALTERNATIVE THERAPY

Alternatives are limited, as the alternative is to not reconstruct the penis and thus close the penis and perform a urethrostomy.

One alternative, if microsurgery is not available but the penis is otherwise "replantable," would be macroscopic approximation of the urethra and corpora. This approach harbors substantial risk for edema, skin necrosis, and sloughing of the glans skin. Often the deeper tissues of the glans survive and will re-epithelialize or can be grafted.

## SURGICAL TECHNIQUE

Microsurgical replantation is carried out using microsurgical techniques (2), with systematic exploration and debridement of the corporal bodies and dorsal neurovascular structures as necessary (Fig. 78.3).

The urethra should be spatulated and reanastomosed first, as this provides stability to the remainder of the repair. A two-layer repair using 6-0 polydioxanone suture (PDS) or 6-0 polyglactin (Vicryl) for the epithelium followed by 5-0 PDS for the spongy erectile tissue is appropriate. Coaptation of the cavernosal arteries is difficult and does not seem to offer any advantage (6). The tunica albuginea of the corpora cavernosa should then be meticulously closed with interrupted 4-0 or 5-0 PDS sutures, as this will further provide stability for the microsurgical anastomoses.

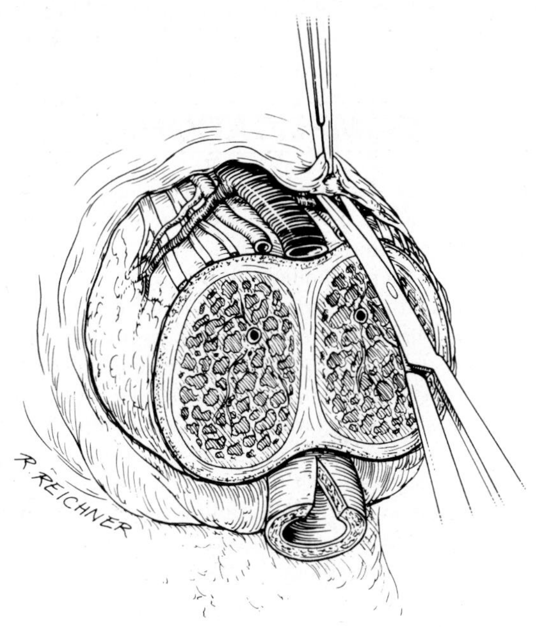


FIGURE 78.3 The urethra, corpora cavernosa, and dorsal neurovascular structures are exposed and minimally debrided. (From Jordan GH, Gilbert DA. Management of amputation injuries of the male genitalia. *Urol Clin North Am* 1989;16:359–367, with permission.)

The dorsal neurovascular structures are repaired next. Both dorsal penile arteries should be anastomosed using 11-0 nylon or polypropylene (Prolene), and the deep dorsal vein is then repaired with 9-0 or 10-0 nylon or Prolene. Following completion of the vascular anastomoses, the dorsal nerve bundles should be reapproximated with 10-0 nylon. The epineurium of each side should be placed in apposition so that fascicular regrowth is facilitated (Fig. 78.4). For distal injuries, fascicular coaptation may be required. These nerves are branches of the pudendal nerve and are responsible for sensation within the glans. The autonomic cavernous nerves branch proximally within the corporal bodies and are not repaired.

Following completion of the microsurgical anastomoses, the dartos fascia should be reapproximated using 5-0 Vicryl sutures and the skin loosely reapproximated using 5-0 or 6-0 Vicryl sutures. Shaft skin should be preserved if at all possible, as initially questionable skin may appear more viable in the postoperative period (Fig. 78.5). A diverting suprapubic cystotomy catheter should be placed and the urethra stented with a small soft silicone catheter. The penis should be immobilized and elevated to facilitate venous and lymphatic drainage. A subcutaneous suprapubic tunnel technique has been described for protection of the replanted penis in the early postoperative period, in cases where there is not adequate skin for coverage (4).

If the microvascular approach to replantation is technically or otherwise not feasible, the penis should be replanted via corporal and urethral reapproximation. The denuded replanted penis may be buried in the scrotum or a subcutaneous suprapubic tunnel as above, followed by delayed liberation with scrotal skin cover, as described by McRoberts et al. (8), or with grafting. Although penile salvage is usually successful via this technique, it obviously requires a second procedure. Covering the penis with scrotal skin is cosmetically less than optimal,

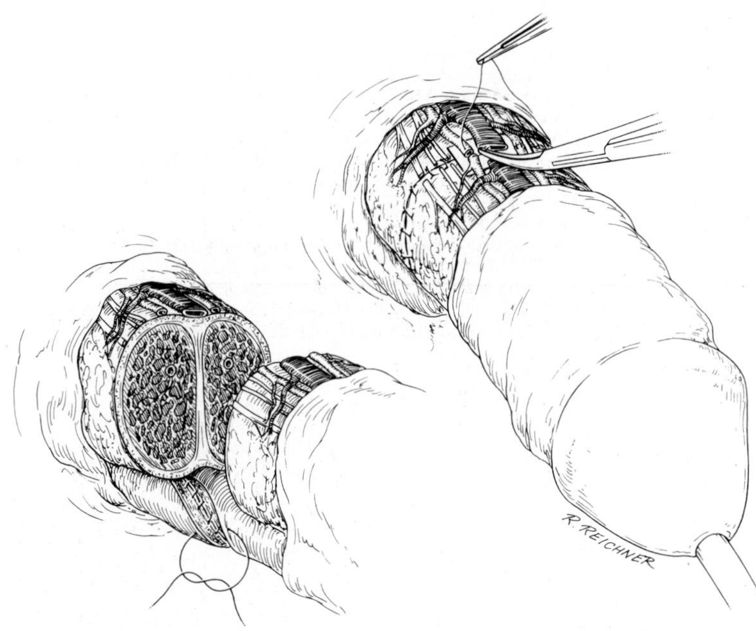


FIGURE 78.4 A two-layer spatulated urethral anastomosis is completed. Microvascular coaptation of the dorsal vein, deep dorsal artery, and dorsal nerves is accomplished. (From Jordan GH, Gilbert DA. Management of amputation injuries of the male genitalia. *Urol Clin North Am* 1989;16:359–367, with permission.)

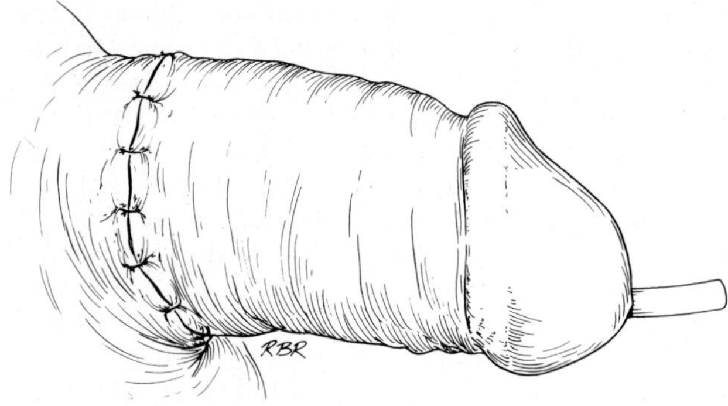


**FIGURE 78.5** Postoperative result. (From Jordan GH, Gilbert DA. Management of amputation injuries of the male genitalia. *Urol Clin North Am* 1989;16:359–367, with permission.)

while grafting the penis provides much more acceptable results. In either case, the shaft sensation will be compromised.

If the amputated penis is absent or too mutilated for replantation, hemostasis should be achieved, followed by spatulation of the neomeatus. The proximal shaft may be buried in the surrounding skin, or the residual corporal stumps may be covered by a split-thickness skin graft. In the unusual circumstance that contamination in the area of the genitalia precludes immediate replantation, temporary ectopic microsurgical implantation (to the forearm) followed by delayed anatomic replantation has been employed successfully (7).

## POSTOPERATIVE MANAGEMENT

The patient is kept on bedrest for approximately 1 week, with urinary diversion continuing for approximately 3 weeks. During this period, the replanted penis should be closely monitored with Doppler and observed for signs of skin slough or decreased glans viability. The stenting catheter may be removed at the 3-week postoperative period, with a voiding urethrogram carried out to document the healing of the urethra. The use of daily aspirin in the postoperative period is recommended. More aggressive anticoagulation is usually not warranted but should be addressed on a case-by-case basis.

## OUTCOMES

Given the uniformly good results of microvascular penile replantation from both cosmetic and functional aspects, this approach should be used if at all possible. If microsurgery is not feasible, macroscopic replantation should still be offered.

## COMPLICATIONS

The frequency of skin necrosis, glans slough, and urethral complications has been reduced with the microvascular approach to replantation. Edema and congestion are common but are usually of a self-limited nature.

Adjuvant treatment with hyperbaric oxygen in the early postoperative period was reported as possibly advantageous to treat the edematous and/or ischemic replanted penis (12).

As with other "free flaps," the successful use of medicinal leeches to treat postoperative venous congestion has been reported (9).

Several reports document the return of partial or complete erectile function in the months following the replantation. Patients who fail to achieve adequate return of erections may still respond to pharmacologic erection therapy.

## *References*


1. Bhanaganada K, Chayavatana T, Pongnumkul C, et al. Surgical management of an epidemic of penile amputations in Siam. *Am J Surg* 1983; 146:376.
2. Cohen BE, May JW, Daly JS, et al. Successful clinical replantation of an amputated penis by microneurovascular repair. *Plast Reconstr Surg* 1977; 59:276.
3. Greilheimer H, Groves JE. Male genital self-mutilation. *Arch Gen Psychiatry* 1979;36:441.
4. Harris DD, Beaghler MA, Stewart SC, et al. Use of a subcutaneous tunnel following replantation of an amputated penis. *Urology* 1996;48:628–630.
5. Jong KP, Jun KM, Hyung JK. Reimplantation of an amputated penis in prepubertal boys. *J Urol* 2001;165:586–587.
6. Jordan GH, Gilbert DA. Management of amputation injuries of the male genitalia. *Urol Clin North Am* 1989;16:359–367.
7. Matloub HS, Yousif NJ, Sanger JR. Temporary ectopic implantation of an amputated penis. *Plast Reconstr Surg* 1994;93:408–412.
8. McRoberts JW, Chapman WH, Ansell JS. Primary anastomosis of the traumatically amputated penis: case report and summary of the literature. *J Urol* 1968;100:751.
9. Mineo M, Jolley T, Rodriguez G. Leech therapy in penile replantation: a case of recurrent penile self-amputation [Review]. *Urology* 2004;63(5): 981–983.
10. Mosahebi A, Butterworth M, Knight R, et al. Delayed penile replantation after prolonged warm ischemia. *Microsurgery* 2001;21:52–54.
11. Tamai S, Nakamura Y, Motomiya Y. Microsurgical replantation of a completely amputated penis and scrotum. *Plast Reconstr Surg* 1977;60:287.
12. Zhong Z, Dong Z, Lu Q, et al. Successful penile replantation with adjuvant hyperbaric oxygen treatment. *Urology* 2007;69(5):983.e3–5.

# CHAPTER 79 ■ VARICOCELE: GENERAL CONSIDERATIONS

CARIN V. HOPPS AND MARC GOLDSTEIN

A varicocele is an abnormal dilation of the veins draining the testis, the internal spermatic veins, that can be palpated through the scrotal skin. While varicoceles are present in 15% of the male population overall, they are present in 35% of men with primary infertility and in 81% of men with secondary infertility (3). Varicocele is the most common etiology of male factor infertility, and varicocelectomy (ligation of the internal spermatic veins) is the most commonly performed surgical procedure for men with infertility. Varicocele is associated with decreased testicular volume, impaired sperm quality, and a decline in Leydig cell function (13). Surgical repair of clinical varicocele has been shown to avert further damage to testicular function, improve spermatogenesis, and improve Leydig cell function. Large varicoceles are associated with greater testicular dysfunction than are small varicoceles, and repair of large varicoceles results in greater improvement in semen parameters when compared with repair of small varicoceles (10).

Varicoceles most commonly occur on the left. Whereas the right internal spermatic vein drains into the vena cava, the left internal spermatic vein drains into the left renal vein and therefore is significantly longer than the right vein, resulting in greater transmission of pressure to the pampiniform plexus. Contributing to increased venous pressure is the position of the left renal vein, which crosses anterior to the aorta and posterior to the superior mesentery artery, potentially causing compression of the renal vein, known as the "nutcracker effect." Retrograde flow of blood into the pampiniform plexus due to incompetent valves within the internal spermatic vein may also contribute to dilation of this venous system.

The pathophysiology by which varicocele impairs testicular function is poorly understood. Of several proposed mechanisms of injury, thermal testicular injury is the hypothesis most supported by animal and human studies. Animal models have demonstrated a clear adverse effect of heat on testicular function. Varicocele is thought to affect thermoregulation of the testis by interfering with the countercurrent heat exchange mechanism within the pampiniform plexus. Although the scrotal location of the testes appears to underscore the importance of temperature regulation, the mechanism by which varicocele causes injury to the testis is likely multifactorial.

## DIAGNOSIS

Varicocele is diagnosed by thorough examination of the scrotal contents with the patient in both the supine and standing positions. Relaxation of the dartos muscle, facilitated by a warm scrotum (we favor a simple heating pad on the scrotum), is essential for proper examination of scrotal contents. Grade I varicocele is palpable with Valsalva maneuver only, grade II is palpable in the standing position, and grade III is visually apparent through the scrotal skin as a "bag of worms." Transscrotal ultrasound is not necessary to diagnose varicocele but may be utilized if physical examination cannot be adequately accomplished or findings on physical examination are equivocal. Internal spermatic vein diameter >3 mm and demonstration of retrograde flow through the vein with Valsalva maneuver on ultrasound are consistent with the diagnosis of clinical varicocele. Varicoceles that do not meet these criteria are defined as subclinical.

## INDICATIONS FOR SURGERY

Most varicoceles are not associated with infertility, decreased testicular volume, or pain and therefore do not require surgical correction. A clinical varicocele in a patient with abnormal semen parameters should be surgically corrected to reverse the process of progressive and duration-dependent decline in testicular function. Repair of subclinical varicocele has not been shown to confer a benefit to the patient with male factor infertility and is not recommended (4). Varicocele associated with ipsilateral testicular atrophy or with ipsilateral testicular pain that worsens progressively throughout the day, but subsides in the recumbent position, should be repaired as well. Varicocele ligation in adolescents with ipsilateral testicular atrophy has been shown to result in a significant increase in testis volume (5), and therefore surgical correction is recommended in this group. Adolescents with small- to moderate-grade varicoceles in the absence of atrophy are followed with yearly examination to assess testicular growth; the occurrence of diminished growth on the side of the varicocele warrants varicocelectomy. A sound argument could be made for repair of all grade III varicoceles in adolescents to conserve testicular function. Approximately 3% of adolescent males have grade III varicoceles.

## ALTERNATIVE THERAPY

For men with infertility, abnormal semen parameters, and clinical varicocele, few alternatives to varicocelectomy are available. Currently utilized nonsurgical techniques include percutaneous radiographic occlusion and sclerotherapy. The retrograde percutaneous approach employs cannulation of the femoral vein and placement of a balloon or coil within the internal spermatic vein. Although this technique is associated with preservation of the testicular artery and lymphatics, it has a high unperformable rate due to difficulty in accessing the internal spermatic vein, and these men ultimately require surgical intervention. Radiographic occlusion is also associated with complications such as migration of embolization material into the renal vein resulting in kidney loss or pulmonary embolization, thrombophlebitis, arterial injury, and allergic reaction to contrast materials. This technique may have a role in the management of varicoceles that persist or recur following open surgical repair to avoid reoperation through scar tissue. Antegrade varicocele occlusion performed by percutaneous cannulation of a scrotal pampiniform vein and injection of a sclerosing agent has been described. This technique is associated with higher performability rates but similar recurrence rates when compared with the retrograde approach, in addition to presenting risk of injury to the testicular artery.

## SURGICAL TECHNIQUE

Ligation of the internal spermatic veins can be approached in several ways. The earliest described technique involved placing an external clamp on the veins through the scrotal skin. Surgical varicocele ligation techniques include retroperitoneal, inguinal or subinguinal ligation, laparoscopic, and microsurgical varicocelectomy.

### Retroperitoneal (Polomo) Approach

The retroperitoneal (Polomo) approach (Fig. 79.1) has the advantage of isolating the internal spermatic veins proximally, near the point of drainage into the left renal vein. At this level, only one or two large veins are present. In addition, the testicular artery has not yet branched and is often separate from the internal spermatic veins. A disadvantage to this approach is difficulty in preserving lymphatics due to the poorly accessible retroperitoneal location of the vessels, leading to a higher incidence of postoperative hydrocele. In addition, a high recurrence rate is observed when the testicular artery is preserved due to preservation of the periarterial plexus of fine veins (venae comitantes), which may dilate with time and present as the source of recurrence. Parallel inguinal or retroperitoneal collaterals originating at the testis and joining the internal spermatic vein cephalad to the level of ligation, in addition to cremasteric veins that are not ligated, may contribute to recurrence. Intentional ligation of the testicular artery has been suggested in children to minimize recurrence, but in adults who present with infertility, ligation of the testicular artery cannot be recommended as this is unlikely to enhance testicular function.

The patient is placed in the dorsal supine position on an operating table. A horizontal iliac incision equidistant from the umbilicus and anterior superior iliac spine is made (7 to 10 cm, depending on the patient's body habitus). The external oblique aponeurosis is incised obliquely. The internal oblique is split 1 cm off the lateral edge of the rectus abdominis, and the transversus abdominis is incised. The peritoneum is dissected free from the abdominal wall and retracted. The spermatic vessels appear adherent to the peritoneum, making it important to remain close to the peritoneum. Continued dissection along the abdominal wall would lead posteriorly to the psoas muscle. Retraction of the peritoneum allows easy identification of the spermatic veins, and in <10% of cases the spermatic artery is clearly visible, isolated from the rest of the spermatic structures, identified, and preserved.

The remainder of the operation depends on the intraoperative findings. In the case of a single vein and no collateral, the

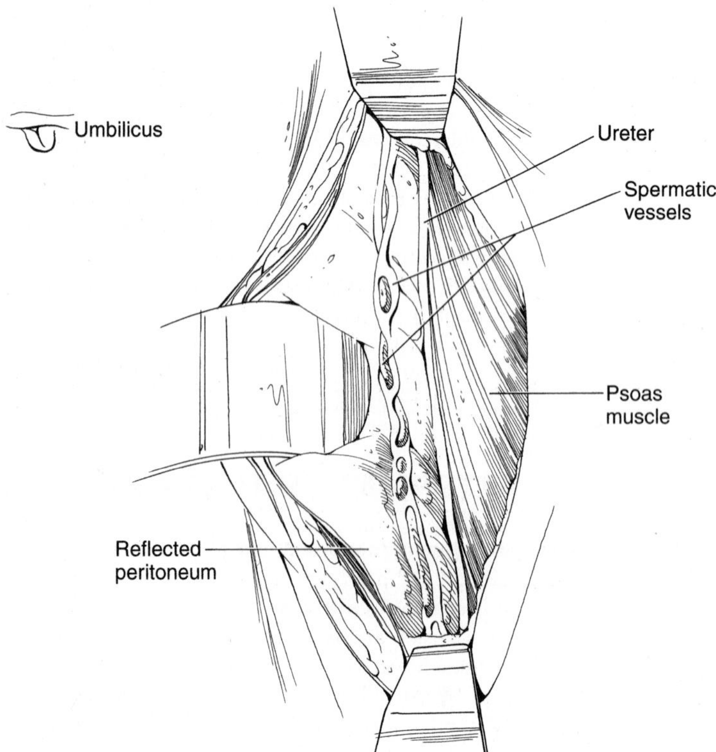


FIGURE 79.1 Modified Palomo retroperitoneal approach for varicocelectomy. The internal spermatic vein is found on the posterior aspect of the peritoneum. It is isolated and divided between ligatures.

artery is identified and will only be preserved when it is not accompanied by a plexus of small veins indissociable from the artery. In the case of multiple veins, the collaterals are identified and all vessels from the ureter to the abdominal wall are ligated. Spermatic vessels are in general inspected over a distance of 7 or 8 cm and ligated by braided, permanent suture material.

After verification of hemostasis, the internal oblique, transversus abdominis, and external oblique aponeurosis are reapproximated with absorbable suture. The Scarpa fascia is closed by a resorbable running suture. The skin is closed in subcuticular manner with absorbable suture.

## Inguinal (Ivanissevich) Approach

The incision is made 2 cm above the symphysis pubica (Fig. 79.2). The external oblique aponeurosis is carefully divided to avoid injuring the underlying ilioinguinal nerve. The cord is mobilized and a Penrose drain is inserted beneath the cord and retracted to gain exposure of the cord. The spermatic fascia is then incised and the vessels are identified. Each vein is isolated, doubly ligated with nonabsorbable suture, and transsected. Intraoperative Doppler may be utilized to identify the testicular artery. After all collaterals are identified, the external oblique aponeurosis is closed with running absorbable suture and the skin is closed in a subcuticular manner.

## Laparoscopic Varicocele Repair

Laparoscopic varicocele repair is a modification of the retroperitoneal technique with similar advantages and disadvantages. The optical magnification afforded through the laparoscope provides the ability to preserve the lymphatics and the testicular artery while ligating the few internal spermatic veins present at this level and the venae comitantes adherent to the testicular artery. Laparoscopic technique introduces a unique set of complications, including injury to bowel, intra-abdominal vessels, and viscera in addition to air embolism and peritonitis, all of which are much more serious than those associated with open varicocelectomy.

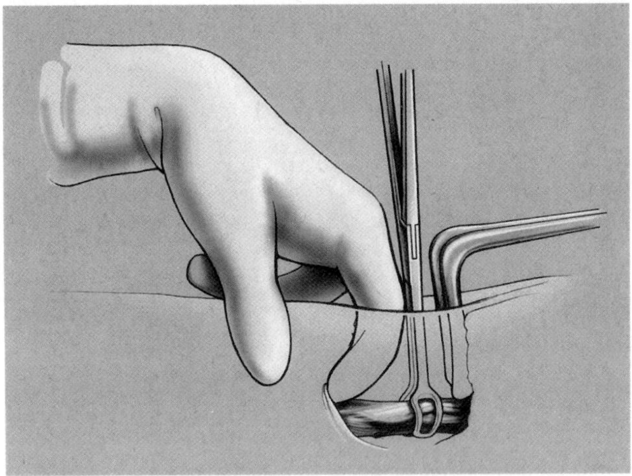

FIGURE 79.3 Subinguinal approach. An index finger is hooked into the external inguinal ring retracting cephalad, while a small Richardson retractor retracts the soft tissues caudad toward the scrotum. The assistant grasps the spermatic cord with a Babcock clamp for elevation of the cord into the wound.

## Microsurgical Varicocelectomy

Microsurgical subinguinal or inguinal varicocelectomy is our preferred approach to varicocele ligation. The spermatic cord is elevated into the incision (Fig. 79.3), providing excellent exposure, and with use of the microscope providing 6× to 25×

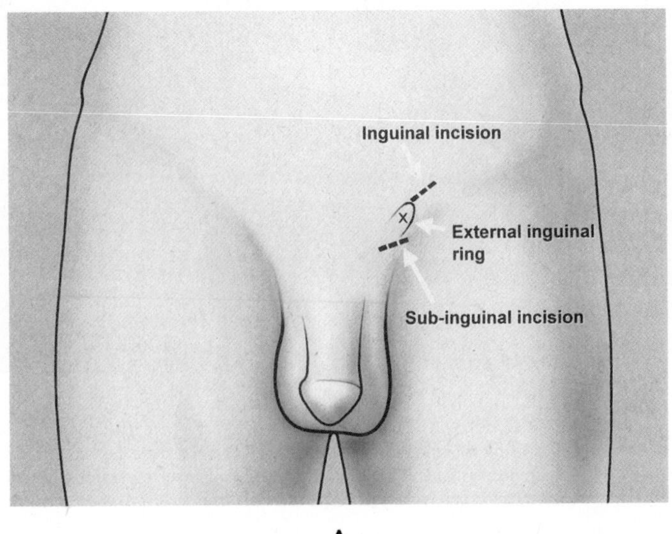


A

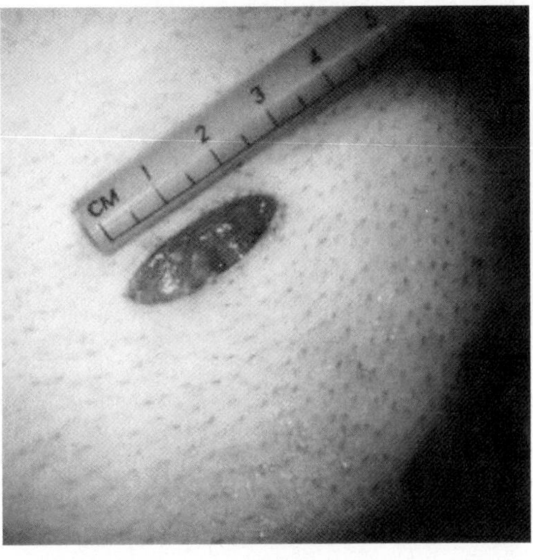


B

FIGURE 79.2 **A:** Position of inguinal and subinguinal incisions. The external inguinal ring can be located by invaginating the scrotal skin with an index finger in a cephalad direction over the pubic tubercle. The location of the ring is marked on the skin. **B:** A subinguinal incision measuring only 2.5 cm in length.

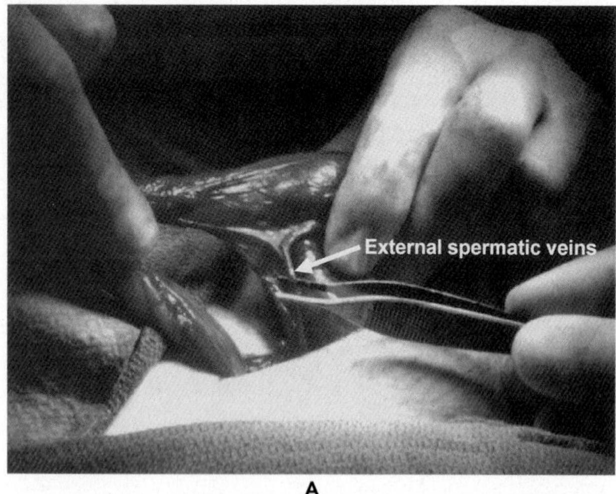


A

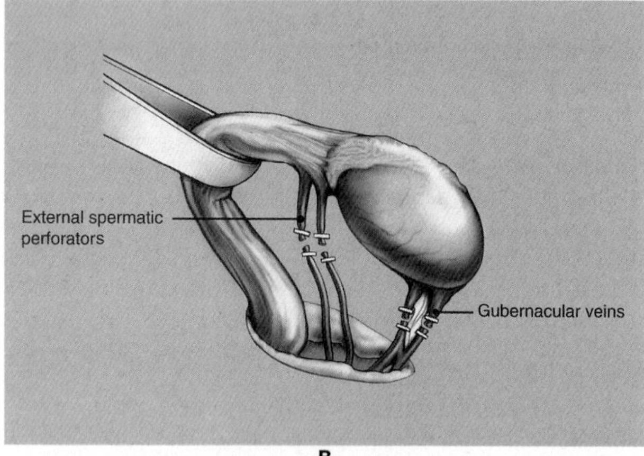


B

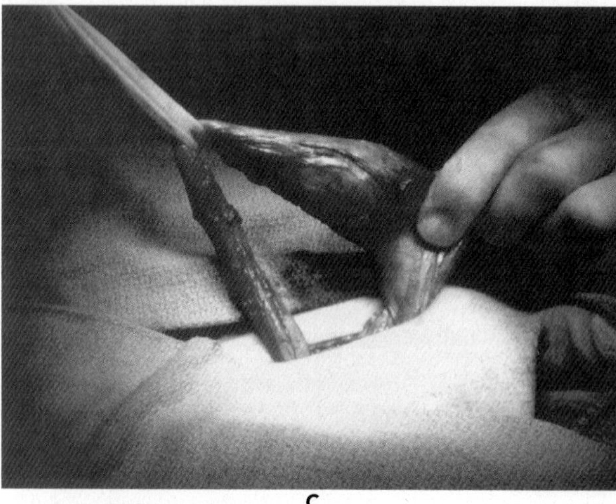

C

FIGURE 79.4 **A:** Following delivery of the testis, the cord and gubernaculum are inspected for extraspermatic collateral veins. **B:** All external spermatic and gubernacular veins are doubly clipped and transected. **C:** The testis and cord following division of these veins. All remaining venous drainage is contained within the cord itself.

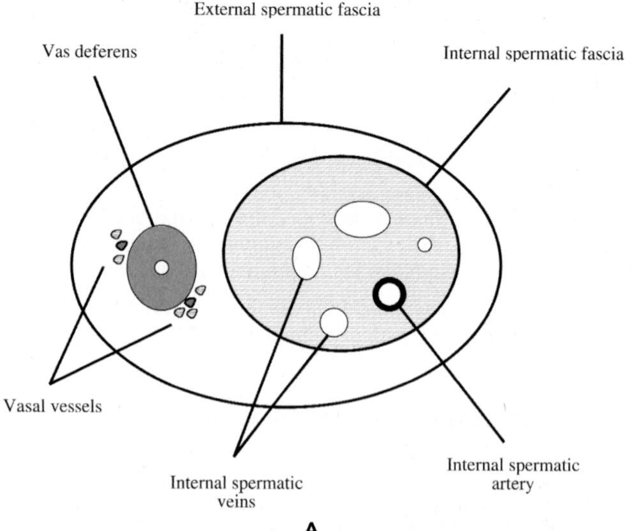


A

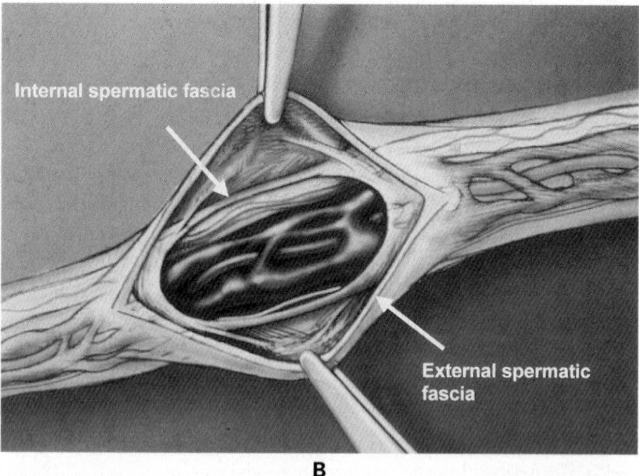


B

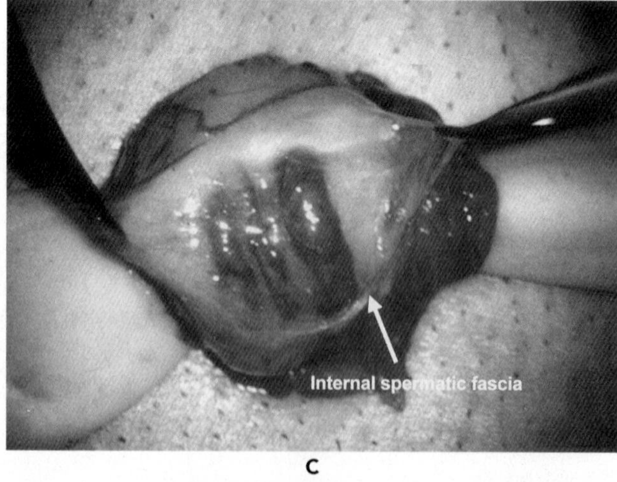


C

FIGURE 79.5 **A:** Diagram of a cross-section of the spermatic cord, illustrating the anatomic relationship between the external and internal spermatic fasciae. A (**B**) diagram and (**C**) intraoperative photo of the spermatic cord with opened external and internal spermatic fasciae.

magnification the small periarterial and cremasteric veins can be readily ligated, as can extraspermatic and gubernacular veins when the testis is delivered into the wound (Fig. 79.4). The external and internal spermatic fasciae are carefully opened to expose the vessels (Fig. 79.5). The testicular artery can be readily identified under the microscope, and preservation of the artery is more likely with enhanced visualization (Fig. 79.6). Lymphatics are also identified and preserved (Fig. 79.7), resulting in a lower incidence of hydrocele postoperatively.

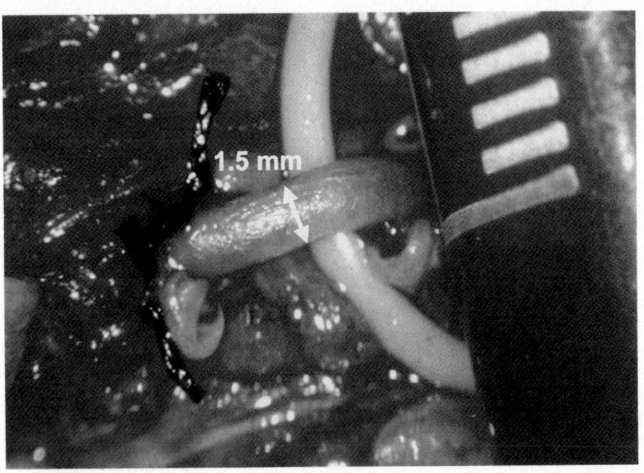


FIGURE 79.6 A vessel loop is placed around the testicular artery for identification throughout the procedure. The artery has been dissected free of all adjacent veins and lymphatics.

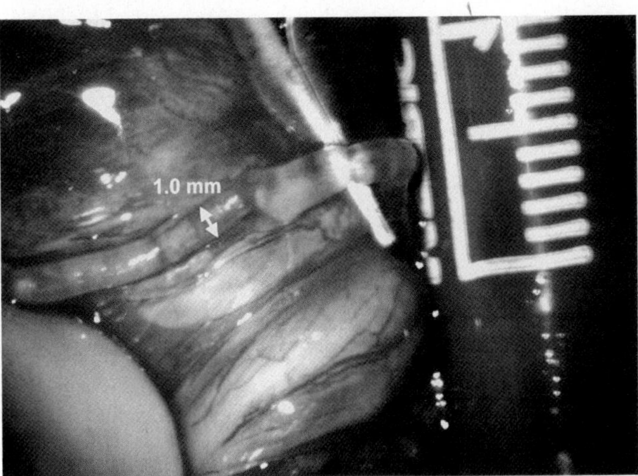


FIGURE 79.7 A lymphatic measuring 1 mm in diameter is visualized under the microscope and preserved.

# OUTCOMES

## Complications

The most common complication following varicocelectomy is hydrocele formation. The incidence of postoperative hydrocele following the nonmicrosurgical technique ranges from 3% to 33% with an average of 7%. Examination of the hydrocele fluid has shown that the fluid characteristics are consistent with obstruction of lymphatics (12). The effect of a hydrocele on sperm function and fertility is uncertain. Nearly half of postoperative hydroceles require surgical correction due to size. Use of magnification to identify lymphatics and preserve them has nearly eliminated the incidence of hydrocele formation (2,8).

Testicular artery injury is a complication of varicocelectomy. Although the testis also receives blood supply from the cremasteric and deferential arteries, ligation of the testicular artery may result in atrophy and/or impaired spermatogenesis. Microscopic technique facilitates identification and preservation of the testicular artery, minimizing the risk of testicular injury (2).

Varicocele recurrence occurs in periarterial, parallel inguinal, midretroperitoneal, or transscrotal collaterals (6). Parallel inguinal collaterals are missed with retroperitoneal repair. Routine inguinal techniques without optical magnification miss scrotal collaterals and small veins adherent to the testicular artery. The microsurgical approach with delivery of the testis is associated with a varicocele recurrence rate <1% when compared with 9% for nonmagnified inguinal techniques (2,8).

## Results

Varicocelectomy has been found to improve sperm concentration, motility, and morphology with a corresponding increase in pregnancy rate. A randomized controlled trial of surgery compared with no surgery (control group) showed that 60% of men who underwent varicocelectomy initiated a pregnancy within 1 year, whereas pregnancy was achieved in only 10% of those couples in which the varicocele went unrepaired (7). The control group then underwent varicocelectomy, and during the second year of the study 44% initiated a pregnancy. A series of 1,500 men who underwent microsurgical varicocelectomy resulted in 43% pregnancy at 1 year and 69% at 2 years when female factors were excluded (2). Varicocelectomy improves semen parameters sufficiently such that for most couples assisted reproductive techniques (ARTs) are either rendered unnecessary or the type of ART necessary to bypass the male factor is downstaged (1). In addition, up to 50% of men with nonobstructive azoospermia will respond to varicocelectomy with return of sperm to the ejaculate (9). In adolescents, a moderate to large varicocele can be responsible for testicular growth retardation, and early ligation of the varicocele may reverse this process (5). Finally, varicocelectomy can increase serum testosterone levels for infertile men with varicoceles (11).

## *References*


1. Çayan S, Erdemir F, Özbey I, et al. Can varicocelectomy significantly change the way couples use assisted reproductive technologies? *J Urol* 2002;167:1749–1752.
2. Goldstein M, Gilbert BR, Dicker AP, et al. Microsurgical inguinal varicocelectomy with delivery of the testis: an artery and lymphatic sparing technique. *J Urol* 1992;148:1808–1811.
3. Gorelick JI, Goldstein M. Loss of fertility in men with varicocele. *Fertil Steril* 1993;59:613.
4. Jarow JP, Ogle SR, Eskew LA. Seminal improvement following repair of ultrasound detected subclinical varicoceles. *J Urol* 1996;155:1287–1290.
5. Kass EJ, Belman AB. Reversal of testicular growth failure by varicocele ligation. *J Urol* 1987;137:475–476.
6. Kaufman SL, Kadir S, Barth KH, et al. Mechanisms of recurrent varicocele after balloon occlusion or surgical ligation of the internal spermatic vein. *Radiology* 1983;147:435–440.
7. Madgar I, Weissenberg R, Lunenfeld B, et al. Controlled trial of high spermatic vein ligation for varicocele in infertile men. *Fertil Steril* 1995;63:120.
8. Marmar JL, Kim Y. Subinguinal microsurgical varicocelectomy: a technical critique and statistical analysis of semen and pregnancy data. *J Urol* 1994;152:1127–1132.
9. Matthews GJ, Matthews ED, Goldstein M. Induction of spermatogenesis and achievement of pregnancy after microsurgical varicocelectomy in men with azoospermia and severe oligoasthenospermia. *Fertil Steril* 1998; 70:71.
10. Steckel J, Dicker AP, Goldstein M. Influence of varicocele size on response to microsurgical ligation of the spermatic veins. *J Urol* 1993;149:769–771.
11. Su LM, Goldstein M, Schlegel PN. The effect of varicocelectomy on serum testosterone levels in infertile men with varicoceles. *J Urol* 1995;154: 1752–1755.
12. Szabo R, Kessler R. Hydrocele following internal spermatic vein ligation: a retrospective study and review of the literature. *J Urol* 1984;132:924–925.
13. World Health Organization. The influence of varicocele on parameters of fertility in a large group of men presenting to infertility clinics. *Fertil Steril* 1992;57:1289.

# CHAPTER 80 ■ HYDROCELE AND SPERMATOCELE

JOHN A. NESBITT

Hydrocele and spermatocele refer to common but abnormal collections of fluid within the scrotum and must be included in the differential diagnosis of scrotal masses. The etiology of each of these masses is different, and both may require surgical intervention for cure. They occur in males of all ages, beginning at birth.

## HYDROCELE

Hydrocele (from the Greek *hydros* for water and *kele* for mass), literally a watery rupture or water in the scrotum, is an abnormal collection of fluid in the tunica vaginalis that may surround the testicle. The fluid is usually amber and is considered to be an exudate. A small amount of fluid, several cubic centimeters, is normally present around the testicle. This fluid is present between layers of the tunica vaginalis and the tunica albuginea covering the testis. About 0.5 cc of fluid is continuously secreted and reabsorbed by this mesothelial layer daily. Several types of hydroceles exist that may be associated with other pathologic findings, including cancer. The majority of hydroceles occur congenitally, and most of these resolve spontaneously during the first year of life. Acquired hydroceles are found later in life. If due to local inflammation, these hydroceles may resolve as the inflammation resolves. Intervention is usually only required for size or discomfort.

During month 3 of gestation, the gubernaculum traverses the inguinal canal from the internal ring, through the external inguinal ring, and out into the scrotum, pulling with it the parietal peritoneal lining of the abdominal cavity (processus vaginalis). Late in the third trimester, the testis leaves its intra-abdominal location, descends along the same route as the gubernaculum through the inguinal canal, and exits the external ring posterolateral to the processus vaginalis. Normally, the segment of the processus vaginalis lying in the inguinal canal obliterates by the time of birth. A portion of the processus is left within the scrotum closely applied to the testicle. This structure is then termed the tunica vaginalis. Persistence of the inguinal portion of the processus may lead to a patent processus vaginalis, a hernia, or a localized portion of fluid lying within the inguinal canal known as a hydrocele of the cord.

Most acquired hydroceles are idiopathic. However, the clinician must be careful to consider other causes, such as trauma, infection, or testicular tumor, when evaluating a patient. Lymphatic obstruction due to ipsilateral inguinal or pelvic surgery may result in a secondary hydrocele. A common surgical cause for hydrocele is renal transplantation. In this scenario, the spermatic vessels and vas deferens are divided on the ipsilateral side, leading to hydrocele development. Epididymitis or orchitis may cause an acute hydrocele that usually resolves with the resolution of the inflammation. Tropical infections, such as filariasis, may produce hydroceles where the tunica thickens due to lymphatic obstruction by the parasites. In these cases, the fluid is usually turbid due to chylous drainage secondary to the lymphatic obstruction. It is generally thought that tense hydroceles are caused by lack of reabsorption of the fluid, and the more flaccid type from excess fluid production.

### Diagnosis

In the pediatric population, hydroceles may present at birth or within the first year of life and are found in about 6% of full-term males. In general, a painless swelling is noticed in the scrotum. The scrotal enlargement may increase or decrease in size if the processus is patent, allowing peritoneal fluid or bowel to enter the scrotum. If the processus is small, only fluid will enter. This persistence of the patent processus allowing the connection from the peritoneal cavity to the scrotum is known as a communicating hydrocele. The change in size may not be apparent to the clinician but will be noticed by the parents.

In acquired hydroceles, the swelling may be accompanied by pain, especially if caused by an inflammatory process. The patient may report an enlargement within the scrotum, a tense sac, or some discomfort within the scrotum that may radiate inguinally or into the ipsilateral flank. The swelling is smooth, confined to the scrotum, and will usually transilluminate if the wall is not too thickened. With somewhat large and tense hydroceles, the testis is not palpable. Because testicular neoplasms may also cause hydroceles, transscrotal ultrasonography is a useful preoperative diagnostic tool for imaging an otherwise inevaluable testicle.

### Indications for Surgery

Surgical intervention is indicated when the hydrocele is symptomatic either due to discomfort or size impairing daily activity. Hydrocelectomy is inappropriate in the face of a testicular neoplasm.

### Alternative Therapy

In congenital hydroceles, the treatment is usually observation, unless the patient has an accompanying hernia. This is an important distinction to make because the latter should be repaired surgically. When the diagnosis is uncertain, some have advocated repair. A period of observation would be appropriate in the absence of other symptoms. Many of these hydroceles will resolve within the first year of life if left untreated.

In acquired hydroceles requiring treatment, the approach is in general considered to be surgical. Various surgical techniques have been described, all of which yield satisfactory results (7). The surgical approach is generally preferred due to the high success and low recurrence rates. Alternative therapies may be considered in symptomatic patients who are poor surgical risks. Hydroceles may be aspirated with some expected temporary pain relief. In addition, a sclerosing agent, such as tetracycline, may be placed within the empty space in an effort to keep the fluid from reaccumulating (2). This treatment has met with mixed results and may be very painful. Other sclerosants have been used, including ethanolamine oleate, polidocanol, sodium tetradecyl sulfate, and phenol. Sclerosing therapy typically requires up to three treatment sessions, and although high success rates have been reported (9), many physicians still reserve this treatment for poor surgical candidates. The recurrence and complication rates associated with sclerotherapy are higher than with the surgical approach, and some side-effects can include infection, impaired fertility, and testicular loss (11). Due to these risks, some authors feel that sclerotherapy is not appropriate for young healthy patients (6).

## Surgical Technique

There are several successful surgical techniques utilized to treat hydroceles. The scrotum is shaved, and, along with the penis, the entire area is cleaned with antiseptic preparation. The approach is usually midline scrotal or transverse between transversely running blood vessels, unless the diagnosis is in question. When neoplasm or hernia cannot be ruled out, the approach should be inguinal. The scrotal incision should be carried down to the tunica vaginalis, where the blue hue of the hydrocele is seen. The hydrocele and testicle may be delivered through the incision. Blunt dissection and use of a surgical sponge will free any surrounding tissue from the hydrocele sac. Once this parietal layer of tunica vaginalis is exposed, one may select the type of procedure to perform. In general, the Lord procedure is suitable for more thin-walled hydroceles, whereas the other described techniques are used with thicker sacs.

### Andrews Procedure

This technique was described in 1907 by Andrews (1) and is referred to as the "bottle operation." A 2- to 3-cm incision is made in the hydrocele sac near the superior portion (Fig. 80.1). The procedure may be completed by tacking the cut edges around the cord structures or leaving the everted sac open. A two-layer wound closure is then accomplished with absorbable suture, such as 2-0 or 3-0 chromic, approximating the skin over the dartos layer.

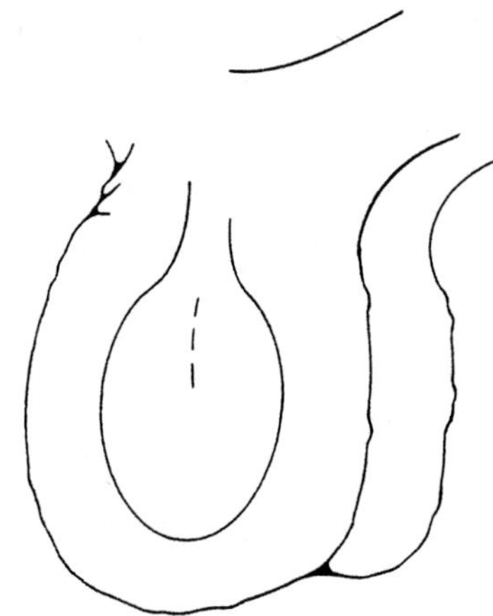

FIGURE 80.1 The Andrews operation. A small incision is made high in the sac prior to eversion of the sac about the cord.

### Jaboulay or Winkleman Procedure

As described by Jaboulay in 1902 (13), this technique involves delivering the testicle through an incision in the tunica. The majority of the sac is then resected, leaving a small cuff along the border of the testicle. After everting the remnant, bleeding may then be controlled rapidly by a running suture closing the free edges around the cord structures (Fig. 80.2). Reapproximation of the edges is done loosely around the cord so as not to compromise the blood supply to the testicle. In another variation of this technique, the parietal tunica vaginalis is resected nearly flush with the testis and epididymis. Electrocautery may be used around the edge to aid in hemostasis, or bleeders may be ligated (Fig. 80.3). The standard two-layer closure is used to close the scrotum.

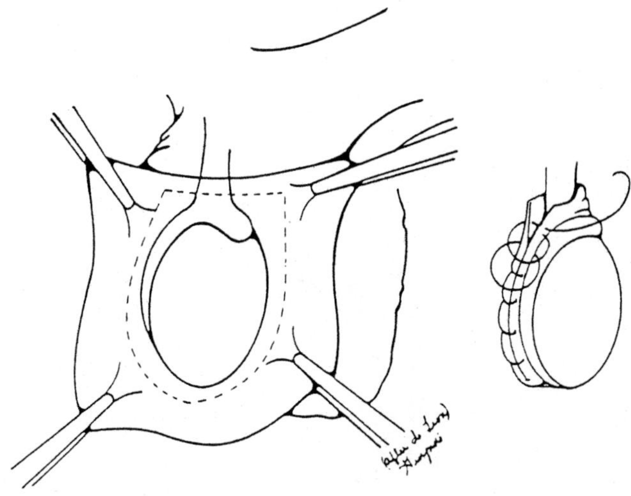

FIGURE 80.2 The Jaboulay or Winkleman technique. The redundant sac is excised, leaving enough room to be loosely closed about the cord. A running suture may be used to close the sac and rapidly control bleeding from the free edges.

### Lord Procedure

In utilizing this plication technique for hydrocelectomy described by Lord in 1964 (8), a small incision is made just large enough to deliver the testis into the field. The parietal layer of the tunica vaginalis is opened without dissection from the dartos layer. With little dissection of the scrotal sac, this procedure is relatively bloodless. Placing the Allis forceps on the cut edges of the open sac allows the testicle to be brought into the wound. Next, the edges are plicated circumferentially with interrupted 2-0 or 3-0 chromic catgut sutures, placing them about 1 cm apart. The bites should be approximately 1 cm as well (Fig. 80.4). As these sutures are tied, the sac will

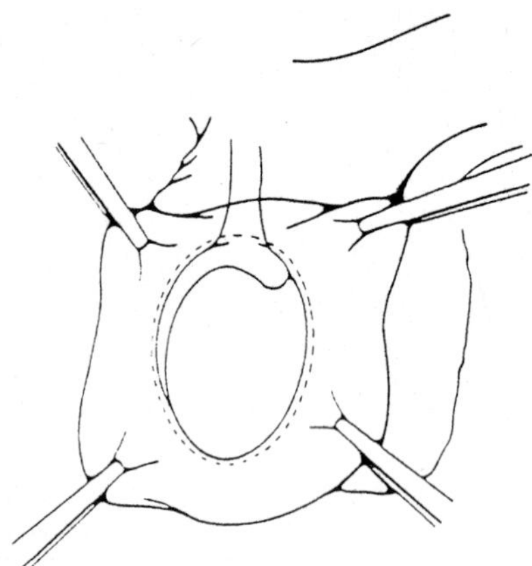

FIGURE 80.3 Alternate technique. The sac is excised nearly flush with the testicle, and the epididymis and bleeders are ligated or fulgurated individually.

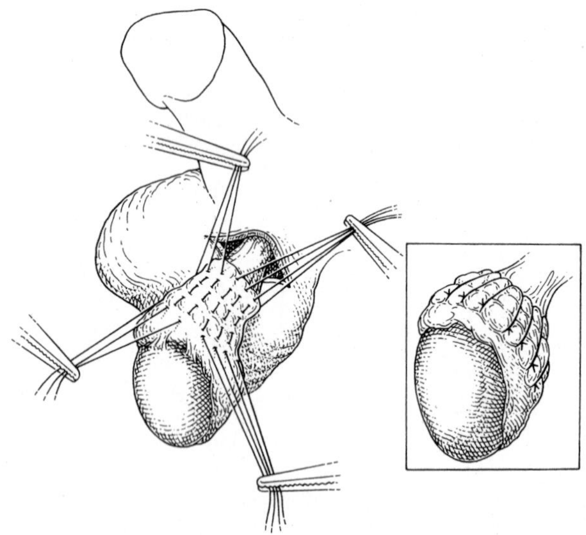

FIGURE 80.4 The Lord operation. The testis is extruded through a small incision placed in the middle of the sac, and interrupted placating sutures are placed in a circumferential fashion. The sutures are tied, and the sac will "accordion" into a collar superior to the testicle.

accordion, forming a collar around the testis and epididymis (Fig. 80.4 inset). Wound closure is accomplished as discussed for the other procedures.

### Inguinal Approach

When a neoplasm is a concern but not definitively diagnosed preoperatively, a Chevassu maneuver may be performed or the Goldstein and Waterhouse modification employed (3). Preservation of the testicle may be accomplished without compromising the cancer operation. Biopsies of the suspicious area may be performed utilizing these techniques and the testicle spared if no cancer is found. These approaches involve exposure through an inguinal incision, clamping the cord with noncrushing clamps, ligating the gubernaculum prior to transection, and cooling the testis with ice slush. The benign testicle is then replaced into the scrotum or a radical orchiectomy performed in the case of malignancy.

In general, any of these procedures may be performed without surgical drainage. When hemostasis is difficult to obtain or the hydrocele particularly large, a small Penrose drain, placed through a separate stab incision in the inferior aspect of the scrotum and left overnight, is useful. This maneuver will also help prevent serous fluid from accumulating in the scrotum postoperatively. Because the scrotum is difficult to dress, fluff dressings held in place by a standard athletic supporter do well in this situation. An ice pack is kept in place for at least 24 hours to help diminish postoperative pain and swelling. Oral analgesics are utilized for several days. Preoperative antibiotics are helpful but not usually continued postoperatively.

# SPERMATOCELE

A spermatocele (from the Greek *spermatos* for sperm and *kele* for cyst or mass) is a cystic structure arising out of the epididymis, rete testis, or ductuli efferentes. These structures are filled with spermatozoa containing fluid that may be milky. These cysts are usually outside the tunica vaginalis and, as with hydroceles, transilluminate easily. They are frequently seen on scrotal ultrasound as an incidental finding and may be present in as many as 30% of males.

The etiology of most spermatoceles is idiopathic, although trauma, infection, or an inflammatory process within the epididymis or scrotum may precede the development of a spermatocele. It is hypothesized that the epididymal ducts become obstructed, causing proximal dilation. The cause of the obstruction is thought to be the seminiferous epithelium continually shedding immature germ cells that are deposited in the efferent ducts (4).

## Diagnosis

Because most spermatoceles are asymptomatic, they are usually discovered incidentally on self-examination or on physical examination by a physician. The typical location within the scrotum is cephalad and sometimes posterior to the testicle. However, spermatoceles may arise from any location on the epididymis. These cystic structures are not usually painful, are round, and have distinct borders. The mass is easily separable from the testis. Scrotal ultrasound may be helpful when the diagnosis is uncertain.

## Indications for Surgery

Most spermatoceles do not require intervention. Painful or large, socially embarrassing spermatoceles may require intervention. Surgery should be entertained when there is a question of diagnosis of a potential tumor. Spermatocelectomy should be avoided in men desiring future fertility.

## Alternative Therapy

In those requiring treatment, the options are aspiration with the use of sclerosing agents or surgery. Results are similar to those of hydrocele.

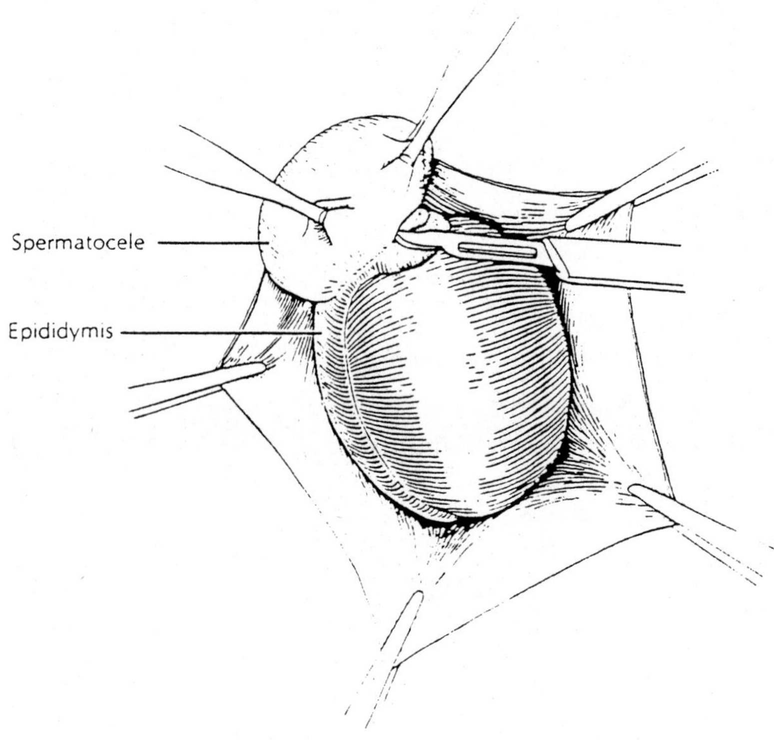


FIGURE 80.5 Spermatocelectomy. The spermatocele is separated from the globus major of the epididymis by sharp dissection and excised.

## Surgical Technique

The spermatocele is approached through the same incision as for the hydrocele. The tunica vaginalis is incised, and the testicle, along with the spermatocele, is delivered into the incision. Utilizing sharp dissection, the cystic structure may be excised or "shelled out" from the epididymis without excessive mobilization of the epididymis or testis (Fig. 80.5). On occasion, an attachment to the epididymis can be identified and ligated or cauterized carefully with minimal trauma (Fig. 80.6). Magnification may be of benefit when fertility is a concern. Hemostasis is accomplished with needle tip cautery or chromic ligatures. The edges of the epididymis are reapproximated or a portion of adjacent fascia or tunica may be used to close the epididymal defect (Fig. 80.6 inset). In some cases it may be necessary to resect a portion of the tunica vaginalis to perform a hydrocelectomy in conjunction with this procedure. Wound closure and postoperative management are similar to those for hydrocelectomy.

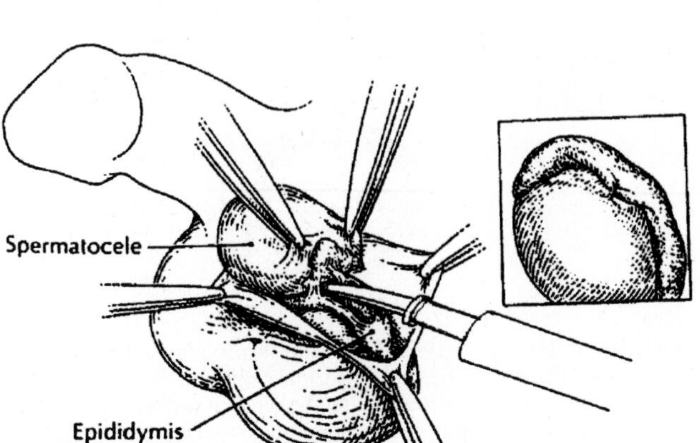


FIGURE 80.6 Attachments to the epididymis are identified, ligated, or cauterized with minimal mobility. The epididymal defect is closed with chromic sutures.

# OUTCOMES

## Complications

The usual surgical complications are seen with these procedures. The most common complication is hematoma, usually within the scrotum. In some cases, testicular atrophy or obstruction of the epididymis (12) or vas deferens may occur (5). Bleeding, wound infection, scrotal abscess, and recurrent hydrocele or spermatocele complete the list of possible complications, but they are much less common. There is some evidence that the Lord procedure for hydrocelectomy has fewer of these complications (10).

## Results

Most patients have a successful outcome with a minimal incidence of recurrence.

## References


1. Andrews EW. The "bottle operation" method for the radical cure of hydrocele. *Am Surg* 1907;46:915–918.
2. Beiko DT, Kim D, Morales A. Aspiration and sclerotherapy vs hydrocelectomy for treatment of hydrocele. *Urology* 2003;4:7808–7712.
3. Goldstein M, Waterhouse K. When to use the Chevassu maneuver during exploration of intrascrotal masses. *J Urol* 1983;130:1199–1200.
4. Itoh M, Li XQ, Miyamoto K, et al. Degeneration of the seminiferous epithelium with aging is a cause of spermatocele? *Int J Androl* 1999;22(2):91.
5. Kiddoo DA, Wollin TA, Mador TR. A population based assessment of complications following outpatient hydrocelectomy and spermatocelectomy. *J Urol* 2004;171:746–748.
6. Ku JH, Kim ME, Lee NK, et al. The excisional, plication, and external drainage techniques: a comparison of the results for idiopathic hydrocele. *Br J Urol Int* 2001;87:82.
7. Landes RR, Leonhardt KO. The history of hydrocele. *Urol Surv* 1967;17: 135.
8. Lord PH. A bloodless operation for the radical cure of idiopathic hydrocele. *Br J Surg* 1964;51:914–1916.
9. Nash JR. Sclerotherapy for hydrocele and epididymal cysts: a five year study. *Br Med J Clin Res* 1984;288(6431):1652.
10. Rodriquez WC, Rodriquez DD, Fortunado RF. The operative treatment of hydrocele: a comparison of four basic techniques. *J Urol* 1981;125:804.
11. Thompson H, Odell M. Sclerosant treatment for hydroceles and epididymal cysts. *Br Med J* 1979;2:704.
12. Zahalsky MP, Berman AJ, Nayler HM. Evaluating the risk of epididymal injury during hydrocelectomy and spermatocelectomy. *J Urol* 2004;171: 2291–2292.
13. Jaboulay M. *Chirurgie des centres nerveux, des viscères et des membres.* Vol 2. Lyon/Paris, 1902:192.


# CHAPTER 81 ■ CONGENITAL CURVATURE

TIMOTHY O. DAVIES AND KURT A. MCCAMMON

Normal erectile function is not only dependent on normal vascular and neurologic function but also requires elasticity and compliance of all tissue layers of the penis. During tumescence the penis begins to fill with blood and the corporal bodies and tunica albuginea reach their limits of compliance, causing rigidity. Patients with straight erections have normal and symmetrical expansion of the tunica albuginea. Those with curvature have an asymmetrical expansion of one aspect of their penis. This could be due to decreased compliance of one aspect of the tunica or foreshortening of one erectile body.

Patients usually present in their late teens to early 30s. Most men cannot remember their penis being straight and have always assumed their curvature was normal. After puberty and onset of sexual activity, they realize that the curvature impedes normal sexual relations. Some patients also notice that their curvature worsens with puberty. On occasion, a patient will present after the age of 30 either having been sexually active but found sex difficult functionally or psychologically or, less commonly, sexually inactive due to the curvature and the embarrassment he feels.

Penile curvature is described as either congenital or acquired. There is some confusion with the terms *congenital curvature* and *chordee without hypospadias*. Some use these terms interchangeably; however, we do not think they are synonymous. This curvature is associated with abnormalities of the ventral tissue planes or the corpus spongiosum.

Devine and Horton (2) proposed a classification system for congenital penile curvature identifying five separate types of curvature. Types I to III can be collectively termed chordee without hypospadias (Fig. 81.1). This refers to an abnormal development of ventral penile tissue with the patient having a normally placed meatus. For patients with type I, none of the surrounding layers are normal and there is malfusion of the corpus spongiosum. Patients with type II curvature have a dysgenic band of fibrous tissue lateral and dorsal to the urethra, which is believed to have formed from the mesenchyme that would have become the Buck and dartos fasciae. In type III congenital curvature, the patient's urethra, corpus spongiosum, and Buck fascia are all developed normally. The abnormality in these patients is in the dartos fascia, which has an elastic band that causes the penis to bend sharply. Not infrequently these patients have a large and prominent mons pubis.

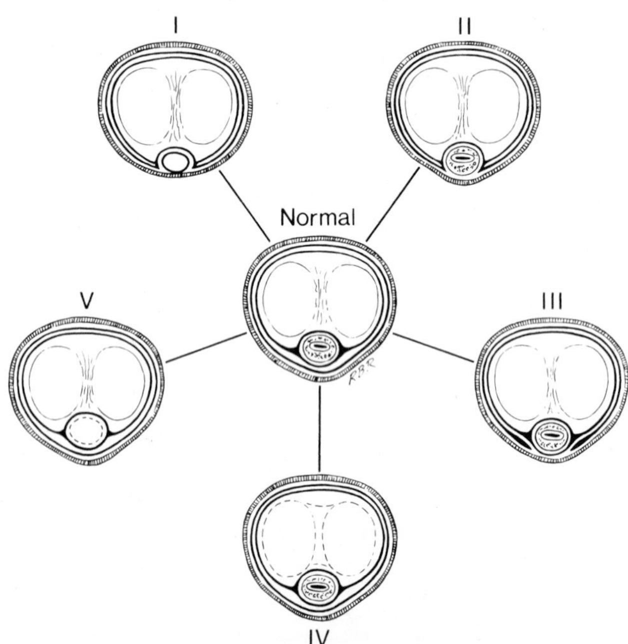


FIGURE 81.1 Cross section of the penis displaying the forms of congenital curvature of the penis. The normal penis is in the center. *Class I*: Epithelial urethra beneath the skin. Dysgenic tissue beneath it represents undeveloped corpus spongiosum, Buck fascia, and dartos fascia. *Class II*: Normal urethra and spongiosum but abnormal Buck and dartos fasciae. *Class III*: Abnormal dartos fascia only. *Class IV*: Normal urethra and fascial layers with abnormal corporocavernosal development. *Class V*: Congenital short urethra (rare). (From Devine CJ Jr, Horton CE. Bent penis. *Semin Urol* 1987;5:252, with permission.)

Type IV curvature is commonly referred to as congenital curvature of the penis by the authors. In type IV penile curvature, development of the urethra, fascial layers, and corpus spongiosum is normal but there is also a relative shortness or inelastic area of the tunica albuginea. Experience with these patients has shown that they have a penis of normal length when flaccid, but when erect the penis may be larger than expected, thought to be due to hypercompliance of the tunica albuginea. Many of these patients will note curvature prior to puberty, but this becomes more accentuated after pubescence and the penile growth spurt that occurs during adolescence.

Type V curvature is the rarest of all types, and some even question whether it exists. This type is known as the congenitally short urethra. The short urethra is not elastic enough or of adequate length, leading to ventral curvature during erections.

## DIAGNOSIS

All patients should undergo a complete history, including an extensive sexual history and physical examination. Complete examination is done to rule out evidence of subclinical fracture or Peyronie disease, which is obviously rare in the younger patient population. Patients are required to supply photographs of their erect penis for documentation of the curvature. The photographs are beneficial in distinguishing between congenital curvature and chordee without hypospadias. Psychological aspects of the disease also need to be addressed. On occasion, patients are evaluated preoperatively by a certified sex therapist and treated as needed.

Patients with chordee without hypospadias usually present with a ventral or ventral-lateral curvature and are noted to have a penis that is normal or shorter than normal in length. As mentioned earlier, these patients also have noted penile curvature throughout their whole life and may note some progression of the curvature during puberty. Many of these patients have abnormalities of the ventral penile skin. This may be a hooded preputial skin or a high insertion of the penoscrotal skin. The deep ventral tissues of the penis seem to be inelastic to examination and stretch. The inelastic tissue that is palpable is the dysgenic tissue that has replaced the Buck and dartos fasciae.

Some of these patients, because of their curvature and smaller-than-average length, have poor self-images. When identified, these are the patients who benefit from psychological counseling preoperatively.

## INDICATIONS FOR SURGERY

Patients who have significant enough curvature to impair their sexual function are candidates for surgery. Surgery for chordee without hypospadias is successful in this patient population, with most curvatures repaired in a single procedure. Many times the curvature is corrected by excising the dysgenic tissue on the ventrum of the penis and mobilizing the corpus spongiosum.

## ALTERNATIVE THERAPY

There are no alternatives to surgery.

## SURGICAL TECHNIQUE

There are a wide variety of surgical procedures to repair congenital curvature, including incision and plication, incision with grafting, and penile disassembly. Most congenital curvatures are straightened completely with incision and plication.

### Incision and Plication

If the patient has been previously circumcised, an incision is made through the circumcision scar. Due to the previous circumcision, there are new patterns of lymph and venous drainage, and an incision proximal or distal to the old scar could lead to marked penile edema. The incision is made down to the superficial layer of the Buck fascia, and the penis is degloved in this plane. Once completely degloved, an artificial erection is created using intravenous normal saline and a high-pressure pump. Perineal pressure may be needed initially, but prolonged pressure is not needed as these patients have normal erectile function. A tourniquet placed at the base of the penis is not recommended as this can mask the proximal extent of curvature.

The artificial erection demonstrates the degree and location of maximal curvature. In patients with ventral curvature, a layer of dysgenic tissue may be noted that includes the Buck and dartos fasciae. This tissue is completely mobilized and excised. Care is taken not to injure the corpus spongiosum, which will need to be detached from the glans to the penoscrotal junction. If injured the urethra is closed primarily. Patients who suffer from a differential elasticity between dorsal and ventral aspects of the corporal bodies may receive some benefit from the excision of the inelastic dysgenic tissue but are rarely straight and often require further maneuvers to straighten the penis. An artificial erection is repeated after this, and if straight the skin is closed (Fig. 81.2).

The options to straighten the penis are to either lengthen the short side with incisions and grafts or to shorten the long side with excisions and/or incisions and plication. In the set of patients for whom penile length is not a major issue, we usually choose to excise and perform plications. The patients recover from plication procedures more quickly, and graft take is not an issue. Although rare, there is a possibility to induce veno-occlusive dysfunction with dermal grafts (Fig. 81.3).

Once it has been determined to proceed with excision of tunica and dorsal plication, the Buck fascia is elevated, incorporating the neurovascular structures via one of two techniques. One approach is to start lateral to the corpus spongiosum and carry the incision medially. The alternative approach is to excise the deep dorsal vein and approach the tunica from the dorsal midline. If done through this approach, after the dorsal vein is excised the inner layer of the Buck fascia is elevated off the tunica, including the dorsal neurovascular structures; this dissection is carried laterally to the corpus spongiosum.

An artificial erection is again performed and the point of maximal curvature identified. The areas of ellipses are identified and marked. Edges of the planned ellipses are apposed with a 3-0 polypropylene (Prolene) suture, and a repeat artificial erection is performed. If this demonstrates adequate straightening, the edges are marked, the suture is removed, and the ellipse of tunica is excised using a sharp scalpel. The

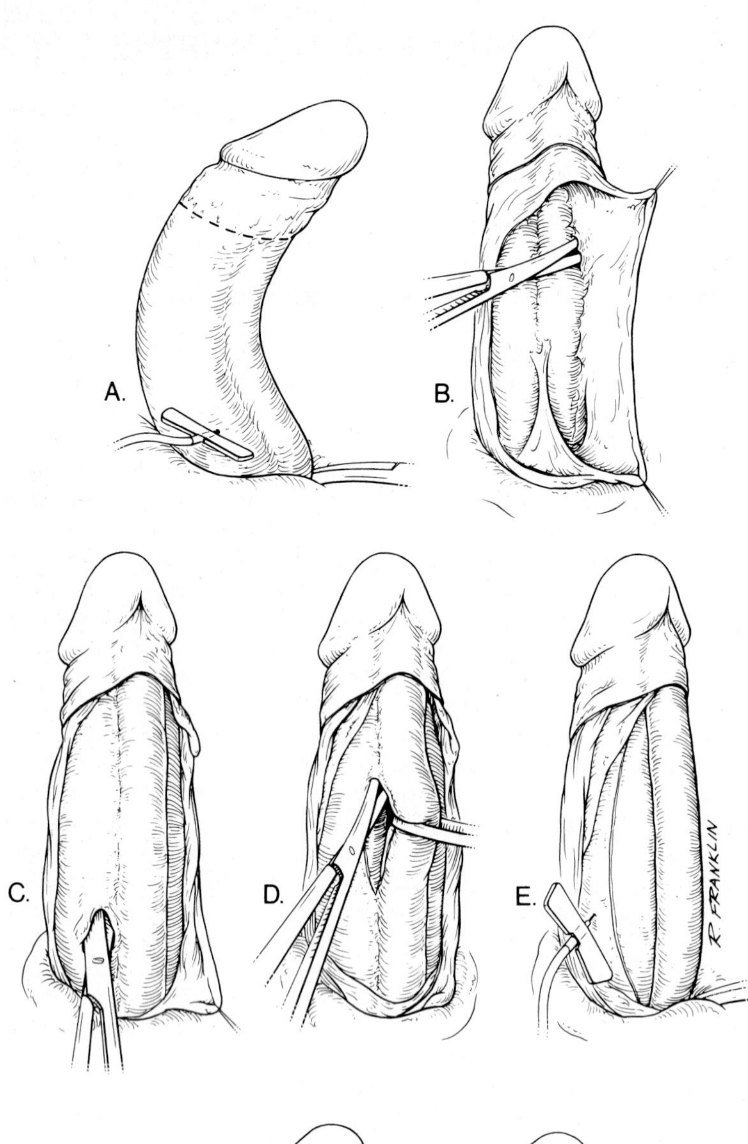


FIGURE 81.2 Surgery for chordee without hypospadias. **A:** Ventral curvature demonstrated with artificial erection. **B:** Dysgenic dartos fascia is elevated and will be excised. **C:** The dysgenic layer of the Buck fascia is undermined by spreading the scissors. **D:** The inelastic fascia is excised as the corpus spongiosum and urethra are mobilized. **E:** Artificial erection demonstrates correction of the curvature.

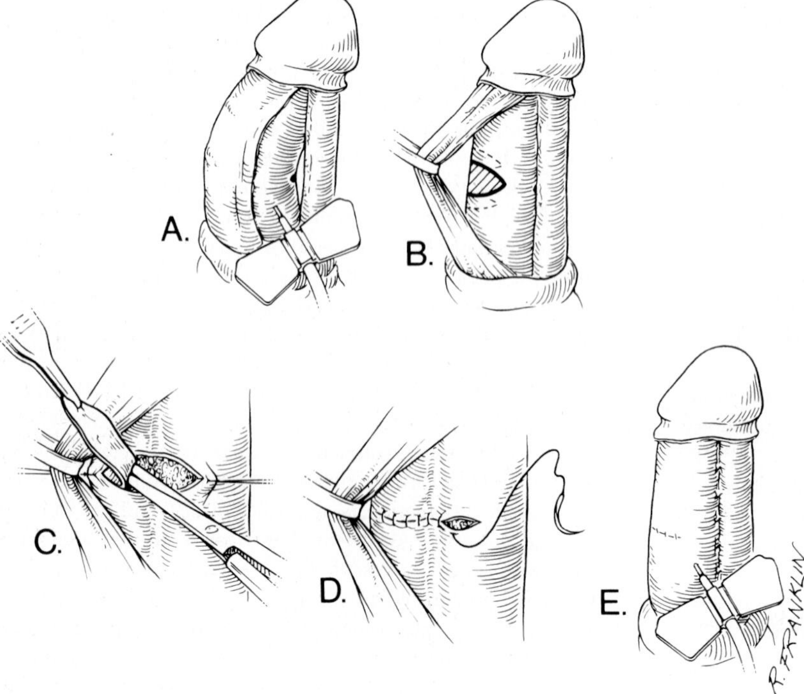


FIGURE 81.3 Surgery for chordee without hypospadias. **A:** A circumcision incision has been made and the urethra has been mobilized by resecting the dartos and Buck fasciae. The needle is in place for an artificial erection. The erection shows continuing chordee. The elastic urethra is not the cause of this curvature. The point of maximum concavity has been marked. **B:** An ellipse of tissue is outlined opposite the point of maximum concavity. As an alternative, two smaller ellipses are shown. **C:** Excision of the ellipse of tunica. Note the tips of the septal strands in the midline. **D:** Closure of the edges of the incision. **E:** Artificial erection revealing a straight penis. When the bend is more complex, ellipses must be excised in other locations. (From Devine CJ Jr, Horton CE. Bent penis. *Semin Urol* 1987;5:4, with permission.)

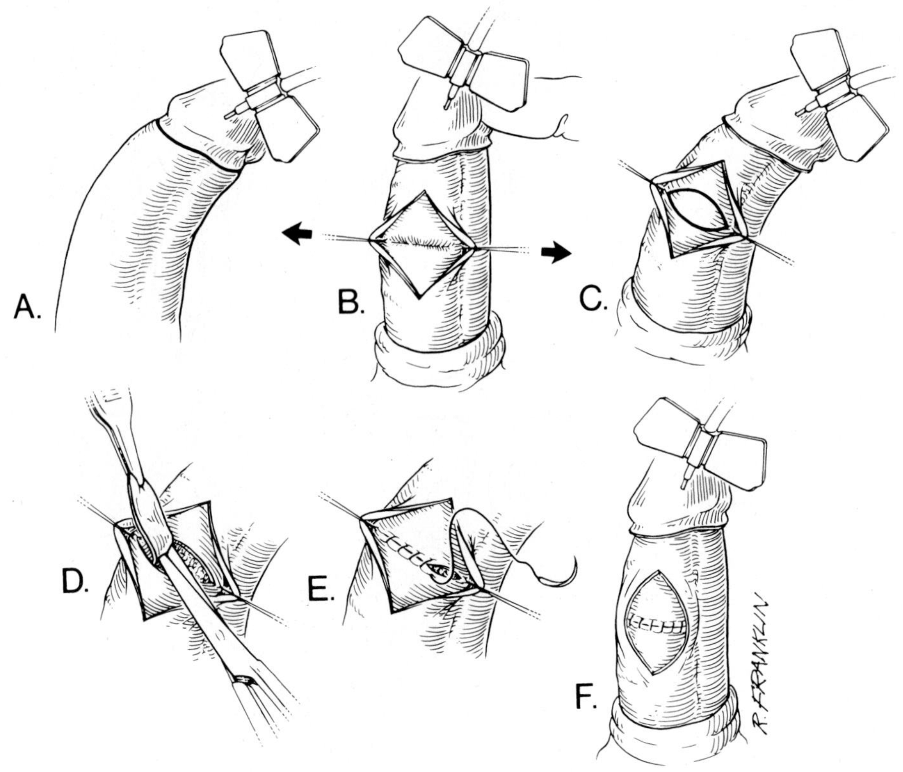


FIGURE 81.4 Congenital lateral curvature. **A:** An artificial erection reveals the curvature. The incision to gain access to the potential ellipse of tissue is marked. **B:** The tunica albuginea has been exposed by mobilizing the Buck fascia, and Prolene sutures have been placed at the dorsal and ventral tips of the potential ellipse. While maintaining the artificial erection, tension is established on the two sutures as the penile shaft is straightened. The fold produced in the tunica is marked. **C:** When the penis is relaxed, this mark defines the ellipse of tunica to be removed. **D:** The tunica is excised. **E:** The edges are approximated. **F:** The penis is straight. The Buck fascia and the skin are closed.

underlying erectile tissue is left undisturbed by staying in the space of Smith. Watertight closure is performed with interrupted 4-0 polydioxanone suture (PDS) and a running 5-0 PDS. An artificial erection is performed after each ellipse is excised to determine results. If the penis is not straight, further ellipses are excised to straighten it.

Once straight, the Buck fascia is closed. Two small suction drains are placed superficial to the Buck fascia. The skin is reapproximated with a 4-0 Vicryl suture, and a small Foley catheter is placed overnight. A bio-occlusive dressing is placed. The Foley catheter is removed on postoperative day 1. One drain is removed in the morning as well, and if output is low, the other is removed that afternoon and the patient is discharged from the hospital.

Patients with lateral curvature may have associated ventral curvature or rarely dorsal curvature. On occasion, patients with lateral curvature may only have lateral curvature. In patients with only lateral curvature, this can be approached through a small incision at the maximal point of curvature. After an artificial erection is obtained, the point of maximal curvature is identified and a small incision is made on the contralateral side at the site of maximal convexity. Again, there is minimal dissection of the dorsal neurovascular structures. After 3-0 Prolene sutures are placed, an artificial erection is performed; if straight, ellipses are excised and closed as previously discussed (Fig. 81.4).

Although uncommon, congenital dorsal curvature is usually approached through a circumcising incision. The corpus spongiosum is partially mobilized so that small incisions in the corpora can be placed just lateral to the ventral midline. The techniques used are those previously described, and the postoperative course is similar to that of the patient with ventral curve.

## Yachia Longitudinal Plication

There are other techniques described for the repair of congenital curvature. Yachia (6,7) described a plication procedure using longitudinal incisions in the tunica albuginea that are closed transversely. The long side is therefore plicated without excising tunica. The procedure is similar to that previously described, with an incision through the previous circumcision scar and complete mobilization (Fig. 81.5).

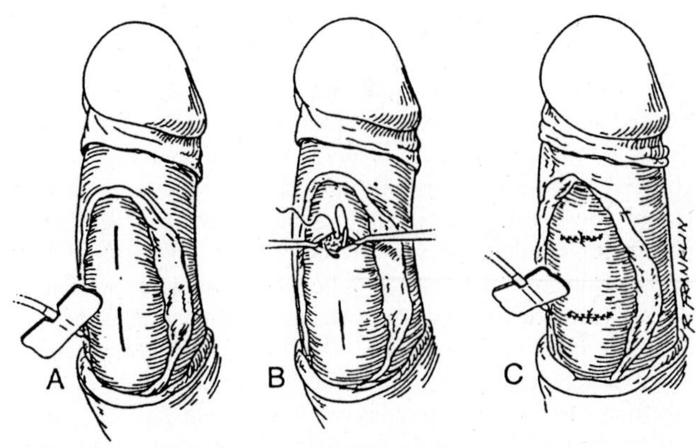


FIGURE 81.5 Technique after Yachia for correction of curvature, in this case a patient with congenital lateral curvature. **A:** The Buck fascia is reflected, exposing the lateral tunica albuginea. **B:** Longitudinal incisions are created at the area of maximal curvature as demonstrated by artificial erection. **C:** The longitudinal closures are closed transversely, with artificial erection demonstrating good straightening of the penis.

## Multiple Parallel Plication

Multiple parallel plication (MPP) is another technique used in the repair of congenital curvature of the penis without excising any tunica albuginea. In the original description, a pharmacologic agent is used to induce an erection. A circumcising incision is performed, the penis is degloved, and the deep dorsal artery and vein are identified. The dorsal neurovascular bundle does not need to be dissected and freed. Multiple deep plication sutures are placed into the tunica albuginea at the point of maximal curvature between the deep dorsal artery and vein using four to six nonabsorbable 3-0 braided sutures. Some of the sutures may not be fully tied down to prevent overcorrection. For patients with lateral or ventral lateral curvature, the sutures are placed more laterally using the same vertical orientation. When the patient has dorsal curvature, a ventral incision is made and the sutures are placed just lateral to the corpus spongiosum (which does not need to be mobilized).

## Penile Disassembly

Perovic et al. (5) proposed a penile disassembly technique in hopes of avoiding penile shortening with the plication procedures. This technique requires complete disassembly of the penis into its component parts, these being the glans cap with its neurovascular bundle dorsally, the urethra ventrally, and the corporal bodies. Unfortunately, this technique only straightened the penis satisfactorily in 68% of patients, and on occasion a plication procedure was required.

## Chordee without Hypospadias

The corpus spongiosum is rarely the limiting factor in these patients, even if they appear to have obvious abnormalities. The curvature in these patients is due mainly to the inelasticity of the ventral aspect of the corporal bodies. After the dysgenic tissue is excised, if there is residual chordee a small incision can be made in the ventral midline of the corporal bodies after an artificial erection is obtained. The erectile tissue is not entered with this incision, and this allows the ventral tunica to move laterally and noticeably straightens the penis. If this is unsuccessful in correcting the curvature, the dorsal neurovascular structures are mobilized and a small ellipse of tunica is excised and closed as discussed earlier (Fig. 81.6).

Some advocate the use of dermal grafts for patients with chordee without hypospadias, especially in those patients with severe chordee or those with a smaller-than-average penis. This approach does not shorten the penis as a plication procedure would, but there are complications associated with it as well. The major concern with placing a dermal graft is the risk of veno-occlusive dysfunction. This is a known complication when using dermis in adult patients with Peyronie disease. Grafting the corpora cavernosa in any patient has the potential for creating erectile dysfunction. The majority of patients seek surgery as young adults, and the occurrence of erectile dysfunction can be devastating. It is thought that the pediatric patient may not develop veno-occlusive dysfunction because no tunica is excised and a much smaller graft is used than in the adult. No long-term studies have been published following these patients into adult life to determine the risk.

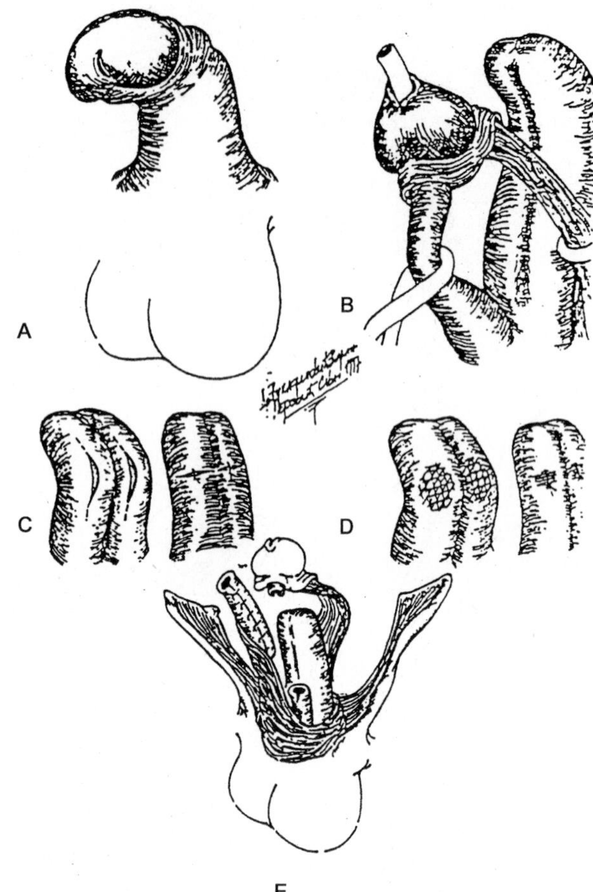

FIGURE 81.6

# OUTCOMES

## Complications

Surgical complications associated with congenital penile curvature surgery are relatively rare. This is in general a healthy population of patients. Complaints of penile shortening and penile irregularity from suture sites are heard. There are also complaints of suture granuloma and sometimes pain at the plication site. Temporary loss of glans sensation has been reported in the past, and there is one report of a patient with permanent loss of sensation. Postoperative erectile dysfunction is extremely rare, and there is one reported case of penile necrosis secondary to a tourniquet; we would not recommend using these.

## Results

The reported success rates of the Nesbitt, Yachia, and incision/plication surgical procedures vary from 85% to 100%. Eight percent of MPP patients were satisfied with their correction, although two of the eight had to undergo a second procedure to correct a residual 15% curvature. All patients did notice the sutures, but only one considered them bothersome.

## References

1. Baskin LS, Lue TF. The correction of congenital penile curvature in young men. *Br J Urol* 1998;81:895–899.
2. Devine CJ, Horton CE. Chordee without hypospadias. *J Urol* 1973; 110: 264–271.
3. Kaplan GW, Brock WA. The etiology of chordee. *Urol Clin North Am* 1981;8:383–387.
4. Kramer SA, Aydin G, Kelalis PP. Chordee without hypospadias in children. *J Urol* 1982;128:559.
5. Perovic SV, Djordjevic MLJ, Djakovic NG. A new approach to the treatment of penile curvature. *J Urol* 1998;160:1123–1127.
6. Yachia D. Modified corporoplasty for the treatment of penile curvature. *J Urol* 1990;143:80–82.
7. Yachia D, Beyar M, Aridagon A, et al. The incidence of congenital penile curvature. *J Urol* 1993;150:1478–1479.
8. Nyirady P, Kelemen Z, Banfi G, et al. Management of congenital penile curvature. *J Urol* 2008;179:1495–1498.

# CHAPTER 82 ■ RECONSTRUCTION OF THE PENIS FOR COMPLICATIONS OF PENILE ENHANCEMENT SURGERY

GARY J. ALTER

Surgery to enlarge the length and girth of the penis has been developed over the past few decades. These procedures were derived from a combination of plastic surgical techniques and urologic reconstructive pediatric and adult surgical operations (1–4). Penile length is increased by releasing the suspensory ligament of the penis followed by the use of penile weights or stretching devices. The girth is increased by either injecting fat into the dartos fascia or by inserting dermal fat grafts or alloplastic cellular matrix grafts such as AlloDerm. Unfortunately, these procedures are often based on faulty concepts or are not performed meticulously, which has led to many complications. The purpose of this chapter is to outline techniques to reconstruct these unfortunate outcomes.

## DIAGNOSIS

A patient may present for reconstruction after only a penile lengthening procedure or also with some girth enhancement. An assortment of deformities can occur (6,7).

### Penile Lengthening

Penile lengthening is achieved by releasing the suspensory ligament of the penis and the postoperative use of penile weights or stretching devices (Fig. 82.1A) (6). A small lower transverse pubic incision is usually used, but many surgeons advance infrapubic skin onto the penis using a V-Y advancement flap (Fig. 82.1B and C) (6,8,9). This theoretically increases penile length and gives the penis the appearance of increased flaccid length. This penile length gain is disputed in most cases, and it can cause the penis to appear either longer or shorter in the flaccid state. The V-Y flap is based distally at the penopubic junction, varying from a small (2- to 3-cm) to a large base. The larger flap encompasses the entire dorsal base of the penis and part of the scrotum, which causes interruption of a significant portion of the proximal penile dartos fascia and skin. The blood supply and lymphatic drainage of the penis are thus partially interrupted, which can cause healing complications such as flap tip loss, poor wound healing with wound dehiscence, and postoperative swelling. Healing problems predispose to hypertrophic or wide scars, which create hairless suprapubic scars and depressions (Figs. 82.2A and 82.3A) (6). The large V-Y flap also advances thick, hair-bearing tissue onto the penis, which frequently creates an unnatural hump at the penile base and the appearance of a low-hanging penis. The penis can appear surrounded by the scrotum (scrotalization) with an overhanging large pubic fat pad, which makes the penis look shorter and hidden. A V-Y flap can also create "dog-ears" at the distal scrotal flap incision. Smaller V-Y advancement flaps cause less frequent problems but have wound and aesthetic complications.

An occasional patient may complain of penile shortening after release of the suspensory ligament. Since there is a dead space between the pubic symphysis and the corpora, it is possible for the corpora to reattach in a shortened position. This dead space can be filled by a proximally or distally based fat flap transposed from the spermatic cord (5). However, most doctors tell the patients to stretch the penis after the release without filling the space.

Penile instability is very rare after suspensory ligament release and usually results from an overly aggressive release of the corporal bodies from the inferior rami of the ischium. If the release is limited to one fingerbreadth on the midline of the pubic symphysis, this will not occur. Dorsal nerve or vessel injuries are prevented by staying directly on the pubic periosteum of the midline of the symphysis with the penis on full stretch and by not releasing the corpora laterally. A mild decrease in the elevation of the erection can occur with release but is not problematic.

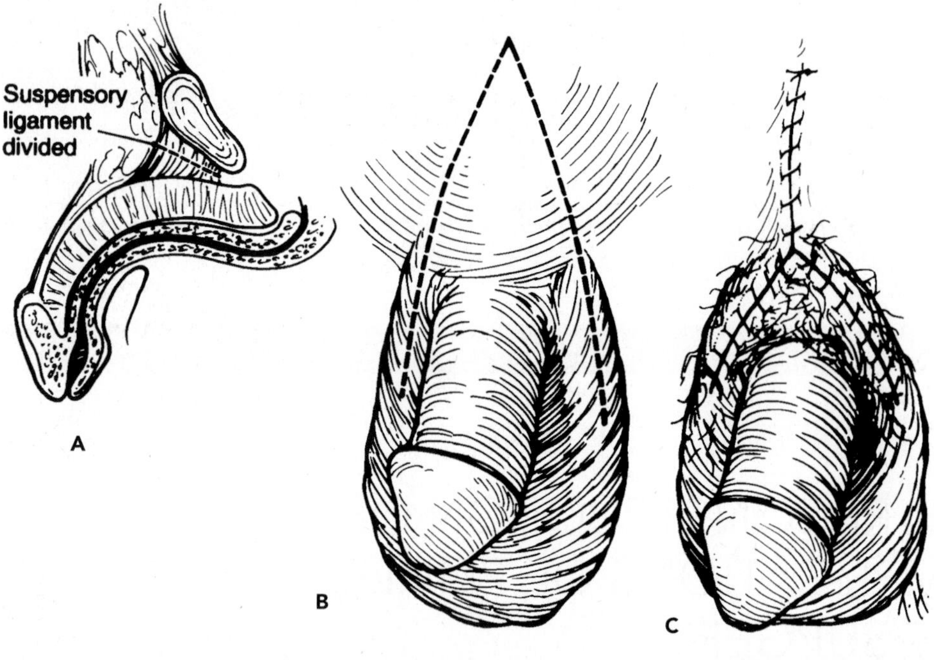


FIGURE 82.1 Method commonly used for penile lengthening that often causes penile deformities. **A:** The suspensory ligament is released. **B:** A large V-Y advancement flap is designed. **C:** The flap is advanced, resulting in hair on the proximal penile shaft, bilateral dog-ears, and a lower-hanging penis.

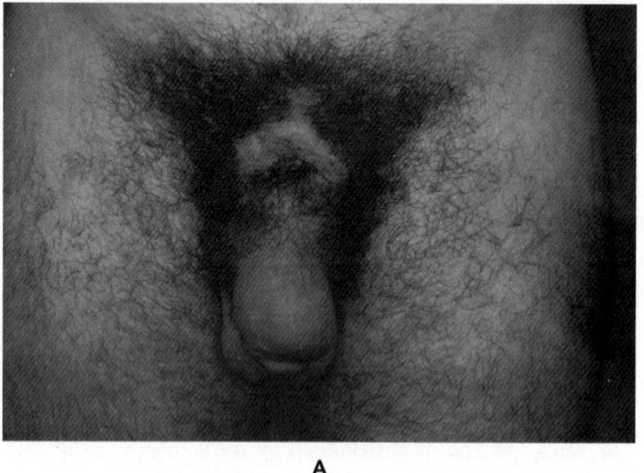


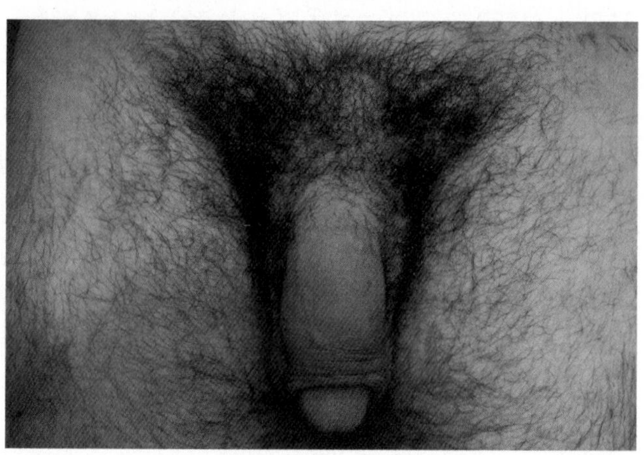


FIGURE 82.2 Patient who had release of the suspensory ligament, a large V-Y advancement flap, and multiple fat injections (same case as in Fig. 82.4). **A:** The deformity shows a low-lying penis, hair on the proximal shaft, bilateral dog-ears at the penoscrotal junction, a shorter-appearing penis, wide pubic scars, and a large amount of fat in the shaft. **B:** Reconstruction after complete reversal of the V-Y advancement flap, correction of V-Y dog-ears, scar revision, selective removal of fat nodules, and contouring of the left side of the penis.

## Fat Injections

Significant complications can occur from autologous fat injections (Figs. 82.2 and 82.3) (6). The penis is a relatively cylindrical structure, so asymmetrical fat absorption can cause severe penile distortion with S-shaped curves, nodules, or liquefied cysts. The larger the amount of fat injected, the greater the chance of deformities. However, a small amount injected may not result in any long-term girth gain. If fat is injected in large amounts, it frequently migrates distally during the initial postoperative period, which causes unsightly fat deposits at the corona. If the fat migrates distally causing penile skin to stretch, and if the patient has a large V-Y flap, then the previously circumcised patient can look uncircumcised. If another circumcision removes this "excess foreskin," then there can be inadequate shaft skin to perform a later reversal of the V-Y advancement flap, thus limiting the reconstructive options.

Patients sometimes complain of inadequate rigidity if a large amount of injected fat survives, since the fat bulk overwhelms the corporal erection. Intercourse difficulty can also occur if large fat injections are combined with a large V-Y flap, since a soft penile shaft is combined with loose penile skin.

## Dermal Fat Grafts

Dermal fat grafts are used for girth enlargement by either inserting dermal fat strips into the dartos along the length of the

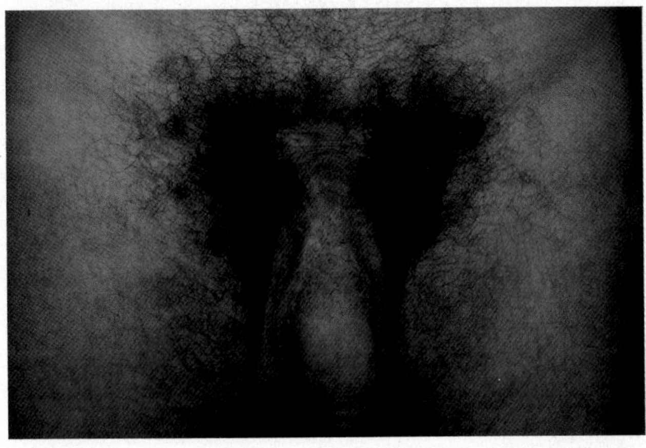

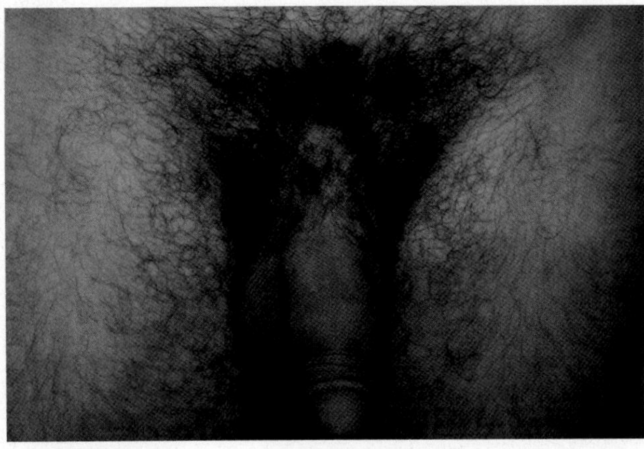

A B

FIGURE 82.3 Patient who had release of the suspensory ligament, a large V-Y advancement flap, and fat injections. **A:** The deformity shows a low-lying penis, hair on the proximal shaft, bilateral dog-ears at the penoscrotal junction, a short-appearing penis, wide pubic scars, and fat in the shaft. **B:** Reconstruction after partial reversal of the V-Y advancement fat, correction of the V-Y dog-ears, scar revisions, and selective removal of fat. Complete reversal of the V-Y flap was not possible due to previous partial loss of a portion of the V-Y flap (Fig. 82.5).

penis or by wrapping sheets of dermal fat around the shaft between the dartos and the Buck fasciae. The grafts are stabilized proximally and distally with sutures to prevent migration. If the grafts do not survive completely and symmetrically, the patient can have fibrosis and firmness. As a result, the patient can complain of loss of penile length, asymmetry, curvature, or firm areas.

### AlloDerm

The use of AlloDerm for girth expansion was motivated by the unpredictability of dermal fat graft "take" with its cosmetically unappealing donor site scars. Layers of AlloDerm are inserted in a plane above the Buck fascia and stabilized proximally and distally. Theoretically, the AlloDerm is a matrix for the ingrowth of tissue and becomes integrated into the area. However, this does not always occur, so the AlloDerm can be isolated within a capsule. The AlloDerm does not stretch, so the patient may complain of loss of length or curvature. Patients may also complain of an unnatural feel of the penis, migration of the AlloDerm, asymmetry, and visual and palpable deformities. Many cases of infected AlloDerm have occurred, resulting in chronic infections and chronic skin sinuses with or without skin loss.

## INDICATIONS AND ALTERNATIVE THERAPY

Secondary surgery should not be performed until at least 6 months after the enlargement operation to allow resolution of swelling, revascularization of tissue, and elimination of induration. The patient must prioritize his reconstructive options and be specific as to his desires. He may want only limited fat removal, partial or no V-Y flap reversal, or minimal scar revisions. Additionally, it may not be possible to correct all deformities at one or multiple operations. The operative plan and probable result are realistically discussed with the patient and often shown while he is standing in front of a mirror. Discussion of expectations and goals is crucial to preventing a hostile patient.

## SURGICAL TECHNIQUE

Most commonly, patients complain of complications of the large V-Y advancement flap. Usually most of the extensive pubic, penile, and scrotal scars is excised (Figs. 82.2B and 82.4) (6). The defect after the excision of the Y scar is much larger than usually anticipated, with the width of the vertical scar often exceeding 5 cm. Ideally, the V flap is re-elevated to near its original previous location, aligning the hair on the V flap with the pubic hair. This will result in an inverted U closure. Determination needs to be made as to the adequacy of shaft skin so that complete reversal of the flap does not shorten the penis (either real or illusory) and restrict an erection. An artificial erection achieved by intracavernosal injection of Prostaglandin $E_1$ helps to determine skin adequacy. Penile skin may be inadequate from a previous circumcision or from flap tip loss from the first procedure. If the skin is inadequate, partial V-Y reversal results in a Y-shaped scar with a shorter vertical limb (Figs. 82.3B and 82.5) (6). No restriction of erection should occur by pulling on the erect penis.

The scrotal dog-ears are excised at this time. Prolonged lymphedema or potential skin loss can occur if the skin and dartos fascia at the penile base are completely circumcised while repairing these scars and dog-ears. The method of closure and dog-ear excision is determined by judging the tightness of the penile skin, taking care not to restrict an erection. If the discrepancy of skin occurs from reversal of the V-Y flap, the dog-ear is usually followed along the lateral scrotum. Alternatively, the dog-ear is excised from the midportion of the lateral side of the incision, which creates a lateral dart instead of following the dog-ear around the penile base (Fig. 82.5B) (6).

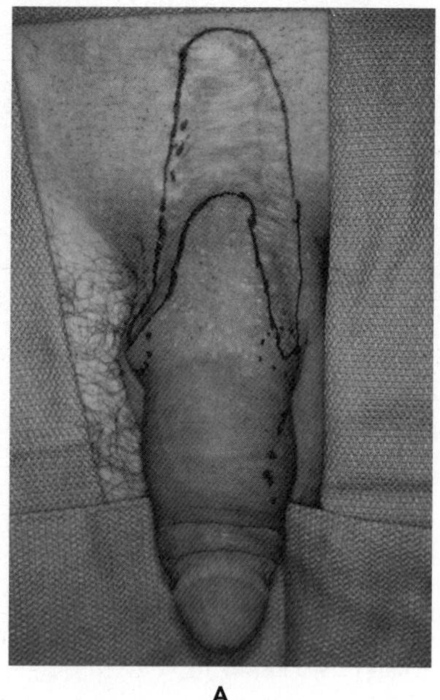

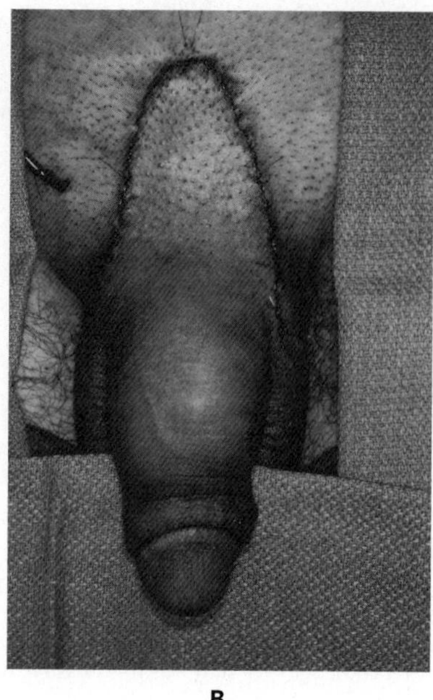

A B

FIGURE 82.4 Complete reversal of V-Y flap (same case as Fig. 82.2). **A:** A scar is marked for excision with solid lines. Fat nodules to be excised are marked by dotted lines on the penis. **B:** Complete reversal of V-Y advancement flap, resulting in a semicircular incision line. Hair on the V-Y flap is aligned with the pubic hair. The marked fat nodules were removed.

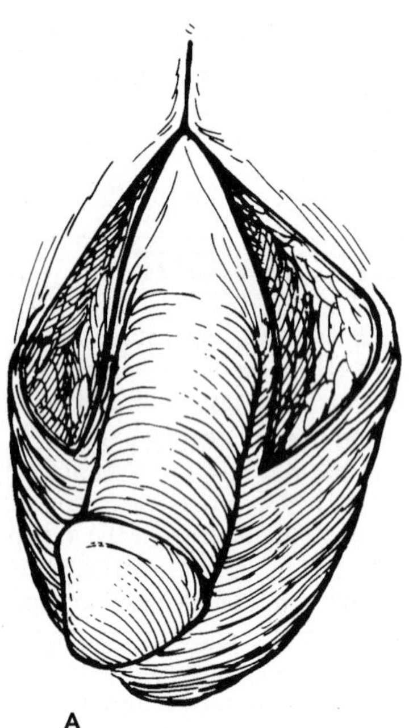

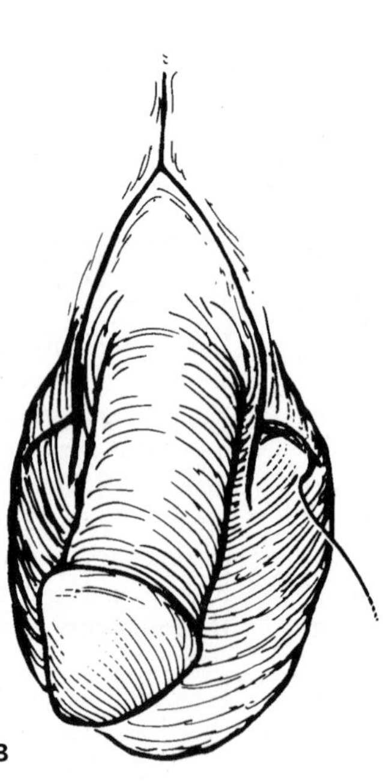

A B

FIGURE 82.5 Diagram of partial reversal of V-Y advancement flap. **A:** The V-Y flap is reversed as much as possible while preserving penile length. A Y-shaped incision line results. **B:** Dog-ears are removed by making lateral darts. They can also be removed by extending the incision along the lateral scrotum.

In order to reduce the risk of redeveloping a hypertrophic scar, closure should be meticulous and without tension. The skin, subcutaneous tissue, and Scarpa's fascia are undermined and then closed in layers. Intradermal buried 4-0 Monocryl sutures are placed, and the skin is closed with a subcuticular suture. A suction drain is used. If the upper limb of the vertical incision pulls, then one of two small Z-plasties can be used to release tension and decrease the risk of a restrictive hypertrophic scar contracture. Even with careful closure, the common junction of the V flap with the vertical closure often has minor healing problems. Also, over time, the pulling of the penis on the incision lines usually causes some stretching of the scars.

If complete V-Y reversal is not possible due to restriction of erection and if a significant dorsal flap hump is present, then the subcutaneous fat on the V flap is conservatively excised to prevent devascularization. This will improve the appearance, but the difference in skin texture and hair growth continues.

The resulting scars are better with the inverted U scar than with the partial V-Y reversal. The reversal and scar revision improve the wide or hypertrophic scars and eliminate the suprapubic concavity. They eradicate the unsightly dorsal penile hump and proximal hair-bearing tissue by redraping the penis with the normal shaft skin and elevating the penis to its normal position. They can also improve or eliminate complaints of penile instability.

Rereleasing the suspensory ligament is performed only if the patient complains of penile shortening. Transposing a fat flap from the lipomatous tissue of the spermatic cord

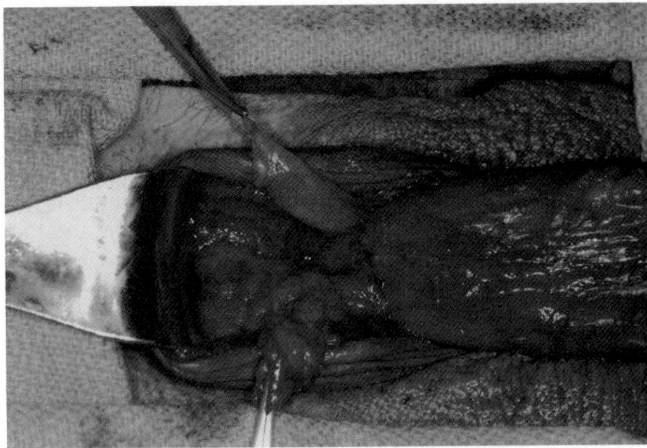

FIGURE 82.6 Bilateral fat flaps from the medial spermatic cords are transposed to the midline to fill the dead space at the penile base.

eliminates the dead space between the corpora and pubic symphysis (Fig. 82.6). The fat flap is dissected off of the cord, divided proximally to leave an intact distal random blood supply, and sutured to the periosteum with 3-0 absorbable sutures.

## Infected Fat

The surgeon should remove fat nodules or contour the penile fat through a limited or complete circumcising incision, a medial raphe incision, or part of the previous V-Y or pubic transverse incision. New incisions on the penile shaft are unsightly and unnecessary. Deforming or firm fat deposits are very conservatively removed and then the residual fat is contoured while leaving as much dartos fascia as possible. It is very important not to overresect fat, which will create an unsightly concavity, so resection is performed in very small increments. Large diffuse fat deposits are usually removed through a circumcision incision (Fig. 82.7). Only rarely will a patient want all of the fat removed. Skin necrosis, chronic lymphedema, or skin attachment to the Buck fascia can occur with overly aggressive removal of the dartos fascia. The goal of fat removal is contouring, not complete fat elimination.

If the patient is undergoing V-Y flap reversal, then simultaneous removal of fat nodules or deforming deposits is limited. If large diffuse fat deposits are removed at the same time as V-Y reversal, then further flap disruption and dartos fascia injury decrease the flap vascularity and possibly prolong edema. Fat is removed through a several-centimeter tunnel on one or

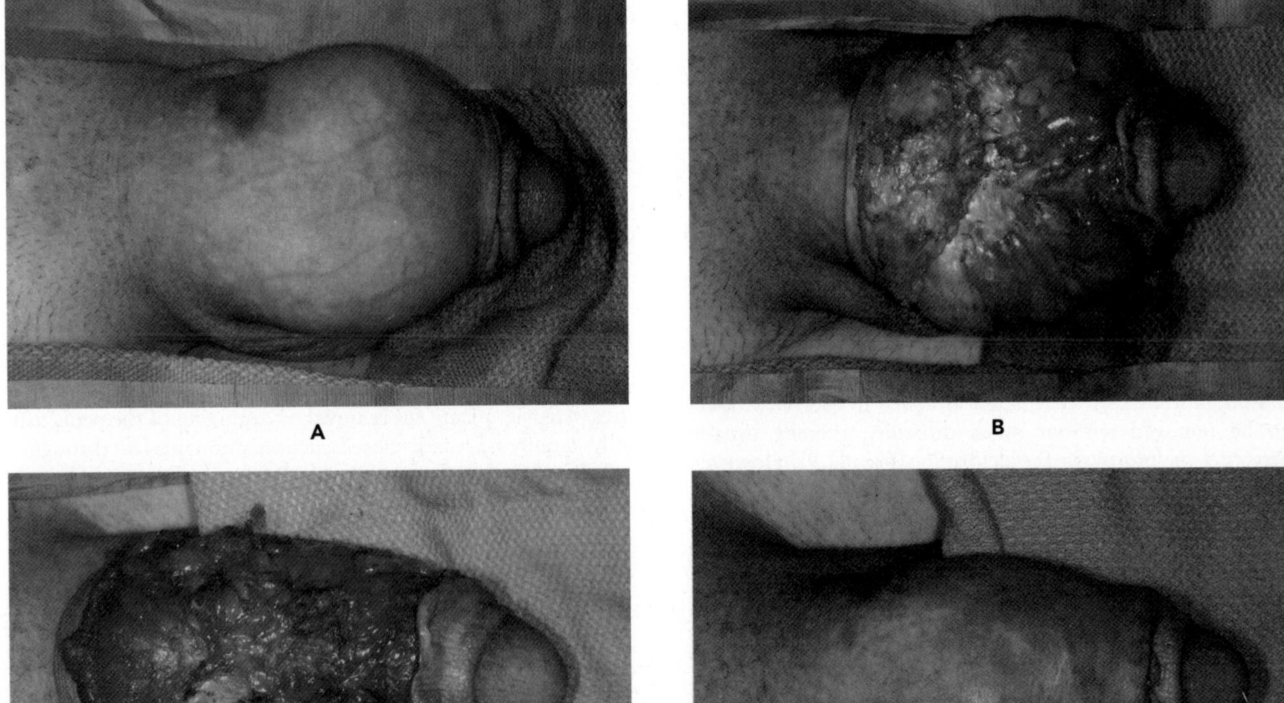


FIGURE 82.7 **A:** Patient with large volume of injected penile fat that is causing obvious convexities. **B:** Circumcision incision reveals diffuse fat deposits. **C:** Residual fat after contouring. Patient did not want complete fat removal. **D:** Penis appearance after closure. It is very difficult to achieve ideal symmetrical contouring.

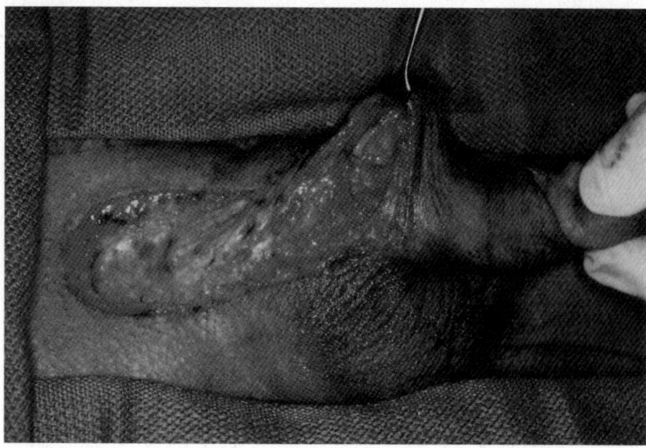

FIGURE 82.8 The fat nodule is removed through a 1- to 2-cm tunnel underneath the V flap, thereby preserving the vascularity of the flap.

both limbs of the distal V-Y incisions without undermining the flap, or through a limited circumcision incision (Fig. 82.8) (6). One side of the penis should be kept relatively inviolate to retain good blood and lymphatic drainage. Degloving of the penis through a circumcision incision and V-Y flap reversal should not be done at the same time. Residual deposits removed at least 6 months later are done through a circumcision, median raphe, or previous incision.

## Dermal Fat Grafts and AlloDerm

The presence of dermal fat grafts and/or AlloDerm creates a different set of problems. Patients complain of penile curvatures, shortening, abnormal texture, chronic infections, and penile distortion. Sometimes patients present after a combination of procedures, such as a V-Y advancement flap and fat injections followed by dermal fat grafts and/or AlloDerm. The graft causing the problems can usually be totally removed through one or a combination of circumcision, median raphe, or pubic incisions. Penile shaft incisions should be avoided. An indurated, scarred graft that is not attached to the Buck fascia can be removed without much difficulty, thereby usually correcting or improving the deformity (Fig. 82.9). However, patients with penile shortening, penile curvature, or chronic infection caused by graft necrosis and subsequent scar contracture may require a difficult dissection. An extensively fibrotic AlloDerm or dermal graft may adhere to the Buck fascia, so extreme care must be taken not to injure the dorsal neurovascular bundles. Loupe magnification is usually necessary. Removal of the scarred dermal graft may eliminate the deformity, curvature, or penile length restriction, but total return of penile length may not occur due to permanent scarring of the skin or of the dartos or Buck fascia. Under rare circumstances, severe fibrosis may require penile plication. The surgeon should preserve as much dartos fascia as possible during graft removal to prevent skin adherence to the Buck fascia.

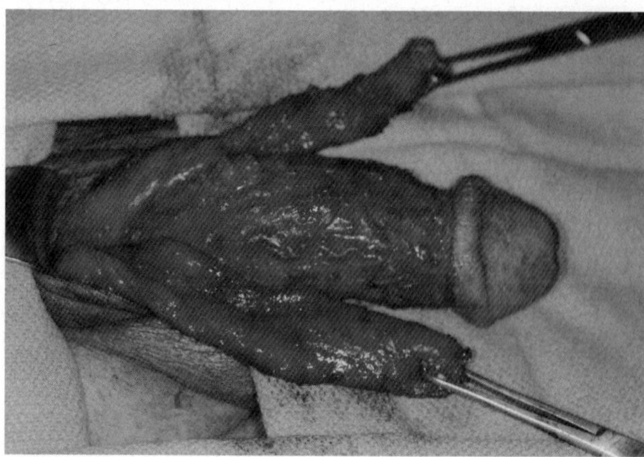

FIGURE 82.9 AlloDerm elevated off the Buck fascia without much difficulty.

A dead space often occurs at the penopubic junction after graft removal. The space must be filled with vascular fat flaps transposed from the medial spermatic cord or other nonadherent vascularized tissue, which will help prevent penile shortening (Fig. 82.6). A closed-suction drain is necessary.

Chronic infections with dermal fat grafts or AlloDerm are often seen. The patient presents with infected sinuses and chronic drainage, erythema, and so forth. Removal of the entire graft is usually recommended. These cases should initially be treated in the short term with antibiotics, but aggressive removal of the dermal grafts and AlloDerm should be done without delay if infection persists. Persistent delay in treatment may complicate the ability of the patient to regain his penile length due to scar contracture of the dartos and Buck fasciae and the skin. These cases can have tragic consequences.

On occasion, dorsal penile skin loss has been seen from both AlloDerm and dermal fat grafts, probably from venous congestion due to stretched dartos fascia and skin combined with a tight dressing. These situations have disastrous consequences. A thick skin graft is needed to maintain the length of the penis or secondary contracture of the wound will cause a short, distorted penis. Unfortunately, the graft has a poor color match, is cosmetically deforming, and may not allow complete length preservation.

The dressing used around the penis after any of these surgeries is crucial to recovery, since it will help prevent hematomas and swelling that can lead to secondary deformities. Any significant fat removal or degloving of the penis usually requires a small closed-suction drain placed through a small pubic stab incision. A thin Duoderm dressing is loosely wrapped around the penis followed by a loose Coban. This dressing is not removed for a minimum of 2 days but frequently longer. It is then replaced with a circumferential loose Tegaderm wrap. Drains are left until they cease draining.

# OUTCOMES

## Complications

Frequently, the patient states that he would just like to return to the appearance of his penis prior to any penile enlargement surgery, but this is usually impossible. Sometimes he just wants to achieve some final girth increase, albeit minor, in order to feel that the enlargement process was not a total loss.

After reversal of the V-Y flap, the patient may have some eventual stretching of the scar so that it does not give the fine line that was present initially. However, there is certainly an improvement in the scar and elimination of the other V-Y deformities.

Despite careful contouring of injected fat, it is extremely difficult to have a smooth penile contour postoperatively. Residual nodules, lumps, concavities, and convexities are common and certainly expected, but the goal is to minimize them as much as possible. Complete removal of all injected fat is to be avoided if at all possible, since restricting bands can form at the penopubic junction and the skin can attach to the Buck fascia. The surgeon should always try to leave some dartos and fat in order to minimize this possibility. Secondary surgery to repair these bands and attachments is not always successful.

Removal of restricting bands and tissue of the penopubic junction from dermal fat grafts or AlloDerm can still result in erectile restriction at the base of the penis from bands and scar tissue. Postoperatively, tissue reaction at the penopubic junction often requires time and multiple Kenalog injections to soften the palpable bands attached to the corpora and penile skin. These usually soften >6 months. On occasion, a limited release of these recurrent bands needs to be performed. Penile weights or stretching devices can also be helpful to prevent scar retraction or regain some length.

## Results

Reconstruction of the complications of these procedures is challenging, requiring an understanding of blood flow, tissue transfer techniques, and plastic surgical principles. These patients are often psychologically devastated when coming for reconstruction, since they started with self-esteem issues that led to their initial penile enlargement operation. Thus, the reconstructions must be done with extreme care in order to regain the patients' penile form and function and psychological health.

The outcome for most patients with reconstruction is usually satisfactory. There is a low complication rate if meticulous technique is used. However, more than one operation is often necessary. The vast majority of these patients are able to resume normal sex lives without being self-conscious after correction of their deformities.

## *References*

1. Johnston JH. Lengthening of the congenital or acquired short penis. *Br J Urol* 1974;46:685.
2. Kelley JH, Eraklis AJ. A procedure for lengthening the phallus in boys with exstrophy of the bladder. *J Pedriatr Surg* 1971;6:645.
3. Kabalin JN, Rosen J, Perkash I. Penile advancement and lengthening in spinal cord injury patients with retracted phallus who have failed penile prosthesis placement alone. *J Urol* 1990;144:316.
4. Rigaud G, Berger RE. Corrective procedures for penile shortening due to Peyronie's Disease. *J Urol* 1995;153:368.
5. Alter GJ. Penile enhancement surgery. *Techniques Urol* 1998;4:70.
6. Alter GJ. Reconstruction of deformities resulting from penile enlargement surgery. *J Urol* 1997;158:2153.
7. Wessells H, Lue TF, McAninch JW. Complications of penile lengthening and augmentation seen at 1 referral center. *J Urol* 1996;155:1617.
8. Long DC. Elongation of the penis [in Chinese]. *Chung-Hua-Cheng-Hsing-Shoa-Shang-Wai-Ko-Tsa-Chih* 1990;6(2):17–19, 7.
9. Roos H, Lissoos I. Penis lengthening. *Int J Aesthetic Restorative Surg* 1994;2:89.

# CHAPTER 83 ■ ILEAL CONDUIT URINARY DIVERSION

MICHAEL C. LEE AND ERIC A. KLEIN

Despite the established role of continent catheterizable and orthotopic voiding urinary diversion techniques, the ileal conduit remains the most common form of urinary diversion performed worldwide. The operation, first described by Bricker in 1950, maintains this popularity in large part because of its applicability to a wide variety of urologic disorders, its tolerability in patients with often significant comorbidities, and its adaptability to almost all patients' anatomic constraints.

## DIAGNOSIS

The ileal conduit may be constructed as part of a reconstruction following extirpative pelvic surgery, such as radical or simple cystectomy and pelvic exenteration, or as a diversion with the bladder left in situ, such as in cases of neuropathic bladder refractory to conservative management. The clinical evaluation in these patients is therefore directed to their bladder pathology.

## INDICATIONS FOR SURGERY

Before choosing an ileal conduit, patients should be counseled on all forms of diversion. Comorbidities such as renal insufficiency (serum creatinine >2.5 mg per dL), bowel disease (inflammatory or malignant), extreme obesity, or neurologic illness that prevents the ability to perform self-catheterization may make incontinent diversion a wise choice. While it was suggested in the past that patients with cardiovascular or pulmonary diseases may do better with the shorter, simpler conduit diversions, newer evidence suggests that perioperative morbidity is equivalent with conduit and continent diversions (12).

## ALTERNATIVE THERAPY

Continent catheterizable or orthotopic voiding diversions are the most common alternatives to conduit diversion. If the aforementioned concerns make conduit diversion preferable to continent diversion, there still exist options regarding the bowel segment to be used and the type of ureteroenteric anastomosis. Jejunal conduits are associated with a higher incidence of metabolic complications, characterized by hypochloremia, hyponatremia, hyperkalemia, and acidosis, but may be the only viable option in certain patients due to previous surgery, irradiation, or concomitant bowel diseases (6).

Colonic conduits, which are thought to be more protective of kidney function by some surgeons due to the ability of colonic conduits to accommodate nonrefluxing anastomoses, may be preferable in children and adults with a longer life expectancy. A transverse colon conduit may be safest in patients who have undergone pelvic irradiation due to its higher intra-abdominal position outside of the radiation field. Another use of colon for conduits is the sigmoid conduit diversion in patients who are undergoing pelvic exenteration, with a transverse colostomy that avoids the potential morbidities of a bowel anastomosis.

Other potential urinary diversions include an ileovesicostomy, which can be used in patients undergoing diversion for reasons other than malignancy and avoids the complications associated with ureteral mobilization and ureteroenteric anastomoses. In patients requiring urinary diversion with life expectancies less than several months, percutaneous nephrostomy tubes should be considered.

## SURGICAL TECHNIQUE

Most patients can tolerate an at-home preoperative regimen of a clear liquid diet 1 to 2 days before surgery, followed by 4 L of polyethylene glycol or two bottles of magnesium citrate on the afternoon before surgery. Broad-spectrum intravenous antibiotics are given at the time of the surgery. The stoma site should be selected after examining the patient in the supine, seated, and standing positions. To best accommodate an appliance, the site should not be too near the anterior superior iliac spine, costal margin, umbilicus, surgical scars, or skin folds. The usual ideal location is just medial to the linea semilunaris on a line between the umbilicus and the anterior superior iliac spine.

Markedly obese patients may require a higher site to allow them to perform stoma care under direct vision. In instances where there is a question regarding the ideal stoma site, ambulatory trials of pouching candidate sites can help determine the optimal location.

Laparoscopic techniques have been reported for the creation of ileal conduits and have been successfully performed with no reported intra- or postoperative complications (10). However, the open approach remains the standard given the technical difficulty and the need to remove the specimen through a minilaparotomy when performing a concurrent cystectomy.

A low midline incision extending from just above the umbilicus down to the symphysis pubica allows for exposure of the bladder for cystectomy as well as bowel exposure for the conduit portion of the procedure. The patient is positioned supine. A Bookwalter-type retractor may be used to retract the bowel from the cystectomy field, and then the blades may be repositioned on the abdominal wall for the conduit procedure. The posterior peritoneum is incised at the pelvic inlet above the iliac vessels, where the ureter can be found coursing over the vessels. The ureters are then dissected with care distally and transected as close to the bladder as possible. A lesser degree of proximal mobilization is also usually necessary. During mobilization of the ureter, care should be taken to maintain its blood supply by leaving a generous amount of periureteral soft tissue. The distal ends of the ureters may be clipped to allow dilatation while the ileal conduit is harvested and prepared.

The terminal ileum is then identified and examined. If signs of inflammatory bowel disease, radiation changes, or insufficient mesenteric length are not present, then this segment is in general preferred for conduit formation. The mesentery is examined by transillumination, and the watershed area between the ileocolic artery and the right colic artery is selected for the distal mesenteric incision. This is typically located 15 to 20 cm from the ileocecal valve, and the preservation of this length of terminal ileum suffices to maintain bile salt and vitamin B12 absorption. The bowel incision is continued proximally into the mesentery to allow the distal end to reach the stoma site without tension. Figure 83.1 demonstrates the isolation of the ileal segment.

The mesentery is again transilluminated, and a relatively avascular site is selected for the proximal incision. The optimal length of the conduit differs from patient to patient due to differences in body habitus and the degree of ureteral mobilization. The longest length of conduit should not exceed the distance between the sacral promontory and the stoma site; usually, if there is adequate left ureteral mobilization, a shorter length than this is optimal. If there is any question regarding the length, one should err on the longer side, as redundant conduit is much easier than insufficient conduit to treat intraoperatively. The conduit and its mesentery are positioned caudal to the rejoined bowel and its mesentery.

Standard hand-sewn or staple techniques are then performed to reestablish bowel continuity. The mesenteric window is also closed with a shallow running suture to prevent internal bowel herniation. Care should be taken during closure of the mesenteric window to avoid ligation of the ileal blood supply, which might compromise the healing of the anastomosis. Sterile towels are placed beneath the isolated ileal conduit, which is irrigated free of enteric contents with an antibiotic solution.

At this point in the procedure, either stoma formation or ureteroenteric anastomosis can be performed. This choice is based on surgeon preference. If ureteral stents are to be used, performing the ureteroileal anastomosis first allows for easier antegrade passage of the stent out of the distal end of the conduit. Creating the stoma first provides for more optimal localization of the ureteroileal anastomotic sites and helps direct the optimal level of the sigmoid mesentery through which the left ureter should be passed.

Construction of the stoma begins with the excision of a circular plug of skin around the preselected stoma site. Dissection is carried down to the anterior rectus fascia, and a cruciate incision is made in this layer. A Kelly clamp is passed bluntly through the rectus muscle after palpating for and avoiding the pulsations of the inferior epigastric artery. The Kelly is then spread to create a hiatus that allows the passage of two fingers; this breadth is usually ideal for not compromising the mesenteric blood flow to the stoma while minimizing the risk of parastomal hernia.

In the standard end stoma ("rosebud") technique, the efferent end of the conduit is grasped and pulled through the abdominal wall defect until the end is 2 to 3 cm above the skin surface. Each of the four tabs of the cruciate incision is then sutured to the bowel serosa, taking care not to pass sutures through the bowel mesentery. Absorbable sutures are then passed through the mucosal edge of the bowel, then the bowel serosa and muscularis deep to the skin edge, and finally through the dermal tissue just deep to the skin edge. Care is taken not to suture the bowel mucosa to the epidermis, as this can lead to mucosal rests that complicate pouching of the stoma. Figure 83.2 shows the technique of suture placement for the end stoma. Four quadrant sutures placed in this manner usually suffice to evert the stoma; additional sutures may be placed for reinforcement.

In obese patients or patients with a short mesentery, a Turnbull loop stoma should be considered. The distal end of the loop is closed with absorbable sutures (if the GIA stapler was used to harvest bowel, no additional closure is needed). An umbilical tape is passed through the mesentery at its border, with the ileum about 3 cm proximal to the end of the conduit. The tape is then grasped and pulled through the

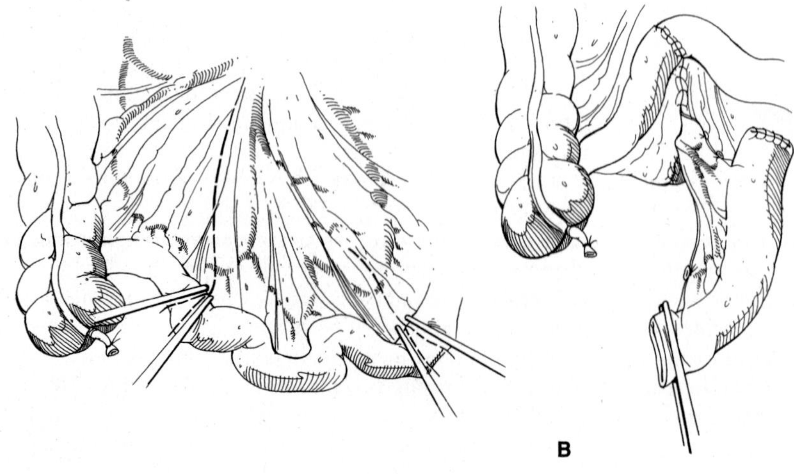


**FIGURE 83.1 A:** The ideal segment of bowel for the ileal conduit spares the terminal 10 to 20 cm of ileum and should require minimal ligation of mesenteric vessels to harvest. **B:** Once isolated, the conduit mesentery is positioned caudal to the bowel mesentery, which is reapproximated with a running silk suture.

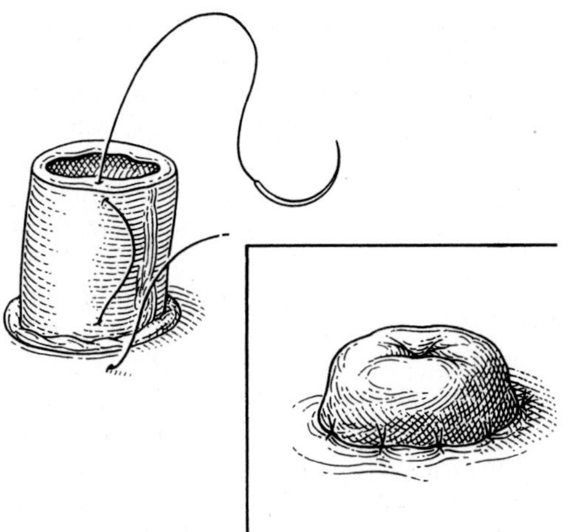

FIGURE 83.2 The end stoma ("rosebud") is everted by passing sutures first through a full-thickness bite at the cut edge, then through the bowel serosa at the skin level, and finally through the dermis.

abdominal wall defect. A stomal rod is in general passed through the umbilical tape defect to prevent stomal retraction; this is then sutured in place and left in for 1 to 2 weeks. The blind end of the loop is positioned cephalad, and the loop is opened transversely nearer to the distal limb. The stoma is then matured using eversion sutures in the same manner described for the rosebud stoma. The technique for end-loop stoma formation is detailed in Fig. 83.3.

A long-term follow-up study comparing the results of these two techniques revealed no major differences in outcome (2). Patients with an end stoma had slightly more ischemic complications, while those with the loop stoma required more frequent repair of parastomal hernias, presumably due to the need for a wider aperture in the abdominal wall.

Principles to consider in the creation of the ureteroenteric anastomoses include the maintenance of an adequate distal ureteral blood supply, the avoidance of tension on the anastomosis, the documentation of malignancy-free status in the distal ureter (if the diversion is performed for cancer), and the avoidance of ureteral kinking. While techniques for nonrefluxing ureteroileal anastomoses have been described (9), the benefits of a nonrefluxing anastomosis have never been conclusively proven. Moreover, these techniques are likely to result in higher rates of anastomotic obstruction and prevent the use of the simple loopogram study in the evaluation of upper-tract pathology after ileal conduit formation. Therefore, the freely refluxing end-to-side (Bricker) and conjoined end-to-end (Wallace) techniques remain the most commonly performed and recommended techniques.

In the Bricker technique, the proximal end of the conduit is either left closed if staples were used in the bowel harvest or closed in two layers with absorbable sutures. The left ureter is passed through a hole created in the sigmoid mesocolon. This hole is typically created at the level of the sacral promontory but may be moved cephalad or caudally to avoid ureteral kinking. A site on the conduit where the ureter lies naturally is incised down to the submucosal layer. The submucosa is grasped with forceps, and a small portion is excised along with its mucosa. The ureter is then spatulated, and a single-layer full-thickness anastomosis is performed with 4-0 or 5-0 interrupted absorbable sutures. Prior to closing the anastomosis, silicone ureteral stents may be placed; these can be guided in through the stoma using a Kelly clamp or a copper suction tip. Anchoring sutures through the ureteral adventitia and the bowel serosa may be placed 1 to 2 cm proximal to the anastomosis. Figure 83.4 demonstrates the ideal locations of the ureteroenteric anastomoses using the Bricker technique.

The Wallace technique involves leaving the proximal end of the conduit open. The ureters are spatulated for a distance slightly greater than the conduit diameter. The posterior edges may be joined side-by-side or end-to-end using two running 4-0 absorbable sutures. One suture is then used to join the back walls of the conjoined ureters and the conduit, after

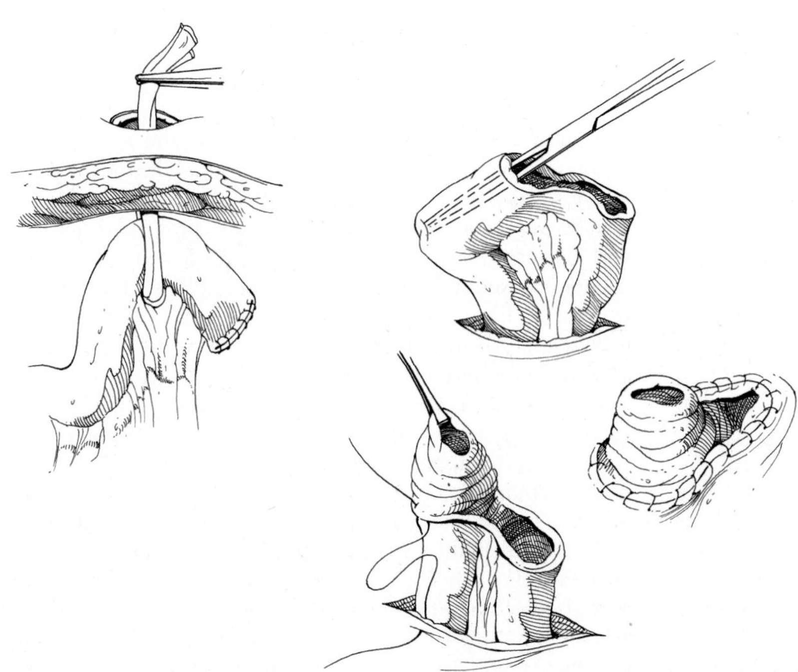

FIGURE 83.3 Creation of the end-loop stoma. The defunctionalized limb is positioned cephalad.

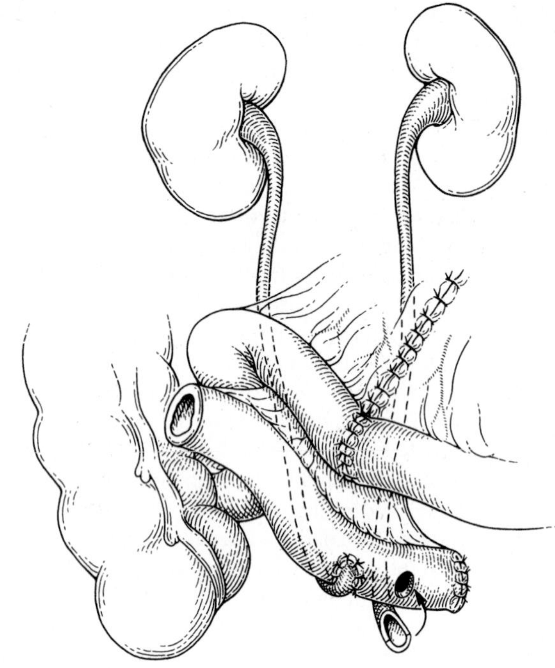

FIGURE 83.4 Ideal placement of the vesicoenteric anastomoses using the Bricker technique. The spatulated ureters should pass under the conduit and lie without tension or kinking.

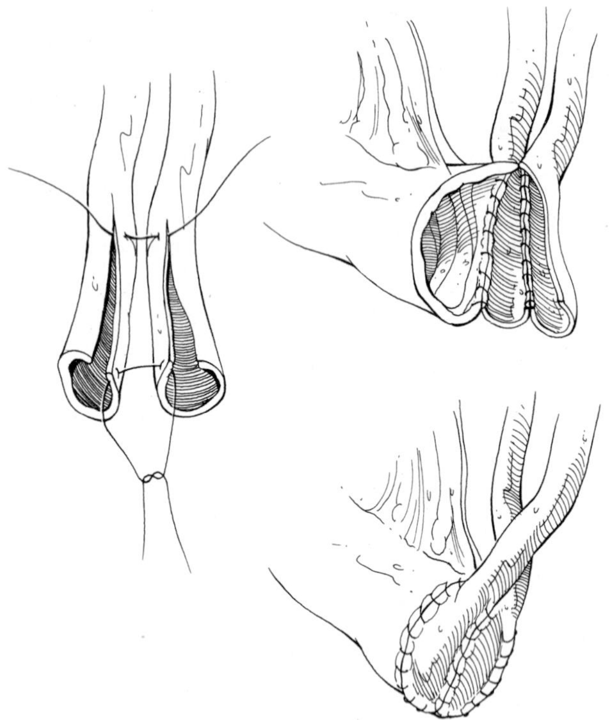

FIGURE 83.5 The side-to-side Wallace technique creates a widely patent vesicoenteric anastomosis at the "butt" end of the conduit.

which the anterior walls are closed. The side-to-side Wallace technique is detailed in Fig. 83.5. Stents may be passed prior to closure of the anterior wall. This technique allows for the rapid creation of a widely patent ureteroileal anastomosis; its theoretical disadvantage is that a process creating obstruction of one ureter (recurrent malignancy, anastomotic stricture) is more likely to cause bilateral obstruction.

After performing the ureteroileal anastomosis, the proximal end of the conduit is retroperitonealized by sewing the cut edges of the peritoneum to the conduit. Closed-suction drains (Jackson–Pratt type) are placed in the area of the ureteroileal anastomoses and maintained for the first few postoperative days.

The return of bowel function is the major determinant of the length of the postoperative hospital stay; this is evidenced by similar lengths of hospitalization for urinary diversion procedures with and without cystectomy. Most patients can expect a hospital stay of 6 to 8 days in centers with well-defined clinical pathways (1). Nasogastric decompression is optional. The conduit also experiences an ileus, and its return of peristalsis parallels that of the small bowel; therefore, some surgeons advocate placement of a cut Foley or Rob-Nel catheter to promote conduit drainage in the first few postoperative days. There is no consensus for the optimal length of ureteral stenting (if it is performed at all); the timing of stent removal is left to the discretion of the surgeon. Jackson–Pratt drains are left in place until the drainage is negligible; if drainage persists at high levels several days postoperatively, the drain fluid should be sent for creatinine analysis to rule out a urine leak. If a rod is left under the stoma, this may be removed prior to discharge.

Counseling and teaching by the enterostomal therapist should begin in the preoperative period and continue during the hospitalization. The patient or his or her caregivers should be competent in all aspects of stoma care prior to discharge. Follow-up care is tailored to the individual patient; in most cases, a periodic serum renal profile is indicated. In patients undergoing cystectomy for malignancy, urine cytology should be followed. The upper tracts can be assessed via a loopogram, avoiding the toxicity of intravenous contrast agents.

# OUTCOMES

## Complications

The mortality rates for cystectomy and diversion have steadily decreased over the years since Bricker's initial description; in a recent series a mortality rate of 0.3% was reported (1).

The most common morbidity causing prolonged hospital stay is ileus (1). This usually resolves quickly with nasogastric decompression; failure to do so after a few days should prompt a diagnostic workup for bowel obstruction. Urine leak at the ureteroileal anastomosis or from the conduit closure and urosepsis are the most common urologic complications of the procedure. Urine leaks can usually be managed successfully with placement of an abdominal drain and percutaneous nephrostomy diversion.

Late complications of ileal conduits are common but usually not severe. Stomal stenosis has been reported in up to 29% of ileal conduits (11); proper stoma construction can decrease this incidence. Definitive treatment includes removal or partial resection of conduit. Parastomal hernias have been reported in 14% of patients with obesity as an independent risk factor (8); stoma relocation may be superior to fascial repair in these cases. Hyperchloremic metabolic acidosis can occur but is rare in well-functioning conduit; the presence of more than a mild acidosis should prompt an evaluation for obstruction or redundancy of the conduit. Alkalinizing agents (sodium bicarbonate) or chloride transport blockers (chlorpromazine, nicotinic acid) can effectively treat this acidosis. Ureteroileal anastomotic strictures are also uncommon (about 6% in older series); these can be successfully managed with dilation with a cutting balloon (about a 50% success rate), with open surgical repair (76% long-term success) (4), or chronic ureteral stents. The Wallace anastomosis has been reported to have a lower stricture rate than the Bricker (7).

Acute pyelonephritis occurs commonly in patients with ileal conduits (18% of patients) (5). Indeed, bacteriuria can be found in up to three-fourths of ileal conduit urine specimens (5). Most of these can be safely observed without treatment, as patients seem to tolerate this chronic colonization well, and few progress to acute pyelonephritis. Infections with *Proteus* or *Pseudomonas* are associated with deterioration of the upper tracts and should therefore be treated.

Deterioration in renal function occurs in a significant portion of patients undergoing conduit diversion; over the long term, 50% of patients have radiographic evidence of functional deterioration at 15-year follow-up, and up to 7% of patients can develop renal failure requiring dialysis (5). Renal function should be monitored periodically, and declines in function should alert the clinician to examine for correctable causes of renal dysfunction.

## Results

The ileal conduit has provided reliable urinary diversion for patients with a variety of underlying illnesses for over 50 years. Continent catheterizable diversions and orthotopic neobladders continue to gain acceptance, and recent studies have focused on quality-of-life outcomes after continent and incontinent diversions. Existing studies are unable to prove that continent reconstruction is superior to conduit diversion (4). Unfortunately, as younger, thinner, and healthier patients undergo continent diversion while older and more frail patients undergo ileal conduit, a real comparison of the quality of life after these procedures will likely never be possible. Still, it is clear that ileal conduit is a simple form of diversion that is well tolerated by most patients and has fewer contraindications than continent diversions. These factors make it likely that the ileal conduit will continue to play a major role in many urologists' practices.

## *References*


1. Chang SS, Baumgartner RG, Wells N, et al. Causes of increased hospital stay after radical cystectomy in a clinical pathway setting. *J Urol* 2002;167:208–211.
2. Chechile G, Klein EA, Bauer L, et al. Functional equivalence of end and loop ileal conduit stomas. *J Urol* 1992;147:582–586.
3. DiMarco DS, LeRoy AJ, Thieling S, et al. Long-term results of treatment for ureteroenteric strictures. *Urology* 2001;58:909–913.
4. Gerharz EW, Mansson A, Hunt S, et al. Quality of life after cystectomy and urinary diversion: an evidence based analysis. *J Urol* 2005;174:1729–1736.
5. Hautmann RE, Abol-Enein H, Hafez K, et al. Urinary diversion. *Urology* 2006;69(1A):17–49.
6. Klein EA, Montie JE, Montague DK, et al. Jejunal conduit urinary diversion. *J Urol* 1986;135:244–246.
7. Kouba E, Sands M, Lentz A, et al. A comparison of the Bricker versus Wallace ureteroileal anastomosis in patients undergoing urinary diversion for bladder cancer. *J Urol* 2007;178:948–949.
8. Kouba E, Sands M, Lentz A, et al. Incidence and risk factors of stomal complications in patients undergoing cystectomy with ileal conduit urinary diversion for bladder cancer. *J Urol* 2007;178:950–954.
9. Leduc A, Camey M, Teillac P. An original antireflux ureteroileal implantation technique: long-term follow-up. *J Urol* 1987;137:1156–1158.
10. Matin SF, Gill IS. Laparoscopic radical cystectomy with urinary diversion: completely intracorporeal technique. *J Endourol* 2002;16:335–341.
11. Dahl DM, McDougal WS. Use of intestinal segments and urinary diversion. In: Wein AJ, Kavoussi LR, Novick AC, et al., eds. *Campbell-Walsh urology*, 9th ed. Philadelphia: Saunders Elsevier, 2007.
12. Parekh DJ, Gilbert WB, Koch MO, et al. Continent urinary reconstruction versus ileal conduit: a contemporary single-institution comparison of perioperative morbidity and mortality. *Urology* 2000;55:852–855.


# CHAPTER 84 ■ TRANSVERSE COLONIC CONDUIT

MARGIT FISCH, RUDOLF HOHENFELLNER, RAIMUND STEIN, AND JOACHIM W. THÜROFF

Since the first publication in 1969 (10), the transverse colonic conduit has been increasingly implemented in patients with urologic or gynecologic malignancies and additional radiotherapy (2,9,11,12). With its cranial position outside the irradiation field, it fulfills the requirement of not being irradiated, which is of utmost importance for a segment to be used for urinary diversion. Not only the transverse segment but also the ascending and descending colon can be used, which offers an adaptation to the individual patient's situation. The ascending and descending colon are located in a retroperitoneal position, as is the sigmoid colon. There are no limitations with regards to short ureters. As part of the colon, the segments offer the option of antirefluxing as well as refluxing ureteral implantation (3,5,8,13) and for positioning of the stoma either to the left or right upper abdomen. In addition, colon can be used either in an isoperistaltic or anisoperistaltic way and is less prone to stoma stenosis than ileum when used for creation of a conduit.

In patients with total damage of the ureters by irradiation or retroperitoneal fibrosis and in patients with recurrent urothelial tumors (7), a direct anastomosis of the conduit to the renal pelvis represents an option (pyelotransverse pyelocutaneostomy) (4).

## DIAGNOSIS

Preoperatively, an intravenous (IV) urography should be performed to evaluate the upper urinary tract. An enema with water-soluble contrast medium should be done to exclude diverticuli or polyps. The bowel is irrigated with Ringer lactate solution (8 to 10 L) via a gastric tube or oral intake of 5 to 7 L of Fordtran solution. The day before surgery, positioning of the stoma should be done. The best position is in the epigastric region; the attached stoma plate has to be checked in sitting, lying, and standing positions of the patient.

## INDICATIONS FOR SURGERY

Indications for transverse colonic conduit include urinary diversion in patients with urologic or gynecologic malignancies and irradiation damage of bowel and distal ureters. Other indications are urinary incontinence in patients with radiation cystitis, complex vesicovaginal and rectovesicovaginal fistulas after irradiation, recurrent retroperitoneal fibrosis, Crohn disease, and unsuccessful primary urinary diversion requiring conversion. Complex cases of prostate cancer with a history of irradiation or brachytherapy, recurrent stenosis of the posterior urethra, and/or fistula formation in addition to a small bladder capacity represent rare indications. In patients with recurrent urothelial tumors, anastomosis of the conduit to the renal pelvices allows direct endoscopic access to the calices. Absolute contraindications for the transverse colonic conduit are irradiation of the upper abdomen, previous extensive colon resection, and ulcerative colitis.

## ALTERNATIVE THERAPY

In young and healthy patients capable of catheterization, a continent transverse pouch (6) represents an alternative.

## SURGICAL TECHNIQUE

Instruments required include a basic kidney set with additional instruments for intra-abdominal surgery, a Siegel retractor, suction, and a basin containing prepared iodine solution for disinfection. Absorbable monofilament sutures like polyglycolic acid 4-0 are used for closure of the conduit and intestinal anastomosis to re-establish bowel continuity as well as to create the stoma. The ureters are implanted using 5-0 and 6-0 sutures. Intraoperatively, a gastric tube (alternatively gastrostomy), a rectal tube, and a central venous catheter are placed.

Access is gained by a median laparotomy. Both ureters are identified at the points where they cross over the iliac vessels and are dissected in the cranial direction. The dissection toward the bladder goes down until the irradiated level is reached. The ureters are cut above the irradiated field where they show good vascularization. There should be capillary arterial bleeding out of the ureteral wall and spontaneous urine efflux. The ureteral stump is ligated, and the cranial end is marked by a stay suture. Depending on the remaining length of the ureters, it is decided which one can be brought to the opposite side by a retromesenteric pull-through. The retromesenteric entrance should be wide enough and the path of the ureter slightly curved in order not to angle or compress it.

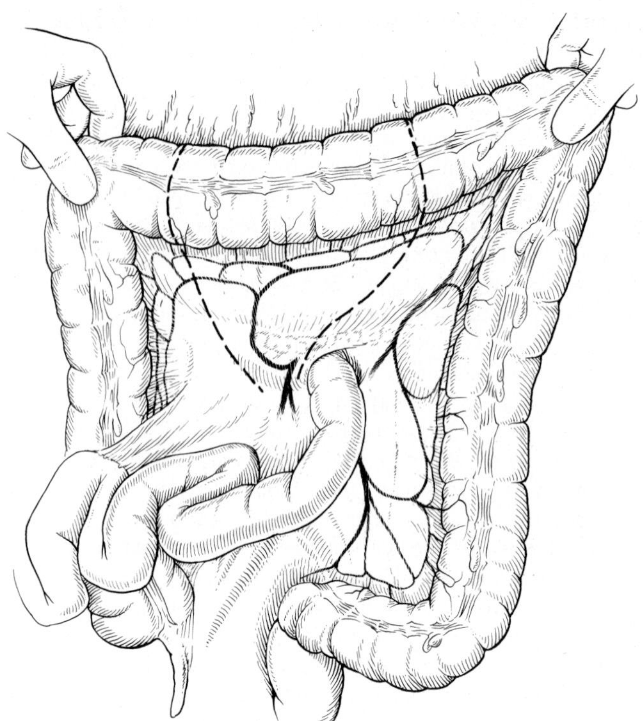

FIGURE 84.1 A bowel segment of approximately 15 cm in length in patients with normal weight is selected, respecting the course of the vessels.

A bowel segment of approximately 15 cm in length in patients with normal weight is selected respecting the course of the vessels (Fig. 84.1). The length of the segment depends on the thickness of abdominal wall. Stay sutures outline the segment. Bowel mobilization differs depending on the segment chosen: If the ascending segment is selected, the right colonic flexure is mobilized. The greater omentum is separated from the transverse colon over a distance of 10 to 15 cm starting at the right side. When the descending colon is chosen, the left colonic flexure has to be mobilized, and the left part of the omentum has to be separated from the transverse colon. The selection of a transverse colonic segment makes it necessary to mobilize both the right and left flexure and to completely separate the greater omentum from the transverse colon.

The mesentery of the selected segment is incised lateral to the supplying artery, and the arcade is divided between mosquito clamps and ligated. The fat is dissected from the seromuscularis of the bowel in the area where the segment will be cut, and bleeding vessels are coagulated. The segment is isolated without the use of clamps so that the bleeding out of the ends can be seen. The segment is cleaned using moist sponges.

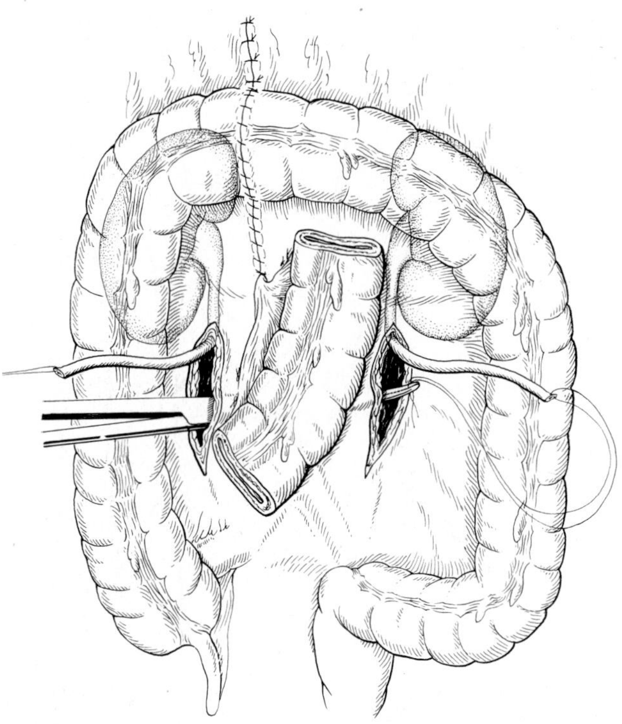

FIGURE 84.2 Bowel continuity is reestablished by a one-layer seromuscular suture using polyglycolic acid 4-0, and the mesenteric slit is closed by running suture.

Bowel continuity is re-established by a one-layer seromuscular suture using polyglycolic acid 4-0, and the mesenteric slit is closed by running suture (Fig. 84.2).

One option for ureteral reimplantation uses the refluxing Wallace technique (13). Both ureters are resected to an adequate length and spatulated over a distance of 3 cm. A stay suture is placed at the 6 o'clock position and a ureteral stent inserted. The first suture for anastomosis of the medial margins of the ureters is placed at the 12 o'clock position and tied later. The anastomosis is performed by a running suture of polyglycolic acid 5-0. The ureteral stents are fixed to the ureteral mucosa (polyglactin 4-0 with short reabsorption time) and subsequently brought out through the conduit. The ureteral plate is then anastomosed to the oral end of the conduit by two running sutures of polyglycolic acid 5-0 (Fig. 84.3A). When the conduit is positioned on the right side and the left ureter is relatively short, it can be implanted antidromically to the right ureter (like the "crossed hands of a ballerina"; Fig. 84.3B).

An alternative method of refluxing ureteral reimplantation is a direct implantation using a "buttonhole" technique. The conduit is longitudinally opened in the area of the taenia libera over a length of 3 to 4 cm starting at the oral end. Two stay sutures are placed at the back wall of the conduit. The mucosa in between is excised and the seromuscular layer incised to create an entrance for the ureter. The ureter is pulled through and implanted by two anchor sutures at the 5 and 7 o'clock positions (polyglycolic acid 4-0) and mucomucous sutures (polyglycolic acid 5-0). A stent is inserted, fixed, and led out through the conduit (Fig. 84.4). The contralateral ureter is implanted in the same manner and the conduit closed.

An antirefluxive ureteral implantation can be performed using the Goodwin–Hohenfellner technique (1). The conduit is longitudinally opened over a length of approximately 4 cm starting from the end chosen for ureteral implantation (proximal end preferable). Four stay sutures are placed to facilitate ureteral implantation. A submucosal tunnel is dissected starting from the end of the conduit (tunnel length, 3 to 4 cm). The bowel mucosa at the end of the tunnel is incised, and the ureter is pulled through the respective submucosal tunnel. After spatulation and resection of the ureter to an adequate length, implantation is performed by one anchor suture at the 6 o'clock position, grasping the seromuscularis of the bowel and all layers of the ureter (polyglycolic acid 5-0). The anastomosis is completed by mucomucous single sutures (polyglycolic acid 6-0).

To secure the ureteral implantation, a 6Fr ureteral stent is inserted in each ureter and fixed to the bowel mucosa

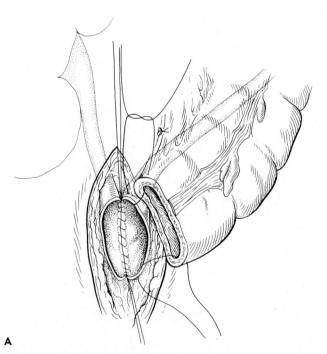

A

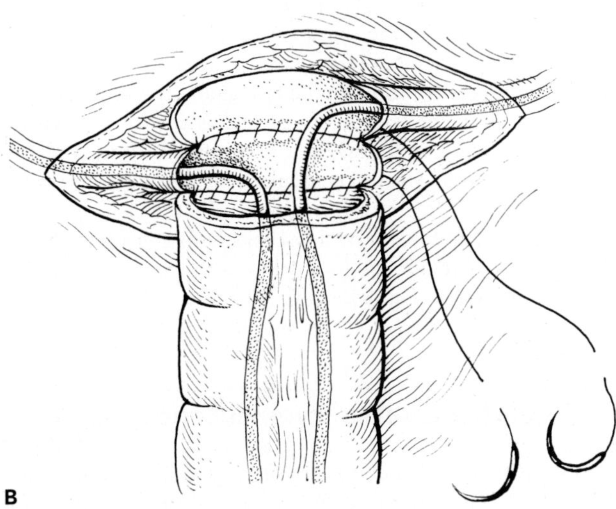

B

FIGURE 84.3 The ureteral plate is then anastomosed to the oral end of the conduit by two running sutures of polyglycolic acid 5-0. **A:** Classical implantation; **B:** Implantation with left ureter in opposite direction to the right.

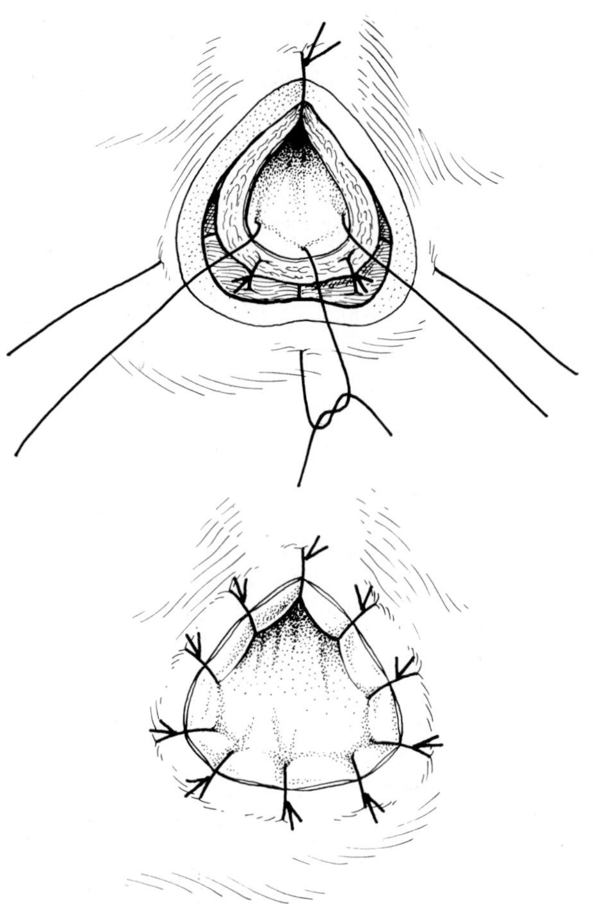

FIGURE 84.4 The mucosa in between is excised and the seromuscular layer incised to create an entrance for the ureter.

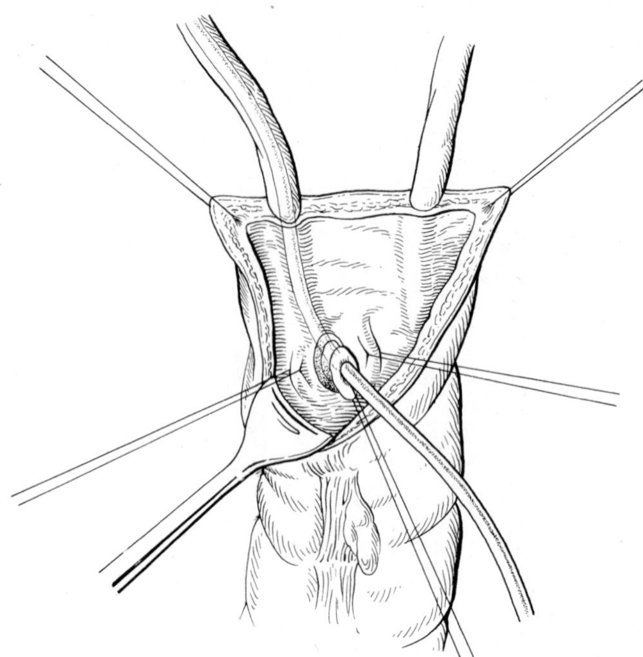

FIGURE 84.5 For implantation of the second ureter, a second tunnel is prepared beside and parallel to the first; the implantation is done in the same way.

(polyglactin 4-0 with short reabsorption time). For implantation of the second ureter, a second tunnel is prepared beside and parallel to the first; the implantation is done in the same way (Fig. 84.5). Both ureteral stents are led out through the aboral end of the conduit. The proximal ends of the conduit and of the incision line in the area of the taenia libera are closed (single seromuscular sutures, polyglyconic acid 4-0).

A circular area of the skin (approximately 3 cm in diameter) is excised. The abdominal fascia is crosslike incised, and the conduit is pulled through the fascial and the skin opening, together with the ureteral stents, by means of two Allis clamps after having freed the distal end of the conduit of fat and epiploic appendages. The seromuscularis of the conduit is fixed to the abdominal fascia by circular single stitches of polyglycolic acid 3-0, and the oral end of the conduit is anastomosed to the skin by circular single stitches of polyglycolic acid 5-0 everting the stoma (Fig. 84.6).

## Pyelotransverse Pyelocutaneostomy

An extensive bowel mobilization is necessary, including caecum, root of the mesentery, the Treitz ligament, and the right and left colonic flexures (Fig. 84.7A). The omentum majus is completely dissected from the transverse colon, and the bursa omentalis is opened. The bowel is exteriorized out of the abdomen. The ureters are cut at the ureteropelvic junction, and the renal pelvis is longitudinally spatulated. A transverse colon segment with a length of 25 to 30 cm and an adequate blood supply is isolated (Fig. 84.7B). After having placed a ureteral stent in a calyx of the right kidney, and fixed it within the renal pelvis (using polyglactin 4-0 with short reabsorption time), an end-to-end anastomosis of the right renal pelvis and the distal end of the conduit is performed using two running sutures of polyglycolic acid 5-0. The ureteral stent is led out through the conduit before the anastomosis is completed. The conduit is brought to the left renal pelvis without tension (Fig. 84.7C). Also on this side, a stent is inserted into the kidney, fixed, and led out through the conduit later. For anastomosis of the renal pelvis with the conduit, the wall of the conduit is incised at the taenia libera over an adequate length, and an end-to-side anastomosis of the renal pelvis and the conduit is done by two running sutures of polyglycolic acid 5-0 (Fig. 84.7D). The stoma formation is identical to the standard technique. In patients with a single kidney, the technique is more simple: a direct anastomosis of the spatulated renal pelvis and the oral end of the isolated bowel segment is performed, and the aboral end is led out through an abdominal stoma created as described previously.

## Surgical Tips

Transilluminating the mesentery with a fiberoptic light source visualizes the vessels and facilitates the selection of the segment

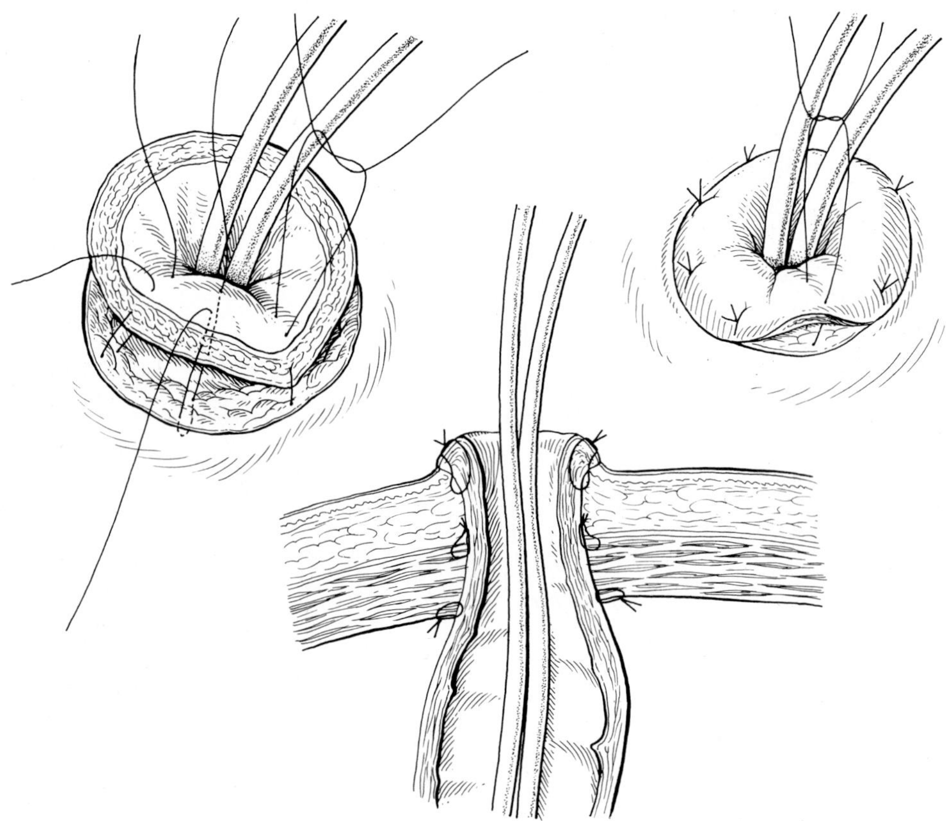

FIGURE 84.6 The seromuscularis of the conduit is fixed to the abdominal fascia by circular single stitches of polyglycolic acid 3-0, and the oral end of the conduit is anastomosed to the skin by circular single stitches of polyglycolic acid 5-0 everting the stoma.

as well as the preparation of the mesenteric slits. When the conduit is positioned on the right side and the left ureter is relatively short, it can be implanted directly to the right ureter (like the crossed hands of a ballerina). This is applicable for the Goodwin–Hohenfellner as well as the Wallace technique. The colonic conduit can be performed so that the urine flow is peristaltic and antiperistaltic and so that the stoma can be alternatively positioned in the right or left upper-abdominal quadrant. For an antiperistaltic application, an extensive mobilization of the Treitz ligament and the descending part of the duodenum becomes necessary; otherwise, compression of the duodenum by the conduit may result. If an isoperistaltic application is preferred, either the right or left colonic flexure can be used for conduit creation. Extraperitonealization of the conduit facilitates revisional surgery, and this can be done through a flank incision. As a result, a transabdominal approach with the need for adhesiolysis can be avoided.

## POSTOPERATIVE CARE

Antibiotics are given for 5 days. As a standard for postoperative care, parenteral nutrition is continued until bowel contractions appear and then gradually reduced. The gastric tube is removed starting from postoperative day 3 after clamping. The rectal tube stays for 3 days. Today, fast-track regimes with early removal of the gastric tube and early oral nutrition are being increasingly implemented. Ureteral stents are loosened after day 9 and removed after day 10, beginning on one side with a check of the kidney by ultrasonography on day 11. Then the second stent is removed. An IV urography demonstrates regular kidney function after stent removal.

The acid-base balance should be checked before the patient is discharged. The patient should be taught about all aspects of stoma care.

## OUTCOME

### Complications and Results

At Mainz University, an incontinent diversion using the transverse conduit was performed in 78 patients. Six of the 78 patients developed early complications requiring revision in 3. Forty-nine of the patients were followed for an average of 81 months. Twenty-two of the 49 patients developed a total of 27 complications, and 11 patients required operative intervention. In the long-term follow-up, the status of the upper-tract dilatation improved or remained stable in 85% of the renal units.

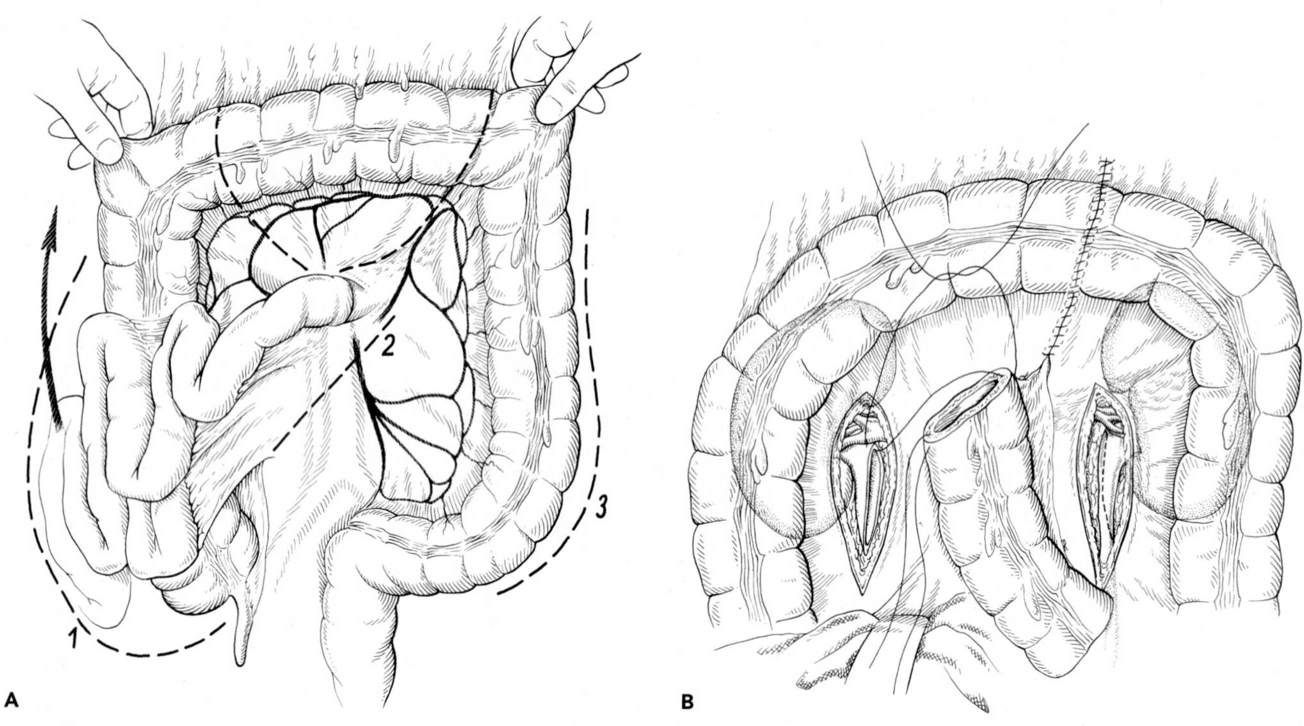


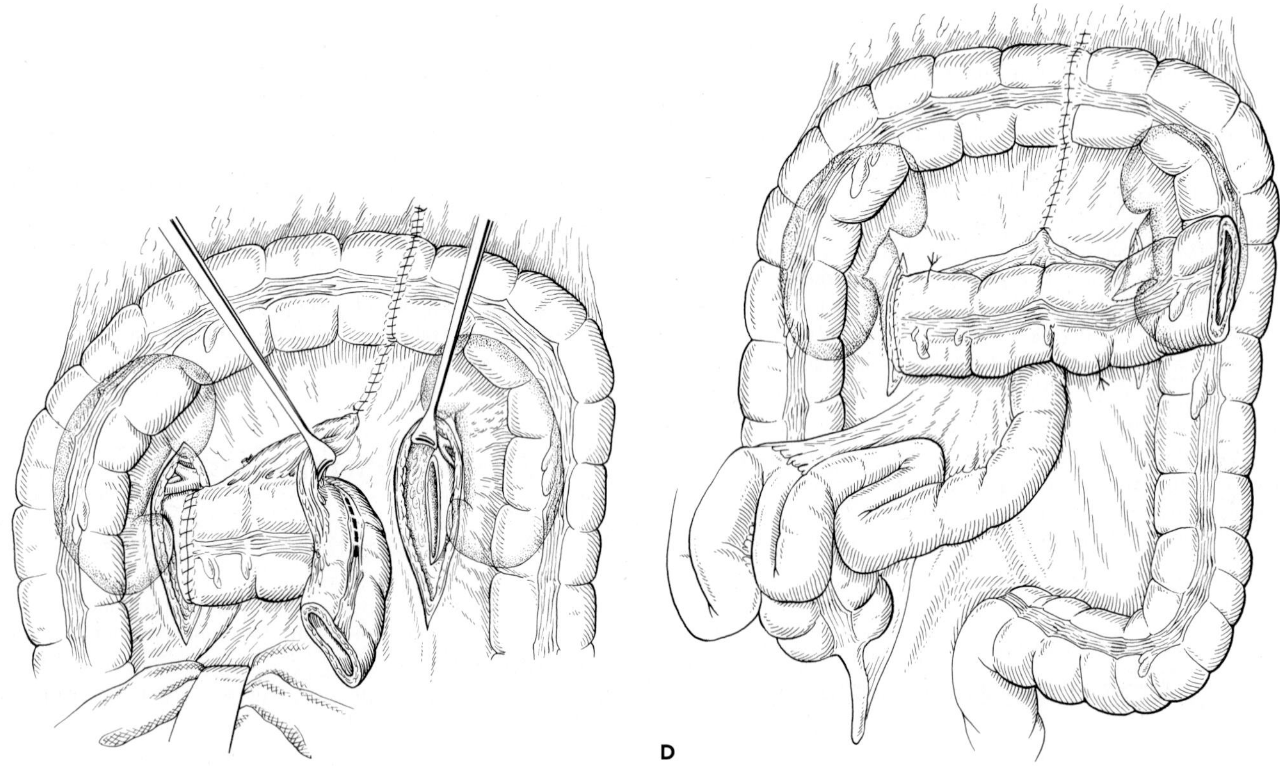


FIGURE 84.7 An extensive bowel mobilization is necessary, including caecum, root of the mesentery, the Treitz ligament, and the right and left colonic flexures.

## *References*

1. Altwein JE, Jonas U, Hohenfellner R. Long-term follow-up of children with colon conduit urinary diversion and ureterosigmoidostomy. *J Urol* 1977;118:832–836.
2. Altwein JE, Hohenfellner R. Use of the colon as a conduit for urinary diversion. *Surg Gynecol Obstet* 1975;140:33–38.
3. Camey M, Le Duc A. L'enterocystoplastie après cystoprostatectomie totale pour cancer de la vessie. *Ann Urol* 1979;13:114.
4. Fisch M, Riedmiller H, Hohenfellner R. Pyelotransverse pyelocolostomy: an alternative method for high urinary diversion in patients with extended bilateral ureter damage. *Eur Urol* 1991;19:142–149.
5. Leadbetter WF, Clarke BG. Five years experience with ureteroenterostomy by the "combined technique." *J Urol* 1954;73:67–82.
6. Leissner J, Black P, Fisch M, et al. Colon pouch (Mainz pouch III) for continent urinary diversion after pelvic irradiation. *Urology* 2000;56: 798–802.
7. Lindell O, Lehtonen T. Rezidivierende urotheliale Tumoren in einzelnieren mit Anschluss eines kolonsegmentes an das nierenbecken. *Akt Urol* 1988; 19:130–133.
8. Mogg RA. Urinary diversion using the colonic conduit. *Br J Urol* 1967; 39:687–692.
9. Morales P, Golimbu M. Colonic urinary diversion: 10 years of experience. *J Urol* 1975;113:302–307.
10. Nelson JH. *Atlas of radical pelvic surgery*. London: Butterworth, 1969.
11. Schmidt JD, Buchsbaum HJ, Jacobo EC. Transverse colon conduit for supravesical urinary diversion. *Urology* 1976;8:542–546.
12. Schmidt JD, Buchsbaum HJ, Nachtsheim DA. Long-term follow-up. Further experience with and modifications of the transverse colon conduit in urinary tract diversion. *Br J Urol* 1985;57:284–288.
13. Wallace DM. Ureteric diversion using a conduit: a simplified technique. *Br J Urol* 1966;38:522–527.


# CHAPTER 85 ■ MANAGING THE PATIENT WITH ORTHOTOPIC BLADDER SUBSTITUTION

URS E. STUDER AND N. BHATTA-DHAR

Orthotopic bladder substitution approximates the original bladder in both location and function. The goal of lower-urinary-tract reconstruction is to create a reservoir that provides a safe and continent means to store and eliminate urine. Over the last 100 years, bowel has been utilized in various ways for bladder substitution, but only with a recent improved understanding of bowel physiology and Laplace's law (pressure = tension/radius) has bowel been successfully applied.

In the 1980s, orthotopic reconstruction became the procedure of choice in selected male patients. The excellent clinical and functional results achieved subsequently motivated an interest in applying orthotopic reconstruction to women (8). This option is now possible because of an improved understanding of female pelvic anatomy as well as the substantiated low risk of urethral recurrence in women. Specific pathological criteria have allowed clinicians to select appropriate female candidates for orthotopic diversion.

Several different bladder substitutes have been developed, some of which are presented in the following chapters. Each of these bladder substitutes has its own specific advantages and disadvantages. Regardless of the type of substitution, an optimal outcome requires a low-pressure, high-compliance reservoir made of detubularized bowel segments with minimal outlet resistance and a preserved sphincter function.

The critical components to good long-term results with any bladder substitute include not only surgical finesse but also a thorough preoperative evaluation, meticulous postoperative care, and patient compliance. Therefore, this chapter is divided into the preoperative, intraoperative, and postoperative periods followed by a discussion of the necessary long-term management of these patients.

## DIAGNOSIS

A thorough preoperative assessment requires that the following factors be evaluated when determining candidacy for bladder substitution (Table 85.1).

### Patient Agreement and Mental Status

Perhaps the single most important factor contributing to a successful bladder substitute is the willingness of a patient to comply with indefinite follow-up. Adequate physical dexterity and a thorough understanding of how one's bladder substitute works are mandatory. In addition, ongoing educational reinforcement is necessary for long-term management and success. A dedicated nurse can facilitate the preoperative assessment

**TABLE 85.1**

PREOPERATIVE CHECKLIST

- Patient agreement to indefinite follow-up
- Adequate mental status, dexterity, and mobility
- Serum creatinine of < 1.5 mg/dL
- Liver function within normal limits
- No evidence of significant bowel disease
- No evidence of tumor in the distal urethra, paracollicular, or bladder neck region
- Continence status

and education, as well as be a useful resource as patients become comfortable with their bladder substitutes.

### Renal Function

The most frequently observed postoperative issues are metabolic acidosis followed by electrolyte abnormalities. The type and severity of these disorders depend on the intestinal segment used, the length of this segment, the time of urine contact with bowel mucosa, and the compensatory renal reserve. While a creatinine level of 1.5 mg per dL is considered the upper limit, some patients with significant creatinine elevations due to primary bladder cancer may recover sufficient function to allow for continent diversion once the obstruction is relieved. Placement of a percutaneous nephrostomy tube in these patients before surgery may provide a better idea of the true renal function (10).

### Hepatic Function

A bladder substitute candidate must have adequate preoperative liver function. The reservoir's continuous contact with urine permits ammonium to shift through the bowel mucosa and into circulation. A urinary tract infection caused by a urease-splitting organism will further increase the ammonium load. With pre-existing liver disease, hyperammonemia results, which can lead to neurologic decompensation and eventual coma (7).

### Bowel Function

Since bowel is needed for a bladder substitute, the impact of a prior bowel resection or a diseased or radiated bowel needs to be considered as it relates to malabsorption or diarrhea. The bowel segment used for the bladder substitute itself needs to be free of any pathology. To minimize vitamin B12 deficiency and diarrhea induced by bile acid, the terminal ileum needs to be preserved. Ileal segments of up to 60 cm can be resected in healthy individuals without any significant consequences provided the ileocecal valve is left intact. When >60 cm of bowel is resected, the risk of malabsorption further increases, and it becomes inevitable if >100 cm is used. If the right colon is preserved, an extended length of colon can be resected without significant malabsorptive side-effects because fluid reabsorption occurs predominantly in the right colon, whereas the left colon serves as a conduit.

### Paracollicular and Bladder Neck Biopsy

Positive biopsies from the paracollicular region in the prostatic urethra or the bladder neck in women (site of bladder substitution anastomosis) indicate a high likelihood of a urethral recurrence. These patients should undergo a primary urethrectomy and be considered for an alternative form of urinary diversion. Prostatic infiltration (superficial or stromal) proximal from the paracollicular site, carcinoma in situ, and multifocal transitional cell cancer confer a higher risk of urethral recurrence (2). However, these findings are not absolute contraindications for a bladder substitution.

### Continence

Incontinence, especially in female patients, may reflect a poorly functioning rhabdosphincter. These patients require urodynamic evaluation, including a urethral pressure profile, since this may identify an etiology and thereby potential treatment options. Severe incontinence is a contraindication to bladder substitution.

## INDICATIONS FOR SURGERY

Orthotopic bladder substitution is generally used in patients who are undergoing radical cystectomy for cancer. Patients must meet the preoperative assessment noted in the Diagnosis section.

## ALTERNATIVE THERAPY

Alternatives to orthotopic bladder substitution include ileal and colon conduits and other continent urinary diversions.

## SURGICAL TECHNIQUE

### Preoperative Period

The preoperative evaluation is the same as that for a radical cystectomy: exclusion of metastases and establishment of medical clearance for surgery. Any significant liver, renal, or bowel pathology must also be fully evaluated to determine candidacy for bladder substitution.

The type of bowel preparation depends on the bowel segment needed for the bladder substitute. Colonic bladder substitutes often require a full mechanical bowel preparation with agents such as Glycoprep. For ileal bladder substitutes, a limited bowel preparation with two enemas late in the afternoon before the day of surgery suffices. For this type of substitute, antegrade rinses of the bowel and neomycin-erythromycin intestinal preparations are avoided. In addition, such preparations can increase the risk of fluid imbalances. In the elderly patient, this can produce cardiovascular instability due to intravascular volume depletion as well potentially place the patient in a catabolic state even prior to surgery.

Subcutaneous deep venous thrombosis prophylaxis is started the evening before surgery and continued postoperatively. It is administered in the upper extremity so as to prevent a pelvic lymphocele. All patients receive perioperative and postoperative prophylactic antibiotics. Also, to prevent a deep venous thrombosis of the lower extremities or bronchopneumonia, patients wear stockings and are taught appropriate exercises by a physiotherapist.

## INTRAOPERATIVE MANAGEMENT

There are certain critical surgical steps that, if adhered to during the cystectomy, will allow for optimal functional results of the bladder substitute (Table 85.2).

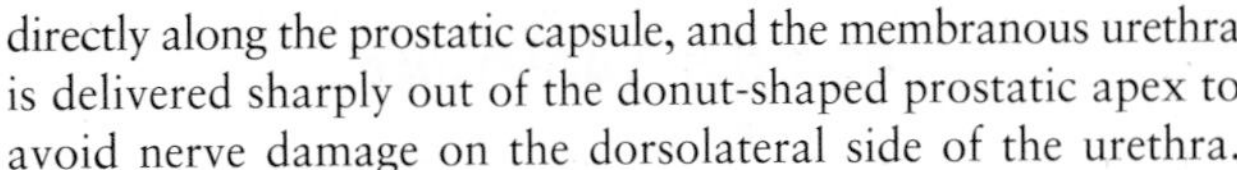

**TABLE 85.2**

INTRAOPERATIVE CHECKLIST

- Antibiotics and compression stockings
- Anatomical pelvic exenteration with attempt of nerve preservation on the non–tumor-bearing side
- Atraumatic dissection with maximum urethral length preservation
- Preservation of periureteric tissue
- Epidural anesthesia stopped 1 hour prior to bowel length measurement
- Preservation of the ileocecal valve and distal 25 cm of ileum
- Small bowel resection limited to under 60 cm
- Ureterointestinal anastomosis should not be obstructive
- Low-pressure reservoir with transected/opened, cross-folded bowel segments, spheroidal in shape
- Ureteric stents and cystostomy tubes placed through the fatty tissue of the bowel mesentery
- Tension-free anastomosis of the reservoir to the urethra
- The anastomosis of the urethra to the bladder substitute is not to the funnel-shaped end of the reservoir

## Preservation of Pelvic Nerves

In general, nerve sparing should be performed on the non–tumor-bearing side and extensive surgery on the tumor-bearing side. It has been shown that nerve-sparing radical cystectomy does have a positive impact on erectile function and urinary continence after bladder substitute (5). For nerve-sparing cystectomy in men, the nerve fibers in the dorsomedial pedicles lateral to the seminal vesicles as well as the paraprostatic neurovascular bundle have to be spared. The pelvic plexus can be preserved by sectioning the dorsomedial pedicle along its ventral aspect, anterolateral to the seminal vesicles, and terminating the dissection at the base of the prostate. A nerve-sparing prostatectomy must also be performed, which requires a lateral approach with incision of the endopelvic and periprostatic fascia and bunching of the Santorini plexus at the level of the prostate and not distal to it. The dorsolateral neurovascular bundle can be separated from the prostatic capsule. The prostatic apex needs to be approached laterally directly along the prostatic capsule, and the membranous urethra is delivered sharply out of the donut-shaped prostatic apex to avoid nerve damage on the dorsolateral side of the urethra.

For nerve sparing in women, the vaginal wall dissection at the cervical level is in the anteroventral plane of the vagina, that is, at the 2 or 10 o'clock position. An empty sponge-holding forceps in the vagina helps facilitate dissection along the whitish vaginal wall. It is important to remain in close contact with the whitish wall of the vagina to ensure that the paravaginal venous plexus is hemostatically controlled and resected with the dorsomedial bladder pedicle. The endopelvic fascia is disturbed as little as possible to minimize damage to the intrapelvic branch of the pudendal nerve, which also contributes to urethral innervation.

## Atraumatic Dissection of the Urethra

To obtain maximum urethral length, sharp, atraumatic dissection of the urethra with minimal use of electrocautery at the prostatic apex in men and the bladder neck in women is required. Preservation of the puboprostatic and pubourethral ligaments and incision of the endopelvic fascia, not at its deepest point, but along the bladder neck in female patients, will allow for further urethral stability and improved continence.

## Ureters

The ureters need to be resected at a safe oncologic distance from the bladder, allowing for removal of periureteral lymphatics that may harbor micrometastases. In addition, by removing most of the proximal ureter, ureteral ischemia is precluded and thereby subsequent stricture formation.

When mobilizing the ureters, the periureteric tissue must be preserved, since this contains the ureters' blood supply. This will also help prevent anastomotic strictures. The left ureter is brought without tension to the right side of the abdomen retroperitoneally by crossing the aorta above the inferior mesenteric artery. An antireflux ureteral anastomosis is not required in low-pressure ileal bladder substitutes (11). Another important point is to pass the ureteral stents through the distal tubular wall where their exit sites are covered with mesenteric fat so as to prevent urine leakage when they are removed (Fig. 85.1).

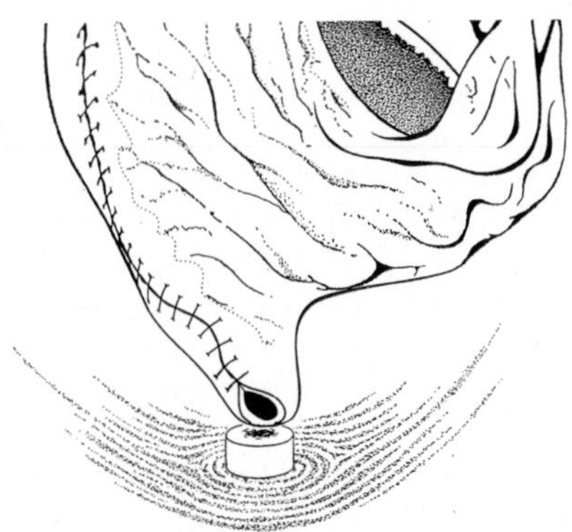

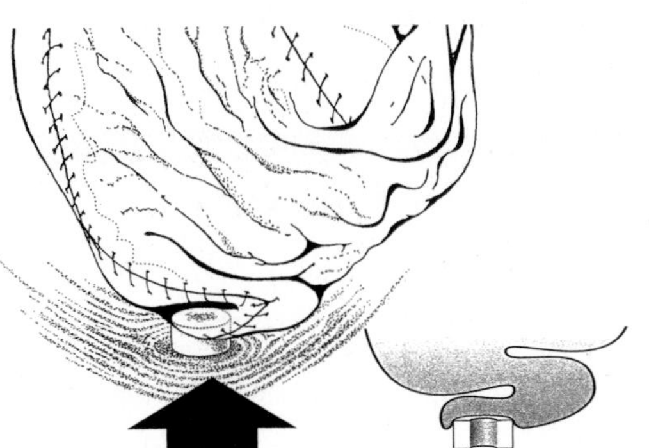

FIGURE 85.1 Placement of cystostomy and ureteric catheters through the fat of the mesentery.

## Bladder Substitute

If small bowel is used for the reservoir, the ileocecal valve and the most distal 25 cm of ileum should be preserved to reduce the associated risk of malabsorption and bile acid–induced diarrhea. One hour prior to bladder substitute construction, administration of anesthetics via the epidural is stopped. This prevents increased muscle tone and activity which results in an artificial shortening of bowel and thereby avoids removal of more bowel than is necessary for reservoir construction.

The reservoir should be spherical to achieve maximum capacity and the lowest possible pressure for the given surface of bowel used. As illustrated by Laplace's law (pressure = tension/radius), intraluminal pressure is low for a given tension, since conversion of a tubular structure into a spherical reservoir increases the radius. Furthermore, the spherical shape obtains maximal capacity while the surface-volume ratio limits the reabsorbing surface and therefore minimizes associated metabolic issues.

It is imperative that the anastomosis of the urethra to the bladder substitute is not to the funnel-shaped end of the reservoir. This error would increase the risk of kinking and obstruction at the anastomotic site, especially when the reservoir is full. To obtain optimal voiding, the anastomosis should sit broadly on the pelvic floor (Fig. 85.2). In addition, all suture material should be absorbable, thereby eliminating any potential nidus for stone formation.

# POSTOPERATIVE MANAGEMENT

During the postoperative period, fluid and electrolyte management predominates; however, it is also important to use this time to educate and encourage patients to become comfortable with their bladder substitute.

## Immediate Postoperative Period

Table 85.3 lists the elements of immediate postoperative care. The suprapubic and transurethral catheters must be flushed and aspirated with normal saline 0.9% every 6 hours. This is needed to prevent mucus buildup, which can block catheters and result in rupture of the bladder substitute. This complication is greatest when bowel activity has resumed but while the catheter is still in situ. Prevention of abdominal distention and return of bowel activity can be accelerated with parasympathomimetic medications (neostigmine) and in smokers with nicotine patches. The ureteral stents should be removed between postoperative days 5 and 7, around the time bowel function returns.

On postoperative day 10 and provided a pouchography documents no evidence of urinary extravasation, the suprapubic tube can be removed. The urethral Foley catheter remains in place for an additional 2 days to provide enough time for the suprapubic tube exit site to heal.

**TABLE 85.3**

IMMEDIATE POSTOPERATIVE CHECKLIST

- Deep venous thrombosis prophylaxis
- Catheters irrigated every 6 hours
- Ureteral stents removed day 5 to 7
- Cystogram day 10 with withdrawal of suprapubic tube if no leakage
- Urethral catheter removed 48 hours after suprapubic tube

## Management of Patients after Catheter Removal

Management after catheter removal is outlined in Table 85.4. After all drains are removed, any bacteriuria should be managed with antibiotics until the urine is sterile. Infected urine can cause reservoir instability with subsequent urinary incontinence as well as increased mucus production, which can lead to increased postvoid residuals and even urinary retention.

Patients must be carefully instructed on how to void. Initially, they are taught to empty the bladder substitute every 2 hours during the daytime in a sitting position by relaxing the pelvic floor and if necessary by also increasing their intra-abdominal pressure. At night, they should use an alarm clock to void every 4 hours. The adequacy of emptying needs to be monitored postvoid with a straight catheterization and/or ultrasound of the reservoir.

Patients without metabolic acidosis (no negative base excess) or those managed with oral sodium bicarbonate are instructed to retain urine thereafter for 3 hours and later for 4 hours in order to obtain a bladder capacity of up to 500 mL. During this exercise, increased bladder substitute pressures may cause incontinence, but the elevated pressures are required to increase the reservoir's capacity. Therefore, patients are advised not to void when they experience such incontinence; otherwise the bladder substitute will never achieve the desired capacity. It is essential to increase the capacity to approximately 500 cc in order to have low-end fill pressures to ensure urinary continence. With increasing capacity, nighttime continence will improve; on the other hand, a bladder

**TABLE 85.4**

POST-CATHETER REMOVAL CHECKLIST

- Antibiotic prophylaxis with a quinolone following catheter removal for 5 days
- All urinary tract infections must be treated
- Proper voiding technique must be taught
- Ensure reservoir is emptying completely with ultrasound and/or in-out catheterization
- Voids are gradually increased from every 2 hours to every 4 hours (at night with the help of an alarm clock)
- Effective sphincter training must be taught and performed regularly
- Measure daily body weight and correct a negative base excess
- Oral fluid intake of 2 to 3 L/day for the first 3 months
- Ileal bladder substitute patients should increase salt consumption for the first 3 months
- Lifelong regular follow-up

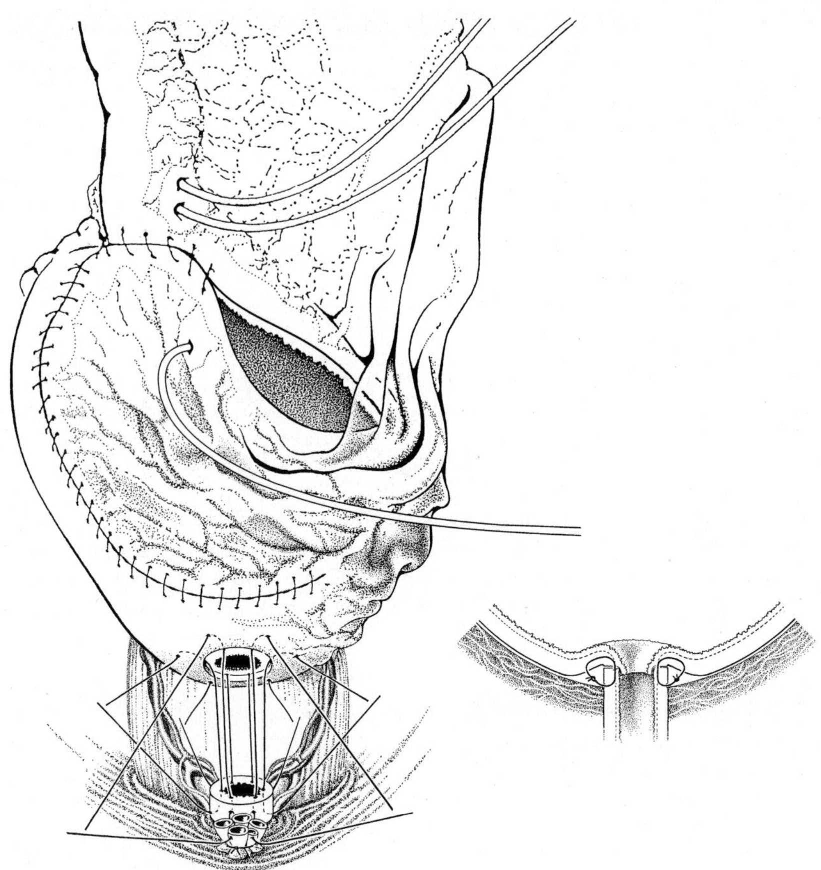

FIGURE 85.2 A funnel-shaped reservoir to urethra anastomosis must be avoided because of the risk of subsequent kinking and outlet obstruction.

substitute capacity of >500 mL should be prevented. Overdistention of the reservoir will result in a floppy pouch unable to adequately empty, increased residual urine, and the potential for urinary retention.

The time required to achieve continence depends on diligent sphincter training, the age of the patient, and achieving intraoperative neural preservation to the urethra and pelvic floor (if oncologically safe). A postvoid dribble incontinence can be prevented by instructing the patient to milk the urethra at the end of each void (1). Daytime continence rates of up to 90% and nocturnal rates of 80% at 12 months can be achieved (6).

Hypercontinence tends to be a problem primarily for female bladder substitute patients. Having an unobstructed outlet with prevention of kinking of the urethra or reservoir can help avoid this concern (Fig. 85.2). The contribution to sphincter function of the intrapelvic pudendal somatic nerves and autonomic branches of the pelvic plexus has not been fully established, but animal studies have demonstrated a pressure increase in the distal urethra after pudendal nerve stimulation and in the proximal urethra after stimulation of the pelvic plexus (3). This suggests that nerve sparing has functional significance for both continence and voiding ability. Using the female sheep model, Strasser and colleagues (9) found marked degeneration of the smooth muscle cells of the proximal urethra after bilateral denervation of an isolated urethra, which reflects the situation in bladder substitute patients. Thus complete autonomic denervation of the urethra in patients undergoing cystectomy and bladder substitute may result in long-term smooth muscle dysfunction. Absence of the tonus-regulating function of the autonomic nerves may lead to a dilation or rigidity of the urethra, resulting in intrinsic sphincter deficiency. A denervated proximal urethra may result in ineffective active relaxation and/or kinking during voiding, and thus incomplete emptying, which necessitates self-catheterization.

Urethral length is also important in the genesis of urinary incontinence, as demonstrated by the following formula: continence = urethral length × closing urethral pressure (12). In female sheep, Strasser et al. (9) showed that maximal urethral closure pressure was markedly decreased in sheep with denervated urethra (18 cm $H_2O$ compared to baseline of 49 cm $H_2O$). If the autonomic nerves are compromised, closing urethral pressure cannot compensate for a shortened urethral length. Theoretically, after resection of the proximal urethra, patients may not leak with increased intra-abdominal pressure because of the intact pudendal nerve pathway but may leak when walking, particularly with a full bladder, because of reduced functional urethral length. Also, sensory innervations of the proximal urethra may influence urinary continence. Division of these nerves may result in loss of the afferent limb of the external sphincter guarding reflex stimulated by urinary leakage into the proximal urethra.

## Metabolic Management

After catheter removal, the patient is at an increased risk for metabolic acidosis, particularly if there is residual urine. In fact, this is the most frequent yet most often underdiagnosed complication associated with bladder substitutes. Jagenburg et al. (4) reported that the iso-osmolality between urine in the reservoir and serum is established within 2 to 6 hours. This explains why, initially, when the urine is hypo-osmolar, the bladder substitute will secrete sodium chloride, resulting in a salt-losing syndrome, hypovolemia, and metabolic acidosis. The resultant dehydration and anorexia may lead to a rapid decrease in body weight; therefore, daily postoperative weight assessment is essential. To prevent this metabolic cascade, patients should increase salt intake (pretzels, chips, etc), primarily because they are also encouraged to consume 2 to 3 L of fluids a day to prevent a metabolic acidosis resulting from highly concentrated acidotic urine (7). With time, the villi will atrophy and this syndrome will become less pronounced.

Both the urologist and the patient should be aware of the symptoms that may arise with a metabolic acidosis (Table 85.5). The base excess can be monitored with a venous blood gas analysis. A negative base excess needs to be corrected. This is usually accomplished with sodium bicarbonate 2 to 6 g daily for ileal bladder substitutes and with potassium citrate for colonic bladder substitutes.

**TABLE 85.5**

**SYMPTOMS OF METABOLIC ACIDOSIS IN PATIENTS WITH BLADDER SUBSTITUTES**

- Fatigue
- Anorexia
- Dyspepsia and heartburn
- Nausea and vomiting
- Weight loss

# OUTCOMES

## Long-Term Follow-up

Meticulous lifelong follow-up is essential for optimal reservoir function and prevention of long-term complications. A suggested schema is illustrated (Table 85.6). A bladder substitute should have no infection, no incontinence, no acidosis, and no

**TABLE 85.6**

**FOLLOW-UP SCHEDULE FOR PATIENTS WITH ILEAL BLADDER SUBSTITUTE**

| MONTHS AFTER SURGERY | 3 | 6 | 12 | 18 | 24 | 30 | 36 | 42 | 48 | 54 | 60 |
|---|---|---|---|---|---|---|---|---|---|---|---|
| Clinical examination | X | X | X | X | X | X | X | X | X | X | X |
| Urine dipstick, urine culture | X | X | X | X | X | X | X | X | X | X | X |
| Weight, blood pressure | X | X | X | X | X | X | X | X | X | X | X |
| Basic blood tests (Hb,Cl,Bic,creat,alk.phos.)[a] | | | | X | | X | | X | | X | |
| Extended blood tests (Hb,Na,K,Ca,Cl,alk.phos.,LDH, Mg,Bic,urea,creat,ALAT,γGT)[a] | X | X | X | | X | | X | | X | | X |
| PSA (only in patients with prostate cancer) | X | | | | X | | | | | | X |
| Folic acid, vitamin B12 | | | | | X | | X | | X | | X |
| Chest X-ray (only if Ca) | | X | X | X | X | | X | | X | | X |
| Bone scan (only if ≥pT3 and any pN+) | | X | X | | | | | | | | |
| Pelvic/abdominal CT scan (only if ≥pT3 and any pN+) | | X | X | | | | | | | | |
| IVU[b] with tomography (only in patients with multifocal and/or carcinoma in situ) | | | X | | X | | X | | | | X |
| Ultrasound of kidneys | X | X | | X | | X | | X | X | X | |
| Ultrasound for residual urine | X | X | X | X | X | X | X | X | X | X | X |
| Urethral lavage | | X | X | X | X | | X | | X | | X |
| Micturition protocol | X | | X | | X | | X | | X | | X |
| Voiding questionnaire | | X | | X | | X | | X | | X | |

[a]Hb, hemoglobin; Cl, chlorine; Bic, ; creat., creatinine; alk.phos., alkaline phosphatase; Na, sodium; K, potassium; Ca, calcium; LDH, L-lactate dehydrogenase; Mg, magnesium; ALAT, alanine aminotransferase; γGT, .

[b]IVU, intravenous urogram.

or minimal postvoid residual urine. Intravenous urogram (IVU) and lavage cytology are used to follow the upper tract and urethra, respectively, for recurrences.

Residual urine should be monitored, recognized early, and promptly managed. The most common reasons for residual urine are protrusion of ileobladder mucosa into the urethra, residual prostatic tissue, and urethral anastomotic strictures. All of these can be managed endoscopically. Permanent indwelling catheters and intermittent straight catheterizations are not adequate therapies and should only be reserved for patients with personal preferences or for nursing purposes.

## *References*


1. Bader P, Hugonnet CL, Burkhard F, et al. Inefficient urethral milking secondary to urethral dysfunction as an additional risk factor for incontinence after radical prostatectomy. *J Urol* 2001;166(6):2247–2252.
2. Freeman JA, Thomas A, Esrig D, et al. Urethral recurrence in patients with orthotopic ileal neobladders. *J Urol* 1996;156(5):1615–1619.
3. Hubner WA, Trigo-Rocha F, Plas EG, et al. Urethral function after cystectomy: a canine in vivo experiment. *Urol Res* 1993;21:45.
4. Jagenburg R, Kock NG, Norlén L, et al. Clinical significance of changes in composition of urine during collection and storage in continent ileum reservoir urinary diversion. *Scan J Urol Nephrol* 1978;49[Suppl]:43–48.
5. Kessler TM, Burkhard FC, Perimenis P, et al. Attempted nerve sparing surgery and age have a significant effect on urinary continence and erectile function after radical cystoprostatectomy and ileal orthotopic bladder substitution. *J Urol* 2004;172(4, Pt 1):1323–1327.
6. Madersbacher S, Möhrle K, Burkhard F, et al. Long-term voiding pattern of patients with ileal orthotopic bladder substitutes. *J Urol* 2002; 167(5): 2052.
7. Mills RD, Studer UE. Metabolic consequences of continent urinary diversion. *J Urol* 1999;161:1057.
8. Stenzl A, Jarolim L, Coloby P, et al. Urethra-sparing cystectomy and orthotopic urinary diversion in women with malignant pelvic tumors. *Cancer* 2001;92(7):1864–1871.
9. Strasser H, Ninkovic M, Hess M, et al. Anatomic and functional studies of the male and female urethral sphincter. *World J Urol* 2000;18(5):324–329.
10. Studer UE, Burkhard FC, Danuser H, et al. Keys to success in orthotopic bladder substitution. *Can J Urol* 1999;6(5):876.
11. Studer UE, Siegrist T, Casanova GA. Ileal bladder substitute: antireflux nipple or afferent tubular segment? *Eur Urol* 1991;20(4):315–326.
12. Weil A, Reyes H, Bischoff P, et al. Modification of the urethral rest and stress profiles after types of surgery for urinary stress incontinence. *Br J Obstet Gynaecol* 1984;91:46–45.


# CHAPTER 86 ■ ORTHOTOPIC URINARY DIVERSION USING AN ILEAL LOW-PRESSURE RESERVOIR WITH AN AFFERENT TUBULAR SEGMENT

STEPHAN JESCHKE AND URS E. STUDER

An ileal low-pressure orthotopic bladder substitute offers several significant advantages over other forms of orthotopic diversion. One is the ease of surgery, as the operation can be performed by any urologist experienced in performing a radical prostatectomy or a cystectomy and ileal conduit (1). The short ileum segment, approximately 55 cm long, that is used to construct this bladder substitute minimizes intestinal malabsorption. The terminal ileum, as well as the ileocecal valve, is preserved. The reservoir is spherical, achieving a maximum volume-to-surface area ratio with maximum capacity from a given bowel segment (2). Another advantage is the isoperistaltic tubular afferent segment with the end-to-side ureteroileal anastomosis at its proximal end. This allows resection of the distal ureters, including the paraureteral lymphatics, at a safe distance from the bladder cancer and reduces the risk of leaving distal ureters behind that may contain carcinoma in situ. Furthermore, the shorter the ureters are, the better the blood supply at their distal end and the lower the risk of ischemic stricturing of the distal ureter. The peristalsis of the afferent ileal segments acts as a dynamic antireflux mechanism. In cases of complicated urethral strictures or urethral tumor recurrence, the afferent tubular segment can easily be transformed into an ileal conduit. By slightly modifying this reservoir, one can also use it for bladder augmentation following subtotal cystectomy in patients with benign bladder pathology.

## DIAGNOSIS

Patients undergoing orthotopic bladder substitution will generally have the diversion as part of a cystectomy for bladder cancer. A full metastatic workup to stage the cancer is important, as well as a cystoscopy to determine the extent of the cancer in the urethra. As is true for all bladder substitutes, specific criteria for selection are related to the disease stage, the renal and liver function, and the patient's willingness to comply with routine follow-up. These criteria are summarized in table 86.1. Adequate renal function as defined by serum creatinine $<1.5$ mg per dL precludes the need for lifelong bicarbonate supplementation.

**TABLE 86.1**

**PATIENT SELECTION CRITERIA FOR CONTINENT URINARY DIVERSION**

- Non-metastatic disease
- Negative biopsies from prostatic urethra (m)/bladder neck (f)
- Adequate renal function (serum creatinine < 1.5 mg/dL)
- Normal liver function
- No active inflammatory bowel disease or previous extensive bowel resection
- Physical and mental ability to live with a bladder substitute
- Compliance to routine follow-up

## INDICATIONS FOR SURGERY

Orthotopic diversion may now represent the procedure of choice in the properly selected patient undergoing cystectomy. However, as with all bladder substitutes, the cancer operation must not be compromised by the orthotopic reconstruction. In addition, the external rhabdosphincter and internal lissosphincter complex and corresponding innervations must be functionally intact. The ileal orthotopic bladder substitute is also particularly well suited for patients in whom the sequelae of ileocecal resection should be avoided.

## ALTERNATIVE THERAPIES

Alternatives to the ileal orthotopic bladder include other forms of diversion, including ileal and colon conduits, continent urinary diversions, and other orthotopic diversions.

## SURGICAL TECHNIQUE

### Cystectomy

Pelvic lymphadenectomy and cystectomy are performed according to standard technique, with slight modifications (3). The external iliac vessels, the obturator fossa, and the hypogastric vessels are freed of all lymphatic, fatty, and connective tissue. Having divided the dorsolateral bladder pedicles containing the superior and inferior vesical vessels along the hypogastric arteries, the pelvic floor fascia is incised and the Santorini plexus is ligated. If possible, the prostatic vessels should be preserved on the non–tumor-bearing side to ensure adequate blood supply to the pelvic plexus and neurovascular bundle.

The ureters are divided where they cross the iliac vessels. This allows en bloc removal of the distal ureters and paraureteral lymphatic vessels, together with the cystectomy specimen. The dorsomedial pedicle is resected along the pararectal-presacral plane on the tumor-bearing side. Whenever possible, care is taken to preserve the hypogastric fibers and the pelvic plexus situated dorsolaterally to the seminal vesicle on the contralateral non–tumor-bearing side. On this side the dissection along the dorsolateral wall of the seminal vesicle is stopped at the base of the prostate. The Santorini plexus is then divided, and the membranous urethra is transected as close as possible to the apex of the prostate by excavating it out of the donut-shaped apex. The neurovascular bundles located dorsolateral to the prostate are also preserved on the non–tumor-bearing side.

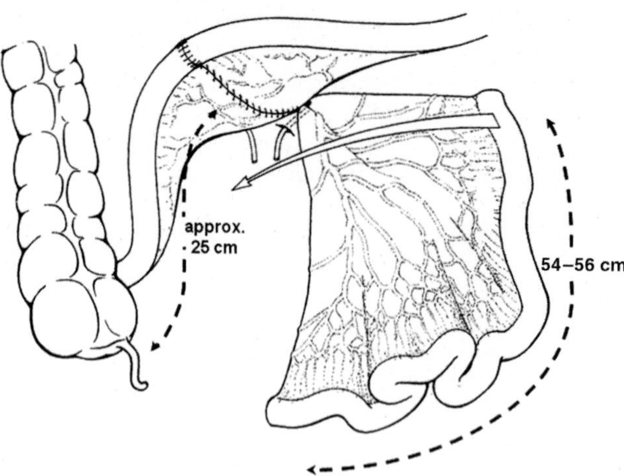


FIGURE 86.1 The 55-cm-long ileal segment for the bladder substitute is isolated 25 cm proximal to the ileocecal valve. Note the different incision depth of the mesoileum proximally and distally, to preserve the blood supply.

### Preparation of the Ileum Segment for the Bladder Substitute

For construction of the reservoir, an ileal segment approximately 55 cm long is isolated 25 cm proximal to the ileocecal valve and bowel continuity is restored (Fig. 86.1). The length of the ileum segment is measured with a ruler in portions of 10 cm along the border of the mesoileum without stretching the bowel. Irritation of the bowel as well as epidural anesthesia with local anesthetics should be avoided since this can increase smooth muscle tone and activity and “shorten” the length of the bowel, which will then be too long after muscle relaxation. The distal mesoileum incision transects the main vessels, whereas the proximal mesoileum incision must be short in order to preserve the main vessels perfusing the future reservoir segment (Fig. 86.1). The mesoileum borders are adapted with a running suture (2-0 polyglycolic acid) in which the mesoileum of the bladder substitute is included (Fig. 86.2). The sutures must be applied superficially, taking care to preserve the blood supply to the bladder substitute. Both ends of the isolated ileal segment are closed by seromuscular running sutures (4-0 polyglycolic acid). The distal end of the ileal segment, approximately 42 to 45 cm long, is opened along its antimesenteric border (Fig. 86.2), leaving a 10- to 12-cm afferent tubular limb for anastomosing the ureters.

### Ureteroileal End-to-Side Anastomosis

The left ureter is mobilized up to the lower pole of the kidney, with care taken to maintain its surrounding blood supply and thereby prevent ischemia. It is then brought without tension to the right side of the abdomen retroperitoneally by crossing the aorta slightly above the inferior mesenteric artery. Note: If the ureters need to be resected close to the kidney (e.g., if there is carcinoma in situ, compromised vascular supply, or previous radiation history), a longer afferent ileal segment can be harvested

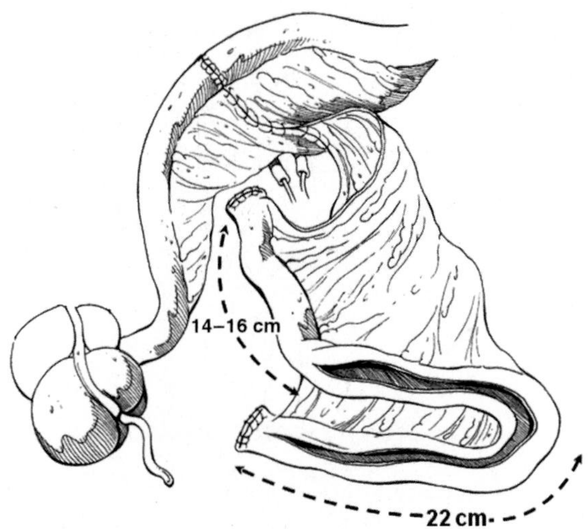


FIGURE 86.2 Closure of the mesoileum incision. Avoid deep sutures in the area joining the mesoileum of the terminal ileum to the mesoileum of the bladder substitute, in order not to compromise circulation. Transpose the afferent ileal segment as shown by the *arrow*.

to bridge the necessary distance. The ureters are spatulated over a length of 1.5 to 2.0 cm. Incisions (2 cm) are made along the paramedian antimesenteric border of the afferent tubular ileal segment by running sutures using the Nesbit technique in an open end-to-side fashion (Fig. 86.3). The anastomoses are placed paramedial to the antimesenteric border at the most proximal portion of the afferent tubular segment. To prevent bowel ischemia between the ureteral anastomosis, the right ureter is placed approximately 1 cm distal to the left ureter.

The ureters are stented with 7Fr or 8Fr catheters. To prevent dislocation of the catheters, a rapidly absorbable suture (5-0 polyglycolic acid) is placed through the ureter and catheter together 3 to 4 cm proximal to the anastomosis. It is tied loosely, to not compromise the ureteral blood supply. The most distal periureteral tissue is sutured to the afferent ileal segment to remove tension on the anastomosis and to cover it. The ureteric catheters are passed through the wall of the most distal end of the afferent tubular segment, where it is covered by some mesoileum. This provides a "covered" canal in the reservoir wall when withdrawing the ureteric splints 4 to 7 days postoperatively.

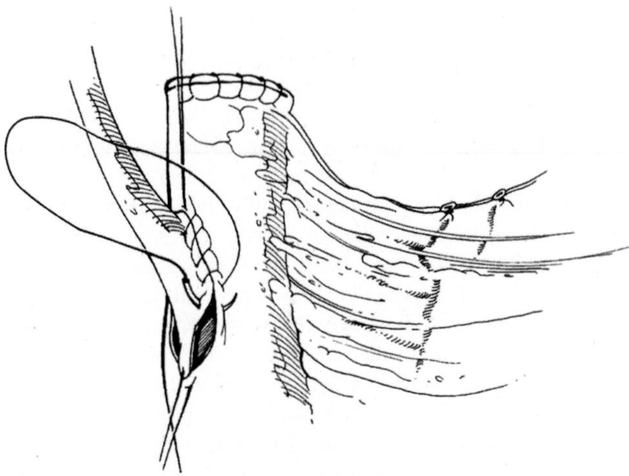

FIGURE 86.3 A ureteroileal anastomosis using a simple end-to-side Nesbit technique with a 4-0 running suture ensures a low stricture rate.

## Construction of the Bladder Substitute and Anastomosis to the Urethra

To construct the reservoir itself, the two medial borders of the opened U-shaped distal part of the ileal segment are oversewn with a single continuous seromuscular layer of 2-0 polyglycolic acid suture (Fig. 86.4). The bottom of the U is folded over between the two ends of the U (Fig. 86.4), resulting in a spherical reservoir consisting of four cross-folded ileal segments. After closure of the lower half of the anterior wall and part of the upper half (Fig. 86.5), the surgeon's finger is introduced through the remaining opening to determine the most caudal part of the reservoir. At this point, a hole 8 to 10 mm in diameter is cut out of the pouch wall, outside the suture line (Fig. 86.6). Importantly, although it may appear easier to perform, it is imperative that the anastomosis of the urethra to the neobladder is not to the funnel-shaped end of the reservoir.

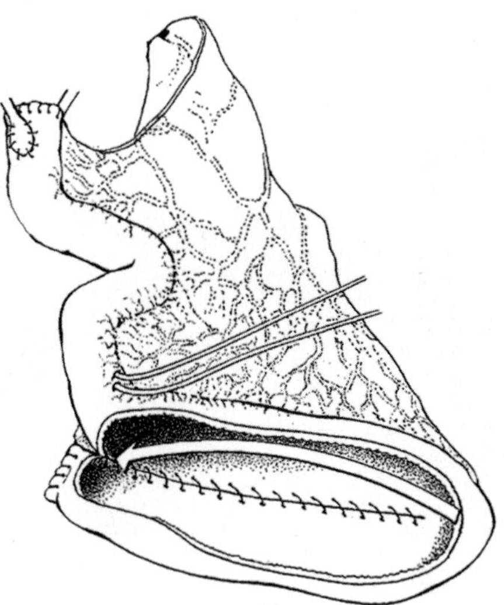

FIGURE 86.4 The two medial borders of the antimesenteric opened U-shaped distal ileum segment are oversewn with a single-layer seromuscular running suture. The bottom of the U is folded over and tied between the two ends of the U.

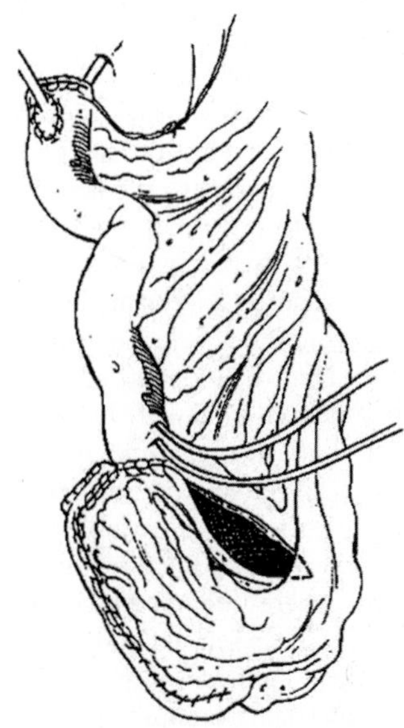

FIGURE 86.5 The caudal half of the remaining reservoir opening is closed completely, and the cranial half partially by a running seromuscular suture.

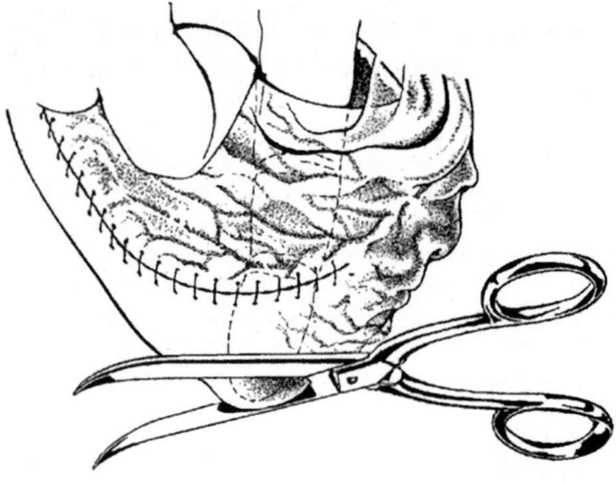

FIGURE 86.6 The surgeon's finger is introduced to determine the most dependent part, and a 8 to 10 mm-diameter hole is excised.

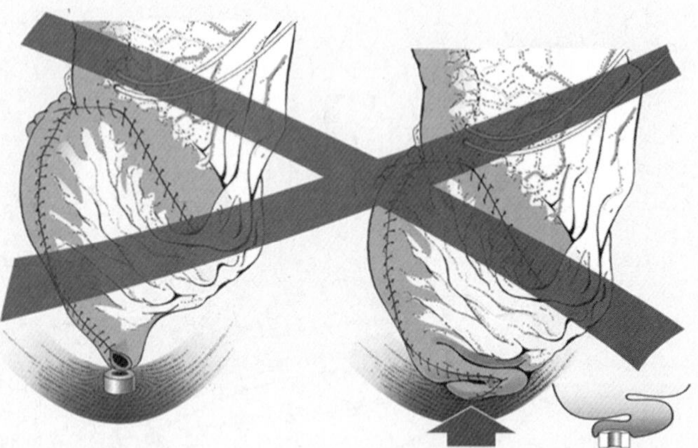

FIGURE 86.7 Anastomosis of the urethra to the neobladder is not made using the funnel-shaped end of the reservoir.

This error would increase the risk of kinking and obstruction at the anastomotic site when the reservoir is full (Fig. 86.7). To achieve optimal voiding, the anastomosis must sit broadly on the pelvic floor. After placement of a silicone 18Fr Foley urethral catheter, six 2-0 Vicryl sutures anastomose the previously made hole in the bladder substitute with the urethra (Fig. 86.8). Two posterior sutures are passed through the Denonvilliers fascia and medial to the neurovascular bundles, two anterolaterally to them through the lateral portion of the urethra, and two anteriorly, taking only a little of the urethra but also through the ligated Santorini plexus. When the urethral sutures are placed, the needle incorporates 3 to 4 mm of the sphincter but exits at the mucosal edges, thereby bringing them close to the mucosal edges of the reservoir. This minimizes tension on the anastomosis and shortening of the urethral length, and it also reduces the incidence of anastomotic strictures. If necessary, the operating table is now flexed to reduce the distance between the bladder substitute and the urethra. In situations where the mesentery is short and the anastomosis between the reservoir and urethra is under tension, careful superficial incisions of the neobladder mesentery will provide for further length. Sutures are loosely tied to prevent cutting, ischemia, and stenosis. Rarely, to prevent undue traction on the anastomosis, two stitches placed lateral to the urethra can fix the bladder substitute to the pelvic floor.

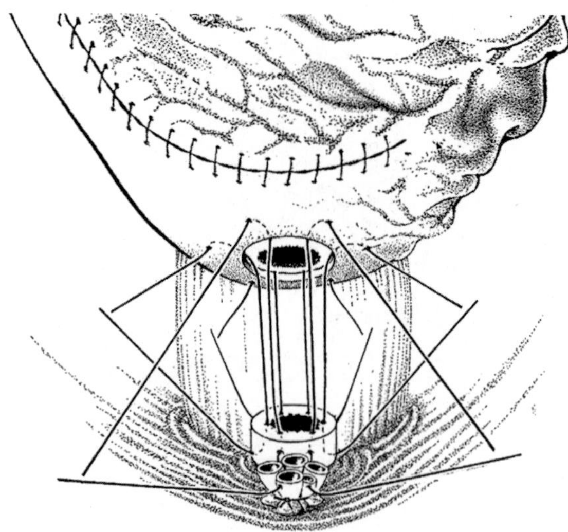

FIGURE 86.8 Six 2-0 Vicryl sutures anastomose the previously made hole in the bladder substitute to the urethra.

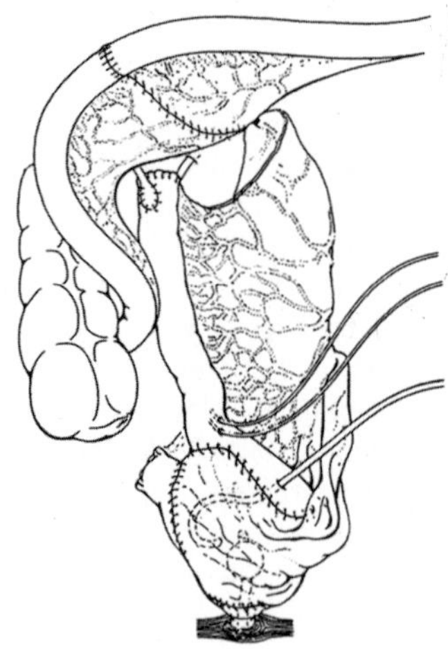

FIGURE 86.9 After insertion of a cystostomy tube into the reservoir, the pouch is closed completely.

Before complete closure of the reservoir, a cystostomy tube is passed through the bladder substitute wall and its exit site is covered with mesenteric fat (Fig. 86.9). The cystostomy tube is withdrawn 10 days postoperatively after exclusion of any leakage by a "pouchography." The indwelling catheter is left on continuous drainage for 2 more days before removal to allow for closure of the cystostomy canal in the reservoir wall.

## Surgical Modifications for Obese Patients

An ileal neobladder can successfully be constructed and brought down into the pelvis of obese patients. A measure of whether the reservoir will work in obese patients is if the bowel at 12 cm from the distal harvested end is able to reach the base of the penis. To ensure this will happen, the following steps should be employed. First, extend the distal mesenteric division deeper into the mesentery; this will provide for increased mobility (Fig. 86.10). In addition, unflex the operating table as much as possible, and if necessary make superficial transverse incisions of the serosa. If there is still tension, then, 12 cm from the distal end, transect a vessel proximal to the Riolan arch (Fig. 86.11). Provided collateral vessels are left

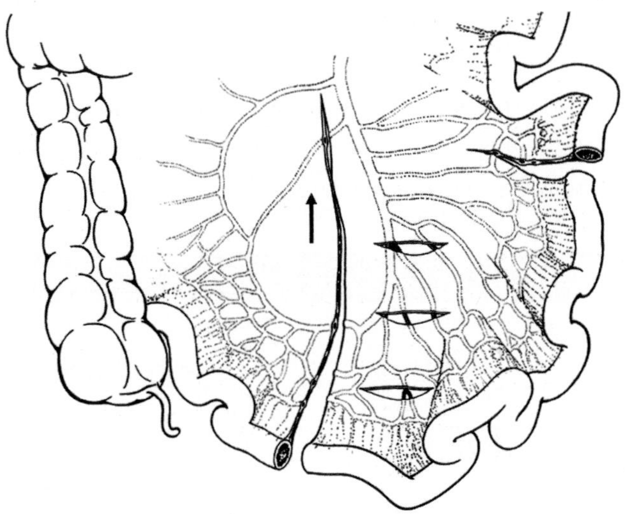

FIGURE 86.10 The distal mesenteric division should be extended deeper into the mesentery.

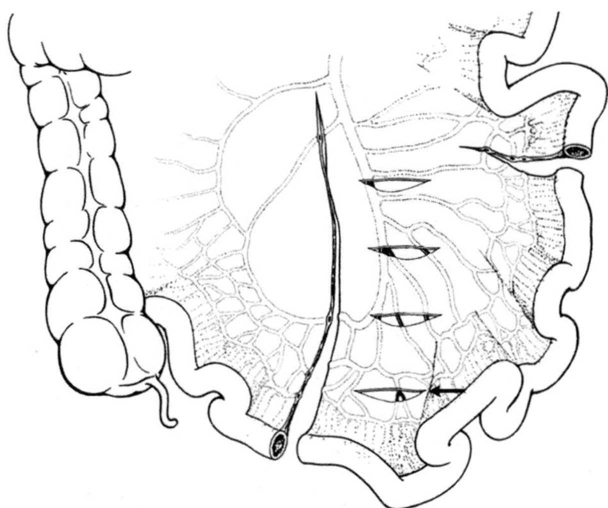

FIGURE 86.11 A vessel proximal to the Riolan arch is transected.

on either side, this will not compromise vascular supply to the reservoir.

## Postoperative Care

Critical components to good long-term results include the ability to create a high-compliance, low-pressure reservoir with an adequate continence mechanism, as well as patient compliance and meticulous postoperative care. Ureteral stents are removed 5 to 7 days after surgery. At 8 to 10 days postoperatively and after pouchography documents no evidence of urinary leakage, the cystostomy tube is removed. The Foley catheter remains for an additional 2 days to provide adequate time for closure of the cystostomy tube exit site from the reservoir wall. Although our patients are on antibiotics, all drains are removed as early as possible to prevent infections. After the patient is drain-free, any bacteriuria is treated with antibiotics until the urine is sterile.

Patients are carefully instructed on how to void. Initially, they are taught to empty the pouch every 2 hours during the daytime in a sitting position by relaxing the pelvic floor and increasing intra-abdominal pressure. At night, they are instructed to use an alarm clock to void every 3 to 4 hours. Initially, the urine is often hypo-osmolar; consequently, the bladder substitute will secrete sodium chloride, resulting in a salt-losing syndrome and therefore hypovolemia and metabolic acidosis. To prevent this series of metabolic events, patients are instructed to consume 2 to 3 L of liquid a day and to increase salt intake, and they are prophylactically placed on sodium bicarbonate (2 to 6 g per day) after ureteral stent removal. These patients are carefully followed with regular assessments of blood gas and body weight.

Patients without metabolic acidosis (no negative base excess) or those managed appropriately with oral intake of sodium bicarbonate are instructed to retain urine for 3 and later for 4 hours in order to obtain a bladder capacity of up to 500 mL. During this exercise, increased pouch pressures may result in incontinence, but the elevated pressures are essential to increase the reservoir's capacity. Therefore, patients are advised to not void when they experience such incontinence; otherwise the bladder substitute will never achieve the desired capacity.

With increasing capacity, nighttime continence will improve; on the other hand, a reservoir capacity of >500 mL should be prevented. Overdistention of the reservoir will result in a floppy pouch that is unable to adequately empty, increased residual urine, and the potential for urinary retention. Residual urine should be monitored, recognized early, and promptly managed. The cause of residual urine needs to be addressed (urethroscopy), and any evidence of outlet obstruction needs to be incised or resected. In addition, bacteriuria should also be appropriately treated. Our patients are followed regularly at every 6 months for 5 years and then at yearly intervals.

# OUTCOMES

## Complications

We recently published our 20-year experience with the ileal neobladder (4). In our experience, early diversion-related complications (within 30 days) occurred in 13% of patients. Pyelonephritis was the predominant complication noted (5.8%). Diversion-related late complications (>30 days) that required rehospitalization were metabolic acidosis, pyelonephritis, and sepsis in 4.4%, 3.9%, and 2.1%, respectively, and urinary retention due to infection and consequent mucus production in 4.5%. Typical late complications requiring surgery were bladder substitute outlet obstruction in 12% and incisional or inguinal hernias in 10%.

## Results

After 20 years' experience and a median follow-up of 32 months in 482 patients, our results are promising. In this series, 93% could void spontaneously at the last visit, and 90% had daytime and 78% nighttime continence with 3- to 4-hour voiding intervals. The remaining 7% were on intermittent self-catheterization or had an indwelling catheter for nursing home reasons. In addition to the correct performance of the above detailed surgical technique, success with this method of substitution demands meticulous postoperative care and follow-up.

## References


1. Benson MC, Seaman EK, Olsson CA. The ileal ureter neobladder is associated with a high success and low complication rate. *J Urol* 1996;155:1585.
2. Casanova GA, Springer JP, Gerber E, et al. Urodynamic and clinical aspects of ileal low pressure bladder substitutes. *Br J Urol* 1993;72:728.
3. Skinner DG. Technique of radical cystectomy. *Urol Clin North Am* 1981;8:353.
4. Studer UE, Burkhard FC, Schumacher M, et al. Twenty years experience with an ileal orthotopic low pressure bladder substitute: lessons to be learned. *J Urol* 2006;176(1):161–166.


# CHAPTER 87 ■ ILEAL NEOBLADDER

RICHARD E. HAUTMANN

During the last 20 years orthotopic reconstruction evolved from "experimental surgery" over "standard of care at larger medical centers" to the "preferred method of urinary diversion" in both sexes. During the last decade the time-honored conduit has given way to the increasingly frequent use of orthotopic reconstruction.

The goal of patient counseling about urinary diversion should be to find the method that will be the safest for cancer control, has the fewest complications in both the short and long term, and provides the easiest adjustment for the patient's lifestyle that is supporting the best quality of life. The paradigm for choosing a urinary diversion has changed substantially, and the proportion of cystectomy patients receiving a neobladder has increased at medical centers to 50%.

## DIAGNOSIS

This procedure is used as an adjunct for reconstruction of the urinary tract, usually following cystectomy. The diagnostic modalities therefore are relevant only to the primary diagnosis that resulted in the plan for the cystectomy. This reconstructive technique is performed following cystectomy, usually for malignant disease. As such, proper diagnostic studies for the underlying disease are important.

## INDICATIONS FOR SURGERY

The primary determining factor for a neobladder is the patient's desire for the procedure. The patient needs a certain motivation to tolerate the initial and sometimes lasting inconveniences of the nocturnal incontinence associated with a neobladder. Most patients readily accept some degree of nocturnal incontinence for the benefit of avoiding an external stoma; but not all patients do, and realistic expectations of the functional outcome are essential for both the surgeon and the patient. The psychologically damaging stigma to the patient who enters surgery expecting a neobladder but awakens with a stoma plays an increasing role in today's surgery.

An absolute contraindication to continent diversion of any type is compromised renal function as a result of long-standing obstruction or chronic renal failure, with serum creatinine >150 to 200 μmol per L. Severe hepatic dysfunction is also a contraindication to continent diversion. Patients with compromised intestinal function, in particular inflammatory bowel disease, may be better served by a bowel conduit. Absolute contraindications to orthotopic reconstruction are all patients who are candidates for simultaneous urethrectomy based on their primary tumor (1–3). The role of relative contraindications and comorbidity is steadily decreasing. However, some of them—like mental impairment, external sphincter dysfunction, or recurrent urethral strictures—deserve serious consideration.

In many cases, the patient's main motivation is to "get out of the hospital as soon as possible" and resume normal, rather sedentary activities. Many frail patients undergoing cystectomy will have less disruption of normal activities with a well-functioning conduit than with an orthotopic reservoir associated with less-than-ideal continence. Patients who have no concern about body image may also be better served with an ileal conduit.

In addition to the above contraindications, patients undergoing cystectomy for cancer have concerns regarding completely resecting the cancer versus preserving the rhabdosphincter. One of the initial deterrents to orthotopic diversion is the risk for urethral recurrence of cancer. The best predictor of the risk for urethral disease is the presence and extent of carcinoma in situ (CIS) in the prostatic urethra, ducts, or stroma. If there is diffuse CIS in the ducts and invasion of the stroma, the risk for urethral disease has historically been 25% to 35%, thus discouraging the use of the urethra. Lesser amounts of CIS confer a lesser degree of risk. Our aggressive approach for neobladder diversion relies only on a frozen section of the urethral margin at the time of surgery. A conservative approach would disqualify a patient with any prostatic involvement. In our view, neither multifocal bladder tumors nor CIS of the bladder is an indication for urethrectomy. The frequency of urethral recurrence after orthotopic diversions is much less than anticipated. Increasing experience with orthotopic reconstruction has made patient selection based on tumor stage less restrictive. Should extensive pelvic disease, a palpable mass, or positive but resectable lymph nodes preclude a neobladder because of the high propensity for a pelvic recurrence or distant relapse?

There is no convincing evidence that a patient with an orthotopic diversion tolerates adjuvant chemotherapy less well or that a pelvic recurrence is any more difficult to manage with a neobladder than after an ileal conduit. Patients can anticipate normal neobladder function until the time of death. Nevertheless, our philosophy respects the patient's desire for a neobladder; if the patient is strongly motivated, he or she gets a neobladder. Even though the patient has a poor prognosis and relapse is likely to occur, we still try to construct the diversion he or she wants. However, all patients should be informed that diversion to the skin either by a continent reservoir or ileal conduit may be necessary due to unexpected tumor extent, and there should be an appropriate stoma site marked on the abdominal wall beforehand.

## ALTERNATIVE THERAPY

The alternatives to orthotopic urinary diversion (neobladder construction) are incontinent cutaneous urinary diversion (percutaneous nephrostomy, pyelostomy, ureterostomy, and bowel conduit urinary diversion), ureterosigmoidostomy, and continent cutaneous urinary diversion. The patient must understand that the choice of a particular form of urinary diversion is primarily a quality-of-life decision and has essentially no impact on the course of the disease necessitating bladder replacement. It is the responsibility of the surgeon who undertakes urinary reconstruction to fully educate the patient about all available forms of reconstruction and their relative benefits and risks. Having been so educated, the patient is prepared to make a truly informed decision.

## SURGICAL TECHNIQUE

No particular bowel preparation is necessary. Intravenous antibiotic coverage is indicated at the time of surgery. Heparin is given subcutaneously peri- and postoperatively as thrombosis prophylaxis.

### Cystectomy

Modifications of pelvic lymphadenectomy and the approach to the pelvic ureter are made to allow for optimum ileal neobladder construction (4). Pelvic lymphadenectomy and cystectomy are performed according to standard technique with slight modifications. Ideally, the ileal neobladder anatomically replaces the native bladder (i.e., it is located extraperitoneally in the pelvic cavity) and ileourethral anastomoses are located extraperitoneally. Depending on tumor stage and location, this goal can be easily achieved by the creation of two large peritoneal flaps obtained from the visceral pelvic peritoneum (Fig. 87.1).

### Modified Pelvic Lymph Node Dissection Following a Standard Laparotomy

Following a standard laparotomy via a lower midline incision, the prevesical space is entered. The space between the bladder and the iliac vessels is opened. The peritoneum is sharply

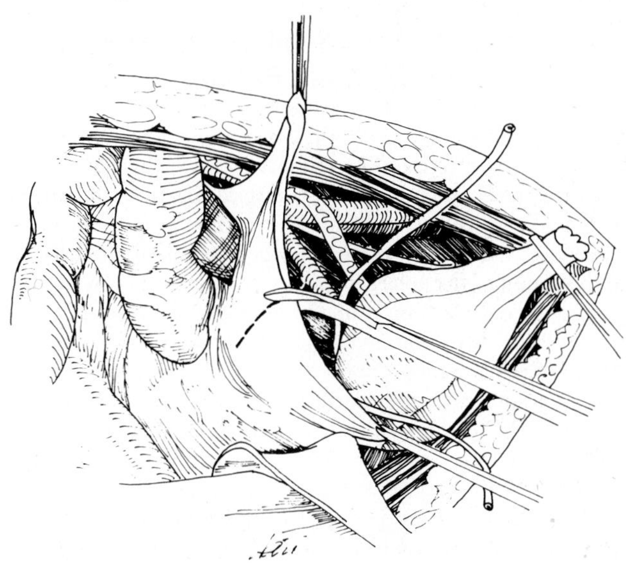

FIGURE 87.1 Modified pelvic lymph node dissection has been completed. Ureters are exposed extraperitoneally. The peritoneum over the bladder is bisected to create two large peritoneal flaps for later total extraperitonealization of the ileal neobladder.

dissected from the anterior abdominal wall, from the ileopsoas region, and from the internal ring. The spermatic cord is freed and looped out of the way with a vessel loop. The dissection is carried distally far enough to reach and resect the large medial retrocrural lymph node of Cloquet near the inguinal canal. The surgeon should stop at the circumflex iliac vein and clear the tissue from the posterolateral aspect of the common and external iliac veins. The bladder is retracted medially to dissect in the obturator fossa, and the important nodal tissue and fat are gently pulled out, clearly exposing obturator vessels and nerves. The peritoneum is mobilized bluntly in a cephalad direction to expose the anterior surface of the ureter.

### Ureteral Mobilization

The standard vertical incision lateral to the sigmoid mesocolon should not be used. The peritoneal sac should be mobilized medially on both sides. The surgeon should continue to locate the ureter extraperitoneally, realizing that it is displaced during exposure because it adheres to the peritoneum (Fig. 87.1). The ureters are mobilized with sufficient periureteral adventitia in a cephalad direction on both sides. A plane is established between the ureter and the lateral pedicles of the bladder. As the ureter and bladder are retracted medially, the lateral pedicle is exposed. Finally, the ureter is clamped distally. Fine-traction sutures are inserted in the proximal surface of the ureter, and it is divided against the clamps with scissors. Then, the ureter is dissected proximally so that about 6 to 9 cm is free.

Depending on tumor stage and location, the bladder is completely extraperitonealized and the peritoneum is bisected over the bladder (Fig. 87.1). If this cannot be done safely, an incision in the peritoneum is made high on the base of the bladder, leaving a peritoneal patch on the posterior bladder wall.

## Approach to the Membranous Urethra in the Male Patient

Urethral preparation with preservation of the continence mechanism is of critical importance when orthotopic diversion is anticipated. Attention to surgical detail is important and deserves special mention. The author believes that the continence mechanism in men may be maximized if dissection in the region of the anterior urethra is minimized. This has led to a slight modification in the technique of the apical dissection in the male patient undergoing orthotopic reconstruction. All fibroareolar connections between the anterior bladder wall, prostate, and undersurface of the pubic symphysis are divided. The endopelvic fascia is incised adjacent to the prostate, and the levator muscles are carefully swept off the lateral and apical portions of the prostate (Fig. 87.2A).

With tension placed posteriorly on the prostate, the puboprostatic ligaments are identified and slightly divided just beneath the pubis and lateral to the dorsal venous complex that courses between these ligaments (Fig. 87.2A). Care should be taken to avoid any extensive dissection in this region. The puboprostatic ligaments should only be incised enough to allow for proper apical dissection of the prostate (Fig. 87.2B). The apex of the prostate and membranous urethra becomes palpable. Several methods can be performed to properly control the dorsal venous plexus. An angled clamp may be passed carefully beneath the dorsal venous complex, anterior to the urethra (Fig. 87.3A and B). The venous complex can then be ligated with a 2-0 absorbable suture and divided close to the apex of the prostate. If any bleeding occurs from the transected venous complex, it can be oversewn with 2-0 polyglycolic acid sutures in a slightly different fashion; the dorsal venous complex may be gathered at the apex of the prostate with a long Allis clamp (Fig. 87.2B).

A 1-0 absorbable suture is then placed under direct vision anterior to the urethra (distal to the apex of the prostate) around the gathered venous complex (Fig. 87.3A and B). This suture is best placed with the surgeon facing the head of the table and holding the needle driver perpendicular to the patient. This maneuver avoids the unnecessary passage of any instruments between the dorsal venous complex and the rhabdosphincter, which could potentially injure these structures and compromise the continence mechanism.

After the complex has been ligated, it can be sharply divided with excellent exposure to the anterior surface of the urethra (Fig. 87.4). Once the venous complex has been severed, the suture can be used to further secure the complex. The suture is then used to suspend the venous complex anteriorly to the periosteum to help re-establish anterior fixation of the dorsal venous complex and puboprostatic ligaments. This may enhance recovery of continence. The anterior urethra is now exposed. Regardless of the technique, the urethra is then incised 180 degrees, just beyond the apex of the prostate (Fig. 87.5). Six 2-0 polyglycolic acid sutures are placed in the urethra circumferentially, carefully incorporating only the mucosa and submucosa of the striated urethral sphincter muscle anteriorly. The urethral catheter is clamped and divided distally. Two sutures are placed, which should incorporate the rectourethrales muscle posteriorly or the caudal extent of the Denonvillier fascia (Fig. 87.6). Following this, the posterior urethra is divided and the specimen is removed.

## Construction of the Reservoir

The light behind the mesentery should be adjusted, and a 60- to 70-cm-long ileal segment should be selected 10 to 20 cm proximally from the ileocecal valve (6,9,10). Spasticity of the

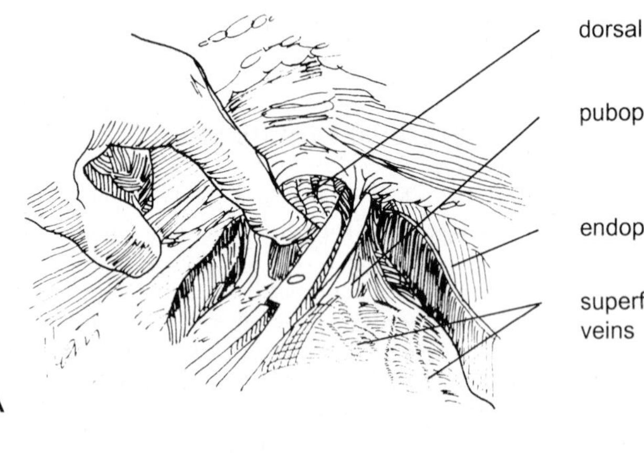


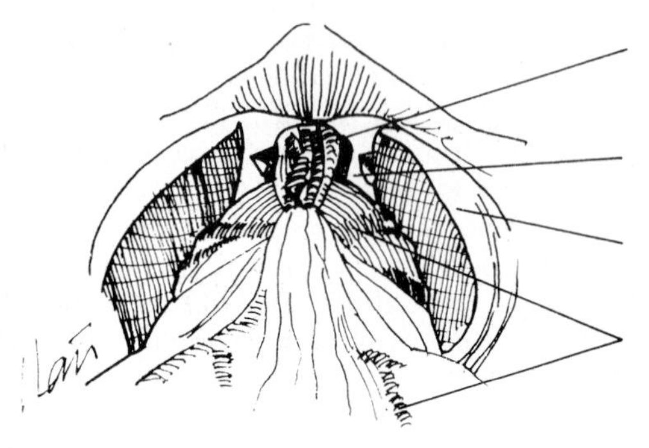


FIGURE 87.2 **A:** The endopelvic fascia adjacent to the prostate is incised. Note that care should be taken not to perform excessive dissection along the pelvic floor levator musculature, which could injure the innervation to the rhabdosphincter. The puboprostatic ligaments are slightly divided, providing excellent exposure to the apex of the prostate and the membranous urethra. **B:** The dorsal venous complex should be gathered with an Allis clamp near the apex of the prostate or with a stitch.

bladder
dorsal vein complex
urethra (ext. sphincter)
catheter
neurovascular bundle
rectum
A
B

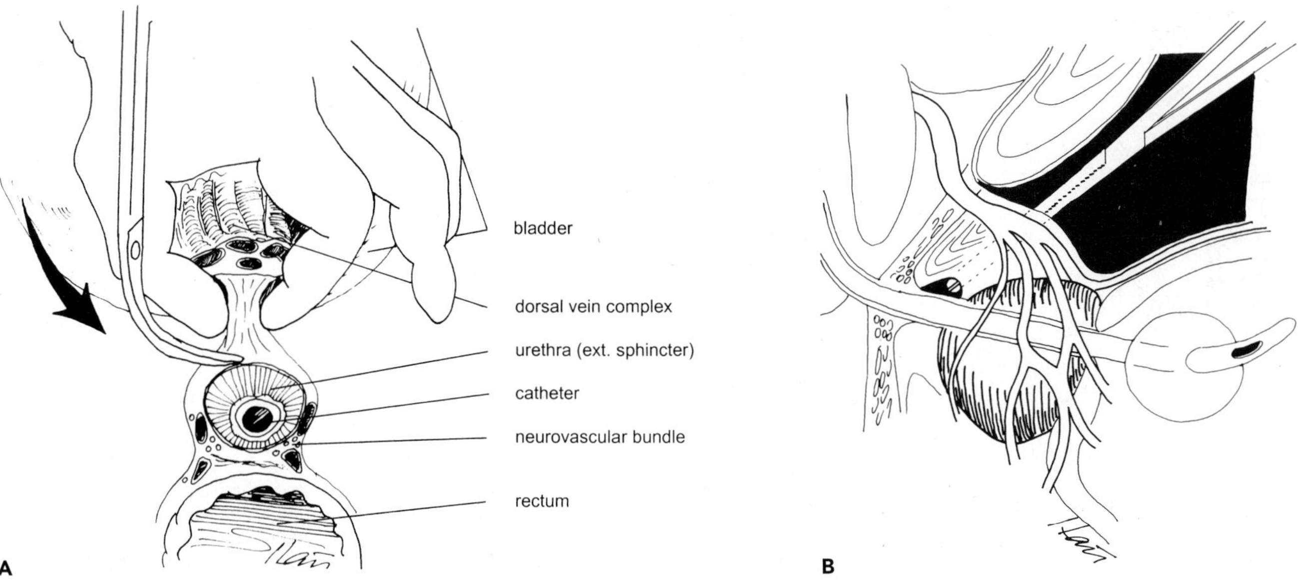

FIGURE 87.3 **A:** The dorsal venous complex may be controlled by carefully passing a clamp between the venous complex (anterior) and the urethra (posterior). **B:** A suture is carefully placed anterior to the urethra and around the gathered venous complex.

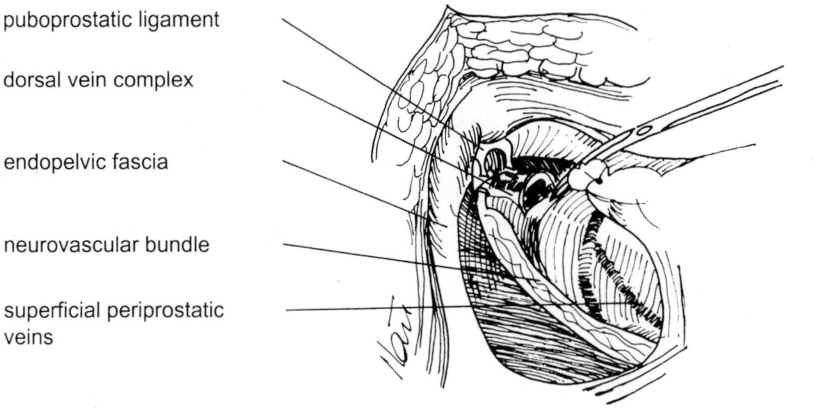

puboprostatic ligament
dorsal vein complex
endopelvic fascia
neurovascular bundle
superficial periprostatic veins

FIGURE 87.4 The venous complex is divided. The previously placed suture can then be used to further secure the dorsal venous complex if any bleeding occurs. The complex is then fixed anteriorly to the periosteum.

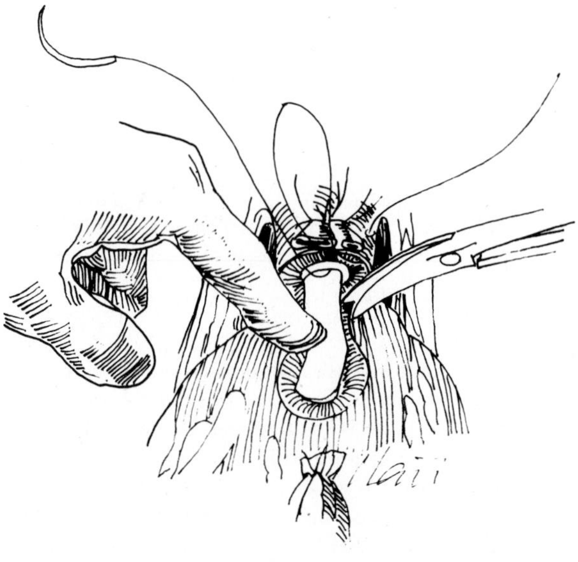

FIGURE 87.5 The anterior urethra is incised 180 degrees just beyond the prostate apex.

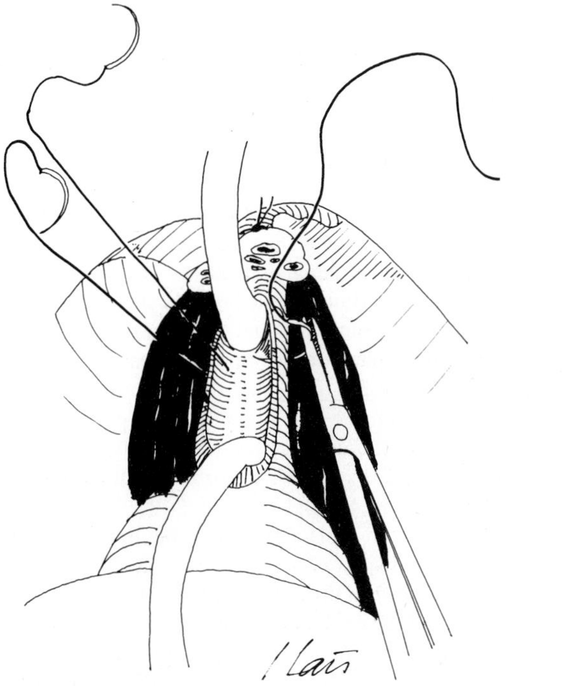

FIGURE 87.6 Placement of urethral sutures and division of the posterior urethral wall.

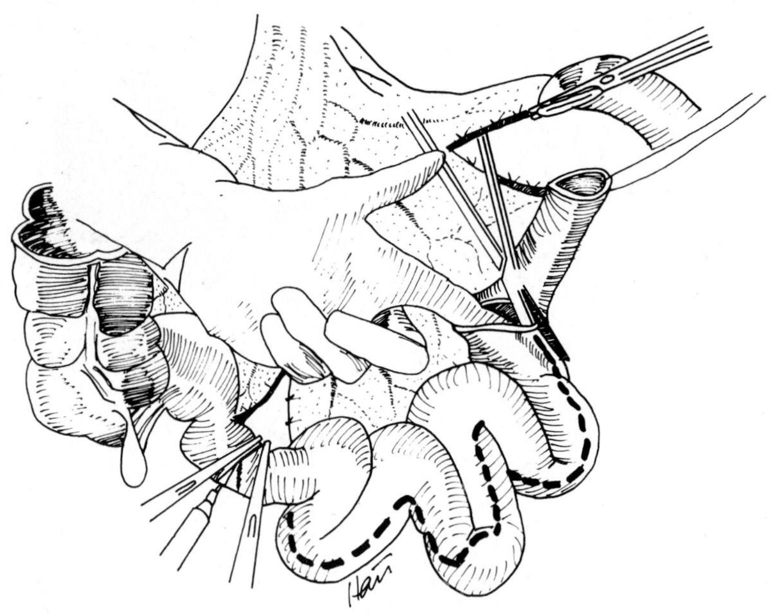

FIGURE 87.7 Selection of the ileal segment with an appropriate vascular supply and antimesenteric incision of ileum, except for the small chimneys on both sides of the W and the intended site of the ileourethral anastomosis *(broken line)*.

bowel or a thick, short mesentery may lead to more bowel than necessary, thus increasing the reservoir capacity. It is helpful to place two temporary stay sutures at the intended resection lines. They can be moved several times if necessary. The most dependable part of the segment should be long enough to reach the top of the symphysis pubica in the skin level. That point should be marked with a suture. This maneuver guarantees that the reservoir will reach the urethral remnant without difficulty. The distal division of the mesentery along the avascular region between the ileocolic artery and the terminal branches of the superior mesenteric artery should extend to the base of the mesentery to provide maximum mobility and sufficient length to reach the membranous urethra. The proximal incision of the mesentery is made as short as possible to provide maximum vascular supply to the ileal segment. The ileum is then divided between bowel clamps. A standard bowel anastomosis is performed and the mesenteric trap is closed. The isolated bowel segment is thoroughly cleaned or rinsed with saline or an iodine solution (Fig. 87.7).

Four lengths of ileum are arranged in the shape of a W with 3- to 5-cm-long chimneys on each side of the W using five to six Babcock clamps. Other than the two chimneys, the bowel is opened on the antimesenteric border except for a 5- to 7-cm section centered around the marking suture, which is opened to close to the antimesenteric border to create a U-shaped flap. Two to 3 cm from the tip of that flap, a buttonhole of all layers is excised from the ileal plate. An ileal plate is formed by sewing together the cut edges of the antimesenteric borders of the W using 2-0 synthetic absorbable sutures (SASs) on a straight needle (Fig. 87.8).

A 22Fr catheter is placed through the buttonhole. For the actual anastomosis, six previously placed double-armed sutures using 3-0 SAS in the urethra are used. The inner sutures are passed through the neobladder outlet in the ileal plate without grasping the ileum, and the corresponding outer sutures grasp the entire ileal wall 5 to 8 mm lateral to the neobladder outlet (Fig. 87.9). This guarantees a wide, ideal, funnel-shaped anastomosis so that mucosa is in direct contact with urethral epithelium. Next, under gentle traction on the transurethral catheter, the ileal plate is manipulated down to the urethral remnant and the knots are tied inside the bowel (Fig. 87.10). The cut edges of the 5- to 7-cm U-shaped flap are sewn together over the catheter. The lower third of the anterior wall of the neobladder is closed, beginning inferiorly with interrupted 3-0 SAS (Fig. 87.11).

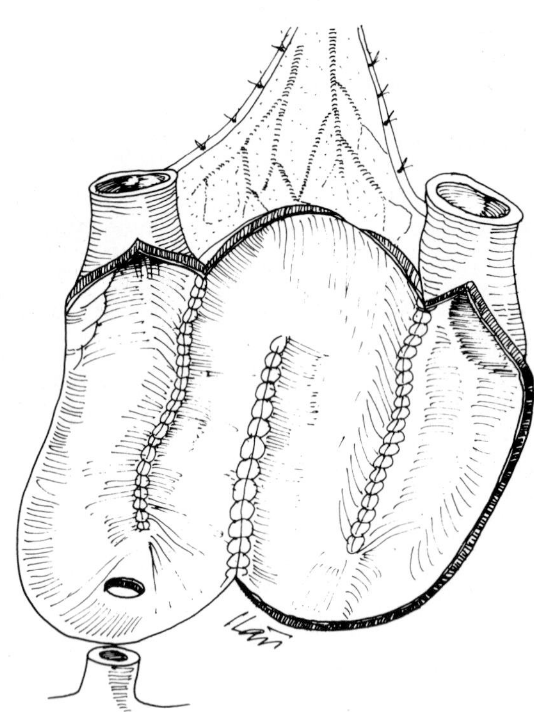

FIGURE 87.8 W-shaped reconfiguration of the intestinal segment after detubularization and asymmetrical incision of the ileal wall at the site of the anastomosis to the urethra, forming a U-shaped flap.

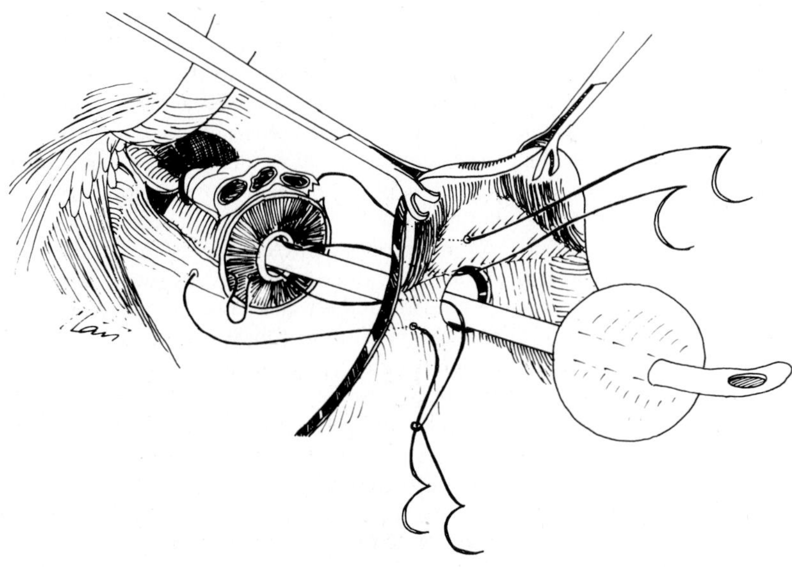

FIGURE 87.9 Ileourethral anastomosis, anterior view.

In 10% of patients, the ileourethral anastomosis may cause some difficulties. Some or all of the following tricks are helpful to overcome this dilemma (Fig. 87.12A and B): loosening the retractor, straightening the operating table, removing the sacral cushion, neutralizing the extended position of the patient, bringing up the perineum with a sponge stick, freeing the cecum and descending colon as in retroperitoneal lymph node dissection (RPLND), moving up the neobladder outlet to the tip of the U-shaped flap, or performing an end-to-end anastomosis after tubularization of the U-shaped flap (Fig. 87.13). Any incisions into the mesentery of the neobladder should be avoided. The neobladder mesentery should not be pulled roughly to the pelvic floor.

## Refluxing Ileoureteral Anastomosis

Controversy exists about the importance of an antireflux mechanism, and the benefits are not easy to define in adults undergoing urinary diversion. It is clear that the need for reflux prevention is not the same as in ureterosigmoidostomy conduit or continent diversion. The rationale for implanting the ureters in an antireflux fashion into orthotopic bladder substitutes or continent reservoirs is to prevent the upper urinary tract from retrograde hydrodynamically transmitted pressure peaks and from ascending bacteriuria. However, the routine of antireflux ureter implantation into intestinal urinary reservoirs was born in the era before the creation of designated low-pressure reservoirs. Reflux prevention in neobladders is even less important than in a normal bladder because there are no coordinated contractions during micturition and there is a simultaneous pressure increase in neobladder, abdomen, and kidney pelvis during the Valsalva maneuver. Using nonrefluxing techniques, the risk of obstruction is at least twice that following a direct anastomosis, irrespective of type of bowel segment used, and half of these strictures require secondary procedures.

Since 1996 we have been using a freely refluxing, open, end-to-side ureteroileal anastomosis, which is the simplest small-bowel surgery and which has reduced our stenosis rate from 9.5% to 1.0%. Further advantages of this chimney modification are the extra length to reach the ureteral stump, the

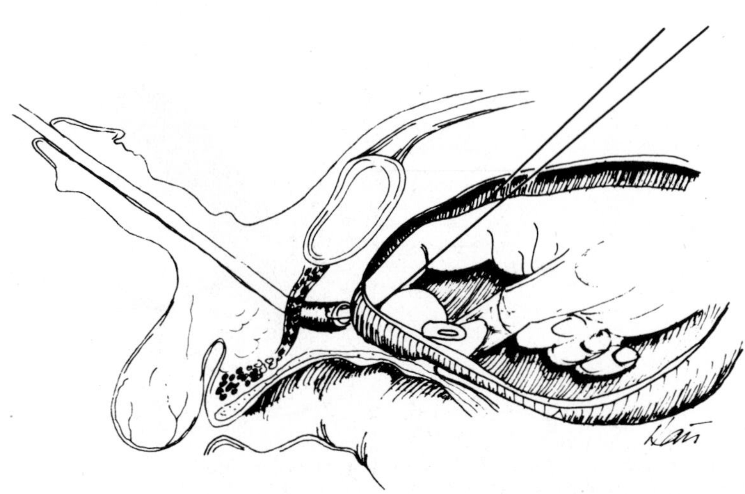

FIGURE 87.10 Lateral aspect of the ileourethral anastomosis. The sutures are tied from inside the ileal bladder.

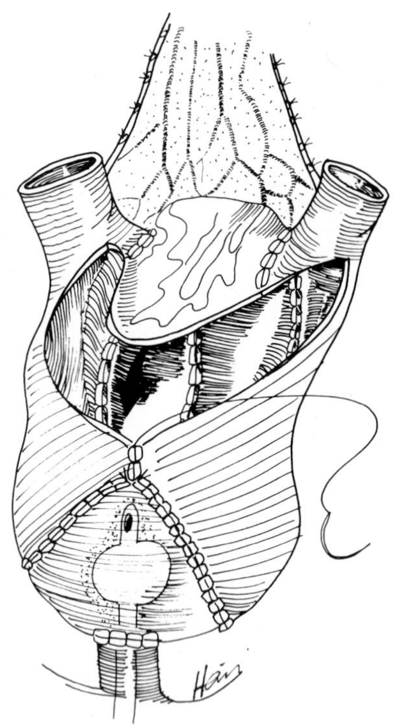

FIGURE 87.11 Closure of reservoir.

ease of surgery far outside the pelvic cavity, a tension-free anastomosis, no risk of ureteral angulation with neobladder filling, and a simplified flank access for revisional surgery.

On each side, the ureters are trimmed as appropriate for their chimney (Fig. 87.14). The ureterointestinal anastomosis can be done extraperitoneally above the common iliac vessels using a Bricker or Wallace (our choice) technique without competing with the bowel mesentery for an anastomotic site (Fig. 87.14). After appropriate ureteral stents are placed, they are brought through the anterior neobladder suture line. The remaining anterior neobladder wall is closed in a T shape with running 3-0 SASs. No cystostomy tube is placed. Two 20Fr silicone drains are placed into the small pelvis.

Using the two large peritoneal flaps from the visceral pelvic peritoneum, this goal can easily been reached (Fig. 87.1). Both flaps are sewn together, except for the portion where the mesentery of the neobladder runs through them. The peritoneal cavity is closed in a standard fashion (Fig. 87.15). Alternatively, the flaps can be sewn to the posterior wall of the neobladder.

Excessive mucus production of the ileal bladder may rarely cause a problem by obstructing the urethral catheter in the postoperative course. Therefore, the ileal bladder is rinsed via the cystostomy with 50 to 100 mL of saline twice a day, starting on postoperative day 5. Routinely, the ureteral stents are removed between postoperative days 7 and 14.

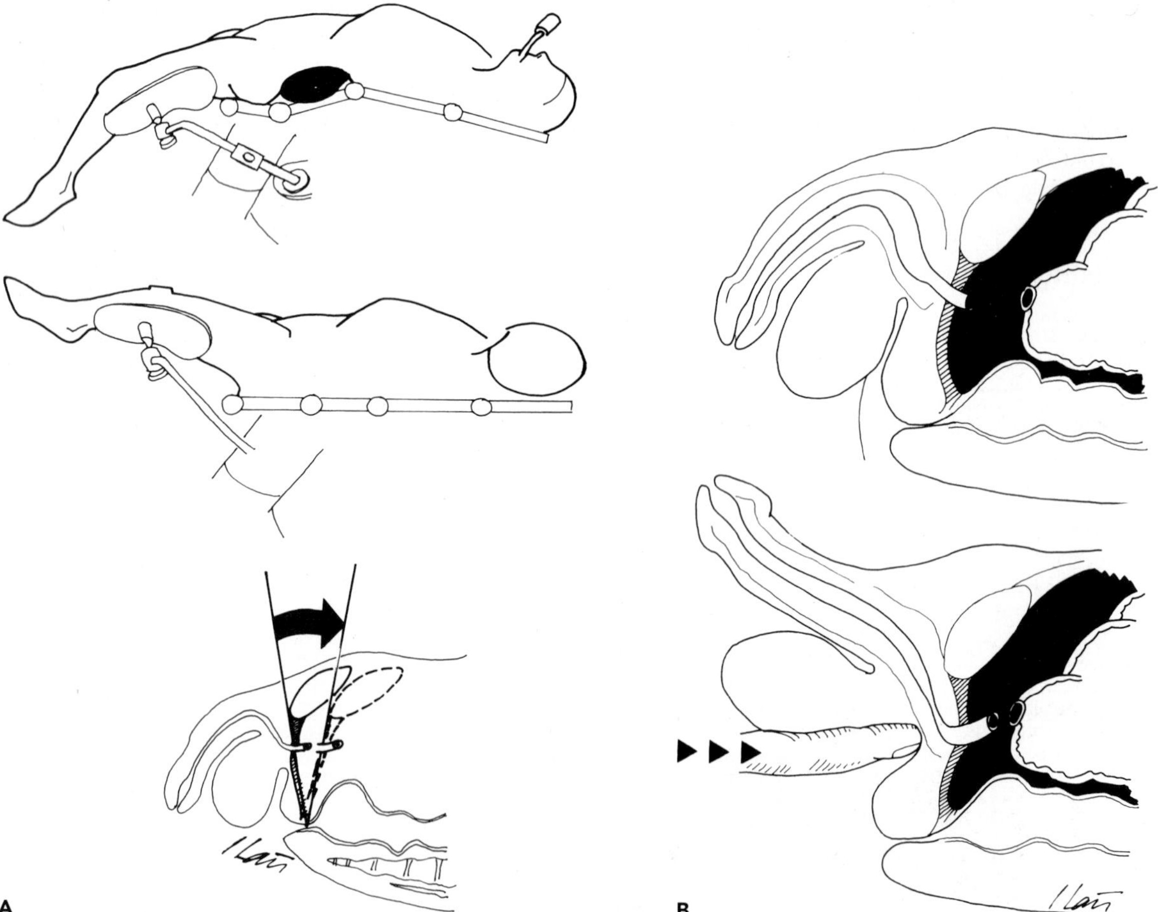


FIGURE 87.12 Methods to get the ileal neobladder to the pelvic floor. **A:** Changing the extended position of the patient to slightly supine and removing the sacral cushion rotate the pelvic floor upward. **B:** Pushing up the perineum with a sponge stick or finger approximates the urethral remnant and neobladder.

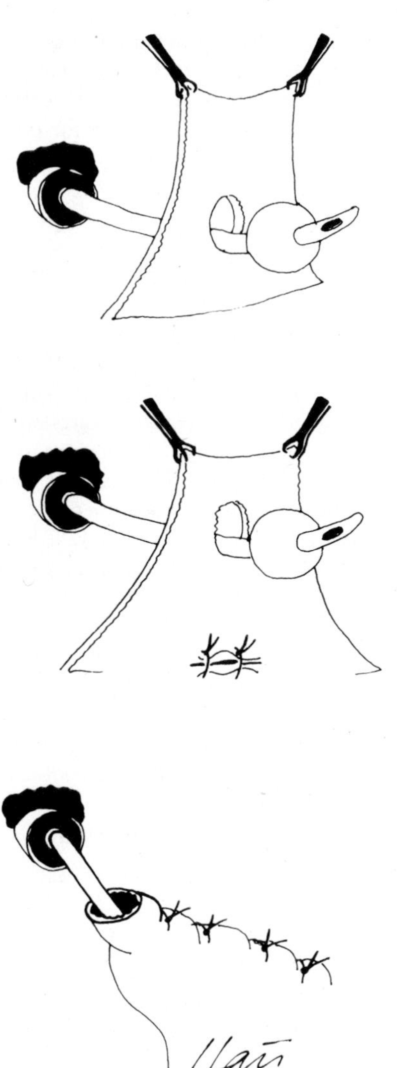

FIGURE 87.13 Moving the neobladder outlet closer to the tip of the U-shaped flap of ileal plate. If this still does not allow tension-free anastomosis, one should tubularize the U-shaped form and perform direct (end-to-end) anastomosis.

As soon as the urine is in contact with the ileal bladder mucosa, reabsorption of urine electrolytes may occur. Therefore, the base excess is checked at weekly intervals for the first 4 weeks and monthly thereafter. Approximately 50% of all patients need temporary alkalinizing therapy.

The urethral catheter is removed between postoperative days 14 and 21, after a cystogram has demonstrated complete healing of the ileourethral anastomosis. Rarely, there is still leakage from the anastomosis. When this is occurs, it is treated by prolonged catheter drainage until the leak has closed spontaneously.

## OUTCOMES

### Complications

The complications of both continent catheterizable reservoirs and orthotopic bladder substitutes in the hands of the most experienced surgeons have been considered in detail (4,7,8).

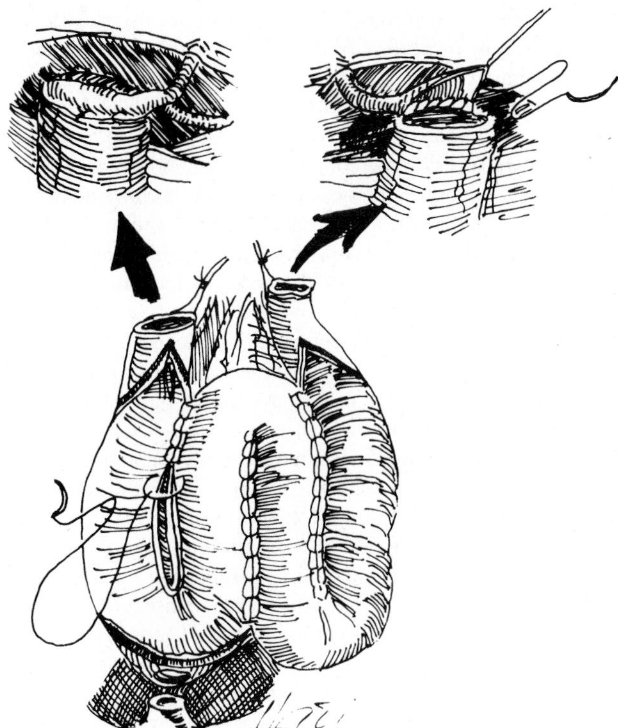

FIGURE 87.14 Refluxing ileoureteral anastomosis using chimneys of a 3- to 5-cm afferent limb on each side.

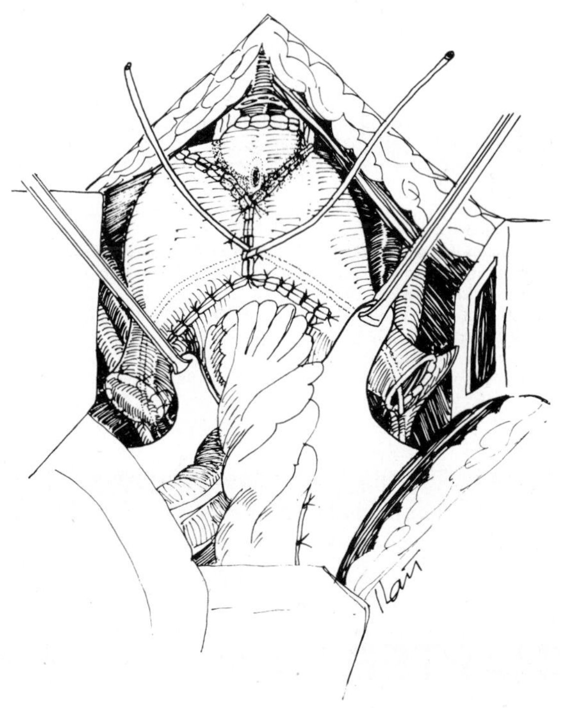

FIGURE 87.15 Completely extraperitoneal localization of the neobladder as well as ileourethral and ileoureteral anastomoses.

Reoperation for early complications overall occurred in 3% of continent catheterizable reservoirs and 7% of orthotopic bladder substitutions. Reoperation for late complications overall occurred in about 30% of continent catheterizable reservoirs and in 13% of orthotopic bladder substitutions (4,7,8). We believe that the morbidity of orthotopic bladder substitutes is actually similar to, or lower than, the true rates of morbidity after conduit formation, contrary to the popular view that conduits are simple and safe.

There are several new complications unknown during the conduit era, including incisional hernias, as a consequence of the Valsalva maneuver: neobladder-intestinal and neobladder-cutaneous fistulas, mucus formation, and neobladder rupture. The secretion of mucus can be dramatically increased.

Spontaneous late rupture of neobladders is a rare but potentially life-threatening complication. In the majority of cases it is secondary to acute or chronic overdistention and bacterial infection. Other factors are minor blunt abdominal trauma or urethral occlusion. Chronic ischemic changes of the neobladder's wall, possibly facilitated by detubularization and the variability of the mesenteric circulation, are additional factors that lead to perforation. The rupture site is typically the upper part of the right side of the reservoir. This is the most mobile part of the reservoir and undergoes the most marked distention during overfilling, which may constitute an additional factor for perforation in this location. There is no reliable procedure to establish the diagnosis. Cystography is misleading in three of four patients with neobladder rupture. A high index of suspicion and early aggressive operative treatment in patients suspected of having a neobladder rupture are instrumental in providing a successful outcome. Prevention of neobladder rupture comprises careful monitoring of neobladder emptying. Physicians must be aware of the risk of rupture. Patients must be encouraged to void regularly, especially at bedtime, and perform clean intermittent self-catheterization to avoid chronic reservoir overdistention. In the event of anesthesia, proper bladder drainage should be performed.

## Results

In some studies, perioperative death occurred in 3% of patients. Neobladder-related early and late complications occurred in 15% and 23% of patients, respectively. Neobladder-related early and late abdominal reoperation rates were 0.3% and 4%, respectively. Perioperative neobladder-unrelated early complications were observed in 33%, and 12% of patients required operative treatment. Late postoperative complications unrelated to the neobladder occurred in 12% of patients, and 5% required open surgical revision. Ninety-six percent of patients voided spontaneously, 4% performed clean intermittent catheterization in some form, and 1.7% performed regular intermittent catheterization. Thirty percent to 40% of women required some form of intermittent catheterization to completely empty their neobladder (6–8). Daytime and nighttime continence was reported as good by 96% and satisfactory by 95% of patients. Unacceptable daytime continence requiring more than one pad per day occurred in only 4% of patients, and only 5% were wetting more than one pad per night.

## *References*


1. Hautmann RE. The ileal neobladder to the female urethra. *Urol Clin North Am* 1997;24:827–835.
2. Hautmann RE. The ileal neobladder. *Atlas Urol Clin North Am* 2001;9: 85–108.
3. Hautmann RE. Urinary diversion: ileal conduit to neobladder [Review]. *J Urol* 2003;169:834–842.
4. Hautmann RE, de Patriconi R, Gottfried H-W, et al. The ileal neobladder: complications and functional results in 363 patients after 11 years of followup. *J Urol* 1999;161:422–428.
5. Hautmann RE, Egghart G, Frohneberg D, et al. The ileal neobladder. *J Urol* 1988;139:39–43.
6. Hautmann RE, Paiss T, de Petriconi R. The ileal neobladder in women: 9 years of experience with 18 patients. *J Urol* 1996;155:76–81.
7. Hautmann RE, Volkmer BG, Schumacher MC, et al. Long-term results of standard procedures in urology: the ileal neobladder. *World J Urol* 2006; 24:305–314.
8. Hautmann RE, Abol-Enein H, Hafez K, et al. Urinary diversion. *Urology* 2007;69 [Suppl 1A]:17–49.
9. Skinner DG, Studer UE, Okada K, et al. Which are suitable for continent diversion or bladder substitution following cystectomy or other definitive local treatment? *Int J Urol* 1995;2[Suppl 2]:105.
10. Studer UE, Hautmann RE, Hohenfellner M, et al. Indications for continent diversion after cystectomy and factors affecting long-term results. *Urol Oncol* 1998;4:172.


# CHAPTER 88 ■ THE PADUA ILEAL BLADDER

FRANCESCO PAGANO AND PIERFRANCESCO BASSI

The Padua ileal bladder (VIP, or "vescica ileale Padovana") was developed as a practical application of the concepts expressed by Camey (3), Bramble (2), Kock (5), and Hinman (4) for the construction of a urinary reservoir employing an intestinal segment: detubularization, reconfiguration, and search for a spherical pouch of adequate capacity.

Large and small bowel nondetubularized segments used as bladder substitutes have been shown to generate significant intraluminal pressures (4,5) and subsequently cause urinary incontinence and/or renal failure. Disrupting directional peristalsis by opening the antimesenteric border of the bowel (detubularization) and folding (reconfiguration) has been proven to significantly decrease intraluminal pressure by making ineffective the bowel contractions. However, a single folding of the intestinal detubularized segment incompletely suppresses the peristaltic activity, as Kock demonstrated: a double folding is necessary for this aim (5). As a consequence, the double-folding Kock principle is the gold standard in constructing a spherical reservoir from a cylindrical bowel segment.

The capacity and the intraluminal pressure of a reservoir also depend on the geometric configuration, as demonstrated by Hinman (4) with geometric considerations: the larger the radius, the larger the volume. From the surgical standpoint, this explains why the double folding produces the largest volume from the same initial intestinal length. Coupling the double folding with the spherical configuration also offers a relevant feature: at the same endoluminal pressure, the larger diameter accommodates a larger volume, according to the Laplace and Pascal laws.

## GOALS

Following the above-mentioned principles, the functional requirements of the Padua ileal bladder were identified in 1990 (6): adequate capacity (300 to 500 mL), low-pressure storage phase (<40 cm of water ), no reflux to upper urinary tract, daytime and nighttime continence, and voluntary as well as easy and complete voiding "per urethram." An intestinal reservoir respecting these requirements should allow the long-term preservation of renal function and provide a reliable control of continence and voiding with satisfactory patient acceptance.

Further features have also been considered. Because urine absorption throughout the intestinal wall is unavoidable, the shortest intestinal segment must be selected to minimize secondary metabolic disorders. An easy-to-perform and quick procedure with a short learning curve is considered highly desirable. Last but not least, from the oncologic standpoint, the neobladder must not interfere with the natural history of the disease and the related treatment(s).

## DIAGNOSIS

Normal renal function is compulsory: however, a dilated upper urinary tract(s) per se does not represent a contraindication to the procedure. A normal urethral closure pressure, evaluated by the urethral pressure profile and the tumor site far from the trigone and the posterior bladder wall, is requested in female patients. To benefit from the procedure, the patient must have intelligence, maturity, and motivation.

## INDICATIONS FOR SURGERY

Any patient, male or female, who is a candidate for a conduit diversion is potentially suitable for bladder substitution as long as an adequate ileal segment is available. Surgical indications include bladder cancers, neurogenic bladder, congenital abnormalities, and refractory interstitial cystitis. From the oncologic standpoint, the only contraindication is a positive urethral margin biopsy: patients with locally advanced bladder cancer (T3 to T4) or with nodal involvement and candidates for adjuvant systemic chemotherapy are also suitable for the procedure.

## ALTERNATIVE THERAPIES

Other urinary diversions, including ileal and colonic conduits, continent urinary diversions, and other forms of orthotopic bladders, are possible alternatives. The patient's health, motivation, and desires, together with the abdominal anatomy, will determine the optimal diversion.

## SURGICAL TECHNIQUE

### Cystectomy

In men, the membranous urethra is managed as in radical prostatectomy and is incised as close as possible to the prostatic apex to preserve the distal urethral sphincter. In selected patients, the nerve-sparing cystoprostatectomy can be performed.

In women, the ureters are dissected and divided distally and the uterine vessels ligated and divided. The peritoneum is circumferentially incised just below the vaginal fundus. The uterus is lifted posteriorly, and the plane between the anterior vaginal wall and bladder is developed toward the bladder neck (Fig. 88.1). In this phase the bladder vessels are ligated and divided with respect of the autonomic nerves that originate from the pelvic plexus and run along the lateral vaginal wall toward the urethra. The bladder neck is identified by filling the catheter balloon to 20 cc and using a slight outward traction. Before the bladder neck incision, a Satinsky clamp is cranially placed to avoid the spilling of urine and tumor cells. The urethral margin is sent for pathological evaluation.

Thereafter the uterus with the ovaries is removed and the vaginal fundus accurately sutured. A 2- by 15-cm strip of

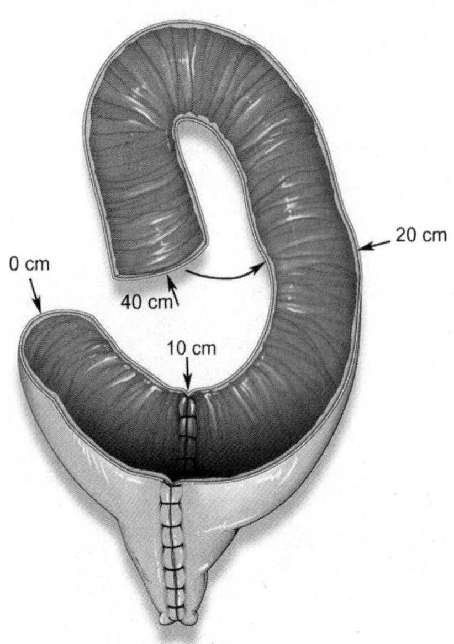


**FIGURE 88.1** Creation of lower funnel

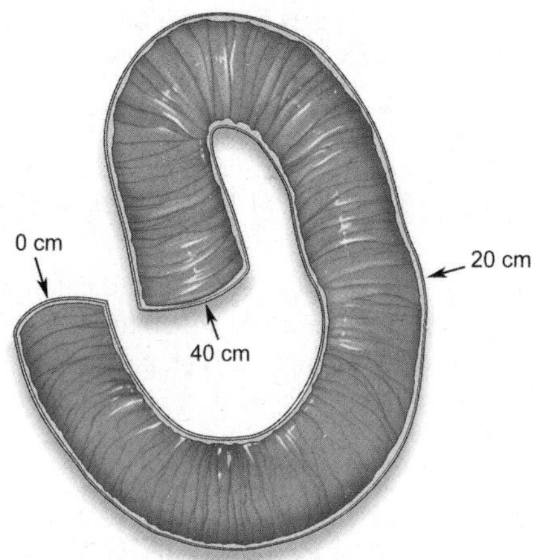


FIGURE 88.2 Detubularization and reconfiguration (scheme).

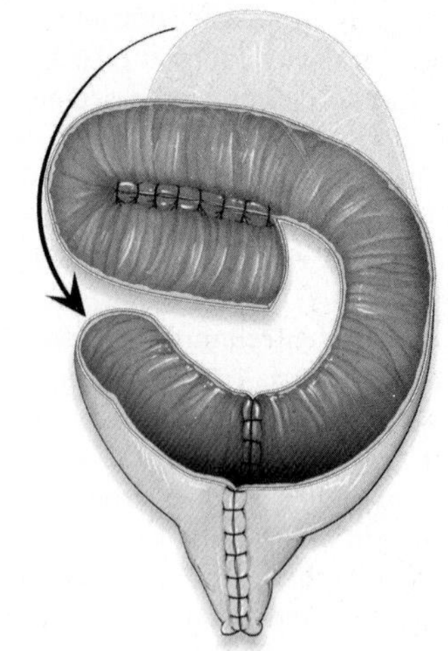

FIGURE 88.4 First folding maneuver.

abdominal fascia is dissected from the laparotomic incision and bilaterally fixed to the sacrum promontory with nonabsorbable sutures and to the vaginal fundus with 2-0 polyglactin sutures, respectively (Fig. 88.2).

## Creation of the Padua Ileal Bladder

A 40-cm ileal segment is isolated, starting at a convenient point 15 to 20 cm proximal to the ileocecal valve (Fig. 88.3). The distal (aboral) mesenteric incision is deepened at the level of the ileocolic artery to obtain better mobility and to allow a tension-free urethrointestinal anastomosis. On the contrary, the proximal (oral) mesenteric incision can be short because it does not contribute to the mobility of the reservoir. The intestinal continuity is restored by an end-to-end anastomosis with surgical staplers.

The entire ileal segment is split open along the antimesenteric border (Fig. 88.4). A lower funnel is created by means of two running sutures, posteriorly and anteriorly, about 5 cm in length in order to make the urethrointestinal anastomosis easier and tension-free (Fig. 88.5). The ileal anastomotic hole is placed at the lowest edge of the funnel: the eversion of the ileal mucosa in the anastomotic hole is recommended. Medially, the proximal loop is folded on itself in a reversed U shape, and the inner opposite borders are sutured side to side to create an upper ileal cup (Fig. 88.6).

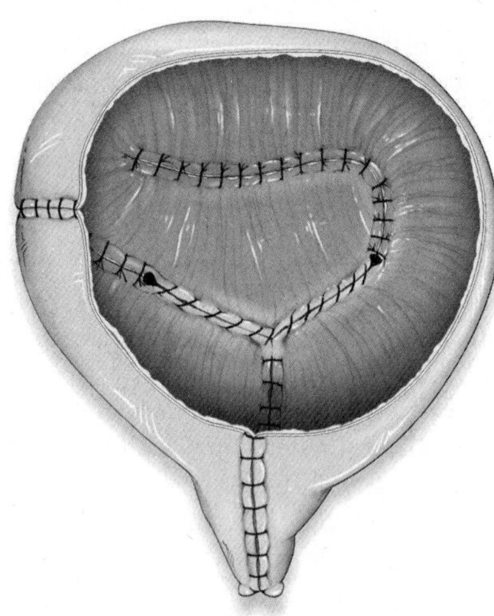

FIGURE 88.5 Ureteral reimplantation: serous-lined intestinal troughs.

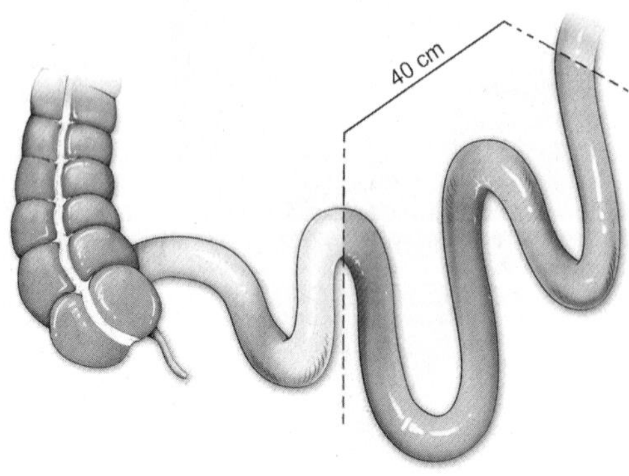


FIGURE 88.3 Isolation of a 40-cm segment of distal ileum.

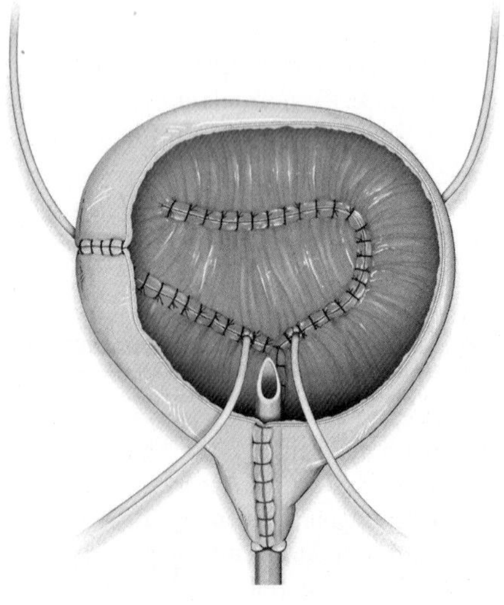

FIGURE 88.6 Ureteral reimplantation: final view.

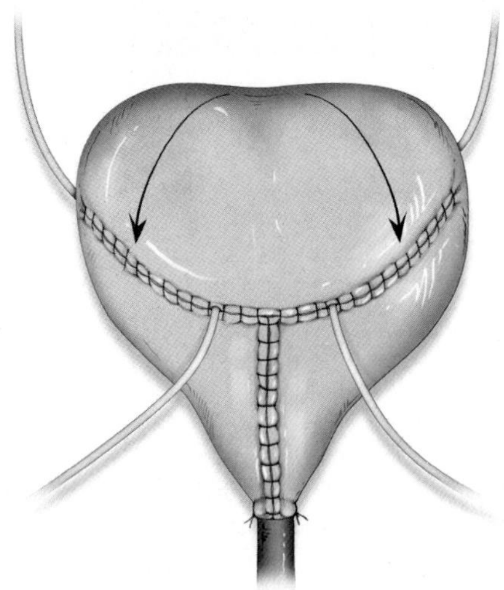

FIGURE 88.7 Second folding maneuver and final view.

The ureteroileal anastomosis with serous-lined extramural reimplantation according to the Abol-Eneim and Ghoneim technique (1) is carried out bilaterally. The edges of two medial intestinal flaps are joined by a running through-and-through suture of 3-0 polyglactin, resulting in the creation of two oblique serous-lined intestinal troughs (Fig. 88.7). The left ureter is brought medially through a suitable mesenteric window in the left mesocolon, providing a downward smooth curve without kinking. Each ureter is then laid into its corresponding trough. A mucosa-to-mucosa anastomosis between the stented (6Fr) and spatulated end of the ureter and the ileal flaps is performed using 4-0 polyglactin suture. The implanted ureters are then covered by approximation and an interrupted 3-0 polyglactin suture is inserted.

When appropriate, a direct non-antirefluxing ureteroileal anastomosis is performed monolaterally or bilaterally: in this case the neobladder is also fixed with 3-0 polyglactin sutures to the ipsilateral psoas muscle. The ureteral stents are fixed to the pouch mucosa close to the ureteral hiatus and secured to their exits (made by stabbing through the anterior wall of the reservoir) using a 4-0 polyglactin suture. The urethroileal anastomosis is performed with six to eight 3-0 polyglactin sutures.

The closure of the reservoir is completed at the anterior aspect by folding downward the upper edge of the ileal cup to obtain a spherical reservoir. A running suture of 3-0 polyglactin is employed for all the suturing of the reservoir. The reservoir is drained by a transurethral 22Fr or 24Fr hematuria catheter.

Parenteral alimentation is supplied until normal bowel function resumes. Wide-spectrum antibiotics are given for 7 days; then quinolones are administered orally as long as the pouch catheter stays in. The rectal and the gastric tubes are left in place for 3 to 4 days or until bowel contractions begin. The ureters are drained by 6Fr to 8Fr or more stents and are removed after 10 days. Radiologic evaluation of the pouch is performed after 12 days. Special attention is paid to train the patient to completely empty the reservoir by abdominal straining and simultaneous perineal relaxation and to develop alternatives to the normal voiding desire.

## OUTCOMES

### Results

The Padova small bowel neobladder procedure was first performed in 1987 (6). Since its first applications, some changes have been sequentially introduced to simplify and shorten the procedure. Initially, the sequence was as follows: ileourethral anastomosis, detubularization, lower funnel, ureteral reimplantation according to the LeDuc technique, posterior reconfiguration, and anterior reconfiguration. The length of the ileal segment was progressively reduced from between 50 and 60 cm to 40 cm. Recently the sequence of maneuvers has been established as follows: detubularization, construction of the lower funnel, posterior reconfiguration, bilateral ureteral reimplantation, incomplete anterior reconfiguration, ileourethral anastomosis, complete reconfiguration, and extraperitonealization of the reservoir. This sequence allows the surgeon to perform the major part of the procedure on the surface of the surgical field, thus reducing the operative time (at present about 2 hours). Because of the unsatisfactory rate of ureterointestinal anastomosis stenoses (7), the LeDuc ureteral reimplantation technique has been abandoned and favorably replaced with the serous-lined extramural reimplantation according to the Abol-Eneim and Ghoneim procedure (1). The procedure can be easily performed in women with satisfactory functional results provided the vaginal axis is respected by a colpopexy.

## CONCLUSIONS

The Padua ileal bladder (VIP, or "vescica Ileale Padovana") is a simple, quick procedure with a short learning curve for the urologist who is accustomed to performing radical cystoprostatectomy, ileal conduit, and antireflux procedures. The procedure provides both sexes a good-capacity, low-pressure, nonrefluxing, and continent reservoir by employing only a 40-cm ileal segment in both men and women. The procedure can be easily customized according to anatomical and oncologic needs.

## *References*


1. Abol-Eneim H, Ghoneim MA. A novel uretero-ileal reimplantation technique: the serous lined extramural tunnel. A preliminary report. *J Urol* 1995;151:1193–1197.
2. Bramble FG. The treatment of adult enuresis and urge incontinence by enterocystoplasty. *Br J Urol* 1982;54:693.
3. Camey M, Richard F, Botto H. Bladder replacement by ileocystoplasty. In: King LR, Stone AR, Webster GD, eds. *Bladder reconstruction and continent urinary diversion*. Chicago: Year Book Medical Publishers, 1987.
4. Hinman F Jr. Selection of intestinal segments for bladder substitution: physical and physiological characteristics. *J Urol* 1988;139:519–524.
5. Kock NG. The development of the continent ileal reservoir (Kock pouch) and application in patients requiring urinary diversion. In: King LR, Stone AR, Webster GD, eds. *Bladder reconstruction and continent urinary diversion*. Chicago: Year Book Medical Publishers, 1987.
6. Pagano F, Artibani W, Ligato P. Vescica ileale Padovana: a technique for total bladder replacement. *Eur Urol* 1990;17:149–154.
7. Pagano F, Bassi P, Artibani W. The Padua ileal bladder (V.I.P., vescica ileale Padovana). *Acta Urol Ital* 1996;10(2):79–83.

# CHAPTER 89 ■ THE T-POUCH ILEAL NEOBLADDER

JOHN P. STEIN AND DONALD G. SKINNER

The goals of urinary diversion have evolved from simply diverting the urine and protecting the upper urinary tracts. Contemporary objectives of urinary diversion should also include a form of reconstruction that provides a safe and continent means to store and eliminate urine, with efforts to improve the quality of life of the patient requiring cystectomy (6). Currently, four reasonable options regarding lower-urinary-tract reconstruction exist: (a) an incontinent cutaneous diversion: the ileal or colon conduit; (b) a continent cutaneous reservoir, requiring catheterization of a cutaneous stoma; (c) a continent rectal reservoir, with storage and elimination of urine via the rectum; and (d) the orthotopic bladder substitute (neobladder), with reconstruction to the native intact urethra.

The evolution of urinary diversion and lower-urinary-tract reconstruction over the past 60 years has been remarkable. Progress should be attributed to advances in medical and surgical improvements but should also be credited to thoughtful and creative surgeons looking to improve upon existing forms of urinary diversion. In 1950, Bricker (2) introduced the ileal conduit, which established a technically simple and reliable form of urinary diversion. The ileal conduit remains even today a commonly performed urinary diversion and a standard to which other forms of urinary reconstruction are compared. Concurrent with Bricker's introduction of the ileal conduit, Gilchrist (3) independently reported on a continent cutaneous form of diversion utilizing the ileocecal valve as the continence mechanism and the terminal ileum as a catheterizable stoma. For various medical reasons, Gilchrist's ileocecal reservoir garnered little support, and the technically simpler Bricker ileal conduit became the urinary diversion of choice for the next several decades.

The concept of a continent cutaneous urinary diversion was eventually reintroduced and popularized in the early 1980s, revolutionizing urinary diversion to a continent cutaneous form of diversion (4). Although patients were relieved from the issues of an external collection device, catheterization of the continent abdominal stoma was required. The continent cutaneous urinary diversion was considered a step forward and an improvement on the standard ileal or colon conduit. These continent reservoirs, however, are technically more challenging, take significantly longer to construct, and are associated with a reoperation rate, particularly the efferent catheterizable limb. Despite the benefits of the continent cutaneous reservoir over an ileal conduit, these aforementioned issues even today have limited the widespread application of this form of urinary diversion.

A natural progression from the continent cutaneous urinary diversion was the orthotopic bladder substitute (neobladder) connected directly to the native intact urethra (6). The orthotopic neobladder resembles the original bladder in location and function. An orthotopic form of reconstruction eliminates the need for a cutaneous stoma and a cutaneous collection device, and it relies on the patients' intact rhabdosphincter continence mechanism (external striated sphincter muscle), thus eliminating the need for intermittent catheterization in most cases and the often plagued efferent limb of the continent cutaneous reservoir. Voiding is effectively accomplished by concomitantly increasing intra-abdominal pressure (Valsalva) with relaxation of the pelvic floor musculature.

Orthotopic reconstruction was initially applied to carefully selected male patients in the mid 1980s with excellent clinical and functional results (6). The positive experience in men subsequently stimulated interest in applying orthotopic reconstruction to women (7). After neuroanatomical dissections provided a better understanding of the continence mechanism in women and defined pathologic guidelines allowed for proper patient selection from a cancer perspective in women, orthotopic reconstruction was subsequently and successfully applied to women in the early 1990s. The majority of both male and female patients undergoing cystectomy today are appropriate candidates for orthotopic reconstruction (6).

From 1982 to 1997, the primary form of urinary diversion at the University of Southern California (USC) was the continent Kock ileal reservoir (Kock pouch) (4,5). The intussuscepted nipple valve provided the continence and antireflux mechanism in the Kock ileal reservoir. The principles of the continent Kock ileal reservoir (cutaneous and orthotopic forms) are sound; however, complications can occur (8). Most complications associated with the Kock ileal reservoir relate to the intussuscepted limb, either the antireflux (afferent limb) or the continent catheterizable (efferent limb) nipple.

A review of our large experience at USC with the Kock ileal reservoir subsequently revealed a 10% complication rate associated with the afferent intussuscepted antireflux nipple in over 800 patients (including the continent cutaneous and orthotopic Kock ileal reservoir) (8). The three most common complications associated with the intussuscepted afferent nipple include (a) stone formation (associated with exposed staples that secure the afferent nipple valve), seen in 5%; (b) afferent nipple stenosis (thought to be caused by ischemic changes resulting from the mesenteric stripping required to maintain the intussuscepted limb), seen in 4%; and (c) extussusception (prolapse of the afferent limb), seen in 1% of patients. Although the majority of these afferent nipple valve complications (60%) can be managed with endoscopic techniques, they nonetheless may result in some morbidity. Approximately 3% of all patients undergoing a continent

Kock ileal reservoir will require an open surgical revision to repair an afferent nipple complication (8).

The need to improve upon the intussuscepted Kock nipple valve became increasingly obvious. Based on reports from Ghoneim's group in Mansoura, Egypt, employing a ureteral serous-lined, extramural tunnel (1), as well as our initial experience with the Mitrofanoff appendiceal subserosal tunnel at USC, we subsequently developed and reported our initial experience with a flap-valve technique called the "T-mechanism" (9). The T-mechanism is a versatile technique that can be applied as an antireflux mechanism as well as a continent mechanism in a cutaneous reservoir (10). Since 1997, we have utilized the T-mechanism as an important modification to the Kock ileal reservoir (11).

The T-mechanism was first successfully incorporated as the afferent antireflux limb of an orthotopic reservoir (T-pouch) (9,11) and subsequently into an afferent antireflux and efferent continence limb of a cutaneous reservoir (double-T-pouch) soon after (10). We believe the flap-valve T-mechanism has eliminated the complications associated with the intussuscepted nipple valve while maintaining an effective antireflux or continence mechanism. The surgical technique of the orthotopic T-pouch ileal neobladder will be described herein.

## DIAGNOSIS

Indications for an orthotopic diversion are related to a functional loss of the bladder for either benign or malignant causes. In the United States, the most common cause is related to bladder cancer requiring radical cystectomy. All diagnostic tests are related to the underlying disease and indication for cystectomy.

## INDICATIONS FOR SURGERY

Any patient who is an appropriate candidate for orthotopic diversion may undergo this procedure. If a patient has a history of bladder cancer, the authors recommend intraoperative frozen section analysis of the proximal urethra. If there is no evidence of tumor on this biopsy and no other contraindications exist, an orthotopic diversion is performed.

## ALTERNATIVE THERAPY

Other forms of urinary diversion may be performed, including various incontinent reservoirs (ureterostomy, conduits), continent cutaneous reservoirs, continent rectal reservoirs, and other orthotopic neobladders.

## SURGICAL TECHNIQUE

The terminal portion of the ileum is used to construct the orthotopic T-pouch ileal neobladder (Fig. 89.1). The distal mesenteric division is best made along the avascular plane of Treves between the ileocolic artery and terminal branches of the superior mesenteric artery. This division extends deep into the avascular portion of the mesentery, which is essential for adequate mobility of the reservoir. The proximal mesenteric division, however, is short and provides a broad vascular blood supply to the reservoir. In addition, a small window of mesentery and a 5- to 7-cm portion of small bowel most proximal to the overall ileal segment are discarded. This helps ensure mobility to the pouch and small bowel anastomosis.

The T-pouch reservoir is created from a 44-cm segment of distal ileum placed in an inverted V configuration. Each limb of the V measures 22 cm. A proximal 8- to 10-cm segment of ileum (afferent limb) is used to form the afferent antireflux T-mechanism. Note: If ureteral length is short or compromised, a longer afferent ileal segment (proximal ileum) may be harvested to bridge the ureteral gap.

The ileum is divided between the proximal afferent ileal segment and the 44-cm ileal segment that will form the reservoir portion of the neobladder. The mesentery between these ileal segments does not need to be incised; this could potentially compromise the blood supply to the afferent limb. There is generally adequate mobility of the afferent ileal segment, which will ultimately be advanced into the serous-lined ileal trough formed by the base (cephalad) of the two adjacent 22-cm segments of ileum.

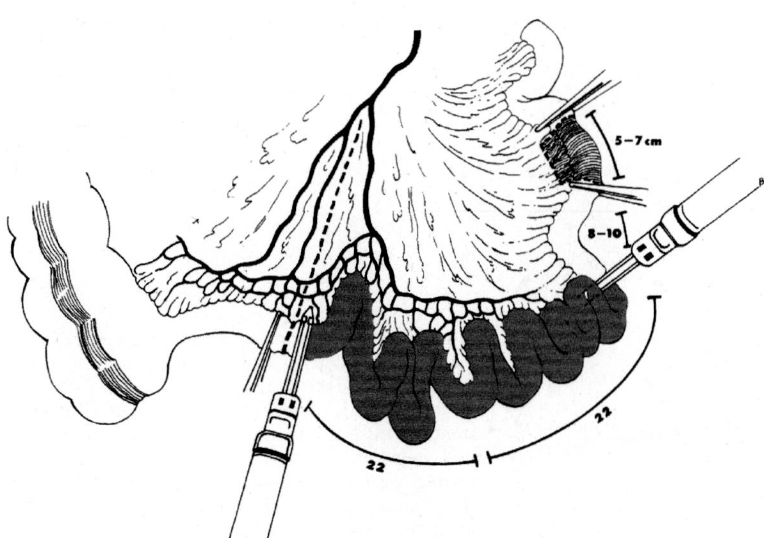


FIGURE 89.1 Designated segments of terminal ileum for construction of the orthotopic T-pouch ileal neobladder. Note that the distal mesenteric division is made between the ileocolic and terminal branches of the superior mesenteric artery, which extends into the avascular plane of the mesentery. In addition, a small window of mesentery and a 5- to 7-cm segment of most proximal small bowel is discarded to allow mobility to the pouch and small bowel anastomosis.

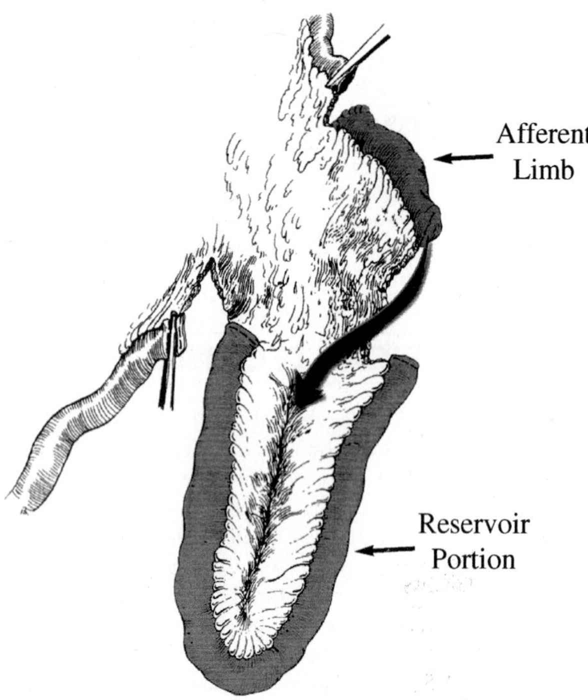


FIGURE 89.2 The T-pouch is constructed from an isolated 44-cm ileal segment (laid out in an inverted V configuration) that forms the reservoir portion of the pouch, and a proximal 8- to 10-cm segment of ileum to form the antireflux limb. The mesentery between the afferent ileal segment and the proximal portion of the 44-cm ileal segment is carefully incised (2 cm) with preservation of the major vascular arcades. Note the serous-lined ileal trough created at the base of the two 22-cm ileal segments where the afferent limb will be advanced *(arrow)*.

The proximal end of the isolated afferent ileal segment is closed with a running Parker-Kerr suture of 3-0 chromic, and a third layer of interrupted 4-0 silk sutures. A standard small bowel anastomosis is performed to re-establish bowel continuity, and the mesenteric trap is closed.

The isolated 44-cm ileal segment is then laid out in an inverted V configuration, with the apex of the V lying caudally toward the feet and with a suture marking a point between the two 22-cm adjacent segments of ileum (Fig. 89.2). The opened end (base) of the V is directed in a cephalad manner toward the head. Note the serous-lined ileal trough formed at the base of the 44-cm segment.

The antireflux (flap-valve) T-mechanism is then created by anchoring the distal 4 cm of the afferent ileal segment into the serous-lined ileal trough formed by the two adjacent 22-cm ileal segments. First, mesenteric windows of Deaver are opened between the vascular arcades (carefully excising mesenteric fat adjacent to the serosa of the ileum, which facilitates the development of these mesenteric windows) for 4 cm proximal to the distalmost portion of the isolated afferent ileal segment (Fig. 89.3). Preserving these arcades (blood vessels) maintains a well-vascularized afferent limb and allows permanent fixation of this portion of the limb into the serous-lined ileal trough with complete preservation of the mesentery and blood supply. Note: Placement of small Penrose drains through each mesenteric window helps identify and facilitates passage of suture through each window.

Next, a series of 3-0 silk sutures are then used to approximate the serosa of the two adjacent 22-cm ileal segments at the base of the V. Note: These sutures are passed through the previously opened windows of Deaver in the afferent ileal limb. This will anchor the 4-cm segment of afferent limb into the serous-lined ileal trough. Specifically, a silk suture is placed into the seromuscular portion of the bowel (adjacent to the mesentery) at the base (most cephalad portion of the V) of one of the 22-cm ileal segments (Fig. 89.4A). The suture is then passed through the most proximal window of Deaver opened in the afferent ileal limb (Fig. 89.4B) and placed in a corresponding seromuscular site of the bowel (next to mesentery) of the adjacent 22-cm ileal segment (Fig. 89.4C). The suture is brought back through the same window of Deaver and tied down (Fig. 89.4D). Generally, two to three silk sutures are placed within each window of Deaver to ensure that the back wall of the reservoir (serous-lined ileal trough) is anchored and does not separate. This process is repeated through each individual window of Deaver until the distal 4 cm of the afferent segment is permanently fixed in the serous-lined ileal trough. We have found that placement of small (1/4–in.) Penrose drains through each window of Deaver facilitates passage of the silk suture back and forth through the mesentery without difficulty. The Penrose drains are systematically removed as the afferent limb is fixed within the serous-lined ileal trough.

In our early experience with the T-pouch, the previously anchored portion of the afferent ileal segment (distal 4 cm) was consistently tapered on the antimesenteric (anterior) border over a 30Fr catheter (Fig. 89.5). Tapering this portion of the

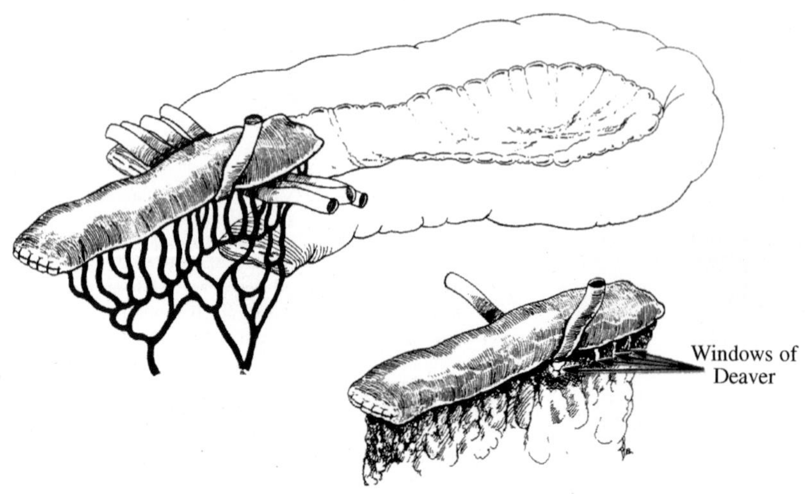


FIGURE 89.3 Creation of the antireflux mechanism. First, four mesenteric windows of Deaver are opened (adjacent to the serosa of the ileum) at the distal 4 cm of the isolated afferent ileal segment. Placement of small Penrose drains through each mesenteric window helps identify and facilitates passage of suture through each (*insert with arrows*). The distal 4 cm of the afferent segment will be anchored into the serous-lined ileal trough formed by the base of the two adjacent 22-cm ileal segments.

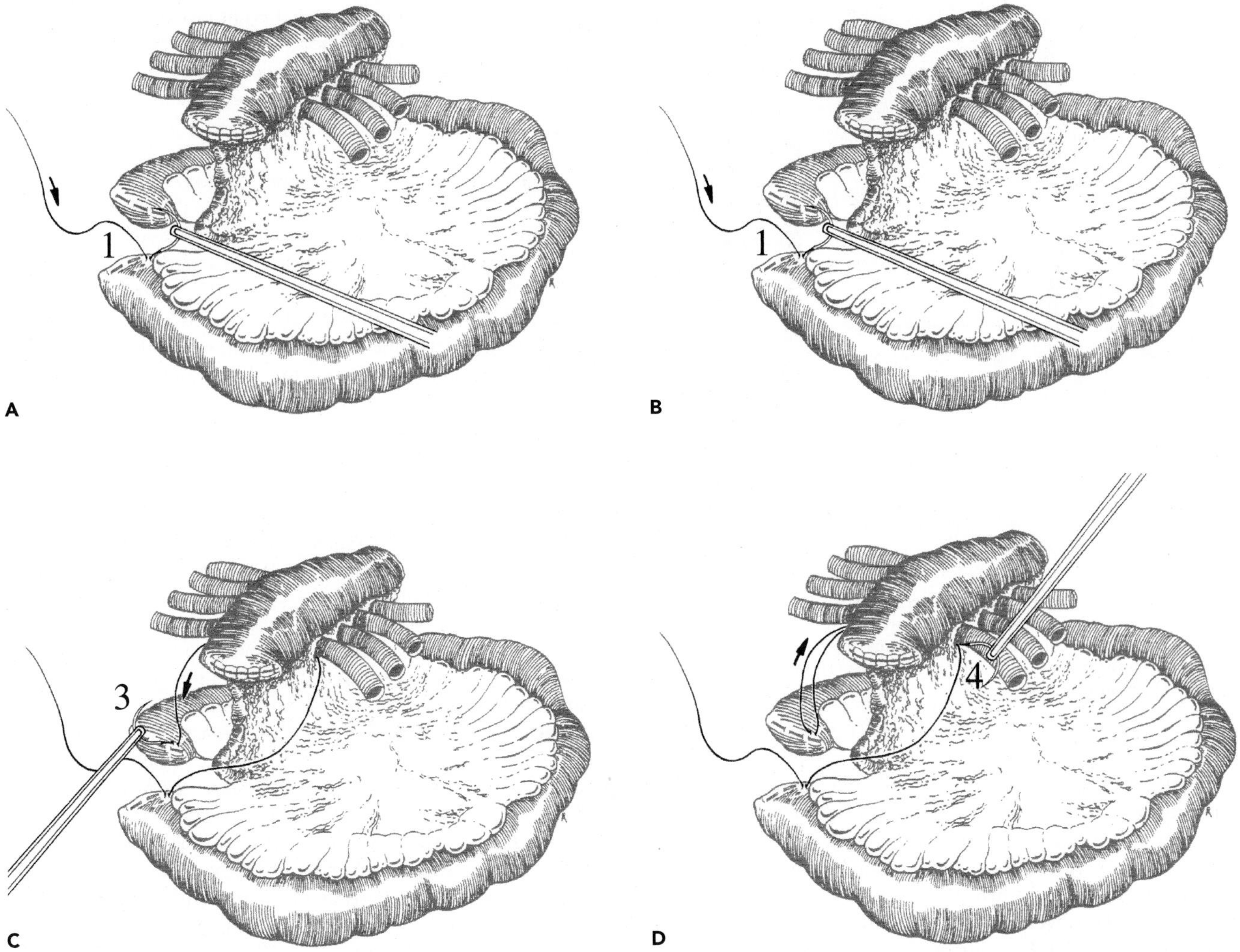

FIGURE 89.4 **A:** A series of interrupted silk sutures are used to approximate the serosa of the base of the two adjacent 22-cm ileal segments. Note that these sutures are brought through the windows of Deaver, facilitated by the use of the Penrose drains. After the silk suture is passed through the window of Deaver (**B**), it is placed in a corresponding site on the adjacent 22-cm ileal segment (**C**). **D:** This suture will then be brought back through the same window of Deaver and tied down.

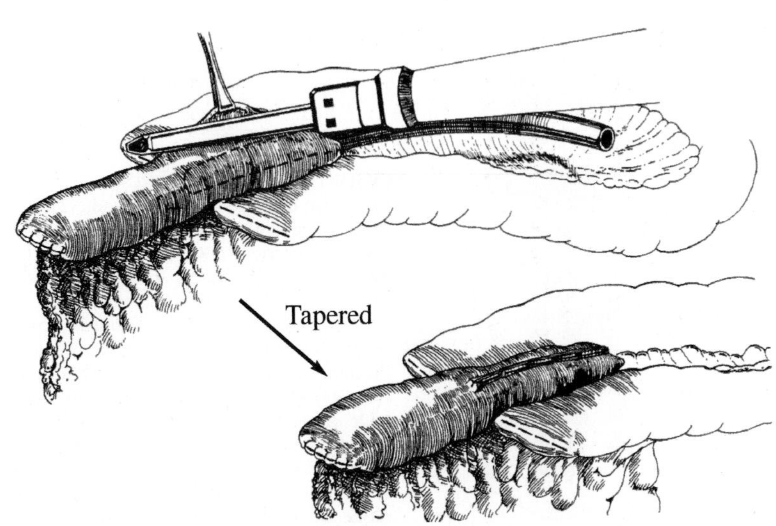


FIGURE 89.5 The previously anchored distal 4-cm afferent ileal segment is tapered over a 30Fr catheter on the antimesenteric border. Since the initial description of the T-pouch, we now selectively taper the afferent limb only in those cases where there is clearly a large diameter of ileum.

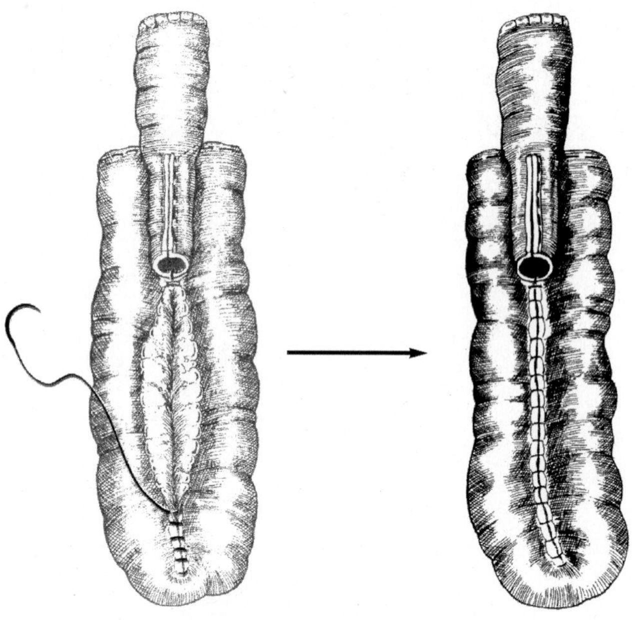

FIGURE 89.6 The two 22-cm ileal segments are joined by a running 3-0 polyglycolic acid continuous suture. Note that this suture is placed adjacent to the mesentery and runs from the apex up to the ostium of the afferent ileal segment. The serosa of the two 22-cm ileal segments is reapproximated.

afferent ileal segment reduces the bulk and lumen of the afferent limb and facilitates later coverage of the anchored afferent limb with ileal flaps. In addition, this tapering of the afferent limb increases the ratio of the tunnel length to the lumen diameter, theoretically providing a more effective flap-valve mechanism. However, we have found that with longer follow-up this tapering may contribute, in a small percentage of patients, to some narrowing and even stenosis at the ostium. Currently, tapering of the afferent limb on the antimesenteric boarder is only performed when the ileum has an obviously large diameter.

After the distal 4 cm of the afferent ileal segment has been anchored into the serous-lined tunnel, the remaining portions of the adjacent 22-cm ileal segments are approximated together with a side-to-side 3-0 polyglycolic acid suture. This suture line simply reapproximates the two ileal limbs and is placed adjacent to the mesentery (Fig. 89.6). This can be performed in a running or interrupted fashion.

Next, starting at the apex of the V, the ileum is opened immediately adjacent to the previously placed serosal suture line using electrocautery. This incision is carried upward toward the ostium of the afferent limb where the afferent limb is anchored (Fig. 89.7A). Once this incision reaches the level of the afferent ostium, the incision is then extended directly lateral to the antimesenteric border of the ileum and carried upward (cephalad) to the base of the ileal segment. An incision is made in similar fashion on the contralateral 22-cm ileal segment (Fig. 89.7B). Once completed, these incisions provide wide flaps of ileum that will ultimately be brought over and cover the anchored afferent ileal segment to create the antireflux mechanism in a flap-valve technique (Fig. 89.7C).

The previously incised ileal mucosa is then oversewn with two layers of a running 3-0 polyglycolic acid suture starting at the apex and running upward toward the ostium of the afferent limb (Fig. 89.8). Once the ostium of the afferent limb is reached, the running suture is tied. An interrupted mucosa-to-mucosa anastomosis is then performed between the ostium of the afferent ileal limb and the incised intestinal ileal flaps with 3-0 polyglycolic acid sutures (Fig. 89.9). The mucosal edges of the ileal flaps are then approximated over the tapered portion of the afferent ileal limb (4 cm) with a running suture in two layers (Fig. 89.10). This suture line completes the posterior wall of the reservoir and creates the effective flap-valve T-mechanism: the serous-lined ileal antireflux limb.

The reservoir is then closed by folding the ileum in half in an opposite direction to which it was opened (Fig. 89.11). This effectively creates a low-pressure, high-capacity urinary reservoir. The anterior wall is closed with a running, two-layer 3-0 polyglycolic acid suture that is watertight (Fig. 89.12). This anterior suture line is stopped just prior to the end of the

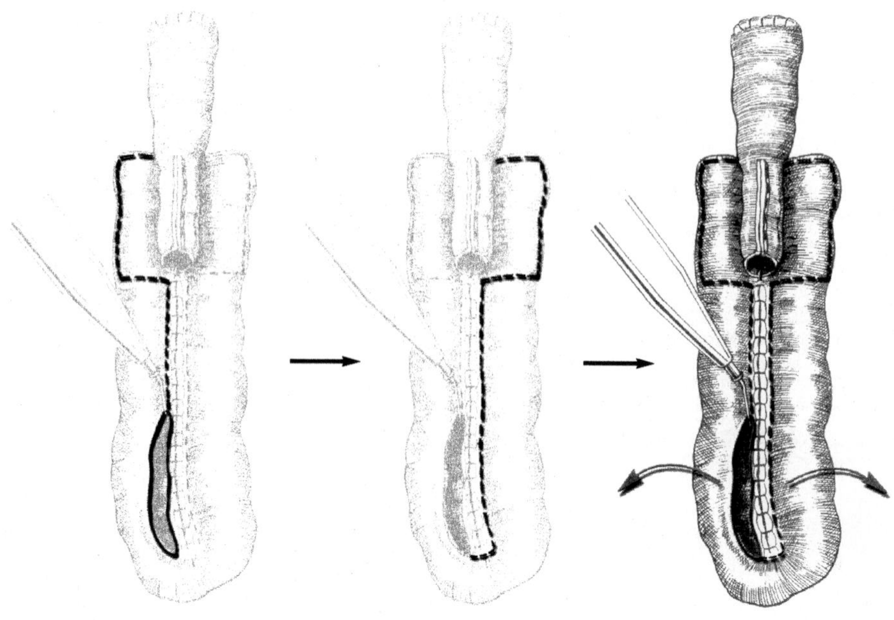

FIGURE 89.7 **A:** The two 22-cm ileal segments are opened immediately adjacent to the serosal suture line beginning at the apex and carried upward to the ostium of the afferent segment. Note: Once this incision reaches the ostium, it is then directed lateral (to the antimesenteric border) and cephalad to the base. The *dotted line* depicts the incision line. **B:** Completing the incision of the bowel. **C:** The incision provides wide flaps of ileum that can easily be brought over and that cover the tapered distal afferent ileal segment to form the antireflux mechanism in a flap-valve technique.

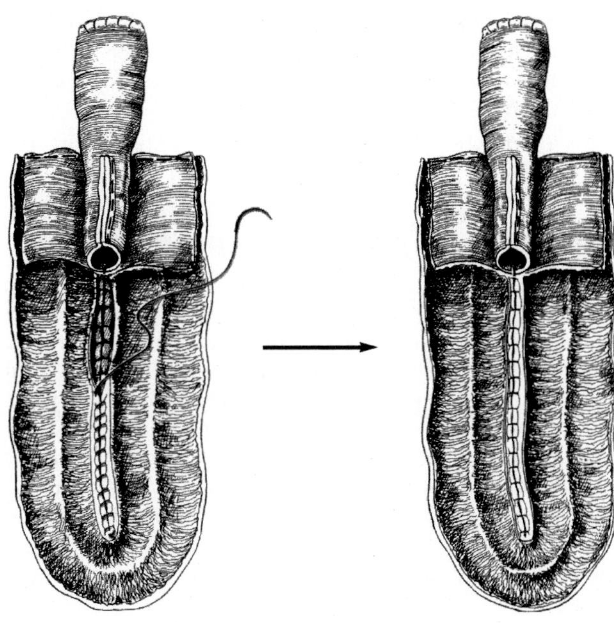

FIGURE 89.8 The incised ileal mucosa is oversewn in two layers beginning at the apex and continuing toward (cephalad) the ostium of the afferent ileal segment.

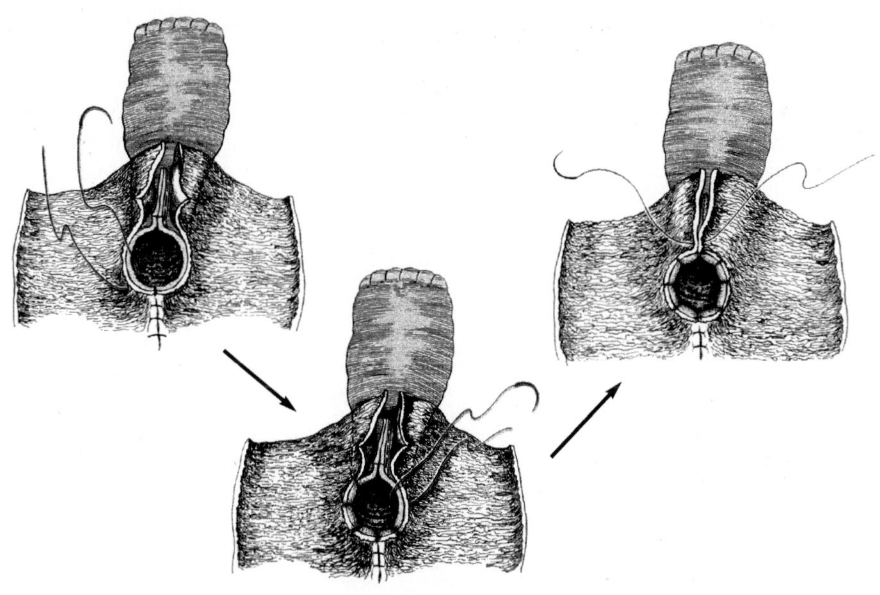

FIGURE 89.9 A mucosa-to-mucosa, ileal-to-ileal anastomosis is performed between the ostium of the afferent segment and the edges of the ileal flaps. Note that this is performed with interrupted 3-0 polyglycolic acid suture with completion of the ileal-to-ileal anastomosis.

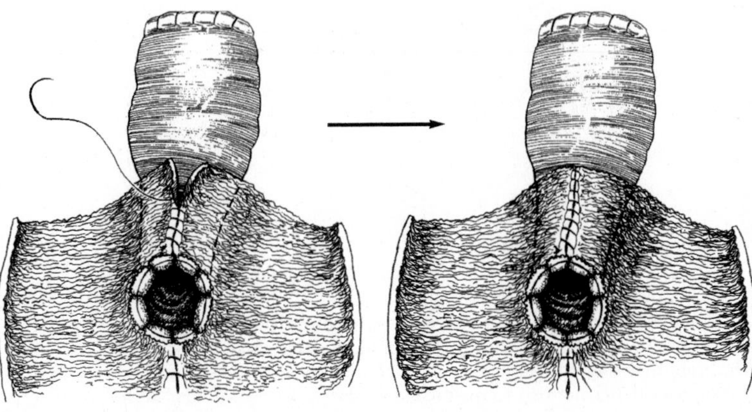

FIGURE 89.10 **A:** The mucosal edges of the ileal flaps are brought over the tapered distal portion of the afferent ileal segment. **B:** Completion of the posterior suture line covering the afferent segment with the ileal flaps. Note: This will exclude the staple line from the reservoir.

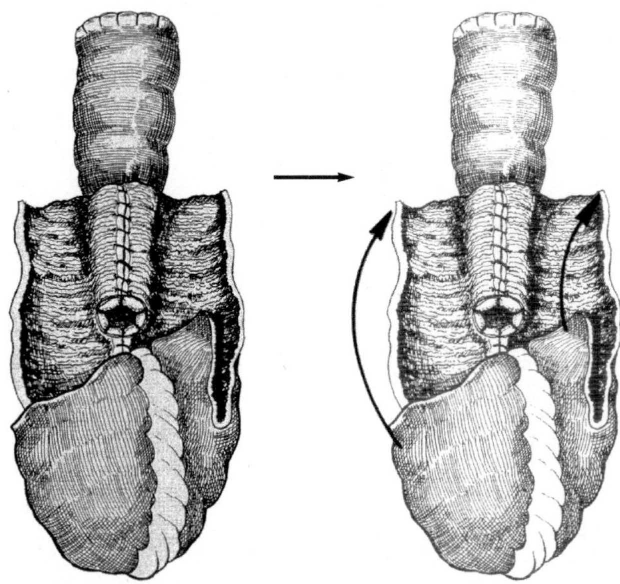

FIGURE 89.11 The T-pouch is folded *(arrows)* and closed in the opposite direction to which it was opened. This manner of folding will create a low-pressure, large-capacity spherical reservoir.

right side to allow insertion of an index finger. This is the most mobile and dependent portion of the reservoir and will later be anastomosed to the urethra.

Once the pouch has been closed, each ureter is spatulated and a standard, bilateral end-to-side ureteroileal anastomosis is performed to the proximal portion of the afferent limb using interrupted 4-0 polyglycolic acid suture. These anastomoses are stented with no. 8 infant feeding tubes that are directed from the ipsilateral renal pelvis (kidney), across the ureteroileal anastomosis through the afferent limb into the reservoir and out the neourethra. A 24Fr hematuria catheter is placed per urethra to provide adequate drainage of the reservoir, and the ureteral stents are secured to the end of the urethral catheter with a 3-0 nylon suture. This step facilitates removal of the stents at approximately 3 weeks along with the urethral catheter. A tension-free mucosa-to-mucosa urethroileal anastomosis is performed.

## OUTCOME AND COMPLICATIONS

From November 1996 through May 2000, 209 patients (169 men [79%], 40 women), with a mean age of 69 years (range, 33 to 93 years) underwent an orthotopic T-pouch ileal neobladder following cystectomy (11). The indication for cystectomy included bladder cancer in 198 patients (95%). The median follow-up for the entire cohort is 33 months (range, 0 to 69 months). Data were analyzed according to perioperative mortality, early (within 3 months) and late diversion-related and diversion-unrelated complications, radiographic evaluation of the upper urinary tract and urinary reservoir, and determination of renal function.

Three patients (1.4%) died during the perioperative period. A total of 63 (30%) early complications occurred, including 53 (25%) diversion-unrelated and 10 (5%) diversion-related. The most common early diversion-unrelated complication was dehydration (10 patients). The most common early diversion-related complication was urine leak in 6 patients. There were no early complications directly related to the antirefluxing T-limb. Late complications occurred in a total of 66 (31%) patients, including 30 (14%) diversion-unrelated and 38 (17%) diversion-related. The most common late diversion-unrelated complication was incisional hernia in 16 patients. Of the 38 late diversion-related complications, the most common were pouch calculi in 17 patients and ureteroileal obstruction in 9 patients. The only late complication directly related to the T-limb was afferent ostial stenosis seen in 4 patients, 3 of whom received adjuvant pelvic radiation.

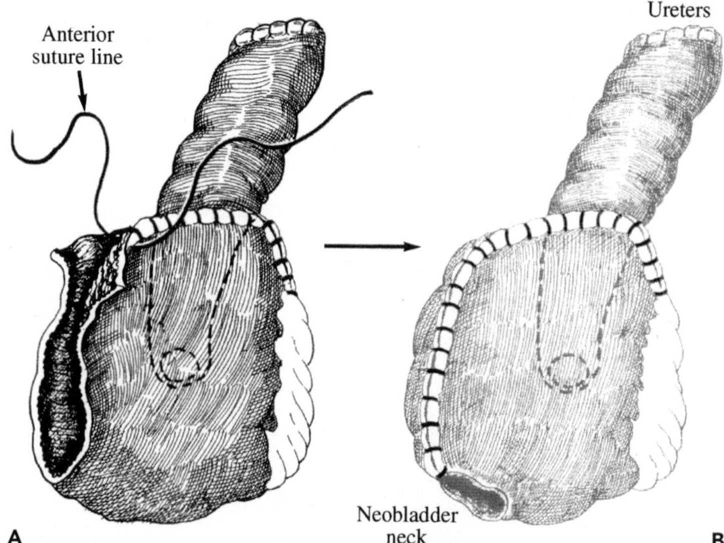


FIGURE 89.12 **A:** The anterior suture line is completed with two layers of a continuous 3-0 polyglycolic acid suture. Note that the anterior suture line is stopped just short of the right side to allow insertion of an index finger, which will be the neourethra. **B:** Completion of the T-pouch. Note that the most mobile and dependent portion of the reservoir will be anastomosed to the urethra following the ureteroileal anastomosis to the proximal portion of the afferent limb.

A total of 181 patients had radiographic evaluation of the upper urinary tract, including 162 (90%) with a normal radiographic study or evidence of decompression postoperatively. An abnormal upper-tract study was seen in 18 patients (10%), including 9 patients with ureteroileal obstruction and 4 with afferent T-limb stenosis. Gravity cystography of the neobladder was normal in 143 of 158 (90%) evaluable patients. Reflux was seen in 15 patients (10%). Renal function as determined by serum creatinine was stable or improved in 96% of patients.

Good daytime and nighttime continence was reported in 87% and 72% of evaluable patients, respectively. Overall, 75% of patients completely voided, while 25% required some form of intermittent catheterization to completely empty their neobladder, including 20% of men and 43% of women.

## DISCUSSION

The development of orthotopic reconstruction was a significant improvement in the evolution of urinary diversion. The importance of preventing the reflux of urinary constituents following orthotopic reconstruction is a controversial subject and remains a topic of significant debate. The authors have been, and continue to be, strong proponents of reflux prevention in patients undergoing lower-urinary-tract reconstruction. It is emphasized that the complications or risks associated with incorporating an antireflux mechanism (i.e., obstruction) should not outweigh the theoretical advantage of reflux prevention. To meet this end, we have been diligent to critically evaluate our antireflux techniques and continually improve upon existing ideas and methods. This evaluation process has subsequently stimulated a change from the intussuscepted nipple of the Kock pouch to the development of the flap-valve T-mechanism, incorporated as an antireflux limb in the orthotopic T-pouch ileal neobladder as well as a rectal reservoir (9,11). This technique provides an effective antireflux mechanism without the complications associated with the intussuscepted nipple. Furthermore, the T-mechanism has been successfully applied as a catheterizable continent mechanism in cutaneous reservoirs, as discussed elsewhere (10).

Many antireflux techniques exist today. The inclusion of an antireflux mechanism in the chronically infected, continent cutaneous reservoir (requiring intermittent catheterization) is still thought to be important and not a source of considerable debate. With increasing popularity and further application of the low-pressure orthotopic reservoir, the issue of reflux prevention has regained attention. Studer and associates (12) advocate a long (20-cm), dynamic, isoperistaltic ileal segment as an afferent limb of an orthotopic neobladder reservoir. Proponents of the isoperistaltic afferent ileal limb argue that radiographic evidence of reflux in a sterile, low-pressure reservoir may not have the same importance and clinical consequence. Furthermore, the complications of late stenosis from the various antireflux techniques could potentially outweigh their theoretical advantage of protecting the upper urinary tract. Others, however, argue that antireflux procedures are not only theoretically inherent in humans but are also critical to preserve or maintain renal function and important in all forms of lower-urinary-tract reconstruction, even orthotopic diversion. Reasons include the fact that patients, even with an orthotopic neobladder, may have colonized bacteriuria. The unexpected patient who requires intermittent catheterization to completely empty the neobladder (which is unpredictable) can also be expected to have colonized bacteriuria with the risk of upper-tract deterioration.

Reflux prevention following orthotopic diversion may become more important as the comprehensive therapy (medical and surgical) for pelvic malignancies improves and patients' life expectancy increases following exenteration and urinary diversion. This may then place patients at further risk for renal deterioration in the future. Subsequently, several novel antireflux mechanisms have been developed to improve on existing techniques and to eliminate or reduce the complications associated with previous antireflux mechanisms, particularly obstruction (9,11). Longer follow-up will be required to accurately evaluate the isoperistaltic afferent limb, as well as these more recent antireflux techniques, to determine if reflux prevention in patients undergoing orthotopic diversion is truly necessary.

From 1982 to 1997, we incorporated the intussuscepted nipple valve as an antireflux mechanism in all forms of continent urinary diversion at USC and as an efferent continence mechanism in patients undergoing a cutaneous Kock ileal reservoir (4,5,7). The basic surgical premise and structural characteristics of the Kock ileal reservoir are sound: a low-pressure, large-capacity reservoir, employing an antirefluxing and continent nipple valve. The Achilles heel of the Kock ileal reservoir, however, remained the intussuscepted nipple valve. Despite several surgical modifications to improve upon the construction of the intussuscepted nipple valve, there remained complications and a reoperation rate (8). The intussuscepted nipple valve needed to be improved.

The so-called T-mechanism is a flap-valve technique that can be applied as an antireflux and continence mechanism in lower-urinary-tract reconstruction (9–11). In general, all flap-valve techniques rely on the dynamic principle that the channeled segment (appendix, ureter, intestine) is fixed and tunneled along the inner wall of the reservoir. As reservoir filling occurs, the channeled segment is compressed against the wall of the pouch and continence or reflux prevention is achieved. This technique is based on similar principles for reimplantation of the ureter into the bladder. Keys to success of the flap-valve technique include an appropriate ratio of tunnel length to lumen diameter. Furthermore, the back wall of the reservoir must be sufficiently capable to allow compression of the tunneled channel as the pouch fills.

The unique aspect of the T-mechanism (antireflux and continence) is the ability to create a reliable and effective flap-valve system. Maintenance of the vascular arcades (opening the windows of Deaver) provides complete preservation of the mesentery and blood supply to the entire limb, thus eliminating problems with ischemia or stenosis of the bowel segment. Permanent fixation of the limb into the serous-lined ileal trough should also eliminate issues associated with prolapse or extussusception of the limb. Importantly, no exposed metallic staples exist within the reservoir, which should reduce the incidence of stone formation, typically associated with exposure of metallic foreign bodies to urine. Furthermore, if necessary, the proximal portion of the afferent limb can be easily lengthened when there is shortened or compromised ureters. A longer proximal afferent segment may be harvested to bridge any ureteral defect and maintain a tension-free ureteroileal anastomosis.

Several technical points regarding the specifics of the construction of the flap-valve T-mechanism (antireflux, continence) deserve mentioning. An effective afferent antireflux valve can be created from 4 cm of ileum anchored within the serous-lined ileal trough. Permanently anchoring the portion of ileum in the serous-lined ileal trough is critical to fix the limb and prevent any valve slippage or prolapse. In addition, the silk sutures used to anchor the valve (passed through the windows of Deaver) should be placed adjacent to the mesentery and should incorporate a generous portion of the seromuscular ileum to prevent separation of the serous-lined ileal trough. This trough forms the so-called "backboard" (posterior wall to the reservoir) of the flap-valve technique, which is critical to antireflux prevention as the reservoir fills. Placement of two to three sutures within each window of Deaver should prevent separation of this trough.

The antimesenteric tapering of the valve was initially described and performed on all patients with this technique. Tapering the afferent limb over a 30Fr catheter was effective in preventing reflux of urinary constituents and in protecting the upper tracts in patients undergoing an orthotopic T-pouch ileal neobladder (11). This effectively increases the ratio of the tunnel length to the lumen diameter and has provided an excellent efferent continence mechanism. However, several patients (2%) with longer follow-up developed some narrowing of the ostium and even stenosis that may be attributed to either some postoperative radiation to the reservoir or possibly to the antimesenteric tapering. We subsequently tapered the T-limb only in those patients with a large ileal diameter and have found that it does not appear to compromise the antireflux mechanism; to date, we have not observed any further issues with stenosis of the afferent limb.

The flap-valve T-mechanism in the T-pouch provides an effective and reliable antireflux mechanism. The long-term results of the T-pouch are yet to be determined; however, the initial and intermediate results have been promising. Furthermore, we believe that this technique can be easily learned with a little experience. The T-mechanism is a very versatile flap-valve technique that can also be applied as a continent mechanism in a cutaneous reservoir (double-T-pouch). We believe that reconstructive surgeons interested in lower-urinary-tract reconstruction should understand this concept and technique to broaden their surgical armamentarium.

## *References*


1. Abol-Enein H, Ghoneim MA. Further clinical experience with the ileal W-neobladder and a serous-lined extramural tunnel for orthotopic substitution. *Br J Urol* 1995;76:558–564.
2. Bricker EM. Bladder substitution after pelvic evisceration. *Surg Clin North Am* 1950;30:1511–1521.
3. Gilchrist RK, Merricks JW, Hamlin HH, et al. Construction of a substitute bladder and urethra. *Surg Gynecol Obstet* 1950;9:752–760.
4. Skinner DG, Boyd SD, Lieskovsky G. Clinical experience with the Kock continent ileal reservoir for urinary diversion. *J Urol* 1984;132: 1101–1107.
5. Skinner DG, Boyd SD, Lieskovsky G, et al. Lower urinary tract reconstruction following cystectomy: experience and results in 126 patients using the Kock ileal reservoir with bilateral ureteroileal urethrostomy. *J Urol* 1991; 146:756–760.
6. Stein JP, Skinner DG. Orthotopic bladder replacement. In: Wein AJ, Kavoussi LR, Novick AC, et al., eds. *Campbell-Walsh urology*, 9th ed. WB Saunders, 2006:2613–2649.
7. Stein JP, Stenzl A, Esrig D, et al. Lower urinary tract reconstruction following cystectomy in women using the Kock ileal reservoir with bilateral ureteroileal urethrostomy: initial clinical experience. *J Urol* 1994;152: 1404–1408.
8. Stein JP, Freeman JA, Esrig D, et al. Complications of the afferent antireflux valve mechanism in the Kock ileal reservoir. *J Urol* 1996;155: 1579–1584.
9. Stein JP, Lieskovsky G, Ginsberg DA, et al. The T pouch: an orthotopic ileal neobladder incorporating a serosal lined ileal antireflux technique. *J Urol* 1998;159:1836–1842.
10. Stein JP, Skinner DG. T-mechanism applied to urinary diversion: the orthotopic T-pouch ileal neobladder and cutaneous double-T-pouch ileal reservoir. *Tech Urol* 2001;7:209–222.
11. Stein JP, Dunn MD, Quek ML, et al. The orthotopic T pouch ileal neobladder: experience with 209 patients. *J Urol* 2004;172:584–587.
12. Studer UE, Danuser H, Thalmann GN, et al. Antireflux nipples or afferent tubular segments in 70 patients with ileal low pressure bladder substitutes: long-term results of a prospective randomized trial. *J Urol* 1996;156: 1913–1917.


# CHAPTER 90 ■ COLONIC ORTHOTOPIC BLADDER SUBSTITUTION

JOACHIM W. THÜROFF AND LUDGER FRANZARING

Orthotopic bladder substitution can be realized from ileum only or from colonic segments either alone or in combination with small bowel segments as a composite reservoir. The rationale of using large bowel for urinary diversion is based on anatomical and functional considerations. Surgical creation of a urinary reservoir from bowel segments generally means transformation of a cylinder into a sphere. The length of bowel to be excluded from the intestinal tract for formation of a reservoir of a given capacity depends only on bowel diameter. Since in the volume formula of a cylinder ($V = \pi r^2 \cdot l$) the radius determines the volume by its second power, the wider the bowel diameter, the less the bowel length required. Thus, large bowel with its wider diameter can contribute a significant capacity to a continent reservoir while excluding only a short length of a functional segment.

Physiologically, fat-soluble vitamins such as vitamin B12 and folic acid as well as biliary acids are absorbed from the entire ileum, but not from colon. Consequently, possible malabsorption syndromes are related only to resection of ileum but not to colon resection. The critical length of ileum resection is >40 cm, at which the risk of secondary malabsorption syndromes starts to increase. These facts should influence choice of bowel segments for reservoir formation in favor of reducing the length of ileum segments for a composite reservoir or of avoiding ileum entirely in an all-colon reservoir.

However, the large bowel is less distensible than small bowel. Although at first this may be regarded as a disadvantage, it may be advantageous, specifically for spontaneous evacuation of an orthotopic bladder substitute in the long run. Intestinal urinary reservoirs start their life at a surgically determined volume that increases over time by gradual distention. During this process, large bowel segments have the advantage that the longitudinal arrangement of taeniae prevents the development of a decompensated substitute megacystis as has been described for ileum reservoirs. In addition, large bowel segments, especially cecum and ascending colon, offer several alternatives for safe and effective antirefluxive ureteral implantation.

The downsides of using large bowel for creation of an orthotopic reservoir have to be weighed against the advantages of large capacity, less malabsorption, less overdistention, and reliable antireflux techniques.

First, many urologic surgeons are not familiar with large bowel surgery and feel uncomfortable with it, specifically when mobilizing the large bowel and performing the bowel anastomosis after resection of the segments for the urinary reservoir. However, generous mobilization of segments as well as rotation of segments may be required to allow a tension-free transposition as an orthotopic reservoir in patients with a deep true pelvis. Surgical techniques using large bowel may also be more time-consuming because adhesions with the greater omentum have to be freed and the bowel anastomosis after exclusion of the segments for urinary diversion has a significantly larger circumference to be sutured than in a small bowel anastomosis.

Finally, the use of large bowel segments may have functional sequaelae as well. All reservoirs that use the ileocecal segment and thus require resection of the ileocecal valve may allow retrograde colonization of the ileum if the ileocecal valve is not reconstructed by an antirefluxing technique of the ileoascendostomy anastomosis.

The different techniques of constructing an orthotopic reservoir, either from large bowel only or in combination with small bowel segments as a composite reservoir, refer to the very same principles of continent urinary diversion: detubularization and spherical reconfiguration. Thus, the success of orthotopic bladder substitution is not confined to selection of small bowel segments; good results have been reported with the ileocecal segment, the right colon, and the sigmoid colon. However, in general, large bowel segments have physiologically decreasing capacity and compliance from proximally to distally, while wall tension and pressure are increasing at the same time. This translates into higher capacity and lower pressure of the cecum and ascending colon as compared to the descending and sigmoid colon. The surgical technique of the Mainz ileocecal pouch as described following in detail may in this context serve as a general example of construction of an ileocolonic composite pouch.

However, one single technique of continent urinary diversion does not fit all patients and all pathologies. Thus, modern concepts of intestinal urinary diversion require surgical versatility instead of stereotypic repetition of fixed surgical strategies.

## DIAGNOSIS

The scope of diagnostic studies is determined by the underlying disease because of which the native bladder has to be substituted. For continent urinary diversion as compared to incontinent diversion, the most important assessment is renal morphology and function. Grossly dilated upper urinary tracts may not drain as well into a continent urinary reservoir as into a conventional zero-pressure conduit diversion. Every intestinal urinary reservoir reabsorbs hydrogen and chloride ions. The resulting metabolic acidosis is generally balanced by respiratory compensation and by an increased renal secretion. As a consequence, renal reserve must be sufficient as judged by a glomerular filtration rate better than a minimum of 50% of the age-related normal global renal function.

The intestinal tract must be evaluated in order to avoid surgical or postoperative problems. Concerning patient history, special attention must be paid to inflammatory bowel disease, prior abdominal surgery or radiation, and related abnormalities of stool and defecation. When large bowel segments are used for continent diversion, contrast enema or coloscopy are mandatory to exclude asymptomatic diverticulosis or tumors of the large bowel.

## INDICATIONS FOR SURGERY

The indications for a colonic orthotopic bladder substitute or a composite reservoir of ileum and colon are not different from those for ileal orthotopic bladder substitution. However, in patients with neurogenic bowel and anal sphincter incompetence, any change in stool consistency secondary to bowel resection bears the risk of worsening pre-existing anal incontinence. Another aspect of all forms of orthotopic bladder substitution, specifically in women, is the risk of urinary retention requiring emptying of the reservoir by intermittent catheterization. Thus, the willingness and ability to perform intermittent self-catheterization have to be determined and possibly practiced preoperatively. This is of special importance in women, patients with neurogenic bladder, and children. Generally, children can perform intermittent self-catheterization of the urethra from about 6 years of age.

## ALTERNATIVE THERAPY

Alternatives to orthotopic bladder substitution with colonic segments are orthotopic ileal neobladders. Alternatives to continent orthotopic bladder substitution are continent cutaneous urinary diversion (e.g., Mainz Pouch I, Indiana Pouch) or continent anal urinary diversion (Mainz Pouch II). Alternatives to continent urinary diversion are incontinent conduit diversions (ileal conduit, sigmoid conduit, transverse colonic conduit).

## SURGICAL TECHNIQUE

The day before surgery the bowel is cleansed either by oral administration with 4 to 6 L of a hyperosmotic nonabsorbable solution (e.g., macrogol) or by irrigation with 8 to 10 L of isotonic saline with a total of 50 mval of potassium chloride added through a nasogastric tube. After irrigation, serum electrolyte concentrations have to be checked and, if necessary, intravenously substituted.

During surgery, the small and large bowel segments that have been excluded for construction of the intestinal urinary reservoir are intubated with a Foley catheter and antegradely flushed with saline until the irrigation fluid turns out clear before they are opened antimesenterically. Perioperative parenteral antibiotic therapy with broad-spectrum antibiotics should include antianaerobic activity. The antibiotics are administered 1 hour before surgery and continued until the fifth to seventh postoperative day.

The patient is positioned supine on the operating table. Radical cystoprostatectomy should adhere to the same principles as radical prostatectomy: that is, to preserve maximum urethral length and, if possible and indicated, to preserve the neurovascular bundles.

For ileocecal orthotopic bladder substitution, the cecum and ascending colon are mobilized beyond the right colonic flexure. Extended mobilization is helpful for later sliding the pouch easily into the small pelvis.

Ten to 15 cm of cecum and ascending colon and about 20 to 30 cm of distal ileum are marked by stay sutures and isolated from bowel continuity. An ileoascendostomy is accomplished either as a sutured single-row, dual-layer (seromuscularis), running end-to-end anastomosis after antimesenteric spatulation of the ileum for adjustment of bowel diameter or as stapled mechanical end-to-side anastomosis of ileum to ascending colon using EEA and TA-55 staplers. The isolated ileocecal segment is intraoperatively irrigated with isotonic saline for further cleansing.

Ascending colon, cecum, and ileum are split open at their antimesenteric borders. The posterior wall of the pouch is completed by side-to-side anastomosis of the ascending colon with the terminal ileal loop and of the latter with the next proximal segment. The anastomosis is performed by single-row, all-layer running sutures of 4-0 polydioxanone with a straight needle. The still open pouch is slid into the small pelvis. For bladder substitution to the bladder neck (benign disease), the pouch is anastomosed with the posterior bladder wall using single-row, all-layer running sutures of 4-0 polydioxanone. For bladder substitution to the urethra after cystectomy, a small vertical buttonhole incision is made at the lowest aspect of the cecal pole and the opened mucosa is everted with a few 5-0 absorbable stitches before anastomosis to the membranous urethra is performed by eight interrupted sutures of 4-0 glykonat (Fig. 90.1). Alternatively, the ileocecal pouch may be created by using G1A staplers with reabsorbable staples (Fig. 90.2).

The ileocecal segments may also be used for creating an orthotopic pouch in the "Le Bag" technique (Fig. 90.3). The right colonic pouch is constructed from cecum and ascending colon (Fig. 90.4). The blood supply of ileocecal reservoirs is based on the ileocolic artery, which always allows tension-free anastomosis to the urethra, specifically if a 180-degree counterclockwise rotation of the pouch around the "insertion" of the ileocolic vessels is performed. In right colonic pouches, with additional blood supply from the right colonic artery, reaching down to the urethral stump may sometimes be more difficult. The blood supply of the sigmoid colon is from the inferior mesenteric and superior rectal arteries (Fig. 90.5). Sigmoid reservoirs thus always easily reach down to the urethral stump (Fig. 90.6).

### Ureteral Implantation

A variety of techniques reflects the surgical challenge to create an antireflux mechanism without obstruction of the ureter. This challenge may be heightened by a number of pathological conditions in the individual patient. Ureters may be dilated, fibrotic, or ischemic secondary to obstruction, previous surgery, or irradiation. Bowel segments may be altered from inflammation, dilatation, or ischemia secondary to inflammatory bowel disease, previous surgery, or irradiation. Mechanical factors (e.g., position changes of the reservoir) or biochemical factors (e.g., effects of urine on the ureteral adventitia or on the intestinal mucosa) may have long-term effects on the whole system.

The rationale of implanting the ureters by an antirefluxive technique into an orthotopic bladder substitute is to protect the upper urinary tracts from retrogradely transmitted pressure peaks and from ascending bacteriuria. However, the standard technique of antirefluxive ureteral implantation into large bowel was conceived from ureterosigmoidostomy, which means diverting urine into a high-pressure reservoir. The debate about the necessity of antirefluxive ureteral implantation into orthotopic low-pressure reservoirs is still not concluded. One argument is that, in contrast to most forms of continent cutaneous diversion, orthotopic reservoirs have the pop-off valve of urethral incontinence when overfilled. Another argument is a supposedly lower bacterial contamination rate as compared to reservoirs that require intermittent catheterization. Nevertheless, antirefluxive ureterointestinal reimplantation is still the method of choice for colonic reservoirs. A variety of surgical techniques is based on different antireflux mechanisms, which have been described, although two general types exist. In one type, the ureter itself is part of the antireflux mechanism, while in the other a bowel-derived antireflux mechanism is interposed between ureter and reservoir.

In any case, for implantation of the ureters into cecum or ascending colon, the left ureter has to be brought into the right retroperitoneum behind the mesentery of the descending colon as for ileal conduit diversion.

Antirefluxive ureteral implantation techniques in which the ureter becomes part of the antireflux mechanism mostly follow the "flap-valve" principle: An oblique entry of the ureter into the reservoir is created with a "tunnel" course that allows transmission of the reservoir pressure onto the ureter and against the seromuscularis of the reservoir. This pressure transmission passively compresses the ureter with rising reservoir pressures. The most frequently utilized principles to

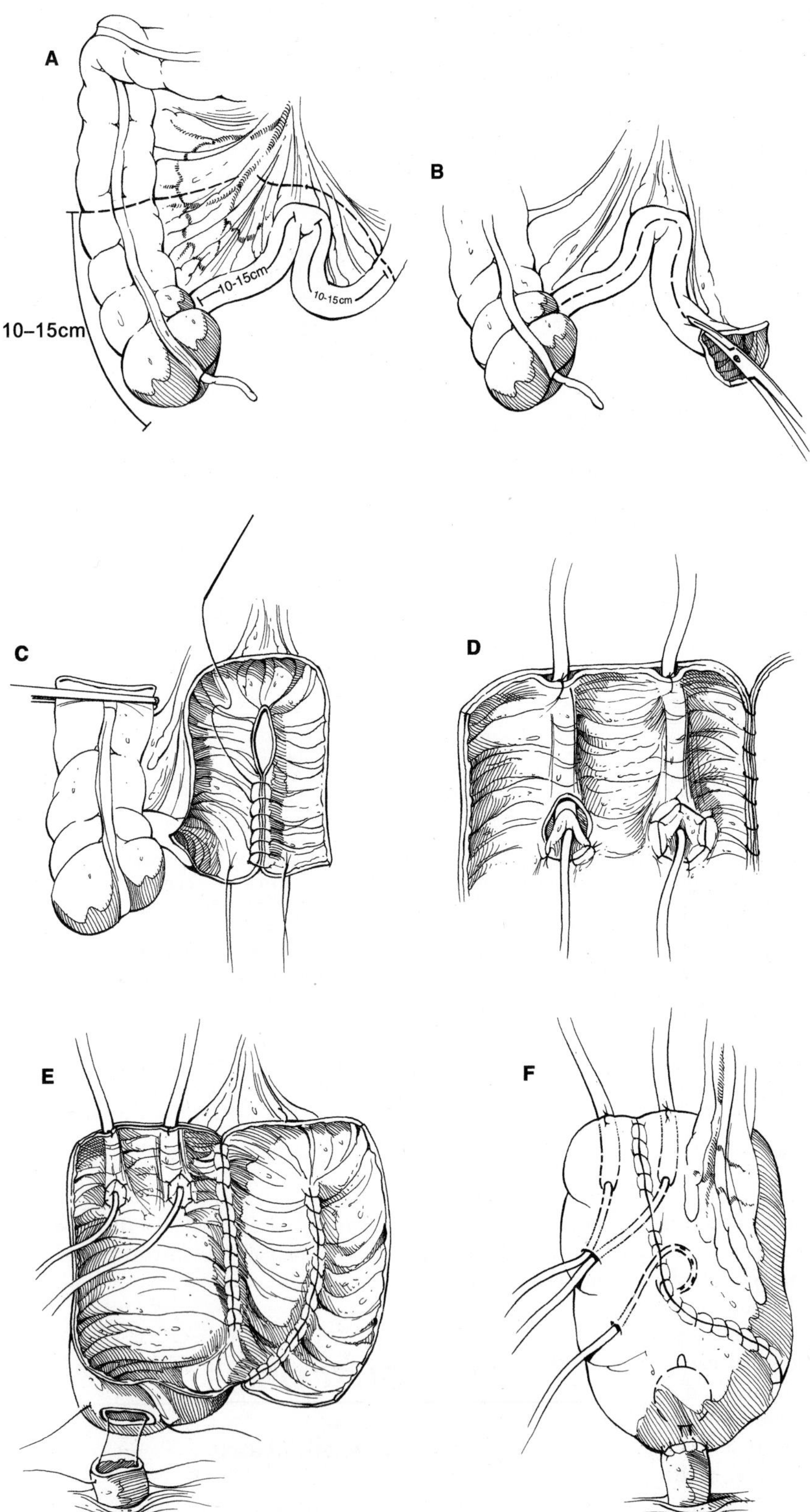


FIGURE 90.1 Construction of the Mainz ileocecal reservoir. **A:** Isolation of the ileocecal segment consisting of 20 to 30 cm of ileum and 10 to 15 cm of cecum and ascending colon. **B:** Antimesenteric opening of the intestinal segments. **C:** Detubularization and reconfiguration of the ileal segment. Note: The ileocecal valve may be left intact. **D:** Submucosal tunnel implantation of the ureters in "open-end" technique into the colonic segment. The term *open end* describes the ureters entering the submucosal tunnel from the resection margin. **E:** Completion of the posterior wall of the pouch by anastomosing the medial margin of the colonic segment to the right margin of the ileal plate. The lowest part of the pouch is anastomosed to the urethra. **F:** Completion of the anterior wall of the pouch by anastomosing the lateral margin of the colonic segment to the left margin of the ileal plate. Drainage of the pouch is secured by a transurethral Foley catheter and a percutaneous pigtail pouchostomy catheter.

transmit the reservoir pressure to the ureter are the submucosal tunnel technique and the seromuscular extramural tunnel technique.

In the submucosal tunnel technique, both ureters are implanted into the colon with a 2- to 3-cm submucosal tunnel. Ureters are anchored with 6-0 glykonat sutures to the muscularis of the bowel wall, and the neo-orifices are established by 6-0 glykonat or 7-0 polyglycolic acid ureteromucosal sutures.

The most common technique of interposition of an antirefluxive mechanism between the urinary reservoir and the ureters

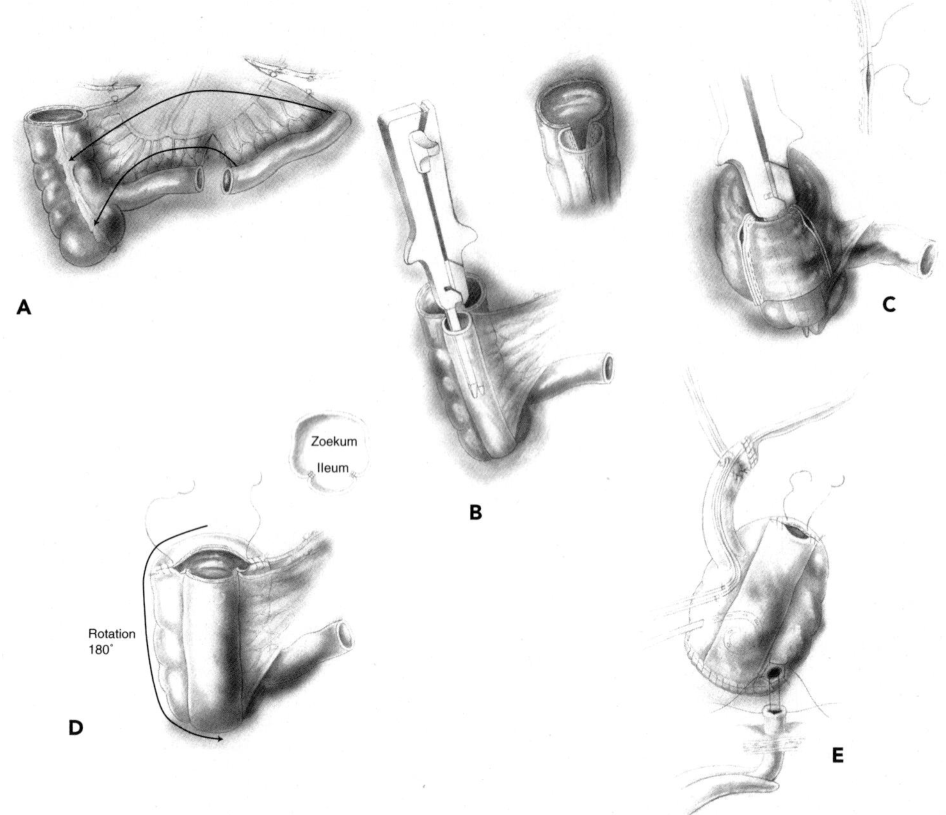


FIGURE 90.2 Construction of an ileocecal reservoir utilizing reabsorbable staples. **A:** Isolation of the ileocecal segment comprising 15 cm of large bowel with 10 cm of prevalvular terminal ileum and an additional 15 cm of ileum. **B:** Alignment of cecum or ascending colon and the separated segment of 15 cm of ileum and one-step antimesenteric opening and side-to-side anastomosis of the large bowel segment and the ileal segment, with the GIA-75 (Autosuture) stapler applying on either side two rows of polyglycolic absorbable staples (copolymer Lactomer). **C:** Eversion of the pouch wall and second stapler application (a third application in the very same way may be required). Gaps between the staple lines are closed with a running 4-0 polydioxanone suture *(insert)*. Note: The 10-cm terminal prevalvular ileum remains intact. **D:** The cranial aspect of the pouch is closed with a running seromuscular 4-0 polydioxanone suture. Then the pouch is rotated 180 degrees counterclockwise. **E:** At the most dependent aspect of the pouch, a vertical buttonhole incision is performed and the pouch is anastomosed to the urethral stump. The left ureter is pulled into the right retroperitoneum above the inferior mesenteric artery, and the ureters are anastomosed to the terminal ileum in an end-to-end (left ureter) and end-to-side (right ureter) technique.

is to take advantage of the antireflux function of the ileocecal valve. The cecum with the ileocecal valve is incorporated in the pouch, and the ureters are anastomosed in an end-to-side (Nesbit) or spatulated end-to-end (Wallace) technique to the terminal prevalvular ileum. Thus, the flow of urine is directed from the ureters into the pouch through the ileocecal valve.

The ureters are intubated with 6Fr or 8Fr stents, and a 10Fr pouchostomy pigtail catheter and a 20Fr transurethral Foley balloon catheter are inserted into the reservoir. The closure of the anterior wall of the pouch is completed in the same way as described previously. However, at the site of a submucosal ureteral tunnel implantation, the pouch is closed by mucosal sutures only to prevent ureteral obstruction at the entry. A 20Fr gravity drain is placed each into the small pelvis and at the ureteral implantation site.

The ureteral stents are removed at day 10 and 11. The transurethral catheter is removed at day 12 when a pouchogram has ruled out extravasation. Residual urine is checked via the pouchostomy catheter when patients void spontaneously. The pouchostomy catheter is removed at residual urine volumes <50 mL. In neurogenic cases, patients are instructed in intermittent catheterization.

## OUTCOMES

### Complications

In the early postoperative months, nonperistaltic contractions of the bowel segments of a Mainz pouch do occur but subside spontaneously with increasing capacity of the pouch. For persistent inadequate compliance or persistent contractions of the pouch, antimuscarinics can be used for pharmacotherapy.

About 60% of patients postoperatively have an asymptomatic metabolic acidosis as judged by blood gas analysis (base excess below −2.5), which is balanced prophylactically by oral alkali substitution (sodium/potassium citrate/bicarbonate).

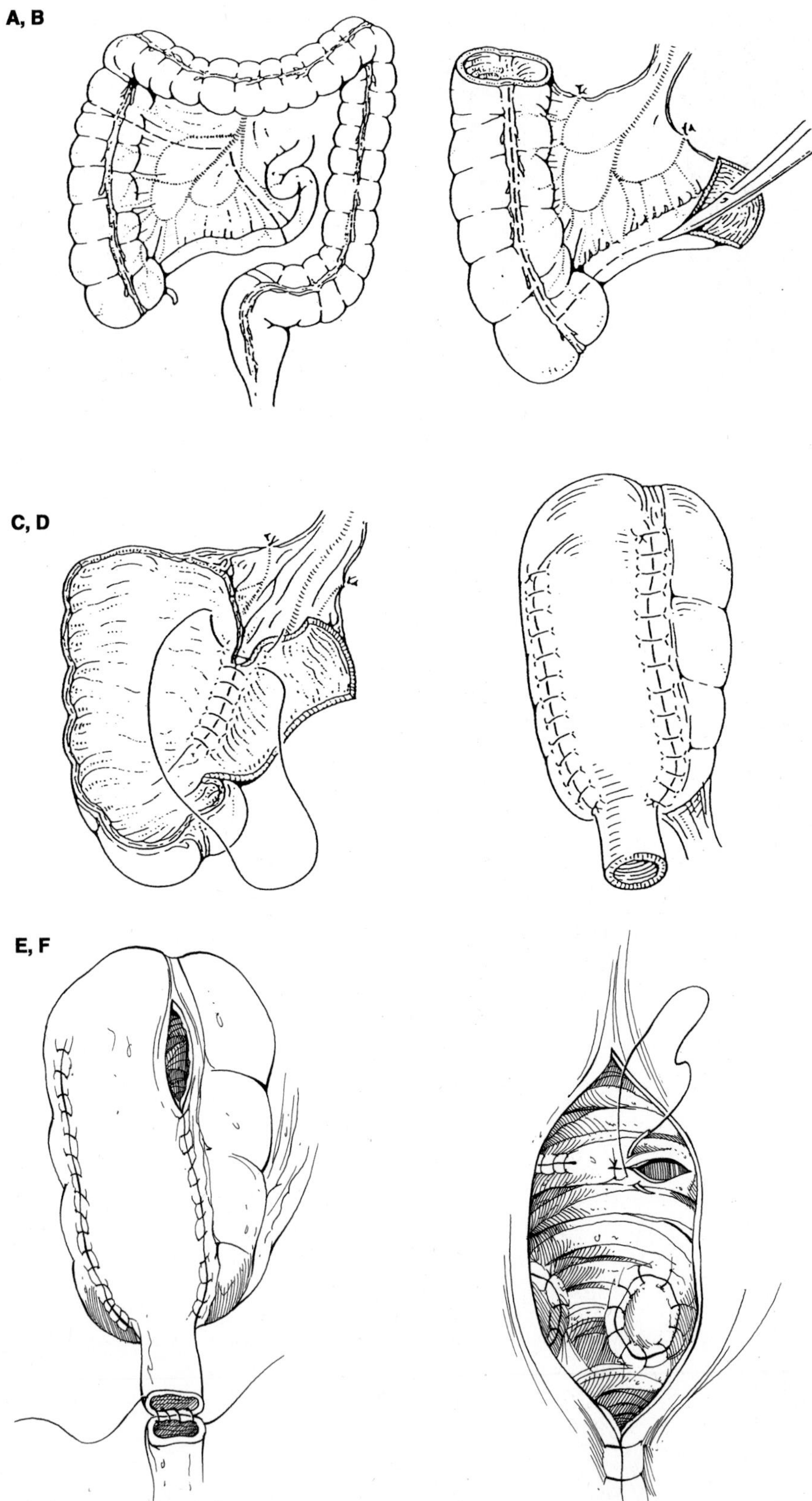


FIGURE 90.3 "Le Bag" procedure. **A and B:** Isolation of the ileocecal segment and antimesenteric opening, leaving the oral end of the ileal segment intact. **C and D:** Detubularization and reconfiguration of the segments into a pouch. A 180-degree counterclockwise rotation brings the oral intact ileum segment down to the urethra. **E:** Ileourethral anastomosis with the oral end of the ileal segment. F: Antirefluxive submucosal tunnel ureter implantation through two separate incisions of the posterior pouch wall (buttonhole technique).

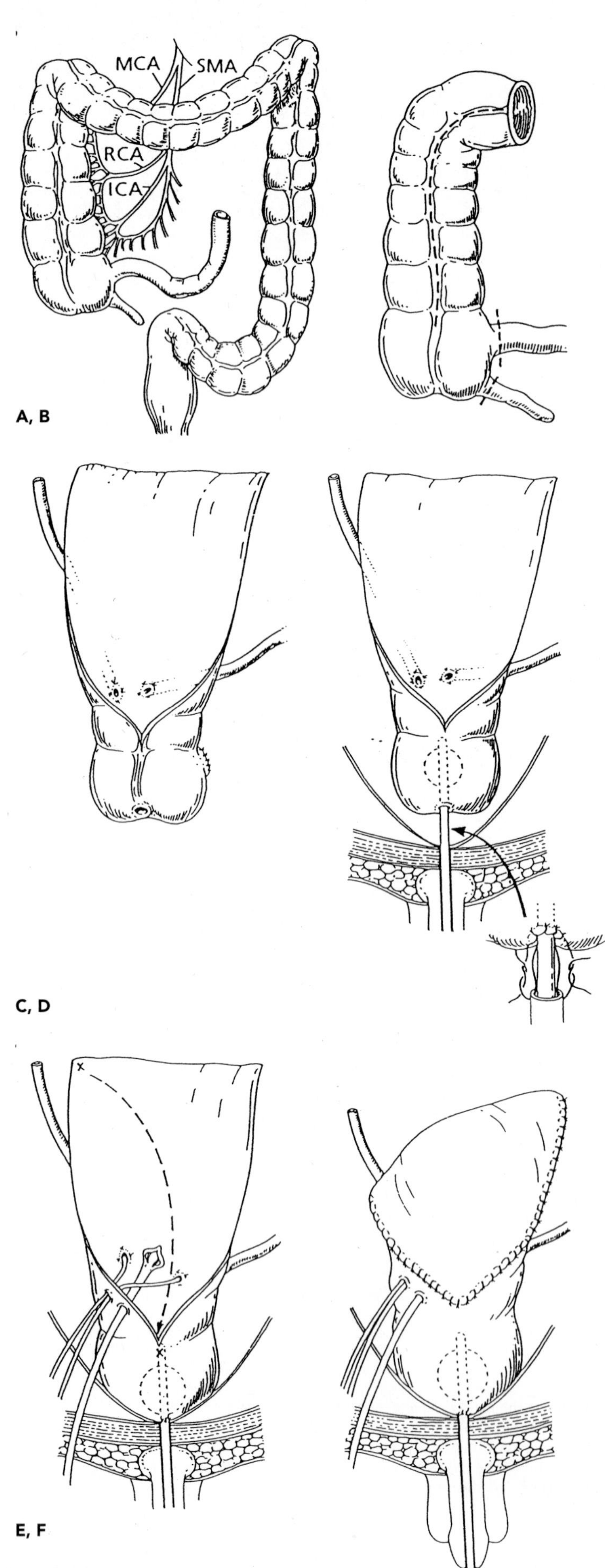


FIGURE 90.4 Construction of a right colonic reservoir. **A and B:** Isolation of a colonic segment consisting of cecum, ascending colon, and the right colic flexure. **C and D:** Opening of the segment through the taenia libera, leaving the cecum intact and anastomosing it to the urethra. **E and F:** The ureters are anastomosed into the colonic segment utilizing the "buttonhole" submucosal implantation technique. This technique describes the ureters entering the submucosal tunnel via a buttonhole incision into the posterior wall of the pouch. Reconfiguration is completed by folding the open cranial segment over the caudal segment and anastomosing both lateral margins.

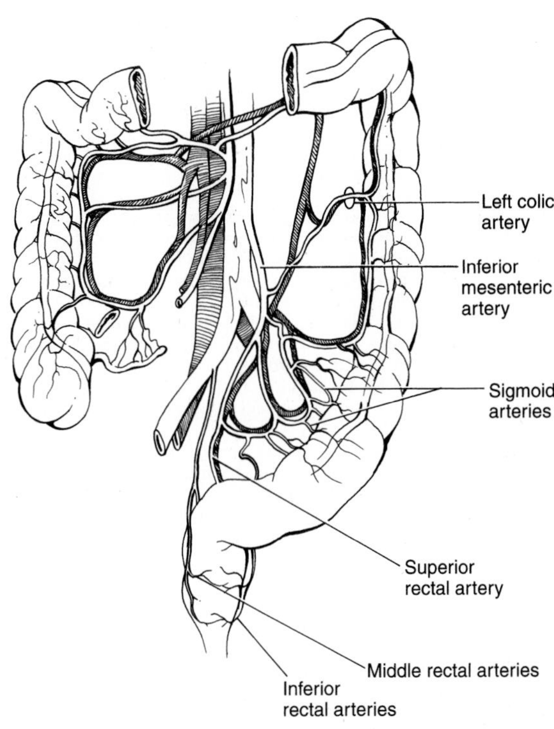


FIGURE 90.5 Vascular supply of the left colon and rectosigmoid.

At present, the risk of secondary malignancies cannot be comprehensively determined. Follow-up examinations must include renal ultrasound and/or intravenous pyelogram, blood gases, and, starting from the fifth postoperative year, pouchoscopy and evaluation of serum cobalamin.

## Results

In general, the outcome criteria for orthotopic bladder substitution by intestine are (a) the function and morphology of the upper urinary tracts, (b) frequency during day and night, (c) continence, and (d) ability to void spontaneously. However, one has to keep in mind that especially continence and the ability for spontaneous micturition may significantly be influenced by the type and quality of surgery preceding the orthotopic substitution itself. Related factors are, for example, preparation of the bladder neck and urethra, sparing of the autonomous nerves, and measures to prevent pouch displacement or kinking. Therefore, functional results attributed to specific kinds of reservoirs actually rely on more factors than the segment(s) of intestine chosen. For ileocecal reservoirs, a ureterointestinal obstruction rate of up to 7% is reported. Continence rates for ileocecal reservoirs vary between 75% and 88% during the day and 67% during the night (6,11). Continence rates for sigmoid colon reservoirs are significantly lower, at 50% (11).

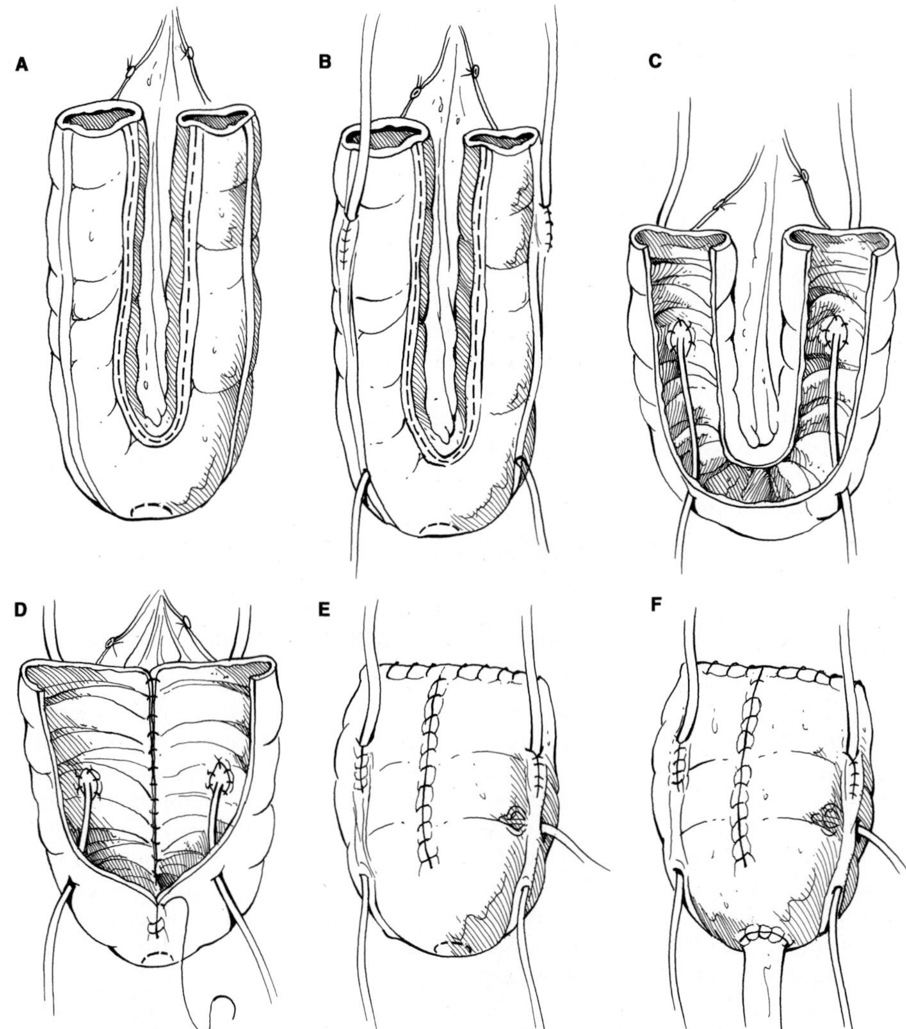


FIGURE 90.6 Construction of a sigmoid colon reservoir (Reddy). **A:** Isolating a segment of about 30 cm of sigmoid colon. **B:** Submucosal tunnel ureteral implantation. **C and D:** Detubularization, U-shaped reconfiguration of the segment, and side-to-side anastomosis of the back wall of the pouch. **E and F:** Completion of the anterior wall of the pouch and anastomosis to the urethra.

## References

1. Ali-El-Din B, El-Sobky E, Hohenfellner M, et al. Orthotopic bladder substitution in women: functional and urodynamic evaluation. *J Urol* 1999; 161:1875–1880.
2. El-Mekresh M, Franzaring L, Wöhr M, et al. Simplified orthotopic ileocecal pouch (Mainz pouch) for bladder substitution. *Aktuelle Urol* 2003; 34:226–230.
3. Hinman FJ. Selection of intestinal segments for bladder substitution: physical and physiological characteristics. *J Urol* 1988;139:519–523.
4. Hohenfellner M, Black P, Linn J, et al. Surgical treatment of interstial cystitis in women. *Int Urogynecol J Pelvic Floor Dysfunct* 2000;11:113–119.
5. Hugonnet C, Danuser H, Springer J, et al. Urethral sensitivity and the impact on urinary continence in patients with an ileal bladder substitute after cystectomy. *J Urol* 2001;165:1502–1505.
6. Kolettis PN, Klein EA, Novick AC, et al. The Le Bag orthotopic urinary diversion. *J Urol* 1996;156:926–930.
7. Leissner J, Stein R, Hohenfellner R, et al. Radical cystoprostatectomy combined with Mainz pouch bladder substitution to the urethra: long-term results. *BJU Int* 1999;83:964–970.
8. Light JK, Engelmann UH. Le Bag: total replacement of the bladder using an ileocolonic pouch. *J Urol* 1986;136:27–31.
9. Linn JF, Hohenfellner M, Roth S, et al. Treatment of intersitial cystitis: comparison of subtrigonal and supratrigonal cystectomy combined with orthotopic bladder substitution. *J Urol* 1998;159:774–778.
10. Reddy PK. The colonic neobladder. *Urol Clin North Am* 1991;18: 609–614.
11. Riedmiller H, Thuroff J, Stöckle M, et al. Continent urinary diversion and bladder augmentation in children: the Mainz pouch procedure. *Pediatr Nephrol* 1989;3:68–74.
12. Santucci R, Park C, Mayo M, et al. Continence and urodynamic parameters of continent urinary reservoirs: comparison of gastric, ileal, ileocolic, right colon, and sigmoid segments. *Urology* 1999;54:252–257.
13. Stein R, Fisch M, Beetz R, et al. Urinary diversion in children and young adults using the Mainz pouch I technique. *Br J Urol* 1997;79:354–361.
14. Stenzl A, Colleselli K, Poisel S, et al. Rationale and technique of nerve sparing radical cystectomy before an orthotopic neobladder procedure in women. *J Urol* 1995;154:2044–2049.
15. Thüroff JW, Alken P, Riedmiller H, et al. The MAINZ pouch (mixed augmentation ileum and cecum) for bladder augmentation and continent diversion. *J Urol* 1986;136:17–26.
16. Thüroff JW, Mattiasson A, Andersen JT, et al. Standardization of terminology and assessment of functional characteristics of intestinal urinary reservoirs. *Neurourol Urodyn* 1996;15:499–511.
17. Turner W, Danuser H, Moehrle K, et al. The effect of nerve sparing cystectomy technique on postoperative continence after orthotopic bladder substitution. *J Urol* 1997;158(6):2118–2122.

# CHAPTER 91 ■ CONTINENT CATHETERIZABLE RESERVOIR MADE FROM ILEUM

HASSAN ABOL-ENEIN AND MOHAMED A. GHONEIM

A substantial number of techniques have been described for the creation of continent cutaneous urinary reservoirs. For construction of such systems three elements are required: a low-pressure compliant reservoir, an antirefluxive ureterointestinal anastomosis, and a continent stoma that allows easy catheterization.

To create a reservoir with high capacity at low pressure, various segments of bowel have been utilized: the ileum, the ileocolonic region, the ascending colon, and the transverse colon. Regardless of the selected bowel segment, detubularization and double folding are basic prerequisites to achieve this goal.

A reliable antirefluxive ureterointestinal anastomosis is necessary, since bacteriuria is a constant feature in these systems and results from intermittent catheterization. The technique employed should provide a unidirectional but nonobstructed flow. The antirefluxing mechanism should not be at the expense of a higher incidence of obstructive complications.

Hinman (7) classified continent outlets into four categories according to the mechanism of their action. These included an antiperistaltic ileal segment (6); imbricated or tapered ileal segments resulting in passive tubular resistance (11); outlets using the pressure equilibration principle, including an ileal spout valve (3), flutter valve (4), inkwell hydraulic valve, intussusception nipple (5), or ileal servomechanism sphincter (8); and flap valves, which are created by the incorporation of tubular structures within the wall of the reservoir, such as the appendix (10), fallopian tubes (12), parts of ileum (13), or tubularized cecal segments (9). Multiplicity of techniques implies that none is optimal. Many of the above techniques rely on an inert or even unphysiologic mechanism, and problems and malfunctions soon appear.

In our proposed technique, we have utilized the ileum for construction of the low-pressure reservoir and a serous-lined tunnel to provide an antirefluxive mechanism (1) as well as to create a reliable continent outlet (2).

## INDICATIONS FOR SURGERY

Any patient who requires bladder replacement is a potential candidate for this operation. The indications of continent cutaneous urinary diversion include the following:

1. ***Pelvic malignancies:*** In patients for whom cystectomy is indicated for bladder cancer or those requiring an anterior pelvic exenteration for other pelvic malignancies.
2. ***Benign indications***: These include neuropathic bladders when conservative measures fail, extensive urethral strictures with damaged urethral sphincter, contracted bladders with compromised urinary continence, complex urinary fistulas affecting the sphincteric mechanism, and some cases of bladder exstrophy with failed attempts of primary repair.

3. *Urinary conversion:* Conversion from other types of urinary diversion, such as ileal conduits in young healthy patients, for patients who develop isolated urethral recurrence following radical cystectomy and orthotopic bladder substitution, and in some cases of ureterosigmoidostomy suffering from intractable metabolic acidosis.

## PATIENT SELECTION AND EVALUATION

Suitable candidates should have reasonable manual dexterity. Motivation to carry out clean intermittent catheterization at regular intervals is necessary. Furthermore, a good prognosis might be expected if the indication to diversion was a pelvic malignancy. Patients who are unfit for prolonged surgery and those with a history of previous bowel resection, short bowel syndrome, or heavily irradiated bowel are among the contraindications for this procedure. Patients with impaired renal function (serum creatinine equal to or >1.8 mg per dL and or creatinine clearance equal to or >40 mL per minute) are unsuitable candidates since metabolic acidosis would be inevitable.

## ALTERNATIVE THERAPY

Alternative techniques of urinary diversion should be discussed with the patient when orthotopic bladder substitution or continent cutaneous reservoirs are contraindicated or unfeasible. These include conduit diversion and anal sphincter–controlled bladder substitutes. The potential postoperative complications, changes in future lifestyle, and long-term sequelae should be clearly explained to the patients.

## SURGICAL TECHNIQUE

### Preoperative Preparation

Since the small bowel is utilized, no specific preparation is necessary. The only requirement is fasting overnight with administration of intravenous fluids to ensure good hydration. Patients with histories of thromboembolic disease or varicose veins should receive a prophylactic dose of heparin (5,000 U subcutaneously) the night before the operation and every 12 hours thereafter until ambulation. Compression leg stockings are also advised. Although the intention is to use a concealed umbilical stoma, a stoma therapist should examine the patient and determine a suitable site for an abdominal stoma. A parenteral broad-spectrum antibiotic is given just before induction of anesthesia and continued postoperatively for 3 days.

### Operative Technique

The patient is put in the supine position with a Trendelenberg tilt. Slight flexion of the knees will further help in the relaxation of the abdominal muscles, facilitate retraction, and provide wider exposure. If total urethrectomy is planned, the patient is put in a slight lithotomy position for access to the perineum. The surgical area to be sterilized and draped extends from the lower chest down to the upper thighs.

A midline incision from the pubis inferiorly to a point halfway between the umbilicus and xyphoid process of the sternum superiorly is generally employed. The incision is encircling the umbilicus by 2 to 3 cm to the left.

The bowel is examined, and a 60-cm-long segment of the terminal ileum is isolated. Backlight transillumination of the mesenteric attachment greatly helps the identification of the arterial arcades supplying the selected segments. The bowel is divided 15 to 20 cm proximal to the cecum in the avascular window of Treves between the ileocolic artery and the terminal branch of the superior mesenteric artery. The ileum is divided proximally in a suitable avascular plane between the superior mesenteric arcades. Continuity of the bowel is re-established by end-to-end anastomosis. The use of an automatic stapler or a hand-sewn technique is a matter of surgeon's preference. The isolated bowel segment is subsequently subdivided into three parts. The middle 40-cm segment is used for construction of the reservoir, the 10-cm oral segment is used for creation of the antireflux mechanism, and the distal 10-cm caudal segment is used for creation of the outlet valve (Fig. 91.1). Great attention is paid to preserving an adequate blood supply for the oral and caudal small bowel segments.

The middle segment is arranged in a W configuration, and its antimesenteric border is incised by a diathermy knife. The edges of the two medial flaps are joined by a single layer of continuous 3-0 polyglactin sutures. The two lateral limbs are left to serve as serous-lined troughs. The oral and caudal short

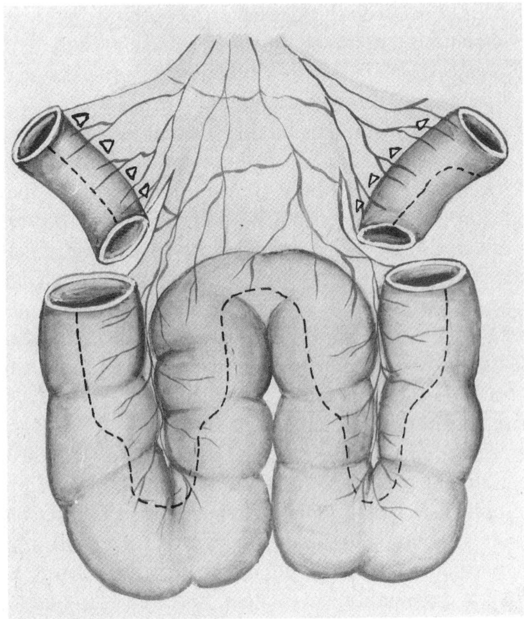

FIGURE 91.1 A 60-cm-long ileal segment is isolated; the 40-cm middle segment is arranged in a W configuration and used for construction of the body of the reservoir, the 10-cm oral segment is used for the antireflux mechanism, and the caudal segment is used for the outlet valve.

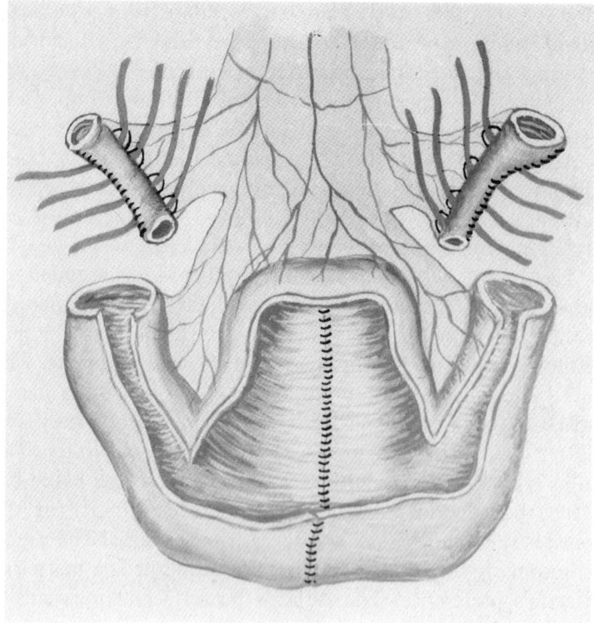

FIGURE 91.2 The bowel segment is incised at the antimesenteric border. The medial flaps are approximated with continuous 3-0 polyglactin sutures. The oral and caudal segments are tapered around a 20Fr catheter. The proximal one-third of the inlet segment is kept untapered. The created mesenteric windows are marked by a strip of vessel loops.

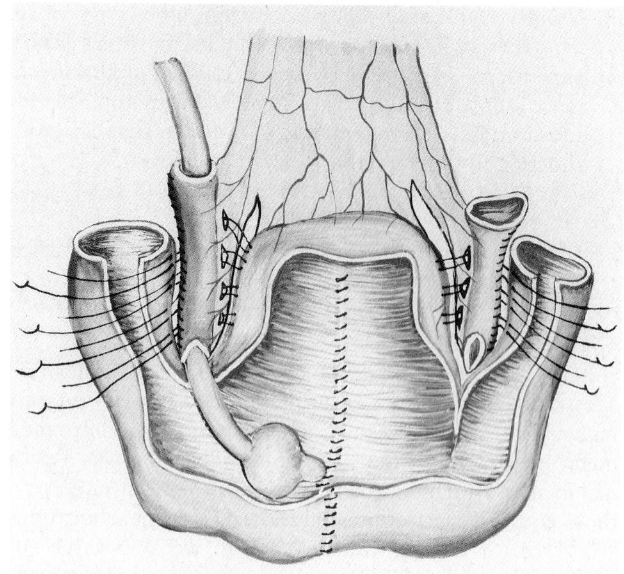

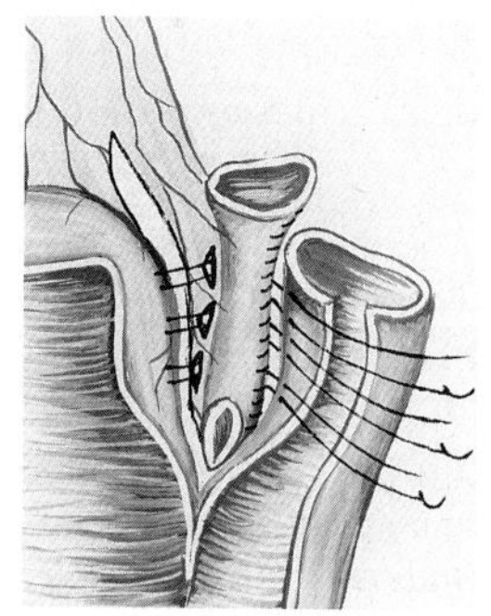

FIGURE 91.3 The tapered ileal segments are fixed and embedded within the serous-lined extramural troughs. The bulky mesentery of the embedded segments is excluded behind the pouch.

segments are tapered around a 22Fr catheter. Bowel tapering could be performed either by simple excision and hand-sewn technique or by using a one-step technique with an automatic gastrointestinal stapler. The proximal one-third of the inlet segment is kept untapered for ureteral anastomosis. Three to four small mesenteric windows close to the mesenteric border are created in between the arterial arcades supplying these segments. Each mesenteric window is marked by a small strip of rubber vessel loop. This step will facilitate easy passage of sutures through the mesenteric window (Fig. 91.2).

Each tapered segment is inlaid in its corresponding serous-lined trough. The two adjacent limbs of each trough are approximated using 3-0 silk seromuscular suture passing through the mesenteric windows and guided by the inserted strips of vessel loops. The tapered ileal segments are fixed and embedded within the serous-lined extramural troughs. Thus, the bulky mesentery of the embedded segments is excluded behind the pouch (Fig. 91.3). The spatulated distal ends of the tapered segments are anastomosed to the tunnel flaps, and the ileal trough is closed in front of the embedded segment using interrupted 4-0 polyglactin sutures (Fig. 91.4).

Two soft siliconized 8Fr to 10Fr stents are threaded through the inlet segment and secured in place by 4-0 chromic gut sutures. The pouch plate is then closed by approximation of the most lateral ileal flaps anteriorly and to the shoulder flap between the inlet and outlet segments (Fig. 91.5).

The skin of the umbilical funnel is raised and separated from the underlying rectus fascia in the midline. A fascial cruciate incision is made that can admit a 20Fr to 24Fr catheter. The invaginated umbilical skin funnel is identified and a suitable button hole is excised. The distal end of the outlet segment is

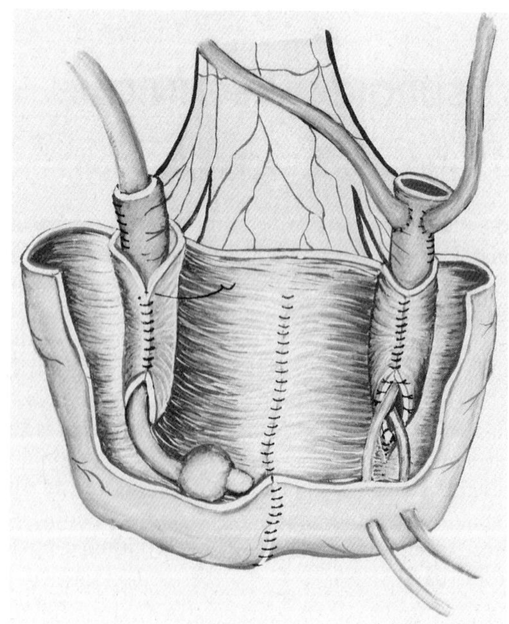

FIGURE 91.4 The spatulated distal ends of the tapered segments are anastomosed to the tunnel flaps, and the ileal trough is closed in front of the embedded segment using interrupted 4-0 polyglactin sutures. Two siliconized stents are threaded through the inlet segment.

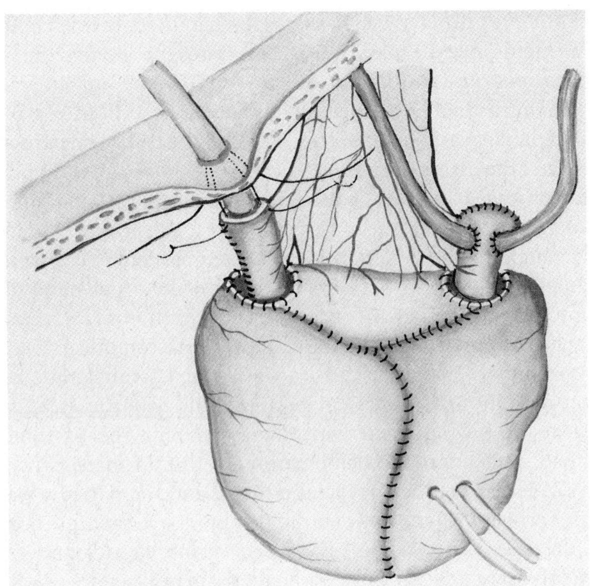

FIGURE 91.5 The pouch plate is closed by approximation of the most lateral ileal flaps anteriorly and to the shoulder flap between the inlet and outlet segments.

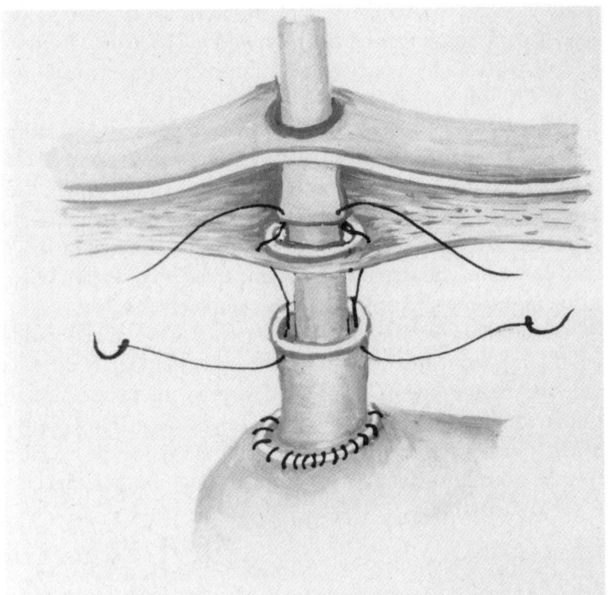

FIGURE 91.6 The edge of the outlet is fixed to the edge of the umbilical skin funnel using interrupted sutures including the rectus fascia.

pulled through the rectus fascia aperture. The edge of the intestinal outlet is fixed to the edge of the umbilical skin funnel using interrupted monofilament 4-0 or 3-0 monocryl sutures including the rectus fascia (Fig. 91.6).

The body of the reservoir wall around the outlet segment is then fixed to the inner aspect of the abdominal wall. Attention is paid to avoid twisting and/or angulation of the outlet segment. This would avoid difficulties in catheterization later.

The reservoir is drained by an 18Fr to 20Fr Foley balloon siliconized catheter fixed through the stoma.

Both ureters are prepared and oriented toward the inlet segment according to the final position of the pouch. The left ureter is passed from left to right through a high, wide enough mesenteric hole created in the left mesocolon. The right ureter comes from right to left in front of the common iliac artery behind the mesentery of the pouch. Tension-free, widely spatulated, stented implantation of the ureters into the inlet segment is then performed. A Wallace, Nesbit, or end-to-end anastomosis could be utilized according to surgical needs, using 4-0 or 5-0 polyglactin sutures.

The ureteral stents are exteriorized through the anterior wall of the reservoir to which they are secured. This will provide almost a dry reservoir during the healing stage.

The pelvic cavity is drained by two 18Fr fenestrated tubes. Only straight gravity drainage is used. Gastric drainage is established using either a nasogastric tube or open gastrostomy.

## An Alternative: Utilization of the Appendix

If the appendix is suitable to serve as an outlet, the ileocecal junction is mobilized sufficiently to ensure a tension-free implantation of the appendix. The appendix is mobilized and detached at its base. The isolated appendix is cut and spatulated at its tip. The lumen is then dilated up to 16Fr to 18Fr using straight dilators. Four windows are created in the mesoappendix. The windows are labeled by rubber vessel loops. The appendix is embedded in the serous-lined trough as described previously (Fig 91.7).

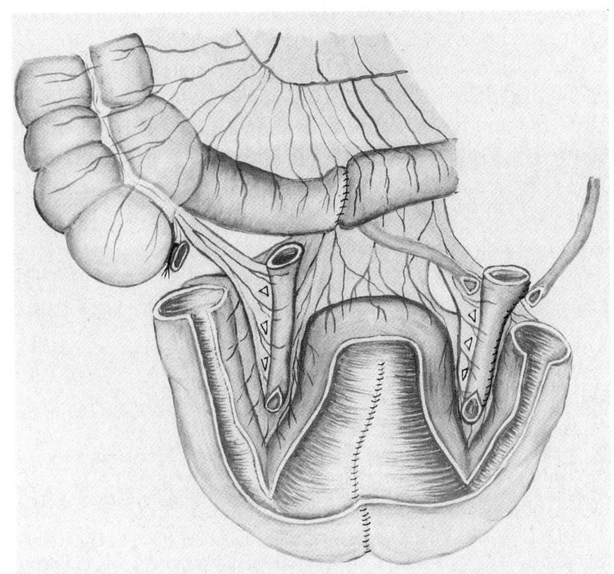

FIGURE 91.7 The appendix is isolated and spatulated at its tip. Four windows are created at the mesoappendix. The appendix is fixed and embedded in the serous-lined trough as previously described.

## POSTOPERATIVE CARE

Parenteral fluids are maintained until bowel habit resumes. Prophylactic antibiotics are given routinely for 5 days. Low-molecular-weight heparin is given for 10 days. The draining tubes are removed when the drainage ceases. The reservoir is irrigated with 30 to 60 mL of normal saline every 8 hours to prevent mucus retention. The ureteric stents are removed after 10 to 12 days postoperatively. The pouch is drained for 21 days before training by intermittent catheter clamping. All patients start self-catheterization 2 days before discharge from the hospital. A 2-hour interval is allowed in week 1, which is increased gradually until the pouch matures. By the end of week 6 most of the patients evacuate the pouch every 4 to 5 hours.

## OUTCOMES

### Complications

In our experience with 101 patients, early complications were observed in 15%. These included urinary leakage (2%), pelvic collections (8%), ureteroileal obstruction (1%), ileus (3%), and wound complications (3%). Small nonsymptomatic pelvic collections need no treatment. Sizable and/or infected symptomatic ones are usually treated by ultrasound-guided needle aspiration with or without an indwelling tube drain. None of these pelvic collections required open drainage. Urinary leakage was an infrequent complication in our series (2%). This complication was due to pouch perforation during catheterization training. Prolonged pouch drainage was required for an additional 2 weeks until healing of the injury occurred. Early evidence of ureteroileal obstruction was observed in one patient. Antegrade fixation of a double-J stent was done for 6 weeks. The stent was removed by pouchoscopy carried out through the umbilical stoma. Gastrointestinal and wound complications were similar to those for other urinary diversion procedures.

Late complications included stomal stenosis at the skin level with catheterization difficulties in 6% of the patients. Two-thirds of them had an appendix stoma. Half of these patients required revisional surgery to widen the mucocutaneous stenotic area using a wedge skin flap technique. In one child it was impossible to pass a catheter into the pouch due to overdistention resulting in angulations of the outlet tract. Under ultrasound guidance, percutaneous insertion of a pigtail catheter was carried out. Once the pouch became empty, outlet catheterization again was easy. Rupture of the pouch was observed in one patient following blunt abdominal trauma. Laparotomy was necessary, and the pouch tear was adequately repaired. Pouch stones were observed in 5% of the patients. All of them were amenable for endoscopic manipulations, but one patient required open pouchlithotomy. The incidence of upper-tract dilatation due to anastomotic stricture was minimal (1%); the stricture was treated by antegrade balloon dilatation. One patient required left nephroureterectomy 3 years following cystectomy due to a renal pelvis tumor. Gravity pouchography demonstrated reflux in three patients (3%). Reflux was asymptomatic in all, and the patients were kept on prophylactic antimicrobial suppressive therapy. None of the operated patients developed metabolic acidosis. All patients were advised to use oral alkali therapy.

### Results

Patients regained their normal lifestyle once healing was completed. Ninety-five percent of our patients were completely dry day and night. The catheterization interval was every 4 to 5 hours during daytime and every 1 to 2 hours at night. The average capacity at 6 months postoperatively was 550 ± 130 mL.

Five patients (5%) had a frequently wet stoma due to failure of the continence mechanism. Two patients were revised. One underwent revision of the continent outlet, and augmentation ileopouchoplasty was required to increase pouch capacity in the other. Two patients preferred frequent catheterization to avoid leakage. The remaining patient fixed a collection device during nighttime and refused further intervention.

Patients have to understand that they have a neobladder constructed from the bowel and that this bladder is different from the native one. The usual desire to micturate and the familiar micturition mechanism no longer exist. However, all patients with a dry, continent outlet stoma enjoy an excellent lifestyle, normal social activities, an accepted body image, and personal satisfaction.

## *References*


1. Abol-Enein H, Ghoneim MA. A novel uretero-ileal reimplantation technique: the serous lined extramural tunnel. A preliminary report. *J Urol* 1994;151:1193–1197.
2. Abol-Enein H, Ghoneim MA. Serous-lined extramural ileal valve: a new continent urinary outlet. *J Urol* 1999;161:786–791.
3. Ashken MH. An appliance free ileocecal urinary diversion: preliminary communication. *Br J Urol* 1974;46:631–634.
4. Askhen MH. Urinary reservoirs. In: *Urinary diversion.* Berlin: Springer-Verlag, 1982:112.
5. Benchekroun A. Continent caecal bladder. *Eur Urol* 1987;3:248–251.
6. Gilchrist RR, Merricks JW, Hamlin HH, et al. Construction of a substitute for bladder and urethra. *Surg Gynecol Obstet* 1950;90:752–760.
7. Hinman F Jr. Functional classification of conduits for continent diversion. *J Urol* 1990;44:27–30.
8. Koff AS, Cerulli C, Wise HA. Clinical and urodynamic features of a new intestinal urinary sphincter for continent urinary diversion. *J Urol* 1989;142:293–296.
9. Lample A, Hohenfellner M, Schultz-Lample D, et al. In situ tunneled bowel flap tubes: 2 new techniques of a continent outlet for Mainz Pouch cutaneous diversion. *J Urol* 1995;153:308–315.
10. Mitrofanoff P. Cystostomie continente trans-appendicularie dans la traitement des vessies neurologiques. *Chir Pediatr* 1980;21:297–300.
11. Rowland RG, Mitchell ME, Bihrle R. The cecoileal continent urinary reservoir. *World J Urol* 1985;3:185–190.
12. Woodhouse CRJ, Malone PR, Cummning J, et al. The Mitrofanoff principle for continent urinary diversion. *Br J Urol* 1989;63:53–57.
13. Zinman L, Libertino JA. Ileocecal conduit for temporary or permanent urinary diversion. *J Urol* 1975;113:317–323.

# CHAPTER 92 ■ CONTINENT CATHETERIZABLE RESERVOIR MADE FROM COLON

HUBERTUS RIEDMILLER AND ELMAR W. GERHARZ

Over the past 15 years there has been an increasing interest in alternatives to the Bricker ileal conduit as a form of urinary diversion. A wide range of techniques are currently available, including orthotopic bladder substitution and continent cutaneous and rectal bladder diversion. The current body of published literature is insufficient to conclude that there is a superior form of urinary diversion in terms of evidence-based medicine. It is quite clear, however, that not all patients are candidates for one type of diversion. The best results are obtained when a comprehensive concept is tailored to the individual patient at a high-volume center with experience in all major types of diversion techniques (4).

## DIAGNOSIS

The most common indication for continent cutaneous diversion is a bladder replacement after anterior pelvic exenteration for malignant disease, followed by functional or morphologic bladder loss for other reasons. Diagnostic modalities therefore should be directed at the underlying pathology and definitive treatment.

## INDICATIONS FOR SURGERY

Despite the recent trend toward orthotopic substitution, continent catheterizable urinary reservoirs remain a good form of diversion. Whereas previous or synchronous urethral transitional cell carcinoma (TCC) is an absolute contraindication to urethral preservation, the role of multifocality, associated carcinoma in situ and of bladder neck and prostatic involvement on urethral recurrence is less well defined. In these cases, continent cutaneous diversion is still a safe alternative in the appropriate patient.

Advanced age (>70 years) with its physiologic deterioration of sphincter competence is another relative contraindication for orthotopic reconstruction; older patients who are otherwise physically fit may well benefit from a continent cutaneous reservoir.

Whenever the native sphincter mechanism is lacking, destroyed, or dysfunctional or urethral catheterization is painful or technically impossible, cutaneous diversion is the only alternative to modified ureterosigmoidostomy and ileal loop. As a salvage procedure in failed exstrophy reconstruction, in other complicated congenital abnormalities of the urinary tract, in neurogenic bladder dysfunction (wheelchair-bound myelomeningocele patients), and in patients with intractable urinary incontinence, severe pelvic traumas, and complicated fistulas, continent cutaneous reservoirs provide excellent results even in extremely complex cases.

Until recently, renal transplant patients were excluded from the benefits of continent urinary diversion. Several authors have, however, reported encouraging experiences with kidney transplantation into continent urinary intestinal reservoirs as a planned two-stage procedure in patients with functional or morphologic bladder loss (see below) (9).

Other factors to consider when deciding on the type of urinary diversion include patient age, prognosis of underlying disease, comorbidity, urinary and anal sphincter competence, manual dexterity, renal function and upper-urinary-tract configuration, and subjective criteria (motivation, compliance, expectation of social support, emotional capability of dealing with clean intermittent catheterization). Patient priorities are considered whenever medically justifiable and technically feasible.

Contraindications of continent urinary diversion include impaired renal function with serum creatinine >2 mg per L, inflammatory bowel disease, large bowel malignancy, or previous history of multiple bowel ablative procedures, with or without a history of diarrhea.

## ALTERNATIVE THERAPY

Alternatives to catheterizable colonic reservoirs include pouches made from ileum (Kock), ileal or colonic conduits, classic and modified ureterosigmoidostomy (e.g., sigma-rectum pouch/Mainz pouch II), or orthotopic neobladder (Camey II, Kock, Hautmann, Studer).

## SURGICAL TECHNIQUE

While there is a broad consensus among reconstructive urologists regarding detubularization and spheric reconfiguration of bowel as a basic principle in the creation of a low-pressure, high-capacity reservoir, the issues of reflux prevention (afferent limb) and continence (efferent limb) are more controversial. The still-growing number of techniques described for achieving continence in urinary reconstruction indicates that a universally applicable procedure with a low complication rate has not yet evolved. The principal methods for construction of a continence mechanism depend on the formation of a nipple valve, utilization of the ileocecal valve, or construction of a flap valve. Among the different techniques, the versatile Mitrofanoff principle (6) has acquired significant popularity, predictably providing continence and allowing easy catheterization in >90% of cases. In 1990, Riedmiller et al. introduced the Mitrofanoff theme to the ileocecal reservoir, significantly facilitating the Mainz pouch procedure (8,12).

When performing a Mitrofanoff, the method of attaching the appendix to the reservoir (reversed, in situ: imbricated, embedded, unaltered), the location of the stoma (umbilicus, lower abdomen), and appropriate alternatives are controversial. It is known that the success of the Mitrofanoff principle is not dependent upon the underlying pathologic condition, the type of tube and its possible peristalsis, the type and configuration of the reservoir, or the patient's age, but rather on the maintenance of a pressure gradient between channel lumen and the reservoir. It is therefore the availability of the required material and the simplicity of a technique that determine its popularity. Recent variations of the Mitrofanoff theme have aimed at its simplification and at reduction of long-term complications.

## Ileocecal Pouch (Mainz Pouch I)

### Intussuscepted Ileal Nipple

After mobilization of cecum, ascending colon, and the right colonic flexure, the mesentery is divided between the right colic and the ileocolic arteries. A 13-cm segment of cecum and ascending colon is isolated along with two equal-sized limbs of distal ileum. If the vermiform appendix is absent, as in cloacal exstrophy, completely obliterated, immobile, insufficient in diameter and length, or has been removed beforehand, we usually isolate an additional portion of ileum measuring 8 to 10 cm (Fig. 92.1A). While the latter is left tubularized, the remaining bowel segment is split antimesenterically. These three opened bowel loops are folded in the form of an incomplete W, and their posterior aspects are sutured to one another to form a broad posterior plate (Fig. 92.1B). Both ureters are implanted into the large bowel segment of the pouch plate, forming submucosal tunnels for reflux prevention (Fig. 92.1C).

The midportion of the intact ileal segment is freed of its mesentery up to a distance of 4 to 5 cm to allow its intussusception (Fig. 92.1D and E). One row of staples is applied to stabilize the intussusception itself (Fig. 92.1F). Thereafter, the intussuscepted nipple is pulled through the intact ileocecal valve and two additional rows of staples are applied to attach the nipple to the ileocecal valve. After the mucosa has been removed from the rim of the intussuscepted nipple and the colonic aspect of the ileocecal valve, their circumferences are sewn together with a running suture.

The bowel is then folded on itself in a side-to-side fashion, thus creating a low-pressure, high-capacity reservoir. Ureteral stents (6Fr or 8Fr) and a 10Fr pouchostomy are led through

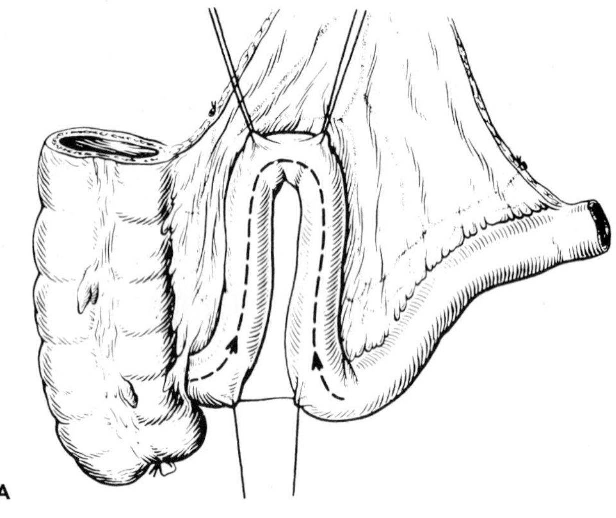


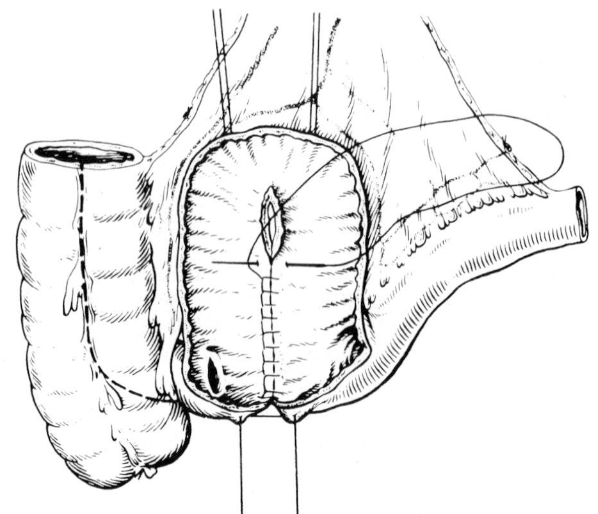


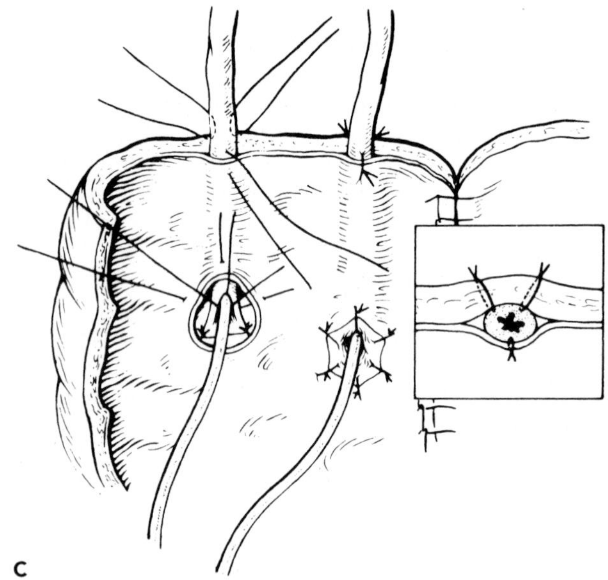


**FIGURE 92.1** Ileocecal pouch (Mainz pouch I) with intussuscepted ileal nipple valve. **A:** Isolation of cecum or ascending colon (13 to 15 cm), two equal-sized ileal loops (13 cm each) for reservoir formation, and an additional ileal segment (8 to 10 cm) for nipple formation. Antimesenteric splitting of the bowel. **B:** Side-to-side anastomosis of the terminal and next proximal ileal loop with subsequent detubularization of the ascending colon. **C:** Antirefluxing ureteral implantation into the colonic portion of the pouch plate using submucosal tunnels (3 cm length) and insertion of 6Fr ureteral stents.

(*continued on next page*)

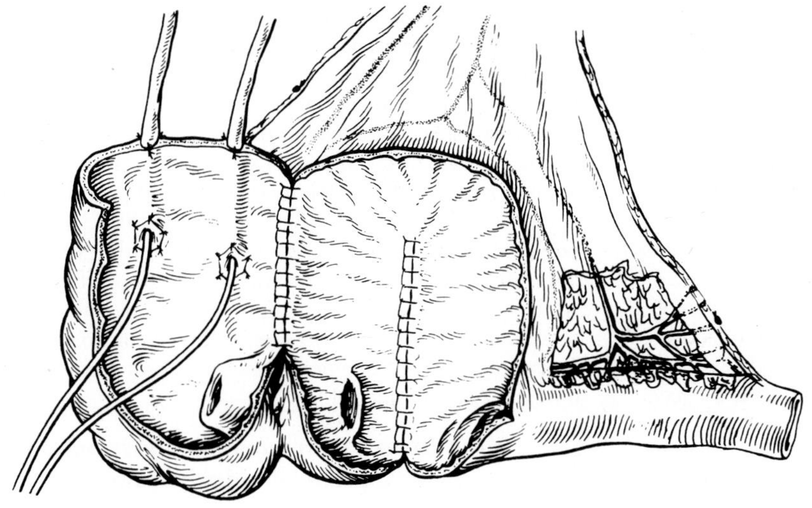

D

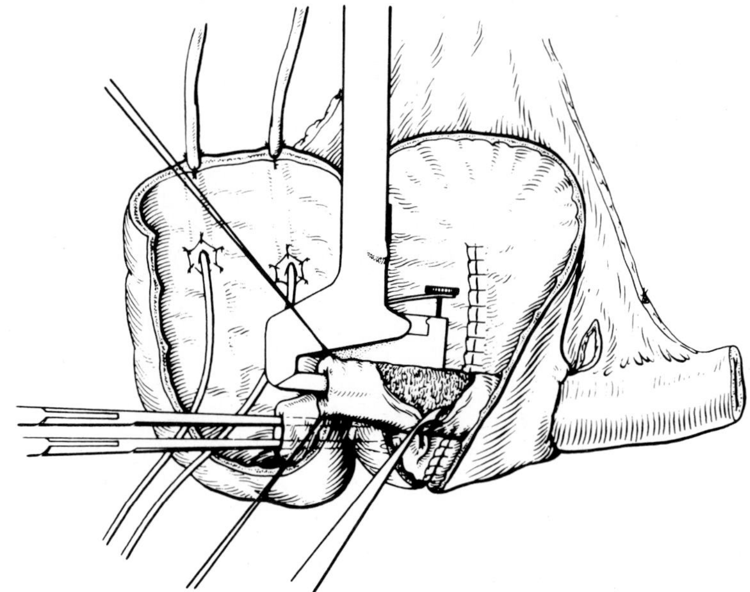

E

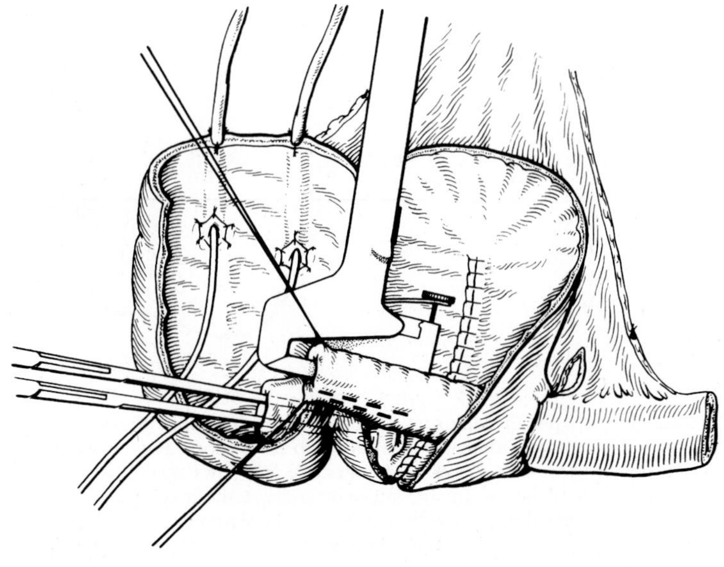

F

FIGURE 92.1 (*continued*) **D:** Removal of mesentery (4 to 5 cm) in the midportion of the oral ileal segment in preparation for intussusception. **E:** Intussusception of the ileal segment and stabilization by applying one row of staples. **F:** The intussuscepted ileal nipple is pulled through the ileocecal valve and two additional rows of staples are used to attach the nipple to the valve. (From Thieme Stuttgart, New York, with permission.)

the abdominal wall at separate sites. The entire pouch is rotated to bring the efferent limb to the region of the umbilicus. A small button of skin is removed from the depth of the umbilical funnel. The pouch is carefully attached to the posterior fascia with interrupted nonabsorbable sutures to prevent the pouch from rotating and kinking. The efferent limb is then connected to the umbilical funnel with interrupted absorbable sutures. In the absence of an umbilicus (as in the case of exstrophy), it is created by tubularizing a V-shaped cutaneous flap and connecting it to the appendicular stump (12).

A vigorous washout regimen is started early in the postoperative course. Ureteric stents are removed after 10 to 14 days. Clean intermittent catheterization is usually started at the end of the third postoperative week after leakage and reflux have been ruled out by pouchogram.

## Appendix Stoma

If the appendix is present and can be dilated to accommodate a 16Fr to 18Fr catheter, it is ideally our first choice as the efferent segment for construction of a continence mechanism. In this case, a 15-cm segment of cecum and ascending colon is isolated along with two equally sized limbs of distal ileum (12 to 13 cm each). The lower 5 cm of the cecum (cecal pole) is left tubularized and intact. The seromuscular layer of the intact cecal pole is divided along the tenia down to the mucosa in a manner analogous to the Lich-Gregoir procedure for vesicoureteral reflux (Fig. 92.2A). By careful dissection of the seromuscular tissue, a broad submucosal bed (5 cm) is created for the appendix. The appendicular mesentery is freed of its excessive fatty tissue. Windows in the mesoappendix are excised between the branches of the appendicular artery without compromising the blood supply (Fig. 92.2B). Anatomic variations of the appendicular artery have to be respected, and an additional branch of the anterior or posterior cecal artery supplying the base of the appendix should be preserved. After the appendix is correctly positioned, the seromuscular layer is closed over the embedded in situ appendix with interrupted 4-0 polydioxanone sutures. A short mobile portion of the distal appendix remains for the creation of the appendicoumbilical stoma (Fig. 92.2C). Formation of the pouch plate, the ureterointestinal anastomosis, and the attachment to the umbilicus follows the same procedure as that for a pouch with an intussuscepted nipple (8).

## Alternative Techniques for Construction of Continence Mechanism

More recent alternative techniques use a small-caliber conduit fashioned from the cecal wall. One technique uses a full-thickness tube lined by mucosa (Fig. 92.3) and the other a seromuscular tube lined by serosa (Fig. 92.4) (5). Other authors have described transversely retubularized ileum (Fig. 92.5) to create a tunneled access into the right colon (7).

## Alternative Techniques for Ureteral Implantation

In dilated, irradiated, or otherwise compromised ureters, ureterointestinal anastomosis may be performed according to a technique that has been described by Abol Enein and Ghoneim (serous-lined extramural tunnel) (Fig. 92.6) (1).

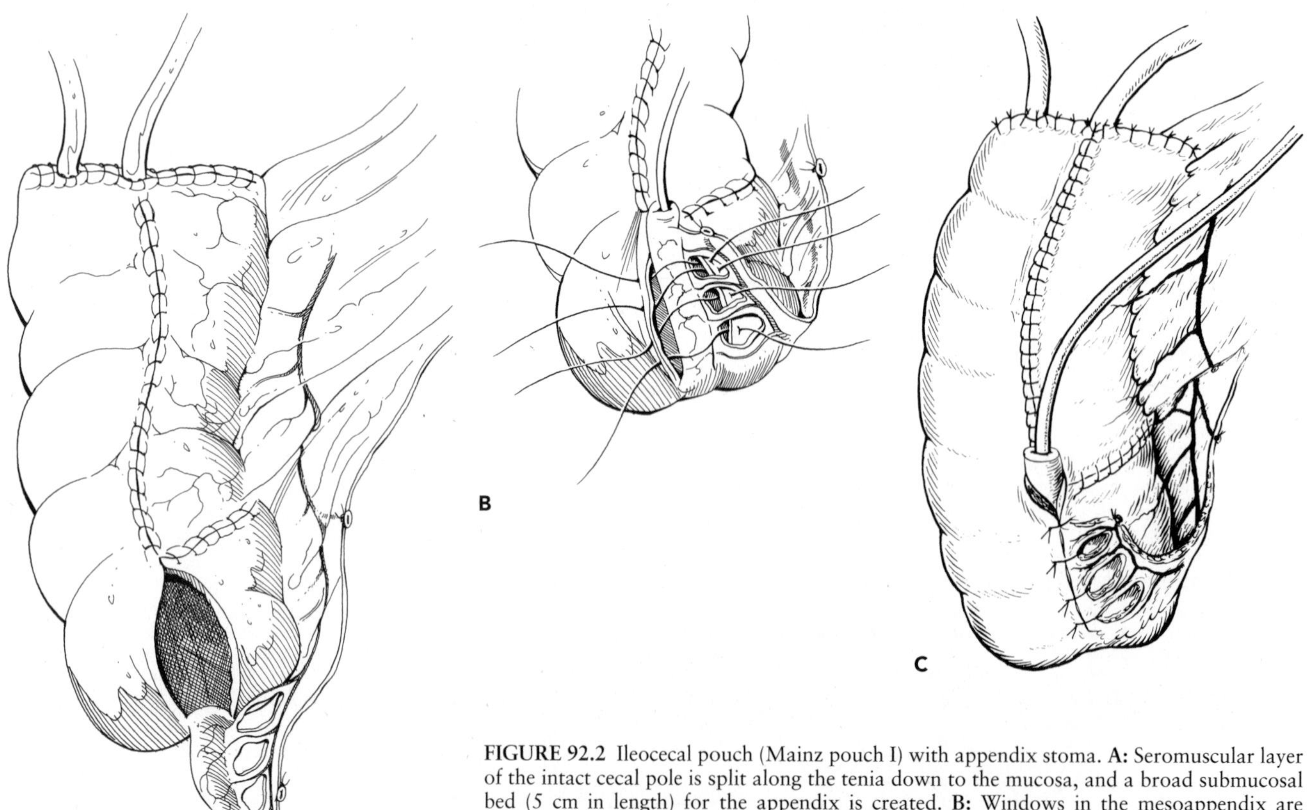


FIGURE 92.2 Ileocecal pouch (Mainz pouch I) with appendix stoma. **A:** Seromuscular layer of the intact cecal pole is split along the tenia down to the mucosa, and a broad submucosal bed (5 cm in length) for the appendix is created. **B:** Windows in the mesoappendix are excised between the branches of the appendicular artery without compromising the blood supply. **C:** After the appendix is correctly positioned, the seromuscular layer is closed over the embedded in situ appendix. (From Thieme Stuttgart, New York, with permission.)

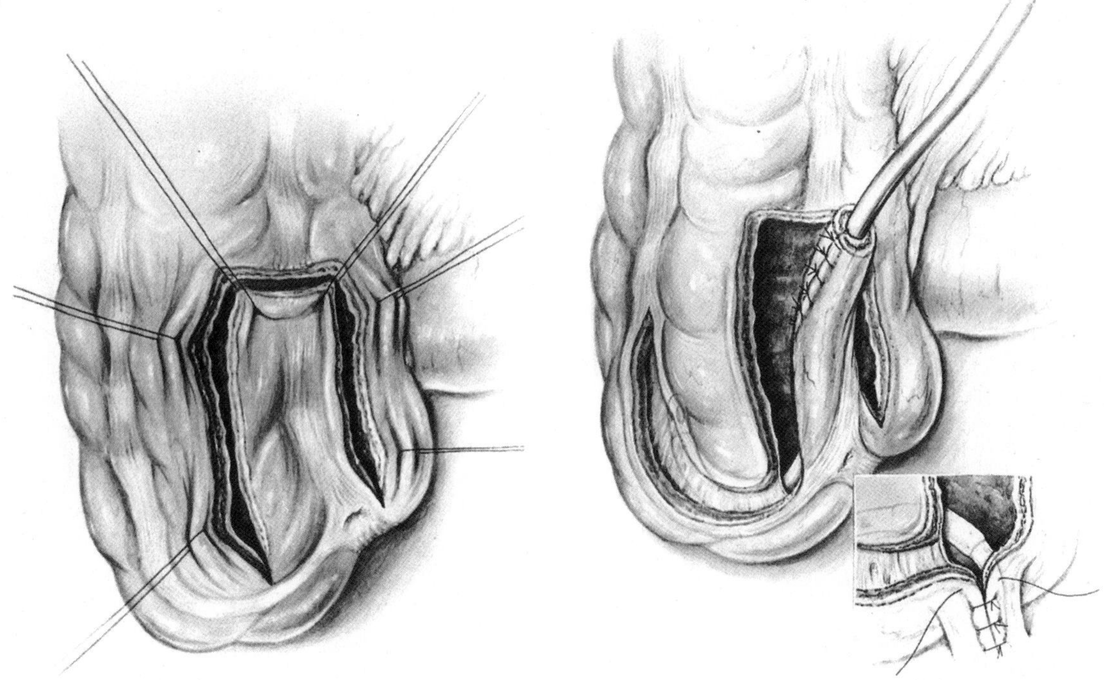


FIGURE 92.3 Full-thickness bowel flap tube. **A:** U-shaped incision (3 × 6 cm) of all layers of bowel wall, resulting in pedicled bowel flap at lower pole of cecum. **B:** Tubularization of pedicled flap over 18Fr Foley catheter and incision of seromuscularis of tenia omentalis (5 cm) for submucosal embedding, starting at pedicle of bowel flap tube. (From Thieme Stuttgart, New York, with permission.)

## Right Colon Pouches with Intussuscepted or Tapered Terminal Ileum

Several other authors use the ileocecal region in continent cutaneous urinary diversion. In contrast to the Mainz technique, they employ the ileum for construction of the continence mechanism but not for creation of the reservoir itself. Other colon pouches using nipple valve configuration for the continence mechanism include modifications from many other centers and differ from one another by only a few features, predominantly related to the technique employed for stabilizing the nipple valve. For example, in the "Tiflis" technique, the continence mechanism is created by tapering and submucosally embedding the terminal ileum (Fig. 92.7) (2).

## Indiana Pouch

Between 25 and 30 cm of cecum and ascending colon and 8 to 10 cm of terminal ileum are isolated (10). The entire colonic segment will be detubularized by incising it along its antimesenteric surface. If an appendix is present, it is removed at this time. Reconfiguration of the opened bowel segment by folding the cephalad end down to the apex of the antimesenteric incision allows the creation of a spheric reservoir (Fig. 92.8A). For construction of the efferent limb and continence mechanism, metal staples are applied sequentially to narrow the efferent limb over a 12Fr straight catheter (Fig. 92.8B). Any excess antimesenteric ileum is then removed. The last row of staples is placed at an angle to prevent stapling into the wall of the cecum. After narrowing the efferent limb, the ileocecal valve area is plicated with five to seven Lembert stitches of 3-0 silk suture (Fig. 92.8C). Care is taken to avoid having the sutures enter the lumen of the bowel. Each Lembert suture is progressively wider than the last. This has the effect of narrowing the ileocecal valve by wrapping cecal wall over the angled staple line. The tightness of the plication sutures is tested by passing an 18Fr catheter through the efferent limb. Once the efferent limb and continence mechanism have been completed and a Malecot catheter has been placed as a cecostomy tube in the dependent portion of the cecum, the reservoir is closed. Both ureters are led in such a manner as to allow alignment with a tenia. A tenial incision is made for each ureter. The ureter is cut obliquely or spatulated, and the site for the ureteral orifice is created by incising the bowel mucosa. The ureteromucosal anastomosis is performed with interrupted sutures of 5-0 synthetic absorbable monofile material. The tenia is reapproximated over the ureter with a nonabsorbable 5-0 suture.

## Colon Pouch (Mainz Pouch III)

Between 15 and 17 cm of transverse colon and either ascending [transverse-ascending pouch (TAP)] or descending colon [transverse-descending pouch (TDP)] (Fig. 92.9A) are required to create a pouch of adequate capacity (350 to 400 mL). Complete mobilization of the right or left colic flexure should be performed to gain adequate colon length for the pouch. The greater omentum is dissected from the transverse colon from right to left in the TAP and vice versa in the TDP. The bowel segment is detubularized antimesenterically, leaving 5 to 6 cm of the oral or aboral end intact for construction of the efferent limb. The terminal segment is tapered over a

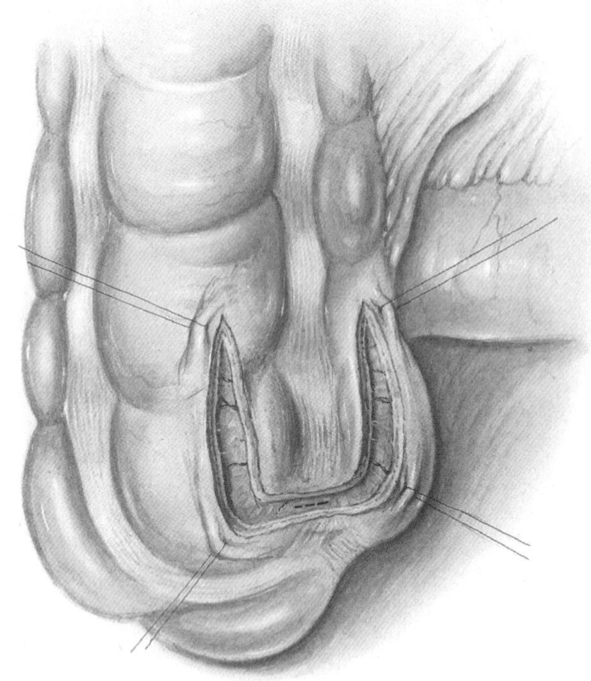


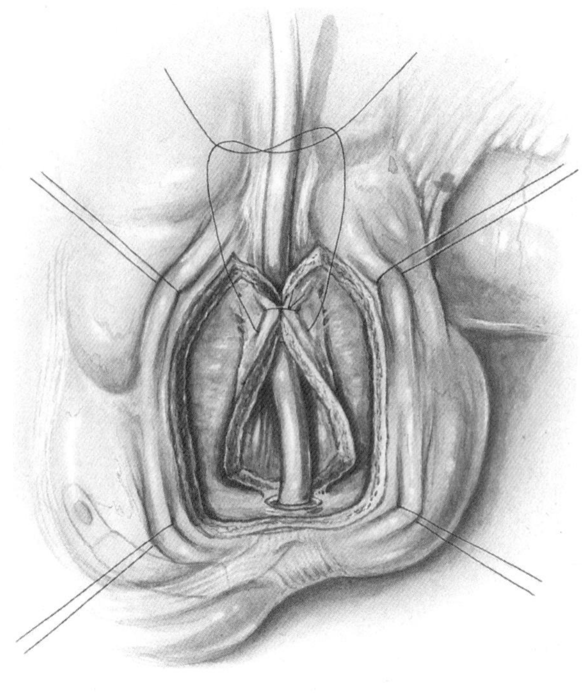


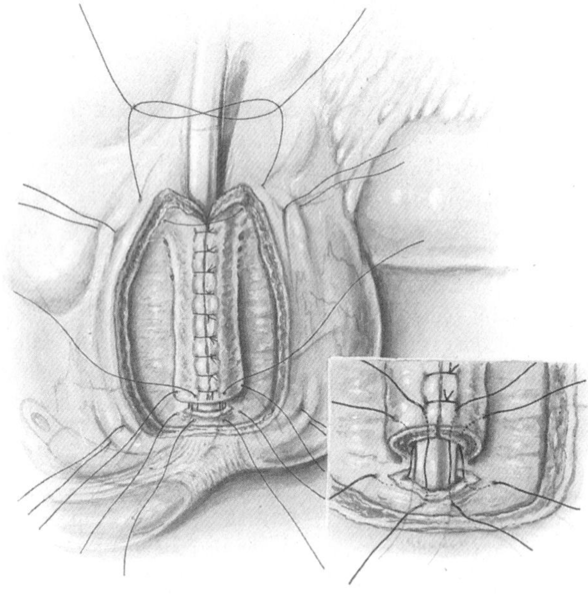


**FIGURE 92.4** Seromuscular bowel flap tube. **A:** U-shaped incision (3 × 5 cm) of seromuscular layer at lower pole of cecum and transverse incision of mucosa (0.5 cm) at the oral end of flap for insertion of 18Fr Foley catheter into lumen of reservoir. **B:** Tubularization of seromuscular bowel flap over 18Fr Foley catheter. **C:** Suturing of anterior circumference of seromuscular tube to margin of mucosa *(inset)*. (From Thieme Stuttgart, New York, with permission.)

18Fr silicone catheter, thus creating a neoappendix (Fig. 92.9B). The mucosa is sewn with polyglycol suture and the seromuscular layer with a nonabsorbable running suture. Easy insertion of the catheter is important, as a shrinkage of approximately 30% has to be allowed for. After the pouch plate is created, antirefluxing ureterointestinal implantation according to Goodwin is performed on both sides of the suture line (Fig. 92.9C). For refluxing ureteral implantation, about 1 cm$^2$ of the bowel mucosa is excised and the seromuscular layer is incised in the shape of a cross. After anchor sutures at the 5 and 7 o'clock positions are placed, a watertight anastomosis with 5-0 Monocryl sutures is performed. Ureteral stents and a 10Fr pouchostomy are led through the abdominal wall at separate sites.

The pouch is closed and the efferent segment is established. Windows are dissected in the mesentery of the tapered colon between the vessels. The efferent limb is then placed in the suture line, and the seromuscular layer of the anterior wall is approximated through the windows in the mesentery (Fig. 92.9D). Our favorite technique comprises isolation of a short segment of jejunum or ileum, which is tapered over a 18Fr Foley catheter and embedded submucosally after incising the tenia of a tubularized portion of the colonic segment. Sutures are led through windows in the ileal mesentery (Fig. 92.10).

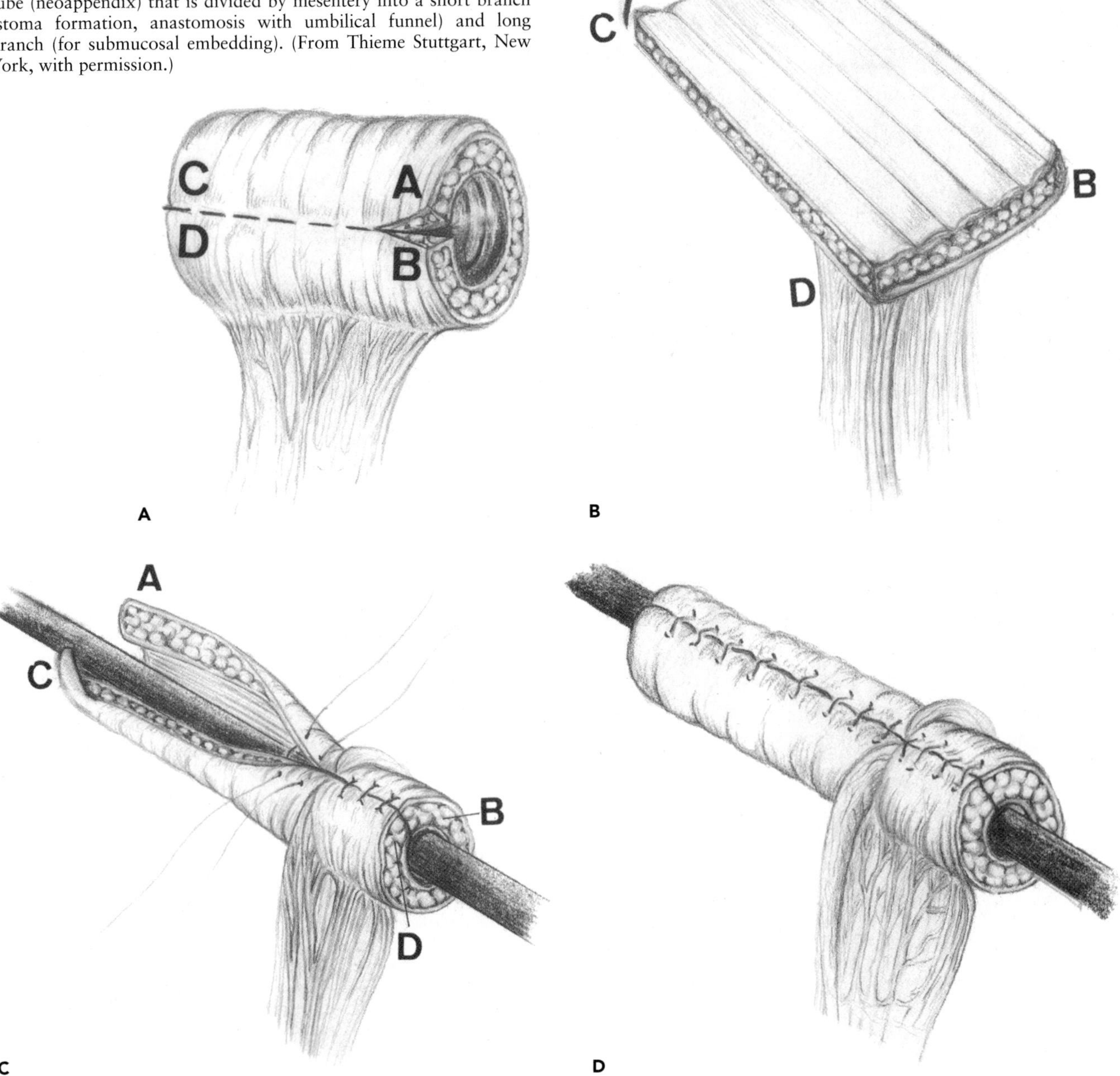


FIGURE 92.5 Yang-Monti technique. **A:** An ileal segment 2.0 to 2.5 cm long is excised and opened longitudinally about 1 cm from mesentery. **B:** The resulting pedicled rectangle (2 × 6 to 7 cm). **C:** Retubularization in transverse direction using interrupted sutures (4-0 chromic catgut or 5-0 polydioxanone), resulting in a small-caliber tube (neoappendix) that is divided by mesentery into a short branch (stoma formation, anastomosis with umbilical funnel) and long branch (for submucosal embedding). (From Thieme Stuttgart, New York, with permission.)

The umbilicointestinal anastomosis is performed in the same fashion as in the ileocecal pouch. Finally, the reservoir is attached to the abdominal wall. The greater omentum is used to cover pouch and bowel. Ureteric stents are removed after 10 to 14 days. Clean intermittent catheterization is started 3 weeks postoperatively (11).

## COMPLICATIONS

While continence using the appendix, once established, is durable with late-onset failure of 1% to 2% at about 4 years, stomal stenosis is seen in between 8% to 28% of patients, depending on the length of follow-up. Although stenosis represents a minor technical problem, the subsequent inability to insert the catheter is a distressing complication with potentially serious consequences in patients in whom the Mitrofanoff channel is the only route of evacuation. In these cases the reservoir must be immediately emptied percutaneously, which is facilitated by fixation of the pouch to the abdominal wall.

Skin stenosis may be dilated, incised, or repaired by open surgery, carefully removing fibrotic tissue. According to our experience, dilatation alone seldom produces a lasting improvement. We therefore tend to intervene early. Although revisions are usually successful, prevention of

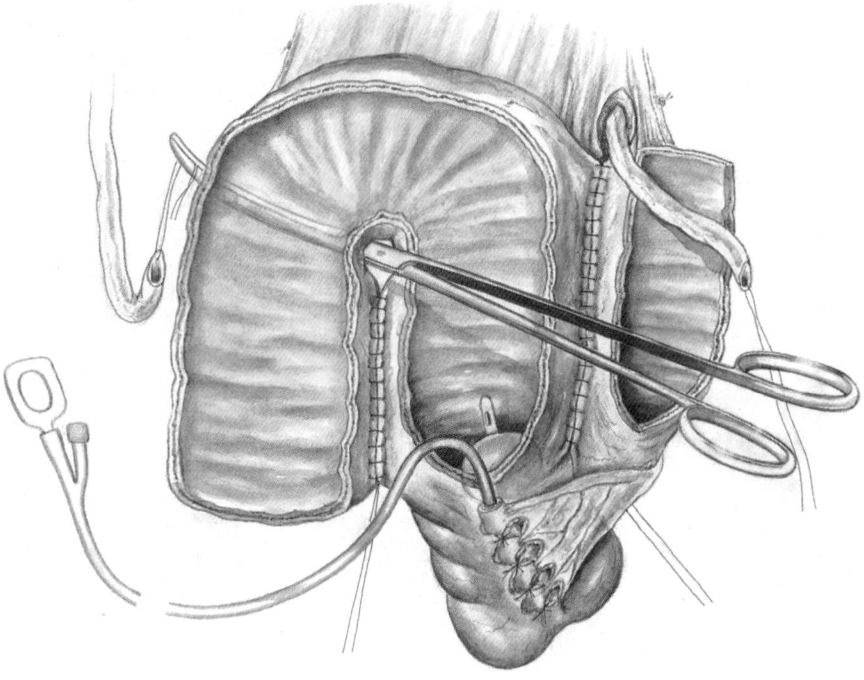

A

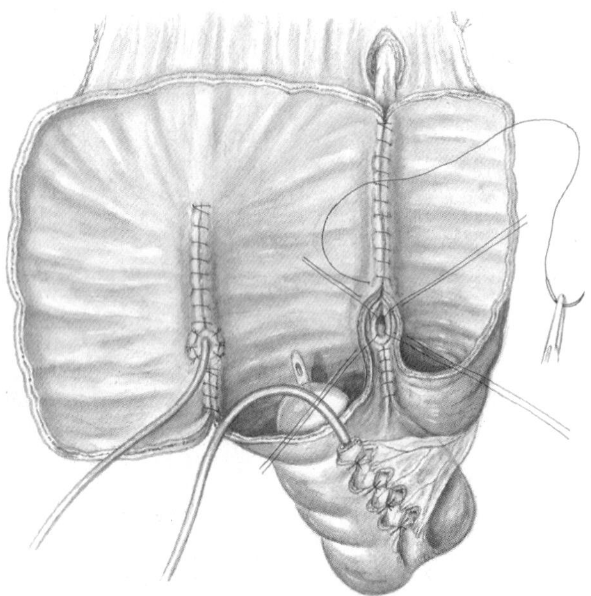

B

**FIGURE 92.6** Ileocecal pouch (Mainz pouch I) with serous-lined implantation of ureters. **A:** In contrast to the original technique, the pouch plate is not created by anastomosing the edges of detubularized bowel segments, but by creating two serous-lined extramural troughs. **B:** The ureters are placed into the serous-lined tunnels and covered by approximating the margins of the detubularization. (From Thieme Stuttgart, New York, with permission.)

stenosis is desirable. Stomal stenosis can be avoided by incorporation of a V-shaped flap of umbilical funnel into the spatulated appendix. To prevent recurrence, we have developed a cone-shaped metal dilator. Its effective length was designed to cover only the known critical segment of the channel. Directly before inserting the catheter for evacuation of the reservoir, the stoma is gently dilated for a few minutes once or twice daily. A similar effect might be produced by occasionally leaving the catheter in the pouch at night.

Metabolic complications are due to either reduction of the absorptive bowel capacity through functional loss of those segments required for reservoir construction or the highly unphysiologic exposure of the reconfigured bowel to urine. Factors that affect solute absorption include the size and segment of bowel used, the time of retention of urine, the concentration of the solutes in the urine, renal function, and the pH and osmolality of the fluid (3).

The most common consequence of intestinal urinary diversion is metabolic acidosis. Depending on definition, diagnostic modality, reservoir characteristics, renal function, and length of follow-up, it has been reported in 20% to 100% of patients after ureterosigmoidostomy, bladder substitution, and continent diversion using ileal and/or colonic segments. There is no proven effect on either bone absorption or childhood growth and development.

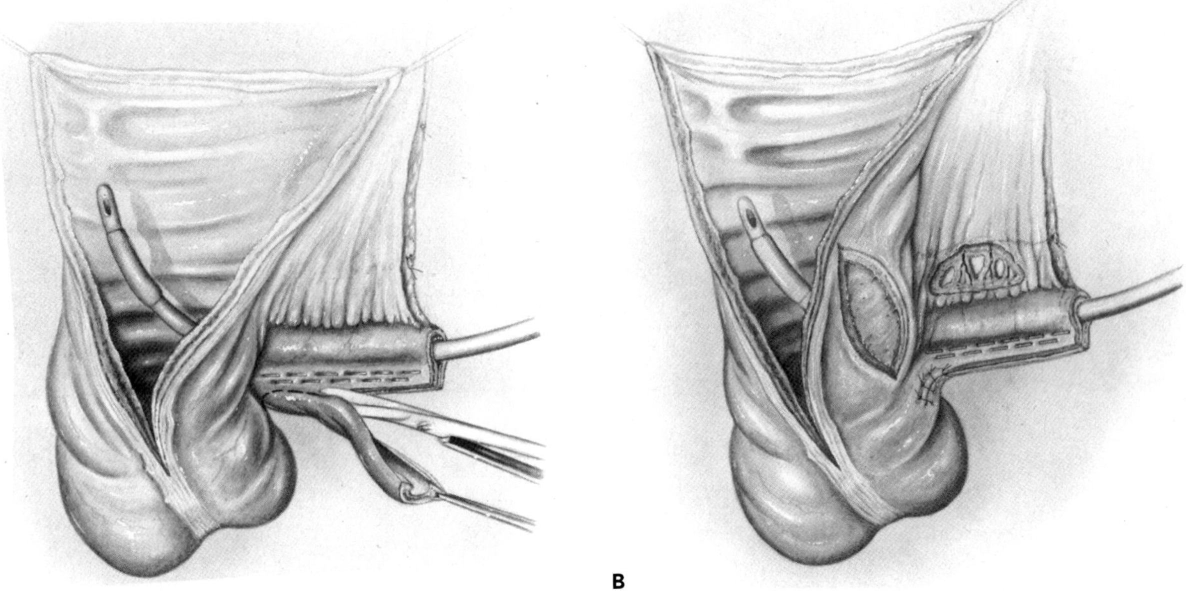


FIGURE 92.7 Tiflis pouch. **A:** Tapering of terminal ileum over a 18Fr Foley catheter with removal of excessive bowel wall. **B:** Incision of seromuscular layers of the cecum adjacent to the terminal ileum in preparation for submucosal embedding. (From Thieme Stuttgart, New York, with permission.)

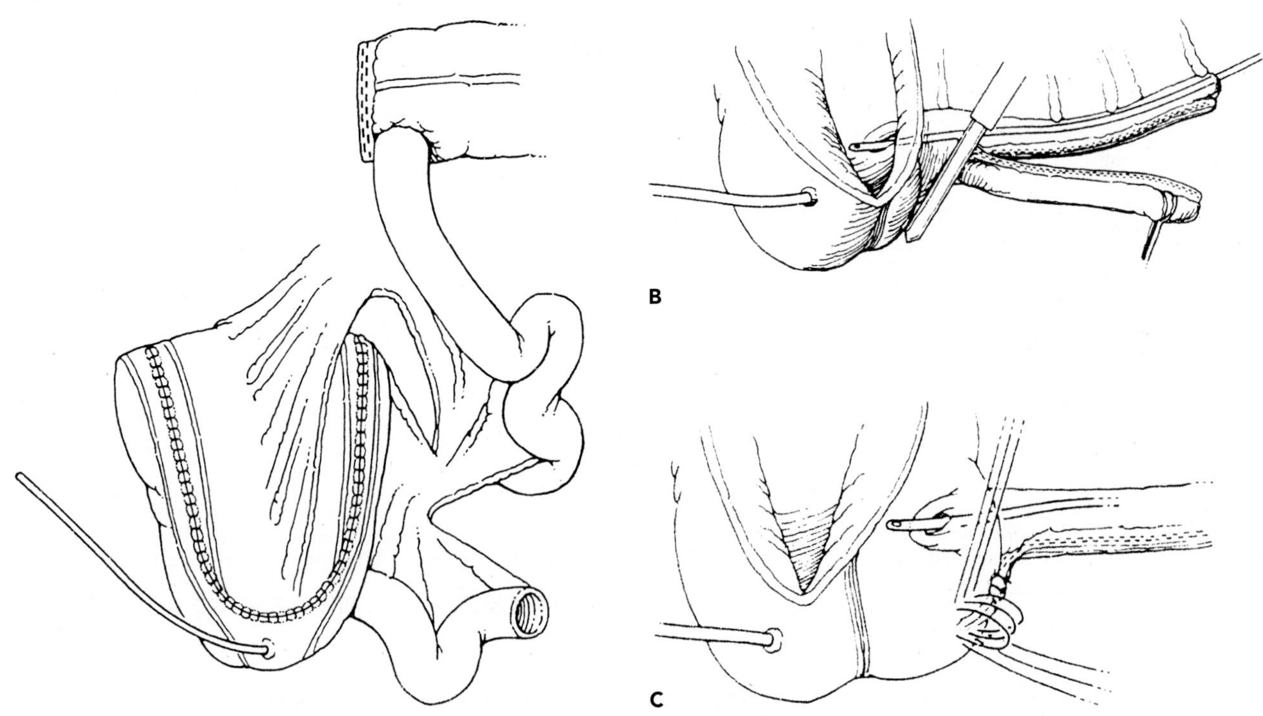


FIGURE 92.8 Indiana pouch. **A:** The cephalad end of the detubularized right colon segment is folded caudally to the apex of the antimesenteric incision. A Malecot catheter is placed in the dependent portion of the cecum prior to closing the reservoir. **B:** A stapler is used to trim away the excess bowel wall of the ileal segment (tapering). **C:** A total of five to seven Lembert sutures are placed to plicate the ileocecal valve.

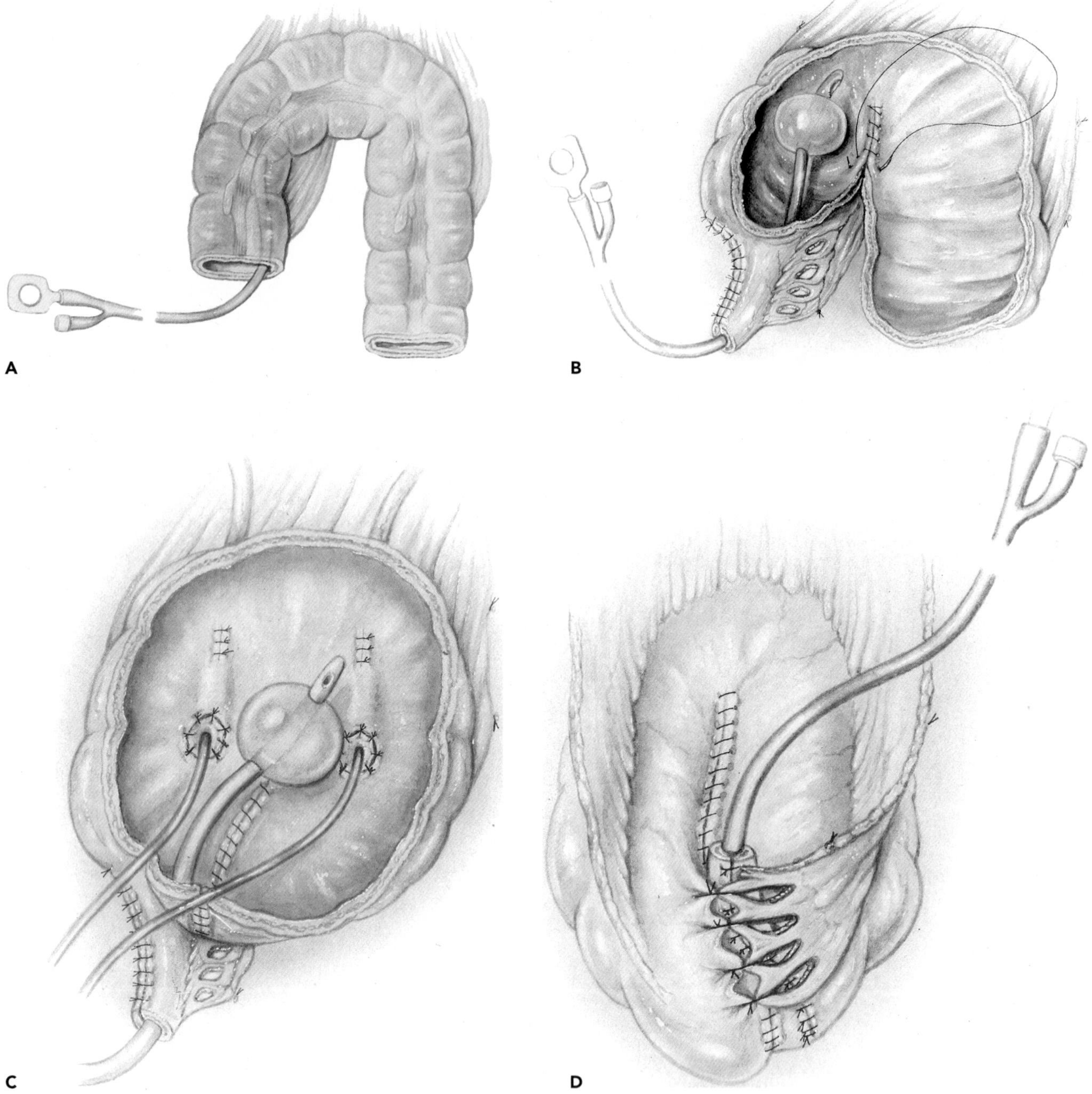


FIGURE 92.9 Colon pouch (Mainz pouch III) with tapered colon as efferent limb. **A:** About 15 to 17 cm of nonirradiated large bowel is isolated for reservoir creation. The oral end with a Foley catheter is used for construction of the efferent limb. **B:** The colonic segment is detubularized and the pouch plate is formed. The oral end is tapered over an 18Fr Foley catheter and windows are made in the mesentery. **C:** The ureters are attached to the posterior pouch wall through a submucosal tunnel. **D:** Pouch formation is completed by closing the anterior wall. The efferent segment is embedded serosa-to-serosa by sutures led through mesenteric windows. (From Thieme Stuttgart, New York, with permission.)

Intestinal urinary reservoirs have an increased propensity to form urinary calculi, predominantly in the lower tract, that tend to recur with an increasing incidence over time. Risk factors include the presence of foreign material (e.g., staples), recurrent and chronic infection, the composition of the urine, mucus production, urinary stasis, and noncompliance with irrigation and catheterization regimes.

Spontaneous rupture or perforation during catheterization has been reported after bladder augmentation, after orthotopic ileal and ileocolonic bladder replacement, and in continent cutaneous reservoirs 4 weeks to >5 years after surgery.

Hypovitaminosis is a well-studied sequela of bowel resection, particularly of vitamin B12, in which patients may develop irreversible neurologic disease following an unrecognized deficiency. Substitution of vitamin B12 is simple and even less expensive than regular analysis. Empirical supplementation should therefore be considered.

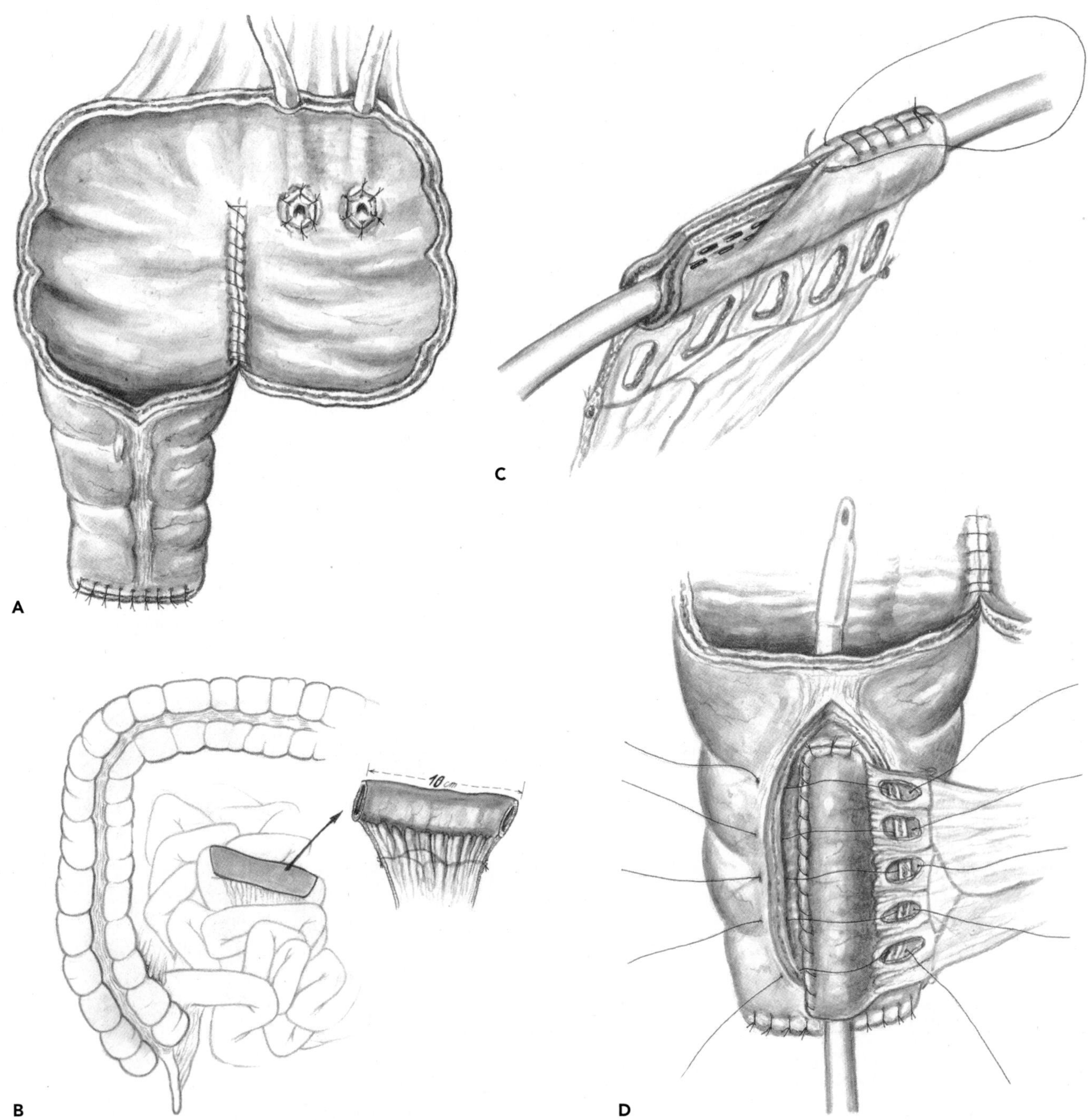


FIGURE 92.10 Colon pouch (Mainz pouch III) with tapered small bowel as efferent limb. **A:** The oral end of the large bowel segment is closed and left intact. **B:** A 10-cm jejunal or ileal segment is isolated with careful preservation of its mesenteric pedicle. **C:** The ileal segment is tapered over an 18Fr Foley catheter, trimming away the excess bowel wall. The tube is formed using a running suture. Windows are created in between the vasculature of the mesentery. **D:** Submucosal embedding of tapered ileum after incision of seromuscular layer of the tenia of the intact colonic segment. Sutures are led through mesenteric windows. (From Thieme Stuttgart, New York, with permission.)

## OUTCOMES

Between 1985 and 2005, a continent cutaneous ileocecal reservoir was created in 977 patients in two high-volume tertiary referral centers (Departments of Urology, Johannes-Gutenberg-University Medical School at Mainz, Bavarian Julius-Maximilians-University Medical School at Würzburg, Germany) (12), reflecting the learning curves of numerous surgeons. The mean age of the patients at the time of surgery was 47.8 years. The most common indication for urinary diversion was bladder replacement after anterior exenteration for pelvic malignancies (69.9%), followed by morphologic or functional bladder loss due to various benign conditions. Mean follow-up was 91.1 months (4.3 to 220.2 months). The vast majority of ureterointestinal anastomoses were performed using a submucosal tunnel [1,470 renal units (RU)]. In 419 patients, the in situ appendix could be embedded submucosally to form a Mitrofanoff type of continence mechanism (43%), while an intussuscepted ileal nipple valve was established in 491 patients (50%). In 56 patients the outlet was created by using other techniques (Figs. 92.3, 92.4, 92.5). Stoma stenosis was the most frequent outlet-related complication, affecting 161 out of 839 patients (19.2%). A reintervention was necessary in 93 of 396 patients (23.5%) with appendix stoma and in 68 of 443 patients (15.3%) with an intussuscepted ileal nipple. While stoma-related complications in patients with appendix stoma could be treated successfully by minor outpatient procedures in the vast majority of cases, management of nipple complications more often required open revision such as refixation of the nipple in the ileocecal valve or at the fascia. Creation of a new outlet became necessary because of ischemic outlet degeneration in 11 patients, including 8 with an appendix stoma and 3 with a nipple valve.

Continence was reported in 96% of the patients with an appendix stoma and in 89.5% of patients with a nipple valve.

Calculus formation was observed in 22 out of 396 patients (5.6%) with an appendix stoma and in 48 out of 443 patients (10.8%) with an intussuscepted ileal nipple.

Ureteral complications are mostly due to anastomotic stricture. Of 1,422 renal units with ureterointestinal reimplantation by submucosal tunnel, 93 (6.5%) developed obstruction at the anastomotic site. Of those, 74 renal units were reimplanted by open surgical revision, and 7 renal units were treated endoscopically by balloon dilatation, incision with the cold knife, or ureteral stent implantation. Eleven renal units had to be removed because of renal deterioration.

In 17 patients with an absent or dysfunctional lower urinary tract, a continent urinary reservoir was created in preparation for renal transplantation (9). In a recent update, follow-up ranged from 3 months to 15 years after kidney transplantation, with serum creatinine values documented between 0.9 and 2.0 mg per dL.

## *References*


1. Abol-Enein H, Ghoneim MA. A novel uretero-ileal reimplantation technique: the serous lined extramural tunnel. A preliminary report. *J Urol* 1994;151:1193–1197.
2. Chanturaia Z, Pertia A, Managadze G, et al. Right colonic reservoir with submucosally embedded tapered ileum: "Tiflis pouch." *Urol Int* 1997;59: 113–118.
3. Gerharz EW, Turner WH, Kälble T, et al. Metabolic and functional consequences of urinary reconstruction with bowel. *BJU Int* 2003;91:143–149.
4. Gerharz EW. Is there any evidence that one continent diversion is any better than any other or than ileal conduit? *Curr Opin Urol* 2007;17: 402–407.
5. Lampel A, Hohenfellner M, Schultz-Lampel D, et al. In situ tunneled bowel flap tubes: 2 new techniques of a continent outlet for Mainz pouch cutaneous diversion. *J Urol* 1995;153:308–315.
6. Mitrofanoff P. Cystostomie continente transappendiculaire dans le traitement des ves-sies neurologiques. *Chir Pediatr (Paris)* 1980;21:297–305.
7. Monti PR, Lara RC, Dutra MA, et al. New techniques for construction of efferent conduits based on the Mitrofanoff principle. *Urology* 1997;49: 112–115.
8. Riedmiller H, Bürger R, Müller S, et al. Continent appendix stoma: a modification of the Mainz pouch technique. *J Urol* 1990;143:1115–1116.
9. Riedmiller H, Gerharz EW, Köhl U, et al. Continent urinary diversion in preparation for renal transplantation: a staged approach. *Transplantation* 2000;70:1713–1717.
10. Rowland RG. Right colon reservoir using a plicated tapered ileal outlet. In: Webster GD, Goldwasser B, eds. *Urinary diversion,* 1st ed. Oxford: Isis Medical Media, 1995:229–235.
11. Stolzenburg JU, Schwalenberg T, Liatsikos EN, et al. Colon pouch (Mainz III) for continent urinary diversion. *BJU Int* 2007;99:1473–1477.
12. Wiesner C, Bonfig R, Stein R, et al. Continent cutaneous urinary diversion: long-term followup of >800 patients with ileocecal reservoirs. *World J Urol* 2006;24:315–318.


# CHAPTER 93 ■ URETEROSIGMOIDOSTOMY: MAINZ POUCH II

MARGIT FISCH, RUDOLF HOHENFELLNER, JÖRG SCHEDE, AND JOACHIM W. THÜROFF

Since the introduction of internal urinary diversion 140 years ago by Simon (11), >60 modifications of ureterosigmoidostomy have been published. It remained the method of choice for urinary diversion until the late 1950s, when electrolyte imbalance and secondary malignancies arising at the ureteral implantation site were described. However, with increased follow-up, secondary malignancies were later reported in all other forms of urinary diversion using bowel (2). The development of new absorbable suture material, modern ureteric stents, antibiotics, and alkalinizing drugs has solved many of the traditional shortcomings of ureterosigmoidostomy and has rekindled the interest in this technique.

At this time continence became a more important issue. Frequency and urgency were often observed, and nighttime incontinence was reported to be high (7,10). Urodynamic investigations showed that bowel contractions with a pressure rise in the bowel/reservoir are responsible for the incontinence (7,10). By interrupting the circular contractions (antimesenteric opening of the bowel and reconfiguration), a low-pressure reservoir can be created, thus improving continence rates and protecting the upper urinary tract. The era of low-pressure anal reservoirs began.

Kock was the first to apply these principles to ureterosigmoidostomy: By an antimesenteric opening of the rectosigmoid and augmentation by an ileal patch, a low-pressure reservoir was created (10). To avoid metabolic disorders, a valve mechanism cranial to the augmentation was formed by invagination of the sigmoid colon. A temporary colostomy was needed to protect the invagination, and the advantage of the low-pressure reservoir was, however, tempered by the complexity of the operative procedure. Reports on similar techniques of augmenting the sigmoid segment with either ileal or ileocecal segments followed.

At the Mainz Medical School, a more simple but equally effective operative procedure for the creation of a low-pressure rectal reservoir was developed, in which the sigmoid-rectal pouch was based on Kocher's description in 1903 (5,6). Although the standard technique describes ureteral implantation into the sigmoid-rectal pouch, the submucous tunnel represents an excellent implantation technique for normal undilated ureters with a low risk of stenosis or reflux. It is, however, associated with an increased complication rate when dilated or thick-walled ureters are present. For these ureters the serosa-lined extramural tunnel as published by Abol-Enein and Ghoneim represents an alternative (1). The technique was first described for the ileal neobladder but is also applicable for the sigmoid-rectal pouch. More recently, modifications of the original technique have been described with good results. With the increased interest in minimally invasive procedures, the technique of the sigmoid-rectal pouch, as with radical cystectomy and urinary diversion, can be completely performed endoscopically (12). The bladder specimen can even be removed transanally through the opened rectosigmoid during pouch creation, thus avoiding an additional incision. Today the techniques of low-pressure anal reservoirs have completely replaced classic ureterosigmoidostomy.

## DIAGNOSIS

The anal sphincter function can be checked by a *water tap enema* (perianal instillation of 200 to 300 mL saline, which the patients should keep for at least 3 hours) and a *rectodynamic investigation* (no incontinence during measurement; anal sphincter profile: resting closure pressure >60 cm $H_2O$, closure pressure under stress >100 cm $H_2O$). The upper tract should be normal as proven by renal ultrasound and intravenous urography or renal function study. An enema with water-soluble contrast medium should be performed to exclude any rectal or sigmoidal anomalies.

## INDICATIONS FOR SURGERY

The sigmoid-rectal pouch is suitable for primary urinary diversion, revision of ureterosigmoidostomy, and conversion of incontinent diversion. The procedure is indicated in patients with functional or actual loss of the urinary bladder. Our main indications are urinary diversion in patients with bladder exstrophy and incontinent epispadias or after radical cystectomy for bladder cancer. The sigmoid-rectal pouch also has been used for treatment of complex ureterovaginal and vesicovaginal fistula. It presents an excellent method of urinary diversion, especially for countries in which catheters or any stoma appliances are difficult to obtain. A competent anal sphincter is a prerequisite for the sigmoid-rectal pouch, as it is for ureterosigmoidostomy. There should be no renal insufficiency (creatinine maximum 1.5 mg per dL) or liver dysfunction.

Contraindications are an incompetent anal sphincter, irradiation of the pelvis, diverticulosis of the sigmoid colon, polyposis, liver dysfunction, and a serum creatinine >1.5 mg/dL.

## ALTERNATIVE THERAPY

Alternatives to the sigmoid-rectal pouch are any other forms of urinary diversion, including bladder substitution, continent cutaneous urinary diversion, and conduit diversion.

## SURGICAL TECHNIQUE

For bowel preparation, oral administration of 4 to 7 L Fordtan solution can be used on the day before the operation (alternatively, 8 to 10 L of Ringer lactate solution via a gastric tube). Metronidazole in combination with a cephalosporin (alternatively, piperacillin sodium) and an aminoglycoside is given at the beginning of surgery. A gastric tube or gastrostomy and a rectal tube are placed. For parenteral nutrition a central venous catheter has to be inserted.

### Classical Ureterosigmoidostomy

After a median laparotomy, the peritoneum is incised lateral to the descending colon and the left ureter is identified. A peritoneal incision is made on the contralateral side lateral to the ascending colon and the right ureter identified. Both ureters are dissected, respecting the longitudinal vessels running inside the Waldeyer sheet. The dissection is extended caudally to the ureterovesical junction. The ureters are cut as distal as possible, and stay sutures are placed at the 6 o'clock position. The ureteral stumps are ligated.

The colon is slightly elevated at the rectosigmoid junction by four stay sutures. After opening of the sigmoid colon over a length of 4 cm by an incision of anterior teniae, four mucosal stay sutures are placed in the mucosa of the posterior aspect of the sigmoid (Fig. 93.1). The bowel mucosa is incised between

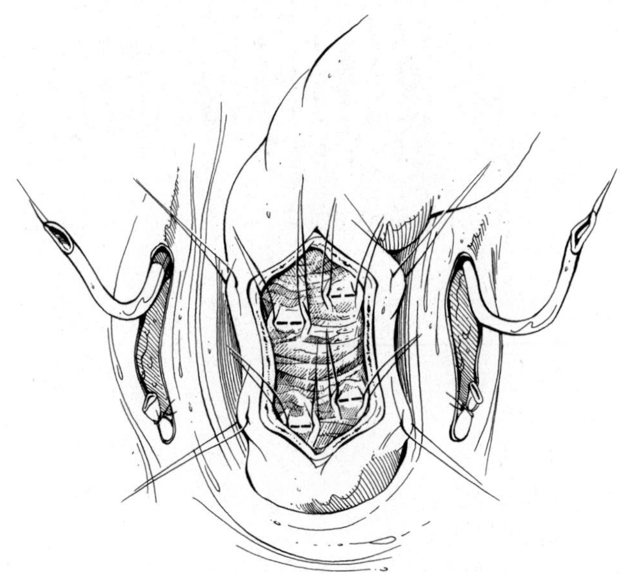

FIGURE 93.1 Open transcolonic ureterosigmoidostomy: Both ureters have been cut at its entrance into the bladder and mobilized. The sites of the planned ureteral implantations in the posterior sigmoid wall are outlined by stay sutures.

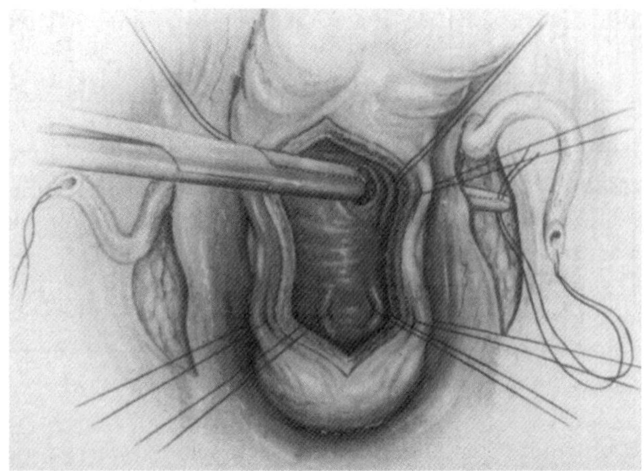

FIGURE 93.2 After incision of the mucosa and a buttonhole type of excision of the posterior bowel wall site, the ureter is to be brought through the intestinal wall; a subperitoneal tunnel is modeled bluntly from this point to the left incision in the peritoneum. The curved clamp is advanced precisely below the peritoneum

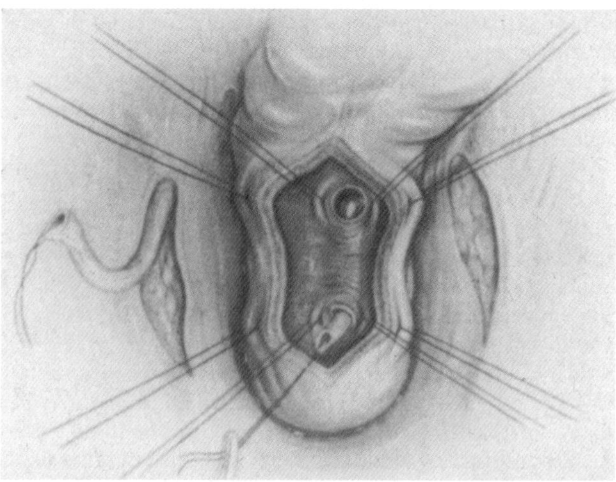

FIGURE 93.3 The ureter has been pulled into the bowel and through a submucous tunnel reaching from the proximal to the distal stay sutures.

the proximal stay sutures, and a buttonhole type of excision of posterior bowel wall is performed. A straight or slightly curved clamp is advanced through the opening, and a tunnel is created by blunt dissection below the visceral peritoneum of the mesosigmoid (Fig. 93.2). The ureter is pulled into the lumen of the intestine. After creation of a submucosal tunnel of about 3 cm in length, the ureter is threaded through this tunnel, avoiding torsion of the ureter (Fig. 93.3). The anterior wall of the ureter is spatulated for a length of 1 cm. For the ureterointestinal anastomosis, an anchor suture is placed at the 6 o'clock position grasping intestinal mucosa and musculature (5-0 polyglactin), and the anastomosis is completed by several ureteromucosal single stitches (6-0 polyglactin). A 6Fr silastic stent is inserted into the ureter and fixed to the mucosa by a polyglactin 4-0 suture (Fig. 93.4). The contralateral ureter is implanted about 3 cm lateral and either proximal or distal to the first anastomosis using the same technique (Fig. 93.5). The ureteral stents are inserted into the rectal tube

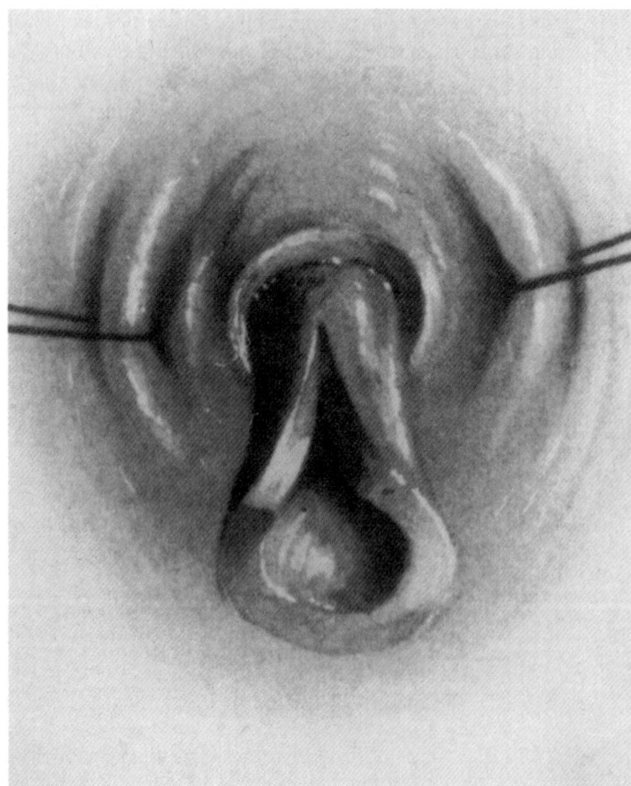



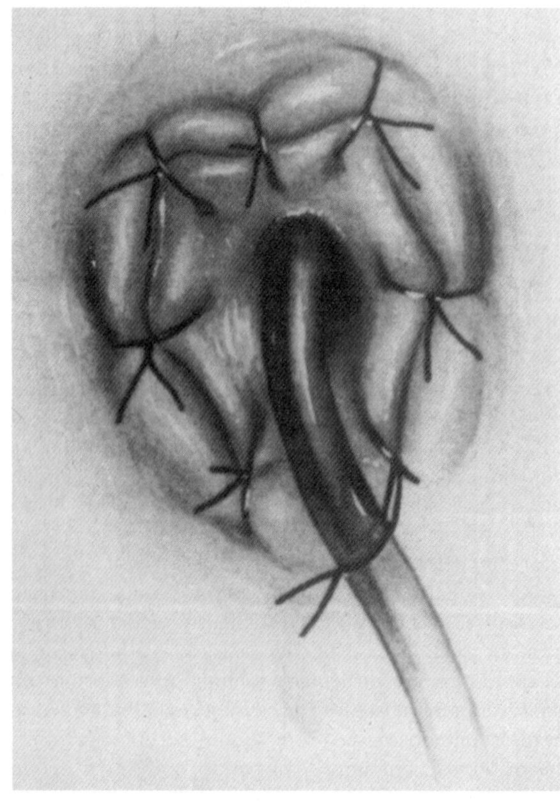



FIGURE 93.4 Spatulation of the anterior wall of the ureter (A) and ureteromucosal anastomosis between ureter and intestinal wall. The ureter is stented (B).

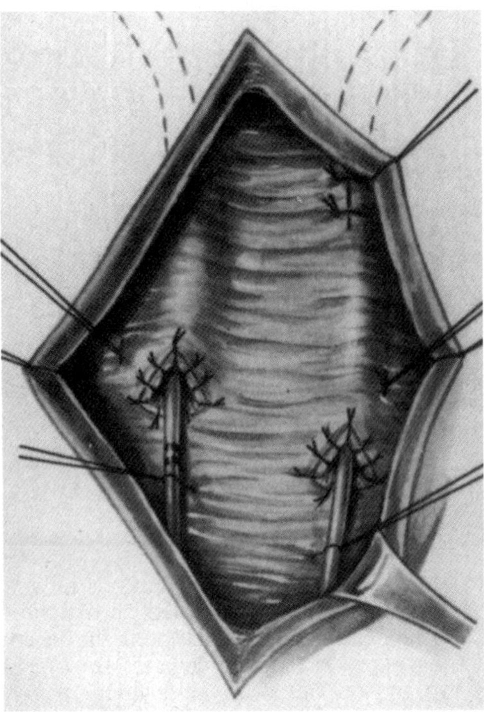

FIGURE 93.5 Identical implantation of the right ureter 3 cm lateral and proximal or distal of the first anastomosis.

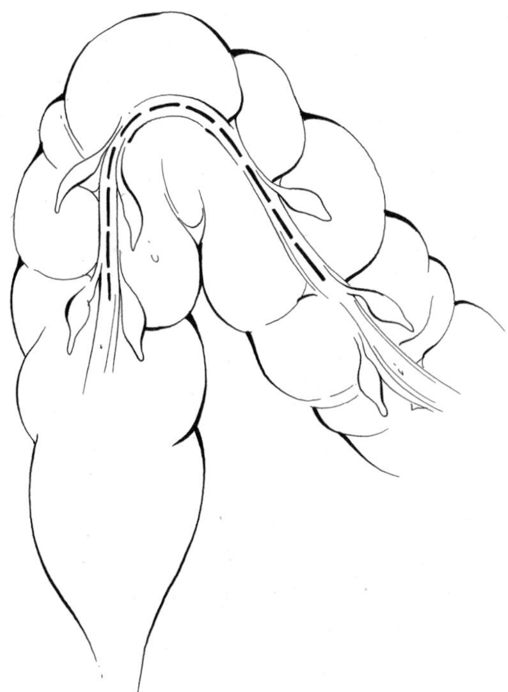

FIGURE 93.6 Identification of the rectosigmoid junction.

and pulled out through the anus. Thereafter, the rectal tube is reinserted.

The anterior sigmoid colon is closed in one layer using interrupted sutures of 4-0 polyglactin or in two layers using running sutures (5-0 polyglactin for the mucosa and 4-0 polyglactin for the seromuscularis). The peritoneal incisions are closed. At the end of the operation separate fixations of the rectal tube and ureteral stents to the skin of the anus are performed (nonabsorbable material).

## Sigmoid-Rectal Pouch (Mainz Pouch II)

Access is gained by a median laparotomy as for ureterosigmoidostomy. The rectosigmoid junction is identified and two stay sutures are placed. The peritoneum is incised lateral to the descending colon and the left ureter is identified. Another peritoneal incision is made lateral to the ascending colon and the right ureter is identified. Both ureters are dissected down to the ureterovesical junction, respecting the longitudinal vessels running inside the Waldeyer sheet. The ureters are cut as distal as possible, stay sutures are placed at the 6 o'clock position, and the ureteral stumps are ligated.

For creation of the pouch, the intestine is opened at the anterior tenia starting from the rectosigmoid junction over a total length of 20 to 24 cm distal and proximal of this point (Fig. 93.6). By placing two stay sutures in the middle of the incision at the right side of the opened rectosigmoid, the intestine is positioned in a shape of an inverted U. The posterior wall of the pouch is closed by side-to-side anastomosis of the medial margins of the U using two-layer running sutures of 4-0 polyglactin for the seromuscular layer and 5-0 polyglactin for the mucosa (Fig. 93.7).

The left ureter is pulled through retromesenterically above the inferior mesenteric artery from the left to the right side (Fig. 93.8). For ureteral implantation, four mucosal stay sutures are placed parallel right and left to the medial running suture. The mucosa is incised, and the seromuscular layer is excised between the two cranial stay sutures to create a wide buttonhole type of opening as an entrance of the ureter into

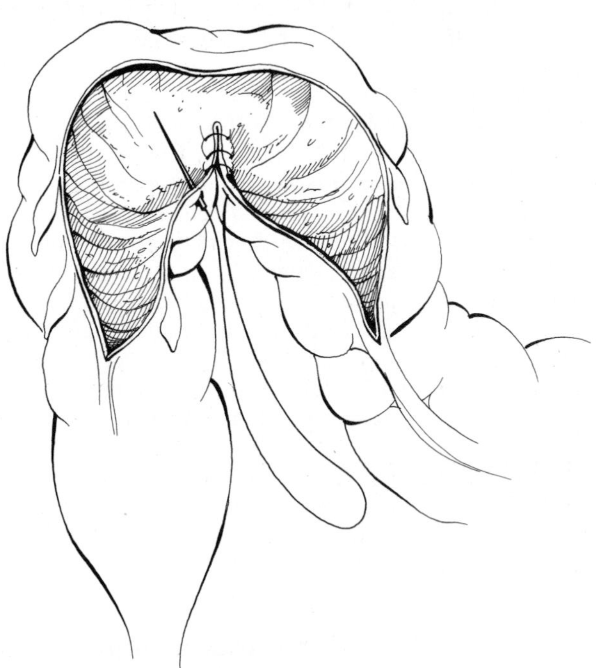

FIGURE 93.7 Opening of the rectosigmoid at the anterior tenia starting from the rectosigmoid junction over a total length of 20 to 24 cm distal and proximal of this point. Side-to-side anastomosis of the medial margins of the cut bowel edges by two-layer closure using running sutures of absorbable synthetic suture material (4-0 for the seromuscular layer and 5-0 for the mucosa).

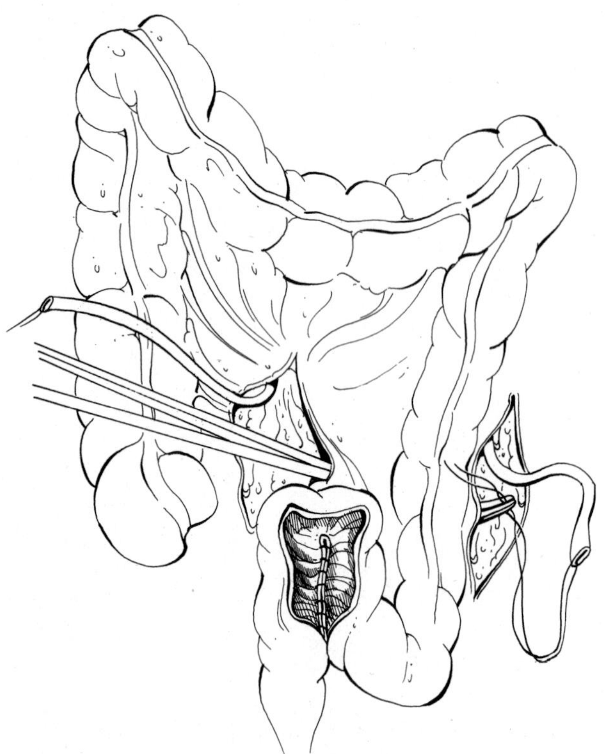

FIGURE 93.8 The left ureter is pulled through retromesenterically to the right side.

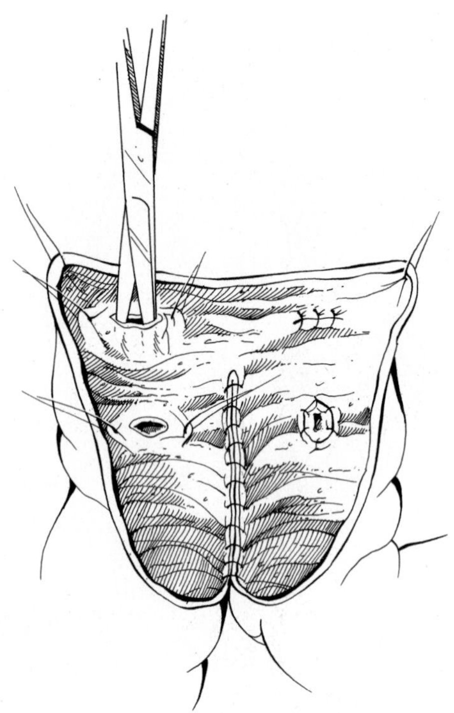

FIGURE 93.9 The left ureter is pulled through retromesenterically to the right side.

the pouch. The dissection of the submucous tunnel starts from this incision downward over a length of 2.0 to 2.5 cm. The mucosa is incised at the distal end of the tunnel and the ureter is pulled into the tunnel. After having resected the ureter to an adequate length, implantation is completed by placing an anchor suture at the 6 o'clock position (5-0 polyglactin) and several interrupted ureteromucosal sutures (6-0 polyglactin). The cranial mucosal incision is closed by a running suture with polyglactin 4-0, which has a short reabsorption time. The contralateral ureter is implanted in the same manner (Fig. 93.9). Next, 6Fr ureteral stents are inserted into the ureters and are pulled out through the anus with the rectal tube, which is afterwards reinserted. The pouch is fixed to the anterior longitudinal band at the sacral promontory in the region of the proximal end of the posterior medial running sutures by two Bassini sutures of 3-0 nonabsorbable suture material (Fig. 93.10). Closure of the anterior pouch wall is performed in two-layer sutures (5-0 polyglactin for the seromuscular and 4-0 polyglactin for the mucosal layer). Alternatively, single-layer closure using interrupted stitches can be used (Fig. 93.11). The peritoneal incisions are closed and the anastomotic site of the pouch is covered by omentum. The rectal tube and the ureteral stents are separately fixed to the skin of the anus (nonabsorbable material).

## Serosa-Lined Extramural Tunnel Ureteral Implantation

Mobilization of the bowel includes the left colonic flexure (in cases of a short sigmoid segment). Dissection of the ureters is identical to the standard technique (Fig. 93.12). An S-shaped sigmoid segment is outlined by stay sutures, with each limb of 10- to 12-cm length, resulting in a total length of 30 to 36 cm (Fig. 93.13). After antimesenteric opening of the S-shaped sigmoid colon (Fig. 93.14) in the area of the anterior tenia, a

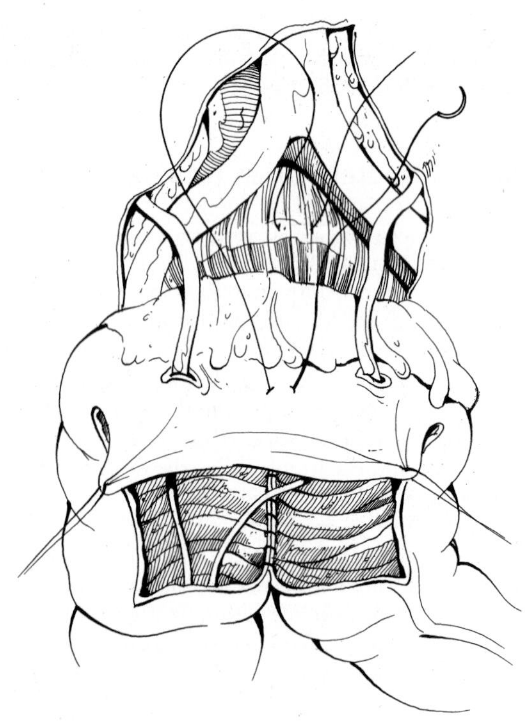

FIGURE 93.10 After a 6Fr stent is inserted in each ureter, which are pulled out through the anus with the rectal tube, the pouch is fixed to the anterior longitudinal band of the spine in the region of the proximal end of the posterior medial running sutures by two Bassini sutures.

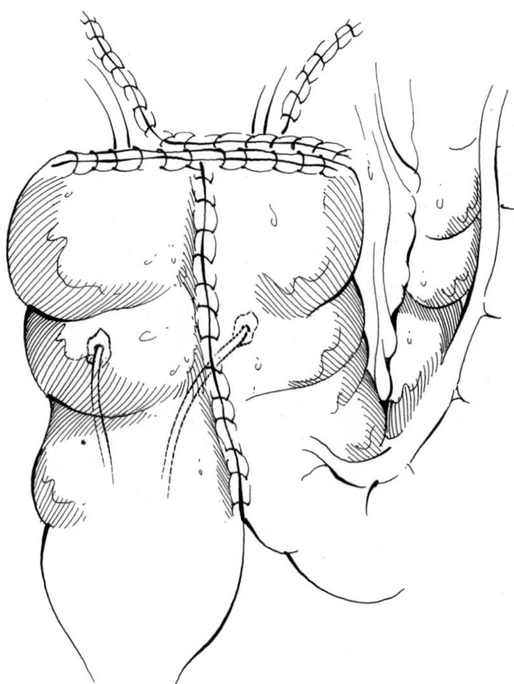

FIGURE 93.11 Closure of the anterior pouch wall by seromuscular single stitches with 4-0 absorbable synthetic suture material. Closure of the peritoneal incisions.

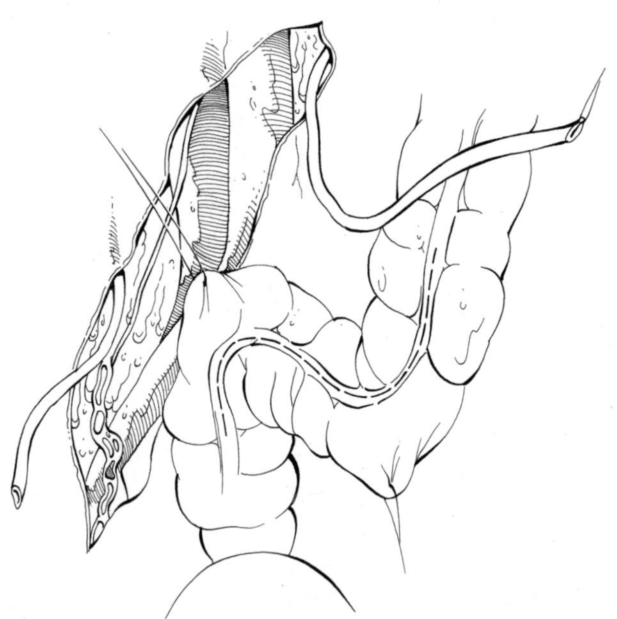

FIGURE 93.12 Right and left paracolonic incision; identification and dissection of the ureters.

side-to-side adaptation of the seromuscularis of both limbs is obtained by single-stitch sutures close to the mesentery (nonabsorbable suture), thereby creating two serosa-lined channels. On the right side an entrance for the right ureter is left at the cranial aspect of the running suture. The mesentery cranial to the left running suture is incised and the left ureter pulled through. The ureters are placed in their respective channels (Fig. 93.15), and the cut edges of the bowel are sutured above

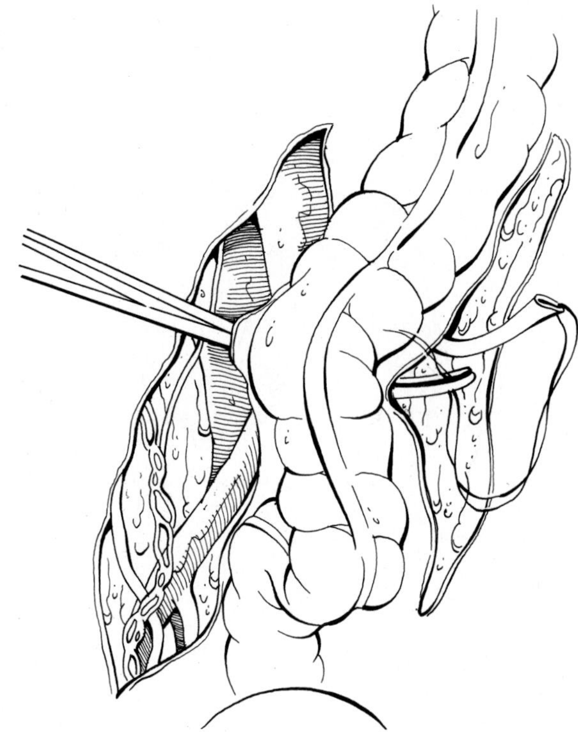

FIGURE 93.13 S-shaped sigmoid segment is outlined by stay sutures. The length of each segment is 10 to 12 cm, starting at the rectosigmoid junction (standard technique), adding another segment of 10 to 12 cm of ascending colon.

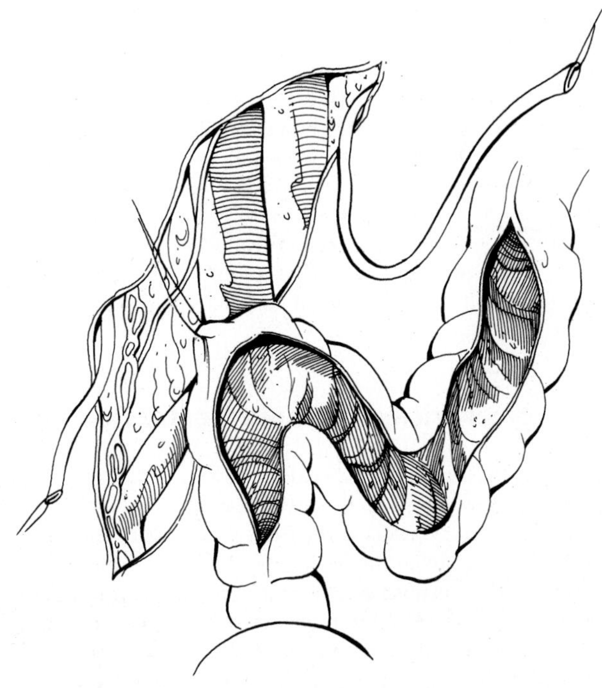

FIGURE 93.14 The marked segments are opened in the area of the anterior tenia. Excision of a mesenteric window for pull-through of the left ureter.

the ureter with a running suture incorporating all layers, thus converting the channel into a tunnel. The length of the tunnel should be four times the diameter of the ureter. For implantation, the ureter is cut at its required length and spatulated.

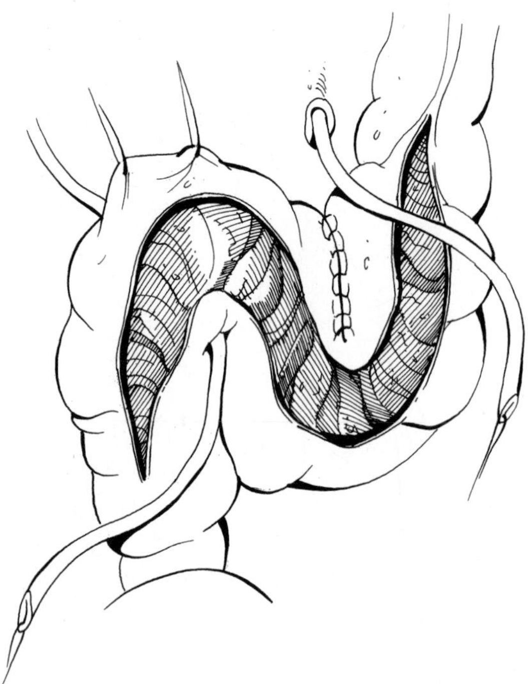

FIGURE 93.15 Side-to-side adaptation of the seromuscularis of the limbs of the S by two interrupted sutures close to the mesentery (4-0 nonabsorbable suture), thereby creating two serosa-lined channels. On the right side, an entrance for the right ureter is left at the cranial aspect of the running suture and the ureter is pulled through. One ureter is placed in each channel created between the segments of the S.

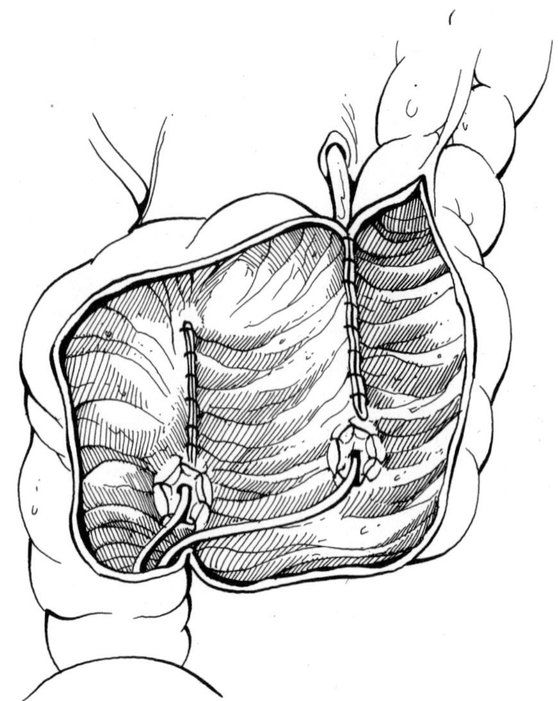

FIGURE 93.16 Ureteral implantation in the area of the continuous suture line. Insertion of ureteral stents.

Four anchor sutures are placed at the 11 and 1 o'clock and the 5 and 7 o'clock positions through all layers of the ureter as well as all layers of the bowel wall (4-0 polyglactin). Ureteromucosal sutures are placed in between the anchor sutures to complete the anastomosis (5-0 polyglactin) (Fig. 93.16). Two ureteral stents are inserted and pulled out through the anus with the rectal tube after having been fixed to the bowel mucosa (4-0 polyglactin). The anterior pouch wall is closed by interrupted seromuscular sutures (4-0 polyglactin) (Fig. 93.17).

## Surgical Tricks (Sigmoid-Rectal Pouch)

When the anastomosis reaches deep down to the rectum, it is easier to suture the pouch starting caudally, as the deepest point of the anastomosis is the most critical part and can be reached more easily at the beginning of the anastomosis.

To facilitate fixation of the pouch to the promontory, one sutured end of the dorsal running suture can be pulled through dorsally outside of the pouch and be tightened with the fixation suture placed in the anterior band at the promontory.

A Bassini needle facilitates placement of the fixation suture through the anterior band of the spine.

During ureteral implantation, sufficient spatulation of the ureters is of utmost importance to avoid a nipplelike protrusion of the ureters.

To drain an incidental hematoma of the submucous tunnel, the mucosa covering the tunnel can be selectively incised at different points.

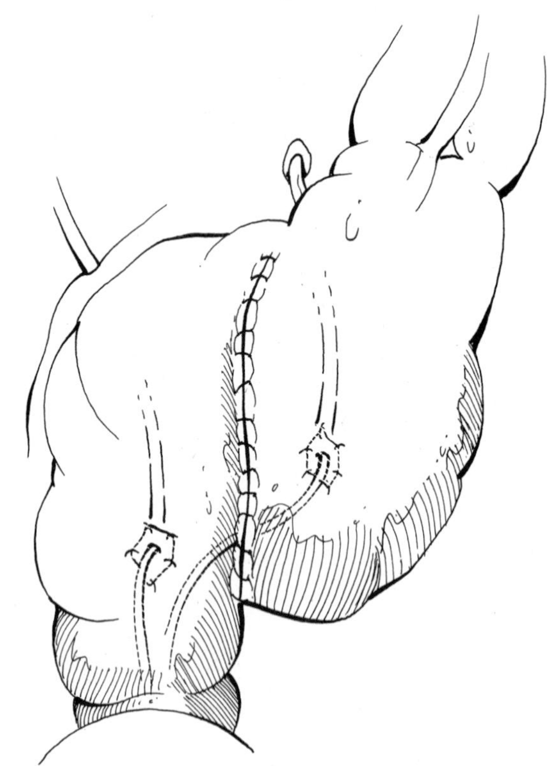

FIGURE 93.17 The stents are pulled through the anus and the pouch is closed.

The S-shaped sigmoid-rectal pouch as created for the ureteral implantation via a serosa-lined tunnel has an ideal and stable position within the pelvis; therefore, no fixation to the promontory is needed.

## OUTCOMES

Of utmost importance for the outcome is patient selection. A functioning anal sphincter is a prerequisite. Also important are technical details such as ureteral implantation, side-to-side anastomosis by two layers, and the fixation at the promontory (classical technique).

Between 1990 and 1999 a sigmoid-rectal pouch was performed in 123 patients (94 adults and 29 children). Mean age was 44 years (10 months to 73 years). Indications were malignancy ($n = 92$), bladder exstrophy and incontinent epispadias ($n = 26$), trauma ($n = 4$), and sinus urogenitalis ($n = 1$). A total of 102 of the 123 patients were followed, with a mean follow-up of 46.2 months (1 to 9 years). Eight patients died during follow-up due to their primary malignant tumor; another 2 died unrelated to the underlying disease. Eleven were lost to follow-up. Four early pouch-related complications were encountered: two dislodged ureteral stents requiring temporary nephrostomy and one ileus treated by operative intervention. One patient developed severe complications as a result of anastomotic leakage from a pouch fistula requiring revision and colostomy. Stenosis at the ureteral implantation site was the most common complication (7%, or 14 renal units). Eleven renal units required surgical reimplantation. During follow-up, pyelonephritis was observed in 3% of patients. Ninety-nine of the 102 patients were completely continent postoperatively; nighttime continence was 95%. The majority of the patients (70 out of 102, or 69%) used alkalinizing drugs to prevent metabolic acidosis.

Between 1991 and 2004 a total of 38 children with a mean age of 5 years underwent a Mainz pouch II procedure. Of these, 33 had bladder exstrophy or incontinent epispadias. In 14 children (37%) urinary diversion was performed after failed primary reconstruction. Thirty-five children could be followed, with a mean follow-up of 112 months (range 5 to 147). All children were continent during daytime, but 3 (8.6%) suffered from nighttime incontinence requiring pads. Six children (15.8%) had developed pyelonephritis, mostly with stenosis of the ureterointestinal anastomosis. Reimplantation of the ureter was required in 10 of 69 renal units (14.4%), in 10.1% due to stenosis, and in 4.3% due to reflux. Early alkali supplementation was initiated in 24 (69%). No secondary malignancies were observed during follow-up.

Concerning quality of life, the Mainz pouch II serves as a satisfying continent urinary diversion for both sexes. No statistically significant differences in functional and symptom scales or global health status were detected between males and females. All scales but diarrhea showed good results, and the outcome was comparable to health-related quality of life in a reference population (4).

## COMPLICATIONS

The main complication is stenosis at the ureterointestinal anastomosis. The incidence in our series was 7% in the whole collective and 10% in the children. Hadzi-Djokic et al. (8) reported a stenosis in 11 out of 220 patients. Hammouda (9) used the serosa-lined extramural tunnel as well as the submucosal tunnel for ureteral implantation in 95 patients and found reflux in 1.6% of renal units and stenosis in 5.3%. Balloon dilatation and endoscopic incision of the stenosis have been described to treat ureterointestinal anastomosis; however, we would recommend open revision with reimplantation.

Pyelonephritis is described in our series (3,8,9) with an incidence of 3.0% to 15.8% and should be treated with antibiotics. Only those patients with recurrent pyelonephritis and a decrease in split renal function require ureteral neoimplantation.

About two-thirds of patients will develop an acidosis with a negative base excess. Early correction (starting from a base excess of −2.5) with alkali supplementation is recommended to avoid further complications, especially in children. Incontinence is a rare complication but can be disastrous. In severe forms a conversion to another form of urinary diversion is required.

To discover secondary malignancies early, endoscopy is recommended starting from the fifth postoperative year.

## *References*


1. Abol-Enein H, Ghoneim MA. A novel uretero-ileal reimplantation technique: the serous lined extramural tunnel. A preliminary report. *J Urol* 1994;151(5):1193–1197.
2. Austen M, Kälble T. Secondary malignancies in different forms of urinary diversion using isolated gut. *J Urol* 2004;172(3):831–838.
3. Bastian PJ, Albers P, Hanitzsch H, et al. The modified ureterosigmoidostomy (Mainz pouch II) as continent form of urinary diversion. *Urologe A* 2004;43(8):982–988.
4. Bastian PJ, Albers P, Hanitzsch H, et al. Health-related quality-of-life following modified ureterosigmoidostomy (Mainz Pouch II) as continent urinary diversion. *Eur Urol* 2004;46(5):591–597.
5. Fisch M, Hohenfellner R. Der Sigma-Rektum Pouch: Eine Modifikation der Harnleiterdarmimplantation. *Akt Urol* 1991;I–IX.
6. Fisch M, Wammack R, Müller SC, et al. The Mainz pouch II (sigma rectum pouch). *J Urol* 1993;149(2):258–263.
7. Ghoneim MA, Shebab-El-Din AB, Ashamallah AK, et al. Evolution of the rectal bladder as a method for urinary diversion. *J Urol* 1981;126(6):737–740.
8. Hadzi-Djokic JB, Basic DT. A modified sigma-rectum pouch (Mainz pouch II) technique: analysis of outcomes and complications on 220 patients. *BJU Int* 2006;97(3):587–591.
9. Hammouda H, Shalaby M, Adelelateef A, et al. Mainz II and double folded rectosigmoid pouches. Experience with 95 patients. *J Surg Oncol* 2006;93(3):228–232.
10. Kock NG, Ghoneim MA, Lycke KG, et al. Urinary diversion to the augmented and valved rectum: preliminary results with a novel surgical procedure. *J Urol* 1988;140(6):1375–1379.
11. Simon J. Ectropia vesica (absence of the anterior walls of the bladder and pubic abdominal parieties); operation for directing the orifices of the ureters into the rectum; temporary success; subsequent death; autopsy. *Lancet* 1852;568.
12. Türk I, Deger S, Winkelmann B, et al. Complete laparoscopic approach for radical cystectomy and continent urinary diversion (sigma rectum pouch). *Tech Urol* 2001;7(1):2–6.

# CHAPTER 94 ■ PALLIATIVE URINARY DIVERSION

BURKHARD UBRIG AND STEPHAN ROTH

The word *palliative* derives from the Latin *palliare*, which means "to cover with a coat." The term *palliative therapy* implies the impossibility of cure. The main goal of palliative urinary diversion is the control or the prevention of symptoms caused by incurable diseases of the urinary tract, usually cancer. In addition to bladder and prostate cancer, advanced cervical, ovarian, breast, or colorectal cancer may interfere with the urinary tract.

Typical symptoms of locally progressive pelvic cancer with impairment of the urinary bladder include urgency, pelvic pain, pyocystis, recurrent gross hematuria, ileus, and fistulas (e.g., vesicovaginal, vesicorectal, cloacal) that may severely compromise quality of life. In a broader sense, palliative treatment for ureteral obstruction may also be considered in this chapter.

## DIAGNOSIS

Diagnosis of incurable pelvic cancer is based on the diagnosis of metastatic disease or local infiltration of adjacent pelvic structures and organs. Diagnostic studies may depend upon the underlying pathology. In general, the detection of distant and locoregional metastases will be achieved with common imaging procedures: computed tomography and/or magnetic resonance imaging and bone scan. Urethrocystoscopy, rectal digital examination, and bimanual palpation of the pelvis by the experienced pelvic surgeon aid in local staging of the primary tumor and reveal important information on resectability.

## INDICATIONS FOR SURGERY

There are no prospective studies that compare bladder-preserving strategy versus palliative cystectomy in locally advanced bladder cancer. However, the clinical course of patients with advanced muscle-infiltrating bladder cancer under a bladder-preserving strategy is often dismal. In a recent study, 24 patients with muscle-infiltrating bladder tumor (mean age 81 years) were treated with bladder preservation for a mean 22.6 months (7). All complained of frequency, urgency, and severe nocturia. The mean hospital readmission rate was eight times per patient. Salvage cystectomy was required in 11 of 24 cases, in 7 alone because of recurrent macrohematuria. Major complications that might have been prevented with early cystectomy were ileus in three cases and an enterovesical fistula in one. All patients in whom the bladder was preserved complained of severe symptoms that reduced the quality of life of their remaining life span (7).

Radical cystectomy with urinary diversion is nowadays a routine procedure with acceptable risk in many urologic departments. Recent reports have proven the feasibility of radical cystectomy with acceptable morbidity and mortality also in octogenarians (5). There is some evidence that radical cystectomy itself, if performed with minimal blood loss and in a time-efficient manner, does not decisively increase the morbidity of the palliative urinary diversion (8,11).

Therefore, in most palliative patients with acceptable surgical risk and good motivation for surgery, radical cystectomy with urinary diversion will be the most suitable option. Nevertheless, the decision will be made on an individual basis between the urologic surgeon and his or her patient. In some borderline cases the risk of the surgical approach is considered too high, either because of a poor general health condition (American Society of Anesthesiologists (ASA) score 3 and 4) or because the operation cannot be considered due to advanced age and limited life expectancy.

## ALTERNATIVE THERAPY

In most patients with locally advanced pelvic cancer, cystectomy or complete pelvic exenteration is the standard option. In a select group of patients with high surgical risk, frozen pelvis, and a short residual life expectancy, supravesical diversion without exenteration may be a viable option that results in good symptom control (12). Indications are infrequent, and results of this strategy have rarely been reported in the literature. Further alternatives to radical cystectomy with urinary diversion are observation, repeated transfusions, or indwelling catheters, depending upon the underlying disease process.

## SURGICAL TECHNIQUE AND OUTCOMES

Palliative urinary diversion will usually be performed with the lowest risk options that are acceptable to the patient. Continent orthotopic or cutaneous diversion will be considered if the patient is suitable and motivated. It may take 3 to 12 months before continence and an acceptable quality of life are attained (4). The presence of (completely resectable)

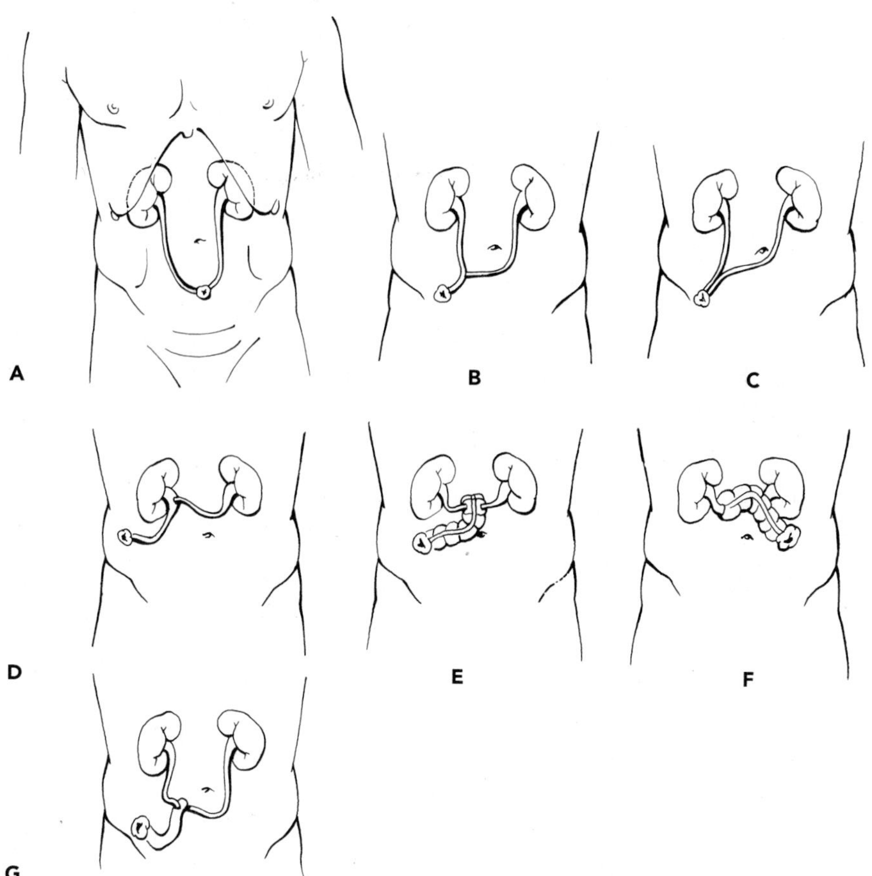


FIGURE 94.1 Supravesical urinary diversion. **A–D:** Cutaneous ureterostomy with (**A**) median or (**B**) lateral stoma, (**C**) transureteroureterostomy, and (**D**) pyeloureteral anastomosis. **E and F:** Transverse colon conduit, with (**F**) anastomosis to the pyelon; (**G**) ileal conduit.

nodal disease does not preclude the placement of an orthotopic bladder substitute (4). In general, conduits will often be preferred in palliative situations. Some patients for whom palliation is the goal may be very poor surgical candidates. Therefore, in these select cases, less elaborate techniques such as cutaneous ureterostomy or nephrostomy placement may also be considered.

## Ileal Conduit

Assuming adequate surgical risk and life expectancy, an ileal conduit is the first choice of many urologists in a palliative situation. Ostomy care is relatively easy, and patients may return to normal activity soon after discharge (Fig. 94.1). An ileal conduit should not be used in patients with short bowel syndrome or inflammatory small bowel disease and in those who have had high-dose radiation to the ileum. The small intestine and ureters are usually within the radiation portals for treatment of pelvic malignancy and may evidence long-term sequelae. Impaired healing of gut anastomosis and scarring with stricture formation of the ureterointestinal anastomosis may occur.

## Sigmoid Colon Conduit

The sigmoid colon is a viable alternative to ileum if the latter cannot be used for conduit construction (see above). However, it should not be used if diseased, if exposed to radiation, or if the internal iliac arteries have been ligated with the rectum still in place. This last condition might lead to rectal sloughing because of compromised rectal blood supply (10). The stoma will usually be placed in the lower left abdominal quadrant (Fig. 94.1).

## Transverse Colon Conduit

The transverse colon is not within the radiation portals commonly used for pelvic malignancies, such as cervical cancer. The blood supply via the middle colic artery is usually ample (10). Indications for the use of transverse colon for conduit construction may be marked radiation fibrosis of the ureters or impaired ureteral mobilization because of frozen pelvis or periureteral lymph nodes. The ureterointestinal anastomosis can be accomplished with very short ureteral stumps. Also, anastomosis with the renal pelvis is feasible (Fig. 94.1). The perioperative mortality rate has recently been reported at 3% (10).

## Bilateral Cutaneous Ureterostomy with Single Stoma

In patients for whom major gut surgery is not advisable, cutaneous ureterostomy is an alternative to transintestinal diversion (Fig. 94.1); operative time is short, and renal function is not a selection factor, while paralytic ileus rarely occurs. Construction of a single stoma in the lateral or midline position is generally feasible and ensures easy care with minimal patient discomfort. Occasionally, though, excessive obesity, extensive paraureteral lymph node involvement, or frozen pelvis makes construction of a single stoma impossible.

Stoma construction is of critical importance. Stomal stenosis rates of 50% and more have been reported (10). Distal spatulation of the ureteral end and plastic augmentation with a V-shaped skin flap as proposed by Rodeck should be considered (8). Stomal stenosis results mainly from ischemia of the distal ureteral end with consequent sloughing and fibrosis. Also, postoperative tension or hyperplastic epithelium at the ureterocutaneous anastomosis may play a role. Firm fixation of the anastomosis to the skin and healing by first intention are essential. The following different techniques have been proposed. Both ureters are guided to the skin and anastomosed with each other and the stomal skin (Fig. 94.1). This can be done by passing one ureter to the contralateral side through the retroperitoneum and behind the descending colon (8). Alternatively, in slender patients, the ureters may be mobilized completely extraperitoneally, led around the peritoneal sac, and conjoined in the midline. An infraumbilical stoma can then be formed (12).

### Transureteral Cutaneous Ureterostomy

One ureter is retroperitoneally led to the other side and anastomosed to the contralateral ureter end-to-side (e.g., with 5-0 Monocryl). This ureter will be guided through the abdominal wall and anastomosed to the skin.

### Transureteropyelocutaneous Ureterostomy

Alternatively, the collecting systems of both renal units have been connected with a high ureteral or pyeloureteral anastomosis (Fig. 94.1). Operative mortality was 1.75%; severe late complications occurred in 10.5%. The most frequent problems arose from the nephrostomy and from stenoses of the ureteropelvic or ureteral anastomosis (9).

### Percutaneous Nephrostomy

Percutaneous nephrostomy is another alternative for supravesical diversion. The advantages are the relative ease with which these can be placed under local anesthesia, but the drawbacks are the need for continuous replacement due to encrustation as well as the propensity for these to become dislodged. Bilateral nephrostomies are sometimes badly tolerated, and usually only the renal unit with better function should be diverted by nephrostomy.

To prevent further flow of urine downstream, additional occlusion of the ureter may sometimes be necessary. Transection and ligation of the ureter with nonabsorbable material may be performed. This may be accomplished by a small flank incision or laparoscopically. If feasible, a unilateral cutaneous ureterostomy may be the better alternative in such cases.

Several percutaneous techniques to obliterate the ureteral lumen have been proposed: butyl-2-cyanoacrylate, detachable balloons, liquid polyacrylonitrile, butyl-2-cyanoacrylate and lipiodol with adjuvant balloon catheter occlusion, electrocautery, and nylon and silicone occlusion devices. Some nephrostomy devices for transient closure of the ureteral lumen have been reported, including modified nephroureteral catheters and balloon occlusion devices. None of these methods has gained wide acceptance.

### Defunctionalization of the Contralateral Unit

If only one kidney is diverted and urine continues to flow downstream from the contralateral kidney, it may be necessary to defunctionalize the latter. Some palliative patients are poor candidates for nephrectomy. In a previously obstructed hydronephrotic kidney with significant parenchymal reduction, ligature and transection of the ureter will usually result in long-term success. Postinterventional paralytic ileus and some pain may be expected during the first postoperative days.

However, in unobstructed kidneys, ligature of the ureter should not be done because of significant pain and spontaneous ureteral recanalization. Usually renal arterial embolization will be considered. Excellent results to stop urine production from the kidney have been reported with transcatheter ablation with a mixture of ethanol and contrast agent and a combination of sponge and coil plugging of the proximal artery: Out of 20 patients, urinary flow ceased after 2 days in 18 patients; 2 required a second session. The authors propose epidural anesthesia, which may also be used in the first 2 postoperative days for pain control. Transient postinterventional paralytic ileus and fever may be expected (1).

## PALLIATIVE TREATMENT OF URETERAL OBSTRUCTION

Common causes of malignant compression of the ureterovesical junction and the prevesical ureter are bladder, prostate, and cervical cancers. Malignant obstruction of the mid- or upper ureter is usually caused by metastatic lymphatic spread as from metastatic breast cancer, lymphatic disease, colon cancer, and cancers of the female internal genitalia. However, even years after radiation therapy, newly arising ureteral obstruction may represent long-term sequelae of radiation and not tumor recurrence.

Indications for treatment should be considered very carefully. Septic episodes, with accompanying persistent pain, are rare in malignant ureteral obstruction if there has been no retrograde endoscopic manipulation. The insertion of a regular double-J stent or a nephrostomy will result in repeated consultations to change the catheters, sometimes under general anesthesia. Any measure carries the risk of infection or dislocation. Many patients are in critical condition, and quality of life should be the main treatment goal.

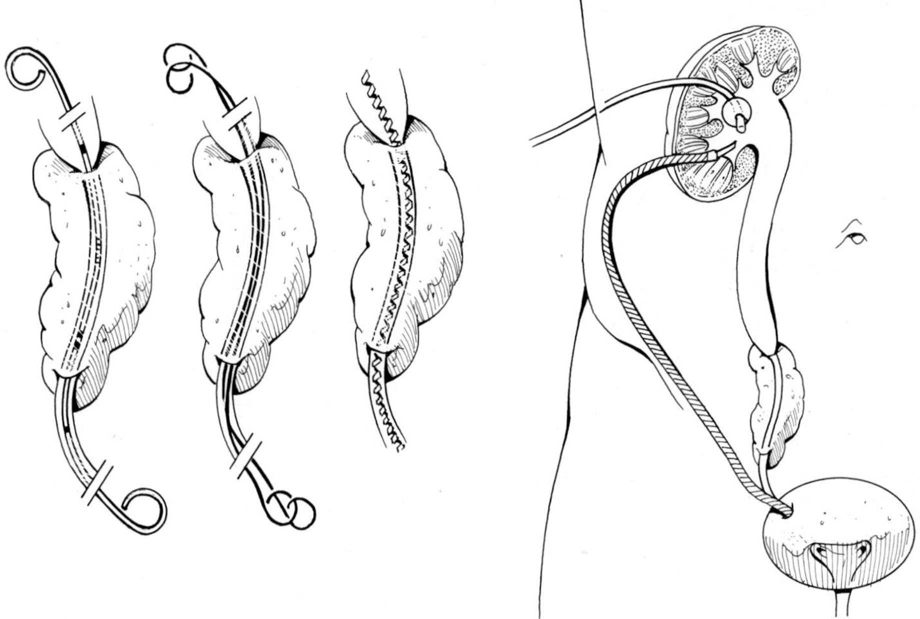

FIGURE 94.2 Endourologic techniques for treatment of malignant ureteric obstruction. A: Ureteral stent. B: Two parallel ureteral stents. C: Metal stent. D: Nephrostomy tube. E: Extra-anatomic prosthetic bypass.

In patients with unilateral ureteral obstruction and sufficient function of the contralateral kidney, one should generally abstain from therapy; however, if nephrotoxic chemotherapy is planned or life expectancy exceeds 1 to 2 years, intervention may be indicated. In patients with bilateral ureteral obstruction and impending renal failure, it is usually sufficient to stent, divert, or bypass only one renal unit (usually the one with better function). In some patients, however, it may be preferable to abstain from any treatment at all. The use of the below-mentioned techniques assumes normal bladder function. Otherwise, supravesical diversion may be discussed.

Retrograde stenting with replaceable double-J stents is often considered the first-line option for relieving ureteral obstruction (Fig. 94.2). Transurethral resection will sometimes be necessary to find the ureteral orifice or intramural ureter hidden in the tumor. In these situations prior antegrade placement of a guide wire or antegrade placement of the stent itself may be very useful. Specific drawbacks of double-J stents are irritative bladder symptoms, stent obstruction, and encrustation—necessitating repeated changes (intervals range from 6 weeks to 6 months, but can be much shorter) and stent migration.

Under conditions of extrinsic compression, hard polyurethane stents are recommended over soft silicone to ensure patency of the stent lumen. Specially developed "tumor stents" are available.

## Two Double-J Stents

Extensive compression from the tumor may lead to malfunction and obstruction of conventional double-J stents. Liu and Hrebinko (6) used two 4.7Fr double-J stents passed simultaneously over guide wires when drainage with a single ureteral stent had failed. The increased stiffness of two stents reduces kinking and luminal compression, and the potential space between the stents likely preserves flow around as well as through them (Fig. 94.2).

## Metallic Mesh Stents

Metallic mesh stents such as the Wallstent have been used with limited success. Epithelial hyperplasia and tumor ingrowth through the mesh have been reported to result in recurrent ureteral obstruction. These stents are virtually unremovable. An alternative might be nickel-titanium shape-memory alloy stents that occupy only the obstructed ureteral segment. These are soft and malleable at 10°C and regain their shape when reheated to 55°C. The tendency to form encrustations is apparently low (3).

## Extra-anatomic Pyelovesical Prosthetic Bypass

In 1992 Desgrandschamps and colleagues introduced their technique of pyelovesical bypass with a composite prosthesis (internal diameter, 18Fr; external diameter, 28.5Fr), and Jabbour et al. (2) reported long-term results with 35 prosthetic ureters in 27 patients, 22 with malignancies. Minor early and late complications were noted in 5 and 3 patients, respectively. No encrustations of the inner silicone lumen were noted, although asymptomatic bacteriuria sometimes was. The 5 surviving patients (4 with renal transplants, 1 with retroperitoneal fibrosis) were followed from 34 to 84 months (mean, 47 months), and the authors found no encrustation, kinking, or obstruction (2). Alternatively, single- or multiple-piece stents with small diameters (7Fr to 11Fr) have been used. Recent data from this work group suggest that quality of life

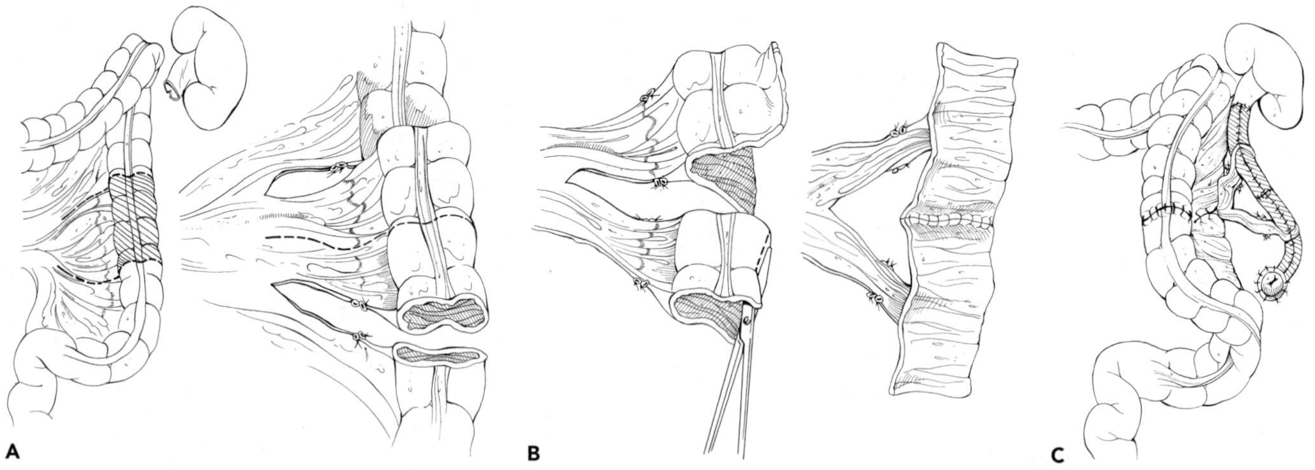


FIGURE 94.3 Combined reconfigured colon segments for incontinent diversion of solitary kidney. **A, B:** A 6-cm segment is excised from the ascending or descending colon. The segment is split in the middle and the rings are opened antimesenterically. When reconfigured, the tube produced will be approximately 18 cm long, suitable for incontinent urinary diversion. **C:** Pyelocolocutaneostomy in a solitary kidney.

in patients with unimpaired bladder function may be better than with conventional nephrostomy tubes.

## Transverse Retubularized Colon Segments

In selected patients, transverse reconfigured colon segments may be used successfully to reconstruct extensive ureteral defects (Figs. 94.3 and 94.4). The successful use of a combination of two such segments has been described to divert solitary kidneys in palliative situations (11). In patients with renal insufficiency or a history of irradiation, this technique may be superior to the use of ileum. An advantage of the colon is its immediate proximity to the ureters bilaterally and its position outside the radiation portals for treatment of pelvic malignancy. Nevertheless, unreconfigured colon has not been widely recruited for ureteral replacement because of its wide diameter: Its large volume when replacing long defects could result in metabolic or septic complications. Surgical access is via flank or pararectal incision, and intraperitoneal surgery is minimal. The colonic segments are taken immediately proximal to the ureteral defect, necessitating little mobilization of the mesenteric pedicle. Metabolic consequences have not been described and should be absent or low, as only minimal amounts of intestine need be isolated (11).

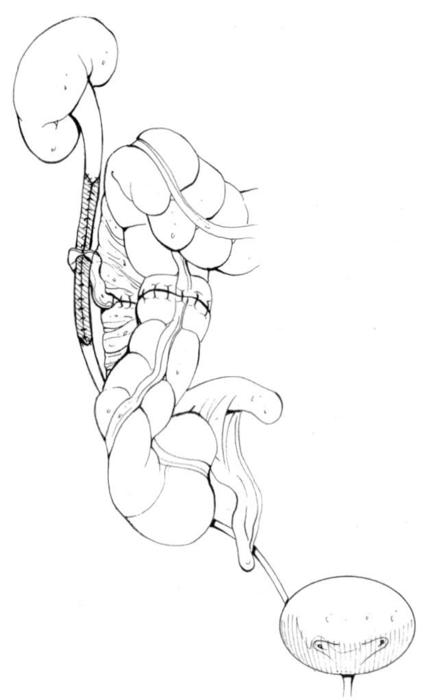

FIGURE 94.4 Interposition of a reconfigured colon segment to repair an extensive ureteral defect.

## *References*

1. De Baere T, Lagrange C, Kuoch V, et al. Transcatheter ethanol renal ablation in 20 patients with persistent urine leaks: an alternative to surgical nephrectomy. *J Urol* 2000;164:1148–1152.
2. Jabbour ME, Desgrandchamps F, Angelescu E, et al. Percutaneous implantation of subcutaneous prosthetic ureters: long-term outcome. *J Endourol* 2001;15:611–614.
3. Kulkarni R, Bellamy E. Nickel-titanium shape memory alloy Memokath 051 ureteral stent for managing long-term ureteral obstruction; 4-year experience. *J Urol* 2001;166:1750–1754.
4. Lebret T, Herve JM, Yonneau L, et al. After cystectomy, is it justified to perform a bladder replacement for patients with lymph node positive bladder cancer? *Eur Urol* 2002;42(4):344–349.
5. Liguori G, Trombetta C, Pomara G, et al. Major invasive surgery for urologic cancer in octogenarians with comorbid medical conditions. *Eur Urol* 2007;51:1600–1605.
6. Liu JS, Hrebinko RL. The use of 2 ipsilateral ureteral stents for relief of ureteral obstruction from extrinsic compression. *J Urol* 1998;159:179–181.
7. Lodde M, Palermo S, Comploj E, et al. Four years experience in bladder preserving management for muscle invasive bladder cancer. *Eur Urol* 2005;47(6):773–778.
8. Lodde M, Pycha A, Palermo S, et al. Uretero-ureterocutaneostomy (wrapped by omentum). *BJU Int* 2005;95(3):371–733.
9. Marx FJ, Laible V. [Ureterotransversopyelostomy with unilateral nephrostomy]. *Urologe A* 1985;24:334–339.
10. Segreti EM, Morris M, Levenback C, et al. Transverse colon urinary diversion in gynecologic oncology. *Gynecol Oncol* 1996;63:66–70.
11. Ubrig B, Waldner M, Roth S. Reconstruction of ureter with transverse retubularized colon segments. *J Urol* 2001;166:973–976.
12. Ubrig B, Lazica M, Waldner M, et al. Extraperitoneal bilateral cutaneous ureterostomy with midline stoma for palliation of pelvic cancer. *Urology* 2004;63(5):973–975.

H. GIL RUSHTON

# CHAPTER 95 ■ NEUROBLASTOMA

W. ROBERT DEFOOR, JR., PRAMOD P. REDDY, AND CURTIS A. SHELDON

Neuroblastoma represents the most common extracranial malignant solid neoplasm of infancy and childhood and the most common intra-abdominal malignancy in the newborn. The biological, genetical, and morphological characteristics of this neoplasm demonstrate heterogeneous behavior. These tumors have a varied clinical course, with reports of spontaneous regression and tumor maturation from malignant to a benign histological form. However, in many cases the disease is progressive (1,2) and exhibits a wide spectrum of morphological differentiation, ranging from primitive (neuroblastoma) to well differentiated (ganglioneuroma), or between these two extremes (ganglioneuroblastoma).

The clinical incidence is approximately 1 in 8,000 to 10,000 children. There are approximately 500 new cases diagnosed each year in the United States; 90% occur in children <7 years old. Cervical and mediastinal lesions tend to present in younger patients (<1 year of age) and tend to have a better prognosis. Neuroblastoma is slightly more common in boys than in girls, with a ratio of 1.2:1, and has been described in familial settings (2). Infants presenting with the following four clinical conditions have a higher incidence of neuroblastoma than the general population: Beckwith–Wiedemann syndrome, Hirschsprung disease, fetal alcohol syndrome, and fetal hydantoin syndrome.

## DIAGNOSIS

The clinical presentation of neuroblastoma is varied and dependent upon the site of the primary tumor, the presence of metastatic disease, the age of the patient, and the production of metabolically active substances. Vasoactive tumors can present with hypertension. The catecholamine urinary metabolites, vanillylmandelic acid (VMA) and homovanillic acid (HVA), are elevated in >80% of patients with a neuroblastoma. An increased VMA/HVA ratio is associated with a better prognosis in localized disease. Other elevated metabolic products can include lactate dehydrogenase (LDH) >1,500 IU/mL, serum ferritin >142 ng/mL, and serum neuron-specific enolase (NSE) >100 ng/mL; these are associated with a poor prognosis.

At least 50% of children with neuroblastoma will have metastatic disease, including spread to the cortical bone, bone marrow, liver, and skin, at the time of initial presentation. Initial evaluation of a child with a suspected neuroblastoma includes random urine for VMA and HVA, chest radiograph, ultrasound of the abdomen, computed tomography (CT) or magnetic resonance imaging (MRI) body scans, radioisotopic bone scan, $I^{131}$-metaiodobenzylguanidine (MIBG) scan, bone marrow aspirate/biopsy from multiple sites, and N-*myc* oncogene copy number of tumor. Serum LDH, ferritin, and NSE are also obtained.

**TABLE 95.1**

**EVANS STAGING SYSTEM**

| Stage of Tumor | Description of Stage |
|---|---|
| I | Tumor confined to the organ of origin |
| II | Tumor extends beyond organ of origin but does not cross the midline; unilateral lymph nodes may be involved |
| III | Tumor extends across the midline; bilateral regional lymph nodes may be involved |
| IV | Distant metastases (skeletal, other organs, soft tissues, distant lymph nodes) |
| IV-S | Stage I or II with remote disease confined to one or more of the following sites: liver, skin, or bone marrow, but without evidence of bone cortex involvement |

From Evans AE, D'Angio GJ, Randolph J. A proposed staging for children with neuroblastoma. Children's Cancer Study Group A. *Cancer.* 1971;27:374–378, with permission.

### Staging Systems

Multiple staging systems have evolved in the management of neuroblastoma. The Evans–D'Angio staging system (Table 95.1) consists of a clinical assessment that describes the initial tumor distribution and incorporates whether the tumor crosses the midline (3). The International Neuroblastoma Staging System (INSS) incorporates many of the important criteria from each of these three staging systems and includes initial tumor distribution as well as its surgical resectability (Table 95.2) (4). The most useful histologic classification is the system described by Shimada (5). This system utilizes the mitosis karyorrhexis index (MKI) of nuclear fragmentation. This system divides the tumors into age-related favorable and unfavorable histologic categories based on whether the tumor exhibits a stroma-rich or stroma-poor appearance (Table 95.3).

## INDICATIONS FOR SURGERY

The management of patients presenting with neuroblastoma varies with the extent of disease at the time of diagnosis, the age of the patient, and the staging criteria used. If the patient

**TABLE 95.2**

**INTERNATIONAL NEUROBLASTOMA STAGING SYSTEM**

| Stage of Tumor | Description of Stage |
|---|---|
| 1 | Localized tumor confined to the area of origin. Complete gross excision, with or without microscopic residual disease. Identifiable ipsilateral and contralateral lymph nodes that are microscopically negative. |
| 2-A | Unilateral tumor with incomplete gross resection. Identifiable ipsilateral and contralateral lymph nodes that are microscopically negative. |
| 2-B | Unilateral tumor with complete or incomplete gross excision. Positive ipsilateral regional lymph nodes. Identifiable contralateral lymph nodes that are microscopically negative. |
| 3 | Tumor infiltration across the midline with or without regional lymph node involvement. Unilateral tumor with contralateral lymph node involvement or midline tumor with bilateral regional lymph node involvement. |
| 4 | Dissemination of tumor to distant lymph nodes, bone marrow, bone, liver, or other organs (except as defined in Stage 4-S) |
| 4-S | Localized primary tumor as defined for Stage 1 or 2 (Stage 2-A or 2-B), with dissemination limited to the liver, skin, or bone marrow |

From Brodeur GM, Seeger RC, Barrett A, et al. International criteria for diagnosis, staging, and response to treatment in patients with neuroblastoma. *J Clin Oncol.* 1988;6:1874–1881, with permission.

**TABLE 95.3**

**SHIMADA PATHOLOGIC CLASSIFICATION**

| | Favorable Histology | Unfavorable Histology |
|---|---|---|
| Stroma rich | Well-differentiated, intermixed appearance | Nodular appearance |
| Stroma poor | | |
| Age <18 mo | Mitosis karyorrhexis index (MKI) < 200/5,000 | MKI < 100/5,000 |
| Age 18–60 mo | MKI > 100/5,000 | MKI > 100/5,000 |
| | Differentiating | Undifferentiated |
| Age >5 yr | None | All |

Shimada H, Ambros IM, Dehner LP, et al. The International Neuroblastoma Pathology Classification (the Shimada system). *Cancer.* 1999;86:364–372, with permission.

has stage I or II disease (with favorable histology), then surgical resection alone can be undertaken with reasonable success. A multimodal approach utilizing chemotherapy, radiation, and surgery is used for advanced disease (stages III and IV).

Surgical intervention ("second-look" laparotomy) after open biopsy is usually performed 13 to 18 weeks after chemotherapy has been administered. During this procedure, surgical resection and dissection may appear to be somewhat easier, especially around vital structures and major blood vessels, because chemotherapy usually makes the tumors smaller and firmer. This rubbery consistency also decreases the risk of rupture and spillage of the tumor that might otherwise be encountered. Intraoperative radiation (IORT) may be utilized and is helpful in reducing the exposure to normal adjacent structures. In advanced-stage tumors radiation therapy is delivered to the tumor bed and regional lymph nodes.

### Neonatal Observation Protocol

For neonatally detected adrenal tumors that are thought to be localized neuroblastoma, an option for close observation without surgical intervention has been proposed. This is based on the experience that many of these lesions may regress or mature spontaneously, and the majority of persistent tumors have favorable biological activity, with a 95% 4-year survival. In addition, there are significant surgical risks of ablative surgery in small or preterm neonates. Consequently, some centers have adopted a "wait-and-see" strategy of management for those detected from prenatal screening. However, each case should be evaluated thoroughly and carefully, with any possible benefit balanced against the morbidity of the diagnosis (6).

## SURGICAL TECHNIQUE

In cases of very large tumors where resection of adjacent organs or intestine might be required, a mechanical bowel preparation is reasonable. The procedure is performed with the patient in a supine position. The patient should be given prophylactic antibiotics (broad-spectrum cephalosporin). Depending on the location and size of the tumor, the surgeon can choose between three different incisions: (a) transverse transperitoneal–supraumbilical incision (for primary tumor of the retroperitoneum), (b) bilateral subcostal chevron incision (for large tumors), or (c) thoracoabdominal incision (for upper abdominal and/or large tumors).

The retroperitoneum is entered by incising the posterior peritoneum along the white line of Toldt. The colon is reflected medially to expose the retroperitoneum. For left-sided tumors the spleen and pancreas are displaced upward and medially. For tumors on the right side the various peritoneal attachments of the liver can be divided to improve exposure. In children with locally metastasizing disease it is sometimes necessary to perform en bloc excision of adjacent organs (i.e., ipsilateral kidney, spleen). Neuroblastomas typically have a friable pseudocapsule; therefore, during dissection it is useful to think of the surgery as aimed at dissecting the patient from around the tumor to decrease the risk of tumor spillage.

Vascular control should be achieved early in the procedure. These tumors often invade the tunica adventitia of large blood vessels; therefore, special care should be taken to identify and spare the blood supply to important visceral structures such as the branches of the celiac axis and superior mesenteric artery. The venous drainage of these tumors is usually constant, with right-sided tumors draining directly into the inferior vena cava. Left-sided tumors drain into the left renal vein and subdiaphragmatic venous tributaries. Regional lymph nodes should be sampled to complete the surgical staging. Once the tumor has been resected, the margins of the tumor bed should be marked with titanium clips to guide radiation therapy. A liver biopsy is indicated if there is clinical or imaging suspicion of disease within the liver; an effort should be made to biopsy the involved area.

In some instances it is not possible to perform primary resection of the tumor; in these cases a wedge biopsy of the tumor should be obtained for histopathological and genetical analysis. Neuroblastoma tissue should be rushed to the lab for processing in a fresh state. Following a good response to chemotherapy, the residual tumor may be successfully removed at a "second-look" procedure (7).

### Laparoscopic (Minimally Invasive) Procedures for Neuroblastoma

Minimally invasive surgery (MIS) procedures are accepted as a safe alternative to open surgery. Its use in children has been increasing rapidly as evidenced by a growing body of literature. The theoretical benefits include decreased surgical stress, decreased postoperative morbidity, decreased use of narcotic analgesics, reduced time to initiation of enteral nutrition, and improved cosmetic appearance. Most importantly, the earlier recovery may reduce the time to initiation of adjuvant therapy. Previously, MIS techniques were reserved for biopsy prior to planned multimodal therapy in diffuse disease; however, there are several contemporary reports in the literature that have described MIS, including the use of the surgical robot, as a safe alternative to open surgery for excision of small localized primary lesions. This has not gained widespread international acceptance; thus, the following discussion is limited to the technique of laparoscopic biopsy.

General anesthesia is induced and the patient undergoes endotracheal intubation. An orogastric or nasogastric tube and urethral catheter are placed. The patient is then positioned in a 45-degree lateral decubitus position. The use of the open Hasson technique is strongly recommended for initial umbilical trocar placement (5 to 12 mm) to lower the risk of visceral or vascular injury associated with the Veress needle technique. A pneumoperitoneum is created, with the pressure maintained at around 12 mm Hg. Two 3- or 5-mm ports are then placed under laparoscopic vision. The retroperitoneum is then dissected using electrocautery and/or a Harmonic Scalpel (Ethicon Endo-Surgery, Ohio).

On the right side, the retroperitoneum may be entered by a transverse incision in the posterior peritoneum to expose the inferior vena cava and the region of the adrenal gland. When operating on a left-sided lesion, the colon should be mobilized; this is achieved by incising the posterior peritoneum along the line of Toldt from the splenic flexure to the pelvic rim. The major vessels surrounding the tumor, such as the inferior vena cava and the renal vein and artery and the adrenal vessels, are mobilized by blunt dissection; this dissection should begin medially and proceeds laterally. Vascular control may be obtained at this time prior to proceeding with the biopsy or excision of the mass.

Once the tumor surface has been adequately exposed, a Tru-cut biopsy of the tumor can be obtained by passing the biopsy needle through one of the 5-mm ports or directly through the abdominal wall and performing the biopsy under visualization. Hemostasis is then obtained. It is recommended that an incisional biopsy be obtained when possible as this minimizes the chances of sampling error and provides the surgical pathologist with adequate quantities of tissue. The tissue specimen is placed in a laparoscopic bag and removed through the umbilical port. The defect may be cauterized, but to achieve complete hemostasis, an absorbable hemostatic agent may be applied to the surface of the tumor. The fascial defect left by the ports is closed with an absorbable suture, and the skin edges are approximated. Some authors advocate that the fascial defect in 5-mm and smaller ports does not require closure because the risk of visceral herniation is low (8). No drains are left at the end of the procedure. To avoid port site recurrence, high-dose adjuvant chemotherapy is given as soon as possible.

## OUTCOMES

### Results

Modern chemotherapy has conferred improved survivability upon many pediatric neoplasms (e.g., Wilms tumor); however, in the case of neuroblastoma chemotherapy has had no such effect. Although a demonstrable initial tumor response is achieved in 70% to 80% of patients, current chemotherapeutic protocols have not effectively increased the cure rate in patients with neuroblastoma. The main purpose of chemotherapy in the management of children with stage II or higher-stage neuroblastoma is to reduce the size of the tumor (permitting surgical excision), to clear the bone marrow of tumor cells, and possibly to produce histological maturation of the tumor.

Figure 95.1 shows a coronal view from an MRI scan of a solitary tumor adjacent to the lower pole of the right kidney. The patient was treated with surgical excision alone and remained free from relapse. Figure 95.2 shows the microscopic pathology from the same mass consisting of small round blue cells typical of neuroblastoma. Patients such as this with Evans stage I or II with favorable histology (low-risk) neuroblastoma do not

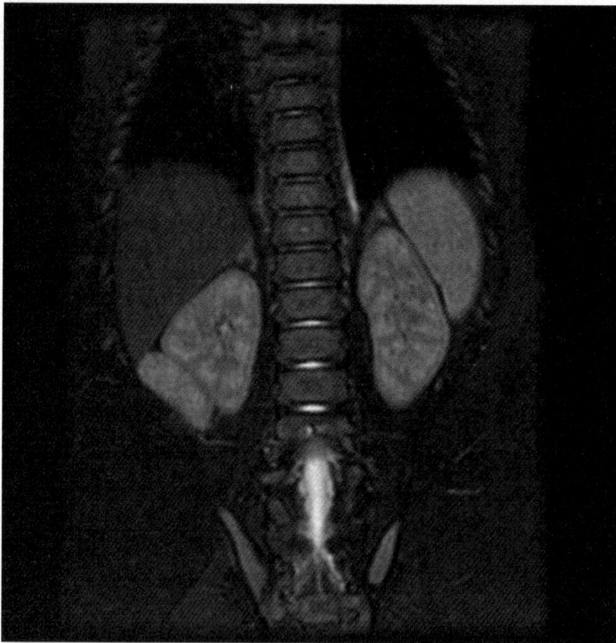

FIGURE 95.1 Coronal MRI scan of a 1-year-old girl found to have a left pararenal mass on a screening ultrasound after a urinary tract infection.

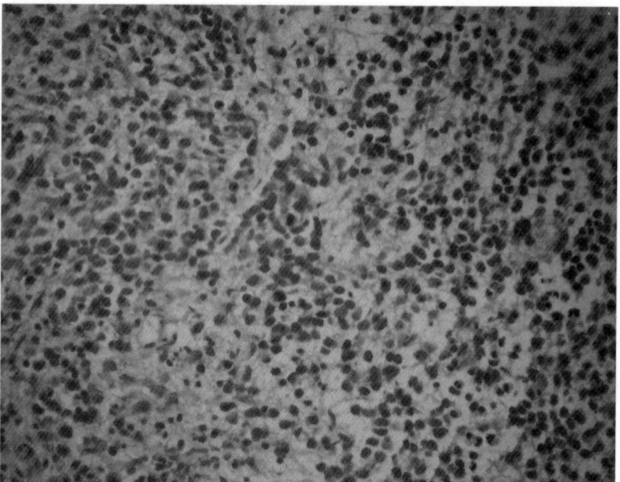

FIGURE 95.2 Microscopical view of lesion excised from patient in Figure 95.1 showing small round blue cells consistent with neuroblastoma.

require adjuvant chemotherapy if the tumor can be surgically excised. Patients with stage II to IV disease and poor prognostic biological factors (intermediate- to high-risk neuroblastoma) should be treated with multiagent chemotherapy, including a combination of carboplatin, doxorubicin (Adriamycin), cyclophosphamide, and etoposide (VP-16) (9).

Clinical experience has demonstrated that neuroblastoma is a radiosensitive tumor. Tumor shrinkage and symptomatic pain relief are often observed after radiation treatment. In patients with advanced neuroblastoma, lymph node metastases, and/or incomplete surgical resection of the primary tumor, chemoradiotherapy appears to improve long-term disease control as compared to chemotherapy alone (10,11). Radiation therapy protocols include delivery of hyperfractionated radiotherapy (2,100 cGy at 150 cGy twice daily). The final setting for external beam treatments is a total body irradiation given as part of a preparative regimen for autologous bone marrow transplantation. IORT is being used to treat patients with advanced-stage disease. Initial reports demonstrate a low complication rate with IORT and a 38% 3-year survival rate in patients with stage IV disease.

The age of the patient and the stage of the disease at the time of diagnosis were the two main independent variables determining the prognosis of children with neuroblastoma. The worst survival data were observed in patients older than 1 year, with stage IV disease, and with metastases to cortical bone (12). Over the years a number of factors have become available to the clinician managing these patients to help determine the prognosis of the individual patient. These factors are presented in Table 95.4. Patients with neuroblastoma detected by urinary screening for VMA and HVA in Japan have a survival rate of 96%, suggesting that most of these tumors spontaneously regress and do not present with clinical disease (13). The intrinsic properties of the tumor itself appear to be the greatest determinant of the eventual outcome of the patient with neuroblastoma. Survival data from the Children's Cancer Group neuroblastoma protocols are presented in Table 95.5 (13).

## Surgical Complications

Among the potential complications of open surgery are vascular injuries that may occur during dissection of the tumor. Others complications include injury to adjacent intraperitoneal organs (e.g., splenic injury, pancreatic injuries), lymphatic leak, brachial plexus injury related to patient positioning, and acute renal failure (secondary to spasm of the renal artery). MIS complications include hypercapnia, hypothermia, surgical emphysema, and electrosurgical complications. Others are gas embolisms, tension pneumothorax, complications of surgical access, Veress needle injury to blood vessels or bowel structures, access failure, bleeding/vascular injury, and visceral injuries. Port site neoplastic recurrences have also been described.

# CONCLUSION

Neuroblastoma is a common pediatric malignancy that remains an enigma because of the high variability in its natural history and behavior. Information on prenatally detected cases and the infant screening programs have clearly demonstrated that some tumors spontaneously regress and may be managed with close observation. A better understanding of the factors influencing tumor regression, tumor differentiation, and tumor–host immunorelations will improve our ability to identify and aggressively treat patients at risk for a poor outcome (14). This knowledge may also allow a decrease in treatment-related morbidity in patients with low-risk tumors. Ongoing clinical trials utilizing retinoic acid and gene therapy may result in the development of additional tools in the clinical armamentarium to better treat neuroblastoma and further improve the prognosis of these patients (15).

**TABLE 95.4**

FACTORS AFFECTING PROGNOSIS OF THE CHILD WITH NEUROBLASTOMA

| Prognostic Factor | Good Prognosis | Poor Prognosis |
|---|---|---|
| Patient age | <1 yr | >1 yr |
| Tumor stage | I, II, IV-S | III, IV |
| Shimada histology | Stroma rich | Stroma poor |
| Site of tumor | Mediastinum, pelvis, neck | Adrenal, celiac axis |
| >10 copies N-*myc* | No | Yes |
| DNA flow cytometry | Hyperdiploid | Diploid |
| Elevated trk-A | Yes | No |
| Elevated serum ferritin | No | Yes |
| Neuron-specific enolase | No | Yes |
| Lactate dehydrogenase | No | Yes |
| Loss of heterozygosity (LOH) chromosome 1p | No | Yes |
| Multidrug-resistant gene | No | Yes |
| Multidrug-resistant protein–gene | No | Yes |
| Somatostatin receptors | Yes | No |
| Vasoactive intestinal peptide secretion | Yes | No |
| MHC class I antigen | Yes | No |
| Detection by screening | Yes | No |

From Grosfeld JL. Neuroblastoma. In: O'Neill JA, Rowe MI, Grosfeld JL, et al., eds. *Pediatric Surgery.* St. Louis, MO: Mosby; 1988:405–419, with permission.

**TABLE 95.5**

SURVIVAL DATA FROM CHILDREN'S CANCER GROUP NEUROBLASTOMA PROTOCOLS

| INSS Tumor Stage | All Ages | Patients <1yr | Patients >1yr |
|---|---|---|---|
| All stages | | 76% | 32% |
| I | 94–99% | | |
| II | 89–96% | | |
| III | 37% | | |
| IV | 12% | 50–75% | 10% |
| IV-S | 90% | | |

INSS, International Neuroblastoma Staging System. From Grosfeld JL. Risk-based management: current concepts of treating malignant solid tumors of childhood. *J Am Coll Surg* 1999;189:407–425, with permission.

## References


1. Evans AE, Gerson J, Schnaufer L. Spontaneous regression of neuroblastoma. *Natl Cancer Inst Monogr* 1976;44:49–54.
2. Grosfeld JL, Rescorla FJ, West KW, et al. Neuroblastoma in the first year of life: clinical and biologic factors influencing outcome. *Semin Pediatr Surg* 1993;2:37–46.
3. Evans AE, D'Angio GJ, Randolph J. A proposed staging for children with neuroblastoma. Children's Cancer Study Group A. *Cancer* 1971;27:374–378.
4. Brodeur GM, Seeger RC, Barrett A, et al. International criteria for diagnosis, staging, and response to treatment in patients with neuroblastoma. *J Clin Oncol* 1988;6:1874–1881.
5. Shimada H, Ambros IM, Dehner LP, et al. The International Neuroblastoma Pathology Classification (the Shimada system). *Cancer* 1999;86:364–372.
6. Fritsch P, Kerbl R, Lackner H, et al. "Wait and see" strategy in localized neuroblastoma in infants: an option not only for cases detected by mass screening. *Pediatric Blood Cancer* 2004;43:679–682.
7. Kumar AP, Wrenn EL Jr, Fleming ID, et al. Preoperative therapy for unresectable malignant tumors in children. *J Pediatr Surg* 1975;10:657–670.
8. Bloom DA, Ehrlich RM. Omental evisceration through small laparoscopy port sites. *J Endourol* 1993;7:31–33.
9. Nitschke R, Cangir A, Crist W, et al. Intensive chemotherapy for metastatic neuroblastoma: a Southwest Oncology Group study. *Med Pediatr Oncol* 1980;8:281–288.
10. Haase GM, LaQuaglia MP. Neuroblastoma. In: Zeigler MM, Azizkhan RG, Weber TR, eds. *Operative Pediatric Surgery.* 1st ed. New York: McGraw-Hill Professional, 2003:1181–1191.
11. Haase GM, O'Leary MC, Ramsay NK, et al, et al. Aggressive surgery combined with intensive chemotherapy improves survival in poor-risk neuroblastoma. *J Pediatr Surg* 1991;26:1119–1124.
12. Grosfeld JL, Baehner RL. Neuroblastoma: an analysis of 160 cases. *World J Surg* 1980;4:29–37.
13. Grosfeld JL. Risk-based management: current concepts of treating malignant solid tumors of childhood. *J Am Coll Surg* 1999;189(4):407–425.
14. Grosfeld JL. Neuroblastoma. In: O'Neill JA, Rowe MI, Grosfeld JL, et al., eds. *Pediatric Surgery.* 5th ed. St. Louis: Mosby, 1998:405–419.
15. Reynolds CP, Kane DJ, Einhorn PA, et al. Response of neuroblastoma to retinoic acid in vitro and in vivo. *Prog Clin Biol Res* 1991;366:203–211.

# CHAPTER 96 ■ WILMS TUMOR

SARAH CONLEY AND MICHAEL L. RITCHEY

Wilms tumor, or nephroblastoma, is the most common solid tumor of childhood. It represents approximately 6% of all childhood cancers in the United States and is the most common primary malignant renal tumor of childhood. The incidence of Wilms tumor is 1 in 10,000 children, with a new case rate of approximately 500 annually in the United States. The incidence has remained stable for the past several decades and is equal among boys and girls (1). The mean age at diagnosis for unilateral Wilms tumor is 36.5 months for boys and 42.5 months for girls. The age of peak incidence for bilateral tumors is lower for both sexes: 29.5 months for boys and 32.6 months for girls.

Most cases of Wilms tumor are sporadic; however, there are certain phenotypical syndromes associated with Wilms tumor (2). These syndromes are divided into overgrowth and non-overgrowth categories. Examples of overgrowth syndromes include Beckwith–Wiedemann syndrome, Perlman syndrome, Sotos syndrome, and Simpson–Golabi–Behmel syndrome. Examples of non-overgrowth syndromes include isolated aniridia, trisomy 18, WAGR syndrome (Wilms tumor, aniridia, genitourinary malformations, and mental retardation), Bloom syndrome, and Denys–Drash syndrome. Wilms tumor is also associated with isolated genitourinary anomalies such as hypospadias, cryptorchidism, and renal fusion. Less than 2% of Wilms tumor cases show familial patterns of inheritance.

The identification of the relationship between Wilms tumor and WAGR syndrome led to the discovery of genes associated with Wilms tumor. The WT1 gene located on chromosome 11p13 encodes a transcriptional factor that serves both tumor-suppressive and developmental regulatory functions (2). Nonmutated WT1 is critical in the early embryogenesis of the genitourinary system. WT1 mutations are present in up to 15% of patients with unilateral Wilms tumors (3). Another genetical mutation associated with Wilms tumor has been designated the WT2 gene, located on chromosome 11p15. Loss of heterozygosity (LOH) at this locus is associated with Beckwith–Wiedemann syndrome.

LOH at chromosome 16q and/or 1p occurs in up to 20% of Wilms tumors (4). These have been shown to be associated with an increased risk for tumor relapse and mortality. In National Wilms Tumor Study (NWTS)-5, patients with stage I or II favorable-histology Wilms tumor (FHWT) and LOH of either 1p or 16q had an increased relative risk of relapse and death compared to patients lacking LOH at either locus. The risks of relapse and death for patients with stage III or IV FHWT were increased only with LOH for both regions.

Nephrogenic rests (NRs) are foci of primitive metanephric tissue that persist into infancy and are found in 1% of infant postmortem kidneys. The presence of NRs in up to 44% of kidneys removed for Wilms tumor suggests that they represent precursor lesions in children genetically predisposed to Wilms tumor. NRs are categorized as either perilobar or intralobar based on their anatomical location within the kidney. Perilobar NRs are observed in kidneys harboring Wilms tumors with WT2 locus deletions, whereas intralobar NRs are more often observed in those with WT1-associated tumors (5). The presence of multiple NRs in the nontumoral portion of a Wilms tumor kidney has been shown to be a risk factor for development of metachronous tumor in the contralateral kidney.

## DIAGNOSIS

More than 90% of children with Wilms tumor present with an asymptomatic abdominal mass discovered incidentally by a family member or physician. The mass may be extremely large relative to the size of the child and is not necessarily confined to one side. Approximately 20% of children with Wilms tumor have hematuria at diagnosis. Gross hematuria warrants further evaluation to rule out tumor extension into the collecting system (6). Other symptoms include fever, anorexia, and weight loss in 10% of patients. Rarely children may present with acute abdominal pain from tumor rupture into the peritoneal cavity or bleeding within the tumor. A persistent varicocele in the supine position or hepatomegaly may be reflective of inferior vena caval obstruction from tumor thrombus. Atrial thrombus may present as hypertension or congestive heart failure.

The preoperative laboratory evaluation of a child with an abdominal mass should include a complete blood count, liver enzymes, and serum electrolytes, including blood urea nitrogen, creatinine, and calcium. There is an 8% incidence of acquired von Willebrand disease in patients newly diagnosed with Wilms tumor. Coagulation studies, including prothrombin time and partial thromboplastin time, may be normal in the presence of von Willebrand disease. This defect can be corrected preoperatively with the administration of 1-desamino-8-D-arginine-vasopressin (DDAVP).

The first radiographic study usually obtained in children with an abdominal mass is an abdominal ultrasound, which can differentiate between solid and cystic masses. Real-time ultrasonography of the renal vein and inferior vena cava (IVC) can evaluate for the presence of tumor thrombus in children with renal tumors. If this study is inconclusive, magnetic resonance (MR) imaging is an excellent modality to assess for venous tumor extension. All patients should undergo computed tomography (CT) of the abdomen and pelvis with oral and intravenous contrast or MR of the abdomen and pelvis with gadolinium. These imaging modalities allow for improved preoperative planning by evaluating for extrarenal spread of disease, the relationship of the tumor to adjacent visceral structures, and the presence of synchronous tumors in the contralateral kidney. Preoperative chest CT is performed to rule out pulmonary metastases.

## INDICATIONS FOR SURGERY

There have been tremendous advances in survival with adjuvant therapy, but surgery remains an integral part of the multimodal approach to treatment of Wilms tumor. Primary radical nephrectomy is the procedure of choice for the majority of patients with unilateral Wilms tumor. Nephron-sparing surgery is preferred for children with bilateral tumors. It may be considered for some children with syndromes known to be at high risk for development of Wilms tumor, particularly if these patients are found to have small tumors on screening studies (7). There are reports of laparoscopic nephrectomy in children with unilateral nonmetastatic Wilms tumor who received preoperative chemotherapy (8). However, the role of laparoscopy prior to chemotherapy may be limited because of large tumor size and risk of intraoperative spillage. Histopathology and tumor stage have been demonstrated to be the key determinants of prognosis in patients with Wilms tumor. Tumor grade is the most important prognostic factor. Assignment of tumor stage (Table 96.1) is based on intraoperative and pathological findings.

The International Society of Pediatric Oncology (SIOP) advocates preoperative chemotherapy for all patients with Wilms tumor regardless of the extent of disease. Preoperative treatment can produce dramatic reduction in the size of the primary tumor, facilitating surgical excision. The SIOP trials have demonstrated that the incidence of tumor rupture is lower after preoperative therapy (9). There is no survival advantage over a primary surgical approach.

The Children's Oncology Group (COG) recommends preoperative chemotherapy in children with bilateral tumors, tumors inoperable at surgical exploration, or IVC extension above the hepatic veins. All other patients are recommended to undergo primary excision of the tumor. This allows precise staging of patients with modulation of treatment for each individual, thereby decreasing the intensity of treatment when possible while maintaining excellent overall survival.

**TABLE 96.1**

**STAGING SYSTEM OF THE CHILDREN'S ONCOLOGY GROUP**

| Stage | Characteristics |
|---|---|
| I | The tumor is limited to the kidney and completely excised. The renal capsule is intact and the tumor was not ruptured prior to removal. There is no residual tumor. The vessels of the renal sinus are not involved. |
| II | The tumor extends beyond the kidney, but is completely excised. There is regional extension of the tumor (i.e., penetration of the renal capsule, extensive invasion of the renal sinus). Extrarenal vessels may contain tumor thrombus or be infiltrated by tumor. |
| III | Residual nonhematogenous tumor confined to the abdomen: lymph node involvement, tumor spillage either before or during surgery, peritoneal implants, tumor beyond surgical margin either grossly or microscopically, or tumor not completely removed. |
| IV | Hematogenous metastases (lung, liver, bone, brain, etc.) or lymph node metastases outside the abdominopelvic region are present. |
| V | Bilateral renal involvement at diagnosis |

## SURGICAL TECHNIQUE

The recommended surgical approach for Wilms tumor is through a transperitoneal transabdominal incision. An extraperitoneal flank incision should be avoided because it does not allow for proper staging. A generous transverse abdominal incision allows for inspection and exploration of the abdominal cavity. The patient is placed in a supine position with mild flexion of the lumbar spine to facilitate the exposure of retroperitoneal structures. The incision is made approximately two fingerbreadths above the umbilicus beginning in the midaxillary line on the side of the neoplasm. The extent to which the incision is extended across the midline will vary with the size of the tumor and amount of exposure needed. The incision may be extended into a thoracoabdominal approach by continuing through the bed of the ninth or tenth rib, if necessary. The muscle layers are divided sequentially to facilitate exposure. The peritoneal space should be opened carefully. The tumor may compress the colon and/or small bowel against the anterior abdominal wall, inadvertently resulting in enterotomy. A thorough exploration of the abdomen is performed. The peritoneal cavity is assessed for evidence of preoperative tumor rupture and peritoneal implants. The liver is carefully examined, as liver metastases may not be identified on preoperative imaging studies. An assessment of tumor extent is performed next, including palpation of the IVC and assessment of regional lymphadenopathy, perinephric extension, and tumor mobility.

In the past, formal exploration of the contralateral kidney was routinely performed in children with presumed unilateral Wilms tumor to rule out synchronous bilateral tumors.

Imaging has improved dramatically over time and very few small contralateral lesions will be missed on preoperative imaging. Long-term outcomes in these cases are favorable (10). Contralateral renal exploration is no longer recommended if preoperative CT or MR demonstrates a normal kidney.

Following exploration of the abdominal cavity, the colon is reflected medially by incising the white line of Toldt. The colonic mesentery is mobilized, with care taken to preserve the colonic vessels that may be draped over the tumor. The colon can then be retracted medially to expose the renal vessels (Fig. 96.1). For right-sided tumors, the posterior peritoneum can be incised up to the base of the mesentery. This will allow reflection of the entire colon and small bowel, which provides excellent exposure of the retroperitoneal vessels. Early ligation of the renal vessels before manipulation is ideal. The renal vessels are identified and encircled individually with vessel loops.

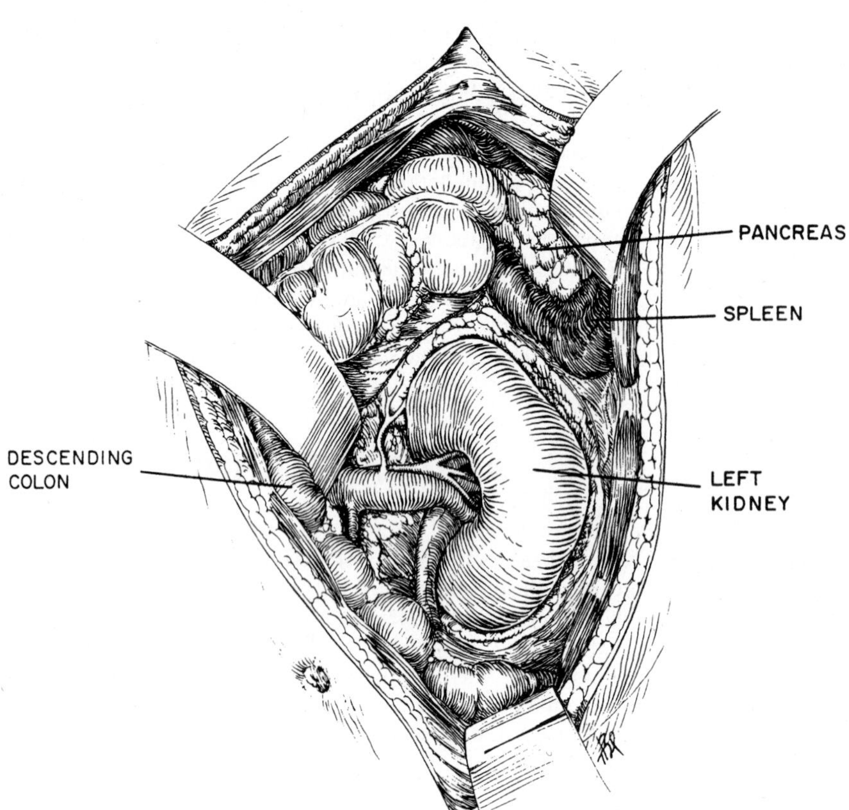


FIGURE 96.1 Descending colon retracted medially after incising of the line of Toldt and mobilizing of the mesocolon off the anterior surface of the tumor.

The artery can be identified with careful retraction of the vein. The renal vein and IVC should be carefully palpated for the presence of Wilms tumor thrombus, which occurs in 4% and 0.7% of patients, respectively. Prior to ligation of the vessels, the contralateral renal vessels and superior mesenteric artery are identified to avoid injury to these structures. Large tumors can significantly distort vascular anatomy. The renal vessels are then doubly ligated and divided. The renal artery should be ligated prior to the renal vein in order to avoid distention of the vein, which can dislodge the ligature. Early ligation of the artery also decreases the theoretical risk of tumor dissemination.

An alternative for management of the renal vein is to place a Satinsky clamp on the vena IVC just proximal to the insertion of the renal vein. This maneuver can be valuable when the vein is short or if there is tumor extension beyond the renal vein. The tumor thrombus is gently milked back prior to placement of the Satinsky clamp. The renal vein is then divided and the venous stump is oversewn with continuous 5-0 Prolene in two layers (Fig. 96.2).

If tumor thrombus is present in the IVC, additional surgical exposure is warranted. Both proximal and distal vascular control is necessary. For minimal thrombus extension below the level of the hepatic veins, the inferior edge of the liver can be retracted to expose the infrahepatic vena cava. For a tumor that extends more cephalad, mobilization of the liver is required. Division of the triangular and coronary ligaments of the liver allows rotation and exposure of the retrohepatic vena cava. Additional exposure can be gained by dividing the lesser hepatic veins. The contralateral renal vein and infrarenal IVC are controlled with vessel loops. The vena IVC is then vertically incised just medial to the entrance of the renal vein. If the thrombus is free floating, it is manually extracted at this point. In many cases, the thrombus is adherent to the wall of the IVC. A Fogarty or Foley balloon catheter can be passed beyond the level of the hepatic veins, then inflated. The catheter is then pulled inferiorly, thus displacing the adherent thrombus into the cavotomy. The vena IVC is allowed to fill by releasing the vessel loops on the distal cava and contralateral renal vein. This will displace the air from within the IVC. The cavotomy is then clamped with a Satinsky clamp and oversewn with a continuous 5-0 Prolene suture (Fig. 96.3). In rare instances, tumor thrombus invades the wall of the IVC, precluding thrombectomy, and this may necessitate partial resection of the IVC.

Patients with IVC extension above the level of the hepatic veins or atrial thrombus remain a difficult surgical challenge. Pretreatment with chemotherapy is usually done. If this fails to shrink the thrombus or if a primary surgical approach is chosen, the procedure may require cardiopulmonary bypass and benefit from a combined abdominothoracic approach with a pediatric cardiothoracic surgeon. Suprahepatic or atrial involvement is best approached through a median sternotomy. This can be performed in conjunction with a subcostal incision or a midline abdominal incision required for nephrectomy.

After the vessels are controlled, a dissection plane is established outside of the fascia of Gerota by sharp and blunt dissection. The perforating vessels can be quite large and should be ligated individually. Gentle manipulation of the tumor should be emphasized. Wilms tumors are very soft and may easily rupture, leading to tumor spill and an increased risk of local recurrence (11).

The ureter is palpated to rule out intraureteral extension before it is divided as distally as possible (6). Formal lymph

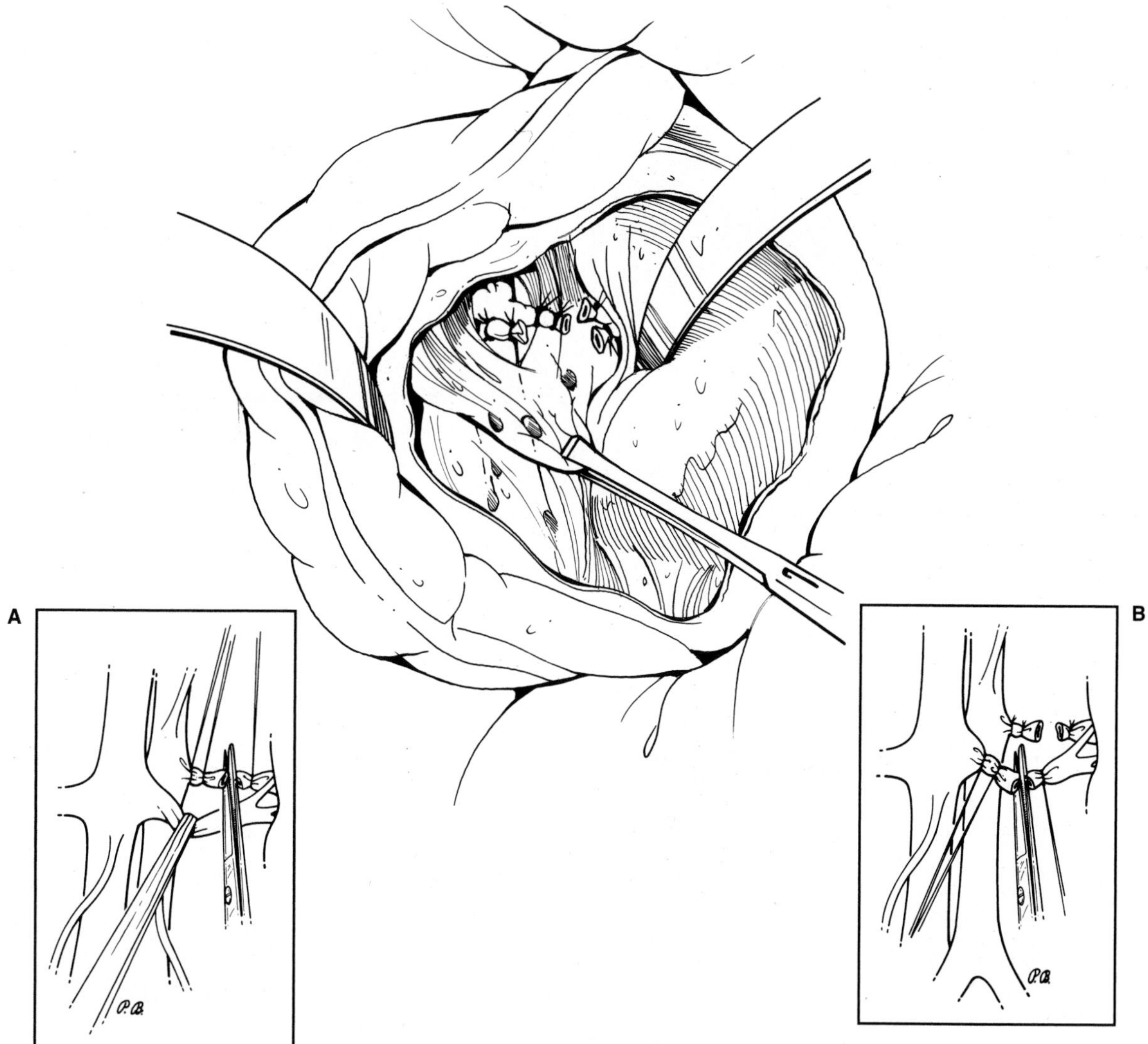


FIGURE 96.2 Mobilization of left-sided Wilms tumor by blunt dissection after ligation and division of the (**A**) renal artery and (**B**) vein.

node dissection is not required, but all suspicious lymph nodes should be biopsied. Lymphatic tissue in the renal hilum and adjacent precaval and preaortic areas is generally removed with the specimen. Failure to sample lymph nodes will mandate increased therapy due to an increased risk of local recurrence secondary to incomplete staging (11). After extraction of the intact tumor, the wound is copiously irrigated and hemostasis is assessed. Drains are not routinely placed unless a portion of the pancreas or liver has been resected. The displaced colon is replaced in the tumor bed.

## Bilateral Tumors

Synchronous bilateral Wilms tumor occurs in 4% to 6% of patients with Wilms tumor (12). Children with bilateral Wilms tumors should not undergo initial radical nephrectomy; rather, they should receive preoperative chemotherapy with the goal of tumor shrinkage and renal preservation. Children treated with preoperative chemotherapy will have more renal units preserved. This is important because the risk of renal failure in patients with bilateral disease approaches 15% at 15 years posttreatment (13).

The proposed COG protocol for patients with bilateral Wilms tumor recommends 6 weeks of chemotherapy prior to surgery. Tumor response is evaluated with CT or MR after 6 weeks.

Patients with tumors amenable to renal-sparing procedures can proceed with surgery. If there has not been a good response, biopsy of the tumor(s) is recommended to determine the histology. Additional chemotherapy is then given, but all patients should proceed to surgical resection within 12 weeks of starting therapy.

At the time of definitive surgery, partial nephrectomy or wedge excision of the tumor is preferred, but only if it will not compromise tumor resection and if negative margins can be obtained. The kidney with the lower tumor burden is addressed first. If complete excision of tumor from this kidney can be performed leaving a viable and functioning kidney, then surgery of the contralateral kidney with more extensive

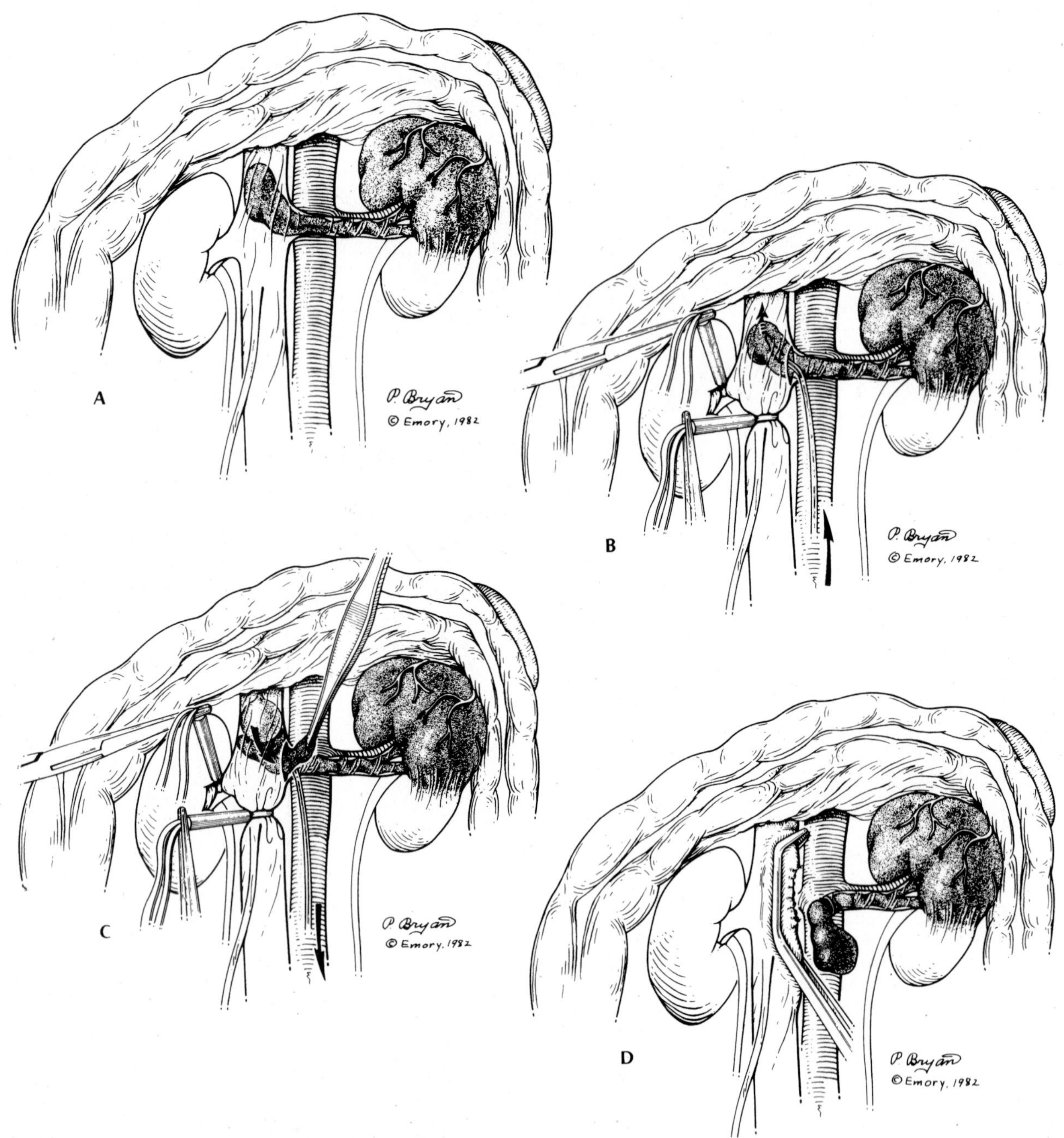


**FIGURE 96.3** Surgical technique to manage tumor extension through the renal vein. **A:** Tumor extension into the vena cava (limited to the infrahepatic level). **B:** After exposure of the vessels, the infrarenal vena cava and contralateral renal vein are controlled with vessel loops and the vena cava is incised vertically at the intersection with the renal vein. **C:** A Fogarty catheter is passed superior to the tumor thrombus and the balloon is inflated. **D:** The vena cava is flushed of air and a Satinsky clamp is placed to allow closure of the cavotomy.

tumor involvement is done. Enucleation of the tumor may be considered in lieu of a formal partial nephrectomy. This will usually be considered for large centrally located tumors where removal of a margin of renal tissue would compromise the vascular supply to the kidney. Even when very large bilateral masses remain after initial chemotherapy, a high percentage of children can be successfully managed with renal-sparing surgery (14). It is easy to underestimate the amount of renal parenchyma that can be salvaged due to compression by the tumor; therefore, renal-sparing surgery should be entertained in all patients.

## POSTOPERATIVE CARE

All clinical trials for children with Wilms tumor strive to tailor treatment to individual risks for tumor recurrence and reduce the overall morbidity of treatment. The latter will allow

**TABLE 96.2**

**RECOMMENDED THERAPY ON CHILDREN'S ONCOLOGY GROUP PROTOCOLS**

| Stage/Histology | Radiotherapy | Chemotherapy |
|---|---|---|
| Stage I FHWT <2 y, <550 g | None | None |
| Stage 1 FHWT, >2 y or >550g | None | Regimen EE-4A |
| Stage II FHWT | None | Regimen EE-4A |
| Stage I or II FHWT and LOH 1p, 16q | None | Regimen DD-4A |
| Stage III FHWT, no LOH 1p, 16q | Yes | Regimen DD-4A |
| Stage I–III focal AHWT | Yes | Regimen DD-4A |
| Stage I diffuse AHWT | Yes | Regimen DD-4A |
| Stage III or IV FHWT and LOH 1p, 16q | Yes | Regimen M |
| Stage IV FHWT pulmonary metastases | | |
| Lesions resected at diagnosis | Yes | Regimen DD-4A |
| Lesions resolve after 6 weeks chemo | None | Regimen DD-4A |
| Lesions persist after 6 weeks chemo | Yes | Regimen M |
| Stage IV FHWT nonpulmonary metastases | Yes | Regimen M |
| Stage II or III diffuse AHWT | Yes | Regimen UH-1 |
| Stage IV diffuse AHWT (no measurable disease) | Yes | Regimen UH-1 |
| Stage IV focal AHWT | Yes | Regimen UH-1 |
| Stage I CCSK | None | Regimen I |
| Stage II or III CCSK | Yes | Regimen I |
| Stage IV CCSK | Yes | Regimen UH-1 |
| Stage I–III MRT | Yes | Regimen UH-1 |
| Stage IV MRT | Yes | Regimen UH-2 |
| Stage IV AHWT (measurable disease) | Yes | Regimen UH-2 |

Regimen EE-4A: Pulse-intensive AMD plus VCR (18 weeks)
Regimen DD-4A: Pulse-intensive AMD, VCR, and DOX (24 weeks)
Regimen M: VCR, AMD, DOX, alternating with CYCLO and ETOP (24 weeks)
Regimen UH-1: CYCLO, carboplatin, ETOP alternating with VCR, DOX, CYCLO (30 weeks)
Regimen I: VCR, DOX, CYCLO alternating with CYCLO, ETOP (24 weeks)
Regimen UH-2: VCR, DOX, CYCLO alternating with CYCLO, carboplatin, ETOP and VCR, irinotecan (30 weeks)
FHWT, favorable-histology Wilms tumor; LOH, loss of heterozygosity; AHWT, anaplastic-histology Wilms tumor; CCSK, clear cell sarcoma of the kidney; MRT, malignant rhabdoid tumor of the kidney; AMD, dactinomycin; VCR, vincristine; DOX, doxorubicin; CYCLO, cyclophosphamide; ETOP, etoposide.

clinicians to reduce treatment-related side effects. Current treatment recommendations of the COG are listed in Table 96.2 (3,15). All renal tumors are eligible for enrollment in COG protocols, including renal cell carcinoma and congenital mesoblastic nephroma.

There are several study arms grouped by risk for recurrence (very low, low, standard, and high). The COG will again examine the role of surgery-only treatment for patients with stage I FHWT weighing <550 g and age <2 years. Children with stage I or II FHWT and LOH of 1p and 16q will undergo treatment with vincristine (VCR), dactinomycin (AMD), and doxorubicin (DOX) without radiotherapy. Patients with stage III FHWT disease without LOH of 1p and 16q are treated with VCR, AMD, and DOX and irradiation of the flank or abdomen. The COG will evaluate a response-based approach for management of children with pulmonary metastases. Those with resolution of the pulmonary lesions on chest CT after 6 weeks of chemotherapy will not be given whole-lung irradiation and will be treated with VCR, AMD, and DOX. Patients who do not have resolution of the pulmonary lesions by week 6 will receive more intensive chemotherapy and pulmonary irradiation. Children with stage I to III focal anaplastic histology Wilms tumor (AHWT) and stage I diffuse AHWT are treated with AMD, VCR, DOX, and abdominal irradiation. Patients with stage II, III or IV (no measurable disease) diffuse AHWT, stage IV focal AHWT, stage IV clear cell sarcoma, and stage I to III malignant rhabdoid tumor will be treated with a new chemotherapy regimen to try to improve overall survival.

# OUTCOMES

## Complications

The most common intraoperative complication of nephrectomy for Wilms tumor is bleeding. Major vascular injuries and injury to other organs are less frequent. Following surgery the most common complication is small bowel obstruction, which occurs in about 5% of patients. The surgical complication rate of nephrectomy for Wilms tumor has declined over the past three decades.

Preoperative chemotherapy may influence surgical complication rates by producing tumor shrinkage. In a report from SIOP, nephrectomy performed after 4 or 8 weeks of chemotherapy was associated with an overall surgical complication rate of 5% (16). A prospective comparison of complications in patients enrolled in the NWTS-5 and the SIOP-93-01 trials demonstrated that the overall complication rate for the SIOP patients was 6.4% compared to 9.8% in NWTS-5 patients (17). There was a much lower incidence of intraoperative tumor spill in the SIOP patients (2.2%) than the NWST-5 ones (15.3%).

A mortality rate of 0.5% related to surgical complications was reported from NWTS-3. However, a higher intraoperative mortality rate of 1.5% has been reported from other centers. The latter may reflect that intraoperative deaths may not be reported to the cooperative groups since study enrollment occurs after surgery. Factors that have been associated with an increased risk for surgical complications are higher tumor stage, tumor size >10 cm, incorrect preoperative diagnosis, thoracoabdominal incision, intracaval tumor extension, and resection of other visceral organs.

## Results

The overall prognosis for children with FHWT is excellent as a result of multimodal therapy. Common sites of recurrence are the lungs, liver, and renal fossa. Tumor histology and clinical stage are the most important predictors of outcome. There is an increased risk for local recurrence in the setting of unfavorable histology and intraoperative tumor rupture (11). Omission of lymph node biopsy also correlates with recurrence and is attributed to understaging. Preventing local recurrence is important as the survival after abdominal recurrence is poor. Current trials continue to refine chemotherapeutic regimens to improve survival, in particular for higher-risk populations with unfavorable histology. The use of biological factors to further stratify patients for therapy may further advance survival and minimize late effects of treatment.

## *References*

1. Breslow N, Olshan A, Beckwith JB, et al. Ethnic variation in the incidence, diagnosis, prognosis, and follow-up of children with Wilms' tumor. *J Natl Cancer Inst* 1994;86:49–51.
2. Dome JS, Coppes JM. Recent advances in Wilms tumor genetics. *Curr Opin Pediatr* 2002;14:5–11.
3. Ehrlich PF. Wilms tumor: progress and considerations for the surgeon. *Surg Oncol* 2007;16:157–171.
4. Grundy PE, Breslow NE, Li S, et al. Loss of heterozygosity for chromosomes 1p and 16q is an adverse prognostic factor in favorable histology Wilms tumor: a report from the National Wilms Tumor Study Group. *J Clin Oncol* 2005;23:7312–7321.
5. Beckwith JB. Nephrogenic rests and the pathogenesis of Wilms tumor: developmental and clinical considerations. *Am J Med Genet* 1998;79: 268–273.
6. Ritchey ML, Daley S, Shamberger R, et al. Ureteral extension in childhood renal tumors: a report from the National Wilms Tumor Study Group (NWTSG). *J Pediatr Surg* 2008;43:1625–1629.
7. McNeil DE, Langer JC, Choyke P, et al. Feasibility of partial nephrectomy for Wilms' tumor in children with Beckwith-Wiedemann syndrome who have been screened with abdominal ultrasonography. *J Pediatr Surg* 2002;37:57–60.
8. Duarte RJ, Denes FT, Cristofani LM, et al. Further experience with laparoscopic nephrectomy for Wilms' tumour after chemotherapy. *BJU Intl* 2006;98:155–159.
9. Tournade MF, Com-Nougue C, Voute PA, et al. Results of the Sixth International Society of Pediatric Oncology Wilms' Tumor Trial and Study: a risk-adapted therapeutic approach in Wilms' tumor. *J Clin Oncol* 1993; 11:1014–1023.
10. Ritchey ML, Shamberger RC, Hamilton T, et al. Fate of bilateral renal lesions missed on preoperative imaging: a report from the National Wilms Tumor Study Group. *J Urol* 2005;174:1519–1521.
11. Shamberger RC, Guthrie KA, Ritchey ML, et al. Surgery-related factors and local recurrence of Wilms' tumor in National Wilms' Tumor Study 4. *Ann Surg* 1999;229:292–297.
12. Horwitz JR, Ritchey ML, Moksness J, et al. Renal salvage procedures in patients with synchronous bilateral Wilms' tumors: a report from the National Wilms' Tumor Study Group. *J Pediatr Surg* 1996;31:1020–1025.
13. Breslow NE, Collins AJ, Ritchey ML, et al. End-stage renal disease in patients with Wilms tumor: results from the National Wilms Tumor Study Group and the United States Renal Data System. *J Urol* 2005;174: 1972–1975.
14. Davidoff AM, Giel DW, Jones DP, et al. The feasibility and outcome of nephron-sparing surgery for children with bilateral Wilms tumor. *Cancer* 2008;112:2060–2070.
15. Dome JS, Cotton CA, Perlman EJ, et al. Treatment of anaplastic histology Wilms' tumor: results from the fifth National Wilms' Tumor Study. *J Clin Oncol* 2006;24:2352–2358.
16. Godzinski J, Tournade MF, deKraker J, et al. Rarity of surgical complications after postchemotherapy nephrectomy for nephroblastoma. Experience of the International Society of Paediatric Oncology—Trial and Study "SIOP-9." *Eur J Pediatr Surg* 1998;8:83–86.
17. Ritchey ML, Godzinski J, Shamberger RC, et al. Surgical complications following nephrectomy for Wilms tumor: prospective study from the National Wilms Tumor Study Group (NWTSG) and the International Society of Pediatric Oncology (SIOP). Unpublished manuscript.

# CHAPTER 97 ■ RENAL FUSION AND ECTOPIA

ROSS M. DECTER

Abnormalities of renal position and fusion predispose to infection, hydronephrosis, stone disease, and, in some instances, neoplasia. Although clinical problems associated with these anomalies present infrequently in urological practice, an understanding of the deviations from standard urological techniques required to address them is important.

The ureteral bud branches from the wolffian duct and extends toward the metanephric blastema during the fourth and fifth weeks of gestation. The ureteral bud induces the metanephric blastema to form the functioning kidney. The exact mechanism of renal ascent is not known, but during normal development the kidneys ascend and rotate. The renal

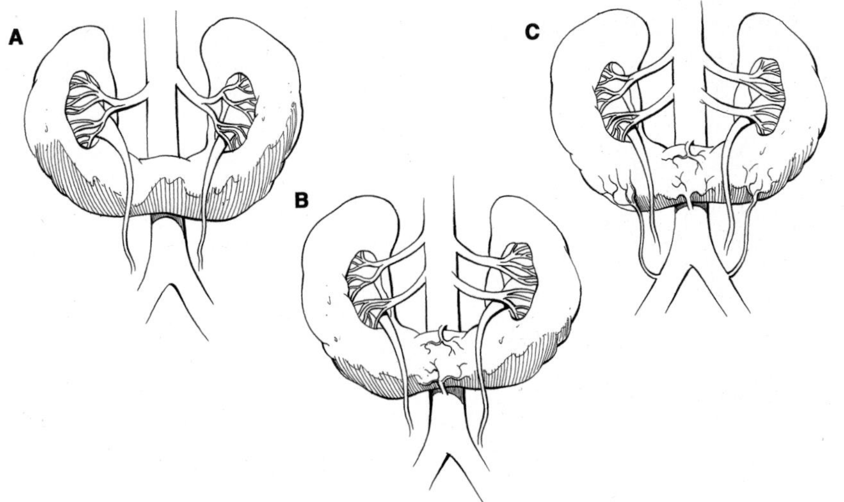


FIGURE 97.1 Three common variants of blood supply in horseshoe kidney. **A:** Single renal arteries arising from the aorta. **B:** Multiple aortic arteries. **C:** Multiple aortic and iliac arteries.

pelvis rotates from its initial anterior position 90 degrees toward the midline until it reaches its final medial position. Migration and rotation occur simultaneously between the fourth and eighth or ninth weeks of gestation. The blood supply to the kidney is derived from successively higher levels of the aorta and its branches during ascent.

The most common anomaly of renal position is malrotation: incomplete rotation of the kidney to its final position. The renal pelvis in a malrotated kidney in general lies anterior to the parenchyma, as opposed to its normal medial location. Simple malrotation of a normally positioned kidney is often an incidental finding. The pyelocaliceal systems of malrotated kidneys are morphologically abnormal, but functionally they usually drain without impairment. Malrotation occurs occasionally in orthotopically positioned kidneys, and it is commonly observed in ectopic kidneys.

Close approximation of the two proliferating renal blastemas prior to significant ascent is a normal embryological finding (1). If there is any disturbance of separation of the closely approximated renal blastemas, fusion anomalies of the kidneys may develop.

The most common fusion anomaly is the horseshoe kidney. The horseshoe kidney in general ascends until the upper border of the isthmus is at the level of the inferior mesenteric artery. Horseshoe kidney occurs in 1 in 400 to 1 in 1,800 births (2). There is a male predominance for the condition (3). The fusion in horseshoe kidney almost always occurs at the lower poles; cases of upper pole fusion are recorded rarely (3). The isthmus of the horseshoe kidney lies just below the inferior mesenteric artery at the L4 vertebral level. The blood supply to these kidneys is variable (Fig. 97.1).

Crossed–fused ectopia is the second most common fusion anomaly. This abnormality occurs when the developing kidney crosses from one side to the other during its ascent or when the ureteral bud from one side crosses to the contralateral side and induces abnormal development of that metanephric blastema. Crossed ectopia with fusion may occur in a variety of forms (Fig. 97.2). Although crossed ectopia occurs most frequently with fusion, the anomaly may occur without fusion (Fig. 97.3).

An ectopic kidney lies outside of the normal position in the renal fossa. The kidney, in simple ectopia, in general lies in the ipsilateral retroperitoneal space at a position that is lower than normal (Fig. 97.4). In crossed ectopia, the kidney crosses the midline and is frequently fused to its contralateral mate. The autopsy incidence of renal ectopia is about 1 in 1,000 cases, and the condition often is totally asymptomatic (4). Reviews of renal ectopia show that the left kidney is affected slightly more frequently than the right. Ectopic kidneys occur bilaterally around 10% of the time, and the most common position of the ectopic kidney is in the pelvis. Pelvic ectopia was reported in about 55% of patients in one series of ectopic kidneys; crossed–fused ectopia occurred in 27%; lumbar ectopia occurred in 12%; non–crossed–fused ectopia occurred in 5% of patients; and a thoracic kidney was recorded only 1% of the time (4). Rarely, a solitary pelvic kidney occurs. This kidney suffers the risk of injury during pelvic surgical procedures and on occasion has been reported as an unusual cause of giant hydronephrosis.

Ectopic kidneys are smaller than their orthotopically positioned mates (5). The blood supply to the pelvic kidney, the most common of the ectopic kidneys, is variable. The arterial supply may arise from the distal aorta or bifurcation, the ipsilateral common iliac, or the hypogastric vessels. In general, the lower the kidney is in its pelvic location, the greater the likelihood that multiple arterial vessels will supply it (6).

# DIAGNOSIS

## Horseshoe Kidney

Historically, 25% to 33% of patients with horseshoe kidneys who survived beyond the newborn period were asymptomatic (3). The advent of prenatal ultrasound screening makes it likely that an even larger proportion of these kidneys are asymptomatic. Patients with symptoms typically present with urinary tract infections (about 50% of the time), an abdominal mass, hematuria, or abdominal pain (approximately 10% each).

The initial diagnostical evaluation in children is usually a renal ultrasound (RUS), and many patients subsequently have intravenous pyelography (IVP) or computed axial tomography (CT). Many adults have an IVP as their initial study. The intravenous pyelographic features of the horseshoe kidney are typical. The renal axis is abnormal, being either vertically

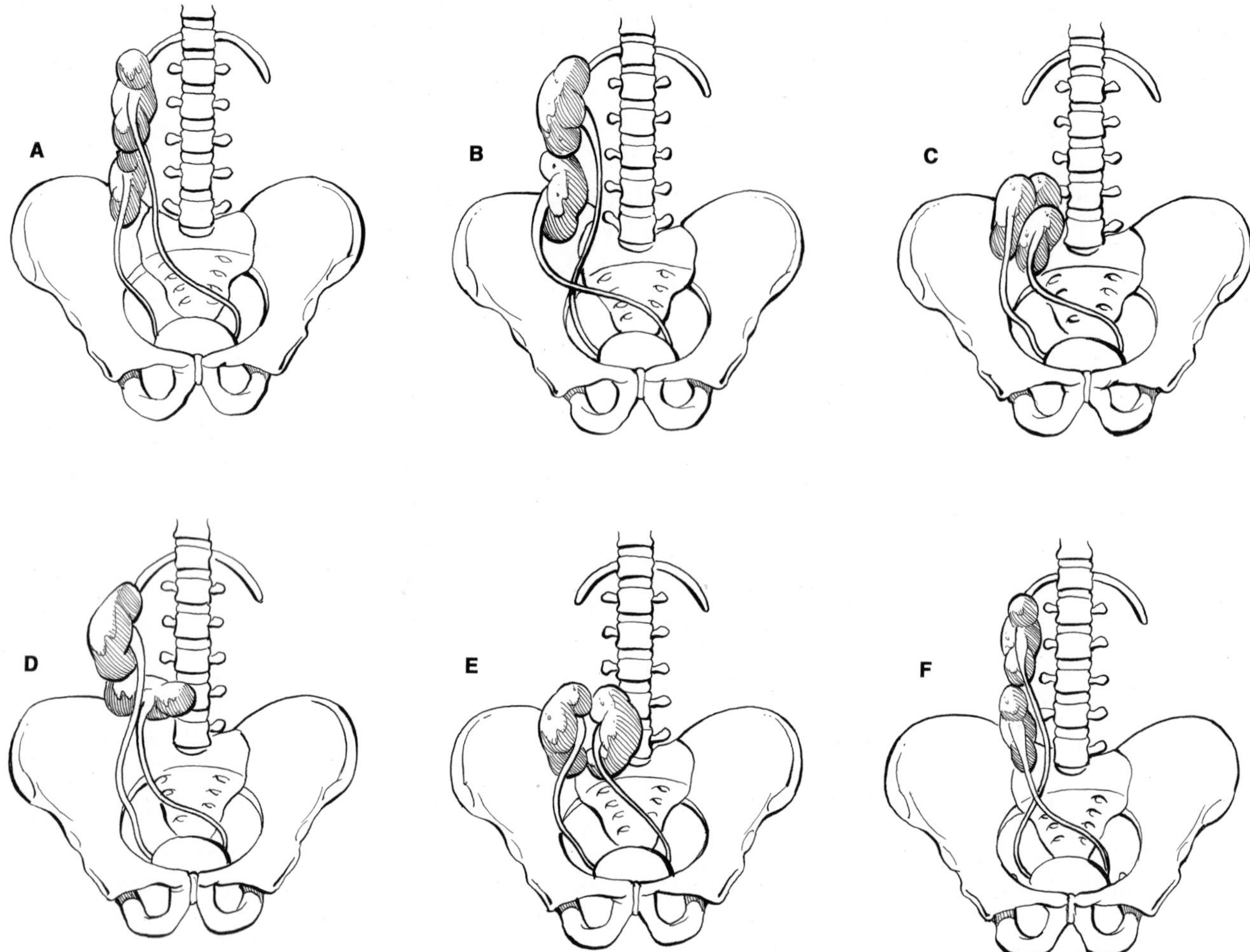


FIGURE 97.2 Six types of crossed renal ectopia with fusion. **A:** Ectopic kidney superior. **B:** Sigmoid or S-shaped kidney. **C:** Lump kidney. **D:** L-shaped kidney. **E:** Disk kidney. **F:** Ectopic kidney inferior. (Modified from McDonald JH, McClellan DS. Crossed renal ectopia. *Am J Surg* 1957;93:995.)

orientated or tilted laterally. The renal pelves tend to be located anteriorly and the ureters course ventral to the isthmus. The lower calices are oriented caudally or even medially as opposed to laterally. Kidneys with fusion anomalies are subject to a high incidence of vesicoureteral reflux, variably reported between 20% and 50%. Voiding cystourethrography (VCUG) is therefore mandated during the evaluation of children with a horseshoe kidney.

The diagnosis of a ureteropelvic junction (UPJ) obstruction in a horseshoe kidney is straightforward when the patient's symptoms lead to a RUS, IVP, or CT that reveals significant pyelocaliectasis. In other instances, with less severe dilation, and especially when there is coexistent stone disease, we find the diuretic renal scan a valuable adjunct in assessing the drainage of these systems and assessing whether the hydronephrosis is functionally significant.

### Ectopic Kidney

Patients with a symptomatic ectopic kidney frequently present with a urinary tract infection, or the ectopic kidney is discovered in the evaluation of abdominal pain. The workup of a palpable abdominal mass and the discovery of the abnormal renal position during the evaluation of other anomalies each account for the diagnosis in about 20% of cases. Hematuria, incontinence, renal insufficiency, and nephrolithiasis are less common presenting complaints. It is important to emphasize that the majority of patients with ectopic kidneys are asymptomatic.

The evaluation in children is usually by RUS, while older patients will in general have an IVP or CT scan. The ectopic kidney can be difficult to detect on the IVP because the pyelocaliceal system often overlies the bony pelvis. Functional evaluation of the ectopically positioned kidney is routinely performed with a renal scan. Ectopic kidneys have a high incidence of associated vesicoureteral reflux, so a VCUG should be a routine part of the evaluation of these patients.

## INDICATIONS FOR SURGERY

The indications for surgical intervention in the ectopic or horseshoe kidney are similar to those in a normally positioned kidney. Pyeloplasty is required in patients with symptomatic UPJ obstruction or when the evaluation suggests that the abnormality at the UPJ may affect ultimate renal function. Symptomatic stone disease needs to be addressed using open, endoscopic, or extracorporeal techniques. If the evaluation

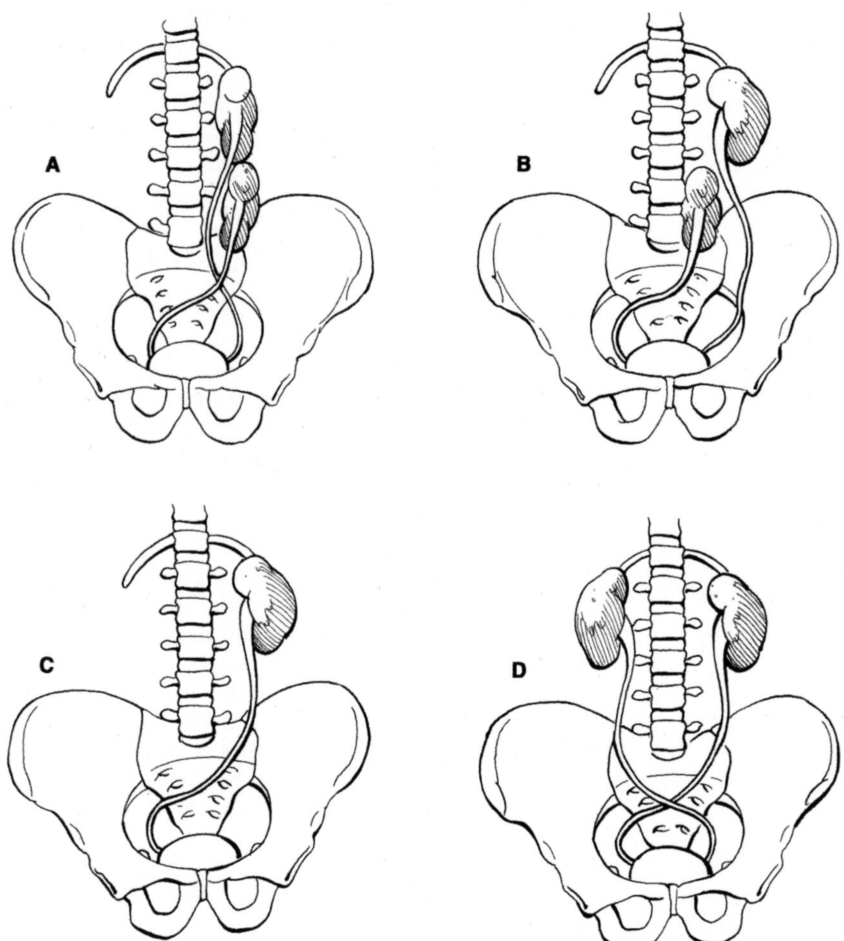


FIGURE 97.3 Types of crossed renal ectopia. **A:** Fused. **B:** Nonfused. **C:** Solitary. **D:** Bilateral. (Modified from McDonald JH, McClellan DS. Crossed renal ectopia. *Am J Surg* 1957;93:995.)

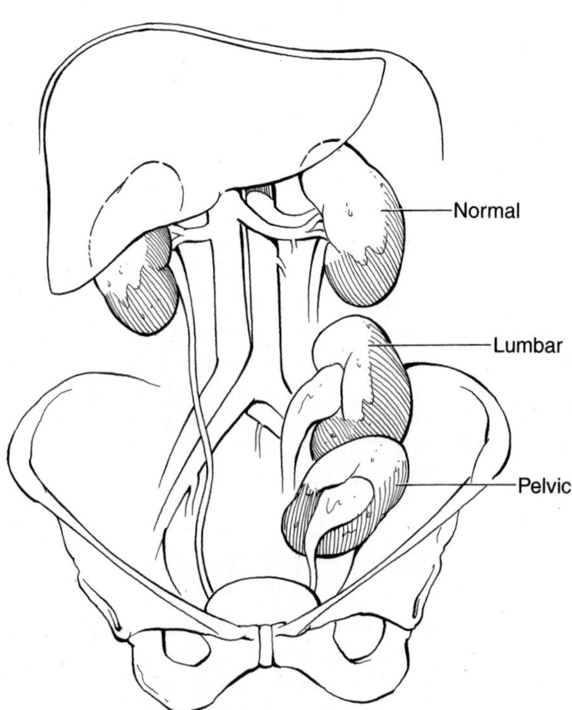


FIGURE 97.4 Location of lumbar and pelvic ectopically positioned kidneys in relation to the normally positioned kidney.

of infections in a horseshoe kidney reveals vesicoureteral reflux, operative management, either subureteral injection of Deflux or ureteral reimplantation, may be mandated if the reflux is of high grade, if it persists, or if prophylaxis fails to prevent infection.

## ALTERNATIVE THERAPY

The alternative to surgical intervention for reflux is nonoperative management, usually consisting of observation either with or without antibiotic prophylaxis.

Surgery is the only viable option for patients with significant UPJ obstruction, significant stones, and tumors.

Endopyelotomy has been utilized to treat UPJ obstruction in horseshoe kidneys. The initial results of endopyelotomy performed in adults by experienced surgeons are encouraging; however, we currently prefer pyeloplasty as the initial procedure for UPJ obstructions in children.

## SURGICAL TECHNIQUE

### Pyeloplasty

Pyeloplasty is the most common open procedure performed on the horseshoe kidney. Division of the isthmus with nephropexy had been considered to be an important part of the procedure, but recent experience suggests that isthmus division or symphysiotomy is rarely necessary in the correction of UPJ obstruction. Pyeloplasty may be performed either open or laparoscopically. Laparoscopic procedures can be accomplished with or without robotic assistance. Although laparoscopic pyeloplasty is becoming more widely practiced, we still favor open surgery in abnormally positioned kidneys.

The surgical exposure of the horseshoe kidney can be achieved through a midline transperitoneal, anteriorly positioned flank extraperitoneal, or transverse transperitoneal approach. We prefer the transverse transperitoneal exposure as it seems to provide the widest exposure with a cosmetically acceptable scar. We perform a retrograde ureteropyelogram at the time of pyeloplasty so we can position the incision accurately. The incision generally extends from the anterior axillary line on the affected side to the midline several centimeters below the umbilicus. It can be extended laterally in either direction if necessary. For a right-sided UPJ obstruction, the posterior peritoneum may be incised medial to the inferior mesenteric, then inferior and laterally along the small bowel mesentery around the cecum, and up along the line of Toldt. The small bowel and cecum can then be reflected upward out of the operative field and packed in the upper abdomen. For a left-sided UPJ obstruction, the sigmoid colon may be mobilized if necessary to afford better exposure. Exposure is maintained with a ring retractor.

Repair of UPJ obstruction in the horseshoe kidney can be performed by a Foley Y–V-plasty or a dismembered pyeloplasty. Although the Foley Y–V repair is nicely suited to the typical high-insertion obstruction seen in horseshoe kidneys (Fig. 97.5D), we prefer the dismembered technique because it provides more flexibility. During the conduct of the pyeloplasty, care must be taken to avoid inadvertent division of small vessels to the parenchyma and excessive dissection of the ureter or pelvis. As much adventitial tissue is left on the ureter as possible, and no vessels to the ureter are sacrificed unless their division is necessary to provide for adequate mobilization.

After the proximal ureter and renal pelvis are adequately exposed using sharp dissection, two stay stitches of 5-0 chromic are positioned in the ureter just below the UPJ (Fig. 97.5). The ureter is divided between these stitches and carefully mobilized. A pelvic flap is then created by orienting a wide-based inverted-V-shaped incision on the renal pelvis, with the apex of the inverted V at the UPJ. The flap is designed such that it will provide a dependent portion of pelvis for the anastomosis. It is important that the base of the V be wide to avoid ischemia of the flap. The flap is opened with tenotomy scissors and the tip is trimmed minimally to smooth the point of the V. The ureter is then positioned so the length and position of the spatulation can be judged. The spatulation is positioned on the posterior aspect of the ureter using Potts scissors such that the ureter will not be twisted when it is laid on the dependent pelvic flap. It is critical that the flap and the spatulated ureter are approximated in a tension-free fashion. If the repair is performed under tension, an anastomotic stricture may result. It is also important that the upper ureter or anastomosis are not compressed by any of the renal vessels, as they may obstruct the repair (7). The anastomosis and dissection are performed with the aid of 2.5× optical magnification. We perform the anastomosis using 7-0 Vicryl in younger children and 6-0 Vicryl in adolescents.

The fact that the ureter is dismembered and freely mobile allows the surgeon to position it so that the ureteral spatulation can extend into a relatively wide portion of the ureter and simultaneously the ureter can be oriented to avoid torsion or redundancy that might kink the ureter distal to the repair. The anastomosis in the dismembered pyeloplasty seems technically easier than the Foley Y–V because the ureter is not fixed at two points.

We begin the anastomosis at the heel, suturing the most dependent portion of the V-shaped incision to the apex of the ureteral spatulation. The initial portion of the anastomosis is performed using interrupted sutures, in general one at the apex and two on either side of the apex. Each stitch must be precisely positioned to avoid postoperative leakage and/or compromise of the lumen. After the apex is anastomosed, the remainder of the pyeloplasty is performed using a running locking 7-0 Vicryl suture up one side of the spatulated ureter and then up the other side. Prior to complete closure, the patency of the anastomosis is tested by passing a 5Fr and 8Fr feeding tube through the repair. No stent or diversion is in general employed in children. A Penrose drain is positioned near the anastomosis and made to exit through a separate stab wound. The abdominal wall closure is performed using running 3-0 or larger PDS. We close the skin with a subcuticular pull-out stitch of 3-0 Prolene. Most children are discharged the day after surgery. The skin suture is removed between 6 and 8 days postoperatively and the drain is removed at that time if drainage is minimal.

## Ureterocalicostomy

A ureterocalicostomy is usually performed to salvage a failed prior pyeloplasty, but it should be considered as the primary procedure for UPJ obstruction when there is a small intrarenal pelvis or in other instances with significant lower-pole caliectasis and thin overlying parenchyma (7) (Fig. 97.6). The ureter is carefully separated from the pelvis as described above, and if feasible a pyelotomy is performed. We find that a finger inserted into the open renal pelvis and positioned in the lower pole calyx aids in the dissection. The parenchyma over the dilated lower-pole calyx is incised with electrocautery; the capsule is incised and the parenchyma resected to allow adequate exposure of the calyx. Hemostasis is achieved using cautery and/or sutures of 4-0 chromic through the edge of the resected parenchyma. The ureter is spatulated and the anastomosis between the ureter and the opened calyx is performed as described in the figure. We divert the urine by using a nephrostomy tube (a 10Fr or 12Fr Malecot catheter) and either a ureteral stent (usually a 5Fr feeding tube) or a double-J stent. A ureterocalicostomy as it would appear in a horseshoe kidney is shown in Figure 97.7.

## Surgery for Tumors

Renal cell carcinoma and renal pelvic tumors are reported in horseshoe kidneys (12). Wilms tumor occurring in a horseshoe kidney represented 0.48% of tumors in the National Wilms Tumor Study; this incidence is about twice that expected in the general population (8). When Wilms tumor involves a horseshoe

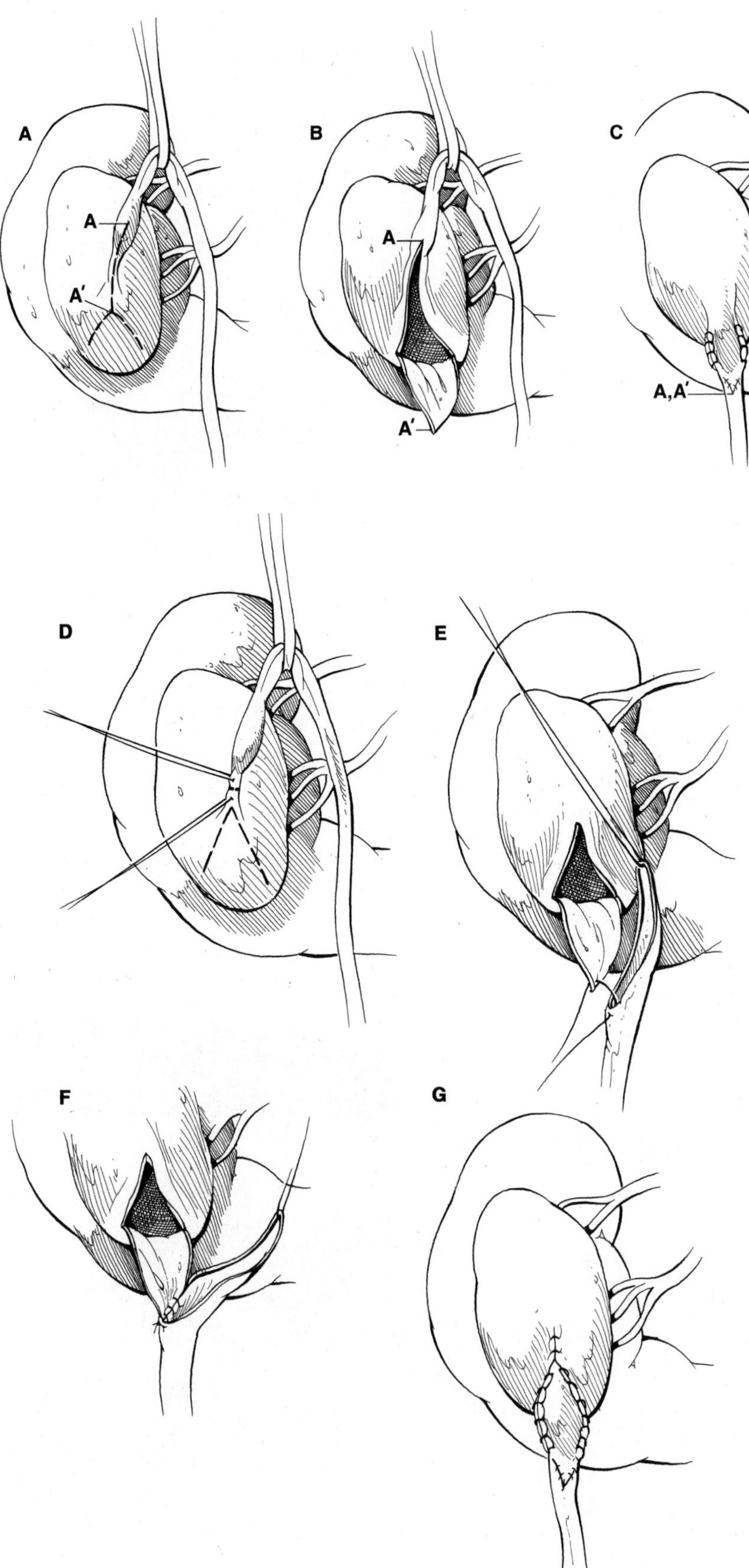


FIGURE 97.5 Pyeloplasty techniques. **A–C:** The Foley Y–V technique. **A:** Broken lines indicate inverted-Y–shaped incision. Stay sutures of 5-0 chromic help define the margins of the incision. **B:** *A'* indicates the tip of the renal pelvic flap. *A* indicates the inferior margin of the ureteral incision. **C:** *A* and *A'* are sutured together with 7-0 Vicryl; as the remainder of the repair is closed, a widely patent dependent anastomosis is created. **D–G:** The dismembered technique. **D:** The ureter is divided distal to the ureteropelvic junction after stay stitches are positioned. The inverted V, indicating the outline of the pelvic incision, is indicated by a broken line. **E:** The ureter has been spatulated after the narrowed segment is excised and the pelvic flap developed. The initial stitch of 7-0 Vicryl is positioned to approximate the most dependent portion of the pelvic flap to the heel of the ureteral spatulation. **F:** Interrupted sutures around the heel are completed. **G:** The running locking sutures extending between the spatulated ureter and pelvis are completed, creating a widely patent anastomosis.

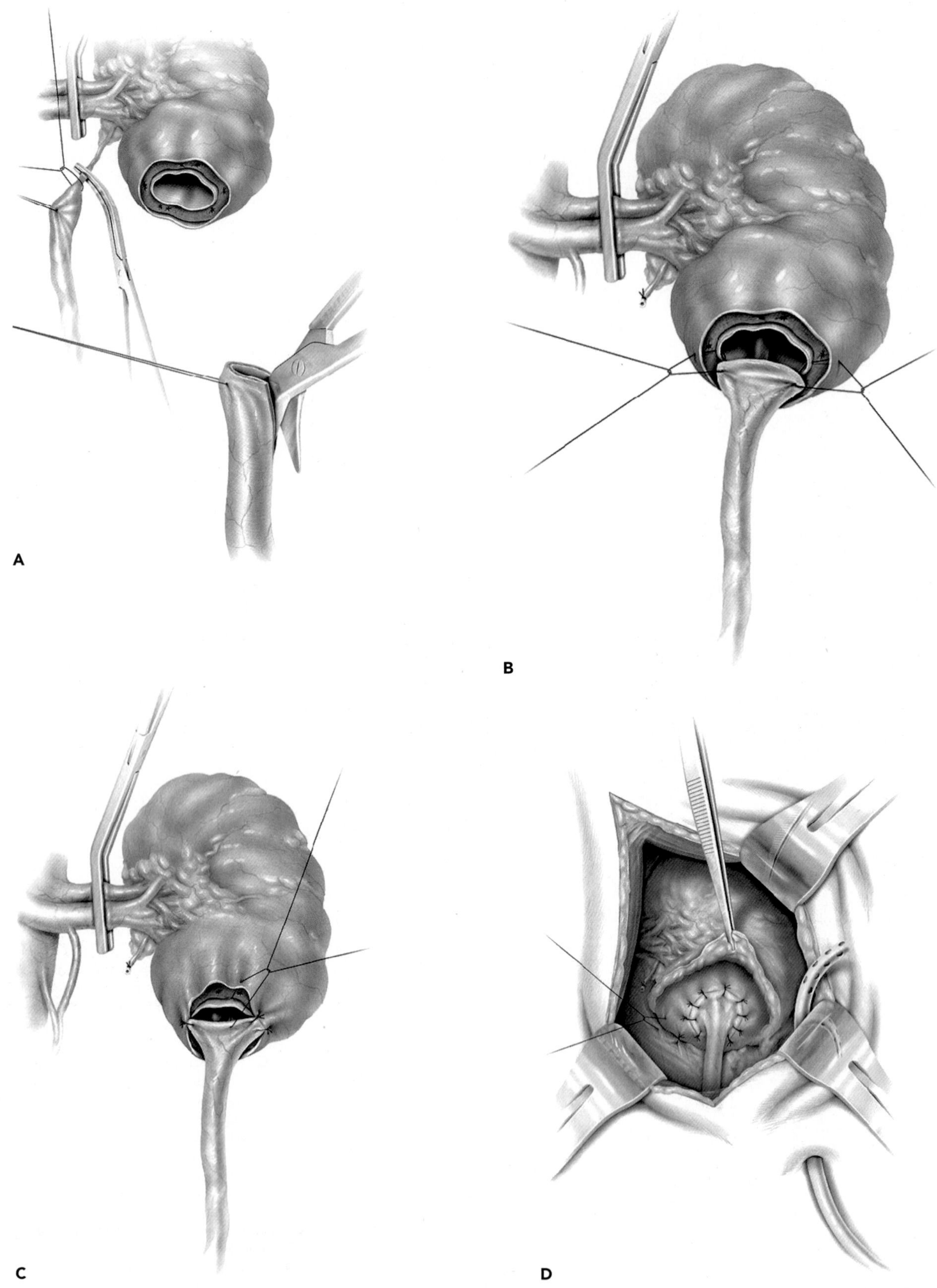


FIGURE 97.6 Ureterocalicostomy for correction of ureteropelvic obstruction after a prior failed pyeloplasty. **A:** The scarred ureter is divided and spatulated widely. Thin cortex over the dilated lower pole calyx has been excised and hemostasis achieved. **B:** The spatulated ureter is anastomosed to the open lower-pole calyx. The sutures of 4-0 chromic catch the capsule, calyx, and ureter (the end of a double-J stent is visualized in the pelvis). **C:** The anastomosis is completed with interrupted sutures. A nephrostomy tube (not visualized) should be used. The surgeon may irrigate through the nephrostomy tube to ensure a watertight repair. **D:** Place one or two nephropexy sutures to obviate kinking of the repair. Replace the perirenal fat and place a perinephric drain. (Modified from Steffens J, Humke U, Haben B, et al. Open ureterocalycostomy. *BJU Int* 2008;101(3):397–407.)

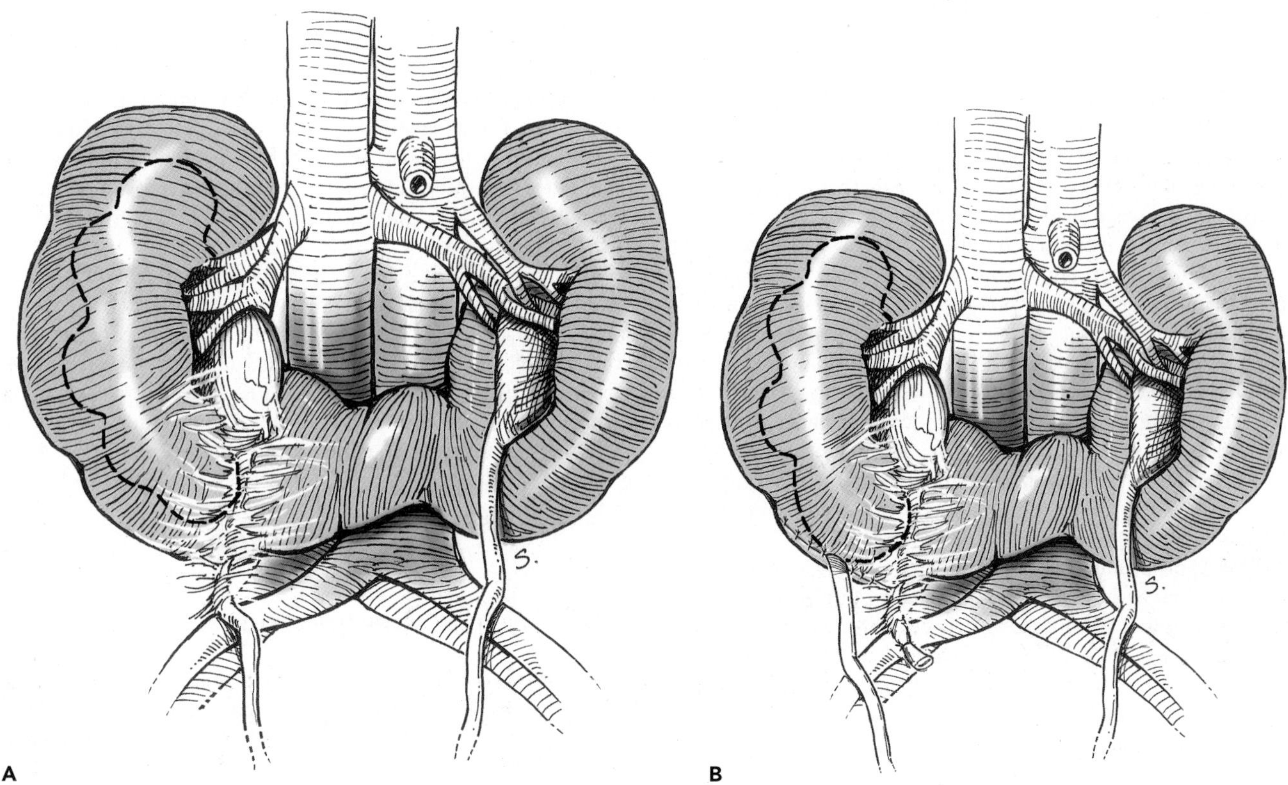


FIGURE 97.7 **A:** Horseshoe kidney with prior failed pyeloplasty; note the dilated intrarenal collecting system. **B:** After ureterocalicostomy, dependent drainage has been achieved. (Modified from Kay R. Ureterocalicostomy as a salvage procedure. *Urol Times* 2001;April:34.)

kidney, the involved portion of the kidney and isthmus are generally resected in the course of removal of the tumor. If the tumor occurs in the isthmus, some authors have recommended bilateral lower-pole heminephrectomy. If the Wilms tumor is bilateral at presentation, management is the same as for bilateral Wilms tumors in orthotopically positioned kidneys.

Tumor surgery of the horseshoe kidney deserves special mention because excision of the involved kidney will necessitate division of the isthmus. If the isthmus is composed of a band of fibrous tissue, it can be readily divided using cautery; however, if it is functioning parenchyma, it must be carefully addressed to avoid excessive blood loss and necrosis of the remaining parenchyma, with the risk of secondary bleed and urinary fistula. The area must be carefully dissected and arteries to the isthmus sequentially occluded with bulldog clamps to assess the line of demarcation. Once this line is established, the capsule is divided sharply and the parenchyma divided. Bleeding from the cut parenchyma is controlled with 4-0 chromic sutures. Any exposed calices are closed with running locking 4-0 or 5-0 chromic sutures, and the capsule and parenchyma are closed with carefully positioned horizontal mattress sutures of 2-0 chromic (Fig. 97.8).

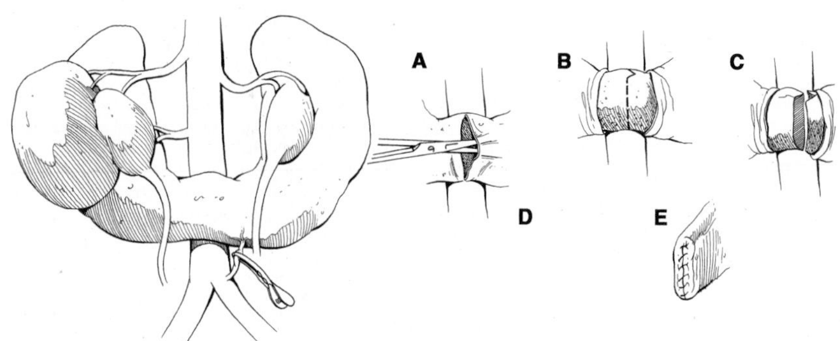


FIGURE 97.8 Division of the isthmus of a horseshoe kidney with a right-sided renal tumor. The isthmus blood supply is from the left iliac. **A:** After identification of the line of demarcation, an incision is made around the capsule of the isthmus. **B:** The capsule is peeled back. **C:** The parenchyma of the isthmus is transected in a wedge fashion to facilitate closure. **D:** Horizontal mattress sutures of absorbable 2-0 material are used to close the parenchyma for hemostasis. **E:** The capsule is closed over the parenchyma with a continuous absorbable suture.

## Stone Surgery in the Horseshoe Kidney

Pyelolithotomy had been utilized in past decades to clear calculi from horseshoe kidneys, but currently, percutaneous and extracorporeal techniques are employed almost exclusively. Extracorporeal shock-wave lithotripsy (ESWL) in the horseshoe kidney has not enjoyed the success rate that it provides in orthotopically positioned kidneys. Most series note the requirement for an increased number of shocks, an increased need for retreatment, and a somewhat decreased stone clearance rate in horseshoe kidneys compared to stones in normally positioned kidneys. One series recorded a 73% stone-free rate in horseshoe kidneys using ESWL after multiple treatments (9). One of the reasons for difficulties treating stones with ESWL is that the anterior position of the stone makes it harder to position the stone at the F2 focus; often, the surgeon will have to employ the blast path to try to fragment the stone. Some investigators have used prone positioning to overcome this problem.

After appropriate CT planning, percutaneous access to the horseshoe kidney is best achieved using an upper-pole posterior calyx. Stones in any calyx can be managed though this access, although often a long nephroscope and flexible instrumentation are required (10,11). Reports comparing ESWL of stones in horseshoe kidneys to percutaneous nephrostolithotomy conclude that the percutaneous technique provides superior stone clearance rates (10).

When calculus disease complicates obstruction of the UPJ in a horseshoe kidney, the stone is removed at the time of pyeloplasty. In these instances, there may be considerably more reaction around the pelvis and ureter, so the use of a nephrostomy tube and ureteral stent is prudent. An antegrade study can be performed 10 to 12 days postoperatively prior to nephrostomy tube removal to confirm drainage through the UPJ and integrity of the repair.

## Surgical Options for the Ectopic Kidney

The ectopic kidney can be affected by any of the processes that occur in a normally positioned kidney. Overall, the evaluation and surgical management of these conditions will follow the lines of those discussed with horseshoe kidney. Reflux, if it mandates operative treatment, is addressed by a standard ureteral reimplantation or, alternatively, subureteral injection of a bulking agent.

On occasion, one has to address the problem of a failed pyeloplasty in a patient who has an ectopic pelvic kidney. Ureterocalicostomy is one alternative in management of this problem; another is the use of a pyelovesicostomy. Pyelovesicostomy has been performed in renal transplant recipients after ureteral loss due to ischemia and/or rejection and has proven to be a viable salvage procedure.

# OUTCOMES

## Complications

Complications of pyeloplasty, such as prolonged urine leakage and poor anastomotic drainage, occur somewhat more frequently in horseshoe kidneys than in normal kidneys. The risk of renal ischemia caused by damage to an aberrant vessel is increased in the horseshoe or ectopically positioned kidney.

## Results

Pyeloplasty in the horseshoe kidney is in general a successful procedure. A higher rate of complications was experienced in the era when division of the isthmus was employed.

## *References*


1. Friedland GW, DeVries P. Renal ectopia and fusion: embryologic basis. *Urology* 1975;5:698–706.
2. Kolln CP, Boatman DL, Schmidt JD, et al. Horseshoe kidney: a review of 105 patients. *J Urol* 1972;107:203–204.
3. Pitts WR Jr, Muecke EC. Horseshoe kidneys: a 40-year experience. *J Urol* 1975;113:743–746.
4. Gleason PE, Kelalis PP, Husmann DA, et al. Hydronephrosis in renal ectopia: incidence, etiology and significance. *J Urol* 1994;151:1660–1661.
5. Dretler SP, Olsson C, Pfister RC. The anatomic, radiologic and clinical characteristics of the pelvic kidney: an analysis of 86 cases. *J Urol* 1971;105:623–410.
6. Dretler SP, Pfister R, Hendren WH. Extrarenal calyces in the ectopic kidney. *J Urol* 1970;103:406–410.
7. Dewan PA, Clark S, Condron S, et al. Ureterocalycostomy in the management of pelvi–ureteric junction obstruction in the horseshoe kidney. *BJU Int* 1999;94:366–368.
8. Neville H, Ritchey ML, Shamberger RC, et al. The occurrence of Wilms tumor in horseshoe kidneys: a report from the National Wilms Tumor Study Group (NWTSG). *J Pediatr Surg* 2002;37:1134–1137.
9. Locke DR, Newman RC, Steinbock GS, et al. Extracorporeal shock-wave lithotripsy in horseshoe kidneys. *Urology* 1990;35:407–411.
10. Gupta M, Lee MW. Treatment of stones associated with complex or anomalous renal anatomy. *Urol Clin North Am* 2007;34:431–441.
11. Jones DJ, Wickham JEA, Kellett MJ. Percutaneous nephrolithotomy for calculi in horseshoe kidneys. *J Urol* 1991;145:481–483.
12. Buntley D. Malignancy associated with horseshoe kidney. *Urology* 1976; VIII:146.

# CHAPTER 98 ■ TRANSURETEROURETEROSTOMY

H. GIL RUSHTON

Ureteral surgery and various conditions, including trauma, stricture, neoplasm, or a previous failed surgical procedure, can render a ureter inadequate for successful ureteroureterostomy or ureteroneocystostomy. Transureteroureterostomy (TUU), first described by Higgins (1) in the 1930s, has gained increased prominence in pediatric urology as a method to compensate for a lacking or defective distal ureter. In some cases, bridging the midureter to the contralateral ureter TUU may salvage a renal unit, especially in cases when an ipsilateral psoas hitch and/or Boari flap are insufficient to accomplish this task. In other situations, TUU can be performed as a salvage procedure following previous failed ureteral surgery (2,3). More recently, TUU has been employed in complex reconstructive procedures that entail harvesting of the distal donor ureter for alternative purposes, including augmentation ureterocystoplasty or as a continent catheterizable conduit (2).

## DIAGNOSIS

In the majority of cases in pediatric urology, TUU is employed as part of a planned reconstruction. The preoperative workup requires thorough assessment of bilateral renal function and drainage, knowledge of the anatomy of both the donor and recipient ureters, and careful evaluation of bladder function. Differential renal function and drainage are the most objectively determined by preoperative MAG-3 renal scintigraphy. Sonography can aid in determining the presence and severity of hydronephrosis. Contrast imaging with intravenous, retrograde, or antegrade pyelography may be necessary in select cases when detailed anatomic definition of the ureters is required. Contrast voiding cystography is the best modality to assess for the presence of vesicoureteral reflux, which when present provides a "free" retrograde ureteropyelogram. In cases involving children with abnormal or neuropathic bladder function, preoperative urodynamics is required to evaluate bladder capacity, compliance, and emptying.

Less commonly in children than in adults, initial recognition of a ureteral injury requiring a TUU occurs intraoperatively during resection of a tumor or during exploration for trauma. Fortunately, in the majority of these cases one can usually anticipate a normal recipient ureter and bladder.

## INDICATIONS FOR SURGERY

The primary goal of a TUU is to reestablish nonobstructive, nonrefluxing drainage of the ureter. Historically, TUU in children has been performed either to salvage a failed ureteral reimplantation or in conjunction with cutaneous ureterostomy for urinary diversion (4–6). Because TUU requires only one ureter for reimplantation, this procedure was commonly employed in the 1980s for urinary undiversion of conduits or in the construction of continent urinary reservoirs (3,7). In the majority of these cases, TUU was used simultaneously with reimplantation of the recipient ureter, many of which required tapering or tailoring, frequently with a psoas hitch and/or bladder augmentation. TUU has also been used as an adjunct to reimplant procedures complicated by an abnormal bladder, which precludes reimplantation of more than one ureter, or as a salvage procedure for failed ureteral reimplantation surgery (3). More recently, indications for TUU have been broadened to allow for harvesting the distal donor ureter to construct a continent ureteral conduit for clean intermittent catheterization or for unilateral ureterocystoplasty in cases where there is sufficient ureteral dilatation (2).

Ureteral reconstruction with TUU may not be possible if there is insufficient donor ureter (approximately one-half the original length) for a tension-free anastomosis. Any disease process that has the potential to affect contralateral renal function or drainage is also a contraindication, such as retroperitoneal fibrosis, high-dose radiation therapy, calculus disease, recurrent pyelonephritis, and urothelial malignancy. Although size disparity between ureters has been regarded as a relative contraindication in the past, successful TUU has been accomplished by use of a longer vertical ureterotomy in the recipient ureter to accommodate a larger-caliber donor ureter (3,5,7).

## ALTERNATIVE THERAPY

Other procedures to be considered in lieu of TUU include ureteroneocystostomy with a psoas hitch or Boari flap, nephropexy to allow ureteroneocystostomy or ureteroureterostomy, ileal substitution, and autotransplantation. Other alternatives to TUU include mitigating or temporizing procedures such as cutaneous ureterostomy, pyelostomy, nephrostomy drainage, and ureteral stenting. Nephrectomy should also be considered in cases of marginal donor renal function.

## SURGICAL TECHNIQUE

The patient is placed supine with such options as kidney rest elevation, retroflexion of the surgical bed, and Trendelenburg positioning to enhance retroperitoneal exposure. A midline vertical incision is usually made in the abdomen, extending

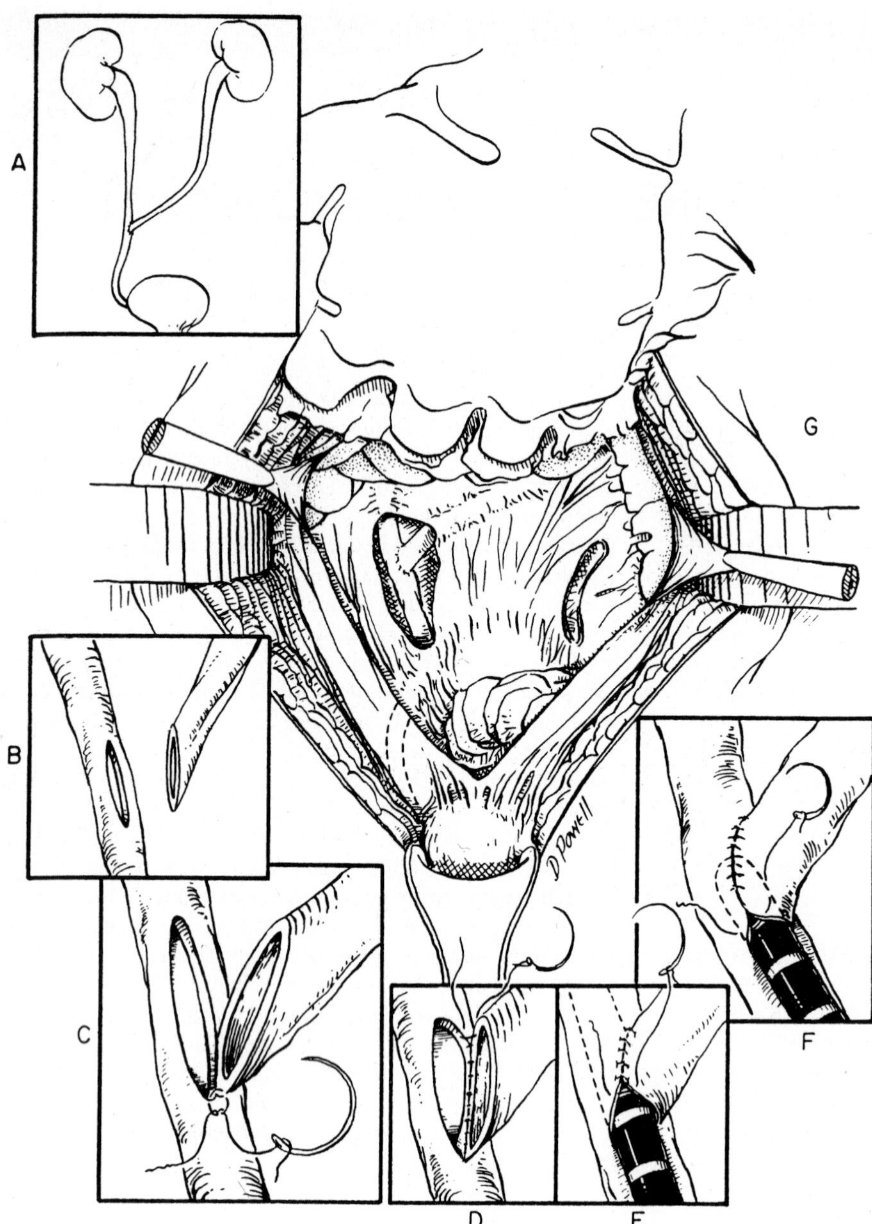


FIGURE 98.1 Transureteroureterostomy (TUU) approached by two incisions in the posterior peritoneum. **A:** Schematic diagram of left-to-right TUU. **B:** The donor ureter is approximated to the vertical ureterotomy on the anteromedial aspect of the recipient ureter. **C and D:** The anastomosis is begun at the apex and is extended to the posterior aspect of the TUU, using either running or interrupted absorbable sutures. **E and F:** The anterior aspect of the anastomosis may be performed over a catheter or feeding tube removed prior to the last stitch. **G:** Completed TUU in situ.

from just above the umbilicus to the pubic symphysis. However, in cases of distal TUU following a failed reimplantation, a Pfannenstiel incision may be sufficient. A choice of exposure approaches is then available.

## Transperitoneal Approach

Wide transperitoneal exposure is indicated in cases that require complex adjunct procedures such as tapered reimplantation of the recipient ureter or bladder augmentation, as well as when there is a long segment of diseased distal donor ureter. This approach would also be preferred when a high TUU is necessary for the distal donor ureter to be used as a continent catheterizable channel or for augmentation of the bladder.

The bowel is packed and retracted superiorly to allow for further dissection. Once the ureters have been visualized as they pass over the iliac vessels, two options for opening the retroperitoneum have been described (8): (a) two 5-cm vertical incisions may be made over the ureters where they cross the iliac vessels, creating a window on each side (Fig. 98.1), and (b) wider retroperitoneal exposure can be achieved through a single curved incision that opens the retroperitoneum from over the left distal ureter, extending across the midline along the small bowel mesentery and cecum, and up the right side along the line of Toldt (Fig. 98.2). This technique allows for more extensive mobilization of the bowel in an upward direction.

Once the ureters are adequately exposed, the retroperitoneal tunnel is created by blunt dissection beneath the posterior peritoneum, anterior to the great vessels and superior to the inferior mesenteric artery (IMA). The angle between the aorta and IMA may kink or even obstruct the donor ureter. The position of the IMA should therefore be noted and

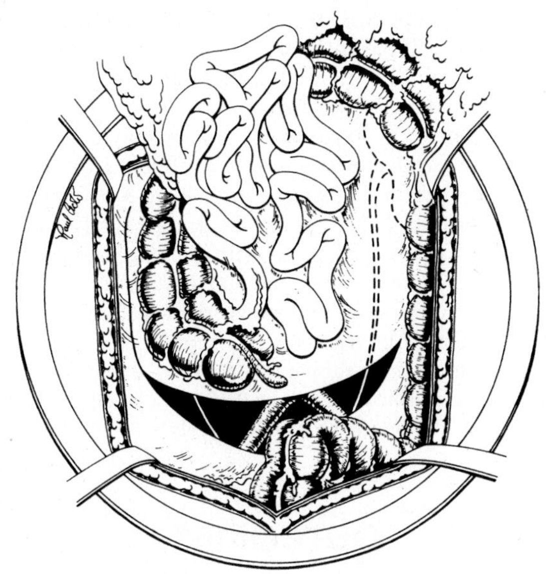

FIGURE 98.2 Approach for single curvilinear incision in the posterior peritoneum to mobilize the bowels and mesentery and expose the retroperitoneum.

avoided in calculating the path of the donor ureter to the contralateral retroperitoneum. Rarely, it may be necessary to ligate the IMA to prevent donor ureteral compression.

## Retroperitoneal Approach

This technique provides the benefit of preventing complications associated with intraperitoneal procedures. The author prefers this approach for a more distal TUU, which requires less mobilization of the donor ureter. Other authors have also described this method as a viable alternative to the transperitoneal approach (9). Most commonly, this approach would be used in salvage procedures for failed ureteral reimplantation.

After the transversalis fascia is incised, the extravesical space is mobilized on each side of the bladder. The ureters are identified crossing beneath the obliterated umbilical arteries. After dividing these vessels with Vicryl or silk ties, the peritoneal sac is retracted superiorly to further expose the retroperitoneum. The peritoneal sac may also be reflected medially to expose the area of interest.

Once adequate exposure of the ureters has been achieved, blunt finger dissection is then used to create an ample retroperitoneal tunnel. In cases of a low TUU using a retroperitoneal approach, the tunnel is created beneath the posterior peritoneum just superior to the posterior wall of the bladder and anterior to the sacral promontory.

## TUU

Adjunct procedures required for the recipient ureter, such as tapering and reimplantation, should be undertaken prior to the anastomosis of the donor and recipient ureter. For a standard TUU, mobilization of the donor should be sufficient to create a tension-free anastomosis. Because preservation of blood supply is essential for the success of TUU, great care is taken to avoid unnecessary disruption of the adventitia. The ipsilateral gonadal vessel may be tied off with a 3-0 silk suture to provide even greater mobilization with adventitial preservation. If even greater donor ureteral length is necessary, the donor kidney may be gently mobilized, moved inferiorly, and pexed to the psoas muscle using interrupted 3-0 Vicryl or 3-0 polydioxanone sutures.

After dividing the donor ureter as distal as possible, a long tagged 4-0 chromic or Vicryl suture is then placed on the most distal aspect of the divided donor ureter to allow the ureter to be brought through the retroperitoneal tunnel. A right-angle clamp can then be passed from the recipient to the donor side to grasp the stay suture on the donor ureter and pull the donor ureter through the tunnel. Care must be taken to avoid twisting or kinking of the ureter, and the ureter should reach easily to the other side without tension.

With respect to the recipient ureter, mobilization should be minimized. To enable touch-free manipulation of the recipient ureter, stay sutures consisting of 4-0 or 5-0 chromic may be placed in the recipient ureteral adventitia, superior and inferior to the intended area of anastomosis. A vertical ureterotomy at least 1.5 cm in length on the anteromedial wall of the recipient ureter is then performed at the site of the anastomosis. The donor ureter is then spatulated to accommodate the recipient ureterotomy. However, spatulation may not be necessary if the donor ureter is sufficiently dilated. The anastomosis is performed using interrupted (Fig. 98.3) or running 4-0 or 5-0 absorbable

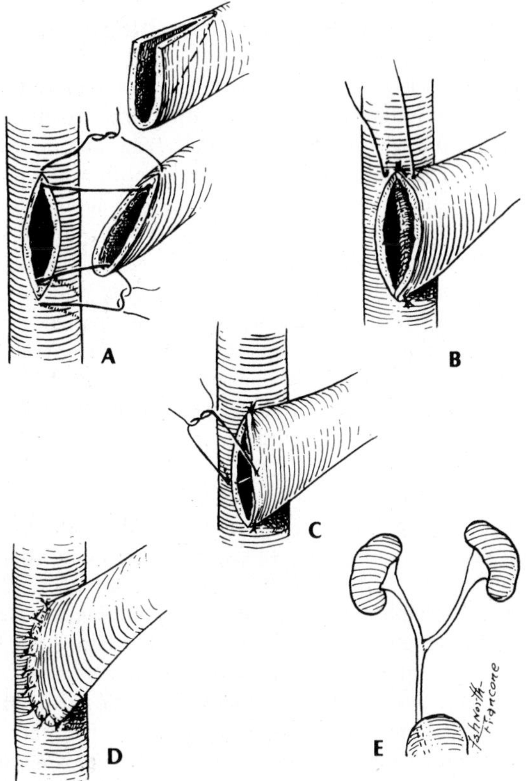


FIGURE 98.3 Transureteroureterostomy (TUU) anastomosis performed with interrupted absorbable sutures. **A and B:** After aligning the distal donor ureteral lumen and recipient ureterotomy, apical sutures are placed and tied. **C:** Subsequent intervening interrupted sutures are placed halfway between previously placed sutures. **D:** Completed anastomosis. **E:** Schematic diagram of completed TUU.

sutures, beginning with the superior and inferior apices, followed by the approximation of the more posterior wall of the anastomosis. At this juncture, a ureteral catheter or infant feeding tube may be helpful in some cases to facilitate the anterior wall anastomosis. This tube may be removed just prior to the final anastomotic stitch (Fig. 98.1).

The use of an indwelling ureteral stent is mandatory only when the recipient ureter distal to the anastomosis has been altered in some fashion, such as in reimplantation. A 5Fr or 8Fr feeding tube or a double-J stent may be used. In addition, nephrostomy drainage of the recipient ureter may be employed if extensive mobilization or tapering of the recipient ureter and/or kidney is required to complete the reconstruction (3). In all cases, it is vital to drain the retroperitoneal space using either a Penrose or closed-suction drain. Furthermore, with the transperitoneal approach it is recommended to close the posterior peritoneum to avoid drainage of urine into the peritoneal cavity. Finally, a suprapubic catheter or urethral catheter should be placed to keep the bladder decompressed, as an overly distended bladder in the early postoperative period may stress the TUU anastomosis.

Approximately 2 months postoperatively the patient should undergo a renal sonogram and/or a diuretic renal scan to assess drainage and/or renal function. Depending on the results, imaging may be repeated in 3 to 9 months until a trend of progression has been established. Renal function by creatinine measurements should also be followed, particularly if these levels were elevated preoperatively.

## Laparoscopic Approach

Laparoscopic TUU has recently been described in children (10). The patient is initially placed in the lithotomy position under general anesthesia for cystoscopy and retrograde pyelogram with stent placement, wire placement, or both in the normal recipient ureter. The patient is then placed supine and redraped. After gaining periumbilical access to the peritoneal cavity, working ports (3 to 5 mm) are placed under laparoscopic vision in the hypogastrium and in the right and left flank. The position is adjusted according to patient size, at the level of the umbilical line and above for infants and older children, respectively. The patient is placed in the Trendelenburg position with the donor ureter side elevated 30 to 45 degrees and the surgeon standing on the opposite side.

The donor ureter is identified at the pelvic brim. The peritoneum is incised and the ureter is dissected distally as close to the bladder as possible, with special care not to damage the vas deferens in male patients. The distal ureter is ligated with an absorbable suture and divided in an oblique fashion. Proximal mobilization of the donor ureter is performed, preserving the periureteral tissue and its vascularization. The surgical table is then turned to elevate the side of the recipient ureter, and the surgeon changes position to the other side. The recipient ureter is exposed at the same level while incising the peritoneum. A tunnel under the rectosigmoid mesentery is created with blunt dissection, bridging the two peritoneal windows.

Once enough space is developed to accommodate the donor ureter free of external compression it is transposed, pulling it through the retroperitoneal tunnel with an atraumatic grasper or a stay suture. If the donor ureter was under tension, further proximal mobilization is performed. Care is taken to avoid twisting or kinking of the donor ureter as it enters the retroperitoneal tunnel. A longitudinal ureterotomy at the medial aspect of the recipient ureter is performed to match the lumen of the donor ureter using laparoscopic sharp KOH Ultramicro suture scissors. The indwelling stent is identified and left in place. The anastomosis is carried out with running 5-0 absorbable monofilament sutures. An abdominal drain is left in the proximity of the anastomosis and exteriorized through one of the port sites. The Foley catheter is removed on postoperative day 2, and the drain is subsequently removed once the patient has voided and urine leakage is ruled out. The double-J stents are removed 2 to 4 weeks postoperatively.

# OUTCOMES

## Complications

Postoperative complications include urinoma, pyelonephritis, prolonged anastomotic drainage, and stricture (11). The risk of any of these complications is heightened by tenuous ureteral blood supply from excessive mobilization or from previous radiation (12). Patients with neuropathic or abnormal bladders may be more at risk for developing new vesicoureteral reflux or distal ureteral stenosis in cases that involve reimplantation of the recipient ureter (13). Early anastomotic obstruction leading to persistent drainage may be initially treated conservatively with placement of a double-J ureteral stent or percutaneous nephrostomy.

Late complications include small-bowel obstruction, but only in cases involving the transperitoneal approach. A TUU performed in the context of neoplasm may suffer from late ureteral obstruction. Subsequent stone disease can potentially obstruct the common segment, rendering the patient anuric and mandating emergent percutaneous nephrostomy drainage. Rarely, compression of the donor ureter by the IMA can develop years after TUU if precautions to avoid the artery during donor ureter tunneling were not taken. However, despite potential problems and the possible need for reoperation, several series have shown that TUU anastomotic revision is rarely, if ever, necessary. Also, donor renal loss due to chronic infection or obstruction has proven infrequent, with rates ranging from 0% to 6% (2,3,5). Recipient kidney loss is even less common, reportedly occurring only after extensive mobilization required in complex reconstructions (3,7).

## Results

Numerous studies have shown excellent results after TUU. Damage to the recipient kidney and ureter has rarely been observed, and successful preservation of both renal units occurs in >90% of cases. TUU performed in the correct setting, with meticulous attention to maintaining ureteral blood supply and a tension-free anastomosis, is clearly an important component of the urologist's repertoire of reconstructive ureteral surgery.

## References


1. Higgins CC. Transuretero-ureteral anastomosis. Report of a clinical case. *J Urol* 1935;34:349.
2. Mure P, Mollard P, Mouriquand P. Transureteroureterostomy in childhood and adolescence: long-term results in 69 cases. *J Urol* 2000;163:946–948.
3. Rushton HG, Parrot TS, Woodard JR. The expanded role of transureteroureterostomy in pediatric urology. *J Urol* 1987;138:357–363.
4. Halpern GN, King LR, Belman AB. Transureteroureterostomy in children. *J Urol* 1973;109:504–509.
5. Hodges CV, Barry JM, Fuchs EF, et al. Transureteroureterostomy: 25-year experience with 100 patients. *J Urol* 1980;123:834–838.
6. Weiss RM, Beland GA, Lattimer JK. Transureteroureterostomy and cutaneous ureterostomy as a form of urinary diversion in children. *Urol Int* 1968;23:103–112.
7. Hendren WH, Hensle TW. Transureteroureterostomy: experience with 75 cases. *J Urol* 1980;123:826–833.
8. Casale A. Transureteroureterostomy. In: *Glenn's Urologic Surgery*, 5th ed. Philadelphia: Lippincott Williams & Wilkins, 1998.
9. Baert L, Claes H. A retroperitoneal approach for transureteroureterostomy: a neglected and forgotten procedure. *Acta Urol Belg* 1990;58(4): 51–58.
10. Piaggio LA, Gonzalez R. Laparoscopic transureterouretostomy: a novel approach. *J Urol* 2007;177:2311–2314.
11. Sandoz IL, Paul DP, MacFarlane CA. Complications with transureteroureterostomy. *J Urol* 1977;117:39–42.
12. Ehrlich RM, Skinner DG. Complications of transureteroureterostomy. *J Urol* 1975;113:467–473.
13. Pesce C, Costa L, Campobossa P, et al. Successful use of transureteroureterostomy in children: a clinical study. *Eur J Pediatr Surg* 2001;11: 395–398.


# CHAPTER 99 ■ PYELOPLASTY

EVAN J. KASS AND KEVIN M. FEBER

Ureteropelvic junction (UPJ) obstruction is a common etiology for hydronephrosis in the neonate and young child. UPJ obstruction has been classically divided into intrinsic, extrinsic, and secondary causes. The most common etiology in an infant is an intrinsic adynamic or atretic segment of ureter that inhibits urine exiting from the renal pelvis (1). This restriction to urine flow can lead to varying degrees of renal pelvic dilation and renal damage. Less common causes of intrinsic obstruction include valvular mucosal folds and persistent fetal ureteral convolutions. Extrinsic obstruction is most often the result of periureteral fibrous bands or aberrant lower-pole vessels. Rarely, severe vesicoureteral reflux with periureteral scarring can be a cause of secondary UPJ obstruction.

## DIAGNOSIS

Historically, most cases of UPJ obstruction were diagnosed in older children who presented with symptoms of flank pain, urinary tract infection, hematuria, and abdominal mass. The widespread utilization of prenatal ultrasound has allowed earlier identification of UPJ pathology in newborns. Children with hydronephrosis persisting on a postnatal ultrasound routinely should have a voiding cystourethrogram to exclude reflux as a possible etiology. When no reflux is present a MAG-3 renogram with Lasix washout allows objective measurement of renal function and drainage. Whitaker antegrade perfusion studies are no longer routinely preformed. The natural history of most children with antenatally detected hydronephrosis is usually benign. Operative intervention is in general reserved for patients demonstrating increasing hydronephrosis, worsening renal function, pain, urinary tract infection, or other symptoms. The role of the Lasix washout half-time remains controversial (2).

## INDICATIONS FOR SURGERY

The indications for pyeloplasty at our institution encompass the following: (i) severe hydronephrosis (Society for Fetal Urology grade III or IV) postnatally and a diuretic renogram of the affected side with <40% differential kidney function and no response to furosemide; (ii) worsening hydronephrosis on serial ultrasound studies; (iii) symptomatic UPJ obstruction with intermittent flank pain; (iv) loss of relative renal function (>10% on serial scans of the affected kidney); or (v) a persistent obstructive half-time on serial diuretic renograms in a child with severe hydronephrosis.

## ALTERNATIVE THERAPY

Any procedure for correction of UPJ obstruction must satisfy four criteria first described by Foley in 1937: (i) formation of a funnel at the UPJ, (ii) dependent drainage, (iii) watertight anastomosis, and (iv) tension-free anastomosis (3). The Anderson–Hynes dismembered pyeloplasty is the most widely used procedure today and is in general applicable regardless of the etiology of obstruction. Access to the UPJ can be achieved from several incisions, including anterior extraperitoneal, flank, and dorsal lumbotomy. These approaches allow excellent exposure to the renal pelvis with minimal morbidity to the child. Anterior transperitoneal incisions are rarely used due to the increased morbidity associated with intraperitoneal bowel manipulation and the possibility of secondary bowel obstruction.

Ureterocalicostomy is another option for children with massive hydronephrosis or those who have failed primary pyeloplasty. A Foley Y- or V-plasty is indicated when there is a

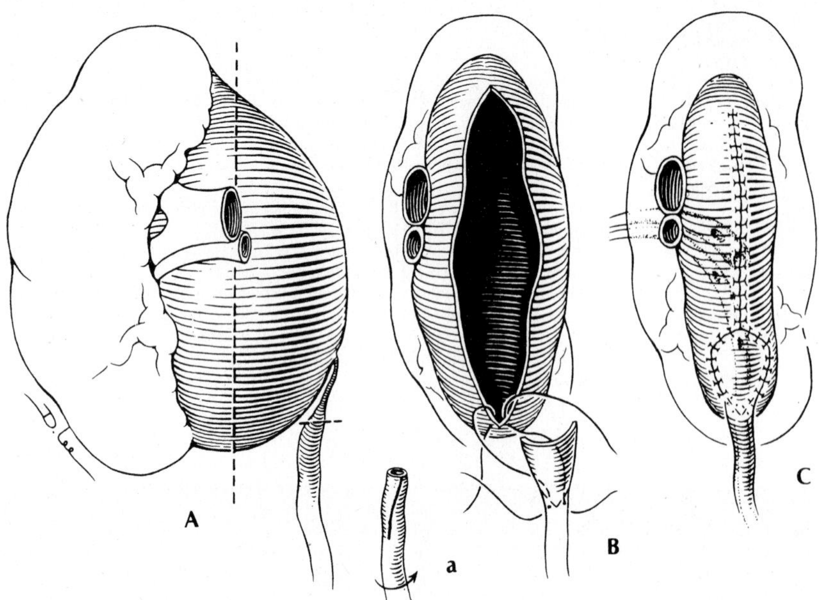


FIGURE 99.1 Dismembered pyeloplasty. A: The renal pelvis is incised, redundant tissue excised, and the ureter divided distal to the atretic segment. B: The ureter is spatulated and brought to the most dependent portion of the pelvis. C: The remaining pelvis is closed with running sutures.

UPJ obstruction secondary to a high insertion of the ureter, which is often found in patients with horseshoe kidney.

The refinement of more minimally invasive technologies has allowed correction of UPJ obstruction with minimal operative morbidity. Antegrade and retrograde endopyelotomy procedures have been successful in older children with UPJ obstruction (4). This technique, however, is associated with decreased success rates and an increased risk of intraoperative and postoperative bleeding.

Laparoscopic and robotic-assisted pyeloplasty procedures are evolving techniques to correct UPJ obstruction. In expert hands, success rates following laparoscopic repairs approach results seen with open pyeloplasty (5). Decreased hospital stay and analgesic requirements have been reported in children undergoing the transperitoneal or retroperitoneal approach with or without robotic assistance (6,7). The drawbacks of the laparoscopic and robotic techniques include increased operative time, expensive surgical instruments that may not be available at all centers, and the need for proficiency in laparoscopic surgery. Although laparoscopic and robotic-assisted pyeloplasty procedures have been gaining popularity, open pyeloplasty with optical magnification continues to be the gold standard, with established long-term results.

## SURGICAL TECHNIQUE

The patient is placed in the flank position and flexed with the use of rolled towels and/or table flexion with elevation of the kidney rest. We make a transverse incision starting just medial to the angle of the 12th rib and carry it anteriorly. The subcutaneous tissues and musculofascial layers are opened with electrocautery. The lumbodorsal fascia in then divided, the peritoneum is mobilized medially, and the fascia of Gerota is opened.

The lower pole and entire renal pelvis are sharply dissected to identify the UPJ to determine the cause of the obstruction. Care is taken in dissection to preserve the blood supply in the periureteral tissues and ureter. Stay sutures are placed just cephalad to the UPJ and in the ureter to minimize handling of the tissues. The renal pelvis is incised circumferentially, decompressing the obstructed collecting system (Fig. 99.1). The proximal ureter is mobilized using the stay suture distal to the obstructing segment to facilitate handling, and the atretic portion is excised. The renal pelvis is trimmed of redundant tissue, the ureter is spatulated for 2 cm, and a 5Fr feeding tube is placed in the ureter. The ureter is then anastomosed to the most dependent portion of the renal pelvis using 7-0 interrupted PDS sutures, and the feeding tube is removed. Optical magnification with a 3.0 to 4.5 × loupe facilitates precise suture placement. Alternatively, 7-0 running sutures can be used, but in infants we prefer interrupted sutures to decrease the purse-string effect and subsequent narrowing of the anastomosis. Care is taken to ensure there is no twisting or kinking of the anastomosis. The remainder of the trimmed upper renal pelvis is closed with a running 6-0 polydioxanone suture.

If the UPJ obstruction is secondary to an accessory lower-pole vessel, the divided ureter is brought anterior to the vessel and anastomosed to the pelvis (Fig. 99.2). Pelvic tailoring is often required in this correction as well.

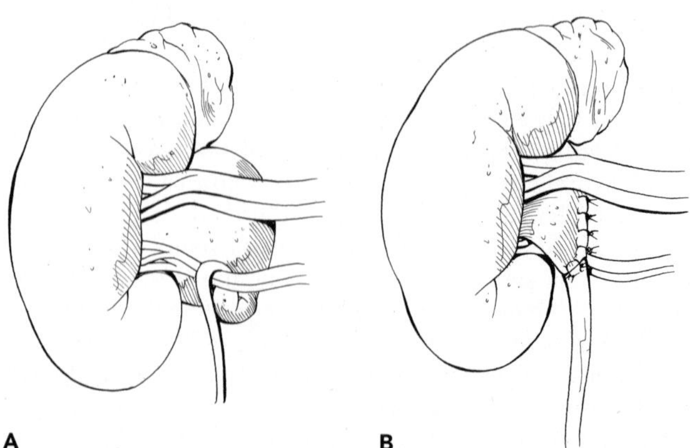


FIGURE 99.2 Dismembered pyeloplasty with accessory vessels. A: Vessels causing ureteral compression and hydronephrosis. B: Anastomosis performed anterior to crossing vessels. Pelvic tailoring as needed.

The placement of intraoperative stents and/or nephrostomy tubes remains controversial, and we do not use either routinely. Whereas some of the early pyeloplasty descriptions used both internal and external drainage, many authorities now believe routine stenting is unnecessary. Stents are indicated in children with poor renal function, those undergoing repeat pyeloplasty, those with a solitary kidney, and those requiring extensive renal pelvic tailoring (4). Disadvantages of percutaneous nephrostomy tubes and ureteral stenting include patient discomfort and need for drain removal either in the office or under a second anesthetic. A 0.25-in Penrose drain is placed in the perirenal space and brought out through a separate, more caudal incision. The musculofascial layers are closed using 3-0 Vicryl. The subcutaneous tissues are closed using 4-0 plain sutures and the skin is reapproximated with 5-0 Monocryl in a subcuticular fashion.

Postoperatively the patient is kept on intravenous antibiotics until the drain in removed, usually on postoperative day 1 or 2. We routinely administer ketorolac 0.5 mg/kg intravenously for the first 48 hours. We have found that it provides excellent pain relief, with the majority of children requiring no parenteral narcotic. Children are typically discharged within 24 hours of surgery. A follow-up ultrasound is done at 3 to 4 weeks postoperatively. If a stent was placed at the time of pyeloplasty, it is removed in 4 to 6 weeks.

## OUTCOMES

### Complications

Most children do very well postoperatively. Significant bleeding, infection, or other morbidity is uncommon. Urinary leakage from the anastomosis can occur and usually resolves spontaneously. When leakage persists or when hydronephrosis increases postoperatively, a ureteral stent can be placed in either an antegrade or retrograde fashion.

### Results

We have found that dismembered pyeloplasty has been shown to successfully relieve pelvic obstruction in >95% of cases.

### *References*


1. Park J. The pathophysiology of UPJ obstruction: current concepts. *Urol Clin North Am* 1998;25:161–170.
2. Kass E. Pediatric hydronephrosis: my approach to management. *Dialog Pediatr Urol* 2002;25:1–2.
3. Foley F. New plastic operation for strictures at the ureteropelvic junction: report of 20 operations. *J Urol* 1937;38:643–372.
4. Ward A. Ureteropelvic junction obstruction in children: unique considerations for open intervention. *Urol Clin North Am* 1998;25:211–218.
5. Tan H. Laparoscopic Anderson–Hynes dismembered pyeloplasty in children using needlescopic instrumentation. *Urol Clin North Am* 2001;28: 43–51.
6. Bonnard A, Fouquet V, Carricaburu E, et al. Retroperitoneal laparoscopic versus open pyeloplasty in children. *J Urol* 2005;173:1710–1713.
7. Lee R, Retik A, Borer J, et al. Pediatric robot assisted laparoscopic dismembered pyeloplasty: comparison with a cohort of open surgery. *J Urol* 2006;175:683–687.


# CHAPTER 100 ■ MEGAURETER

J. CHRISTOPHER AUSTIN AND DOUGLAS A. CANNING

Megaureter, or wide ureter, is an unusual congenital anomaly of the urinary tract. We define megaureter as a ureter that is 8 mm or greater in diameter. Megaureter is classified into three categories: (a) refluxing megaureter, (b) obstructed megaureter, and (c) nonobstructed, nonrefluxing megaureter. Urologists further subdivide megaureters into primary and secondary types, with the secondary types resulting from an abnormality such as posterior urethral valves, high-volume vesicoureteral reflux or neuropathic bladder resulting in higher detrusor pressure, or less commonly an acquired condition such as external compression of the ureter from a mass lesion. Primary megaureters, in contrast, are isolated abnormalities of the ureter or ureterovesical junction resulting in a wide ureteral lumen.

Prior to the widespread use of screening prenatal ultrasonography, most children with megaureters presented with urinary tract infection, flank pain, urolithiasis, abdominal mass, or hematuria. Today, most cases are detected in asymptomatic infants with hydroureteronephrosis in utero. This earlier presentation has led to changes in the approach to management.

The pathophysiology of obstructive megaureters lies not within the dilated ureter but in the distal nondilated segment. This segment of ureter fails to effectively propagate the wave of peristalsis as it descends down the ureter. This segment is not usually narrowed compared with the normal ureter. When the bolus of urine is propagated to the aperistaltic segment, only a portion of the urine passes into the bladder; the remainder is reflected back up the ureter in a yo-yo fashion. This causes the characteristic appearance of the ureter with fusiform dilation affecting the distal ureter more severely. When the amount and force of the bolus are sufficiently large that it dilates the entire ureter and reaches the renal pelvis, hydronephrosis may develop as well.

## DIAGNOSIS

Differentiating an obstructed megaureter from a nonrefluxing, nonobstructed megaureter can be difficult. These ureters demonstrate a spectrum of severity rather than separate conditions. The diagnostic workup depends on the presenting signs and symptoms and may vary from patient to patient. For the child with prenatal hydronephrosis, the usual evaluation includes a renal/bladder ultrasound, a voiding cystourethrogram (VCUG), and a renal scintigram (renal scan). Hydroureteronephrosis is identified with the renal ultrasound. The dilated ureter is usually visible in the pelvis and is often posterolateral to the bladder. If the ureter is dilated beyond the level of the trigone, an ectopic ureter may be present rather than a primary megaureter. The VCUG separates children with refluxing megaureters from those without reflux. The renal scan in the newborn should be performed with mercaptoacetyl triglycine (MAG-3) with diuretic washout. The scan will estimate the relative function of each kidney and measure the effectiveness of renal clearance of radiotracer from the collecting system. In the past, the $t_{1/2}$ (time required for half of the radiotracer to clear from the renal pelvis) had been used as an indicator of obstruction. However, in practice, the use of the $t_{1/2}$ alone to estimate obstruction is not always reliable. Because the clearance is variable based on the patient's prestudy hydration level, age, renal function, and response to the diuretic, we prefer to follow trends in the relative renal function, reserving surgery for those with increasing $t_{1/2}$ or decreasing relative renal function.

In children who are symptomatic, the presenting symptom determines the workup. Hematuria, rarely noted in children with megaureter, is normally evaluated initially with a renal/bladder ultrasound. The finding of hydroureteronephrosis should be followed by a renal scan or intravenous pyelogram. If there is suspicion of renal or ureteral stone, a noncontrast computed tomography scan should be performed. The renal scan may be required to provide a baseline estimate of relative renal function.

If the anatomy is unclear, magnetic resonance (MR) imaging or MR urography may be useful in distinguishing primary megaureters from ectopic ureters. If there is impaired function of the affected kidney and the child is undergoing surgical correction, cystoscopy should be performed at the beginning of the reconstructive procedure to evaluate the position of the ureteral orifice. The orifice is normally positioned in an obstructed megaureter. If an ectopic ureter is present, the trigone on the affected side will be distorted and the ectopic orifice will not be located at the trigone.

## INDICATIONS FOR SURGERY

Relative indications to proceed with surgical repair include poor initial relative function (<40% of differential renal function by renal scan), progressive hydronephrosis, decreasing function (>10%) in serial renal scans, persistent severe hydroureteronephrosis, bilateral megaureters, or the development of symptoms such as pain or urinary tract infection localized to the side of the megaureter. In some cases, we consider infants with a poorly functioning kidney for alternative approaches to primary repair, given the infant's small, thin-walled bladder and the technical difficulties of reimplanting a hydronephrotic ureter into the infant bladder. Options in this case include a staged reconstructive approach with temporary diversion to an end-cutaneous ureterostomy, construction of a refluxing ureteral reimplantation, or, rarely, diverting pyelostomy should be given consideration instead of primary surgical repair (1,2).

We usually operate on children with megaureter who present with symptoms of intermittent flank pain or urinary tract infection. Prior to surgery, we evaluate the child for voiding dysfunction. Rarely, children develop a secondary megaureter from high-pressure bladder storage that is transmitted to the ureter and renal pelvis. Ureteral dilation can be detected in association with neuropathic bladder dysfunction, posterior urethral valves, or severe voiding dysfunction. Appropriate treatment of the posterior urethral valves or the bladder dysfunction may result in improvement or resolution of ureteral dilation. Failure to recognize bladder dysfunction before planning surgery leads to persistent obstruction or postoperative vesicoureteral reflux.

## ALTERNATIVE THERAPY

Because most patients are asymptomatic and identified as part of an in utero ultrasound, most children with primary megaureters do not require surgical correction. Ureteral dilation does not always equal obstruction. Dilation in some boys and girls may represent the residuum of in utero obstruction that has resolved. The long-term experience at the Children's Hospital of Philadelphia has been that the majority of children with megaureter maintain renal function and ureteral dilation often improves with time. In a series of 27 children with megaureters treated conservatively with a mean follow-up of 6.8 years, hydronephrosis completely resolved in 53% and was improved or stable in the rest. Only 10% of patients required surgical correction, while 90% were followed with serial radiologic studies. A single patient from this cohort developed progression of hydronephrosis and diminished function at age 14 (3). Likewise, in a series of 53 patients with 67 megaureters, only 17% required surgery for poor initial function or progressive loss of function; in addition, the dilation completely resolved by ultrasound in 34% (4). These two series suggest that the majority of megaureters can be managed conservatively. Because of the rare risk of late decompensation, children with persistent hydronephrosis require extended follow-up.

## SURGICAL TECHNIQUE

The surgical correction is similar for refluxing and obstructed megaureters. Obstructed megaureters have a distal ureteral segment of variable length with a normal or narrowed caliber that does not contract normally and should be excised. Refluxing megaureters are dilated to the level of the ureterovesical junction. Distal segment excision is not always required.

The child is positioned supine on the operating room table. In boys, the lower abdomen and genitalia are fully prepared and draped. Females are placed in a mild frog-legged position

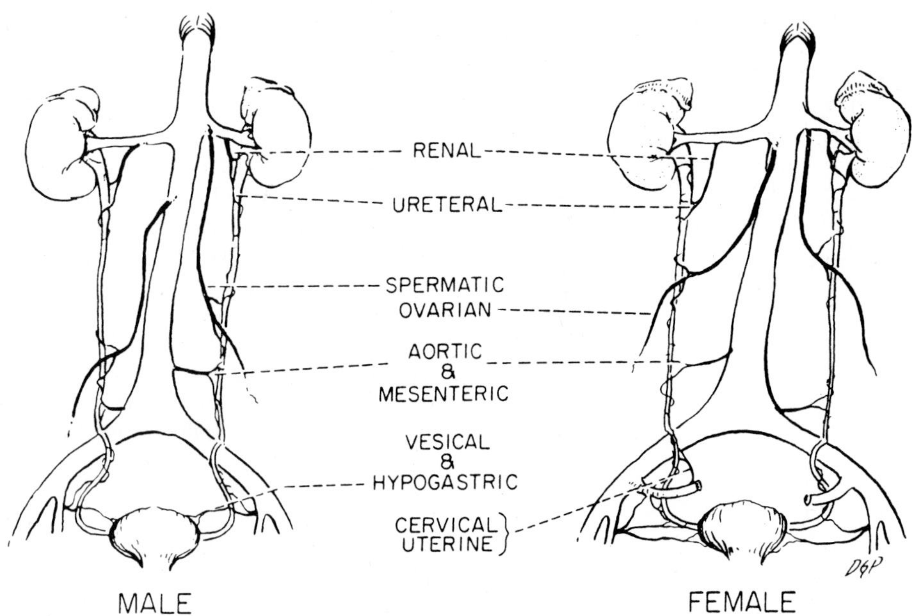


**FIGURE 100.1** Major arterial supply to the ureter. It is not necessary to sacrifice any medially based blood supply for primary megaureter repair.

with gel bolsters under the knees to permit intraoperative access to the urethra if needed. The bladder may be left full during the initial surgical exposure. A Pfannenstiel incision is made in the abdominal skin crease. The rectus fascia is opened along the course of the incision and the flaps of fascia are elevated off the muscle superiorly to just below the umbilicus and inferiorly to the pubis. The rectus muscles are separated in the midline. The space of Retzius is entered, exposing the bladder.

## Intravesical Approach

At this point, depending upon the surgeon's preference, the dissection of the ureter begins either intravesically or through an extravesical exposure. It has been our preference to begin intravesically. The bladder is opened via a midline cystotomy. The bladder dome is packed with damp sponges and a Dennis–Brown retractor is placed to provide exposure of the trigone. A 5Fr feeding tube is passed up the ureter and secured at the orifice with a 4-0 suture. The urothelium surrounding the orifice is divided using electrocautery. With the mucosa divided circumferentially, the ureteral catheter is gently pulled to expose the medial and inferior attachments of the trigonal musculature. These attachments are divided with electrocautery. At this point the dissection proceeds to carefully divide the muscular attachments of the ureter through the plane of Waldeyer's sheath. This dissection will free the distal ureter, which should have a normal or narrowed caliber. The surgeon should recognize the blood supply of the ureter, as shown in Figure 100.1. As the dissection proceeds more proximally, the blood supply of the ureter originates from medial branches of the hypogastric (male) or cervical (female) arteries. These vessels should be preserved, as should the longitudinal blood supply, by taking care to prevent dissection too close to the ureteral wall. When the ureter is free from its detrusor attachments, the mobilization should proceed extravesically. The ureter at this point can be passed through the bladder wall, and the dissection proceeds more proximally. When the dilated region of the ureter is reached, dissection should continue until an adequate length for reimplantation has been mobilized, again paying attention to the previous outlined principles for preserving the blood supply. An ischemic distal ureter may lead to fibrosis and obstruction.

At this point the surgeon must decide whether to taper the ureter. In general, if the lumen of the ureter is significantly larger than 16Fr it should be tapered prior to reimplantation. There are two techniques used to taper the size of the ureter: (a) excisional tapering and (b) tapering by folding. We will review the three most commonly used procedures. The goal of tapering is to provide a distal ureter with a small enough diameter that postoperative vesicoureteral reflux will be prevented with a reasonable length of intramural tunnel. The tapering needs to extend for only a short distance beyond the bladder wall rather than the whole length of the ureter. The dilation of the proximal ureter should improve postoperatively with the relief of obstruction and/or reflux. The decision to perform an excisional versus a folding technique depends on the preference of the surgeon and the size and thickness of the ureter. Folding a very dilated, thick wall ureter will create a large amount of bulk, making the creation of the submucosal tunnel difficult. In general, the taper should not be aggressive. In a bladder that functions well, reflux is less hazardous than persistent obstruction.

Excisional tapering (Fig. 100.2) begins with carefully examining the ureter. Without twisting the ureter, the surgeon observes the pattern of blood supply to the ureter. In most cases, the longitudinal ureteral vessels are predominately along the medial aspect of the ureter. Usually, the excised segment of ureter is taken from the opposite side along the lateral border. The distal nondilated ureteral (aperistaltic) segment is excised. A 16Fr catheter is passed up the ureter. With this

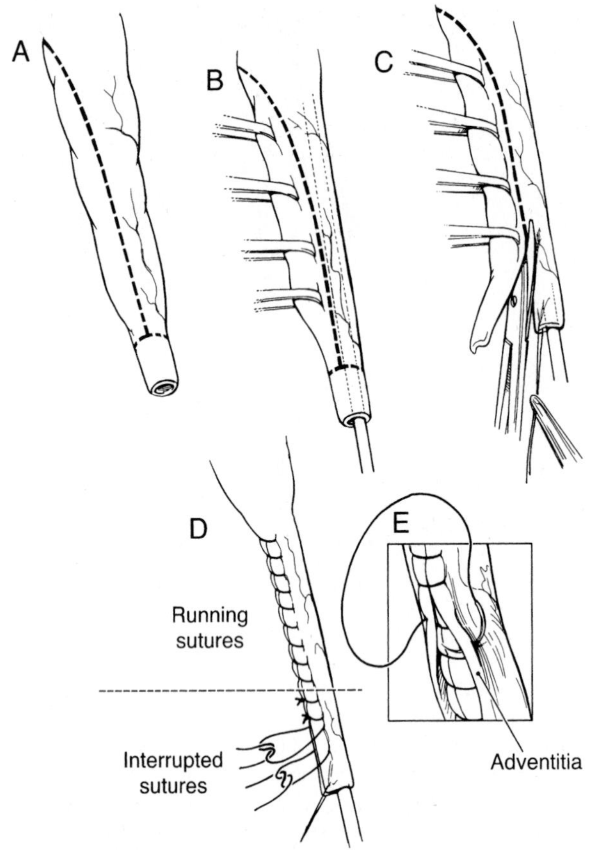


FIGURE 100.2 **A and B:** The wedge of ureter to be excised is secured with Allis or Hendren clamps. **C:** The outlined segment of ureteral wall is excised sharply. **D and E:** The ureter is closed in two layers. Distally, interrupted sutures are placed to allow for trimming of the end of the ureter at the time of reimplantation.

in place, the wedge to be excised is identified and outlined. Aggressive tailoring may result in obstruction. The process of excising and suturing the ureter will result in considerable contraction of the ureteral lumen. The tailored segment should gradually widen as the ureter is reconstructed proximally. The ureter is then closed. The mucosa and the muscularis of the ureter are closed with absorbable interrupted or running fine suture. A second layer if desired may incorporate the muscularis and adventitia with a series of interrupted absorbable fine sutures. The ureter is then reimplanted in a cross-trigonal fashion. If possible, the suture line should be positioned facing the detrusor muscle to prevent the development of a ureterovesical fistula and reflux. The 12Fr catheter is replaced with a 5Fr or 8F feeding tube or a double-J stent. The advantage to leaving an open-ended ureteral catheter is that a retrograde ureteral study can be performed postoperatively to demonstrate ureteral drainage, and the catheter can be removed in the office. The internal stent is easy to care for and leaves the patient free of external tubes; however, it requires a general anesthetic for removal. All tapered reimplants should be stented, regardless of which type of stent is used.

There are two techniques commonly employed for tapering by ureteral folding: (a) Starr plication and (b) the Kaliscinski technique. Both techniques are similar to excisional tapering with regard to the length of ureter to be narrowed and the choice of the segment of the wall based upon the intrinsic blood supply. Starr plication (Fig. 100.3) reduces the diameter of the ureter by infolding the ureteral wall with interrupted Lembert sutures of 5-0 polyglyconate or polydioxan. The tapering begins proximally and gradually reduces the caliber of the ureter until the diameter approaches that of the 12Fr catheter. Care should be taken to ensure the wedge of folded ureter stays in the same position of the ureteral wall as you proceed distally and does not spiral from lateral to medial as the sutures are placed more distally. The ureter is reimplanted with the plication sutures facing the detrusor muscle as was described with excisional tapering. The Kaliscinski technique (Fig. 100.4) begins with a running horizontal mattress suture of 5-0 or 6-0 chromic that runs the length of the segment to be tapered, creating a defunctionalized wedge of ureter that is then wrapped around the ureter and secured posterior with interrupted absorbable sutures. The ureter is reimplanted with the imbricated segment against the muscularis. Again, ureteral stents are placed in both repairs as with excisional tapering.

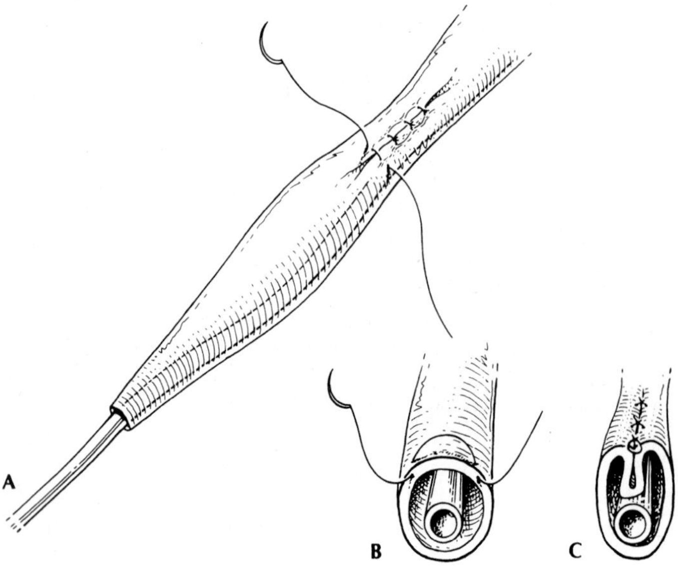


FIGURE 100.3 **A:** Starr plication of the ureter suture to infold the ureter. **B:** Cross section to show placement of Lembert-type sutures. **C:** Cross section after ligation of sutures.

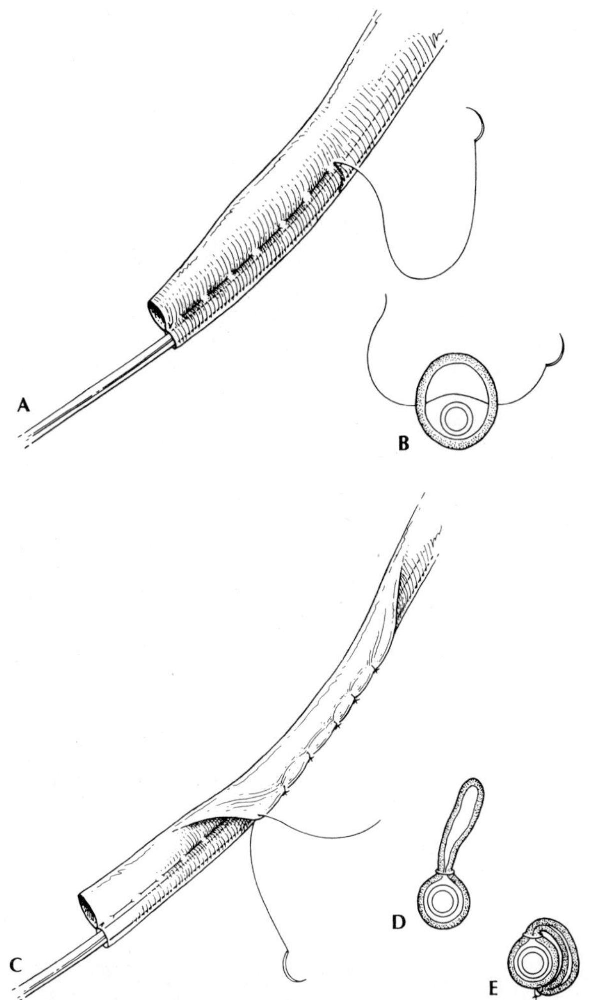


FIGURE 100.4 Kaliscinski technique of ureteral imbrication. **A:** Placement of cobbler's stitch to exclude a major portion of the ureteral lumen. **B:** Same in cross section. **C:** After ligation. **D:** Excluded portion of the ureter is folded over and wrapped around the intubated ureter. **E:** Final appearance in cross section.

## Extravesical Approach

Several authors have reported good results with the extravesical approach to megaureter repair (5,6). We avoid this technique in bilateral megaureter. In cases of bilateral megaureters, a high rate of voiding dysfunction postoperatively has been reported that may require intermittent catheterizations for a period following surgery. A Foley catheter is placed at the beginning of the procedure. The catheter may be attached with a Y-connector for intraoperative filling and emptying. The ability to regulate the bladder volume aids in the dissection. The incision and initial approach is identical as for the intravesical approach until the bladder is exposed. The dissection then proceeds into the lateral extravesical space. The obliterated umbilical artery is divided to expose the ureter. The ureter is carefully dissected free and encircled with a vessel loop. The ureter is dissected distally to the ureterovesical junction. With the bladder full, a detrusorotomy is made in a line extending from the bladder neck cephalad and circumscribing the detrusor adjacent to the ureter. The length of the incision should be 3 to 4 cm.

The ureter is freed from all detrusor attachments, keeping the mucosal attachments intact. The edges of the detrusor incision are then dissected free of the urothelium to form flaps that can be closed over the ureter. If the urothelium is perforated during the dissection it can be repaired with 6-0 or 7-0 chromic. The most distal region is ligated and the ureter divided proximal to the ligature. The aperistaltic segment of the ureter is resected. The dilated ureter is then tapered as necessary. An indwelling stent is placed if the ureter is tapered. The bladder is partially emptied and the ureter is then directly anastomosed to the urothelium at the distal apex of the detrusorotomy using 5-0 absorbable sutures. With this accomplished, the distal ureter is fixed to the detrusor with 5-0 polyglyconate horizontal mattress sutures at the apex. The detrusor is then closed over the ureter with 4-0 polydioxan sutures. The hiatus should be approximated, but not closed too tight. A Foley catheter is left indwelling postoperatively and a Penrose drain is placed during closure.

## Staged Approach

Although repair of megaureters has been performed safely in newborns and young infants, there is a reasonable concern about reimplanting a markedly dilated ureter into the thin bladder wall of an infant (1,7). In some infants where severe dilation and diminished relative function (<35%) exists, end-cutaneous ureterostomy is a good alternative to reimplantation with tapering (7). The infant bladder often empties with high pressure, and postponing the definitive reimplantation while decompressing the obstructed ureter may reduce complications. In this case an end-cutaneous ureterostomy (technique presented in Chapter 93) is performed and the distal stump is resected. This provides reliable decompression of the kidney and allows for improvement in the degree of ureteral dilation prior to reimplantation. In some cases the ureterectasis recovers enough to avoid the need for tapering. In addition, if the initial function is poor and the kidney fails to recover following decompression, a nephrectomy rather than reimplantation may be preferred. This temporary measure will allow the reimplantation to be delayed until the infant is older. The takedown of the ureterostomy and ureteral reimplantation is usually done when the child is 12 to 18 months old and can be performed intravesically or extravesically.

# POSTOPERATIVE CARE

A Foley catheter is usually left in place for 24 to 48 hours. The external stent is left in place for 10 to 14 days. Children are discharged from the hospital on prophylactic antibiotics. Contrast injection of external stents at low pressure by gravity infusion with antibiotic coverage is performed to document drainage. If there is not prompt drainage around the stent, it is left for another 10 to 14 days and the study is repeated. Internal stents are removed 4 to 6 weeks postoperatively. Patients are evaluated with a renal ultrasound 1 month after surgery or stent removal. If hydronephrosis is not improved, a renal scan should be obtained. A VCUG and renal scan should be performed 3 months after surgery, and the ultrasound is repeated at 1 year.

## OUTCOMES

### Complications

The most common complication related to surgery for megaureters is new or persistent reflux. This complication is more common when the surgery is performed for refluxing megaureters than for obstructed megaureters. Management options include observation with prophylaxis, endoscopic injection, and surgical revision. Obstruction is a rare complication, with reported rates of 0% to 4% (4,5,7). It should be initially evaluated endoscopically as on occasion a synechia has been reported to narrow the orifice. Strictures can be assessed by retrograde pyelography. Initial management with dilation and stenting may be successful, but failures will require an open revision.

### Results

Most series report success rates >90% (1,7–9). In a series of infants treated with reimplantation, 20% had reflux postoperatively; however, with time a few patients had spontaneous resolution of their reflux, lowering the rate to 12.5% (10). Extravesical reimplants had rates of postoperative reflux similar to intravesical rates (12%). When performed bilaterally for megaureters, two thirds of patients treated with extravesical reimplantation required intermittent catheterization for a period of 1 to 4 months (5).

### *References*


1. Vereecken RL, Proesmans W. A review of ninety-two obstructive megaureters in children. *Eur Urol* 1999;36:342–347.
2. Lee SD, Akbal C, Kaefer M. Refluxing ureteral reimplant as temporary treatment of obstructed megaureter in neonate and infant. *J Urol* 2005;173:1357–1360.
3. Shukla AR, Cooper JR, Patel RP, et al. Prenatally detected primary megaureter: a role for extended followup. *J Urol* 2005;173:1353–1356.
4. Liu HY, Dhillon HK, Young CK, et al. Clinical outcome and management of prenatally diagnosed primary megaureter. *J Urol* 1994;152:914–917.
5. McLorie GA, Jayanthi VR, Kinaham TJ, et al. A modified extravesical technique for megaureter repair. *Br J Urol* 1994;74:715–719.
6. Perovic S. Surgical treatment of megaureters using detrusor tunneling extravesical ureteroneocystostomy. *J Urol* 1994;152:622–625.
7. Perdzynski W, Kalicinski ZH. Long-term results after megaureter folding in children. *J Pediatr Surg* 1996;31:1211–1217.
8. Rabinowitz R, Barkin M, Schillinger JF, et al. The influence of etiology on the surgical management and prognosis of the massively dilated ureter in children. *J Urol* 1978;119:808–813.
9. Fretz PC, Austin JC, Hawtrey CH, et al. Long-term outcomes analysis of Starr plication for primary obstructed megaureters. *J Urol* 2004;172:703–705.
10. Peters CA, Mandell J, Lebowitz RL, et al. Congenital obstructed megaureters in early infancy: diagnosis and treatment. *J Urol* 1989;142:641–645.


# CHAPTER 101 ■ PRUNE BELLY (TRIAD) SYNDROME

DAVID B. JOSEPH

Triad syndrome—the clinical association of a thin flaccid abdominal wall, undescended testes, and bladder hypertrophy with hydroureters—was originally described in 1895 by Parker (1). Shortly thereafter, Osler presented a similar constellation of findings in a child he described as having the appearance of "a wrinkled prune" (2). From that point, "prune belly" has unfortunately become synonymous with this syndrome. This clinical manifestation is also known as the Eagle–Barrett syndrome and the abdominal muscular deficiency syndrome. By classic description, the triad syndrome occurs in boys. However, 5% of patients are girls presenting with similar physical findings, with the obvious exception of the gonadal abnormality. The incidence of triad syndrome occurs in 1 of every 30,000 to 50,000 live births. Most cases are sporadic, although a familial occurrence has been described (3).

Approximately three quarters of children with classic triad syndrome will have other associated anomalies. Urethral abnormalities, including atresia and megalourethra, have been reported but are not required as part of the triad. Urethral atresia is usually associated with a patent urachus. The most common skeletal abnormality is a thoracic deformity resulting in a protruded upper sternum, depressed lower sternum, and splayed ribs. Other less frequent skeletal deformities include talipes equinovarus, congenital hip dislocation, calcaneus valgus, polydactyly, syndactyly, arthrogryposis, scoliosis, and lordosis. Intestinal malformations are noted in approximately one third of children and most often are due to defective fixation or malrotation of the midgut. Cardiac atrial or ventricular septal defects, patent ductus, and teratology of Fallot have been reported in approximately 15% of children (3).

## DIAGNOSIS

The diagnosis of triad syndrome can be established in utero with fetal sonography. However, similar findings can be seen in a fetus with posterior urethral valves or the megacystis–megaureters syndrome. Close inspection for thinned or absent abdominal wall musculature should hedge the differential diagnosis to that of the triad syndrome. In utero diagnosis allows for a planned neonatal investigation. Triad syndrome is often obvious at birth with the pathognomonic physical findings of a loose, lax, wrinkled abdominal wall; flared chest; and undescended testes.

Several classifications of the triad syndrome have been established based on severity and initial clinical presentation. There is no single classification system that incorporates the total spectrum of this syndrome. For practical purposes, children can be grouped into severe, moderate, or mild presentations. With a severe presentation, survival is often limited by significant respiratory compromise due to pulmonary immaturity and dysplasia, as well as extensive renal dysplasia, resulting in a Potter-like syndrome. Children described with moderate involvement have combined renal and respiratory insufficiency, mandating close observation and early intervention to minimize the sequelae of pulmonary and renal compromise. The combination of increased bilateral renal echogenicity on sonography, chronic urinary tract infections (UTIs), and a nadir serum creatine of >0.7 mg/dL are prognostic for renal failure (4). Monitoring of the urinary system is necessary to prevent progressive renal deterioration due to stagnation of urinary flow, UTIs, and possible urinary tract obstruction. Urinary tract reconstruction may play an important role in limiting long-term morbidity. Children with mild involvement do not suffer from respiratory or renal compromise. While long-term follow-up is necessary, operative intervention is often limited to orchiopexy and abdominal wall reconstruction.

A team approach consisting of a pediatric urologist, neonatologist, nephrologist, pulmonologist, and cardiologist is required to maximize the outcome. The initial cardiorespiratory status of the neonate must be established. The baby should undergo a chest X-ray and, when indicated, cardiac sonography. Urologic evaluation commences with abdominal sonography and a baseline chemistry profile. Both the upper and lower urinary tract should be assessed. Attention should be placed on the degree of hydronephrosis, the volume of renal parenchyma, and its echogenicity. Often, there will be a disproportionate degree of distal ureteral dilation and megacystis compared to dilation of the proximal ureter and kidney. On occasion, a marked transition of ureteral dilation is noted. If the infant is clinically stable with normal renal function and is voiding per urethra or draining through a patent urachus, further diagnostic testing can be placed on hold.

Children with renal insufficiency require further imaging to differentiate renal dysplasia and stagnant urine flow from true obstruction. The MAG-3 renal scan has limitations in the newborn period but still provides the most objective data. The voiding cystourethrogram can assess vesicoureteral reflux and the effectiveness of bladder emptying. The neonate with triad syndrome and hydroureteronephrosis is susceptible to bacteriuria and can quickly become symptomatic. Bacteriuria is often

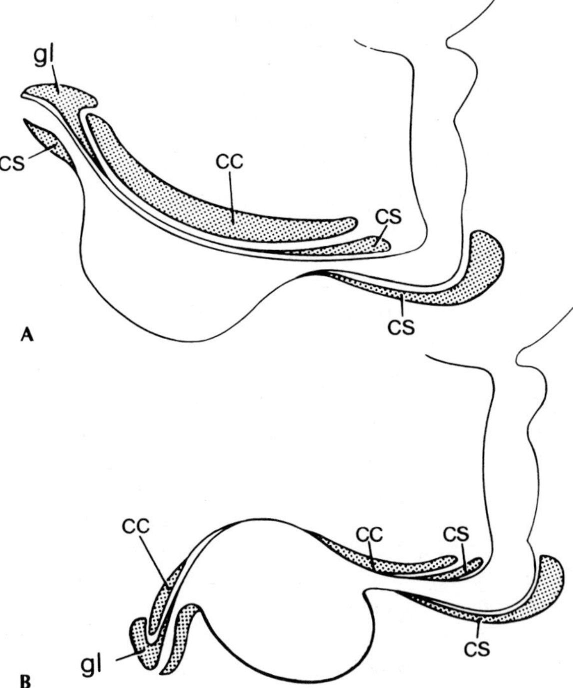


FIGURE 101.1 **A:** Scaphoid megalourethra. Corpora spongiosum (*CS*) is deficient throughout the ventral aspect of penile urethra. Corpora cavernosum (*CC*) is normal. **B:** Fusiform megalourethra. Both corpora spongiosum and cavernosum are deficient. Glans (*gl*) is normal in both variants.

persistent and difficult to clear. Therefore, it is of utmost importance that any invasive lower urinary tract imaging be performed in a sterile environment, with the child receiving pre- and postprocedural antibiotics.

Megalourethra has been classified as scaphoid and fusiform (Fig. 101.1). The more common scaphoid defect is confined to the penile portion of the corpus spongiosum, resulting in a variable length of massively enlarged ventral, anterior urethra similar in appearance to a saccular diverticulum. The fusiform variety encompasses a defect of the corpus spongiosum and deficiency of one or both of the corpus cavernosum, resulting in circumferential ballooning of the urethra and generalized penile flaccidity. Megalourethra is usually an isolated defect but can present with upper urinary tract changes, including hydronephrosis, vesicoureteral reflux, and renal dysplasia. It has been reported to occur with the triad syndrome, which may represent a continuation of the abnormal mesodermal theory of development related to the triad syndrome.

## INDICATIONS FOR SURGERY

Each child presents with a unique constellation of problems resulting in its own set of considerations and requires individualized care (5). Therefore, no one treatment plan is appropriate for all children. In general, operative management can be divided into three broad areas: reconstruction of the urinary system, reconstruction of the abdominal wall, and transfer of the intra-abdominal testes to the scrotum.

## Urinary Tract Reconstruction

Controversy surrounds the need for aggressive urinary tract reconstruction. Early aggressive operative intervention for all children is countered by the fact that renal dysplasia may be inherent, thus preventing any intervention from improving the functional status. In addition, imaging studies depicting significant hydroureteronephrosis do not always correlate with obstruction or the potential for symptoms, and hydroureteronephrosis by itself does not mandate reconstruction. Urinary tract reconstruction is beneficial in a child who has a component of obstructive uropathy and has been shown to have improved renal function with decompression of the urinary system. Reconstruction is also of benefit in the child who has progressive hydroureteronephrosis associated with increasing renal compromise and in the child who has recurrent symptomatic UTIs due to stagnant urine flow.

Urinary diversion plays an initial temporary role in the management of acute renal failure or sepsis. Often, children with urethral atresia or obstruction will present with a patent urachus, effectively emptying their lower tract. Infants with associated posterior urethral abnormalities resulting in obstruction or poor bladder decompression, who are not candidates for intermittent catheterization, benefit from a vesicostomy. A vesicostomy, however, may not adequately drain the upper urinary tract due to a relative obstruction of the ureter at the level of the bladder or poor urinary transport secondary to a highly compliant, adynamic ureter. Vesicostomy should be undertaken only when bladder catheterization has been shown to be effective. Otherwise, temporary diversion of the upper urinary tract will be required. Nephrostomy tube drainage is helpful to stabilize an acute problem but its long-term effectiveness is limited, resulting in a need for a more formal upper urinary tract diversion. There is a theoretical advantage in performing upper tract diversion as proximal as possible. This should maximally relieve stress to the kidney and limit stagnation of urine in a dilated tortuous ureter. However, there is often a disproportionate degree of distal versus proximal ureteral dilation that can prevent easy access of the proximal ureter.

It is compelling to perform a reduction cystoplasty during urinary reconstruction in a child with triad syndrome. However, long-term follow-up has not shown an objective advantage (6,7). With time, the bladder will often regain its large size and lose its tone, resulting in inadequate emptying. For these reasons, it is not practical to proceed with reductive cystoplasty as the primary indication for urinary reconstruction. If a large, poorly contracting bladder results in inadequate urinary emptying, intermittent catheterization would be a more appropriate form of initial management. However, when undertaking formal upper tract reconstruction and ureteral tailoring, reductive cystoplasty is practical and may provide limited improved bladder emptying.

## Reconstruction of the Abdominal Wall

Several techniques have been devised to maximize the cosmetic benefits of abdominal wall reconstruction in children with triad syndrome. There is evidence indicating that the muscular defect is more pronounced centrally and caudally. Initial reconstructive efforts were based on removal of this abnormal tissue. While the appearance of the abdomen was improved, it was not ideal and resulted in a transverse incision and loss of the umbilicus. Monfort described preservation of the umbilicus, and others have added various modifications (8–10). Based on this approach, abdominal wall reconstruction now allows for an excellent cosmetic and functional outcome (11). The benefit of abdominal wall reconstruction is dependent on the degree of abdominal wall laxity. The timing for this procedure should be based on the need for other operative intervention. If it is obvious that the child will not require upper urinary tract reconstruction, abdominal wall reconstruction can be undertaken at any time. If, however, there is the potential for upper urinary tract reconstruction, abdominal wall reconstruction should be deferred until the time of that intervention.

## Orchiopexy

The timing for orchiopexy can be individualized based on the child's need for urinary reconstructive surgery. If urinary reconstructive surgery is required, orchiopexy can be performed at the same time. If urinary reconstructive surgery is not required, then the timing and approach are variable. Placement of the testes within the scrotum is important for maintaining hormone function, allowing for pubertal development and sexuality, but unfortunately fertility is not improved (12). Biopsies of testes have shown a Sertoli-cell-only feature prohibiting future fertility.

## Urethral Reconstruction

Correction of the megalourethra is dependent on presenting symptoms of urinary dribbling and/or urinary infections. Most often operative correction is undertaken because of the unusual appearance of the megalourethra. Urethral tapering is an appropriate treatment.

# ALTERNATIVE THERAPY

Alternative therapy relates to conservative medical management and observation. The floppy abdominal wall and poor musculature can be supported with use of an elastic corset.

# SURGICAL TECHNIQUE

## Vesicostomy

A vesicostomy is placed between the symphysis and umbilicus. A 2- to 3-cm incision is made down to the rectus fascia. A triangular segment of fascia is removed, which will help limit problems of stenosis. The rectus is separated, the space of Retzius is entered, and the dome of the bladder is identified along with the urachus and umbilical ligaments. The bladder is opened in this region to decrease the risk of prolapse. The bladder wall is secured to the rectus fascia with 4-0 polyglactin sutures and the bladder epithelium is approximated to the skin with 4-0 chromic gut.

## Distal Cutaneous Ureterostomy

When there is minimal proximal dilation, a low distal cutaneous ureterostomy provides adequate decompression with relief of stagnated urine flow and stabilization of renal function. The ureter can be approached from a small (2.5-cm) incision placed in a lower inguinal location. The muscles are split to enter the retroperitoneum. The ureter may have the appearance of bowel due to its large size. When in doubt, a 21-gauge needle should be passed, aspirating contents to confirm urine. Once confirmed, the ureter is opened at the level of the obliterated umbilical artery. The size of the ureter usually prevents postoperative stenosis, allowing for either an end or loop ureterostomy. An advantage of distal diversion is noted at the time of definitive urinary reconstruction: the proximal urinary system will have remained uncompromised, allowing for easier mobilization and greater flexibility when tailoring the ureter.

## Ureteral Reconstruction

When definitive primary urinary reconstruction is necessary, the initial approach to the ureter can be extravesical. The ureter is isolated at the level of the bladder and proximal dissection ensues. If there is an obvious transitional phase noted on imaging between the dilated distal ureter and the normal proximal ureter, the dissection should be continued proximal to the transition point. During dissection, the adventitial tissue surrounding the ureter is preserved to prevent devascularization. All of the distal ureter is excised when there is adequate length for the proximal ureter to be reimplanted in the bladder in a standard fashion or with the assistance of a psoas hitch.

If total proximal and distal ureteral tailoring is necessary due to massive dilation, full mobilization of the ureter will be required. This can be accomplished via a retroperitoneal approach, but in most children it is helpful to enter the peritoneum and reflect either the descending or ascending colon along the white line of Toldt. The dilated ureter is often exceedingly redundant and tortuous. Straightening of the ureter without devascularization is required. The functional capability of the ureter for peristalsis and transmission of urine into the bladder parallels the degree of hydroureter. Therefore, ureteral tapering may enhance urinary flow into the bladder. Multiple techniques exist for ureteral tailoring, including ureteral imbrication and formal ureteral excision as with any megaureter (Fig. 101.2). Ureteral imbrication is appropriate for marginally dilated ureters. But, when massive ureteral dilation is present, which is usually the reason for reconstruction, formal excision is preferred, eliminating the bulky tissue that results from the large imbricated ureter.

The ureter is tapered loosely over either a 10Fr or 12Fr catheter, depending on the child's age and size. The excised ureteral segment may need to take an unconventional course to preserve adequate blood supply to the tailored ureter. If a large, redundant renal pelvis is present in association with a dilated proximal ureter, a reduction pyeloplasty should be performed in line with the ureteral excision. Preservation of the proximal ureteral blood supply is mandatory.

After excision, the ureter and renal pelvis are closed in a two-layer technique using absorbable sutures. The first running suture line is 5-0 or 6-0 chromic gut, polydioxanone, or polyglactic acid, directly apposing the mucosa and muscularis of the ureter. The second layer reapproximates the adventitial tissue using the same suture material. Both running layers are discontinued a few centimeters from the distal end of the ureter. The very distal portion of the ureter is closed with interrupted sutures. This allows for excision of the distal ureter without interruption of the running suture line. Enough ureteral length should be preserved to allow for a tunneled antirefluxing ureteroneocystostomy in all cases. A ureteral stent will remain for 5 to 10 days postoperatively.

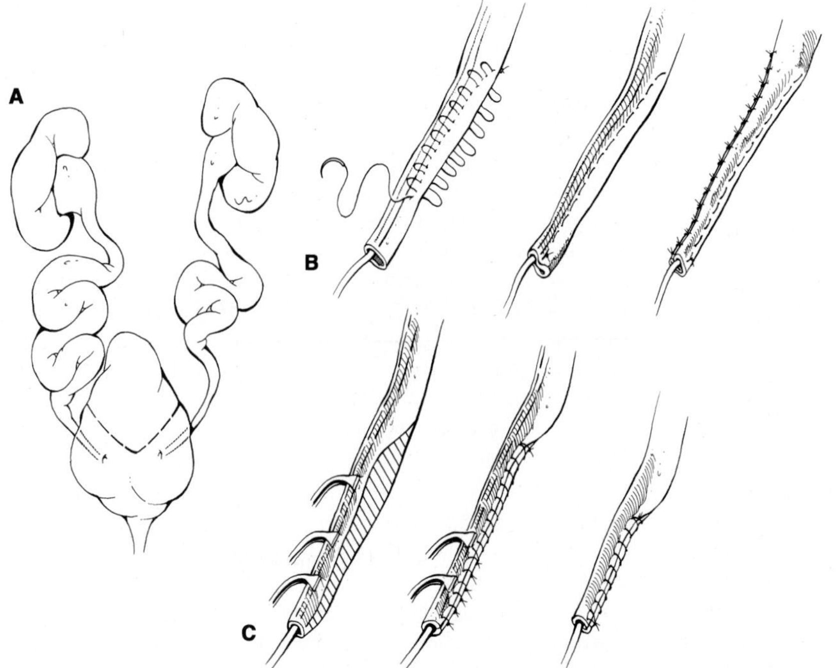


FIGURE 101.2. **A:** The tortuous dilated ureter is carefully straightened without compromising blood supply. The redundant portion is excised and the remaining distal segment tapered if necessary. **B:** Ureteral folding over a 10Fr or 12Fr ureteral catheter. **C:** Formal ureteral tapering with excision and closure. *Note*: The continuous running closure stops 1 to 2 cm from the end of the segment, followed by interrupted suture placement, allowing for excision of the distal end of the ureter without compromising the running closure.

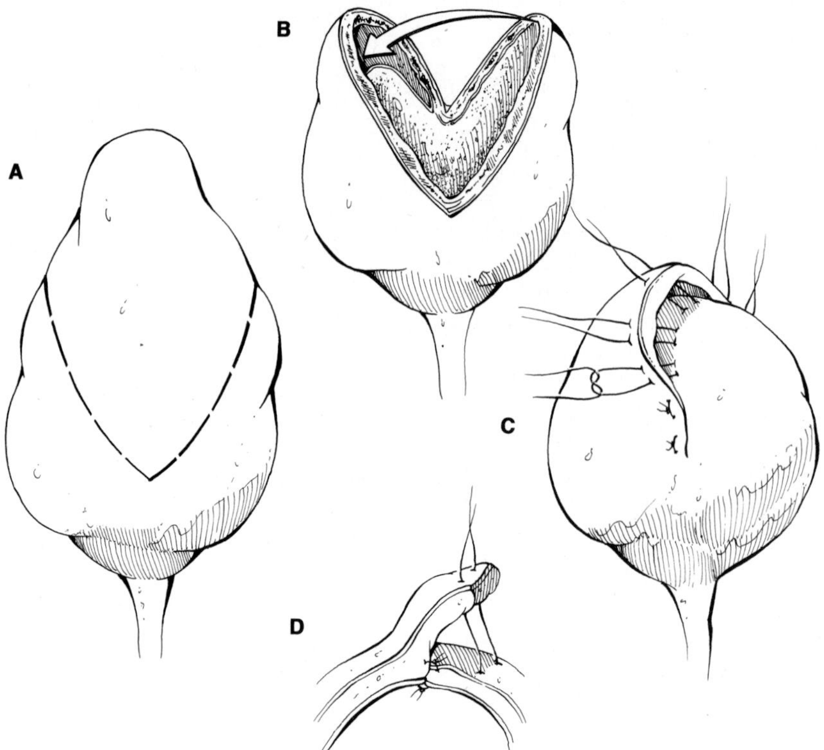


FIGURE 101.3 Reduction cystoplasty. **A:** The dome of the bladder, including any urachal remnant, is removed. **B:** A 2- to 3-cm mucosal strip is then removed from one portion of the bladder. **C and D:** The bladder is closed with overlapping suture lines.

## Reduction Cystoplasty

Reductive cystoplasty should include the urachus and the majority of the dome of the bladder (Fig. 101.3). A 2- to 3-cm strip of mucosa is removed from one side of the bladder wall, allowing for a reinforced overlapping suture line. The bladder is closed in three independent layers using a running suture of 3-0 chromic gut, polydioxanone, or polyglactic acid. A suprapubic tube is inserted for postoperative monitoring regarding the effectiveness of bladder emptying.

## Abdominal Wall Reconstruction

The Monfort approach begins with a midline incision from the tip of the xiphoid process carried inferiorly, circumscribing the umbilicus, leaving an adequate umbilical island of tissue, and ending at the symphysis pubis (Fig. 101.4). A full-thickness skin flap is created bilaterally, elevating the subcutaneous fat from the underlying fascia. The dissection is continued laterally to the anterior axillary line. Often, there will be variability and asymmetry of muscular development. Care must be taken not to enter the peritoneum while mobilizing the skin flaps, in particular in areas where the fascia is relatively thin. An incision is then made lateral to the superior epigastric artery through the fascia, entering the peritoneum. The incision is continued lateral and parallel to the course of the superior and inferior epigastric arteries from the costal margin to the symphysis pubis. The fascia is then elevated and the contralateral superior and inferior epigastric arteries are identified. A second parallel incision is made lateral to these arteries. The central fascial bridge with the umbilical island is now supported by both sets of epigastric arteries. The two lateral incisions provide excellent exposure for orchiopexy and major urinary tract reconstruction when required.

At the time of abdominal closure, the lateral fascia wall is secured to the central fascial strip with a running 2-0 or 3-0 polyglactin suture. The lateral fascia can be scored with the cautery along the intended suture line to enhance adherence. The edge of the lateral fascia is then overlapped and secured in the midline with figure-of-eight suture placement using 2-0 or 3-0 polyglactin sutures. This pants-over-vest closure provides additional ventral support. Two flat 7Fr suction drains are placed between the fascia and the subcutaneous space. The skin flaps are then tailored, removing the excess, allowing for a midline and periumbilical closure. The skin flap is closed in multiple layers, securing the subcutaneous tissue with 4-0 plain gut sutures. The epithelial edge is reapproximated with a running subcuticular suture of 4-0 or 5-0 polyglactin. The drains remain in place for 2 or 3 days for decompression of the dead space. An alternative laparoscopic-assisted approach may allow for improved abdominal wall plication and simultaneous orchiopexy (13).

## Orchiopexy

The testicle is usually found closely associated with a dilated distal ureter and should be released from the ureter in order to determine whether it can be delivered into the scrotum without

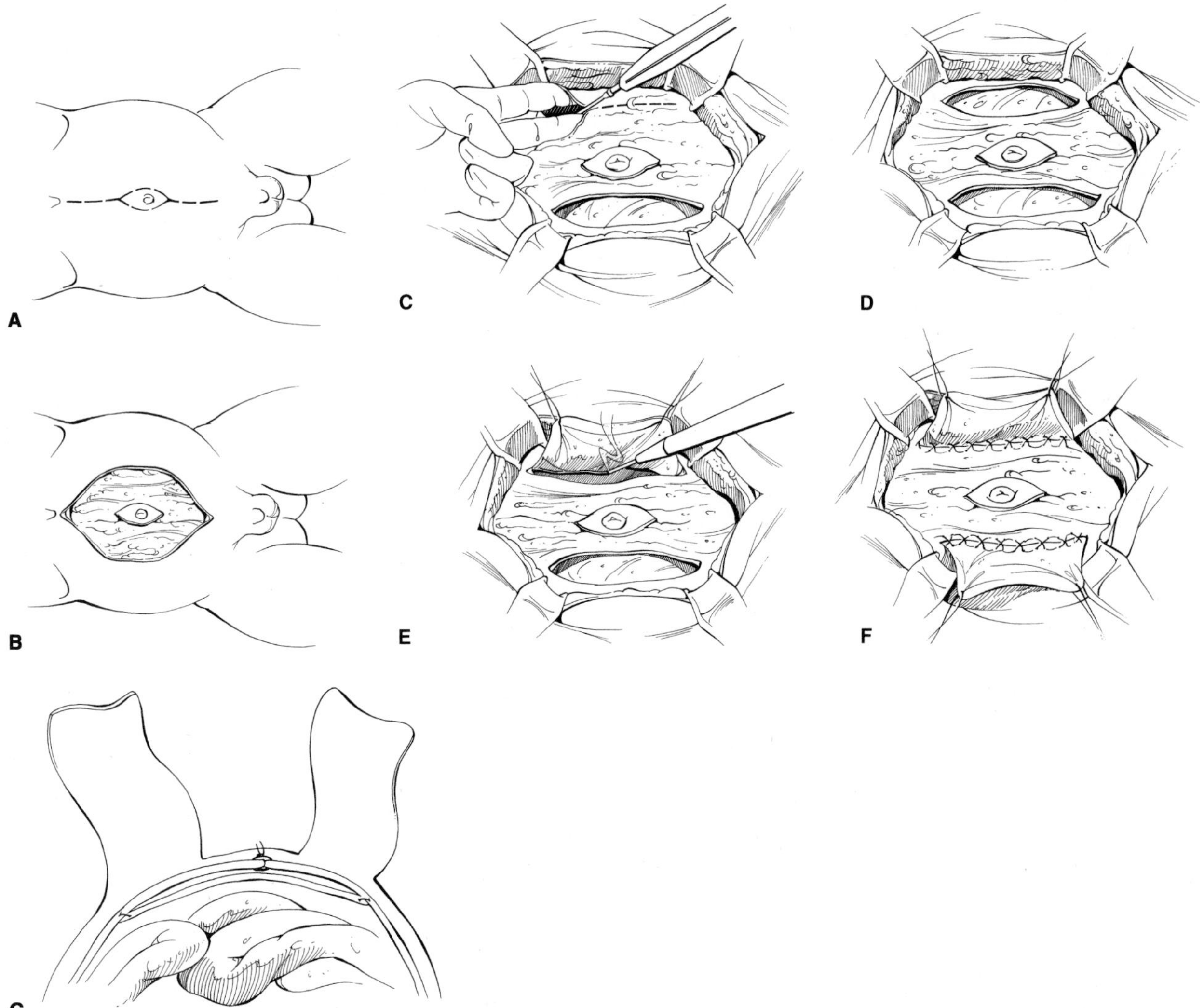


FIGURE 101.4 **A:** An incision is begun at the xiphoid, circumscribing the umbilicus, and carried down to the pubis. **B:** Skin flaps are then elevated, dissecting between the subcutaneous fat and the fascial layer. The lateral extension is the anterior auxiliary line. **C and D:** The umbilicus is supported by the central fascial bridge. Incisions will be made into the peritoneum lateral to the epigastric vessels. The central fascial bridge is easily manipulated to allow for excellent intra-abdominal exposure. **E:** At the time of closure, a line is scored on the peritoneal surface of the fascia. **F:** The central fascial strip is then secured laterally to the scored fascia line with a running suture of 2-0 or 3-0 polyglactin. **G:** The lateral fascia is then secured in the midline above and below the umbilicus with 2-0 or 3-0 polyglactin. Centrally, the fascia is secured directly to the umbilicus. This allows for an overlapping reinforced fascial wall closure. Subcutaneous tissue is closed with 3-0 or 4-0 plain gut and the skin with a running subcuticular 4-0 or 5-0 polyglactin suture.

sacrifice of the gonadal artery. If orchiopexy is undertaken early, particularly within the first 6 months of life, there is often adequate vascular length to deliver the testicle directly into the scrotum without transection of the gonadal artery (5). After the testicle is separated from the ureter, an incision is made in the peritoneum lateral to the gonadal artery and directed to the internal ring. A second incision medial to the gonadal vessels is made in the peritoneum and continued caudally along the course of the vessels and vas deferens. It is important not to disrupt the vascular supply of the peritoneal pedicle running on both sides of the vas deferens. If it becomes apparent that the testes will not reach into the scrotum after mobilization, the gonadal artery is sacrificed to obtain adequate length for the testicle to be delivered in the scrotum, as described by Fowler and Stephens (14). The blood supply to the testes is maintained by the vasal artery and small anastomotic channels within the peritoneal flap. A tunnel is then made into the scrotum and an incision placed inferiorly in the scrotum to create a dartos pouch. A clamp is passed from the scrotum to the inguinal canal. The testicle is grasped, pulled down through the tunnel, and delivered to the scrotum. Care must be taken not to twist or place the peritoneal pedicle on tension. If desired, the testicle can be secured to the dartos tissue with a 5-0 polydioxanone suture. When the orchiopexy is approached as an independent procedure it can be undertaken laparoscopically.

## Urethral Reconstruction

Urethral reconfiguration is most effective by formal excisional tapering, as described by Nesbitt (Fig. 101.5). An incision is made in line with the previous circumcision or beneath the

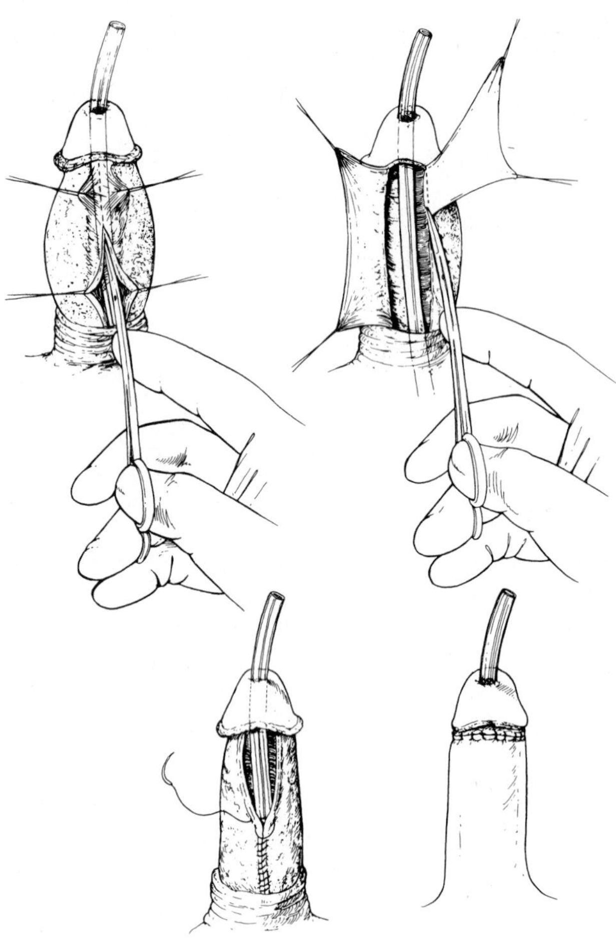

FIGURE 101.5 Nesbitt reduction urethroplasty for megalourethra. **A:** The urethra is opened vertically in the midline, followed by excision of the lateral redundant tissue (**B**). **C:** Reconstruction is carried out over a 12Fr catheter using two layers of running suture. **D:** The penile skin is reapproximated to the coronal margin circumferentially.

coronal sulcus if the patient is uncircumcised. The penile shaft skin is then mobilized to the base of the penis. The anterior urethral wall is usually thin and poorly supported, and care needs to be taken to prevent inadvertent entrance into the urethra. The urethra is split in the midline ventrally. The redundant portion of the urethra is excised and the urethra is reapproximated over a 10Fr or 12Fr catheter, depending on the child's age. The urethra is closed in two layers using 6-0 or 7-0 polydioxanone or polyglactic acid sutures. The glanular urethra is usually patent and the reconstruction is limited to the penile shaft. Because of poor development of the spongiosum it may be difficult to achieve additional tissue for a second layer of coverage. The penile shaft skin is then secured to the coronal tissue with 6-0 chromic sutures. A urethral stent or catheter is placed for 7 days. The penis is dressed with the personal technique used for a hypospadias repair.

A variant of megalourethra is the "megameatus with an intact prepuce" (MIP). This is corrected using standard hypospadias techniques (Fig. 101.6). The glans is infiltrated with a mixture of 1:200,000 epinephrine for hemostasis. Parallel incisions are made lateral to the urethral plate and extended into the glans, creating two glanular wings. The incisions are continued along the shaft of the penis and connected beneath the urethral meatus. The urethra is then tubularized over an 8Fr, 10Fr, or 12Fr catheter using 6-0 or 7-0 polyglactic or polyglycolic acid sutures. The glans is closed in the midline, reapproximating the deep tissue with 6-0 Vicryl and the epithelium with 6-0 chromic. The penile shaft skin is brought up and the excess excised and then reapproximated to the coronal ring. A urethral stent or catheter can be positioned for 7 days, depending on the length of the defect. The penis is dressed as above.

# OUTCOMES

## Complications

Ureteral devascularization resulting in ischemia and subsequent obstruction can occur if attention has not been paid to the ureteral blood supply. The risk of bowel obstruction is present as in any intra-abdominal procedure. Testicular ischemia and atrophy due to a single-stage Fowler–Stephens procedure has been reported to occur in 30% of children. This can be decreased with a staged approach (12). More importantly, ischemia may be prevented with early orchiopexy, eliminating the need for sacrificing the gonadal vessels.

The cosmetic appearance following urethral tapering is good and limited only by any residual corpora cavernosa deficiency. Postvoid dribbling can be abolished and the risk of urinary infections due to stagnant urine can be diminished. The most common complication is that of a urethral fistula due to limited spongiosum tissue for a multiple-layer closure. The circumferential degloving of the penis with subsequent reapproximation of the penile shaft skin to the corona will limit fistula formation. The greatest risk for a fistula is located at the level of the ventral coronal sulcus.

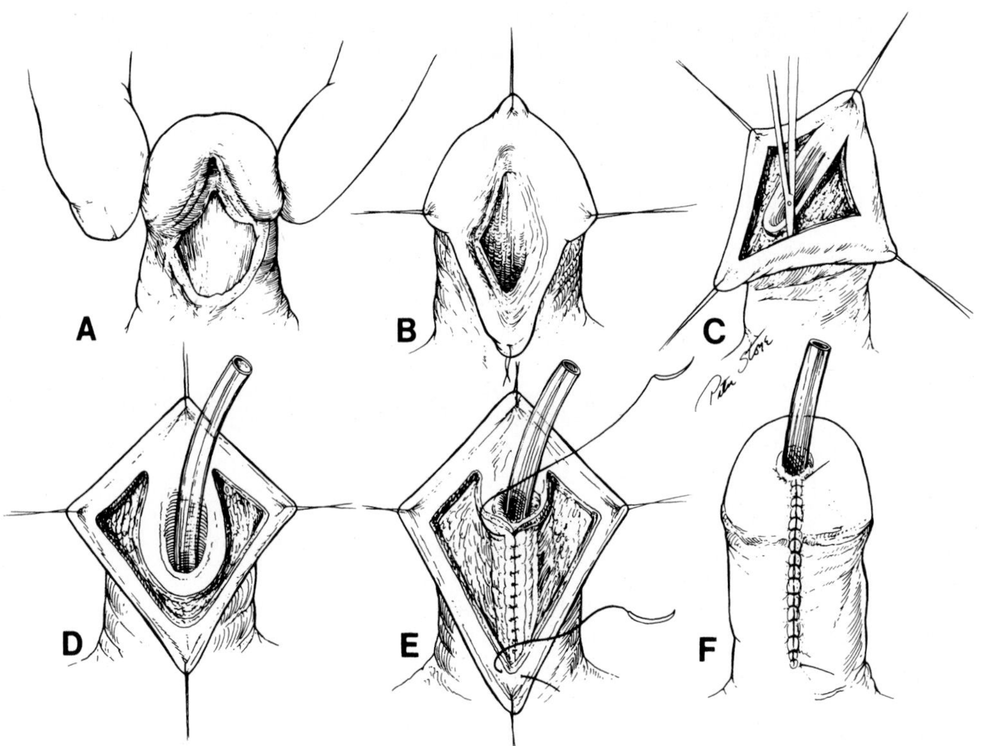


FIGURE 101.6 **A:** Pyramid procedure for repair of the megameatus with intact prepuce variant of hypospadias. **B and C:** Stay sutures are placed and the urethra is mobilized sharply. **D and E:** The urethra is tubularized in a two-layer technique. **F:** Subcutaneous glandular tissue is reapproximated and the skin closed.

## Results

The results of urologic reconstruction can be very gratifying in the initial postoperative period, in particular the cosmetic appearance of the abdomen and improvement in upper urinary tract drainage. Voiding function may become more effective due to the benefits of abdominal wall reconstruction and reduction cystoplasty (11). However, with time there can be an increase in both bladder size and ureteral dilation. This is often due to ineffective voiding and is independent of bladder reduction. For those reasons, long-term follow-up of the urinary tract is required. Patients should be prepared for the potential need for intermittent catheterization. Because of normal sensation, children are often unwilling to cooperate with urethral catheterization. Placement of an appendicovesicostomy should be considered if catheterization appears to be a realistic possibility at the time of urinary reconstruction. An appendicovesicostomy provides excellent access to the bladder in a normally sensate child.

## *References*

1. Parker RW. Absence of abdominal muscles in an infant. *Lancet* 1895;23:1252.
2. Oster W. Congenital absence of the abdominal muscles with distended and hypertrophied urinary bladder. *Bull Johns Hopkins Hosp* 1901;12: 331–335.
3. Strand WR. Initial management of complex pediatric disorders: prunebelly syndrome, posterior urethral valves. *Urol Clin North Am* 2004;31: 399–415.
4. Noh PH, Cooper CS, Winkler AC, et al. Prognostic factors for long-term renal function in boys with the prune-belly syndrome. *J Urol* 1999;162: 1399–1401.
5. Woodard JR. Prune-belly syndrome: a personal learning experience. *BJU Int* 2003;92:10–11.
6. Bukowski TM, Perlmutter AD. Reduction cystoplasty in the prune-belly syndrome: a long-term follow-up. *J Urol* 1994;152:2113–2116.
7. Kinahan TJ, Churchill BM, McLorie GA, et al. The efficiency of bladder emptying in the prune-belly syndrome. *J Urol* 1992;148:600–603.
8. Bukowski TM, Smith CA. Monfort abdominoplasty with neoumbilical modification. *J Urol* 2000;164:1711–1713.
9. Ehrlich RM, Lesavoy MA, Fine RN. Total abdominal wall reconstruction in the prune-belly syndrome. *J Urol* 1986;136:282–285.
10. Montfort G, Guys JM, Boccoardo A, et al. A novel technique for reconstruction of the abdominal wall in the prune belly syndrome. *J Urol* 1991; 146:639–640.
11. Smith CA, Smith EA, Parrott TS, et al. Voiding function in patients with the prune-belly syndrome after Monfort abdominoplasty. *J Urol* 1998; 159:1675–1679.
12. Patil KK, Duffy PG, Woodhouse RJ, et al. Long-term outcome of Fowler-Stephens orchiopexy in boys with prune-belly syndrome. *J Urol* 2004;171: 1666–1669.
13. Franco I. Laparoscopic-assisted modification of the Firlit abdominal wall plication. *J Urol* 2005;174:280–283.
14. Fowler R, Stephens FD. The role of testicular vascular anatomy in the salvage of high undescended testis. *Aust NZ J Surg* 1959;29:92–106.

# CHAPTER 102 ■ CHILDHOOD RHABDOMYOSARCOMA

HSI-YANG WU AND HOWARD M. SNYDER III

The management of rhabdomyosarcoma (RMS) remains the most controversial topic in pediatric urological oncology. While all agree that a combination of surgery, chemotherapy, and radiotherapy is best, the optimal timing and extent of the three treatment modalities remain unclear. It is useful to remember three key points: (i) chemotherapy cures microscopical disease, (ii) residual mass does not equal disease, and (iii) radiotherapy renders pathology very difficult to read.

Twenty percent of RMS cases involve the bladder, prostate, vagina, or paratesticular area. The incidence of RMS peaks between ages 2 to 4 and ages 15 to 19. The tumor is nonencapsulated, grows rapidly, and spreads to regional lymph nodes as well as hematogenously. The Intergroup Rhabdomyosarcoma Study (IRS) Group initiated studies in the United States in 1972 to achieve better survival with less morbidity. The Children's Oncology Group (COG) has taken over responsibilities for these trials, and is currently investigating new chemotherapeutic options such as irinotecan (1). Patient survival, which was only 40% to 73% prior to chemotherapy, has improved to 86% in IRS IV with VAC (vincristine, dactinomycin, and cyclophosphamide) (2). During the same time, the surgical approach has changed from initial exenterative surgery to organ-preserving surgery following chemotherapy. The functional bladder salvage rate has risen from 25% to approximately 60% with this change in management.

RMS consists of small, blue, round cells, arising from undifferentiated mesoderm, with a microscopical appearance of spindle cells resembling fetal skeletal muscle. Embryonal pathology accounts for 90% of genitourinary RMS cases. Embryonal pathology is more favorable than alveolar pathology, which tends to occur in extremities. Sarcoma botyroides ("bunch of grapes") is a polypoid form of embryonal pathology.

## DIAGNOSIS

Bladder and prostate primaries present with urinary retention and gross hematuria and tend to be located at the trigone and bladder neck. Often, determining the organ from which the tumor arose can be difficult. Vaginal primaries present with vaginal bleeding or an introital mass and tend to occur on the anterior vaginal wall. Paratesticular primaries present with a painless scrotal mass. The preoperative evaluation can be carried out with ultrasound, computed tomography (CT), or magnetic resonance imaging (MRI) (T2 weighting). The retroperitoneum is best evaluated with CT or MRI. Metastatic workup is completed with a chest X-ray, liver function tests, bone scan, and bone marrow biopsy.

**TABLE 102.1**

**PREOPERATIVE STAGING**

| |
|---|
| T1: Confined to organ of origin, a: ≤5 cm, b: >5 cm |
| T2: Extension or fixed to surrounding tissue, a: ≤5 cm, b: >5 cm |
| N0: Regional nodes clinically negative |
| N1: Regional nodes clinically positive |
| Nx: Unknown |
| M0: No distant metastasis |
| M1: Metastasis present |
| Stage I: Vaginal and paratesticular RMS, any T, any N, M0 |
| Stage II: Bladder/prostate RMS, T1a or T2a, N0 or Nx, M0 |
| Stage III: Bladder/prostate RMS, (T1a or T2a) and N1, M0, *OR* (T1b or T2b), any N, M0 |
| Stage IV: Any tumor with M1 |

**TABLE 102.2**

**POSTOPERATIVE GROUPING**

| |
|---|
| Group 1: Localized disease, completely excised, no microscopical residual |
| A: Confined to site of origin, completely resected |
| B: Infiltrating beyond site of origin, completely resected |
| Group 2: Total gross resection |
| A: Gross resection with microscopical local residual |
| B: Regional disease with involved lymph nodes, completely resected with no microscopic residual |
| C: Microscopical local and/or nodal residual |
| Group 3: Incomplete resection or biopsy with gross residual |
| Group 4: Distant metastases |

The IRS studies included both preoperative staging and postoperative grouping (2) (Tables 102.1 and 102.2). The IRS I–III studies grouped patients based on completeness of resection, introducing biases (shifting patients from group 1 to group 3) that are not seen with the use of the tumor–node–metastasis (TNM) system in IRS IV and V.

## INDICATIONS FOR SURGERY

During the initial procedure, adequate tissue for a definitive diagnosis should be obtained and, if possible, one should remove the tumor without removing the affected organ (with the exception of paratesticular RMS, where the testis is removed with the tumor inguinally). If excision is not possible, primary chemotherapy should be given. In follow-up staging, a biopsy is needed during the "second-look" operation because residual mass does not always represent tumor: the cancer can involute more rapidly than the supporting stroma. Definitive surgery aims to do a good radical but pelvic-organ–sparing operation if possible. If microscopical residual disease is found, it is treated with brachytherapy or external-beam radiotherapy. Exenteration is reserved for patients who fail this protocol of chemotherapy, conservative surgery, and radiotherapy. In Europe, the approach is to give primary chemotherapy without initial local control (radiotherapy or surgery) and offer local therapy based on the initial chemotherapy response (3).

## ALTERNATIVE THERAPY

The use of surgery or radiotherapy as definitive local control remains a difficult choice. In favor of radiotherapy, it has been remarkably successful in decreasing the need for radical surgery to achieve a cure. However, the difficulty with radiotherapy and bladder RMS is that because the tumors tend to be located at the bladder neck, even the lowest dose (41 Gy) that the radiation oncologists are willing to deliver may significantly risk urinary continence. Current attempts at limiting radiation toxicity to adjacent organs involve both conformal radiotherapy and brachytherapy. The long-term risk of radiation vasculitis, which is inevitably progressive, as well as possible bony pelvis deformity in these children is another issue to consider. Therefore, one must sometimes weigh whether preserving a bladder without an outlet is better than removing the bladder entirely (4). The final issue is that postradiation artifact makes subsequent biopsy very difficult to interpret, so it would make sense to delay radiation until the patient is free of gross disease.

## SURGICAL TECHNIQUE

For bladder and prostate RMS, we will summarize the surgical options available after the initial biopsy has shown RMS, the patient has received chemotherapy, and the choice has been made to use surgery to achieve local control. For vaginal and paratesticular RMS, we will review the overall surgical approach starting with the initial resection.

### Bladder

The approach to partial or total cystectomy is similar to that for muscle-invasive transitional cell carcinoma (see Chapters 23 and 24). We will highlight the technical points that are unique to the management of bladder RMS.

The initial step after opening the abdomen is to examine the retroperitoneum. While we do not perform a full retroperitoneal lymphadenectomy because there is no therapeutic benefit, any suspicious lymph nodes along the vessels between the obturator fossa and the renal veins are removed. The next step is to properly stage the tumor by obtaining multiple frozen-section biopsies of the bladder around the area of the tumor. If these are negative and the tumor is amenable to partial cystectomy with a 2- to 3-cm margin, then the bladder does not need to be entirely removed. RMS is a nonencapsulated, infiltrative tumor, so adequate margins are necessary.

If the tumor extends down the urethra, then the symphysis should be split to gain better access. After completing distal dissection of the urethra, the symphysis is closed with long-term absorbable sutures. With this improved exposure, it is also possible to perform a nerve-sparing dissection (see Chapter 33), although follow-up potency data are not yet available. The placement of brachytherapy catheters for afterloading (to treat microscopical positive margins if needed) should be considered.

Following cystectomy, we have often placed Dexon mesh across the abdomen to hold the intestines out of the pelvis at the level of the sacral promontory. This is done by attaching it to the sacral promontory and wrapping it around the sigmoid. This serves to prevent adhesion of the bowel to the raw surface of the pelvis until it has re-epithelialized, and if postoperative radiation is necessary for microscopical residual disease it limits the exposure of the bowel to the radiation field. Currently, pelvic exenteration is reserved for patients who have failed both chemotherapy and radiotherapy and who have tumors that invade both the bladder and the rectum.

The final surgical decision is whether to proceed with continent urinary reconstruction at the same time. We have taken the approach that it is not necessary to perform the reconstruction at the same time unless the patient is both motivated and able to perform clean intermittent catheterization to drain a urinary reservoir. For younger patients who are not ready to manage a urinary reservoir, we have either brought up the remaining bladder plate with ureterovesical junctions intact as a vesicostomy or performed low end-cutaneous ureterostomies, with the ureters placed side by side as a single stoma on the abdomen.

### Prostate

The approach is similar to that for localized prostatic adenocarcinoma (see Chapter 33). Again, no follow-up on nerve-sparing procedures is yet available. Splitting the symphysis is useful as it is essential to remove the urethra to the midbulbar level, and the placement of brachytherapy catheters for afterloading (to treat microscopical positive margins if needed) should be considered.

### Vagina

The patient is placed in the lithotomy position and the pelvis and vagina are prepared. For the initial resection, vaginoscopy is helpful in defining the limits of the tumor. Stay sutures and a small weighted vaginal speculum are helpful for exposure, as is a headlight for vision. Sharp excision of the tumor is carried out, staying away from the external sphincter, urethra, and bladder neck. The vaginal mucosa is closed with interrupted absorbable sutures. Hysterectomy is rarely carried out because uterine tumors are rare and tend to present in older girls (>10 years old).

## Paratestis

The testis and adnexa are removed via inguinal orchiectomy (see Chapter 62). Frozen section of the proximal cord should reveal no tumor. The key step is to avoid making a scrotal incision for a solid paratesticular mass because, while chemotherapy often cures residual disease, some cases have required hemiscrotectomy due to tumor infiltration. Retroperitoneal lymph node dissection is carried out for all boys with stage I disease older than age 10, regardless of the findings on abdominal CT. The technique is identical to that used for retroperitoneal involvement by testicular tumors (see Chapter 63). Again, sympathetic nerve-sparing techniques can be used to maintain ejaculation, but no follow-up data are currently available. For boys under age 10, the retroperitoneum is imaged by CT or MRI, and if there is no gross disease then retroperitoneal lymph node dissection is not performed. Chemotherapy has been shown to adequately clear microscopical disease (30% to 40% incidence).

## Postoperative Decisions

Review of the pathology may reveal persistent rhabdomyoblasts in a patient who has received as much chemotherapy as can safely be given. Currently, there is debate concerning the malignant potential of these cells, which represent matured rhabdomyoblasts (5). Normally, resection of the involved organ is carried out. If this would require destruction of a functional bladder, observation with frequent radiological follow-up may be an option to consider.

# OUTCOMES

## Results

### Bladder and Prostate

Bladder and prostate RMS has a 2.5:1 male predominance. IRS III included intensified chemotherapy (dactinomycin, etoposide) and 6 weeks of radiotherapy, increasing the functional bladder salvage rate from 25% to 60%. The initial procedure consists of percutaneous, endoscopic, or transrectal biopsy of the mass, followed by chemotherapy. In IRS IV, VAC was shown to be as effective as two other three-drug regimens (VIE/VAE: ifosfamide, etoposide) (2). On a "second-look" procedure, half of patients were managed with biopsy, 30% had partial cystectomy, 13% had cystoprostatectomy, and the remainder had either cystectomy or prostatectomy alone (6). For persistent disease, group 2 was treated with 41 Gy and group 3 was treated with 50 Gy. At 24 weeks, a third operative evaluation was performed with consideration for exenteration. Patients with embryonal pathology had an 83% 3-year failure-free survival, compared to 40% in those with alveolar pathology. All patients with group 4 (metastatic) prostate disease died. Renal function, as assessed by serum blood urea nitrogen and creatinine, was normal in 95%, although 29% of patients had abnormal renal scans (7). Bladder function (as assessed by questionnaire) was normal in only 40% of patients (6).

In a larger international series, 48% of patients underwent biopsy alone, 30% had partial cystectomy, and 21% had complete cystectomy. Of male patients, only 24% underwent prostatectomy. Bladder function was normal in 69% of patients treated with biopsy alone and 73% of patients who underwent partial cystectomy. Neither of these series utilized urodynamic studies to fully evaluate bladder function. Renal function was abnormal in 40% of patients, and bowel function was abnormal in 13% (8).

### Vagina

Surgery and chemotherapy cure most cases of vaginal RMS. In the overall IRS I–IV experience, 42% of patients were treated with surgery and chemotherapy, 19% required additional radiotherapy, 21% were treated with biopsy and chemotherapy alone, and 12% were managed with biopsy, chemotherapy, and radiotherapy (9). In IRS IV, only 19% of patients required wide excision of the tumor. Primary treatment with VAC chemotherapy is usually successful, and a biopsy 8 to 12 weeks after chemotherapy is recommended. Pelvic lymph node dissection is not necessary. Radiotherapy should be used only for persistent disease or relapse (10). Rhabdomyoblasts on biopsy are evidence of chemotherapy response, and therefore further chemotherapy, instead of resection, is the proper treatment (5).

### Paratestis

Paratesticular RMS has two peak incidences: in the 3- to 4-month-old boy and in the teenager. Scrotal ultrasound will confirm the paratesticular primary, which should then be resected along with the testis in a radical inguinal orchiectomy. Serum β-human chorionic gonadotropin and α-fetoprotein levels should be obtained to confirm that the mass is not a testicular primary. Thirty percent to 40% of patients will have metastases to the retroperitoneum. The biological activity of the tumor is different between the neonate and the teenager (90% vs. 63% failure-free survival at 3 years). In previous studies, all patients underwent retroperitoneal lymph node dissection (RPLND) (2). However, Olive et al. (11) showed in 1984 that of 19 patients with clinical stage I disease, 17 were cured with adjuvant chemotherapy alone. This showed that chemotherapy can clear microscopical retroperitoneal disease, making RPLND unnecessary. In IRS IV, RPLND was not recommended, leading to a significant understaging of disease and a decrease in failure-free survival rates because patients with negative CT scans did not receive radiation. Thirty percent of those patients who were clinically stage I and over at 10 years of age required retreatment. Because the outcome for stage I disease in those under 10 years of age was so good in IRS IV, those patients who are <10 years old and have stage I disease and negative abdominopelvic CT are treated with VA (vincristine, dactinomycin) only in IRS V, whereas all patients with stage I disease who are 10 years or older undergo RPLND regardless of CT findings. Group 2 tumors (positive lymph nodes on pathology) are treated with radiotherapy and VAC. The 3-year failure-free survival rate was 81% for group 1 tumors overall, but those patients >10 years old had only a 63% survival rate (2).

## Complications

The majority of patients have acute toxicity from the chemotherapy: 90% developed myelosuppression, 55% developed significant infections, and renal toxicity was seen in 2% (2). Most relapses occur within 3 years of initial diagnosis (12). Late recurrences can occur in patients who are treated with chemotherapy alone. Of 883 patients, 10 developed a secondary cancer. Patients with pre-existing renal abnormalities were at a higher risk of death (5% vs. 1%). Relapse in group 3 patients (incomplete resection) was associated with a 22% chance of 3-year survival, compared to 41% in group 1 or 2 patients (localized disease or total gross resection) (2). Twenty-nine percent required sex hormone replacement and 11% were shorter than expected (4). If radiotherapy has been used, there is an increased risk of a secondary neoplasm, often another sarcoma, in the radiation field.

## *References*


1. Ferrer FA, Isakoff M, Koyle MA. Bladder/prostate rhabdomyosarcoma: past, present, and future. *J Urol* 2006;176:1283–1291.
2. Crist WM, Anderson JR, Meza JL, et al. Intergroup Rhabdomyosarcoma Study—IV: results for patients with nonmetastatic disease. *J Clin Oncol* 2001;19:3091–3102.
3. Flamant F, Rodary C, Rey A, et al. Treatment of non-metastatic rhabdomyosarcoma in childhood and adolescence. Results of the second study of the International Society of Paediatric Oncology: MMT84. *Eur J Cancer* 1998;34:1050–1062.
4. Raney B, Heyn R, Hays DM, et al. Sequelae of treatment in 109 patients followed 5 to 15 years after diagnosis of sarcoma of the bladder and prostate. *Cancer* 1993;71:2387–2394.
5. Arndt CAS, Hammond S, Rodeberg D, et al. Significance of persistent mature rhabdomyoblasts in bladder/prostate rhabdomyosarcoma. Results from IRS IV. *J Pediatr Hematol Oncol* 2006;28:563–567.
6. Arndt C, Rodeberg D, Breitfeld PP, et al. Does bladder preservation (as a surgical principle) lead to retaining bladder function in bladder/prostate rhabdomyosarcoma? Results from Intergroup Rhabdomyosarcoma Study IV. *J Urol* 2004;171:2396–2403.
7. Paidas CN. Results of rhabdomyosarcoma of the bladder and prostate: is bladder preservation successful? Presented at the Section on Surgery, American Academy of Pediatrics meeting, Chicago, 2000.
8. Raney B, Anderson J, Jenney M, et al. Late effects in 164 patients with rhabdomyosarcoma of the bladder/prostate region: a report from the International Workshop. *J Urol* 2006;176:2190–2195.
9. Arndt CAS, Donaldson SS, Anderson JR, et al. What constitutes optimal therapy for patients with rhabdomyosarcoma of the female genital tract? *Cancer* 2001;91:2454–2468.
10. Andrassy RJ. Modern approach to rhabdomyosarcoma of the vagina and uterus. Presented at the Section on Surgery, American Academy of Pediatrics meeting, Chicago, 2000.
11. Olive D, Flamant F, Zucker JM, et al. Paraaortic lymphadenectomy is not necessary in the treatment of localized paratesticular rhabdomyosarcoma. *Cancer* 1984;54:1283–1287.
12. Pappo AS, Anderson JR, Crist WM, et al. Survival after relapse in children and adolescents with rhabdomyosarcoma: a report from the Intergroup Rhabdomyosarcoma Study Group. *J Clin Oncol* 1999;17:3487–3493.


# CHAPTER 103 ■ VESICOURETERAL REFLUX

MARK R. ZAONTZ

Considering that vesicoureteral reflux (VUR) was first recognized during the time of Galen (150 A.D.), not much progress was noted until the beginning of the 20th century. Young (1) and later Sampson (2) noted that those patients with both normal ureterovesical junction and ureteral path through the bladder did not have VUR. It was not until the 1950s that the strong relationship between VUR and pyelonephritis was recognized by Hutch (3). His work demonstrated the pathologic anatomy that underlies VUR and led to successful surgical correction of this entity. His pioneering work was also instrumental in making the voiding cystourethrogram (VCUG) part of the evaluation in patients with urinary tract infection (UTI) as well as hydronephrosis.

Until the 1980s, the treatment for reflux was largely surgical, with cure rates approaching 98%. However, multicenter studies have shown that lower grades of reflux had high spontaneous resolution rates and these patients could be followed at least initially with medical management using prophylactic antibiotics and yearly reassessment. Higher grades of reflux are associated with a higher incidence of renal scarring and lower rates of spontaneous resolution.

Surgical correction of reflux may not prevent progression of reflux nephropathy when present, although corrected reflux in general prevents new renal scarring. Reflux in the presence of sterile urine in general does not cause renal damage, although reflux in the presence of UTI can lead to renal scarring.

Boys in general present with higher reflux grades than girls of the same age, but boys also have a higher spontaneous resolution rate than girls. Studies showing that circumcised boys with low grades of reflux rarely get UTIs or related morbidity have led to a nonoperative algorithm in this group of patients.

Reflux is commonly linked with voiding dysfunction in children. Recent evidence using urodynamics and biofeedback techniques has shown high spontaneous cure rates for refluxing children with concomitant voiding dysfunction. Conversely, children with significant voiding dysfunction have higher failure rates from conventional surgery than those with normal bladder function.

Sampson (2) in the early 1900s proposed a flap-valve mechanism for the ureterovesical junction that was corroborated by Gruber (4), who found that those ureters with shorter intravesical segments were more prone to have reflux and therefore have a defective flap-valve mechanism. Stephens and Lenaghan (5) added that the deficiency of the intravesical ureter's longitudinal muscle with or without a deficiency in ureteral tunnel length was also responsible for the reflux phenomenon. From a surgical perspective we have learned that a 5:1 ratio of ureteral tunnel length to ureteral lumen diameter is necessary to prevent reflux.

While most cases of reflux are congenital in nature and considered primary reflux, increased intravesical pressure due to anatomic bladder outlet obstruction or functional causes such as neuropathic bladder/voiding dysfunction may lead to what is termed secondary reflux.

## DIAGNOSIS

Today, thanks in great part to common antenatal screening, reflux is often diagnosed prior to the development of a urinary infection and, as a result, pyelonephritis may be avoided by promptly beginning prophylaxis just after delivery. Presenting symptoms in neonates may include malaise, fever, vomiting, diarrhea, or failure to thrive. Toddlers and young children may have more typical symptoms, such as fever, frequency, urgency, dysuria, foul-smelling urine, incontinence, or abdominal and/or back discomfort.

It is critical that a urine culture be obtained in all cases of suspected UTI. A urinalysis alone is unacceptable as it only alludes to the presence of UTI and at best is only 80% accurate in diagnosis. Radiographic evaluation is indicated after the first UTI in boys of any age and in all preadolescent girls. Further, any girl with a febrile infection or recurrent UTIs should be studied regardless of her age. Workup for UTI should include an ultrasound of the kidneys and bladder as well as a VCUG. In cases where screening is needed for siblings or children of known refluxers, a renal ultrasound and nuclear cystogram (NVCUG) for girls and a fluoroscopic VCUG for boys is recommended. Recently, there has been discussion of alternative initial evaluation of the first febrile UTI by performing a $^{99m}$Tc-labeled dimercaptosuccinic acid (DMSA) scan to see if the kidney has been engaged in the infection. If the scan is negative, then a VCUG can be obviated. However, a second febrile UTI would still warrant a VCUG. Once reflux is diagnosed, it is graded according to the International Study Classification (Fig. 103.1) (6). This system is based on the radiographic appearance of the ureter and collecting system during a VCUG. Follow-up studies are in general done using nuclear cystography at yearly intervals to assess the resolution or progression of reflux.

Ultrasound appears to be relatively accurate in determining the presence or absence of renal scars in low-grade reflux patients. However, in those with higher-grade reflux a "normal" renal ultrasound may miss significant renal scarring. The DMSA scan is to date the best available study to assess focal pyelonephritis and renal scarring.

Cystoscopy has little value in predicting the presence or cessation of reflux based on ureteral orifice configuration or location. Factors such as tunnel length or the presence of incomplete versus complete duplication anomalies will guide the surgeon to choose an appropriate technique, open or endoscopic.

## INDICATIONS FOR SURGERY

Indications for surgical correction of VUR include an older patient, higher grade of reflux, presence of renal damage, noncompliance with prophylaxis, and the family's concerns with respect to repeated invasive testing and long-term prophylaxis. Findings from the International Reflux Study lend support toward surgical intervention in grade III and IV refluxers, with the majority of these patients failing to resolve their reflux (7). Other studies have supported these findings, with rates of resolution of reflux ranging from 10% to 33% in patients with grade IV reflux (8,9). Surgery is in general recommended for grade V reflux because of the low likelihood of spontaneous resolution.

Girls should not be allowed to go into puberty with reflux due to the increased risk and morbidity of pyelonephritis during pregnancy. Recurrent breakthrough urinary infection

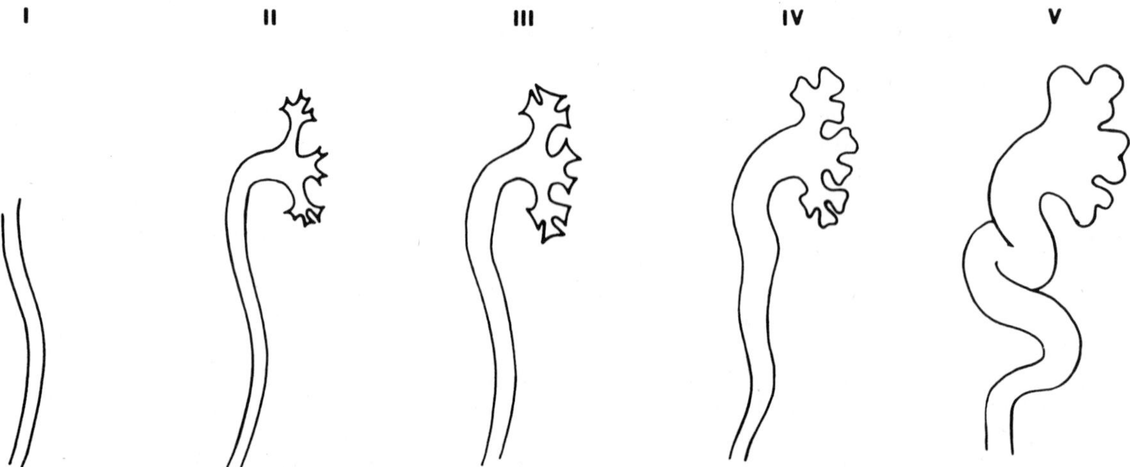


FIGURE 103.1 International classification of vesicoureteral reflux. Grade I, into the nondilated ureter; grade II, into the pelvis and calices without dilation; grade III, mild to moderate dilation of the ureter, renal pelvis, and calices with minimal blunting of the fornices; grade IV, moderate ureteral tortuosity and dilation of the pelvis and calices; grade V, gross dilation of the ureter, pelvis, and calices and loss of papillary impressions and ureteral tortuosity.

while on adequate antibiotic prophylaxis is the sine qua non for surgical intervention because otherwise these children are at high risk for renal damage.

## ALTERNATIVE THERAPY

There are several factors that must be taken into consideration for appropriate management: reflux grade, presence/degree of renal scarring, patient age, presence or absence of bladder outlet obstruction, compliance of the patient/family on prophylactic antibiotics, ability to remain infection-free while on prophylaxis, and presence/absence of associated voiding dysfunction. Reflux may spontaneously resolve, and the peak time for resolution is between 5 and 7 years of age. The lower the grade of reflux, the higher is the likelihood for spontaneous resolution. Unilateral reflux is statistically more likely to resolve than bilateral reflux. Medical management consists of antibiotic prophylaxis, usually a sulfa-based compound or nitrofurantoin at bedtime. In addition to antibiotics, bladder training in cases of dysfunctional voiding is instituted. This is designed to improve bladder emptying at regular intervals, obviate bladder-sphincter dyssynergia, and have minimal postvoid residual. This may require a variety of teaching aids and the use of pharmacotherapy such as anticholinergics and/or alpha antagonists. In addition, urodynamics and biofeedback may be used in selected cases. Equally important is to improve bowel function/evacuation in the presence of constipation.

## SURGICAL TECHNIQUE

Once the decision is made for surgical intervention, there are a myriad of operative procedures available depending on one's preference and comfort level. The existing techniques are divided into endoscopic, extravesical, intravesical, a combination of intravesical and extravesical approaches, and laparoscopic correction.

### Endoscopic Surgery

Teflon was the first bulking agent used for endoscopic correction of reflux. Although the results were encouraging, later studies showed that there was migration of the Teflon particles to the lung, lymph nodes, and brain as well as the finding of granuloma formation; this resulted in the search for more biocompatible bulking agents (10). These have included both autologous agents (fat, blood, human collagen, bladder muscle cells, and ChondroGEL) and nonautologous agents (silicone, BioGlass, polyvinyl alcohol, and dextronomer microspheres). Deflux (dextronomer microspheres) is at present approved by the U.S. Food and Drug Administration for use as a bulking agent. Endoscopic surgery technique for reflux will be discussed in another chapter.

### Extravesical Approach

Lich (11) and Gregoir (12) in the 1960s separately developed the extravesical approach to correct reflux. Further modifications of this approach have yielded success equal to that of the intravesical techniques (13). The benefits of this procedure are several: (a) The surgery is performed outside of the bladder mucosa and as such avoids gross hematuria and irritable postoperative voiding problems such as urgency symptoms and bladder spasms, (b) catheter drainage of the bladder is brief, (c) wound drains are avoided, and (d) ureteral stents are eliminated. A further advantage of this technique is that hospital stay is brief, averaging 1.5 days in my hands, thus decreasing overall hospital costs.

Prior to the incision, after the patient is prepared and draped, the bladder is catheterized and the bladder filled to about one third to one half of its estimated capacity with sterile saline. This allows for easier dissection when separating the detrusor muscle from the mucosa. The bladder may be further filled or emptied depending on the surgeon's preference during the procedure. The surgical procedure for detrusorrhaphy begins similarly to the intravesical approach with a Pfannenstiel incision. A Dennis–Browne retractor is then placed over moistened gauze pads and the bladder is carefully mobilized and rotated anteromedially, exposing the appropriate perivesical space. Care should be taken to avoid entering the peritoneum during this maneuver. Placing an appropriate-sized Deaver retractor to help keep the rotated bladder in place will greatly facilitate locating the obliterated hypogastric vessel. This vessel is tied off with 3-0 polyglycolic acid suture and the most lateral tie is clamped to help expose the ureter, which lies just beneath this vessel. In cases of bilateral detrusorrhaphy, the obliterated hypogastric vessel need not be tied off but simply recognized for ease of finding the underlying ureter. This minimal dissection technique, as well as limiting the dissection of the extravesical submucosal tunnel, may help prevent significant nerve denervation and avoid postoperative urinary retention. The ureter is carefully mobilized and encircled with a vessel loop (Fig. 103.2). The ureter is freed up to its entry point into the bladder. During this maneuver the Deaver retractors may need to be reset such that the ureter is in the middle of the operative field throughout the procedure. A tennis racket incision is made around the ureteral detrusor hiatus and deepened until the ureter is only attached to its connection with the mucosa. The incision is then extended such that a 3- to 5-cm trough is created. All vessels encountered during this dissection are tied off with 4-0 or 3-0 polyglycolic acid suture. Dissection carefully proceeds down to the mucosa and great care is exercised to avoid making a rent in the bladder

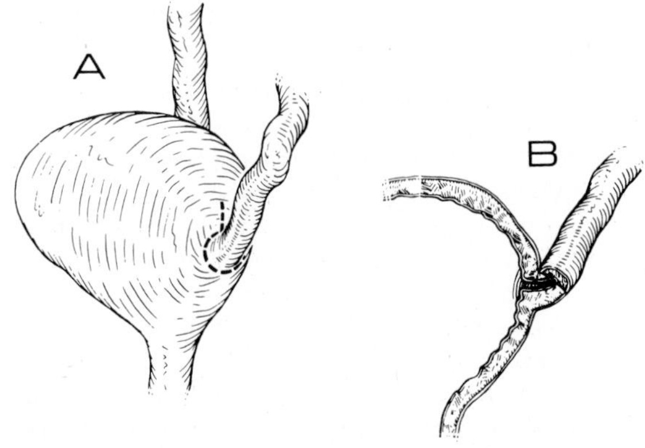


**FIGURE 103.2 A:** After ureteral mobilization, detrusor is incised (*dotted lines*) at level of ureteral hiatus. **B:** Sagittal section demonstrates ureteral hiatus.

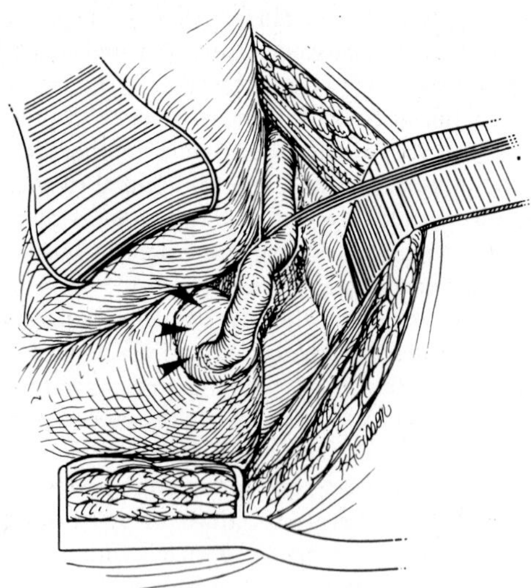

FIGURE 103.3 Ureter contiguous with detrusor mucosa (*arrowheads*).

(Fig. 103.3). If this occurs, immediately close the defect with the 6-0 chromic catgut. Place stay sutures of 3-0 polyglycolic acid on the detrusor edges to facilitate dissection of the mucosa off the detrusor muscle. The mucosal dissection should be generous enough to allow the ureter to easily sit in the newly created trough and permit the detrusor muscle to be closed over the ureter without tension. Prior to this step, further dissection is performed toward the bladder neck beyond the distalmost detrusor incision to allow placement of the advancement sutures. Once completed, the ureteral orifice is advanced on the trigone toward the bladder neck with a pair of "vest-type" sutures of 4-0 chromic catgut (Fig. 103.4). The first limb of the sutures is through the detrusor (outside/in). The sutures enter the detrusor at the distal limit of the trigonal musculature and exit in the plane between the mucosa and detrusor. The second limb of the suture is through the ureteral muscle, and the final limb of the suture is back through the detrusor (inside/out). Tying the pair of vest sutures advances and anchors the ureteral orifice distally and creates a new longer submucosal tunnel. The remaining detrusor defect is closed over the ureter in two layers; the first is a running layer and the second is an interrupted Lembert suture, both using 4-0 polyglycolic acid suture. Care must be exercised to avoid making the ureteral hiatus too snug. The exit point for the ureter should be able to admit a hemostat between the detrusor and the ureter easily (Fig. 103.5). No perivesical drains or ureteral stents are used, and the Foley catheter is removed the following morning.

Complete and incomplete ureteral duplication may also be approached extravesically. Cystoscopy at the time of surgery is recommended to visualize the ureteral orifice location with respect to location and proximity to each other as well as distance to the bladder neck. This information will aid in determining if detrusorrhaphy is feasible or if another technique is more appropriate.

Finally, as we continue to push the envelope into minimally invasive procedures, the extravesical technique can also be approached in selected patients via a small transverse inguinal incision to achieve access to the ureter. In these cases, I find it advantageous to first cystoscope the patient and pass a temporary ureteral stent up the refluxing ureter to aid in initial

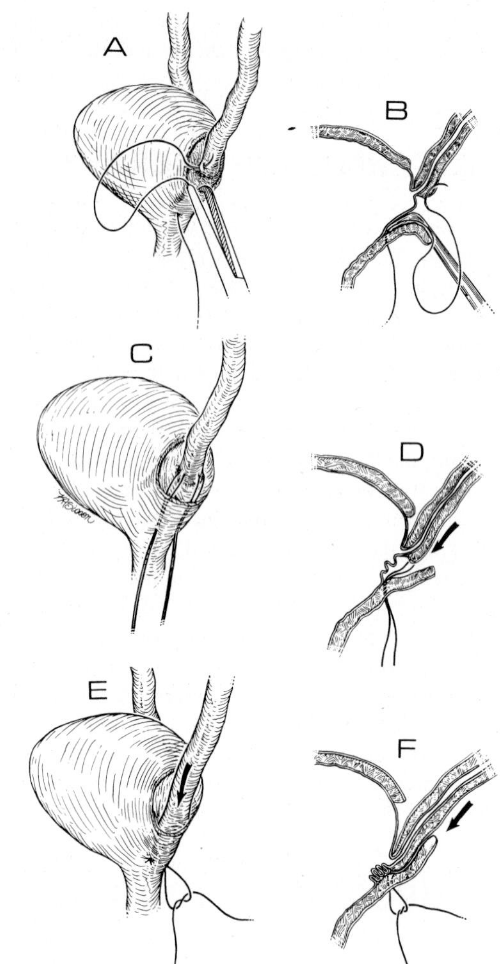


FIGURE 103.4 **A:** Bladder mucosa is elevated off bladder wall muscle and vest-type sutures are placed. **B:** Sagittal section shows suture passing between undermined mucosa and detrusor. **C:** Alignment of vest sutures after placement. **D:** Sagittal section demonstrates appropriate positioning of sutures. **E:** Tying vest sutures advances and anchors ureter onto trigone. **F:** Sagittal section of ureteromeatal advancement.

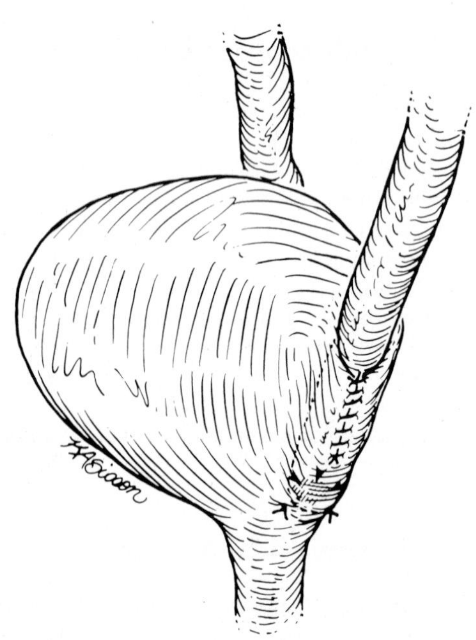

FIGURE 103.5 Closure of detrusor flaps over ureter allows for long submucosal tunnel and completes detrusorrhaphy.

identification. The procedure is otherwise essentially the same as already described, although some institutions are obviating the advancement portion of the procedure, making this technique that much simpler.

## Intravesical Approach

One of the earlier and still highly popular and successful techniques to correct reflux is the Politano–Leadbetter approach (14). This procedure is performed entirely intravesically and avoids mobilization of the bladder as seen in the extravesical approach. Once the bladder is exposed via the technique described for the extravesical approach, it is opened in the midline between 3-0 chromic catgut stay sutures. The bladder is packed with moist 4 × 8-inch gauze pads to allow superior retraction of the bladder and easier exposure of the ureteral orifices. This is further facilitated with the placement of a Dennis–Browne retractor with the curved blades actually within the bladder over moist sponges. The ureteral orifice is identified and intubated with a 5Fr feeding tube and secured with 4-0 or 5-0 silk sutures to allow tenting of the ureter by pulling on the feeding tube. As with all intravesical repairs the ureter is mobilized in similar fashion (Fig. 103.6). An incision is made to score the mucosa around the orifice. This can be done with a scalpel, tenotomy scissor, or, as I prefer, the cutting current of the Bovie, which provides a precise incision. Carefully, using long tenotomy scissors, vascular forceps, Kittner dissector, a right-angle clamp, and judicious use of the cautery unit, the muscular attachments to the ureter are taken down. As the dissection proceeds proximally, I have employed the use of a number 3 Freer elevator along the posterior surface of the ureter, which further aids in mobilization. It is critically important to stay outside of the adventitia of the ureter to avoid devascularization during its dissection. As the peritoneum is encountered, it is generously swept back off the ureter to avoid injuring the bowel during the relocation of the ureter. A hernia retractor or a very thin Deaver helps to better expose the peritoneum and extravesical attachments to the ureter. Take care in the male patient to avoid injury to the vas deferens.

After completion of ureteral mobilization, the surgeon may choose one of several procedures to complete the ureteral reimplantation. The Politano–Leadbetter repair employs a suprahiatal approach (Figs. 103.7 and 103.8). A submucosal tunnel is created from the old hiatus superiorly, long enough to achieve a 5:1 ratio of submucosal tunnel to ureteral diameter. I like to use 135-degree blunt-tip Metzenbaum scissors to facilitate this maneuver and avoid tearing the bladder mucosa. Once the desired tunnel length is achieved, the new hiatus is developed by making a small incision directly on top of a right-angle clamp. Using a stay suture or the feeding tube, the mobilized ureter is passed from the old hiatus to the new

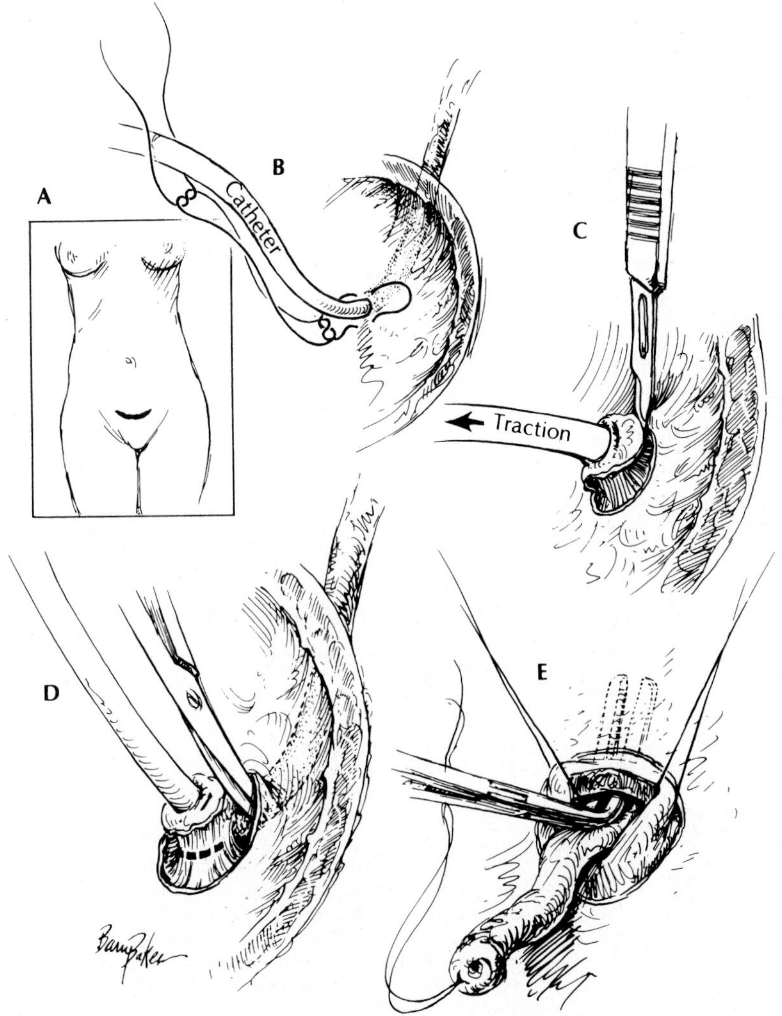


**FIGURE 103.6** Intravesical mobilization of ureter. **A:** Low transverse incision. **B:** A 3.5Fr or 5.0Fr polyethylene tube and traction suture. **C:** Incision around meatus with mucosal cuff using long-handled knife. **D:** Cutting and blunt dissection of muscle of superficial trigone. **E:** Extravesical mobilization with right-angle clamp and Kittner dissector.

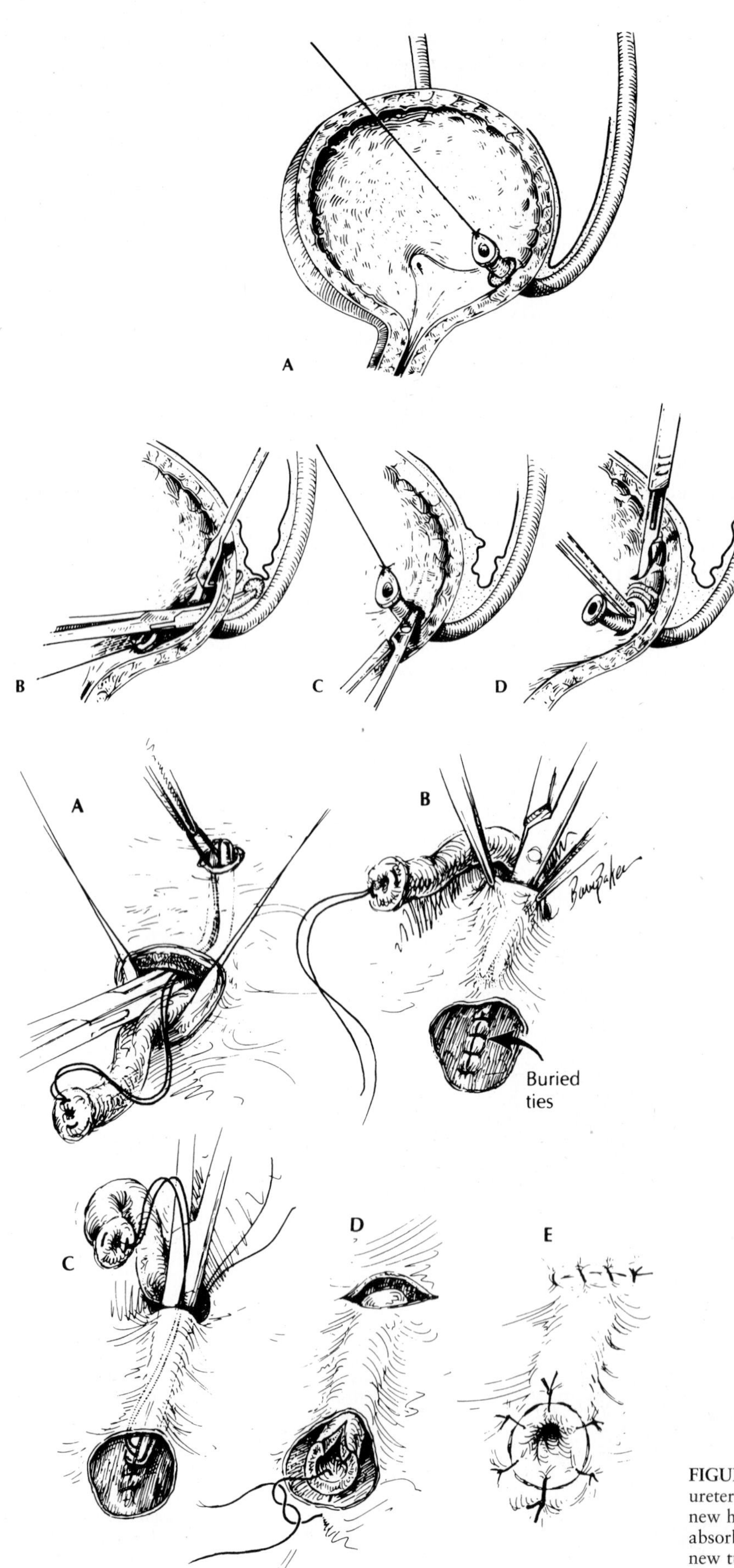


FIGURE 103.7 Politano–Leadbetter repair. **A:** Mobilization of intravesical ureter. **B:** Dissection of peritoneum with Kittner dissector. **C:** Development of submucosal tunnel. **D:** Creation of the new hiatus.

FIGURE 103.8 Politano–Leadbetter repair and details of ureteral reimplant. **A:** The ureter is brought through the new hiatus, and the old hiatus is closed with interrupted absorbable suture. **B:** The ureter is brought through the new tunnel (**C**), spatulated if necessary (**D**), and sewn in place with interrupted absorbable suture (**E**).

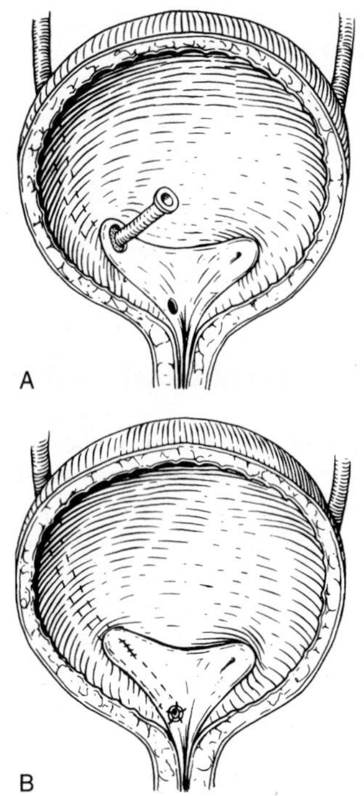


FIGURE 103.9 Glenn–Anderson repair. (From Walker RW. Vesicoureteral reflux. In: Gillenwater JY, Grahhack JR, Howards SS, et al., eds. *Adult and Pediatric Urology*, vol 2. St. Louis: Mosby–Year Book, 1996, with permission.)

hiatus, care being taken to avoid twisting, kinking, or angulating the ureter as well as avoiding the peritoneum. The old hiatus is repaired with 4-0 chromic catgut. The ureter is then brought through the new tunnel. The old meatus is then trimmed up and spatulated if necessary. The distal and posterior lip of the ureter is anchored first with a deep suture of 4-0 or 5-0 chromic catgut to the mucosa and muscular layers of the bladder. The remaining anastomosis is performed with the same suture for a mucosal-to-mucosal approximation. Leaving a ureteral stent is at the surgeon's preference. In general, I assess how the urine output appears from the reimplanted ureteral orifice. If there is copious drainage, I do not leave a stent. If I am uncomfortable with urine drainage or there is significant edema at the orifice, a stent is left and brought out through a separate stab wound in the bladder and secured there with a chromic catgut suture. Then, a separate stab wound is made to bring the stent out through the skin and secured there with 4-0 nylon. Likewise, if I have to taper the ureter a stent is left in place for 4 to 7 days postoperatively. I close all bladders in three layers using running 4-0 chromic catgut for the mucosa, muscularis, and seromuscular layers. This has allowed me to avoid leaving any perivesical drains when the ureters are not stented. A Foley catheter remains in the bladder for 1 or 2 postoperative days.

The Glenn–Anderson procedure (Fig. 103.9) (15), in comparison to the Politano–Leadbetter, is an infrahiatal repair and develops a submucosal tunnel toward the bladder neck (Fig. 103.10). It is in particular advantageous when there is good distance between the native ureteral orifice and the bladder neck such that an appropriate tunnel length can be obtained. Adequate mobilization of the ureter is paramount to achieve satisfactory success rates. If the tunnel length appears too

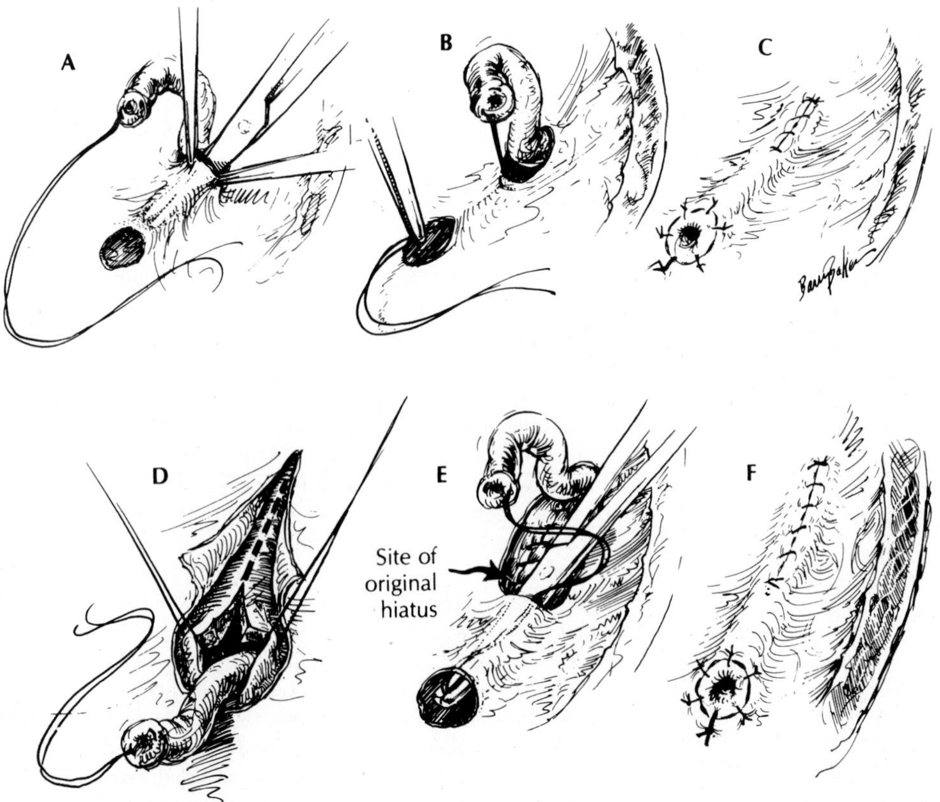


FIGURE 103.10 Glenn–Anderson repair: details of ureteral reimplantation. **A:** Tunnel made toward bladder neck. The ureter is brought through the tunnel (**B**) and sewn in place (**C**). An alternative, similar to the Mathison technique, allows enlargement of hiatus (**D**) and results in longer repair (**E and F**).

short on initial inspection, moving the hiatus more superiorly will allow for satisfactory tunnel creation. Advantages of the Glenn–Anderson technique are that the entire procedure is done under direct vision and it creates a relatively straight tunnel with an easily catheterized ureter.

The transtrigonal approach (Cohen) (16) is similar to the Glenn–Anderson procedure with the exception that the ureter is transposed across the trigone (Fig. 103.11). This is in particular useful in small-capacity and neurogenic bladders where an appropriately long tunnel is critical to success. The ureteral course created is an extension of the natural direction of the ureter; thus, it carries a low risk of ureteral kinking and obstruction. If bilateral reimplant is necessary, it is important to create separate tunnel paths for each ureter. Always remember to close the hiatus with absorbable 4-0 chromic catgut. Leave enough room for a hemostat or right-angle clamp to be interposed between the ureter and the approximated detrusor muscle to avoid obstruction at the hiatus. A potential disadvantage of the Cohen technique is the difficulty of ureteral access postoperatively. These patients may need percutaneous access for any future procedures.

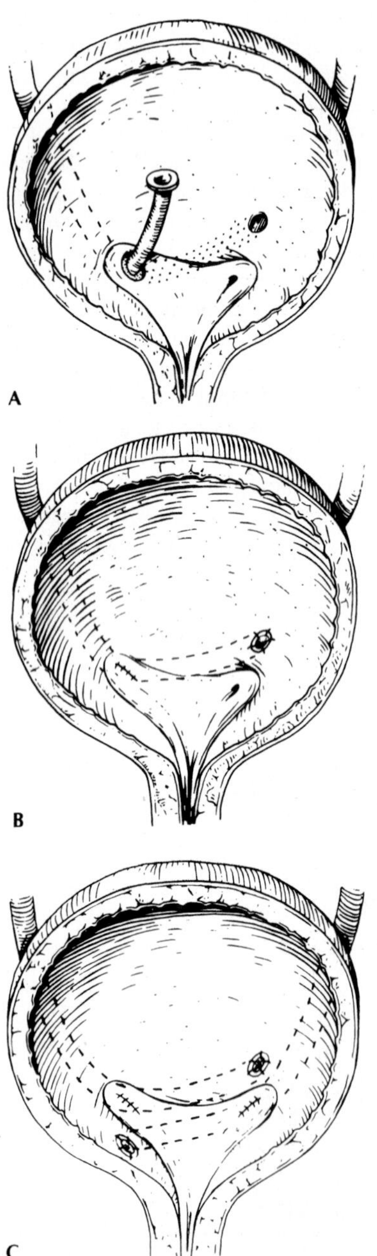


FIGURE 103.11 Cohen technique of ureteral reimplantation. Cross-trigonal tunnel, with the stippled area (A) sewn in place with interrupted sutures (B). C: Bilateral reimplants easily accomplished. (From Walker RW. Vesicoureteral reflux. In: Gillenwater JY, Grayhack JT, Howards SS, et al., eds. *Adult and Pediatric Urology*, vol 2. St. Louis: Mosby–Year Book, 1996, with permission.)

## Ureteral Duplication

Determining whether the ureteral duplication is complete or incomplete guides operative considerations. In the absence of a ureterocele, an intravesical complete duplication can be approached extravesically as well as intravesically. The key to intravesical surgery is to mobilize the duplicated ureters as one unit because their blood supply at the bladder level is intertwined within a common sheath (Fig. 103.12). This will avoid unnecessary devascularization. The technique chosen for reimplant can be any of the intravesical repairs mentioned. In cases of a complete duplication, an ipsilateral ureteroureterostomy is an attractive alternative. In situations where there is an associated ectopic ureter with a salvageable renal moiety, separate ureteral tunnels should be created.

One tip that I have found useful to aid in freeing up the ureter and also with submucosal dissection for all of the intravesical techniques is the use of 1% lidocaine (Xylocaine) with a 1:100,000 epinephrine solution. This is injected periureterally at the orifice and along the proposed subepithelial tunnel using a 26-gauge needle. This minimizes bleeding and provides ease of dissection in a readily defined plane.

## Intra–Extravesical Approach

The Paquin technique (Fig. 103.13) (17) is a commonly used repair and has the advantage over the Politano–Leadbetter approach of doing the complete procedure under direct vision, thus avoiding the potential risk of peritoneal injury. The approach to the ureter is extravesical, similar to that described in detrusorrhaphy. When the ureter is mobilized to the level of the detrusor hiatus, a right-angle clamp is used to clamp the ureter and then the distal stump is oversewn after the ureter has been divided using polyglycolic acid suture. Alternatively, the bladder may be opened in the midline and the ureteral orifice circumscribed and mobilized from within the bladder. The ureter should be intubated with a 5Fr or 8Fr feeding tube and secured with a suture prior to mobilization. The ureter is then passed extravesically, taking care to avoid the peritoneum, which should be swept off the posterior lateral bladder wall. If ureteral tailoring is warranted, it is performed at this point of the procedure. If a longer tunnel is needed and ureteral length is suspect, consider a psoas hitch at this time as well (Fig. 103.14). Using two fingers inside the bladder, bring the bladder up to the psoas muscle tendon, where it should sit under no tension. Place interrupted figure-of-eight sutures of heavy chromic or polyglycolic acid from the tendon of the psoas to the bladder wall just lateral to where the new ureteral hiatus will be situated. Avoid the genitofemoral nerve running along the psoas muscle during this

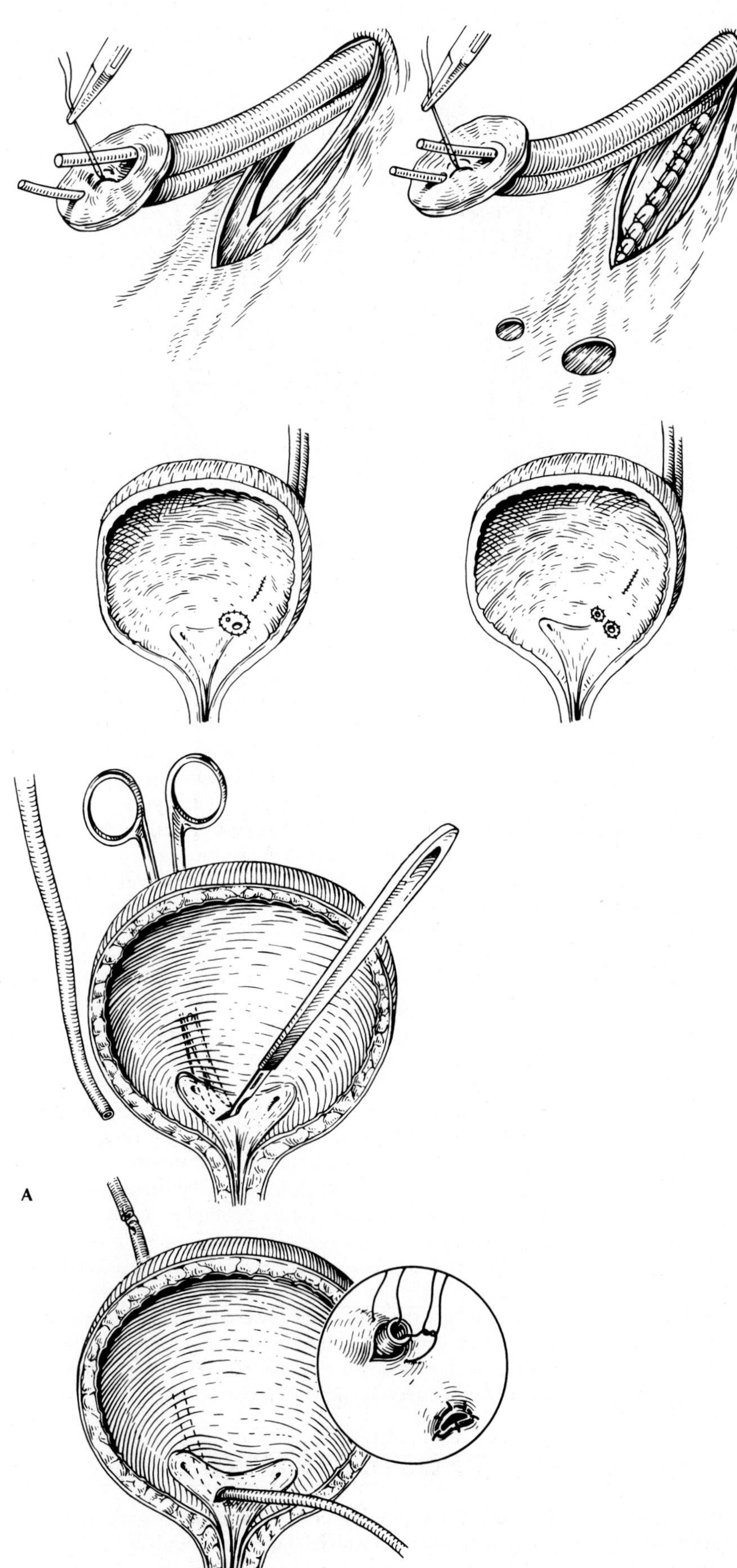


FIGURE 103.12 Reimplantation of duplex ureters.

FIGURE 103.13 Paquin repair.

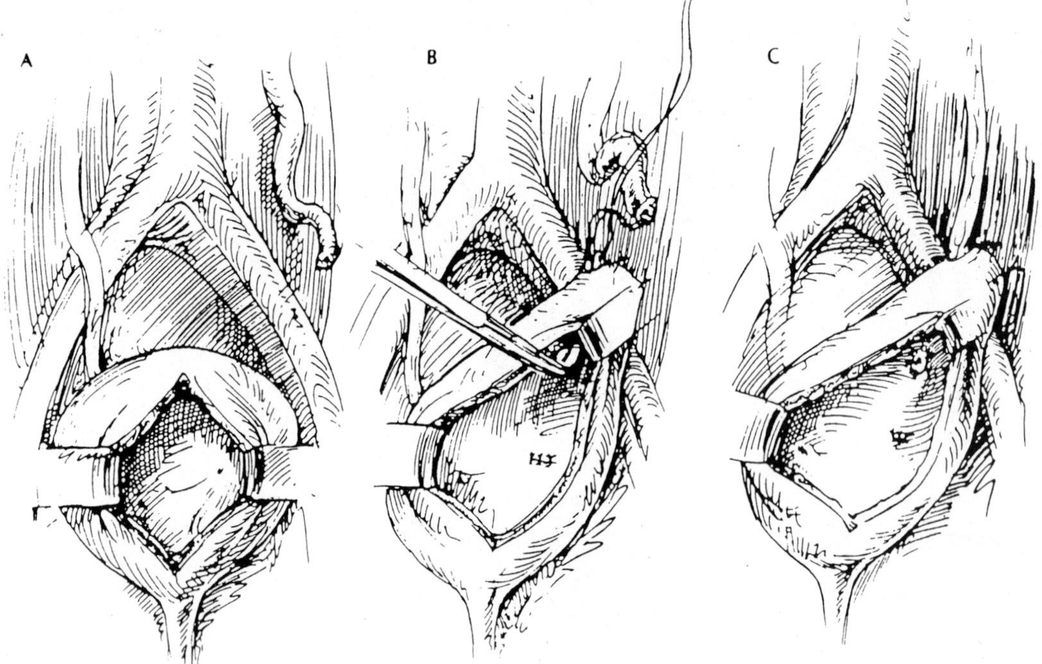


FIGURE 103.14 Bladder mobilized and sutured to psoas over iliac vessels by psoas hitch. **A:** Blunt dissection and exposure of psoas tendon and iliac vessels. **B:** Psoas hitch with interrupted absorbable sutures. **C:** Completed reimplant. Long submucosal tunnel to prevent reflux is shown. (From Ehrlich RM, Melman A, Skinner DG. The use of the vesicopsoas hitch in urologic surgery. *J Urol* 1978;119:324, with permission.)

maneuver. Likewise, the vas deferens in boys and the fallopian tubes in girls must be protected.

A submucosal tunnel is created as described for the Politano–Leadbetter repair. The ureter is brought through the new hiatus, under the subepithelial tunnel, and secured in its new location. Care is taken to avoid twisting or kinking the ureter as it is brought back intravesically. As with all of the intravesical techniques, after the final ureteral anastomosis is complete, a 5Fr feeding tube should easily pass up through the reimplanted ureter to the kidney.

## Laparoscopic Repair

The modern era of laparoscopy has brought forth many new and innovative techniques. These new procedures have been designed to decrease morbidity and hospital costs as well as speed patient recovery. Among these is the laparoscopic extravesical ureteral reimplant. Designed to emulate the Lich–Gregoir repair, this repair is at present utilized in few centers specializing in laparoscopic technique. This particular repair requires two surgeons and can be performed intraperitoneally or retroperitoneally. The technique for intraperitoneal access has been well described. In the pediatric population, access to the peritoneum should be performed using an open technique. I do this using the 10-mm Hassan trocar to avoid intraperitoneal injury. Once the pneumoperitoneum is created, three other trocars are placed. A second 10-mm trocar (instruments) is placed 1 to 5 cm above the infraumbilical site (camera) on the opposite side of the refluxing ureter in the midclavicular line. Two 5-mm trocars are placed in the left and right midclavicular lines at the level of the anterior superior iliac spine for dissecting instruments and retraction. The operating room table is rotated away from the refluxing side to shift the peritoneal contents and bladder away from the operative location. The peritoneum is incised over the iliac vessels, where the obliterated hypogastric artery is recognized. The ureter is identified (Fig. 103.15), grasped with a Babcock-type instrument, and tented up to allow dissection and mobilization of the ureter for 3 or 4 cm proximal to its detrusor insertion. This will allow placement of the ureter within a trough that is to be created. Next, using electrocautery the muscle layer of the bladder is incised for approximately 3 cm proximal to the ureterovesical junction. Spreading carefully with scissors will expose the mucosa. Dissection continues for the length of the tunnel until the mucosa bulges throughout the incision. The ureter is placed in the trough and the detrusor edges are approximated and the ureter is advanced with a fixation suture at the distalmost part of the trough. The remaining detrusor defect is closed over the ureter with either absorbable polydioxanone suture or staples. A Foley catheter is left overnight.

At present, laparoscopic correction of reflux takes longer than traditional repairs and the incisions made are actually more unsightly than the single lower-abdominal incision done for open surgery. The instruments used are more costly. As a whole, the laparoscopic repair is not yet as cost-effective as either open surgery or endoscopic correction.

# POSTOPERATIVE CARE

The patient stays on prophylactic antibiotics until reflux has been shown to be resolved. An ultrasound of the kidneys and bladder is usually done 4 to 6 weeks after surgery to assess for occult hydronephrosis and hydroureter. Assuming

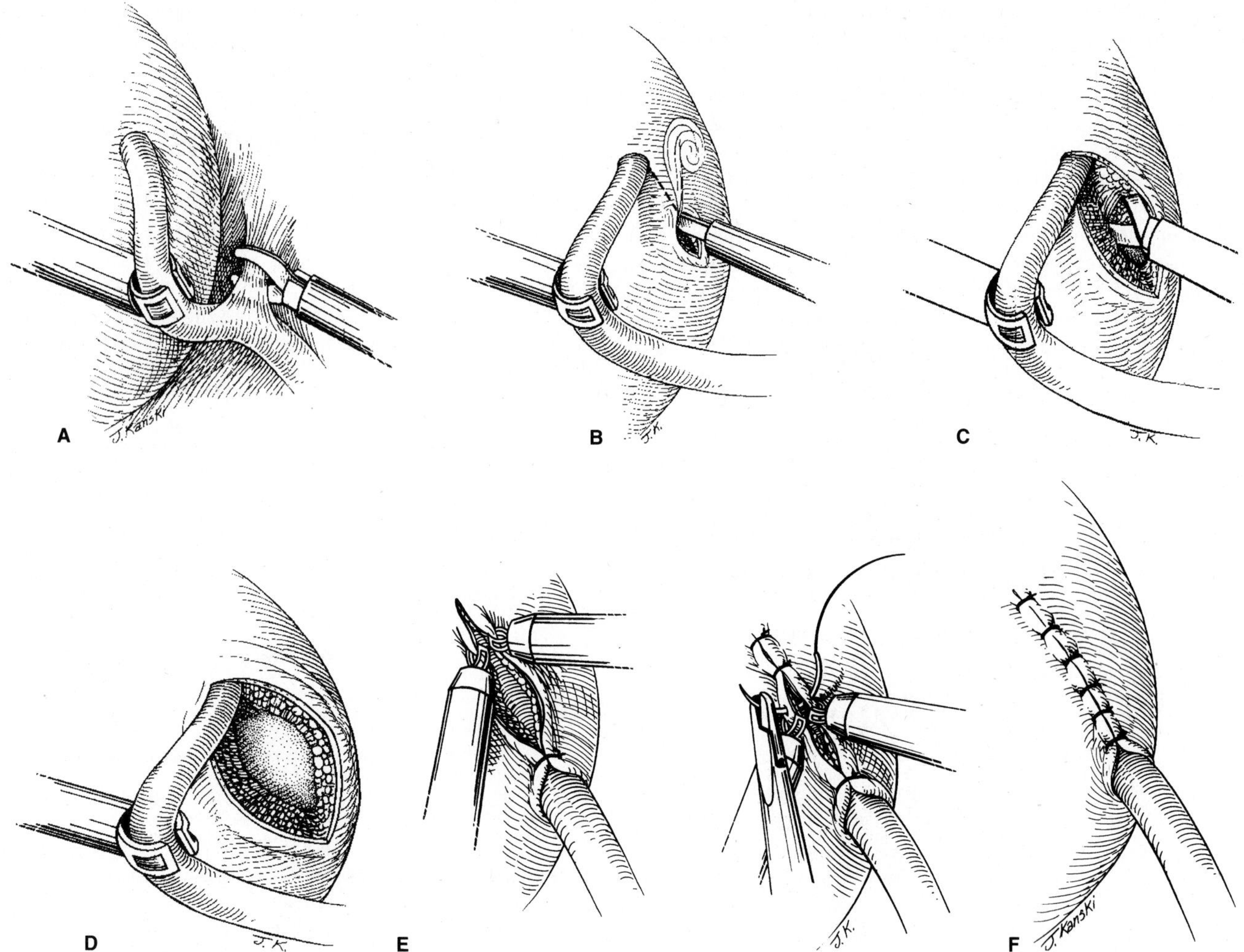


FIGURE 103.15 Laparoscopic reimplant. **A:** Ureteral mobilization. The obliterated umbilical artery is identified and traced distally until the ureter is seen. The ureter is grasped gently and the periureteral tissue dissected bluntly toward the ureterovesical junction. **B–D:** Creation of bladder wall trough. Bladder wall is incised with electrocautery 3 cm proximal to the ureterovesical junction. Muscle fibers are gently cut and spread. Dissection is complete when mucosal tissue bulges outward. **E:** After placing the ureter in the trough-grasping instruments, the superior aspect of the bladder wall is wrapped around the ureter and a suture placed proximally, immobilizing the ureter in the trough (*left*). Remaining sutures are placed throughout the length of the tunnel (*right*). **F:** Completed repair. (From Atala A, Keating M. Vesicoureteral reflux. In: Walsh PC, Retik AB, Wein A, et al., eds. *Campbell's Urology*, vol 2. Philadelphia: WB Saunders, 1997, with permission.)

the ultrasound is normal, a follow-up VCUG or nuclear cystogram is performed 3 months later to assess the surgical result. If reflux is no longer present, I routinely repeat a renal ultrasound 1 year later to make sure that anatomically all is well. Should known renal scarring be present, then yearly urinalysis, blood pressure measurements, and periodic ultrasounds are recommended.

## OUTCOMES

### Complications

Fortunately, the success rates for open surgery to correct reflux approach 98% for nondilated ureters and those with normal bladder function. In cases with dilated ureters, significant voiding dysfunction, neuropathic bladder, and anatomic conditions such as prune belly syndrome and posterior urethral valves, the success rates diminish somewhat. Previously unrecognized bladder and bowel dysfunction is the most common cause of postoperative problems and needs to be vigorously addressed. The most common complication is persisting reflux on the operative side or contralateral reflux of a previously nonrefluxing ureter. In most cases observation is the treatment of choice as the vast majority of these patients will have spontaneous resolution of reflux within 1 year. Always look for voiding or bowel dysfunction in any case of persistent reflux. If the recurrent reflux is high grade, then most likely there was a technical failure such as not creating a long enough tunnel or insufficient ureteral mobilization. These cases frequently require reoperation. Always treat any voiding problems first.

Ureteral obstruction is fortunately a rare complication of reflux surgery and frequently is transient in nature, resulting from postoperative bladder spasms, edema, or blood clots. Hence, it is not unusual to see some mild renal or ureteral dilatation in the first few weeks after surgery on sonography.

Should problems persist, ureteral stenting or percutaneous nephrostomy will help temporize the situation until resolution occurs spontaneously or surgical reimplantation is performed. Higher-grade obstructions usually present with a variety of symptoms such as flank pain, fever, nausea, vomiting, and ileus. These are due to angulation, obstruction at the hiatus, extravasation (of a tapered ureter), or ureteral ischemia with resultant stricturing. Urinary diversion or stenting is paramount in these situations and redo reimplantation required. If the remaining ureter is too short to reimplant in the standard fashion, consider a psoas hitch or a transureteral ureterostomy.

Bladder diverticula are usually the result of a defect in the closure of the muscular hiatus at the original procedure. If the diverticula is wide-mouthed and drains well in the absence of obstruction or reflux, then observation is all that is needed. In the presence of ureteral pathology or poor drainage of the diverticula, surgical correction is necessary.

## CONCLUSIONS

Surgical management of VUR is highly successful if performed for the right indications and if one adheres to the proper principles of good surgical technique. There are a myriad of corrective techniques available, each with their respective advantages and disadvantages. It is up to the individual surgeon to decide what works best in his or her hands after analyzing the available information on the respective patient.

## *References*


1. Young HH, Wesson MB. The anatomy and surgery of the trigone. *Arch Surg* 1921;3:1.
2. Sampson JA. Ascending renal infection with special reference to the reflux of urine from the bladder into the ureters. *Johns Hopkins Hosp Bull* 1903;14:334.
3. Hutch JA. Vesicoureteral reflux in the paraplegic: cause and correction. *J Urol* 1952;68:457.
4. Gruber CM. A comparative study of the intravesical ureters (ureterovesical valves) in man and in experimental animals. *J Urol* 1929;21:567.
5. Stephens FD, Lenaghan D. The anatomical basis and dynamics of vesicoureteral reflux. *J Urol* 1962;87:669.
6. International Reflux Study Committee. Medical versus surgical treatment of primary vesicoureteral reflux. *Pediatrics* 1981;67:392–400.
7. Weiss R, Duckett J, Spitzer A, on behalf of the International Reflux Study in Children. Results of a randomized clinical trial of medical vs. surgical management of infants and children with grades III and IV primary vesicoureteral reflux (United States). *J Urol* 1992;148:1667.
8. Duckett JW. Vesicoureteral reflux: a conservative analysis. *Am J Kidney Dis* 1983;3:139–144.
9. Skoog SJ, Belman AB, Majd M. A nonsurgical approach to the management of primary vesicoureteral reflux. *J Urol* 1987;138:941.
10. Aaronson IA, Rames RA, Greene WB, et al. Endoscopic treatment of reflux: migration of Teflon to the lungs and brain. *Eur Urol* 1993;23:394.
11. Lich R Jr, Howerton LW, Davis LA. Recurrent urosepsis in children. *J Urol* 1961; 86:554.
12. Gregoir W, Van Regemorter GV. Le reflux vesico-ureteral congenital. *Urol Int* 1964;18:122.
13. Zaontz MR, Maizels M, Sugar EC, et al. Detrusorrhaphy: extravesical ureteral advancement to correct vesicoureteral reflux in children. *J Urol* 1987;138:947–949.
14. Politano VA, Leadbetter WF. An operative technique for the correction of vesicoureteral reflux. *J Urol* 1958;79:932–941.
15. Glen JF, Anderson EE. Technical considerations in distal tunnel ureteral reimplantation. *J Urol* 1978;119:194.
16. Cohen SJ. The Cohen reimplantation technique. *Birth Defects* 1977; 13:391.
17. Paquin AJ. Ureterovesical anastomosis. The description and evaluation of a technique. *J Urol* 1959;82:573.


# CHAPTER 104 ■ ENDOSCOPIC TREATMENT OF VESICOURETERAL REFLUX

WOLFGANG H. CERWINKA AND ANDREW J. KIRSCH

Approximately 1% of children are diagnosed with vesicoureteral reflux (VUR), a condition that promotes pyelonephritis and may lead to renal scarring and hypertension. VUR is one of several treatable risk factors, such as dysfunctional elimination, in the development of urinary tract infection (UTI). The goal of VUR treatment is to prevent pyelonephritis and to preserve renal function. Antibiotic prophylaxis is initiated in most children irrespective of VUR grade. Surgical management, indicated in cases of breakthrough UTIs and/or persistence of VUR, comprises ureteral reimplantation and endoscopic injection. In 1981 endoscopic injection for VUR was introduced as an investigational method and the first clinical experience was published in 1984 (1,2). Over the last 20 years, injection techniques, injectable agents, and consequently treatment success rates have significantly improved (3). The success rate of outpatient endoscopic treatment of VUR approaches that of open ureteral reimplantation and offers considerable advantages to patients and parents such as lower morbidity (e.g., pain, scar), fewer complications, and reduced cost. Consequently, an apparent trend from reimplantations toward injection treatments has been observed over the last several years.

## DIAGNOSIS

VUR is diagnosed by nuclear cystography or voiding cystourethrography (VCUG) and graded from I to V. This grading system bears clinical significance not only for spontaneous resolution, but also for treatment method and outcome. VCUGs performed with a single cycle of filling and voiding show false negatives in approximately 20%; for improved sensitivity, cyclic VCUGs consisting of three voiding cycles are recommended. VCUG as a means to detect VUR is indicated in various clinical scenarios. The current guidelines recommend VCUGs for children of both sexes and all ages after the first febrile UTI or subsequent UTIs if the previous VCUGs did not demonstrate VUR. Approximately 40% of children with febrile UTIs are subsequently diagnosed with VUR. Children who experience recurrent febrile UTIs without evidence of VUR by VCUG may suffer from occult VUR. It is conceivable that despite negative conventional VCUG, occult VUR is clinically significant. One method to diagnose occult VUR is the positional instillation of contrast cystography (PICC). The tip of the cystoscope is positioned at the ureteral orifice and contrast instilled at full flow with a pressure of 80 cm of water. A patient is designated PICC-positive if contrast is seen in the ureter, without the need to grade occult VUR. An alternative approach for the diagnosis of occult VUR is hydrodistention of the distal ureter, thus avoiding the use of contrast and ionizing radiation. The degree of hydrodistention was shown to correlate with the presence of occult reflux. VCUGs are recommended in patients with multicystic dysplastic kidneys because of the condition's association with contralateral VUR in 15% to 20%. Antenatal hydronephrosis, even when it resolves postnatally, will be associated with VUR in 20%. Screening siblings or parents implies a 30% to 65% chance of VUR. VUR may be incidentally discovered by a VCUG obtained for reasons other than febrile UTIs, such as posterior urethral valves, patent urachus, or suspected bladder rupture. The obligation to diagnose VUR in asymptomatic patients (no history of febrile UTIs, prenatally diagnosed hydronephrosis, sibling screening) has been questioned because the natural history of asymptomatic VUR may be benign and treatment not necessary.

The "top-down approach" in the management of UTI attempts to distinguish clinically significant from insignificant VUR by evaluating kidneys for pyelonephritis and/or scarring with DMSA scans performed within weeks of the onset of acute pyelonephritis. A positive DMSA scan is an indication for VCUG and consequently 50% of "unnecessary" VCUGs can be avoided. However, many patients suffering from the significant morbidity of recurrent febrile UTIs without detectable renal injury are missed. At this time, this approach is rarely used and should be considered investigational until long-term data become available.

While VCUGs and nuclear cystographies both apply ionizing radiation to a field that includes the gonads, in cases of prolonged nonoperative management of VUR, nuclear cystography is often preferred because it utilizes a lower radiation dose. Magnetic resonance voiding cystourethrography (MRVCU) became a potential alternative to conventional VCUG with the advent of near real-time magnetic resonance fluoroscopy. In comparative studies, MRVCU demonstrated inferior sensitivity (76%) and specificity (90%) to conventional VCUG and has limitations, such as incomplete voiding of some infants and young children secondary to sedation. Although technically feasible, it seems unlikely that MRVCU will gain widespread acceptance.

## INDICATIONS FOR SURGERY

Endoscopic treatment using Deflux is U.S. Food and Drug Administration (FDA) approved for VUR grades II to IV in single or duplex ureters and for cases of initial endoscopic treatment failure; however, it has been applied to all VUR scenarios. While open ureteral reimplantation may be a good treatment option after failed injection therapy, endoscopic treatment has been successfully employed after failed ureteral reimplantation (Table 104.1). Current evidence does not suggest that antireflux surgery of any means reduces the incidence of renal scarring or end-stage renal disease. Valuable goals of VUR treatment are to prevent UTIs, particularly pyelonephritis, to avoid long-term antibiotic prophylaxis, and to reduce the need for distressing VCUGs and radiation exposure. Proponents of the endoscopic approach will argue that decreasing the incidence of UTIs is the main goal of therapy. Recurrence, while possible, may occur in the absence of symptoms and be viewed as subclinical, similar to an individual with VUR diagnosed after a sibling screen or for fetal hydronephrosis. Proponents of the open surgical approach will argue that ureteral reimplantation provides a permanent cure of VUR and is worth the increased morbidity to achieve this goal. In terms of reducing the risk of UTI, endoscopic treatment may achieve this goal as well as or better than open surgery, and there are no long-term data on the radiographic results of open surgery (4,5).

The indications for ureteral reimplantation and endoscopic treatment are with few exceptions identical and include persistent VUR after a period of observation, new renal scarring, breakthrough UTIs, and poor compliance with antibiotic prophylaxis. When surgical options are discussed with parents, a significant preference for endoscopic treatment becomes apparent (6,7). While endoscopic injection has focused on the treatment of primary VUR, it was largely avoided for cases of complex VUR (i.e., VUR associated with functional or anatomic abnormalities such as neurogenic bladder or megaureters). In general, endoscopic treatment is emerging as the treatment modality of choice for VUR, whereas ureteral reimplantation remains reserved for cases of failed injection therapy, significant anatomic abnormalities (e.g., large paraureteral diverticula, ectopic ureters, megaureters), and surgeon's or parents' preference.

## ALTERNATIVE THERAPY

Most patients diagnosed with VUR are started on antibiotic prophylaxis irrespective of grade. Antibiotic prophylaxis may be continued for several years until VUR resolution or significant grade reduction or if it is deemed clinically insignificant. The presumed benefits of antibiotic prophylaxis, prevention of pyelonephritis, and avoidance of surgery have been challenged by recent studies demonstrating increased bacterial resistance and failure to protect against UTIs. Observation off antibiotics was consequently proposed as an alternative management option. However, at the current time, observation protocols in young patients who are at risk for renal injury (<4 years of age)

TABLE 104.1

SUCCESS RATES OF ENDOSCOPIC TREATMENT FOR PRIMARY AND COMPLEX VESICOURETERAL REFLUX

| Reference | Indication | Bulking Agent | Volume (mL) | Ureters | Follow-Up (months) | Success (%) |
|---|---|---|---|---|---|---|
| Elder JS et al., 2006 | Various | Various | 0.2–1.7 | 8,101 | Variable | 85 |
| Capozza N et al., 2004 | Various | Various | 0.2–2.2 | 1,694 | 12–204 | 77 |
| Kirsch AJ et al., 2004 | Various | Dx/HA | 0.5–1.5 | 119 | 3–12 | 92 |
| Kirsch AJ et al., 2006 | Various | Dx/HA | 0.8–2.0 | 139 | 3–18 | 93 |
| Van Capelle JW et al., 2004 | Primary | PDMS | 0.2–2.0 | 311 | 3–110 | 75 |
| Kajbafzadeh AM et al., 2006 | Primary | Ca hydroxylapatite | 0.4–0.6 | 364 | 6 | 69 |
| Yu RN et al., 2006 | Primary | Dx/HA | 1.0 | 162 | 2–26 | 93 |
| Puri P et al., 2006 | Various | Dx/HA | 0.2–1.5 | 1101 | 3–46 | 96 |
| Lorenzo AJ et al., 2006 | Various | PDMS | | 351 | 72 | 72 |
| Pinto KJ et al., 2006 | Primary | Dx/HA | | 86 | 3 | 84 |
| Perez-Brayfield M et al., 2004 | Neurogenic bladder | Dx/HA | 0.4–2.0 | 9 | 3 | 78 |
| Läckgren G et al., 2007 | Voiding dysfunction | Dx/HA | | 74 | 12 | 83 |
| Elmore JM et al., 2006 | Failed initial injection | Dx/HA | 1.0–1.5 | 53 | 3 | 89 |
| Perez-Brayfield M et al., 2004 | Failed reimplantation | Dx/HA | 0.4–2.0 | 19 | 3 | 88 |
| Kitchens D et al., 2006 | Failed reimplantation | Dx/HA | 0.7–3.8 | 20 | 19 | 83 |
| Campbell JB et al., 2006 | Renal transplantation | Dx/HA | | 11 | | 55 |
| Molitierno JA et al., 2007 | Duplicated ureter | Dx/HA | 0.8–2.8 | 63 | 1.3 | 85 |
| Cerwinka WH et al., 2007 | Paraureteral diverticulum | Dx/HA | 0.8–1.8 | 20 | 6.6 | 81 |
| Chertin B et al., 2007 | Ureterocele | Various | | 44 | 1–21 | 91 |

Meta-analysis by Elder JS et al., 2006, summarizes results until 2003. More recent series are listed here. Success after one or several treatments in some studies.
Dx/HA, dextranomer/hyaluronic acid; PDMS, polydimethylsiloxane.

or who have shown a propensity for recurrent pyelonephritis should be considered investigational.

Treatment of concomitant dysfunctional elimination (i.e., constipation and/or voiding dysfunction) reduces the risk of UTIs in patients with VUR. Surgical intervention comprises open ureteral reimplantation (extravesical and intravesical), laparoscopic ureteral reimplantation, and endoscopic treatment. Ureteral reimplantation has a success rate of 95% to 99% for grade I to IV and 80% for grade V VUR. Persistent or recurrent VUR after surgical treatment may be treated in an identical fashion or with an alternative method (i.e., reimplantation or endoscopic injection). A second injection was shown to be highly successful in patients after initial endoscopic treatment failure (90%); however, a third injection in general yields low success (34% to 50%) and is not recommended. Older patients with persistent VUR and no other risk factors (e.g., worsening VUR grade, renal scarring, dysfunctional elimination) often remain asymptomatic and may be taken off antibiotic prophylaxis (8). However, parents should be warned of the risks of pyelonephritis and its associated morbidity that may be seen during sexual activity and pregnancy.

## SURGICAL TECHNIQUE

Numerous injectable bulking materials have been utilized and abandoned over time in search of a nonimmunogenic, noncarcinogenic, biocompatible, and biodegradable agent. Teflon, the first bulking material used for the treatment of VUR, was abandoned in pediatric urology in the United States because of the material's propensity to migrate to distant organs and to form granulomas; however, carcinogenesis of Teflon has not been reported. Silicone also demonstrates distant migration and granuloma formation. Its carcinogenic potential has been controversial but is most likely unsubstantiated. Glutaraldehyde cross-linked bovine collagen demonstrates a lower degree of absorption as compared to native collagen and can cause allergic reactions even in patients with a negative skin test. Several new bulking agents are currently under investigation, such as inorganic materials and autologous tissue. The latter is nonimmunogenic; however, cell harvest and/or cell culture are time-consuming and expensive.

Dextranomer/hyaluronic acid copolymer (Deflux) is easy to inject and is biodegradable with stable implant volume, and its relatively large particle size prevents distant migration. It has been used as an injectable material in pediatric urology since 1995 and is currently the first-choice injectable agent due to its safety and efficacy (9). Deflux implants in animal tissue were shown to undergo time-dependent histopathological changes. The initial phase was dominated by an ingrowth of granulation tissue, a foreign body giant cell reaction, and the formation of a surrounding capsule. In the later phase, cellular elements became largely replaced by a collagen-rich matrix, whereas the capsule remained unchanged. These findings were confirmed in patients who had failed endoscopic injection and proceeded to ureteral reimplantation. Besides biological properties, cost of bulking agents, and surgeon's experience, the choice may ultimately depend on approval by administrative agencies, such as the European Medicines Agency or the FDA.

The endoscopic method currently achieving the highest success rates is the double hydrodistention implantation technique (HIT) (Fig. 104.1). The patient is placed in the low dorsal lithotomy position and antibiotic prophylaxis is given. Cystoscopy is performed with a pediatric cystoscope equipped with an offset lens. An offset lens permits direct passage of the needle in line with the ureter without bending the needle. The bladder is filled to less than half capacity to permit visualization of the ureter and avoid tension within the submucosal layer of the ureter secondary to overdistention. Hydrodistention (HD) is performed with the tip of the cystoscope placed at the ureteral orifice (UO) and a pressured stream is achieved by placing the irrigation bag approximately 1 meter above the bladder on full flow. HD of the distal ureter serves two purposes: it allows visualization of the intraureteral injection site and assessment of treatment progress (i.e., ureteral coaptation). The needle is passed into the UO and inserted at the mid-ureteral tunnel at the 6 o'clock position. Sufficient bulking agent is injected to produce a bulge, which initially coapts the detrusor tunnel, while a second implant within the most distal intramural tunnel leads to coaptation of the UO (approximately 1 to 1.5 mL). Rarely, if the two intraureteric submucosal injections (double HIT method) fail to coapt the ureter, a classic STING (supraureteric injection of Teflon) is needed to achieve coaptation. The latter two injection sites are used more commonly in complex or redo cases (Fig. 104.2). HD is performed after each injection to monitor treatment progress; when HD ceases to dilate the UO, appropriate coaptation has been achieved.

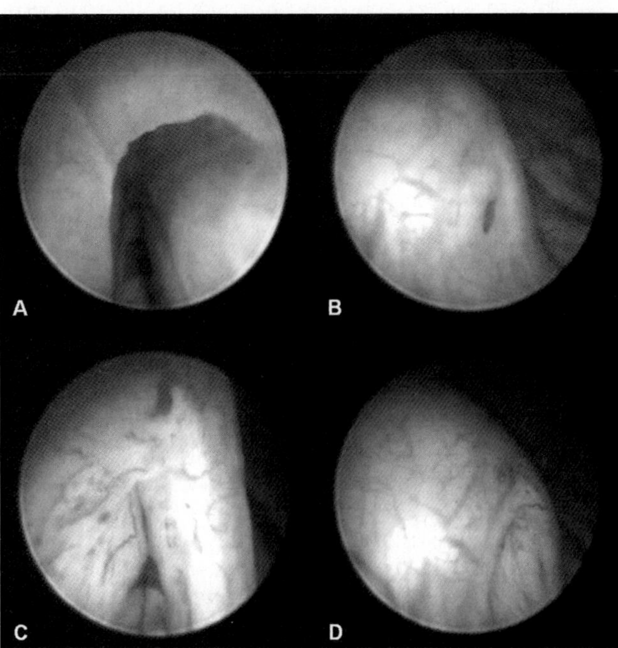


FIGURE 104.1 Endoscopic treatment of vesicoureteral reflux (double HIT technique). **A:** Proximal intraureteric injection. **B:** Coapted intramural ureter. **C:** Distal intraureteric injection. **D:** Coapted ureteral orifice.

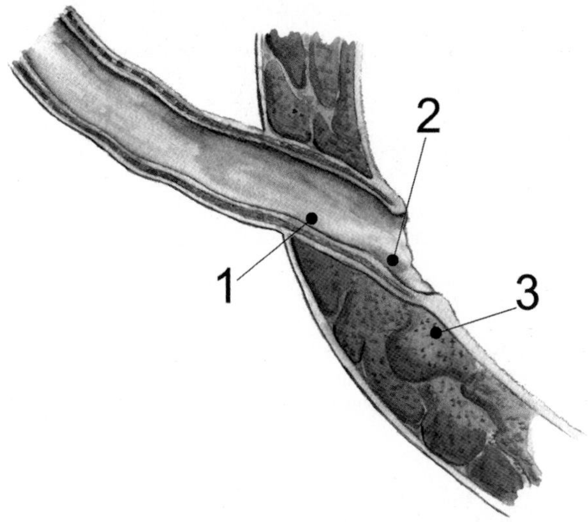


FIGURE 104.2 Needle placement algorithm for the endoscopic treatment of vesicoureteral reflux. The double hydrodistention implantation technique uses sites 1 and 2; site 3 (subureteric injection of Teflon) is rarely used.

In general, all procedures are performed on an outpatient basis and all patients receive preoperative antibiotic prophylaxis, which is continued until resolution of VUR has been confirmed. Radiographic success is defined as grade 0 VUR on a postoperative VCUG, 1 to 6 months after a single treatment. Patients are then followed clinically on an annual basis to determine clinical success and recurrence.

## OUTCOMES

Outcome of endoscopic treatment for VUR has been evaluated in several large series (Table 104.1). Most studies included both primary and complicated cases of VUR. Interpretation of and comparison among these studies are confounded by different inclusion criteria (e.g., with or without complex VUR, grade I, grade V), varying lengths of follow-up, definitions of success, and single versus multiple injections. Nevertheless, most current series report cure rates of >85%. Age, gender, and bilaterality of VUR have not been shown to predict treatment outcome. While the STING technique yields lower success rates with higher grades of VUR, the HIT method achieves similar outcomes across all VUR grades up to grade V. Endoscopic treatment of complicated VUR has been evaluated in smaller series and success rates vary significantly depending

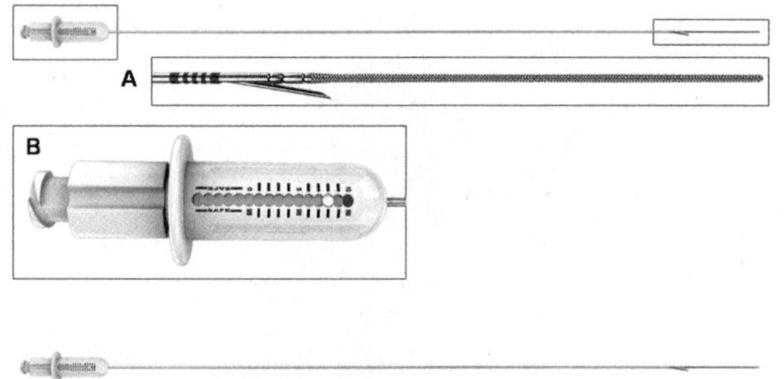

FIGURE 104.3 Retractable injection needle guide (Injekt, Cook Urological, Spencer, IN). A: Flexible wire is placed into the ureter and the needle is advanced submucosally. B: Depth gauge allows needle advancement in 1-mm increments.

on the associated pathologies (Table 104.1). In general, cure rates for complex cases of VUR are lower than for primary VUR. Treatment of VUR associated with neurogenic bladder or voiding dysfunction was shown to yield acceptable outcomes. Endoscopic injection has been successfully employed in patients who failed either ureteral reimplantation or initial injection. Injection after failed reimplantation or second injection will be curative in most instances, whereas a third injection has been shown to be far less successful (10). Refluxing ureters of transplanted kidneys in symptomatic patients may be treated endoscopically. Although this approach is curative in only half the cases, it represents an attractive alternative to open surgery in the setting of immune compromise and reduced wound-healing properties. VUR associated with anatomical abnormalities (e.g., duplex ureters, paraureteral diverticula, and ureteroceles), previously thought to be contraindications for endoscopic treatment, was recently shown to be amenable to injection treatment.

There are many factors that may affect the success of the procedure. Preoperative (i.e., patient selection), intraoperative (i.e., injection technique, injected volume), and postoperative variables have been shown to correlate with treatment outcome. Postoperatively, failures may result from Deflux displacement (implant migration), disruption (mucosal breach), or dissolution (decrease in implant volume). Success may be improved with the HIT method when performed by an experienced surgeon familiar with the subtleties of the technique. New technologies will continue to improve the success of endoscopic injection. For example, a prototype of a new retractable injection needle guide (Injekt, Cook Urological, Spencer, IN) has been developed to reproduce the double HIT method and reduce the learning curve (Fig. 104.3). New biologic injectable agents are also under study.

## COMPLICATIONS

In comparison to ureteral reimplantation, endoscopic VUR treatment offers major advantages to patients and parents. The procedure generally lasts <15 minutes and is performed on an outpatient basis. While cure rates are approaching those of open ureteral reimplantation, significant complications are rare. Endoscopic treatment entails greater patient convenience, lower morbidity (e.g., pain, abdominal scar), and reduced cost (11). Consequently, a significant parental preference for endoscopic treatment is evident (6,7). A recent study demonstrated that both patients and parents viewed injection therapy as the least bothersome aspect of VUR treatment, followed by antibiotic prophylaxis and VCUG (5).

The most common complications following endoscopic treatment of VUR are new contralateral VUR (2.3% to 17.3%) and treatment failure. Less than 4% of children complain of flank pain or emesis several hours after the procedure and all respond to analgesics. Gross hematuria, urinary retention, or febrile UTIs have not been observed. The most significant potential complication of endoscopic treatment for VUR includes a 0.6% risk of ureteral obstruction (12). Factors that may increase the risk of obstruction include bladder dysfunction and markedly dilated ureters. Patients with recurrent VUR often remain asymptomatic, and those without risk factors for pyelonephritis such as young age, voiding dysfunction, or significant history of UTIs may be taken off antibiotic prophylaxis (8).

## *References*


1. Matouschek E. Die Behandlung des vesikorenalen Refluxes durch transurethrale Einspritzung von Teflonpaste. *Der Urologe Ausgabe A* 1981; 20:263–264.
2. O'Donnell B, Puri P. Treatment of vesicoureteric reflux by endoscopic injection of Teflon. *Br Med J (Clin Res)* 1984;289:7–9.
3. Kirsch AJ, Perez-Brayfield M, Smith EA, et al. The modified STING procedure to correct vesicoureteral reflux: improved results with submucosal implantation within the intramural ureter. *J Urol* 2004;171:2413–2416.
4. Jodal U, Smellie JM, Lax H, et al. Ten-year results of randomized treatment of children with severe vesicoureteral reflux. Final report of the International Reflux Study in Children. *Pediatr Nephrol* 2006;21:785–792.
5. Stenberg A, Läckgren G. Treatment of vesicoureteral reflux in children using stabilized non-animal hyaluronic acid/dextranomer gel (NASHA/DX): a long-term observational study. *J Pediatr Urol* 2007;3:80–85.
6. Ogan K, Pohl HG, Carlson D, et al. Parental preferences in the management of vesicoureteral reflux. *J Urol* 2001;166:240–243.
7. Capozza N, Lais A, Matarazzo E, et al. Treatment of vesico-ureteric reflux: a new algorithm based on parental preference. *BJU Int* 2003;92:285–288.
8. Cooper CS, Chung BI, Kirsch AJ, et al. The outcome of stopping prophylactic antibiotics in older children with vesicoureteral reflux. *J Urol* 2000; 163:269–272.
9. Stenberg A, Läckgren G. A new bioimplant for the endoscopic treatment of vesicoureteral reflux: experimental and short-term clinical results. *J Urol* 1995;154:800–803.
10. Elder JS, Diaz M, Caldamone AA, et al. Endoscopic therapy for vesicoureteral reflux: a meta-analysis. I. Reflux resolution and urinary tract infection. *J Urol* 2006;175:716–722.
11. Kobelt G, Canning DA, Hensle TW, et al. The cost-effectiveness of endoscopic injection of dextranomer/hyaluronic acid copolymer for vesicoureteral reflux. *J Urol* 2003;169:1480–1484.
12. Vandersteen DR, Routh JC, Kirsch AJ, et al. Postoperative ureteral obstruction after subureteral injection of dextranomer/hyaluronic acid copolymer. *J Urol* 2006;176:1593–1595.

# CHAPTER 105 ■ URETEROCELES

RICHARD N. YU, CHESTER J. KOH, AND DAVID A. DIAMOND

Ureteroceles are congenital cystic dilations of the intravesical submucosal ureter. They are more commonly found in female children and are almost exclusively diagnosed in whites. Approximately 10% of these children have bilateral ureteroceles. Ureteroceles may be "orthotopic" and contained entirely within the bladder, or "ectopic" and partially situated at the bladder neck or urethra. An orthotopic ureterocele is typically associated with a single collecting system, while an ectopic ureterocele is usually associated with the upper-pole moiety of a kidney with complete ureteral duplication.

## DIAGNOSIS

Increasingly, ureteroceles are diagnosed by prenatal ultrasonography, which can demonstrate both the intravesical cystic dilation as well as the corresponding hydronephrosis. These patients should undergo a comprehensive postnatal urological evaluation and be placed on prophylactic antibiotics, which may help to prevent future urinary tract infections (UTIs) (1). However, for many children the diagnosis of ureterocele is made only after a UTI or urosepsis. Ureteroceles can also present as a palpable abdominal mass, usually representing a hydronephrotic kidney, or as a vaginal mass, which represents prolapse of an ectopic ureterocele. Large ureteroceles may even lead to obstruction of the bladder neck or of the contralateral ureteral orifice, which may result in bilateral hydronephrosis.

In general, ultrasonography is the first radiological study obtained in diagnosing ureteroceles. In addition to the intravesical cystic dilation, ureteroceles are usually seen with duplex collecting systems, with the ureterocele being associated with hydronephrosis of the upper-pole moiety.

A voiding cystourethrogram (VCUG) is essential in the evaluation of the patient with a ureterocele because of the high incidence of concomitant ipsilateral and contralateral vesicoureteral reflux. In addition to the reflux, VCUG can demonstrate the size and location of the ureterocele.

Currently, the dimercaptosuccinic acid (DMSA) renal scan provides the most precise estimates of the differential renal function between each kidney, as well as of the associated upper pole's contribution to the overall renal function. DMSA scans may even detect lower-moiety abnormalities that may not have been demonstrated by ultrasonography (2).

Intravenous urography (IVU) is less commonly used in the modern evaluation of ureteroceles. However, in cases of unusual urinary tract anatomy IVU may be helpful in the delineation of previously undefined anatomy. Severe hydroureteronephrosis associated with a ureterocele may lead to lateral deviation of the upper pole away from the spine.

## INDICATIONS FOR SURGERY

The goals of surgical treatment should be the preservation of renal function, elimination of obstruction and reflux, prevention or elimination of infection, and maintenance of urinary continence (3) while minimizing surgical morbidity. The main factors to consider in developing an individual treatment plan should be patient age, patient's clinical presentation, ureterocele size and anatomy, presence of reflux and UTI, and function of the involved renal segments.

## ALTERNATIVE THERAPY

The anatomy and clinical presentations of children with ureteroceles vary widely. Therefore, each child should have an individualized treatment plan as no single method of surgical repair is appropriate for all cases. Table 105.1 lists some therapeutic options for patients with ureteroceles.

## SURGICAL TECHNIQUE

Techniques that preserve functional upper-pole moieties are listed below. However, in many instances the upper pole has little to no contribution to the overall renal function and upper-pole ablative techniques, also described below, may be indicated.

**TABLE 105.1**

**URETEROCELE THERAPEUTIC OPTIONS**

| URETEROCELE THERAPEUTIC OPTIONS |
|---|
| Upper-pole preservation |
| Endoscopic incision of the ureterocele |
| Complete lower-tract reconstruction (excision of ureterocele with ureteral reimplantation) |
| Ureteroureterostomy/ureteropyelostomy |
| Upper-pole ablation |
| Upper-tract approach (upper-pole nephrectomy and partial ureterectomy) |
| Complete reconstruction |

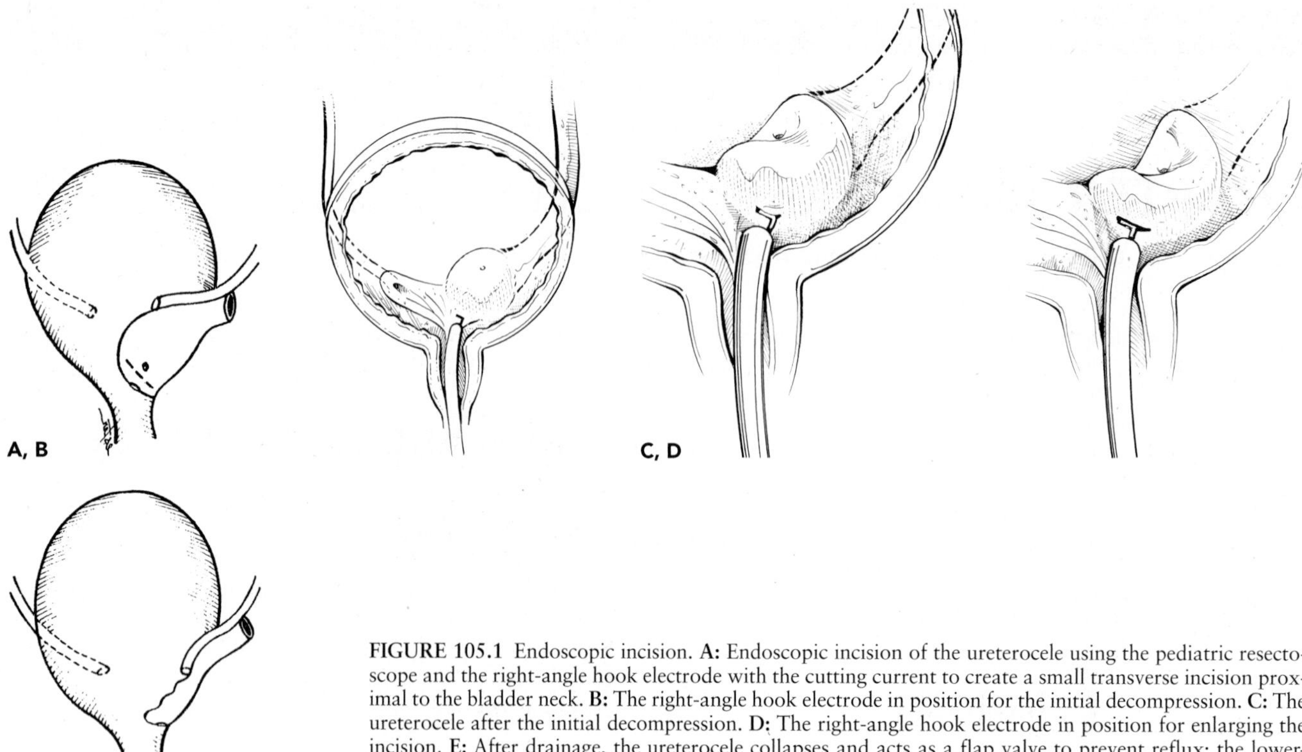


FIGURE 105.1 Endoscopic incision. **A:** Endoscopic incision of the ureterocele using the pediatric resectoscope and the right-angle hook electrode with the cutting current to create a small transverse incision proximal to the bladder neck. **B:** The right-angle hook electrode in position for the initial decompression. **C:** The ureterocele after the initial decompression. **D:** The right-angle hook electrode in position for enlarging the incision. **E:** After drainage, the ureterocele collapses and acts as a flap valve to prevent reflux; the lower-pole ureter lies over the collapsed ureterocele.

## Upper-Pole Preservation

### Endoscopic Incision of the Ureterocele

The goal of endoscopic incision of ureteroceles is to decompress the ureterocele in a minimally invasive manner while minimizing the risk of postincision vesicoureteral reflux and the need for further urinary tract reconstruction (4). This technique can be used in infants if infant-sized endoscopic equipment is available and should be used to drain obstructive urinary systems in any ureterocele patient with urosepsis. Blyth et al. recommended the use of a 3Fr Bugbee wire electrode (using the cutting current) to incise the roof of the ureterocele through its full thickness near its base and proximal to the bladder neck (5). A new unobstructed intravesical ureteral orifice will be created, and the roof of the collapsed ureterocele can act as a flap-valve mechanism to prevent reflux. While the Bugbee electrode has been a widely utilized instrument for ureterocele puncture, it has limitations, primarily that following initial decompression enlargement of the puncture site is difficult. Therefore, we prefer to use the pediatric resectoscope and the right-angle hook electrode with the cutting current, which allows one to make a clean transverse incision and enlarge it by placing the hook into the original incision and withdrawing under vision (Fig. 105.1). Magnification with the use of video projection helps improve the accuracy of the incision. Making the incision as distal and as close to the bladder neck as possible should reduce the risk of postoperative reflux into the corresponding ureter. The adequacy of the incision can be confirmed by the presence of a jet of urine from the ureterocele or by visualization of the urothelium inside the ureterocele. The major advantage of the endoscopic incision is that it can be done on an outpatient basis, without the need for hospitalization.

### Complete Lower-Tract Reconstruction (Excision of Ureterocele with Ureteral Reimplantation)

For excision of the ureterocele and common sheath reimplantation of upper- and lower-pole ureters, a Pfannenstiel incision is made and the bladder is opened (Fig. 105.2). The lower-pole and contralateral ureters are intubated with 5Fr feeding tubes, and multiple circumferential stay sutures are placed. A circumferential incision is made around the perimeter of the ureterocele with electrocautery and the wall of the ureterocele and its

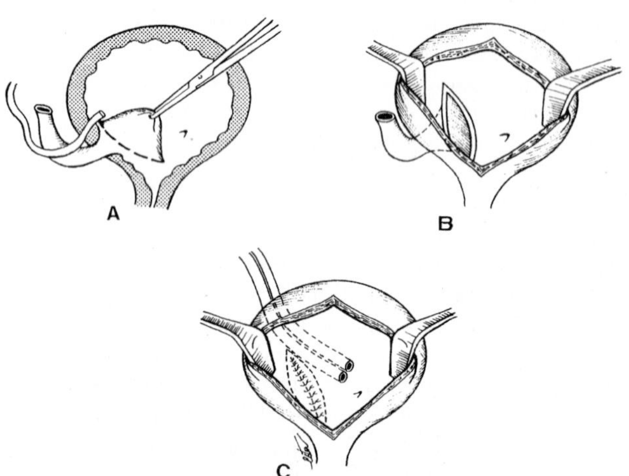


FIGURE 105.2 Complete lower-tract reconstruction. **A:** After the bladder is opened, multiple circumferential stay sutures are placed around the ureterocele to assist with the excision. **B:** All ureters should be intubated with 5Fr feeding tubes for identification of the ureters during the dissection. **C:** After excising the ureterocele, the posterior bladder wall is repaired with running 3-0 absorbable sutures and the ureters are reimplanted into a generous tunnel.

associated upper-pole ureter are dissected away from the thinned posterior muscular wall of the bladder, incorporating the lower-pole ureter in the dissection. All attempts should be made to avoid injury to the sphincteric mechanisms at the bladder neck during the distal dissection of the ureterocele. The upper- and lower-pole ureters are dissected as a common sheath to avoid injury to the blood supply of both ureters. After excising the distal ureterocele, the dilated upper-pole ureter often requires tapering. The thin posterior bladder wall is repaired by imbrication of adjacent muscle with running 3-0 absorbable sutures to provide sufficient muscle backing for the reimplanted ureters. An unoperated portion of the bladder floor is selected and the ureters are reimplanted as a common sheath into a generous ureteral tunnel.

### Ureteroureterostomy/Ureteropyelostomy

In upper urinary tract anastomotic techniques, the dissection of the upper tracts should be kept to a minimum, and mobilization should be directed toward the upper-pole ureter, so that distortion of the adjacent lower-pole ureter can be avoided. Because the upper-pole ureter is usually larger than the lower-pole ureter, generous spatulation of the ureters during ureteroureterostomy may be necessary for an optimal end-to-side anastomosis. Furthermore, a feeding tube should be passed distally into the ureterocele to decompress it.

## Upper-Pole Ablation

### Upper-Tract Approach (Upper-Pole Nephrectomy and Partial Ureterectomy)

In many cases, the upper pole associated with the ureterocele has minimal or no contribution to the overall renal function. The upper-tract approach (upper-pole nephrectomy and partial ureterectomy) should lead to the relief of obstruction, prevention of recurrent infection, and resolution of the reflux that is present in about half of these patients. This approach should result in the decompression of the ureterocele, hopefully with resolution of the ipsilateral lower-pole reflux, because the trigone will be returned to a more normal configuration. This usually eliminates the need for lower-tract reconstruction with a potentially difficult bladder neck and urethral dissection (3).

For the upper-pole heminephrectomy, we suggest the use of the flank or laparoscopic approach, which offers superior access to the upper-pole vessels. With either approach, care should be taken to avoid excessive traction upon the kidney to avoid damage to the viable lower pole. In many cases, the upper pole resembles a dysplastic nubbin, and early division of the upper-pole ureter with upward traction on the proximal portion of the transected ureter usually helps in the definition and manipulation of the upper pole (Fig. 105.3). After the upper-pole vessels are sequentially ligated, demarcation of the upper-pole parenchyma should become apparent. We recommend the use of a no. 15 blade or electrocautery around the upper-pole parenchyma, which usually results in a wedge-shaped defect. During the dissection of the upper-pole parenchyma, the plane of dissection should remain as close as possible to the upper-pole ureter to avoid injury to the vascular supply of the lower-pole ureter. After the upper-pole nephrectomy, the wedge-shaped defect is closed with interrupted 3-0 chromic sutures in a vertical mattress fashion to achieve effective hemostasis.

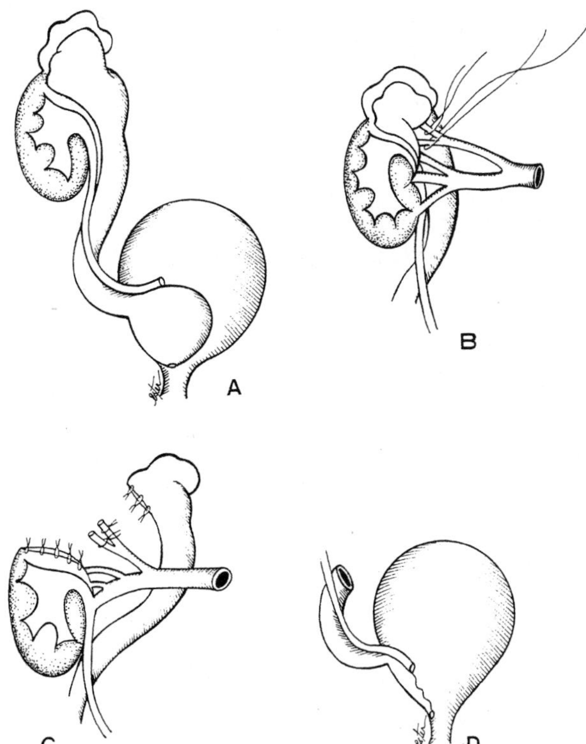


FIGURE 105.3 Upper-pole partial nephrectomy and partial ureterectomy. **A:** This procedure is commonly used for a duplex system with a nonfunctioning upper pole and minimal or absent ipsilateral reflux. **B:** The upper-pole ureter is transected early after a stay suture has been placed proximally. Upward traction on the proximal portion of the transected ureter assists in the manipulation of the upper pole during the partial nephrectomy. **C:** After removal of the upper pole, the wedge-shaped kidney defect is repaired with 3-0 chromic sutures in a vertical mattress fashion. **D:** This approach should result in the decompression of the ureterocele, with the return of the trigone to a more normal configuration.

## Complete Reconstruction

In certain instances, a complete reconstruction may be indicated where both an upper-tract repair and a lower-tract reconstruction are performed via separate incisions in a single stage. These situations include the presence of high-grade reflux into the ipsilateral lower-pole ureter or the presence of lower-pole reflux associated with a large, everting ureterocele and a nonfunctioning upper pole. Depending on the amount of upper-tract function, either an upper-pole nephrectomy with partial ureterectomy or a ureteropyelostomy (as described above) is performed for the upper-tract repair. Lower-tract reconstruction is also performed, which involves excision of the ureterocele with reimplantation of the ureters as a common sheath, as previously described.

# OUTCOMES

## Complications

Excision of the ureterocele with ureteral reimplantation achieves the goal of upper-tract drainage. However, the disadvantage of this approach is the morbidity associated with bladder surgery, including hematuria, bladder spasm, and catheter drainage. Extensive distal dissection also carries the risk of bladder neck and sphincteric injury, which may jeopardize urinary continence (6).

## Results

Endoscopic incision of the ureterocele may be the only surgical procedure required for many patients. For infants, endoscopic incision may be used as a temporizing measure that achieves early decompression. Secondary surgery, if necessary, can be performed electively when the child is older. If the ureterocele is orthotopic, one can expect high rates of decompression and low rates of de novo reflux and the need for secondary procedures (7). On the other hand, ectopic ureteroceles are associated with a high rate of secondary surgery and a significant incidence of postoperative reflux after endoscopic incision. Therefore, patients with ectopic ureteroceles may be best served by more definitive reconstruction, even those <1 year of age (8).

The upper-tract approach, which includes upper-pole nephrectomy and partial ureterectomy, is usually reserved for the patient with an upper pole that provides little or no contribution to the overall renal function and mild or absent ipsilateral reflux. This approach has the advantage of avoiding the lower-tract complications noted previously.

For patients who are at significant risk for requiring a second procedure with some of the approaches detailed previously, such as those patients with large, ectopic ureteroceles or high-grade ipsilateral reflux, complete upper- and lower-tract reconstruction in a single stage has the advantage of expediency (9).

## *References*


1. Upadhyay J, Bolduc S, Braga L, et al. Impact of prenatal diagnosis on the morbidity associated with ureterocele management. *J Urol* 2002;167:2560–2565.
2. Connolly LP, Connolly SA, Drubach LA, et al. Ectopic ureteroceles in infants with prenatal hydronephrosis: use of renal cortical scintigraphy. *Clin Nucl Med* 2002;27:169–175.
3. Schlussel RN, Retik AB. Ectopic ureter, ureterocele, and other anomalies of the ureter. In: Walsh PC, ed. *Campbell's Urology*, 8th ed. Philadelphia: WB Saunders, 2002:2022–2034.
4. De Filippo RE, Bauer SB. New surgical techniques in pediatric urology. *Curr Opin Urol* 2001;11:591–596.
5. Blyth B, Passerini-Glazel G, Camuffo C, et al. Endoscopic incision of ureteroceles: intravesical versus ectopic. *J Urol* 1993;149:556–560.
6. Coplen DE, Duckett JW. The modern approach to ureteroceles. *J Urol* 1995;153:166–171.
7. Hagg MJ, Mourachov PV, Snyder HM, et al. The modern endoscopic approach to ureterocele. *J Urol* 2000;163:940–943.
8. Husmann D, Strand B, Ewalt D, et al. Management of ectopic ureterocele associated with renal duplication: a comparison of partial nephrectomy and endoscopic decompression. *J Urol* 1999;162:1406–1409.
9. Scherz HC, Kaplan GW, Packer MG, et al. Ectopic ureteroceles: surgical management with preservation of continence—review of 60 cases. *J Urol* 1989;142:538–543.


# CHAPTER 106 ■ URACHAL ANOMALIES AND RELATED UMBILICAL DISORDERS

LESLIE T. MCQUISTON AND ANTHONY A. CALDAMONE

During bladder development, the urogenital sinus is initially contiguous with the allantois. When the lumen of the allantoic duct becomes obliterated, the urachus remains, connecting the bladder to the umbilicus (Fig. 106.1A,B). It continues to elongate as the fetus grows. The urachus is a muscular tube, with a length ranging from 3 to 10 cm and a diameter of approximately 8 to 10 mm, that extends from the dome of the bladder to the umbilicus. It has three distinct tissue layers: (a) an epithelial-lined lumen with cuboidal or transitional epithelium, (b) an intermediate connective tissue layer, and (c) an outer smooth muscle layer. In the adults, the urachus lies between two layers of umbilicovesical fascia along with the umbilical ligaments and the remnants of the obliterated umbilical arteries. This fascial investment tends to contain the spread of urachal disease between the peritoneum and transversalis fascia (Fig. 106.1C).

The urachus normally closes or involutes at approximately 32 weeks' gestation, and urachal anomalies in general represent an abnormality in this process. These anomalies are characterized as patent urachus, urachal cyst, urachal sinus, and urachal diverticulum (Fig. 106.2) (1). Of these anomalies, urachal cysts (45%) and sinuses (37%) are the most commonly identified (2).

## DIAGNOSIS

In general, the diagnosis of urachal anomalies requires clinical suspicion and a thorough physical examination. Further evaluation in patients with periumbilical drainage should include a sinogram, and those with a periumbilical mass should undergo

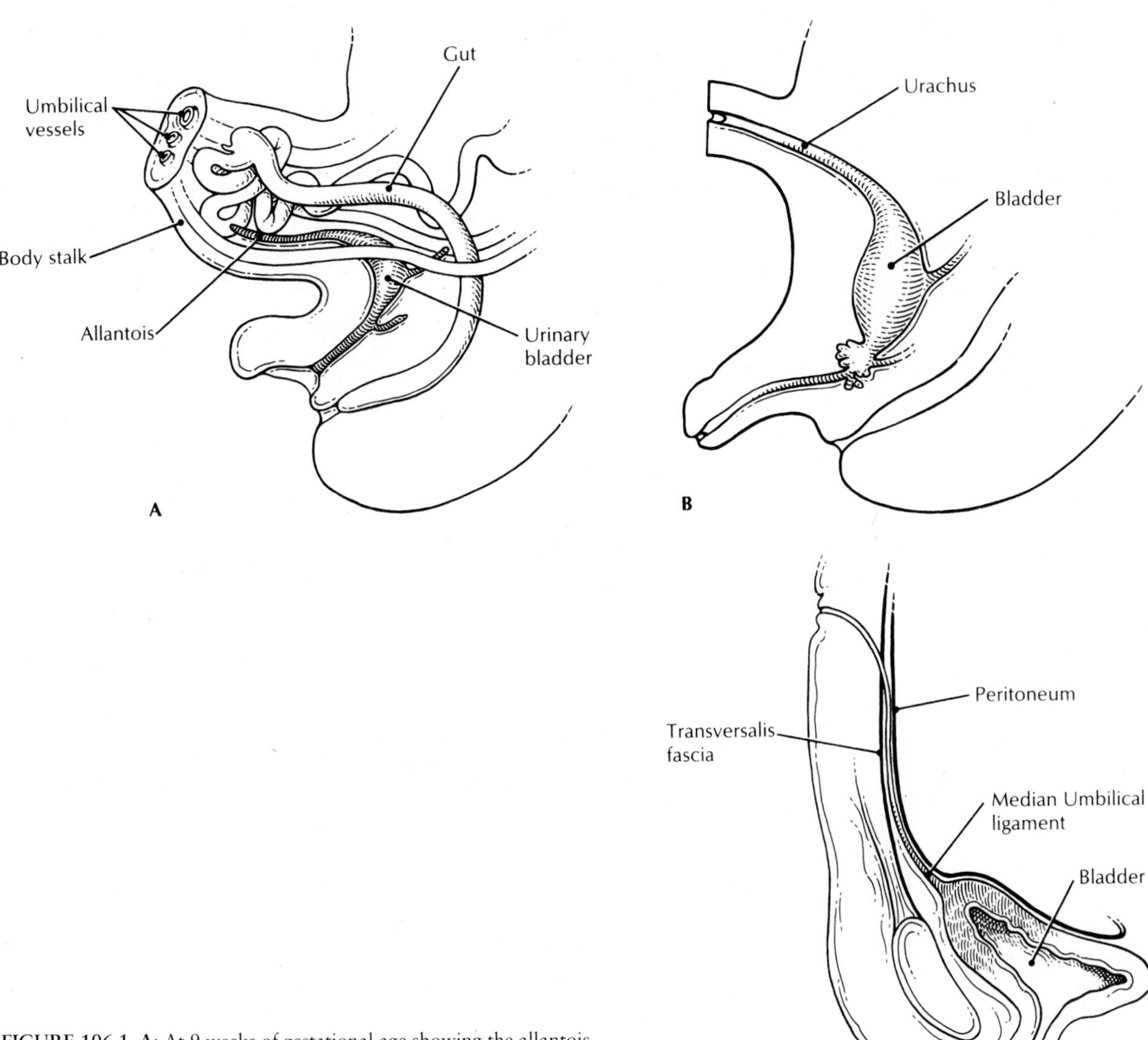


**FIGURE 106.1 A:** At 9 weeks of gestational age showing the allantois extending into the body stalk. **B:** At 3 months' gestation, the urachus connects to the dome of the bladder. **C:** The urachus persisting as the median umbilical ligament in the adult.

ultrasonographic imaging. A voiding cystourethrogram may be required in only selected patients (2,3).

Complete failure of the urachal lumen to close results in an open connection between the bladder and the umbilicus. Patients present with umbilical leakage of urine and often a protruding tissue mass (Fig. 106.3). The leakage may be more obvious during times of increased intra-abdominal pressure such as crying, coughing, or straining. The fluid may be analyzed for urea and creatinine to confirm its urinary quality. Two factors thought to contribute to a persistent patent urachus are bladder outlet obstruction and failure of the bladder to descend into the pelvis (4,5). With regard to bladder outlet obstruction, distal urinary obstruction is thought not to be the only causative factor because normally the urachus closes developmentally before the urethra becomes tubularized (6). In addition, only 14% of patients with patent urachus demonstrate bladder outlet obstruction clinically, and it is uncommon for a patent urachus to be associated with posterior urethral valves. The diagnosis may be confirmed with a sonogram, although a voiding cystourethrogram may be more useful because it may rule out bladder outlet obstruction concurrently. Alternatively, methylene blue or indigo carmine may be instilled in either the bladder or the umbilical opening and detected in the umbilicus or bladder, respectively. The differential diagnosis for patent urachus includes patent omphalomesenteric duct, urachal sinus, omphalitis, granulation of a healing umbilical stump, and infected umbilical vessel.

Segmental or incomplete closure of the urachal lumen may result in the formation of a urachal cyst (Fig. 106.4). The cyst usually forms in the proximal or lower third of the urachal remnant near the bladder (7). Usually, the cyst is lined with transitional epithelium and filled with serous fluid, but mucinous contents have been described. In general, urachal cysts are small and asymptomatic. Symptoms such as pain, redness with localized swelling, and tenderness below the umbilicus may occur with infection and may be accompanied by chills, fever, irritative voiding symptoms, hematuria, and pyuria.

A B C D

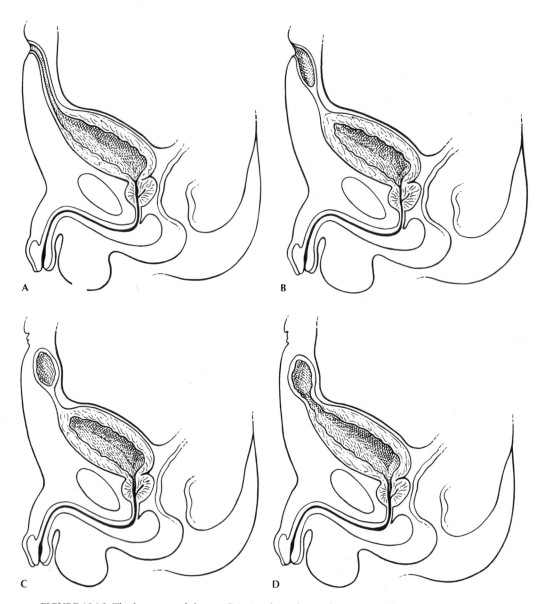

FIGURE 106.2 The four types of abnormalities involving the urachus. **A:** Complete patency to the umbilicus. **B:** A blind-ending urachal sinus open at the umbilicus but not complete to the bladder. **C:** A urachal cyst without communication to either the umbilicus or the bladder. **D:** Simple diverticulum from the dome of the bladder.

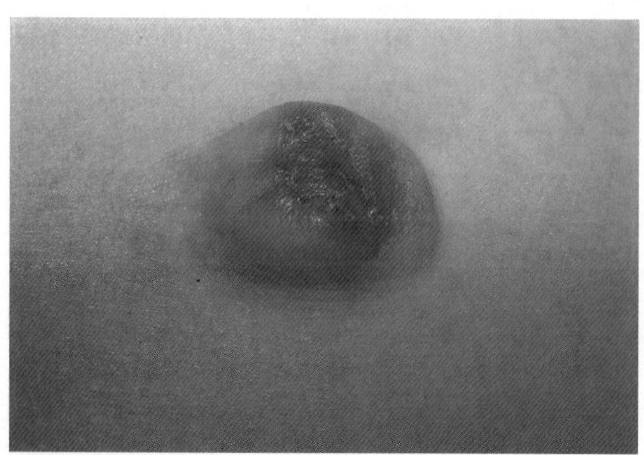

FIGURE 106.3 Patent urachus.

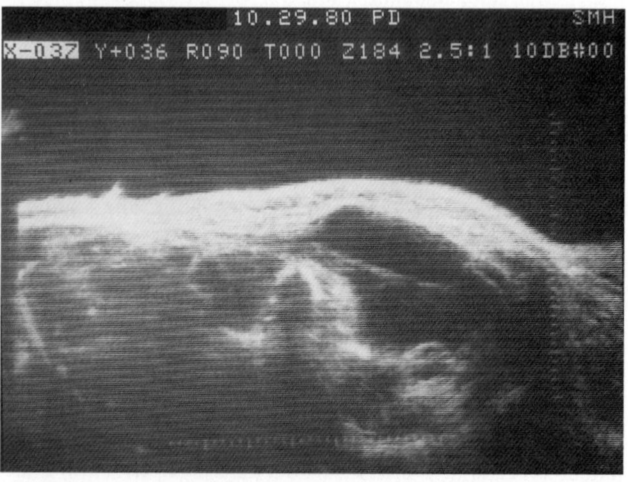


FIGURE 106.4 Abdominal ultrasound that demonstrates an infected urachal cyst.

Alternatively, symptoms may arise as the result of mass effect due to a large urachal cyst. These patients present with a sensation of abdominal fullness or pain, a mass, or irritative voiding symptoms due to compression of the bladder. Diagnosis is most easily confirmed by ultrasound or computed tomography (CT).

Incomplete closure of the urachus may also result in a urachal sinus. This may be the result of a urachal cyst that extended either to the bladder or to the skin for drainage. Some urachal sinuses may alternate and at first drain at the umbilicus and then later into the bladder. Presenting symptoms may include periumbilical redness and tenderness with intermittent drainage, umbilical irritation or granulation tissue, or symptoms of urinary tract infection. Clinical suspicion of a urachal sinus may be confirmed by a sinogram or ultrasound. A cystogram may show an irregular area at the dome of the bladder. Cystoscopy may demonstrate an inflamed area at the dome that may extrude purulent drainage.

A urachal diverticulum results from failure of closure of the urachus adjacent to the bladder, leaving a wide-mouth diverticulum at the dome of the bladder. The urachal diverticulum may or may not be associated with bladder outlet obstruction, as has been often reported in patients with prune belly syndrome. In general, aside from treatment for any coexisting bladder outlet obstruction, the urachal diverticulum requires no specific management as it usually drains well.

Omphalomesenteric disorders may be confused with urachal anomalies. The omphalomesenteric duct is a fetal structure that connects the yolk sac and the gut. Incomplete closure of this tubular structure may lead to a patent omphalomesenteric duct, an omphalomesenteric sinus, or an omphalomesenteric cyst. A patent duct may be characterized by the drainage of intestinal fluid or fecal material. A sinogram should demonstrate a connection to the gastrointestinal tract.

Malignant lesions of the urachus are rare; however, the cancer risk does increase with advancing adult age (8). The most common sign of urachal cancer is hematuria. Patients may also present with a suprapubic mass, abdominal pain, irritative voiding symptoms, or mucus in the urine. The diagnosis may be made by identification of a filling defect at the dome of the bladder with calcifications on intravenous urogram or cystogram, CT, and cystoscopy with transurethral biopsy. Adenocarcinoma is the most common malignancy; however, sarcoma and transitional cell carcinoma have been reported (9).

## INDICATIONS FOR SURGERY

Surgical management is central to the treatment of urachal anomalies with the exception of infants under 6 months of age, in whom the anomalies may resolve spontaneously, and the wide-mouth diverticulum, which in general requires no treatment (10). In the patient with a persistently patent urachus beyond 6 months of age, surgical excision is recommended because of the risk of recurrent infections, stone formation, and persistent umbilical drainage, excoriation, and pain.

Urachal cysts that are symptomatic due to size or infection also merit surgical treatment. Incidentally discovered small, asymptomatic urachal cysts may be excised at the time of discovery or watched for the development of symptoms or progressive enlargement. With infected cysts, initial antibiotic therapy with possible drainage followed by delayed excision may be required. Similarly, in the case of the urachal sinus initial treatment should focus on the eradication of any infection before excision is undertaken.

Treatment of urachal malignancy follows the principles of treatment for any malignancy of the bladder and is discussed elsewhere in this book.

## SURGICAL TECHNIQUE

For the patent urachus, urachal cyst, alternating urachal sinus, or urachal diverticulum requiring correction, the patient is placed in a supine position. If possible, a small catheter, guide wire, or probe is placed through the patent urachus (Fig. 106.5). If nothing will pass, the tract may be stained with methylene blue for later identification. A Foley catheter should be placed in the bladder and the bladder distended with sterile saline to bring the anterior bladder wall up to the abdominal wall and, in doing so, push the peritoneum cephalad.

The urachus may be approached via a vertical midline incision or a transverse infraumbilical incision one-half to two-thirds the distance from the symphysis pubis to the umbilicus. Although the transverse infraumbilical incision will result in excellent exposure, alternatively a vertical midline incision along the course of the urachus may be more direct and can allow for extension to the umbilicus in a cosmetic fashion, should this be required because of difficulty in procuring the umbilical end of the urachus or for any additional necessary procedures. The rectus fascia is opened and the dome of the bladder is identified. The urachus is identified and isolated. Once the proximal portion of the urachus is delineated, it is resected along with a small cuff of bladder to prevent a residual diverticulum. The bladder is then closed in two layers. Dissection then proceeds toward the umbilicus. The operation is facilitated by identifying the proper plane of dissection between the peritoneum posterior to the urachus and the posterior rectus fascia, which is anterior to the urachus. In this same plane will lie the obliterated umbilical arteries, which may be ligated proximally on the bladder wall or distally at the umbilicus.

Infected urachal remnant structures, such as urachal cyst or sinus, may present a more challenging dissection. In fact, it is sometimes advisable to drain a large infected urachal cyst initially percutaneously and allow a period for antibiotic therapy to reduce the local inflammation. Smaller infected urachal cysts or sinuses, however, can be managed safely as a single procedure. With these infected remnants, it may be impossible to dissect the urachus away from contiguous structures. For instance, a larger portion of the bladder may need to be removed with the infected urachal cyst. Similarly, one may find it impossible to separate the infected cyst or sinus from the underlying peritoneum. One should be extremely careful in identifying adherent loops of bowel that may have been involved in the inflammatory process and could easily be injured.

Once the urachus is completely dissected distally it is excised or ligated at its obliterated point. The goal is to remove all urachal tissue and leave the umbilicus intact. If an umbilical hernia is present, it may be corrected concurrently. A catheter may be left in the bladder and a drain in the prevesical space postoperatively at the surgeon's discretion.

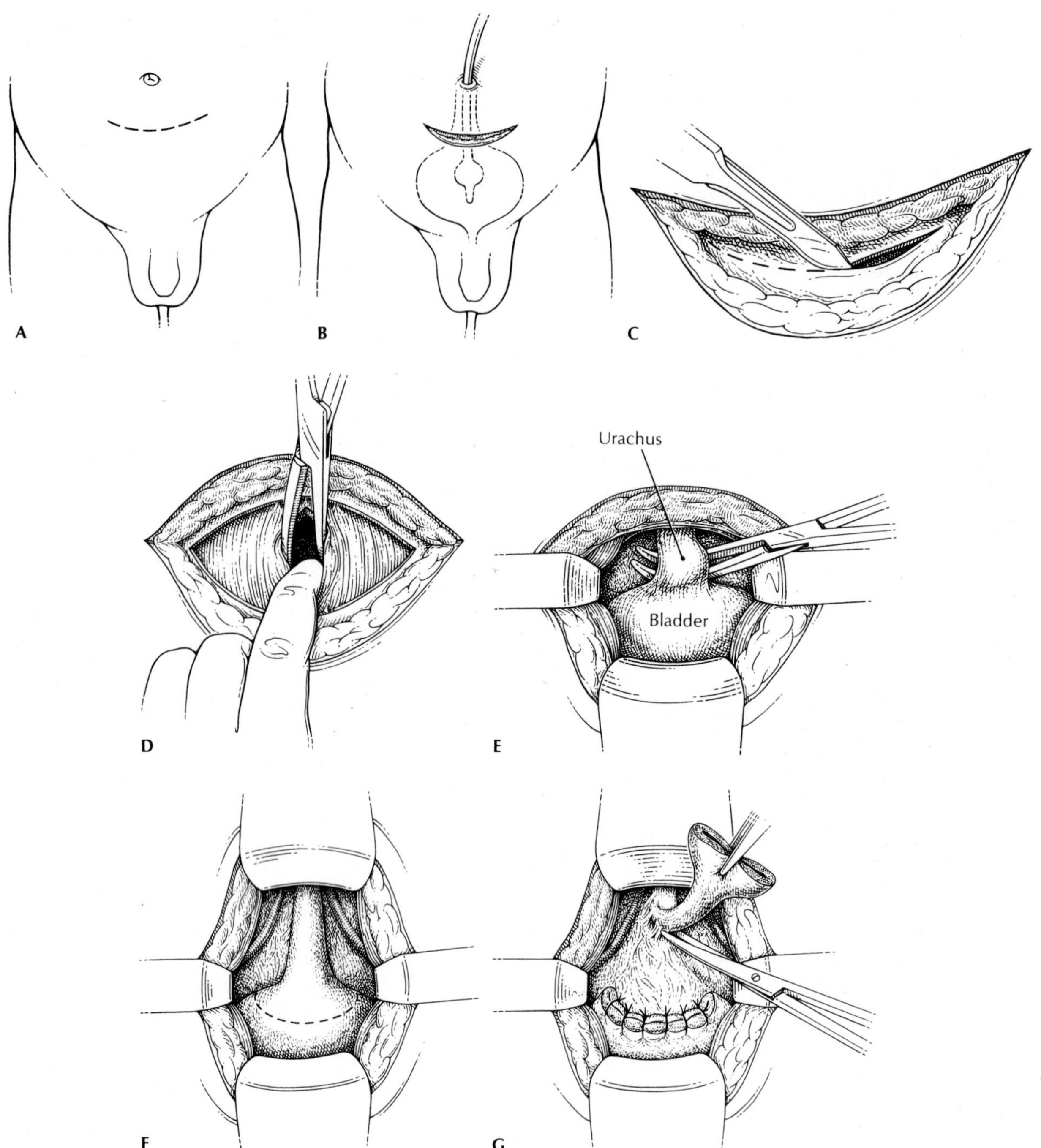


FIGURE 106.5 **A and B:** Typical transverse infraumbilical approach to the urachus. The catheter through the urachus can aid in identification of a patency. **C and D:** The fascia is divided transversely and the rectus muscle is parted in the midline, remaining preperitoneal. **E:** The urachus or urachal remnant can be separated from the peritoneum and identified in its proximal and distal extent. **F and G:** The urachus is resected with a cuff of bladder and the bladder closed in a watertight fashion. The urachus is removed completely out to the umbilicus if necessary.

For the urachal sinus draining at the umbilicus, dissection is begun by circumscribing the sinus, again with the goal of preserving as much of the umbilicus as possible. The obliterated umbilical arteries are ligated as they are encountered. The tract is dissected to its termination and excised, and the area is drained because the sinus tract is usually infected.

An alternative to open surgical treatment is laparoscopic treatment. Laparoscopic treatment, including robotic treatment, has been reported in both children and adults with excellent visualization and access to the urachal remnant (Fig. 106.6) (11,12). Port placement may vary by surgeon preference; however, in general, the first port is placed using open Hasson technique in the midline halfway between the umbilicus and the xiphoid process, and two additional ports are placed under direct vision on each anterior axillary line just above the umbilicus, creating an angle of approximately 45 degrees between

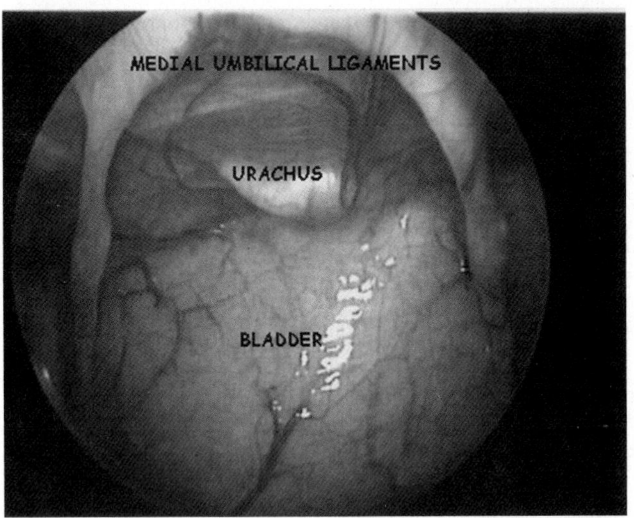


**FIGURE 106.6** Typical view of the bladder and urachus during laparoscopy with a 30-degree telescope, showing the urachus, bladder, and medial umbilical ligaments.

the working ports. The procedure then follows the principles as outlined previously for open surgery.

## OUTCOMES

### Complications

Postoperative complications include persistent urinary drainage, which can be managed by prolonged bladder catheter drainage, and infection, which is generally superficial and responds well to antibiotic therapy. With laparoscopic procedures, the reported complications are most often port-related, and therefore, open Hasson technique for initial port placement is recommended.

### *References*


1. Bauer SB, Retik AB. Urachal anomalies and related umbilical disorders. *Urol Clin North Am* 1978;5:195.
2. Yiee JH, Garcia N, Baker LA, et al. A diagnostic algorithm for urachal anomalies. *J Pediatr Urol* 2007;3(6):500–504.
3. Galati V, Donovan B, Ramji F, et al. Management of urachal remnants early in childhood. *J Urol* 2008;180(4 supp):1824–1826.
4. Hinman F. Surgical disorders of the bladder and umbilicus of urachal origin. *Surg Gynecol Obstet* 1961;113:605–614.
5. Nix JT, Menville JG, Albert M, et al. Congenital patent urachus. *J Urol* 1958;79:264.
6. Schreck WR, Campbell WA III. The relation of bladder outlet obstruction to urinary–umbilical fistula. *J Urol* 1972;108:641–643.
7. Persutte WH, Lenke RR, Kropp K, et al. Antenatal diagnosis of fetal patent urachus. *J Ultrasound Med* 1988;7:399–403.
8. Ashley RA, Inman BA, Routh JC, et al. Urachal anomalies: a longitudinal study of urachal remnants in children and adults. *J Urol* 2007;178(4 pt 2): 1615–1618.
9. Sheldon CA, Clayman RA, Gonzalez R, et al. Malignant urachal lesions. *J Urol* 1984;131:1–8.
10. Cilento BG, Bauer SB, Retik AB, et al. Urachal anomalies: defining the best diagnostic modality. *Urology* 1998;52:120–122.
11. Khurana S, Borzi PA. Laparoscopic management of complicated urachal disease in children. *J Urol* 2002;168:1526–1528.
12. Yamzon J, Kokorowski P, DeFilippo RE, et al. Pediatric robot-assited excision of urachal cyt and bladder cuff. *J Endourol* 2008; 22(10):2385–2388.


# CHAPTER 107 ■ VESICAL NECK RECONSTRUCTION

JOHN C. POPE IV AND JOHN H. MAKARI

Prior to toilet training, the functions of the lower urinary tract include storage of urine at low pressure and good emptying. The result is protection of the upper tract and avoidance of urinary tract infection. Adequate outflow resistance is not necessary during that time, but is eventually critical to achieve urinary continence, another ultimate function of the lower tract. Congenital anomalies resulting in inadequate outflow resistance, and thus failure to achieve urinary continence, can in general be divided into two groups based on pathophysiology. In the first group there is an anatomic or developmental abnormality where the bladder outlet is malformed and incapable of providing adequate resistance. This group would include patients with bladder exstrophy, bilateral single ectopic ureters, persistent cloaca, and rarely an extensive ureterocele. In the second, more common, group involving neurogenic dysfunction, the outlet is normally developed from an anatomic standpoint, but abnormal neurologic control results in inadequate function.

## DIAGNOSIS

When urinary continence is not achieved in children, the critical evaluation is video urodynamic study of the bladder and outlet. Parameters that need to be evaluated include sphincteric function, outflow resistance, detrusor function, and bladder compliance.

Monitoring of external urinary sphincter activity is helpful during studies of storage and emptying. Perineal surface electrodes are most widely used to evaluate the activity; however, in children with neurogenic dysfunction who tolerate placement, a concentric needle electrode or dual electrodes placed through a 25-gauge needle increase accuracy.

The functional length and pressure of the external sphincter are important and can be measured with urethral pressure profilometry. This measurement is technically challenging in a small child and there are no adequate standard nomograms for urethral pressure profilometry to use in pediatric patients. Continuous monitoring of the urethral pressure during filling in the area of maximum resistance may demonstrate an etiology of incontinence. Some surgeons also use leak point pressure to evaluate outflow resistance during passive filling and performance of Valsalva maneuvers. Simultaneous fluoroscopic observation is advantageous.

Detrusor function should be evaluated by the cystometrogram, synergistic relaxation of the external sphincter on electromyography, urinary flow rate, and measurement of postvoid residual urine. Bladder compliance should also be evaluated with the detrusor pressure measured as the bladder is filled with warm saline or contrast (37°C) at a rate equal to or <10% of estimated or known bladder capacity. Such filling minimizes irritation of the bladder, which may artifactually increase bladder pressure. Other artifacts that affect the measurement of compliance such as urinary infections or low urethral resistance should be eliminated to obtain the best results.

Before reconstructive surgery on the bladder is considered, the status of the patient's upper urinary tract should also be evaluated. Standard evaluation includes renal ultrasonography and serum electrolytes, including creatinine. If hydronephrosis is present, renography should be obtained to rule out obstruction. Vesicoureteral reflux should be sought on voiding cystourethrography, often at the time of video urodynamic evaluation. Any upper-tract obstruction or reflux should be corrected at the time of lower urinary tract reconstruction.

Unfortunately, no test ensures that a patient will be able to void spontaneously and empty well after outlet reconstruction with or without bladder augmentation. All patients must be prepared to perform clean intermittent catheterization before considering reconstruction. The native urethra should, therefore, be examined for the ease and discomfort of catheterization.

## INDICATIONS FOR SURGERY

If urinary continence is not achieved at an appropriate age in patients with congenital anomalies, and the patient has failed behavioral regimens such as timed voiding, had urodynamics, and failed all medical regimens and other conservative therapies (e.g., intermittent catheterizations), then surgical intervention should be considered. It is critical to ensure that the bladder is a compliant storage reservoir prior to any reconstructive procedure on the lower urinary tract. Increasing outflow resistance in the presence of inadequate bladder capacity would put the patient at significant risk for upper-tract deterioration and febrile urinary tract infection. Determining the commitment of the patient and family to achieve a good result with reconstructive surgery, including a willingness to perform intermittent catheterization if necessary, is critical.

## ALTERNATIVE THERAPY

In few areas of reconstructive urology are there as many choices to consider as for bladder neck repair and as little consensus as to which repair is appropriate for a given patient or setting. One reason for the variety of choices is the wide range of patients and problems for which the procedures are used. In some cases, the procedure to increase outflow resistance may logically be chosen based on particular patient considerations, but the experience and confidence of the surgeon with a given technique also may play a significant role in the choice.

Conceptually, techniques to increase outflow resistance may be considered as one of two general types. The first set of repairs is used to improve the function of the native outlet, while the second set is designed to repair the anatomy and functionally alter the outlet. Several procedures that may provide benefit and are occasionally used include urethral suspensions, injection of bulking agents, artificial sphincters, and obliteration of the bladder neck.

One of the first bladder neck repairs to function in such a manner was the urethral suspension described by Marshall, Marchetti, and Krantz and since modified by numerous surgeons. While these procedures have been successful in treating stress urinary incontinence among neurologically normal female patients, they have had minimal effect and are rarely indicated for pediatric patients with congenital anatomic anomalies of the outlet or neurogenic dysfunction.

Recently, transurethral injection of bulking agents has been tried to improve the function of the existing outlet. Initially, the use of polytetrafluoroethylene and later, the use of bovine collagen were reported. More recently, the availability of dextranomer/hyaluronic acid copolymer has renewed interest in injection therapy for increasing bladder outlet resistance and for correction of sphincteric incontinence. Injection therapy is relatively simple and avoids any incision, but has met with limited results for significant outlet anomalies (1). Further, the durability of this approach is a concern, as declining rates of dryness and/or improvement are observed even years after treatment (2). Injection therapy may, however, be useful after primary repairs in patients who have some persistent incontinence (2,3).

The most definitive procedure to improve the function of the outlet as it exists is placement of an artificial urinary sphincter. This group of procedures would seem appropriate for patients with a normal or near-normal outlet from an anatomic standpoint and to have little role for patients with significant anatomic anomalies such as bladder exstrophy or bilateral single ectopic ureters.

The ultimate procedure to increase outlet resistance is division of the bladder neck. Effective closure requires extensive mobilization of the bladder and bladder neck away from the urethra with interposition of omentum between. It must be accompanied by construction of a continent abdominal wall stoma for bladder catheterization and effectively moves the reconstruction into the realm of continent urinary diversion. Division of the bladder neck has in general been reserved for complex patients who have failed multiple prior procedures to effectively increase outflow resistance; however, it may be performed in select patients as primary definitive management.

Extremely high success rates have been reported for both primary or secondary management when the previous principles are followed (4).

# SURGICAL TECHNIQUE

## Fascial Sling for Bladder Neck Suspension

In adults, fascial slings may be performed transvaginally, and a small patch of fascia is secured with suspension sutures. In pediatric patients with congenital anomalies, fascial slings have in general been placed from above, often at the time of bladder augmentation. Before placement, the pelvic floor is cleared of overlying fatty tissue and a 2-cm incision made through the endopelvic fascia on either side of the bladder neck and proximal urethra (Fig. 107.1A). This area may be identified by palpation of a transurethral catheter and balloon seated at the bladder neck. Using blunt dissection, a plane is developed between the bladder neck and vagina in girls or rectum in boys (Fig. 107.1B). This plane may at times be more easily developed from the cul-de-sac by dissecting behind the bladder and ureters from above. With a difficult dissection it may be useful to open the bladder, in particular if bladder augmentation is planned.

Once the proper plane is developed and the appropriate length of graft determined, a rectus abdominis fascial strip 1 cm in width and appropriate in length is harvested. The fascia may be taken in either a vertical or horizontal fashion depending on the initial incision. Fascia from other sites has been utilized but requires a second incision. Autologous cadaveric tissue or biodegradable scaffolds may also be used.

All of the grafts are in general brought though the rectus muscle and anterior rectus fascia on either side and approximated to the anterior rectus fascia using permanent sutures (Fig. 107.1C). If long enough, the two limbs of the sling may also be approximated to each other superficial to the fascia. In patients with stress incontinence, the sling is placed tightly enough to maintain the proximal urethra and bladder neck in the appropriate anatomic position. Too snug of placement in such a setting may impede spontaneous voiding. When used for patients with neurogenic dysfunction who will not rely on spontaneous voiding, the sling may be pulled up more tightly to improve compression of the bladder neck and proximal urethra. If intermittent catheterization will be performed postoperatively through the native urethra, intraoperative catheterization should be repeated frequently to make sure the fascial sling is not placed so tightly as to impede catheterization.

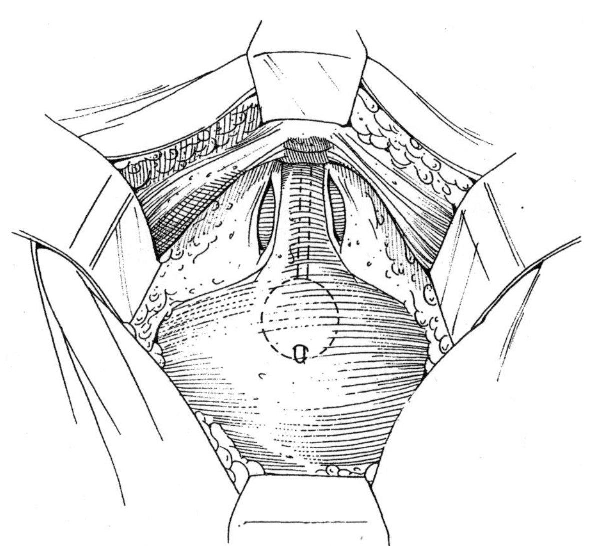

A

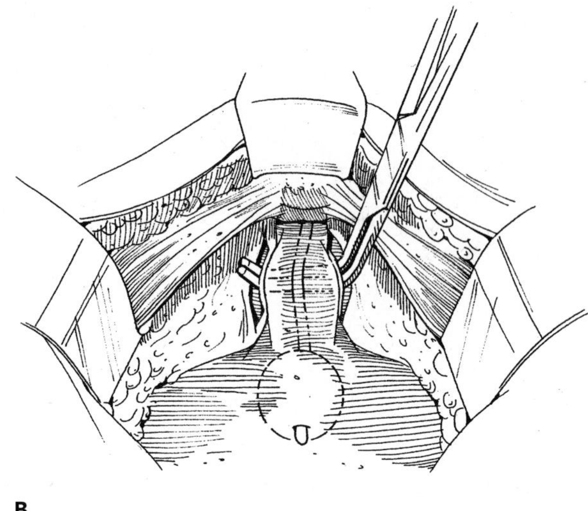

B

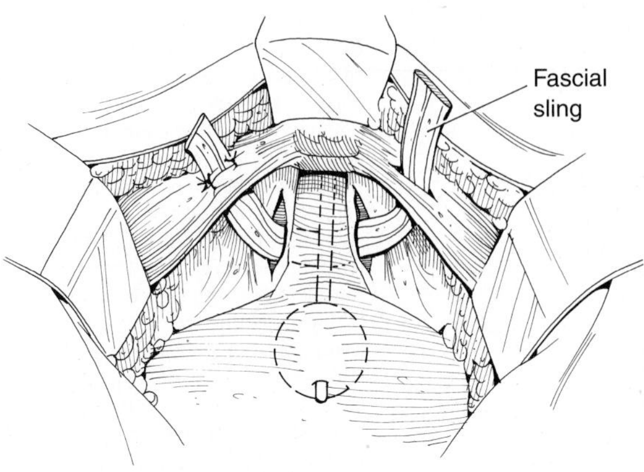


C

FIGURE 107.1 Pubovaginal sling. **A:** The endopelvic fascia is cleared of fatty tissue and a 2-cm incision made on either side of the urethra. A Foley catheter through the urethra may be palpated for identification of the urethra and bladder neck. **B:** The plane between the posterior urethra and anterior vagina is carefully developed using a right-angle clamp. **C:** A fascial strip 1 cm wide is passed through the anterior rectus fascia and rectus muscle lateral to the midline incision. It is secured on the left to the anterior fascia. The sling is then passed behind the bladder and will be brought through the right rectus muscle and fascia to be secured at the proper tension.

## Young–Dees–Leadbetter Bladder Neck Repair

Often done after bladder exstrophy closure, the procedure is typically performed through a lower midline incision. For patients with epispadias who do not require augmentation, the reconstruction may be done through a Pfannenstiel incision. The anterior bladder is opened. This incision is carried as far distally into the proximal urethra as possible. Splitting of the intersymphyseal band with subsequent closure may allow closure and tapering of the proximal urethra. Virtually all exstrophy patients require antireflux surgery, and typically the ureteral hiatus is initially quite low in the bladder. The ureters are mobilized and reimplanted into the bladder 3 to 4 cm more cephalad in location. Typically, the ureters are reimplanted with a cross-trigonal technique, although the tunnels may even be angled upward in a cephalad direction from the new hiatus. A 12- to 15-mm-wide strip of mucosa is preserved in the posterior midline of the urethra and bladder trigone for reconstruction of the neourethra. Parallel incisions through mucosa are made on either side of this strip and the triangles of trigone mucosa on either side are excised (Fig. 107.2A). Submucosal infiltration of dilute epinephrine in those two areas may aid in excision and decrease bleeding. The midline strip of mucosa and the subsequent neourethra are typically made 4 to 6 cm long, depending on how much proximal urethra is exposed and reconstructed. The midline strip is tubularized over an 8Fr catheter using absorbable sutures to approximate the edges. This tubularization may be done with interrupted or running absorbable sutures but should be tension free (Fig. 107.2B). Small purchases of the adjacent superficial muscle of the trigone may be included with the mucosa for strength. The closure is easier to begin distally and finished cephalad. The lateral flaps of trigone muscle are then wrapped over the neourethra in an overlapping fashion. To do so without tension, the muscle must be incised transversely at the cephalad margin of the mucosal excision. One flap of muscle is wrapped over the neourethra and approximated to the underside of the other muscle flap using interrupted, absorbable mattress sutures. The second flap of muscle is then wrapped over the first and approximated to the outside of the muscle, again with absorbable sutures (Fig. 107.2C). A soft urethral catheter is left in place during healing but should be secured so as to avoid tension on the neourethra. Ureteral stents or catheters are often left in place because of potential edema. The bladder is closed in two layers.

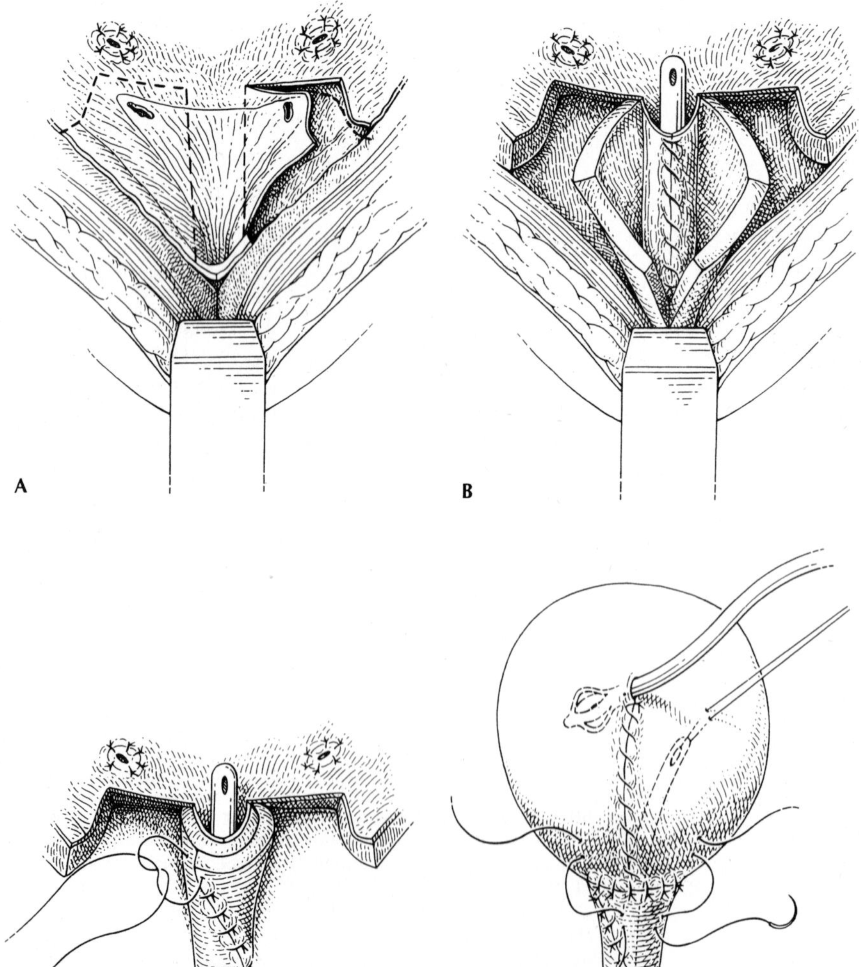


**FIGURE 107.2** Young–Dees bladder neck repair. **A:** The trigone mucosa is incised to leave a posterior, central strip of mucosa 15 mm wide. The triangles of mucosa on either side are excised. The ureters have previously been reimplanted in a more cephalad position. **B:** The central mucosa strip is tubularized using a running absorbable suture. **C:** The lateral trigone muscle flaps are closed in an overlapping fashion around the neourethra. **D:** After completion of the bladder and urethral closure, several pairs of suspension sutures secure the urethra and bladder to the underside of the intersymphyseal band and lower abdominal wall.

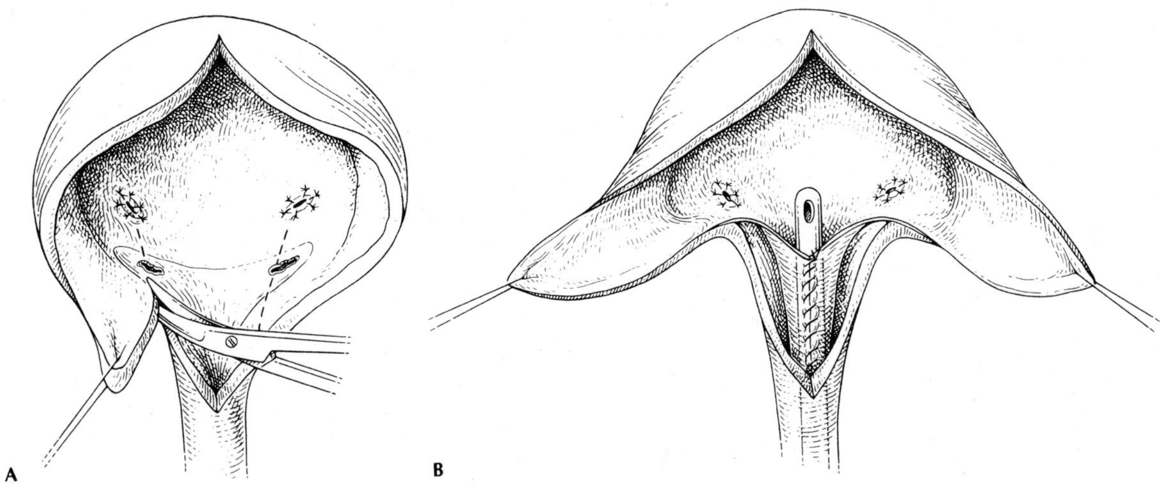


FIGURE 107.3 Leadbetter modification of Young–Dees–Leadbetter bladder neck repair. **A:** Full-thickness parallel incisions are made through the trigone mucosa and muscle, leaving a central strip 15 mm wide. **B:** The mucosa of the neourethra is tubularized using a running absorbable suture. The muscle is then closed. The lateral flaps of trigone are left in continuity with the bladder.

If bladder augmentation is required, the bladder should be closed to itself for a short distance from the urethra prior to applying the bowel segment. A clear demarcation between the neourethra and bladder can often be seen after closure. Care should be taken that there is effective closure of the urethra and bladder at this junction. The bladder may tend to kink over the urethra at that level, and the neourethra and new bladder neck should be suspended to the undersurface of the intersymphyseal band and lower abdominal wall using several pairs of sutures as described for the Marshall–Marchetti–Krantz procedure (Fig. 107.2D).

Alternatively, Leadbetter described full-thickness, parallel incisions through the trigone mucosa and muscle on either side of the central strip. These incisions, again made 12 to 15 mm apart, are started distally at the old bladder neck and continued in a cephalad direction for 4 to 5 cm (Fig. 107.3A). The central strip of mucosa is tubularized with interrupted or running absorbable sutures. The muscle of the central strip is closed as a second layer. If the incision through the muscle is made slightly wider than on the mucosa, the muscle may be approximated in an overlapping manner but to a lesser degree than that described by Young and Dees. The lateral triangles of full-thickness trigone are left in continuity with the bladder and included in that closure (Fig. 107.3B).

## Kropp Urethral Lengthening Procedure

The bladder is exposed through a lower midline incision and the bladder neck is identified by palpation of a catheter placed through the urethra. A rectangular, full-thickness strip of anterior bladder is marked and incised. This strip is based at the bladder neck and should be left in continuity with the urethra (5). The incised strip measures 6 cm in length and 2 cm in width (Fig. 107.4A). Stay sutures placed at the cephalad corners of the strip aid in mobilization. The bladder cephalad to the strip is opened in the midline. After anterior incision, the catheter is pulled over the pubis to expose the posterior bladder neck. This allows identification of the ureteral orifices, which are catheterized. If reflux is not present and the space between the orifices is adequate for urethral tunneling, ureteral reimplantation may not be necessary. The ureteral stents are often left in place for 4 to 5 days due to edema. Posterior incision of the mucosa at the bladder neck is performed using cutting current with the electrosurgical cautery to completely separate the neourethra from the bladder at the mucosal level. Further dissection through the posterior muscle in the midline is performed to allow smooth tubularization of the neourethra. Posterolateral musculoadventitial tissue at the 5 and 7 o'clock positions is left intact so that the bladder remains anchored in a caudal position. This eventually ensures that the tubularized neourethra reaches well into the bladder lumen to achieve an effective flap valve.

The anterior bladder flap in continuity with the urethra is tubularized by approximating the mucosa and then the muscle with continuous absorbable sutures (Fig. 107.4B). This closure is again begun distally and continued in a proximal or cephalad direction.

A submucosal tunnel is developed from the posterior bladder neck to a position several centimeters above the interureteric ridge (Fig. 107.4C). The more cephalad portion of this tunnel is easily developed from above and the more distal or caudal portion is typically developed from the bladder neck (Fig. 107.4D). This tunnel must be made wide enough that the neourethra can be brought through in a nice smooth course. Care must be taken that there is no kink whatsoever at the entrance of the neourethra into the bladder at the area of the old bladder neck. Any kinking at that level will result in difficult catheterization.

Alternatively, the mucosa in the posterior midline may be incised for the entire length for the proposed tunnel. The mucosa on either side is then mobilized to create a wide trough into which to place the urethra. The mucosa from either side is then approximated to the adventitia of the neourethra and will eventually grow to cover it completely. The tubularized neourethra should not be redundant in length relative to the submucosal tunnel to minimize the risk of difficult catheterization. If necessary, excess length may be excised. The proximal end of the neourethra is approximated to the bladder mucosa at its orifice with interrupted absorbable suture (Fig. 107.4E).

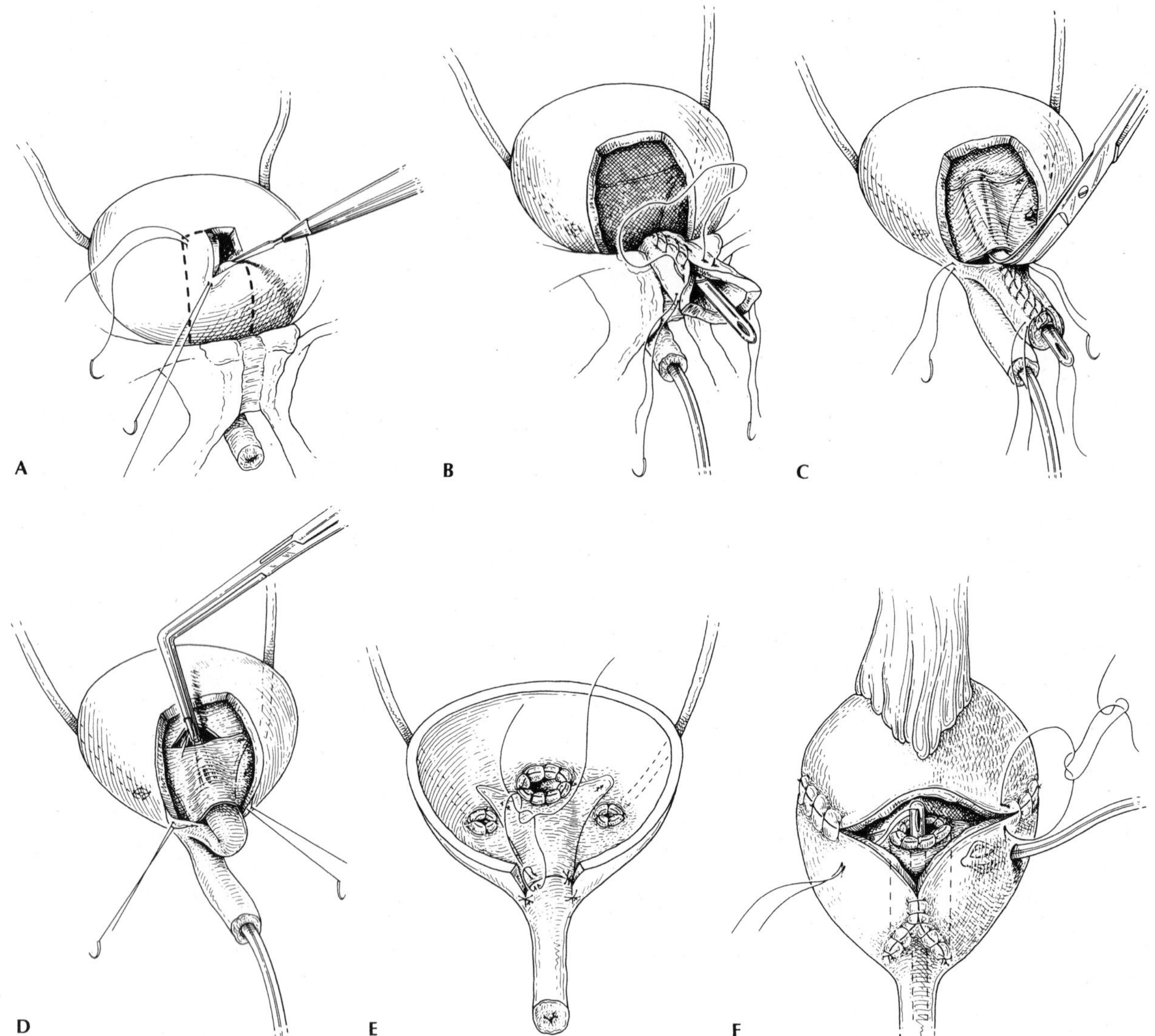


FIGURE 107.4 Kropp procedure for urethral lengthening. **A:** A 6 × 2-cm flap of anterior bladder is mobilized in continuity with the urethra. **B:** The flap is tubularized. **C:** The posterior mucosa is incised transversely at the bladder neck and a tunnel created for the neourethra from the old bladder neck to a position above the interureteric ridge. **D:** The neourethra is brought through the tunnel, taking care that it does not kink. Note that the posterolateral musculoadventitial tissue is intact and keeps the bladder anchored distally. **E:** The proximal end of the neourethra is trimmed flush with its orifice in the bladder. The end is approximated to the vesical mucosa circumferentially. **F:** The bladder is carefully closed distally by approximating the bladder muscle and mucosa to the adventitia of the neourethra. The neourethra extends well into the lumen of the bladder to create an effective flap valve. Bladder augmentation is performed when necessary.

Distally, the lateral and anterior bladder is securely approximated to the adventitia and muscle of the urethra (Fig. 107.4F). This closure should be performed as distally as possible on the urethra to avoid foreshortening of the tunnel within the bladder. Ease of catheterization through the neourethra should be tested at each step of reconstruction and any problems addressed when noted. If augmentation of the bladder is necessary, the incision is extended and the peritoneal cavity entered. A short segment of distal bladder should be closed to itself up from the urethra prior to placing the segment for augmentation. A soft urethral catheter is left in place per urethra during healing. The catheter should be secured so as to avoid any pressure on the reconstructed urethra. The catheter is usually left in place for 4 to 6 weeks during healing, often with a suprapubic cystotomy tube as well. After a static cystogram demonstrates no leakage and good healing, self-catheterization may begin.

## Pippi Salle Urethral Lengthening Procedure

In an effort to achieve the effective flap valve created with the Kropp procedure while decreasing the risk for problems with catheterization, Salle et al. (6) described a modification for urethral lengthening. The anterior bladder wall flap is used as an

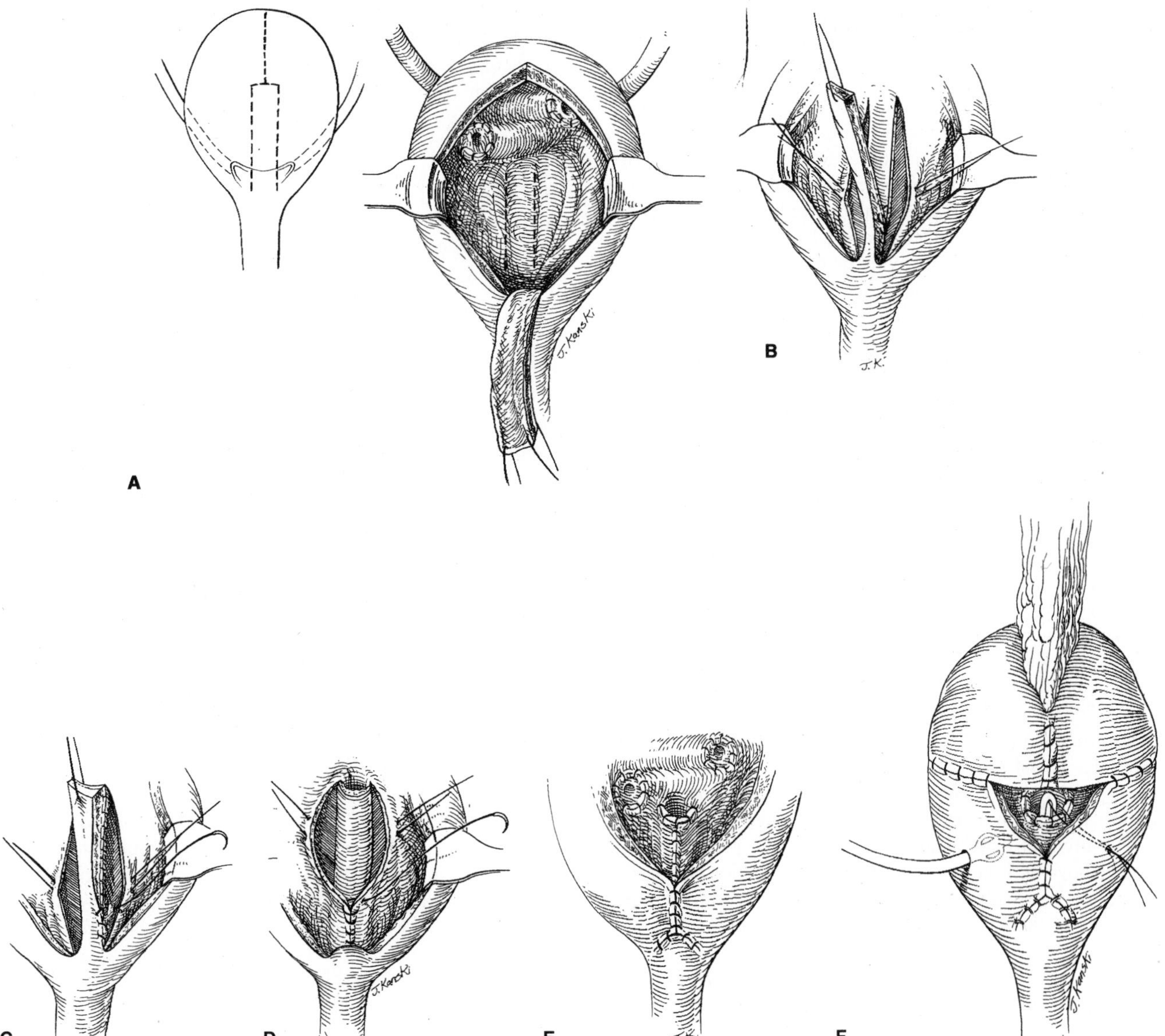


FIGURE 107.5 Pippi Salle procedure for urethral lengthening. **A:** A full-thickness, anterior bladder flap 5 × 1 cm is marked and incised. Parallel incisions through the trigone mucosa posteriorly leave a central strip of similar length and width. **B:** The lateral trigone mucosa is mobilized to cover the neourethra. The mucosa of the anterior flap is approximated to the edge of the central mucosal strip using a running absorbable suture. **C:** The muscle of the anterior flap is approximated to the superficial trigone muscle on either side of the mucosal closure. **D:** The lateral mucosa is closed over the neourethra. **E:** The distal bladder is closed to itself and carefully to the urethra. **F:** Bladder augmentation is performed when necessary.

onlay and eventually contributes half of the circumference of the neourethra. Therefore, a full-thickness anterior bladder flap 5 × 1 cm is mobilized in continuity with the bladder neck (Fig. 107.5A). One millimeter of mucosa on either side is excised to avoid overlapping suture lines. Two parallel incisions through the mucosa of the trigone are made so as to leave a central strip of mucosa 8 to 10 mm in width and 5 cm in length. The lateral trigone mucosa on either side is mobilized to eventually close over the neourethra. The mucosa of the anterior flap is approximated to the midline strip of trigone mucosa using a running absorbable suture started distally (Fig. 107.5B). The muscle of the anterior flap is approximated to the superficial muscle on either side of the central mucosa (Fig. 107.5C). The trigone muscle on either side of the posterior mucosal strip may be incised superficially to provide an edge to which to sew the muscle of the anterior flap. Closure of the lateral mucosa of the trigone over the reconstructed neourethra creates a flap valve and a neourethra with an intact posterior wall (Fig. 107.5D,E). Distally, the muscle and mucosa of the bladder neck are approximated to the lateral and anterior adventitia and muscle of the neourethra as distally as possible. Proximally, the neourethra should extend well into the lumen of the bladder to create an effective flap-valve mechanism for continence. The neourethra and ureters are often stented temporarily in a manner similar to that described for the Kropp procedure (Fig. 107.5F).

## OUTCOMES

In the pediatric population, fascial slings have been used most extensively in patients with neurogenic sphincter incompetence. Long-term success with slings in that population has varied greatly, from 40% to 100%. Success rates have varied so much that it is not clear that any particular modification of the sling configuration results in any difference in terms of continence. Fascial slings have been used more extensively and with better results in girls with neurogenic dysfunction, in whom the continence rate may reach 75% (7). The primary factor predictive of success has been concomitant enterocystoplasty to ensure a compliant bladder. Placement does not in general interfere with the ability to perform intermittent catheterization, which is usually necessary in the patient population.

The Young–Dees–Leadbetter bladder neck repair has been used most commonly in the classic staged reconstruction for bladder exstrophy. Continence with spontaneous voiding has been achieved in up to 80% of patients with exstrophy and may be even higher for patients with epispadias (8). Other authors have reported a lower continence rate, and even among patients considered dry, clinical and urodynamic problems related to poor emptying may exist (9). When used for patients with neurogenic dysfunction and denervated sphincter muscle, the procedure initially resulted in continence in approximately 25% of patients, but the rate can be improved to almost 70% if combined with bladder augmentation (10,11). Due to the high percentage of additional procedures required, the repair has in general fallen out of favor for patients with neurogenic dysfunction. Reliable catheterization through the urethra after a Young–Dees–Leadbetter repair may be difficult.

The urethral lengthening procedures have primarily been used in boys with neurogenic bladder dysfunction. Using the technique described by Kropp, continence has been achieved in 75% to 90% of such patients (5,12). Difficulty with catheterization has been reported in 40% of male patients in some series, although that incidence may be lowered when the posterior urethra is not totally transected (12). Because of concerns about the potential problem with catheterization, some surgeons prefer routine construction of a continent catheterizable stoma (13). A significant incidence of new reflux has been apparent in some series using the Kropp technique (13). Using the modification by Salle et al., less trouble with catheterization in male patients has been noted, although continence rates have not been quite as high (14,15). Urethrovesical fistula and partial necrosis of the intravesical neourethra have on occasion resulted in incontinence after the repair, and widening the base of the anterior flap at the level of the bladder neck may decrease those problems.

### Complications

Relatively common clinical problems after bladder neck reconstruction include urinary tract infection and bladder stones. Both may occur in exstrophy patients after Young–Dees–Leadbetter bladder neck repair due to poor emptying (9), but they are even more common among patients with neurogenic dysfunction requiring intermittent catheterization, in particular if bladder augmentation has been performed. The urethral sling and the artificial urinary sphincter possess unique complications that are related to their periurethral placement or mechanical and synthetic characteristics. Urethral erosion, although the rate is low with fascial slings and 5% to 15% with artificial urethral sphincters, is most commonly related to infection. Erosion is a leading cause for permanent failure of the artificial urinary sphincter. Additionally, mechanical problems or tissue atrophy at the cuff lead to artificial urinary sphincter revision rates of approximately one in four in modern series (16).

It is important to perform routine surveillance for hydronephrosis of the upper urinary tract with ultrasonography after any form of bladder neck repair. This is particularly true among patients with neurogenic dysfunction if they have not undergone bladder augmentation. Even if the bladder appeared adequate prior to outlet reconstruction, up to one quarter of patients may develop bladder hostility after an increase in outlet resistance, which may silently threaten the kidneys (17).

## *References*


1. Perez LM, Smith EA, Parrott TS, et al. Submucosal bladder neck injection of bovine dermal collagen for stress urinary incontinence in the pediatric population. *J Urol* 1996;156:633–636.
2. Lottmann HB, Margaryan M, Lortat-Jacob S, et al. Long-term effects of dextranomer endoscopic injections for the treatment of urinary incontinence: an update of a prospective study of 61 patients. *J Urol* 2006;176:1762–1766.
3. Cole EE, Adams MC, Brock JW 3rd, et al. Outcome of continence procedures in the pediatric patient: a single institutional experience. *J Urol* 2003;170:560–563.
4. Jayanthi VR, Churchill BM, McLorie GA, et al. Concomitant bladder neck closure and Mitrofanoff diversion for the management of intractable urinary incontinence. *J Urol* 1995;154:886–888.
5. Kropp KA, Angwafo FF. Urethral lengthening and reimplantation for neurogenic incontinence in children. *J Urol* 1986;135:533–536.
6. Salle JL, McLorie GA, Bagli DJ, et al. Urethral lengthening with anterior bladder wall flap (Pippi Salle procedure): modifications and extended indications of the technique. *J Urol* 1997;158:585–590.
7. Perez LM, Smith EA, Broecker BH, et al. Outcome of sling cystourethropexy in the pediatric population: a critical review. *J Urol* 1996;156:642–646.
8. Gearhart JP, Matthews R. Exstrophy–epispadias complex. In: Wein AJ, Kavoussi LR, Novick AC, et al., eds. *Campbell-Walsh Urology*, 9th ed., vol. 4. Philadelphia: Saunders Elsevier, 2007:3497–3553.
9. Yerkes EB, Adams MC, Rink RC, et al. How well do patients with exstrophy actually void? *J Urol* 2000;164:1044–1047.
10. Donnahoo KK, Rink RC, Cain MP, et al. The Young-Dees-Leadbetter bladder neck repair for neurogenic incontinence. *J Urol* 1999;161:1946–1949.
11. Leadbetter GW Jr. Surgical reconstruction for complete urinary incontinence: a 10- to 22-year followup. *J Urol* 1985;133:205–206.
12. Belman AB, Kaplan GW. Experience with the Kropp anti-incontinence procedure. *J Urol* 1989;141:1160–1162.
13. Snodgrass W. A simplified Kropp procedure for incontinence. *J Urol* 1997;158:1049–1052.
14. Rink RC, Adams MC, Keating MA. The flip-flap technique to lengthen the urethra (Salle procedure) for treatment of neurogenic urinary incontinence. *J Urol* 1994;152:799–802.
15. Salle JL, McLorie GA, Bagli DJ, et al. Modifications of and extended indications for the Pippi Salle procedure. *World J Urol* 1998;16:279–284.
16. Kryger JV, Gonzalez R, Barthold JS. Surgical management of urinary incontinence in children with neurogenic sphincteric incompetence. *J Urol* 2000;163:256–263.
17. Bauer SB, Reda EF, Colodny AH, et al. Detrusor instability: a delayed complication in association with the artificial sphincter. *J Urol* 1986;135:1212–1215.

# CHAPTER 108 ■ SURGERY FOR POSTERIOR URETHRAL VALVES

ROSALIA MISSERI AND KENNETH I. GLASSBERG

A posterior urethral valve (PUV) is the most common cause of congenital bladder outlet obstruction in boys. It is associated with a dilated posterior urethra, poor urinary stream, and incomplete bladder emptying. Bilateral hydroureteronephrosis of varying degrees is almost always present and frequently accompanied by vesicoureteral reflux and/or bladder diverticula.

## DIAGNOSIS

With the widespread use of antenatal ultrasound, PUVs are often diagnosed prenatally. The condition is suspected in utero when a male fetus is found to have bilateral hydroureteronephrosis and a thick-walled bladder that does not empty completely on sonography. In addition, there may be a keyhole deformity noted on sonography. This is noted when a dilated bladder and posterior urethra is seen. In severely affected fetuses, oligohydramnios, pulmonary hypoplasia, and Potter syndrome may occur. Newborns may present with abdominal masses representing a distended bladder or hydronephrotic kidney, dry diapers, nonspecific gastrointestinal symptoms, respiratory distress, or urinary ascites. Younger boys usually present with urinary tract infection, respiratory distress, abdominal distention, sepsis, or azotemia, while older boys may present with dysfunctional voiding symptomatology, incontinence, poor urinary stream, urinary tract infections, or hematuria.

If a PUV is suspected in an infant, prophylactic antibiotics should be initiated and the bladder should be drained with a 5Fr or 8Fr feeding tube securely taped in place with a clear transparent dressing. Positioning is best confirmed with an abdominal radiograph as the tube may coil in the dilated posterior urethra. The feeding tube is left in place until a voiding cystourethrogram (VCUG) is obtained to make the diagnosis. In patients with severe hydroureteronephrosis and/or azotemia, the catheter should be left in place until the azotemia resolves/stabilizes and hydroureteronephrosis improves.

The VCUG of a boy with a PUV will reveal a posterior urethra that appears dilated, often taking on a "shield shape" or squared-off appearance. The bladder neck is often clearly demarcated and may appear as a thick collar, and the urethra distal to the obstruction will appear less full than normal (Fig. 108.1).

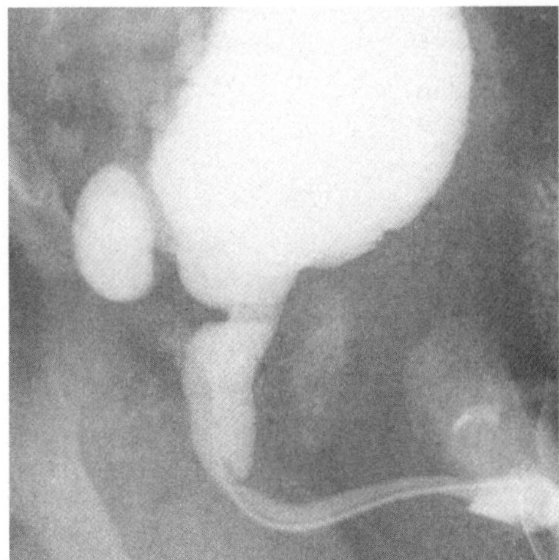

FIGURE 108.1 Voiding cystourethrogram of newborn with posterior urethral valves. Note the dilated posterior urethra and bladder diverticulum.

## INDICATIONS FOR SURGERY

Today, most valve ablation is accomplished transurethrally. Some controversy still exists as to what to do once the bladder has been drained with a catheter (Fig. 108.2). For severe hydronephrosis, some report better long-term outcomes when these infants are temporarily diverted, while most feel that primary valve ablation is the treatment of choice (1). For those who believe temporary diversion is best, many methods of vesical and supravesical diversion of the obstructed bladder exist.

## ALTERNATIVE THERAPY

There is no effective alternative to surgical therapy.

## SURGICAL TECHNIQUE

### Transurethral Valve Ablation

Valve ablation is most commonly accomplished transurethrally. The size of the infant's fossa navicularis usually limits the size of cystoscope that may be used. Typically, a 7.5Fr or 8.5Fr scope is used in infants, while a larger scope may be used in older children. The cystoscope should be well lubricated and advanced under direct vision. Gentle dilation of the distal urethra may be required to advance the cystourethroscope. With the bladder full and applying gentle suprapubic pressure, the valve leaflets are more easily seen coming off the verumontanum and extending distally to fuse anteriorly (Fig. 108.3). The goal of valve ablation is to disrupt the leaflet, hence destroying the obstruction.

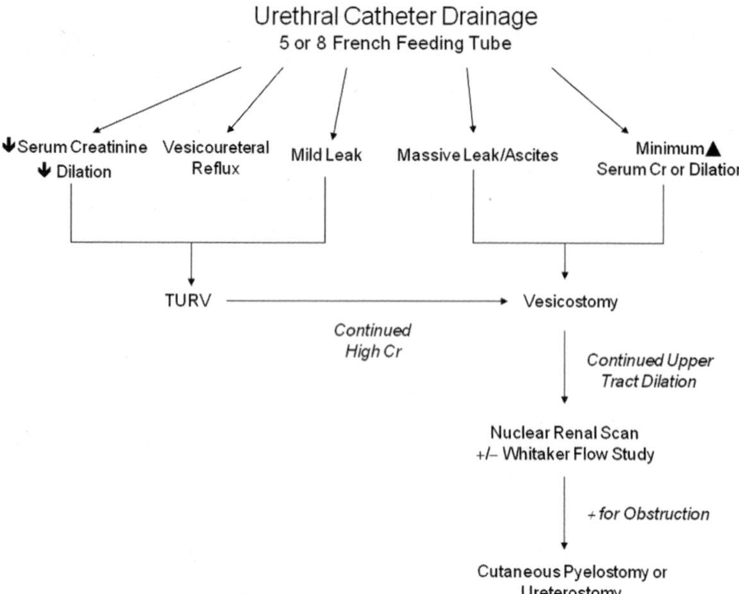


FIGURE 108.2 Proposed management of posterior urethral valves.

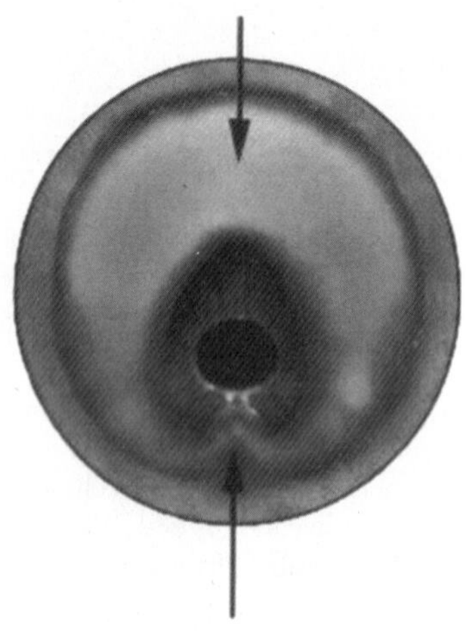


FIGURE 108.3 Cystoscopic appearance of type 1 posterior urethral valve.

A PUV may be ablated or incised in several ways. It may be ablated using a 3Fr Bugbee electrode through a cystoscope. Alternatively, the wire insert of a 3Fr ureteral catheter with the distal end connected to electrocautery may be used. Once in position the wire is advanced and pushed into the valve at the 5 and 7 o'clock positions while employing a cutting current of 20 to 25 W. (Note that power settings may vary from machine to machine.) When using cautery care must be taken to ensure that thermal energy is targeted at the valves alone. This may be particularly useful if the infant resectoscope is too large for the child's urethra.

Using a small pediatric resectoscope, the valves are incised with a right-angle hook, loop electrode, or hook-shaped cold-knife. When using a loop electrode, a narrow, more oblong loop is preferable to a wider, more circular loop. Some debate exists as to the best location for valve incision. Williams et al. (2) preferred incising at the 12 o'clock position, while Gonzales (3) advocated cutting at the 4, 8, and 12 o'clock positions. However, most prefer incising at the 4 to 5 o'clock and 7 to 8 o'clock positions using a hook-shaped cold knife or with the cutting current set at 20 to 25 W pure cut.

Lasers such as the neodymium:YAG have also been employed for PUV ablation. Additional methods of PUV ablation have also been described for use in patients with small-caliber urethras. With the advent of smaller scopes, perineal urethrostomy is now rarely necessary for valve ablation. Zaontz and Firlit (4) have described percutaneous antegrade ablation of PUV as well as antegrade incision of PUV in infants with small-caliber urethras.

Once the valves are endoscopically ablated the bladder should be cystoscoped to evaluate for diverticula, trabeculations, and the appearance of the ureteral orifices. A full stream should be noted at the end of the procedure while applying gentle pressure to the suprapubic area. A small urethral catheter is left in place for 1 to 2 days following the procedure or until an elevated creatinine nadirs. A VCUG may be performed after the catheter is removed to assess the success of the procedure. Timing of the VCUG is determined by the surgeon based on his or her confidence in the adequacy of ablation. A VCUG and urodynamics or preferably videourodynamics should be delayed no >6 to 8 weeks after ablation. If there is suspicion of inadequate ablation or continued obstruction, "second-look" cystoscopy with ablation of residual leaflets should be considered. If the child is found to have diminished compliance or detrusor hyperactivity, anticholinergic therapy should be considered. Anticholinergic therapy may also be instituted immediately after valve ablation or prior to closure or reversal of vesical or supravesical diversion.

## Vesicostomy

While most patients with PUV are treated with primary valve ablation, a vesicostomy may be useful in neonates whose urethra will not accommodate a cystoscope or in those whose creatinine rises despite adequate valve resection.

With the patient in the supine position the lower abdominal skin is prepared and draped in the typical fashion. The procedure is more easily performed with a full bladder. A 2-cm transverse incision is then made midway between the pubic symphysis and umbilicus. The rectus fascia is exposed and a 2 × 2-cm cruciate incision is made. Alternately, a triangle or circle of rectus fascia measuring 2 cm may be excised. One must remember that the size of the fascial opening ultimately determines the caliber of the stoma. The rectus muscles are then retracted laterally, exposing the bladder. A 3-0 suture is placed near the dome of the bladder and used for traction. Using the traction suture the bladder is mobilized superiorly. The peritoneum is gently swept off the superior aspect of the bladder. Additional cephalad sutures may be placed in a stepwise fashion to help bring the dome into the surgical field. Care is taken to avoid the peritoneal contents. With gentle traction one should be able to visualize the urachus or obliterated hypogastric artery.

The vesicostomy may be created in one of two ways. In the first method, a stay suture is placed proximal to the urachus. The urachus is then transected and excised. In the second method, the portion of the bladder cephalad to the urachal remnant is used as the site for the vesicostomy. The bladder is incised and the fascial edges are sewn to the outer bladder wall using 3-0 or 4-0 polyglactin sutures approximately 0.5 to 1 cm from the opening created in the bladder. The vesicostomy should be calibrated to 24Fr or large enough to allow passage of the surgeon's fifth digit. If the fascial defect is too large, interrupted 3-0 polyglactin sutures may be used to narrow the opening. The edges of the detrusor are then sewn to the skin using 4-0 polyglactin sutures in an interrupted fashion. If the skin incision is wider than the stoma created, the skin is approximated with a suture of choice (Fig. 108.4).

The decision to close a vesicostomy should be made only once bladder dynamics have been assessed and a plan for

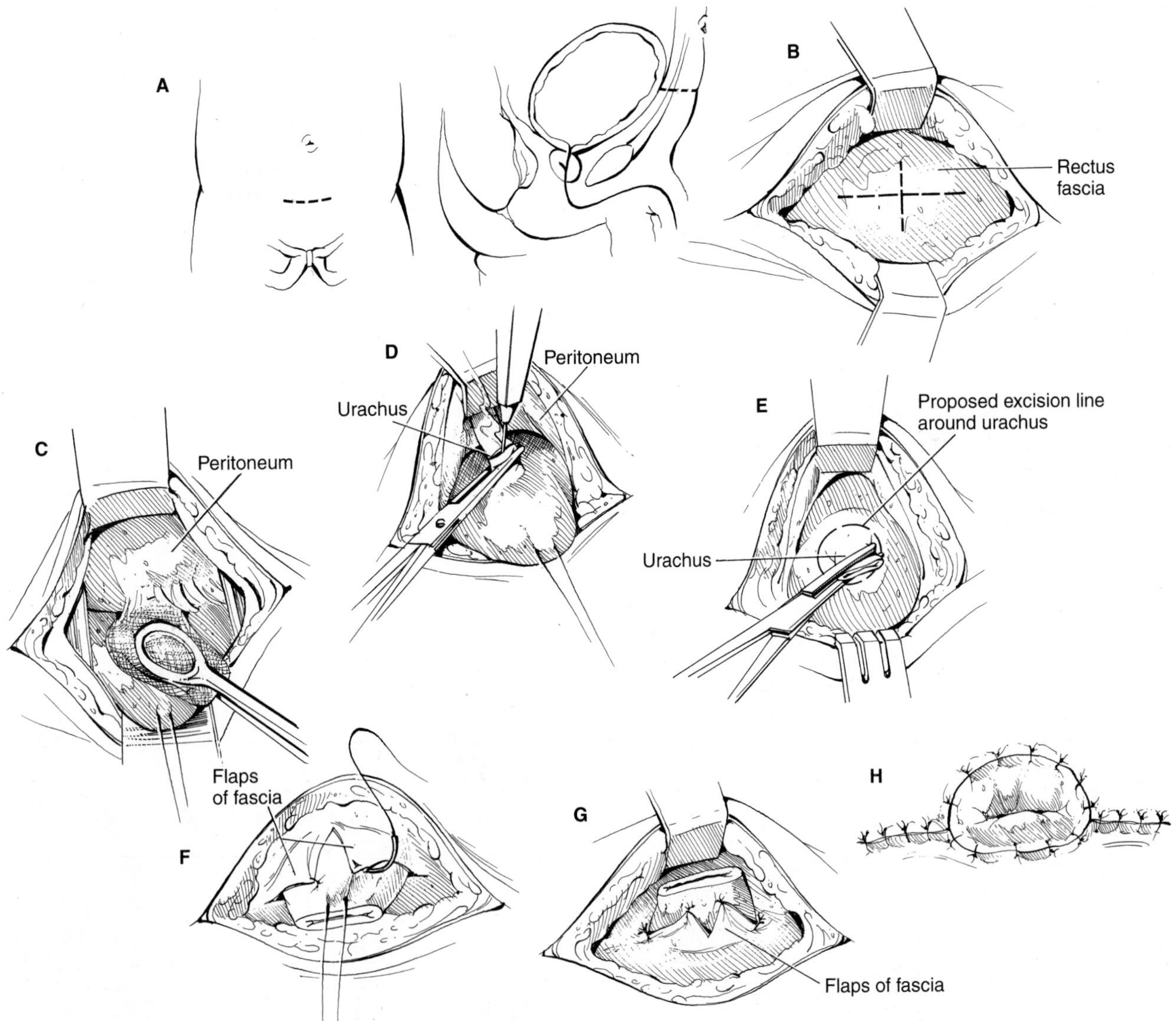


FIGURE 108.4 Blocksom vesicostomy. **A:** A 2-cm transverse incision is made midway between the pubic symphysis and umbilicus. **B:** A 2 × 2-cm cruciate fascial incision is made. **C:** Using the traction suture the bladder is mobilized superiorly. The peritoneum is gently swept off the superior aspect of the bladder. **D:** The urachus is incised and the bladder is further mobilized. **E:** The urachus is excised. **F and G:** The outer bladder wall is sewn to the edges of the incised rectus fascia. **H:** The edges of the detrusor are sewn to the skin. (Modified from Belman AB, King LR. Vesicostomy: useful means of reversible urinary diversion in selected infant. *Urology* 1973;1:208–213.)

permanent therapy has been devised. Ultimately, the timing of closure is dictated by the surgeon's philosophy. Some believe an empty bladder becomes a contracted bladder, while others close vesicostomies just prior to the expected time of potty training.

Initially, an adequate-size balloon catheter is placed into the stoma of the vesicostomy. With the balloon inflated, an elliptical skin incision is made around the stoma. The subcutaneous and perivesical tissues are dissected circumferentially around the vesicostomy. Next, 3-0 chromic stay sutures are placed through the bladder wall approximately 1 cm cephalad and 1 cm caudad to the stoma. The skin and protruding portion of the bladder are excised. The previously placed catheter is removed and a urethral catheter is placed for bladder drainage. The bladder defect is then closed in two layers: a running 4-0 chromic suture is used to reapproximate the bladder mucosa, followed by interrupted or running 3-0 polyglactin or chromic sutures as a second layer. The remainder of the wound is closed in a standard fashion.

## Supravesical Diversion

### Cutaneous Pyelostomy

The decision to proceed with a supravesical diversion remains controversial, and it is rarely used. To safely perform a cutaneous pyelostomy, the renal pelvis should be sufficiently dilated to avoid tension on the renal pelvis as it is pulled toward the abdominal wall. A dilated renal pelvis also ensures that dissection can be carried out away from the ureteropelvic junction (UPJ).

The renal pelvis may be approached in several ways, including a dorsal lumbotomy or a subcostal extraperitoneal approach. A surgeon may use the approach he or she is most comfortable with. Despite the limited exposure that a dorsal lumbotomy incision affords, it is excellent for visualization of the renal pelvis and upper ureter. The procedure avoids a muscle-splitting incision and may produce less postoperative pain.

After the patient is intubated, he should be placed in the prone position on the operating room table. Cushions should then be placed under the chest and just superior to the anterior superior iliac spines. The landmarks include the 12th rib superiorly, the iliac crest inferiorly, and the lateral border of the sacrospinalis medially. A vertical incision with or without a slight curve at its distal end is made approximately one-third to one-half the distance between the 12th rib and the iliac crest. Alternatively, an oblique incision may be made along the Langer lines (Fig. 108.5). Care should be taken to avoid

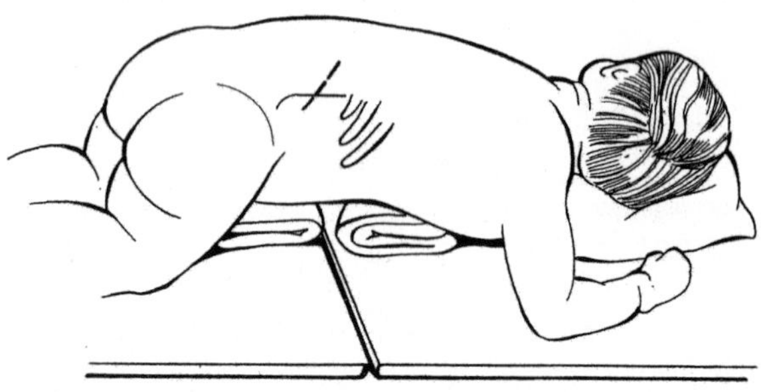

FIGURE 108.5 Positioning for dorsal lumbotomy and possible skin incisions. The *solid line* represents our incision of choice; the *broken line* represents a suitable alternative.

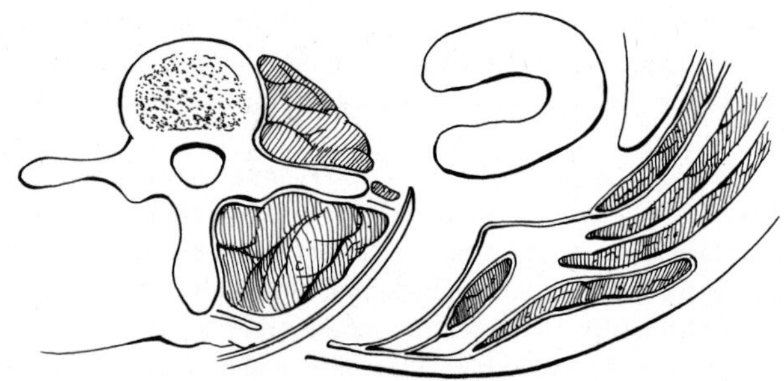

FIGURE 108.6 Fascial incision through lumbodorsal fascia lateral to the sacrospinalis and quadratus lumborum, avoiding the division of muscles.

injuring the subcostal neurovascular bundle. The lumbodorsal fascia is exposed by elevating the skin and subcutaneous tissues for about 3 cm on either side of the incision so that a vertical fascial incision may be comfortably made. The posterior layer of the lumbodorsal fascia is incised vertically 2 cm lateral to the midline. The sacrospinalis muscle is then retracted medially. This exposes the middle layer of the lumbodorsal fascia, which is incised at the lateral border of the quadratus lumborum. Retracting the quadratus lumborum medially, the anterior layer of the lumbodorsal fascia is exposed (Fig. 108.6). This layer and the transversalis fascia are then incised between the subcostal and iliohypogastric nerves. The perinephric fat should then be in view. The kidney should be located in the superomedial part of the wound.

Once the fascia of Gerota is entered, the dilated renal pelvis is identified and rotated anteromedially. The surgeon must assess if the pelvis can comfortably reach the skin. If not, a very proximal portion of the ureter may be brought out to serve the same purpose. Care should be taken to avoid dissection near the UPJ so as to avoid the possibility of a future UPJ obstruction. Two 3-0 chromic traction sutures are placed on the posterior aspect of the renal pelvis away from the UPJ. Using a scalpel a 3-cm incision is made. The full thickness of the renal pelvis is sutured to the posterior corner of the skin incision using multiple interrupted 4-0 polyglactin sutures (Fig. 108.7). The pyelostomy should be calibrated to approximately 20Fr to avoid future stenosis or prolapse. Once the planned procedure

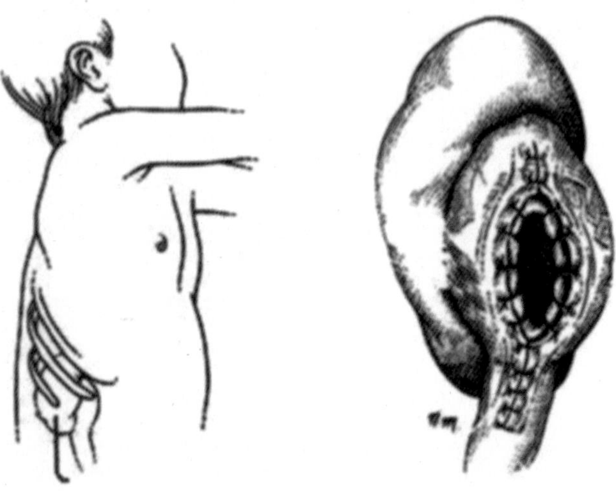

FIGURE 108.7 Cutaneous pyelostomy (sutures at the skin level).

has been performed, the posterior layer of the lumbodorsal fascia is reapproximated with 3-0 polyglactin sutures and the skin is then closed with either a subcuticular suture or skin staples.

### High Cutaneous Loop Ureterostomy

This method is typically employed when the renal pelvis is not large enough for a cutaneous pyelostomy to be performed. The initial steps for a high cutaneous ureterostomy are similar to that for a cutaneous pyelostomy. The ureter is brought to skin level. Two 4-0 polyglactin sutures are placed in the upper ureter approximately 5 mm from each other. Using a scalpel a 2-cm vertical ureterotomy is created. The abdominal musculature is closed on either side and behind the loop of ureter. Care is taken to avoid strangulating the ureter. The incised ureteral margins are sewn to the skin using interrupted 4-0 polyglactin sutures. The final product is a double-barreled ureteral stoma (Fig. 108.8).

Loop ureterostomies maintain continuity of part of the ureter, therefore decreasing the likelihood of disruption of ureteral blood supply and possibly making closure of the ureterostomy simpler.

### Pelvioureterostomy-en-Y (Sober Loop Ureterostomy)

The Sober Y ureterostomy allows some urine to drain into the bladder, thus avoiding a completely defunctionalized bladder that may eventually become contracted (5). It is not the procedure of choice in critically ill patients as it is more extensive and time consuming than other forms of diversion, and it is best used in patients with redundant tortuous ureters. The ureter is mobilized from the level of the kidney to the level of the true pelvis. The ureter is divided at a point where the lower ureteral segment comfortably reaches the renal pelvis. The upper ureter that remains in continuity with the renal pelvis is brought out to the flank caudad to the flank incision. The proximal end of the lower portion of the transected ureter is anastomosed to the renal pelvis. This is done in an end-to-side fashion after creating a pelviotomy at a point that will not cause ureteral kinking. The anastomosis is performed using a 6-0 or 7-0 polyglactin suture in a running fashion (Fig. 108.9). The flank incision is closed in the standard fashion. A small Penrose drain may be temporarily placed. Initially, most urine will drain via the ureterostomy. Over time, increasing amounts of urine will drain into the bladder.

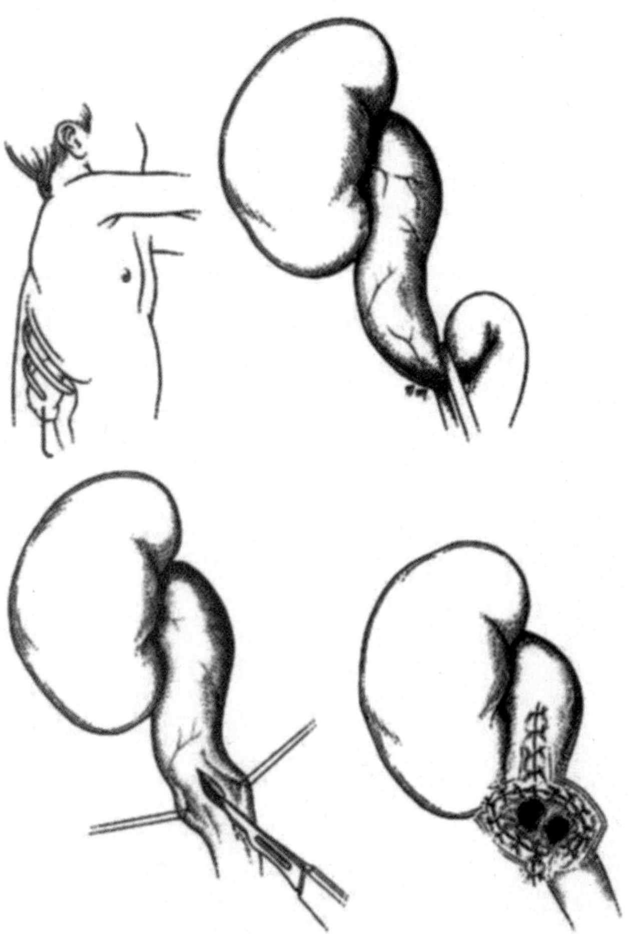

FIGURE 108.8 Loop cutaneous ureterostomy (sutures at the skin level).

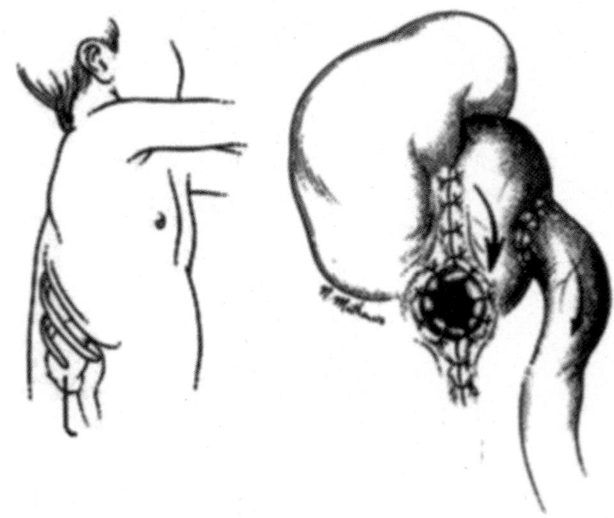

FIGURE 108.9 Pelvioureterostomy-en-Y (Sober ureterostomy).

### End Cutaneous Ureterostomy

To successfully perform a cutaneous ureterostomy, the ureter must be sufficiently thick-walled and dilated. Preservation of the ureteral blood supply is essential. The ureter should be approached extraperitoneally via either a low abdominal incision or a Gibson incision. The ureter should be carefully dissected from the level of the sacral promontory to the bladder with care to avoid stripping the ureter's adventitia. Once dissected, a thick vessel loop or Penrose drain should be placed around the ureter. One should estimate whether the ligated ureter will comfortably reach the anterior abdominal wall at the right or left lower quadrant. Once satisfied with this, the ureter is clamped and cut. The distal segment is ligated using a 3-0 polyglactin suture. A 3-0 polyglactin stay suture is placed on the cut end with care to avoid the ureter's medial blood supply (Fig. 108.10).

The cutaneous stoma is then created. Stomas should be placed in the right or left lower quadrant for ease of stomal fit in the event an appliance will be used. Once the site of the stoma has been determined, a V-shaped incision is made and taken down through the subcutaneous tissues and rectus sheath. Using the previously placed stay suture, the ureter is gently brought through the incision. If the ureter seems

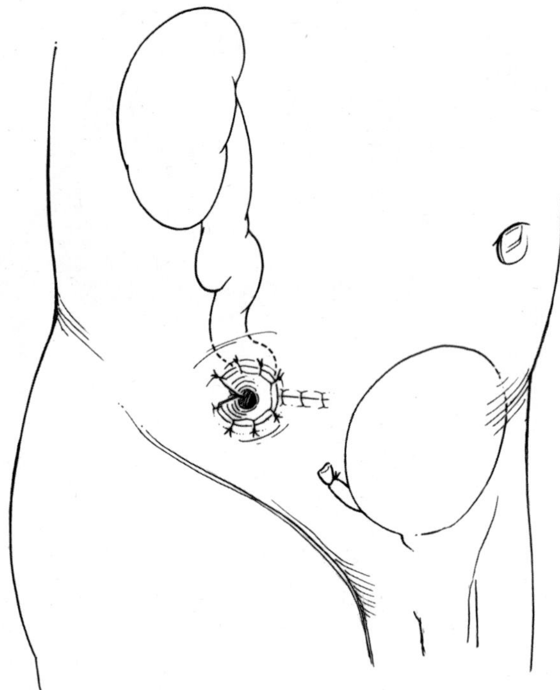

FIGURE 108.10 End ureterostomy (sutures at skin level). (From Indiana University School of Medicine, Office of Visual Media, with permission).

stretched, additional mobilization may be necessary. The ureter is then spatulated medially to avoid its blood supply. The apex of the spatulated ureter is then sewn to the apex of the skin incision using a 4-0 polyglactin suture. The ureter is then sewn to the other angles of the skin incision and additional sutures are placed circumferentially.

Bilateral end ureterostomies may be brought to the midline or either lower quadrant. The medial wall of each ureter is incised approximately 3 cm. The apexes of the incised ureters are sewn to each other using a two-armed 5-0 polyglactin suture. The incised walls of the ureters are then sewn to each other in a running fashion.

### Closure of Supravesical Diversions

To close a cutaneous pyelostomy, an elliptical skin incision is made around the stoma. The portion of pelvis that has been exteriorized is trimmed so that healthy renal pelvic edges may be approximated. Using a 6-0 polyglactin suture in a running fashion the renal pelvis is closed in a transverse fashion. The UPJ should be inspected to ensure that no kinking has occurred secondary to pyelostomy closure.

To close a loop ureterostomy, an elliptical skin incision is made in the skin surrounding the stoma. The proximal and distal ureteral segments are adequately mobilized. The fibrotic exposed portions of the ureter are excised, while trying to maintain the continuity of the ureter's back wall and blood supply. The remaining ureteral margins are then spatulated and closed in a transverse fashion using a 6-0 polyglactin suture (Fig. 108.11). Again, one must ensure that no angulation or narrowing of the ureter has occurred. A temporary indwelling ureteral stent may be placed to bridge the anastomosis.

A Sober ureterostomy may be reversed by excising the stoma at the skin level along with the limb of ureter used to create the cutaneous ureterostomy. The dissection is taken down to the level of the renal pelvis. The defect in the renal pelvis is closed using a 6-0 polyglactin suture in a running watertight fashion.

## OUTCOMES

### Complications

Cutaneous vesicostomies may be complicated by early or late prolapse of the dome or posterior bladder wall in up to 17% of patients. To prevent prolapse the most cephalad portion of the bladder or the urachus should be used as the site for the vesicostomy. By employing this portion of the bladder, the peritonealized part of the dome becomes immobilized, decreasing the risk of prolapse. The stomal opening itself should be no larger than 2 cm. The final stoma should calibrate to 24Fr. Excessive mucosal eversion should not be mistaken for

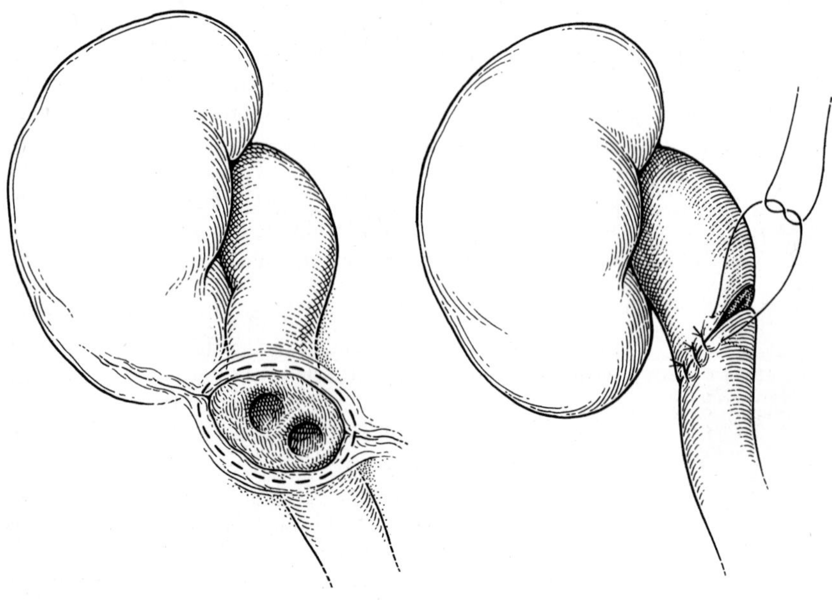

FIGURE 108.11 Takedown of loop cutaneous ureterostomy.

prolapse. Despite its appearance, no intervention is necessary for excessive eversion.

If the vesicostomy does not appear to be draining well and there is evidence of large amounts of residual bladder urine or large amounts of urine are voided by urethra, the suspicion of stomal stenosis should be raised. Stomal stenosis rates of 3% to 12% have been reported (6). The stenosis may be secondary to a small fascial opening or excessive tension on the vesicocutaneous anastomosis. Continuous drainage of urine into a diaper commonly may lead to peristomal dermatitis. Prolonged, severe dermatitis may ultimately lead to stomal stenosis. This can be prevented by air drying the skin or applying topical ointments used for diaper rash. Fungal superinfections may occur and are treated with antifungal creams and powders.

Some infants, particularly those with persistent vesicoureteral reflux, may have recurrent urinary tract infections despite patent vesicostomy and small bladder residuals. These children may benefit from intermittent catheterization through their vesicostomies.

The most common complication associated with pyelostomy is chronic skin irritation and dermatitis. As in other forms of diversion, chronic bacteriuria is also common. Less common complications of pyelostomy include stomal stenosis and prolapse of the renal pelvis. Chronic bacteriuria has been found in approximately two thirds of patients with ureterostomies and is the most common complication in this group. Stomal stenosis occurs in 11% to 70% of patients undergoing end cutaneous ureterostomies (7). The incidence of stenosis and obstruction is related to the caliber of the ureter used as well as the type of stoma created. Chronic skin irritation may also result in scarring and stenosis.

### Results

Despite the ease of performing a vesical diversion and its effectiveness in relieving bladder outlet obstruction, controversy exists regarding both its necessity and ultimate effects on bladder function (1,3).

## ANTERIOR URETHRAL VALVES

Anterior urethral valves occur 10 times less frequently than posterior urethral valves and may be located anywhere along the anterior urethra. In most cases, an anterior urethral valve is actually a congenital urethral diverticulum with the lip of the diverticulum preventing antegrade flow of urine. The bulging diverticulum may further obstruct the urethra by compressing the lumen. These children present with symptoms similar to those with a PUV, including varying degrees of hydroureteronephrosis; however, many also present with penile ballooning. As with PUV, the diagnosis is also made on VCUG. A renal ultrasound should be performed to complete the evaluation. Cystourethroscopy may miss the valve due to the retrograde flow of fluid during the procedure.

The obstruction is relieved endoscopically. The distal lip is incised using a hook or right-angle wire electrode. If unsuccessful, the diverticulum may be excised and the urethra reconfigured. Staged urethroplasty may be the best treatment option when faced with a large urethral diverticulum. Management of the hydroureteronephrosis would be similar to that in a patient with a PUV.

### *References*


1. Glassberg KI. The valve bladder syndrome: 20 years later. *J Urol* 2001;166:1406–1414.
2. Williams DI, Whitaker RA, Barratt TM, et al. Urethral valves. *Br J Urol* 1973;45:200–205.
3. Gonzales ET Jr. Posterior urethral valves and other anomalies. In: Walsh PC, Retik AB, Vaughan ED Jr, et al, eds. *Campbell's Urology.* 7th ed. Philadelphia: WB Saunders, 1998:2069–2091.
4. Zaontz MR, Firlit CF. Percutaneous antegrade ablation of posterior urethral valves in infants with small caliber urethras: an alternative to urinary diversion. *J Urol* 1986;136:247–248.
5. Sober I. Pelvioureterostomy-en-Y. *J Urol* 1972;107:473–475.
6. Skoog SJ. Pediatric vesical diversion. In: Graham SD, Glenn JF, eds. *Glenn's Urologic Surgery.* 5th ed. Philadelphia: Lippincott Williams & Wilkins, 1998:871–878.
7. Burstein JD, Firlit CF. Complications of cutaneous ureterostomy and other cutaneous diversion. *Urol Clin North Am* 1983;10:433–443.


# CHAPTER 109 ■ HYPOSPADIAS

LAURENCE S. BASKIN

Hypospadias is defined by three major anatomic defects: (i) the abnormal location of the urethral meatus, (ii) penile curvature, and (iii) abnormalities of the foreskin. The objective in treating patients with hypospadias is to reconstruct a straight penis for normal coitus and place the new urethral meatus on the terminal aspect of the glans to allow a forward-directed stream. There are five basic steps for a successful hypospadias outcome: (i) orthoplasty (straightening), (ii) urethroplasty, (iii) meatoplasty and glanuloplasty, (iv) scrotoplasty, and (v) skin coverage. These various elements of surgical technique can be applied either sequentially or in various combinations to achieve a surgical success (1).

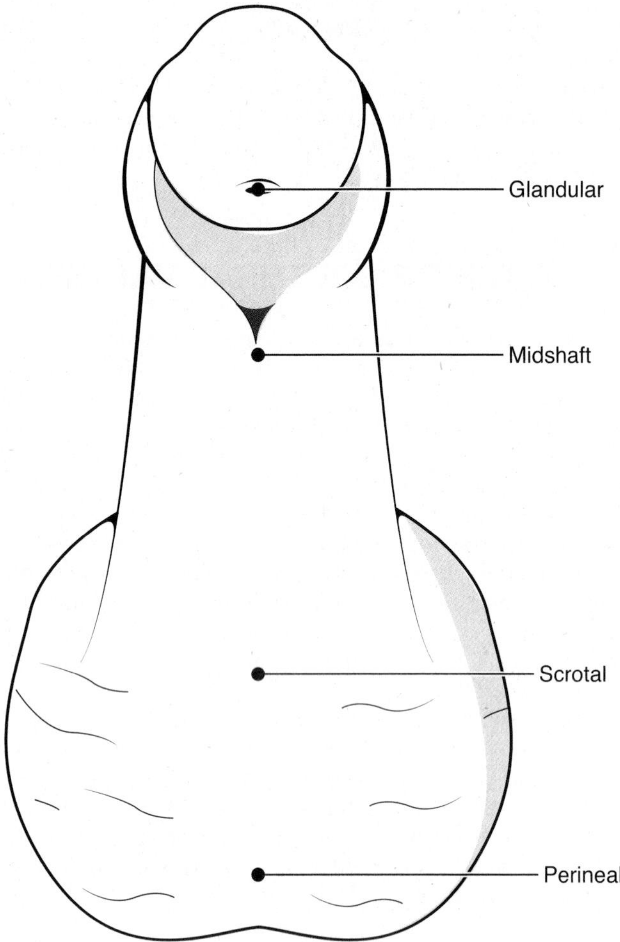


FIGURE 109.1 Location of the hypospadias meatus. Glandular, midshaft, scrotal, and perineal.

# DIAGNOSIS

## Meatal Abnormalities

Hypospadias is characterized by an abnormality in location and configuration of the urethral meatus (Fig. 109.1). The urethral meatus may be ventrally placed just below a blind dimple at the normal meatal opening on the glans or so far back in the perineum that it appears as a "vaginal" hypospadias. Most patients present with the urethral meatus somewhere between these extremes. The meatus is encountered in a variety of configurations in form, diameter, elasticity, and rigidity. It can be fissured in both transverse and longitudinal directions or can be covered with delicate skin. In the case of the megameatus intact prepuce, the distal urethra is enlarged, tapering to a normal caliber in the penile shaft. Often, there is an orifice of a periurethral duct located distal to the meatus that courses dorsal to the urethral channel for a short distance. It is blind ending and does not communicate in any way with the urinary stream. The periurethral duct corresponds with the sinus of Guérin or the lacunae of Morgagni. Unless these ducts are inadvertently closed, leading to a blind-ending epithelial pouch, they are of no clinical consequence.

## Skin and Scrotal Abnormalities

The skin of the penis is radically changed as a result of the disturbance in the formation of the urethra. Distal to the meatus, there is often a paucity of ventral skin, which may contribute to penile curvature. The frenulum is always absent in hypospadias. Vestiges of a frenulum are sometimes found inserting on either side of the open navicular fossa.

The skin proximal to the urethral meatus may be extremely thin, so much so that a catheter or probe passed proximally is readily apparent through a tissue-paper thickness of skin. When it is present, it abrogates the use of perimeatal skin flaps in repairs.

The urethral plate extending from the hypospadiac meatus to the glanular groove may be well developed. Even with a meatus quite proximal on the shaft, this normal urethral plate is quite elastic and typically nontethering. Artificial erection demonstrates no ventral curvature in these situations. A normal urethral plate may be incorporated into the surgical repair. However, if the urethral plate is underdeveloped, it will act as a tethering fibrous band that bends the penis ventrally during artificial erection. When this fibrous chordee tissue is divided, the penis will frequently straighten.

Normally, the genital tubercle should develop in a cranial position above the two genital swellings. The penis may be caught between the two scrotal halves and become engulfed with fusion of the penoscrotal area. The boundary between the penis and the scrotum may be formed by two oblique raphes that extend from the very proximal meatus to the dorsal side of the penis.

## Penile Curvature

The curvature of the penis is caused by deficiency of the normal structures, most commonly on the ventral side of the penis. It has been labeled *chordee*; however, this term implies a strand of connective tissue stretched like a cord between the meatus and glans, which is rarely found in practice. Penile curvature can be from skin deficiency, a dartos fascial deficiency, a true fibrous chordee with tethering of the ventral shaft, or deficiency of the corpora cavernosa on the concave side of the penis (2).

There are occasional reports of other penile anomalies that represent variations of the embryologic defect causing hypospadias. They can be characterized as a defect in the course of the urethra, such as congenital urethral fistula, and a group characterized by curvature of the penis without hypospadias, or so-called chordee without hypospadias.

# SURGICAL TECHNIQUE

## Hypospadias Training

Success is directly related to the experience of the surgeon. For a successful result in hypospadias repair, the penile tissues must be handled with great care. Experience in mobilizing and rotating skin flaps is needed, as are the minutiae involved in plastic surgical techniques. It is not enough to review pictures and follow descriptions; training in the techniques is essential. Knowledge of a few methods is not enough, because the one used must be the best for the individual situation of the child.

A pediatric urology fellowship is the appropriate place to become competent in hypospadias surgery.

## Preoperative Evaluation

Because hypospadias is an isolated anomaly, the entire genitourinary tract does not require evaluation. The absence of one gonad, perineal hypospadias, severe chordee, or a bifid scrotum suggests a disorder of sex development and requires genotypic evaluation. If both gonads are not palpable, consider the possibility of congenital adrenal hyperplasia in a phenotypic female.

## Age for Operation

Select a time between 6 and 9 months for surgery. At this age the infants are also easiest to manage, are not walking and remain in diapers. Babies appear to have fewer bladder spasms and require smaller doses of pain medication. They do not seem to remember the surgery as teenagers and adults. Parenteral testosterone may be administered to increase the size of the penis and especially the size and vascularity of the prepuce should it be needed for proximal and perineal hypospadias repair. Give 25 to 50 mg intramuscularly, repeated once or twice at 3-week intervals, before the operation.

## Outpatient Repair

An uncomplicated hypospadias operation can be done without hospital admission. Parents and children should visit the surgeon sometime before the date of surgery for history taking and examination, as well as for instructions in feeding and preoperative care. The surgeon and nurse should give considerable support to the parents because of their need to know what to expect. At this visit surgeons can explain the procedure, hand out suitable booklets describing details, and obtain informed consent. They can also review the postoperative catheter care and medications.

## Nerve Block

A caudal nerve block placed by the anesthesia team is an excellent form of postoperative pain control. A good alternative is a penile nerve block. To place a penile nerve block in an infant, use 3 to 4 mL of 0.5% long-lasting bupivacaine mixed with 1% of quick-acting lidocaine. Inject it at the base of each crus just below the notch of the symphysis, or vertically in the midline deep to the notch of the symphysis, with a 1-1/2-inch 25-gauge needle. When placed at the beginning of an operation it will reduce the amount of general anesthesia required and will provide anesthesia that will last well into the postoperative period.

## Surgical Hints

### Hemostasis

For hemostasis use 1% lidocaine with 1:100,000 epinephrine and inject it through a 27-gauge needle within the glans and the area of abortive spongiosum. Wait 7 minutes for it to act. This vasoconstrictor will reduce the bleeding during the dissection, but if the operation is prolonged beyond 90 minutes, rebound vasodilation can be expected. Remember that halothane anesthesia sensitizes the heart to catecholamines, thus promoting arrhythmias. Avoid electrocoagulation as much as possible; if it is necessary, use a bipolar cautery or touch a monopolar cautery to only the forceps unit set at a low current. Once the skin flaps are applied, bleeding improves, and a pressure dressing will usually ensure hemostasis. On rare occasion the use of a tourniquet that is typically used for artificial erections can facilitate hemostasis.

### Artificial Erection

To induce a saline-induced erection, place a sterile rubber band around the base of the penis and snug it with a hemostat. Introduce a 25-gauge butterfly needle into the corpus cavernosum. Gently distend the penis with injectable normal saline solution; avoid overdistention. Maintain the erection during evaluation of the chordee. After the chordee has been corrected, create a second erection to check penile alignment.

### Local Urinary Diversion in Children

Diversion of urine away from the suture lines has always been a problem in children because any indwelling tube, particularly one terminating in a balloon, induces bladder spasms that force urine around it into the repair. This disrupts the suture line and leads to formation of fistulas. Besides, the lumen of a balloon catheter is small compared to that of a straight catheter, especially a plastic one.

Many techniques have been tried to minimize these problems with diversion. The simplest method for infants, one that combines stenting with drainage, is to insert a fine silicone tube, such as 6Fr peritoneal shunt tubing or neurosurgical tubing with its wand-like end, into the bladder through the urethra and fasten the end to the glans in one or two places with nonabsorbable sutures.

Alternately, place a 6Fr Kendall catheter of soft Silastic, with a Luer-loc at the end, to prevent internal migration and to allow irrigation. Whatever intubation system is used in infants, collect the urine in a double diaper. For older boys use a urethral balloon catheter; tape it to the abdomen so that it cannot disturb the ventral glans repair. Drainage should be continued for 4 to 7 days for distal and penile shaft repairs and 7 to 10 days for more severe hypospadias repairs.

## Dressings

Apply a dressing to immobilize the area, to reduce edema, and to prevent the formation of a hematoma. Use transparent and permeable absorbent plastic film (Tegaderm or OpSite) applied over Telfa or tincture of benzoin. Let the catheter drain into an outer diaper. The dressing may be removed in 2 to 3 days after a few warm baths at home. Once the dressing has been removed use petroleum jelly on the diaper to keep the repaired penis from sticking, typically for 4 to 5 days.

## Setup for Operation

### Instruments

Select instruments designed for delicate handling of tissues. A reasonable list would include loupe magnification, genitourinary

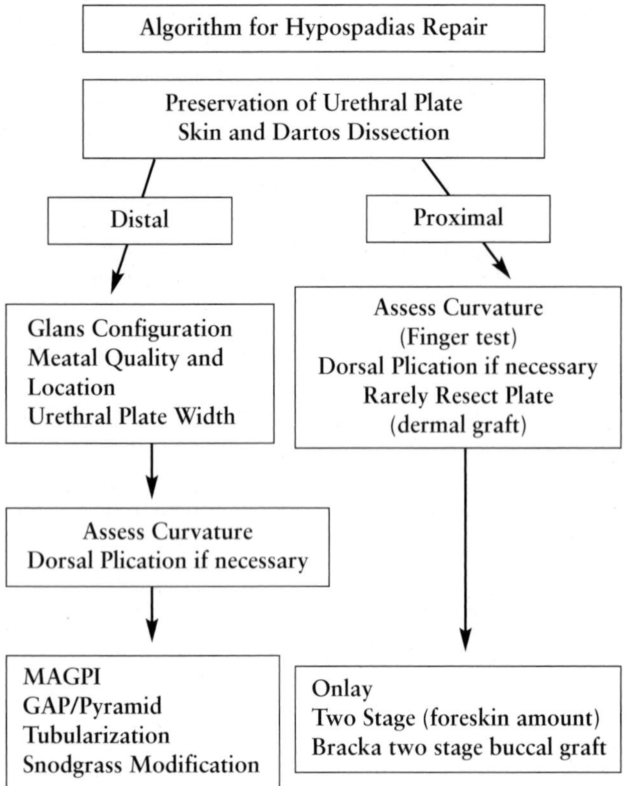


FIGURE 109.2 Algorithm for hypospadias repair.

fine and microsurgery sets, microsurgical knife (Weck), toothed and nontoothed forceps (Adson), fine Allis clamps, fine clamps, two pairs of Bishop–Harmon forceps or 0.5 platform forceps, sharp small tenotomy scissors, iris scissors, microtip Castroviejo scissors, microtip Castroviejo needle holders, plastic needle holders and ring retractor (Scott/Lone Star), and hooks. Also have available bougies á boule, 5Fr and 8Fr infant feeding tubes, rubber bands, a marking pen, a 25-gauge butterfly needle and syringe, and a hand-held Bovie, or an ophthalmic electrocautery. Have fine sutures of appropriate sizes and types at hand but unopened—for example, 5-0 Prolene on a C-1 tapered needle for glans traction, 7-0 PDS and Vicryl for urethroplasty, and 6-0 PDS for the skin.

## Selection of the Operative Technique

Figure 109.2 presents an algorithm for the reconstruction of hypospadias. A tried-and-true approach is to start each repair by preserving the urethral plate, dissecting the skin to the penile scrotal junction, and assessing for the presence of penile curvature. If curvature is not present or is mild to moderate and amenable to dorsal plications, then a one-stage approach is typically successful. The specific repair is now dependent on the meatal configuration and the surgeon's preference (1).

### Meatal Advancement and Glanuloplasty

The hypospadiac penis that is amenable to meatal advancement and glanuloplasty (MAGPI technique) is characterized by a dorsal web of tissue within the glans that deflects the urine from either a coronal or a slightly subcoronal meatus (3). Once the patient is asleep, the urethra itself must have a normal ventral wall, without any thin or atretic urethral spongiosum. The urethra also must be mobile so it can be advanced into the glans (Fig. 109.3).

### Glans Approximation Procedure

The glans approximation procedure (GAP) is applicable in a small subset of patients with anterior hypospadias who have a wide and deep glandular groove (4). These patients do not have a bridge of glandular tissue that typically deflects the urinary stream, as seen in patients who would be more appropriately treated with the MAGPI procedure. In the GAP procedure, the wide-mouth urethra is tubularized primarily over a stent (Fig. 109.4). Ventral glanular tilt, meatal retraction, and splaying of the urinary stream can result from the inappropriate use of the MAGPI technique in these circumstances.

### Tubularized Incised Plate Urethroplasty (Snodgrass)

Historically, if the urethral groove was not wide enough for tubularization in situ, such as in the GAP or Thiersch–Duplay procedure, then an alternative approach such as the Mathieu or, for more severe hypospadias, a vascularized pedicle flap was performed. Recently the concept of the incision in the urethral plate with subsequent tubularization and secondary healing has been introduced by Snodgrass (5) (Fig. 109.5). Short-term results have been excellent, and this procedure is enjoying extensive popularity. One appealing aspect is the slit-like meatus that is created with the dorsal midline incision. More recently, this technique has been applied to more posterior forms of hypospadias. Theoretically, there is concern about the possibility of meatal stenosis from scarring as occurs in patients with urethral stricture disease, where direct-vision internal urethrotomy often leads to recurrent stricture. However, reports of meatal stenosis have been rare. In hypospadias, the native virgin tissue with excellent blood supply and large vascular sinuses seems to respond to primary incision and secondary healing without scar. The tubularized incised plate (TIP) urethroplasty is conducive to preservation of the foreskin (6). To preserve the foreskin the incision is made only on the ventrum; therefore, patients with significant penile curvature are not candidates for this procedure. A three-layer closure of the prepuce prevents foreskin fistulas. The fact that the foreskin cannot be used as a de-epithelialized flap theoretically increases the chance for urethra fistula.

## Treatment of Posterior Hypospadias

### The Urethral Plate

Duckett has popularized the concept of preservation of the urethral plate, which is now standard practice for anterior as well as more severe posterior hypospadias surgery (7,8). The urethral plate serves as the dorsal urethral wall, and the ventral urethra is created by a vascular onlay flap of tissue from the inner prepuce. Extensive experience has shown that the urethral plate is rarely the cause of penile curvature. The concept of preserving the urethral plate yet undermining the plate and exposing the corporal bodies with the idea that chordee

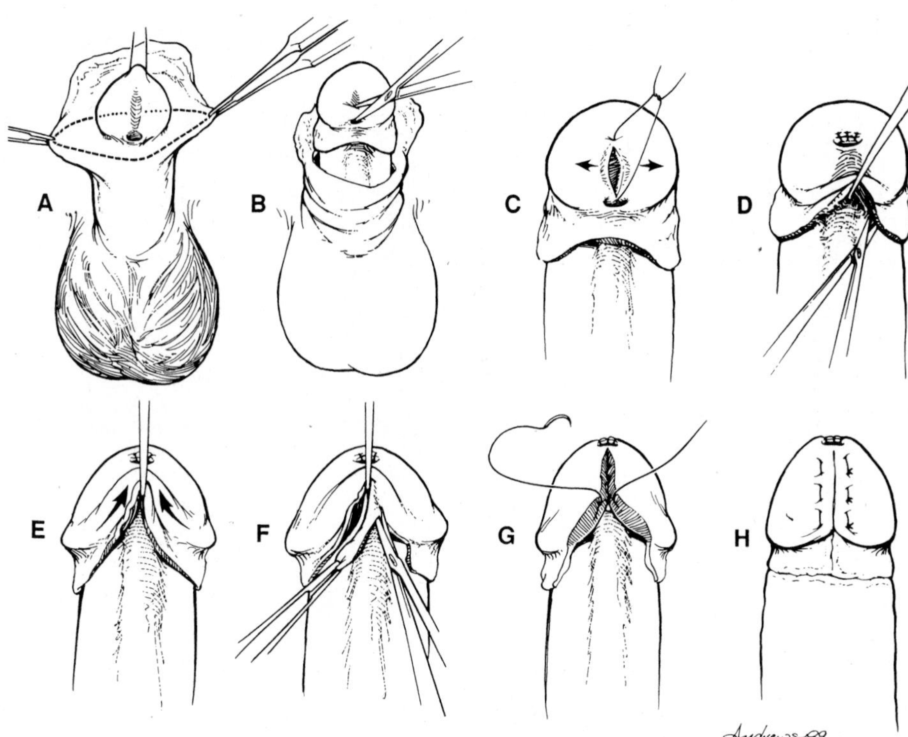


FIGURE 109.3 Meatal advancement with glanduloplasty (MAGPI) procedure. Note the proximal location of the initial circumcising incision in relation to the urethral meatus (**A**). The dorsal meatotomy is as shown (**B and C**). The glans is then detached from the lateral margin of the corpus spongiosum and the side of the corpora cavernosa (**D**). The edge of the glans on either side that will be approximated ventrally is identified (**E**). The triangle of skin between these two points and the urethral meatus is excised completely (**F**). Dissection must stay right on the skin because the urethra here is usually thin and easily entered. Excising this skin allows exposure of the glans tissue which can now be reapproximated into a conical shape to complete reconstruction with the meatus in a terminal position (**G and H**).

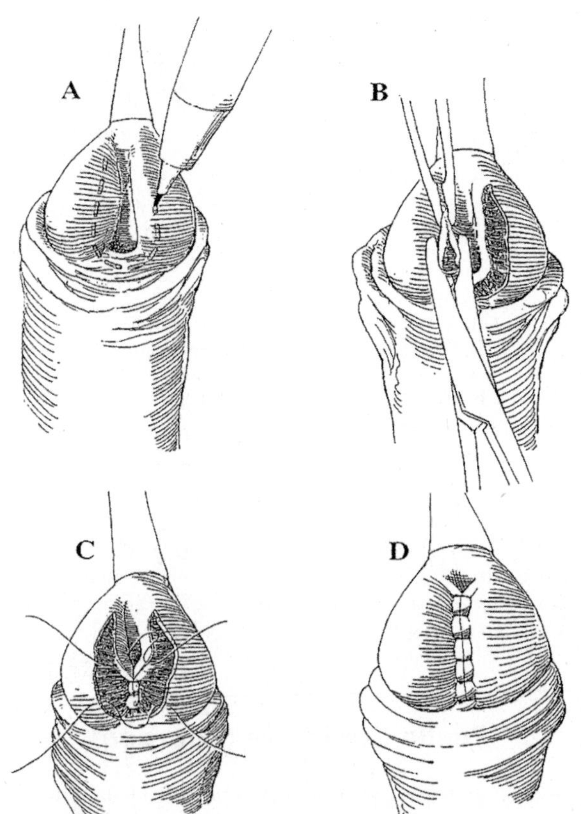


FIGURE 109.4 Glans approximation procedure (GAP) hypospadias technique. **A:** Initial incision. **B:** Exposure of the glans mesenchyme by de-epithelialization of tissue, which is critical for a two-layer glans closure, allowing for good support of the urethroplasty. **C:** Tubularization of the neourethra, followed by glans closure. **D:** The completed repair. (Reproduced with permission from Grossfeld J, O'Neill J, Coran A, Fonkalsrud, E. *Pediatric Surgery*, 6th ed. Elsevier, 2006.)

tissue could be released has not held true. In fact, careful anatomic studies have shown an extensive network of blood vessels supplying the urethral plate in the hypospadiac penis, and lifting of the urethral plate defeats the purpose of preservation by violating this intricate blood supply (9). At present, in the majority of cases of posterior hypospadias, including perineal hypospadias, the urethral plate can be preserved and a vascularized flap used in an onlay fashion. In the rare case when the urethral plate needs to be resected, a two-stage technique can be employed (see below).

## Onlay Island Flap

The blood supply to the hypospadias preputial tissue is reliable and easily delineated. The abundance of cutaneous tissue on the dorsum of the penis is vascularized in a longitudinal fashion. For posterior hypospadias, all cases are approached by initially leaving the urethral plate intact. This includes patients with and without penile curvature. This technique can be applied to penile shaft as well as scrotal and perineal hypospadias. The intact dorsal plate essentially avoids complications of proximal stricture, and the excellent blood supply has decreased the fistula rate to approximately 5% to 10% for all cases of onlay island flap hypospadias repair (Fig. 109.6) (7). Long-term results with the onlay island flap have been very durable. For very severe hypospadias, the prepuce can be designed in a horseshoe style to bridge extensive gaps.

## Two-Stage Hypospadias Repair

An alternative approach for severe hypospadias is to transfer the dorsal prepuce to the ventrum after correction of penile curvature (Fig. 109.7). In severe cases the urethral plate may need to be resected to correct chordee. Dermal grafting may be required, and performing a urethroplasty on top of the healing graft is not suggested. Byars flaps can be rotated from the dorsum, setting up ventral coverage for subsequent

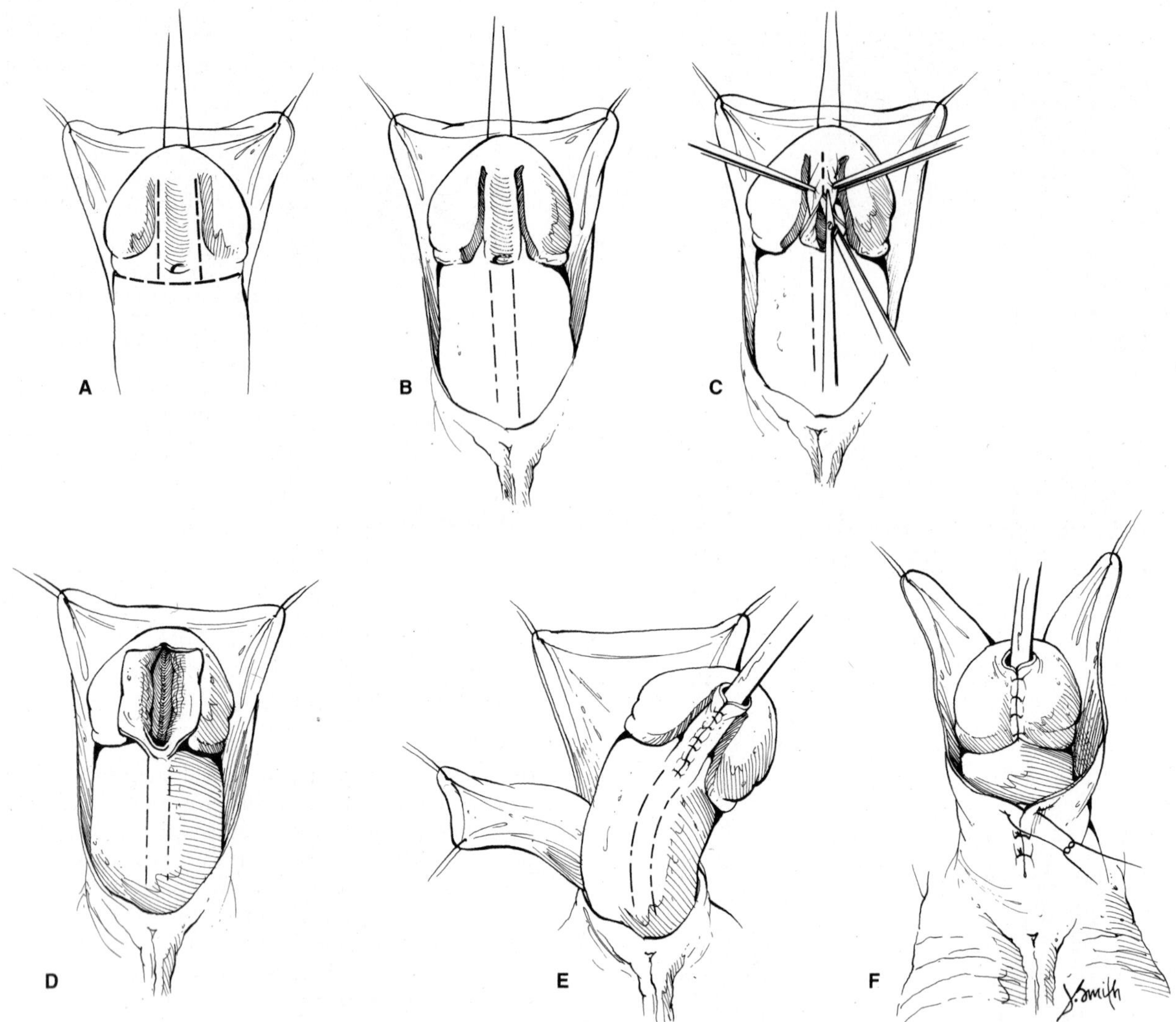


FIGURE 109.5 Tubularized, incised plate (TIP) urethroplasty. **A:** *Horizontal line* indicates circumscribing incision to deglove penis. *Vertical lines* show junction of urethral plate and ventral glans. **B:** Parallel incisions separate urethral plate from glans. **C:** Midline incision of urethral plate from meatus to granular tip. **D:** Incision has widened and deepened the urethral plate. **E:** Plate tubularized over 6Fr stent. Dorsal subcutaneous tissues are rotated ventrally to cover the repair. **F:** Midline closure of glans wing, mucosa collar, and ventral shaft skin.

urethroplasty (10). The second stage is performed at least 6 months after the first stage. To facilitate the urethroplasty within the glans, during the first stage dorsal skin is tucked within the glans wings. Subcutaneous secondary coverage of the reconstructed urethra is performed to prevent fistula.

### Bracka Buccal Two-Stage Repair

For patients with prior surgery or with severe hypospadias, Bracka has described a buccal free graft two-stage repair (11). In the first stage the penis is straightened and the scarred urethra is discarded (Fig. 109.8). Buccal mucosa is harvested from either the check or lip and grafted to the prepared bed (12). Extensive quilting of the graft is performed to prevent hematoma from lifting off the buccal mucosa. During the first stage, glans wings are mobilized in preparation for the creation of a slit-like meatus during the second stage. The second-stage urethroplasty is undertaken at least 6 months after the first stage. In the second stage excess buccal tissue is trimmed off the glans, setting up a two-layer glans closure. The buccal mucosa is rolled into the new urethra and subcutaneous tissue is used for secondary coverage.

## Penile Curvature (Chordee)

Correction of penile curvature has also evolved along with the concept of preservation of the urethral plate. Based on anatomic studies of the human fetal penis, a simpler approach placing dorsal midline plication sutures in the nerve-free zone at 12:00 is now advocated (9). The midline dorsal plication avoids the need for mobilization of the neurovascular bundle (Fig. 109.9). The midline plication can be applied to mild and moderate to severe degrees of curvature. If more than two rows of plication sutures or greater than four permanent sutures are

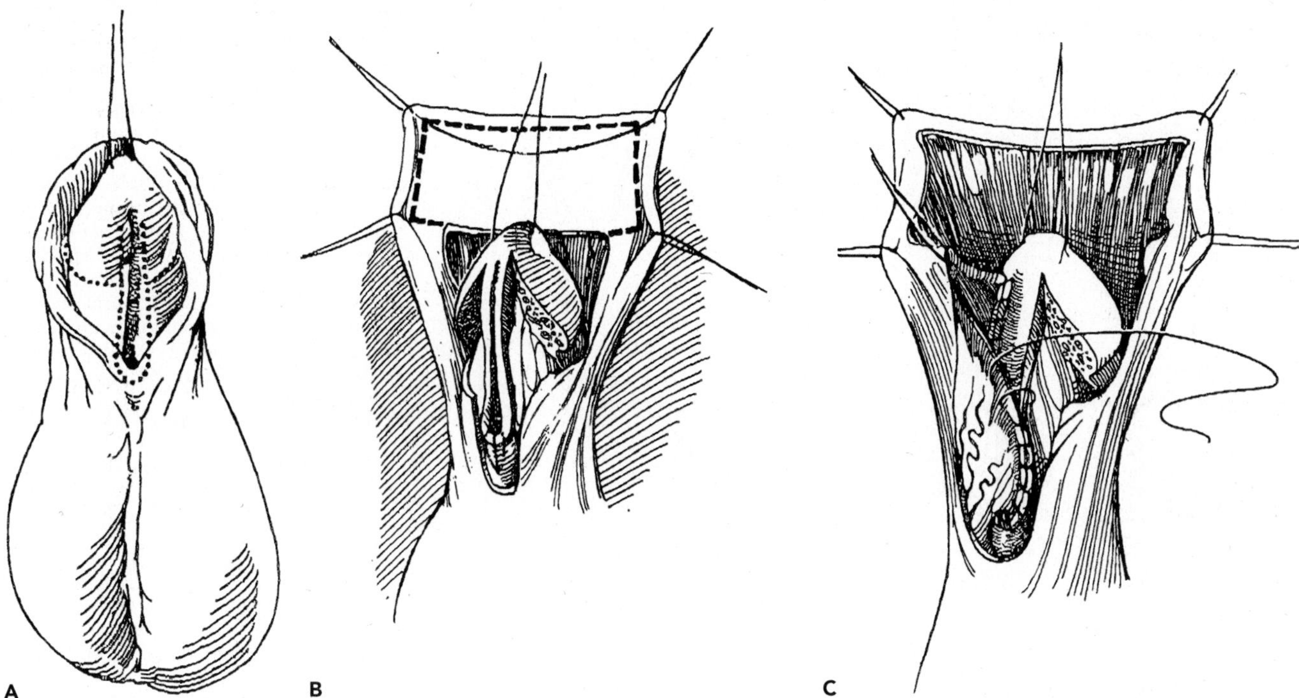


FIGURE 109.6 Onlay island flap **A:** Penile hypospadias. **B:** Preservation of the urethral plate and rectangular outline of the onlay flap. **C:** Onlay of preputial island flap onto urethral plate.

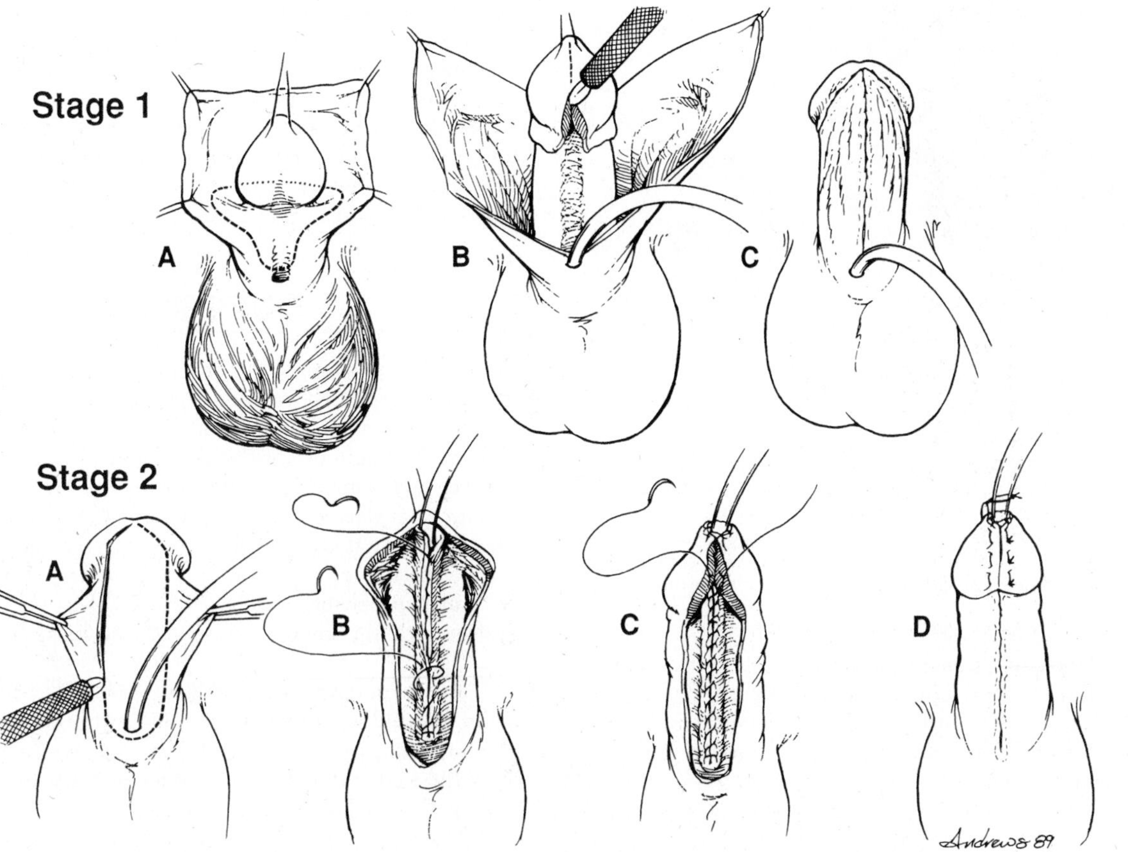


FIGURE 109.7 Two-stage repair. Stage 1: The unfolded foreskin is brought out to the tip of the incised and mobilized glanular wings (B). Delicate sutures reapproximate the skin in the midline and fix the skin to the corpora cavernosa (C). Stage 2: A sufficient strip of skin is outlined (A). Dissection of the shaft skin is lateral and away from the neourethra. Two layers of inverting sutures are used to close the neourethra (B). If the prepuce has been positioned sufficiently distal at the first stage, a normally positioned meatus with good ventral glandular support can be achieved (C). Any excess shaft skin is excised, but the dartos layer is preserved (de-epithelialization) to drape across the neourethral suture line (D).

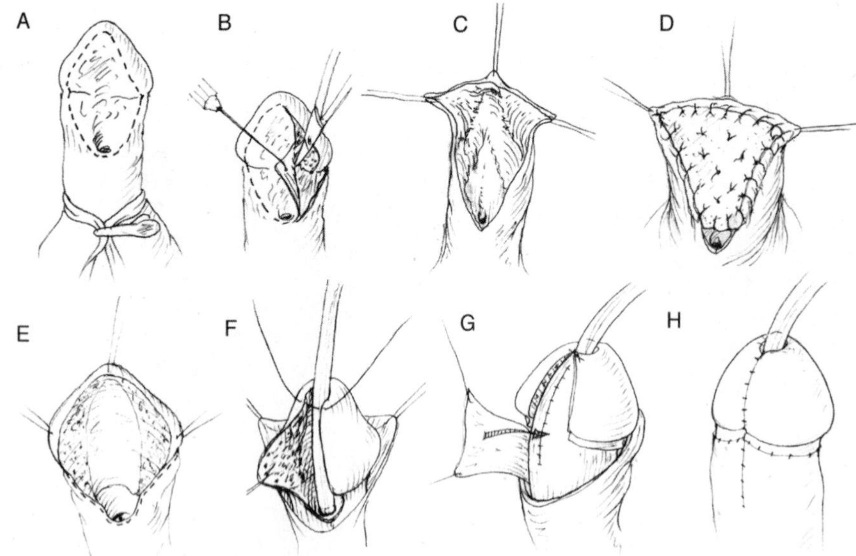


FIGURE 109.8 Schematic two-stage Bracka buccal hypospadias repair. First stage: **A:** Patient with a midshaft hypospadias and a paucity of available skin after multiple previous hypospadias repairs. **B:** Resection of scar tissue. **C:** Mobilization of glans wings **D:** Buccal free graft quilted into the resected scar. Second stage after 6 months of healing. **E:** Exposure of glans mesenchyme and trimming of buccal graft for subsequent urethroplasty. **F:** Urethroplasty. **G:** Secondary de-epithelialized pedicle coverage of the urethroplasty. **H:** Two-layer glansplasty and completed repair. (Reproduced with permission from Grossfeld J, O'Neill J, Coran A, Fonkalsrud E. *Pediatric Surgery*, 6th ed. Elsevier, 2006.)

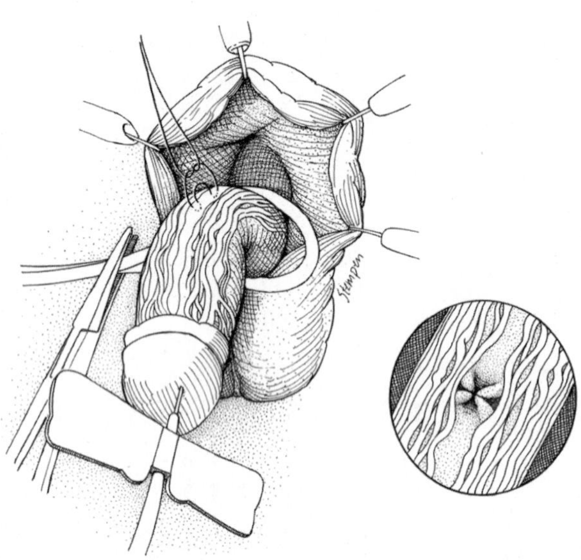

FIGURE 109.9 Midline dorsal plication technique. In this technique, plication sutures are placed in the tunica albuginea in the 12 o'clock position, which is free of both nerves and vascular structures. This technique involves a minimum amount of manipulation to the penis. It is not necessary to incise into the corporeal body or extensively mobilize the fascia of Buck. A maximum of two rows of parallel plications at the 12 o'clock position can be placed for correction.

necessary, then an alternative approach such as complete resection of the urethral plate and possible dermal grafting should be considered. During artificial erection, if the chordee cannot be corrected with your "finger," the midline dorsal plication is not advised.

## Postoperative Problems

Bladder spasms not only cause the child to move about in response to pain, but also force urine through the repair. Give analgesics and antispasmodics, such as oxybutynin (Ditropan). Recommend a suitable diet, because the antispasmodic regimen may result in constipation and lead to straining and urine leakage.

Bleeding is an infrequent problem. A compressive sandwich dressing will resolve the problem in all but the rare patient. In selected cases, give a broad-spectrum antibiotic such as trimethoprim (Septra) or a cephalosporin, and continue it for a few days after the tubing has been removed. Should postoperative erections in older boys become a problem, use amyl nitrate ampules or diazepam sedation to reduce them.

See the patient 6 weeks and 1 year after the repair. Re-evaluate after potty training and at puberty to confirm patient satisfaction and the absence of fistula, stenosis, diverticulum, recurrent chordee, and cosmetic issues.

# OUTCOMES

Results today, cosmetically and functionally, are better than those in the past. The use of a one-stage hypospadias repair at an early age with a low complication rate encourages our current positive outlook for this condition. Curvature correction with the aid of an artificial erection is extremely important for ensuring satisfactory sexual function. With the placement of the urinary meatus at the tip of the glans, the infertility potential has been improved unless the patient has other coexisting testicular problems. Evidence shows that the neourethra grows with the child, and subsequent repairs are seldom necessary.

Early hypospadias repair with minimal hospitalization helps to avoid separation anxiety and castration fears. We can now counsel parents confidently that there is an excellent outlook for a good cosmetic, functional, and emotional result in boys with all degrees of hypospadias.

## Complications

Complications occur after 10% to 30% of hypospadias operations. These include meatal retraction, urethrocutaneous fistula formation, meatal stenosis, urethral stricture, development of a diverticulum (sometimes with hair, followed by stones), and persistent chordee. Of these, strictures, fistulas, and urethral diverticula account for most of the late problems. These complications should be managed at least 6 months from the time of the initial surgery.

## PRACTICAL CONCLUSIONS

Hypospadias should be repaired within the first year of life, preferably at 4 to 6 months of age. Pain control and catheters seem better tolerated and the baby's lack of mobility simplifies postoperative care.

A terminal slit-like meatus should be the goal, with or without preservation of the foreskin, depending on parental preference. Preservation of the urethral plate creates the best possible chance to recreate normal urethral anatomy by incorporating the abortive spongiosum into the repair. Midline dorsal plication is safe and effective for the correction of penile curvature in the majority of patients (placing more than two rows of sutures is a sign that another technique, such as dermal grafting, is indicated). In the small percentage of patients who require resection of the urethral plate, a two-stage approach is generally warranted. Vascularized pedicle onlay flaps are successful in primary and redo hypospadias surgery. De-epithelialized vascular flaps should be used as a second layer for all urethroplasties. Patients with a paucity of skin are best managed with the Bracka two-stage buccal repair. Coronal fistulas require a redo glansplasty.

Surgical volume correlates with successful outcomes.

## *References*


1. Baskin LS, Ebbers MB. Hypospadias: anatomy, etiology, and technique. *J Pediatr Surg* 2006;41(3):463–472.
2. Baskin L, Duckett J, Lue T. Penile curvature. *Urology* 1996; 48(3): 347–356.
3. Duckett J. MAGPI (meatal advancement and glanuloplasty): a procedure for subcoronal hypospadias. *Urol Clin North Am* 1981;8:513–520.
4. Zaontz MR. The GAP (glans approximation procedure) for glanular/coronal hypospadias. *J Urol* 1989;141(2):359–361.
5. Snodgrass W. Tubularized, incised plate urethroplasty for distal hypospadias. *J Urol* 1994;151(2):464–465.
6. Snodgrass WT, Koyle MA, Baskin LS, et al. Foreskin preservation in penile surgery. *J Urol* 2006;176(2):711–714.
7. Baskin LS, Duckett JW, Ueoka K, et al. Changing concepts of hypospadias curvature lead to more onlay island flap procedures. *J Urol* 1994; 151(1): 191–196.
8. Duckett JW. The current hype in hypospadiology. *Br J Urol* 1995; 76(Suppl 3): 1–7.
9. Baskin LS, Erol A, Li YW, et al. Anatomical studies of hypospadias. *J Urol* 1998;160(3, Pt 2):1108–1015.
10. Retik AB, Bauer SB, Mandell J, et al. Management of severe hypospadias with a two-stage repair. *J Urol* 1994;152(2, Pt 2):749–751.
11. Bracka A. Hypospadias repair: the two-stage alternative. *Br J Urol* 1995; 76(Suppl 3):31–41.
12. Baskin LS, Duckett JW. Buccal mucosa grafts in hypospadias surgery. *Br J Urol* 1995;76(Suppl 3):23–30.


# CHAPTER 110 ■ COMPLETE PRIMARY REPAIR FOR EXSTROPHY

RICHARD W. GRADY

Bladder exstrophy is a congenital anomaly that has characteristic external physical manifestations; the diagnosis of exstrophy is usually made immediately after birth, although it can be detected antenatally. The anterior portion of the bladder and/or urethra and abdominal wall structures are deficient, and the pubic symphysis is widely separated from the midline in the exstrophy anomalies (Fig. 110.1); the bladder and urethra are herniated ventrally. The exstrophic defects are typically found in isolation; other organ systems are only infrequently affected. However, children with exstrophy typically have an anteriorly located anus. Female genital anatomy is altered, with a more vertically oriented vaginal opening after closure and a wider and shorter vagina than normal. The anterior component of the penis is also foreshortened in males compared to the general population.

## DIAGNOSIS

In some situations, the diagnosis may be made antenatally, although many affected fetuses are not suspected to have exstrophy before birth (1). In Gearhart's review of 29 antenatal studies of 17 children born with exstrophy (2), only 3 were identified before delivery despite the presence of findings to suggest the diagnosis. Ultrasonography can reliably detect exstrophy before the twentieth week of gestation (2,3). The absence of the bladder is a hallmark of exstrophy. Ultrasonographic findings of exstrophy also include a semisolid mass protruding from the abdominal wall, an absent bladder, a lower abdominal protrusion, an anteriorly displaced scrotum with a small phallus in male fetuses, normal

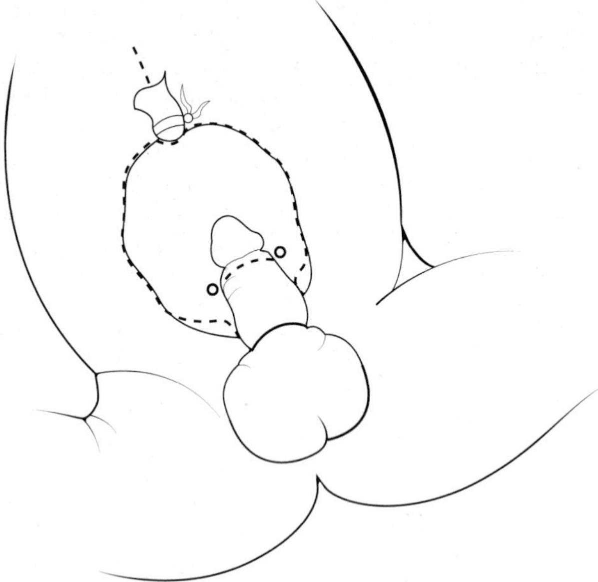

FIGURE 110.1 Initial dissection, inferior view. *Dashed lines* indicate lines of dissection. Note that the lines of dissection proceed around the umbilicus and superior to it. The line of dissection also extends subcoronally around the ventral aspect of the penis. See Fig. 110.2 for another view of the initial lines of dissection.

kidneys in association with a low-set umbilical cord, and an abnormal iliac crest widening.

Subtle findings such as low umbilical cord insertion and the location of the genitalia will only be seen if the fetus is examined in a sagittal alignment with the spine (4). Because exstrophy affects the external genitalia, the diagnosis is easier to make in males than in females. Iliac crest widening can also be seen during the routine prenatal evaluation of the lumbosacral spine that is performed to evaluate for myelomeningocele. The iliac angle will be about 110 degrees rather than the 90 degrees that is normally seen (4). Since urine production is normal for these fetuses, amniotic fluid levels should be normal.

Prenatal diagnosis allows optimal perinatal management of these infants. The infants can be delivered near a pediatric center equipped to treat babies with this unusual anomaly. Of equal importance, antenatal diagnosis also allows the parents the opportunity to discuss early management of the patient. The early counseling should include the expertise of a pediatric urologist experienced in the treatment of bladder exstrophy. Patients with exstrophy can have a satisfactory long-term outcome and life expectancy with appropriate management.

## INDICATIONS FOR SURGERY

Exstrophy anomalies are nonlethal; children with exstrophy can survive untreated into adulthood (5). However, significant morbidity exists with these conditions if they are left untreated, including total urinary incontinence, bladder and kidney infections, skin breakdown, and tumor formation in the bladder plate. The surrounding skin around the exposed exstrophic bladder is often inflamed secondary to urine contact dermatitis, loss of skin integrity from constant wetness, and secondary infection. In contrast, when these patients receive effective surgical and medical treatment, they can lead productive, healthy lives with minimal morbidity from their underlying urologic abnormality.

## SURGICAL TECHNIQUE

Primary goals for exstrophy reconstruction include preservation of kidney function, urinary continence, low-pressure urinary storage, volitional voiding, and functional and cosmetically acceptable external genitalia. Secondary goals for reconstruction include minimization of urinary tract infections, adequate pelvic floor support, minimization of the risk for malignancy associated with the urinary tract, minimization of the risk for urinary calculi, and adequate abdominal wall fascia.

Surgical reconstruction of exstrophy and epispadias represents one of the most significant challenges for physicians who specialize in the urologic care of children. Over the last 15 years, a novel surgical reconstructive approach has been developed for the exstrophy-epispadias complex. In the late 1980s Mitchell (6) devised an anatomic approach that integrated epispadias and exstrophy repair. This operation evolved out of a technique developed for the treatment of epispadias: the complete penile disassembly technique. By employing this technique, the surgeon permits the tissue deformation in exstrophy to return more closely to an anatomically normal position. We have used this approach exclusively for the surgical treatment of newborns with exstrophy since 1990. This operation or its principles are also useful in some reoperative repairs or delayed repairs for exstrophy.

### Preoperative Care

After delivery, to reduce trauma to the bladder plate, the umbilical cord should be ligated with silk suture rather than a plastic or metal clamp. A hydrated gel dressing may be used to protect the exposed bladder from superficial trauma. This type of dressing is easy to use, keeps the bladder plate from becoming desiccated, and stays in place to allow handling of the infant with minimal risk of trauma to the bladder. Plastic wrap is an acceptable alternative. Dressings should be replaced daily, and the bladder should be irrigated with normal saline with each diaper change. A humidified air incubator may also minimize bladder trauma.

We routinely use intravenous antibiotic therapy in the pre- and postoperative period to decrease the risk for infection following reconstruction. We also perform preoperative ultrasonography to assess the kidneys and to establish a baseline examination for later ultrasonographic studies. Preoperative spinal sonographic examination should be considered if sacral dimpling or other signs of spina bifida occulta are noted on physical examination.

### Operative Considerations

Ideally, the primary exstrophy closure is performed in the newborn period. We routinely use general inhalation anesthesia. However, nitrous oxide should be avoided during primary closure as it may cause bowel distention, which decreases surgical exposure during the operation and increases the risk of wound dehiscence. Some advocate the use of nasogastric tube drainage to decrease abdominal distention in the postoperative period, but we do not routinely use it postoperatively. We do routinely place an epidural catheter to reduce the inhaled anesthetic requirement during the operation. Tunneling the catheter may reduce the risk for infection if it is left in for prolonged periods after surgery.

For patients older than 3 days or newborns with a wide pubic diastasis, we perform anterior iliac osteotomies. Osteotomies assist closure and enhance anterior pelvic floor support, which may improve later urinary continence.

Factors that appear to be important in the operative period include use of osteotomies in selected cases and for newborn closures >48 hours after birth to decrease the tension on the repair, ureteral stenting and bladder drainage catheters placed intraoperatively for use in the postoperative period to divert urine, avoidance of abdominal distention, and use of intraoperative antibiotics.

## Complete Primary Repair for Exstrophy Surgical Technique: Boys

After standard preparation of the surgical field, we place transversely oriented traction sutures into each of the hemiglans of the penis. We then mark the lines of dissection (Figs. 110.1 and 110.2). Care is taken in marking these lines to exclude dysplastic tissue at the edges of the exstrophic bladder and bladder neck. This is particularly important at the bladder neck, where dysplastic tissue left in the continuity may impair later bladder neck function. Following this, we place 3.5Fr umbilical artery catheters into both ureters and suture them in place with 5.0 chromic sutures. Bladder polyps are removed prior to beginning the dissection, since these will act as space-occupying lesions after the bladder is reconstructed (Fig. 110.2). Initial dissection begins superiorly and proceeds inferiorly to separate the bladder from the adjacent skin and fascia, since it is usually easiest to identify tissue planes in this location. We use tungsten fine-tip electrocautery (Colorado tip) during this dissection to reduce blood loss. The umbilical vessels may be ligated if necessary. We also incise the periumbilical skin circumferentially at this time. The umbilicus will be moved superiorly to a more anatomically normal location and will be later used as the location to bring out the suprapubic catheter (Figs. 110.3 and 110.4).

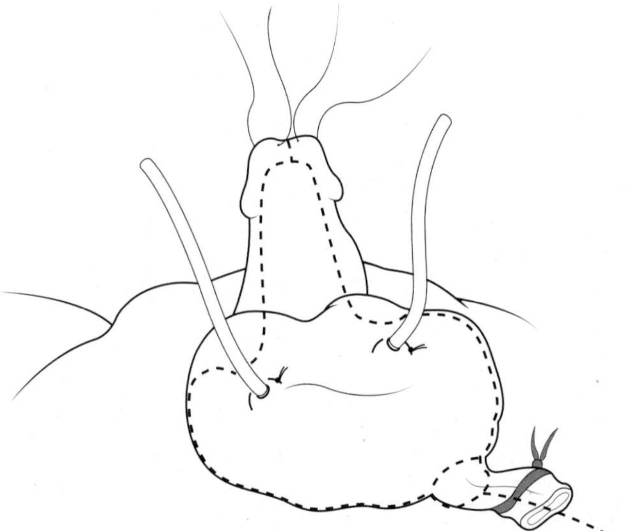

FIGURE 110.2 View of lines of dissection from above. The urethral dissection is carried along the lateral aspect of the urethral plate.

### Penile/Urethral Dissection

Traction sutures placed into each hemiglans of the penis aid in dissection at this point in the operation (Fig. 110.2). The sutures will rotate to a parallel vertical orientation (Fig. 110.5) because the corporal bodies will naturally rotate medially after they are separated from the urethral wedge (urethral plate plus underlying corpora spongiosa). We begin the penile dissection along the ventral aspect of the penis as a circumcising incision (see line of dissection in Fig. 110.1). This step precedes dissection of the urethral wedge from the corporal bodies because it is easier to identify the plane of dissection above the Buck fascia ventrally (Fig. 110.6). The Buck fascia is deficient or absent around the corpus spongiosum; as the dissection progresses medially to separate the urethra from the corpora cavernosa, the plane shifts subtly from above the Buck fascia to just above the tunica albuginea. It is important to recognize this. Failure to adjust the plane of dissection will carry the dissection into the corpus spongiosum; this will result in excessive, difficult-to-control bleeding during the deep ventral dissection of the urethral wedge from the corporal bodies.

Applying methylene blue or brilliant green to the urethra can help identify the plane between urothelium and squamous epithelium. We routinely inject surrounding tissues with 0.25% lidocaine and 1:200,00 U per mL epinephrine to improve hemostasis. This may assist the dissection. Shallow incisions are made laterally along the dorsal aspect of the urethra to begin the dissection (Fig. 110.7). Sharp dissection is required to develop the plane between the urethral wedge and the corporal bodies. Careful dissection will preserve urethral width and length. This is particularly important because the urethra is often too short to reach the glans penis once the bladder has been moved into the pelvis.

Careful lateral dissection of the penile shaft skin and dartos fascia from the corporal bodies will avoid damaging the laterally located neurovascular bundles on the corpora of the epispadic penis. The lateral dissection on the penis should be superficial to the Buck fascia because of the lateral location of the neurovascular bundles in the epispadic penis.

### Complete Penile Disassembly and Deep Dissection

Once a plane is established between the penis and the urethral wedge (Fig. 110.8), the penis may be disassembled into three components: (a) the right and (b) left corporal bodies with their respective hemiglans and (c) the urethral wedge (urothelium with underlying corpora spongiosa). This is done primarily to provide exposure to the intersymphyseal band and to allow adequate proximal dissection. We have found that the easiest plane of dissection to completely isolate the corporal bodies is proximal and ventral (Fig. 110.9). The plane of dissection should be carried out at the level of the tunica albuginea on the corpora. After a plane is established between the urethral wedge and the corporal bodies, this dissection is carried distally to separate the three components from each other (Fig. 110.10). Complete separation of the corporal bodies

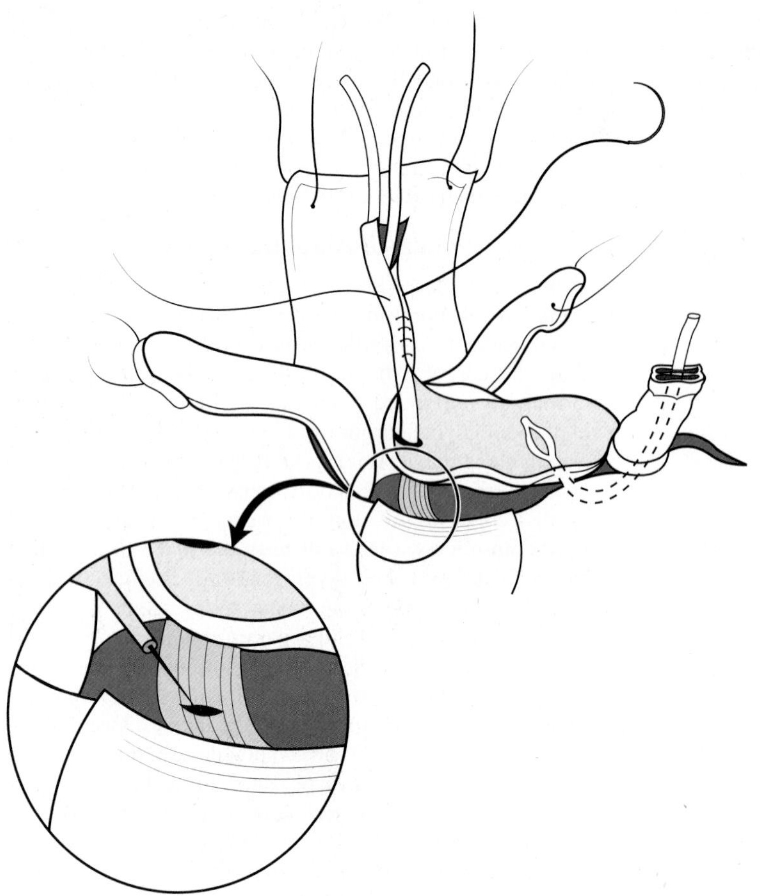

**FIGURE 110.3** The exposure for deep dissection is optimal after complete separation of the corporal bodies. It is crucial to adequately divide the intersymphyseal band *(inset)* to allow the bladder and urethra to move posteriorly.

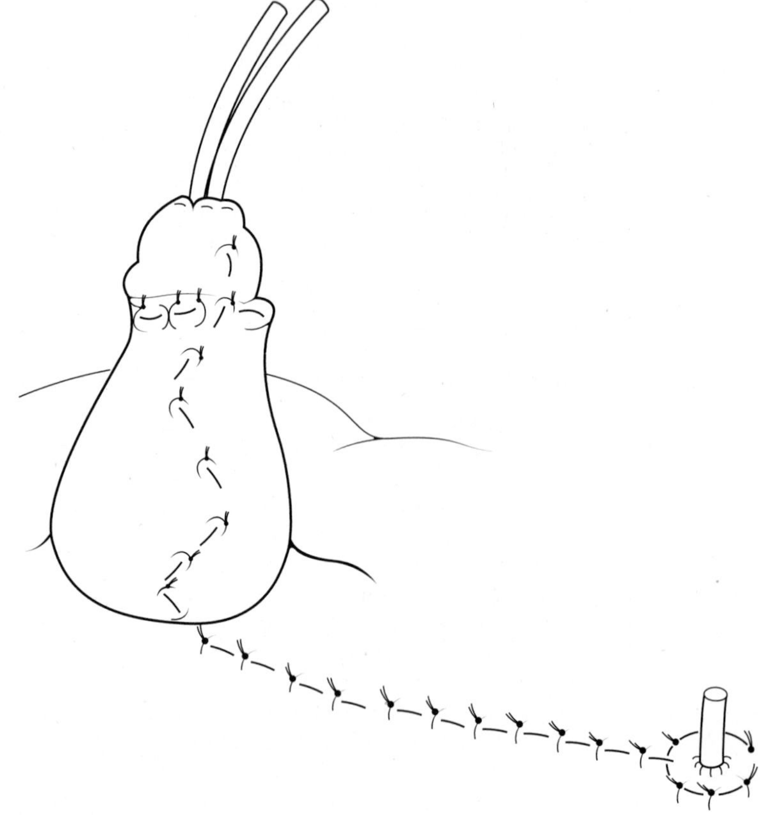

**FIGURE 110.4** To adequately cover the penis dorsally, Z-plasty incisions may be necessary. We also employ tacking sutures dorsally *(inset)*.

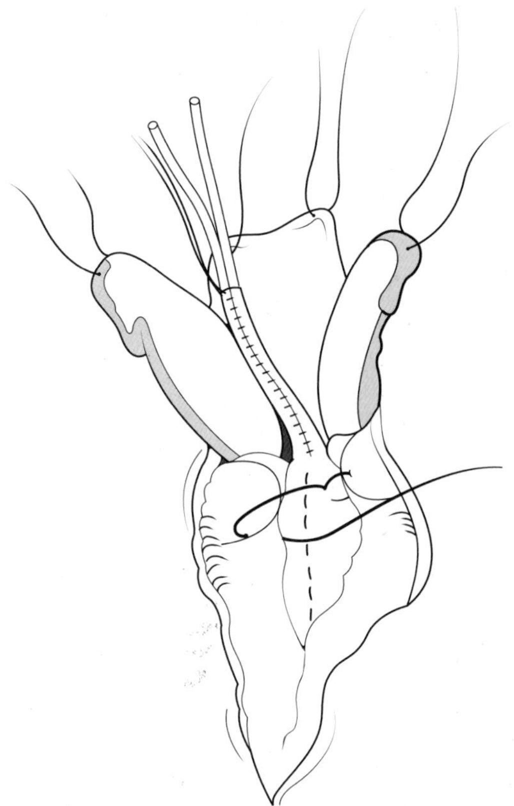

FIGURE 110.5 The urethra and bladder are reapproximated in a two-layer closure.

increases exposure to the pelvic diaphragm for deep dissection. The corporal bodies may be completely separated from each other because they exist on a separate blood supply (Figs. 110.9 and 110.10). It is important to keep the underlying corpora spongiosa with the urethra; the blood supply to the urethra is based on this corporal tissue, which should appear wedge-shaped after its dissection from the adjacent corpora cavernosa. The urethral/corpora spongiosa component will later be tubularized and placed ventral to the corporal bodies. Paraexstrophy skin flaps should not be used with this technique because this maneuver will place the blood supply to the distal urethra at risk. Because the bladder and urethra are moved posteriorly in the pelvis as a unit (with a common proximal blood supply), division of the urethral wedge is counterintuitive to the intent of the repair. In some cases, a male patient will be left with a hypospadias that will require later surgical reconstruction. The urethra and corporal bodies do not always have to be separated; occasionally the urethra is long enough and the bladder mobile enough to preserve the connection between them while still effectively carrying out the deep pelvic dissection that is integral to this repair.

After separating the components distally, the urethral dissection is carried proximally to the bladder neck. Exposure to the pelvic diaphragm is optimized by complete separation of the urethra and corporal bodies (Fig. 110.10). This creates the surgical exposure to perform the deep incision of the intersymphyseal band required to move the bladder and urethra posteriorly. When dissecting the urethral wedge from the corporal bodies medially, the dissection plane is on the tunica albuginea of the corpora cavernosa (Fig. 110.9). This medial dissection should be carried down through the intersymphyseal band (the condensation of anterior pelvic fascia and ligaments) (Fig. 110.3 inset).

Deep incision of the intersymphyseal band posterior and lateral to each side of the urethral wedge is absolutely necessary to allow the bladder and bladder neck to achieve a posterior position in the pelvis. This dissection should be carried until the pelvic floor musculature becomes visible. Failure to adequately dissect the bladder and urethral wedge from these surrounding structures will prevent posterior movement of the bladder in the pelvis and create anterior tension along the urethral plate.

## Primary Closure

Once the intersymphyseal band is adequately incised and the bladder and urethral wedge are adequately dissected from the surrounding tissues, the bladder and urethra can be

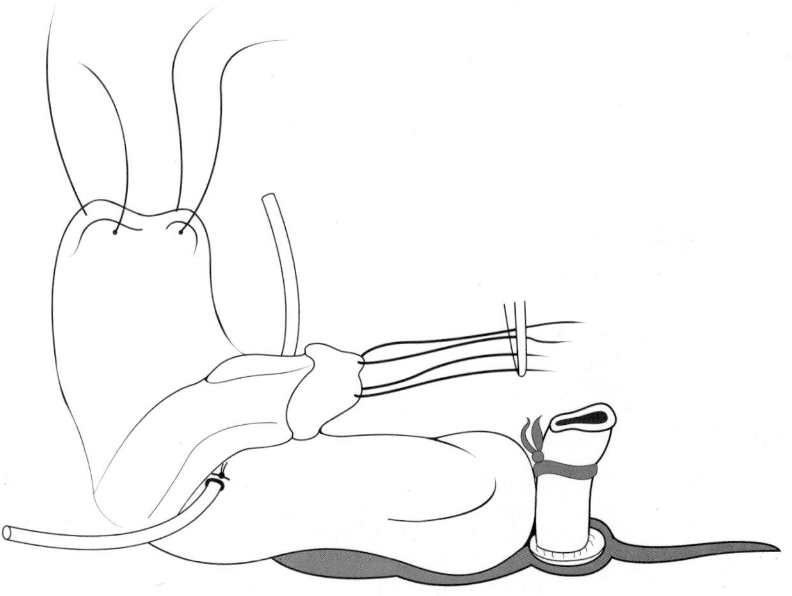

FIGURE 110.6 Ventral dissection is initiated most easily below the glans with a circumcising incision. The dissection may be carried proximally.

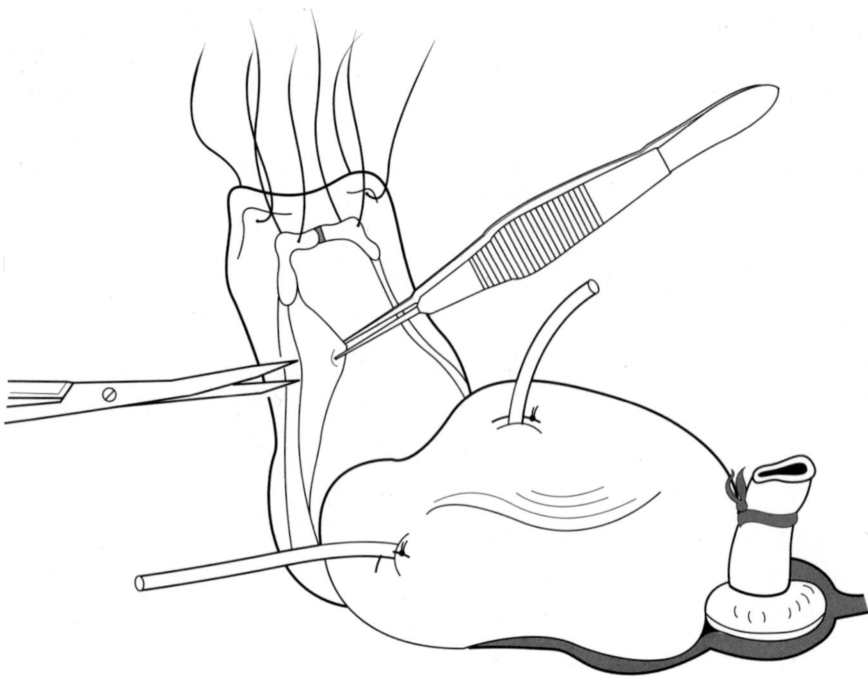

FIGURE 110.7 The urethra is dissected from the corporal bodies. This plane of dissection is developed from both a ventral and lateral perspective using sharp dissection.

reapproximated. This portion of the repair is straightforward and anatomic. To provide urinary drainage, we place a suprapubic tube and bring it out through the umbilicus. We then perform a primary closure of the bladder using a three-layer closure with monofilament absorbable suture (i.e., Monocryl and Vicryl). The urethra is tubularized using a two-layer running closure with monofilament and braided absorbable suture (Fig. 110.5). Because of the previous deep dissection, we can position the tubularized urethra ventral to the corpora in a tension-free fashion. If the urethra cannot be positioned ventrally without creating tension, it is likely that a deeper incision is required into the intersymphyseal band and pelvic fascia.

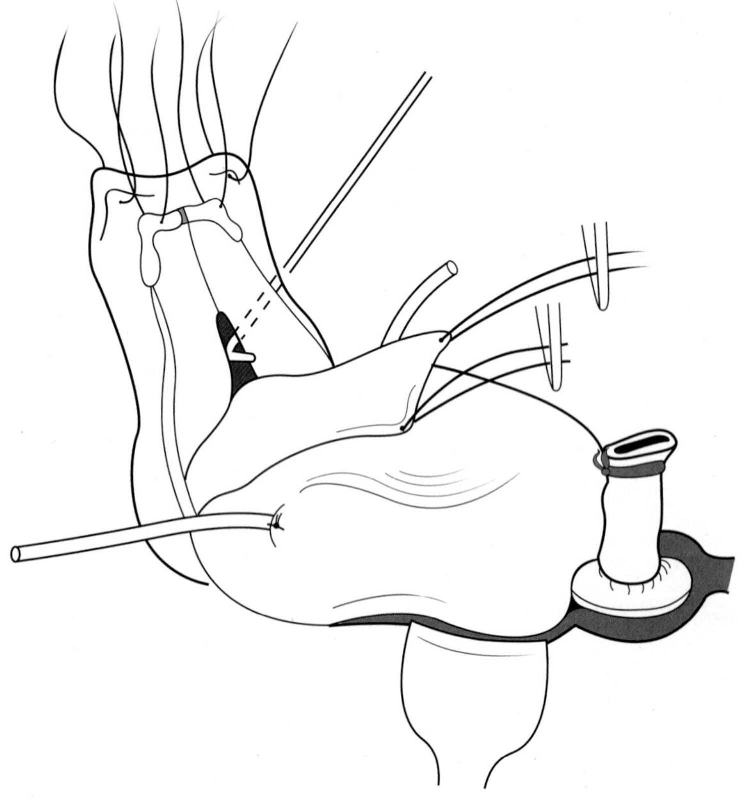

FIGURE 110.8 Disassembly of the corporal bodies from the urethra and corpora spongiosa (the urethral wedge) can often be most easily begun at the position depicted here. The dissection is carried distally to completely separate the glans penis.

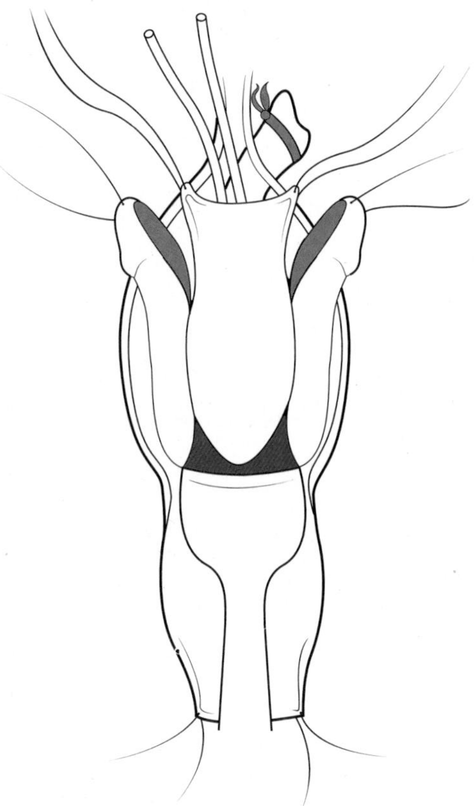

FIGURE 110.9 Perineal view of complete disassembly. Notice depth of dissection.

We reapproximate the pubic symphysis using two no. 1 polydioxanone interrupted sutures placed in a figure-of-eight fashion. Knots are left anteriorly to prevent suture erosion into the bladder neck (Fig. 110.11). The rectus fascia is reapproximated using an interrupted or running 2-0 polydioxanone suture (PDS). We also place interrupted 6-0 PDSs along the dorsal aspect of the corporal bodies to reapproximate them (Fig. 110.12). We provide penile skin coverage by using either a primary dorsal closure or reversed Byars flaps if needed. The skin covering the abdominal wall is reapproximated using a two-layer closure of absorbable monofilament suture.

The corporal bodies will rotate medially with closure (Fig. 110.11). This rotation will assist in correcting the dorsal deflection and can be readily appreciated by observing the new vertical lie of the previously horizontally placed glans traction sutures. Occasionally, significant discrepancies in the dorsal and ventral lengths of the corpora will require dermal graft insertion to correct chordee.

If there is adequate urethral length, the urethra may be brought up to each hemiglans ventrally to create an orthotopic meatus (Fig. 110.12). We reconfigure the glans using interrupted mattress PDSs followed by horizontal mattress sutures of 7-0 monofilament suture to reapproximate the glans epithelium. The neourethra is matured with 7-0 braided polyglactin suture similar to our standard hypospadias repair. When needed, we also perform glans tissue reduction to create a conical-appearing glans and to eliminate the furrow between the glans halves. Tacking sutures are placed ventrally and dorsally to prevent penile shaft skin from riding over the corporal bodies and "burying" the penis (Figs. 110.4 and 110.13).

In our hands, the urethra lacks enough length to reach the glans in about half the cases. In this situation we mature the urethra along the ventral aspect of the penis to create a hypospadias. This can be corrected at a later date as a second-stage procedure (7). We often leave redundant shaft skin ventrally in these patients to assist in later penile reconstructive procedures.

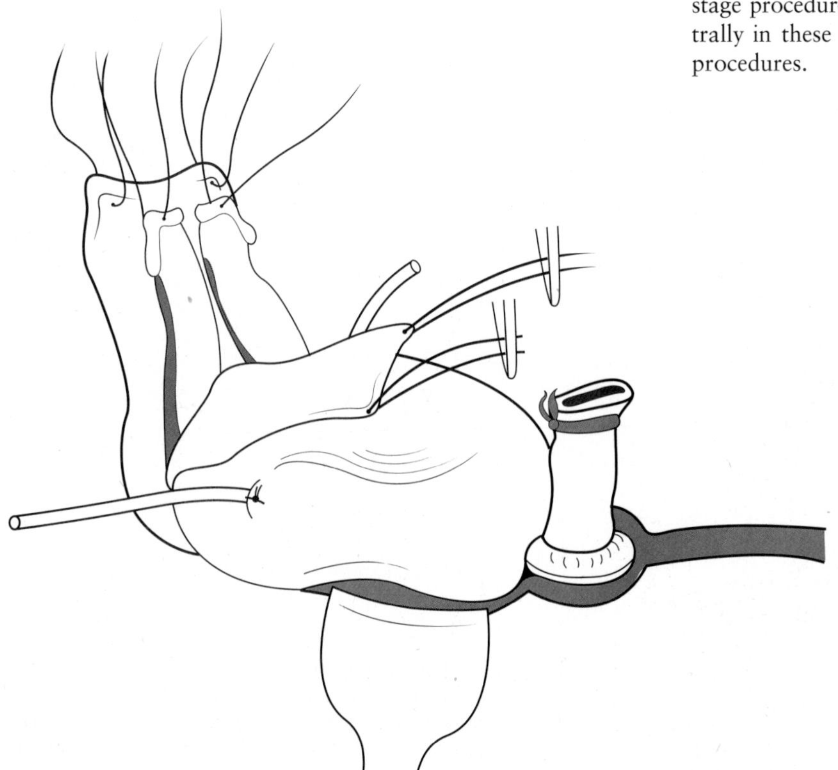

FIGURE 110.10 The urethra and corporal bodies are separated distally to allow deep dissection of the pelvic floor musculature.

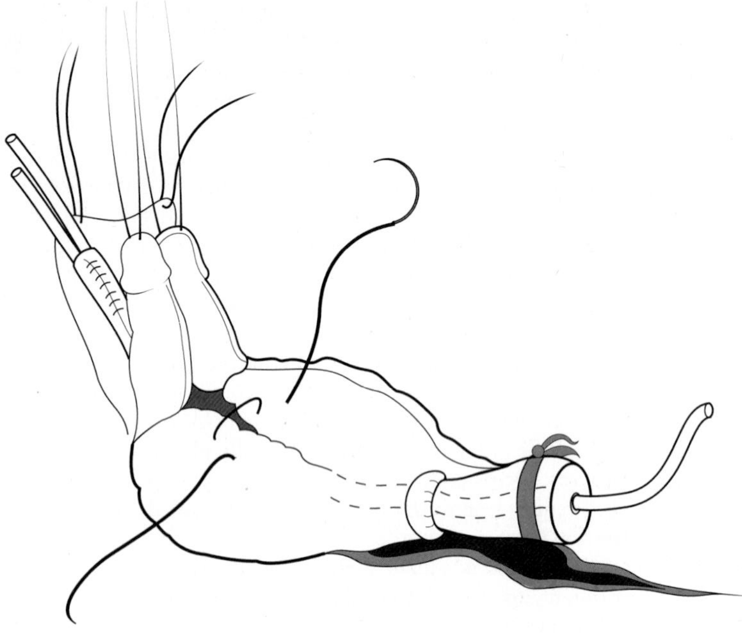

**FIGURE 110.11** After the bladder and urethra are reconstructed, these structures will move posteriorly. The urethra will assume a more normal anatomic position. The pubic symphysis is reapproximated with two figure-of-eight sutures.

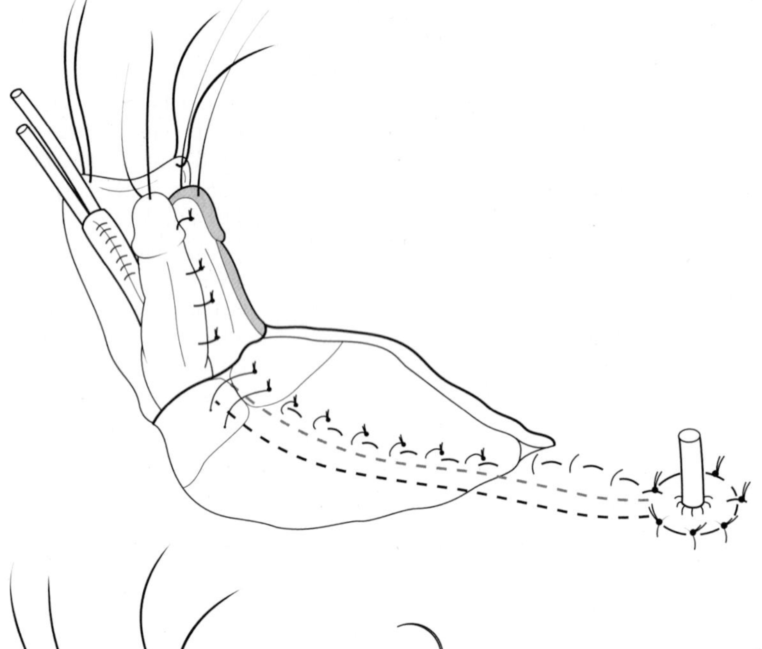

**FIGURE 110.12** The corporal bodies will rotate medially so that the neurovascular bodies are located medially. The suprapubic tube can be brought out through the umbilicus. The umbilicus is moved superiorly to a more normal anatomic location.

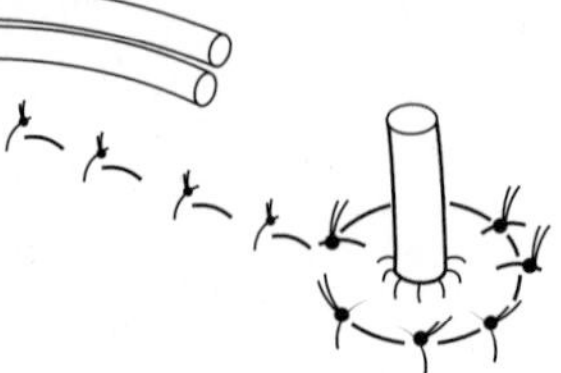

**FIGURE 110.13** The ventral shaft skin is secured to the base of the penis to prevent the penile shaft skin from riding over the body of the penis. The ureteral catheters are brought out through the urethra.

## The Primary Repair Technique: Girls

The principles of this single-stage technique are similar in boys and girls. After preoperative antibiotics are given, the patient is prepared and draped in a sterile field. We mark the planned lines of incision (Fig. 110.14) with the bladder neck, urethra, and vagina mobilized as a unit. We perform this dissection with a tungsten-tip electrocautery (Colorado tip) to minimize tissue damage while achieving hemostasis. The appropriate plane of dissection is found anteriorly along the medial aspect of the glans clitoris and proceeds posteriorly along the lateral aspect of the vaginal vault (Fig. 110.15). The vagina is mobilized with the urethra and bladder neck. Dissection along the vaginal wall extends quite laterally. Placement of a hemostat in the vaginal vault will help with retraction to identify the plane of dissection. The urethra and bladder neck should not be dissected from the anterior vaginal wall, as this will compromise the blood supply to the urethra. During the posterior lateral dissection, the intersymphyseal band will be encountered and should be deeply incised to allow the urethra and bladder neck to move posteriorly. The posterior limit of the dissection is reached when the pelvic floor musculature is exposed and the bladder, bladder neck, and urethra can move into the pelvis without tension.

Following adequate dissection, the vagina, urethra, and bladder neck are moved posteriorly using a Y-V plasty if the vagina is anteriorly located (Fig. 110.16). The urethra is then tubularized using a two-layer closure of absorbable suture. Prior to the urethral closure, we routinely place a suprapubic tube to provide postoperative urine drainage. The pubic symphysis is reapproximated using two figure-of-eight no. 1 PDSs (Fig. 110.17). Osteotomies may be necessary when a wide pubic diastasis prevents a low-tension reapproximation of the pubic symphysis or if the patient is older than 48 to 72 hours old. We use anterior iliac osteotomies in these situations. The rectus fascia can then be closed in the midline. We

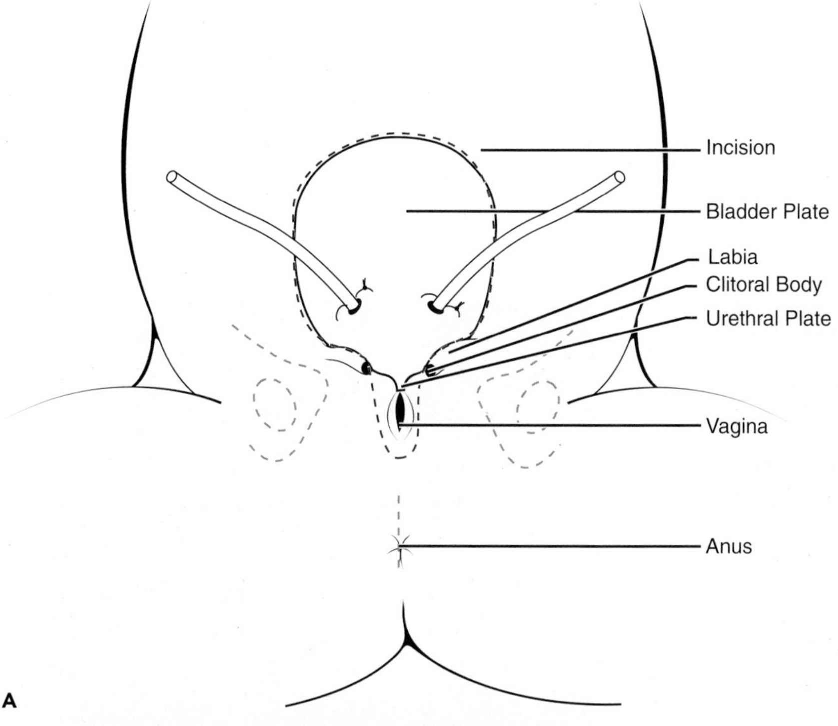


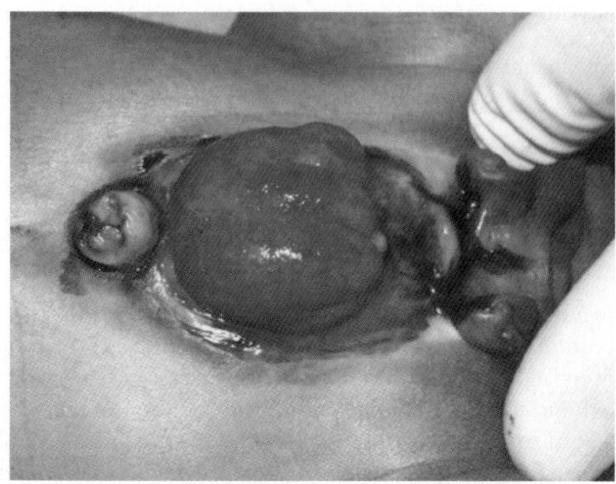


FIGURE 110.14 A: Schematic diagram of lines of incision for complete primary repair of a female infant with bladder exstrophy. This concept has been applied to the repair of female epispadias in the adjacent photograph (B), demonstrating lines of incision for an infant girl with epispadias. Note the posterior extent of dissection to allow movement of the vagina, bladder neck, and urethra as a unit posteriorly.

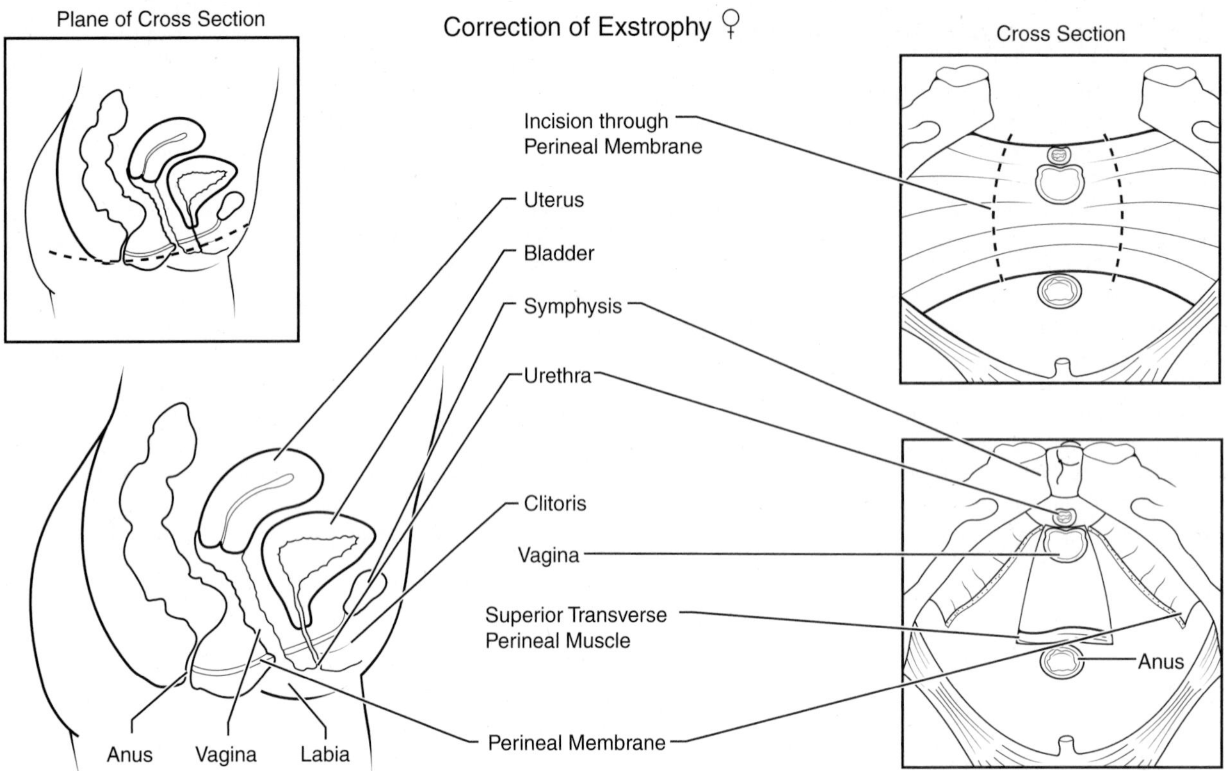


FIGURE 110.15 The plane of dissection lies adjacent to the urethra and vaginal vault *(dashed lines in upper right cross-sectional view)*.

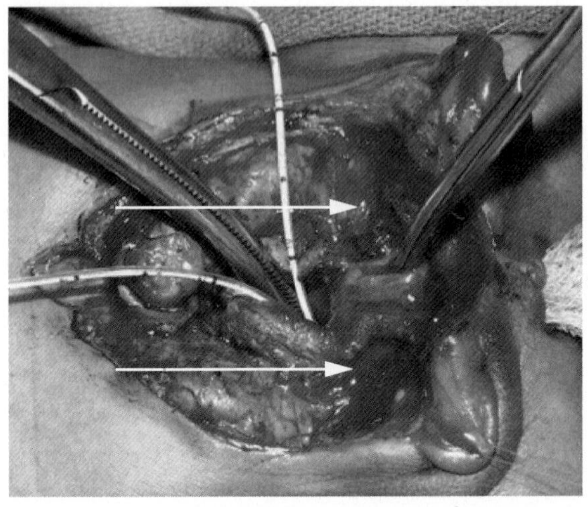

FIGURE 110.16 The intersymphyseal band is incised laterally *(white arrows)* to allow the urethra, bladder, and vaginal vault to move posteriorly as a unit.

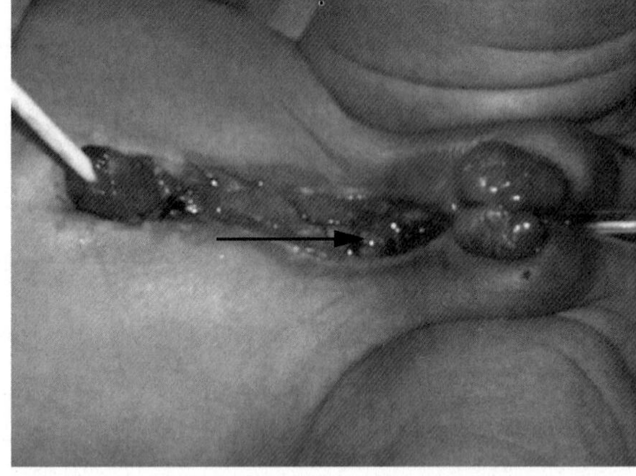

FIGURE 110.17 The pubic symphysis is reapproximated *(arrow)*. With adequate dissection, the pubic symphysis can be reapproximated with minimal compressive effects on the urethra and bladder.

mature the neourethra with 5-0 Vicryl sutures and reapproximate the bifid clitoris by denuding the parts medially so that they fuse together after suturing with 7-0 Maxon suture (Fig. 110.18). The labia majora should be advanced posteriorly to the perineum at this time as well. A Z-plasty skin closure aids in skin closure. A simplified monsplasty technique described by Pippi-Salle et al. (8) provides a satisfactory aesthetic result to the introital area and can be applied at the time of the primary repair.

## Adjunctive Aspect of Repair

Inguinal hernias are commonly associated with exstrophy in both male and female patients. The majority of these hernias occur indirectly. They arise as a consequence of enlarged internal and external inguinal rings combined with compromised fascial support and lack of obliquity of the inguinal canal. In a review of patients from the Toronto Sick Children's Hospital,

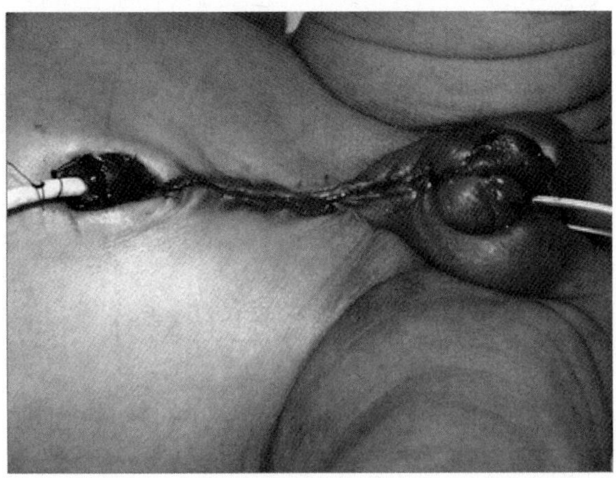

FIGURE 110.18 Final reconstruction demonstrates apposition of the labia and clitoral bodies. Denuding the epithelium on the clitoris medially improves the cosmetic results postoperatively.

56% of classic male exstrophy patients and 15% of classic female exstrophy patients developed inguinal hernias over a 10-year period (9). The authors recommended that these hernias be repaired at the time of primary bladder closure to prevent incarcerated hernias, which could affect up to 50% of these patients in the first 2 years of life. Reinforcement of the transversalis and internal oblique fascia during hernia repair decreases the incidence of later direct inguinal hernias. Umbilical hernias, as a contiguous defect with the bladder plate, also uniformly occur with exstrophy and are repaired at the time of the primary repair.

## POSTOPERATIVE CARE

The patient must be immobilized to decrease lateral stresses on the closure after the primary reconstructive procedure for exstrophy. A number of options exist for this purpose. We prefer to use a spica cast for 3 weeks to prevent external hip rotation and to optimize pubic apposition, which can facilitate early discharge and home care (Fig. 110.19). Modified Buck traction has been used by many groups with success. A posterior lightweight splint can be used in newborns when the child is out of traction to maintain hip adduction. We have stopped using Buck traction because spica casts are easier for the families to care for at home. External fixation devices have also been used with success (10). Fixator pins for these devices should be cleaned several times a day to reduce the chance for infection. Internal fixation may be necessary in older patients.

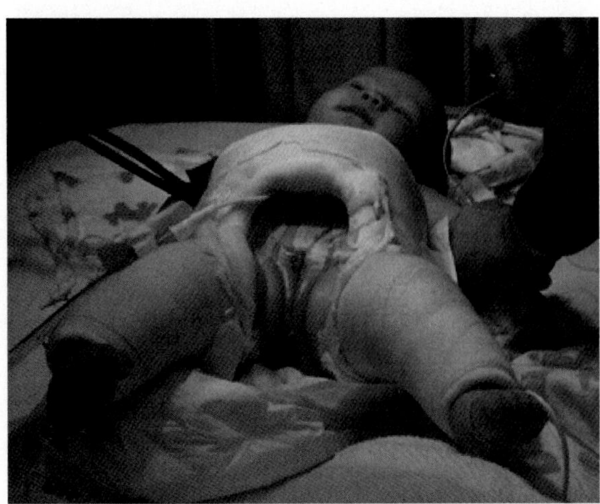

FIGURE 110.19 Use of a spica cast postoperatively to immobilize the pelvis and prevent hip abduction.

Because of the high incidence of vesicoureteral reflux, we prescribe low-dose suppressive antibiotic therapy for all newborns after bladder closure. This is continued until the vesicoureteral reflux is corrected or resolves spontaneously. Some surgeons perform neoureterocystotomies at the time of initial closure. The success of this approach has not been reported.

Postoperative factors that appear to directly impact the success of initial closure include postoperative immobilization, use of postoperative antibiotics, ureteral stenting catheters, adequate postoperative pain management, avoidance of abdominal distention, adequate nutritional support, and secure fixation of urinary drainage catheters.

## OUTCOMES

### Complications

Complications can occur with this form of exstrophy closure. The most commonly reported complication is urethrocutaneous fistula formation (at the penopubic angle dorsally) in males. These fistulas will often close spontaneously. They may initially be managed conservatively by providing urinary diversion via catheter drainage. If the fistula does not close after conservative management, the bladder and urethra should be examined cystoscopically for the possibility of obstruction at the bladder neck or urethra.

Other complications have been reported following a primary reconstructive technique. These include atrophy of the corpora cavernosa and urethra. These complications can occur if the blood supply to the corporal bodies or urethral wedge is damaged during dissection or during closure (11). Similar complications have been described following the initial stage of a staged reconstruction (12). In experienced hands, such complications are unusual and underscore the importance of involving surgeons experienced in the surgical management of these patients in their care.

If a child develops chronic bladder and kidney infections following exstrophy closure, he or she should be evaluated for possible outlet obstruction. We routinely maintain our patients on suppressive antibiotic therapy because of the high incidence of vesicoureteral reflux in this population.

### Results

Since 1989 we have performed this operation for 36 children with the exstrophy-epispadias complex in a prospective fashion. This series represents a treatment group who underwent the CPRE technique to construct classic bladder exstrophy ($n$ = 31) or proximal or female epispadias ($n$ = 5). Twenty-three of these children underwent this operation in the first 48 hours of life. Mean follow-up for the original group of patients that we reported in 1999 is 85 months. Mean follow-up for the entire series is 68 months.

Daytime continence with volitional voiding was achieved in 77% of boys and girls 4 years old or older. Primary urinary continence was achieved by 18% of boys and 36% of girls without the need for bladder neck reconstruction. Complications occurred in 13% of the children in the entire series; 81% of the children demonstrated mild or no hydronephrosis following this operative technique (13).

Hammouda (14) reported a series of 33 cases. They achieved continence in 72% of the patients with minimal complications, mirroring the results at our institution. Hammouda (14) has also used the complete penile disassembly technique for 42 patients with excellent functional results.

Borer et al. (15) at Boston Children's Hospital have performed detailed urodynamic studies for 23 children with exstrophy who have been closed using the complete primary repair technique. In a comparison with patients closed using a staged approach, these children demonstrated universal bladder stability, bladder capacities within the expected range, and normal sphincter electromyogram (EMG) activity, suggesting no neuromuscular compromise of the pelvic floor. Further, magnetic resonance imaging studies in this group suggest that urinary control is improved as pelvic floor anatomy becomes more normal in appearance (16).

## *References*

1. Skari H, et al. Consequences of prenatal ultrasound diagnosis: a preliminary report on neonates with congenital malformations. *Acta Obstet Gynecol Scand* 1998;77(6):635–642.
2. Gearhart JP, et al. Criteria for the prenatal diagnosis of classic bladder exstrophy. *Obstet Gynecol* 1995;85(6):961–964.
3. Mirk P, Calisti A, Fileni A. Prenatal sonographic diagnosis of bladder extrophy. *J Ultrasound Med* 1986;5(5):291–293.
4. Sanders R. Prenatal diagnosis of bladder and cloacal exstrophy and related conditions. In: Gearhart MJ, ed. *The exstrophy-epispadias complex: research concepts and clinical applications*. New York: Kluwer Academic/Plenum Publishers, 1999:5–8.
5. O'Kane HO, Megaw JM. Carcinoma in the exstrophic bladder. *Br J Surg* 1968;55(8):631–635.
6. Grady RW, Mitchell ME. Complete primary repair of exstrophy. *J Urol* 1999;162(4):1415–1420.
7. El-Sherbiny MT, Hafez AT. Complete repair of bladder exstrophy in boys: can hypospadias be avoided? *Eur Urol* 2005 47(5):691–694.
8. Cook AJ, Farhat WA, Cartwright LM, et al. Simplified mons plasty: a new technique to improve cosmesis in females with the exstrophy-epispadias complex. *J Urol* 2005;173(6):2117–2120.
9. Husmann DA, McLorie GA, Churchill BM, et al. Inguinal pathology and its association with classical bladder exstrophy. *J Pediatr Surg* 1990;25(3): 332–334.
10. Sponseller PD, et al. Anterior innominate osteotomy in repair of bladder exstrophy. *J Bone Joint Surg Am* 2001;83-A(2):184–193.
11. Gearhart JP. Complete repair of bladder exstrophy in the newborn: complications and management. *J Urol* 2001;165(6, Pt 2):2431–2433.
12. Gearhart J. Complete repair of bladder exstrophy in the newborn: complications and management. *BJU Int* 2000;85[Suppl 4]:74 (abstract 150).
13. Shnorhavorian M, Mitchell M, Redel M, et al. Long-term followup of complete primary repair of exstrophy: the Seattle experience. *J Urol* 2008; 180(4 Suppl):1615–1619; discussion 1619–1620.
14. Hammouda HM. Results of complete penile disassembly for epispadias repair in 42 patients. *J Urol* 2003;170(5):1963–1965; discussion 1965.
15. Borer JG, et al. Bladder growth and development after complete primary repair of bladder exstrophy in the newborn with comparison to staged approach. *J Urol* 2005;174(4, Pt2):1553–1557; discussion 1557–1558.
16. Gargollo PC, et al. Magnetic resonance imaging of pelvic musculoskeletal and genitourinary anatomy in patients before and after complete primary repair of bladder exstrophy. *J Urol* 2005;174(4, Pt 2):1559–1566; discussion 1566.

# CHAPTER 111 ■ BLADDER EXSTROPHY AND EPISPADIAS

THOMAS E. NOVAK AND JOHN P. GEARHART

Bladder exstrophy is a rare, severe congenital defect that affects the lower urinary tract, genitalia, abdominal wall, and pelvis. The reported incidence ranges from 1:10,000 to 1:50,000 live births, with boys being affected five to six times more frequently than girls (1). Bladder exstrophy is usually an isolated defect, and in its classic form, associated chromosomal abnormalities or defects of the central nervous system, heart, and digestive tract are extremely uncommon.

Until the middle of the 19th century, bladder exstrophy was treated primarily nonsurgically. Early forms of repair focused on abdominal wall closure using skin flaps for partial reconstruction, leaving a fistula to attach a urinal for dryness. Trendelenburg recognized that pubic reapproximation would not only prevent prolapse of the reconstructed bladder but also be crucial to achieve continence. Although his theoretical assumptions were correct, his surgical efforts were not successful (2). Early failures lead to an abandonment of interest in primary closure with a shift toward urinary diversion. In 1942, Hugh Hampton Young performed the first successful primary closure of a female exstrophy patient (3). Although similar reports about continent, primary closures were published in the same era, the numbers were small and most surgeons were not able to reproduce these favorable results. Both Jeffs (4) and Cendron (5) published their description about successful staged anatomic reconstruction in the mid-1970s, and their pioneering work set the standard for the modern staged repair of exstrophy (MSRE). Grady and Mitchell (6) subsequently developed the complete primary repair of exstrophy (CPRE), in which the primary closure is combined with a complete penile disassembly and epispadias repair.

While older techniques have evolved and alternative approaches have been developed, the primary objectives of modern exstrophy management remain consistent:

1. Secure closure of the abdominal wall, pelvis, bladder, and urethra
2. Reconstruction of a functional and cosmetically acceptable penis in the male and external genitalia in the female
3. Urinary continence, preferably via urethral voiding, with preservation of renal function

The complex embryology and genetics of exstrophy are not well understood. A number of theories have been proposed, which include premature rupture of the cloacal membrane, arrested mesenchymal ingrowth, and failure of cranial yolk sac progression during development (1). In its classic form, bladder exstrophy describes the condition in which an exteriorized bladder template develops in association with a diastasis of the pubic symphysis. This pubic separation results in characteristic genital and pelvic abnormalities. The pubic diastasis is found in association with foreshortened, externally rotated anterior pubic rami and a wide pelvic inlet. The perineum is short and broad and there is anterior displacement of the anus. The appearance of the genitalia varies by gender. In boys, the urethra lies in an epispadiac position, splayed open on the dorsal surface of the corporal bodies. The pubic diastasis results in corporal shortening and severe dorsal chordee. The testes are usually descended, but inguinal hernias are extremely common (especially in boys). In girls, the pubic diastasis results in an absence of a mons pubis, with a bifid clitoris and lateral displacement of the labia. Girls usually present with a bifid clitoris and a short vagina that often has a stenotic orifice. In isolated epispadias, which can be viewed as the least severe form of exstrophy, the bladder is closed and covered by a normal abdominal wall, but the pubic separation and genital abnormalities persist. Degrees of epispadias vary in a manner analogous to hypospadias from the very proximal "complete" epispadias in which the urethra is open through the bladder neck, to minor distal variants. A number of other exstrophy variants have been described (7).

## DIAGNOSIS

The definitive diagnosis of bladder exstrophy is made by recognition of the characteristic physical examination findings at the time of birth. Diagnosis by prenatal ultrasound is becoming more common with advances in sonographic techniques. Ultrasound findings include an absence of bladder filling, an anterior abdominal mass, a low-set umbilicus, abnormal widening of the iliac crests, and an anteriorly displaced scrotum with a small phallus in male fetuses (8). The differential diagnoses include cloacal exstrophy, omphalocele, and gastroschisis. Children with a prenatal diagnosis of exstrophy should be delivered at term via cesarean section. The principal implication of prenatal diagnosis of exstrophy is that most parents will seek early counseling regarding the nature of the disease and will temporarily relocate, if necessary, to a center with experience in exstrophy management. Some parents ultimately decide to terminate their pregnancies. The regionalization of complex surgical care such as that required for exstrophy patients is the subject of current debate and outcomes research.

## INDICATIONS FOR SURGERY

Historically, some children with bladder exstrophy have survived without surgical reconstruction. As mentioned previously, the earliest attempts at treatment focused on providing a suitable drainage apparatus that would help to manage chronic wetness and odor. Because of the rarity of the condition, it is unlikely that a prospective study will ever compare observation to reconstruction. The importance of treating this condition, however, can be inferred from several studies that have investigated the profound negative impact of urinary incontinence and sexual dysfunction on quality of life and social and psychological well-being (9,10). Furthermore, it is known that chronic exposure of the exposed bladder mucosa to the environment results in painful ulceration and metaplastic and ultimately neoplastic changes (11). It seems reasonable to conclude that all children with exstrophy deserve surgical treatment and that every attempt should be made to deliver this to even underprivileged populations whose medical capabilities are deficient.

## ALTERNATIVE THERAPY

### Urinary Diversion

A number of different urinary diversion techniques have been used historically with success in the management of exstrophy/epispadias (12). Although incontinent conduits are rarely indicated in contemporary pediatric practice, reconstructive urologists should be comfortable with their construction. Ureterosigmoidostomy was the first successful continent diversion performed in an exstrophy patient, and continence rates without the need for intermittent catheterization are very good (13). The role of ureterosigmoidostomy has decreased with the application of anatomic reconstructions, but it is still used in some centers today. The Mainz II pouch is a modification of the ureterosigmoidostomy that reconfigures the sigmoid into a theoretically lower-pressure reservoir, thereby promoting continence and renal preservation (12). Long-term concerns over the potential for malignancy at the ureterocolonic anastomosis and renal deterioration are cause for ongoing postoperative surveillance. Urinary diversion remains an important salvage approach in children who fail anatomic reconstruction.

### Anatomic Reconstruction

The modern staged repair of exstrophy will be described in detail as performed at Johns Hopkins. Alternate anatomic reconstructions have been proposed and are used in some centers. Grady and Mitchell developed the one-stage closure in the newborn period, which combined primary closure of the bladder, urethra, abdomen, and pelvis with epispadias repair using the complete penile disassembly technique. Proponents of CPRE believe that this approach will promote bladder growth and better continence outcomes by initiation of bladder cycling early on (6). Schrott (14) describes bladder closure, ureteral reimplantation, epispadias repair, and bladder neck reconstruction in the newborn period, applying the same technique to even older children without osteotomies. Primary newborn exstrophy closure followed by subsequent combined bladder neck reconstruction and epispadias repair has been described by Baka-Jakubiak (15). The combination of bladder closure with modified Cantwell–Ransley epispadias repair has been reported in a series of delayed and secondary exstrophy closures (16).

# SURGICAL TECHNIQUE

## Preoperative Considerations

A type and screen with baseline complete blood count and coagulation studies should be obtained. A plain film of the pelvis allows for precise measurement of the pubic diastasis. A baseline renal/bladder ultrasound is recommended to establish the presence of both units and for purposes of later comparison. The use of cross-sectional imaging (computerized tomography/magnetic resonance imaging) is investigational. The umbilical cord should be ligated with a heavy silk suture. If a plastic cord clamp was used initially, this should be changed in order to prevent it from irritating the bladder mucosa. Likewise, the bladder template should be kept moist with periodic saline irrigation and covered with either a hydrated gel or Saran-type dressing. Petroleum-based gauze dressings are discouraged as they may dry and denude the mucosa when removed. Latex precautions are recommended as many of these children will develop latex sensitivity or allergy later in life.

## Timing and Staging

Modern staged closure has defined strict criteria for the selection of patients suitable for this approach. The technique includes early bladder, posterior urethral, and abdominal wall closure, usually with pelvic osteotomy in the newborn period, subsequently followed by an early epispadias repair at 6 months of age after intramuscular testosterone stimulation. Around age 4 to 5 years a competent bladder neck is reconstructed along with bilateral ureteral reimplantation, when adequate bladder capacity is reached and the child demonstrates the maturity necessary to participate in a postoperative voiding program (17).

Successful initial bladder and posterior urethral closure is the most important factor for achieving eventual urinary continence and sufficient bladder capacity. The primary objective in initial, functional closure is to convert the bladder exstrophy into a complete epispadias with incontinence with balanced posterior outlet resistance that preserves renal function but stimulates bladder growth. The size and the functional capacity of the detrusor muscle are ultimately the most important determinants of success (18). In the presence of a small, fibrotic bladder template without elasticity or contractility, the operation should be deferred until adequate template growth has taken place. If sufficient size is not reached 4 to 6 months after birth, alternative options should be considered. Inguinal hernia repairs should be considered early if the closure is delayed in order to guard against incarceration during this time interval.

The role of pelvic osteotomy performed at time of initial closure ensures a tension-free approximation of the bladder, posterior urethra, and abdominal wall, placement of the urethra deep within the pelvic ring, enhancing bladder outlet resistance, and finally aligning the large pelvic floor muscles to support the bladder neck. Usually, osteotomies are not needed in the patient <72 hours old with malleable pubic bones that are easily brought together in the midline by medial rotation of the greater trochanters. However, if the pubic bones are >4 cm apart or unable to be reapproximated without tension, osteotomies are mandated to ensure a secure closure.

## Osteotomy

The bilateral anterior innominate and vertical iliac osteotomy has been used in our institution because it has numerous advantages over the posterior approach. The patient is placed in a supine position, preparing and draping the lower body below the costal margins and placing soft absorbent gauze over the exposed bladder. The pelvis is exposed from the inferior wings inferiorly and the pectineal tubercle and posteriorly to the sacroiliac joints. The periosteum and sciatic notch are carefully elevated and a Gigli saw is used to create a transverse innominate osteotomy exiting anteriorly at a point halfway between the anterosuperior and the anteroinferior spines (Fig. 111.1). This osteotomy is created at a slightly more cranial level than that described for a Salter osteotomy to allow placement of external fixator pins in the distal segments. Also, the posterior ileum may be incised from the anterior approach in an effort to correct the deformity more completely. This is important because anatomic studies have shown that the posterior portion of the pelvis is also externally rotated in patients with exstrophy, and as patients age they lose the elasticity of their sacroiliac ligaments. An osteotome is used to create a closing wedge osteotomy vertically and just lateral to the sacroiliac joint. The posterior iliac cortex is kept intact and used as a hinge (Fig. 111.2). Two fixator pins are placed in the inferior osteotomized segment and two pins are placed in the wing of the ilium superiorly. Radiographs are obtained to confirm pin placement, soft tissues are closed, and the urologic procedure is performed. At the conclusion of the exstrophy closure, external fixators are applied between the pins to hold the pelvis in a correct position.

Radiographs are taken 7 to 10 days postoperatively. If the diastasis has not been completely reduced, the right and left sides can be gradually approximated using the fixator bars over several days. Light longitudinal Buck skin traction is used to keep the legs still. The patient remains supine in traction for approximately 4 weeks to prevent dislodgement of tubes and destabilization of the pelvis. The external fixator is kept on for approximately 6 weeks, until adequate callus is seen at the site of osteotomy. The pins are removed under light sedation at the bedside. Postoperatively, newborns undergoing closure without osteotomy are immobilized in modified Bryant traction for 4 weeks with the hips in 90 degrees of flexion.

Staged pelvic closure in the setting of an extreme (>8 cm) pubic diastasis has been described with good results in a series of children with both classic and cloacal exstrophy. In this approach, osteotomies are performed in conjunction with interfragmentary pin placement during the initial procedure. The pelvis is then gradually reduced under sedation at the bedside over the next several weeks, and ultimately the pubis is secured with an interpubic stainless steel plate that is placed at the time of bladder and urethral closure (19).

The use of spica casting and mummy wrapping for immobilization following exstrophy closure has been described. In our experience, these techniques are associated with higher rates of complications and inferior surgical outcomes and are

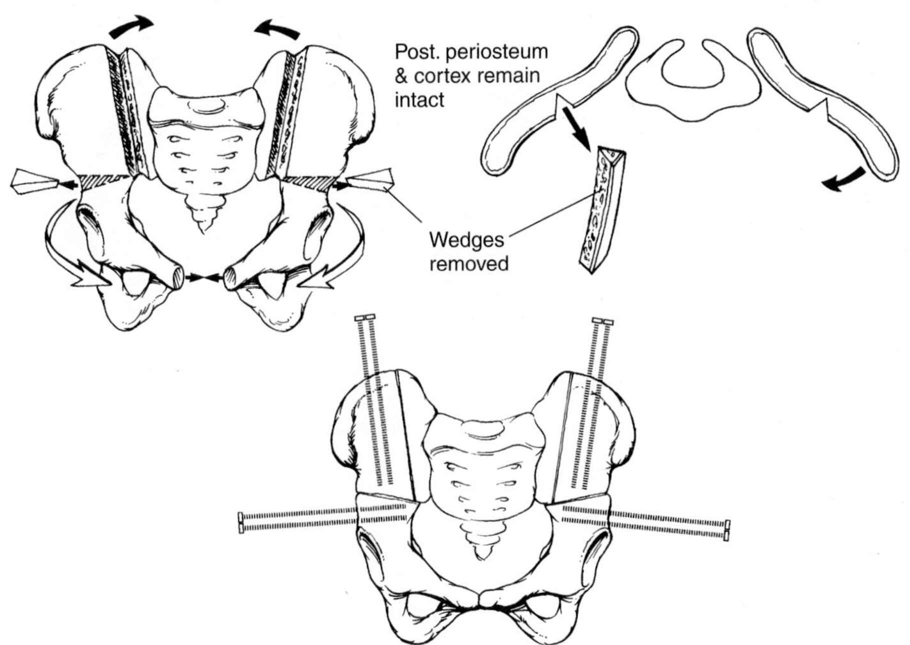


FIGURE 111.1 Combined transverse anterior innominate and anterior vertical iliac osteotomies with pin placement and preservation of the posterior periosteum and cortex. (Drawings by Timothy Phelps after Leon Schlossberg. ©2002 Brady Urological Institute, with permission.)

not recommended (20). Okubadejo (21) reviewed the orthopedic complications of exstrophy management in 624 patients from Johns Hopkins: 26 complications were noted (4%), of which four were identified as being specifically caused by traction.

## Bladder, Posterior Urethral, and Abdominal Wall Closure

The various steps in primary bladder closure are illustrated in Figure 111.2. A strip of mucosa 2 cm wide, extending from the distal trigone to below the verumontanum in the boy and to the vaginal orifice in the girl, is outlined for prostatic and posterior urethral reconstruction (Fig. 111.2A). With the advent of the modified Cantwell–Ransley epispadias repair, the urethral plate should not be incised unless the length of the urethral groove from the verumontanum to the glans is so short that it interferes with eventual penile length and produces dorsal angulation. In this situation, the urethral groove is lengthened. Figures 111.2B to 111.2D show marking of the incision from just above the umbilicus down around the junction of the bladder and the para-exstrophy skin to the level of the urethral plate. The appropriate plane is entered just above the umbilicus and a plane is established between the rectus fascia and the bladder (Fig. 111.2E,F). The umbilical vessels are doubly ligated and incised and allowed to fall into the pelvis. The peritoneum is taken off the dome of the bladder, to be deeply placed into the pelvis at the time of closure. The plane is continued caudally down between the bladder and rectus fascia until the urogenital diaphragm fibers are encountered bilaterally. With electrocautery, these urogenital diaphragm fibers between the bladder neck, the posterior urethra, and the pubic bone are taken sharply down to the levator hiatus in their entirety (Fig. 111.2F). A double-pronged skin hook can be inserted into the pelvic bone and pulled laterally to accentuate the urogenital diaphragm fibers. If this maneuver is not performed adequately, the vesicourethral unit will be brought anteriorly with pelvic closure in an unsatisfactory position for later reconstruction.

If the decision is made to transect the urethral groove, then it is cut distal to the verumontanum with continuity maintained between the thin, mucosa-like non–hair-bearing skin adjacent to the posterior urethra and bladder neck and the skin and mucosa of the penile glans. Flaps in the area of thin skin are subsequently moved distally and rotated to reconstruct the urethral groove, resurfacing the penis dorsally. The corporal bodies are not brought together because later Cantwell–Ransley epispadias repair requires the urethral plate to be brought underneath the corporal bodies. If the urethral plate is left in continuity, it must be mobilized up to the level of the prostate to create as much urethral and penile length as possible. Apparent penile lengthening is achieved by exposing the corpora cavernosa bilaterally and freeing the corpora from their attachments to the suspensory ligaments. After the urogenital diaphragm is completely incised bilaterally, freeing the bladder neck and urethra well from the pubis, the mucosa and muscle of the bladder and the posterior urethra well onto the penis are closed in the anterior midline (Fig. 111.2G). The resulting orifice should be easily passed by a 12Fr sound, creating enough resistance to aid in bladder adaptation and prevent prolapse but not too much to cause outlet resistance altering the upper tracts. A second layer is closed if possible (Fig. 111.2H). Bladder drainage is achieved using a suprapubic nonlatex Malecot catheter for 4 weeks. The urethra is not stented to prevent necrosis. Ureteral stents are left in place for 10 to 14 days, until swelling goes down.

By applying gentle pressure over the greater trochanters bilaterally, the pubic bones are approximated in the midline. A horizontal mattress suture of no. 2 nylon is placed between the fibrous cartilages of the pubic rami and tied anteriorly to the pubic closure to avoid the neourethra (Fig. 111.2I,J). A second stitch is placed caudal to the insertion of the rectus fascia if possible for added support. Should the sutures work loose or cut through the tissues during subsequent healing, the anterior placement of the knot of the horizontal mattress suture ensures that it will not erode through into the urethra. A V-shaped flap of abdominal skin at a point corresponding to

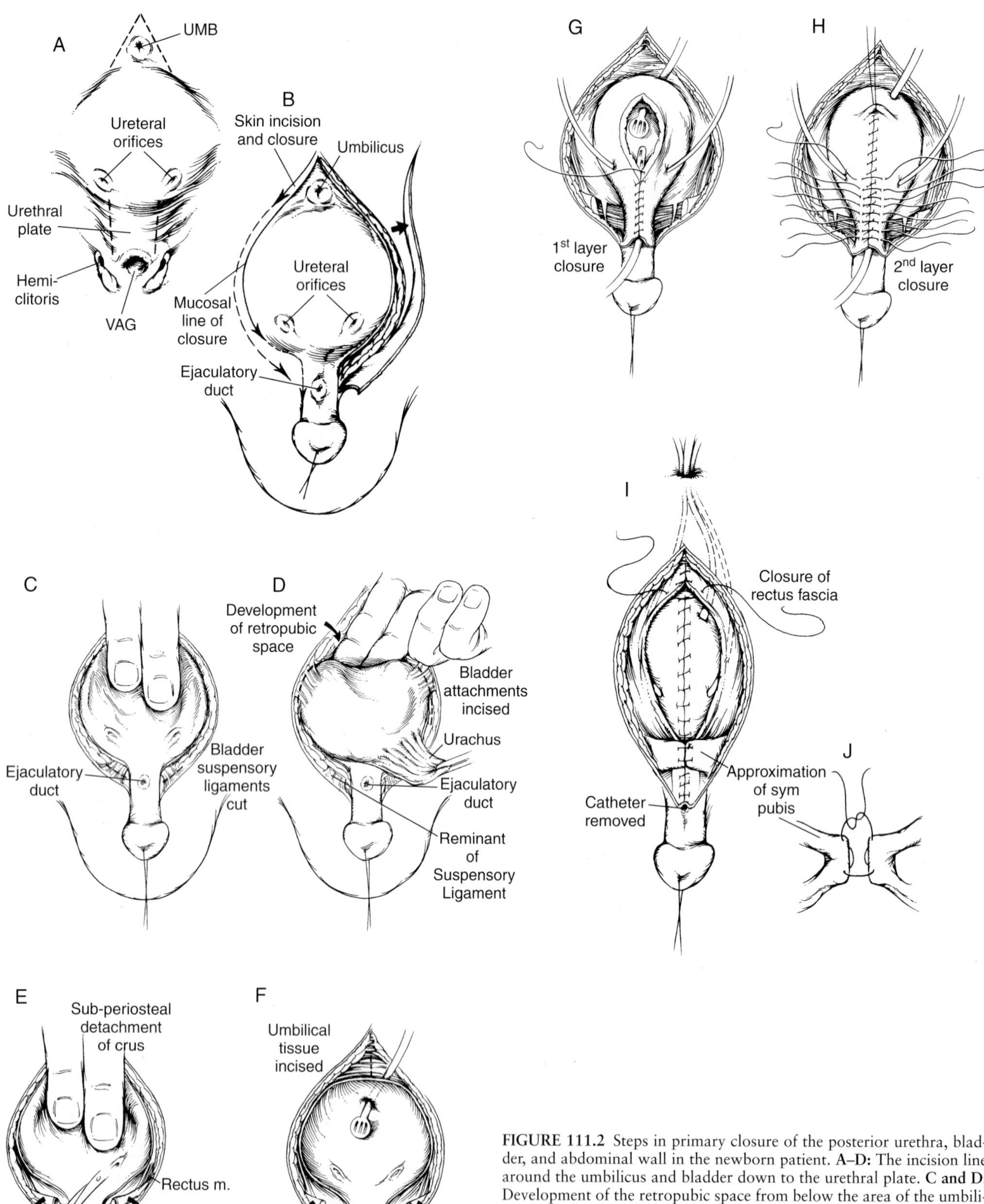


FIGURE 111.2 Steps in primary closure of the posterior urethra, bladder, and abdominal wall in the newborn patient. **A–D:** The incision line around the umbilicus and bladder down to the urethral plate. **C and D:** Development of the retropubic space from below the area of the umbilical insertion to facilitate separation of the bladder from the rectus sheath and muscle. **E and F:** Medial extension of the rectus muscle attaching behind the prostate to the upper border of the urogenital diaphragm, which together with the anterior corpus is freed from the pubis by deep incision. **G and H:** Ureteral stent placement and layered closure of the bladder wall. **I and J:** A horizontal mattress suture is tied on the external surface of the pubic symphysis and exit of the ureteral and suprapubic tube at the site of the neoumbilical opening. (Drawings by Timothy Phelps after Leon Schlossberg. ©2002 Brady Urological Institute, with permission.)

the normal position of the umbilicus is tacked down to the abdominal fascia, and the drainage tubes exit this neoumbilicus.

Postoperatively, before suprapubic tube removal the bladder outlet is calibrated to ensure free passage of urine. Repeated ultrasound examinations are obtained before discharge and every 3 months to check for upper-tract dilatation and residual urine. Continuous, prophylactic antibiotic therapy is advised to prevent upper-tract infection from ureteral reflux. Yearly gravity cystograms under anesthesia are performed to receive quality information about reflux and, more importantly, bladder capacity. For successful continent procedures a minimal bladder capacity of 100 cc is needed (18). An increase in bladder capacity is seen after epispadias repair, which is why the bladder neck procedure is performed after the urethral reconstruction.

## Epispadias Repair

Four key concerns have to be addressed: (a) a functional and cosmetically pleasing penis, (b) correction of dorsal chordee, (c) urethral reconstruction, and (d) penile skin closure and glandular reconstruction. In patients undergoing delayed repair or reclosure, a combined epispadias/exstrophy closure using the modified Cantwell–Ransley repair is possible.

The modified Cantwell–Ransley repair is begun by placing a nylon suture through the ventral glans for traction. A meatal advancement and glanuloplasty incorporated (MAGPI) incision is made in the urethral plate distally and closed with 6-0 polyglycolic sutures in a transverse fashion to flatten the distal urethral plate and advance the urethra to the tip of the phallus (Fig. 111.3A). The reconstructed neourethra will be in excellent glandular position once the wings are closed. Next, incisions are made over two parallel lines marked previously over the dorsum of the penis that outline an 18-mm-wide strip of urethral mucosa extending from the prostatic urethral meatus to the tip of the glans (Fig. 111.3A). Triangular mucosal areas of the dorsal gland are excised adjacent to the urethral strip, and thick glandular flaps are constructed bilaterally. Lateral skin flaps are mobilized and undermined.

A Z-incision of the suprapubic area permits exposure and division of the suspensory ligament and old scar tissue from the initial exstrophy closure. The ventral skin is taken down to the level of the scrotum (Fig. 111.3B). Care is taken to preserve the mesentery to the urethral plate, which arises proximally and extends upward between the corpora as a blood supply to the urethral plate. The corpora are dissected ventrally on the surface of the Buck fascia. The plane is followed closely bilaterally until one exits on the dorsum of the penis between the corpora spongiosum and the corporal body (Fig. 111.3C).

After placement of loops, the urethral plate is dissected just on the corporal bodies to the level of the prostate and the glans, respectively (Fig. 111.3D). Care is taken to leave the most distal 1-cm attachment of the mucosal plate to the glans intact. The neurovascular bundles are dissected free from the corporal bodies only if rotating the corpora over the urethra does not straighten the penis. The urethral strip is closed in a linear manner from the prostatic opening to the glans over an 8Fr silicone stent with 6-0 polyglycolic sutures. Afterward, the corporal bodies are incised at the point of maximal curvature, leaving a diamond-shaped defect (Fig. 111.3E). The corpora are then closed over the neourethra with two running sutures of 5-0 polydioxanone (PDS), with the adjacent areas of the diamond sutured to each other (Fig. 111.3F). The now ventrally placed urethra is secured in place with further 5-0 polyglycolic acid sutures between the corpora, especially at the coronal level (Fig. 111.3G–I). The glans wings are subcuticularly closed with 5-0 and the glans epithelium with 6-0 polyglycolic acid. Finally, the ventral skin is brought up and sutured to the ventral edge of the corona, while the flaps provide coverage of the dorsum. The skin as well as the Z-plasty at the base of the penis is reapproximated with interrupted 5-0 or 6-0 polyglycolic acid sutures (Fig. 111.3J,K). The silicon stent is secured and left for 10 to 12 days.

In girls the mons and external genitalia are reconstructed at the time of initial exstrophy closure. The bifid clitoris is denuded medially and brought together in the midline, along with labia minora reconstruction, creating a fourchette.

Postoperatively it is critical to control pain and bladder spasms to prevent urine extravasation and fistula formation. This is best achieved by preoperative placement of a caudal epidural catheter and the administration of anticholinergic medication. At the time of discharge, the postoperative plastic occlusive dressing is left intact and the patient is supplied with oral broad-spectrum antibiotics, pain medications, and antispasmodics.

## Continence and Antireflux Procedure

The bladder is opened through a transverse incision at the bladder neck with a vertical incision (Fig. 111.4A). Figure 111.4 depicts a Cohen transtrigonal ureteral reimplantation or a cephalotrigonal reimplantation for either moving the ureter across the bladder above the trigone or, if the ureters are too low, moving them on the upper aspect of the trigone (Fig. 111.4B). The modified Young–Dees–Leadbetter procedure is begun by selecting a posterior strip of mucosa 15 to 18 mm wide and 30 mm long that extends from the midtrigone to the prostate or posterior urethra (Fig. 111.4C). The bladder muscle lateral to the mucosal strip is denuded of mucosa and sponges, soaked in 1:200,000 epinephrine, and applied to control bleeding for better visualization. Tailoring of the muscle triangles is aided by multiple small incisions on the free edge bilaterally that allow the area of reconstruction to assume a more cephalic position (Fig. 111.4D). A transverse, full-thickness muscular incision is not performed as described in the original Young–Dees–Leadbetter procedure because there is a significant risk of denervation and ischemia for the bladder neck. The edges of the mucosa and underlying muscle are closed with interrupted sutures of 4-0 polyglycolic acid (Fig. 111.4E). The adjacent denuded muscle flaps are overlapped and sutured firmly in place with a 3-0 polydioxanone to provide reinforcement of the bladder neck and urethral reconstruction (Fig. 111.4F,G). Two or three of the overlapping sutures are left long, brought through the rectus fascia, and tied as bladder suspension to elevate the bladder neck (Fig. 111.4G). An 8Fr urethral stent may be used during construction but is removed afterward. Exposure is essential for the creation of a continent bladder neck. Therefore, if visualization of the posterior urethra is problematic, the

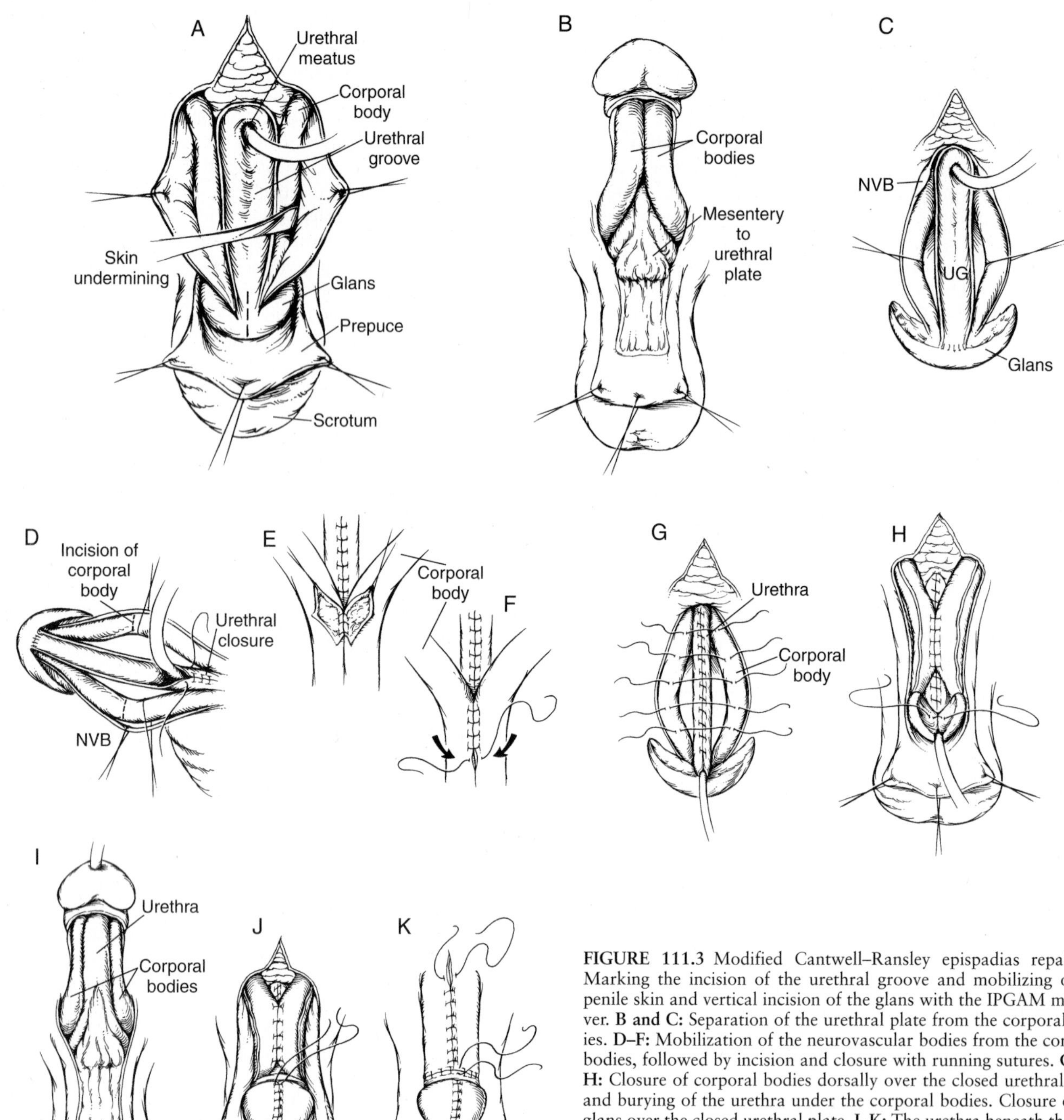


FIGURE 111.3 Modified Cantwell–Ransley epispadias repair. **A:** Marking the incision of the urethral groove and mobilizing of the penile skin and vertical incision of the glans with the IPGAM maneuver. **B and C:** Separation of the urethral plate from the corporal bodies. **D–F:** Mobilization of the neurovascular bodies from the corporal bodies, followed by incision and closure with running sutures. **G and H:** Closure of corporal bodies dorsally over the closed urethral plate and burying of the urethra under the corporal bodies. Closure of the glans over the closed urethral plate. **I–K:** The urethra beneath the corporal bodies and the mesentery is coming from the foreskin. The ventral foreskin is split and sewn to the corporal margin and to itself in the midline. (Drawings by Timothy Phelps after Leon Schlossberg. ©2002 Brady Urological Institute, with permission.)

intrasymphyseal bar has to be cut and afterward approximated with 0 PDS nylon sutures. In this case the child should be immobilized postoperatively.

The ureteral stents are removed after 10 to 12 days and the suprapubic catheter is clamped after 3 weeks, for no longer than 1 hour for the first time. After residual-free voiding is achieved, the suprapubic catheter is removed. The patient is followed up with frequent bladder and renal ultrasounds in the first few months.

# OUTCOMES

## Complications

Failure of the closure is marked by dehiscence, prolapse, or outlet obstruction. It is possible that these complications are underreported secondary to patients changing surgeons following an initially undesirable outcome. Osteomy is recommended at the

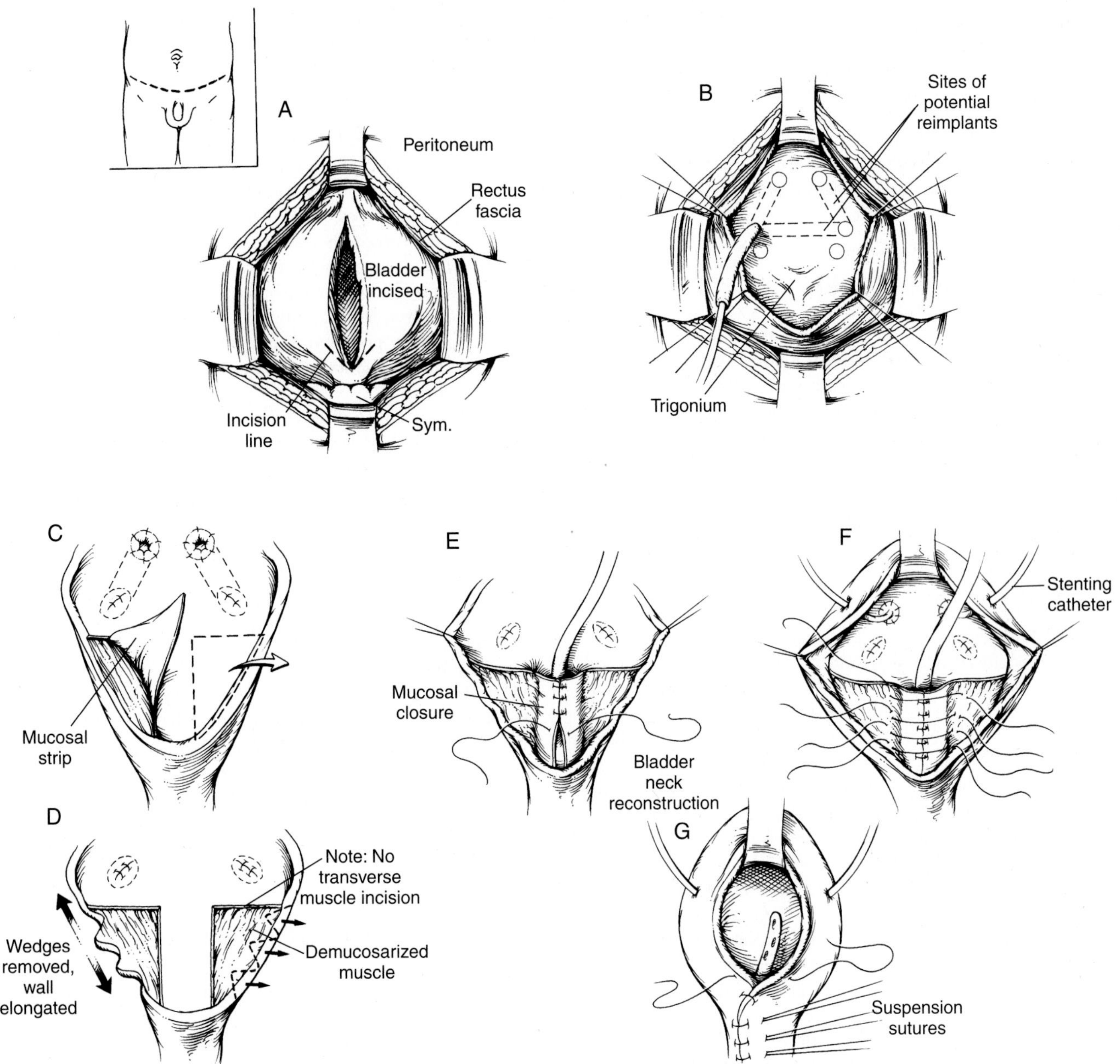


**FIGURE 111.4** Modified Young–Dees–Leadbetter bladder neck repair. **A:** Vertical bladder incision with transverse extension distally. **B and C:** Ureteral mobilization for ureteral reimplantation. **C–E:** Use of mucosal trigone strip to form the bladder neck and prostatic urethra. Lengthening of the denuded muscle triangles by several incisions. Note: No transverse muscle incision. **E–G:** Double-breasted closure and exact suture placement of the bladder neck reconstruction. The bladder neck and urethra are unstented at the end of the operation. (Drawings by Timothy Phelps after Leon Schlossberg. ©2002 Brady Urological Institute, with permission.)

time of secondary closure in all cases. Outlet obstruction may develop early following removal of the urethral catheter. Surveillance of residual volumes and upper-tract dilation with ultrasound is important following removal of the urethral catheter and prior to removing the suprapubic tube. The development of pyelonephritis is likewise a cause for evaluation of the bladder outlet following primary closure. In some cases, calibration and temporary catheter replacement are sufficient. We prefer to calibrate under anesthesia with a cystoscope because this allows for precise catheter placement if needed.

The incidence of urethrocutaneous fistulas following Cantwell-Ransley epispadias repair is 19% at 3 months (22). Some of these will close spontaneously. The majority, however, will require operative repair as an outpatient procedure. Residual chordee is a common indication for revision surgery, usually as an adolescent, prior to becoming sexually active.

It is clear that the bladder needs time to adjust to the increased resistance added by the reconstructed bladder neck. Bladder spasms and detrusor instability are expected and should be treated with oral anticholinergics. The biggest challenge of the child and the parents after bladder neck reconstruction is the initiation of a voiding trial. If the child cannot void, an 8Fr catheter is placed under anesthesia and left in place for 5 days and the voiding trial is initiated again. Ultimately, if the child is not dry for a period of 3 hours during the day within 12 months of the operation, the bladder neck reconstruction has failed. Multiple options are available for these children to achieve future continence, but few will void through their urethra.

## Results

The success or failure of the initial closure is highly associated with long-term functional results. Bladders that dehisce or prolapse and require repeat closure are not likely to grow and reach the capacity needed for bladder neck reconstruction. In a review of 23 patients with one or more failed closures, we found that only 6 children reached sufficient capacity for bladder neck reconstruction, with a success rate of 50% (23). The use of osteotomy in conjunction with pelvic and lower extremity fixation has produced the best success rates at our institution and is recommended for all closures beyond the first 72 hours of life (i.e., delayed or secondary closures) (20). A recent presentation of long-term outcomes from the Seattle Children's experience with CPRE reported dehiscence in 2 of 41 patients closed primarily and during the newborn period (24). In a comparable group of 194 primary MSRE closures at Johns Hopkins, 63 of which had simultaneous osteotomy, there were 4 failures (2 dehiscence and 2 prolapse) (25). Interpretation of continence rates requires consideration for the definition applied and the manner in which the child voids/empties. The ultimate goal remains continence, day and night, with volitional voiding and stable renal function. Daytime dry intervals vary in the literature from 1 to 3 hours. "Social" continence refers to an adequate daytime dry interval with bedtime wetness. The use of catheterizable stomas, with or without bladder augmentation and additional outlet procedures such as artificial urinary sphincters, slings, or bladder neck, should likewise be noted when reviewing published continence rates. Chan et al. (26) reported complete and social continence rates of 77% and 91%, respectively, with urethral voiding following bladder neck repair in children treated exclusively at Johns Hopkins. Preoperative bladder capacity measured under anesthesia appears to be the primary determinant of success in these patients. Patients with capacities >100 mL are good candidates for modified Young–Dees–Leadbetter procedures (18). A small number of children have been reported to attain continence following CPRE without additional surgery at the bladder neck. Comparable continence outcomes of children undergoing CPRE with subsequent Mitchell bladder neck repair have been recently reported (24). Like the MSRE, the results of bladder neck repair following CPRE appear to be related to a successful primary closure, and in one report this was highly associated with the use of osteotomy (17). There are a number of options for salvage procedures in patients who fail bladder neck repair. Ultimately, however, several series have reinforced the fact that very few of these children will obtain continence with volitional voiding (27,28). Upper-tract dilation following exstrophy closure is common, as most of these children have significant degrees of vesicoureteric reflux. Long-term poor renal outcomes are uncommon following ureteral reimplantation at the time of continence surgery in the MSRE.

It is important to differentiate between functional and cosmetic outcomes of genitoplasty. Cosmetic outcomes rely on subjective patient interpretation. From a cosmetic standpoint, VanderBrink (29) recently reported a 92% esthetic satisfaction rate in 65 male patients undergoing genitoplasty for exstrophy/epispadias. Nineteen revision procedures were required to obtain this outcome. The majority of these cases were treated with a Cantwell–Ransley technique. From a functional standpoint, prospective studies of sexually active adults are needed to ascertain this long-term outcome. North et al. (30) recently reported International Inventory of Erectile Function (IIEF-15) and Female Sexual Function Inventory (FSFI) scores for a group of adult exstrophy males and females, respectively. When compared to controls, adult males with exstrophy reported similar scores for erection, orgasm, desire, and satisfaction. Females, on the other hand, had poor sexual satisfaction and lower scores when compared to controls in all FSFI domains. The reason for this gender dichotomy is not clear.

# CONCLUSION

The modern treatment of bladder exstrophy can be quite successful in experienced hands. A successful initial closure can place the child on the road to eventual continence and volitional voiding, while failed closures are likely to result in a less satisfactory outcome that often involves augmentation or continent diversion. These surgeries should be performed in exstrophy centers if at all possible in order to give the child born with this major birth defect the best chance at a good quality of life.

## *References*

1. Gearhart J, Mathews R. Exstrophy/epispadias. In: *Campbell-Walsh Urology* 9th ed. Philadelphia: Saunders, 2007.
2. Trendelenburg F. The treatment of ectopia vesicae. *Ann Surg* 1906;44:981.
3. Young H. Exstrophy of the bladder: the first case in which a normal bladder and urinary control have been obtained by plastic operations. *Surg Gynecol Obstet* 1942;74:729.
4. Jeffs RD. Functional closure of bladder exstrophy. *Birth Defects Original Article Series* 1977;13(5):171–173.
5. Cendron J. [Bladder reconstruction. Method derived from that of Trendelenbourg]. *Ann Chir Infant* 1971;12(6):371–381.
6. Grady RW, Mitchell ME. Complete primary repair of exstrophy. *J Urol* 1999;162(4):1415–1420.
7. Lowentritt BH, Van Zijl PS, Frimberger D, et al. Variants of the exstrophy complex: a single institution experience. *J Urol* 2005;173(5):1732–1737.
8. Gearhart JP, Ben-Chaim J, Jeffs RD, et al. Criteria for the prenatal diagnosis of classic bladder exstrophy. *Obstet Gynecol* 1995;85(6):961–964.
9. Wilson CJ, Pistrang N, Woodhouse CR, et al. The psychosocial impact of bladder exstrophy in adolescence. *J Adolesc Health* 2007;41(5):504–508.
10. Diseth TH, Emblem R, Schultz A. Mental health, psychosocial functioning, and quality of life in patients with bladder exstrophy and epispadias: an overview. *World J Urol* 1999;17(4):239–248.
11. Novak TE, Lakshmanan Y, Frimberger D, et al. Polyps in the exstrophic bladder. A cause for concern? *J Urol* 2005;174(4 Pt 2):1522–1526.

12. Cain M, Metcalfe P, Rink R. Urinary diversion. In: Docimo S, ed. *Kelalis-King-Belman Textbook of Clinical Pediatric Urology*. 5th ed. London: Informa, 2007:911–946.
13. Stockle M, Becht E, Voges G, et al. Ureterosigmoidostomy: an outdated approach to bladder exstrophy? *J Urol* 1990;143(4):770–774.
14. Schrott K. Komplette einzeitige Aufbauplastik der Blasenekstrophie. In: Schreiter F, ed. *Plastisch-rekonstruktive chirurgie in der urologie*. Stuttgart: Georg Thieme-Verlag, 1999:430–438.
15. Baka-Jakubiak M. Combined bladder neck, urethral and penile reconstruction in boys with the exstrophy-epispadias complex. *BJU Int* 2000;86(4):513–518.
16. Baird AD, Mathews RI, Gearhart JP. The use of combined bladder and epispadias repair in boys with classic bladder exstrophy: outcomes, complications and consequences. *J Urol* 2005;174(4 Pt 1):1421–1424.
17. Gearhart JP, Baird A, Nelson CP. Results of bladder neck reconstruction after newborn complete primary repair of exstrophy. *J Urol* 2007;178(4 Pt 2):1619–1622.
18. Baird AD, Nelson CP, Gearhart JP. Modern staged repair of bladder exstrophy: a contemporary series. *J Pediatr Urol* 2007;3(4):311–315.
19. Mathews R, Gearhart JP, Bhatnagar R, et al. Staged pelvic closure of extreme pubic diastasis in the exstrophy-epispadias complex. *J Urol* 2006;176(5):2196–2198.
20. Meldrum KK, Baird AD, Gearhart JP. Pelvic and extremity immobilization after bladder exstrophy closure: complications and impact on success. *Urology* 2003;62(6):1109–1113.
21. Okubadejo GO, Sponseller PD, Gearhart JP. Complications in orthopedic management of exstrophy. *J Pediatr Orthop* 2003;23(4):522–528.
22. Surer I, Baker LA, Jeffs RD, et al. The modified Cantwell-Ransley repair for exstrophy and epispadias: 10-year experience. *J Urol* 2000;164(3 Pt 2):1040–1042.
23. Gearhart JP, Ben-Chaim J, Sciortino C, et al. The multiple reoperative bladder exstrophy closure: what affects the potential of the bladder? *Urology* 1996;47(2):240–243.
24. Shnorhavorian M, Grady R, Andersen A, et al. Long-term follow-up of the complete repair of exstrophy: the Seattle Children's experience. American Academy of Pediatrics NCE, San Francisco, 2007.
25. Schaeffer A, Purves T, King J, et al. Complications of primary newborn closure of classic bladder exstrophy. American Academy of Pediatrics NCE, San Francisco, 2007.
26. Chan D, Jeffs RD, Gearhart JP. Determinants of continence in the bladder exstrophy population: predictors of success? *Urology* 2001;57(4):774–777.
27. Cervellione RM, Bianchi A, Fishwick J, et al. Salvage procedures to achieve continence after failed bladder exstrophy repair. *J Urol* 2008;179(1):304–306.
28. Burki T, Hamid R, Duffy P, et al. Long-term followup of patients after redo bladder neck reconstruction for bladder exstrophy complex. *J Urol* 2006;176(3):1138–1141.
29. VanderBrink BA, Stock JA, Hanna MK. Esthetic outcomes of genitoplasty in males born with bladder exstrophy and epispadias. *J Urol* 2007;178(4 Pt 2):1606–1610.
30. North A, Nelson C, Gearhart J, et al. Patient-reported sexual and reproductive function among adults born with classic bladder exstrophy. American Academy of Pediatrics NCE, San Francisco, 2007.

# CHAPTER 112 ■ CONGENITAL ANOMALIES OF THE SCROTUM

SEAN T. CORBETT AND DAVID R. ROTH

Isolated congenital anomalies of the scrotum, including inclusion cysts, the bifid or hypoplastic scrotum, penoscrotal transposition, and webbed penis, are unusual. Most often these anomalies are found in association with other abnormalities: penoscrotal transposition and bifid scrotum with hypospadias, bifid scrotum and scrotal ectopia with exstrophy, and scrotal hypoplasia with cryptorchidism. When these anomalies occur in conjunction with other genital abnormalities, the scrotum can be surgically repaired with excellent results at the time of the procedure to correct the primary anomaly. It is important, however, that neonatal circumcision be avoided in boys with genital anomalies because the prepuce may be required for reconstruction of the penis and its presence will allow greater flexibility for the surgeon.

## DIAGNOSIS

The diagnosis of scrotal congenital anomalies is made by physical examination. Rarely do these anomalies occur as solitary lesions, and the patient should be appropriately evaluated for associated anomalies. The physician should examine the scrotum for its relative position to the penis, rectum, and median raphe. The appearance of the scrotum should be noted with attention to symmetry and distribution of its rugations. The testes, penis, urethra, and rectum should be inspected to ensure that they are normal.

## INDICATIONS FOR SURGERY

Timing of the surgical repair of urogenital anomalies is important with regard to feasibility of the surgery, safety of the surgery to the patient, and the psychological impact of the anomaly and surgery. Because congenital scrotal anomalies do not interfere with urinary function, repair can be scheduled at the time that is most appropriate for the infant and most convenient for parents and physicians. Technically, from the surgeon's point of view, there is little to be gained by delaying surgery beyond the child's fourth to sixth month because by that time the genitalia have developed to sufficient size for easy reconstruction. With optical magnification and the standardization of fine sutures, excellent results can be expected even in the very young child. In addition to the degree of scrotal development, the safety of anesthetics has always been a concern in determining the minimum age at which an operation seems appropriate. However, as a result of the proliferation of specially trained and dedicated pediatric anesthesiologists, the anesthetic complication rate has reached a nadir at approximately 3 months of age. To delay repair beyond that time is no longer necessary in centers dedicated to pediatric surgery.

Psychological concerns limit the opposite end of the time spectrum (1). The child's anxiety concerning hospitalization, gender identity, and subsequent sexual development must be considered. If genital surgery is performed before the child is 18 months of age, he neither remembers the surgery nor associates the experience with an abnormality of his penis or scrotum. Therefore, a window (4 to 18 months) exists for surgery, limited on the younger side by both anesthetic and technical concerns and on the older side by memory and psychological issues. Parents need to determine a time during that 14-month period that is best for their schedules. Because most of these surgical repairs require only external relocation of skin, they usually can be performed on an outpatient basis and only rarely with a hospital stay of a single night. A further consideration is that it is easier for parents to care postoperatively for a boy who is younger and not yet walking.

Certain technical points are relevant to all of these operations and warrant mentioning. For instance, optical magnification has proved to be very useful. Several companies now make loupes in powers of 2.5× to 4.5× that practitioners have found to be invaluable when performing delicate surgery on the genitalia. Also helpful are the fine (6-0 to 8-0) absorbable (plain, chromic) sutures, which are excellent materials with which to repair a child's scrotum. They do not have to be removed and are absorbed quickly, so skin tracks are unlikely to form. The use of tissue expanders for progressive skin dilatation, as in the cases of hypoplastic/absent scrotum, has offered a viable alternative to myocutaneous flaps, which often result in a poor cosmetic result in the pediatric population. Finally, prophylactic antibiotics are seldom necessary in uncomplicated cases with the prepubertal child.

## ALTERNATIVE THERAPY

There are no alternatives to surgical correction of the congenital anomaly. On the other hand, nontreatment is an option, and reconstructive surgery can be delayed until the boy can participate in the decision to proceed. The psychological advantage of earlier surgery would need to be weighed against the importance of allowing the youngster to be involved in the decision-making process.

## SURGICAL TECHNIQUE

### Bifid Scrotum

Isolated bifid scrotum is rare. When it occurs, the corpus spongiosum appears to be continuous with a prominent median raphe of the scrotum, a fibrous band that separates and divides the scrotum into two individual parts. Surgical reapproximation of the two hemiscrotums can be achieved after excision of the fibrous midline band. The underlying urethra must be preserved and allowed to fall away from the dense band. This requires mobilization of each hemiscrotum to the extent that it can be elevated and moved medially to the midline. Closure is accomplished in at least two layers. Deep absorbable sutures allow fixation and reconstruction of the midline. Fine absorbable sutures should be used to close the skin. In general, interrupted simple sutures are used, but a running subcuticular closure may also be utilized.

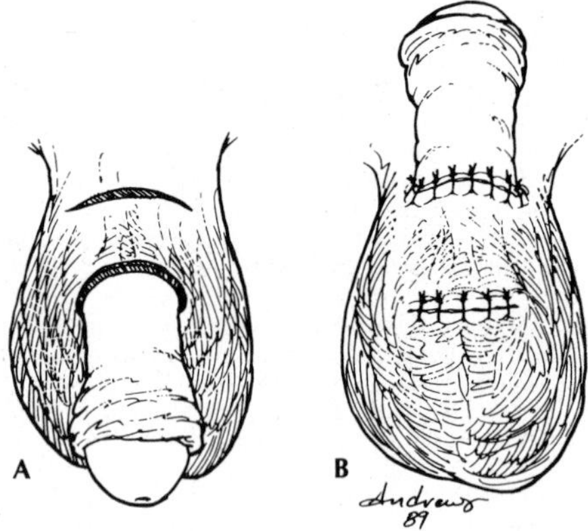


FIGURE 112.1 **A:** In the moderately severe case of penoscrotal transposition, the phallus is circumscribed and freed of supporting tissue. An incision is made cephalad to the base of the phallus. **B:** The penis can then be brought back through the new opening and the skin sutured about it. The original opening is then sewn closed.

### Penoscrotal Transposition

Various degrees of penoscrotal transposition exist, ranging from the complete form, in which the scrotum is actually anterior and cephalad to the base of the penis, to incomplete forms, in which the penis emerges from the center of the scrotum, and the milder forms, in which only the superior edges of the scrotum lie anterior to the penis. For correction of the anomaly, the two hemiscrotums are mobilized, swept inferiorly and medially, and sutured together. It may be necessary to transpose the penis cephalad to the scrotum. This can be achieved by using a skin bridge (Fig. 112.1) or by dividing the abnormal scrotum in its midline cephalad and caudal to the phallus and swinging both halves below the penis (Fig. 112.2) (2). Some authors suggest leaving a segment of skin intact cephalad to the penis to avoid jeopardizing the vascularity and lymphatic drainage of the penile shaft skin. Other authors advocate the creation of a

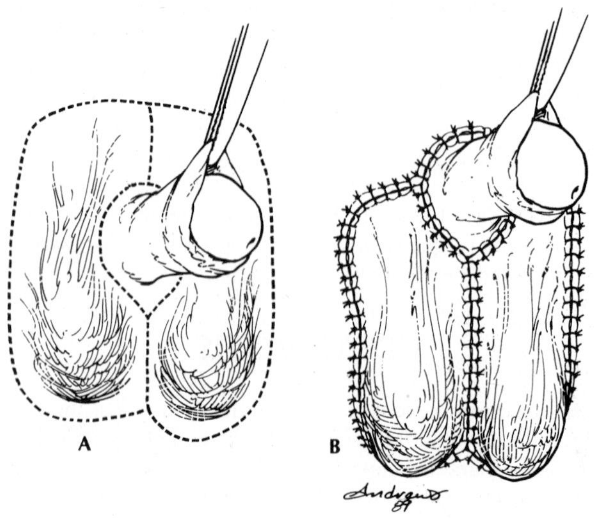


FIGURE 112.2 **A:** In the more severe case of penoscrotal transposition, each hemiscrotum is circumscribed. **B:** Once each side is freed to rotate caudally and medially the two portions are sewn together. Some authors suggest leaving a bridge of skin cephalad to decrease the possibility of a vascular insult.

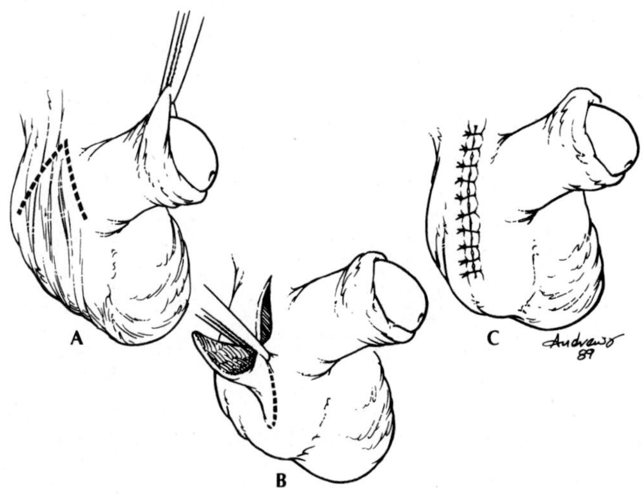


FIGURE 112.3 **A and B:** In the mild case of penoscrotal transformation, a V-shaped wedge of ectopic scrotal skin is excised. **C:** The defect is then closed, thereby eliminating the ectopic scrotal skin.

suprapubic buttonhole through which the penis can be delivered (3,4). For less severe cases of penoscrotal transposition, the wedge of ectopic scrotal skin is removed and the resultant defect closed, thereby eliminating the problem (5). This approach is most appropriate when there is incomplete mild penoscrotal transposition (Fig. 112.3). The penoscrotal angle can be recreated by anchoring sutures applied to the underlying fascia and corresponding skin. Fixation of the penopubic angle can also be performed in a similar fashion. The anchoring sutures may have the additional benefit of stabilizing penile length (6,7).

## Scrotal Hypoplasia

Scrotal hypoplasia is almost always restricted to boys with cryptorchidism. A limited course of androgen stimulation (testosterone enanthate 2 mg/kg intramuscularly) will induce scrotal development and enlargement in addition to increasing penile length and glans circumference (8). This allows easier surgical placement of either a testis or prosthesis in the poorly developed scrotum at the time of inguinal surgery for the undescended testis. The hormonal treatment should be undertaken only in conjunction with either an orchiopexy or placement of a testicular prosthesis because the effects of the testosterone are temporary; if the scrotum is not distended, it may revert to its hypoplastic appearance. In severe cases of scrotal hypoplasia or the rare case of congenital scrotal agenesis, tissue expanders may be used as another alternative where there is inadequate space for the testis or prosthesis. The expanders can be used to progressively dilate the scrotum to an adequate size (3). Placement of a testicular prosthesis before puberty is not routinely advocated as these children will outgrow their prosthesis and need a larger size at a later date.

## Scrotal Ectopia

Although less common than either scrotal transposition or a bifid scrotum and usually associated with cloacal exstrophy, scrotal ectopia on occasion is found in the otherwise normal child (9). The ectopic scrotal tissue can be found on the inner aspect of the thigh or caudal and inferior to the external inguinal ring. Often, the ipsilateral testis can be found within the ectopic tissue. Correction is accomplished by relocating the ectopic tissue, by way of a flap or graft, or by utilizing the normally positioned contralateral hemiscrotum as a reservoir for both gonads and discarding the ectopic tissue (10). The latter can be accomplished by stretching local tissue either primarily or after pretreatment with parenteral testosterone enanthate (2 mg/kg intramuscularly). The ectopic scrotal tissue in that case can then be excised.

## Webbed Penis

In boys with a webbed penis, scrotal skin is tethered to the ventrum of the penile shaft. This tethering produces a web of skin stretching from the penis to the scrotal base. The webbed penis causes no problem during childhood. However, as the scrotal skin is hair-bearing, future intercourse could be difficult or uncomfortable. Therefore, a webbed penis should be corrected during infancy. A modified circumcision can often correct the defect. The circumcision incision is brought more distal than normal on the ventrum, thereby preserving all penile shaft skin possible in that location. After the inner preputial skin is excised, the additional length on the ventrum allows the scrotum to fall away from the glans and penis. If necessary, skin from the dorsum can be mobilized and swept ventrally to provide additional shaft skin (Fig. 112.4). A second type of repair can be performed by incising the web transversely and closing it longitudinally, thereby separating the penis from the median raphe of the scrotum. A circumcision should be considered at the same time because it facilitates the approximation of the skin (Fig. 112.5).

In more severe cases of webbed penis, a U-shaped incision is made about the phallus (11). This releases the penis from the dependent scrotum. Flaps are developed to allow ventral closure of the penis with fine absorbable sutures. The scrotum is closed in a side-to-side manner (Fig. 112.6). In a manner

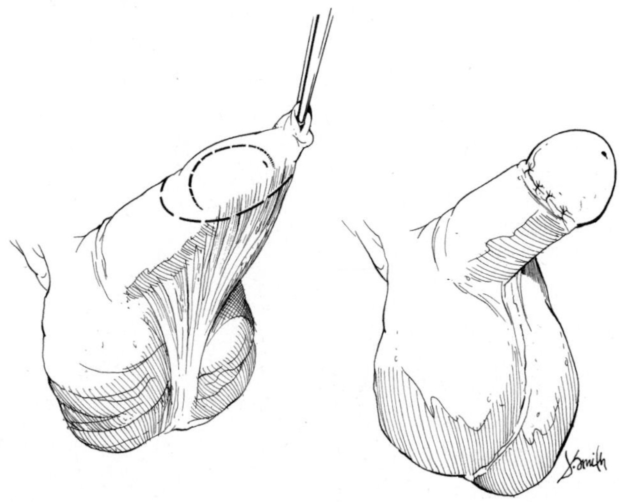

FIGURE 112.4 In the mildly webbed penis, a modified circumcision may be all that is required. With the ventral incision made at the phimotic band, the ventral skin can be repositioned to cover the penile shaft appropriately.

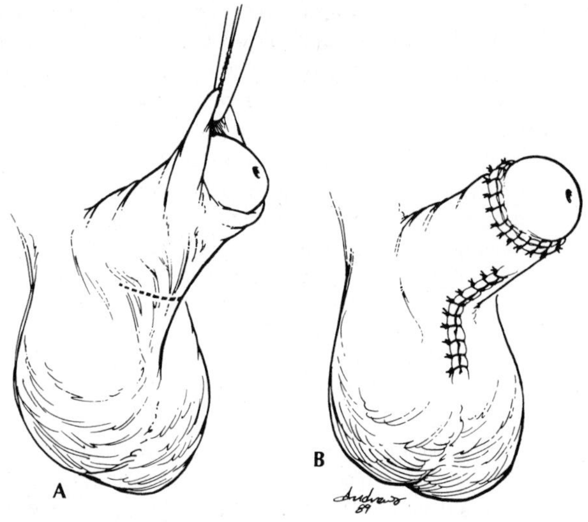


FIGURE 112.5 In the moderately webbed penis, the defect can be repaired by (**A**) transversely incising the web and (**B**) closing it longitudinally. As in the mild cases, a modified circumcision incision with preservation of all the ventral skin can be helpful in recovering the penile shaft.

similar to cases of penoscrotal transposition, the penoscrotal angle can be recreated by the placement of anchoring sutures securing the skin to the underlying fascia.

### Scrotal Inclusion Cysts

Midline scrotal inclusion cysts are in general dermatoid in origin and can be managed by local excision (12). However, care must be taken not to confuse these with the sinus associated with an imperforate anus. Both are located in the median raphe and can be multiple. Because cysts can lead to calculi formation or infection, local excision should be considered.

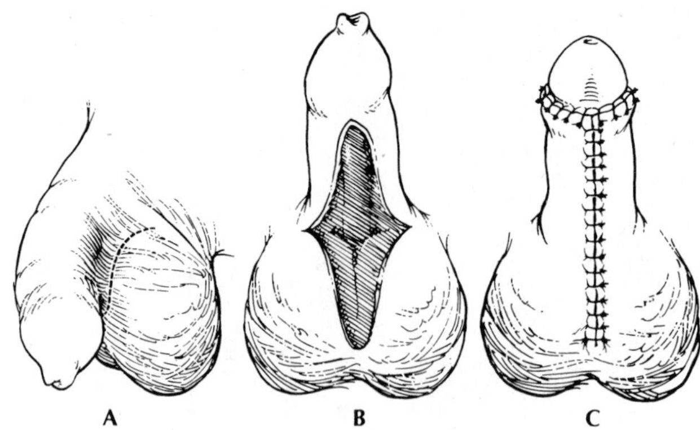


FIGURE 112.6 **A:** In a severely webbed penis, an incision is made between the penis and scrotum. **B:** Skin flaps are elevated in all directions so that the surgical defect can be closed. **C:** A two-layer closure is used to stabilize and approximate the skin and underlying tissues.

## OUTCOMES

### Complications

Complications from these surgeries are in general uncommon. Superficial infections can be treated with antibiotics.

### Results

The cosmetic results of this surgery are usually excellent.

## *References*

1. Schultz JP, Klykylo WM, Wacksman J. Timing of elective hypospadias repair in children. *Pediatrics* 1996;97:590–594.
2. Glenn JF, Anderson EE. Surgical correction of incomplete penoscrotal transposition. *J Urol* 1973;110:603–605.
3. Janoff DM, Skoog, SJ. Congenital scrotal agenesis: description of a rare anomaly and management strategies. *J Urol* 2005;173:589–591.
4. Kolligian ME, Franco I, Reda EF. Correction of penoscrotal transposition: a novel approach. *J Urol* 2000;164:994–997.
5. Redman JF. The surgical correction of incomplete scrotal transposition associated with hypospadias. *J Urol* 1983;129:565–567.
6. Borsellino A, Spagnoll A, Vallasciani S, et al. Surgical approach to concealed penis: technical refinements and outcome. *Urology* 2007;69: 1195–1198.
7. Casale AJ, Beck SD, Cain MP, et al. Concealed penis in childhood: a spectrum of etiology and treatment. *J Urol* 1999;162:1165–1168.
8. Gearhart JP, Jeffs RD. Use of parenteral testosterone therapy in genital reconstructive surgery. *J Urol* 1987;138:1077–1078.
9. Lamm DL, Kaplan GW. Accessory and ectopic scrota. *Urology* 1977;9: 149–153.
10. Spears T, Franco I, Reda EF, et al. Accessory and ectopic scrotum with VATER association. *Urology* 1992;40:343–345.
11. Perlmutter AD, Chamberlain JW. Webbed penis without chordee. *J Urol* 1972;107:320–321.
12. Hamada Y, Sakiyama H, Nakashima K, et al. Median raphe cysts and canal of the penis. *Eur Urol* 1982;8:312–313.

# CHAPTER 113 ■ PEDIATRIC CRYPTORCHIDISM, HYDROCELES, AND HERNIAS

KENNETH G. NEPPLE AND CHRISTOPHER S. COOPER

Between 3% and 5% of full-term boys are born with an undescended testicle. Often associated with the undescended testicle is a patent process vaginalis that predisposes to hydrocele and hernia formation. The urologist treating the infant with an undescended testicle must therefore be familiar with the anatomy (Fig. 113.1) and operative techniques employed in treating this common condition. This familiarity assists with orchiopexy and hydrocele and hernia repair.

## CRYPTORCHIDISM

Cryptorchidism includes the strict definition of a hidden or nonpalpable testicle as well as a testicle that is undescended but palpable in the inguinal canal. True undescended testicles stop along the normal path of descent into the scrotum. They may remain in the abdominal cavity (least common), in the

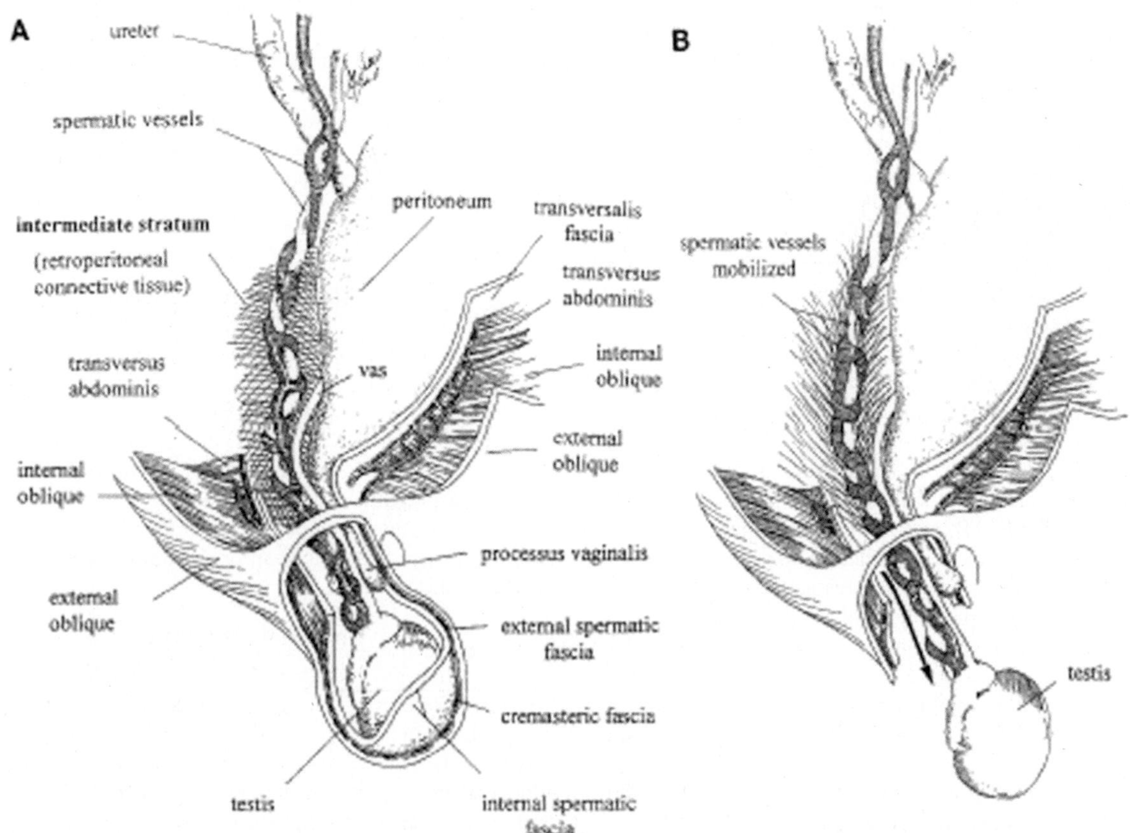


FIGURE 113.1 Anatomy of inguinal orchiopexy. **A:** Relationship of the vas deferens, spermatic vessels, and processus vaginalis to investing fascial layers. The transversalis fascia is contiguous with internal spermatic fascia. **B:** With tension applied to the cord (*arrow*), the orientation of the fibers of the intermediate stratum investing the retroperitoneal spermatic cord is changed so that fibers become parallel to cord structures. Freeing the vas and vessels from this investing fascia is the most important step in achieving distal testicular displacement. (From Hutcheson JC, Cooper CS, Snyder HM III. The anatomical approach to inguinal orchiopexy. *J Urol* 2000;164:1702–1704, with permission.)

inguinal canal (canalicular), or just outside the external ring (suprascrotal, most common). Testes may also pass through the external ring and then be located ectopically, most commonly in a superficial inguinal pouch. The incidence of undescended testicles increases from 3% to 5% in full-term infants to 30% in premature infants. Low birth weight has also been shown to be a predictor of cryptorchidism, independent of gestational age. Most of these testicles descend within the first 6 months of life, and by 1 year of age the prevalence is 1%. The left testicle is affected more often, and 1% to 2% of children with cryptorchidism will have both testicles affected. Twenty percent of boys who present with cryptorchidism have one nonpalpable testis. Of nonpalpable testes, 20% are intra-abdominal, 40% are canalicular, scrotal, or ectopic testes, and 40% are atrophic or absent.

## Diagnosis

The diagnosis of cryptorchidism relies on the physical examination. Absence of an identifiable testicle with ultrasound, computed tomography, or magnetic resonance imaging does not prove testicular agenesis and therefore does not alter the need for surgical exploration. The testicular examination in the infant and young child requires two hands and patient relaxation. One hand is placed near the anterior superior iliac spine and the other on the scrotum. The first hand is swept from the anterior iliac spine along the inguinal canal to gently express any retained testicular tissue into the scrotum. Placing soap on the fingertips of the palpating hand may improve the sensitivity of palpation. A true undescended or ectopic inguinal testis may slide or "pop" under the examiner's fingers during this maneuver. A low ectopic or retractile testis will be felt by the second hand as the testis is milked toward the scrotum by the first hand. To distinguish a retractile testicle, the testicle is brought into the scrotal position; holding it in place for at least 1 minute fatigues the cremaster muscle. After this maneuver, a retractile testicle remains in the scrotum, whereas an ectopic or undescended testis immediately springs out of the scrotum. If a testis cannot be palpated in the inguinal canal or the scrotum, or in the typical ectopic sites, evaluation for a nonpalpable testis must be performed.

A child with bilateral nonpalpable testes should undergo hormonal evaluation for testicular absence (1). Elevations in luteinizing hormone (LH) and follicle-stimulating hormone (FSH) and absence of detectable müllerian inhibiting substance (MIS) suggest testicular absence (2). Testicular absence is confirmed by a negative human chorionic gonadotropin (HCG) stimulation test. The HCG stimulation test is performed by the administration of intramuscular HCG (2,000 IU per day for 3 to 4 days) (3). Raised gonadotropin levels (FSH and LH) *and* a lack of a testosterone rise from HCG indicate bilateral absent testes and a formal surgical exploration is not necessary. When one or both components are lacking or there is detectable MIS, surgical exploration is warranted.

## Indications for Surgery

Treatment of the undescended testicle offers the possibility of improved fertility, correction of patent processus vaginalis, prevention of testis torsion, and improvement in body image. There is controversy whether orchiopexy decreases the risk of malignancy, but placement of an undescended testicle in the scrotum assists physical examination of the testis. Because histologic changes related to fertility occur in the undescended testicle as young as 1 year of age and spontaneous descent rarely occurs after 6 months of age, the optimal time for surgical correction is around 6 months of age.

Almost 90% of undescended testes have an associated patent processus vaginalis. If a patient with cryptorchidism presents with an incarcerated or strangulated inguinal hernia, repair at the time of presentation along with orchiopexy should be undertaken. Otherwise, the hernia should be repaired at the time of orchiopexy. Occult inguinal hernia in patients with untreated undescended testis can present at any time with the typical symptoms or complications, including incarceration.

## Alternative Therapy

Hormonal therapy is an option in the treatment of cryptorchidism because the condition may be related to hypogonadotropic hypogonadism. HCG is the only hormone approved for use in the treatment of cryptorchidism in the United States. Side effects of administration of HCG include enlargement of the penis, growth of pubic hair, increased testicular size, and aggressive behavior during administration. The likelihood of success with hormonal therapy is greatest for the most distal undescended testes or for testes that have been previously descended (4). Some suggest that hormonal therapy is effective only for retractile and not truly undescended testes (5). Although hormonal therapy may not be effective in achieving testicular descent, it may improve fertility in cryptorchid boys (6).

## Surgical Technique

Prior to any surgical intervention, the patient is re-examined while under anesthesia because on occasion a retractile testicle descends under anesthesia or a previously nonpalpable testicle becomes palpable. A bimanual examination with a finger in the rectum may permit detection of an intra-abdominal testicle. For a palpable testicle an open inguinal approach is performed. For the nonpalpable testicle in a child a laparoscopic approach is preferred, but an open inguinal approach may be performed.

### Inguinal Orchiopexy

Preoperative antibiotics (cefazolin 25 mg/kg) are administered and operating loupes can be used for magnification. A 3- to 4-cm incision along the lines of Langer is made in a groin crease one third of the way between the pubic tubercle and the anterior superior iliac spine (Fig. 113.2). The incision is carried through subcutaneous fat and the fascia of Scarpa to the level of the anterior aspect of the inguinal canal using Metzenbaum scissors. Overlying fat and fascia are cleared off the external oblique fascia to its lateral shelf. An ectopic testicle may be visualized exiting through the external ring. The external ring is visualized and the anterior aspect of the inguinal canal is incised by nicking the fascia with a scalpel blade. An incision placed too far medial makes cord

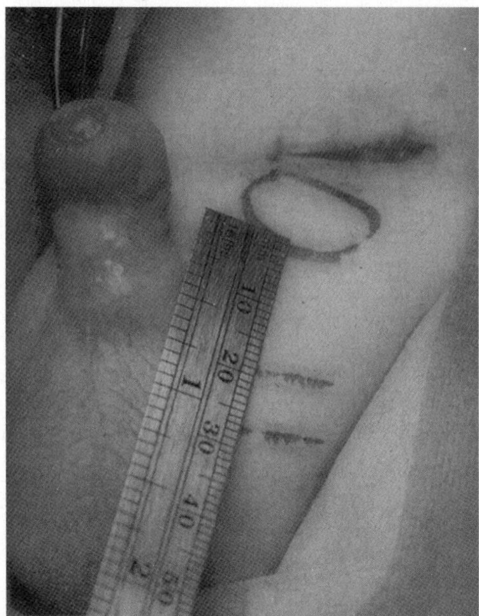

FIGURE 113.2 Incision for left orchiopexy.

identification more difficult, while an incision too far lateral makes fascia closure more difficult. Metzenbaum scissors with the tips facing upward are inserted into the nick and used to spread the adjacent tissue away while taking care to identify and protect the underlying ilioinguinal nerve. The roof of the inguinal canal is then opened along the course of its fibers downward toward and through the external ring. The spermatic cord is identified and elevated and dissected free of the anterior cremaster fibers using blunt dissection and DeBakey forceps. If no cord structures are identified, attention is turned to the level of the internal ring, and by application of abdominal pressure and retraction in the internal ring frequently a testicle may be identified just inside the internal ring. If no testicle is identified, the peritoneum is opened and a search is made for either a testicle or a blind-ending vas and vessels (see below). Blind-ending spermatic vessels must be identified to confirm absence of a testicle as a blind-ending vas does not guarantee testicular absence.

After identification of the testicle and spermatic cord in the canal, the gubernaculum is divided sharply after placement of 4-0 Vicryl sutures. Placement of a hemostat on the proximal end for traction provides a means of manipulating the testicle and cord structures safely. Care must be taken at this point to avoid a long-looped vas deferens that sometimes extends distally. Elevation of the cord permits blunt sweeping dissection of the inferior cremaster fibers proximally to the level of the internal ring. By placing a retractor in the internal ring and pulling the cord and attached peritoneum medially, the surgeon gains access to the retroperitoneal space along the lateral aspect of the internal ring, which is enveloped in the endopelvic fascia. The cord and peritoneum may then be swept anterior and medial with blunt dissection in the retroperitoneal space.

The intermediate stratum, an extension of connective tissue that envelopes the spermatic vessels and vas deferens in the retroperitoneum, is located between the inner striatum (connective tissue of the peritoneum) and the outer striatum (transversalis fascia). As the vas joins the vessels in the inguinal canal, the

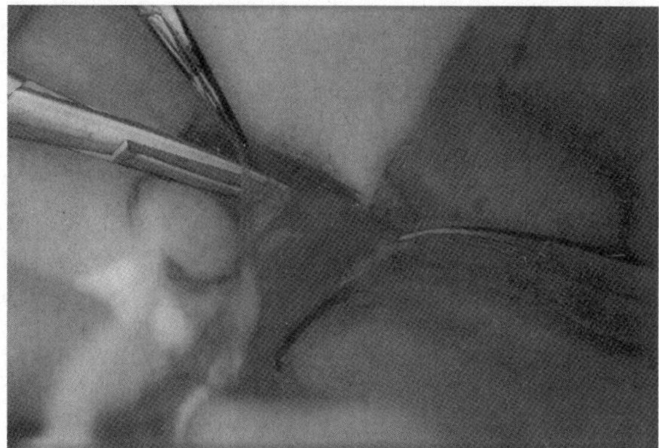

FIGURE 113.3 Isolation of cord structures during orchiopexy.

fibers of the intermediate stratum attenuate and the structures (vas, vessels, processus vaginalis) are enveloped by the internal spermatic fascia, which is an extension of the transversalis fascia from the floor of the inguinal canal. To free the remaining anterior and medial retroperitoneal attachments to the spermatic vessels and vas deferens, the internal spermatic fascia must be divided, allowing separation of the processus and contiguous peritoneum from the vas and vessels and complete access to the retroperitoneum (Fig. 113.3).

With a nonpatent processus vaginalis, a hemostat providing anterior traction on the tip of the peritoneal reflection permits dissection of the underlying cord from the internal spermatic fascia binding it to the peritoneum. With a patent processes vaginalis, the posterior cord is exposed, the internal spermatic fascia is swept off the cord structures, and the processus vaginalis is freed to the level of the peritoneum. The processus vaginalis is incised and the edges can be held and the processus can be flattened and readily dissected from the underlying cord. The processus is twisted and ligated at the level of the peritoneum with a 3-0 or 4-0 Vicryl suture.

The anterior and medial retroperitoneal attachments to the cord may be approached by placing a retractor anterior to the vessels in the internal ring, allowing the bands of the retroperitoneal fascia to be bluntly dissected from the vessels to obtain increased cord length. The beginning of the retroperitoneum is marked by the divergence of the vas medially and inferiorly. The circumferential dissection of the vessels can be extended in the retroperitoneum up to the level of the renal hilum if the need arises to gain additional cord length so the testicle can reach the scrotum without tension. True skeletonization of the vas and vessels should be avoided as this can lead to testicular atrophy. The limiting factor on length is most often the spermatic vessels rather than the vas deferens (Fig. 113.4). To gain additional length a Prentiss maneuver can be performed by using a right angle to puncture through the floor of the inguinal canal near the pubic tubercle and then passing the testicle directly under the transversalis fascia towards the scrotum, in effect moving the course of the vessels toward the midline with alignment of the internal and external rings.

With an absent testicle, blind-ending vas and vessels may be encountered in the inguinal canal. The tubular structures in the canal must be traced proximally to the internal ring, where the divergence of the vas and vessels helps the surgeon positively identify the spermatic vessels. With identification of blind-ending spermatic vessels, no further exploration for a

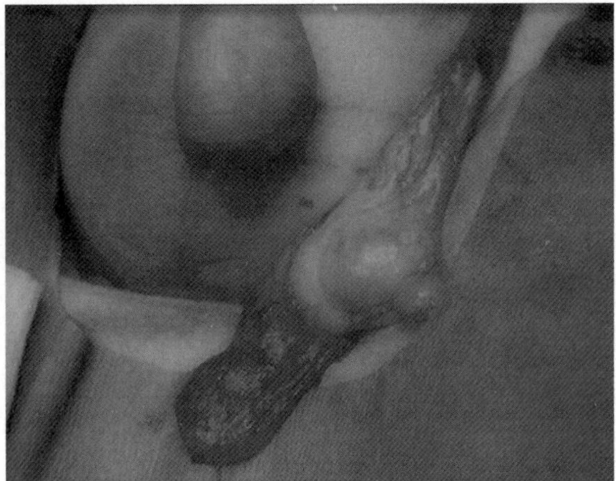

FIGURE 113.4 After dissection, adequate spermatic cord length is demonstrated.

testis is indicated. However, a blind-ending vas deferens is not sufficient reason to stop the exploration because there are patients with a wide separation of the vas and an intra-abdominal testis. When no spermatic cord structures are identified in the inguinal canal, the dissection is carried to the internal ring and into the retroperitoneum. If no structures are identified, the peritoneum is opened and the testicle or blind-ending spermatic vessels are sought.

Repeat inguinal exploration for a failed orchiopexy is associated with scar tissue surrounding the testicle and spermatic cord causing adherence to the underside of the external oblique fascia. Following the inguinal incision, the testicle should be identified and freed from surrounding scar tissue. Once this is accomplished, the cord can usually be freed along its posterior aspect extending through the inguinal canal. No attempt is made to dissect the cord from the scar extending along its anterior surface and the overlying external oblique fascia. By cutting the fascia along the medial and lateral sides of the cord and then connecting these incisions above the internal oblique muscle, a strip of fascia is left attached to the cord as described by Cartwright et al. (Fig. 113.5). The peritoneum may then be opened and the spermatic vessels freed as described above. At the peritoneal level there is rarely any significant scar tissue.

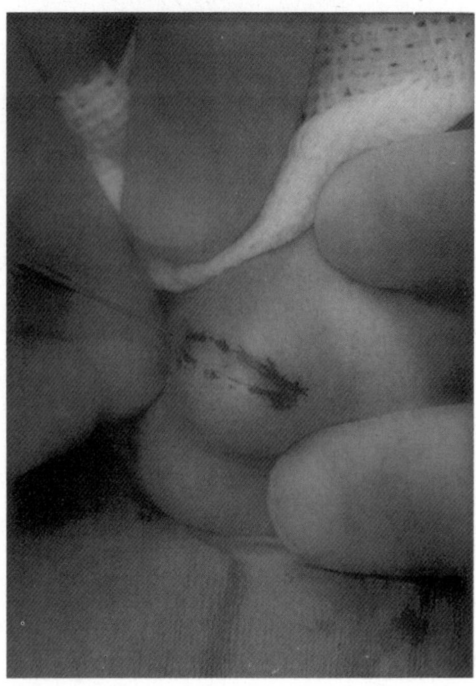

FIGURE 113.6 Incision for subdartos pouch.

## Scrotal Fixation (Subdartos Pouch)

Multiple methods have been described for fixing the testis to the scrotum, although the subdartos pouch is our preferred method because it avoids transparenchymal sutures. Following a transverse incision in the hemiscrotum (Fig. 113.6), a pocket for the testicle is created by dissecting the scrotal skin superiorly and inferiorly from the adherent underlying dartos using Ragnell orchiopexy scissors (Fig. 113.7). Care must be taken not to develop the pouch too lateral or too inferior because this could result in an ectopic testis location. The testicle is exposed by opening the tunica vaginalis. A testicular biopsy is not routinely indicated. Once adequate cord length has been obtained, the testicle is passed down from the inguinal incision using a hemostat attached to the gubernaculum. The testicle is brought through the dartos and placed in the pouch, taking care to avoid any torsion of the cord. For additional security, the inlet

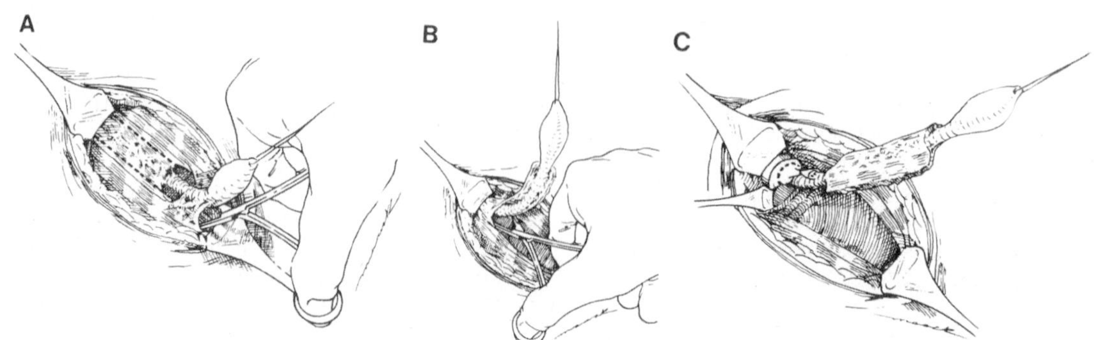


FIGURE 113.5 Reoperative orchiopexy demonstrating external oblique fascial incisions lateral and medial to the cord structure. The adherent scar tissue is dissected with the spermatic cord and no attempt is made to dissect the spermatic cord from the scar. (From Cartwright PC, Velagapudi S, Snyder HM III, et al. A surgical approach to reoperative orchiopexy. *J Urol* 1993;149:817–818, with permission.)

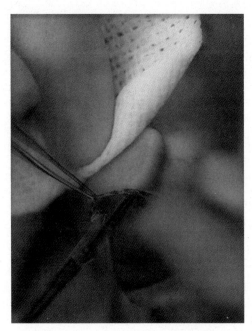

FIGURE 113.7 Creation of dartos pouch using Ragnell orchiopexy scissors.

into the pouch may be narrowed with a single polyglycolic acid suture at a diameter less than that of the testis but not so narrow as to compromise the blood supply of the testis. A small portion of the parietal tunica vaginalis or spermatic cord adventitia is incorporated into this stitch for further fixation. The use of an absorbable suture may heighten the inflammatory reaction around the testis and create a greater degree of scarring and fixation. The scrotal skin is then closed with subcuticular sutures (Fig. 113.8). For the inguinal incision, the fascia is closed with interrupted 3-0 Vicryl suture, taking care not to close the external ring too tightly, followed by closure of the subcuticular tissue with 4-0 Vicryl and skin with absorbable suture. For postoperative pain control, anesthesia can administer a caudal block, or a local nerve block with 0.25% Marcaine can be performed by the surgeon just prior to closure.

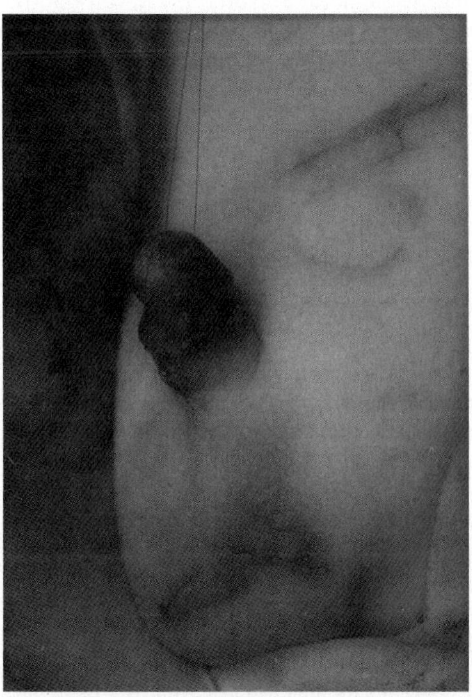

FIGURE 113.8 Successful orchiopexy shows both testes in the scrotum.

## Transperitoneal Orchiopexy

Open transperitoneal orchiopexy has been in large part replaced by laparoscopic exploration. In cases where an open approach is undertaken, an incision is made transversely or in the midline with subsequent intraperitoneal exploration. The spermatic vessels may be dissected free from their attachments cephalad to the level of their origin/insertion. With intra-abdominal testicles, this dissection should leave a broad leaf of peritoneum attached to the vas deferens along the medial aspect in case transection of the spermatic vessels is required (see below). A new external inguinal ring is created lateral to the pubic tubercle to provide the most direct route into the scrotum.

Despite a high retroperitoneal dissection, some testicles may not reach a scrotal location due to short spermatic vessels. Often, these testicles can be identified after opening the peritoneum by applying traction to the testicle and observing minimal caudal displacement and no redundancy in the spermatic vessels. In this case the surgeon must consider either bringing the testicle down as low as possible, with an anticipated reoperative orchiopexy in 6 to 12 months, or Fowler–Stephens orchiopexy, with transection of the spermatic vessels with immediate or secondary orchiopexy. A Fowler–Stephens bleeding test involves occluding the spermatic vessels for 5 minutes with atraumatic bulldog clamps and then incising the tunica albuginea toward the testicular upper pole and watching for testicular bleeding. If there is adequate bleeding a Fowler–Stephens orchiopexy is performed by ligating the spermatic vessels while a broad-based medial pedicle of peritoneum and the vas deferens are mobilized. This procedure relies on collateral blood flow to the testicle from the vas deferential artery, a branch of the inferior vesical artery, and cremasteric vessels, which branch off the inferior epigastric artery. Spermatic vessel ligation should not be done for a failed previous inguinal orchiopexy or when the vas has been skeletonized during initial orchiopexy because the collateral blood supply along the vas deferens will have been compromised and is unreliable.

An alternative is the staged testicular vessel transection orchiopexy, which involves ligation at the initial stage without mobilization to provide time for vasal collateral blood supply development. After several months, at the second stage the vessels are divided and the testicle is brought into a scrotal location after a dissection similar to that described above. A final option that is rarely utilized is testicular autotransplantation with anastomosis to the inferior epigastric artery and vein by an experienced microvascular surgeon.

## Scrotal Orchiopexy

The high transscrotal incision for testicular mobilization including ligation of an associated inguinal hernia through one incision has been applied to primary and secondary cryptorchidism, although the increased technical difficulty of inguinal herniorrhaphy and concern for gaining adequate cord length through this approach have limited its popularity. The scrotal approach may be especially suited to ectopic or ascended testes, including those that have failed prior orchiopexy. Bassel et al. (7) recently reported that scrotal incision orchiopexy was highly successful in a select group of children with palpable undescended testis that can be brought down following induction of anesthesia to the scrotum with caudal traction by the surgeon. The processus vaginalis is dissected free of cord structures and, if patent, then high suture ligation is performed. An alternative procedure is a low scrotal incision, with addition of an inguinal incision if a patent processus is encountered. A scrotal incision is made and blunt dissection is used to expose the processus vaginalis. The processus is opened and then the testis is delivered. The processus is probed and, if patent, an inguinal incision is made.

## Outcomes

### Complications

Retraction is the most common complication of orchiopexy and usually occurs secondary to an incomplete initial dissection and tension on the testicle. It is possible that some cases of retracted testicle after an orchiopexy occur because of dislodgement of the testis from the scrotum. To prevent this possibility, straddle toys are avoided for at least 3 weeks following the operation.

The most significant complication is testicular atrophy, which occurs in 1% to 2% of cases of orchiopexy, while complete devascularization of the testis is rare. The dissection of the testicular vessels and/or postoperative swelling and inflammation can result in ischemic injury with subsequent testicular atrophy. The failure rate with orchiopexy is 8% for distal undescended testes and 26% for intra-abdominal undescended testes (8). Other potential complications include ascent of the testis requiring reoperative orchiopexy, infection, bleeding, ilioinguinal nerve injury, or damage to the vas deferens.

### Results

Successful therapy, as defined by a viable testis positioned in the scrotum, is dependent on the preoperative anatomic position of the testis. Success rates are 74% for the abdominal testis, 87% for canalicular, and 92% for those distal to the external ring. Success rates for various operative techniques are 89% for the standard inguinal orchiopexy, 67% for Fowler–Stephens, 77% for staged Fowler–Stephens, 81% for transabdominal, 73% for two-stage, and 84% for microvascular (9). All of these results suggest an advantage to maintaining intact vessels where possible.

Paternity rates among men who had attempted to father children were 65%, 90%, and 93% in men with bilateral cryptorchidism, unilateral cryptorchidism, and normally descended testicles, respectively (10). If only one testis is undescended, the sperm count will be subnormal in 25% to 33% and the serum FSH concentration will be slightly elevated (11, 12). The presence of these abnormalities suggests that both testes are abnormal, perhaps congenitally, although only one fails to descend. If both testes are undescended, the sperm count usually will be severely subnormal and the serum testosterone may be reduced (12).

# HYDROCELE/HERNIA

A hydrocele consists of a collection of fluid in the tunica vaginalis around the testicle. In children this is almost always found in association with a patent processus vaginalis that permits flow of peritoneal fluid into the tunica vaginalis (communicating hydrocele). An indirect inguinal hernia forms when bowel or any other tissue from the abdominal cavity protrudes into the patent processus vaginalis. Between 0.8% and 4.4% of newborns and up to 30% of premature infants have an inguinal hernia. Boys are six times more likely than girls to have a hernia and right-sided hernias occur twice as frequently as left-sided hernias, with bilateral hernias occurring about 10% of the time.

## Diagnosis

Children with a hydrocele or hernia present with swelling in the groin and scrotum/labia. This swelling can be persistent or intermittent and may not be observed by the physician. Often, it is noted by the parents only when the child is crying or straining and the intra-abdominal pressure is elevated. In this case, the diagnosis depends on a reliable history from the parents describing the intermittent groin and scrotal swelling. Older children may be examined while standing and performing a Valsalva maneuver to increase the intra-abdominal pressure. Rarely children will present with large abdominoscrotal hydroceles that cross the internal inguinal ring and contain an intra-abdominal component resulting in a palpable abdominal mass.

With increasing size of the hydrocele, the testicle becomes more difficult to palpate and often is not palpable. Usually, a hydrocele becomes narrow at the level of the internal ring and the examiner is able to detect this narrowing and get above the swelling. With a hernia, the swelling extends through the internal ring. The fluid in a hydrocele sac will transilluminate; however, bowel can also be transilluminated, making this a nonspecific finding for either a hydrocele or a hernia. Ultrasonography may help define the testicle and rule out any testicular pathology, as well as help differentiate a hydrocele from a hernia.

## Indications for Surgery

The majority of infant hydroceles resolve by 18 months of age as the patent processus obliterates. If a hydrocele persists beyond 18 months, then it is unlikely to undergo spontaneous resolution and surgical treatment is indicated. When the fluid in a hydrocele sac is easily reduced, it suggests the size of the patent processus vaginalis is larger than with a hydrocele that does not have easily reducible fluid. This examination finding and a history of waxing and waning size of the hydrocele may serve as an indication for surgical correction before 18 months of age.

A healthy child presenting with an incarcerated hernia should undergo attempts at manually reducing the hernia. This may require sedation and placement of the child in the Trendelenburg position. Once the hernia is reduced, surgical correction should be performed within the next several days because an inguinal hernia will not resolve spontaneously and the child is at risk for repeat incarceration. If the hernia is not reducible, an emergent operation should be performed. Preterm infants with a reducible hernia may be observed during their stay in the intensive care unit until they are thought to be medically stable enough to undergo a surgical procedure.

Because of the high incidence of a contralateral patent processus, some surgeons routinely explore the contralateral groin during hernia surgery. We do not routinely explore the contralateral groin as there is only a 20% chance of developing a clinical contralateral hernia. Some physicians will perform laparoscopy through the hernia sac and examine the contralateral inguinal ring to determine if a contralateral groin exploration and hernia repair is required, and others will perform a pneumoperitoneum and feel for crepitance in the contralateral groin as an indication to operate on this side.

## Alternative Therapy

There are no alternative therapies.

## Surgical Technique

A similar inguinal incision is made for indirect hernias or communicating hydroceles as previously described in surgical technique of inguinal orchidopexy. After the inguinal canal is opened, the cremaster fibers may be spread off the anterior aspect of the spermatic cord. The bulging shiny hernia sac or patent processus vaginalis, which is typically located anterior and medial, is identified and grasped with a hemostat. By elevation of the hernia sac the cord is brought up and freed from surrounding cremaster attachments, permitting the surgeon's finger to be placed beneath the entire spermatic cord and hernia sac. Extensive dissection of cremasteric fibers need not be performed. The sac is teased off the underlying cord by breaking apart the internal spermatic fascia that encases the cord structures and the hernia sac. As this is done, the cord structures are separated from the hernia sac by passing a hemostat from lateral to medial and spreading at a 90-degree angle to separate cord from hernia sac. When the cord structures are completely freed, the sac is transected and then dissected up to the internal inguinal ring. It is important to identify the internal spermatic fascia and break this down so that when the sac is twisted and ligated, the cord structures will not become incorporated.

The hernia sac is twisted and high ligation is performed with two 4-0 Vicryl sutures and divided close to the level of the internal ring. The distal sac or hydrocele is then delivered along with the testicle into the wound, and the sac is opened down to the level of the testicle, taking care not to injure the cord structures. The authors routinely evert and sew the hydrocele sac behind the cord or testis in a Bottle technique with an absorbable suture to prevent the possible reformation of the hydrocele. Repair of the dilated internal inguinal ring may be required and is accomplished by approximation of the transversalis fascia to itself at the level of the internal ring, taking care not to strangulate the cord. The conjoined tendon may also be sutured to the shelving edge of the inguinal ligament. The testicle is then drawn back into the scrotum with traction on the scrotal skin and gubernaculum. The external oblique aponeurosis and wound are then closed with 3-0 Vicryl suture as described above.

## Outcomes

### Complications

Recurrence or persistence of the hernia or hydrocele may occur if the patent processus is not well ligated. Injury to the underlying spermatic and/or vas deferens vessels may result in testicular atrophy. Displacement of the testicle to an extrascrotal location may occur after surgery. To prevent this complication, every hydrocele and hernia repair should be concluded by confirmation of the testis location in its normal dependent scrotal position.

## *References*


1. Jarow JP, Berkovitz GD, Migeon CJ, et al. Elevation of serum gonadotropins establishes the diagnosis of anorchism in prepubertal boys with bilateral cryptorchidism. *J Urol* 1986;136:277–279.
2. Lee MM, Donahoe PK, Silverman BL, et al. Measurements of serum müllerian inhibiting substance in the evaluation of children with nonpalpable gonads. *N Engl J Med* 1997;336:1480–1486.
3. Grant DB, Laurance BM, Atherden SM, et al. hCG stimulation test in children with abnormal sexual development. *Arch Dis Child* 1976;51:596–601.
4. Kaleva M, Arsalo A, Louhimo I, et al. Treatment with human chorionic gonadotropin for cryptorchidism: clinical and histological effects. *Int J Androl* 1996;19:293–298.
5. Rajfer J, Handelsman DJ, Swerdloff RS, et al. Hormonal therapy of cryptorchidism. A randomized, double-blind study comparing human chorionic gonadotropin and gonadotropin-releasing hormone. *N Engl J Med* 1986;314:466–470.
6. Demirbilek S, Atayurt HF, Celik N, et al. Does treatment with human chorionic gonadotropin induce reversible changes in undescended testes in boys? *Pediatr Surg Int* 1997;12:591–594.
7. Bassel YS, Scherz HC, Kirsch AJ. Scrotal incision orchiopexy for undescended testes with or without a patent processus vaginalis. *J Urol* 2007;177:1516–1518.
8. Docimo SG. The results of surgical therapy for cryptorchidism: a literature review and analysis. *J Urol* 1995;154:1148–1152.
9. Hutcheson JC, Cooper CS, Snyder HM III. The anatomical approach to inguinal orchiopexy. *J Urol* 2000;164:1702–1704.
10. Lee PA, Coughlin MT. Fertility after bilateral cryptorchidism. Evaluation by paternity, hormone, and semen data. *Hormone Res* 2001;55:28–32.
11. Lipshultz LI, Caminos-Torres R, Greenspan CS, et al. Testicular function after orchiopexy for unilaterally undescended testis. *N Engl J Med* 1976;295:15–18.
12. Werder EA, Illig R, Torresani T, et al. Gonadal function in young adults after surgical treatment of cryptorchidism. *Br Med J* 1976;4:1357–1359.

# CHAPTER 114 ■ LAPAROSCOPIC MANAGEMENT OF THE UNDESCENDED TESTICLE

DANIELLE D. SWEENEY, MICHAEL C. OST, AND STEVEN G. DOCIMO

Cryptorchidism is defined as the absence of a testicle; one that is not present in the scrotum, or one that cannot be manipulated into the scrotum on physical examination. These testicles may be truly absent, due to agenesis or intrauterine torsion, or more commonly, they may have not completed their normal path of descent into the scrotum. This condition is reported in 3.4% to 5.8% of full-term boys, and the incidence decreases to about 1% at year one of life (1). Cryptorchidism is reported to be bilateral in 10% of cases (2).

Of the boys diagnosed with cryptorchidism, as many as 20% will have a nonpalpable testis (3). In this subset of patients, testicles may be absent, intra-abdominal, or within the inguinal canal (canalicular). Prior to the 1970s, surgical management of the nonpalpable testicle consisted of inguinal exploration with extension of the dissection into the peritoneum if a testis, nubbin, or blind-ending vessels could not be identified. However, Cortesi (4) described using diagnostic laparoscopy for nonpalpable testis in 1976, revolutionizing the diagnosis and surgical management of the undescended testicle. This technique has become the gold standard for the diagnosis of the intra-abdominal testis, and in urology for its surgical management.

## PREOPERATIVE ASSESSMENT

Upon the initial evaluation, a thorough history and physical examination must be obtained. Antenatal as well as maternal history for the use of gestational steroids or hormones should be elicited, as well as the birth history and physical examination at the time of delivery. The presence of palpable gonads, hypospadias, genital surgery, or inguinal herniorrhaphy should be noted, as well as a family history of cryptorchidism or other urologic syndromes.

A careful physical examination in a nonthreatening, warm environment, with warm lubricant, is crucial to identifying a subtle but palpable testicle. In children with a referral to a urologic specialist for an undescended testicle, approximately 80% will have a palpable testicle on examination (5). Contralateral testicular size should be documented to assess for compensatory hypertrophy in cases of nonpalpable or atrophic testis.

## DIAGNOSTIC ASSESSMENT

In general, radiographic imaging in the evaluation of cryptorchidism is not cost-effective or warranted. Radiologic testing, including inguinal/abdominal ultrasound, magnetic resonance imaging or magnetic resonance angiography, herniorrhaphy, venography, and arteriography, has been shown to have limited value in detection or localization of nonpalpable testicles (5,6). Even when a good examination is not obtained in the office setting, examination under anesthesia at the time of surgical exploration is generally more cost-effective than preoperative radiographic imaging (7). Surgical intervention, either open or laparoscopic, has been the only modality proven to accurately diagnose, localize, and concurrently treat the nonpalpable testicle (7). Hormonal therapy has been used to promote testicular descent; however, this is best reserved for those with bilateral nonpalpable testis and is unlikely to be cost-effective in those with unilateral cryptorchidism (8). In patients with bilateral nonpalpable testicles and a phenotypically male appearance, it is very important to rule out congenital adrenal hyperplasia and other intersex conditions.

## SURGICAL INTERVENTION

### Timing of Surgery

Optimal timing of surgery should be prior to the child's second birthday, and ideally between 6 and 12 months of age, since spontaneous testicular descent has been noted as late as 4 to 6 months of age. The overall goals of orchiopexy are to preserve testicular function and fertility, to relocate the testicle to the scrotum for easier neoplasm examination, and to prevent testicular torsion and trauma. In some cases, there is a psychological benefit of relocating the testicle to its anatomically correct position.

At birth, the undescended testis has been shown to have normal histology; however, delayed germ cell development has been described in the older infant, and this appears to be progressive over time. Histology correlates with testicular position, with worse features seen in higher testicles.

Early surgical intervention has been shown to improve testicular growth (9) and adult Leydig cell function (10). In children over the age of 2, the decision to perform an orchiopexy versus orchiectomy is based on the risks and benefits of the testicle to the individual. In prepubertal children the usefulness of androgen production must be considered, especially in cases of a solitary testicle. In postpubertal presentation of the undescended testis, sperm are rarely noted (11) and the testes are at significant risk for malignant change, leading some authors to recommend orchiectomy in all healthy, postpubertal cryptorchid males under 50 years of age (12).

## Diagnostic Laparoscopy

The indications for diagnostic and therapeutic laparoscopy are identical to the goals of open surgical management: to determine if a testicle is present and viable, and if so, to relocate the testicle into the scrotum. Historically, laparotomy was performed to localize an intra-abdominal testis or diagnose blind-ending vessels if cord vessels were not observed on initial inguinal exploration. This was most often accomplished with a high inguinal (i.e., Jones incision) or Pfannenstiel incision. It is now standard practice at most centers to proceed with diagnostic laparoscopy when the testicle is nonpalpable. Approximately 10% of boys with nonpalpable testis are found at the time of diagnostic laparoscopy to have blind-ending vessels, indicating the absence of testicular tissue (7).

During diagnostic laparoscopy for the nonpalpable testis, there are three scenarios that may be encountered. If blind-ending vessels and vas deferens are present proximal to the internal ring, a vanishing testis is diagnosed and no further action is required. If the vessels and vas deferens are present and appear to enter the internal ring, then inguinal or scrotal exploration is warranted. The final scenario includes the presence of an intra-abdominal testis, which can be located in a variety of positions. At this point the surgeon will need to assess which therapeutic modality is the most appropriate for treatment.

Recent studies report blind-ending cord structures or an intra-abdominal testis found during laparoscopic evaluation of nonpalpable testis between 31% and 83% of the time (7,13). Barqawi et al. (13) reviewed 27 patients who had undergone previous negative inguinal exploration and reported that 67% had a viable intra-abdominal or inguinal testicle. Cisek et al. (7) reported that laparoscopic findings precluded unnecessary abdominal exploration in 13% of cases and that the typical surgical incision for inguinal exploration would have left the surgeon compromised in 66% of the cases. In many of these patients, diagnostic laparoscopy can eliminate the need for further exploration or facilitate open or laparoscopic orchiopexy.

Ultimately, the decision to proceed with an inguinal or laparoscopic abdominal exploration depends on the surgeon's confidence in the physical examination. However, the evidence clearly suggests that if an initial open inguinal exploration is inconclusive, laparoscopic exploration should be the next step in the diagnosis and treatment of the nonpalpable testis. Our current protocol is to perform an examination under anesthesia. If any tissue suggestive of a scrotal nubbin is felt, then open scrotal exploration is performed. If this is negative or inconclusive, only then do we perform laparoscopic exploration.

## Laparoscopic Orchiopexy

The driving force behind the success of laparoscopic orchiopexy has been the need to improve upon the technique of open orchiopexy for the high undescended testis. In a meta-analysis of open orchiopexy techniques, Docimo (14) reported success rates by type of procedure (inguinal 89%; Fowler–Stephens 67%; staged Fowler–Stephens 77%; transabdominal 81%; two-stage 73%; microvascular 84%) and concluded that the high failure rates left significant room for improvement. Bloom (15) started the era of therapeutic laparoscopy with clip ligation of the spermatic vessels in preparation for an open second-stage Fowler-Stephens orchiopexy. Jordan and Winslow (16) extended the technique to introduce laparoscopic orchiopexy. Lindgren (17) reported a 93% success rate in the treatment of 44 nonpalpable testes in 36 patients with no evidence of testicular atrophy. In a large multi-institutional analysis, Baker et al. (18) reported excellent success rates superior to that of historical open orchiopexy and no significant difference in success or complication rates between low- and high-volume centers. When compared to open orchiopexy, laparoscopic orchiopexy is a successful approach with low risk in the management of the impalpable, undescended testicle.

During diagnostic laparoscopy for nonpalpable testis, if a testicle is present, it is evaluated for size and location. If the testicle appears to be atrophic or grossly abnormal, then orchiectomy should be considered. If the testicle appears relatively normal, the ability to mobilize it to the scrotum is assessed, based on the distance of the testicle to the internal inguinal ring and redundancy of the spermatic vessels.

Deciding whether to perform a single-stage procedure leaving the vessels intact or to perform a one- or two-stage Fowler–Stephens procedure has been challenging since no specific set of criteria has been determined. As part of the decision-making process, intraoperative measurement of the distance between the testis and the internal ring, observation of the cord anatomy, or assessment of the ability of the intra-abdominal testicle to reach the opposite inguinal ring after dissection can be helpful. Baker et al. (18) reported the incidence of testicular atrophy after primary laparoscopic (2.2%), one-stage Fowler–Stephens (22%), and two-stage Fowler– Stephens (10%) orchiopexy. When counseling preoperatively, parents or guardians should be aware of the approximately 8% to 25% risk of testicular atrophy associated with performing an orchiopexy regardless of operative technique (14). Ultimate "success" of laparoscopic orchiopexy will therefore be measured by maintenance of the testicle in proper scrotal position without evidence of atrophy. Equally important is avoiding the rare complications possible during this laparoscopic procedure. In light of this, it is critical to know the different steps that will maximize successful outcomes.

### Diagnostic Laparoscopy Technique

Prior to obtaining access, re-examination of the patient in an anesthetized state is essential. Approximately 18% of boys with a previously nonpalpable testis will have a palpable testis when examined under anesthesia (7). In the instance of a unilateral nonpalpable testicle, assessment of the size and length of the contralateral testicle may be helpful in predicting if the intra-abdominal testicle is present. A contralateral palpable testicle length exceeding 2 cm and an average volume exceeding 2 cc for example, have been cited as being predictive of monorchia in over 90% of cases (19), although not reliably enough to forgo exploration.

An open dialogue with the anesthesia team is essential. Inhaled $NO_2$ should be avoided in order to avoid bowel distention, and an oral gastric tube should be inserted to maximize visualization in the abdomen. After induction of general anesthesia, the patient is secured to the bed in the supine position with his arms tucked, and the legs are placed in a slightly abducted position. The patient is secured to the bed with wide tape at the level of the chest and low thigh. Care is taken to place the tape without tension over the chest and legs and not to restrict ventilation. Adequate space should

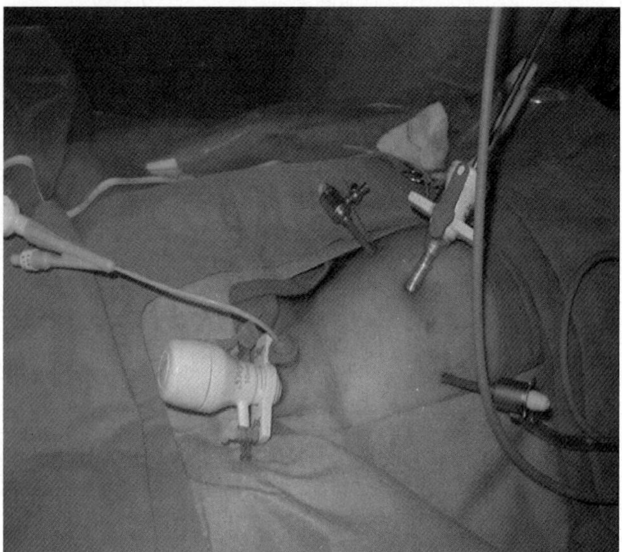

FIGURE 114.1 Preferred setup for a left single-stage laparoscopic orchiopexy. A 5-mm radial dilating trocar is placed at the umbilicus. Two 3-mm working ports are placed lateral to the rectus muscles just inferior to the umbilicus. Care is taken to avoid injury to the epigastric vessels. In the event a larger port is needed to accommodate a clip applier, a 5-mm trocar would be used on the contralateral side to ligate the testicular vessels. A 10-mm scrotal port is placed in the final stage of the case when the mobilized intra-abdominal testicle is delivered into the scrotum.

also be left for access to the scrotum. Securing the child to the table permits Trendelenburg or laterally rolled positions. When preparing and draping the patient, plan for an open procedure and drape accordingly. In the sterile field an appropriately sized Foley catheter is placed. Figure 114.1 demonstrates the preferred setup and trocar placement for performing a laparoscopic orchiopexy.

Access into the peritoneum is achieved in an open fashion at the umbilicus. Blind access for pneumoperitoneum with a Veress needle or trocar is less commonly used in the pediatric population as an overly compliant abdomen may increase the risk of injury to intra-abdominal structures. It is our preference to use the Bailez technique for open access (20), modified to employ the use of a radially dilating trocar. In our current technique a 2-0 Vicryl suture is placed in the umbilicus to provide continual anterior tension. A 3-mm hidden infraumbilical incision is made in the skin and a scissor is then used at an approximately 15- to 20-degree angle cephalad to cut through the umbilical fascia into the underlying adherent peritoneum. Alternatively, the rectus fascia and underlying peritoneum may be entered sharply at 90 degrees under direct vision.

For the umbilical camera port, we utilize a 5-mm radially dilating trocar to accommodate a 5-mm camera with a 0-degree lens. The child is placed in Trendelenburg position and the abdomen is insufflated at 1 to 2 liters/minute to a pressure of 10 to 12 cm $H_2O$. A general survey of the abdomen is undertaken, inspecting the underlying bowel for injury that might have occurred during port placement. Next, attention is focused on the evaluation of the pelvis. If an instrument is needed to aid in the inspection, a 3-mm port is placed on the ipsilateral side of the nonpalpable testis, lateral to the rectus and just caudal to the umbilicus. An atraumatic 3-mm instrument may then be used to sweep bowel cephalad. Placement of an additional 3- or 5-mm trocar on the contralateral side (lateral to the rectus and just caudal to the umbilicus) is reserved for the need of an additional working port or use of a 5-mm clip applier. Clinical circumstances in which this would be necessary include if an atrophic nubbin is to be excised, and if a viable testicle is found far from the internal ring and a staged Fowler-Stephens orchiopexy is to be performed.

In the case of a unilateral undescended testicle, the internal ring of the descended testicle is examined first to gain an appreciation of the anatomy. Possible findings on inspecting the affected side of the "nonpalpable" testicle may include blind-ending vessels, cord structures entering the internal ring, or an intra-abdominal testis. Note the status of the processus vaginalis: most undescended testicles are associated with a patent processus.

## Blind-Ending Testicular Vessels

Blind-ending gonad vessels indicate a "vanishing" testicle. This is the result of in utero testicular torsion that is either an intra-abdominal or intrascrotal event. Vessels will have a "horse tail" appearance; they diverge, do not exit the internal ring, and do not supply obvious testicular tissue (Fig. 114.2). If found during exploration, no further investigation is needed and the procedure is terminated. It is important to note that the finding of a blind-ending vas deferens during laparoscopy is insufficient to conclude the absence of testicular tissue. Further cephalad inspection toward the aortic origin of the gonadal vessels is then necessary.

## Cord Structures Entering the Internal Ring

Cord structures may be visualized entering a closed internal ring or a patent processes vaginalis (open ring) (Fig. 114.3). In the instance of a closed internal ring, a groin or scrotal exploration may be performed (Fig. 114.4). If a patent processus vaginalis is present, the laparoscope may be used to inspect the inguinal canal antegrade. Alternatively, gentle manual retrograde pressure can be placed over the inguinal canal in an attempt to push groin contents (viable testicle versus nubbin) intra-abdominally. In the instance of a nubbin or

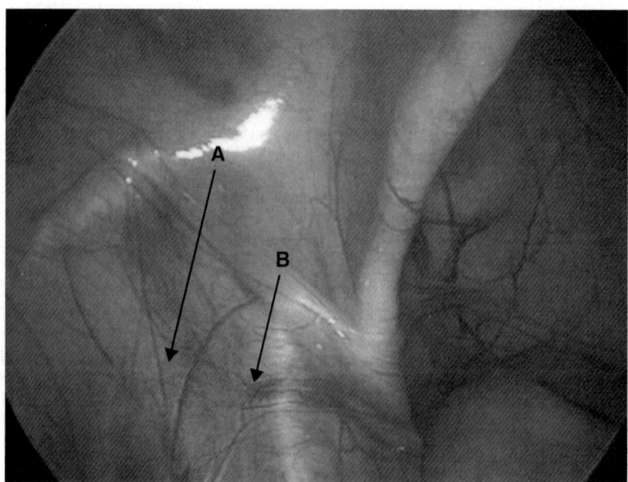


FIGURE 114.2 Finding blind-ending and divergent testicular vessels (A) is evidence of a vanishing testicle. The sole finding of a blind-ending vas (B) is insufficient evidence to conclude that there is absence of ipsilateral testicular tissue.

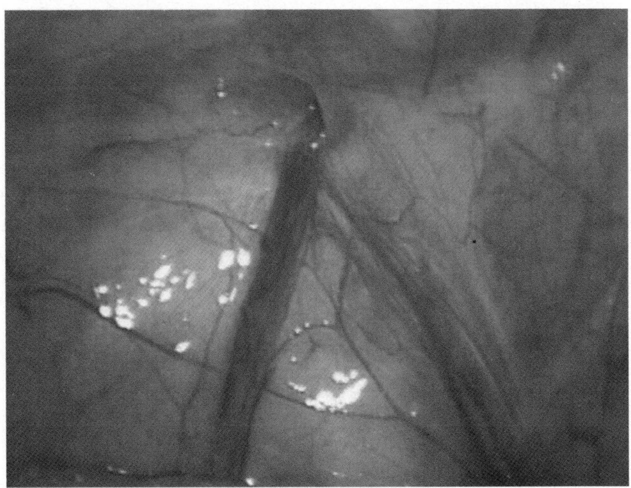

FIGURE 114.3 Laparoscopic view of a left patent processus vaginalis (hernia) with normal cord structures exiting the internal rings. Left groin exploration revealed a high viable intracanalicular testicle. Inguinal orchiopexy with hernia sac ligation was performed.

testicular remnant, laparoscopic orchiectomy is performed. This is accomplished by either clipping or dividing the cord contents or using a 5-mm instrument designed to seal and divide smaller vessels (i.e., LigaSure or Harmonic Scalpel). The specimen is grasped and removed from the contralateral 5-mm port. This incision can be widened as needed by spreading the fascia with any clamp while under direct vision from the camera port.

## INTRA-ABDOMINAL TESTIS

There are three minimally invasive reconstructive options to address an intra-abdominal testicle: (i) primary laparoscopic-orchiopexy, (ii) one-stage laparoscopic Fowler–Stephens orchiopexy, and (iii) two-stage laparoscopic Fowler–Stephens orchiopexy. Laparoscopic orchiectomy is reserved for an intra-abdominal nonviable testis (atrophic nubbin) or a testis that cannot be brought into the scrotum based on an extreme ectopic location (retrovesical, pararenal, pararectal), limiting blood supply length. Older children (>10 years of age) found to have an intra-abdominal testis may be better served with a laparoscopic orchiectomy, provided the contralateral testicle is intrascrotal. Although an intra-abdominal testicle may remain hormonally active indefinitely, spermatogenic potential tends to decline after 18 months.

The initial measured distance of the testicle from the internal ring will determine which laparoscopic approach should be utilized and is therefore a predictor of success rates. "Peeping testes" or those located in close proximity to the internal ring (<2 cm away) can usually be mobilized into the scrotum in a single stage without dividing the testicular vessels (Fig. 114.5). It is important to counsel parents that intra-abdominal ectopic testes and those located >2 cm from the internal ring are at increased risk for surgical failure.

## SINGLE-STAGE LAPAROSCOPIC ORCHIOPEXY

In 1991, Bloom (15) reported using laparoscopy to ligate the testicular vessels in the first stage of a Fowler-Stephens approach. Jordan and Winslow (16) further advanced the role of laparoscopy as a therapeutic modality when they reported the first laparoscopic orchiopexy. There have been many subtle variations described for performing this procedure (21).

### Establishing a Peritoneal Pedicle Flap

Following abdominal access, insufflation, and additional trocar placement, as outlined above, attention is focused on the ipsilateral testicle and internal ring. Figure 114.6 demonstrates the surgical "map" needed to mobilize a triangular flap of peritoneum demarcated by the testicular vessels laterally and vas deferens medially. The preliminary goal is to create two continuous peritoneotomies parallel to the testicular vessels and vas in order to mobilize the testicle on a well-vascularized peritoneal pedicle.

The testicle, epididymis, and extent of vasal descent distally into the inguinal canal are evaluated. It is critical from the onset to define the gubernacular attachments and identify a long-looping vas, if present. Scissors are used in the preliminary dissection. Care must be taken not to activate cautery in proximity to the vessels and vas. The first peritoneotomy is made lateral to the testicular vessels at the most proximal position. The incision is directed toward the internal

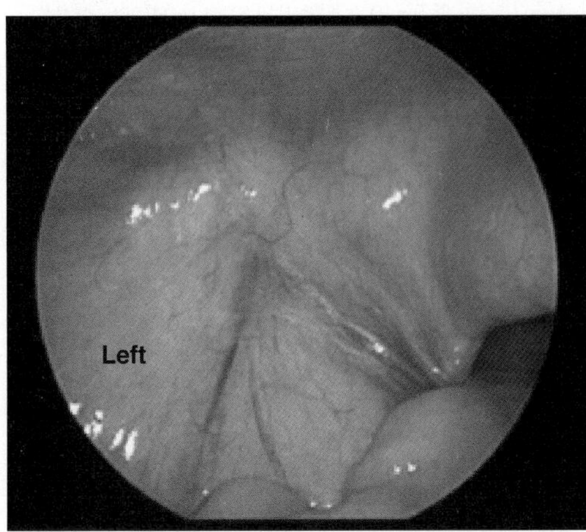


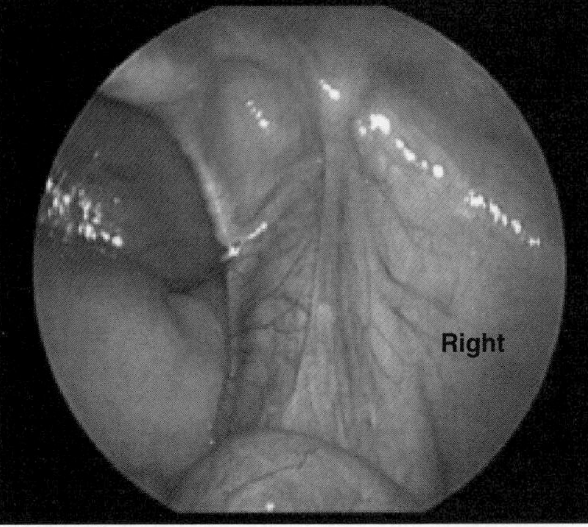


FIGURE 114.4 Bilateral closed processus vaginalis with normal cord structures exiting the internal rings. This morbidly obese 8-year-old boy underwent exploratory laparoscopy for a "nonpalpable" left testicle. The findings on diagnostic laparoscopy of cord structures exiting the left internal ring proceeded to a left groin exploration. A high viable intracanalicular testicle was found and open orchiopexy was performed.

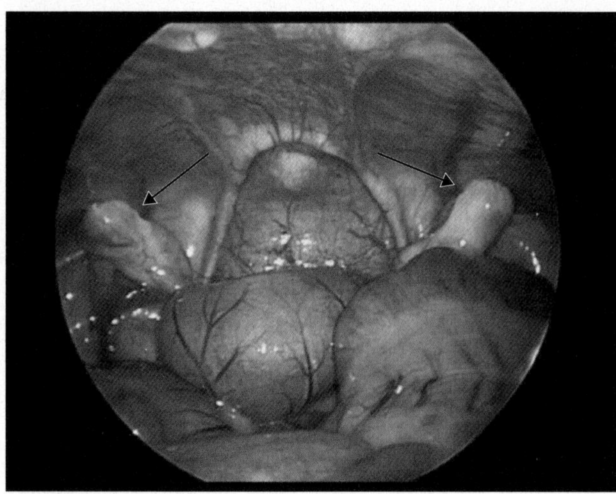

FIGURE 114.5 Bilateral intra-abdominal "peeping" testicles at the internal rings in a 6-month-old with nonpalpable gonads. Bilateral single-stage laparoscopic orchiopexies were performed.

ring. Often after the first incision, pneumoperitoneum will diffuse into the plane between the peritoneum and pelvic side wall. In this regard, $CO_2$ can aid in isolating the peritoneum to be dissected.

The second line of dissection will again begin at the level of the internal ring distally but will parallel the vas medially. Care is taken not to injure the iliac vessels and ureter that lie beneath the vas. It is also critical that dissection is not performed within the distal triangular area enclosed by the gonadal vessels and vas (Fig. 114.7). Critical collateral microvasculature within this flap will flow from the vasal artery to the testicle and should be maintained if possible. This is especially relevant if a single-stage Fowler–Stephens orchiopexy is performed; dividing the testicular vessels and interrupting collateral blood flow will invariably lead to testicular atrophy. Widely mobilizing the peritoneal flap laterally and medially leaves only the distal gubernacular attachments. A window is created distally, allowing the gubernaculum to be divided while visualizing the course of the vas deferens. An indication that dissection has maximized the flap length is that the testicle can reach the contralateral internal ring without tension. The ipsilateral ring is not closed since there is not an increased risk for a clinically significant hernia to develop. The patent processus is ablated by the peritoneal incisions, division of the gubernacula, and, if necessary, incision of the anterior peritoneum. Subsequently, peritoneal regrowth obliterates the previously patent tract.

## Creating a Neoinguinal Hiatus and Testicular Delivery into the Scrotum

Various methods to deliver the testicle into the scrotum have been described. It is our belief that the testis may be most safely and effectively delivered to the scrotum using 2- or 3 mm instruments and a radially dilating trocar system (22). A 12-mm ipsilateral scrotal incision is first made and a subdartos pouch is created. A 2-mm laparoscopic grasper is placed through the ipsilateral 3-mm lateral trocar directed toward the scrotal incision. Care is taken to place the instrument over the pubis and between the medial umbilical ligament and epigastric vessels. The surgeon's free hand should palpate the pubic area and scrotal incision to ensure the instrument is being guided over the pubis and through the scrotal incision. After the instrument is passed through the scrotum, the Foley catheter is checked for hematuria. A bladder injury, which is very rare, would most likely occur during this step of the procedure. Proper placement of the instrument in the position described above should minimize the risk of this complication (Fig. 114.8). The step sheath is then passed onto the end of the 2- or 3-mm instrument ex vivo and brought through the scrotum. The 5- or 10-mm trocar obturator, depending on the size of the testicle, is then inserted, creating the neoinguinal hiatus. A locking grasper is introduced into the abdomen through the scrotal trocar and the testicle is grasped at the gubernaculum and then delivered into the scrotum (Fig. 114.9). It is imperative for the surgeon to personally monitor the tension on the cord during scrotal delivery so the vessels are not avulsed.

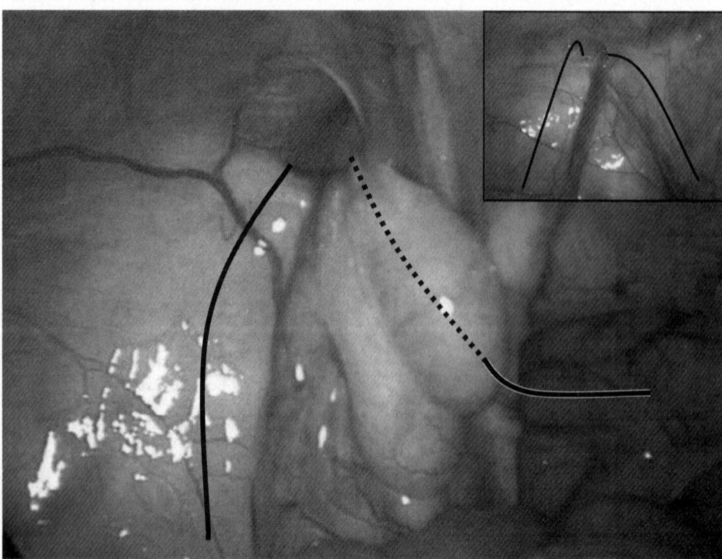

FIGURE 114.6 A left intra-abdominal testicle in an 8-month-old boy at the internal ring. The *dark lines* represent where peritoneotomies are made parallel to the testicular vessels (lateral) and vas deferens (medial) in order to mobilize the testicle on a vascularized peritoneal pedicle flap. The insert shows the same landmarks when an nonpalpable intracanicular testicle is milked into the abdomen and then mobilized via laparoscopic orchiopexy.

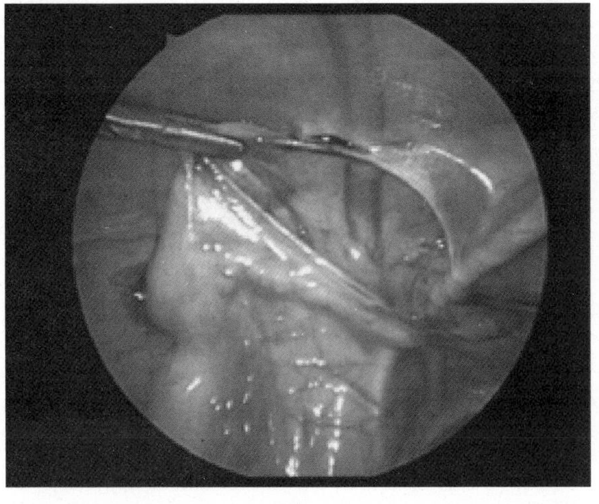

A

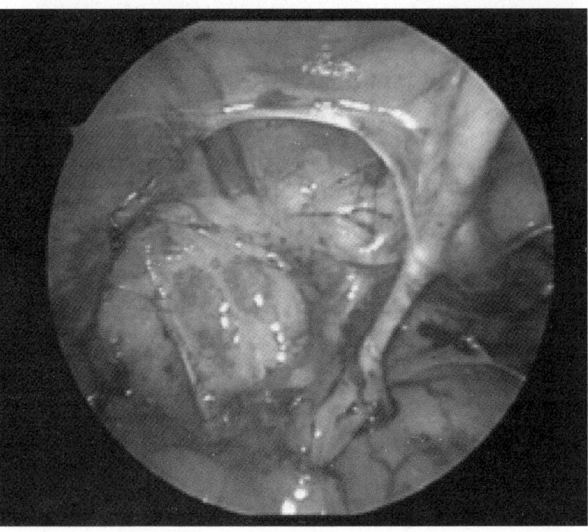

B

FIGURE 114.7 After lateral mobilization, medial dissection follows the course of the vas deferens (**A**). Collateral paravasal blood supply to the testicle is visualized. Cephalad traction following release of the distal gubernacular attachments (**B**) demonstrates the extent of the peritoneal flap and clarifies the boundaries where the neoinguinal hiatus is to be created between the inferior epigastric vessels and the medial umbilical ligament.

## Gaining Additional Cord Length and Securing the Testicle

After delivering the testicle into the scrotum, if there is tension and/or additional length is needed, further dissection can be carried out laterally and cephalad toward the kidney. In most instances the cord length will still be inadequate and additional maneuvers are required. An option at this point is to divide the peritoneum overlying the testicular vessels to provide extra cord length and release any remaining tension (Fig. 114.10). If incising the peritoneum has not helped, consideration can be given to dividing the testicular vessels, therefore performing a one-stage Fowler–Stephens orchiopexy. The contralateral 3-mm port must be upsized to a 5-mm port in order to accommodate a clip applier. Consideration must be given to

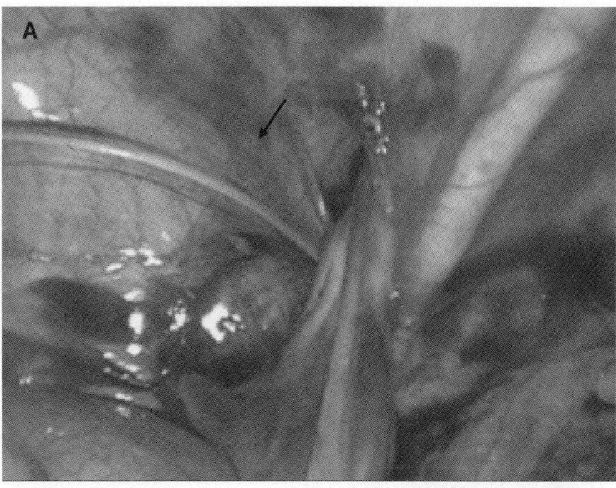


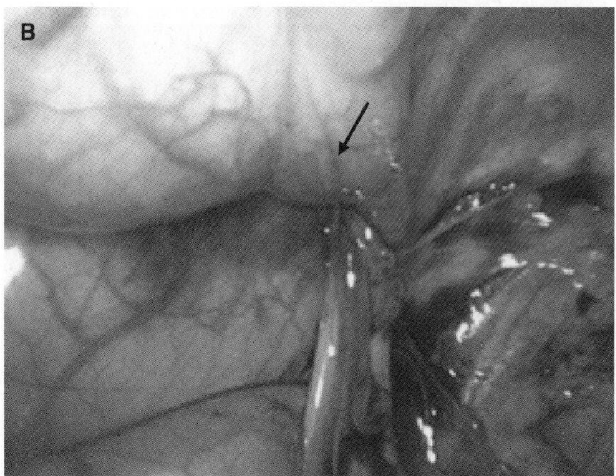


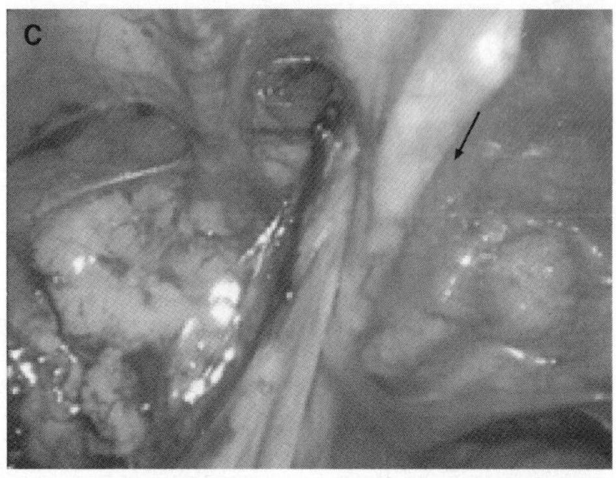


FIGURE 114.8 During delivery of the testicle into the scrotum, the bladder edge (*arrows*) is at risk for perforation. The risk is increased if the neoinguinal hiatus is not created anterior to the pubis and lateral to the medial umbilical ligament. Following delivery of the testicle medial to the ligament in a right laparoscopic orchiopexy, there was concern that the bladder was perforated (**A**). Filling the bladder demonstrated no evidence of a leak (**B**). After delivery of the testicle through a 12-mm scrotal trocar in the final stage of a left laparoscopic orchiopexy, there is little concern of a bladder injury. The neohiatus was created in a plane lateral to the medial umbilical ligament and medial to the epigastric vessels (**C**).

the higher risk of testicular atrophy after a one-stage Fowler–Stephens maneuver.

When the testicle lies tension-free in the scrotum, the orchiopexy can be completed (Fig. 114.11). The testicle is harnessed in the dartos pouch and the scrotal skin is closed by any of the preferred technique(s) utilized by the surgeon.

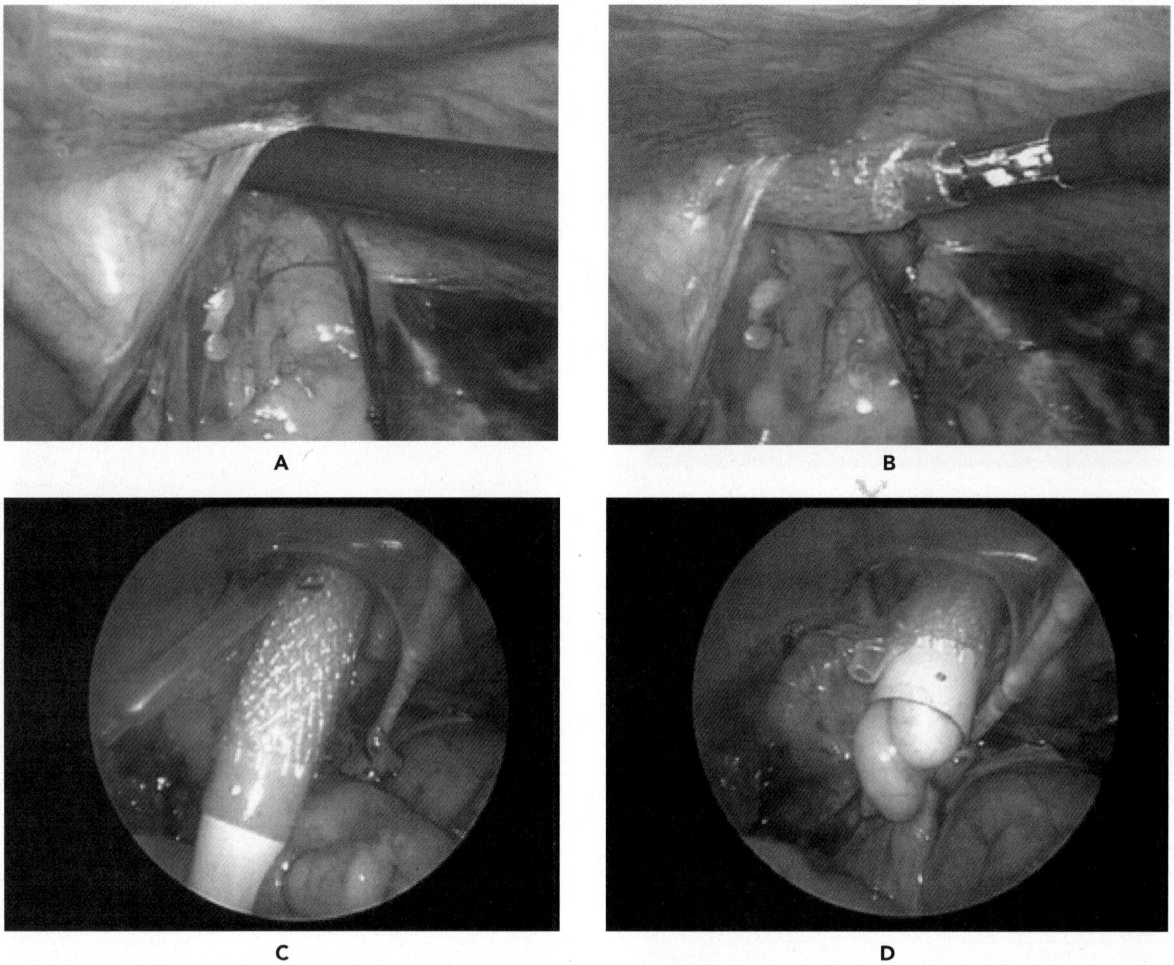

A B

C D

FIGURE 114.9 Delivering the testicle into the scrotum requires developing a neohiatus (A–C) to facilitate passage of the testicle, epididymis, and cord structures into the scrotum without resistance. This technique minimizes the risk of an avulsion injury (D).

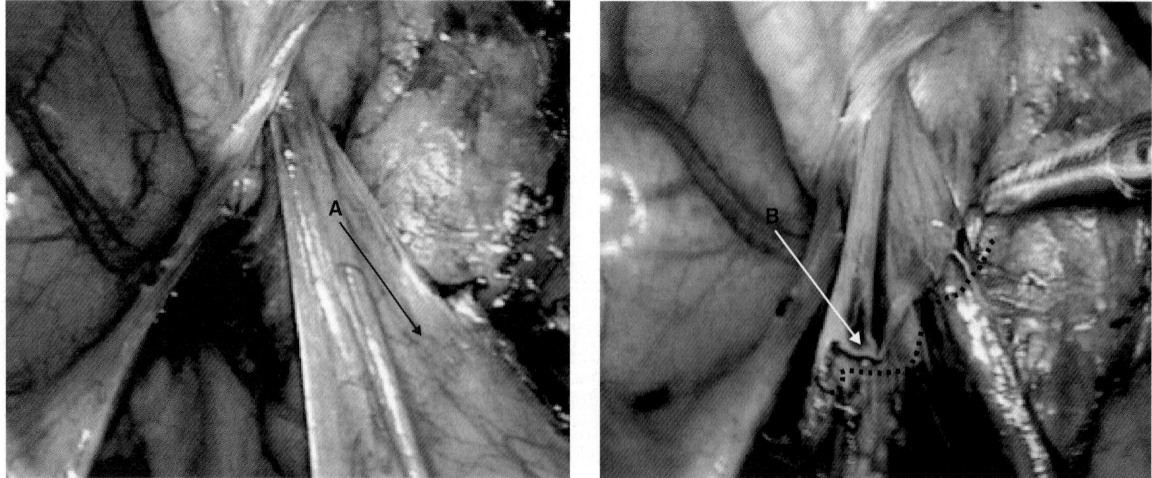


FIGURE 114.10 Delivering the testicle into the scrotum provides the traction and assistance of a "third arm." If there is tension and/or additional length is needed, further dissection can be carried out laterally and cephalad. The peritoneum overlying the testicular vessels (A) may also be divided (B) to release tension and provide extra cord length.

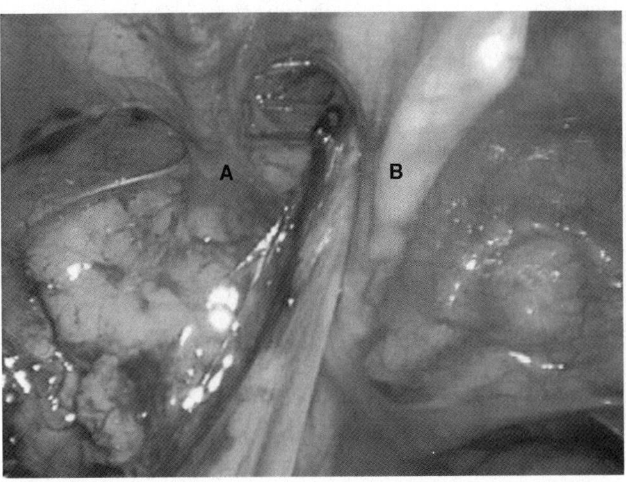


**FIGURE 114.11** Antegrade view of a left neoinguinal hiatus created between the inferior epigastric vessels (**A**) and the medial umbilical ligament (**B**). The testicle is fixed to the scrotum after maximal length on the cord has been reached without residual tension.

## Closure and Exiting the Abdomen

The abdomen is surveyed a final time and the pneumoperitoneum pressure is lowered. Any occult bleeding should be identified and addressed at this time. While maintaining pneumoperitoneum, the two lateral ports are removed sequentially and inspected for bleeding. The fascial layers of these trocar sites are closed with 2-0 Vicryl sutures through the fascia. The laparoscopic view is maintained on the port sites during closure to ensure that it is airtight and free of any intra-abdominal contents (i.e., bowel or omentum). Through the umbilical port the pneumoperitoneum is evacuated. Larger tidal volumes given by the anesthesiologist and mild abdominal pressure help with the expulsion of $CO_2$. The umbilical trocar and camera are removed while inspecting for bleeding. Final fascial stitches are placed in the umbilical port, the skin is closed, and dressings are applied.

# SECOND-STAGE FOWLER–STEPHENS PROCEDURE

As a general rule, the further the intra-abdominal testicle lies from the internal ring (i.e., >2 cm) the higher the likelihood that a staged procedure is necessary. Staging the procedure will enable delivery of the testicle into the scrotum without tension and at a decreased risk for atrophy. This may be accomplished by ligating the testicular vessels by using a 5- mm stapler through the contralateral port (Fig. 114.12). A laparoscopic second-stage Fowler–Stephens orchiopexy will be performed approximately 6 months later, when collateral blood flow from the deferential artery has matured.

# BILATERAL NONPALPABLE TESTES AND LAPAROSCOPIC ORCHIOPEXY

Bilateral nonpalpable testicles in a newborn should raise the suspicion of an intersex condition, especially with coincidental genital ambiguity (i.e., proximal hypospadias). Other possibilities include bilateral anorchia or bilateral intra-abdominal testis. It is urgent to institute a workup to rule out life-threatening intersex conditions such as congenital adrenal hyperplasia (CAH). Once an intersex disorder has been excluded, endocrine studies, including a human chorionic gonadotropin (hCG) stimulation test and or serum müllerian inhibitory substance (MIS), will be useful in differentiating anorchia from bilateral nonpalpable testis (23). Regardless of such laboratory findings, however, exploratory laparoscopy will be needed for a gonadal biopsy, gonadectomy, or orchiopexy (Fig. 114.13). Bilateral laparoscopic orchiopexies can be performed simultaneously or at separate procedures, depending on perceived risk of atrophy.

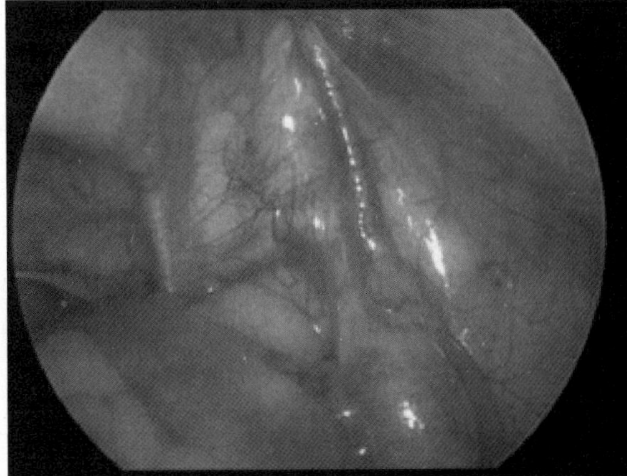

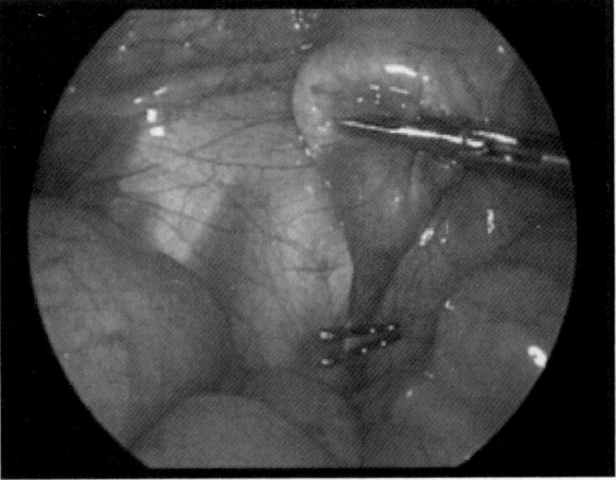

**FIGURE 114.12** A right intra-abdominal testicle in a 9-month-old boy was found >2 cm from the internal ring. The testicular vessels were clipped in the first stage of a two-stage Fowler–Stephens reconstruction. Note that clips are applied without dissecting the peritoneal attachments free from the vessels.

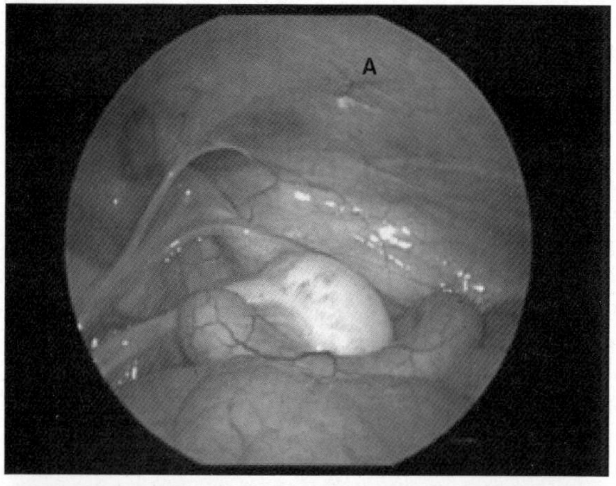


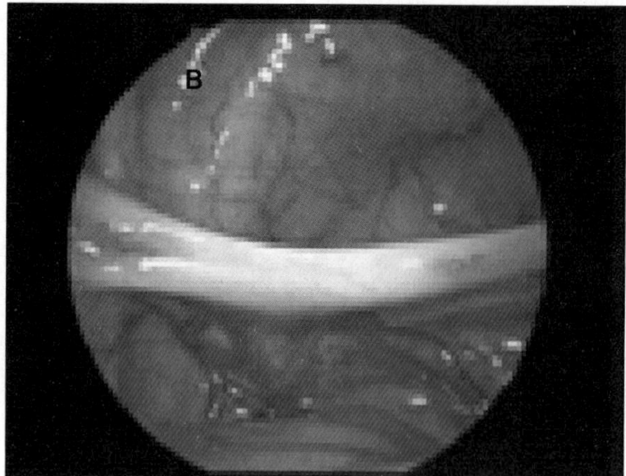


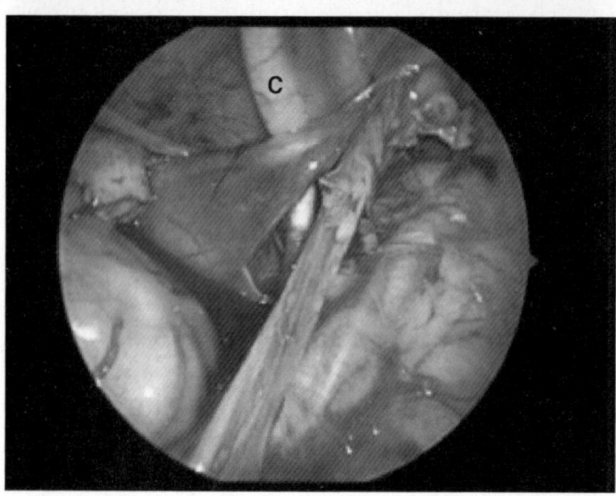


FIGURE 114.13 Eight-month-old XY phenotypic boy with bilateral undescended testicle and müllerian inhibiting substance (MIS) deficiency. MIS hormone level was 0.1 ng/mL (normal 48–83). Diagnostic laparoscopy revealed bilateral intra-abdominal testicles (**A**) with müllerian (uterus) and wolffian (vas) structures intimately associated (**B**). Left laparoscopic orchiopexy was performed, aided by releasing the contralateral round ligament (**C**).

## COMPLICATIONS

Complication rates in contemporary series of adult laparoscopic procedures range from 12% to 16% (24). Although the same issues reported in the adult literature are experienced in children, there is little published information regarding laparoscopic complication rates in the pediatric population, particularly in the urologic literature. However, the number of complications associated with laparoscopic orchiopexy compares quite favorably to that of an open approach. In a large multi-institutional review, Baker et al. (18) reported a major complication rate of 3.0% and a minor complication rate of 2.0%. Major complications that have been reported include acute testicular atrophy, bowel perforation, cecal volvulus, vascular injury, bladder perforation, ileus, laceration of the vas, testicular vessel avulsion, and wound dehiscence/infection.

The prevention of complications associated with laparoscopy starts with proper positioning and padding to reduce the risk of neuromuscular injuries. Although injuries are less likely to occur with pelvic laparoscopy, extremes in table positioning are often necessary. Close attention to placement of straps and/or tape and adequate padding should limit positioning-related injuries. As in adults, abdominal visceral injuries related to access are encountered; however, an understanding of the unique anatomic aspects of the pediatric abdominal wall can decrease these risks. The pediatric abdomen requires less force for entry, so penetration injury to the abdominal viscera can easily occur. The smaller pediatric working space also sets up the potential for injury to the visceral structures from the laparoscopic working elements.

For this reason, open peritoneal access has been associated with fewer complications than when a Veress needle is used. As previously mentioned, we prefer to gain access using an open technique. Surgical planning and an appreciation for the anatomic landmarks within the pelvis will aid in avoiding complications. During testicular mobilization, care must be taken to avoid injury to the vas, testicular, femoral, and iliac vessels and the ureter. When mobilizing the vas on the medial aspect of the peritoneal flap, these structures lie directly posterior and medial (Fig. 114.14). In general, complications can be limited by careful intra-abdominal mobilization, using cautery in short bursts, and execution of meticulous technique. The laparoscopic approach facilitates this by allowing extensive and high retroperitoneal mobilization of the testicular vessels in an atraumatic manner.

Today the learning curve for pediatric laparoscopy is decreasing as trainees are entering the field with far more laparoscopic experience gained during general urology residency.

## CONCLUSIONS

Laparoscopic orchiopexy is now commonplace in the pediatric urologist's armamentarium, since evolving from a diagnostic procedure to the surgical treatment of choice when managing the intra-abdominal testicle. The option of what type of procedure to be performed is reflective of the intra-abdominal positioning of the testicle and its distance from the internal

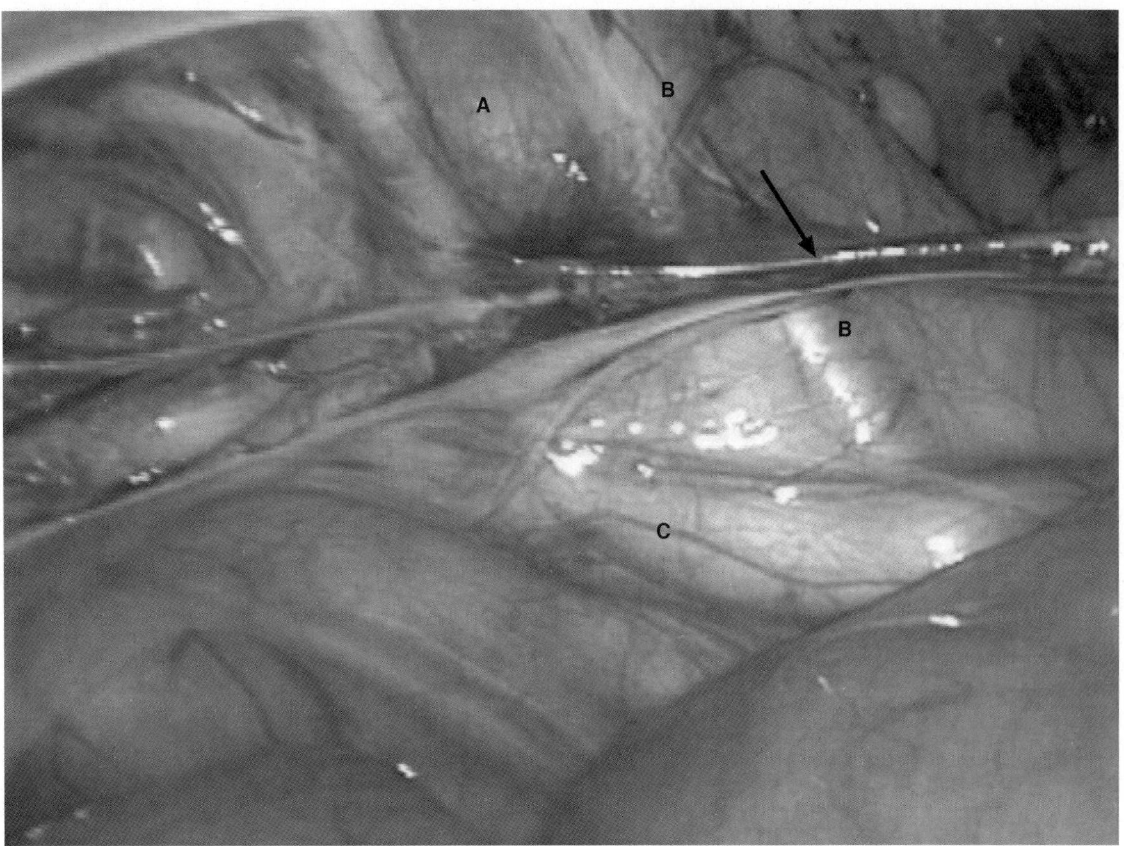


FIGURE 114.14 Pelvic view during a right laparoscopic orchiopexy. During medial mobilization of the vas deferens, the cord structures (*arrow*) are held cranially and laterally. Care must be taken not to injure the iliac vein (A), iliac artery (B), or ureter (C), which lie immediately posterior to the mobilized peritoneal flap.

ring. Success rates for these techniques are comparable to or better than those reported in open series. Maintaining a mobilized testicle on a wide peritoneal flap free from tension is the key to maintaining scrotal position and minimizing the risk of testicular atrophy. Although there is a learning curve associated with this minimally invasive technique, it is surmountable.

## *References*


1. Berkowitz GS, Lapinksi RH, Dolgin SE, et al. Prevalence and natural history of cryptorchidism. *Pediatrics* 1993;92:44–49.
2. Scorer CG, Farrington GH. *Congenital Deformities of the Testis and Epididymis* New York: Appleton-Century-Crofts, 1971.
3. Cendron M, Huff DS, Keating MA, et al. Anatomical, morphological and volumetric analysis: a review of 759 cases of testicular maldescent. *J Urol* 1993;149:570–573.
4. Cortesi N, Ferrari P, Zambarda E, et al. Diagnosis of bilateral abdominal cryptorchidism by laparoscopy. *Endoscopy* 1976;8:33–34.
5. Hrebinko HL, Bellinger MF. The limited role of imaging in managing children with undecended testes. *J Urol* 1993;150:458–460.
6. Kanemoto K, Hayashi Y, Kojima Y, et al. Accuracy of ultrasonography and magnetic resonance imaging in the diagnosis of nonpalpable testis. *Int J Urol* 2005;12:668–672.
7. Cisek LJ, Peters CA, Atala A, et al. Current findings in diagnostic laparoscopic evaluation of the nonpalpable testis. *J Urol* 1998;160:1145-1150.
8. Docimo SG. Re: Is human chorionic gonadotropin useful for identifying and treating nonpalpable testis? *J Urol* 2001;166:1010–1011.
9. Nagar H, Haddad R. Impact of early orchiopexy on testicular growth. *Br J Urol* 1997;80:334–335.
10. Lee PA, Coughlin MT. Leydig cell function after cryptorchidism: evidence of the beneficial result of early surgery. *J Urol* 2002;167:1824–1827.
11. Rogers E, Teahan S, Gallagher H. The role of orchiectomy in the management of postpubertal cryptorchidism. *J Urol* 1998;159:851–854.
12. Oh J, Landman J, Evers A, et al. Management of the postpubertal patient with cryptorchidism: an updated analysis. *J Urol* 2002;167:1329–1333.
13. Barqawi AZ, Blyth B, Jordan GH, et al. Role of laparoscopy in patients with previous negative exploration for impalpable testis. *Urology* 2003; 61:1234–1237.
14. Docimo SG. The results of surgical therapy for cryptorchidism: a literature review and analysis. *J Urol* 1995;154:1148–1152.
15. Bloom DA. Two-step orchiopexy with pelviscopic clip ligation of the spermatic vessels. *J Urol* 1991;145:1030–1033.
16. Jordan GH, Winslow BH. Laparoscopic single-stage and staged orchiopexy. *J Urol* 1994;152:1249–1252.
17. Lindgren BW. Laparoscopic orchiopexy: procedure of choice for the nonpalpable testis? *J Urol* 1998;159:2132–2135.
18. Baker LA, Docimo SG, Surer I, et al. A multi-institutional analysis of laparoscopic orchidopexy. *BJU Int* 2001;87:484–489.
19. Belman AB, Rushton HG. Is an empty left hemiscrotum and hypertrophied right descended testis predictive of perinatal torsion? *J Urol* 2003;170: 1674–1676.
20. Docimo SG. Re: Experience with the Bailez technique for laparoscopic access in children. *J Urol* 2004;171:806.
21. Docimo SG, Moore RG, Adams J, et al. Laparoscopic orchiopexy for the high palpable undescended testis: preliminary experience. *J Urol* 1995; 154:1513–1515.
22. Ferrer FA, Cadeddu JA, Schulam P, et al. Orchiopexy using 2-mm laparoscopic instruments: 2 techniques for delivering the testis into the scrotum. *J Urol* 2000;164:160–161.
23. Jarow JP, Berkovitz GD, Migeon CJ, et al. Elevation of serum gonadotropins establishes the diagnosis of anorchism in prepubertal boys with bilateral cryptorchidism. *J Urol* 1986;136:277–179.
24. Cadeddu JA, Wolfe JS, Nakada S, et al. Complications of laparoscopic procedures after concentrated training in urological laparoscopy. *J Urol* 2001; 166:2109–2111.

# CHAPTER 115 ■ PEDIATRIC LAPAROSCOPIC PYELOPLASTY

PASQUALE CASALE AND WALID A. FARHAT

Historically, open pyeloplasty has been the standard treatment for congenital or acquired ureteropelvic junction (UPJ) obstruction in adults and children, with overall success rates of 90% to 100% (1). Although endopyelotomy and retrograde dilation are alternative methods of managing UPJ obstruction in children (2), the success of these two procedures is inferior to that reported for conventional dismembered pyeloplasty (3). Advances in technology have enabled the introduction of laparoscopic and robot-assisted laparoscopic pyeloplasty over the last few years.

Laparoscopic pyeloplasty was introduced in adults in 1993 (4). In the initial reports, the operative time ranged from 3 to 7 hours, but the procedure has gradually gained in popularity and acceptance, with a reported success rate of over 95% (5).

## DIAGNOSIS

Approximately 1% of prenatal ultrasounds detect hydronephrosis in the fetus. In 50% of these cases, UPJ obstruction causes the condition. UPJ obstruction is more common in male patients and affects the left kidney more often than the right. About 10% to 30% of cases occur in both kidneys (bilaterally) (6). Congenital abnormalities are the most common cause of UPJ obstruction in children. The condition often results from an abnormality in the muscles that surround the UPJ, causing an intrinsic narrowing. It may also be caused by an abnormality in the structure or position of the ureter, such as a high insertion onto the renal pelvis. Lower-pole renal blood vessels crossing over the ureter can cause an obstruction as well. Other etiologies are compression of the ureter caused by inflammation, retroperitoneal fibrosis, kidney stones, or scar tissue from previous surgery to correct UPJ obstruction. Symptoms are typically seen in older children but can be seen in infants; they include back or flank pain, hematuria, failure to thrive, flank mass, and pyelonephritis.

Neonatal patients are evaluated for the obstruction using renal ultrasound and diuretic renography. Magnetic resonance urography is also an option, and a voiding cystourethrogram (VCUG) might be utilized to rule out vesicoureteral-associated reflux.

## INDICATIONS

The indications for laparoscopic pyeloplasty are similar to those for an open pyeloplasty and include increasing hydronephrosis, progressive deterioration of renal function, recurrent urinary tract infection, and persistent pain. The introduction of refined instrumentation and more experience with intracorporeal suturing allows reconstructive laparoscopy to be implemented in the pediatric population, with multiple techniques of pyeloplasty described in the literature (7). One of the earliest descriptions of the transperitoneal Anderson–Hynes laparoscopic pyeloplasty in pediatric patients by Tan (8) recommended that it should not be performed in children <6 months of age. The advent of improved 3-mm instrumentation and laparoscopic telescopes has allowed better suture manipulation and visualization, making it feasible even in infants <6 months of age (9). The key point to performing a laparoscopic pyeloplasty in the infant is based on the geometry of the patient's body habitus. A triangle is constructed utilizing the umbilicus as the apex, with the remaining points being lateral to the ipsilateral rectus muscle subcostal and at the level of the anterior superior iliac spine.

Yeung et al. (10) reported their initial experience with retroperitoneal laparoscopic pyeloplasty in 13 children, 1 requiring open conversion. The mean operative time was 143 minutes (range 103 to 235 minutes). El-Ghoneimi (11) reported on 50 retroperitoneal laparoscopic pyeloplasties in children aged between 22 months and 15 years. Conversion to open surgery was necessary in four cases due to technical difficulties during suturing. Mean hospital stay was 2 days, and return to full activities occurred within 5 days of surgery. The longer time needed for the retroperitoneal approach is almost certainly related to the limited working space, which renders suturing more difficult.

As laparoscopic pyeloplasty is technically challenging, this procedure was initially restricted to those medical centers with advanced laparoscopic surgeons, and long-term outcome data are still being evaluated. With increasing experience, however, laparoscopic pyeloplasty in children is more commonly being considered as the initial treatment for UPJ obstruction. This procedure maintains the benefits of the endoscopic approaches, including decreased postoperative pain, short hospitalization, and reduced postoperative recovery time, while demonstrating success rates comparable to those of the conventional open approach (12,13).

## ALTERNATIVE THERAPY

Open pyeloplasty remains the gold standard, with a high success rate for a flank, dorsal lumbotomy, or anterior muscle-splitting incision. Proponents have shown that this procedure can be done without an indwelling ureteral stent and with simple percutaneous drainage.

Endopyelotomy and retrograde dilation are also alternative methods of managing UPJ obstruction in children. Endopyelotomies are performed in the same fashion as in adults either by a percutaneous approach or ureteroscopically in a retrograde manner. The long-term success rate of endopyelotomy is less than with the standard open or laparoscopic approaches (8,9). Retrograde dilation has virtually no role in pediatrics due to its high failure rate, requiring a subsequent procedure (14).

## SURGICAL TECHNIQUE AND STEPS

Initial cystoscopy and ureteric stenting is left to the discretion of the surgeon and may not be necessary (10,15). An indwelling Foley catheter is placed to gravity drainage.

Positioning of the patient is crucial as it facilitates optimal ergonomics for the surgeon and increased access to the operative space. For both a transperitoneal and retroperitoneal approach, the patient is placed in a lateral or semilateral decubitus position in close proximity to the posterior edge of the table. The table is flexed, the kidney rest is elevated, appropriate padding is applied, and the patient is secured with 2-inch tape and a safety belt. An option for the retroperitoneal approach described by Yeung et al. (10) is a modified semiprone position with the left flank up or a 45-degree right lateral decubitus position (for right-sided obstruction) to allow the subsequent ureteropelvic anastomosis using the right hand (for a right-handed surgeon). Another option utilized for the transperitoneal approach is to place the patient supine with a slight 30-degree rotation of the ipsilateral side. The patient is then secured to the table with 2-inch silk tape (Fig. 115.1). The table can then be rotated as needed after visualization of the intraperitoneal field. This approach can be utilized on the left side, allowing the colon to stay lateral to the left kidney so a transmesenteric window is unobstructed.

### Retroperitoneoscopic Approach

Appropriate placement of the trocars is of the utmost importance, and three or four laparoscopic ports are inserted at the surgeon's discretion. Retroperitoneal access is achieved through the first trocar incision, which is 15 mm long and

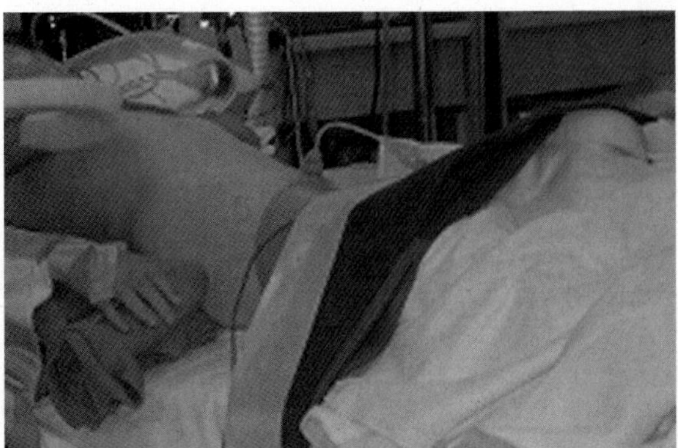

FIGURE 115.1 Supine positioning for transperitoneal approach in left-sided and bilateral cases.

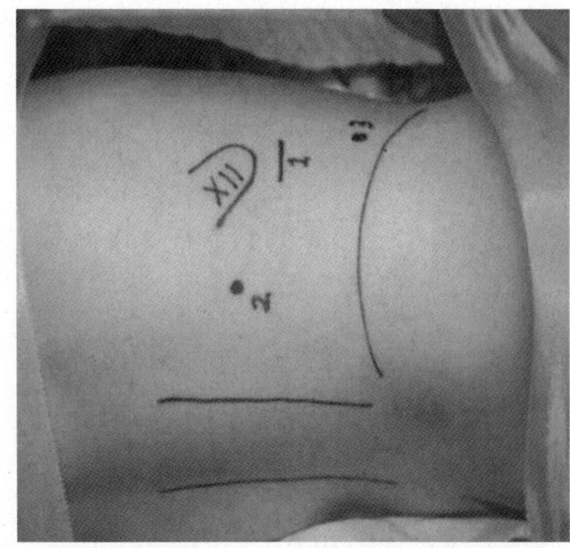

FIGURE 115.2 Port placement for retroperitoneal approach.

10 mm from the lower border of the tip of the 12th rib (Fig. 115.2). Our preferred method to achieve access to the retroperitoneal space is that the Gerota fascia is approached by a muscle-splitting blunt dissection, then opened under direct vision. A working space is created by gas insufflation dissection, and the first trocar is fixed with a pursestring suture applied around the deep fascia to ensure an airtight seal. Another approach to create the retroperitoneal space is a modification of Gaur balloon technique to dissect the retroperitoneum. Two index fingers of a powder-free surgical glove are placed one inside the other and ligated onto the 5/10-mm trocar sheath. The dissection is then performed by instilling 500 mL of warm saline through the insufflation channel of the trocar. After completed dissection, the trocar is reinserted without the balloon and pneumoretroperitoneum is established (maximum pressure 12 mm Hg, or age dependent). A 5- or 10-mm 0-degree telescope is inserted through the first trocar. A second 3-mm trocar is inserted posteriorly near the costovertebral angle, while the third 3-mm trocar is inserted 10 mm above the top of the iliac crest at the anterior axillary line. To avoid transperitoneal insertion of this trocar, the working space is fully developed and the deep surface of the anterior wall muscles identified before the trocar is inserted. The insufflation pressure is <12 mm Hg and the flow rate of $CO_2$ is progressively increased from 1 to 5 L/min.

The kidney is approached posteriorly, the Gerota fascia is incised parallel to the psoas muscle, and the perirenal fat is dissected to reveal the lower pole of the kidney, in which the renal pelvis is first identified and then mobilized. The UPJ is identified and minimally dissected to free the UPJ from connective tissue, and small vessels are divided after bipolar electrocoagulation. The anterior surface of the UPJ is cleared to identify any polar crossing vessels. In order to dissect the UPJ adequately with minimal trauma, stay sutures of 5-0 Prolene are placed at the UPJ for easy manipulation (Fig. 115.3).

The traction sutures not only help to mobilize the UPJ but also facilitate the alignment of the ureter to the trocar axis so that spatulation and suturing are easily accomplished.

Once complete dissection of the UPJ is done, the renal pelvis is partly divided by scissors at the most dependent part,

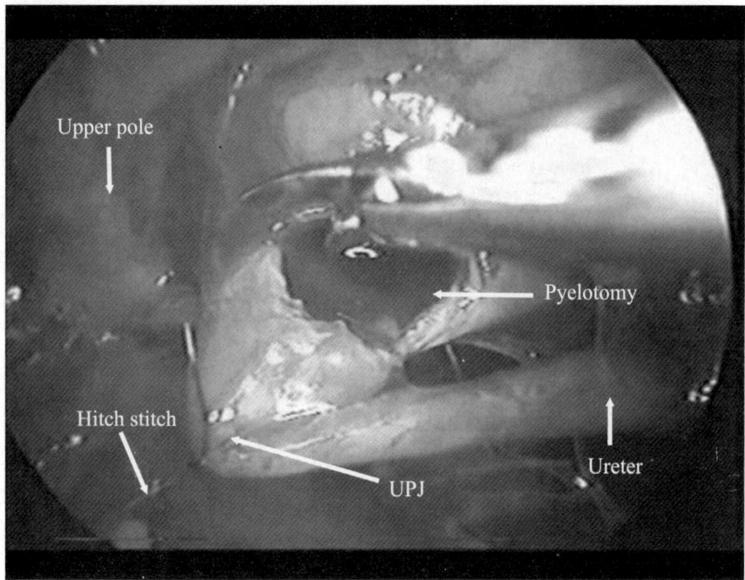


FIGURE 115.3 Retroperitoneal view of 5-0 suture as a hitch stitch at the right UPJ.

and then the ureter is partly divided and spatulated. At all times, the anterior surface of the kidney is left adherent to the peritoneum so that the kidney is retracted medially away from the anastomosis. Nevertheless, if inadvertent dissection of the kidney anteriorly is performed, a fourth trocar (3 mm) is inserted lateral to the lumbosacral muscles near the iliac crest to facilitate medial retraction on the kidney.

The pelviureteric anastomosis begins using 6-0 polydioxanone sutures and a tapered 3/8 circular needle. To facilitate passage of the needles through the 3-mm trocars, needles may be flattened out in the shape of a ski and lubricated. The first suture is placed from the most dependent portion of the pelvis to the most inferior point or vertex of the ureteric spatulation. In the initial few cases, the suture is tied using the intracorporeal technique with the knots placed outside the lumen. In order to facilitate the suturing part of this procedure, two 6-0 undyed polydioxanone sutures 6 cm in length were tied together and one was colored utilizing a surgical marker, thus eliminating a cumbersome step of tying intracorporeally. Once the ureter is approximated to the pelvis, the UPJ is maintained on traction and the suture line stabilized. Once half of the anastomosis is accomplished, a 4.7Fr polyurethane ureteral stent is inserted through the suture line to the bladder at the end of the anterior-layer reconstruction. Our preferred method for this is through a percutaneous placement of a 12Fr angiocatheter; however, the stent can also be inserted through the costovertebral trocar (Fig. 115.4). To ascertain the position of the stent in the bladder, retrograde filling of the bladder with methylene blue saline is done. The stent remains indwelling for 4 to 6 weeks. Perirenal drainage in the form of a Penrose drain is used. The Foley catheter is left in situ in all patients for 24 hours after surgery. Prophylactic antibiotics (third-generation cephalosporin) are routinely prescribed.

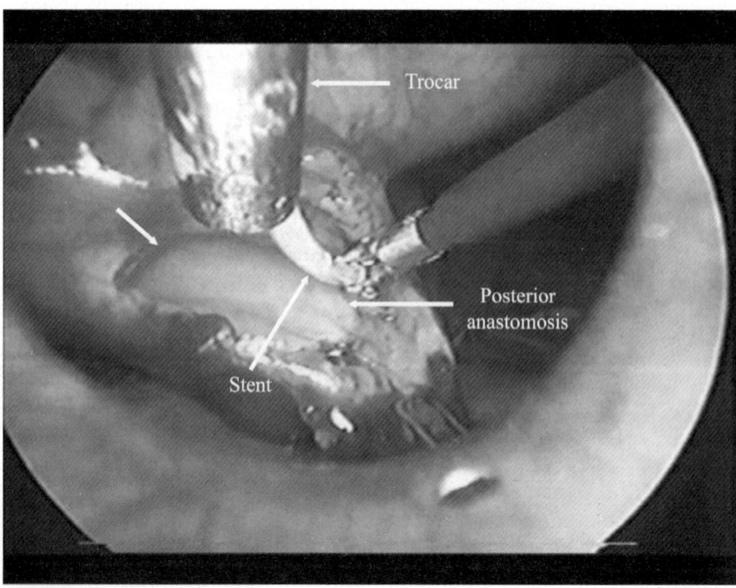


FIGURE 115.4 Retroperitoneal view of the double-pigtail ureteral stent inserted through a trocar traversing the ureter antegrade.

## Transperitoneal Approach

The first trocar is placed at the umbilicus either through a small open technique or after insufflation with a Veress needle. Utilization of 3- or 5-mm trocars depends on the patient size. In patients under a year of age, 3-mm trocars are sufficient. However, in any age group, 5-mm trocars with 3-mm instrumentation have been proven the easiest for suture passage in our experience. The abdomen is insufflated with low pressures and high flow to accommodate for suture passage and potential loss of pneumoperitoneum. A 3- or 5-mm 0-degree telescope is inserted through the first trocar. A second trocar is inserted subcostally lateral to the ipsilateral rectus muscle, while the third trocar is inserted 10 mm above the top of the iliac crest lateral to the ipsilateral rectus muscle. A transmesenteric window is performed if the UPJ obstruction is on the left kidney. If the UPJ obstruction is on the right, the colon is mobilized to expose the UPJ (Fig. 115.5).

The UPJ is identified and mobilized as just described above for the retroperitoneal approach with stay sutures and a hitch stitch. The hitch stitch is placed through the anterior abdominal wall, traversing the renal pelvis, then back through the anterior abdominal wall. It is held in place with a clamp to allow traction control to lift and relax the pelvis as necessary. Once complete dissection of the UPJ is done, the renal pelvis is partly divided by scissors at the most dependent part, and then the ureter is partly divided and spatulated.

The anastomosis and percutaneous stent placement are performed as described in the previous section on retroperitoneoscopic pyeloplasty (Fig. 115.6). The stent remains indwelling for 4 weeks. No perirenal drainage is used. The Foley catheter is left in situ in all patients for 24 hours after surgery. Prophylactic antibiotics (third-generation cephalosporin) are routinely prescribed until the catheter is removed. The patients are placed on prophylactic antibiotics until the stent is removed.

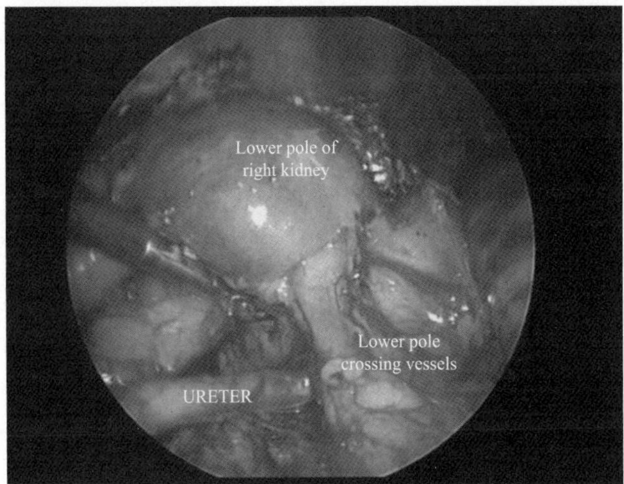


FIGURE 115.5 Transperitoneal view of right lower-pole crossing vessels.

## Special Considerations

Although various reconstructive methods of laparoscopic pyeloplasty such as dismembered or Y–V-plasty have been reported, it remains to be determined which methods are most appropriate for which cases of obstruction. For instance, when an aberrant crossing vessel is identified, the polar vessel is dissected and dismembered pyeloplasty is performed to enable the UPJ transposition. After placing the stay suture, the ureter is completely divided and the UPJ and pelvis are delivered anterior to the vessels with the help of the stay suture. In some retroperitoneoscopic cases when we encounter a long segment of obstruction that precludes the creation of a tension-free anastomosis, we perform a

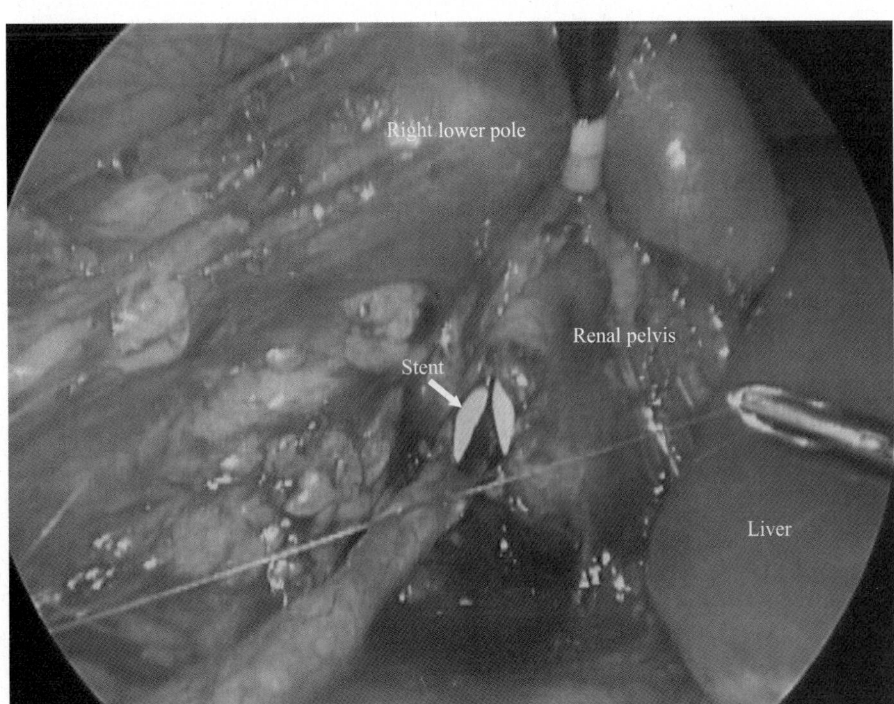


FIGURE 115.6 Completed posterior anastomosis and stent in place. The stent was placed percutaneously after completion of the posterior anastomosis as described.

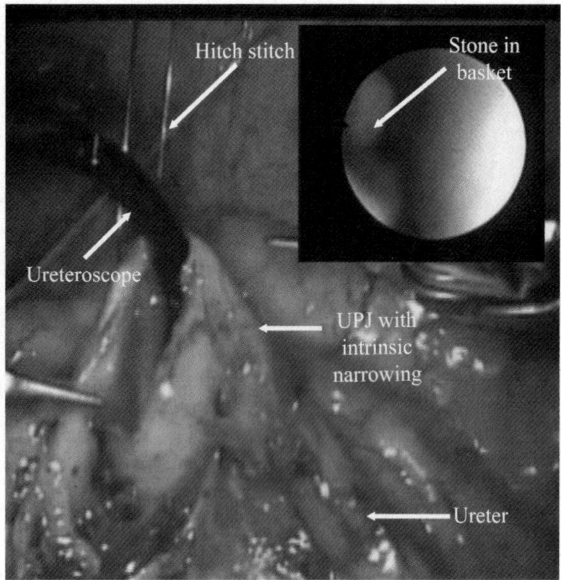


FIGURE 115.7 Concomitant stone extraction. Note the insert showing the ureteroscopic view seen during the procedure. The stone is extracted with a basket though an accessory port.

transperitoneal laparoscopic approach, and a Y–V-plasty can be performed more readily. A concomitant caliceal or renal calculus that cannot be easily accessed via a laparoscopic procedure is not an absolute contraindication if access to the stone is possible using ureteroscopy through one of the access trocars (Fig. 115.7).

## OUTCOMES

Although controversy still goes on concerning which laparoscopic approach to choose (i.e., transperitoneal or retroperitoneal), arguments to advocate one approach over another are more theoretical than true evidence-based criteria. We believe that surgeons who have started with laparoscopic nephrectomy using a retroperitoneal approach will be able to naturally extend the indications to pyeloplasty without changing their habits. Nevertheless, the longer time needed for the retroperitoneal approach is probably related to the limited working space, which makes suturing more difficult.

It is true that the gold standard of pediatric open renal surgery is the retroperitoneal approach and that minimal invasive surgery should follow the same rules (16). The major advantage of the retroperitoneoscopic approach is that it provides a direct access to the UPJ without interference with intra-abdominal structures. Furthermore, the complication of urine leakage would be better tolerated in the retroperitoneal space than in the intraperitoneal cavity. However, in our experience with the transperitoneal approach with stenting, the rate of urinary leakage from the anastomosis into the abdominal cavity has disappeared.

Laparoscopic pyeloplasty in children has been demonstrated to be feasible and to have satisfactory results (8,11,16,17). Although there are only a few published series on the long-term outcomes to date, the short-term data suggest that outcomes are similar to those of open pyeloplasty in children (11,12).

When comparing the gold standard open approach to the laparoscopic approach (16), the mean operative time was significantly shorter in the open surgery group versus the laparoscopy group (96 minutes [range 50 to 150] versus 219 [range 140 to 310], $p < 0.0001$). On the other hand, the mean postoperative use of analgesics and hospital stay were less in the laparoscopy group. The major disadvantage of the laparoscopic approach is that it is clearly a technically challenging and lengthy surgical procedure because of the high proficiency required for intracorporeal suturing. Although automated devices that facilitate suturing (18) are available, the need for accurate suture placement and unavailability of small sizes for pediatric application preclude their use. Development of novel alternatives to suturing, such as fibrin glue and laser welding, may enhance the utilization of the laparoscopic approach; however, the results with these methods alone have not yet matched the success of conventional sutures in providing adequate tensile strength of the anastomosis (19).

### Complications

Potential complications include bleeding, wound infection, hernia at the port site, thermal damage to tissues or organs, trocar or insufflation needle damage to viscera or vessels, persistent leakage of urine, stent migration, reobstruction (transient and persistent), and urinary tract infection with stent in place.

## CONCLUSIONS

Reports on the retroperitoneal approach in laparoscopic pyeloplasty are less common, despite wide use of this approach in laparoscopic nephrectomy. In our experience, the retroperitoneal approach has been difficult in the following scenarios: (i) children under 15 kg with extremely large renal pelvis and (ii) previous violation of the retroperitoneal space. For a relatively long obstructed UPJ segment associated with a hydronephrotic extrarenal pelvis, several flap pyeloplasty techniques, such as a Culp–Deweerd spiral, Scardino–Prince vertical flap, and a dismembered tubularized renal pelvic wall flap described by Kaouk et al., have been performed (19).

The level of difficulty of manipulation certainly increases in the retroperitoneal space, but we believe that difficulty of manipulation in the retroperitoneal space can be overcome with improvement in operative skill, especially in ambidextrous suturing technique. This approach has some advantages. First, it can avoid dissemination of urine into the peritoneal cavity. Second, it can theoretically minimize the risk of injury to intraperitoneal organs.

The success rate of laparoscopic pyeloplasty is equal to that of conventional open pyeloplasty. Transperitoneal and retroperitoneal approaches are reported to have comparable outcomes (11). We believe that laparoscopic dismembered pyeloplasty for UPJ obstruction in infants is technically possible and that an indwelling stent is helpful but not mandatory.

## *References*


1. Brooks JD, Kavoussi LR, Preminger GM, et al. Comparison of open and endourologic approaches to the obstructed ureteropelvic junction. *Urology* 1995;46:791–795.
2. Tan HL, Najmaldin A, Webb DR. Endopyelotomy for pelvi-ureteric junction obstruction in children. *Eur Urol* 1993;24:84.
3. Ahmed S, Crankson S, Sripathy V. Pelviureteric obstruction in children: conventional pyeloplasty is superior to endo-urology. *Austr N Z J Surg* 1998;68:641.
4. Kavoussi LR, Peters CA. Laparoscopic pyeloplasty. *J Urol* 1993;150: 1891–1894.
5. Ben Slama MR, Salomon L, Hoznek A, et al. Extraperitoneal laparoscopic repair of ureteropelvic junction obstruction: initial experience in 15 cases. *Urology* 2000;56:45–48.
6. Schwab CW 2nd, Casale P. Bilateral dismembered laparoscopic pediatric pyeloplasty via a transperitoneal 4-port approach. *J Urol* 2005;174(3): 1091–1093.
7. Casale P, Grady RW, Joyner BD, et al. Comparison of dismembered and nondismembered laparoscopic pyeloplasty in the pediatric patient. *J Endourol* 2004;18(9):875–878.
8. Tan HL. Laparoscopic Anderson-Hynes dismembered pyeloplasty in children. *J Urol* 1999;162(3 Pt 2):1045–1048.
9. Kutikov A, Resnick M, Casale P. Laparoscopic pyeloplasty in the infant younger than 6 months: is it technically possible? *J Urol* 2006;175(4): 1477–1479.
10. Yeung CK, Tam YH, Sihoe JD, et al. Retroperitoneoscopic dismembered pyeloplasty for pelvi-ureteric junction obstruction in infants and children. *BJU Int* 2001;87:509–513.
11. El-Ghoneimi A. Laparoscopic management of hydronephrosis in children. *World J Urol* 2004;22:415.
12. Bauer JJ, Bishoff JT, Moore RG, et al. Laparoscopic versus open pyeloplasty: assessment of objective and subjective outcome. *J Urol* 1999;162:692–695.
13. Soulie M, Thoulouzan M, Seguin P, et al. Retroperitoneal laparoscopic versus open pyeloplasty with a minimal incision: comparison of two surgical approaches. *Urology* 2001;57:443–447.
14. Tan HL, Roberts JP, Grattan-Smith D. Retrograde balloon dilatation of ureteropelvic obstructions in infants and children: early results. *Urology* 1995;46:89.
15. Munver R, Sosa RE, Del Pizzo JJ. Laparoscopic pyeloplasty: history, evolution, and future.*J Endourol* 2004;18:748–755.
16. Bonnard A, Fouquet V, Carricaburu E, et al. Retroperitoneal laparoscopic versus open pyeloplasty in children. *J Urol* 2005;173:1710–1713.
17. Peters CA, Schlussel RN, Retik A. Pediatric laparoscopic dismembered pyeloplasty. *J Urol* 1995;153:1962–1965.
18. Chen RN, Moore RG, Kavoussi LR. Laparoscopic pyeloplasty. Indications, technique, and long-term outcome. *Urol Clin North Am* 1998;25:323–330.
19. Kaouk JH, Kuang W, Gill IS. Laparoscopic dismembered tubularized flap pyeloplasty: a novel technique. *J Urol* 2002;167(1):229–231.


# CHAPTER 116 ■ PEDIATRIC LAPAROSCOPIC NEPHRECTOMY AND PARTIAL NEPHRECTOMY

GLENN M. CANNON, JR., AND RICHARD S. LEE

Since the initial description of a laparoscopic heminephrectomy in a 14-year-old by Jordan and Winslow in 1993 (1), a large amount of literature has been devoted to laparoscopic renal ablative surgery in children. With its decreased length of stay, decreased postoperative opioid requirements, improved cosmesis, and equivalent operative times to open surgery, laparoscopic nephrectomy and partial nephrectomy have become widespread procedures in pediatric urology. In a cost analysis from the United Kingdom, the laparoscopic approach to nephrectomy in children was 54% less expensive than the open approach (2). Currently, robotic systems such as the da Vinci Surgical System (Intuitive Surgical, Sunnyvale, CA) are being utilized for more complex reconstructive procedures such as partial nephrectomy. Future research will determine its utility as compared to conventional laparoscopy.

## DIAGNOSIS

Children with prenatal or postnatal hydronephrosis and/or febrile urinary tract infection are often imaged with renal ultrasound, voiding cystourethrogram (VCUG), and possibly radionucleotide renal scanning. If there is no evidence of vesicoureteral reflux (VUR), nuclear renography is performed to determine if there is significant obstruction and/or salvageable function. If a clinically significant nonfunctioning renal moiety (e.g., <5% to 10% function by dimercaprosuccinic acid study) is identified, nephrectomy or partial nephrectomy may be considered. Further imaging is usually not warranted, unless there is a history of a continued day and night wetting and possible ureteral ectopia. In these instances MRI urography may be beneficial. In cases of a renal mass, abdominal CT or MRI is typically obtained to further delineate the mass. In all cases, particular attention should be paid to vascular anatomy, the presence and appearance of the contralateral kidney, the presence and appearance of the ipsilateral and contralateral adrenal glands, and any degree of lymphadenopathy.

## INDICATIONS FOR SURGERY

Indications for laparoscopic nephrectomy or partial nephrectomy in children include nonfunctioning kidney, upper- or lower-pole moieties with duplicated collecting systems, or renal mass. Typical causes include obstruction, reflux, or ureteral ectopia. Symptoms can possibly include pain, hypertension, infections, or stone formation. Laparoscopy can also be applied when bilateral nephrectomy is required of nonfunctioning kidneys causing hypertension, infections, or nephrotic syndrome prior to renal transplantation. Removal of potentially malignant renal masses is not usually approached in a laparoscopic fashion in children.

## ALTERNATIVE THERAPY

Open nephrectomy or partial nephrectomy is the alternative to a laparoscopic approach. Percutaneous renal ablative procedures such as cryogenic and radiofrequency ablation are not performed in children. An open procedure may be considered if the kidney is large or extensive intra-abdominal adhesions are present. Retroperitoneal laparoscopy can be considered if there is a history of previous abdominal surgery, and transperitoneal laparoscopy can be considered if there is a history of retroperitoneal open surgery.

## SURGICAL TECHNIQUE

The following descriptions refer to laparoscopic partial nephrectomy in children. Specific mention is made when the steps of the procedure differ from the performance of a complete nephrectomy. Otherwise, the steps are identical. Although ultimately the surgical approach will be chosen by an individual surgeon's comfort level and experience, Borzi and Yeung (3) proposed selecting an approach based on the specific type of procedure performed. Reporting an experience of 179 laparoscopic procedures, they recommended a posterior retroperitoneal approach for isolated renal excision without extended ureterectomy, a lateral retroperitoneal approach for complete ureterectomy or access to horseshoe and pelvic kidneys, and a transperitoneal approach when complete moiety excision with lower urinary reconstruction is planned.

### Transperitoneal Approach

Preoperatively, patients receive a clear liquid diet for 24 hours and a rectal suppository the night before surgery. Depending on surgeon preference, cystoscopy is performed prior to the start of the partial nephrectomy. A ureteral stent can be placed in the nonfunctioning moiety to assist in identification if necessary. A bladder catheter and orogastric tube are placed.

The affected side is elevated by a 30-degree wedge, and the patient is carefully secured to the operating table. The table is rotated to flatten the patient's abdomen. With the patient's abdomen flat, transperitoneal port access is gained using either a Veress needle or with the modified Hasson technique. A camera port (12 mm) is placed at the umbilicus (Fig. 116.1). A second port is placed superior to the umbilicus in the midline approximately 10 cm from the umbilical port. A third working port (5 or 8 mm) is positioned at the anterior superior iliac spine laterally at a 45-degree offset and 10 cm from the umbilical port. If necessary, a fourth 5-mm port is placed. The fourth port is often helpful in right-sided cases to lift the liver edge and expose the upper pole of the kidney. The table is angled to raise the affected side into a 60-degree flank position. If the da Vinci Surgical System is utilized, the robot is positioned on the ipsilateral side of the patient and angled over the shoulder. The three robotic arms are then engaged to the laparoscopic ports. A 30-degree lens is used in the down position.

The kidney is exposed by medial reflection of the colon. The ureter from the nonfunctioning moiety (or the single ureter for a complete nephrectomy) is identified and mobilized as distally as the iliac vessels. The nonfunctioning ureter is divided. If there is no VUR the distal end can be left open. If there is VUR, the distal ureter is ligated with an absorbable stitch. The affected pole is manipulated by using the divided proximal ureter as a handle (Figs. 116.2 and 116.3).

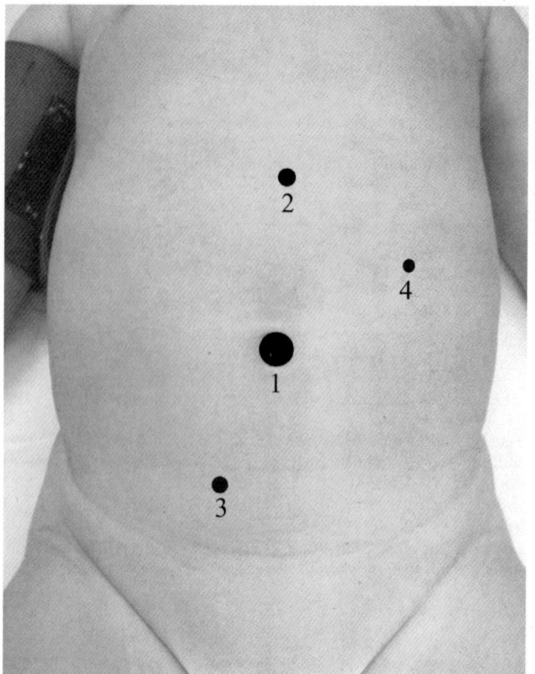


FIGURE 116.1 Port placement for a left-sided laparoscopic nephrectomy and partial nephrectomy.

The proximal nonfunctioning ureter is mobilized and passed posterior to the main renal hilum. During this mobilization, the nonfunctioning ureter is dissected away from the remaining ureter by mobilizing the adventitia of the nonfunctioning ureter toward the remaining ureter. This maneuver is critical to preserve the blood supply of the remaining ureter.

The nonfunctioning ureter is mobilized to the kidney and the Gerota fascia is opened. The ureter is passed posterior to the main renal hilum. Suprahilar, cephalad traction on the ureter should provide access to the upper-pole (nonfunctioning) hilum. If the blood supply is not clearly identified, laparoscopic bulldogs may be placed on the presumed upper-pole vessels. A clear demarcation between the upper and lower pole should be visible. The upper-pole vessels are clipped and divided. The renal pelvis of the nonfunctioning moiety is separated from the normal parenchyma using blunt dissection to better identify the demarcation between the functioning and nonfunctioning moiety. Large hydronephrotic moieties can be opened to help delineate the separation between the upper and lower pole. The nonfunctioning moiety is excised using electrocautery or the harmonic scalpel along the line of vascular demarcation. Any collecting system injuries to the remaining pole should be closed with an absorbable suture. Perirenal fat is used as a bolster prior to closing the cut surface of the remaining moiety with 4-0 absorbable monofilament suture.

If a complete nephrectomy is to be performed, after the ureter is divided and Gerota fascia open, the renal vessels are dissected and divided using clips or an endovascular stapler. The kidney is mobilized and removed.

After inspection for hemostasis, a retroperitoneal drain is placed and the specimen is removed through the camera port. If

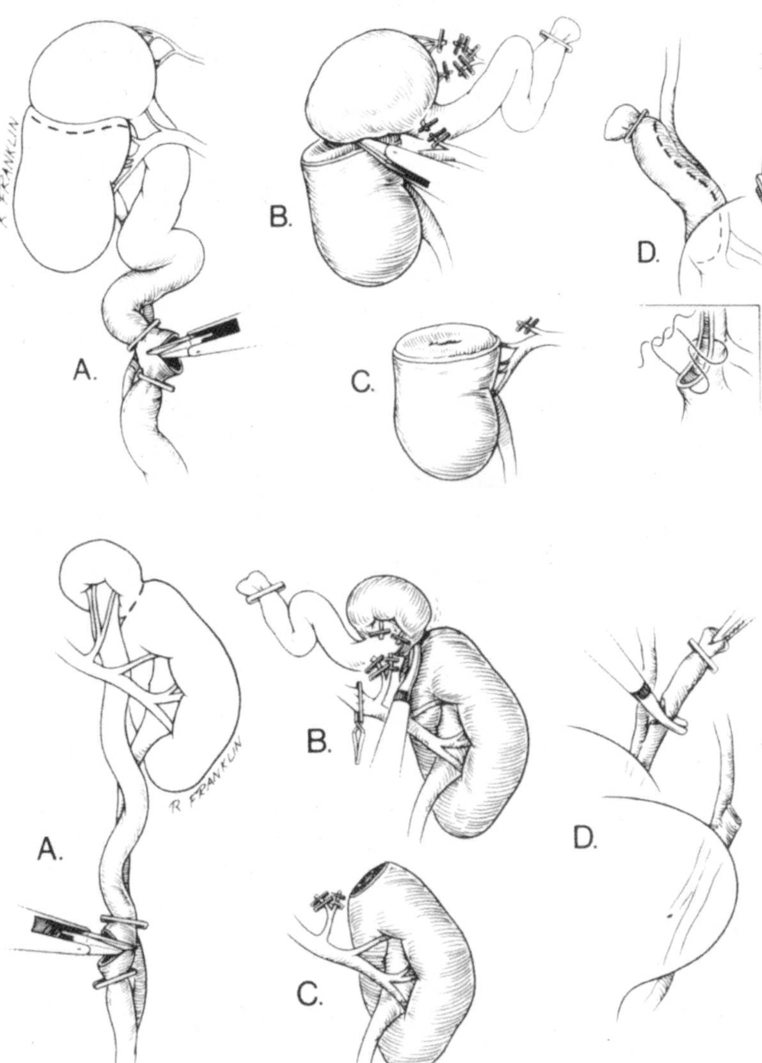


FIGURE 116.2 Laparoendoscopic right upper-pole partial nephroureterectomy. **A:** The ureter is clipped and divided in the region of the midureter. **B and C:** The ureter has been dissected from beneath the main renal pedicle and the upper-pole vasculature has been clipped. The hydronephrotic cap is dissected off with the parenchyma minimally divided. **D:** The ureter is left attached as the remaining wall of the ureter is dissected and ligated at the bladder wall.

FIGURE 116.3 Laparoendoscopic left upper-pole partial nephroureterectomy. **A:** The ureter is clipped and divided in the region of the midureter and dissected in a rostral direction. **B and C:** The upper-pole segmental vessels are clipped and the cap of the kidney allowed to demarcate. The plane of amputation is marked, an endoscopic bulldog is applied to the major pedicle, and the upper-pole cap is amputated. **D:** The ureter is dissected in a caudal direction to the point of the common vascularity and there amputated with the stump left open.

a complete nephrectomy is performed, a drain is typically not placed. Local anesthetic is injected into the port sites. Most patients, if not all, do not require epidural analgesia. The bladder catheter is removed on the first or second postoperative day, depending on whether further bladder work is required. The drain is removed when there is minimal drainage. The patient is discharged when comfortable with diet and oral analgesics.

## Retroperitoneal Approach

Retroperitoneal access to the kidney can be obtained by either a prone or a flank approach. The posterior prone retroperitoneal approach has been recommended for children with end-stage renal disease who may require immediate peritoneal dialysis (4). In the prone approach, initial retroperitoneal access is gained at the costovertebral angle using an open technique. Balloon inflation to 15 to 20 mm Hg of pressure is utilized to dissect and create the retroperitoneal space. Working ports are placed under direct vision inferior to the camera port and just above the iliac crest (Fig. 116.4). In this position, the kidney will move anterior by gravity, thereby exposing the hilar vessels. The psoas muscle is identified as a landmark. During nephrectomy, exposure and dissection of the hilum are performed first

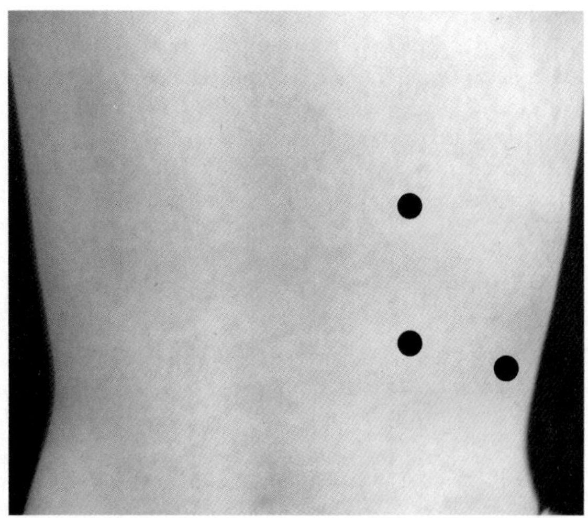

FIGURE 116.4 Port placement for right-sided prone retroperitoneal laparoscopic renal surgery.

with subsequent identification and division of the ureter. In partial nephrectomy, minimal mobilization of the remaining vessels and moiety should be performed to prevent vasospasm of the remaining moiety. The affected vessels should be divided and the nonfunctioning moiety removed as in the transperitoneal approach. The ureter is used as a handle to manipulate and isolate the affected moiety. Collecting system injuries should be closed appropriately, and the edges of the remaining moiety may be sutured together for further hemostasis. A retroperitoneal drain is typically left in place.

The flank approach is similar except that the working space is developed with the camera port just below the tip of the twelfth rib. The working ports are placed along a transverse line with the camera medially and laterally after dissection of the peritoneum from the anterior abdominal wall. The remainder of the procedure is identical to that of the prone approach.

## OUTCOMES

Janetschek et al. (5) presented the first series of pediatric laparoscopic heminephrectomy. In 12 cases, 7 upper renal poles were removed for ectopic refluxing megaureter and obstructive ureteroceles. Five lower poles were removed for reflux nephropathy. Their blood loss was minimal (10 to 30 mL), there were no complications, and mean operative time was 222 minutes. Horowitz et al. (6) later reported a series of 14 laparoscopic upper-pole heminephrectomies with a mean operative time of 100 minutes.

To assess for potential benefits of laparoscopic renal ablative surgery over open procedures, Robinson et al. (7) retrospectively compared 22 consecutive partial nephrectomies of which 11 were performed laparoscopically and 11 performed open in a nonrandomized fashion. Although the mean operative time was significantly longer for the laparoscopic group (200 minutes vs. 114 minutes), there was no difference in mean hospital stay. Patients in the laparoscopic group had a significantly lower opioid requirement than the open group. Piaggio et al. (8) compared intraperitoneal laparoscopic partial nephrectomy to an open retroperitoneal approach. They noted that length of hospitalization was shorter in the laparoscopic group and stated that the procedure is feasible even in infants under 6 months of age.

Success in laparoscopic partial nephrectomy has also been reported via a retroperitoneal approach. Castellan et al. (9) also reported their experience utilizing both transperitoneal and retroperitoneal heminephrectomy. Their overall complication rate was 10%, which included urine leak, pneumothorax, urinary tract infection, and hypertension. Lee et al. (10) performed an age-matched comparison of pediatric patients undergoing retroperitoneal laparoscopic partial nephrectomy to open surgery. Compared to open partial nephrectomy, the laparoscopic approach was eventually associated with equivalent operative times, significantly shorter length of stay, and less postoperative opioid requirements.

## COMPLICATIONS

The most severe complication that can occur during laparoscopic nephrectomy and partial nephrectomy is a major vascular injury. This is most likely to occur during trocar insertion or during the hilar dissection. Trocar injuries may be prevented by using an open approach. Meticulous attention must be paid during the hilar dissection. The vascular anatomy needs to be clearly defined prior to division of the renal vessels. When endovascular staplers are utilized, the surgeon must confirm that only the renal vessels are included within the stapler.

Other complications can include bowel injury, bleeding, infection, or urine leak resulting in urinoma formation. Bowel injuries can occur with inadvertent trocar placement or during dissection secondary to instrument handling or electrocautery misuse. Urine leaks are often discovered by elevated postoperative drain output. They are often managed with bladder decompression, with or without ureteral stent placement. Asymptomatic postoperative retroperitoneal fluid collections can be observed. Symptomatic retroperitoneal fluid collections may require percutaneous drainage and assessment for creatinine. A late complication that can occur is loss of function in the ipsilateral remaining moiety, eventually resulting in hypertension or worse loss of the moiety. If severe, this may require completion nephrectomy. This complication may be prevented with meticulous dissection and minimal mobilization of the hilum and kidney of the functioning moiety to prevent any intimal vascular injury or vasospasm.

As experience with laparoscopic nephrectomy and heminephroureterectomy increases, operative time and estimated blood loss can improve. Yucel et al. (11) retrospectively reviewed their experience with laparoscopic ablative renal surgery performed by one surgeon over a 6-year period. In the fourth year of their experience, they noted a statistically significant improvement in operative time for laparoscopic nephrectomy and in estimated blood loss for laparoscopic heminephroureterectomy. They concluded that their experience should continue to encourage pediatric urologists to perform laparoscopic renal surgery.

## *References*


1. Jordan GH, Winslow BH. Laparoendoscopic upper pole partial nephrectomy with ureterectomy. *J Urol* 1993;150(3):940–943.
2. Cervellione RM, Gordon M, Hennayake S. Financial analysis of laparoscopic versus open nephrectomy in the pediatric age group. *J Laparoendosc Adv Surg Tech A* 2007;17(5):690–692.
3. Borzi PA, Yeung CK. Selective approach for transperitoneal and extraperitoneal endoscopic nephrectomy in children. *J Urol* 2004;171(2,Pt 1): 814–816; discussion 816.
4. Gundeti MS, Patel Y, Duffy PG, et al. An initial experience of 100 paediatric laparoscopic nephrectomies with transperitoneal or posterior prone retroperitoneoscopic approach. *Pediatr Surg Int* 2007;23(8):795–799.
5. Janetschek G, Seibold J, Radmayr C, et al. Laparoscopic heminephroureterectomy in pediatric patients. *J Urol* 1997;158(5):1928–1930.
6. Horowitz M, Shah SM, Ferzli G, et al. Laparoscopic partial upper pole nephrectomy in infants and children. *BJU Int* 2001;87(6):514–516.
7. Robinson BC, Snow BW, Cartwright PC, et al. Comparison of laparoscopic versus open partial nephrectomy in a pediatric series. *J Urol* 2003;169(2): 638–640.
8. Piaggio L, Franc-Guimond J, Figueroa TE, et al. Comparison of laparoscopic and open partial nephrectomy for duplication anomalies in children. *J Urol* 2006;175(6):2269–2273.
9. Castellan M, Gosalbez R, Carmack AJ, et al. Transperitoneal and retroperitoneal laparoscopic heminephrectomy—what approach for which patient? *J Urol* 2006;176(6,Pt 1):2636–2639; discussion 2639.
10. Lee RS, Retik AB, Borer JG, et al. Pediatric retroperitoneal laparoscopic partial nephrectomy: comparison with an age matched cohort of open surgery. *J Urol* 2005;174(2):708–711; discussion 712.
11. Yucel S, Brown B, Bush NC, et al. What to anticipate with experience in pediatric laparoscopic ablative renal surgery. *J Urol* 2008;179(2):697–702; discussion 702.

# CHAPTER 117 ■ UROGENITAL SINUS AND CLOACAL ANOMALIES

JEFFREY A. LESLIE AND RICHARD C. RINK

Anomalies of the urogenital sinus occur on a spectrum ranging from a mild distal communication between the urethra and vagina to a very complex confluence between the urethra, vagina, and rectum. For this last-mentioned complex group a distal common channel for all of these structures drains to a single perineal opening (Fig. 117.1A). The clinical presentation of this single opening results from persistence of the cloaca and is essentially a severe urogenital sinus abnormality with a high imperforate anus (Fig. 117.1B). In addition to a more bizarre and diverse internal anatomy, patients with cloacal anomalies have a high incidence of other serious midline congenital anomalies. Important elements of baseline evaluation and surgical management of urogenital sinus and cloacal anomalies are discussed in detail in this chapter.

Urogenital sinus abnormalities (no rectal involvement) in general occur in one of two forms: pure urogenital sinus anomalies and females with disorders of sexual development (DSD, formerly known as intersex) conditions. The latter group is much more common. In these children surgical management must address not only the urinary and vaginal communication but also the virilization of the clitoris and labia.

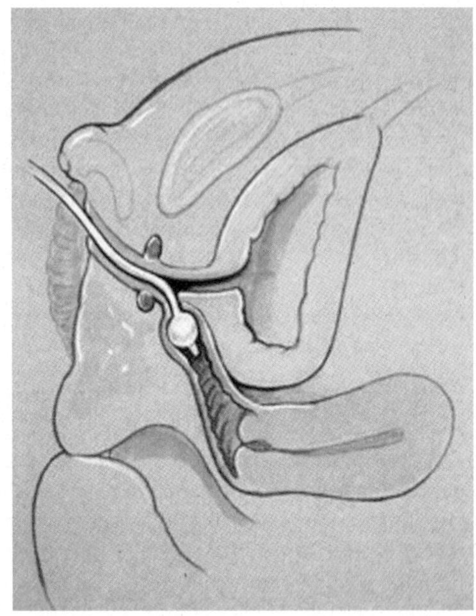

A

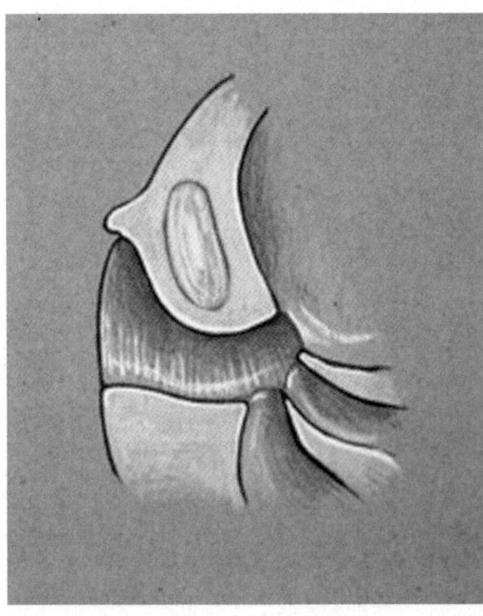

B

FIGURE 117.1 **A:** Urogenital sinus. The confluence of the vagina with the urethra is near the bladder neck and thus "high." A Fogarty catheter is in the vagina. **B:** Cloacal anomaly with the urethra, vagina, and rectum all exiting a single perineal opening.

## DIAGNOSIS

The majority of children with urogenital sinus abnormalities are detected at birth due to genital ambiguity. The initial evaluation in this group of children requires a team approach to gender identification with appropriate rapid chromosomal and endocrinologic studies. The history and physical examination are often helpful in establishing a correct diagnosis. Congenital adrenal hyperplasia (CAH) secondary to 21-hydroxylase deficiency is by far the most common etiology. Some children may be identified antenatally on ultrasound by noting a fluid-filled mass (distended vagina) posterior to the bladder and indeterminant genitalia. Persistence of the cloaca is suspected in utero when large fluid-filled pelvic structures are noted associated with bilateral hydroureteronephrosis, oligohydramnios, and ascites. A 46 XX karyotype is found. Hydrometrocolpos due to retention of urine and secretions results in upper-tract distention, and ascites occurs due to retrograde flow through the genital tract into the peritoneum. The rectum and bladder may also be filled with urine, giving rise to the other fluid-filled structures.

Prematurity and multiple congenital defects are common in children with cloacal anomalies. Initial evaluation of these children should therefore include medical stabilization and evaluation for midline abnormalities. Abdominal distention is common and may result in respiratory embarrassment. Cardiac, renal, and upper gastrointestinal anomalies and spinal dysraphism are frequently identified. Although these infants are uniformly female, ambiguity of the genitalia may occur and should be investigated. A single perineal opening is noted anteriorly, and the anus is absent. The perineum is in general flat with variable amounts of labial tissue mounded around the anterior orifice. Occasionally, a prominent phallic structure is found. The buttocks are often poorly developed, and the sacrum may be deficient on abdominal plain film.

Renal ultrasound reveals anomalies of number and fusion. Magnetic resonance imaging (MRI) clarifies the complex pelvic relationships, evaluates the structural quality of the sphincter complex, and defines the anatomy of the lumbosacral spine and distal spinal cord. A gender assignment committee is convened to determine gender identity. The child must be stabilized. Genitography is of utmost importance to help determine the anatomy (i.e., length of common sinus, location of vaginal confluence, status of bladder, presence or absence of vesicoureteral reflux, or vaginal duplication). Patients with cloacal anomalies will show communication between the urogenital tract and rectum, and vesicoureteral reflux is commonly identified. Ultrasonography of the pelvis and kidneys is also of help to identify the uterus, ovaries, and any vaginal distention, or, in the case of cloacal anomalies, it may reveal hydronephrosis or increased echogenicity suggestive of renal dysplasia. The adrenal glands in CAH may be prominent with a cerebriform appearance. MRI of the pelvis is an excellent tool to determine pelvic anatomy and note the presence of lumbosacral spinal cord anomalies that may be present.

Pure urogenital sinus anomalies are in general not detected early because of normal external genitalia. These patients are usually found at puberty with hydrometrocolpos or difficulty with tampon insertion. Some children are identified earlier with incontinence and urinary tract infection (UTI) from urine pooling within the vagina. Those with pure urogenital sinus anomalies are also more likely to have other organ system abnormalities than those with a urogenital sinus associated with DSD.

## INDICATIONS FOR SURGERY

It is important for the reader to understand that there is a great deal of controversy surrounding feminizing genitoplasty. There are proponents of (a) very early neonatal reconstruction, (b) delayed postpubertal reconstruction (this usually involves vaginoplasty), and (c) no surgery unless the patient requests it. There are obvious advantages and disadvantages to each of these approaches. All children with genital ambiguity should be evaluated promptly by a gender assignment team consisting of a neonatologist, geneticist, endocrinologist, pediatric urologist, and psychiatrist who are all working with and for the child and family. For the purposes of this presentation we will assume that the family and gender assignment team agree to proceed with surgery. It is our belief that early reconstruction is most appropriate with all three steps (clitoroplasty, vaginoplasty, and labioplasty) completed in a single stage. A revisional vaginoplasty is often needed at puberty due to stenosis of the introitus, which should be conveyed to the parents preoperatively. This is usually a minor procedure. In the rare situation of the very small and very high vagina, it may be more appropriate to postpone the vaginoplasty until the child is pubertal. Delayed postpubertal vaginoplasty, however, could easily be done by the same techniques described in this chapter.

## DECOMPRESSION THERAPY

While most of those with a urogenital sinus undergo reconstruction in the first few months, the complex nature of cloacal anomalies and their high incidence of other congenital defects, may necessitate a delay in formal reconstruction while the child is stabilized. Certainly, temporary diversion of the gastrointestinal tract by colostomy is essential, and decompression of the urinary tract may be required. This may be done by clean intermittent catheterization, but if this is not adequate, a temporary cutaneous vesicostomy may be necessary. Rarely a vaginostomy is needed, but this is a last resort as it tethers the vagina to the abdominal wall, making later vaginoplasty difficult. In the current era of Malone antegrade continence enema (MACE appendicocecostomy) procedures to achieve fecal continence, nearly all will ultimately undergo complete reconstruction, including a rectal pull-through.

## SURGICAL TECHNIQUE

All children with a very high vaginal confluence or a cloacal anomaly receive a polyethylene glycol electrolyte solution bowel preparation and prophylactic parenteral antibiotics preoperatively. Those with a low to midlevel confluence receive only a preoperative enema and broad-spectrum antibiotics.

Endoscopy is performed with the child in the lithotomy position. This is one of the most important steps in reconstruction, as it defines the level of vaginal confluence and allows identification of any other lower genitourinary pathology, such as vaginal duplication, ectopic ureter, and so forth. We believe that the distance of the vagina from the bladder neck is the most critical aspect and dictates the type of vaginoplasty. Endoscopy also allows placement of a Fogarty catheter into the vagina, which is left indwelling with the balloon inflated. Correct placement is confirmed by repeating endoscopy. The Fogarty balloon will aid in identification of the vagina during the reconstruction. A separate small Foley catheter is passed into the bladder.

Historically, urogenital sinus surgery has been performed with the child in the lithotomy position. While this position is acceptable, we have found it much easier to prepare the entire lower portion of the body circumferentially to allow access to the abdomen and perineum and to allow the child to be supine or prone (Fig. 117.2A and B). The supine portion of the procedure is done with the child "frog-legged," with the buttocks elevated on towels. This position dramatically improves visualization for the surgical assistants. By far the most common group of patients with a urogenital sinus anomaly to require surgical reconstruction is the group with congenital adrenal hyperplasia, who have not only a urogenital sinus but also virilization of their external genitalia. This includes clitoral hypertrophy, absence of the labia minora, and anteriorly placed labia majora. Therefore, most patients will undergo clitoroplasty, labioplasty, and vaginoplasty.

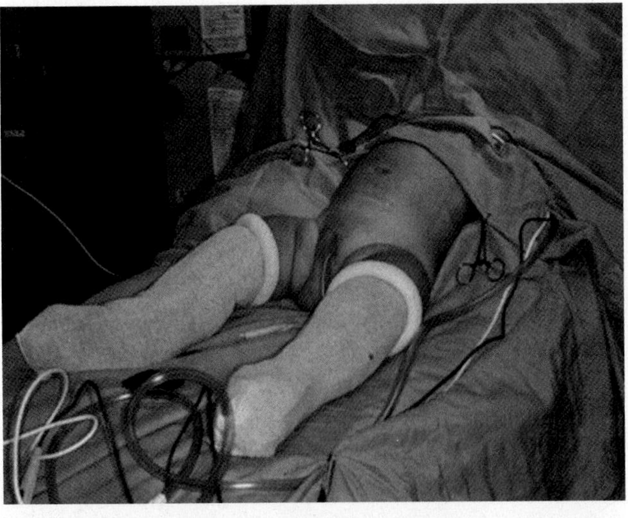

A

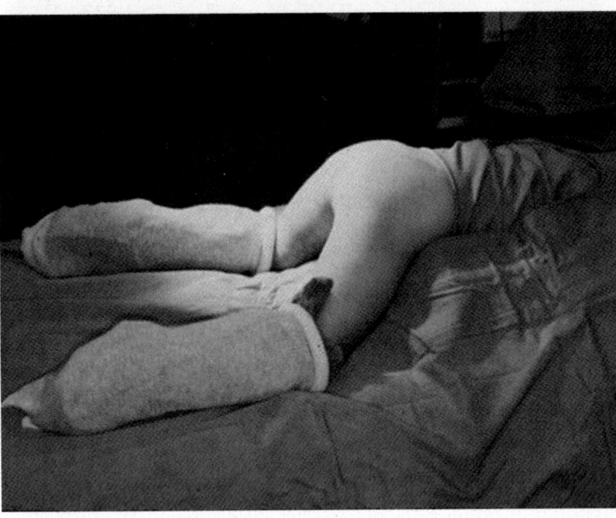

B

FIGURE 117.2 Total lower body preparation. **A:** Supine position allows access to perineum and abdomen. **B:** Child has been rotated prone, allowing access for a posterior sagittal approach.

## Clitoroplasty

In cases of genital ambiguity the operation begins with placement of a traction suture in the glans clitoris. Using a skin scribe, the proposed incisions are outlined as shown in Fig. 117.3. Historically, a very wide-based inverted U-shaped perineal flap has been created. Improved cosmesis occurs, however, if the flap has a narrower base similar to an omega, avoiding the appearance of a triangular introitus. After injecting 0.5% lidocaine with 1:200,000 epinephrine subcutaneously along the proposed suture lines, the clitoroplasty is begun. The initial incision is carried out dorsally well proximal to the glans to preserve the inner preputial layer for a clitoral hood. The entire clitoris is degloved by creating a plane between the Buck's fascia and the dartos circumferentially. Ventrally, the incision is carried around the urogenital sinus meatus. The rounded apex of the perineal flap should extend to near the meatus. This flap is elevated with its underlying subcutaneous and adipose tissue to expose the urogenital sinus. Dorsally, the suspensory ligament is divided and the bifurcation of the corporal bodies is exposed ventrally. With the entire clitoris now exposed, a tourniquet is placed at its base. A vertical ventral midline incision is made along the entire length of each corporal body to the glans (Fig. 117.4A). The erectile tissue is exposed and excised, with care taken not to injure the Buck's fascia, the tunica albuginea, the neurovascular bundle, or glans. This is performed bilaterally from the glans to the level of the bifurcation (Fig. 117.4B). The proximal end of each corporal body is oversewn with 4-0 polyglycolic acid sutures to prevent bleeding. With the Buck fascia folded, the glans is now secured to the corporal stumps with 4-0 polydioxanone sutures. We had previously sutured the glans to the pubis but found that this technique prevents appropriate concealment of the glans. At times the glans is quite large, but one should resist aggressive glans reduction. If any reduction is done, it should only occur on the ventral aspect of the glans to prevent loss of sensation (1).

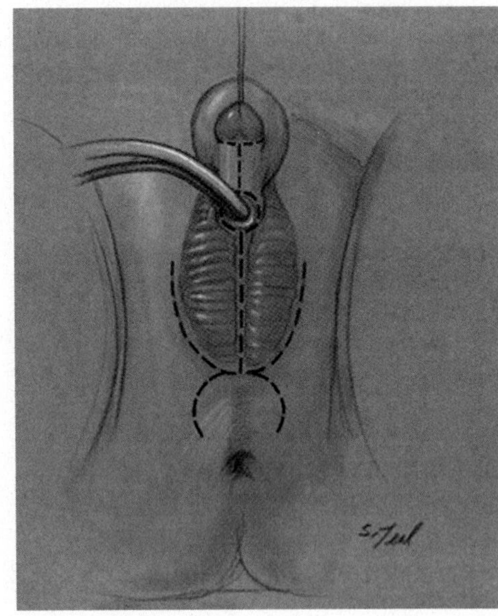

FIGURE 117.3 Proposed initial incisions. Notice the omega-shaped perineal flap. The meatus is encircled.

## Vaginoplasty

The most complex component of reconstruction of the urogenital sinus is the vaginoplasty. While multiple techniques of vaginal reconstruction have been described, they all fall in general into four types: (a) cut-back vaginoplasty, (b) flap vaginoplasty, (c) pull-through vaginoplasty, and (d) vaginal replacement. The type of vaginoplasty is determined by the location of the confluence between the vagina and the common urogenital sinus.

The *cut-back vaginoplasty* is applicable only for minor labial fusion and is in fact contraindicated for any true urogenital sinus anomaly. In this procedure the sinus is opened with a midline vertical incision that is then closed transversely in a Heineke-Mikulicz fashion. It is of historical significance only and will not be addressed further.

### Low Vaginal Confluence

For the low confluence a *flap vaginoplasty* is performed. This procedure leaves the vagina in the same anatomic location but

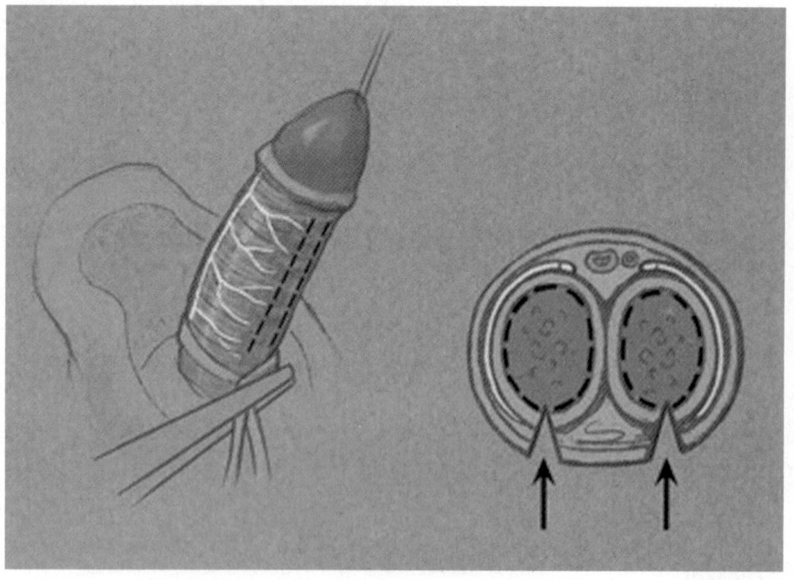

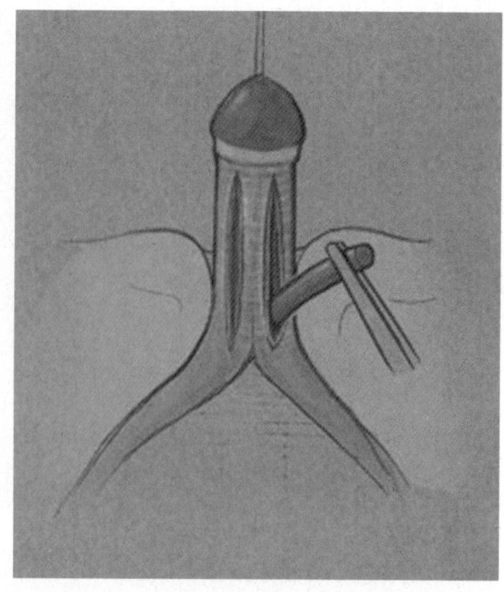

A B

FIGURE 117.4 Clitoroplasty. **A:** The longitudinal incisions must be ventrally placed to avoid injury to the neurovascular supply. **B:** The erectile tissue is removed. There is no excision of any of the tunic, and the neurovascular pedicles are never manipulated.

opens the sinus to provide a larger common opening for the urethra and vagina. It is contraindicated in patients with a high vaginal confluence. The previously elevated perineal flap must be long enough to allow a tension-free anastomosis to the normal-caliber proximal vagina. Redundancy of the flap, however, will create a lip of tissue at the introitus. The exposed ventral aspect of the sinus is opened in the midline, and the incision is carried through the narrowed distal one third of the vagina into the normal-caliber proximal vagina. It is very important to open into the normal-caliber vagina to prevent later vaginal stenosis. It is also noteworthy that the flap vaginoplasty does not change the vaginal location or confluence but merely exposes the vagina by widely opening the introitus. Because the anterior and lateral aspects of the vagina are untouched, stenosis is less common.

### High Vaginal Confluence

If the vaginal confluence is near the bladder neck, a flap vaginoplasty is contraindicated, as it will result in severe female hypospadias with urine pooling. Deep spatulation of the sinus and posterior vagina may permanently open and injure the sphincteric mechanism. Therefore, a *pull-through vaginoplasty* is required, which allows a complete separation of the vagina from the sinus. The sinus is closed in layers to create a urethra, and the vagina is brought to the perineum. In this technically demanding procedure, the vagina is completely separated from the sinus. The dissection of the anterior wall of the vagina from the urethra and bladder neck is the most difficult part of the procedure, and if not done with care and excellent exposure it may result in injury to the urethra or sphincteric mechanism. The initial portion of this procedure is identical to the flap vaginoplasty. It is important to expose the entire posterior wall of the vagina by dividing the bulbospongiosus muscle and sweeping the rectum posteriorly. The sinus is opened in the midline until the Fogarty balloon is exposed in the vagina. At this time we rotate the patient to the prone position and elevate the posterior wall of the vagina with a malleable retractor, providing excellent exposure of the anterior wall of the vagina and its confluence with the urethra (2). Stay sutures on the vagina are very helpful. With the vagina separated from the urethra and sinus, the opened sinus is closed in layers over a catheter, allowing the sinus to become the urethra. Unfortunately, "pull-through" is at times a misnomer: Even following complete circumferential vaginal mobilization, the vagina may not reach the perineum. In these situations the perineal flap will create the distal posterior vaginal wall and the anterior wall can be created by either a preputial or labial flap. In extreme situations, bowel interposition may be required to create the distal vagina. A Penrose drain is left in the vagina, and the Foley remains in the urethra.

## Labioplasty

Having completed the clitoroplasty and vaginoplasty, only the labial reconstruction remains. The phallic skin is unfurled and divided in the midline longitudinally (similar to Byar flaps), stopping short of the base to allow a clitoral hood (Fig. 117.5A). These skin flaps are now sutured in place inferiorly along either side of the vagina to create labia minora. The anteriorly displaced labia majora are mobilized posteriorly by making lateral incisions in a Y–V fashion (Fig. 117.5B). The mobilized labia majora are now sutured to the labia minora and to the apex of the perineal flap. This step moves the labia posteriorly to their normal location on either side of the vagina.

## Cloacal Anomalies

Surgical management of children with cloacal anomalies occurs in several important steps, but the formal reconstruction is best performed in a single stage. Neonates require early diverting colostomy. Hendren (3) prefers a right colostomy to leave adequate distal length and an intact blood supply for

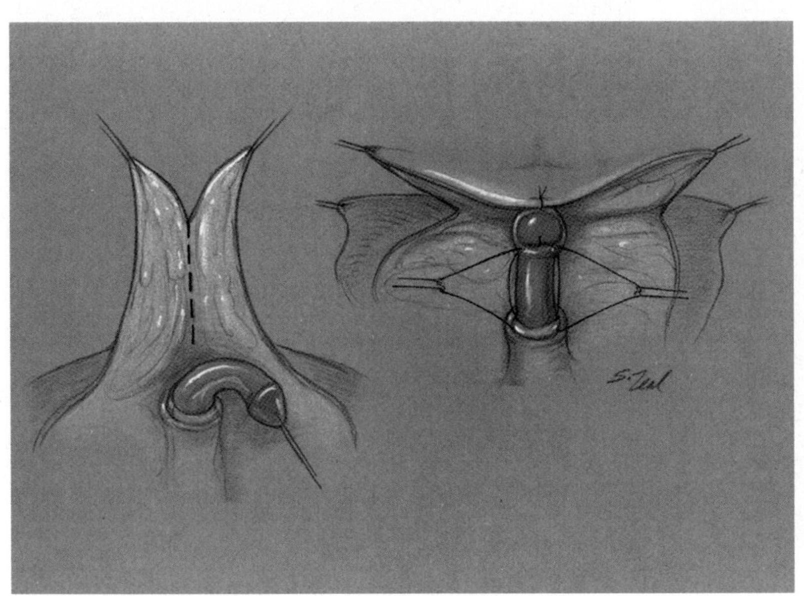

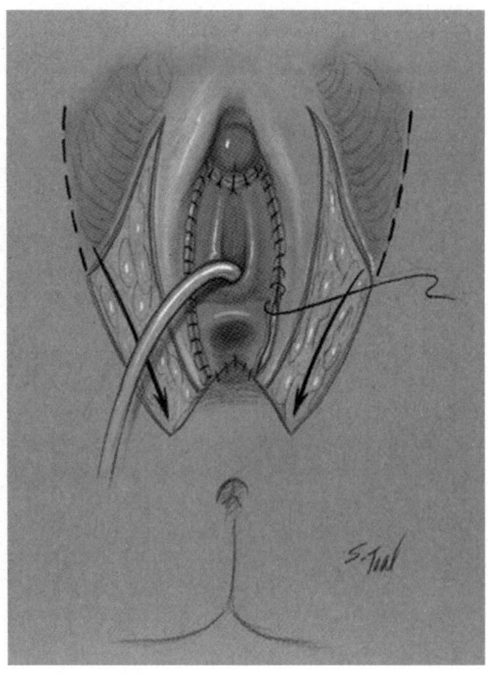

A B

FIGURE 117.5 **A:** The phallic skin is divided in the midline and used to create labia minora. The incision should stop well short of the base to allow creation of a clitoral hood. **B:** Y-V plasty of the labia majora moves the labia inferiorly to place the urethra and vagina between the labia in a more normal location.

subsequent rectal pull-through. A long distal colonic segment, however, can allow persistent retention of urine in the mucus fistula and result in refractory hyperchloremic metabolic acidosis. Preliminary mapping of the anorectal sphincter complex provides prognostic information for future rectal pull-through.

Decompression of the genitourinary tract is performed during endoscopic investigation of the cloacal anatomy. Inspissated mucus and meconium debris are drained. Because the bladder neck and vagina are often closely related, the vagina passively retains voided urine. If vaginal voiding is a problem, intermittent catheterization of the common channel will allow decompression, with the catheter most likely entering the vagina rather than the bladder. Poor emptying is suspected in children with persistence of hydronephrosis postnatally. Alternatively, if the common channel is narrow and more urthrallike, it can be opened distally to facilitate voiding. If the above measures fail, cutaneous vesicostomy is performed. Cutaneous vaginostomy allows free drainage but tethers the vagina anteriorly and complicates the subsequent vaginoplasty.

Severe anomalies of other organ systems should be corrected early. Other urinary tract abnormalities that may compromise long-term renal function should be addressed. Colonization of the urinary tract is common, but symptomatic infections mandate aggressive therapy. Assuming that all other congenital issues have been satisfactorily addressed, formal repair of the cloaca with the Peña posterior sagittal anorectovaginourethroplasty (PSARVUP) is planned for 6 to 12 months of age. This demanding procedure should be completed in a single stage, capitalizing on the virgin tissue planes for both anorectal and urogenital reconstruction.

The initial preparations for repair of the persistent cloaca are similar to those described above for the high-confluence urogenital sinus. After a circumferential lower-body preparation and endoscopic placement of Fogarty catheters in the vagina(s) and rectum and a Foley catheter in the bladder, the patient is placed prone on the chest and pelvic rolls. The sphincter complex is stimulated, and the optimal positions for the anus, perineal body, vagina, and urethra are marked. The perineum is incised in the midline from the tip of the spine to the posterior margin of the single perineal orifice. The sphincteric muscles are split in the midline and tagged to facilitate subsequent reconstruction. The rectal communication is sharply dissected off the common channel, and the distal colon is mobilized for pull-through. Occasionally abdominal exploration is required to achieve adequate rectal mobilization. At this time the entire urogenital system is circumferentially mobilized toward the perineum by the Peña technique of *total urogenital mobilization*. Even if this maneuver cannot bring the vagina to the perineum, it does improve exposure to the confluence for completion of a pull-through vaginoplasty. Duplicate vaginas are often encountered and are combined by division of the vertical septum. Vaginal agenesis or atresia requires bowel interposition for vaginoplasty, and again this is best performed at the time of rectal pull-through and urethroplasty.

## Total and Partial Urogenital Mobilization

*Total urogenital mobilization (TUM)*, described by Peña in 1997 (4), entails complete circumferential dissection of the intact urogenital sinus, urethra, and vagina from the pubis (Fig. 117.6A). This was originally proposed for cloacal anomalies but has since been often applied to those with a urogenital sinus only. TUM allows the midlevel vagina to be moved to the perineum easily, thus avoiding a *pull-through* vaginoplasty, and while the high-confluence vagina may still require a *pull-through* vaginoplasty, the separation of the vagina from the urinary tract is much more easily performed.

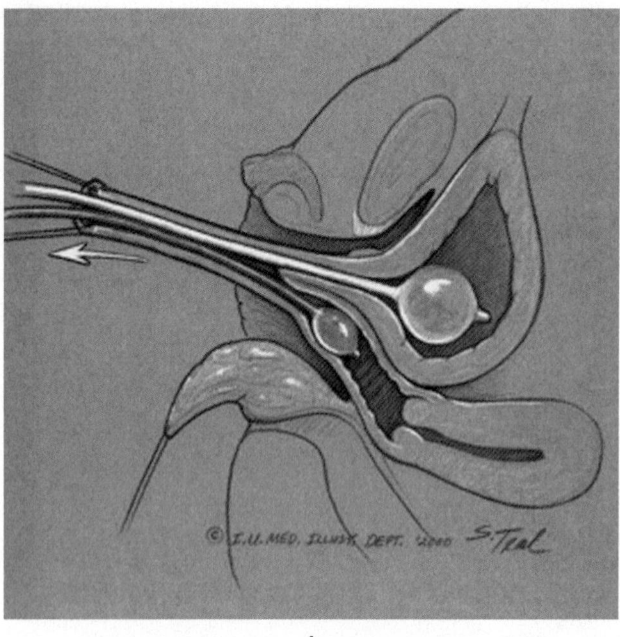


A

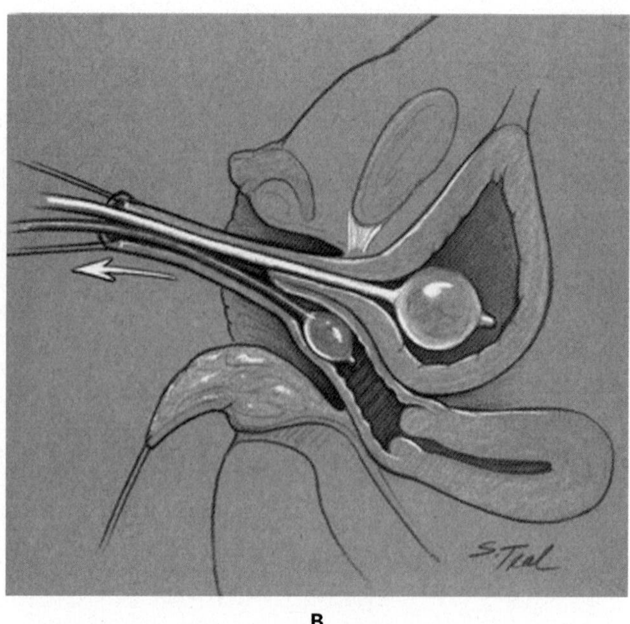


B

FIGURE 117.6 **A:** Total urogenital mobilization. Complete circumferential mobilization of the intact sinus with the dissection well above the pubis. **B:** Partial urogenital mobilization. The anterior dissection ceases at the pubourethral ligament.

The initial incisions are similar to those described previously, but the urogenital sinus is mobilized intact off the corporal bodies and is carried out between their bifurcation through the pubourethral ligament. At this time the dissection is continued posteriorly in the midline, separating the rectum from the posterior wall of the vagina. The Fogarty balloon within the vagina is palpated, and an incision is made into the vaginal wall posteriorly near the confluence. If the vagina reaches the perineum, no further dissection is performed and instead partial urogenital mobilization (PUM) is used. In Peña's original description the mobilized sinus was amputated, but Rink et al. (5) have shown that this is important tissue to save for the reconstruction. If the vagina does not reach the perineum, then the sinus is mobilized between the corporal bifurcation and off the pubis (TUM). When these avascular attachments from the pubis are divided, the sinus moves toward the perineum. If the sinus is near the perineum, we still believe a flap vaginoplasty should be performed to prevent vaginal stenosis. The redundant sinus is then split ventrally to create a mucosa-lined vestibule (Fig. 117.7A and B) (6). Recently, we described splitting the sinus laterally to create a posterior vaginal wall (Fig. 117.8) (7). This is also a form of *flap vaginoplasty,* but

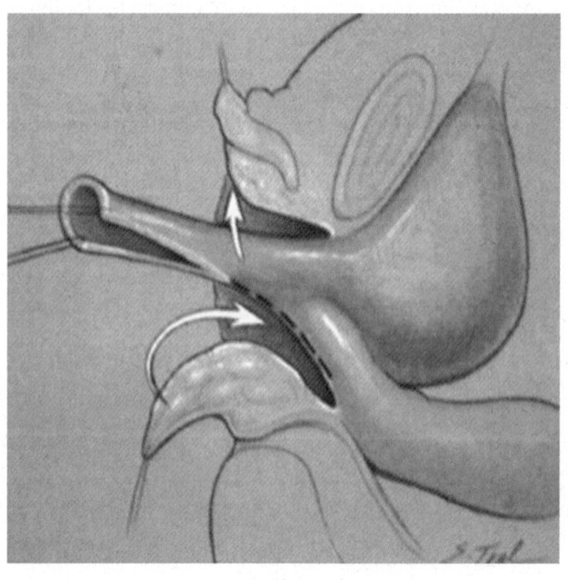


A

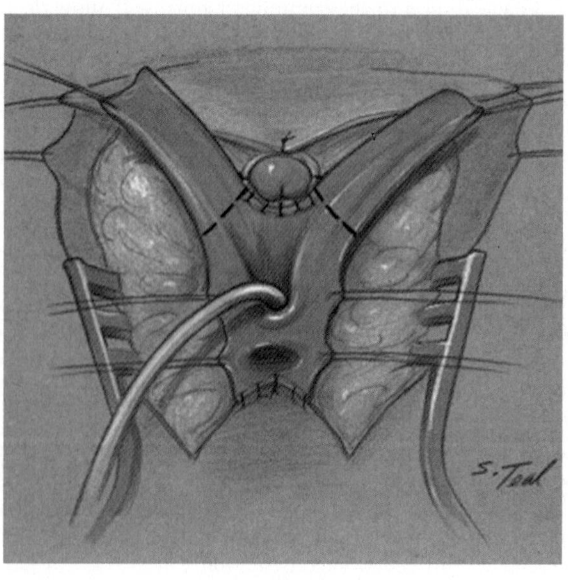


B

FIGURE 117.7 Low confluence with flap vaginoplasty. **A:** The mobilized sinus is opened on the ventral side. **B:** The opened sinus provides a mucosal-lined vestibule.

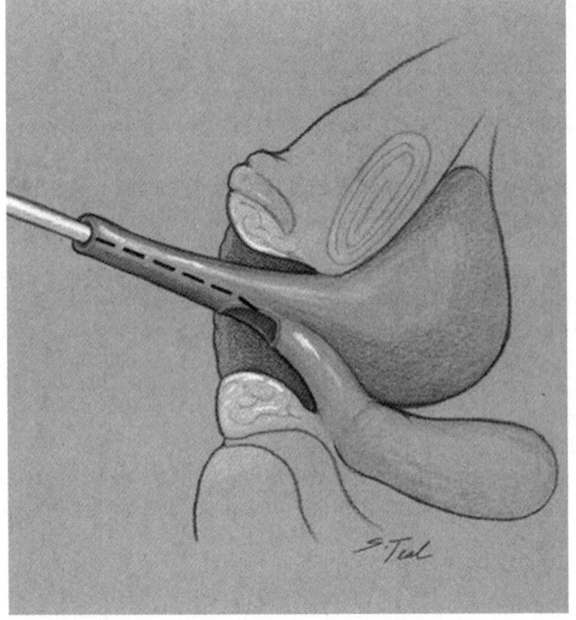

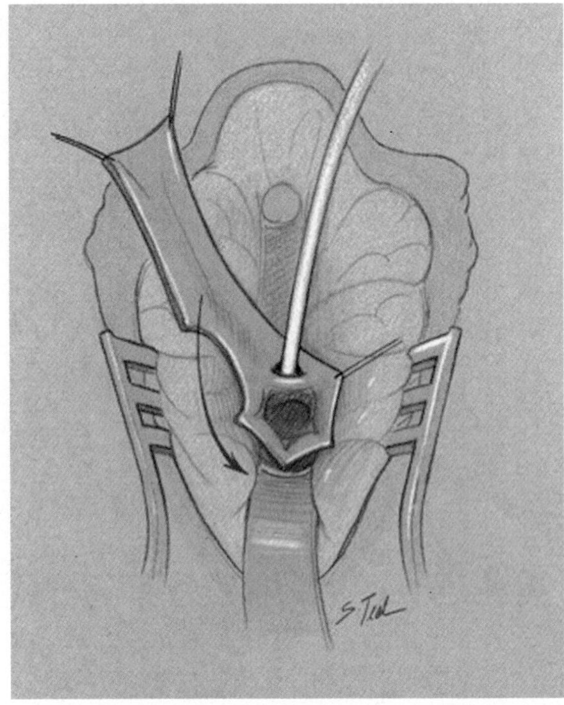

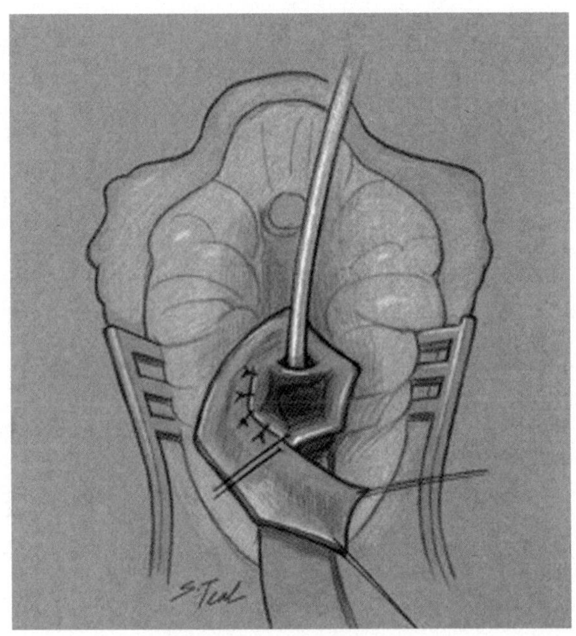

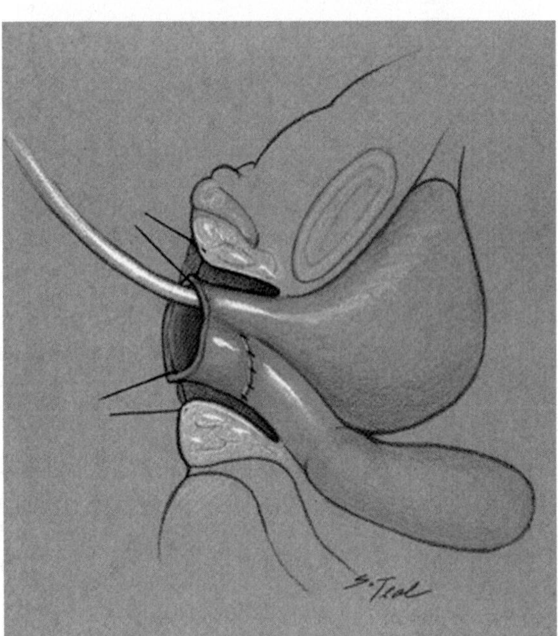

FIGURE 117.8 The mobilized sinus is split laterally to allow rotation of the flap to create a posterior vaginal wall.

the posterior flap is native urogenital tissue rather than perineal skin. If the vagina is high following the TUM, then the vagina is separated from the sinus as described previously for a pull-through vaginoplasty. This vaginal separation is again more easily achieved by placing the patient prone over chest rolls. The mobilized sinus is split dorsally, and the opened sinus is rotated to create an anterior vaginal wall (Fig. 117.9).

Due to concerns for potential sphincteric injury from aggressive retropubic dissection, Rink et al. (8) described *partial urogenital mobilization* (PUM). In the PUM, the dissection anteriorly ceases at the pubourethral ligament (Fig. 117.6B). We believe this procedure is less risky yet still allows use of the mobilized tissue for improved cosmesis and function as described previously for the TUM. In the majority of urogenital sinus anomalies, PUM is adequate to exteriorize the vagina when combined with a flap vaginoplasty.

## OUTCOMES

This is a time of widespread evaluation of all aspects of feminizing genitoplasty. There is little agreement on any component, including the timing of the procedure or even the necessity of some aspects, such as clitoroplasty. While virtually

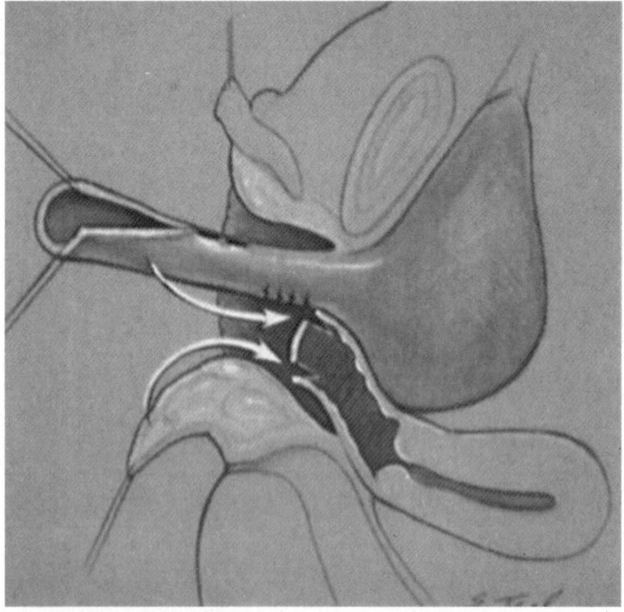

FIGURE 117.9 The sinus is opened dorsally for a pull-through vaginoplasty and rotated to create an anterior vaginal wall.

all surgeons believe they achieve excellent cosmetic results, blinded studies have questioned this. Unfortunately, there are few data available on long-term results from current surgical techniques. There is debate about both the psychological aspects of having genital surgery and the psychological aspects of not having the surgery and growing up with genital ambiguity. Clitoroplasty is controversial, as no one knows if it is a clinical problem to have an enlarged clitoris, and there remains a concern that even modern techniques may alter sensation. Should the parents make the decision about early surgery, or should it be postponed until the patient can decide? If the latter, then what are the social implications of growing up with ambiguous genitalia? Virtually all agree that the vagina must be exposed to allow egress of menstrual fluid, but when this should be done remains controversial. Early TUM results are promising, and incontinence does not seem to be a problem in children who are otherwise neuroanatomically normal. And while the procedure is technically easier, the long-term results may show that sphincteric injury with incontinence or stress incontinence from moving the bladder neck inferiorly occurs with unacceptable frequency. Early PUM results are similarly promising. All neurologically normal children older than 2 who have undergone PUM in our hands are dry and voiding (9). Long-term data are lacking, of course, as these techniques are relatively new and have been applied mainly to young girls. These issues are complex and will only be solved by long-term prospective multi-institutional studies. We believe that virtually all CAH patients can be treated with a PUM technique, avoiding the more aggressive TUM.

From an anatomic and cosmetic standpoint, surgical reconstruction of cloacal anomalies is now satisfactory in the majority of cases. Unfortunately, the functional success of the urinary and rectal elements of the reconstruction also depends upon sacral nerve function and the quality and innervation of the sphincteric complexes. The bladder neck and intrinsic sphincter may be inherently deficient with a high confluence. No natural plane exists between the bladder neck or trigone and the vagina, and therefore the continence mechanism may be further compromised as the vagina is dissected off the bladder neck. The external sphincter may also be congenitally deficient or may be injured during reconstruction. Due to abnormal sacral nerve function, these patients may require intermittent catheterization or further reconstruction, such as outlet resistance enhancement or augmentation cystoplasty, to achieve continence (9).

Outcomes of vaginoplasty in cloacal anomalies are as reported with the high-confluence urogenital sinus. Total urogenital mobilization appears to reduce the incidence of stenosis and the need for a pull-through procedure, although long-term pubertal follow-up is pending. Introital revision may be required at puberty after vaginoplasty in infancy.

One of the most important issues in functional outcome after repair of a persistent cloaca is the long-term preservation of renal function. Many of these children have congenital renal dysplasia related to vesicoureteral reflux and/or in utero infravesical urinary tract obstruction. Persistent postnatal hydronephrosis should be aggressively addressed with diversion if necessary. Chronic renal failure may occur even in the fortunate subset of patients who achieve a normal nadir creatinine in infancy (10). This is usually due to abnormal lower-urinary-tract dynamics. Therefore, even after apparently successful lower-urinary-tract reconstruction, these patients require urodynamic evaluation and vigilant monitoring to prevent upper-urinary-tract deterioration due to silent bladder dysfunction.

## *References*


1. Rink RC, Adams MC. Feminizing genitoplasty: state of the art world. *J Urol* 1998;16:212–218.
2. Rink RC, Pope JC, Kropp BP, et al. Reconstruction of the high urogenital sinus: early perineal prone approach without division of the rectum. *J Urol* 1997;158:1293–1297.
3. Hendren WH. Cloacal malformations: experience with 105 cases. *J Pediatr Surg* 1992;27:890–901.
4. Peña A. Total urogenital mobilization—an easier way to repair cloacas. *J Pediatr Surg* 1997;32:263–268.
5. Rink RC, Metcalfe PD, Cain MP, et al. Use of the mobilized sinus with total urogenital mobilization. *J Urol* 2006;176:2205–2211.
6. Rink RC, Yerkes EB. Surgical management of female genital anomalies, intersex (urogenital sinus) disorders and cloacal anomalies. In: Gearhart JP, Rink RC, Mouriquand PDE, eds. *Pediatric urology*. Philadelphia: WB Saunders, 2001.
7. Rink RC, Cain MP. Urogenital mobilization for urogenital sinus repair. *Br J Urol Int* 2008;102:1182–1197.
8. Rink RC, Metcalfe PD, Kaefer M, et al. Partial urogenital mobilization: a limited proximal dissection. *J Pediatr Urol* 2006:3(5):351–356.
9. Rink RC, Leslie JA, Kaefer M, et al. Outcomes and risk factors in urogenital mobilization. Data presented at meeting of American Academy of Pediatrics. San Francisco, Oct. 2007.
10. Warne SA, Wilcox DT, Ledermann SE, et al. Renal outcome in patients with cloaca. *J Urol* 2002;167:2548–2551.

# CHAPTER 118 ■ SURGERY TO CORRECT AMBIGUOUS GENITALIA (46XX DISORDER OF SEXUAL DEVELOPMENT)

ANTHONY J. CASALE

*Ambiguous genitalia* and *intersex* are historical terms used to describe a congenital condition where the appearance of the genitalia is neither classically male nor female. Modern nomenclature has been proposed to replace the old, and this group of disorders is now described as disorders of sexual development (DSD). The condition affects both external genitalia (phallus, labia, scrotum, and introitus) and internal reproductive structures (vagina, urethra, urogenital sinus). In these cases there is usually a conflict between the genetic sex, gonadal sex, and apparent gender as based on genital appearance. The genital appearance may be gender neutral and give little indication of the genetic or gonadal sex. On the other hand, the genitalia may have an appearance more consistent with the opposite gender, as with females with severely virilized congenital adrenal hyperplasia (CAH). When patients with these conflicts reach adulthood they face significant hurdles in both reproduction and sexual activity.

The historical goal of surgery for ambiguous genitalia has been to provide the child with genitalia that have the appearance of and are functional as either male or female gender and that are consistent with the genetic and gonadal sex when possible. *Feminizing genitoplasty* is the term used to describe a series of surgical procedures designed to create classic female genitalia from a truly ambiguous genital state. This surgery has usually been applied to female patients with partially masculinized genitalia, and in those cases surgery brings the genetic, gonadal, and genital sex back into alignment. Rarely, this surgery has been used to reassign the gender of genetic and gonadal male patients with what was felt to be inadequate phallic tissue to the female gender. It is this later group of patients who have had more difficulties with gender dissatisfaction, and their experience has brought the principle of gender assignment under question. This chapter will discuss the technical aspects of feminizing genitoplasty.

Society dictates that the appearance of the infant's genitals and therefore its apparent gender is the subject of great and urgent interest for the immediate and extended family and friends, making ambiguous genitalia a cause of intense concern and confusion for all. It is this powerful interest that has driven physicians and families to treat the condition as an emergency, even though there are often no immediate health risks. The historical approach to this issue has been to assign gender based on several factors, including the potential for reproduction, the technical limits of surgical reconstruction (i.e., our limited ability to create a male phallus without adequate corpora), and the belief that gender was determined by genital appearance and role assignment in childhood. The validity of this approach has recently been questioned and is the subject of widespread study at this time. At present, intrauterine and postpartum androgen exposure of the central nervous system seems to be the dominant factor in determining gender identity. Exactly how to reliably measure the gender of the brain remains an unsolved question.

Genital ambiguity is a result of an abnormality in sexual determination resulting from a defect in genetic, gonadal, or genital tissue differentiation and has been classified historically into four categories: female pseudohemaphrodite (now called 46XX DSD), male pseudohemaphrodite (46XY DSD), mixed gonadal dygenesis (sex chromosome DSD), and true hermaphrodite (ovotesticular DSD). Female genital reconstruction, also called feminizing genitoplasty, is restricted to female pseudohemaphrodite (46XX DSD), mixed gonadal dygenesis (sex chromosome DSD), and true hermaphrodite (ovotesticular DSD) individuals who have the potential to have normal female sexual function. CAH is a form of 46XY DSD and is by far the most common condition causing ambiguous genitalia. CAH is responsible for over 70% of cases of ambiguous genitalia and the vast majority of patients treated with feminizing genitoplasty.

Candidates for feminizing genitoplasty have two distinct problems: (i) the fusion of their internal reproductive system with the urinary tract as a urogenital (UG) sinus with a single external orifice and (ii) the virilization of the external genitalia, with fused labioscrotal folds and clitoral enlargement. The internal anatomy can cause problems by pooling of urine within the vagina and uterus and inadequate vaginal drainage for secretions and menses. There is no adequate external vaginal orifice for sexual intercourse. Infants with a UG sinus may present with urinary infection or an abdominal mass from a poorly drained vagina or uterus. Today many present on prenatal ultrasound screening that reveals a dilated bladder, vagina, or upper urinary tract. The external genitalia are a concern primarily for sexual function and the potential psychological damage that may result from gender ambiguity.

There have been great advances in the surgical technique of feminizing genitoplasty over the past half-century, resulting in more normal appearance and sexual function. Despite apparently successful surgery, some adult patients have expressed profound dissatisfaction with their childhood genital reconstruction and gender. Because of this concern, more long-term outcome studies that include all patients with these rare conditions must be undertaken in order to understand the most

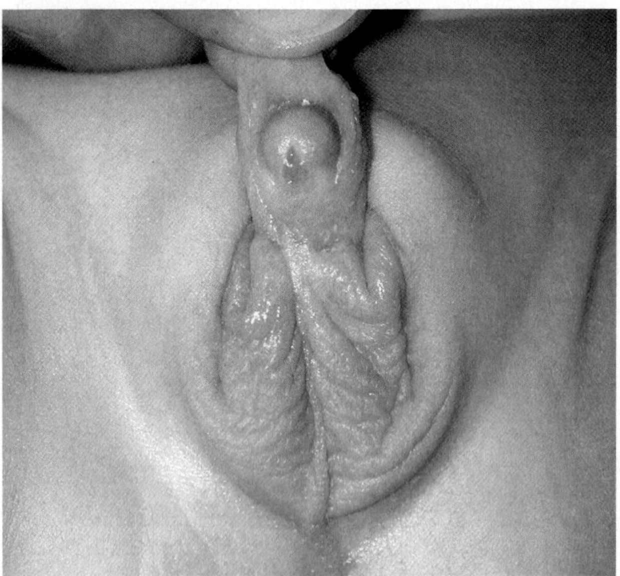

FIGURE 118.1 This intersex female patient demonstrates labial/scrotal fusion and a hypertrophied phallus with a distal urogenital sinus opening.

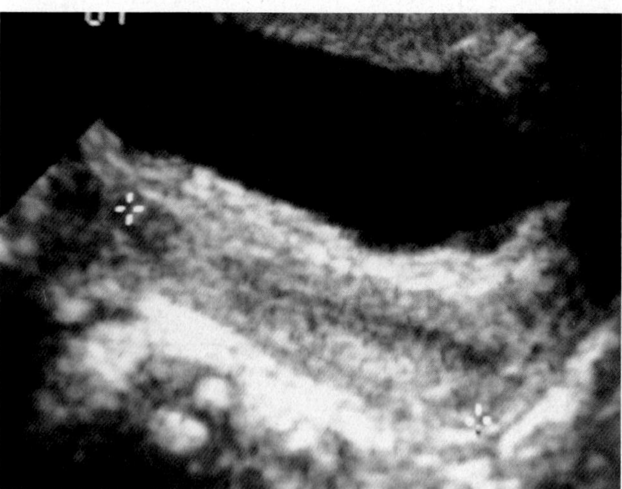

FIGURE 118.2 Pelvic ultrasound demonstrates the uterus in the midline position posterior to the urinary bladder.

appropriate management of these complex patients. The challenge of these studies is to make them comprehensive in surveying medical, sexual, and psychological health.

The first task for the physician faced with a child with intersex is to correctly diagnose the underlying condition responsible for the appearance of the genitalia. A team including a pediatric urologist, pediatric endocrinologist, neonatologist, and either pediatric psychologist or psychiatrist provides the best approach for this complex process.

The first step in diagnosis is a thorough physical examination. The initial caregivers in the nursery are usually alerted to the possibility of gender ambiguity if the phallus is small or curved and if the labioscrotal folds are partially fused (Fig. 118.1). The pediatric urologist should then document the length and diameter of the phallus and the position and number of external perineal openings, including the position of any potential urogenital orifices as well as the rectum. The state of fusion of the labioscrotal folds and their location are important, as is the presence or absence of palpable gonads. The presence of a palpable gonad almost always is consistent with male gender. Hyperpigmentation of the labioscrotal skin is common in cases of CAH. The blood pressure should be measured carefully because of the threat of hypertension with CAH.

Chromosomal studies should be sent immediately. In the immediate newborn period the presence of functioning testicular tissue can be determined by measuring serum testosterone, which is elevated in the first few days of life. CAH is diagnosed by finding elevated plasma levels of 17-hydroxyprogesterone and androstenedione and urine levels of pregnanetriol and 17-ketosteroids. CAH can be a life-threatening condition because adrenal insufficiency commonly causes salt wasting leading to hyponatremia and hyperkalemia and could result in lethargy, vomiting, and eventual hypotension.

Imaging studies of the infant should include a pelvic ultrasound looking for the presence of a uterus and retrograde injection of contrast into the UG sinus (genitogram) to identify the presence of a vagina and uterus. The uterus can usually be identified on pelvic ultrasound of the newborn as a 1-cm solid midline mass just posterior to the bladder (Fig. 118.2). The uterus can often be identified on a genitogram with a cervical impression outlined by the contrast in the vagina.

During the initial investigation the family is advised to delay naming the child and reporting the child's gender to others until the gender is established, and to state only that the child had some developmental problems that need to be investigated. It is during this period that the gender assignment team should carefully educate and counsel the family about the nature of their child's problem and the limitations and potential inherent in the exact condition. The family should be prepared to face the options of therapy, including reconstructive surgery, so that when the diagnosis is clear they can make an informed decision. This is a difficult and often painful process for both family and team, and it is critical that every option be explored and discussed with the family and that this counseling is documented in the medical record.

There are actually two decisions to be made by the parents: the gender that they will raise the child and whether to have reconstructive surgery. Gender decisions have always been considered urgent, while surgical reconstruction decisions may be made later as long as there is not a health concern because of inadequate drainage of urine. The medical team must explain the surgical options, including advantages, risks, and potential complications of delaying surgery, performing the external genital reconstruction (clitoroplasty), and performing the internal genital reconstruction (urogenital sinus repair).

## TIMING OF SURGERY

Once the decision for feminizing genitoplasty has been made, the timing of the procedure is of some importance. In cases of CAH, glucocorticoid and mineralocorticoid replacement therapy will diminish androgen production by the adrenal and lead to partial reversal of the clitoral hypertrophy. For this reason the external genital surgery should be delayed until at least 6 months of age. In some cases hormone replacement therapy decreases the size of the clitoris so that surgery on this structure is not necessary. Since most complaints about childhood genital surgery involve dissatisfaction with clitoral reconstruction, most surgeons have currently limited this surgery to the most extreme cases of enlargement and with the family's clear support. Some surgeons have refused to perform clitoral reconstructive surgery altogether. The decision about clitoral reconstruction is the most difficult issue to face in the care of these children and must be considered carefully by the family and medical team.

Some surgeons prefer to delay reconstruction of the internal structures until adolescence if the child does not have problems with urine retention and urinary tract infections because historically patients who had reconstruction early in life might require a secondary procedure at adolescence to correct vaginal stenosis. On the other hand, those children who have early reconstruction need only dilations or simple revisions of the vagina at adolescence, in contrast to the child who delays the major reconstruction until later in life. We prefer to do a complete reconstruction at 6 months of age and explain to the family that a second minor procedure may be needed later.

## PREOPERATIVE EVALUATION

Each child suspected to have ambiguous genitalia should have a complete anatomic, endocrine, and genetic evaluation. A karyotype is necessary not only to determine the correct genetic sex but to look for other chromosomal errors that may be present. A complete endocrine evaluation should focus on potential gonadal function as well as concerns related to the endocrinopathy of CAH.

A comprehensive definition of the anatomy is imperative in planning for and accomplishing the reconstruction. The upper urinary tract should be imaged with ultrasound and, if the kidneys are not normal, a diuretic (Lasix) renal scan. The lower urinary tract should be imaged with a retrograde genitogram (Fig. 118.3). This is performed by placing a catheter in

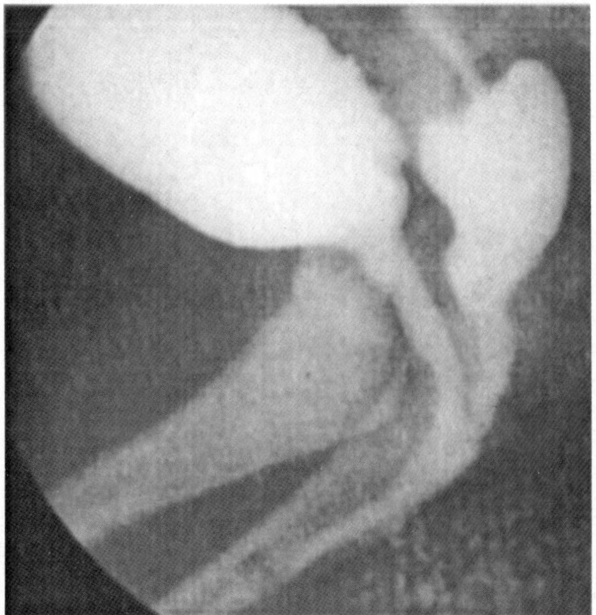

FIGURE 118.3 Genitogram demonstrates confluence of the urethra anteriorly and vagina posteriorly. Note cervical impression at the apex of the vagina and contrast within the cervix.

the most distal portion of the UG sinus and injecting contrast while imaging from the anterior, lateral, and oblique perspectives. This gives the surgeon important information about the length of the UG sinus, the point of confluence of the vagina and urethra, and their relative lengths and position within the pelvis. The level of this confluence, either high (UG sinus over 3 cm) or low (UG sinus <3 cm), ultimately determines the surgical approach. Further imaging of the pelvic organs may be necessary in complex cases and can be done with magnetic resonance imaging or computerized tomographic scanning with good visualization.

Finally, an examination under anesthesia is needed, including cystoscopy and vaginoscopy. It is often easier to measure the length of the UG sinus and determine the height of the confluence with the scope than with imaging. The length of the UG sinus can be measured by placing the tip of the scope at the point of confluence and marking the scope at the level of the external meatus. When the scope is withdrawn, the length of the UG sinus is estimated by measuring the distance from the mark on the barrel to the tip of the scope. These measurements of the UG sinus, vagina, and urethra, along with the position of the confluence of all three, are important in order to plan what techniques may be necessary for repair.

## SURGICAL POSITIONING

Most of the surgery for ambiguous genitalia can be performed in the lithotomy position. The lithotomy position is ideal for the clitoroplasty and reconstruction of the labia and introitus. The lithotomy position, however, does not always provide adequate exposure of the higher forms of urogenital sinus. Hendren and Atala (1), Peña (2), and Rink and Adams (3) have demonstrated the superior exposure provided by the posterior prone approach to the pelvic organs. We follow Hendren's recommendations to prepare the patient circumferentially while applying sterile wrapping to the lower legs to allow the patient to be turned from the lithotomy to the prone position as necessary during the operation. It is wise to have all positioning options available for this challenging surgery. Surgery usually begins in the lithotomy position and the clitoroplasty is done first, followed by the vaginoplasty, and finally the labioplasty.

## SURGICAL TECHNIQUE

### Repair of the External Genitalia

#### Clitoroplasty

Once the decision has been made to surgically reconstruct the clitoris, the goal of clitoroplasty is to reduce the size of the enlarged clitoris to one that is within the range of normal for females. Modern clitoroplasty developed after Mollard et al. (4) realized that the erectile tissue of the corpora was primarily responsible for the large size of the organ and that it caused problems during sexual engorgement. The glans clitoris must be preserved for sensation, but the corpora should be shortened. Mollard mobilized the neurovascular bundle that supplied the glans and excised the corpora from the level of their union at the pubis to the distal tip. He then sewed the glans

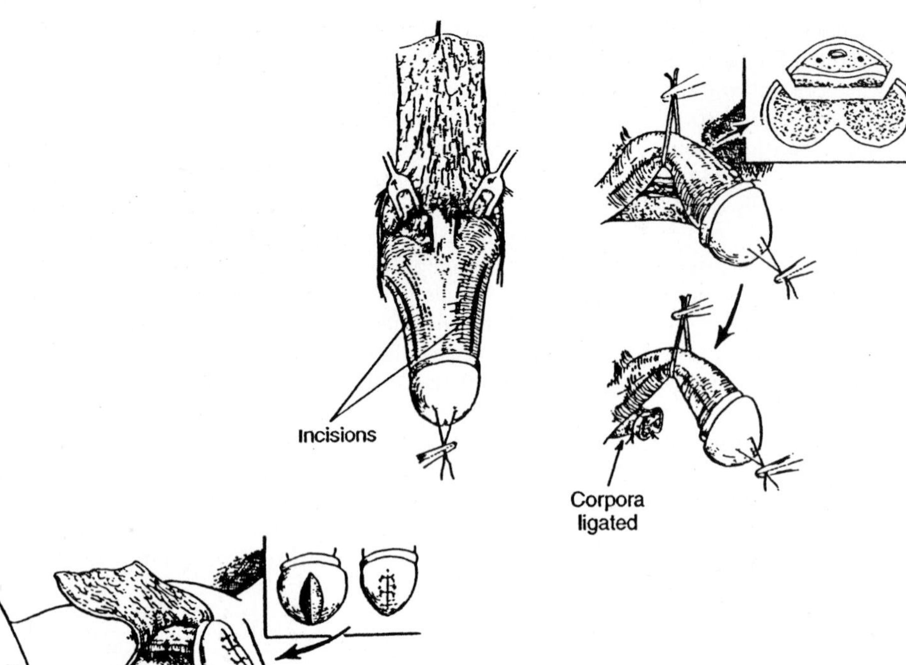


FIGURE 118.4 Corporotomy incisions are extended from the 10 and 2 o'clock positions laterally from just below the corona to 0.5 cm above the pubis. The corporal bodies are ligated at their base and the bodies excised, leaving the dorsal strip of fascia, including the neurovascular bundles, preserved with the glans.

back to the stumps of the corpora cavernosa, resulting in a functional clitoris that could become engorged to an appropriate size and was sensate. The dissection of the neurovascular bundle is somewhat difficult and can potentially lead to compromise of the nerves or infarction, so we prefer a variant of the Mollard procedure that was described by Gonzales and Fernandes (5).

A circumferential incision is made on the clitoris just proximal to the coronal sulcus and the clitoris is degloved from skin and subcutaneous tissue. The urethral plate and rudimentary corpus spongiosum may be divided distally and dissected with the subcutaneous tissue or just mobilized from the corpora cavernosa while leaving it attached both proximally and distally. We prefer to divide the urethral plate from the glans during this dissection. Incisions are made in the tunica albuginea of the corpora at the 2 and 10 o'clock positions using needle-point electrocautery. These incisions are extended and joined across the ventral aspect of the corpora at the subcoronal level distally and 0.5 cm above the pubis proximally (Fig. 118.4). The dorsal tunica albuginea (including the enclosed neurovascular bundle) is dissected from the erectile tissue and remaining tunica of the corpora. The erectile tissue bodies and their ventral and lateral fascia can be dissected from the dorsal fascia and excised. A 4-0 polyglycolic acid suture can be used to ligate each corporal body at its base. The rim of fascia on the glans can be sewn to the fascia on the stumps of the corpora with 4-0 suture to reseat the glans and stabilize it. The dorsal fascia, which contains the neurovascular bundle, is allowed to fold under the skin cranial to the glans. The urethral plate, which was previously separated from the glans, can now be shortened and partially split in the midline to flatten the introitus and to shorten the distance from the vagina to the clitoris (Fig. 118.5).

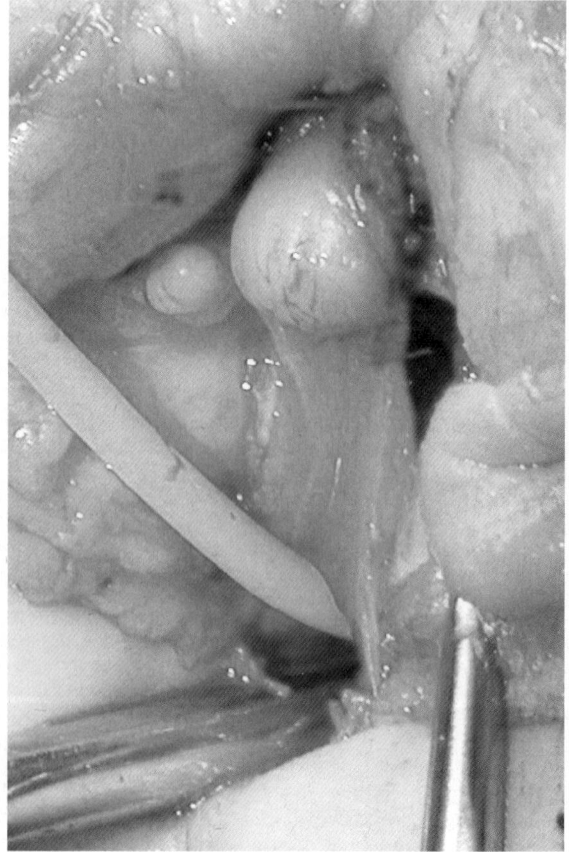

FIGURE 118.5 The urethral plate is used to shorten the distance between the clitoris and the vagina, producing a more normal introitus.

The glans clitoris is often quite large, and several procedures have been described to reduce its size. We have preferred not to decrease the overall size of the glans but instead to conceal some of the dorsal glans with the glans hood. A small patch of the dorsal glans epithelium at the base can be excised, leaving the erectile tissue intact, and the glans hood can be sewn to this area and allowed to fold over the remainder of the glans. This leaves the glans with its full erectile capability, leaves it accessible, and covers it appropriately with a skin hood.

### Labioplasty

The goal of labioplasty is to create a normal-appearing and normal-functioning female perineum and introitus. The shaft skin and dorsal prepuce of the clitoris can be utilized to form the labia minora and to fashion a clitoral hood. The original skin incision had degloved the clitoris and left all skin based on the dorsal pedicle. This skin can then be split in the midline for approximately two thirds of its length (Fig. 118.6). At the proximal end of the incision a transverse incision is made and curved proximally at each end for a few millimeters to develop a flap that is used for the clitoral hood. The two long sides of the shaft skin are folded to form long, thin, vertical two-sided flaps that will form the labia minora. The horizontal central flap is folded under itself to form a two-sided hood for the clitoris. The clitoral hood is sewn to the base of the dorsal aspect of the clitoris and around each side to the approximate 3 and 9 o'clock positions. Each of the three flaps is sewn into shape using 5-0 absorbable suture.

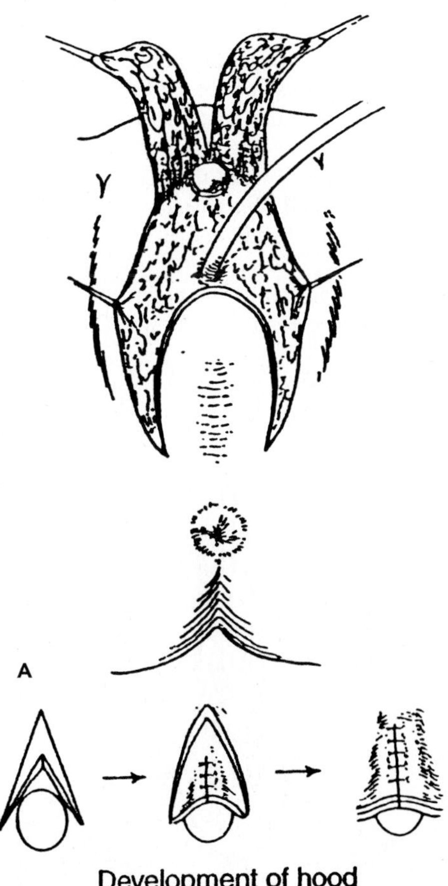


FIGURE 118.6 The dorsal preputial skin is split in the midline and reconfigured to create a clitoral hood.

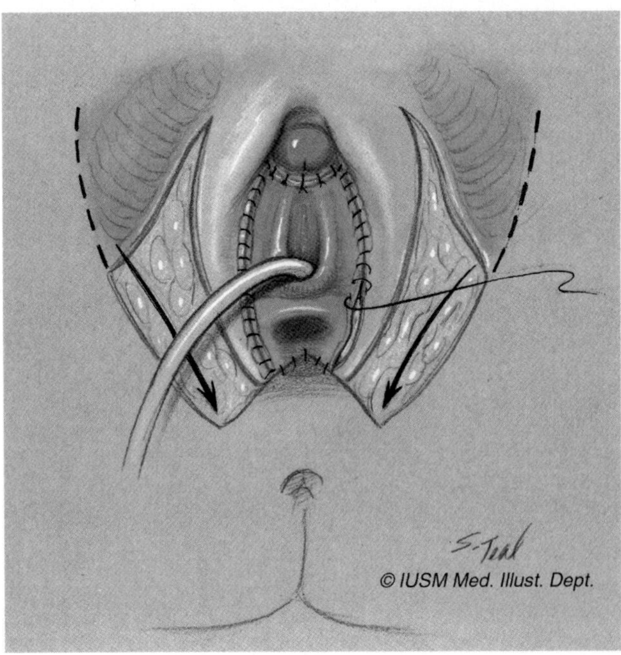


FIGURE 118.7 The dorsal preputial skin flaps are mobilized laterally and advanced toward the vagina. There, they are sewn to the lateral edge of the urethral plate as a labial flap. The labioscrotal folds are then sewn to the lateral edge of the labia minora to form labia majora.

The labia minora are created with the two lateral strips of shaft skin. They are dissected on their pedicles to allow them to extend to the vagina or midperineum (Fig. 118.7). They are then sewn to the lateral aspect of the urethral plate, which now lies in the midline between vagina and clitoris. A three-way stitch is used to fasten the labia minora to the introitus and to narrow their base so that they maintain their character and their base does not spread and flatten. The labioscrotal folds are then sewn to the labia minora to form the labia majora. All sutures are absorbable 4-0 and 5-0, and while some suture lines can be created using a running 5-0 suture, any point of potential tension, such as at corners, should be fixed with an interrupted 4-0 skin suture.

## Repair of the Urogenital Sinus

### Low-Confluence Urogenital Sinus

The goal of urogenital sinus reconstruction is to create separate functional openings for the urinary and genital tracts. The low-confluence UG sinus has a long urethra and vagina that join near the perineal surface, resulting in a short common channel or sinus (Fig. 118.8). There are two good options for managing these anomalies. John Lattimer introduced the posterior flap vaginoplasty in 1964, and it is still a useful technique.

A U-shaped incision is made in the perineum with the open end facing caudally and the proximal point at the orifice of the UG sinus. This incision isolates a posteriorly based skin flap (Fig. 118.9). This flap was originally designed to be wide-based but it needs to be no wider than half of the circumference of the proposed vagina (a 1- to 1.5-cm flap in infants). The excellent blood supply of the tissue allows a narrower flap, which results in a more normally functional and cosmetic introitus.

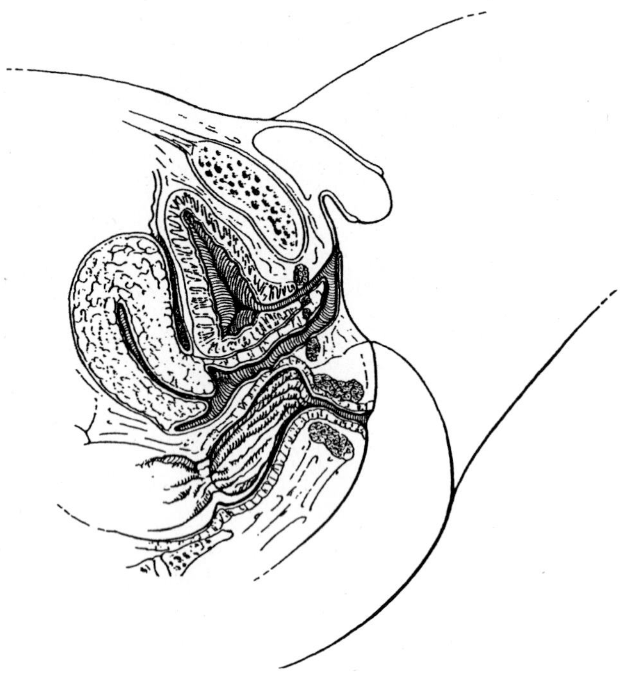

FIGURE 118.8 This illustration demonstrates a low-confluence urogenital sinus with a short common urogenital sinus channel draining the urinary bladder and vagina.

Once the skin flap is isolated, it is mobilized from the deeper tissue and folded back to expose the caudal wall of the UG sinus (Fig. 118.10). A fine-tipped hemostat can be placed in the orifice and the sinus split using electrocautery in the midline to the level that exposes the confluence of the sinus vagina and urethra. The vagina is split as deep as the apex of the posterior skin flap will reach. With a catheter in the urethra, the posterior skin flap is sewn in position starting at the apex and using interrupted absorbable 4-0 sutures. This advancement of the flap into the sinus and vagina both widens the introitus and the vagina and reorients the vagina into a more vertical position, improving passive drainage (Fig. 118.11).

The other option for the low UG sinus is a limited total urogenital mobilization (TUM) technique as described originally by Peña (2). This is a relatively simple technique and is initiated by a circumferential incision around the UG sinus orifice (Fig. 118.12). This dissection is continued around the sinus while providing constant traction on the sinus with multiple stay sutures. The entire sinus vagina and urethra can then be mobilized caudally, delivering the confluence of the urethra, vagina, and sinus to the level of the perineal skin (Fig. 118.13). Peña originally described this technique for use in cloacal reconstruction and stressed that the dissection must extend high in the pelvis, but this is not always necessary in the low-confluence UG sinus. The dissection can be considered complete when the confluence is at the level of the perineum.

If the vagina and urethra reach the appropriate level and are wide enough to be functional, then the distal UG sinus can be amputated and discarded (Fig. 118.14). If the vagina is too narrow, the posterior wall of the vagina can be split and a posteriorly based perineal skin flap can be inserted to widen it.

## High-Confluence UG Sinus

The high-confluence UG sinus with a short urethra and vagina and a long common urogenital sinus channel is much more of a challenge to reconstruct because of the position of the confluence high within the pelvis and the relative lack of suitable tissue for reconstruction. In this condition the urethra and vagina are short and tethered far from the introitus by soft tissue attachments within the pelvis.

Early attempts to repair these children were made using techniques that were more suitable for low-confluence variants, and this fact may explain many of the poor surgical results now apparent in older patients. The posterior flap repair, which was very useful for less severe cases, did not provide enough length to reach the high confluence and left the child with a short, hypospadiac urethra and inadequate tissue to reconstruct the vagina to the introitus. Hendren pioneered the dissection separating the bladder and vagina, allowing the vagina to be advanced toward the perineum. This dissection between the urinary and genital tract is very difficult and can result in vesicovaginal fistula and bladder dysfunction. Even with the vagina completely dissected from the posterior bladder, it often would not reach the perineum, and the gap was bridged with complex skin flaps that were sometimes less than ideal.

Peña's TUM procedure is a perineal-based approach that is based on circumferential dissection of the UG sinus, vagina,

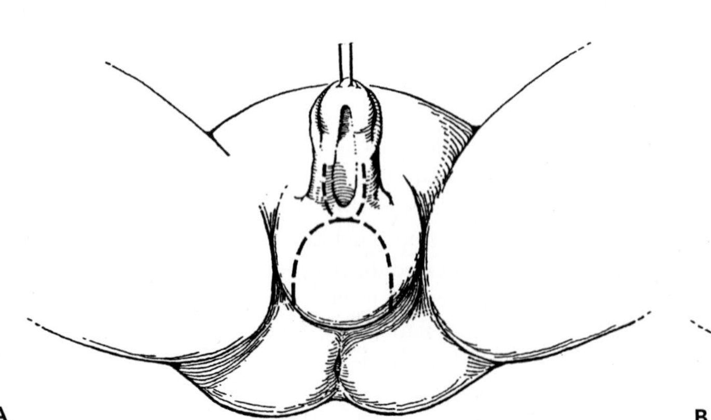


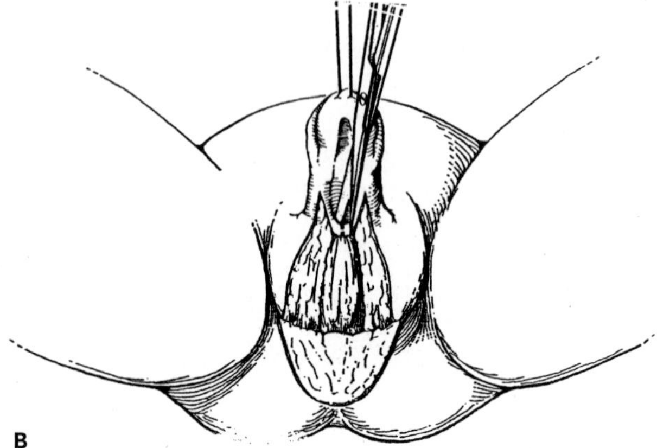


FIGURE 118.9 Inverted-U incision produces a posterior-based perineal skin flap used to reconstruct the posterior wall of the vagina.

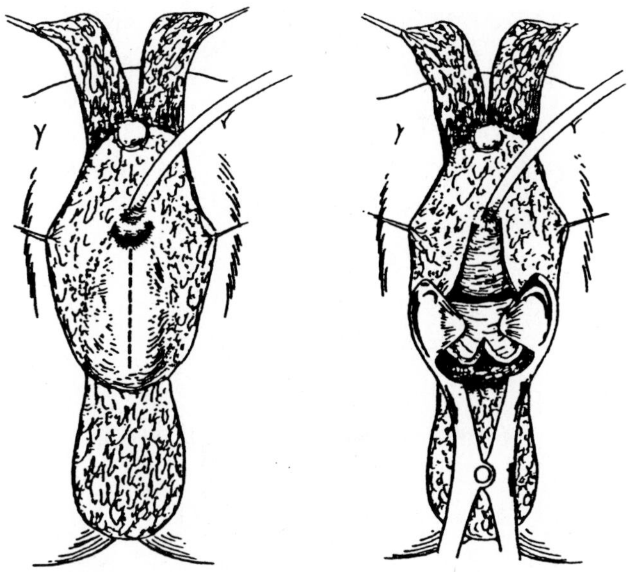

FIGURE 118.10 The caudal portion of the urogenital sinus is exposed by deflecting the perineal skin flap inferiorly. The sinus can then be mobilized intact or split in the midline ventrally to the level of the vagina in a very low-confluence case.

and urethra and advancement of these structures toward the perineal surface. This approach leaves the child with a urethra of normal length by lowering the bladder and vagina in the pelvis. The TUM also lowers the proximal vagina and uterus in the pelvis, allowing the vagina to be reconstructed with less outside tissue. The TUM has become an important tool in the reconstruction of children with UG sinus, particularly those with a high confluence.

The initial circumferential dissection around the UG sinus is performed just as with the lower-confluence variant. Multiple stay sutures are placed and the dissection can be performed in the lithotomy position. Unlike the lower-confluence UG sinus, those who have a high confluence need much more extensive dissection to allow the vagina to come close enough to the perineum for satisfactory reconstruction. The dissection usually must reach the level of the pubis both anterior and posterior to the UG sinus.

If the vagina and urethra reach the appropriate level and are wide enough to be functional, then the distal UG sinus can be amputated and discarded (Fig 118.14). This is usually not the case, however, and the distal vagina is usually too narrow. In this case the vagina can be divided from the sinus, dissected away from the urethra and bladder, and split in the midline dorsally. The mobilized sinus can also then be split in the midline dorsally and the sinus can be folded back on itself ventrally and advanced into the vagina as a flap to widen the vagina. If the vagina is still too narrow, the posterior vaginal wall can be split as well and a posteriorly based perineal skin flap can be inserted (Fig. 118.11). The TUM has allowed UG sinus reconstruction and minimized the need to perform the difficult dissection between bladder and vagina.

We prefer to approach the child with high UG sinus as an individual who may need various techniques for successful repair. The options are TUM, mobilization of the vagina from the urethra/bladder, and various flaps to augment the vagina from either the UG sinus tissue or perineal skin. The less severe cases may need only TUM and a posterior skin flap, while the most severe cases need all techniques in order to have a successful outcome.

Dressing and drains are strictly up to the surgeon and the difficulty of the procedure. A simple genitoplasty may need only antibiotic ointment or, at most, overnight catheter drainage. More complex procedures always merit catheter drainage of the bladder, and complex vaginoplasties may be aided with a vaginal Penrose drain or in some cases a pressure dressing of fluffed gauze and elastic tape crisscrossing the perineum. Some surgeons believe in keeping these patients in bed and relatively immobile for 48 hours, but we often allow them to move about at will and to be held by their mother immediately after surgery.

# OUTCOMES

## Complications

The most common complication of genitoplasty is bleeding, both immediate and delayed. The tissue is very vascular and the use of injected dilute epinephrine during the procedure may be helpful. Late bleeding may originate from the corpora

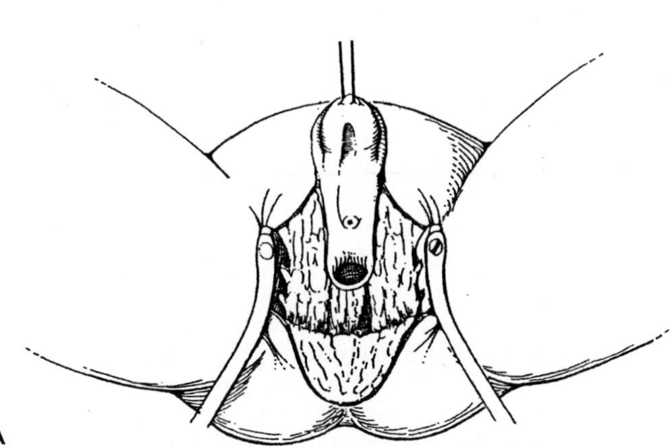



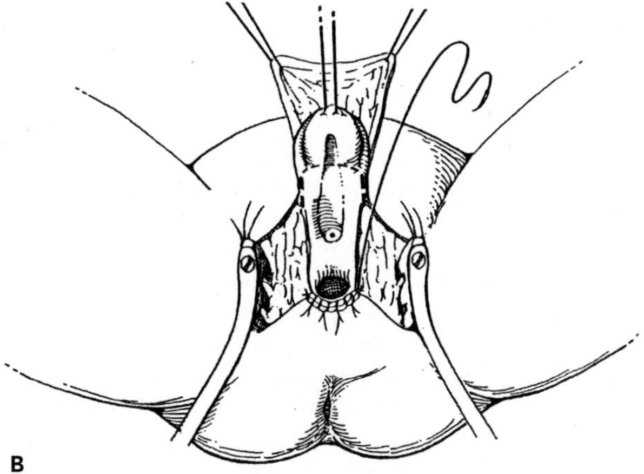



FIGURE 118.11 Advancement of the perineal skin flap widens the posterior wall of the introitus and reorients the vagina in a more vertical plane.

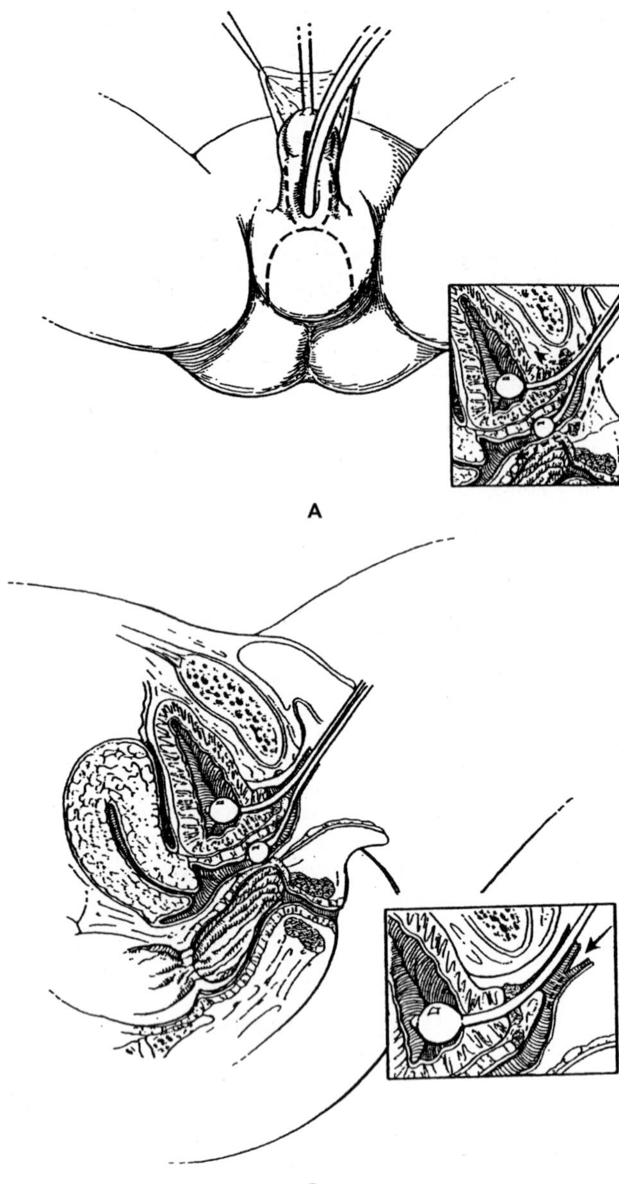

FIGURE 118.12 Total urogenital sinus mobilization (TUM) for the urogenital sinus begins by circumferential dissection around the common channel. With cranial dissection the entire sinus can be mobilized and delivered to the level of the perineal skin. If the vagina reaches the perineum easily, the excess sinus can be amputated. If the vagina is narrow, it can be split in the midline posteriorly and the posterior perineal skin flap inserted as part of the posterior vaginal wall.

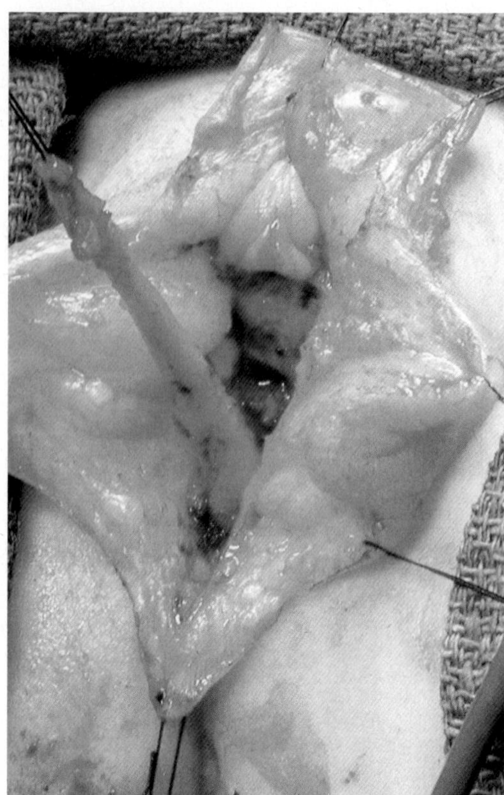

FIGURE 118.13 Total urogenital sinus mobilization for the high urogenital sinus requires a more extensive circumferential cranial dissection that takes down all the attachments to the pubic bone.

cavernosa or vaginal wall and can usually be controlled with pressure dressing. Pressure dressing must be carefully applied since it is possible to cause vascular compromise of the glans clitoris in the immediate postsurgical period.

The neurovascular pedicle of the glans clitoris can be injured during the original dissection. This potential injury is minimized by leaving the entire dorsal fascia, including the bundles, intact during and after dissection. Infections in the urine or wound are also possible but uncommon. It is not unusual to find a small dehiscence of the wound at the posterior apex of the labial incisions due to tension from movement. These heal without surgical intervention. They can be bathed normally and dressed with antibiotic ointment. The skin stress in this area is the prime reason to close with longer-lasting absorbable sutures.

## Results

At this time surgical results are consistently good in terms of appearance and potential for function. There are, however, few long-term outcome data for feminizing genitoplasty, and the studies that have been done are, by necessity, evaluating the surgical technique that was in fashion 25 years ago. The techniques have improved, and while we can see superior cosmetic and functional results in young children and adolescents treated more recently, we still need to observe and evaluate these patients as they mature.

The question of gender assignment is one of great importance and intense study at this time. While it is necessary to learn from our patients, we must learn from all of them and not focus on only those who have been dissatisfied with their treatment. We now know that gender identity is much more complex than to be dependent on genital appearance and gender roles. While we must continuously re-evaluate our management of these difficult problems, we should not lose faith in the ability of surgery to create urogenital structures that can function normally and have an appearance consistent with the classic norm of the human body. Feminizing genitoplasty, like all surgery, has demonstrated that the most difficult question remains the choice of the correct procedure for the proper patient.

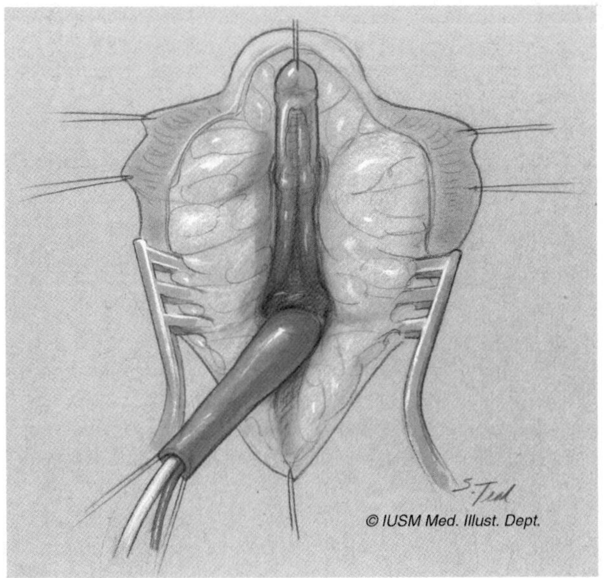


A

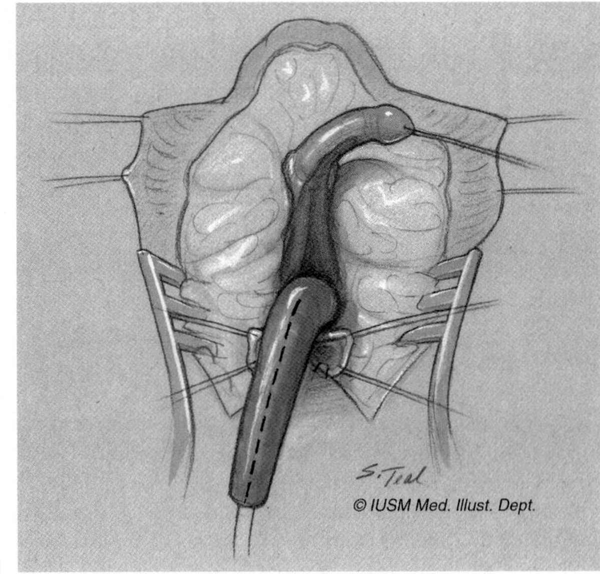


B

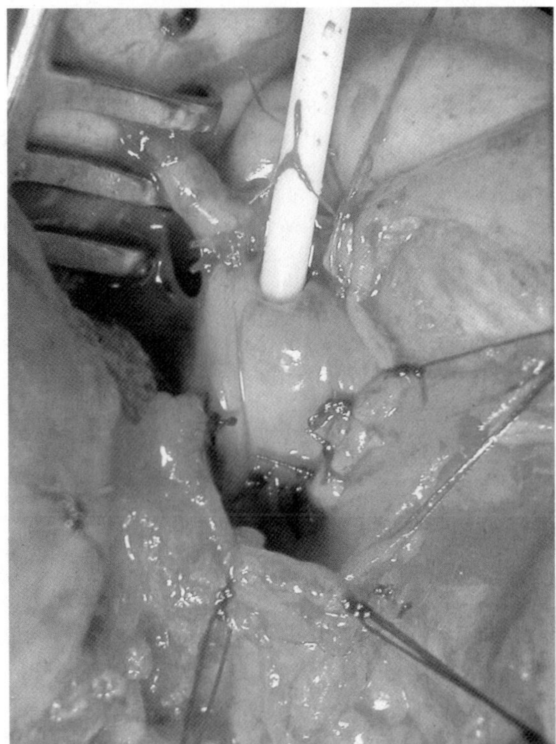

C

FIGURE 118.14 If the vagina does not reach the introitus easily, additional length can be obtained by splitting the urogenital sinus wall dorsally and folding the sinus mucosa back onto itself and inserting it as part of the anterior vaginal wall.

## *References*


1. Hendren WH, Atala A. Repair of high vagina in girls with severely masculinized anatomy from the adrenogenital syndrome. *J Pediatr Surg* 1995; 30:91–94.
2. Peña A. Total urogenital mobilization: an easier way to repair cloacas. *J Pediatr Surg* 1997;32:263–268.
3. Rink RC, Adams MC. Feminizing genitoplasty: state of the art. *World J Urol* 1998;16:212–218.
4. Mollard P, Juskiewenski S, Sarkissian J. Clitoroplasty in intersex: a new technique. *Br J Urol* 1981;53:371–373.
5. Gonzalez R, Fernandes ET. Single-stage feminization genitoplasty. *J Urol* 1990;143:776–778.

Fortunoff S, Lattimer JK, Edson M. Vaginoplasty technique for female pseudohermaphrodites. *Surg Gynecol Obstet* 1964;118:545.

Passerini-Glazel G. A new one-stage procedure for clitorovaginoplasty in severely masculinized female pseudohermaphrodites. *J Urol* 1989;142: 565–568.

Ludwinkowski B, Oesch Hayward I, Gonzalez R. Total urogenital sinus mobilization: expanded applications. *BJU Int* 1999;83:820–822.

Schober JM. Long-term outcomes and changing attitudes to intersexuality. *BJU Int* 1999;83:39–50.

Aaronson IA. The investigation and management of the infant with ambiguous genitalia: a surgeon's perspective. *Curr Problems Pediatr* 2001; 31:168–194.

Lee PA, Houk CP, Ahmed SF, et al. Consensus statement on management of intersex disorders. *Pediatrics* 2006;118:e488–e500.

# CHAPTER 119 ■ CIRCUMCISION

IRENE M. MCALEER AND GEORGE W. KAPLAN

Currently about 1.2 million newborn boys in the United States are circumcised annually, making circumcision probably the most commonly performed surgical procedure on boys or men (1,2). The incidence of circumcision in the United States is highest in whites (88%) and less frequent in African Americans (73%) and Hispanics (42%) (2). The frequency of newborn circumcision is much lower in other countries, such as Canada (35%) and Australia (10%), and is generally much <8% in Europe and most parts of Asia (1).

## DIAGNOSIS

No diagnostic studies are needed preoperatively. Comorbidities, such as excessive prematurity, inherited or transient bleeding disorders associated with infancy, and congenital abnormalities of the skin such as epidermolysis bullosum and of the penis such as exstrophy, hypospadias, penoscrotal webbing, or micropenis, would all mitigate against circumcision, particularly routine newborn circumcision (Fig. 119.1).

## INDICATIONS FOR SURGERY

Circumcision is often performed in the neonatal period, infancy, or childhood for cultural or religious reasons and is also performed after the newborn period, when phimosis, paraphimosis, balanoposthitis, or sexually transmitted diseases are more prevalent. Medical benefits to the boy circumcised in infancy include reduced urinary infections in infancy (3), decreased incidence of sexually transmitted disease (2,4,5), and marked reduction in the incidence of penile carcinoma (6), but these benefits must also be weighed against the risks of the procedure: bleeding, infection, and poor outcome (7).

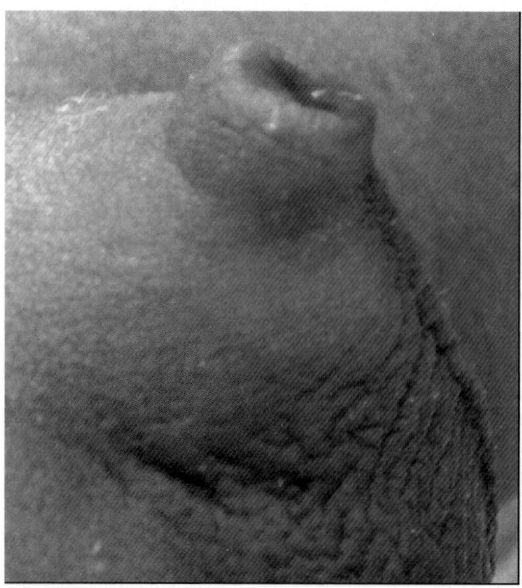

FIGURE 119.1 Webbed penis with paucity of shaft skin.

The American Academy of Pediatrics in 1999 (8) concluded that there were benefits from neonatal circumcision but the benefits gained did not warrant universal routine circumcision. Conversely, there are some opponents who feel that neonatal circumcision is never warranted (9).

Recently, with the increased incidence of human immunodeficiency virus (HIV) in sub-Saharan Africa of epidemic proportions, where over 90% of HIV-positive men in Africa acquire the virus through vaginal intercourse, clinical trials of adult male circumcision in large groups of men have found a reduced risk of >50% in the populations studied (Kenya, Uganda, South Africa). Even though the risk behavior of the circumcised men was no different from the uncircumcised men, the risk of contracting HIV was substantially decreased (2,5). In the uncircumcised man, the inner preputial skin has more Langerhans cells with densely concentrated CD4 receptors needed by HIV for entry into the body than do the glans, outer preputial skin, or penile shaft skin; as a result, the inner preputial skin, which is retracted and telescoped during intercourse, facilitates HIV entry into the body (2,5).

Because circumcision is so common, there are a number of misguided ideas and practices that have crept into American medical practice leading to some circumcisions being done for reasons that are not completely medically sound. At birth the prepuce, in over 90% of infants, is fused to the glans and is not retractable. As studied by Gairdner in 1949 (10), the foreskin progressively retracts on its own with age, so that only 10% of 3-year-olds will have nonretractable foreskins, and Oster et al. (11) found that only 1% of 17-year-olds will not have retractable foreskins. It is not necessary for parents or physicians to retract the prepuce as retractability occurs with penile growth, erection, and smegma formation; the smegma that forms will generally spontaneously be discharged from under the prepuce and does not need to be removed. Balanoposthitis is not a mandatory indication for circumcision in children as the prepuce in that area of the penis after such an episode will be permanently separated from the glans and should not produce recurrences of balanoposthitis. Forcible retraction of the prepuce causes the child pain and can produce paraphimosis or a dense cicatrix and perhaps subsequent balanitis xerotica obliterans (BXO) (Fig. 119.2).

Phimosis becomes pathologic when the opening of the foreskin develops a tight cicatrix usually caused by BXO. According to Shankar and Rickwood (12), BXO represents the one absolute indication for circumcision. BXO is a chronic dermatologic

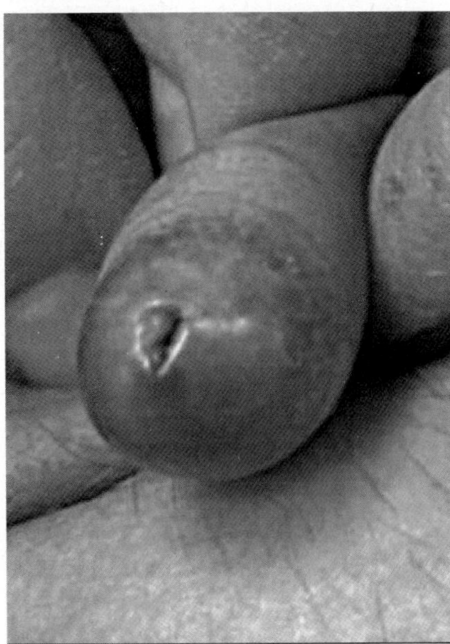

FIGURE 119.2 Photo of pathologic phimosis due to balanitis xerotica obliterans.

condition, analogous to lichen sclerosus et atrophicus, of the glans and prepuce but can also involve the meatus and the anterior urethra, especially if the glans is extensively involved (13).

Most of the series where BXO is reviewed have found that most of the patients affected are older boys, primarily those whose ages range from 5 to 15 years old (12–15). Previously, it was thought that the incidence of BXO was relatively rare in boys (range from 0.6% to 6%) (12,15), but recent reviews have shown that the BXO occurs more frequently in boys than previously reported. Circumcision is thought to be about 96% curative of BXO, but it is concerning that in more obese boys, especially those with prominent pubic fat, more severe disease is prevalent and recurrent (13).

## ALTERNATIVE THERAPY

Observation, intermittent medical treatment for balanoposthitis, and dorsal slit are common alternatives to circumcision. Recently the use of topical steroid creams, typically 0.1% triamcinolone or 0.05% betamethasone cream (16–18), to the preputial opening for about 4 to 8 weeks has successfully treated phimosis and obviates the need for circumcision in 85% to 87% of boys reported to be using the steroid preparations.

Paraphimosis occurs when the prepuce is retracted behind the glans penis and, because the preputial orifice is tight, becomes trapped in this position after it is retracted, with resultant swelling of the glans that prevents its reduction. If untreated, paraphimosis can lead to infection, significant penile swelling and pain, and occasionally loss of penile tissue. The edema can often be reduced by injecting hyaluronidase into the edematous tissue, thereby allowing for easier reduction of the paraphimosis. Many healthcare providers are unlikely to inject anything into such a swollen and painful penis, so an easy and effective treatment for the paraphimotic edema

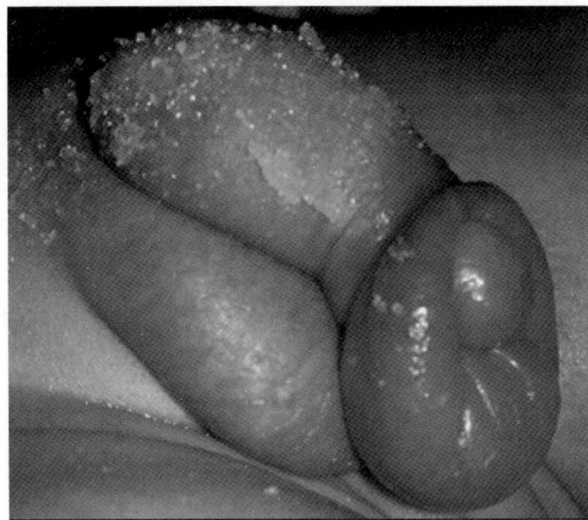

FIGURE 119.3 Photo of paraphimosis with topical granulated sugar.

is to place granulated sugar over the swollen penile tissue, with a resultant osmotic gradient pulling the fluid out. Another alternative to reduce swelling is the application of ice (Fig. 119.3). The paraphimosis is reduced by grasping the penis between the second and third fingers of both hands and pulling the shaft skin distally while simultaneously applying cephalad pressure with both thumbs. If this maneuver is unsuccessful, a dorsal slit is necessary to open the phimotic constriction ring. Circumcision can be performed after the inflammation and edema have resolved and should not be attempted at the time that the acute paraphimosis is present.

## SURGICAL TECHNIQUE

The goal of the operation is to remove an adequate amount of the prepuce such that the glans is exposed and balanoposthitis, phimosis, BXO, and paraphimosis are prevented. Too much or too little skin should not be removed, as the former can tether the penis and on occasion produce chordee, while the latter may produce continued risks of phimosis or paraphimosis.

All circumcisions should take place with an anesthetic: during the newborn period, local anesthesia with 1% lidocaine is generally used with or without topical anesthesia (EMLA 2.5% to 2.5% lidocaine–prilocaine). EMLA should be used cautiously as methemoglobinemia can occur in newborns. In older children and adolescents, general anesthesia is usually used. The penis is cleaned and draped and the foreskin retracted by taking down all the adhesions between the glans and the inner preputial skin. If a dense phimosis prevents this retraction, a dorsal slit may be necessary as a preliminary maneuver by placing one blade of a straight clamp inside the preputial sac in the dorsal midline (ensuring that the blade is not within the urethral meatus) and then placing the other blade on the outer skin. The clamp is closed and left in place for a few minutes, crushing the tissue and producing temporary hemostasis, and then the crushed area is incised with scissors. Marking the coronal ridge (as seen through the shaft skin) in ink helps identify where to place the circumferential incision about the shaft skin. In the adult or older child the proposed line of incision in the inner preputial sac is marked with ink about 3 to 4 mm below the coronal sulcus.

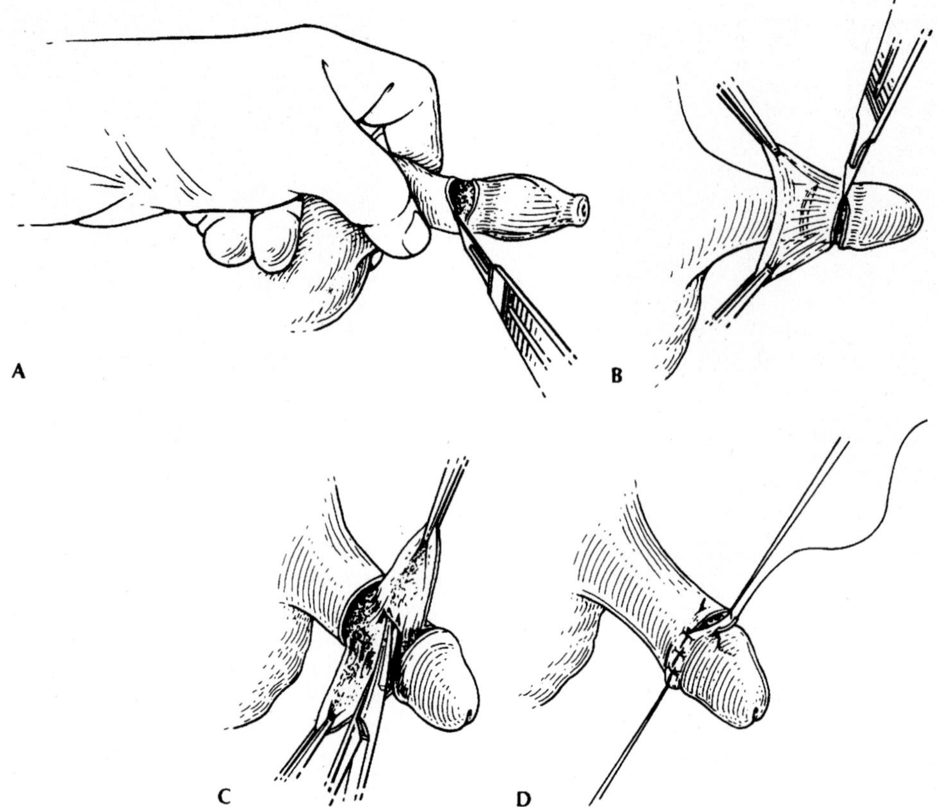


FIGURE 119.4 A: An incision is made on the shaft. B: A second incision is made below the coronal sulcus. C: Removing the excessive preputial skin. D: The wound edges are coapted and sutured together.

A common method of excising the prepuce, called a "sleeve technique," is performed by incising the two previously marked lines of incision circumferentially about the penis and dividing the tissue between the layers. Hemostasis is secured generally with judicious use of cautery, although vessels can also be individually ligated. The skin and the inner preputial epithelium are then coapted with fine absorbable sutures (Fig. 119.4).

Alternatively, an older method involves putting the prepuce on stretch by applying a hemostat to the dorsal and ventral aspects of the preputial orifice. The area of the shaft skin previously marked as overlying the coronal ridge is pulled forward beyond the tip of the glans and a straight clamp is applied, taking care to ensure that the glans is not included in the clamp. The prepuce distal to the clamp is amputated with a knife, the clamp is removed, hemostasis is secured, and the skin edges are coapted.

With the advent of synthetic tissue adhesives such as Dermabond (2-octyl cyanoacrylate, Ethicon), circumcisions can be performed quickly and safely with good cosmetic results in most children with minimal surgical time, few if any sutures required, and minimal tissue handling, thereby decreasing postsurgical swelling and possibly postsurgical pain (19).

## Dermabond Circumcision

Either a typical sleeve circumcision is performed or a Gomco clamp is used to prepare the tissue for the adhesive, which is applied directly to the apposed penile shaft and coronal skin edges. Acceptable surgical results have been obtained as long as the skin edges are closely approximated and the adhesive is not extensively used on subcutaneous tissue (Fig. 119.5).

## Neonatal Circumcision

In newborns, circumcisions performed without anesthesia previously were common. However, local anesthesia using an agent such as lidocaine or bupivacaine as a dorsal penile block or, more importantly, a ring block at the base of the penis can alleviate most of the pain experienced by the newborn at the time of the circumcision. The anesthetic dose must be adjusted for the weight of the patient.

In newborns, circumcision is in general accomplished using some type of device. The common devices in use in the United States are the Gomco clamp, the Plastibell, and the Mogen clamp. The methodology for the Gomco clamp and Plastibell is similar. After local anesthesia has been provided and the skin cleansed, the area of the coronal ridge is marked as previously described, followed by a dorsal slit being performed. The Gomco device has three parts—a bell of variable size that fits over the glans, a plate, and a screw that completes the assembly. After the dorsal slit is performed and all the adhesions are released, the bell is then placed over the glans; a safety pin placed through the distal corners of the previously incised prepuce that keeps the edges aligned may be helpful. Then the plate is placed over the glans, the shaft skin is pulled up until the marked area can be seen emerging from the hole in the

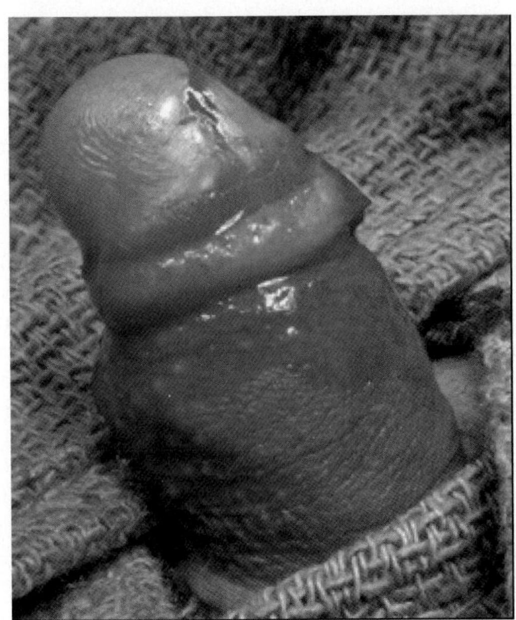

FIGURE 119.5 Photo of circumcision using 2-octyl-cyanoacrylate (Dermabond).

plate, and then the screw is placed and tightened. The device is left in situ for several minutes and the prepuce distal to the plate is then excised with a knife. Electrocautery must never be applied to the Gomco device, as this has resulted in total necrosis of the penis. The device is then removed, reversing the order in which it was applied. By loosening the screw, the plate can be disengaged from the bell and removed. The cut skin edges of the penis are then gently teased over the edge of the bell to ultimately remove the bell and complete the circumcision; rarely are sutures needed for hemostasis for this type of clamp circumcision (Fig. 119.6).

The Plastibell follows the same principles as the Gomco device. After the bell is applied, a heavy string is tied over a groove at the base of the bell at the level of the previously marked area on the shaft. The distal prepuce is then excised. The stem distal to the bell is snapped off, leaving a plastic ring under the inner preputial epithelium. In roughly 1 week, the skin distal to the ligature sloughs and the ring comes off spontaneously.

The Mogen clamp is a clothespin-like device, and the methodology of its application is akin to the older open surgical method described above. After the skin is cleansed and the area of the coronal ridge as seen through the shaft skin is marked with ink, the adhesions between the glans and the

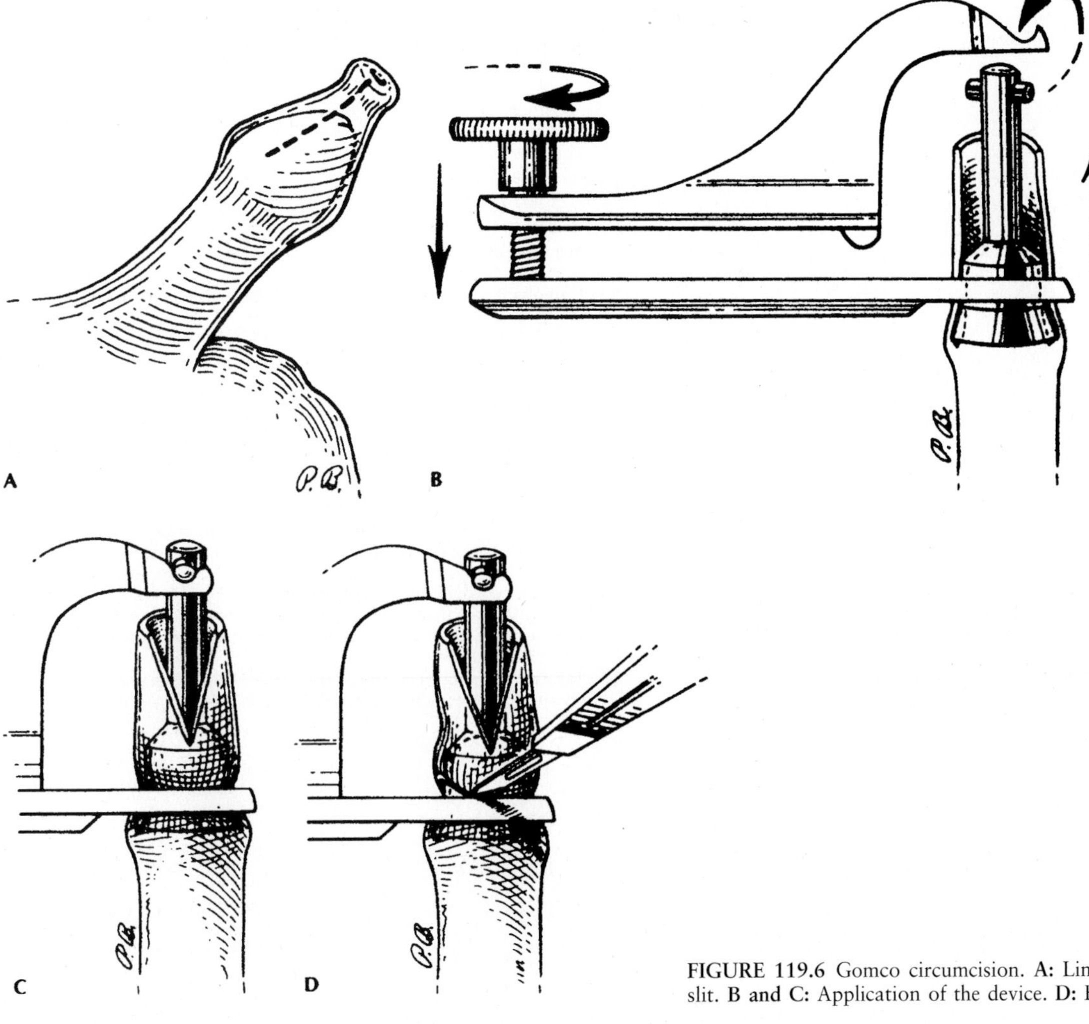

FIGURE 119.6 Gomco circumcision. **A:** Line of incision for dorsal slit. **B and C:** Application of the device. **D:** Excision of the prepuce.

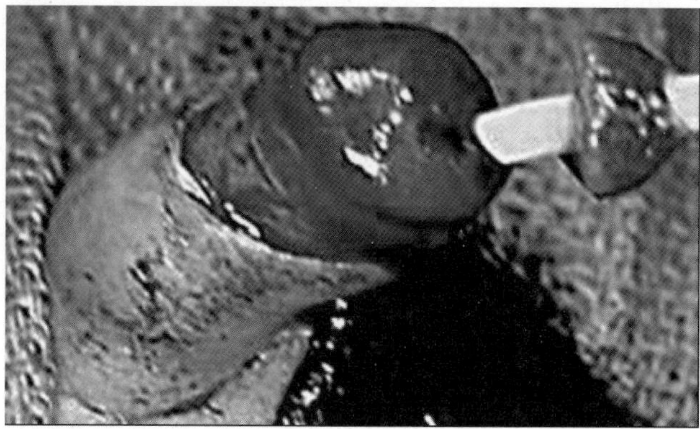

FIGURE 119.7 Traumatic amputation of portion of glans from Mogen clamp circumcision.

inner prepuce are lysed with a blunt probe. It is usually not necessary to perform a dorsal slit when using the Mogen clamp. The prepuce is pulled distally and the clamp applied, taking care to ensure that the glans is not included in the clamp. The clamp is closed and left in situ for a few moments. The prepuce distal to the clamp is excised and the clamp is removed. This type of clamp device is the easiest to use by those first performing neonatal clamp circumcisions, but it is the one most likely to have associated complications, typically partial or complete amputation of the glans if the glans is inadvertently enclosed in the clamp and cut when the tissue in the clamp is incised (20) (Fig. 119.7).

# OUTCOMES

## Complications

Occasionally complications do occur, but most are minor and rarely portend a bad result. Bleeding is the most frequent complication and occurs in approximately 0.1% of cases. Most episodes of bleeding are minor and respond to pressure alone. Some require cautery or suture for control, particularly in the area of the frenulum. Most infections are minor and superficial, manifested by redness and occasionally purulence at the circumcision site that usually responds to local wound care. A common complication of neonatal circumcision is meatal stenosis, probably produced by a chemical meatitis from ammoniacal urine exposure on the tip of the penis while the patient is still wearing diapers. Serious complications, fortunately, are rare but include recurrent phimosis, wound separation, major tissue loss, concealed penis, skin bridges between the shaft and the glans, inclusion cysts, urethrocutaneous fistula, and loss of some of the glans or, extremely rarely, all of the penis.

## Results

A circumcision should remove a sufficient amount of the prepuce so that the glans is exposed, significantly reducing the risk of developing phimosis, paraphimosis, BXO, or balanoposthitis.

## *References*


1. Alanis MC, Lucidi RS. Neonatal circumcision: a review of the world's oldest and most controversial operation. *Obstet Gynecol Surv* 2004;59(5): 379–395.
2. Morris BJ. Why circumcision is a biomedical imperative for the 21st century. *Bioessays* 2007;29:1147–1158.
3. Wiswell TE, Hachey WE. Urinary tract infection and the uncircumcised state: an update. *Clin Pediatr* 1993;32:130–134.
4. Parker SW, Stewart AJ, Wren MN, et al. Circumcision and sexually transmissible disease. *Med J Aust* 1983;2:288–290.
5. Kahn JG, Marseille E, Auvert B. Cost-effectiveness of male circumcision for HIV prevention in a South African setting. *PLoS Med* 2006;3(12): e517.
6. Persky L, deKernion J. Carcinoma of the penis. *CA Cancer J Clin* 1986;36: 258–273.
7. Kaplan GW. Complications of circumcision. *Urol Clin North Am* 1983; 10:543–549.
8. American Academy of Pediatrics Task Force on Circumcision. Policy statement. *Pediatrics* 1999;103:686–693.
9. Schoen EJ. The status of circumcision of newborns. *N Engl J Med* 1990; 322:1308–1312.
10. Gairdner D. Fate of the foreskin: a study of circumcision. *Br Med J* 1949; 2:1433–1437.
11. Huntley JS, Bourne MC, Munro FD, et al. Troubles with the foreskin: one hundred consecutive referrals to paediatric surgeons. *J R Soc Med* 2003; 96:449–451.
12. Shankar KR, Rickwood AMK. The incidence of phimosis in boys. *BJU Int* 1999;84:101–102.
13. Gargollo PC, Kozakewich HP, Bauer SB, et al. Balanitis xerotica obliterans in boys. *J Urol* 2005;174:1409–1412.
14. Kiss A, Kiraly L, Kutasy B, et al. High incidence of balanitis xerotica obliterans in boys with phimosis: prospective 10-year study. *Pediatr Dermatol* 2005;22(4):305–308.
15. Yardley IE, Cosgrove C, Lambert AW. Paediatric preputial pathology: are we circumcising enough? *Ann R Coll Surg Engl* 2007;89:62–65.
16. Zampieri N, Corroppolo M, Camoglio F, et al. Phimosis: stretching methods with or without application of topical steroids? *J Pediatr* 2005;147: 705–706.
17. McGregor TB, Pike JG, Leonard MP. Pathologic and physiologic phimosis: approach to the phimotic foreskin. *Can Fam Physician* 2007;53:445–448.
18. Berdeu D, Sauze L, Ha-Vinh P, et al. Cost-effectiveness analysis of treatments for phimosis: a comparison of surgical and medicinal approaches and their economic effect. *BJU Int* 2001;87:239–244.
19. Elmore JM, Smith EA, Kirsch AJ. Sutureless circumcision using 2-octyl cyanoacrylate (Dermabond): appraisal after 18-month experience. *Urology* 2007;70(4):803–806.
20. Taeusch HW, Martinez AM, Partridge JC, et al. Pain during Mogen or Plastibell circumcision. *J Perinatol* 2002;22:214–218.

# CHAPTER 120 ■ AUGMENTATION CYSTOPLASTY IN CHILDREN

HANS G. POHL

*Dedicated to W. H. Hendren, M.D., whose creative use of intestine in urologic reconstruction I have been honored to observe.*

Neuropathicity, bladder outlet obstruction, or embryologic abnormalities may result in a bladder too small or too overactive to provide normal storage of urine. The goal of augmentation cystoplasty in the pediatric patient is to provide a sufficiently capacious reservoir that stores urine at low pressure and as a result improves urinary continence and prevents upper urinary tract deterioration.

## DIAGNOSIS

Evaluation should include imaging of the upper tracts, urodynamic evaluation and evaluation of the bladder outlet, and urine culture. In the child with no prior history of bowel resection or gastrointestinal comorbidity, it is in general not necessary to evaluate the intestinal tract. However, radiologic imaging is essential with intestinal atresia, intestinal malrotation, and imperforate anus because it is likely that anatomic abnormalities or prior surgical intervention would obviate the use of specific bowel segments.

## INDICATIONS FOR SURGERY

The majority of pediatric patients requiring augmentation cystoplasty have small-capacity, noncompliant, or overactive bladders as a result of neuropathicity (from myelodysplasia or traumatic spinal cord injury) or myogenic failure (from posterior urethral valve). Occasionally, augmentation cystoplasty is required in order to provide adequate bladder volume in cases of classic exstrophy, cloacal exstrophy, and cloacal malformations. Bladder dysfunction should initially be treated with anticholinergic medications and clean intermittent catheterization (CIC) in an effort to diminish uninhibited bladder contractions, improve compliance, and provide regular and effective bladder emptying. When urodynamic evidence exists that nonoperative measures have failed, augmentation cystoplasty is indicated. Intravesical storage pressure that has been demonstrated to be >40 cm $H_2O$ is the most robust indication for augmenting the bladder. Incontinence and urinary tract infections, with or without vesicoureteral reflux (VUR), are associated symptoms that may benefit from enterocystoplasty. However, a thorough evaluation is warranted in order to ascertain what type of augmentation to perform and whether a secondary procedure is indicated in addition to enterocystoplasty to provide continence and/or prevent upper tract deterioration. Since the combination of urinary infection, detrusor hyperreflexia, and VUR poses a significant risk for renal scarring, antireflux surgery should be considered at the time of augmentation cystoplasty when reflux is high grade or recurrent symptomatic urinary infection has occurred. However, reimplanting ureters into a thick-walled bladder is challenging technically and has been associated with postoperative ureteral obstruction, leading some to consider augmentation without ureteral reimplantation. When children with neuropathic bladders and VUR have undergone augmentation cystoplasty alone, VUR has resolved or been significantly downgraded without the need for reimplantation even in high-grade VUR (1) (Table 120.1). If bladder outlet surgery is entertained in conjunction with enterocystoplasty, the incontinence procedure should be performed prior to opening the peritoneal cavity in order to minimize insensible fluid loss.

**TABLE 120.1**

**RESOLUTION OF VESICOURETERAL REFLUX FOLLOWING AUGMENTATION CYSTOPLASTY ALONE IN PATIENTS WITH NEUROPATHIC BLADDER DYSFUNCTION**

| | | *None* | *I* | *II* | *III* | *IV* | *V* |
|---|---|---|---|---|---|---|---|
| Nasrallah and Aliabadi, *J Urol.*, 1991 | Preop | | | 5 | 6 | 8 | 1 |
| | Postop | 12 | 1 | | | | |
| Pereira et al., *J Urol.*, 1994 | Preop | | | | 4 | | 14 |
| | Postop | 13 | | 1 | | | 2 |

## ALTERNATIVE THERAPY

Alternatives are either continued medical management or urinary diversion.

## SURGICAL TECHNIQUE

Preoperative preparation must include a thorough review of the anticipated goals of the surgery with the parent and patient, when he or she is an older child or adolescent. During this meeting, the family's ability to comply with the postoperative care of a bladder augmented with bowel must be assessed. When CIC has been performed preoperatively, the postoperative catheterization and irrigations are more readily adhered to (2). Urinary infection, bladder calculi, or perforation may result when routine emptying and augment cleansing are not performed regularly. Table 120.2 outlines the most common complications of augmentation cystoplasty in the early and late postoperative period.

There is no ideal segment of bowel for augmentation cystoplasty; each has a set of characteristics that are advantages or liabilities depending on the clinical scenario (Table 120.3). It should be noted that none of these complications are seen following ureterocystoplasty, making it the ideal tissue for bladder augmentation. However, it is a procedure ideally performed in a patient with a severely dilated ureter that subtends a nonfunctioning kidney.

Bowel cleansing is typically performed prior to augmentation cystoplasty (Table 120.4). While expedited bowel cleansing protocols (or complete omission) are replacing standard regimens in adults, there are few studies in children demonstrating a significant benefit in the absence of preoperative bowel cleansing. Considering that the majority of children who will undergo augmentation cystoplasty have ventriculoperitoneal shunts that are prone to infection, there appears to be a rationale to continuing the practice of preoperative clean-outs (3).

The patient is positioned supine on the operating table. General anesthesia with endotracheal intubation is mandatory; however, if no spinal abnormality exists that contraindicates the use of an epidural catheter, consideration should be given to regional anesthesia as well. The surgical field is prepared and draped from the xiphoid process inferiorly,

**TABLE 120.2**

**TYPES OF COMPLICATIONS FOLLOWING PEDIATRIC AUGMENTATION CYSTOPLASTY**

| Preoperative Counseling and Informed Consent |
|---|
| Bleeding (pelvic hematoma) |
| Infection (more common after colonic than ileal anastomosis) |
| Small bowel obstruction |
| Urinary leak |
| Ureteral stricture |
| Vesicoureteral reflux |
| Bladder calculi |
| Metabolic abnormalities |
| Poor somatic growth |
| Hematuria–dysuria syndrome |
| Excoriation around stoma site |

**TABLE 120.3**

**COMPARISON OF GASTROINTESTINAL SEGMENTS IN PEDIATRIC AUGMENTATION CYSTOPLASTY**

| | Advantages | Disadvantages |
|---|---|---|
| **Ileum** | Most compliant<br>Less mucus | Diarrhea<br>Vitamin $B_{12}$ deficiency<br>Short mesentery<br>Hyperchloremic acidosis<br>Poor muscle backing |
| **Sigmoid** | Readily mobilized<br>Easily implanted<br>Good muscle backing | Unit contractions<br>Lower compliance<br>Mucus<br>Hyperchloremic acidosis<br>perforation risk |
| **Ileocecal** | Valve as antireflux/continence mechanism<br>Good-capacity reservoir<br>Constant blood supply | Diarrhea<br>Not always available<br>Contractile |
| **Stomach** | Short gut/radiation<br>Chloride pump<br>Minimal mucus<br>Fewer infections<br>Ease of implantation<br>Good muscle backing | Hypochloremic alkalosis<br>Rhythmic contractions<br>Hematuria–dysuria |

TABLE 120.4

COMMONLY UTILIZED BOWEL CLEANSING PERFORMED PRIOR TO AUGMENTATION CYSTOPLASTY

| *GoLytely-Based Bowel Preparation* | | |
|---|---|---|
| Weight (kg) | Vol. infused every 10 min (cc) | Total vol. infused (cc) |
| <10 | 80 | 1,100 |
| 10–20 | 100 | 1,600 |
| 20–30 | 140 | 2,200 |
| 30–40 | 180 | 2,900 |
| 40–50 | 200 | 3,200 |
| >50 | 240 | 4,000 |
| Neomycin base 25 mg/kg × 3 | | |
| Erythromycin base 20 mg/kg × 3 | | |
| Saline enemas until clear | | |

including the genitalia. A Foley catheter is inserted urethrally. A midline incision is created beginning at the symphysis pubis and extending superiorly toward the umbilicus. Retraction can be provided by an Omni or Bookwalter retractor. In order to avoid the insensible loss of heat and water from peritoneal surfaces, it is recommended that any concomitant procedures on the bladder or bladder neck be performed through a limited incision that does not enter the peritoneal space.

When a continent diversion is not planned, a midline cystotomy suffices to prepare the bladder for augmentation. Ureteral reimplants can be easily performed at this point (Fig. 120.1). However, when a continent catheterizable stoma is planned, either a paramedian or transverse cystotomy should be considered since these incisions create bladder flaps that facilitate the creation of a long submucosal tunnel for the appendix or ileal tube. Regardless of the bladder incision created, it must be sufficiently long to open the bladder widely. If the cystotomy is too short, the augmented segment may behave as a diverticulum, thus facilitating urinary stasis and stone formation. Once the bladder has been prepared, the midline incision is carried above the umbilicus and the peritoneum is entered.

## Ileocystoplasty

Ileum is by far the most popular segment used for bladder augmentation. The segment, 20 to 25 cm long, is based on a pedicle that is supplied by branches of the superior mesenteric artery and that is sufficiently mobile to be brought into the pelvis (Fig. 120.2). On occasion an abnormally thick, fatty, or short mesentery can limit mobility of the vascular pedicle, thus necessitating extensive division of the mesentery posteriorly. The terminal 15 to 20 cm of ileum, as measured from the ileocecal valve proximally, is spared in order to retain bile salt absorption, thus preventing steatorrhea and vitamin $B_{12}$ deficiency (Fig. 120.3). The portion of ileum to be used is measured and 5-0 silk sutures are used to mark the proximal and distal limits of resection. Prior to dividing the mesentery, the vascular supply to the isolated segment should be observed by transillumination and the proposed incisions in the mesentery marked. Beginning at the mesenteric border of the bowel, the mesentery is divided between pairs of fine hemostats and the vascular arcades are ligated with 5-0 silk suture ties. The bowel is then divided between atraumatic bowel clamps that have been applied at the proximal and distal limits of resection. Once the ileal segment reaches into the pelvis without tension on the vascular pedicle, no further mesenteric division is needed. An ileoileal anastomosis is performed cephalad to the isolated ileal segment and the mesenteric trap is closed. The bowel clamps are removed and a thorough lavage of the ileal segment is performed with sterile saline. The segment is folded 180 degrees and the adjoining serosal surfaces are sutured with 4-0 PGA. The antimesenteric border of the ileal segment can then be opened using scissors or the cutting current

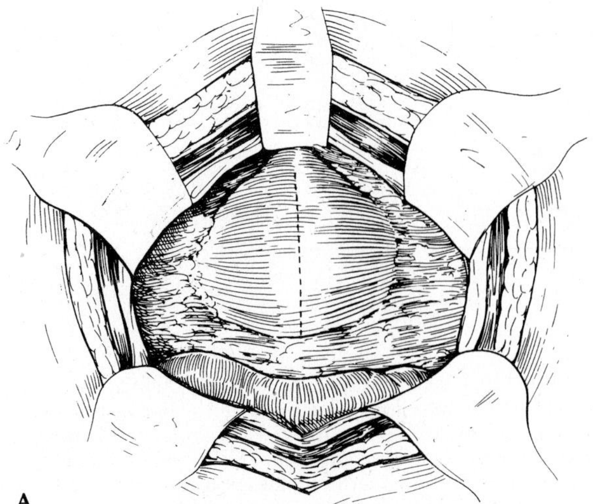


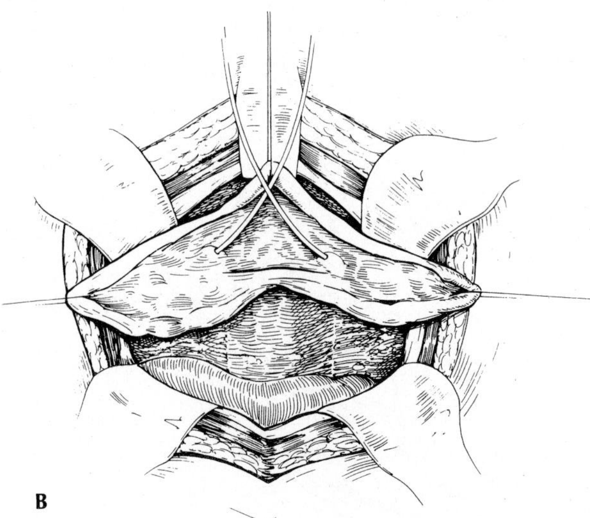


FIGURE 120.1 **A:** Preparation of the bladder for "clam" augmentation cystoplasty. **B:** Sagittal incision is made to create two bladder flaps.

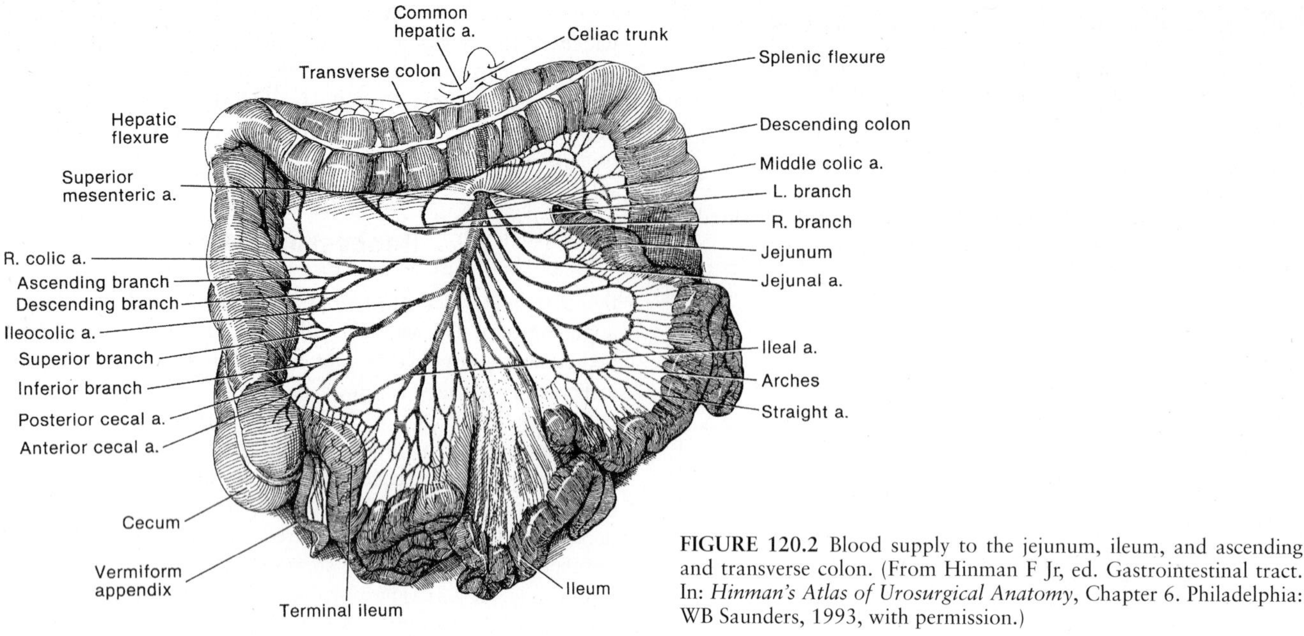


FIGURE 120.2 Blood supply to the jejunum, ileum, and ascending and transverse colon. (From Hinman F Jr, ed. Gastrointestinal tract. In: *Hinman's Atlas of Urosurgical Anatomy*, Chapter 6. Philadelphia: WB Saunders, 1993, with permission.)

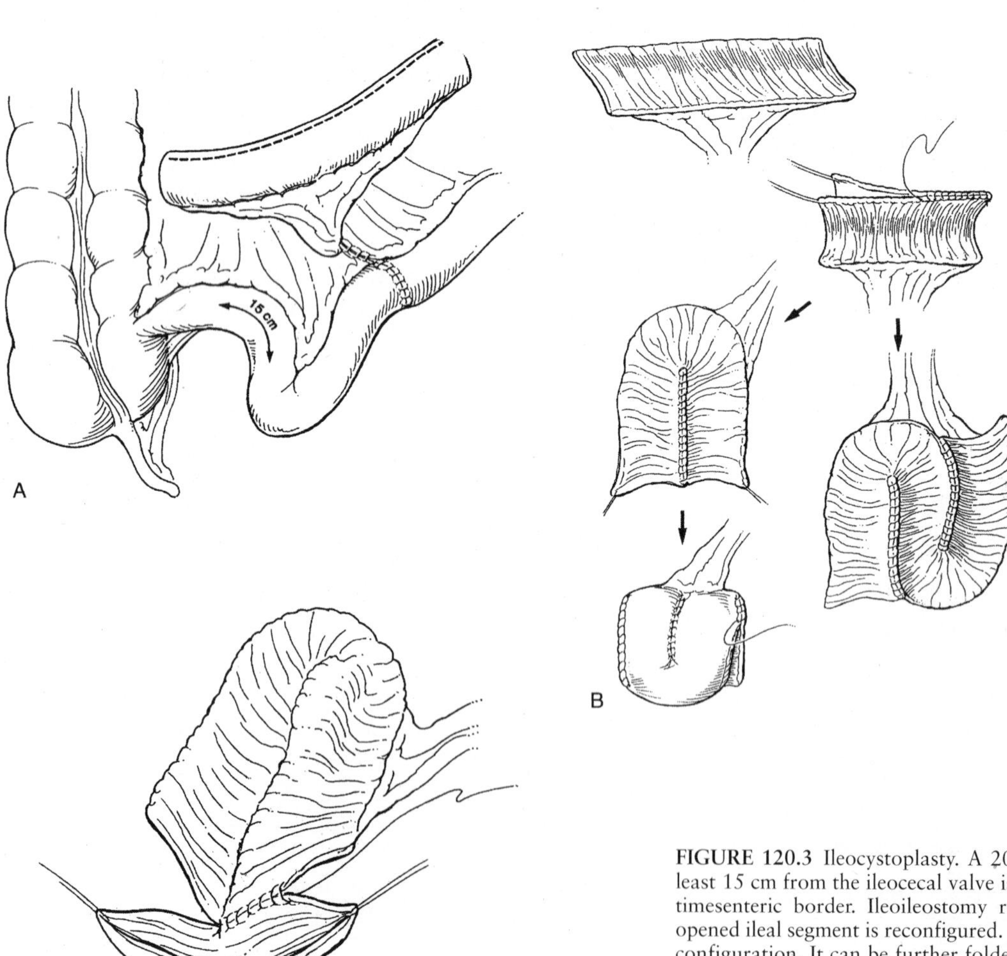

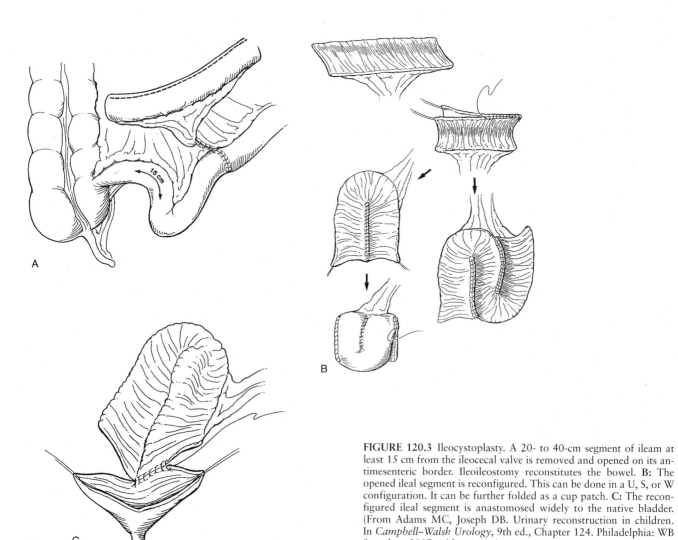

FIGURE 120.3 Ileocystoplasty. A 20- to 40-cm segment of ileam at least 15 cm from the ileocecal valve is removed and opened on its antimesenteric border. Ileoileostomy reconstitutes the bowel. **B:** The opened ileal segment is reconfigured. This can be done in a U, S, or W configuration. It can be further folded as a cup patch. **C:** The reconfigured ileal segment is anastomosed widely to the native bladder. (From Adams MC, Joseph DB. Urinary reconstruction in children. In *Campbell–Walsh Urology*, 9th ed., Chapter 124. Philadelphia: WB Saunders, 2007, with permission.)

with little concern for bleeding, which usually ceases spontaneously. An optional second suture line is created by placing 4-0 PGA through the full thickness of the bowel wall in a continuous fashion. Once the ileal cap has been formed, it is anastomosed to the opened bladder beginning at the most posterior portion of the bladder incision. Hemostatic clamps may be left on the short ends of the tied sutures in order to identify the most posterior limit of the anastomotic line, thus facilitating placement of the second, reinforcing suture layer between the serosal surfaces of the bladder and ileum. A suprapubic catheter is placed through the bladder wall prior to completion of the first anastomotic closure.

## Right Colocystoplasty and Mainz Enterocystoplasty

Enterocystoplasty with a segment of ascending colon is based on vascular supply from the ileocolic artery (Fig. 120.2). Dissection begins at the inferior edge of the cecum and progresses cephalad along the line of Toldt, the peritoneal reflection lateral to the right colon. At the hepatic flexure, the hepatocolic ligament must be divided. Next, the omental attachments to the colon are divided and the omentum is packed into the left upper quadrant with moist laparotomy sponges. The ascending colon is divided at the watershed between the ileocolic and right colic arteries, approximately midway between the cecum and hepatic flexure. The ileum is divided close to the ileocecal valve. An ileocolonic anastomosis is performed and the mesenteric trap is closed. If the appendix will not be used to create a continent catheterizable stoma, an appendectomy is performed at this point. The bowel is folded 180 degrees and the serosal surfaces are sutured with 4-0 PGA. The bowel is incised along its antimesenteric border and the edges are sutured full thickness with 4-0 PGA placed in a continuous fashion. The resulting colonic plate is folded once again. This time the full-thickness suture line is placed first and reinforced with a second continuous line of 4-0 PGA. The resulting cup is inverted and anastomosed to the bladder opening as described for the ileocystoplasty. An alternative approach that has gained wide popularity is the Mainz augmentation, in which 15 to 30 cm of terminal ileum is isolated in continuity with the right colon and detubularized, anastomosed to each other, and sutured to the cystotomy (Fig. 120.4).

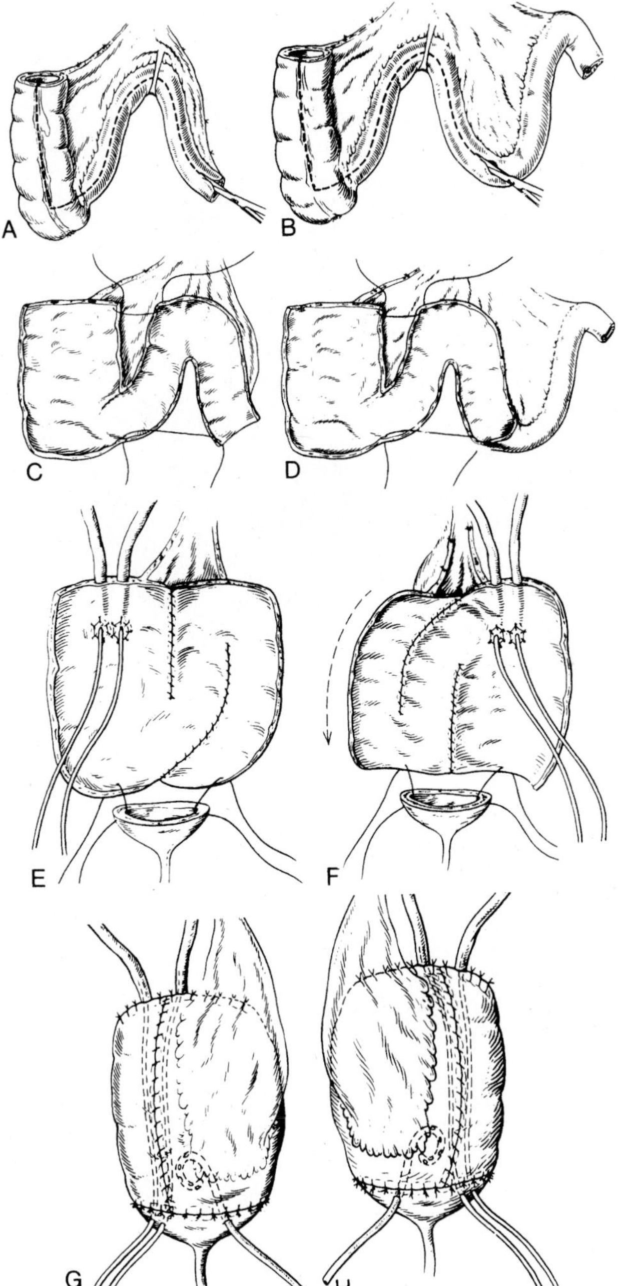


FIGURE 120.4 Mainz Ileocecocystoplasty. **A and B:** The ileal segment is twice the length as the cecal segment. **C and D:** It is opened on the antimesenteric border. **E and F:** The ureters can be opened into the opened cecal segment if necessary. **G and H:** The ileocecal segment is anastomosed to the native bladder. (From Thuroff JW, et al. The Mainz pouch. In: King LR, Stone AR, Websterm GD, eds. *Bladder Reconstruction and Continent Urinary Diversion*. Chicago: Year Book, 1987, with permission.)

## Sigmoidocystoplasty

Since the diameter of the sigmoid is much greater than that of the ileum, a shorter segment is necessary in order to perform a successful augmentation cystoplasty. The isolated segment derives its blood supply from the sigmoid branches of the inferior mesenteric artery (Fig. 120.5). A mesenteric incision is created proximally and distally and bowel clamps are applied to minimize fecal soiling. The sigmoid is divided and a sigmoidosigmoidostomy performed lateral to the mesentery of the isolated segment (Fig. 120.6). It is advisable for each surgeon to standardize the side where he or she performs the sigmoidosigmoidostomy in the event that reoperation is necessary in the future. Two methods are available for anastomosing the bowel segment to the bladder. In the first, the proximal and distal ends of the segment are closed and the bowel is opened along its antimesenteric border and sutured to the bladder opening. In the second, the bowel is opened along its antimesenteric border first, then folded 180 degrees into a U shape prior to suturing it to the bladder. The latter method likely disrupts the high unit contractions of the sigmoid more than the first; however, it requires that a greater length of sigmoid be isolated.

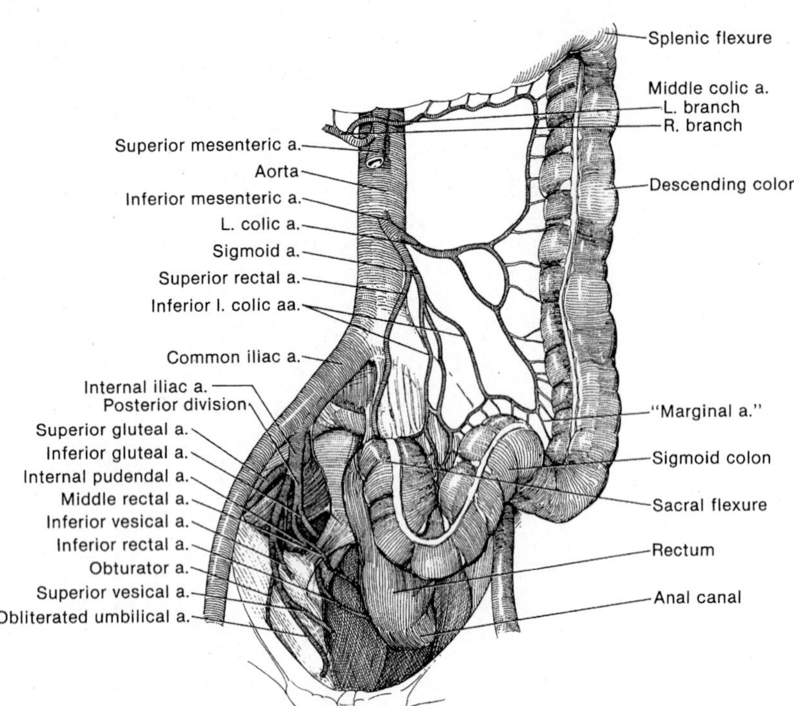


**FIGURE 120.5** Blood supply to the descending and sigmoid colon and rectum. (From Hinman F Jr, ed. Gastrointestinal tract. In: *Hinman's Atlas of Urosurgical Anatomy*, Chapter 6. Philadelphia: WB Saunders, 1993, with permission.)

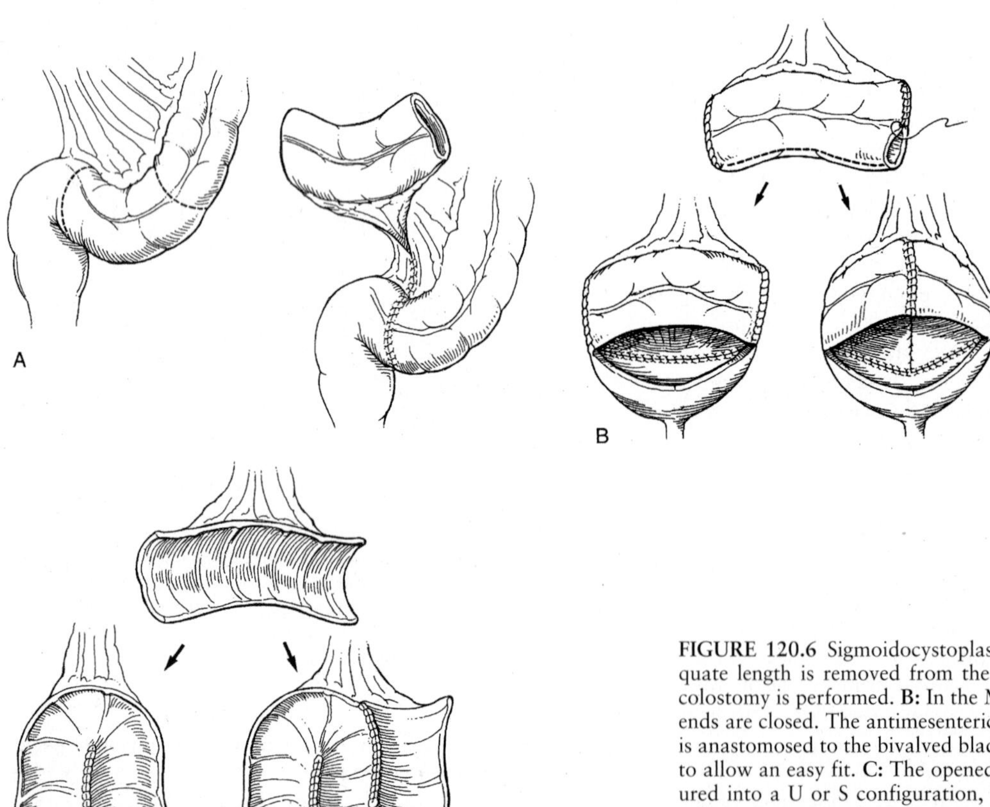


**FIGURE 120.6** Sigmoidocystoplasty. **A:** A sigmoid segment of adequate length is removed from the gastrointestinal tract and a colocolostomy is performed. **B:** In the Mitchell technique, the two opened ends are closed. The antimesenteric border is incised and the segment is anastomosed to the bivalved bladder. It may be rotated 180 degrees to allow an easy fit. **C:** The opened sigmoid segment can be reconfigured into a U or S configuration, which may lower pressure. (From Adams MC, Joseph DB. Urinary reconstruction in children. In *Campbell–Walsh Urology*, 9th ed., Chapter 124. Philadelphia: WB Saunders, 2007, with permission.)

## Gastrocystoplasty

The bladder may be augmented with a gastric segment derived from either the antrum or the body of the stomach. When antral gastrocystoplasty is performed, the enteric stream is reconstructed using a Billroth I anastomosis (gastroduodenostomy). This procedure is now rarely performed in children because resection of the antrum has been associated with delayed gastric emptying, gastric dumping syndrome, and feeding difficulties. Currently, most surgeons prefer the use of the stomach body instead. A segment between 10 and 20 cm is marked along the greater curvature of the stomach and drawn as a rhomboid that extends toward the lesser curvature, ending 1 cm from the edge so as not to interrupt branches of the vagus nerve. Two arterial supplies exist to the greater curvature of the stomach: (i) the right gastroepiploic artery, derived from the right gastric artery, and (ii) the left gastroepiploic artery, from the splenic artery (Fig. 120.7). If the right gastroepiploic artery is chosen, the gastric segment should be obtained from higher on the greater curvature, lower if based on the left (Fig. 120.8). The gastroepiploic arteries supply the stomach with anterior and posterior branches that must be divided before the segment can be excised from the stomach. Atraumatic intestinal clamps are applied in parallel at the proposed incision sites on the stomach. Alternatively, an intestinal stapling device can be used to divide the stomach; however, the staples must be removed later. The vascular pedicle must be retroperitonealized in order to prevent internal hernia formation. A window is created in the transverse mesocolon that accepts the gastric augment and its vascular pedicle. The segment is passed posterior to the mesocolon and exits a second window that has been created in the small bowel mesentery inferiorly. If the vascular pedicle is too short, additional branches between the gastroepiploic artery and the stomach must be divided. The stomach is sutured to the bladder beginning along the posterior aspect of the cystotomy.

## Ureterocystoplasty

Unlike enterocystoplasty, ureterocystoplasty does not require a midline transperitoneal incision. The entire procedure can be performed retroperitoneally through a flank incision, to perform the nephrectomy and harvest the proximal portion of the ureter, and a Pfannenstiel incision, through which the augmentation is performed. Only a midline incision should be considered when two functioning kidneys exist, since a transureteroureterostomy will be required in order to re-establish continuity of the upper urinary tract after the distal ureter has been harvested (Fig. 120.9). Following the nephrectomy, careful mobilization of the ureter from its retroperitoneal location includes dissection of all surrounding adventitia away from the peritoneal lining toward the ureter itself. The ureter is then passed into the pelvis. A midline cystotomy is created such that the posterior portion of the incision includes the ureterovesical junction. The ureter, too, is incised along its anterior aspect. A spherical reservoir can be created by folding the proximal end of the ureter toward the cystotomy in an inverted U and suturing the adjoining edges of the ureter to itself. The remainder of the anastomosis between the ureter and the bladder is performed as in enterocystoplasty, beginning at the posterior aspect of the cystotomy and proceeding in an anterior fashion. Drainage tubes are placed through the native bladder muscle tissue.

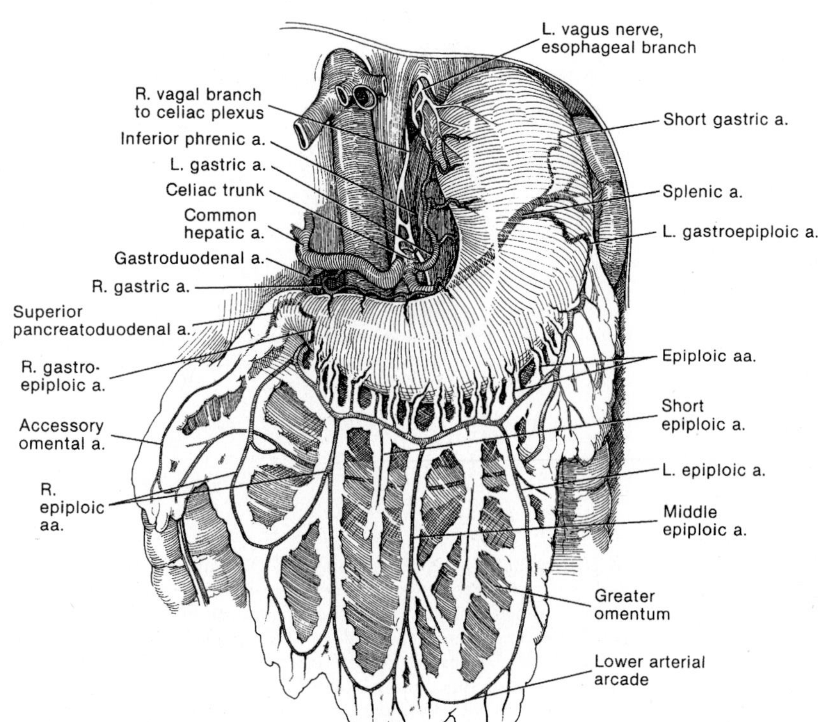


FIGURE 120.7 Blood supply to the anterior aspect of the stomach and greater omentum. (From Hinman F Jr, ed. Gastrointestinal tract. In: *Hinman's Atlas of Urosurgical Anatomy*, Chapter 6. Philadelphia: WB Saunders, 1993, with permission.)

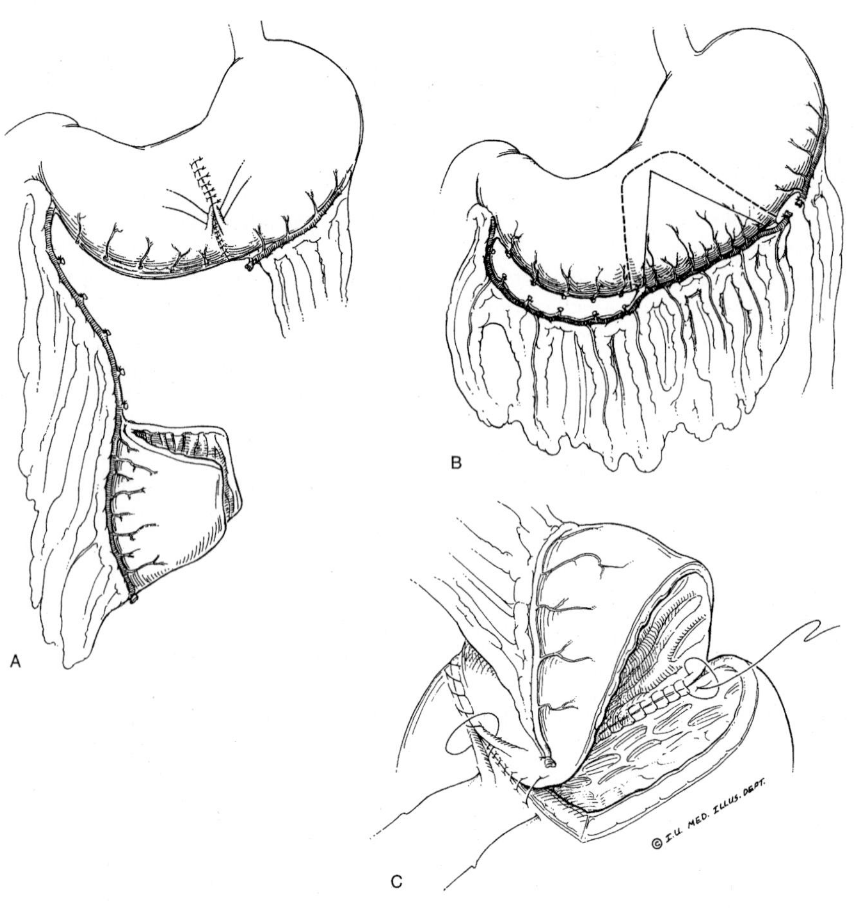


FIGURE 120.8 Gastrocystoplasty using the body of the stomach. **A:** A gastric segment of the body is mobilized on the right gastroepiploic artery. The left vessel may also be used; neither vessel as a pedicle should be free-floating through the peritoneum. **B:** A longer gastric segment along the greater curvature with a wider apex provides more surface area for augmentation. **C:** The gastric segment is anastomosed to the bivalved bladder with the mucosa inverted. (From Adams MC, Joseph DB. Urinary reconstruction in children. In *Campbell–Walsh Urology*, 9th ed., Chapter 124. Philadelphia: WB Saunders, 2007, with permission.)

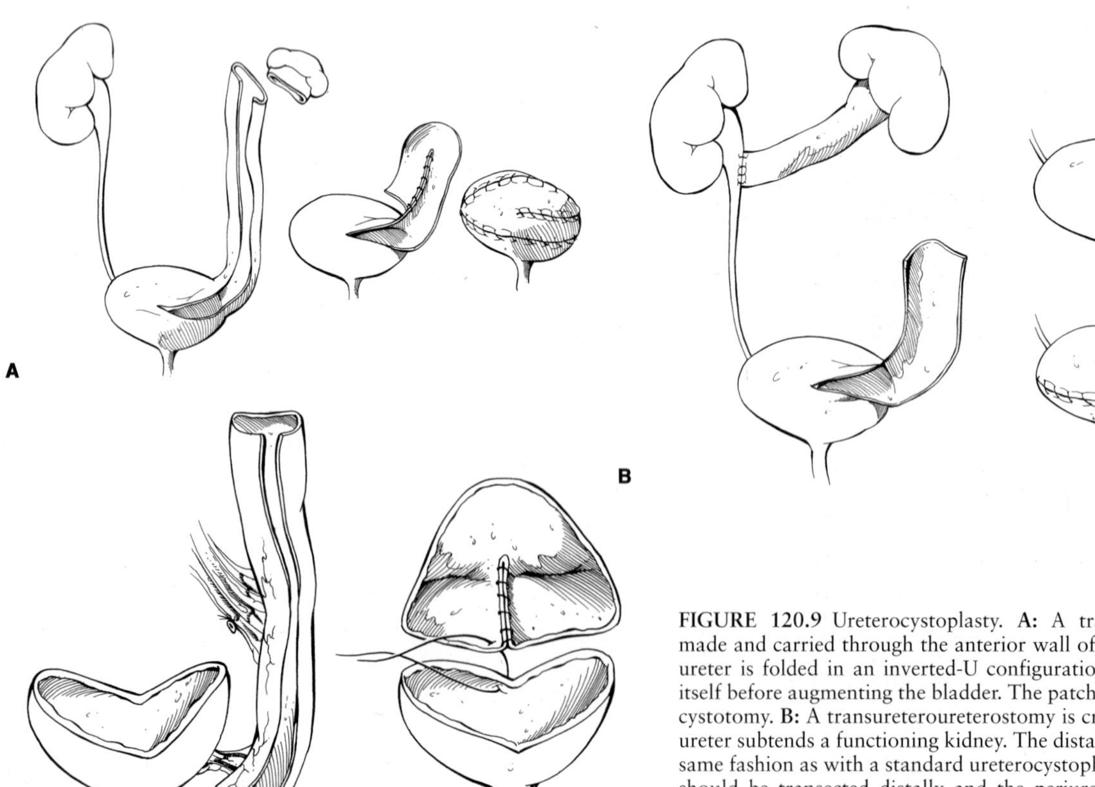


FIGURE 120.9 Ureterocystoplasty. **A:** A transverse cystotomy is made and carried through the anterior wall of the dilated ureter. The ureter is folded in an inverted-U configuration and anastomosed to itself before augmenting the bladder. The patch is folded over onto the cystotomy. **B:** A transureteroureterostomy is created when the dilated ureter subtends a functioning kidney. The distal ureter is treated in the same fashion as with a standard ureterocystoplasty. **C:** Ectopic ureters should be transected distally and the periureteral adventitial tissue preserved as a vascular pedicle to the ureter. An inverted-U shape is created in order to perform the augmentation.

## Urinary and Abdominal Drainage Following Augmentation Cystoplasty

If an incontinence procedure has not been performed, an appropriately sized urethral Foley catheter is used. However, since the retention balloon can cause pressure necrosis of the bladder neck following incontinence procedures, some surgeons would instead use a Robnel catheter or Silastic feeding tube, which may be secured with 3-0 silk sutures passed through the bladder and abdominal wall and tied over a cotton bolster. Additionally, a suprapubic Malecot catheter should be placed through a separate incision in the native bladder and brought out through the anterior abdominal wall. It is advised that this tube in particular be secured with 3-0 nylon sutures, since it will remain until after a cystogram has demonstrated a healed anastomosis and the patient is successfully catheterizing the reconstructed bladder, approximately 3 weeks. Irrigation with sterile saline should be instituted on postoperative day 3 in an effort to cleanse the newly augmented bladder free of the copious amounts of mucus that the enteric segments produce. A closed-system vacuum drain is employed briefly following surgery and removed when minimal peritoneal drainage exists. In patients with ventriculoperitoneal shunts, cerebrospinal fluid can be confused for persistent urinary drainage; it can be discriminated by its lower creatinine level than urine.

# OUTCOMES

## Gastrointestinal Effects

The two most likely gastrointestinal complications following augmentation cystoplasty in children are diarrhea and vitamin $B_{12}$ deficiency (each in up to 23%). Small bowel obstruction may occur in approximately 3% of patients and is no more likely with any one particular segment of bowel. Gastrocystoplasty is associated with a greater risk for small bowel obstruction as a function of the difficulty in retroperitonealizing the vascular pedicle to the gastric patch. The potentially free-floating pedicle can permit internal herniation of bowel loops that in later stages compromises vascularity to the gastric patch itself.

Diarrhea, a complication most often found following the use of the ileocecal valve (up to 23%), may also be seen after standard ileocystoplasty, although less frequently (11%). For this reason, use of the ileocecal valve is not advocated when other segments will serve just as well. The sigmoid, for instance, dilates and lengthens as a consequence of constipation, thus affording the surgeon a more redundant segment with which to augment. An additional advantage of sigmoid is its proximity to the bladder.

Vitamin $B_{12}$ deficiency can be avoided by limiting the length of small bowel harvested and in particular by preserving the terminal 20 cm of ileum, the major site of $B_{12}$ absorption. Ileocecal augmentation cystoplasty carries a greater risk for vitamin $B_{12}$ deficiency (23%) as compared with standard ileocystoplasty (11%), yet one is unlikely to encounter this deficiency at all since in the majority of circumstances a limited portion of nonterminal ileum is employed.

## Metabolic Effects

### Ileocystoplasty and Colocystoplasty

Despite the incorporation of intestine into the urinary tract, its absorptive and secretory capacity is retained: chloride, ammonium, hydrogen ions, and organic acids are readily absorbed and bicarbonate ions are secreted into the urine. The resultant hyperchloremic metabolic acidosis is driven by the absorption of ammonium ions that are followed by chloride in an attempt to maintain electroneutrality. Acidosis is rarely seen in patients with normal renal function, and any measurable increase in serum chloride and decrease in serum bicarbonate is subtle. Mild cases of metabolic acidosis can be managed with oral sodium bicarbonate (1 to 3 mEq/kg/day) with the goal being an increase in serum bicarbonate to a value >20 mEq/L. Severe acidosis requires intravenous administration of bicarbonate, usually as dextrose 5% with one-quarter normal saline and 50 mEq/L of sodium bicarbonate. Hyperchloremic metabolic acidosis may occur following augmentation with ileum, cecum, colon, or sigmoid but is most common following sigmoidocystoplasty.

Use of jejunum is associated with a pattern of metabolic derangement distinct from any other segment of bowel: a hypochloremic, hyponatremic, hyperkalemic metabolic acidosis. For this reason, it is recommended that jejunum not be used in pediatric augmentation cystoplasty, especially when renal function is poor.

As a consequence of the net secretion of chloride and hydrogen ions across the gastric mucosa, augmentation with stomach results in a hypochloremic metabolic alkalosis in 3% to 24% of the patients. This effect can be used to advantage in patients with renal dysfunction and acidemia, who will demonstrate decreased serum chloride and increased serum bicarbonate following gastrocystoplasty. In those patients whose renal dysfunction is characterized by a concentrating defect, gastrointestinal illness with vomiting can precipitate significant alkalosis that must be treated with intravenous fluid containing sodium chloride. Milder cases can be treated with oral salt supplementation, or inhibitors of histamine-2 (i.e., cimetidine) or the gastric acid $H^+/K^+$ ATPase pump (omeprazole). It has also been reported that alkalosis occurs in the absence of gastrointestinal illness and may still be severe enough to require resection of a portion of the gastric segment. Alternatively, addition of ileum may balance the metabolic abnormality.

## Bladder Compliance

The immediate goal of augmentation cystoplasty should be that intravesical storage pressure decreases well below the threshold of 40 cm $H_2O$, thus averting progressive upper tract deterioration. Although any gastrointestinal segment can provide a sufficiently compliant augment if it is very long and fully detubularized, most authors agree that, for a given length of bowel, ileum provides the greatest compliance of any segment. Of 323 patients who had undergone enterocystoplasty in one large review, 6% required an additional augmentation because of persistently elevated intravesical pressure. Colocystoplasty and gastrocystoplasty patients were 10 times more likely to need a repeat procedure as compared with those having undergone an ileocystoplasty (4).

## Urinary Tract Infection

Regardless of the segment chosen, persistent bacteriuria is common following augmentation cystoplasty, occurring in up to 95% of patients. The Indiana group reported symptomatic urinary tract infection in 23% of ileocystoplasties, 17% of colocystoplasties, 13% of cecocystoplasties, and only 8% of gastrocystoplasties, which suggests that bacterial colonization may be impeded by the reduced urine pH in bladders augmented with stomach (5). Symptomatic cystitis may be more likely when CIC is performed sporadically and incompletely or when mucus and stones serve as a nidus for colonizing bacteria.

## Calculi Formation and Mucus Production

The reported incidence of bladder calculi has ranged between 8% and 52% of patients following augmentation cystoplasty, yet the occurrence of bladder calculi may not be a specific complication of augmentation cystoplasty (6,7). Instead, poor patient compliance with CIC, colonization with urea-splitting bacteria, and the presence of mucus to serve as a nidus for the aggregation of salts may be the trifecta that results in calculus formation. By virtue of lesser mucus production and bacteriuria than either ileum or colon, stomach is least likely to be associated with bladder calculi. Mucus production from ileal segments does decrease over time as a result of villous atrophy, a feature not characteristic of colonic epithelium.

## Bladder Perforation

Perforation is the most serious complication of augmentation enterocystoplasty, and patients may present critically ill despite few localizing signs and symptoms. The condition should immediately be suspected when an augmented patient presents with fever and abdominal pain no matter how mild the symptoms; shoulder pain secondary to diaphragmatic irritation from urine in the peritoneal cavity has also been reported. Which gastrointestinal segment carries the greatest risk of perforation is debatable (8). Any child is potentially at risk irrespective of the segment used. The underlying etiology for all perforations is believed to be ischemia within the bowel wall as a consequence of either overdistention from infrequent emptying or high-pressure contractions or even reconfiguration by detubularization (9).

Patients suspected of having bladder perforation should undergo fluid resuscitation and receive intravenous broad-spectrum antibiotics and Foley catheter drainage while the evaluation is underway. A standard cystogram may miss up to 33% of bladder perforations; therefore, computerized tomography cystograms are advocated. While some have successfully employed nonoperative management, surgical exploration with resection of necrotic tissue and primary closure of the defect should be performed in a gravely ill patient, or when the patient fails to improve during nonoperative management (10).

## Hematuria–Dysuria Syndrome

This syndrome, occurring in 9% to 70% of patients who have undergone a gastrocystoplasty, presents with perineal pain, dysuria, hematuria, and skin excoriation around either the urethral meatus or the stoma of a catheterizable channel (11). A recent study of 10 children with hematuria–dysuria identified a positive correlation between the presence of infecting *Helicobacter pylori*, reduced urine pH, and the presence of symptoms following gastrocystoplasty (12). The authors recommend evaluating all patients who are under consideration for a gastric augment for the presence of *H. pylori* and treating the infection before performing surgery. Oral therapy with histamine-2 or $H^+/K^+$ ATPase blockers should be helpful in symptomatic patients. If prolonged catheterization is anticipated, then bladder irrigations should be performed with a sodium bicarbonate–containing solution.

## *References*

1. Woods C, Atwell JD. Vesico-ureteric reflux in the neuropathic bladder with particular reference to the development of renal scarring. *Eur Urol* 1982; 8:23–28.
2. Joseph DB, Colodny AH, Mandell J, et al. Clean, intermittent catheterization of infants with neurogenic bladder. *Pediatrics* 1989;84:778–782.
3. Yerkes EB, Rink RC, Cain MP, et al. Shunt infection and malfunction after augmentation cystoplasty. *J Urol* 2006;165(6, pt 2):2262–2264.
4. Mitchell ME, Piser JA. Intestinocystoplasty and total bladder replacement in children and young adults: follow-up in 129 cases. *J Urol* 1987;138: 579–584.
5. Rink RC, Hollensbe D, Adams MC. Complications of bladder augmentation in children and comparison of gastrointestinal segments. *AUA Update Series* 1995;14:122–127.
6. Barroso U, Jednak R, Fleming P, et al. Bladder calculi in children who perform clean intermittent catheterization. *BJU Int* 2000;85:879–884.
7. Khoury AE, Salomon M, Doche R, et al. Stone formation after augmentation cystoplasty: the role of intestinal mucus. *J Urol* 1997;158:1133–1137.
8. Rink RC. Bladder augmentation. Options, outcomes, future. *Urol Clin North Am* 1999;26:111–123.
9. Pope JC, Albers P, Rink RC, et al. Spontaneous rupture of the augmented bladder: from silence to chaos. Proceedings of the Annual Meeting of the European Society of Pediatric Urology, Istanbul, Turkey, 1999.
10. Slaton JW, Kropp KA. Conservative management of suspected bladder rupture after augmentation enterocystoplasty. *J Urol* 1994;152:713–715.
11. Leonard MP, Dharamsi N, Williot PE. Outcome of gastrocystoplasty in tertiary pediatric urology practice. *J Urol* 2000;164:947–950.
12. Celayir S, Goksel S, Buyukunal SN. The relationship between *Helicobacter pylori* infection and acid–hematuria syndrome in pediatric patients with gastric augmentation, II. *J Pediatr Surg* 1999;34:532–535.

# CHAPTER 121 ■ THE MITROFANOFF PROCEDURE IN PEDIATRIC URINARY TRACT RECONSTRUCTION

MARK P. CAIN

The Mitrofanoff principle offered a major advancement to continent urinary reconstruction for children and adults. Earlier innovations—including clean intermittent catheterization (CIC), bladder augmentation, and a variety of bladder neck tightening procedures—created the foundation that made continent bladder reconstruction possible. The technically difficult problem was creating a bladder outlet that was tight enough to ensure continence but wide enough to allow reliable catheterization over a lifetime. In addition, many of these patients have physical disabilities that prevent easy access to the urethra, making independent urethral catheterization challenging. The concept of a continent catheterizable abdominal channel was introduced by Paul Mitrofanoff in 1980 (1) and has since been widely adopted as an integral part of urinary tract reconstruction for continence in most pediatric centers worldwide. This principle involves creation of a flap-valve continence mechanism for a conduit that is tunneled into a low-pressure urinary reservoir that can then be catheterized and emptied via an abdominal stoma (Fig. 121.1).

There are multiple surgical options for creating the Mitrofanoff channel. Appendicovesicostomy has by tradition been used because of the availability and the reliable blood supply, adequate lumen for catheterization, and supple muscular wall. Long-term follow-up has shown that appendicovesicostomy provides a durable channel with minimal late complications (2,3). In the absence of a suitable appendix, or in conditions where the appendix is used for an alternate procedure (such as for a Malone antegrade continence enema [MACE channel]), there are several other options that have been described. The most reliable alternatives have been the Monti–Yang ileovesicostomy, ureterovesicostomy, and continent bladder tube.

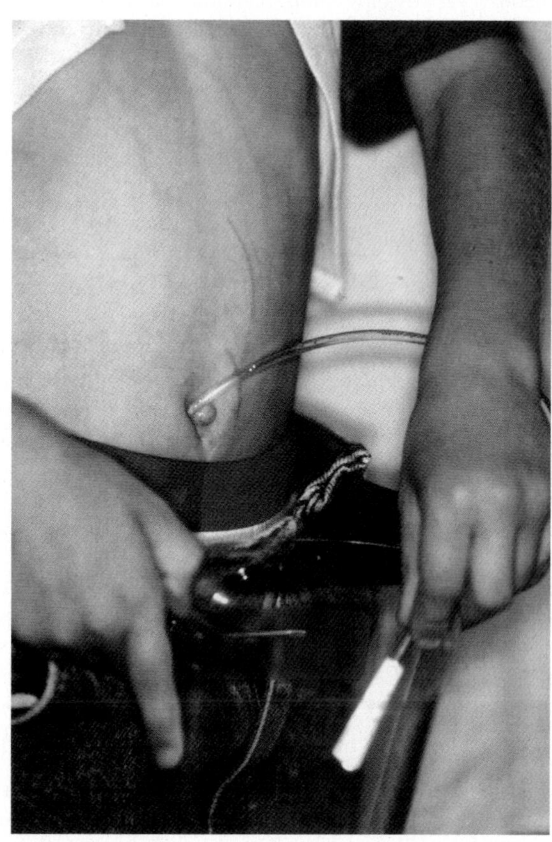

**FIGURE 121.1** Umbilical Mitrofanoff stoma allowing catheterization in the sitting or standing position.

## DIAGNOSIS

The Mitrofanoff procedure can be performed with essentially any underlying bladder pathology. The most frequent diagnosis for children undergoing the procedure is neuropathic bladder, usually due to myelomeningocele. This procedure has also been described for reconstruction in patients with exstrophy–epispadias, cloacal anomalies, prune belly syndrome, posterior urethral valves, and other conditions. Although many of these children will require a bladder outlet procedure to provide urinary continence, some will have an intact and continent bladder outlet and the Mitrofanoff channel will provide an alternative to urethral catheterization. This is especially useful in wheelchair-bound patients who cannot access their perineum independently and also in patients with normal urethral sensation, in whom catheterization can be traumatic both physically and psychologically.

## INDICATIONS FOR SURGERY

In the past, the primary indication for bladder reconstruction was for upper urinary tract preservation. In the era of aggressive use of anticholinergics and intermittent catheterization in young patients, the more common indication for a Mitrofanoff channel is for urinary continence and convenient, independent bladder management for the patient. All patients should undergo a trial of CIC to demonstrate that they are reliable and able to comply with a daily routine prior to bladder reconstruction.

## ALTERNATIVE THERAPY

The most common alternative to continent bladder reconstruction with a Mitrofanoff stoma is anticholinergic therapy with clean intermittent urethral catheterization. With careful attention to catheterization schedules and fluid intake, social dryness can be achieved in many patients with neuropathic bladder and other underlying bladder pathology without the need for surgical intervention.

Less frequently used alternatives are long-term incontinent cutaneous vesicostomy and conduit urinary diversion. Although these are both considered suboptimal in the era of continent urinary reconstruction, there will be a subset of patients who are unable to care for themselves because of physical, mental, or psychosocial problems, and the incontinent diversion provides a safer long-term option for these patients.

In the rare patient with a completely nonusable bladder, a continent urinary reservoir with a continent catheterizable channel is another alternative.

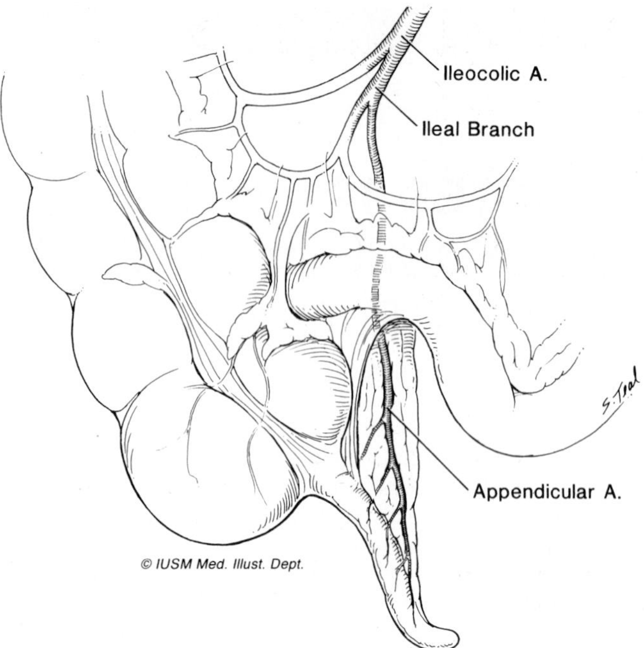


FIGURE 121.2 Vascular anatomy of appendicular artery.

## SURGICAL TECHNIQUE

All patients are admitted the day before surgery for intravenous antibiotics to sterilize the urinary tract and for a mechanical and antibiotic bowel preparation. This is particularly important for patients with ventriculoperitoneal shunts, who have a risk of shunt infection. Potential sites for stomal location should be determined preoperatively, with the patient in the sitting and supine position.

Surgical exposure is usually obtained through a midline transabdominal incision that is carried around the umbilicus to leave enough fascia to close the abdomen without compromising an umbilical stoma. A lower transverse Pfannenstiel incision will also allow adequate exposure for both bladder augmentation and the Mitrofanoff stoma in thin patients. Laparoscopy has been used to assist in mobilization of the appendix and colon, allowing a smaller abdominal incision to complete the reconstruction without compromising exposure.

### Appendicovesicostomy

The right colon is mobilized beyond the hepatic flexure to allow maximal freedom of the appendiceal mesentery. If the appendix is retrocecal in location it is mobilized carefully from the cecal attachments with extra caution to avoid injuring the appendiceal artery, which is a branch of the ileocolic artery (Fig. 121.2). In some cases there is significant peritoneal inflammation due to the presence of a ventriculoperitoneal shunt, and the peritoneal incision must be carried medial to the ileocecal valve to adequately mobilize the appendix. When the length of appendix is inadequate, it can be extended by incorporating a segment of distal cecum as described by Cromie et al. (4). Prior to detaching the appendix, the bladder is mobilized to ensure that the bladder and appendix can easily reach the chosen site for the abdominal stoma without tension. The bladder is then opened to the left of the midline for a right lower-quadrant appendicovesicostomy or in a wide U-shaped anterior bladder incision for an umbilical stoma. The appendix is detached from the cecum either sharply or with a stapling device, and the cecum is closed with absorbable and permanent sutures. The mesentery to the appendiceal artery can be freed from the cecal mesentery to allow complete mobilization of the appendix if needed (Fig. 121.3). The terminal end of the appendix is then opened and irrigated with antibiotic solution, and a 12Fr catheter is passed to ensure that the appendix has an adequate lumen. If necessary the appendix can be gently dilated with serial sounds. If bladder augmentation is to be performed, the segment of bowel is isolated,

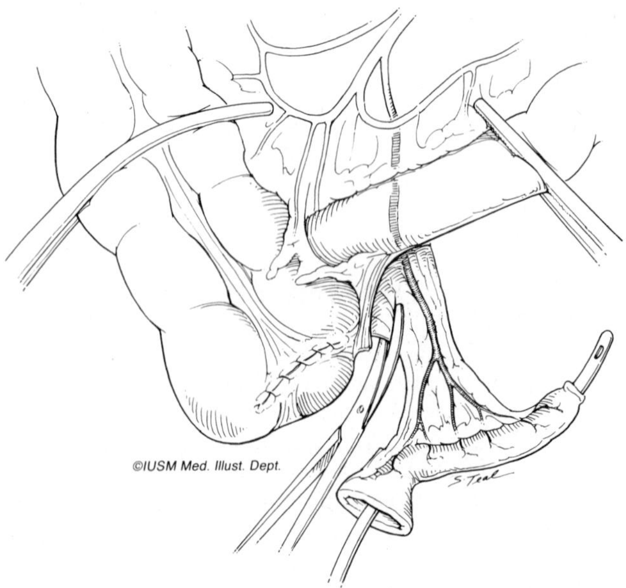


FIGURE 121.3 The mesentery to the appendix can be mobilized carefully, taking care not to injure the appendicular artery.

harvested, and reconfigured appropriately. If an additional segment of intestine is required for the Mitrofanoff (e.g., Monti–Yang) channel, it can be harvested simultaneously. The site of the bladder hiatus is then selected, again ensuring that it can easily reach the posterior abdominal wall fascia without tension. The site of the hiatus is opened wide enough to allow the appendix to pass without any tension, and a vessel loop is passed through the hiatus for traction. A submucosal bladder tunnel is then created using sharp dissection. Placing several traction sutures on the bladder to flatten out the posterior bladder wall facilitates this dissection. The orientation of the tunnel should be directed away from the bladder outlet and trigone to prevent painful catheterization postoperatively. The tunnel length should be at least 2.5 cm in length. It is occasionally helpful to inject 1:200,000 epinephrine along the path of the submucosal tunnel to facilitate the dissection and minimize bleeding. The terminal end of the appendix is then passed through the bladder hiatus and submucosal tunnel. The appendix is spatulated and secured distally with two 4-0 absorbable sutures incorporating full-thickness bites of the appendix and detrusor muscle and mucosa. The remainder of the anastomosis is completed using 4-0 or 5-0 absorbable sutures, securing the bladder mucosa to the appendix. The appendix is also secured at the level of the bladder hiatus using several 4-0 absorbable sutures. The channel is catheterized with a 12Fr or 14Fr catheter to ensure that it passes easily across the hiatus and submucosal tunnel. The stomal site is then selected, taking care to ensure that the bladder hiatus can reach the posterior fascia without tension. A U-shaped (umbilical) or V-shaped skin incision is made at the stomal site, and the flap is freed sharply to the level of the fascia. A cruciate incision is made in the fascia and widened to allow passage of an index finger. The appendix is then brought through the fascial opening and the appendiceal/bladder hiatus is secured to the posterior fascial wall using 3-0 absorbable sutures, taking care not to angulate or compress the appendiceal mesentery (Fig. 121.4). This maneuver ensures a short, straight extravesical appendix channel. The cecal end of the appendix is then spatulated on the antimesenteric side, and if there is redundant appendix it is amputated. The stomal anastomosis is secured using interrupted 4-0 absorbable sutures (Fig. 121.5).

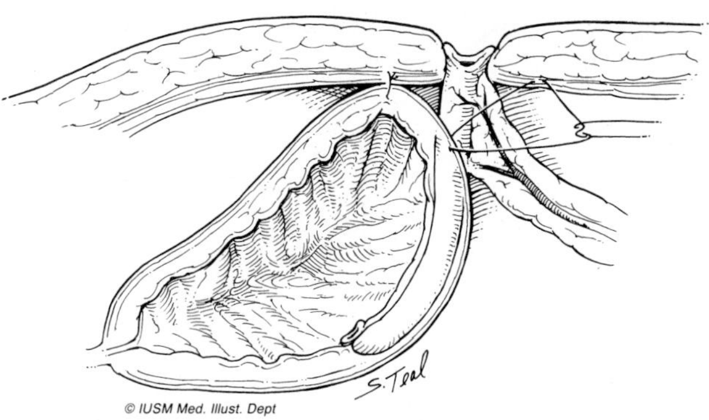


FIGURE 121.4 The bladder is secured to the posterior abdominal fascia to avoid redundancy in the extravesical channel, which can be a source of late catheterization problems.

The stoma is then catheterized multiple times with the bladder both distended and empty to ensure that there is no angulation in the channel. A 12Fr catheter is left indwelling for 3 weeks before initiating intermittent catheterization.

When both Mitrofanoff and MACE channels are indicated, and the appendix is of adequate length to create both channels, it can be split, with the majority of the mesoappendix left intact with the Mitrofanoff segment, basing the blood supply to the appendiceal stump off the cecal artery. In some cases the appendix is too short to use for both channels, but in this circumstance the appendix can still be used for both channels, utilizing one of the described stapling techniques to extend the appendix into the cecum for the MACE channel (5,6).

## Monti–Yang Ileovesicostomy

The concept of retubularized ileum as a replacement for the appendicovesicostomy was introduced in 1997 (7,8), and it has quickly become the ideal alternate to appendix as a choice for the Mitrofanoff channel. Large series with longer follow-up have confirmed the equivalent outcomes for the Monti–Yang channel and appendicovesicostomy (9). The growing indications for and use of the MACE channel have led to

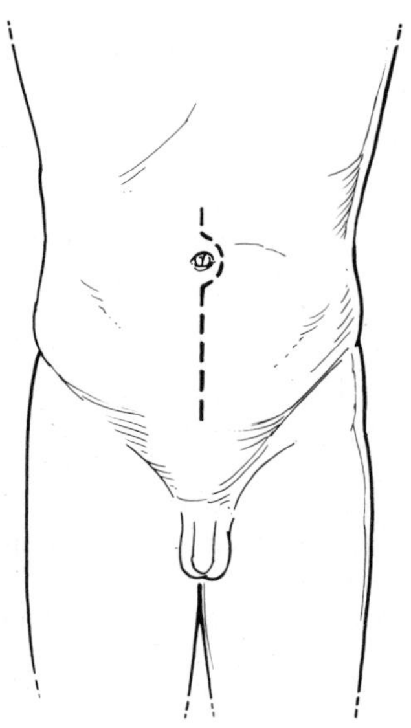

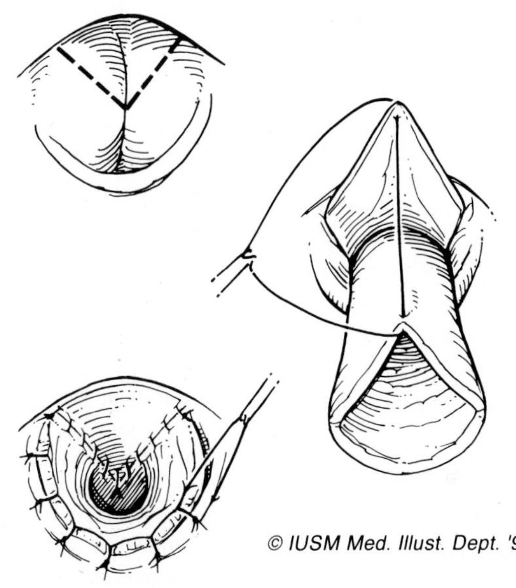


FIGURE 121.5 The skin stoma is completed by securing the wide-based V flap of skin into the spatulated channel.

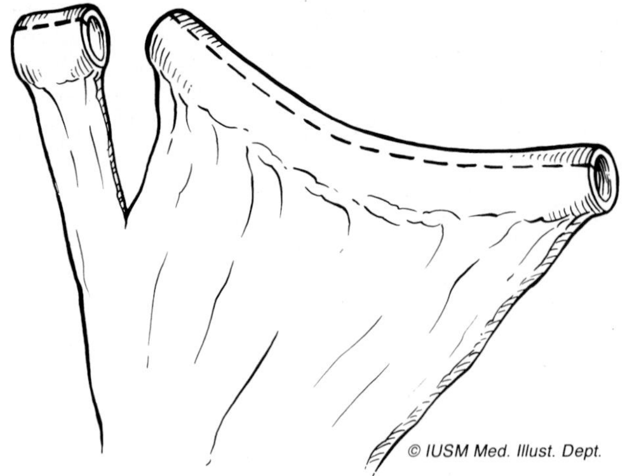


FIGURE 121.6 A 2.5- to 3-cm segment of ileum is harvested, distal to the segment of intestine to be used for augmentation (if indicated).

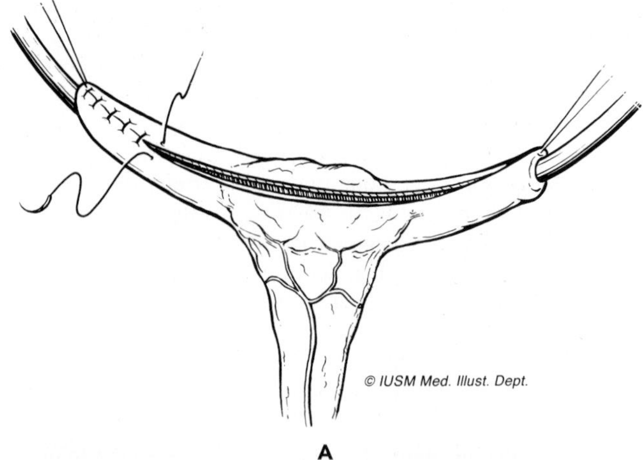


A

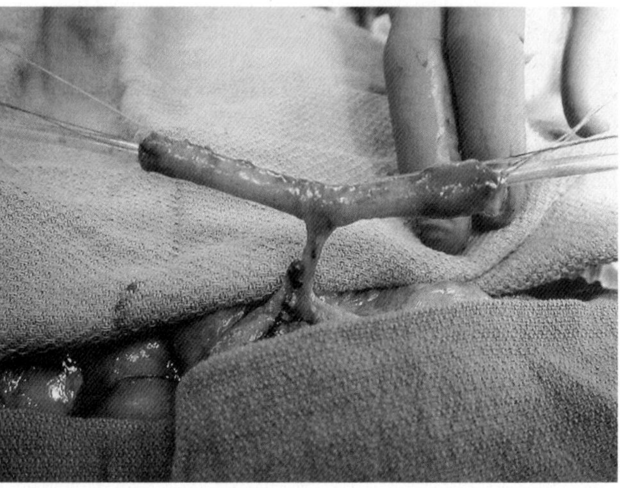

B

FIGURE 121.8 A: The channel is closed with two layers of absorbable sutures. The stomal end is either closed with interrupted sutures or not closed to allow adequate spatulation at the skin stoma. B: Operative photo of completed Monti channel.

preservation of the appendix for the appendicocecostomy stoma and the need for alternatives for a bladder channel. Because many of the children will also undergo bladder augmentation at the time of reconstruction, the Monti–Yang channel can be easily constructed from a segment of the bowel harvested for augmentation.

A 2.5- to 3-cm segment of intestine is harvested with a well-vascularized segment of mesentery (Fig. 121.6). If ileal augmentation is planned, the Monti–Yang segment can be easily harvested from the distal end of the segment with a shared mesentery. The ileal segment is opened on the antimesenteric side (Fig. 121.7). It can be opened slightly off the midline to provide a longer segment for implanting into the bladder. The opened segment is then retubularized transversely in two layers over a 14Fr catheter. The bowel mucosa is approximated with running 5-0 or 6-0 absorbable sutures and the muscular layer is closed with running or interrupted 4-0 absorbable sutures (Fig. 121.8). The stomal end is not closed initially, providing wide spatulation of the antimesenteric side of the tube for later stomal anastomosis. The technique of implanting the tube into the bladder and creating a stoma is identical to that for appendicovesicostomy (Fig. 121.9). The Monti–Yang tube can be created out of any segment of intestine with good results. If there is inadequate bladder volume for creation of a submucosal tunnel,

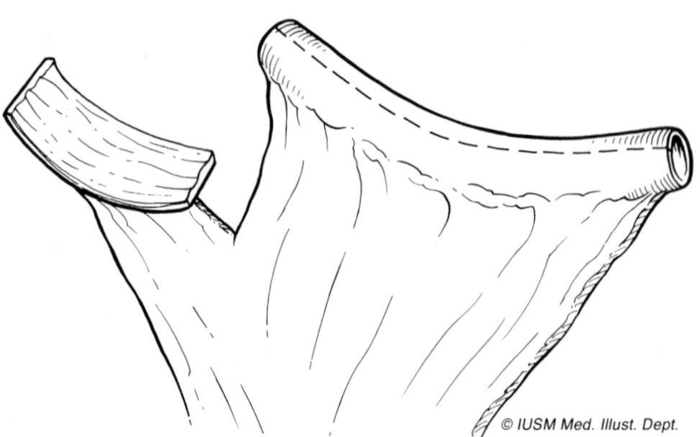


FIGURE 121.7 The Monti segment is detubularized on the antimesenteric side. This incision can be between the 9 and 12 o'clock positions depending on the desired length of intravesical tunnel.

the tube can be implanted into a segment of bowel using an extravesical technique. Care must be taken to secure the entire tunnel length to the posterior fascial wall to prevent breakdown of the thin muscular backing during repetitive bladder filling, with the potential for late incontinence. A 12Fr catheter is left across the channel for 3 weeks before initiating intermittent catheterization. The Monti channel can also be used for the MACE channel, with two channels created side by side (Fig. 121.10).

When the Monti channel does not provide adequate length for the extravesical section to reach the abdominal stomal site without tension, then two Monti tubes can be reconfigured and connected (the "double Monti"). This can provide a longer limb to reach the skin stoma but also introduces additional postoperative complications of diverticulum, angulation, and perforation at the anastomosis of the two channels (10). To avoid this complication, Casale (11) described a long ileovesicostomy technique using a single piece of bowel to create a channel 10 to 14 cm in length. This technique involves a 3.5- to 4-cm segment of bowel that is isolated on its mesentery and divided into two equal segments for approximately 80% of the bowel circumference, leaving the two segments attached on the

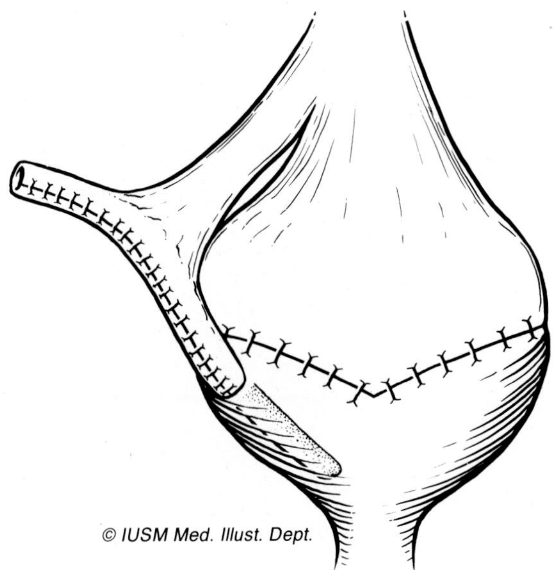


FIGURE 121.9 The Monti channel can be brought out either to a lower-abdominal stoma or to the umbilicus. The mesentery is mobilized from the pedicle of the bladder augmentation to provide a tension-free skin anastomosis.

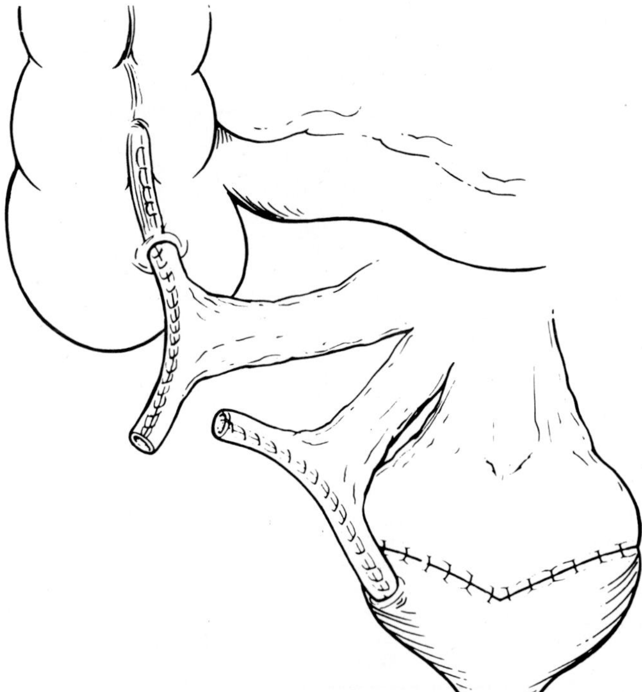

FIGURE 121.10 The "dual Monti," utilizing a Monti channel for both the Malone antegrade continence enema and Mitrofanoff channels.

mesenteric side. The two loops of intestine are opened close to the mesentery on opposite sides, allowing the bowel to unfold in opposite directions, creating a long flat plate of intestine that can be retubularized after trimming the redundant lateral edges. Late follow-up has demonstrated comparable results between the Monti and Casale-Monti, with the exception of slightly higher open revision rates for the longer spiral Monti placed

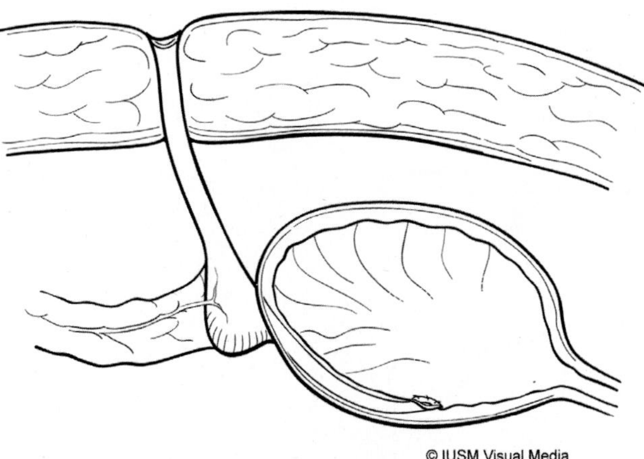


FIGURE 121.11 Diverticula in channel directly outside the bladder hiatus. This complication occurs from repetitive difficult catheterization due to a long and tortuous extravesical portion of the Mitrofanoff channel.

in the umbilicus, presumably due to extravesical channel elongation and tortuosity over time and development of a perihiatal diverticulum (Fig. 121.11) (12).

## Continent Vesicostomy

Small subsets of patients require creation of only a catheterizable bladder channel without bladder augmentation or other intra-abdominal procedures. These patients are good candidates for extraperitoneal continent vesicostomy. The largest reported experience is using the procedure described by Cain and Rink (13) utilizing an intravesical submucosal-mucosal–lined tunnel to create the continence mechanism. This procedure has been successfully used with a variety of underlying bladder pathologies.

The bladder is opened to allow creation of either a midline or lateral full-thickness bladder flap (Fig. 121.12A). Incisions are extended intravesically, leaving a 2.5-cm plate of mucosa. The mucosa is sharply dissected off the underlying detrusor muscle laterally and medially to allow tension-free mucosal closure (Fig. 121.12B). The intra- and extravesical mucosal tube is created over a 14Fr catheter with running 6-0 absorbable suture (Fig. 121.12C). The detrusor muscle of the extravesical portion of the tube is then closed with 4-0 absorbable sutures (Fig. 121.12D). The continence mechanism is then created by closing the lateral edges of the bladder mucosa over the mucosal tube using running 5-0 absorbable suture (Fig. 121.12E). The stoma can be created in either the lower abdomen or umbilicus. An indwelling 12Fr catheter is left in place for 3 weeks.

## Ureterovesicostomy

The ureter can be used as a catheterizable channel but has been less popular than bowel channels due to the additional upper urinary tract reconstruction required and the higher risk of skin stenosis and stomal leakage (14,15). When there is a unilateral nonfunctioning kidney with a nonrefluxing distal

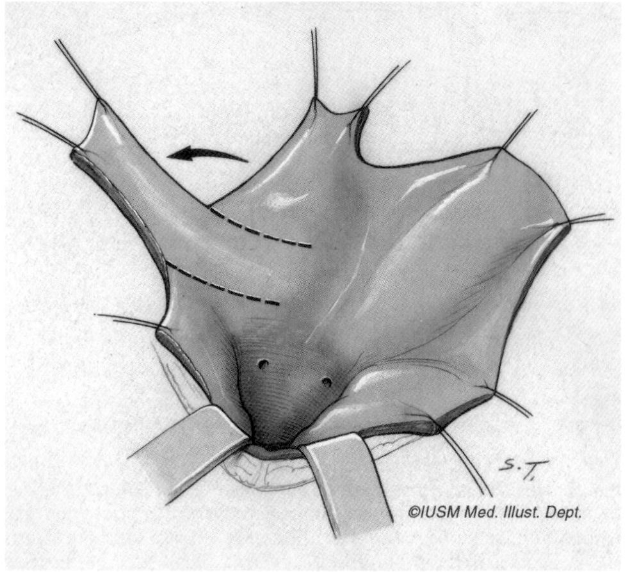


A

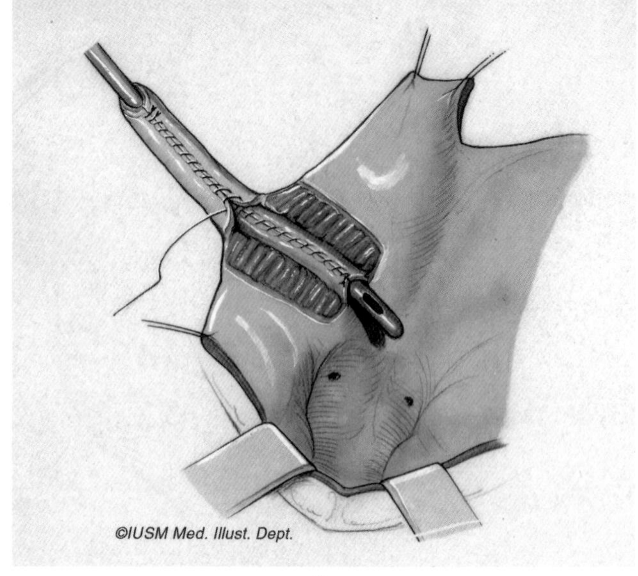


D

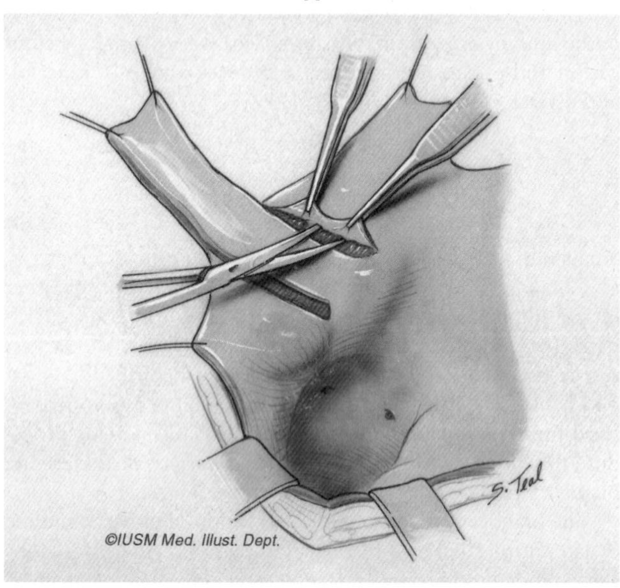


B

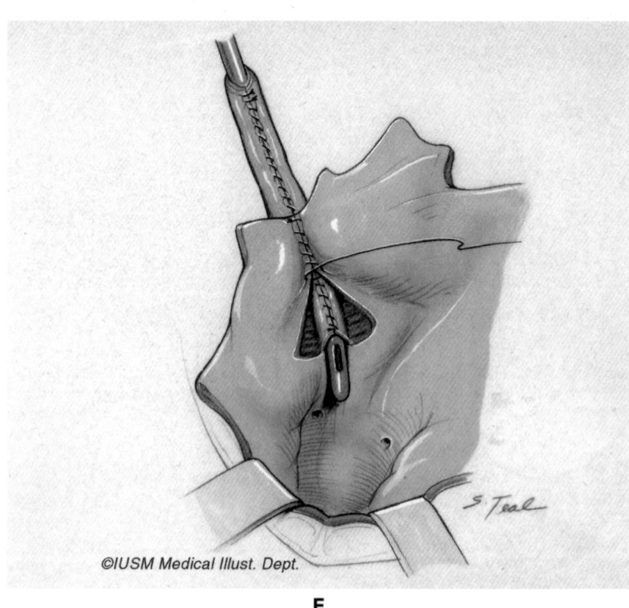


E

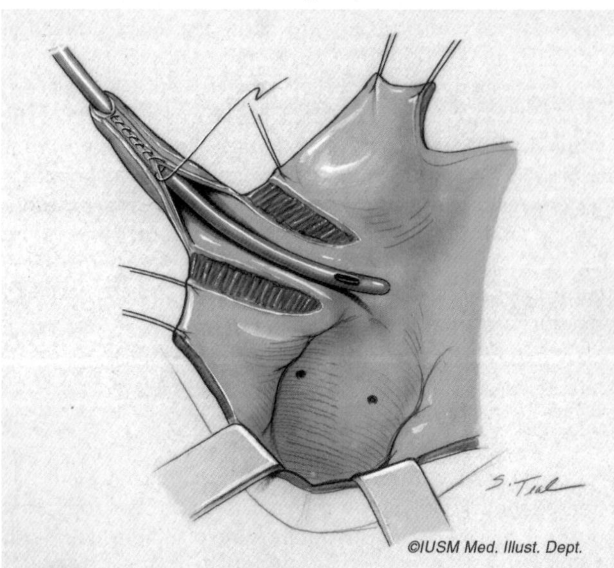


C

FIGURE 121.12 **A:** A 2.5-cm full-thickness bladder tube is harvested with adequate length to reach an abdominal stomal site. **B:** Intravesical mucosal incisions are made, leaving a 2.5-cm mucosal strip. The mucosal incisions should extend approximately 2.5 cm into the bladder. The lateral mucosal edges are mobilized sharply. **C:** The mucosal channel is closed using running 6-0 suture. **D:** The detrusor muscle of the extravesical portion of the bladder tube is closed with running 4-0 suture. **E:** The lateral mucosal edges are closed over the intravesical mucosal tube to create the continence mechanism.

ureter, a ureteral channel should be considered, but this unfortunate situation should be avoidable in the present era of careful management of these patients from early in life. Several reports have also documented successful distal ureteral reimplantation at the time of the ureterovesicostomy. Obviously, careful mobilization of the ureter to prevent proximal and distal stenosis is an important technical factor.

# OUTCOMES

## Complications

Potential complications of the Mitrofanoff channel are listed in Table 121.1. The most common complication is stomal stenosis, occurring in 10% to 20% of channels in most series. The continent vesicostomy has a much higher rate of stenosis than either appendix or Monti–Yang channels. A short period of passive catheter dilation for 7 to 10 days will avoid the need for surgical intervention in some patients. If necessary, revision of the stoma with a well-vascularized flap of skin is usually successful to manage significant stenosis.

Difficulty catheterizing the channel can occur secondary to angulation, perforation/false passage, or stenosis of the channel. Initially this should be treated conservatively with endoscopic placement of an indwelling catheter for 1 to 2 weeks. On occasion reoperation will be necessary, and the patient and surgeon should be prepared to replace the entire tube if required.

Complications will usually occur within the first year but may occur many years after construction of a Mitrofanoff channel, and long-term follow-up with these patients is mandatory, especially when the Mitrofanoff channel is the sole means to empty the bladder (2,16).

**TABLE 121.1**

COMPLICATIONS OF MITROFANOFF CHANNEL

| |
|---|
| Stomal stenosis |
| Stomal incontinence |
| Difficulty catheterizing channel |
| Intra-abdominal adhesions |
| Shunt infection |
| Abdominal abscess |
| Painful catheterization |
| Prolapsed stomal mucosa |
| Peristomal hernia |
| Wound dehiscence/infection |

## Results

Most large series have reported long-term success in up to 96% to 98% of Mitrofanoff channels (2,17). Because appendicovesicostomy has been used since the initial description of the procedure, there are better long-term data for this specific procedure, which has been shown to be durable over long periods of intermittent catheterization. We recently reported our results using the Monti–Yang channel in 199 consecutive patients, achieving 97% success with an average of 3 years of follow-up, which was identical to our experience with appendicovesicostomy (9). Because of the short continence zone required with the mucosal flap-valve technique for continent vesicostomy, there has been nearly 100% success with this procedure with respect to stomal continence.

Failure to obtain continence can be due to an inadequate submucosal tunnel, a fistula into the Mitrofanoff tube, breakdown of the muscular backing to the submucosal tunnel (especially when implanted into a bowel segment), or poor bladder compliance/high intravesical pressure. In many instances, the underlying problem will be the bladder, and any patient with a failed Mitrofanoff should undergo repeat urodynamic studies of the bladder and a trial of anticholinergics. We have had good success with reimplanting a previously constructed channel at the time of secondary bladder augmentation when the initial Mitrofanoff channel has failed because of changing bladder dynamics.

## *References*

1. Mitrofanoff P. Cystostomie continent trans-appendiculaire dans le traitement des vessies neurologiques. *Chir Pediatr* 1980;21:297.
2. Harris CF, Cooper CS, Hutcheson JC, et al. Appendicovesicostomy: the Mitrofanoff procedure—a 15-year perspective. *J Urol* 2000;163:1922–1926.
3. Liard A, Seguier-Lipszyc E, Mathiot A, et al. The Mitrofanoff procedure: 20 years later. *J Urol* 2001;165:2394–2398.
4. Cromie WJ, Barada JH, Weingarten JL. Cecal tubularization: lengthening technique for creation of catheterizable conduit. *Urology* 1991;37:41–42.
5. Herndon CDA, Cain MP, Casale AJ, et al. The colon-flap/extension Malone antegrade colonic enema: an alternative to the Monti-MACE. *J Urol* 2005;174(1):299–302.
6. Sheldon CA, Minevich E, Wacksman J. Modified technique of antegrade continence enema using a stapling device. *J Urol* 2000;163:589–591.
7. Cain MP, Casale AJ, Rink RC. Initial experience using a catheterizable ileovesicostomy (Monti procedure) in children. *Urology* 1998;52:870.
8. Monti PR, Lara RC, Dutra MA, et al. New techniques for construction of efferent conduits based on the Mitrofanoff principle. *Urology* 1997;49:112–115.
9. Dussinger AM, Cain MP, Casale AJ, et al. Appendico-vesicostomy versus Monti ileovesicostomy for Mitrofanoff channel: the Indiana experience in over 300 patients. *J Urol* 2006;175:250–251.
10. Narayanaswamy B, Wilcox DT, Cuckow PM, et al. The Yang-Monti ileovesicostomy: a problematic channel? *Br J Urol* 2001;87:861–865.
11. Casale AJ. A long continent ileovesicostomy using a single piece of bowel. *J Urol* 1999;162:1743–1745.
12. Leslie JA, Cain MP, Kaefer M, et al. A comparison of the Monti and Casale (spiral Monti) procedures. *J Urol* 2007;178:1623–1627.
13. Cain MP, Rink RC, Yerkes EB, et al. Long-term follow up and outcome of continent catheterizable vesicostomy using the Rink modification. *J Urol* 2002;168:2583–2585.
14. Castellan MA, Gosalbez R, Labbie A, et al. Outcomes of continent catheterizable stomas for urinary and fecal incontinence: comparison among different tissue options. *BJU Int* 2005;95:1053–1057.
15. Mor Y, Kajbafzadeh AM, German K, et al. The role of ureter in the creation of Mitrofanoff channels in children. *J Urol* 1997;157:635–637.
16. Thomas JC, Dietrich MS, Trusler L, et al. Continent catheterizable channels and the timing of their complications. *J Urol* 2006;176:1816–1820.
17. Cain MP, Casale AJ, King SK, et al. Appendicovesicostomy and newer alternatives for the Mitrofanoff procedure: results in the last 100 patients at Riley Childrens's Hospital. *J Urol* 1999;162:749.

# SECTION IX ■ LAPARASCOPIC

LEONARD G. GOMELLA

# CHAPTER 122 ■ BASIC PRINCIPLES OF LAPAROSCOPY: TRANSPERITONEAL, EXTRAPERITONEAL, AND HAND-ASSISTED TECHNIQUES

GAURAV BANDI AND LEONARD G. GOMELLA

Laparoscopic surgery is being increasingly utilized for management of urologic conditions that were traditionally managed by open surgery (1–3). Chapters 124 to 136 include laparoscopic procedures commonly performed by urologists in the United States. This chapter provides the foundation for any laparoscopic procedure and describes techniques to enter the intra- or extraperitoneal space, insufflate, place viewing and access ports (including hand-assist devices), and exit the abdomen. This chapter outlines the basic laparoscopic techniques and principles utilized for the other laparoscopic procedures described in this edition, including robotically assisted procedures.

## INDICATIONS FOR SURGERY

Laparoscopy provides a minimally invasive approach to many standard open surgical procedures. Benefits to laparoscopic intervention may include reduced analgesia, shorter hospital stay, faster return to normal activity, and enhanced cosmesis.

**Absolute contraindications** to transperitoneal laparoscopy include inability to tolerate general anesthesia or pneumoperitoneum (i.e., severe cardiac or pulmonary disease), intestinal obstruction and/or substantial distention, massive hemoperitoneum or hemoretroperitoneum, generalized peritonitis, abdominal wall infection, uncorrectable coagulopathy, or advanced intra-abdominal malignancy. **Relative contraindications** include morbid obesity, prior abdominal or pelvic surgery, large abdominal wall hernias, marked organomegaly, and pregnancy. This list, in general, also applies to extraperitoneal and hand-assisted laparoscopic procedures. Contraindications to extraperitoneal laparoscopy also include prior surgery or inflammation in the extraperitoneal space.

## ALTERNATIVE THERAPY

All patients undergoing laparoscopic surgery should be informed of the alternate approaches available (including open surgery and nonsurgical approaches) and the team's experience with the specific procedure. The patient must also be informed that the procedure may be terminated or converted to a hand-assisted or an open approach due to failure to progress or management of complications at any point during the intraoperative or postoperative course. Patients often view laparoscopic surgery so favorably that they may expect to have no discomfort and immediately return to full activities. The patient must understand that interventional laparoscopy is still a surgical procedure with some of the inconveniences and complications associated with any operation. The patient needs to be aware of both complications unique to laparoscopy (e.g., fatal gas embolism, problems owing to hypercarbia, postoperative crepitus, pneumothorax, electrosurgical bowel injury) and procedure-specific complications (e.g., adjacent organ injury).

Although transperitoneal laparoscopy can be performed for the majority of urologic procedures, significant complications, such as bowel or vascular injuries, can occur when utilizing the transperitoneal approach. Extraperitoneal laparoscopy decreases the risk of visceral and vascular injury and may decrease the incidence of shoulder-tip pain, trocar site hernias, postoperative ileus, and adhesions, thereby resulting in slightly more rapid postoperative recovery. It is also associated with decreased alteration in cardiac and pulmonary function and may be especially beneficial in patients with previous transperitoneal surgery. Limitations to the extraperitoneal approach include limited working space, unique anatomic orientation, and a steeper learning curve. Excessive fat in the extraperitoneal space may obscure the anatomy, especially in the retroperitoneum. The limited retroperitoneal working area requires accurate placement of secondary ports and may make entrapment of large masses and intracorporeal suturing difficult. Although there is some evidence to suggest that there may be more $CO_2$ absorption in the extraperitoneal space, in general it can be managed by aggressive ventilation.

Hand-assisted laparoscopy was devised in part to overcome the learning curve of conventional laparoscopy. Hand-assisted laparoscopy has now been applied to many surgical scenarios and has been reported to provide many of the same advantages as "pure" laparoscopy in terms of patient recovery and morbidity (4,5). The hand-assisted approach can offer some additional benefits over pure laparoscopic techniques: it allows tactile feedback, it may facilitate dissection in challenging cases, it may reduce operative times, the hand is a more facile retractor and dissector than standard rigid instruments, and specimens can be easily removed intact. Hand-assisted laparoscopy bridges the gap between standard open skills and advanced laparoscopic skills and may be important for training purposes as the ability to perform rapid hand exchanges is possible. Drawbacks of hand-assisted laparoscopy include the creation of a more noticeable (albeit small) incision, the potential for a slower recovery than pure laparoscopy, and the increased risk of wound-related complications.

# SURGICAL TECHNIQUE

## Patient Preparation

Careful patient selection and identification of possible relative and absolute contraindications are vital to a successful outcome of any laparoscopic procedure. A meticulous past history and physical examination are the initial steps in patient evaluation for possible laparoscopic surgery following the same criteria established for any other significant open surgical procedure. Patients with severe chronic obstructive pulmonary disease and significant cardiac histories should undergo further evaluation. Serum type and screen are sufficient for diagnostic laparoscopy or procedures associated with a low chance of major hemorrhage (e.g., varicocelectomy). More extensive laparoscopic procedures (e.g., nephrectomy, prostatectomy) may require type and hold or type and ready depending on the surgeon's experience. For extraperitoneal laparoscopic surgery, no bowel preparation is needed. For transperitoneal laparoscopic procedures, a light mechanical bowel preparation can be given in an effort to decompress the bowel. Usually, a clear liquid diet and a Dulcolax suppository or half a bottle of magnesium citrate the day before the procedure is sufficient. A full mechanical and antibiotic bowel preparation should be considered if one anticipates encountering dense intra-abdominal adhesions or if the surgery involves entering the bowel.

The role of each operating room personnel (including surgeon, assistants, nurses, anesthesiologist, and other support staff) should be clearly defined and established for each laparoscopic case. Detailed information on laparoscopic instrumentation is available elsewhere, and specific instrumentation may be needed for the growing list of specialized procedures (6). The positioning of the monitors depends on the type of the procedure to be performed. For pelvic surgery, a single monitor at the foot is usually sufficient; for procedures such as nephrectomy and adrenalectomy, monitors on either side of the bed are recommended. All equipment must be fully functional and in operating condition before any laparoscopic procedure is started. A separate tray with open laparotomy instruments must be ready for immediate use in the event of complications or problems necessitating conversion to open surgery.

Positioning of the patient depends primarily on the laparoscopic procedure to be performed. Careful attention to detail during patient positioning, including adequate padding of bony prominences and securing the patient to the table, is critical for table repositioning during the procedure and avoiding neuromuscular complications. Advances in padding and table-mounted accessories have enabled the use of newer devices (e.g., gel pad, lateral support, bean bag), which, when used appropriately, can markedly decrease the incidence of iatrogenic neuromuscular injuries.

General endotracheal anesthesia is essential for interventional laparoscopy. Nitrous oxide anesthesia is discouraged as it may cause bowel distention. An orogastric tube and a Foley catheter should be placed prior to any transperitoneal laparoscopic surgery to decompress the bowel and bladder, respectively, thereby decreasing the chance of injury during insufflation and initial trocar placement and facilitating visualization during surgery. Deep venous thrombosis prophylaxis can be achieved by utilizing pneumatic compression stockings or by administration of subcutaneous heparin preoperatively. The field should always be prepared widely should there be need to convert to an open procedure. In some procedures it is of advantage to extend the preparation to the knees and to drape the external genitalia into the surgical field to ensure access to the urethra for instrumentation (e.g., prostatectomy, cystectomy).

## Transperitoneal Access: Closed Technique

Initial pneumoperitoneum can be established using a Veress needle for most transperitoneal laparoscopic procedures and for many hand-assisted procedures. The Veress needle has a spring-loaded, blunt-tipped obturator to help prevent injury. The site of Veress needle entry depends on the position of the patient and the type of the procedure performed. With the patient in supine position, the patient is placed in the 10- to 20-degree Trendelenburg position and the entry into the abdominal cavity can be performed at the inferior or superior margin of the umbilicus. The umbilicus is the central point of the peritoneal cavity, making it an ideal observation site. Here, the abdominal wall is only two layers thick (fascia and peritoneum) and easy to traverse percutaneously (Fig. 122.1). If the patient is in a lateral decubitus position, then the Veress needle is passed two fingerbreadths medial and two fingerbreadths superior to the anterior superior iliac spine. Other potential insertion sites when the patient is either supine or in a lateral decubitus position are the Palmer point (i.e., subcostal in the midclavicular line on the right side) and the corresponding site on the left side.

Placement of the Veress needle into the abdominal cavity is a blind procedure with potential for injury to the underlying structures. If the patient has undergone prior surgery, open entry using the Hasson technique is considered the safest method (see following). A small incision is made at the Veress needle entry site. The abdominal wall can be elevated by grasping the periumbilical area with a sponge or with towel clamps. These maneuvers may raise the umbilicus up and away from the intestines but, more importantly, stabilize the abdominal wall. The needle is grasped like a dart along the shaft to limit its excursion into the abdominal cavity, with the angle of entry directed slightly caudad into the pelvis. Two distinct "pops" are felt as the needle passes through the fascia and peritoneum. It is important to traverse the layers of the abdominal wall in a near-perpendicular fashion to avoid "bouncing off" the peritoneum and remaining in the preperitoneal space. The umbilicus lies directly over the right iliac vessels, just below the aortic bifurcation at L4-L5 (Fig. 122.1). Deep penetration with the needle directly posteriorly could produce vascular injury.

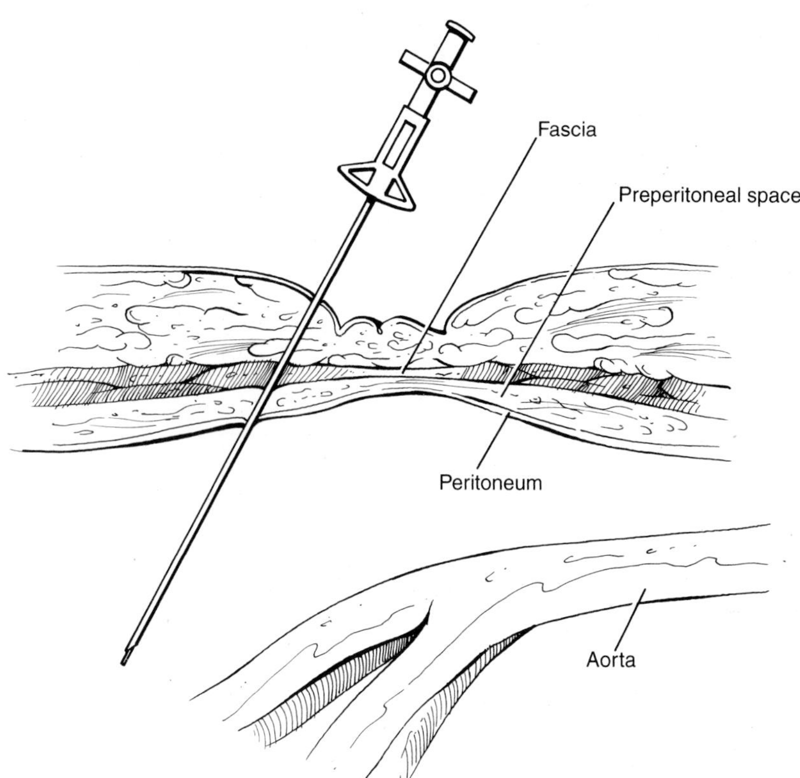


**FIGURE 122.1** The Veress needle is most often placed at the inferior or superior aspect of the umbilicus. The needle is directed into the hollow of the pelvis, below the bifurcation of the great vessels.

Once the needle is in the peritoneal cavity, confirmatory tests are performed prior to insufflation, although none is foolproof. These include:

1. *Color test*: Aspiration of colored (red, yellow, green, brown) or malodorous fluid suggests improper placement.
2. *Drop test*: Apply a drop of saline inside the hub of the needle and lift the abdominal wall. If in proper position, the drop will enter the abdomen due to the negative intraperitoneal pressure.
3. *Advancement test*: If the needle has truly just entered the peritoneal cavity, then the surgeon ought to be able to advance the needle 1 cm deeper without the tip meeting any resistance.
4. *Modified Palmer test*: Inject 10 mL of saline into the needle and attempt to aspirate. Inability to aspirate suggests the fluid has dispersed into the abdomen and the needle is in correct position.
5. *Initial pressure reading <8 mm Hg*. The insufflator is turned on with no flow to obtain a pressure reading.
6. *A decrease in pressure with elevation of the abdominal wall.*

If perforation of a viscus occurs, the needle should be removed and discarded. A new needle may then be inserted at another location or the surgeon may choose to obtain open access using the Hasson technique (see detailed in a later section). Once insufflation has been completed and the primary trocar has been introduced, the injury can be examined with the laparoscope and a decision made as to the appropriate management. If blood appears, the Veress needle should be withdrawn slightly. Its positioning should be retested, the pneumoperitoneum established, and the injury inspected for possible repair. Because of the small size of the Veress needle, the majority of these injuries do not require open operative intervention.

Once proper needle placement is verified, $CO_2$ insufflation should be started at a "low flow" (1 L/min) to maintain a pressure of <8 mm Hg. A high initial pressure with a low flow suggests improper needle placement. Once insufflation is underway, the abdomen should be observed to assure that a symmetrical pneumoperitoneum is developing. Monitor the insufflation by percussion over the liver, noting the characteristic dull echo tone that indicates proper insufflation. If the distention appears correct and 0.5 L has entered the abdomen, increase to "high flow" (usually >2 L/min). Initially, the abdomen is insufflated to 15 to 20 mm Hg to provide maximum distention and assist with atraumatic placement of the early trocars. An adult abdomen will typically require 3 to 6 L of $CO_2$ to create an adequate pneumoperitoneum, while children may require as little as 1 to 1.5 L. The working pressure should be decreased to 12 to 15 mm Hg after all trocars are placed to limit barotrauma.

If preperitoneal insufflation occurs, an attempt can be made to open the peritoneum with laparoscopic scissors and guide the tip of the trocar beneath it. $CO_2$ gas is then insufflated into the true peritoneal cavity, compressing the preperitoneal gas. Alternatively, evacuation of the preperitoneal space with a needle and syringe and reinsertion of the needle at the same or another site (i.e., superior umbilical position) may be attempted. Simply compressing the abdomen will disperse the $CO_2$ within the preperitoneal space. Open access (Hasson technique) can be used if these techniques are unsuccessful.

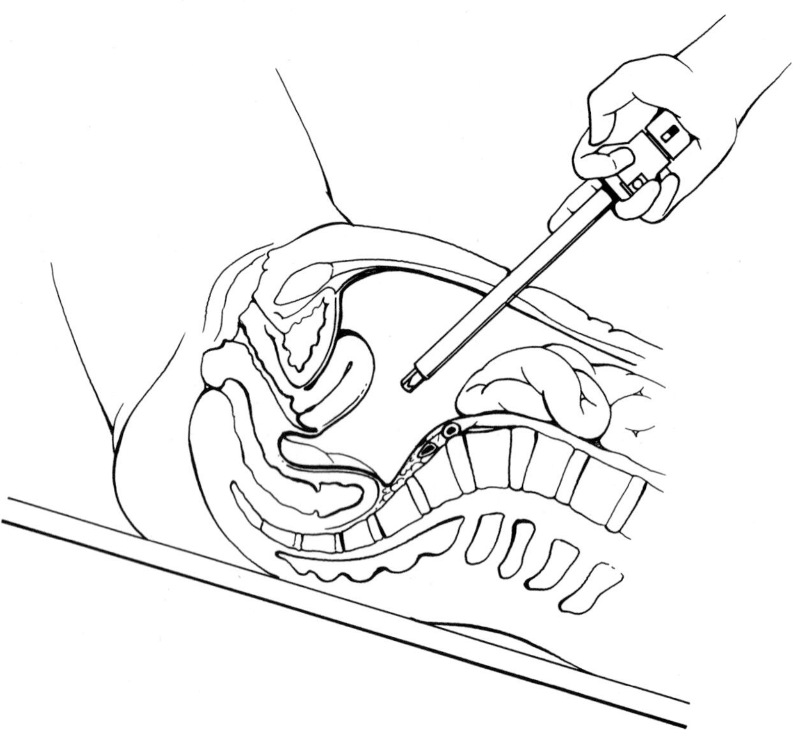

FIGURE 122.2 Primary shielded trocar is held with a finger along the shaft to limit the depth of entry of the trocar.

## Primary Trocar Placement

Once the pneumoperitoneum is established, the Veress needle is removed and the primary (laparoscope) trocar is inserted. Nondisposable and disposable trocars are available. The trocar designation refers to the size of the instrument that can be inserted into the trocar and not the overall diameter of the trocar. Sizes range from 3 to 20 mm in diameter and 5 to 15 cm in length. A 5- or 10-mm trocar is used in adults to allow passage of the laparoscope. The incision site used for the Veress needle should be enlarged and the subcutaneous tissue spread to the fascia using a hemostat. The skin incision should be sufficient to allow the trocar to pass without resistance. Press the end of the trocar on the skin to create an impression that serves as a guide for the size of the incision. Insert a trocar with firm, steady pressure and a gentle twisting movement. A finger can be held along the shaft to serve as a brake from pushing the trocar in too far (Fig. 122.2). Pressure should be applied using the arm and elbow only. Direct the trocar toward the site of interest within the peritoneum to avoid torque from the abdominal wall during the rest of the case (Fig. 122.2). The abdominal wall can be lifted and stabilized with hemostats (Fig. 122.3).

Noncutting dilating trocars and visualizing trocars have largely replaced the bladed/sharp-tipped and shielded metal trocars. After the skin incision is made, the laparoscope is placed into one of the visualizing trocars. Using pressure, a gentle twisting motion penetrates the layers of the abdominal wall, monitored under direct visualization of the tip through the laparoscope. The stopcock on the trocar can be left open during insertion, causing a rush of gas to escape ("whoosh test"), suggesting intraperitoneal placement. The $CO_2$ insufflator is connected to the stopcock on the trocar and insufflation is resumed. Working pressure of the pneumoperitoneum is 10 to 12 mm Hg, but an initial pressure of 15 to 20 mm Hg is needed until all the trocars are placed to ensure a "tense" pneumoperitoneum. White-balance the camera and explore the abdomen to assess for possible injury by the Veress needle or trocar. The chance of a serious injury at the time of the insertion of the primary trocar is much greater than with the Veress needle.

Lens fogging is caused by passage of the room-temperature laparoscope into the warm, humid abdomen. As the laparoscope warms during the procedure, fogging becomes less

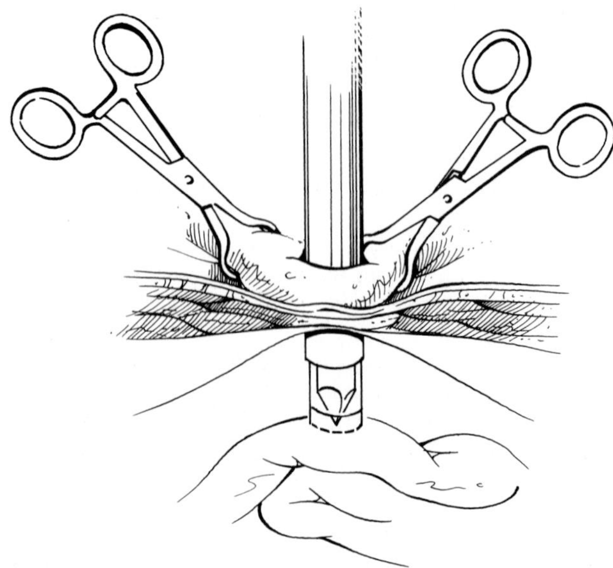

FIGURE 122.3 The abdominal wall can be stabilized with towel clips placed on either side of the umbilicus during primary trocar insertion.

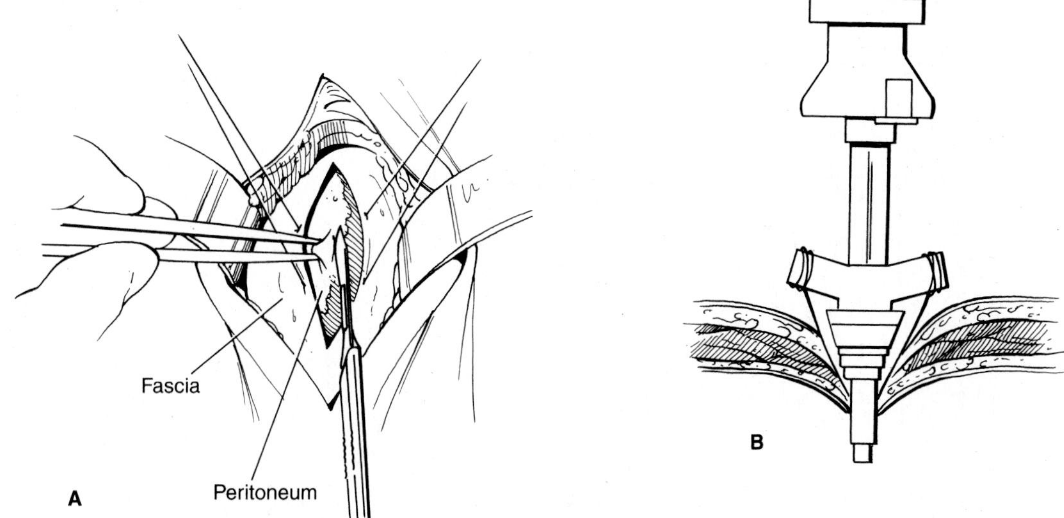


FIGURE 122.4 **A:** Open laparoscopy using the Hasson technique. The peritoneum is entered under direct vision. **B:** A blunt-tipped Hasson-style trocar is secured using the stay sutures.

problematic. Fogging can be reduced by heating the laparoscope before insertion in warmed sterile saline, applying antifogging solutions, and limiting the time the scope is removed from the abdomen. If fogging or debris covers the lens, it can be wiped on a clean bowel; touching fat or a blood-tinged surface may leave a film on the laparoscope. The contact time on the tissue should be limited as the laparoscope tip can become quite warm. Heated circuits connected to the insufflation tubing and newer laparoscope systems with imaging or heating chips at the distal end can also reduce this fogging.

## Transperitoneal Access: Open "Hasson" Technique

Many surgeons use this as the primary access for all patients. Open access (Hasson technique) is also useful both for correcting preperitoneal insufflation and in the patient at high risk for multiple adhesions. The advantage is that entry into the peritoneal cavity is under direct vision, minimizing the risk of injury; however, it requires a larger incision and increases the chances of port-site gas leakage during the procedure.

An infraumbilical incision is made and two stay sutures are placed through the fascia on either side. The fascia and peritoneum are directly visualized and opened (Fig. 122.4A). After visual and digital confirmation of entry into the peritoneal cavity, the stay sutures are repositioned and the Hasson cannula is advanced through the incision into the peritoneal cavity. The stay sutures are either attached to the cannula to hold it in position (Fig. 122.4B), if needed, or secured with hemostats for use during closure. Insufflation tubing is attached to the Hasson-style trocar, and immediately "high flow" can be selected.

## Secondary Trocar Placement

The number, size, and sites of the secondary trocars depend on the procedure to be performed, the patient's anatomy, and the surgeon's preference. The secondary trocars should be oriented toward the surgical site to provide tension-free maneuverability of the laparoscopic instruments. Their configuration should be planned so that neither the tips nor handles of the cannulas cross or come into close contact with one another, respectively ("crossing swords" and "rollover"), such that adequate working space is provided for all instruments to be used during a particular procedure. A general rule is to place secondary trocars in the midline or at least 8 cm from the midline in adults to avoid the rectus sheath (Fig. 122.5). If the rectus muscle is penetrated by a trocar, there is an increased risk of bleeding. Trocar placement for specific procedures is noted in the appropriate chapters that follow. At least one larger secondary trocar (10 or 10/11 mm) is usually placed to allow the passage of needles and larger instruments such as a linear endovascular stapler and clip appliers and to allow removal of specimens. Extended-length trocars are available if patients have particularly thick abdominal walls.

The placement of secondary or "working" trocars can be carefully monitored externally and internally to reduce the risk of injury. After full pneumoperitoneum is achieved, the selected site for the secondary trocar is gently pushed with the index finger while the site is observed through the laparoscope. The room is darkened and the light from the laparoscope is used to transilluminate the anterior abdominal wall to confirm that there are no underlying vessels or bowel. A skin incision of appropriate diameter to accommodate the trocar is made. It is useful to spread the subcutaneous tissue down to fascia with a clamp until the impression of the clamp tip is visible on the peritoneum. The trocar is introduced with the same technique described for the primary trocar except that the progress into the abdomen is followed on the monitor. Newer trocars have intrinsic stability threads that limit accidental removal. Suturing trocars to the skin using a heavy silk tether to prevent accidental removal during the case may be needed occasionally. The robotic surgical systems have specific trocars that should be used that mechanically connect to the robotic arm to allow control of the instrument more precisely.

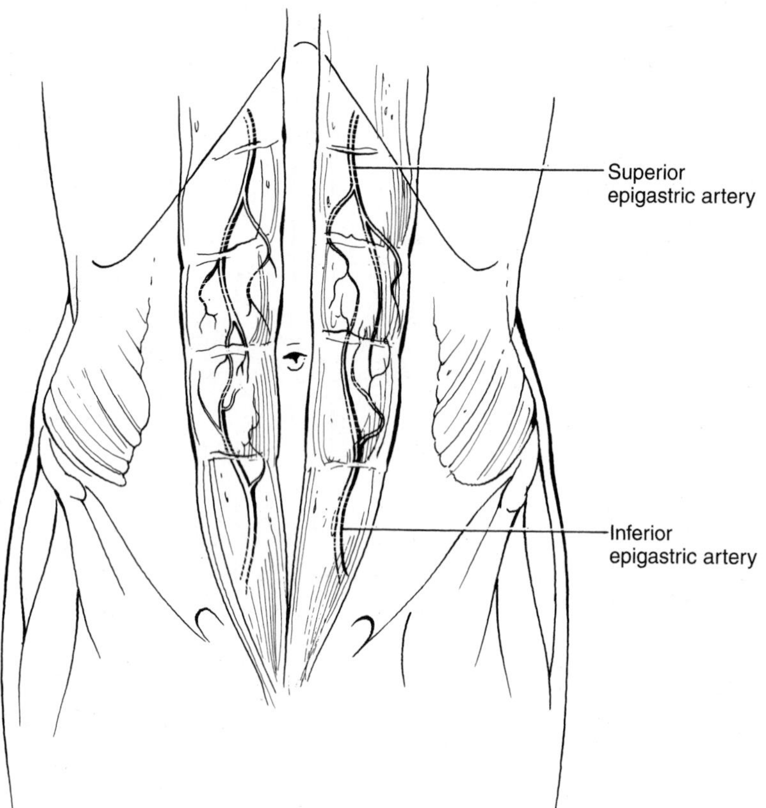


FIGURE 122.5 Secondary trocars should be placed in the midline (linea alba) or at least 8 cm from the midline to avoid injury to the rectus or the epigastric vessels.

## Trocar Removal

At the end of the procedure, the pneumoperitoneum should be lowered to 5 mm Hg or less to observe for any bleeding that may have been tamponaded by the working pressure. A brief survey of the abdomen should verify that there was no injury outside the operative field. Trocar sites should be examined prior to and after removal of the sheaths for bleeding or herniation. During trocar removal and fascial closure, bowel can become trapped along the trocar pathway. Trocar removal and suturing should always be observed laparoscopically; 10 mm and larger trocars require fascial suturing in adults.

Fascial closure can be accomplished by a variety of techniques. A 0 or 2-0 absorbable suture (i.e., Vicryl) on a small curved needle (i.e., CT-3 or UR-6) can be used to close the fascia externally. Fascial edges are grasped with either a toothed forcep or Scanlon clamps. Army-Navy retractors facilitate exposure. Laparoscopic closure needles (i.e., Endo Close, US Surgical, Norwalk, CT) are also available that are similar to a Stamey-style needle. A free 0 or 2-0 absorbable suture is engaged and passed percutaneously along the side of the trocar, through the fascia, and into the abdominal cavity using laparoscopic guidance. (Note: If stability threads were used to secure the trocar, they may interfere with passage of the closure device. Release the thread and slide it out of the incision while maintaining the trocar in the abdominal cavity.) The end of the suture is held with a laparoscopic grasper while the spring-loaded end is depressed to release the suture (Fig, 122.6). The closure device is then passed on the opposite side of the trocar, with the free end of the suture placed in the end of the needle using laparoscopic guidance. Once engaged, the device is withdrawn with the attached end of the suture. The trocar is removed and the ends of the suture are tied from the outside using laparoscopic control. Another

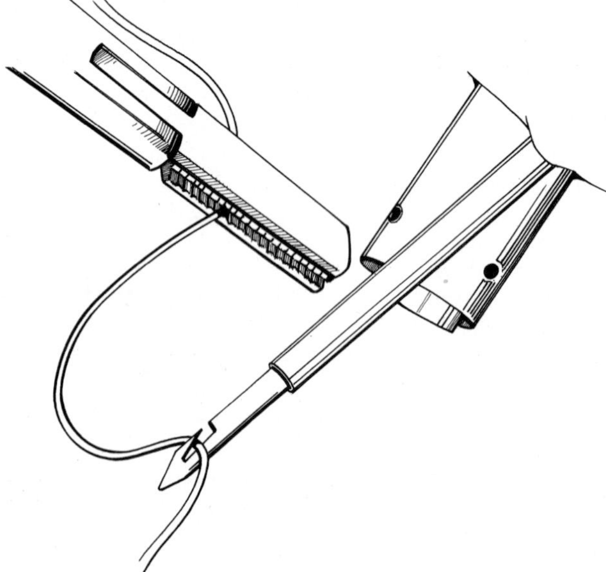

FIGURE 122.6 One technique to close the trocar site uses a device such as the Endo Close fascial closure needle. Here, the 2-0 absorbable suture has been passed into the abdomen alongside the trocar. The suture is grasped and the needle is withdrawn and passed on the opposite side of the trocar.

closure method utilizes the Carter-Thomason suture-passing device (Inlet Medical, Eden Prairie, MN). A suture guide (5 or 10 mm) device is placed into the trocar site and the suture-passing device is loaded with a 2-0 absorbable suture and the suture passed inside. The suture is released, the needle is placed in the opposite hole, and the suture is retrieved and removed through the opposite guide hole. The guide is removed and the suture is tied from outside the body.

After fascial sutures have been placed in all 10-mm port sites, each 5-mm port is removed under endoscopic control at 5 mm Hg pressure. Then each of the non-endoscope-bearing 10-mm ports can be removed under endoscopic control, and the fascial suture can be tied and the closure inspected endoscopically. The final 10-mm port is removed with the endoscope in place to assess for any bleeding along the tract. In this manner, each port is visually assessed for any bleeding at 5 mm Hg, thereby precluding the possibility of removing a port and missing an injured vessel. After removal of all ports, the $CO_2$ is allowed to pass out passively through the 5-mm port sites. This will reduce postoperative shoulder pain due to diaphragmatic irritation from the $CO_2$ gas. If pneumoscrotum is present, this should also be manually decompressed at this time.

The skin site should be thoroughly irrigated prior to closure. Herniation is most often associated with trocars larger than 10 mm, and when it does occur it is often due to a wound infection rather than improper fascial closure. Skin sites are closed with either subcutaneous sutures reinforced by Steri-Strips or with a skin adhesive.

## RETROPERITONEAL LAPAROSCOPY

This is often called "retroperitoneoscopy" and is used most often for renal and adrenal procedures. Following the usual preparation for transperitoneal laparoscopy, the patient is placed in a standard flank position. A 2-cm transverse skin incision is made just anterior to the tip of the 12th rib in the midaxillary line. An alternate site for the skin incision is the triangle of Petit approximately two fingerbreadths above the anterior superior iliac spine (Fig. 122.7). The posterior layer of the thoracolumbar fascia is identified and two stay sutures are positioned. The flank muscles are split to the anterior thoracolumbar fascia; two additional stay sutures are positioned. The anterior layer of thoracolumbar fascia is incised and the retroperitoneal space is entered. Index finger palpation of the belly of the psoas muscle posteriorly and the Gerota fascia-covered inferior pole of the kidney anteriorly confirms proper entry into the retroperitoneal space (Fig. 122.8). The index finger is employed to digitally create a space in this precise location and to sweep the peritoneum away anteriorly.

Simple extraperitoneal insufflation will cause the $CO_2$ gas to track along fascial planes and will not develop the extraperitoneal space. Balloon dissection of this space is the key to performing any procedure in this area. Gaur was the first to describe balloon distention of the extraperitoneal space using a simple device consisting of a surgical glove finger mounted on a red rubber catheter secured with a silk tie (7,8). Several commercially available trocar-mounted balloons are now available. An advantage of these devices is that the inflation

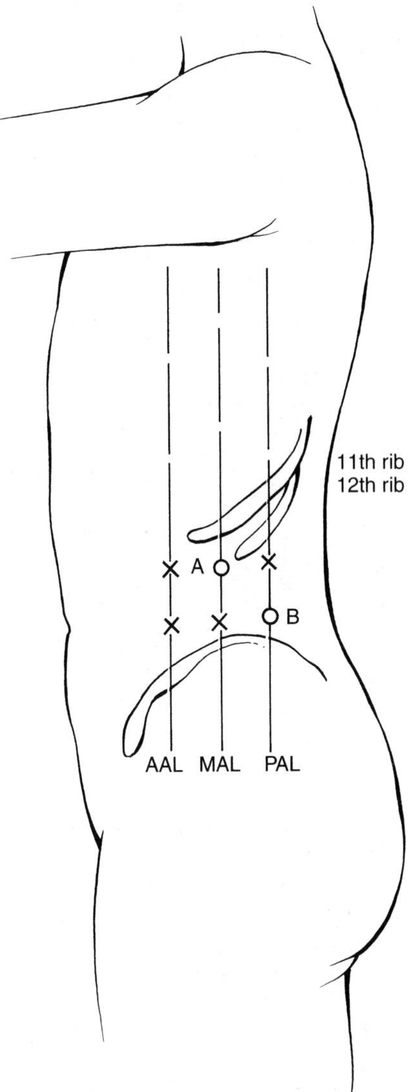


FIGURE 122.7 For retroperitoneal procedures, the initial trocar is placed (**A**) 1 to 2 cm from the tip of the 12th rib or (**B**) in the triangle of Petit, 1 to 2 cm above the anterior superior iliac spine. Additional ports can be placed as needed between the posterior and anterior axillary lines.

and distention of the space can be laparoscopically monitored through the clear balloon. The degree of balloon dilation varies with the patient's body habitus: 1 to 1.2 L of normal saline or room air is average in adults. The balloon is kept inflated for 5 minutes. After balloon removal a blunt-tipped trocar is inserted into the retroperitoneum. Visualization of the psoas muscle confirms proper balloon dilation of the retroperitoneum. The peritoneal envelope may be further mobilized with sweeping motions of the laparoscope. If difficulty is encountered mobilizing the peritoneum, an operating laparoscope can be used to pass a blunt-tipped dissector into the retroperitoneum.

The secondary ports can then be inserted under manual or laparoscopic control. For manual port placement, the laparoscope and cannula are removed and the index finger of the left hand (for a right-handed surgeon) is introduced into the retroperitoneum. An "S-shaped" retractor is inserted into the

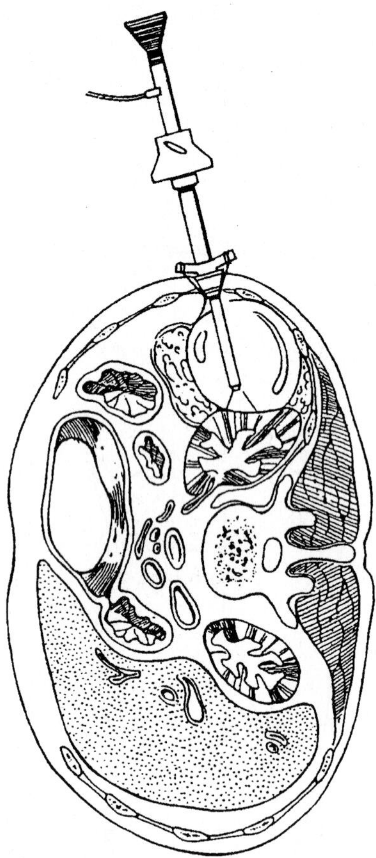

FIGURE 122.8 Technique of trocar-mounted balloon dissection of the retroperitoneal space.

retroperitoneum in such a manner that it lies immediately in front of the finger (i.e., the retractor is cradled by the finger). The fingertip mobilizes and retracts the peritoneum away from the abdominal wall; the S-retractor prevents inadvertent trocar injury to the surgeon's finger. With the surgeon's right hand, the secondary trocars are inserted under bimanual control, with the aim being to introduce the trocar onto the S-shaped retractor. Secondary trocars are placed based on the procedure to be performed. Typical placement for retroperitoneal procedures is demonstrated in Figure 122.7. No trocars are positioned behind the posterior axillary line.

## PELVIC EXTRAPERITONEAL LAPAROSCOPY

Bladder neck suspension, hernia repair, radical prostatectomy, and pelvic lymph node dissection can be approached through the pelvic extraperitoneal space. Patient preparation and positioning are identical to transperitoneal laparoscopy.

A vertical skin incision is made 1 to 2 cm below the inferior umbilical crease to avoid the confluence of the anterior and posterior rectus sheaths at the umbilicus. For procedures such as bladder neck suspension where lateral exposure at the level of the iliac vessels is not needed, the incision is made in the midline about one-third the distance below the umbilicus, between the umbilicus and pubis. The tissues are spread with a clamp to the anterior rectus sheath. Two absorbable 0 (i.e., Vicryl) stay sutures are placed in each side of the midline. Next, the anterior rectus sheath is incised along the linea alba between the sutures. The two bellies of the rectus muscle are separated by blunt dissection to expose the posterior sheath and a finger is passed behind the rectus and above the posterior sheath. Blunt finger dissection is carried out in a caudal direction until the area of the pubis symphysis is reached. At this distal location, the fascia transversalis is punctured with the fingertip, and gentle side-to-side digital dissection is performed in the prevesical space, posterior to the pubic bone. A balloon dilator lubricated with sterile jelly is inserted in this predeveloped space and distended to create an adequate working space. Balloon dilation effectively displaces the prevesical fat and reflects the peritoneum cephalad (Fig. 122.9). The balloon is left inflated for several minutes, deflated, and inflated a second time. The balloon is initially inflated in the midline and then reinflated on either side to further expand the working area. The balloon is removed and a 10-mm Hasson-style cannula or a Bluntport is placed. The extraperitoneal space is insufflated with $CO_2$ at 15 mm Hg to facilitate secondary trocar

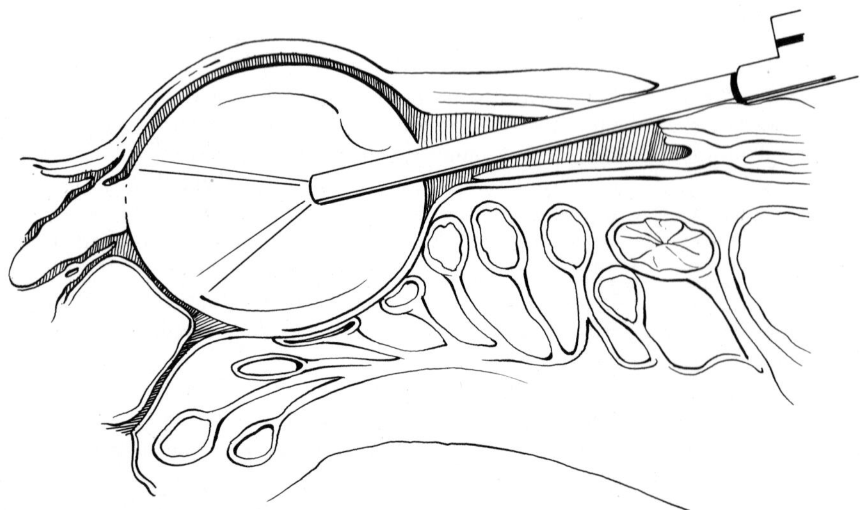

FIGURE 122.9 Technique of trocar-mounted balloon dissection of the preperitoneal space.

placement. Inspection of the preperitoneal space usually confirms adequate dissection of the prevesical space.

Additional trocars are placed under direct vision using a triangular, diamond-, fan-, or W-shaped configuration. Ensure that the lateral trocars do not traverse the peritoneal cavity and they are beyond the peritoneal reflection. Unlike with retroperitoneoscopy, the occurrence of a peritoneotomy during extraperitoneoscopy may interfere with the performance of subsequent extraperitoneal dissection, and conversion to a transperitoneal technique may be required. After the secondary trocars are placed, pneumoextraperitoneum is reduced to 10 to 12 mm Hg for the remainder of the procedure as prolonged high-pressure insufflation may cause tracking of the gas into the subcutaneous tissues.

## HAND-ASSISTED LAPAROSCOPY

Hand-assisted laparoscopy usually begins with the creation of an open incision that is approximately equal in length (in cm) to the surgeon's glove size, avoiding the use of a "blind" Veress needle access. The exact positioning of the incision depends upon the planned procedure, the body habitus of the patient, and surgeon preference (see subsequent chapters for details). The most common sites for hand-port placement include midline, subcostal, and lower quadrant incisions. Once the peritoneal cavity has been entered, the inside surface of the anterior abdominal wall is inspected for the presence of adhesions, which can be taken down sharply. After the hand-assist device is placed, a blunt cannula is passed through the hand-assist device and the abdomen can be insufflated at a high flow rate. Alternatively, a Veress or Hasson pneumoperitoneum may be initially established, and the hand-assist device can then be placed under endoscopic monitoring. After pneumoperitoneum is attained, the surgeon's nondominant hand is passed into the abdomen and additional secondary ports can be rapidly and safely placed using the intra-abdominal hand to palpate the tip of the trocar and hence guide its entry into the abdomen. Use of brown gloves and Ioban (3M, St. Paul, MN) "sticky drape" is recommended to decrease glare and to waterproof the surgeon's hand respectively. A sterile, water-soluble lubricant applied to the back of the surgeon's hand ensures smooth entry and exit through the hand-assist device.

Recent advances in hand-assist devices have made these instruments easier to place and more comfortable for the surgeon. The newer devices rely on compression against the peritoneal surface and body wall to remain in position. The GelPort (Applied Medical, Rancho Santa Margarita, CA) employs a sleeve that is passed into the abdominal cavity and pulled out through the incision. An inner ring holds the sleeve in place. The sleeve is then rolled on an outer ring that rests on the anterior abdominal wall. The GelPort covering is then attached to the outer ring. The entire two-piece system (Fig. 122.10A) is relatively easy to assemble once the incision has been established in the abdominal wall. The Lap Disc (Ethicon Inc., Cincinnati, OH) consists of three rings connected by a silicone membrane (Fig. 122.10B). The lower and middle rings bridge the abdominal wall, while the upper ring rotates on the middle, acting as an iris to seal the device around the surgeon's hand. The Omniport (Advanced Surgical Concepts, Wicklow, Ireland) is a balloon-like device that anchors itself as one piece across the abdominal wall (Fig. 122.10C). The inflated device also creates a seal between itself and the surgeon's wrist. The device has a smaller footprint (12 cm), but it must be deflated and reinflated each time a hand is exchanged, which loses the pneumoperitoneum.

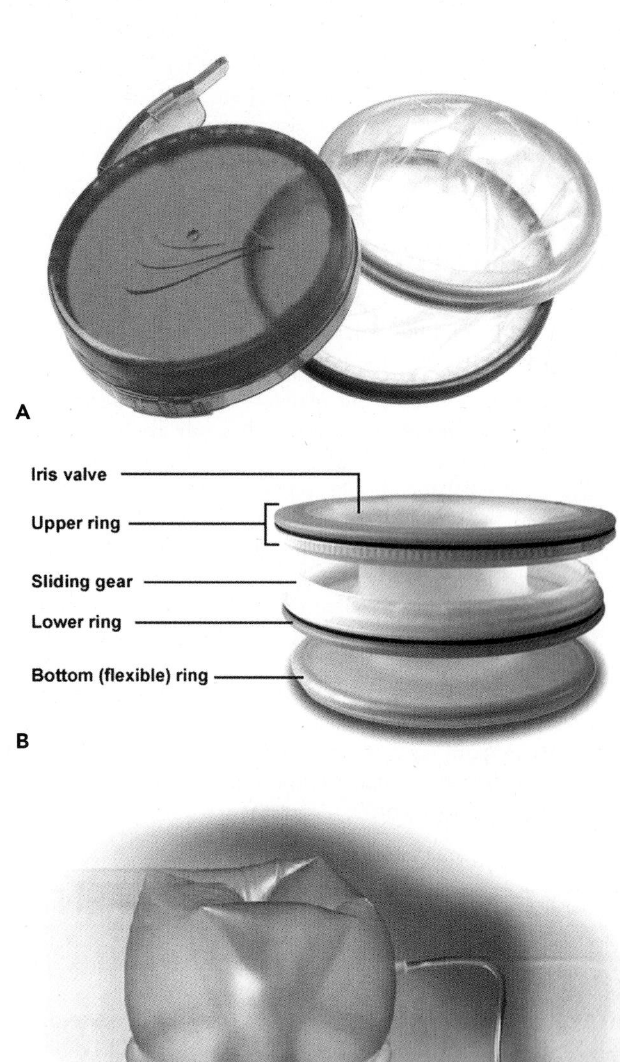


FIGURE 122.10 Devices for hand-assisted laparoscopy. **A:** The third-generation two-piece GelPort is relatively easy to assemble and provides an adequate seal around the surgeon's wrist while minimizing fatigue. **B:** The Lap Disc consists of three rings connected by a silicone membrane. The lower and middle rings bridge the abdominal wall, while the upper ring rotates on the middle, acting as an iris to seal the port around the surgeon's hand. **C:** The Omniport hand-assist device.

Prior to beginning the dissection, laparotomy pads can be preplaced into the abdominal cavity and used to blot any bleeding during the dissection. It is, of course, imperative to remove these pads prior to exiting the abdomen, and a helpful reminder system should be created with the rest of the operating room staff instead of relying solely upon sponge counts. Exiting the abdomen should be carried out with the secondary sites being closed under direct visualization through a port placed in the hand-assist device. The hand site is closed in the standard fashion.

# PEDIATRIC LAPAROSCOPY

Most principles of adult laparoscopy can be applied to the pediatric population, with the following exceptions:

1. In younger children, the bladder is an intra-abdominal structure, requiring more care with lower abdominal trocar placement.
2. The peritoneal membrane is loosely attached to the abdominal wall, making it potentially difficult to pass a Veress needle. Many authors advocate an open access technique for *all* children.
3. The total $CO_2$ to insufflate the abdomen is in general 1 to 3 L. Pressures should be kept lower than in adults (8 to 10 mm Hg).
4. The 5-mm trocars are commonly used in children and the sites *must* be sutured at the end of the case.
5. Many standard laparoscopic instruments will be either too large or long for pediatric procedures, thereby requiring specialized equipment.

# POSTOPERATIVE MANAGEMENT

Patients undergoing limited laparoscopic procedures like varicocelectomy and diagnostic laparoscopy may be discharged the same day. More extensive procedures may require a short hospital stay. Orogastric tubes are removed in the operating room but may be left in longer if bowel surgery was performed. The Foley catheter is removed either while the patient is still in the operating room (pneumoperitoneum <2 hours) or later in the day or the next morning (pneumoperitoneum >2 hours) unless a prostatectomy or cystectomy was performed. Antibiotics are continued over 24 hours and laboratory values are obtained in a standardized manner postoperatively. The patient ambulates within 12 hours of surgery and pneumatic compression stockings are utilized for deep venous thrombosis prophylaxis until the patient is fully ambulatory.

Depending on the procedure, clear liquids can be given after the effects of anesthesia have cleared. Diets can then be advanced as tolerated. For more extensive procedures (i.e., nephrectomy), it may be necessary to advance the diet more slowly. Parenteral analgesia is given as needed on the day of surgery and is usually replaced by oral pain medication on the first postoperative day. The requirement for postoperative analgesics is usually minimal; excessive pain should raise the suspicion of a complication. Patients should be advised that delayed postoperative bruising is on occasion encountered.

# OUTCOMES

Outcomes for contemporary laparoscopic interventions are reviewed for each specific procedure in the appropriate chapter.

## Complications

Although a Veress needle injury of a major blood vessel, bladder, or gastrointestinal tract can be managed expectantly, significant perforation with a trocar should be managed by immediate laparotomy and repair. The trocar and sheath should be left in place while opening the abdomen. In selected instances, laparoscopic repair may be appropriate but often requires significant advanced skills.

Vascular injury within the abdominal wall, especially the inferior epigastric vessels, can be managed by a through-and-through suture placed on a bolster using a Stamey-style needle or laparoscopic closure device; it is removed after 24 to 48 hours.

Anesthetic problems can be caused by the absorption of $CO_2$ or the physiologic effects of the pneumoperitoneum. Both the intra- and extraperitoneal surfaces can readily absorb $CO_2$ and this may cause hypercarbia. End-tidal $CO_2$ monitoring by the anesthesia team can often identify this problem before it becomes clinically significant. Increasing the minute ventilation, use of positive end-expiratory pressure, and reduction of intra-abdominal pressure to 10 mm Hg can usually keep the blood $CO_2$ levels in a safe range. High intra-abdominal pressure (prolonged periods above 15 to 20 mm Hg) can lead to barotrauma. The initial sign may be hypotension owing to decreased cardiac output secondary to an acute drop in venous return caused by compression of the vena cava. High pressures can also result in subcutaneous emphysema that can exacerbate hypercarbia, and on occasion cause pneumomediastinum and pneumothorax. The surgeon should desufflate the abdomen, and once the hemodynamic changes have been reversed, reinitiate the pneumoperitoneum at 10 mm Hg. Transient oliguria may occur in patients with increased intra-abdominal pressures, and the urge to aggressively hydrate the patient should be avoided.

Life-threatening gas embolism is rare and most often caused by direct insufflation of $CO_2$ gas into a vessel by the Veress needle. Subtle collection of $CO_2$ gas in the venous system through an open vessel can rarely occur. The first sign of intravascular insufflation is acute cardiovascular collapse. The diagnosis is usually made by the anesthesiologist based on an abrupt increase of end-tidal $CO_2$ accompanied by a sudden decline in oxygen saturation and then a marked decrease in end-tidal $CO_2$. Sometimes, a "millwheel" precordial murmur can be auscultated. The treatment is immediate cessation of insufflation and prompt desufflation of the peritoneal cavity. The patient is turned into a left lateral decubitus position and hyperventilated with 100% oxygen. Advancement of a central venous line into the right heart with subsequent attempts to aspirate gas may rarely be helpful.

In a recent review of 2,775 diverse urologic laparoscopic procedures, the current overall complication rate was 22.1% and the mortality rate was 0.07%. Transfusions were required in 4.7% of procedures, while open conversion was necessary in only 2.7% (9). The majority were identified in the postoperative period (79%) and were classified as minor (72%). Although each individual procedure had its own characteristic profile of complications, the four most commonly identified complications were vascular injuries (2%), postoperative bleeding requiring blood transfusion (1.8%), ileus that prolonged hospital stay >48 hours (1.6%), and wound infection (1%).

Laparoscopic surgery can be more technically demanding and time-consuming than open surgical intervention. Proper patient selection, formal training, the surgeon's experience, and working with others who are involved with laparoscopic surgery appear to be the best determinants for a successful outcome in urologic laparoscopy (10).

## *References*


1. Gomella LG, Albala DM. Laparoscopic urological surgery: 1994. *Br J Urol* 1994;74:267–273.
2. Hedican SP. Laparoscopy in urology. *Surg Clin North Am* 2000;80: 1465–1485.
3. Jackson CL. Urologic laparoscopy. *Surg Oncol Clin North Am* 2001;10: 571–578.
4. Nakada SY, Fadden P, Jarrard DF, et al. Hand-assisted laparoscopic radical nephrectomy: comparison to open radical nephrectomy. *Urology* 2001;58: 517–520.
5. Wolf JS Jr, Merion RM, Leichtman AB, et al. Randomized controlled trial of hand-assisted laparoscopic versus open surgical live donor nephrectomy. *Transplantation* 2001;72:284–290.
6. Eichel L, McDougall EM, Clayman RV. Basics of laparoscopic surgery. In *Campbell-Walsh Urology* Philadelphia: Saunders-Elsevier, 2007.
7. Gaur DD. Laparoscopic operative retroperitoneoscopy: use of a new device. *J Urol* 1992;148:1137–1139.
8. Gaur DD, Rathi SS, Ravandale AV, et al. A single-centre experience of retroperitoneoscopy using the balloon technique. *BJU Int* 2001;87: 602–606.
9. Permpongkosol S, Link RE, Su LM, et al. Complications of 2,775 urological laparoscopic procedures: 1993 to 2005. *J Urol* 2007;177:580–585.
10. See WA, Cooper CS, Fisher RJ. Predictors of laparoscopic complications after formal training in laparoscopic surgery. *JAMA* 1993;270:2689–2692.


# CHAPTER 123 ■ LAPAROSCOPIC PELVIC AND RETROPERITONEAL LYMPH NODE DISSECTION

HOWARD N. WINFIELD AND WILLIAM J. BADGER

The gold standard for accurate lymph node assessment in both prostate and testicular cancer continues to be lymphadenectomy. While imaging modalities such as computerized tomography (CT) and magnetic resonance imaging (MRI) may detect moderate- to large-volume metastatic disease, many microscopic or small lymph node metastases are not identified with the current limitations of CT and MRI sensitivity (1). With continued refinements in laparoscopic and robotic instrumentation and techniques, the gold-standard lymphadenectomy can be performed with equal efficacy and decreased morbidity when compared to the open approach.

## LAPAROSCOPIC PELVIC LYMPH NODE DISSECTION

Laparoscopic pelvic lymph node dissection (L-PLND) for staging of prostate cancer was first described in 1991 by Schuessler et al. (2). Recently, the importance of pelvic lymphadenectomy has been questioned for patients undergoing radical prostatectomy. The arguments against pelvic lymphadenectomy include stage migration, an increasing percentage of patients with a low prostate-specific antigen (PSA) level and tumor stage, and the practice of omitting lymphadenectomy in low-risk patients (PSA <10 ng/mL and/or Gleason score <7). In patients with high-risk prostate cancer (clinical stage T2c, serum PSA level >10 ng/mL, and Gleason score >7), however, there is an approximately 38% risk of lymph node metastasis (3).

### Diagnosis

L-PLND is an additional diagnostic procedure considered after definitive diagnosis of prostate cancer through biopsy or transurethral resection of the prostate.

### Indications for Surgery

L-PLND is now rarely indicated as an independent staging procedure for prostate cancer. L-PLND should be considered in patients with clinical stage T2b or T3a cancer of the prostate whether surgery or radiation therapy is being considered; stage T1b cancer with Gleason sums of 7 or more; PSA levels >20 ng/mL; or suspicious lymph nodes visualized on CT that are not amenable to guided needle biopsy. Additionally, patients scheduled to undergo perineal prostatectomy, brachytherapy, external-beam radiotherapy, or laparoscopic/robotic prostatectomy who have a risk of node positivity >25% should undergo pretreatment L-PLND or simultaneous L-PLND.

Malignancies other than prostate cancer may be staged with L-PLND, including bladder, urethral, and penile cancers. Patients with transitional cell carcinoma of the bladder with an enlarged pelvic lymph node on imaging may undergo L-PLND if the lymph node is inaccessible to other minimally invasive biopsy techniques (CT-guided biopsy). In patients with urethral and penile cancers, sampling of enlarged pelvic nodes may confirm the presence of metastatic disease and guide the treatment course. Patients with metastatic disease may proceed directly to chemotherapy and avoid the morbidity of radical surgery, which would inadequately treat the underlying disease.

Patients with inability to tolerate general anesthesia or pneumoperitoneum, morbid obesity, numerous previous abdominal or pelvic surgeries, or large aortic or iliac aneurysmal disease are not considered good candidates for any laparoscopic or robotic surgery.

## Alternative Therapy

Open pelvic lymphadenectomy historically has been the gold standard for lymph node removal. CT or MRI scanning can be utilized in combination with percutaneous biopsy for sampling of enlarged lymph nodes.

Some authors advocate an extended PLN dissection in patients with carcinoma of the prostate. This dissection reaches above the bifurcation of the common iliac artery and includes all external iliac, obturator, and hypogastric lymph nodes. A recent series reported that 45.5% of the detected metastases were exclusively located outside of the typically sampled obturator fossa (4). Others advocate the use of radioisotope-guided sentinel lymph node dissection. In one series of this approach, 71.4% of the detected metastases were exclusively located outside of the typically sampled obturator fossa (5). Both the extended lymph node dissection and sentinel lymph node dissection can be performed laparoscopically.

## Surgical Technique

Preoperative counseling should include a discussion of the risks, benefits, and alternatives to L-PLND. Although impractical to list all possible complications, the most common injuries should be mentioned, as well as the risk of conversion to an open procedure. Informed consent should be obtained and documented.

On the day prior to surgery, the patient takes only clear fluids by mouth. This preparation helps to maintain good hydration as well as decompress the bowel to aid in pelvic intraoperative exposure. All patients receive a single dose of intravenous antibiotics within 30 minutes of incision. Antiembolic pneumatic compression boots are placed and activated throughout the procedure. After adequate anesthesia is obtained, a Foley catheter and orogastric tube are placed in the bladder and stomach, respectively. Patients are placed in the supine position with well-padded arms tucked at the side. We utilize a split-leg operating table (Maquet), which allows abduction of the legs but without the need for lithotomy (Fig. 123.1). With this approach, the assistant may stand between the patient's legs during L-PLND. A padded chest strap is used to secure the patient to the table as the Trendelenburg position will be required.

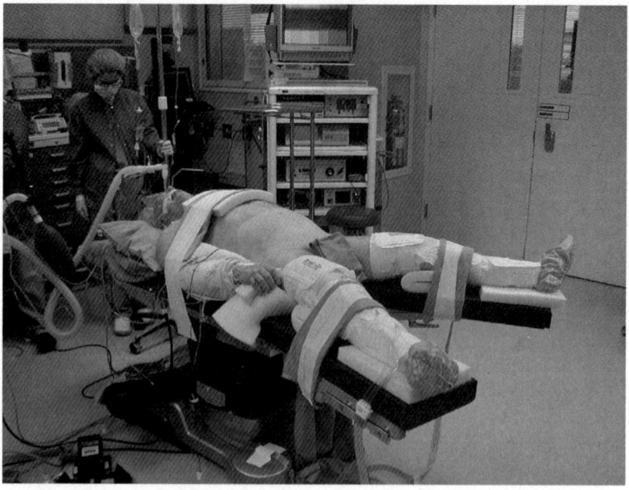

FIGURE 123.1 Split-leg operating table (Maquet) allows abduction of the legs without the need for lithotomy.

### Transperitoneal Approach

Pneumoperitoneum is achieved by insertion of a Veress needle at the superior or inferior crease of the umbilicus, and carbon dioxide is insufflated to an initial pressure of 20 mm Hg. A 10/11-mm trocar sheath unit can then be placed by enlarging the Veress needle puncture site. Alternatively, the open Hasson technique can be utilized at the same location to obtain pneumoperitoneum. Immediate laparoscopy with a 10-mm or 5-mm 30-degree lens should be performed to rule out iatrogenic injuries. Two options for trocar configuration include a four-trocar diamond-shaped configuration or a five-trocar inverted-U-shaped configuration as in laparoscopic radical prostatectomy (Fig. 123.2). After all laparoscopic ports are placed,

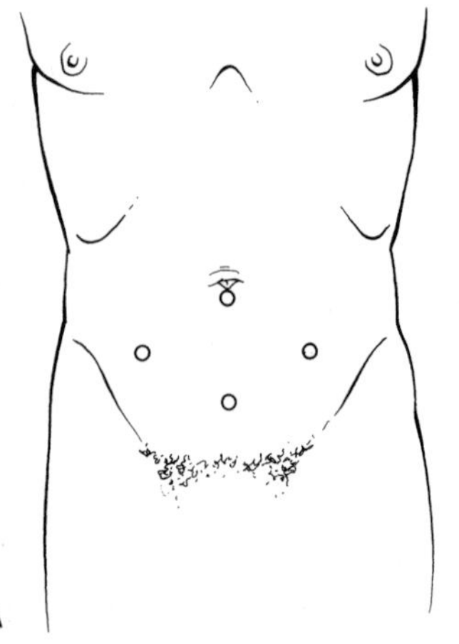

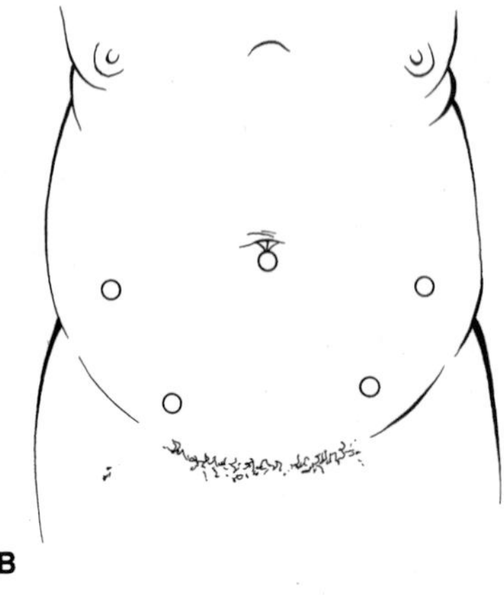

FIGURE 123.2 **A:** The standard diamond configuration for trocar placement with the laparoscope placed in the subumbilical position. **B:** The horseshoe configuration is useful for obese patients.

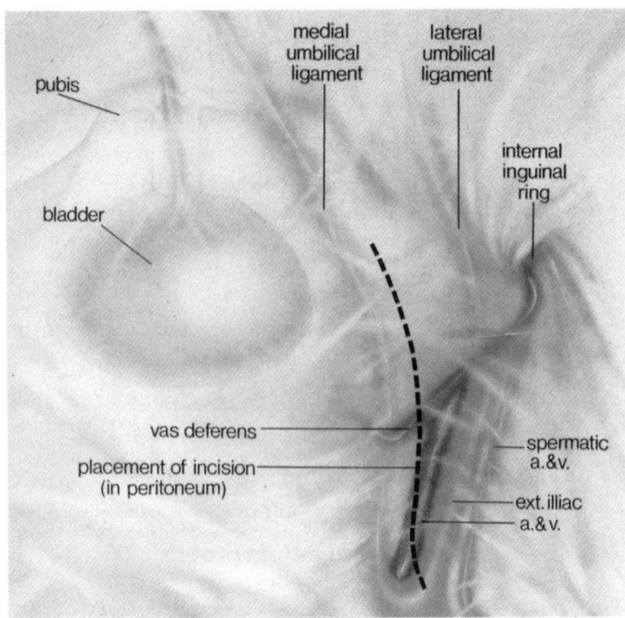


FIGURE 123.3 The initial peritoneal incision is made between the obliterated umbilical artery (medial umbilical ligament) and the internal inguinal ring. (From Gomella LG, Kozminski M, Winfield HN, eds. *Laparoscopic Urologic Surgery*, 1st ed. Philadelphia: Raven Press, 1994:117, with permission.)

pneumoperitoneum is decreased to 15 mm Hg and the patient is placed in 15-degree Trendelenburg with upward lateral rotation of the side to be operated. The combination of Trendelenburg and lateral rotation allows the loops of bowel to fall away from the area of dissection over the iliac/obturator regions. Any bowel adhesions should be carefully mobilized to facilitate the dissection. On the left side it is not uncommon to require takedown of the sigmoid flexure as it often protrudes toward the internal inguinal ring. The posterior peritoneal membrane is incised longitudinally and immediately lateral to the medial umbilical (obliterated umbilical) ligament from the pubis to the bifurcation of the iliac vessels (Fig. 123.3). The incision is directed just medial to the pulsating external iliac artery. The vas deferens will be exposed after the posterior peritoneum is incised. The vas deferens should be isolated, coagulated, and divided. It should be noted that the ureter is closely approximated to the peritoneum at, or just proximal to, the bifurcation of the common iliac artery.

The fibrolymphatic tissue adherent to the external iliac vein is elevated and dissected from the anterior and medial aspect of the vein. The incised edge of the lymph node packet is grasped and retracted medially, and a relatively avascular plane between the lymph node packet and lateral pelvic sidewall is identified and dissected bluntly. Any small perforating vessels are identified, controlled with bipolar cautery, and divided. Dissection is carried proximally to the iliac bifurcation and distally to the pubis. By retracting the lymph node packet medially, the obturator nerve and vessels can be identified and avoided. After securing the distal extent of the lymph node packet, the packet is then retracted cranially to separate it from the obturator vessels and nerves. Hemoclips or bipolar cautery is used to control lymphatics and vessels at the most proximal and distal extent of the dissection. The lymph nodes can usually be removed as a single packet and extracted either through the 12-mm trocar or by placing them in the entrapment sack.

### Extraperitoneal Approach

A 2-cm infraumbilical incision is made and carried through the rectus and transversalis fascia. Stay sutures are placed in the incised rectus fascia and a preperitoneal plane is digitally enlarged. A balloon inflation device is inflated to 800 to 1,000 mL, then deflated and removed. A Hasson-type or balloon cannula is inserted and secured. Carbon dioxide is insufflated to 15 mm Hg to allow for the remaining port placement. Care should be taken to avoid traversing the peritoneal membrane to prevent intraperitoneal insufflation leakage and possible bowel injury. After the port placement under visual or digital guidance, the procedure proceeds as described previously for the transperitoneal L-PLND. Ensuring careful lymphostasis with the extraperitoneal approach is essential to prevent the risk of postoperative lymphocele formation due to the lack of a peritoneal window to vent lymph fluid leakage.

## Complications

Most complications related to pelvic lymph node dissection are either a consequence of trocar placement or vascular injury. An accessory obturator vein is often encountered arising from the distal aspect of the external iliac vein. When present, this vessel must be controlled and divided, or avoided, when managing the distal extent of the lymph node packet. Dissection deep to the obturator nerve can result in bleeding from the obturator vessels. Bleeding from the obturator vessels can be managed using a hemoclip or bipolar electrocautery, but bleeding from the iliac vessels can be more difficult to manage laparoscopically. Pressure to an iliac vessel injury should be applied immediately and maintained for several minutes, along with the use of hemostatic agents such as oxidized regenerated cellulose or fibrin sealants. Bleeding from a small venous injury may be controlled with this maneuver, but for a larger injury an attempt can be made to secure the opening with either hemoclips or sutures. Prompt conversion to open surgery and repair may be required if these attempts are unsuccessful.

Great care must be taken to avoid undue traction, electrothermal injury, or transection of the obturator nerve throughout the procedure. Avoid accidental injury to the obturator nerve by identifying its course before application of hemoclips on vessels or lymphatics.

Postoperative lymphocele and deep venous thrombosis are the two major morbidities associated with open PLND. With L-PLND, postoperative lymphoceles are less common (6). A transperitoneal laparoscopic approach allows continuous drainage of lymphatic fluid into the peritoneal cavity in the event of a lymphatic leak. Regardless of the approach, however, lymphatic fluid loculations have been reported. Deep venous thrombosis is relatively uncommon after L-PLND owing to the steep Trendelenburg position and avoidance of venous compression of the iliac veins that can occur when using a fixed retractor system during open surgery. One comparative study found a lower total complication rate with L-PLND (0%) compared with open PLND (21%) (7).

Despite the excellent outcomes of L-PLND, the true indications for L-PLND continue to decrease, primarily due to advances in prostate cancer screening with a shift toward earlier diagnosis and lower-stage and -grade disease.

# LAPAROSCOPIC RETROPERITONEAL LYMPH NODE DISSECTION

Due to its minimally invasive approach, laparoscopic retroperitoneal lymph node dissection (L-RPLND) may be part of a new treatment paradigm for patients with clinical stage I nonseminomatous germ cell tumors. L-RPLND offers a highly accurate and reliable method of evaluating the presence and extent of retroperitoneal lymph node metastases. Refinements in laparoscopic surgical technique and instrumentation have allowed for the performance of this minimally invasive procedure with low morbidity.

## Indications for Surgery

The use of RPLND primarily involves patients found to have nonseminomatous germ cell tumors, as 20% to 30% of these patients with clinical stage I disease may have retroperitoneal lymph node metastases. Of more concern are patients with stage T2 to T4 primary tumors, evidence of lymphovascular invasion, and embryonal cell carcinoma, who are in general believed to be at an even higher risk of retroperitoneal and systemic relapse (8–10). Although the literature is replete with controversy concerning the use of chemotherapy versus RPLND, surgery is often advocated as a staging, and possibly curative, procedure for such patients. Under these circumstances RPLND is performed in a unilateral template fashion to preserve antegrade ejaculation. L-RPLND has been used as an alternative to open RPLND in this select patient group. However, upon pathologic confirmation of metastatic disease following L-RPLND, patients are then upstaged and given chemotherapy in most series. Thus, the therapeutic effectiveness of L-RPLND alone in such cases is untested. As such, L-RPLND should currently be considered a diagnostic procedure. However, used as such, this minimally invasive procedure aids in identifying patients with pathologic stage I nonseminomatous testis tumors who can safely be spared chemotherapy. L-RPLND is also utilized in stage IIa and IIb patients to demonstrate lymph node metastasis prior to administering chemotherapy. The general indications for L-RPLND are shown in Table 123.1.

## Alternative Therapy

Alternative treatment approaches for patients with stage I nonseminomatous germ cell tumors include open RPLND, chemotherapy, and active surveillance.

**TABLE 123.1**

**INDICATIONS FOR LAPAROSCOPIC RETROPERITONEAL LYMPH NODE DISSECTION**

- Clinical stage I, IIa, and IIb nonseminomatous testicular cancer
- Negative testis tumor markers
- No absolute contraindications to laparoscopic surgery
- Residual isolated abdominal or pelvic mass after chemotherapy in the presence of negative testis tumor markers

## Surgical Technique

On the day prior to surgery, the patient undergoes a mechanical bowel preparation, which includes a clear liquid diet and one gallon of GoLYTELY. Type and cross-matching is done for two units of blood. Janetschek et al. (11) also recommend that a low-fat diet be started 1 week prior to and continued for 2 weeks after surgery to minimize chylous ascites. The patient should have nothing by mouth after midnight on the night prior to surgery.

RPLND for patients with stage I nonseminomatous germ cell tumors involves either right- or left-sided template surgery, depending on the testis involved with disease. Nerve-sparing templates are now used, which yield virtually a 100% chance of maintaining antegrade ejaculation (Fig. 123.4) (12). Surgery for each template will be described.

### Transperitoneal Approach

**Right-Sided Template.** The patient is positioned on the operating table with the right side elevated 45 degrees upward. This allows for both supine and lateral decubitus positioning as needed. Trendelenburg or reverse Trendelenburg positioning can then be used as indicated. In general, trocar ports are 5 to 12 mm and placed in a midline vertical arrangement (Fig. 123.5).

The initial step in L-RPLND is to gain wide exposure of the retroperitoneum. Dissection is begun along the white line of Toldt from the level of the cecum to the hepatic flexure. Cephalad, this incision is carried above the level of the transverse colon and lateral to the duodenum (Kocher maneuver) along the vena cava up to the level of the hepatoduodenal ligament.

The duodenum and the head of the pancreas are further mobilized medially until the anterior surfaces of the vena cava, aorta, and left renal vein crossing the aorta are completely exposed. The peritoneal incision is also carried laterally around the liver toward the triangular ligaments, allowing for medial and superior retraction of the liver. This mobilization is necessary to ensure adequate exposure of the inferior vena cava and renal vessels. Inferiorly, the incision is extended along the spermatic vessels to the level of the internal inguinal ring. Dissection is also extended around the cecum and upward along the root of the mesentery, allowing for medial mobilization of these structures. At this point, the dissection has exposed the entire right-sided template. This template includes all preaortic tissue between the left renal vein and the inferior mesenteric artery, the interaortocaval nodes, and all tissue on the ventral and lateral surfaces of the vena cava extending laterally to the ureter. The template is bounded superiorly by the right renal vessels and inferiorly where the ureter crosses the iliac vessels. The template extends posteriorly to the level of the lumbar vessels. There is recent evidence to suggest that dissection posterior to the lumbar vessels within the template is not necessary in clinical stage I patients as no tumor was found in any patients undergoing laparoscopic lymphadenectomy that included this region (12). However, this finding requires corroboration by further studies.

After the entire template has been exposed, dissection is begun inferiorly where the spermatic vessels enter the internal inguinal ring. Typically, one should identify a nonabsorbable stitch, left at the time of radical orchiectomy, that signifies the

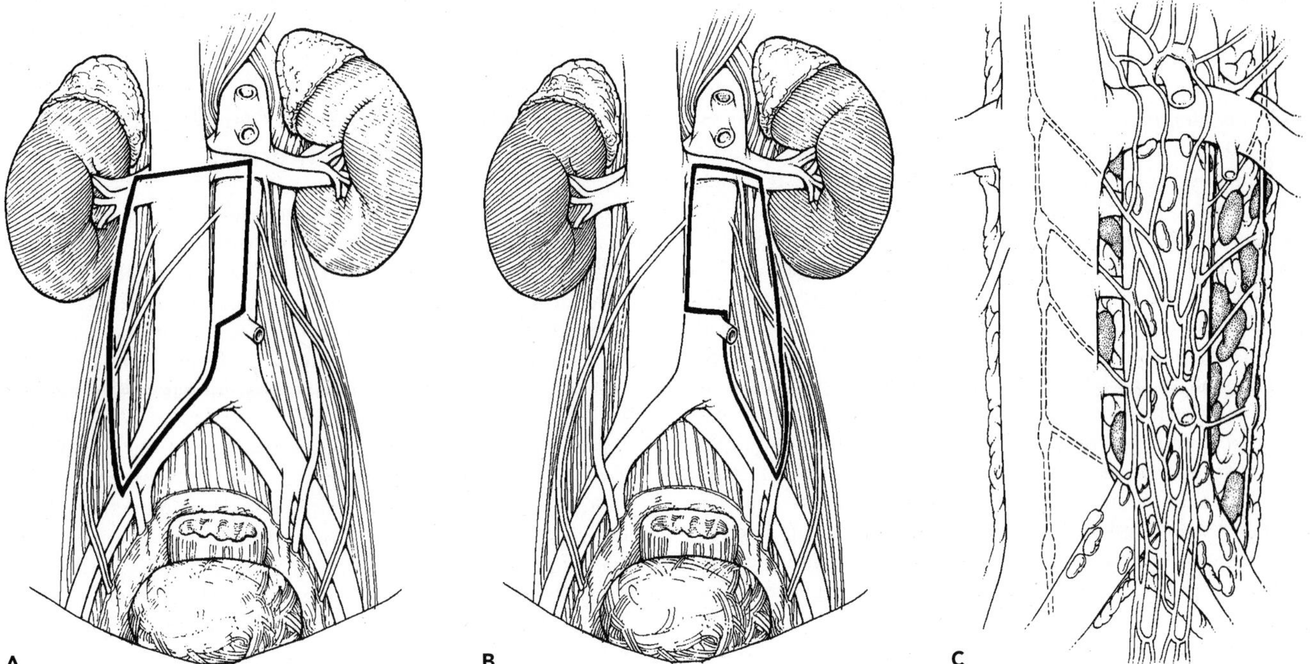


FIGURE 123.4 **A:** Template for right modified nerve-sparing retroperitoneal lymph node dissection (RPLND). **B:** Template for left modified nerve-sparing RPLND. **C:** Anterior view of retroperitoneal sympathetic fibers. (From Foster RS, Donohue JP. *Nerve-Sparing RPLND*. AUA Update Series, vol. 15. Dallas, TX: AUA, 1993, lesson 15, with permission.)

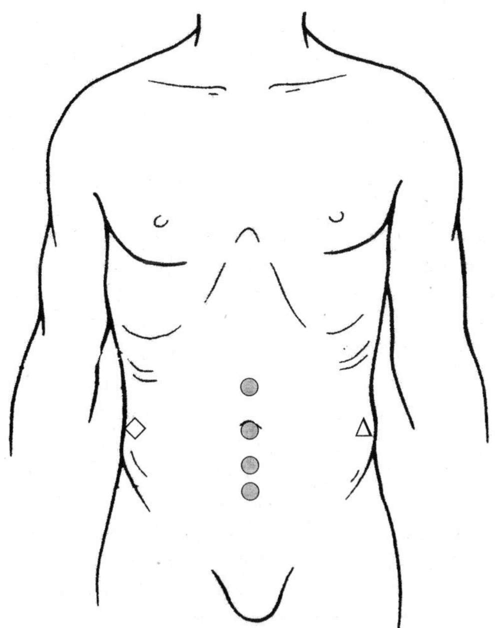

Legend

● = 10/11 mm port.

◇ = 5 mm port for right L-RPLND in anterior axillary line.

Δ = 5 mm port for left L-RPLND in anterior axillary line.

FIGURE 123.5 Trocar placement for transperitoneal laparoscopic retroperitoneal lymph node dissection. (From Clayman RV, ed. *Laparoscopic Urology*. St. Louis, MO: Quality Medical Publishing, 1993:272–308, with permission.)

distal margin of this dissection. The testicular vein is then dissected up to its insertion into the vena cava. Careful dissection is required where the spermatic vein joins the inferior vena cava to prevent inadvertent disruption and bleeding. The testicular artery is clipped and transected where it crosses the inferior vena cava.

Next, the lymphatic tissue overlying the great vessels is dissected free. The lymphatic tissue on the anterior surface of the inferior vena cava is divided, and the anterior and lateral surfaces of the inferior vena cava are dissected free of lymphatic tissue from the level of the renal vessels going inferiorly to where the ureter crosses the iliac vessels. It is important that the left renal vein has already been clearly identified and exposed to prevent injury to this structure during this part of the dissection. The lymphatic tissue overlying the common iliac artery, starting at the level where the ureter crosses it, is dissected free, moving in a cephalad direction until the origin of the inferior mesenteric artery is reached. Cephalad to this artery, the lymphatic tissue is divided toward the lateral border of the aorta so that all tissue anterior to this vessel is freed and included with the specimen. If not already done so, during this part of the dissection the testicular artery is clipped at its insertion into the aorta. This dissection is continued cephalad until the right renal artery, traversing the interaortocaval space, is identified, which marks the superior border of the template. The interaortocaval lymphatic tissue is now excised, with its posterior border being the level of the lumbar vessels. Great care must be taken with retraction of the great vessels as vascular injury may result in hemorrhage that is difficult to control by laparoscopic means. Lumbar vessels may need to be sacrificed to ensure retrieval of all lymphatic tissue. All sympathetic nerve fibers should be spared, if possible. With the medial and superior borders of the template freed, attention is paid to the lateral border along the ureter. After the ureter has been identified, all lymphatic tissue medial to it is freed, beginning where the ureter crosses over the common iliac artery and proceeding cephalad to the level of the renal vessels, where the most cephalad portion of the dissection has already been completed. The posteriorly located lumbar vessels may also be encountered during this portion of the dissection. They should be clipped and divided only when needed to facilitate removal of lymphatic tissue. At this point the lymphatic packages are completely free. They are placed in a specimen bag and removed. Obvious tumor or suspicious fibrolymphatic tissue should be sent for pathologic frozen-section interpretation. The colon and duodenum are then repositioned to their normal anatomic positions.

**Left-Sided Template.** The patient is placed on the operating table with the left side elevated 45 degrees upward. All other aspects of positioning and port placement (except now for left-sided dissection) are similar to that as described for right-sided dissection. Dissection is begun by incising the white line of Toldt on the left side, from the splenic flexure to the pelvic brim. The incision is extended distally along the spermatic vein all the way to the internal inguinal ring, where a nonabsorbable stitch, left at time of radical inguinal orchiectomy, should be identified. Superiorly, the dissection is carried medially around the splenic flexure just below the edge of the spleen. At this point the colon is mobilized medially until the entire anterior surface of the aorta is exposed. The entire length of the spermatic vein, from the renal vein to the internal inguinal ring, is dissected free and removed. The left renal vein is identified and freed along its anterior and inferior surface at this point of the dissection. The ureter, which defines the lateral border of the dissection, is then identified. All lymphatic tissue is dissected free from the ureter from the level of the renal hilum to where the ureter crosses the common iliac artery. Then, starting where the ureter crosses (the inferior border of the template) the common iliac artery, all lymphatic tissue is dissected free from the lateral surface of this blood vessel. From here the dissection is continued cephalad along the lateral surface of the aorta to the level of the inferior mesenteric artery. This artery is preserved during this dissection. Cephalad to the inferior mesenteric artery all lymphatic tissue on the anterior and lateral surfaces of the aorta is removed. Dissection is continued in this manner up to the level of the renal vein. All lymphatic tissue associated with the renal vein is now dissected free. If there is a lumbar vein inserting into the posterior surface of the renal vein it must be divided to dissect free all lymphatic tissue. As a final step, the lymphatic package is dissected free posteriorly. The lymphatic tissue is separated from the lumbar vessels. The lymphatic package is then removed.

## L-RPLND for Stage II or III Disease after Chemotherapy

L-RPLND has in general been performed only in a unilateral fashion, and there is only limited experience of L-RPLND being performed for stage II or III tumors after chemotherapy. In such cases L-RPLND may be performed when there has been a good response to chemotherapy where only smaller tumors/masses (5 cm or less) remain, and tumor markers have returned to normal. In such cases, dissection is carried out in a similar fashion as described for the unilateral templates involved but focusing primarily on resection of the residual tumor mass. Those with experience in such cases have noted that, due to chemotherapy, although tissue planes are more difficult to identify, mobilization of the bowel and identification of the tumor is possible. Due to the desmoplastic reaction typically seen after chemotherapy, careful dissection is required as tumor/residual tissue may be adherent to blood vessels. Janetschek et al. (11) noted that teratomas are usually well delineated, but other types of tumor-free residual tissue may be adherent to surrounding venous structures. All vascular branches from the tumor must also be carefully dissected out, clipped, and transected.

## Retroperitoneal Approach

Since the introduction of the balloon dissecting technique by Gaur, the laparoscopic retroperitoneal approach has been used for a variety of urologic procedures. Rassweiler et al. (13) reported use of this technique for L-RPLND in 17 cases. This technique differs from transperitoneal L-RPLND in how access and exposure are obtained. The essential features of this technique include placing the patient in the flank position without Trendelenburg. On the side of dissection a small incision (<2 cm) is made in the lumbar (Petit) triangle between the 12th rib and the iliac crest. Blunt dissection is then used to identify the peritoneal membrane and create the retroperitoneal space (Fig. 123.6). The retroperitoneal space can be expanded by use of either balloon dilating devices (commercial or homemade), or through further dissection with the surgeon's finger. Surgeons who develop the retroperitoneal space with finger dissection place the secondary ports under digital guidance before placing a 12-mm port through the initial incision. When the retroperitoneal space is developed with a balloon dilating device, a 10-mm trocar is placed through the existing incision. Placement of secondary trocars is then performed under laparoscopic guidance (Fig. 123.7). Once the laparoscopic ports are in place and pneumoretroperitoneum is stable, a wide longitudinal incision of the fascia of Gerota is created for optimal exposure of the retroperitoneum. L-RPLND is then performed using the same template and landmarks as described for transperitoneal L-RPLND.

Use of this approach for L-RPLND, to date, is limited. Authors with considerable experience with retroperitoneoscopy reporting on use of this technique classified retroperitoneal L-RPLND as difficult. Others have described extraperitoneal L-RPLND by an anterior approach.

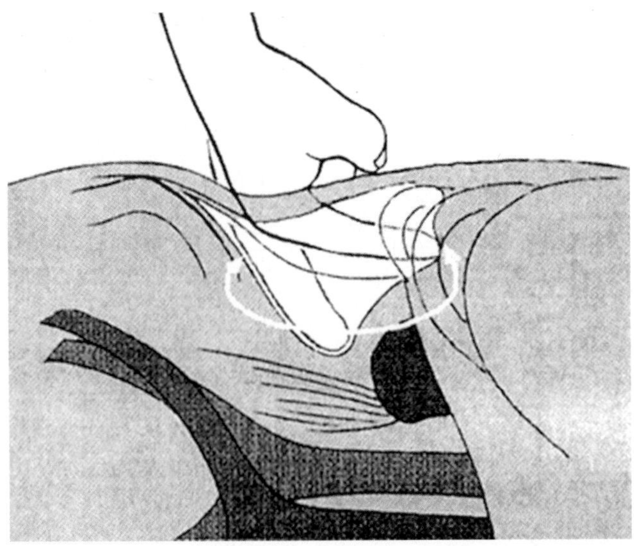

FIGURE 123.6 Blunt dissection of retroperitoneal space with index finger pushing peritoneum medially; the working space is created between the lumbar aponeurosis and renal (Gerota) fascia. (From Janetsckek G. Laparoscopic retroperitoneal lymph node dissection. *Urol Clin North Am* 2001;28:107–114, with permission.)

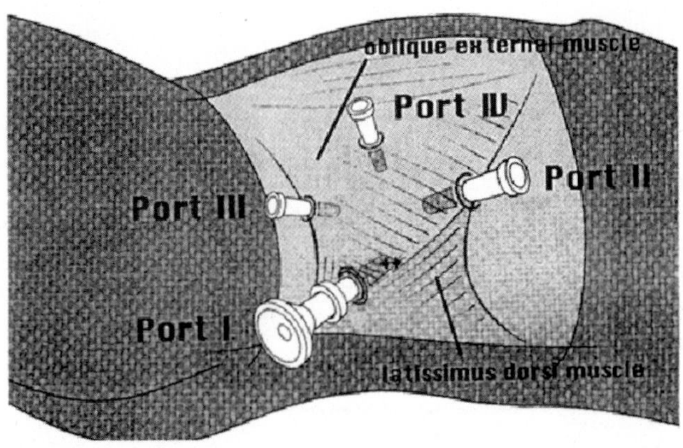


FIGURE 123.7 Port placement for laparoscopic retroperitoneal lymph node dissection (L-RPLND). Surgeon stands at the backside. *Port I*, 12 mm for laparoscope; *port II*, 10 mm for right hand of surgeon; *port III*, 5 mm for left hand; *port IV*, 5 mm for assistant.

# POSTOPERATIVE CARE

In an otherwise uncomplicated case, the orogastric tube may be removed at the end of the operation. Ambulation is initiated on the following morning, after which time the indwelling urethral catheter and pneumatic compression stockings may be discontinued. Diet is advanced on postoperative day 1. After the first 24 hours oral analgesics ordinarily suffice for pain control.

# OUTCOMES

## Complications

The predominant approach to L-RPLND has been by a transperitoneal route. The data presented here relate to L-RPLND performed by this technique. Potential complications associated with L-RPLND most often relate to intraoperative hemorrhaging. Other complications specifically related to this procedure include lymphocele formation and chylous ascites. The cumulative major (0.7%) and minor (7.8%) complication rates (intraoperative and postoperative) of this minimally invasive procedure are reasonable. Patients undergoing L-RPLND are likely to experience fewer pulmonary complications than those undergoing open surgery by midline or thoracoabdominal incisions. Janetschek et al. (11) noted the presence of chylous ascites in 21% of patients who underwent L-RPLND for persistent stage IIb tumor/mass. The authors believe that this complication is not related to surgical technique, as all lymphatic tissue was clipped, but rather to the brief time to oral intake after L-RPLND compared to open RPLND. All such cases resolved with conservative measures (low-fat/medium-chain triglyceride diet). In the hands of experienced laparoscopists, complications specifically related to laparoscopy, such as bowel injury due to trocar insertion or intraoperative manipulation, are less likely.

The largest contemporary series reported that only 3 of 103 patients required conversion to an open surgery because of injury of a small aortic branch, the renal vein in a horseshoe kidney, and a left renal vein ventral to the aorta in one patient each (12). There were four intraoperative vascular complications, including lacerations of the vena cava, renal vein, and a lumbar vein. The authors noted that three of the vascular complications were laparoscopically controlled with compression, clips, and fibrin glue; a left renal vein injury was controlled by laparoscopic suturing. Minor postoperative complications included asymptomatic lymphocele in three patients, genitofemoral nerve irritation in one patient, and a single spontaneously resolving retroperitoneal hematoma. Normal antegrade ejaculation was reported in 100 (97%) patients.

## Results

A summation of the worldwide experience with L-RPLND is shown in Table 123.2 (high-volume centers with 10 or more reported procedures). Review of 311 patients with follow-up for an average 44 months revealed 1 (0.3%) local recurrence and 12 (3.9%) distant recurrences; the solitary local recurrence occurred in the contralateral surgical field (12). Positive lymph nodes were demonstrated in 80 (25.7%) patients, and they were subsequently treated with chemotherapy. A 3.5% open conversion rate is reasonable for this complex procedure. Antegrade ejaculation was maintained in 99%. Longer follow-up of a larger number of patients is still needed to assess the diagnostic efficacy of this procedure.

A major point of discussion relating to L-RPLND is whether this procedure is simply a diagnostic procedure or may also be considered therapeutic. As the vast majority of patients found to have retroperitoneal tumors at the time of L-RPLND received adjunctive chemotherapy, it is not possible to determine the potential therapeutic efficacy of this procedure. L-RPLND has been used in a therapeutic fashion for a limited number of patients who underwent chemotherapy and had a persistent retroperitoneal mass. Janetschek et al. (11) described a group of 59 patients (stage IIb, 43 patients; stage IIc, 16 patients) who underwent chemotherapy, had persistent retroperitoneal mass, and subsequently underwent

**TABLE 123.2**

**WORLDWIDE EXPERIENCE WITH LAPAROSCOPIC RETROPERITONEAL LYMPH NODE DISSECTION FOR CLINICAL STAGE I DISEASE AT HIGH-VOLUME CENTERS WITH >10 REPORTED CASES**

| Study | Number of patients | Number node-positive patients | Mean follow-up (mo) | Mean operating time (min) | Conversion | Complications | | Antegrade ejaculation (%) | Recurrences | |
|---|---|---|---|---|---|---|---|---|---|---|
| | | | | | | Minor | Major | | Local | Distant |
| Albqami and Janetschek, 2005 | 103 | 26 | 62 | 217 | 3 | 9 | 3 | 100 | 1 | 4 |
| Castillo et al., 2004 | 96 | 18 | 34 | 138 | 4 | 9 | 5 | 100 | NR | 4[a] |
| Rassweiler et al., 2000 | 34 | 6 | 40 | 247 | 1 | 5 | 3 | 97.1 | 0 | 2 |
| Bhayani et al., 2003 | 29 | 12 | 72 | 258 | 2 | 2[b] | NR | 96.6 | 0 | 2 |
| LeBlanc et al., 2001 | 20 | 6 | 15 | 230 | 0 | NR | 0 | 100 | 0 | 0 |
| Corvin et al., 2005 | 18 | 7 | 16.7 | 232 | 0 | 1 | 0 | 100 | 0 | 0 |
| Correa et al., 2007 | 11 | 5 | 6 | 323 | 1 | 2 | 0 | 90 | 0 | 0 |
| *Total* | 311 | 80 (25.7%) | 44 | 205 | 11 (3.5%) | 28 (9.0%) | 11 (3.5%) | 99 | 1 (0.3%) | 12 (3.9%) |

NR, Not reported
[a]Did not report location of recurrences
[b]Only reported minor postoperative complications

L-RPLND. These patients all had normalization of tumor markers and a reduction of tumor size after chemotherapy. Of these patients, 21 had mature teratomas, 36 had necrosis and fibrosis only, 1 had active tumor, and 1 had seminoma. The one patient with active tumor received two additional cycles of chemotherapy and has remained disease-free. One patient with stage IIb disease had recurrence at 24 months outside of the surgical margin that was excised laparoscopically; the node contained only mature teratoma. L-RPLND is believed to be therapeutic in the 18 patients with mature teratoma. At a mean follow-up of 35 months, there have been no relapses in this group.

## *References*


1. Borley N, Fabrin K, Sriprasad S, et al. Laparoscopic pelvic lymph node dissection allows significantly more accurate staging in "high-risk" prostate cancer compared to MRI or CT. *Scand J Urol Nephrol* 2003;37:382–386.
2. Schuessler WW, Vancaillie TG, Reich H, et al. Transperitoneal endosurgical lymphadecentomy in patients with localized prostate cancer. *J Urol* 1991; 145:988–991.
3. Partin AW, Mangold LA, Lamm DM, et al. Contemporary update of prostate cancer staging nomograms (Partin tables) for the new millennium. *Urology* 2001;58:843–848.
4. Lattouf JB, Beri A, Jeschke S, et al. Laparoscopic extended pelvic lymph nose dissection for prostate cancer: description of the surgical technique and initial results. *Eur Urol* 2007;52:1347–1355.
5. Jeschke S, Beri A, Grull M, et al. Laparoscopic radioisotope-guided sentinel lymph node dissection in staging of prostate cancer. *Eur Urol* 2008;53: 126–133.
6. Solberg A, Angelsen A, Bergan U, et al. Frequency of lymphoceles after open and laparoscopic pelvic lymph nose dissection in patients with prostate cancer. *Scand J Urol Nephrol* 2003;37:218–221.
7. Herrell SD, Trachtenberg J, Theodorescu D. Staging pelvic lymphadenectomy for localized carcinoma of the prostate: a comparison of 3 surgical techniques. *J Urol* 1997;157:1337–1339.
8. Bosl GJ, Bajorin DF, Sheinfeld J, et al. Cancer of the testis. In: DeVita VF Jr, Hellman S, Rosenberg SA, eds. *Cancer* Philadelphia: lippincott Williams & Wilkins, 2001:1491–1518.
9. Heidenreich A, Sesterhenn IA, Mostofi FK, et al. Prognostic risk factors that identify patients with clinical stage I nonseminomatous germ cell tumors at low risk and high risk for metastases. *Cancer* 1998;83:1002–1011.
10. Sogani PC, Perrotti M, Herr HW, et al. Clinical stage I testis cancer: long term outcome of patients on surveillance. *J Urol* 1998;159:855–858.
11. Janetschek G, Peschel R, Bartsch G. Laparoscopic retroperitoneal lymph node dissection. *Atlas Urol Clin North Am* 2000;8:71–90.
12. Albqami N, Janetschek G. Laparoscopic retroperitoneal lymph node dissection in the management of clinical stage I and II testicular cancer. *J Endourol* 2005;19:683–692.
13. Rassweiler JJ, Frede T, Lenz E, et al. Long-term experience with laparoscopic retroperitoneal lymph node dissection in the management of low-stage testicular cancer. *Eur Urol* 2000;37:251–260.

# CHAPTER 124 ■ LAPAROSCOPIC NEPHRECTOMY AND PARTIAL NEPHRECTOMY

JAMES A. BROWN

Standard transperitoneal and retroperitoneal laparoscopic nephrectomy (LN) were first performed in 1990, and their partial nephrectomy (PN) counterparts followed in 1993 and 1994 (14). Hand-assisted laparoscopic nephrectomy (HALN) was subsequently introduced in 1997.

Equivalent 5-year cancer cure rates combined with decreased morbidity and recovery time have made LN the current standard of care for surgically treating renal malignancies in industrialized countries. Laparoscopy is also the standard today for performing nephrectomy for benign disease. While open partial nephrectomy (OPN) remains the standard of care, laparoscopic partial nephrectomy (LPN) is increasingly being performed at high-volume medical centers of laparoscopic surgical excellence, and at these centers outcomes approach those of OPN. However, concerns regarding warm ischemia time, control of hemorrhage, urinary extravasation, complications, and difficulties in technique training and propagation have promoted ongoing and wide-ranging refinements to the LPN procedural technique.

## DIAGNOSIS

Renal masses are identified during radiologic imaging of patients with hematuria or abdominal or flank discomfort. Additionally, patients are increasingly identified incidentally. Tumors are typically characterized and staged using abdominopelvic computerized tomography (CT) or magnetic resonance imaging (MRI) scan and chest radiography. Preoperative blood work includes metabolic panels including serum creatinine, liver function studies, alkaline phosphatase, and calcium. If the latter two studies are elevated or if the patient has bone pain or other evidence of metastases, a bone scan will be performed. Brain imaging is selectively obtained in patients with cerebral symptoms or evidence for metastasis. Nuclear renography is utilized in patients with renal insufficiency or if there is concern regarding the function of the contralateral kidney.

## INDICATIONS FOR SURGERY

Simple nephrectomy is indicated for benign conditions such as chronic pyelonephritis, nephrosclerosis, multicystic dysplastic kidney, postrenal transplantation or renovascular hypertension, reflux or obstructive nephropathy, and symptomatic acquired renal cystic or autosomal dominant polycystic kidney disease (ADPKD). Radical nephrectomy is indicated for tumors worrisome for malignancy.

Almost all nonfunctioning kidneys and stage T1 and T2 tumors can be removed laparoscopically. Hand-assisted laparoscopy (HAL) is a viable alternative for any case where nephrectomy or PN is indicated. HALN is a particularly useful alternative for urologists with limited laparoscopic surgical experience. Additionally, HALN may be advantageous compared to standard LN in cases of donor nephrectomy, nephroureterectomy, tumors >10 cm, and severe perinephric scarring secondary to prior surgery or infection (e.g., xanthogranulomatous pyelonephritis). Difficult standard laparoscopic operations can be converted to HAL rather than open procedures by the surgeon comfortable with HAL.

Hand-assisted LPN (HALPN) and LPN have differing advantages and disadvantages. LPN minimizes incision length and morbidity. It further allows for more facile suturing and needle handling. HALPN has the advantage of allowing for tumor palpation, which may increase surgeon comfort during tumor excision. It further allows for the selective performance of polar PN with hand compression rather than hilar clamping. In this situation, HALPN may minimize the overall renal injury from the procedure, and if a positive surgical margin occurs, a repeat resection might be performed with less risk for additional renal impairment (5). This is not the case after LPN or HALPN using hilar clamping.

## ALTERNATIVE THERAPY

Open radical nephrectomy (ORN) and OPN may be performed. Cryoablation (CA) and radiofrequency ablation (RFA) are also therapeutic alternatives, particularly for patients who are elderly or who have significant medical comorbidities, hereditary forms of renal cancer, or multiple tumors. These ablative procedures can be performed percutaneously with CT or MRI guidance and laparoscopically. Tumor enucleation may be considered in patients with severe renal insufficiency, a solitary kidney, multiple tumors, or a tumor in a difficult location (e.g., central, hilar). Lastly, observation alone may be reasonable for patients with small tumors, cystic masses, advanced age, or poor health.

## PATIENT PREPARATION

A formal bowel preparation is not routinely performed, but a clear liquid diet the day before surgery augmented by a Dulcolax suppository or an oral saline cathartic (e.g., magnesium citrate or Fleet Phospho-Soda) is often employed. One gram of cefazolin (Ancef) is administered preoperatively.

Deep venous thrombosis prevention with subcutaneous heparin (5,000 U 2 hours prior to procedure and continued every 12 hours postoperatively until the patient is ambulatory) and/or pneumatic compressive stockings are used.

## PATIENT POSITIONING

Under general anesthesia, intravenous access and endotracheal intubation are obtained with the patient supine. Orogastric and Foley catheters are inserted to decompress the stomach and bladder. The patient is then placed in a modified (30- to 70-degree) lateral decubitus position, with the umbilicus over the break in the table. For retroperitoneoscopic procedures, the patient is placed in or closer to the true lateral decubitus position. An axillary roll is placed, the table is flexed as necessary (usually minimally compared with open flank surgery), and a bean bag or padding is positioned to support the buttocks and flank. Pillows are placed between the flexed lower and straight upper leg. The upper arm rests on a well-padded arm board (or pillows) without tension on the brachial plexus. Three-inch tape is used to secure the patient around the hips, shoulders, and thighs to ensure stability when rolling the table to facilitate bowel retraction (Fig. 124.1).

## SURGICAL TECHNIQUE

### Transperitoneal Radical or Total Nephrectomy

#### Access

Although various insufflation techniques can be used, most urologists use a Veress needle. It is commonly inserted at the level of the umbilicus lateral to the ipsilateral rectus muscle. The abdomen is insufflated to 15 mm Hg. Some surgeons prefer a pressure of 20 mm Hg during the trocar placement. Typically a 10- or 12-mm trocar is placed lateral to the rectus at the level of the umbilicus using a visual obturator trocar (e.g., Visiport, AutoSuture or Optiview, Ethicon Endo-Surgery). Once the peritoneum has been entered, the intraperitoneal contents are inspected for injury or adhesions. Trocar site placement varies significantly based on surgeon preference and patient body habitus. Most surgeons prefer the laparoscope ("camera") port positioned between the working ports, which is the author's preference. Some place it caudad to the working ports. Many surgeons use a 30-degree laparoscope placed through an umbilical port, with working ports widely spaced in the subxiphoid midline and the far lateral abdomen (anterior axillary line, umbilical level), creating a 90-degree angle in relation to the umbilical trocar. Other surgeons place the working ports closer to the umbilical trocar, keeping them at least 10 cm apart. Others reduce the angle of the working ports in relation to the umbilicus to approximately 60 to 70 degrees, creating a trocar "diamond" configuration. Alternatively, one can use a 0-degree laparoscope placed through a trocar lateral to the rectus muscle and just cephalad to the umbilicus, with the working ports shifted slightly cephalad and laterally, respectively, to maintain at least 10-cm or five-fingerbreadths distance between trocars. A 5-mm trocar is often placed in the far lateral (anterior to posterior axillary line) position for retraction, and another 5-mm trocar is often placed below the xiphoid process for right-sided procedures to elevate the liver using a locking grasper attached to the lateral abdominal wall. Obese patients or patients with protruberant abdomens will need to have the trocars shifted laterally to maintain effective working angles into the retroperitoneum.

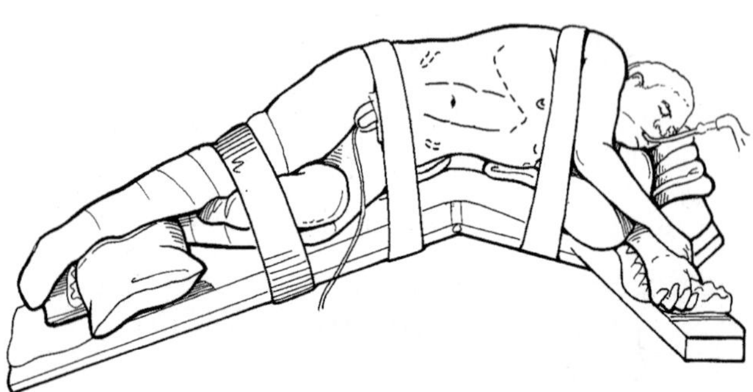

**FIGURE 124.1** The patient is placed in a modified (70-degree) lateral decubitus position, with the umbilicus over the break in the table. (From Figure 11.3 in Bishoff JT, Kavoussi LR, eds. *Atlas of laparoscopic retroperitoneal surgery*. Philadelphia: WB Saunders, 2000, with permission.)

#### Reflection of the Colon

The ipsilateral ascending or descending colon must be mobilized to gain access to the kidney and renal hilum. The parietal peritoneum is first incised medial to the line of Toldt, approximately 1 cm lateral to the mesenteric fat lying lateral to the colon. This incision is carried from the iliac vessels to the level of the spleen (left) or liver (right). Atraumatic graspers are used in the nondominant hand to provide countertension, and a hook electrode, Endoshears (scissors), or harmonic scalpel is used in the dominant hand to perform the dissection. Endoshears are particularly useful when dissecting in close proximity to bowel and when tissue planes are relatively avascular. Selective use of monopolar cautery through the instrument or use of a bipolar grasper in the nondominant hand allows for an efficient and elegant dissection by an experienced surgeon. Conversely, the harmonic scalpel excels at maintaining hemostasis when tissue planes are more vascular, and it is an excellent blunt-tipped dissection tool. Less experienced surgeons and surgeons in training may find the harmonic scalpel an easier tool to master. For left-sided procedures, many surgeons advocate carrying the peritoneal incision above the spleen laterally, allowing the spleen to fall medially with the pancreas and colon. Others prefer to carry the peritoneal incision through the phrenicocolic ligament to the spleen but then carry the dissection medially, leaving the spleen suspended on a "hammock of peritoneum caudad to the spleen and extending to the left abdominal sidewall," (Fig. 124.2). The splenophrenic attachments are left intact while the splenocolic and then renocolic fascial attachments are divided in layers until the descending colon is fully mobilized medially and the left gonadal vein is visible.

For right-sided procedures, the peritoneum just lateral to the ascending colon is divided and carried to the level of the liver. This peritoneal incision is also carried medially, staying approximately 1 cm away from the lateral border of the colonic hepatic flexure. This incision then proceeds cephalad to approximately 1 cm below the liver and back laterally

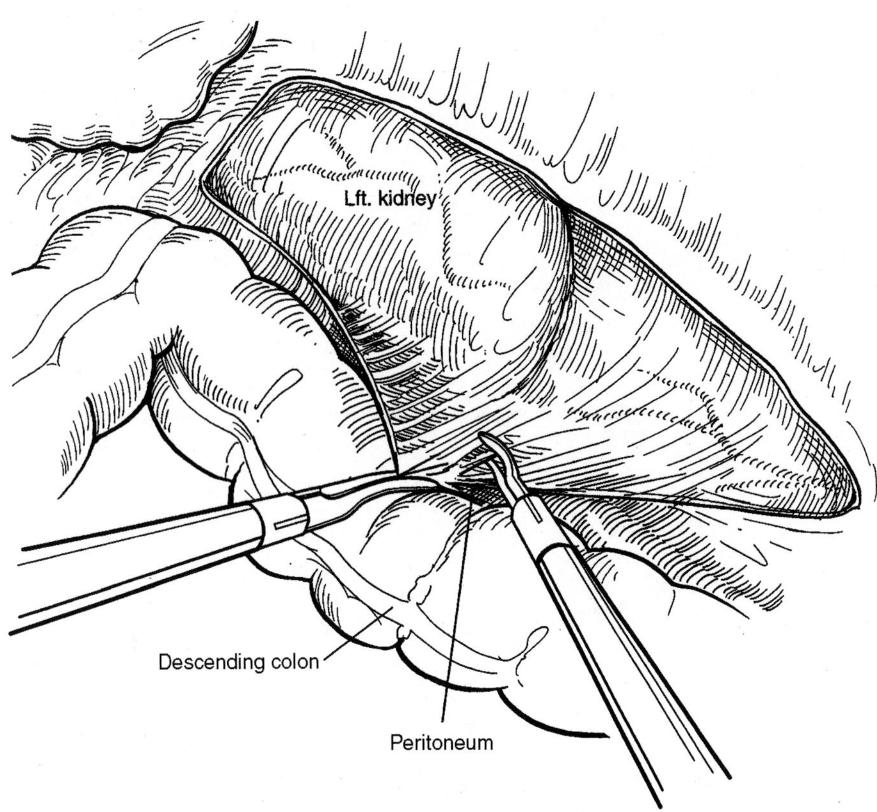


FIGURE 124.2 Mobilization of the colon using medial traction to demonstrate and divide attachments. (From Figure 4.8 in Bishoff JT, Kavoussi LR, eds. *Atlas of laparoscopic retroperitoneal surgery*. Philadelphia: WB Saunders, 2000, with permission.)

along the inferior surface of the liver to the sidewall. This approach will leave a wedge-shaped area of peritoneum covering the anterior aspect of the right kidney (Fig. 124.3). Once the ascending colon is mobilized medially, the duodenum is subsequently identified and a fascial incision is made approximately 1 cm lateral to its second stage. A Kocher maneuver is performed to move the duodenum medially. Third, the inferior vena cava (IVC) is exposed by incising the fascia and dissecting along its lateral border. For both left- and right-sided procedures, care is taken to preserve the lateral attachments of the kidney to prevent it from falling medially, inhibiting dissection of the renal hilum and the medial aspect of the Gerota fascia.

### Gonadal Vein Dissection

Once the colon is fully mobilized, the gonadal vein is identified. Many urologists find the gonadal vein to be the "gateway" for initiating the nephrectomy portion of the procedure and carrying the dissection to the renal hilum. For left-sided nephrectomies, the fascia overlying the gonadal vein is divided and this dissection is carried cephalad to the renal vein. Care must be taken to dissect anterior to the gonadal vein to prevent injuring small gonadal venous tributaries or hilar vessels. The harmonic scalpel is useful for dividing these fascial attachments and maintaining hemostasis. This will allow for exposure of the anterior aspect of the left renal vein and subsequently the adrenal vein. The adrenal vein may be dissected using the harmonic scalpel or a gently curved dissector (e.g., Maryland). It is subsequently cauterized (e.g., with a paddle bipolar instrument), clipped (e.g., with Hem-O-Lock clips), and divided. The gonadal vein is then divided 1 to 2 cm below the renal vein in a similar fashion. It is included with the

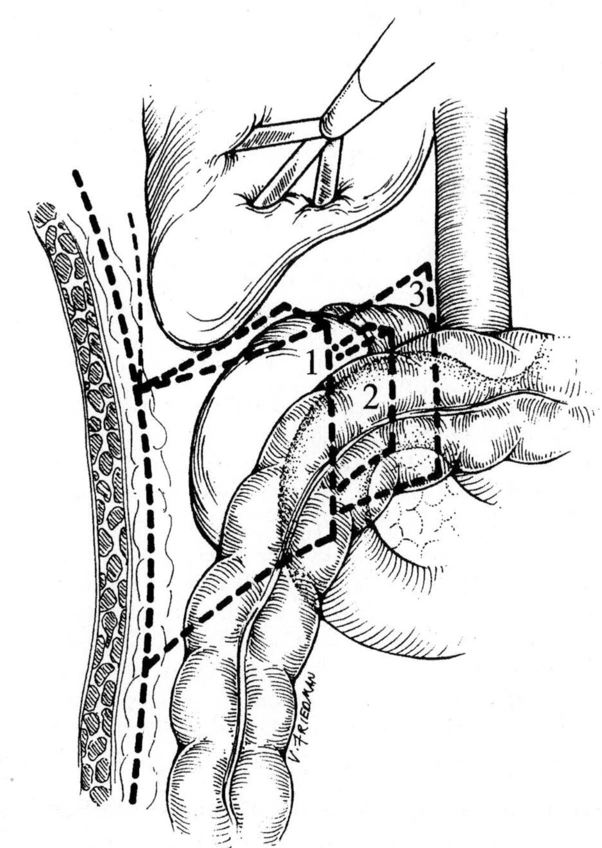


FIGURE 124.3 Diagram of the right-sided nephrectomy demonstrating the wedge-shaped configuration. The numbers refer to the three distinct levels of dissection along the medial aspect of the kidney: colon, duodenum, and inferior vena cava.

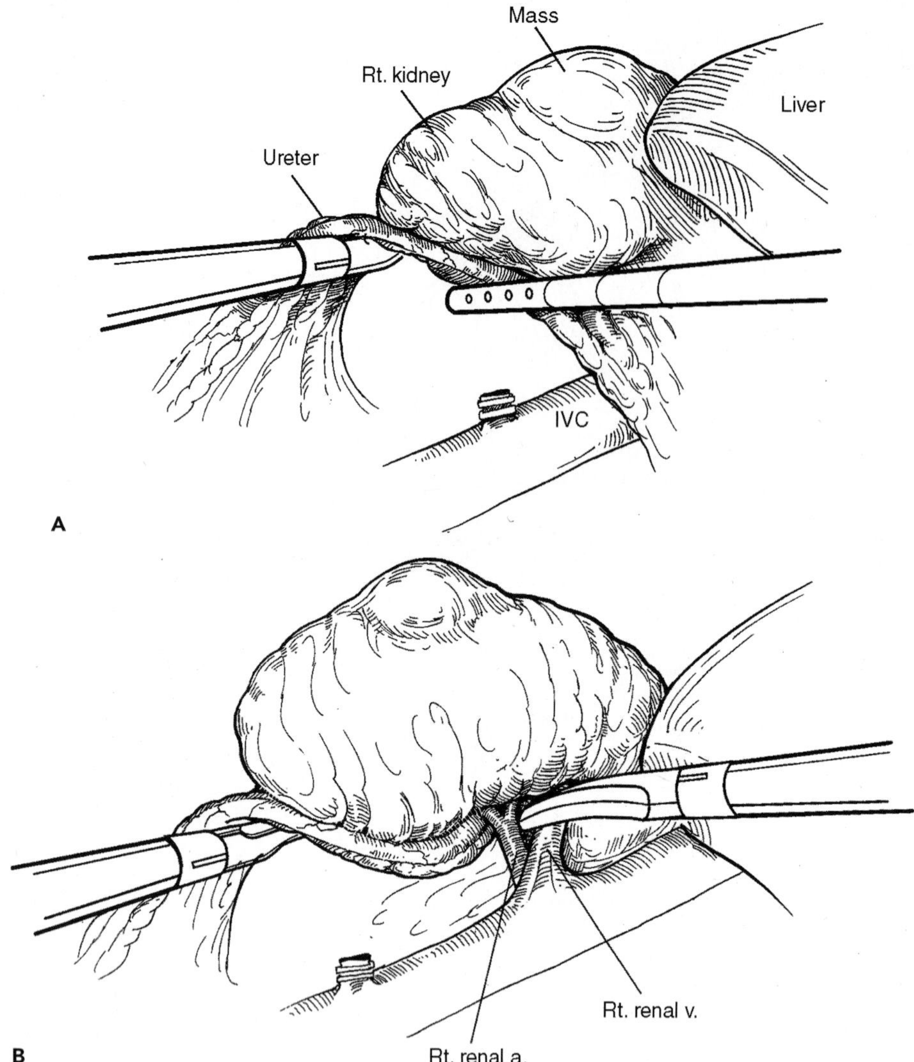


FIGURE 124.4 Elevation of ureter and tail of the Gerota fascia (**A**) to allow dissection to and exposure of renal vessels (**B**). (From Figures 5.8 and 5.9 in Bishoff JT, Kavoussi LR, eds. *Atlas of laparoscopic retroperitoneal surgery*. Philadelphia: WB Saunders, 2000, with permission.)

radical nephrectomy specimen, particularly for large and lower-pole tumors. For right-sided procedures, the fascia over the gonadal vein may similarly be divided along the course of the vein up to its junction with the IVC. The right gonadal vein may, particularly for large tumors, be divided and removed with the specimen. Conversely, the dissection can be made just lateral to the right gonadal vein for smaller mid- and upper-pole tumors. The plane of dissection between the gonadal vein and the tail of the Gerota fascia (containing the ureter) is developed, and the latter is elevated anterolaterally (using a laparoscopic Kitner, atraumatic grasper, or suction device) to allow dissection to the renal hilum via an inferoanterior approach (Fig. 124.4).

## Dissection of Ureter and Tail of the Gerota Fascia

For right-sided procedures, the ureter and tail of the Gerota fascia are elevated anterolaterally and the dissection carried along the gonadal vein to the IVC cephalad and to the iliac vessels caudad. For left nephrectomies, the dissection of the ureter and medial tail of the Gerota fascia is often performed after dividing the left adrenal and gonadal veins, if a true radical nephrectomy is to be performed. The adrenal gland and gonadal vein are spared when performing a simple nephrectomy or in select cancer patients. The tail of the Gerota fascia is mobilized medial to the gonadal vein from the renal hilum to the iliac vessels.

## Securing the Renal Blood Vessels

Firm anterolateral elevation of the lower pole is critical in order to facilitate dissection of the hilum. This is accomplished by placing a laparoscopic Kitner or atraumatic grasping instrument under the tail of the Gerota fascia, the ureter, and the lower pole and lifting to the abdominal sidewall. With the hilum on tension, a harmonic scalpel, suction instrument, hook electrode, dissector (e.g., Maryland), or Endoshears can be used to dissect out the renal artery and vein and any necessary tributaries (e.g., lumbar or accessory vessels). Lymphatic vessels and fascial attachments inferior to and occasionally encasing the renal artery must be divided bluntly or sharply. Once adequate vessel exposure (at least a 1- to 2-cm space) is created, an endovascular gastrointestinal anastomosis (GIA) stapler is used to divide first the renal artery and then the vein. Alternatively, a series of at least three Hem-O-Lock clips may be applied to the renal artery, dividing it approximately 1 cm lateral to the clips. In cases of severe perihilar fibrosis or if individual vessel isolation is difficult, en bloc endovascular GIA stapler division of both the artery and vein simultaneously is effective (17). Hilar side branches (gonadal, adrenal, lumbar, and accessory) may be ligated and divided in a variety of ways. Cauterization with either the LigaSure device or three overlapping deployments of a standard paddle bipolar cautery is effective. Standard titanium or locking polymer Hem-O-Lock clips may be used. The author favors sequential paddle bipolar cauterization of the vessel and placement of a Hem-O-Lock clip on the stay side of the vessel if it won't be in the path of the endovascular GIA stapler when dividing the renal vessels.

### Upper-Pole Isolation

Once all hilar vessels have been divided, the dissection is carried superiorly. For right radical nephrectomies (RNs), the adrenal vein must be identified, ligated, and divided. Hem-O-Lock clips, preferably two on the stay side, or an endovascular GIA stapler may be used. The remaining suprarenal attachments and middle suprarenal arteries are divided with the harmonic scalpel or stapler (Fig. 124.5). A similar dissection can be performed for left RNs, separating the adrenal from the aorta and diaphragm. Alternatively, for simple nephrectomies and selectively for small, non-upper-pole renal tumors (with a normal ipsilateral adrenal gland on preoperative abdominal CT or MRI imaging and intraoperative exam), the adrenal gland can be spared by placing the kidney on caudad traction and dividing the attachments between the adrenal gland and upper pole, staying adjacent to the adrenal. At this point, if it hasn't been performed previously, the ureter is clipped and divided and any remaining posterior or lateral attachments are divided by rotating the kidney as necessary.

### Organ Entrapment

Benign kidneys may be morcellated in a durable entrapment sac, but malignant kidneys should be removed intact. The risk for tumor spillage and the loss of histologic staging information virtually always outweigh the morbidity benefits of minimizing the extraction incision. The kidney is placed into a deployable entrapment sack (e.g., Endocatch II, US Surgical) and then brought out through an incision extended from a 12-mm trocar site. Alternatively, the specimen may be removed through a Pfannenstiel incision. Trocar sites larger than 5 mm should have a fascial closure suture (e.g., interrupted 0 Vicryl) placed prior to specimen extraction. The Carter-Thomason device facilitates placement of these fascial sutures.

## Hand-Assisted Laparoscopic Nephrectomy

### Access

For left HALN, a 7-cm supraumbilical midline incision is made extending into or skirting the umbilicus. It is useful to place a 0 Vicryl suture through the anterior rectus fascia and peritoneum at the midline of the incision bilaterally in order to elevate the abdominal wall to facilitate placement of the intraperitoneal portion of the laparoscopic hand port (e.g., GelPort, Applied Medical; or Lap Disc, Ethicon Endo-Surgery). These current third-generation devices have a narrower base than their predecessors, facilitating subsequent placement of trocars in slender patients. With a 0-degree laparoscope placed through a 12-mm trocar within the device, the peritoneum is inspected for adhesions. Under direct vision or under fingertip control, 12-mm trocars are then placed lateral to the rectus muscle (midclavicular line) and also approximately two fingerbreadths off the tip of the twelfth rib (anterior axillary line). Both trocars are positioned at the level of the hand port device (Fig. 124.6). A 5-mm trocar is

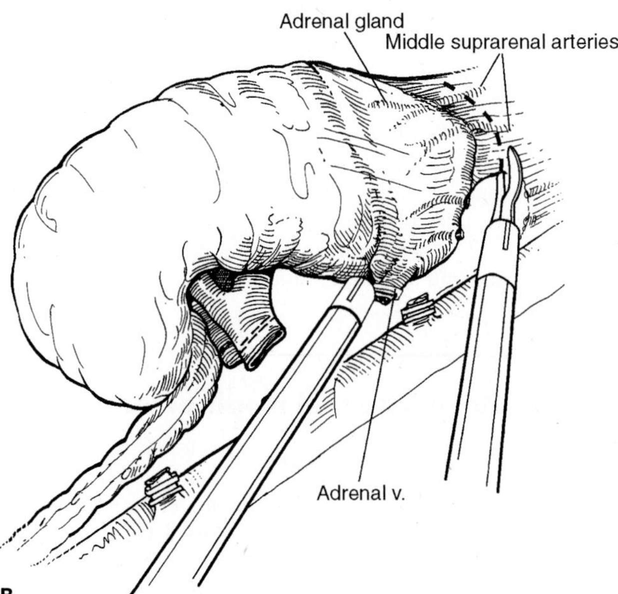


FIGURE 124.5 Adrenal gland excision with a right radical nephrectomy specimen. (From Figure 5.14B in Bishoff JT, Kavoussi LR, eds. *Atlas of laparoscopic retroperitoneal surgery*. Philadelphia: WB Saunders, 2000, with permission.)

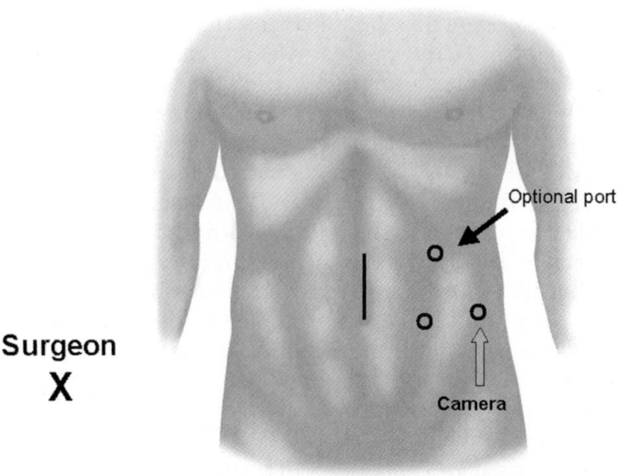


FIGURE 124.6 Hand-assisted laparoscopy port placement for left renal surgery. An optional 5-mm trocar may be placed cephalad (shown) or caudad to two 12-mm trocars placed at the level of the hand port or umbilicus.

selectively placed in the left lower quadrant, approximately 10 cm below the 12-mm trocars or along the costal margin, to use for retraction.

Right-sided HALN procedures may be performed by the left-handed or ambidextrous surgeon with ports placed in a mirror image fashion to the left-sided procedure. Alternatively, the hand port may be placed in the right lower quadrant through a 7-cm muscle-splitting incision. It may also be moved further caudad in the midline using a paraumbilical incision. This will allow room for placement of the laparoscope and the working and liver retraction trocars in the upper right quadrant and abdominal midline, cephalad to the hand port.

### Procedure

A damp laparotomy sponge, useful for hemostasis, is initially carried into the abdomen while inserting the hand. The obvious and only significant difference between HALN and standard LN is the use of the hand for palpation and retraction. Some standard laparoscopic urologic surgeons find the HAL technique cumbersome and find that their hand is "in the way." They are able to use retraction instruments more effectively than an intraperitoneal hand. Conversely, expert HAL surgeons become adept at utilizing their intraperitoneal hand in ways that gain them additional exposure beyond what they can obtain with standard laparoscopic instruments. Initially, the colon is reflected using a harmonic scalpel or Endoshears, while providing medial bowel traction with the fingertips. The hand is then placed in a "C-shaped" configuration while operating within the central space between the fingers and thumb.

For a left HALN, fingertips provide gentle tension and countertension, respectively, on the spleen or kidney and colon while the splenocolic and then renocolic attachments are divided. As the bowel is increasingly mobilized, it may be elevated anteriorly with the hand to facilitate separation of the colonic mesentery from the anterior aspect of the Gerota fascia. The gonadal vein and subsequently renal vasculature are dissected and handled as described for LN. The back of the wrist and hand assist with retraction of the colon to expose the hilum. The fingertips flatten and provide simultaneous cephalad, lateral, and inferomedial tension, facilitating renal vessel dissection and division. The lower pole, ureter, and tail of the Gerota fascia are elevated anteriorly by placing the index and middle fingers posteriorly and lifting anteriorly. The fourth finger may be placed cephalad to the renal vein to further rotate the renal artery into view (Fig. 124.7). Palpation is used to confirm location of the aorta and renal artery or arteries. The remainder of the procedure is accomplished in a similar fashion to standard LN. A simpler, less expensive entrapment sack (Cook Urologic, Spencer, IN) is introduced for specimen extraction. It is unrolled on top of the spleen with the posterior opening of the sack flattened across the body wall using the fifth fingertip to fixate it medially and a grasping instrument to hold it laterally. The third and fourth fingers of the intraperitoneal hand hold the anterior aspect of the sack open, and the thumb and index finger "feed" the kidney into the sack. The neck of the sack is tightened and the specimen is removed through the hand port incision. The incision may be extended as necessary for specimens too large to pass. The retroperitoneum is irrigated and

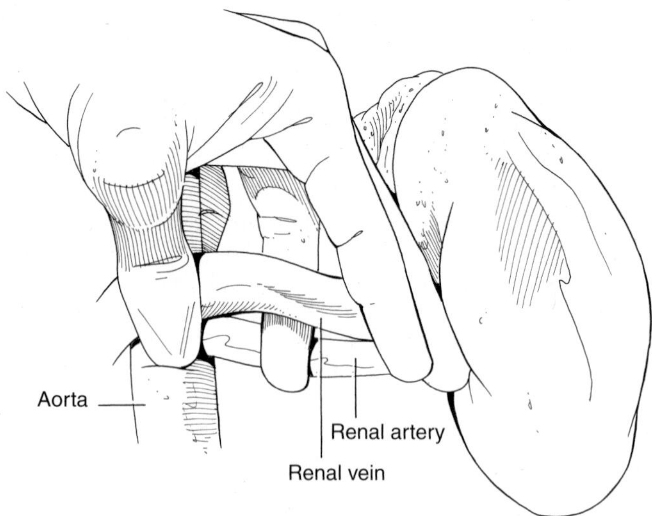


**FIGURE 124.7** Finger and hand position during left renal hilar dissection.

the incisions are closed. The midline hand port incision is closed with interrupted figure-of-eight no. 1 absorbable monofilament sutures (Maxon or polydioxanone).

Right HALN may be performed using a mirror image technique, with the right hand placed within the peritoneum, or the right-handed surgeon may place the left hand in the abdomen. The procedure is accomplished as described for the standard right LN technique, using the hand to provide tension and countertension. The surgeon will often facilitate the hilar dissection by lifting the lower pole anteriorly with a retractor. This will free up the hand to encircle and flatten the hilum, palpating and placing the artery and vein on stretch. This will promote rapid isolation and division. The adrenal gland may be palpated, as can the hilar lymphatics and the liver. The HALN technique is particularly useful if significant perihilar lymphadenopathy is present and for very large tumors impinging on either the IVC or aorta, where a safe dissection plane may be difficult to identify with standard laparoscopy. The subcutaneous tissues are injected with a mixture of 0.25% Marcaine and 1% lidocaine prior to approximating the subcuticular layer with 4-0 Monocryl suture. Sterile bandages are applied to the trocar sites. Injecting these sites prior to port placement may provide additional analgesic benefit. The hand port incision is covered with a small gauze dressing and Tegaderm and the trocar sites with sterile bandages.

## Retroperitoneal Nephrectomy

### Access

A 2-cm incision is made just below the tip of the twelfth rib in the midaxillary line. A Kelly clamp is used to separate the subcutaneous fat and expose the flank musculature. The muscle is bluntly divided, and the underlying thoracolumbar fascia is pierced to enter the pararenal fat of the retroperitoneum. "S" type or Army-Navy retractors are used for exposure, and a fingertip is inserted and rotated 360 degrees in order to palpate the psoas muscle and confirm an appropriate retroperitoneal location. A balloon dilator is introduced and filled to 800 cc with room air. During insufflation, a 10-mm laparoscope may be introduced to view the dissection. A 10-mm blunt-tipped cannula is introduced with 30 cc of air in the balloon (US Surgical). After tightening the outer ring sponge to compress the balloon against the inner abdominal wall, the retroperitoneum is insufflated to 15 to 20 mm Hg. Of note, some surgeons alternatively make the incision midway between the iliac crest and the tip of the twelfth rib in the posterior axillary line. Additionally, a visual obturator trocar with a 10-mm 0-degree laparoscope may be used instead to enter the retroperitoneal space. Entry must be at a 10-degree anterior angle. Angling too far posteriorly will injure the quadratus or psoas musculature, whereas too anterior of a trajectory may allow entry into the peritoneum or cause colon injury.

### Procedure

After obtaining retroperitoneal entry, blunt dissection is performed using only the scope. Anteriorly, the peritoneum is swept medially, exposing the transversalis fascia. Once peritoneal dissection off the abdominal wall is complete, accessory ports are placed in the upper and lower midaxillary line and a 5-mm trocar is placed in the anterior axillary line (Fig. 124.8). Some surgeons eliminate the lower midaxillary line port (three-port approach), while others maintain this trocar and add another anterior to it (five-port approach).

If balloon dilation was effective, the kidney should be displaced anteriorly. The psoas muscle is cleaned of fat and the dissection is carried cephalad and medially until the pulsating renal artery is visualized. The Gerota fascia is incised and the renal hilum is dissected, clipping the artery and stapling the vein with the endovascular GIA stapler. For left-sided nephrectomy, the posterior ascending lumbar vein may be encountered prior to viewing the artery. It should be dissected, clipped with Hem-O-Lock clips, or cauterized and divided. Circumferential dissection of the Gerota fascia is performed. On the right side, cephalad dissection will lead to the adrenal vein, which will be clipped or cauterized and divided. The adrenal vein will also typically be divided during left nephrectomy. The ureter is doubly clipped and divided, followed by division of the remaining retroperitoneal attachments. The specimen is entrapped in a deployable sack and removed through the initial port site by extending the incision horizontally anterior to the tip of the twelfth rib. Morcellation of benign kidneys can be performed in an impermeable sack (e.g., LapSac, Cook Urologic, Spencer, IN).

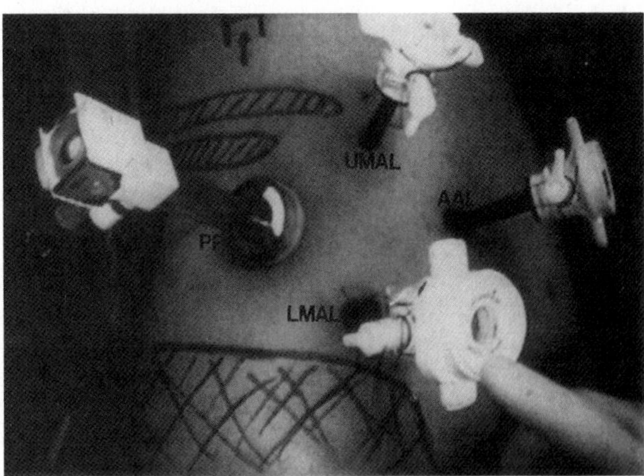


FIGURE 124.8 Port placement during right retroperitoneoscopic renal surgery. The primary port *(PP)* is inserted by the open (Hasson) technique caudad to the tip of the twelfth rib. The 12-mm lower midaxillary line *(LMAL)* port is placed 2 to 3 cm cephalad to the iliac crest. The 5-mm anterior axillary line *(AAL)* port is placed at the level of the PP. The 5-mm upper midaxillary line *(UMAL)* is placed near the tip of the eleventh rib. Care must be taken to avoid transpleural placement of this trocar.

The peritoneal cavity may be entered during anterior dissection of the Gerota fascia, but it does not necessitate conversion to a transperitoneal technique. Conversion to a transperitoneal laparoscopic or open flank nephrectomy approach can be performed in difficult cases. Similar to the transperitoneal technique, the retroperitoneum is inspected for hemostasis with $CO_2$ pressure at 3 to 4 mm Hg prior at end of the case. The port sites will not require fascial closure but are irrigated, and the skin is closed with 4-0 subcuticular suture.

## Transperitoneal Partial Nephrectomy

Access and renal exposure are similar to transperitoneal LN. The renal hilum is identified. At this point the operation will vary somewhat, depending on the PN technique that is employed. In most instances, the renal artery and vein are carefully dissected. The Gerota fascia is then opened horizontally across the anterior midpole, and the perirenal fat is reflected off the capsule. Some surgeons open the Gerota fascia along the lateral margin of the kidney. Fat is reflected until the tumor is visualized and then exposed, leaving it covered with fat. Endoshears or the harmonic scalpel is used to separate the fat from the capsule, with care taken not to get subcapsular. Intraoperative sonography is performed, if available, to assess the depth of the tumor and rule out additional tumors.

The major challenges of laparoscopic nephron-sparing surgery are difficulty performing regional hypothermia (cold ischemia), difficulty maintaining hemostasis if hilar clamping is avoided, and difficulty completing the procedure within a 30-minute warm ischemic period. Previously, numerous techniques were used in an effort to perform simultaneous tumor resection and hemostasis. These included the use of electrocautery, the Cavitron ultrasonic surgical aspirator, the endovascular GIA stapler, the argon bean coagulator, topical agents, ultrasonic energy, microwave thermotherapy, and cable tie compression (32). A 5- to 10-mm rim of normal parenchyma is marked by scoring the renal capsule with electrocautery using the hook electrode. The excision is initiated by dissecting perpendicularly into the kidney along the pyramidal lines. A meticulous effort is made to avoid dissecting too superficially into the pseudocapsule or the tumor itself. The tumor is removed with a 5-mm to 1-cm margin of normal parenchyma. The parenchymal defect is inspected to ensure hemostasis, and if necessary the closure is augmented with adjuvant coagulation (e.g., argon beam) or topical agents (e.g., fibrin glue). These nonhilar clamping PN techniques have been only partially effective in preventing perinephric hemorrhage. They are currently used only selectively, by some surgeons, on polar or very exophytic tumors. More recently, most surgeons have moved toward an LPN technique more closely mimicking the OPN technique, including hilar clamping and parenchymal closure. Although efforts have been made to replicate the regional hypothermia caused by ice slush in open surgery, this has been difficult in the laparoscopic setting due to the technologic and logistical difficulties involved. Efforts to cool the kidney during laparoscopy are further hindered by the flow of room temperature $CO_2$.

Currently, surgeons typically clamp both the renal artery and vein with laparoscopic bulldog clamps, and without cold ischemia rapidly resect the tumor with laparoscopic scissors. This approach causes less tissue distortion than the use of the harmonic scalpel, bipolar cautery, or "hot scissors" (which are ineffective at preventing bleeding or urine leakage) and allows for a more accurate inspection for a positive surgical margin or an opening into the collecting system. Most surgeons attempt to close large (>5mm) urothelial defects with figure-of-eight absorbable sutures (e.g., 4-0 Moncryl). Lapra-Ty clips (Ethicon, Cincinnati, OH) are used by some to speed this process. An interrupted sutured closure of the capsule, often bolstered, is then performed over a Surgicel or Gelfoam sponge (Fig. 124.9). The closure is often augmented by hemostatic agents (e.g., Tisseel or FloSeal) placed directly into the defect or impregnated in the Gelfoam. A roll of Surgicel may also be placed into the defect prior to reapproximating the capsule. Pledgets of numerous materials, including fat, surgical wrapped Gelfoam, and Gore-Tex (W.L. Gore and associates) have been used. The author has also found bovine pericardium to be effective. The bulldog clamps are released and hemostasis assessed. The retroperitoneum is irrigated and aspirated. If hemostasis is adequate at an insufflation pressure of <5 mm Hg, then the perinephric fat is reapproximated. It may be sutured or held in position with clips. A closed system drain (e.g., Jackson-Pratt) is placed outside of the Gerota fascia and away from the renal parenchymal closure. The specimen is placed in a deployable entrapment sack if not done previously and extracted. The incisions are closed.

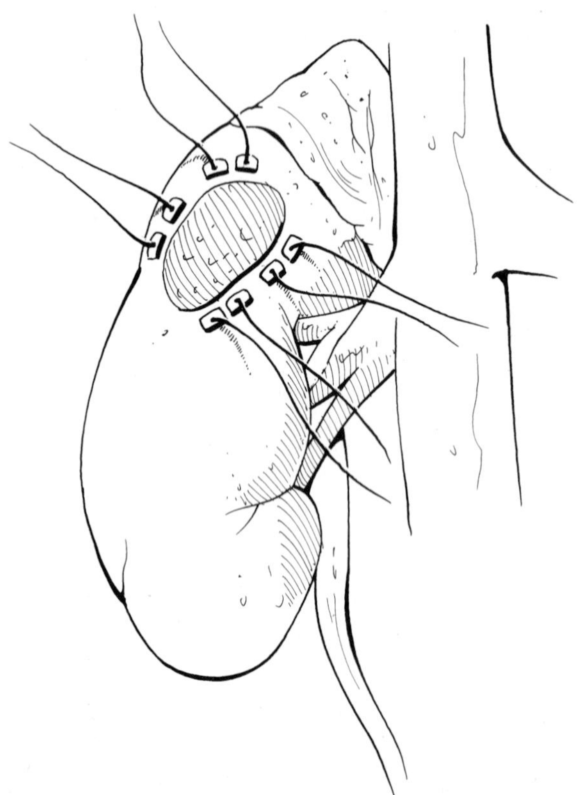

FIGURE 124.9 Resection bed of a right upper-pole tumor. Fibrin glue-impregnated Gelfoam is placed into the defect. Pledgeted interrupted sutures are then used to reapproximate the renal capsule.

## Hand-Assisted Laparoscopic Partial Nephrectomy

The access and renal exposure are similar to HALN. The main disadvantages of HALPN compared to standard laparoscopic PN are that a 7-cm incision is virtually never required to extract the specimen, it may be risky to provide hemostatic control with hand compression alone, and suturing "one-handed" may be difficult. There is further concern regarding increased renal damage due to "intermittent" vascular occlusion, which may occur with hand compression alone. HALPN proponents claim that this technique more closely mimics what many urologic oncologists do during OPN. The hand is used for tumor palpation during tumor excision and may be selectively used to provide hemostasis without hilar clamping. In this situation, the interpolar and opposite polar blood flow will likely be maintained throughout the case, and overall renal recovery and function are likely better. Another advantage is the relative ease of ice slush application through the hand port if hilar clamping is used.

Intraoperative sonography may be used during HALPN to confirm the findings of palpation. The margins of dissection are marked and the specimen excised sharply, using the hand to carefully retract and palpate the tumor during the process. For exophytic polar lesions, a "fibrin glue bandage" of Gelfoam impregnated with Tisseel fibrin sealant (Baxter U.S.) may be used. Prior to this, argon beam coagulation may be used as an adjunct to promote hemostasis. This can be applied through a 5-mm trocar with periodic venting of increased pressure. The "bandage" can be "welded" to the capsule with the argon beam. An unfurled Surgicel dressing may be draped over the "bandage" and around the kidney. The specimen is sent for frozen section analysis to confirm negative margins.

For central or hilar tumors, vascular clamping is employed, and an interrupted parenchymal closure over a "fibrin glue bandage" or rolled Surgicel, similar to the closure described for LPN, is utilized. For both LPN and HALPN, ureteral stents may be positioned in the renal pelvis at the initiation of the case to allow for injection of methylene blue to assess for urothelial defects. The need for this and further the need to close urothelial openings prior to closing the renal parenchyma/capsule has been questioned, and the author does not place a ureteral stent prior to PN and only closes large (≥5-mm) urothelial gaps that occur under hilar clamping control. Once hemostasis is ensured and the specimen removed through the hand port, the incisions are closed.

### Retroperitoneoscopic Partial Nephrectomy

Access and renal exposure are as described in the description of retroperitoneoscopic nephrectomy. This technique is typically performed only by true LPN experts when treating small posterior renal tumors. Hilar dissection and clamping are performed selectively. Excision of the tumor is performed as described for transperitoneal LPN with negative margins confirmed and the defect covered with a fibrin glue bandage if shallow (cortex) or closed with interrupted capsular/parenchymal sutures if deeper (e.g., into the renal medulla). Of note, the limited space within the retroperitoneum makes suturing difficult, and most laparoscopic surgeons prefer to perform LPN transperitoneally. The specimen is entrapped in a deployable sack and removed, followed by hemostasis confirmation, drain placement, and closure.

## POSTOPERATIVE CARE

Postoperative care is similar regardless of the laparoscopic approach, and, with the exception of drain placement for PN, it is similar for nephrectomy and PN patients. Ketorolac (Toradol) 15 mg every 6 hours as requested is typically prescribed for 36 hours. Oral narcotics are made available if necessary. A clear liquid diet is resumed immediately and advanced as tolerated. The patient ambulates on postoperative day 1 and is typically discharged in the evening or the following morning. Parenteral antibiotics are discontinued on postoperative day 1. Oral analgesics are prescribed upon discharge. Dulcolax suppositories are given as necessary for postoperative constipation, and patients are discharged taking a stool softener (e.g., Colace). For PN, the drain is removed when the volume has decreased to <60 to 100 mL per day. If a question exists regarding a urinary leak, a drain fluid creatinine level is obtained.

## OUTCOMES

### Laparoscopic Nephrectomy

In order for LRN to replace ORN as the standard of care, it has to provide equal cancer control with improved patient morbidity and convalescence at comparable operative efficiency. While the latter two issues have been well demonstrated, the remaining most important question is that of long-term cancer control. Several series have now reported overall 5-year disease-free and cancer-specific survival rates for both LRN and HALRN at or over 90%. All have confirmed that the oncologic efficacy of LRN and HALRN is equivalent to that of ORN (8,10,16,26).

In 2007 the Cleveland Clinic reported a 5-year 81% overall and a 90% cancer-specific survival for their LRN cohort compared to a 6-year 79% overall and 92% cancer-specific survival for their ORN cohort. The mean tumor size was 6 cm (5.8 and 6.2 cm, $p = 0.44$). Blood loss and operative times were lower in the LRN cohort (8). Other recent studies have continued to demonstrate that perioperative outcomes, including operative time, blood loss, postoperative analgesia requirements, length of hospital stay, and duration of convalescence, largely favor LRN. However, postoperative convalescence varies widely in patients undergoing laparoscopic kidney procedures. A randomized controlled single-center trial comparing laparoscopic (transperitoneal) with open (flank) simple and radical nephrectomy demonstrated similar, rapid operative times (105 and 93 minutes, $p = 0.4$) in both groups (Burgess) (7). Blood loss, complications, and mortality rates were also similar. The LRN cohort had less postoperative pain returned to normal activity 20 days earlier.

### Laparoscopic Partial Nephrectomy

In 2006 researchers from Johns Hopkins retrospectively reviewed and reported on 143 stage T1 N0 M0 patients who underwent LPN (85) or OPN (58) between 1996 and 2004, with a mean follow-up of 40 +/− 18 months (25). They observed 5-year 91.4% disease-free and 93.8% actuarial survival rates in the LPN cohort and 97.6% and 95.8% rates, respectively, in their OPN cohort. They reported that survival analysis revealed no significant differences and that midrange oncologic results were comparable for pT1 N0 M0 tumors. The Cleveland Clinic subsequently reported their 5-year follow-up outcomes in 2007 (18). One final surgical margin in 37 cancer cases was positive. A single local recurrence (2.7%) and no distant recurrences were identified. Overall and cancer-specific survival rates of 86% and 100%, respectively, were observed. Median serum creatinine levels increased from 0.9 mg per dL preoperatively to 1.0 mg per dL postoperatively. They concluded that these excellent results are comparable to OPN and that LPN is an established alternative at their center. Despite these promising results, they acknowledge that OPN remains the standard of care for small, resectable, solid renal masses and that LPN is an evolving standard.

What then is the current standard LPN technique in this evolving process? The Cleveland Clinic proposed in 2005 that preoperative ureteral catheterization, laparoscopic renal ultrasonography, en bloc renal hilar vascular pedicle clamping, tumor excision with cold Endoshears, pelvicalyceal suture repair, and parenchymal closure over Surgicel bolsters with application of a biologic hemostatic agent and selective use of ice slush for renal hypothermia in cases with anticipated long warm ischemia times is the standard. Others have challenged that a ureteral catheter is not necessary with experience for tumors <4.5 cm and that suture renorrhaphy is not necessary if the renal sinus or collecting system is not entered, given that fibrin glue products will provide adequate hemostasis (3,15). Recently, the Cleveland Clinic group also stated that omitting bolster renorrhaphy may be reasonable, even for select central tumors (33).

## COMPLICATIONS

### Laparoscopic Nephrectomy

Laparoscopy is the current surgical standard for routine simple and radical nephrectomy due to equivalent cancer control and complication rates with decreased patient morbidity and convalescence. Even when laparoscopic nephrectomy has been expanded to treat complex situations, equivalent or nearly equivalent low complication rates have been observed. It is now not only feasible but increasingly reasonable for an experienced laparoscopic surgeon to selectively use LN to treat patients with large stage T2 tumors, stage pT3b tumors, hilar lymphadenopathy, kidneys needing autotransplantation, bilateral renal tumors, horseshoe kidneys, autosomal polycystic kidney disease (ADPKD), xanthogranulomatous pyelonephritis, profound obesity, and even level II caval thrombi (30). Although da Vinci (Intuitive, Sunnyvale, CA) robotic-assisted laparoscopic surgery has little role in routine LN, it may have a future role in certain complex procedures, such as caval thrombectomy.

Technologic malfunction may cause surgical complications and is an important area of concern for laparoscopic surgery. Recent complications secondary to malfunction of polymer self-locking (Hem-O-Lock) clips are an example (21). Bleeding, delayed exploration, and even death were reported in several patients undergoing LN. The Hem-O-Lock clip is thus no longer recommended for laparoscopic donor nephrectomy renal vessel ligation. This will hopefully stimulate the future development of an inexpensive and improved vessel-grasping and ligating clip.

Of importance, complications do occur at an increased rate during a surgeon's initial learning curve. Improvements in training and skills distribution throughout the urologic community are therefore needed. Although LN has made great inroads into the academic centers, its adoption into private, community practice has lagged behind (1). Laparoscopic-naïve open renal surgeons currently in practice need to remember that a significant time investment in retraining is required to work through an approximately 20-case learning curve (6). It is also critical that new technology does not inappropriately supersede a more appropriate operative procedure, as is highlighted by concerns that LRN may be inappropriately replacing PN in the treatment of small renal tumors (22). Lastly, reassessment of the complications and morbidity of techniques as they evolve is necessary. It is possible that future developments in open and HAL surgery, such as minimization of incision lengths, alteration of incision locations, and improved analgesia, may minimize current LN advantages and warrant re-evaluation of the appropriate role of various surgical procedures. Also, future expansion of indications for nephron-sparing renal surgery could diminish the role of LRN.

## Laparoscopic Partial Nephrectomy

Whereas equivalent LRN and ORN complication rates are now commonplace, the same is not true for LPN. In 2002 the Cleveland Clinic reported that LRN had morbidity advantages over OPN, but OPN had the long-term renal function advantage (20). The following year, they reported that LPN has a greater positive surgical margin rate (3% versus 0%, $p = 0.1$) and intraoperative complication rate (5% versus 0%, $p = 0.02$) than OPN (12). Subsequent efforts have been made to demonstrate the utility and safety of LPN. Feasibility and near-equivalent outcomes have been demonstrated in obese patients, centrally located and hilar tumors, solitary kidneys, cystic masses, pT2–pT3b tumors, and kidneys with multiple tumors or renal arteries. Retroperitoneoscopic PN has also demonstrated equivalent outcomes, but it is considered a more difficult operation than transperitoneal PN due to decreased working space.

In a John Hopkins University series, a 15% overall conversion rate of LPN to LRN (13.6%, 35 patients) and LPN to open surgery (1.6%, 4 patients) was observed among 257 operations started as LPN (27). A fourfold increased rate of conversion was noted in patients over 70 years old or with tumors >4 cm. In a review of the Cleveland Clinic's first 200 LPN cases, one third (66) had complications (28). These included a 9.5% (19) hemorrhage and a 4.5% (9) urine leakage rate, 8 of which required double-J stent placement with (2) or without (6) percutaneous drain placement. Two (1%) patients required open conversion and 4 (2%) reoperation. In a subsequent report, a 1.7% renal artery pseudoaneurysm rate in 345 cases was observed, and all 6 patients were effectively treated with percutaneous embolization. Similar LPN complication rates have also been reported from other centers. Importantly, Gill et al. (13) reduced their hemorrhagic complication rate from 12% to 3% by applying gelatin matrix thrombin sealant (FloSeal) to the PN defect prior to sutured renorrhaphy over a Surgicel bolster. They addressed urinary extravasation by running the defect bed with 2-0 Vicryl and testing the repair with gentle injection of indigo carmine through a ureteral catheter. A more recent 200-case series of LPN at the Cleveland Clinic had a complication rate approaching the level observed with OPN (31).

Despite improvements, there remain four principal concerns with LPN: (a) controlling hemostasis, (b) obtaining negative margins (particularly during the learning curve), (c) avoiding lengthy (>30 minutes) warm ischemic times and renal injury, and (d) treating large, complex, or centrally located tumors.

Regarding hemorrhage, the more central or endophytic the tumor, the greater the risk (5). Upper-pole tumors may also create hemostasis challenges. Numerous efforts to prevent bleeding can be categorized as follows: (a) improvement in PN defect closure, (b) energy application, (c) use of hemostatic agents or glues, and (d) superselective embolization prior to LPN. The first category includes use of Lapra-Ty or Hem-O-Lock clips and temporary defect packing. The second category includes use of a saline-irrigated KTP laser, water jet, TissueLink floating ball monopolar device, and radiofrequency coagulation prior to PN. Examples of the third category are gelatin matrix thrombin (FloSeal), fibrin gel (Tisseel), bovine serum albumin (BioGlue), cyanoacrylate glue (Glubran), and autologous fibrin glue.

In a review of positive surgical margins, Breda et al. (4) identified a 2.4% overall rate in 855 U.S. and European LPN procedures. However, surgeons in their initial 30 cases of LPN or HALPN may have positive margin rates ≥10% (23). Fortunately, a large combined review from centers of excellence demonstrated that a positive margin does not necessarily indicate residual disease (25). Nevertheless, efforts to prevent positive margins during LPN should continue.

Warm ischemia >30 minutes has historically been considered detrimental to renal recovery. Recent studies have found that up to 60 minutes may be well tolerated by the human kidney, and a review of LPN patients at Johns Hopkins observed no significant relationship between warm ischemia and creatinine change and no statistically significant increase in serum creatinine postoperatively (2). There is, however, contradictory evidence that the renal damage caused by warm ischemia >30 minutes is only partially reversible. A Cleveland Clinic study observed increased risk of renal dysfunction with warm ischemic times >30 minutes, advanced age, or pre-existing azotemia (9). Porcine studies have found that clamping the renal artery was beneficial in protecting the kidney only during OPN but not during LPN. Importantly, efforts to identify a practical method of creating laparoscopic renal hypothermia have been numerous, yet none have become widely utilized. "On demand" hilar clamping has been recently proposed, and efforts to address this problem will undoubtedly continue.

Given the complexity of standard LPN, surgeons have developed innovative approaches, such as the use of suspension traction sutures, to facilitate tumor exposure, dissection angles, and defect closure (24). As expected, several groups have investigated the potential of da Vinci robot-assisted LPN. Surgeons from the National Institutes of Health successfully treated 14 complex tumors including hilar location (5), endophytic (4) and multiple tumors (3) with robotic LPN (29). It is possible that the da Vinci robot will, like robotic prostatectomy, decrease the learning curve, allow for more facile suturing and tumor excision, and greatly increase the propagation of this procedure into the urologic community.

In conclusion, LN is the current standard of care in many industrialized countries. LPN outcomes now closely approach those of OPN at elite centers. However, even at these centers, OPN remains the gold standard due to shorter ischemic times, slightly better retained renal function (99.6% versus 97.9% at 3 months), reduced postoperative complications, and decreased subsequent procedures (11). The eventual fate of LPN hinges upon how well future technologic and procedural modifications address these concerns and how well renal tumor ablative procedures perform over the long term.

## *References*


1. Best S, Ercole B, Lee C, et al. Minimally invasive therapy for renal cell carcinoma: is there a new community standard? *Urology* 2004;64:22–25.
2. Bhayani SB, Rha KH, Pinto PA, et al. Laparoscopic partial nephrectomy: effect of warm ischemia on serum creatinine. *J Urol* 2004;172:1264–1266.
3. Bove P, Bhanyan SB, Rha KH, et al. Necessity of ureteral catheterization during laparoscopic partial nephrectomy. *J Urol* 2004;172:458–460.
4. Breda A, Stepanian SV, Liao J, et al. Positive margins in laparoscopic partial nephrectomy in 855 cases: a multi-institutional survey from the United States and Europe. *J Urol* 2007;178:47–50.
5. Brown JA, Hubosky SC, Gomella LG, et al. Hand-assisted laparoscopic partial nephrectomy for peripheral and central lesions: a review of 30 consecutive cases. *J Urol* 2004;171:1443–1446.
6. Brown JA, Shah S, Siddiqi K, et al. Incorporation of hand-assisted laparoscopic nephrectomy into an academic training program: an assessment of the utility of a 3-month minifellowship. *J Laparoendosc Adv Surg Tech A* 2007;17:435–439.
7. Burgess NA, Koo BC, Calvert RC, et al. Randomized trial of laparoscopic v open nephrectomy. *J Endourol* 2007;21:610–613.
8. Columbo JR, Haber GP, Aron M, et al. Oncological outcomes of laparoscopic radical nephrectomy for renal cancer. *Clinics* 2007;62:251–256.
9. Desai MM, Gill IS, Ramani AP, et al. The impact of warm ischaemia on renal function after laparoscopic partial nephrectomy. *BJU Int* 2005;95: 377–383.
10. Eskicorapci SY, Teber D, Schulze M, et al. Laparoscopic radical nephrectomy: the new gold standard surgical treatment for localized renal cell carcinoma. *Sci World J* 2007;7:825–836.
11. Gill IS, Kavoussi LR, Lane BR, et al. Comparison of 1800 laparoscopic and open partial nephrectomies for single renal tumors. *J Urol* 2007;178: 41–46.
12. Gill IS, Matin SF, Desai MM, et al. Comparative analysis of laparoscopic versus open partial nephrectomy for renal tumors in 200 patients. *J Urol* 2003;170:64–68.
13. Gill IS, Ramani AP, Spaliviero M, et al. Improved hemostasis during laparoscopic partial nephrectomy using gelatin matrix thrombin sealant. *Urology* 2005;65:463–466.
14. Gillenwater JY, Grayhack JT, Howards SS, et al., eds. *Adult and pediatric urology*, 3rd ed. Mosby-Year Book, 1996.
15. Johnston WK, Montgomery JS, Seifman BD, et al. Fibrin glue v sutured bolster: lessons learned during 100 laparoscopic partial nephrectomies. *J Urol* 2005;74:47–52.
16. Kawauchi A, Yoneda K, Fujita A, et al. Oncologic outcome of hand-assisted laparoscopic nephrectomy. *Urology* 2007;69:53–56.
17. Kouba E, Smith AM, Derksen JE, et al. Efficacy and safety of en bloc ligation of renal hilum during laparoscopic nephrectomy. *Urology* 2007;69: 226–229.
18. Lane BR, Gill IS. 5-Year outcomes of laparoscopic partial nephrectomy. *J Urol* 2007;177:70–74.
19. Matin SF, Dhanani N, Acosta M, et al. Conventional and hand-assisted laparoscopic radical nephrectomy: comparative analysis of 271 cases. *J Endourol* 2006;20:891–894.
20. Matin SF, Gill IS, Worley S, et al. Outcomes of laparoscopic radical and open partial nephrectomy for the sporadic 4cm. or less renal tumor with a normal contralateral kidney. *J Urol* 2002;168:1356–1359.
21. Meng MV. Reported failure of the polymer self-locking (Hem-o-lok) clip: review of data from the Food and Drug Administration. *J Endourol* 2006;20:1054–1057.
22. Miller DC, Hollingsworth JM, Hafez KS, et al. Partial nephrectomy for small renal masses: an emerging quality of care concern? *J Urol* 2006; 175:853–857.
23. Nadu A, Mor Y, Laufer M, et al. Laparoscopic partial nephrectomy: single center experience with 140 patients—evolution of the surgical technique and its impact on outcomes. *J Urol* 2007;178:435–439.
24. Orvieto MA, Chien GW, Tolhurst SR, et al. Simplifying laparoscopic partial nephrectomy: technical considerations for reproducible outcomes. *Urology* 2005;66:976–980.
25. Permpongkosol S, Bagga JS, Romero FR, et al. Laparoscopic versus open partial nephrectomy for the treatment of pathological T1N0M0 renal cell carcinoma: a 5-year survival rate. *J Urol* 2006;176:1984–1988.
26. Permpongkosol S, Chan DY, Link RE, et al. Laparoscopic radical nephrectomy: long-term outcomes. *J Endourol* 2005;19:628–633.
27. Rais-Bahramis, Lima GC, Varkarakis IM, et al. Intraoperative conversion of laparoscopic partial nephrectomy. *J Endourol* 2006;20:205–208.
28. Ramani AP, Desai MM, Steinberg AP, et al. Complications of laparoscopic partial nephrectomy in 200 cases. *J Urol* 2005;173:42–47.
29. Rogers CG, Singh A, Blatt AM, et al. Robotic partial nephrectomy for complex renal tumors: surgical technique. *Eur Urol* 2007 *(Epub ahead of print)*.
30. Romero FR, Muntener M, Bagga HS, et al. Pure laparoscopic radical nephrectomy with level II vena caval thrombectomy. *Urology* 2006;68: 1112–1114.
31. Simmons MN, Gill IS. Decreased complications of contemporary laparoscopic partial nephrectomy: use of a standardized reporting system. *J Urol* 2007;177:2067–2073.
32. Walsh PC, Retik AB, Vaughan ED, et al., eds. *Campbell's urology*, 8th ed. Philadelphia: WB Saunders, 2002.
33. Weight CJ, Lane BR, Gill IS. Laparoscopic partial nephrectomy for selected central tumours: omitting the bolster. *BJU Int* 2007;100:375–378.

# CHAPTER 125 ■ LAPAROSCOPIC NEPHROURETERECTOMY

SCOTT G. HUBOSKY AND MICHAEL D. FABRIZIO

Malignant urothelial tumors of the upper urinary tract account for about 5% to 10% of all renal tumors and 5% of all urothelial tumors. These lesions are relatively rare and have an observed peak incidence of 10 per 100,000 per year (1). The most common location of these lesions is the renal pelvis, followed by the distal ureter, the midureter, and finally the proximal ureter. Tumors of the renal pelvis are almost twice as common as tumors in the ureter. Bilateral involvement of malignant urothelial tumors of the upper urinary tracts occur in 2% to 5% of spontaneous cases. Upper tract lesions are seen in 2% to 4% of patients with primary urothelial carcinoma of the bladder.

## DIAGNOSIS

Hematuria and dysuria are the most common symptoms. Often flank pain is present in those with upper tract obstruction, but sometimes asymptomatic hydronephrosis is seen. Patients presenting with ureteral stricture in the absence of overt benign etiologies should be seriously considered for ureteroscopy and biopsy. However, a filling defect is the usual initial finding on a dedicated upper tract imaging study. Rarely, patients will present with urosepsis and hydronephrosis necessitating percutaneous nephrostomy tube placement. An antegrade nephrostogram can also demonstrate filling defects consistent with upper tract tumors (Fig. 125.1). Biopsy is suggested since filling defects are nonspecific findings and because tumor grade will dictate the management strategy.

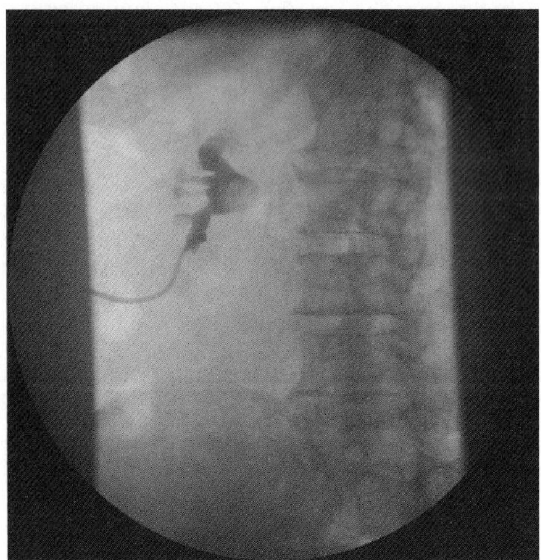

FIGURE 125.1 Antegrade nephrostogram demonstrating a filling defect in the renal pelvis. This patient presented with urosepsis and hydronephrosis.

## INDICATIONS FOR SURGERY

Many variables, including tumor size, location, and grade and extent of disease, need to be considered before choosing a surgical therapy. Additionally, the functional status of the renal unit in question as well as the presence or absence of a contralateral kidney will help guide management decisions. Kidneys with cortical thinning and marginal functional status are likely better treated with nephroureterectomy. Patients with solitary renal units may choose conservative renal-sparing strategies and accept lower cancer-free rates in order to avoid the morbidity associated with dialysis following nephroureterectomy (2). Absolute contraindications for laparoscopic nephroureterectomy include uncorrected coagulopathies, active untreated abdominal wall infection, or significant hemoperitoneum. Relative contraindications include a history of multiple abdominal surgeries or locally advanced disease, both of which may require conversion to open surgery.

## ALTERNATIVE THERAPY

Radical nephroureterectomy is considered the gold-standard therapy for malignant lesions of the upper urinary tracts. This entails removal of the kidney within the fascia of Gerota along with the entire length of ipsilateral ureter, including en bloc resection of the intramural ureter and ureteral orifice with surrounding bladder cuff. More conservative alternatives exist and were initially reserved for patients in whom nephroureterectomy would be contraindicated, such as patients with solitary kidneys, renal insufficiency, or significant comorbidities. Endoscopic procedures such as ureteroscopy and percutaneous nephroscopy can be considered for those patients with low-grade, low-stage malignancies who are willing to undergo rigorous surveillance schedules. With high 5-year survival rates in patients with low-grade tumors, the utilization of ureteroscopy (3) and percutaneous nephroscopy (4) has been extended to patients with low-grade, low-stage disease with a normal contralateral kidney. Radical nephroureterectomy remains the mainstay of treatment for high-grade disease. Many advocate this approach even in patients with solitary kidneys, although others accept percutaneous or ureteroscopic procedures and cite the benefit of avoiding dialysis morbidity against lower disease-specific survival rates. Urologists who treat upper tract urothelial lesions were surveyed about how they treat high-grade lesions in a solitary kidney. Among those responding, 34% favored a nephroureterectomy with the subsequent need for dialysis, while 30% and 27% chose to treat the patient with ureteroscopy or percutaneous resection, respectively (5). Although not curative, endoscopic options are attractive in order to minimize gross hematuria and obstruction in these patients in an effort to improve quality of life. Clayman et al. (6) reported the first laparoscopic nephroureterectomy (LNU) in 1991. In stark contrast to open nephroureterectomy (ONU), which requires either two separate incisions or a single lengthy incision, early series of both LNU and hand-assisted laparoscopic nephroureterectomy (HALNU) very quickly showed a benefit with respect to length of hospital stay, narcotic requirement, and convalescence (6–8). Short- and intermediate-term oncologic outcomes for LNU and HALNU have shown equivalence to ONU, and recently long-term oncologic outcomes with median follow-up of 74 months (range 60 to 148 months) have shown a 5-year disease-specific survival of 68%, comparing well with many ONU series (9). An admitted limitation of this retrospective case series was a small patient population ($n$ = 39), and other large series must be reported before definitive equivalence is determined.

## SURGICAL TECHNIQUE

Just as in ONU, it is useful to consider separate approaches for the kidney and the distal ureter in LNU. There are multiple acceptable laparoscopic approaches to the kidney that have been described, including transperitoneal, retroperitoneal, and hand-assisted techniques. The choice of technique for renal excision is based primarily on the surgeon's preference and training. All three approaches have the important advantage of avoiding a flank incision or an upward extension of a midline incision. HALNU can be used primarily or as an alternative to standard laparoscopic technique if advanced or bulky disease is present.

Multiple options exist for excision of the distal ureter, and currently no consensus has been established as to the optimal method (Table 125.1). Despite the diverse list of options for techniques available, one clear principle shared by all authors is the absolute need to completely resect the entire ipsilateral ureter with a cuff of bladder. Earlier studies demonstrated upwards of 30% recurrence rates when remnants of ureter are left behind after incomplete nephroureterectomy for upper tract urothelial carcinoma (10).

In addition, other factors must be considered in choosing a technique for the distal ureter (Table 125.2). The presence of synchronous bladder tumors mandates maintenance of a closed system and precludes transvesical placement of instruments or formal cystotomy to expose the trigone. Ideally, transurethral resection of bladder tumor (TURBT) should be performed at a separate setting in order to clear the bladder of any overt tumors. Knowledge of the primary tumor location in the upper urinary tract is also critical for surgical planning. The presence of tumor in the distal or intramural ureter typically leads to an open distal ureterectomy with either an intravesical or extravesical approach. The need for repositioning and safety of the contralateral ureteral orifice must also be considered.

**TABLE 125.1**

**DESCRIBED TECHNIQUES FOR DISTAL URETERAL EXCISION TO ACCOMPANY LAPAROSCOPIC NEPHROURETERECTOMY**

- Open approach (intravesical or extravesical approach)
- Pure laparoscopic approach with stapling of distal ureter and bladder cuff (8)
- Transvesical laparoscopic detachment and ligation technique (17)
- Transurethral resection of ureteral orifice (TURUO)
- Intussusception
- Extravesical en bloc distal ureterectomy with bladder cuff during hand-assisted laparoscopic nephroureterectomy (28)
- One-port transvesical endoscopic cuff technique (26)
- Robot-assisted laparoscopic nephroureterectomy (29)

**TABLE 125.2**

**CONSIDERATIONS IN SELECTING A METHOD FOR DISTAL URETERECTOMY**

- Opportunity for complete excision of distal ureter and bladder cuff
- Location of primary tumor and any other synchronous upper tract lesions
- Presence of any synchronous bladder tumors
- Presence of pelvic lymphadenopathy
- History of pelvic radiation
- Body habitus
- Safety of the contralateral ureteral orifice
- Need for patient repositioning

### Transperitoneal Laparoscopic Radical Nephroureterectomy

The authors prefer a transperitoneal conventional laparoscopic approach, which allows for a larger working space, while the retroperitoneal approach usually allows for faster access to the hilum.

Preoperative evaluation should include a computerized tomography (CT) urogram to define the location of the upper tract lesion, to evaluate for any existing lymphadenopathy or overt local disease extension, and to define the anatomy of the renal vasculature. It is our preference to have biopsy information about the lesion in question, which also allows an opportunity to evaluate and treat any synchronous bladder tumors. Additional preoperative workup includes chest radiography, serum electrolytes, complete blood count, liver function tests, and coagulation studies. No formal bowel preparation is instituted, but magnesium citrate solution is given the day before surgery and the patient is asked to stay on a diet of clear liquids that day as well.

After the adequate administration of general anesthesia, an orogastric tube and Foley catheter are placed. This helps to minimize any inadvertent trocar injuries to distended viscera. Spontaneous compression boot devices and intravenous antibiotics are given prior to induction. The patient is placed in a modified decubitus position with the operative side up and propped 30 to 45 degrees from the horizontal plane. A blanket roll is placed under the shoulders and hips in order to help support this position. An axillary roll is also placed at this time. The top of the patient's iliac crest should align with the top of the kidney rest on the operating room table. The table is then flexed about 20 to 30 degrees in order to help maximize the space between the costal margin and the anterior superior iliac spine. The ipsilateral arm is brought across the torso and supported either with pillows or preferably an elevated arm rest. The contralateral arm is placed on the usual arm board perpendicular to the operating table. Pillows are placed between the legs. The downside leg is flexed at the knee and all pressure points must be adequately padded. The patient is then carefully secured to the table with 3-inch tape at the level of the shoulders, hips, and legs just above the knees. This position is then checked for stability.

Access to the peritoneal cavity is achieved with a Veress needle placed in the area of the ipsilateral midclavicular line between the umbilicus and the anterior iliac crest. Alternatively, the Veress needle can be placed just superior to the umbilicus and pointed in the cephalad direction. Gentle injection of saline and failure to aspirate any abdominal contents through the needle help ensure that no bowel or vascular structures have been entered. Carbon dioxide insufflation is commenced and opening pressures should be <10 mm Hg until the abdomen is symmetrically distended. Insufflation is maintained at a pressure of 15 to 20 mm Hg for the case.

Typically a three-port technique is employed, with the occasional additional 5-mm port added as necessary to help with retraction (Fig. 125.2). After pneumoperitoneum is achieved, a 1-cm incision is made in the midclavicular line at the level of the umbilicus. A 10- to 12-mm port is inserted with the use of a zero-degree 10-mm laparoscopic lens. This allows for direct visualization of the initial port placement and the peritoneal cavity is easily identified upon entry. The abdominal contents are surveyed. The second 10- to 12-mm port is placed at the umbilicus using a periumbilical incision. Finally, the third port is placed between the umbilicus and the xiphoid process. For right-sided cases an additional 5-mm port is added just off the tip of the 12th rib to allow for upward retraction of the liver. If colonic retraction is necessary, an additional 5-mm port can be placed in the midline between the umbilicus and the pubic symphysis.

## Left Laparoscopic Radical Nephroureterectomy

The 10- to 12-mm umbilical port is used to place a 10-mm, 30-degree laparoscope, and the surgeon works with instruments through the lateral and subxiphoid ports. Many electrosurgical ligation devices are available, but we prefer to use monopolar electrosurgical scissors and a 10-mm LigaSure device. Alternatively, the harmonic scalpel is also useful. Laparoscopic bipolar forceps are very useful in controlling small points of bleeding, especially around the hilum.

Initial survey of the abdominal contents will allow identification of vital structures, including the colon, spleen, and iliac vessels. The kidney, although not directly visible, is easily palpable with the laparoscopic instruments. Laparoscopic DeBakey instruments are very useful in providing countertraction and help in identification of the white line of Toldt. A combination of sharp and blunt dissection is utilized to reflect the colon from the splenic flexure down to the level of the internal ring. This includes division of the phrenocolic and splenorenal ligaments. Division of splenophrenic ligaments allows for upward retraction of the spleen and better exposure to the anterior surface of the kidney. Once the colon is mobilized, the colorenal ligaments are easily identified. The colonic mesentery must be dissected free from the anterior surface of the fascia of Gerota. A subtle color difference in the fat of these two structures is appreciable and helps direct the surgeon to the correct plane of dissection. Mesenteric fat is a lemon-yellow shade, while the fat around the fascia of Gerota is more of a pale-white color. Division of the colorenal ligaments must be achieved in order to expose the renal hilum. Dissection of these ligaments usually proceeds from inferiorly to superiorly.

Next the psoas muscle is identified off the lower pole of the kidney, and the psoas tendon is usually easily recognized. Within the confines of retroperitoneal fat the gonadal vein and ureter should be identified. The ureter is now secured, with care to leave surrounding adventitia for adequate achievement of a good surgical margin. At this point in the dissection, the ureter can be traced as inferiorly as possible, which will facilitate later complete distal ureterectomy with bladder cuff excision. After this is achieved, attention can be returned to the renal dissection.

Careful elevation of the ureter allows for upward retraction of the undersurface of the kidney, lower pole, and hilar structures. Tracing the gonadal vein superiorly helps identify the inferior aspect of the renal vein. Just as in open surgery, a

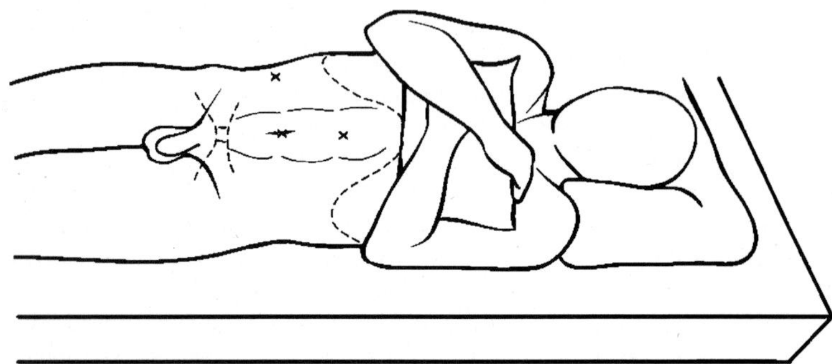

FIGURE 125.2 Port placement for laparoscopic nephroureterectomy. The camera is placed in the umbilical port and the surgeon works through the other two ports, making use of triangulation to optimize visualization and ergonomics. To better access the distal ureter, an additional port can be placed in the midline between the umbilicus and pubic symphysis.

split-and-roll technique is employed by gently grasping the surrounding adventitia, pulling away from the vein and carefully splitting the adventitia with laparoscopic scissors in order to expose the anterior surface of the vein. Once the anterior surface is exposed, hilar fat around the vein must be carefully dissected out. This is achieved by gently grasping surrounding adventitia and hilar fat with a laparoscopic DeBakey grasper, which provides excellent countertraction and allows one to sweep the edge of the vein free with a blunt suction-irrigator device. Ultimately, all tributaries of the left renal vein can be carefully dissected out this way, including the gonadal, lumbar, and adrenal veins. The laparoscopic DeBakey should be able to be easily placed behind any vein prior to its division. The 10-mm LigaSure device provides for safe division of the gonadal, adrenal, and lumbar veins without the use of clips. This allows for easier future placement of the Endo-GIA vascular stapling device across the main renal vein without having to consider the avoidance of surrounding clips. Some surgeons feel the 10-mm LigaSure device is too large or cumbersome to secure some of the left renal vein tributaries, and this is sometimes the case, especially with the lumbar vein. In this event, the tributaries can be taken with clips, as described by many authors. Of the tributaries of the left renal vein, the gonadal is usually encountered and taken first, followed by the lumbar vein. If adrenalectomy is planned, then the adrenal vein should be taken as well.

Once the renal vein is mobilized and its tributaries are divided as needed, the renal artery is usually identified just posterior and superior to the vein. Gentle upward traction of the kidney allows for identification of the renal artery from a posterior position. A combination of sharp and blunt dissection is used to free the edges of the artery, and ultimately this structure is taken with a 10-mm endoscopic GIA stapler with 2.5-mm or 2.0-mm staples. The vein is taken in a similar fashion.

After hilar division, the kidney can be retracted superiorly and any remaining posterior or lateral attachments are divided. If the adrenal gland is being taken, then superior medial attachments are carefully taken down with either an endo-GIA stapler or the LigaSure device. Care must be taken to avoid the tail of the pancreas. The kidney should be freed from all attachments at this point and should still remain with the ureter intact and attached.

## Right Laparoscopic Radical Nephroureterectomy

Laparoscopic port placement is essentially a mirror image of the right side. An additional 5-mm port is almost always needed to help with retraction of the liver. This additional port is well placed just off the tip of the 12th rib. Care must be taken not to place this additional port too close to the iliac crest, as this will limit the ability to point the trocar in the necessary cephalad direction. Once the liver is retracted anteriorly, the upper pole of the right kidney is easily seen and the ascending colon is easily swept medially after taking down the white line of Toldt. Great care must be taken to identify and avoid the duodenum, which is readily seen after the colon is mobilized. We strongly advocate performance of a laparoscopic Kocher maneuver with cold laparoscopic scissors. A laparoscopic DeBakey grasper is very helpful in providing countertraction for the overlying adventitia anterior to the duodenum. The duodenum is easily swept medially once the overlying adventitia is carefully incised. The inferior vena cava is readily identified once the duodenum is dissected free. With upward traction of the posterior portion of the kidney, the renal vein is identified and dissection is similar to that for the left side.

## Hand-Assisted Laparoscopic Nephroureterectomy

Hand-assisted laparoscopy greatly facilitates LNU due to the versatility of the approach in addressing the distal ureter and the fact that the hand speeds ureteral mobilization, especially in cases of inflamed or adherent ureters. Many HALNU series have been reported in the literature and demonstrate good oncologic control and safety parameters (7,11–13). The hand port not only allows for the nephrectomy portion of the case but is also used in performing complete ureteral dissection with excision of bladder cuff. The port placement for left HALNU is shown in Figure 125.3. In a left-sided case, the surgeon inserts the left hand with use of any of the available hand ports. This is done through a 7-cm midline incision that starts at the umbilicus and extends downward. This is slightly lower than the midline incision used for hand-assisted laparoscopic nephrectomy (HALN). A 10- to 12-mm port is placed just lateral to the rectus muscle at the level of the hand port, and this supports the laparoscope. A second 10- to 12-mm port is placed about two fingerbreadths anterior to the tip of the 12th rib. In a left HALNU, the surgeon uses the right hand to operate the laparoscopic instruments. After the nephrectomy portion of the case, the opposite hand is placed in the hand port position and attention is turned toward the distal ureter. The left hand is then used to operate laparoscopic instruments as the ureter is dissected down to the bladder hiatus. An additional 5-mm port can be placed in the midline below the hand port to aid in medial retraction of the bladder. The intracorporeal hand allows for multidirectional ureteral traction until the ureter is followed all the way down to the bladder. Under direct vision the bladder is entered superiorly and medially to the ureteral orifice. The Foley

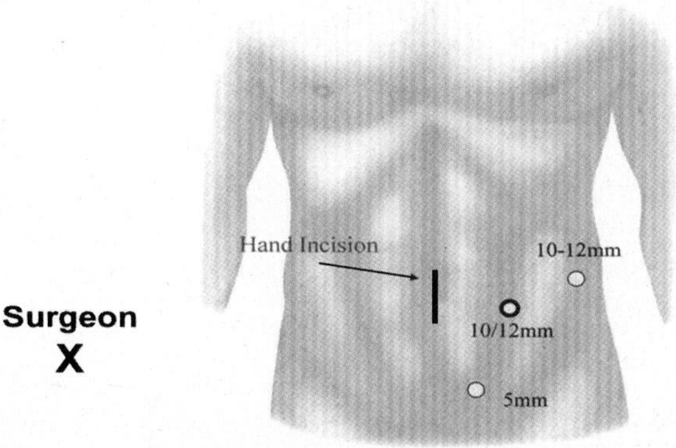


FIGURE 125.3 Port and hand-assist device placement for left hand-assisted laparoscopic nephroureterectomy.

catheter balloon should be readily visible, as should be the contralateral ureteral orifice. The cystotomy can be left open or sutured closed. The entire specimen is then removed in an entrapment sack through the midline hand incision. In addition to this method, the midline hand incision can be extended down to the pubic symphysis if the surgeon prefers an open approach to distal ureterectomy. This results in a midline incision from the umbilicus to the pubic symphysis, which may be considered large by many laparoscopic surgeons but is still well tolerated and much less invasive than two separate incisions or a midline incision spanning the distance from xiphoid to pubic symphysis.

## Surgical Approaches to the Distal Ureter

There is no clear consensus for the ideal minimally invasive approach to the distal ureter during LNU or HALNU. No prospective randomized trials exist comparing the various techniques, and the number of cases is relatively small, making level 1 evidence unavailable. Numerous retrospective surgical series have been published and many make use of different techniques as the specific patient situation dictates. Perhaps the consensus should be that no single technique is ideal in every situation.

In choosing a technique, the location of the primary tumor and any other synchronous tumors must be known. While many distal ureteral techniques will be successful for tumors in the renal pelvis or proximal ureter, they may be completely inappropriate for tumors located primarily in the distal ureter (Fig. 125.4). The following descriptions are of the most popular techniques found in the current literature.

### Open Approach

An open approach to the distal ureter is still considered the gold standard from an oncologic viewpoint. It is probably the most appropriate technique when the primary lesion is in the distal ureter. The approach is versatile and can be combined with a conventional laparoscopic renal excision, whether performed via the transperitoneal or retroperitoneal route. It can also be performed in concert with HALNU. The presence of an open incision is acceptable by most who perform LNU or HALNU due to the preference for intact specimen removal, which is essential in determining the need for adjuvant chemotherapy in higher-stage disease.

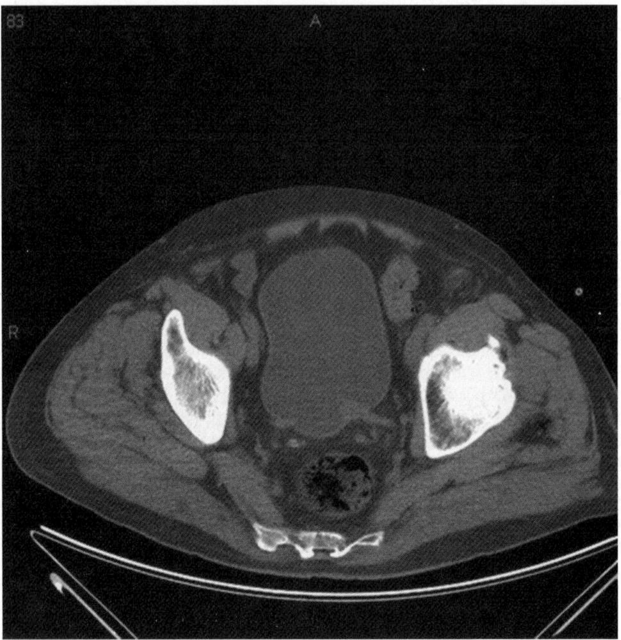

FIGURE 125.4 Computerized tomography scan demonstrating a distal ureteral tumor in the left intramural ureter, thus confirming the importance of acknowledging tumor location.

During LNU or HALNU the ureter should be dissected as inferiorly as possible, which is usually at least to the level of the iliac vessels. If HALNU is being performed, then the midline hand incision should be extended to the pubic symphysis. If conventional LNU is performed, then a variety of options are available, including a lower midline incision, a Pfannenstiel incision, or a Gibson incision. If there is difficulty with ureteral dissection laparoscopically, then a Gibson incision may be used, which can be extended to reach the upper mid- to proximal ureter if needed. If a partial flank position is employed for the LNU, the lower abdominal incision can be fashioned by merely rotating the table, thus avoiding the need for patient repositioning.

Access to both the peritoneal cavity and retroperitoneum is possible through the three incisions mentioned above and is utilized depending on the approach to the kidney. Once the ureter is identified, it should be clipped distal to the primary tumor to minimize downward migration of any tumor cells. As the ureter is followed into the pelvis, the vas deferens or round ligament will be encountered and should be taken. It is possible to spare the vas deferens in young men, although this can compromise exposure. Classic open descriptions of distal ureterectomy direct the surgeon to isolate and divide the superior vesicle artery as it crosses the ureter (14). The medial umbilical ligament should also be identified and divided to maximize exposure to the distal ureter as it enters the detrusor.

In order to resect the bladder cuff and ureteral orifice, an intravesical or extravesical approach can be employed. If the intravesical route is chosen, an anterior cystotomy is performed with the bladder full. The trigone and ureteral orifice are readily visualized. A 5Fr feeding tube can be inserted into the affected ureteral orifice and stitched to the surrounding bladder urothelium. This allows for upward and radial retraction of the intraluminal ureter as the urothelium is scored with needle-tip electrocautery. The intramural ureter is identified and resected out of the surrounding detrusor muscle until perivesical adipose tissue is seen. The kidney, ureter, and bladder cuff are then completely removed en bloc through the skin incision after being placed in an entrapment sack. The resected ureteral orifice can be closed through the bladder in layers with absorbable suture. Finally, the anterior cystotomy is closed in layers, also with absorbable suture. A Jackson-Pratt drain is placed in the perivesical space. No suprapubic tube is necessary, and a Foley catheter is kept in place for 4 days and then removed after a cystogram is performed. The main advantage of an intravesical approach is complete visualization of both the affected and contralateral ureteral orifices. This lends to complete resection of the intramural ureter with bladder cuff and safe preservation of the contralateral orifice. A closed system is not maintained, however, and a cystoscopy should be done prior to nephroureterectomy to ensure no synchronous bladder tumors are present.

An extravesical approach can also be used in which the distal ureter is dissected free of detrusor down to the ureterovesical junction. With upward traction on the ureter, the ureteral orifice is stretched away from the urothelium of the bladder and a right angle is clamped down. The ureteral orifice is then transected and the posterior bladder oversewn. The advantage of this technique is maintenance of a closed system and avoidance of anterior cystotomy. The disadvantages are potentially difficult exposure, predisposing to incomplete resection of the affected intramural ureter, and no direct visualization of the contralateral ureter, which may be inadvertently resected or sewn over. The administration of indigo carmine to the patient intravenously after sewing over the posterior cystotomy can give reassurance of the status of the contralateral ureteral orifice if blue urine is seen in the Foley collection bag.

### Pure Laparoscopic Approach with Stapling of Distal Ureter and Bladder Cuff

This technique involves conventional laparoscopic nephrectomy with extended dissection of the ureter deep within the pelvis. An additional lower midline abdominal port is required to complement those traditionally placed in a triangular fashion for nephrectomy (15). The umbilical port always supports the camera. During kidney and proximal ureteral dissection, the upper midline and lateral ports are used. The lower midline and lateral ports are utilized during mid- and distal ureteral mobilization. Dissection is performed until the entire intramural ureter is made extravesical. Ultimately, a GIA endovascular stapler with an articulating head is used to come across the ureterovesical junction while the ureter is placed on upward tension (Fig. 125.5). This separates the distal ureter from the bladder and simultaneously closes the bladder. Morcellation has been performed in cases with proximal lesions or low-grade disease. Alternatively, the specimen can be placed in an entrapment sack and removed through a small incision.

Cystoscopic unroofing was initially described with this technique using a flexible cystoscope and Bugbee electrocautery (8). The Bugbee was used to score around the ureteral orifice and a portion of the intramural ureter. Some accounts of this technique involve using a 5-cm-long ureteral dilating balloon placed in the intramural ureter. Cautery then incises the intramural ureter over the balloon in the 12 o'clock position up to but not through the ureterovesical junction. After extensive distal ureteral dissection, the ureter is retracted upward, putting the intramural ureter and orifice on stretch. A laparoscopic endo-GIA stapler is fired across the detrusor, incorporating the intramural ureter and orifice with the specimen. Simultaneous flexible cystoscopy can be performed to ensure safety of the contralateral ureteral orifice. According to the authors, after an extravesical recurrence, they modified the technique to perform unroofing of the ureteral orifice after nephrectomy and staple ligation of the distal ureter. More often than not, an orifice is seen cystoscopically and unroofed until a staple line is seen, which is then coagulated with a rollerball electrode. Using a porcine model, the authors verify that viable cells are definitely found within the staple line of the bladder. They also report no recurrences of urothelial carcinoma within their series, which has up to 13 years follow-up. Furthermore, no stone formation has been noted after a mean of 27 months of follow-up on the titanium staples, which remain in contact with urine. The authors concede that if urothelial carcinoma is known to be present in the distal ureter, then an alternative strategy such as open distal ureterectomy is warranted (16).

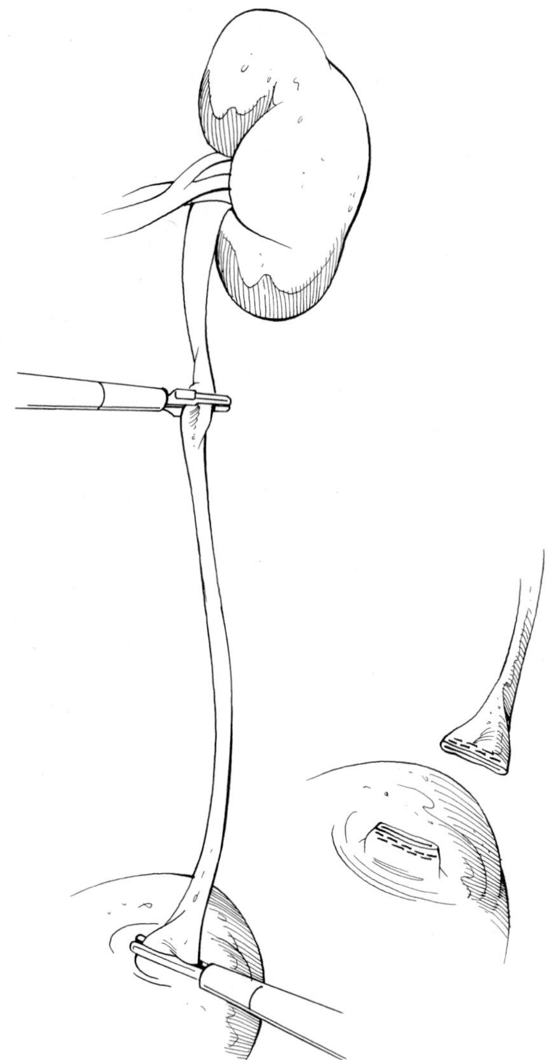

FIGURE 125.5 Pure laparoscopic nephroureterectomy with distal ureter and bladder cuff taken with stapling technique. Articulating heads on the stapler and upward traction on the ureter allow for optimal placement.

### Transvesical Laparoscopic Detachment and Ligation Technique

This technique was developed at the Cleveland Clinic in 1999 and requires formal cystoscopy in the dorsal lithotomy position prior to LNU. With a full bladder and a rigid cystoscope viewing the inside of the bladder, two 5-mm balloon-tipped laparoscopic ports are placed suprapubically into the bladder from above (17,18). A 2-mm endoloop is inserted through one of the suprapubically placed trocars from above. Through the cystoscope, a 5-mm ureteral catheter is placed through the endoloop and into the affected ureteral orifice. A grasper is placed through the second suprapubic port to provide traction on the ureteral orifice while a Collins knife is used to score the affected orifice and intramural ureter. When perivesical adipose tissue is exposed, the ureteral catheter is removed just after the endoloop is secured around the dissected intramural ureter. No formal closure of the bladder is performed, and the Foley catheter is left for 2 weeks.

Possible advantages include intact en bloc excision of the intramural ureter under direct vision and observation of the endoloop tie. Disadvantages include the need for repositioning, fluid extravasation with suprapubically placed laparoscopic ports, and a significant learning curve. The authors of this technique admit it should not be used when there is distal or intramural ureteral tumor or active bladder tumors. Additionally, they advise caution in morbidly obese patients and those with a history of pelvic radiation.

### Transurethral Resection of Ureteral Orifice (TURUO) (Pluck Technique)

This technique involves aggressive transurethral resection around the ureteral orifice until adipose tissue is seen. This is done prior to LNU, at which point the distal ureter is then plucked out of the bladder using upward traction on the ureter. Every attempt is made to clip the ureter as soon as possible to avoid urine draining down the ureter and into the retroperitoneum. The bladder is typically not closed. This procedure has fallen out of practice by most due to the concern of leaving a portion of intramural ureter after the pluck maneuver. Also, tumor seeding of the retroperitoneum has been reported after this maneuver (19). TURUO should also not be performed in the setting of distal, intramural, or perimeatal lesions and is best avoided in patients with active bladder lesions.

## OUTCOMES

In the 1990s various urologic procedures for cancer treatment were adapted to a laparoscopic form in the endeavor to provide equivalent cancer control with less morbidity via smaller incisions. This has definitely been the case with LNU. Early case series reported on the feasibility of the procedure and reported mostly perioperative data and short-term oncologic results. As multiple laparoscopic series have matured we now have intermediate and some long-term data with respect to cancer outcomes (Table 125.3). The series with the longest follow-up for LNU has a median follow-up of 100 months, with a range of 60 to 148 months (20). In this series 26 patients were followed and the distal ureter was addressed either with TURUO or with an open approach if distal ureteral tumors were present. The authors report 72% cancer-specific survival at 7 years, which they compared to a contemporary open series showing 82% cancer-specific survival at 7 years. There was no statistical difference in survival between the two groups. A larger series has also been recently reported in which 39 patients were followed for a median of 74 months (range 60 to 148 months), and 68% cancer-specific survival was noted at 5 years (9). Of note, 80% of these patients had high-grade disease preoperatively. These series show equivalent cancer control with respectable follow-up and compare well to ONU series in the literature (21,22).

Complications are seen in LNU and HALNU that are common to other laparoscopic renal procedures. A recent meta-analysis of reported complications during various laparoscopic renal procedures identified 56 published series each containing at least 20 patients (23). Among these renal procedures were LNU and HALNU. Access-related complications occurred in <0.5%. Intraoperative complications included hemorrhage in 1.4%. Bowel injury, solid organ injury, diaphragmatic injury, and neuromuscular injury were all seen in <0.5% of cases. Postoperative complications included ileus in 1.5%, deep vein thrombosis in 0.7%, and bowel obstruction and incisional hernia in <0.5%. Among the various laparoscopic renal procedures reviewed, LNU ranked highest in both frequency for neural injuries from positioning and for postoperative complications. This is not entirely surprising, given that LNU can be a relative lengthy procedure and is usually performed in elderly patients with multiple comorbidities.

An obviously distressing complication of LNU is that of laparoscopic port site seeding. Fortunately this is a rare occurrence, and there are seven reported cases, which represent an approximately 1.6% incidence (24). The majority of these cases have been high-grade disease in which the specimen was extracted without an entrapment sack or the sack was ruptured during specimen removal. In one case, a ureteral stent placed previously during ureteroscopic biopsy was seen extruding from the renal pelvis during subsequent LNU (25). The authors cautioned against overly aggressive ureteroscopic biopsy, although no evidence of retroperitoneal recurrence was seen.

**TABLE 125.3**

ONCOLOGIC RESULTS OF CONTEMPORARY LAPAROSCOPIC AND OPEN NEPHROURETERECTOMY SERIES

| Series | *n* | Method | Distal Ureter | Cancer-Specific Survival | Median Follow-up (mo) | Local Recurrence Rate |
|---|---|---|---|---|---|---|
| Muntener 2007 (9) | 39 | LNU | Stapling, open | 68% | 74 | 5% |
| Bariol 2004 (20) | 26 | LNU | Open, TURUO | 72% | 100 | 4% |
| Matin 2005 (27) | 60 | LNU | TDL, stapling, open | 85% | 23 | 7% |
| Chung 2007 (7) | 39 | HALNU | Open | 89% | 48 | 3% |
| Wolf 2005 (13) | 54 | HALNU | TURUO, | 94% | 12 | 8% |
| | | | TEC | 86% | 24 | |
| | | | | 80% | 36 | |
| Bariol 2004 (20) | 40 | ONU | | 82% | 96 | |
| Hattori 2006 (21) | 60 | ONU | | 81% | 35 | |
| Hsueh 2006 (22) | 77 | ONU | | 72% | 60 | |

LNU, laparoscopic nephroureterectomy; HALNU, hand-assisted laparoscopic nephroureterectomy; ONU, open nephroureterectomy; TURUO, transurethral resection of ureteral orifice; TDL, transvesical detachment and ligation; TEC; transvesical endoscopic cuff.

## References


1. Messing EM. Urothelial tumors of the urinary tract. In: Walsh PC, Retik AB, Vaughan ED, et al., ed. *Campbell's Urology*, 8th ed. Philadelphia: Saunders, 2002:2765–2773.
2. Soderdahl DW, Fabrizio MD, Rahman NU, et al. Endoscopic treatment of upper tract transitional cell carcinoma. *Urol Oncol* 2005;23:114–122.
3. Chen G, Bagley DH. Ureteroscopic management of upper tract transitional cell carcinoma in patients with normal contralateral kidneys. *J Urol* 2000;164:1173–1176.
4. Liatsikos EN, Dinlenc CZ, Kapoor R, et al. Transitional cell carcinoma of the renal pelvis: ureteroscopic and percutaneous approach. *J Endourol* 2001;15:377–383.
5. Razdan S, Johannes J, Cox M, et al. Current practice patterns in urological management of upper tract transitional cell carcinoma. *J Endourol* 2005;19:366–371.
6. Clayman RV, Kavoussi LR, Figenshau RS, et al. Laparoscopic nephrourerterectomy: initial case report. *J Laparoendosc Surg* 1991;1:343–349.
7. Chung SD, Chueh SC, Lai MK, et al. Long term outcome of hand-assisted laparoscopic radical nephroureterectomy for upper tract transitional carcinoma: comparison with open surgery. *J Endourol* 2007;21:595–599.
8. McDougall EM, Clayman RV, Elashry O. Laparoscopic nephroureterectomy for upper tract transitional cell carcinoma: the Washington University experience. *J Urol* 1995;154:975–980.
9. Muntener M, Nielsen ME, Romero FR, et al. Long-term oncologic outcome after laparoscopic radical nephroureterectomy for upper tract transitional cell carcinoma. *Eur Urol* 2007;51:1639–1644.
10. Strong DW, Pearse HD, Tank ES, et al. The ureteral stump after nephroureterectomy. *J Urol* 1976;115:654–655.
11. Brown JA, Strup SE, Chenven E, et al. Hand-assisted laparoscopic nephroureterectomy: analysis of distal ureterectomy technique, margin status and surgical outcomes. *Urology* 2005;66:1192–1196.
12. Munver R, Del Pizzo JJ, Sosa RE. Hand-assisted laparoscopic nephroureterectomy for upper tract transitional cell carcinoma. *J Endourol* 2004;18:351–358.
13. Wolf JS, Dash A, Hollenbeck BK, et al. Intermediate followup of hand assisted laparoscopic nephroureterectomy for urothelial carcinoma: factors associated with outcomes. *J Urol* 2005;173:1102–1107.
14. Hinman F Jr. Kidney excision (nephroureterectomy). In: Hinman F Jr. *Atlas of Urologic Surgery.* 2nd ed. Philadelphia: Saunders, 1998:1013–1015.
15. Jarrett TW, Chan DY, Cadeddu JA, et al. Laparoscopic nephroureterectomy for the treatment of transitional cell carcinoma of the upper urinary tract. *Urology* 2001;57:448–453.
16. Venkatesh R, Rehman J, Landman J, et al. Determination of cell viability after laparoscopic tissue stapling in a porcine model. *J Endourol* 2005; 19:744–747.
17. Gill IS, Soble J, Miller S, et al. A novel technique for management of the en bloc bladder cuff and distal ureter during laparoscopic nephroureterectomy. *J Urol* 1999;161:430–434.
18. Gill IS, Sung GT, Hobart MG. Laparoscopic radical nephroureterectomy for upper tract transitional cell carcinoma: the Cleveland Clinic experience. *J Urol* 2000;164:1513–1522.
19. Arango O, Bielsa O, Carles J, et al. Massive tumor implantation in the endoscopic resected area in modified nephroureterectomy. *J Urol* 1997;157: 1893–1896.
20. Bariol SV, Stewart GD, McNeill SA, et al. Oncological control following laparoscopic nephroureterectomy. *J Urol* 2004;172:1805–1808.
21. Hattori R, Yoshino Y, Gotoh M, et al. Laparoscopic nephroureterectomy for transitional cell carcinoma of the renal pelvis and ureter: the Nagoya experience. *Urology* 2006;67:701–705.
22. Hsueh TY, Huang YH, Chiu AW, et al. Survival analysis in patients with upper tract transitional cell carcinoma: a comparison between open and hand-assisted laparoscopic nephroureterectomy. *BJU Int* 2006;99:632–636.
23. Pareek G, Hedican SP, Gee JR. Meta-analysis of the complications of laparoscopic renal surgery: comparison of procedures and techniques. *J Urol* 2006;175:1208–1213.
24. Rassweiler JJ, Schulze M, Marrero R, et al. Laparoscopic nephroureterectomy for upper tract transitional cell carcinoma: is it better than open surgery? *Eur Urol* 2004;46:690–697.
25. Ong AM, Bhayani SB, Pavlovich CP. Trocar site recurrence after laparoscopic nephroureterectomy. *J Urol* 2003;170:1301.
26. Gonzalez CM, Batler RA, Schoor RA, et al. A novel approach towards resection of the distal ureter with surrounding bladder cuff during hand assisted laparoscopic nephrouretetectomy. *J Urol* 2001;165:483–485.
27. Matin SF, Gill IS. Recurrence and survival following laparoscopic radical nephroureterectomy with various forms of bladder cuff control. *J Urol* 2005;173:395–400.
28. McGinnis DE, Trabulsi EJ, Gomella LG, et al. Hand-assisted laparoscopic nephroureterectomy: description of technique. *Tech Urol* 2001;7:7–11.
29. Nanigian DK, Smith W, Ellison LM. Robot-assisted laparoscopic nephroureterectomy. *J Endourol* 2006;20:463–466.


# CHAPTER 126 ■ LAPAROSCOPIC RENAL PROCEDURES: RENAL CYSTECTOMY, BIOPSY, AND NEPHROPEXY

CHAD A. LAGRANGE AND STEPHEN E. STRUP

Laparoscopic surgery has become the standard of care for many renal procedures. The benefits of laparoscopic renal surgery, including less postoperative pain, shorter hospitalization, and quicker recovery, have led surgeons to apply this technique to many different types of renal procedures. Renal pathology such as renal cyst disease and nephroptosis, which were historically performed using an open approach, can be effectively treated in a laparoscopic fashion. In addition, procedures traditionally performed percutaneously, such as renal biopsy, can be performed laparoscopically, which may offer the advantages of increased effectiveness and decreased risk in certain high-risk patients.

## LAPAROSCOPIC RENAL CYSTECTOMY

Simple cysts are the most common lesions of the kidney. It is estimated that 50% of the adult population have renal cysts. The incidence of cysts increases with age; simple renal cysts occur with an incidence of at least 20% by age 40 years and 33% by age 60 years (1).

## Diagnosis

The diagnosis of renal cysts was traditionally made during intravenous urography with tomography. Today, ultrasound (US) and computerized tomography (CT) are the principal diagnostic tools, and most cysts are incidental findings. Occasionally, a patient with a very large simple cyst may present with vague abdominal or flank discomfort and fullness on physical examination. However, most patients are asymptomatic.

The sonographic criteria for simple cysts are absence of internal echoes, increased through-transmission of sound, and a sharply defined simple wall. On CT, simple cysts are sharply marginated, nonenhancing, and clearly demarcated from surrounding renal parenchyma with no calcifications. The attenuation values should be in the range of water (−10 to +20 Hounsfield units). On magnetic resonance imaging (MRI), simple cysts appear as round, homogenous, and low intensity (dark) on T1-weighted images and increased intensity (bright) on T2-weighted images.

## Indications for Surgery

Occasionally, patients who present with flank pain are discovered to have no other etiology on radiographic evaluation for their complaint either than a large simple cyst, and they may be candidates for therapy. Large parenchymal cysts or peripelvic/parapelvic cysts can also cause obstruction leading to pain. Depending on the symptoms, size, site, location, presence of infection, and suspicion of malignancy, the following renal cystic disorders can be managed laparoscopically:

1. Renal cystic masses (i.e., Bosniak type IV, cystic renal cell carcinoma): laparoscopic nephrectomy or partial nephrectomy
2. Indeterminate cystic masses (i.e., Bosniak type II or III): laparoscopic exploration and management
3. Bosniak type I and II renal cysts, large (>10 cm) and symptomatic: laparoscopic cystectomy, decortication, or marsupialization
4. Renal hydatid cysts: same as above
5. Peripelvic or parapelvic cysts: same as above
6. Autosomal dominant polycystic kidney disease (ADPKD): cyst decortication

## Alternative Therapy

Aspiration and injection of sclerosing agents is a safe and effective solution. This is usually the initial course of management for symptomatic renal cysts. Aspiration of cysts may also prove to be a diagnostic maneuver to examine the effect on the patient's symptoms, and if the cyst and pain recur then the relationship between the two is solidified. Reported success rates of cyst aspiration and sclerosis range from 75% to 97%, with complication rates between 1.3% and 20% (2,3). Another alternative is open surgical marsupialization, which can be performed when more conservative approaches fail or laparoscopic surgery is contraindicated.

## Surgical Technique

### Retroperitoneal Approach

Standard positioning and preparation are carried out with the patient in the flank position. Port placement is depicted in Figure 126.1. A 1.5-cm incision is made at the tip of the 12th rib and dissection is carried down to the lumbodorsal fascia, which is then pierced with a tonsil clamp to enter the retroperitoneal space. Finger dissection is then performed along the psoas muscle to mobilize the posterolateral aspect of the kidney. A 10- to 12-mm visual balloon dissector trocar is then placed and the space is dilated. The dilating balloon is then removed and a blunt-tip balloon trocar is placed. Pneumoretroperitoneum is established to 15 mm Hg and a 5-mm trocar is placed in the posterior axillary line below the 12th rib. A third trocar is inserted approximately two fingerbreadths above the iliac crest in the anterior axillary line. Laparoscopic ultrasound may be used in cases where cysts are difficult to locate. An additional instrument for dissection and countertraction of large cysts can be placed via a 5-mm trocar midway between the iliac crest and the 12th rib in the posterior axillary line.

Once the cyst is exposed from beneath the perinephric fat, the fluid is aspirated and sent for cytology. A gallbladder needle or Orandi-type needle can be used to accomplish the aspiration. The free wall of the cyst is then excised with dissecting scissors, harmonic scalpel, or hook and sent for pathologic analysis (Fig. 126.2). The wall should be incised as close to parenchyma as possible without entering the parenchyma. The parenchymal base of the cyst is then examined for evidence of neoplastic change using cup biopsy forceps to perform frozen-section analysis. The edges of the cyst are cauterized and hemostasis is verified after the pneumoretroperitoneum has been lowered to 5 mm Hg. The argon beam coagulator can be used to quickly paint over any raw bleeding surfaces of parenchyma or cyst wall. If the argon beam coagulator is used, care should be taken to vent the entering argon gas to prevent overpressure and barotrauma.

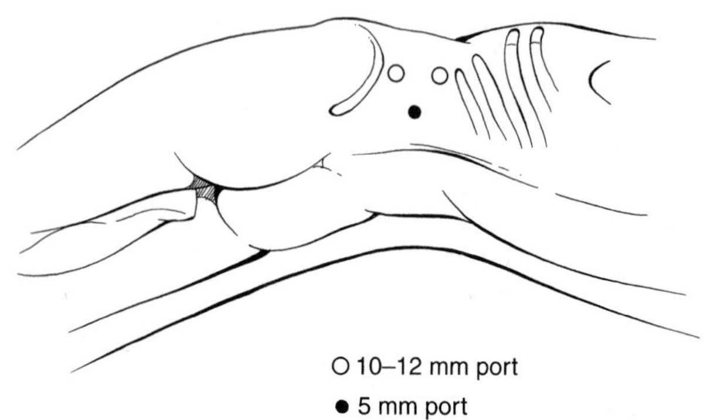


FIGURE 126.1 Port placement for retroperitoneoscopic kidney surgery, such as nephropexy, renal cystectomy, and biopsy.

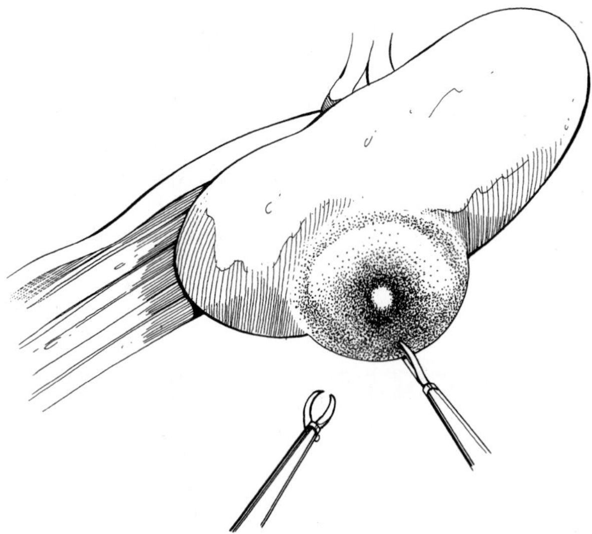

FIGURE 126.2 Renal cyst exposed and ready for excision.

Fibrin glue with or without oxidized cellulose can be applied for refractory areas of bleeding.

### Transperitoneal Approach

The transperitoneal laparoscopic approach is ideal for treating anterior renal cysts, either simple or multiple. The usual technique is laparoscopic marsupialization. This technique has also been reported to treat symptomatic ADPKD (4). Under general anesthesia, with the patient in a 45-degree lateral flank position, pneumoperitoneum is established at the umbilicus. A 10-mm port is placed under laparoscopic visualization lateral to the umbilicus on the affected side in the lower quadrant. A third 5-mm trocar is placed in the midline halfway between the xiphoid process and umbilicus. A fourth trocar may be necessary for retraction in some cases and can be placed either in the lower midline or close to the xiphoid in the midline. The colon is reflected medially and the fascia of Gerota is incised. The perinephric fat around the cyst is dissected cleanly. In cases of polycystic disease, the kidney must be entirely mobilized inside the fascia of Gerota. Once again, the cyst fluid can be aspirated with a needle and sent for cytology. The cyst can then be unroofed as detailed above and its walls and base carefully inspected. Then, a portion of the cyst wall may be attached to the mobilized edge of peritoneum with either a clip or suture to ensure communication with the peritoneal cavity and decrease the likelihood of recurrence.

If the cyst is extremely large, another technique is to fashion a window using dissecting scissors. Retroperitoneal fat or omentum can then be packed into the cyst, thus making it unnecessary to remove a large amount of cyst wall. If during any cyst unroofing, excision, or marsupialization there is concern that the collecting system has been entered, indigo carmine can be administered intravenously or a preoperative ureteral catheter can be placed in complex cases for retrograde irrigation with methylene blue. No drains are necessary postoperatively.

## Results

In most cases, a transperitoneal laparoscopic approach is used. Mean operative time is 89 to 164 minutes in most series, with a mean blood loss of <100 mL (5,6). Procedures performed on peripelvic cysts tend to be more complicated, with longer operative times and higher blood loss. Length of stay in the hospital averages 1 to 2 days.

## Complications

Bleeding is always a possible complication of laparoscopic renal cystectomy. However, this has not been noted in the several reported series. Reaccumulation of cyst fluid is uncommon, ranging from 3% to 4% (5,6). This can occur when the window fashioned in the cyst wall reapproximates. Nieh and Bihrle (7) demonstrated that the use of fat was helpful in maintaining the patency of the marsupialization window. Other rare complications include prolonged ileus, delayed hemorrhage, urinary fistula, and nerve paresthesia.

# LAPAROSCOPIC KIDNEY BIOPSY

Renal biopsy is an invaluable diagnostic procedure for determining the etiology of renal dysfunction. While percutaneous renal biopsy has been proven to be safe and effective, some clinical circumstances mandate the use of other techniques for obtaining kidney biopsies.

## Diagnosis

Renal biopsy is most often performed by nephrologists in a percutaneous fashion. The indication is usually hematuria, proteinuria, or renal insufficiency, especially when a glomerular pathology is suspected.

## Indications for Surgery

US-guided percutaneous kidney biopsy is the most common technique performed. Improved imaging techniques such as US and CT and smaller-gauge biopsy devices have further reduced the contraindications to percutaneous ("blind") renal biopsy. However, some clinical circumstances such as severe hypertension, bleeding diathesis, anticoagulation, morbid obesity, and difficult renal anatomy dictate the use of more controlled access and better visualization of the kidney during biopsy. Hence, laparoscopic renal biopsy can be of great clinical value.

## Alternative Treatments

As mentioned, percutaneous needle biopsy by US or CT guidance is the most common method of performing kidney biopsy. Open kidney biopsy through a subcostal or dorsal lumbotomy incision can also be performed.

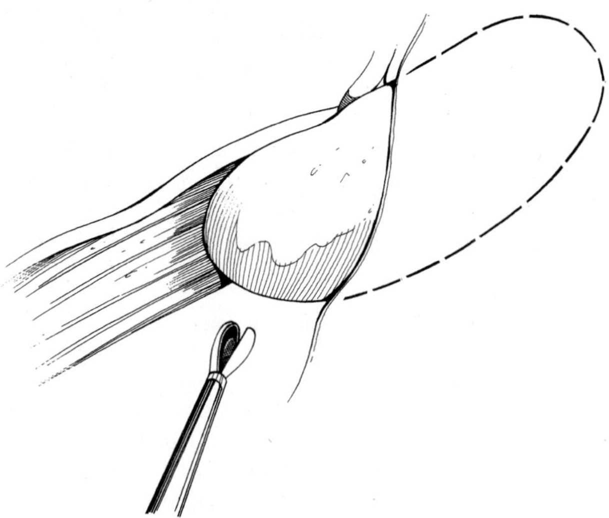

FIGURE 126.3 Lower pole of kidney exposed with spoon forceps or cold-cup biopsy forceps used to take biopsy.

## Surgical Technique

Preoperative US, CT, or MRI can help characterize the kidney and better identify its location to adjacent structures during surgery. The procedure is ideally performed through a retroperitoneal approach. Patient preparation and positioning are identical to that described for laparoscopic retroperitoneal cystectomy (Fig 126.1). However, in many cases only a camera port and single instrument port are necessary. Minimal blunt dissection through the perinephric fat to expose the lower pole of the kidney is then performed. Laparoscopic US may be necessary in some cases to identify the lower pole of the kidney. Cold-cup biopsy forceps or spoon forceps are used to obtain several samples of tissue, and these are sent to the pathologist for frozen-section analysis to confirm adequate tissue sampling (Fig. 126.3). A large-core Tru-cut-type biopsy needle can also be passed through a trocar or percutaneously to obtain the sample.

Hemostasis can be achieved with electrocautery or an argon beam coagulator, and if necessary the sites can be packed with oxidized cellulose (8). The retroperitoneal pressure should then be lowered to 5 mm Hg and the biopsy sites and dissected space examined for hemostasis. The port-site fascial defects can be closed with Vicryl suture or left open since the procedure is exclusively retroperitoneal.

Most patients can be discharged the same day or within 24 hours. However, many patients have coexisting medical problems that may require longer stays.

## Outcomes

Adequate tissue samples are obtained in 96% to 100% of patients in the largest reported series. The mean operative time and estimated blood loss is between 90 and 123 minutes and 25.9 and 67 mL (8,9). The majority of patients are discharged from the hospital within 24 hours.

## Complications

Overall, complications related directly to the procedure are rare because of the direct visualization of the biopsy site for hemostasis and accurate tissue sampling. The reported incidence of delayed bleeding after laparoscopic renal biopsy is 3% to 4% (8,9). Other less common complications are related to visceral injury during access to the retroperitoneum or inadvertent biopsy of other organs.

# LAPAROSCOPIC NEPHROPEXY

Nephroptosis is a condition of great historical interest. It is classically defined as descent of the kidney >5 cm (or two vertebral bodies) when moving to the upright position. The condition is much more common in female patients and more commonly affects the right kidney, but it can be bilateral in up to 20% of cases. Most patients are thin women. Nephroptosis may be an incidental finding and should be treated only when associated with symptoms. Pain is believed to be a result of acute obstruction and/or renal ischemia upon standing due to the hypermobile kidney.

## Diagnosis

Historically, the diagnosis of symptomatic nephroptosis was limited to symptomatology and physical examination. Currently, many diagnostic modalities are available. An intravenous pyelogram with the patient in the supine and standing position is the initial test. The hypermobile kidney will descend in the upright position and might become hydronephrotic. Color Doppler ultrasonography with measurement of resistive indices (RI) in the supine and upright position may also be helpful. A reduction in RI may be seen when moving from the supine to upright position, signifying a decrease in renal perfusion (10). A nuclear renal scan in the sitting position is useful in detecting an obstructive pattern after renal descent, as well as diminished blood flow to the kidney when the patient is erect. However, some facilities may not have the proper nuclear imaging systems to perform upright scans.

## Alternative Therapy

Laparoscopic nephropexy has become the procedure of choice for the correction of nephroptosis. Open nephropexy and its variants are also options.

## Surgical Technique

The surgical management of nephroptosis is controversial and variable. Many historical options exist, ranging from pexy and slings to other organs, ligaments, or the 12th rib. Current techniques usually employ suture fixation to the

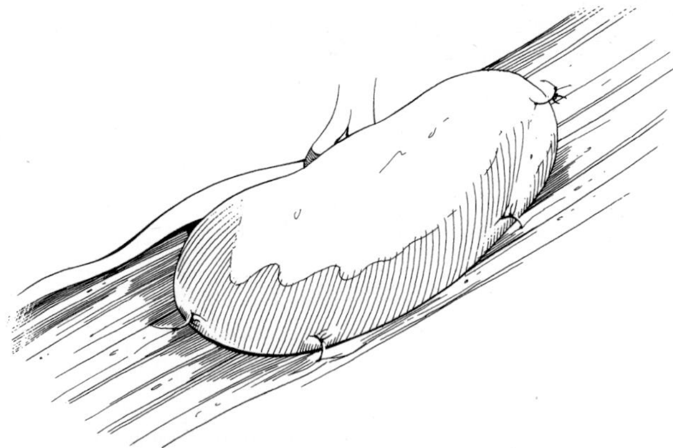

FIGURE 126.4 Nonabsorbable sutures placed through renal capsule and then psoas fascia on upper pole of kidney (medially, superiorly, and laterally).

psoas and/or quadratus lumborum fascias. In general, the techniques require complete mobilization of the kidney inside the fascia of Gerota down the renal capsule, with sutures placed directly through the fascia.

A transperitoneal approach is the most commonly reported access. The patient is positioned in full flank position, unless performing bilateral nephropexy, in which the patient is positioned supine and the bed tilted side to side to access each kidney. A three-port midline approach is generally used. The kidney is completely mobilized inside the fascia of Gerota and the fascia of the psoas muscle is identified. The operating table is then moved to a head-down position, which causes the mobile kidney to be positioned as cephalad as possible. Beginning at the upper pole, three interrupted nonabsorbable 3-0 sutures are then placed along the lateral margin of the kidney (upper, middle, and lower) through the renal capsule and then through the psoas fascia (Fig. 126.4). Care should be taken not to place the sutures too deeply into the renal parenchyma to prevent bleeding. In addition, the genitofemoral nerve running along the psoas fascia should not be entrapped. Intracorporeal suturing can be simplified by the use of Lapra-Ty clips (Ethicon Endosurgery, Cincinnati, OH) to secure sutures instead of tying knots.

The retroperitoneal laparoscopic approach provides a direct route to the kidney and may be useful in patients with prior intra-abdominal surgery. However, working space is sometimes limited, making complete kidney mobilization difficult. Creation of the retroperitoneal space is performed as previously described, and nephropexy proceeds as described above. The procedure can be performed on an outpatient basis or the patient may be admitted for 24-hour observation. Follow-up erect and supine radiographic studies are generally performed in 6 to 12 weeks.

## Outcomes

Success rates are quite high for laparoscopic nephropexy and are comparable to historical open series. Resolution of symptoms occurred in 80% to 100% of patients in published laparoscopic nephropexy series (11–13). Correlation of resolution of symptoms with resolution of renal descent on postoperative imaging appears high. In one series of 31 retroperitoneoscopic nephropexies, complete symptom resolution was present in 83% of patients and 87% of patients had no evidence of persistent renal descent on radiographic studies postoperatively (14).

## Complications

The most feared complication is failure to resolve symptoms. However, as noted above, failure is uncommon. Other complications include bleeding from the renal parenchyma and postoperative ileus.

## *References*


1. Kissane JM. The morphology of renal cystic disease. *Perspect Nephrol Hypertens* 1976;4:31–63.
2. Morgan C Jr, Rader D. Laparoscopic unroofing of a renal cyst. *J Urol* 1992;148(6):1835–1836.
3. Munch LC, Gill IS, McRoberts JW. Laparoscopic retroperitoneal renal cystectomy. *J Urol* 1994;151(1):135–138.
4. Dunn MD, Portis AJ, Naughton C, et al. Laparoscopic cyst marsupialization in patients with autosomal dominant polycystic kidney disease. *J Urol* 2001;165(6 Pt 1):1888–1892.
5. Atug F, Burgess SV, Ruiz-Deya G, et al. Long-term durability of laparoscopic decortication of symptomatic renal cysts. *Urology* 2006;68(2): 272–275.
6. Roberts WW, Bluebond-Langner R, Boyle KE, et al. Laparoscopic ablation of symptomatic parenchymal and peripelvic renal cysts. *Urology* 2001; 58(2):165–169.
7. Nieh PT, Bihrle W 3rd. Laparoscopic marsupialization of massive renal cyst. *J Urol* 1993;150(1):171–173.
8. Shetye KR, Kavoussi LR, Ramakumar S, et al. Laparoscopic renal biopsy: a 9-year experience. *BJU Int* 2003;91(9):817–820.
9. Gimenez LF, Micali S, Chen RN, et al. Laparoscopic renal biopsy. *Kidney Int* 1998;54(2):525–529.
10. Strohmeyer DM, Peschel R, Effert P, et al. Changes of renal blood flow in nephroptosis: assessment by color Doppler imaging, isotope renography and correlation with clinical outcome after laparoscopic nephropexy. *Eur Urol* 2004;45(6):790–793.
11. Marcovich R, Wolf JS Jr. Laparoscopy for the treatment of positional renal pain. *Urology* 1998;52(1):38–43.
12. McDougall EM, Afane JS, Dunn MD, et al. Laparoscopic nephropexy: long-term follow-up, Washington University experience. *J Endourol* 2000;14(3):247–250.
13. Plas E, Daha K, Riedl CR, et al. Long-term followup after laparoscopic nephropexy for symptomatic nephroptosis. *J Urol* 2001;166(2):449–452.
14. Rassweiler JJ, Frede T, Recker F, et al. Retroperitoneal laparoscopic nephropexy. *Urol Clin North Am* 2001;28(1):137–144.

# CHAPTER 127 ■ LAPAROSCOPIC ABLATION OF SMALL RENAL MASSES

ILIA S. ZELTSER AND DAVID E. McGINNIS

As a result of the widespread use of cross-sectional imaging techniques, most incidentally discovered renal tumors are small and locally confined and represent a low-stage renal cell carcinoma (T1a) (1). Long-term oncologic outcomes of open partial nephrectomy have demonstrated that these small tumors (<4 cm) can be treated with nephron-sparing techniques with cancer control outcomes that are equivalent to those of radical nephrectomy (2). Since the development of laparoscopic partial nephrectomy (LPN) in 1993, several centers of excellence have successfully utilized this technique to treat small renal masses. In fact, recent data of the 5-year outcomes of LPN revealed disease-free survival rates of over 90%, with minimal compromise of renal function (3).

Yet despite the excellent outcomes of nephron-sparing surgery (NSS), the widespread adoption of this technique by the urologic community outside of the centers of excellence has been slow. A recent survey of the Surveillance, Epidemiology, and End Results (SEER) registry showed a significant underutilization of NSS in the treatment of small renal masses. Only 42% of the tumors <2 cm were treated with NSS in the 2000–01 time period, and for the treatment of tumors 2 to 4 cm, NSS was employed in a mere 20% of cases (4). The significant technical difficulty of LPN may be responsible for this trend. Furthermore, as compared to open partial nephrectomy, LPN is associated with a longer renal ischemia time and a higher urologic complication rate, even in the most experienced hands.

Thermoablative technologies were introduced to minimize the morbidity of partial nephrectomy, particularly in infirm, elderly patients with multiple comorbidities. Cryoablation (CA) and radiofrequency ablation (RFA) are the two most commonly used energy sources, and both can be applied percutaneously or laparoscopically. The main limitation of in situ ablation is that the tumor is not excised and therefore the pathologic confirmation of complete tumor removal is lacking. Instead, the adequacy of ablation is confirmed by the absence of tumor enhancement on follow-up imaging. Despite this limitation, excellent midrange oncologic efficacy of both CA and RFA has now been demonstrated.

## DIAGNOSIS

Renal malignancy is suspected when a solid renal mass is visualized on renal ultrasound, computerized tomography, or magnetic resonance imaging. Diagnosis is usually established when a clear enhancement of the lesion is seen during the nephrographic phase following administration of an intravenous contrast agent. Cystic lesions of the kidney are suspected to have a high malignant potential when they exhibit coarse calcifications, thick outer wall, irregular shape, thickened internal septations, and enhancing mural nodules (Bosniak category III and IV lesions).

## INDICATIONS FOR SURGERY

Laparoscopic renal ablation is generally indicated for the treatment of suspicious renal masses measuring 4 cm or less in diameter (T1a lesions). Treatment of larger tumors would also be considered for patients with solitary kidneys, renal insufficiency, inherited renal carcinoma syndromes with multiple synchronous renal tumors, and bilateral disease.

Irreversible coagulopathy is the only absolute contraindication to laparoscopic RFA and CA. Large tumors, cystic tumors, and those located in the renal hilum or adjacent to the pelvis or ureter are relative contraindications. Laparoscopic ablation is also relatively contraindicated in patients who are unable to tolerate abdominal insufflation. A transperitoneal laparoscopic approach may be relatively contraindicated in patients who have multiple adhesions secondary to previous abdominal surgery or a history of peritonitis, but a retroperitoneal approach may be considered in these cases. Both RFA and CA can be used to treat exophytic as well as completely endophytic renal masses. Care should be taken to make sure that endophytic lesions to be treated laparoscopically can be well visualized by ultrasound, since they may not be visible on the surface of the kidney. If an endophytic lesion is not visible on ultrasound, then it is not a candidate for laparoscopic ablation. Selection of the approach (intraperitoneal versus retroperitoneal versus percutaneous) depends on the tumor location, the patient's health status, and the surgeon's expertise. Laparoscopic ablation is generally preferred for anterior and lateral tumors or tumors excessively close to vital structures (e.g., bowel, spleen, major vessels, collecting system), although even posterior tumors can be treated following adequate mobilization of the kidney or a retroperitoneal approach.

## SURGICAL TECHNIQUE

### RFA Mechanism of Action

RFA utilizes a monopolar alternating electrical current with the frequency within the radio segment of the electromagnetic spectrum. The current flows between the grounding pad and the RFA probe. Heat is generated as a result of ionic agitation of the tissue around the probe, and cell death is achieved when the temperature within a tumor and a small rim of the surrounding tissue rises over 60°C. High temperatures produce occlusion of the microvasculature and destruction of the cellular cytoskeleton, causing tissue ischemia and impaired DNA replication and ultimately resulting in a predictable zone of coagulation necrosis around the RF electrode (5).

Based on the type of the feedback loop modulating energy delivery to the probe, there are two types of RF generators: impedance-based (Valleylab, Boulder, CO, or Boston Scientific, Natick, MA) and temperature-based (RITA Medical Systems, Mountain View, CA). The feedback loops are designed to prevent an overly rapid tissue heating, which would produce charring and increase tissue resistance, thus decreasing the ablation zone.

## Cryotherapy Mechanism of Action

Cell death secondary to rapid severe freezing occurs by several mechanisms. Extracellular ice formation results in movement of water out of the cell and leads to changes in intracellular pH, protein denaturation, and mechanical disruption of the plasma membrane followed by intracellular ice formation. Delayed tissue effects are due to the injury to the microvasculature resulting in tissue hypoxia, endothelial cell damage, edema, platelet aggregation, and thrombosis, culminating in coagulative necrosis (6). Recently, apoptosis and gene-regulated cell death were identified as another mechanism of tissue disruption following freezing (7). It is generally accepted that a temperature of −20°C must be achieved to ensure cytotoxic effects of CA. It is not clear whether passive thawing between freezing cycles has greater tissue effects than active rapid thawing. However, it is generally accepted that a double freeze–thaw cycle with ice-ball extension beyond the tumor margin should be utilized in clinical practice (8). Cryoablation probes range from large 5-mm probes to 3.4-mm probes to currently available 1.47-mm needles (Galil Medical, Yokneam, Israel, or Endocare, Irvine, CA). Smaller probes were designed to allow for a nontraumatic placement through the body wall and the renal capsule, more precise tumor targeting, and minimal bleeding following cryoprobe removal. The third-generation machines utilize argon for freezing and helium for active thawing.

Routine laboratory studies are obtained and include serum electrolytes, creatinine, liver function tests, and coagulation profile. Urine culture is sent, and culture-specific antibiotics are started in those with positive cultures. A chest radiograph and an electrocardiogram are performed per the discretion of the anesthesiologist. Patients taking aspirin, clopidogrel (Plavix), warfarin (Coumadin), large doses of vitamin E, or other anticoagulation agents are instructed to discontinue them 5 to 7 days prior to the intervention, although they may resume them immediately after RFA or at the surgeon's discretion after CA. A parenteral antibiotic with good coverage of skin flora is given within an hour of starting the procedure.

## Laparoscopic RFA

A transperitoneal approach is utilized for anterior and upper-pole tumors. The retroperitoneal approach is reserved for lateral and posterior lesions when percutaneous RFA is not possible or available. Basic laparoscopic techniques are described in Chapter 123.

1. After antiembolic stockings are placed and general anesthesia is induced, the bladder is drained with a Foley catheter and the patient is positioned in the modified flank position for the transperitoneal approach and in the standard flank position when retroperitoneal RFA is planned.
2. For transperitoneal ablation, the abdomen is insufflated with a Veress needle or via a Hasson technique, and three transperitoneal laparoscopic trocars are placed in the same configuration as for a laparoscopic nephrectomy. Access to the retroperitoneal space can be obtained using a visual obturator trocar or an open technique where a surgeon's finger is inserted through a 10-mm incision at the tip of the 12th rib and the plane over the psoas muscle is bluntly developed. The retroperitoneal space can be enlarged with a dilating balloon or bluntly developed with sweeping motions of the laparoscope.
3. For transperitoneal ablations, the dissection starts with incising of the white line of Toldt as the colon is reflected medially off the fascia of Gerota. Obviously, this step is not required during a retroperitoneal approach.
4. The fascia of Gerota is opened and the perinephric fat is dissected off the renal capsule to identify the tumor. Dissection of the opposite side of the kidney is also performed to create a space for ultrasonic confirmation of probe placement.
5. Laparoscopic renal ultrasound is then used to define tumor margins. Ultrasound is critical in defining the margins of partially or completely endophytic renal tumors.
6. The location on the abdominal wall allowing the most perpendicular path of the probe to the tumor is identified. The probe is inserted through the abdominal wall and the kidney is then manipulated so that the probe enters the lesion at a right angle to the most exophytic point of the tumor. The probe is inserted into the tumor and the tines are deployed to encompass a diameter extending 5 to 10 mm beyond the visualized margin of the tumor. Tine placement is confirmed with laparoscopic ultrasound (Fig. 127.1).

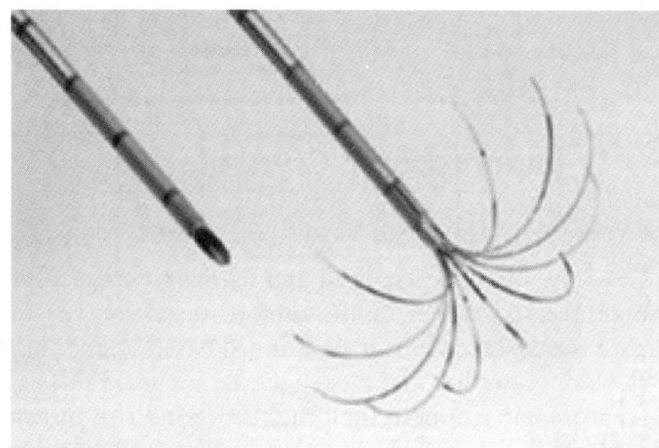

FIGURE 127.1 Example of the tines being deployed from the end of an radiofrequency ablation probe.

TABLE 127.1

**RADIOFREQUENCY ABLATION PROTOCOL UTILIZING STARBURST XL (RITA) PROBE**

| Tumor Size | Length of Treatment Cycle (min) | Number of Cycles |
|---|---|---|
| <1 cm | 3 | 1 or 2 |
| 1–2 cm | 5 | 2 |
| 2–3 cm | 7 | 2 |
| 3–4 cm | 8 | 2 |

From: Ogan K, Jacomides L, Dolmatch BL, et al. Percutaneous radiofrequency ablation of renal tumors: technique, limitations, and morbidity. *Urology* 2002;60(6):954–958.

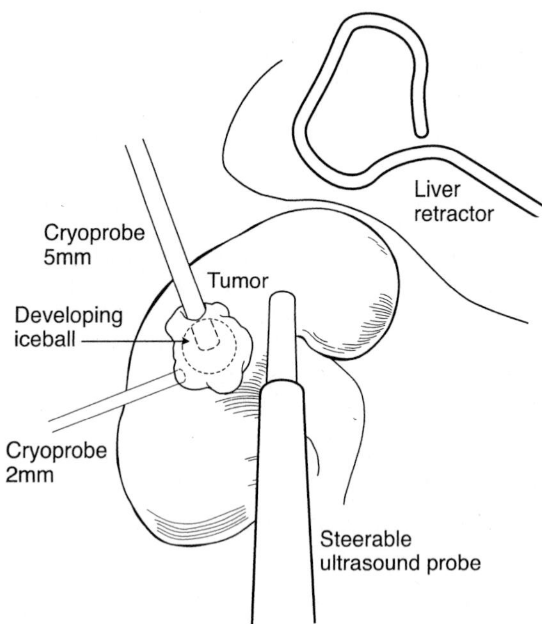


**FIGURE 127.2** During laparoscopic transperitoneal cryoablation a 5-mm diamond flex triangle retractor (Genzyme Surgical) can be used to retract the liver while the ultrasound and laparoscope are used to visualize the procedure.

7. Two cycles of RFA are performed. The duration of each ablation cycle is determined by the size of the tumor (Table 127.1).
8. Once ablation is completed, the probe is removed and biopsies of the tumor with a laparoscopic 5-mm toothed biopsy forceps are taken. Performing the biopsy following rather than before the ablation minimizes bleeding, reduces the potential for tumor seeding, and provides adequate tissue sample for accurate diagnosis.
9. The biopsy site on the surface of the kidney is examined: usually no or minimal bleeding results. Mild bleeding can be controlled by application of FloSeal (gelatin–thrombin matrix, Baxter, Deerfield, IL) hemostatic sealant; however, occasionally argon beam or electrocautery coagulation may be needed.
10. Colon is replaced in its normal anatomic position and the incised edges of peritoneum are approximated with clips or intracorporeal suturing. The abdomen is desufflated and the trocars are removed.
11. The postoperative care is the same as for a laparoscopic nephrectomy.

Patients are followed with contrast-enhanced computerized tomography or magnetic resonance imaging. Successful ablation is confirmed by the absence of contrast enhancement within the tumor and a narrow rim of normal parenchyma. It is important to emphasize that the RFA lesion will persist on the follow-up scans, although it may contract slightly. Endophytic lesions may retract from the renal parenchyma, with a narrow rim of fat infiltrating the margin.

## Laparoscopic Cryoablation

Steps 1 through 5 are identical to those of laparoscopic RFA.

6. Once the tumor is localized and its margins are defined, core needle biopsies or the tumor are taken. The ideal path for the cryoprobe is determined based on the path of the biopsy needle. The biopsy needle is passed through a laparoscopic trocar to limit the theoretical risk of tumor seeding. For tumors 2 cm or less, a single 4.8-mm probe is positioned centrally within the tumor and the proper location is confirmed with ultrasound (Fig. 127.2). For larger lesions three 1.47-mm probes are triangulated within the tumor so that the resulting ice balls overlap and encompass the tumor margins.
7. Two freeze–thaw cycles are performed and freezing is continued until the ice ball extends about 5 mm to 1 cm beyond the tumor margin. Extension of the ice ball is monitored continuously with ultrasound. Temperature monitoring may be utilized as well to ensure uniform tumor destruction. Eighteen-gauge thermocouples may be placed within the tumor or at the tumor margin, and temperatures below −20°C must be registered to ensure uniform cell death.
8. After the second thaw cycle, the cryoprobes are removed and FloSeal or Endoavitene plug (Davol, Cranston, RI) may be applied into the puncture sites to help with hemostasis. To avoid tumor cracking, complete thawing of the tumor must be achieved before the probe is removed.
9. Colon is replaced in its normal anatomic position and the incised edges of peritoneum are approximated with clips or intracorporeal suturing. The abdomen is desufflated and the trocars are removed.
10. The postoperative care is the same as for a laparoscopic nephrectomy.

Radiographic appearance of successful CA shows lack of gadolinium or intravenous contrast enhancement within the cryolesion, although a small rim of enhancement may be seen on early scans. This rim gradually disappears and is thought to represent reactive changes in the area of sublethal injury and interstitial hemorrhage along the periphery of the cryolesion. Following cryoablation, some cryolesions will demonstrate gradual reduction in size, with a mean decrease in diameter of 75% at 3 years.

TABLE 127.2

SELECTED OUTCOMES OF LAPAROSCOPIC RADIOFREQUENCY ABLATION (RFA) AND CRYOABLATION (CA)

| Study | Modality | Access | No. of Tumors | Follow-Up (mo) | Radiographic Recurrence |
|---|---|---|---|---|---|
| Cestari et al., 2004 (12) | CA | Laparoscopy | 37 | >6 | 0/35 |
| Stein and Kaouk, 2007 (13) | CA | Laparoscopy | 66 | >60 | 3/66<br>5-year CCS, 98% |
| Wen and Nakada, 2006 (14) | CA | Laparoscopy | 57 | 12.5 (1–42) | 2/57 |
| Park et al., 2006 (10) | RFA | Laparoscopy | 39 | 26 (12–36) | 0/39 |
| Hwang et al., 2004 (15) | RFA | Laparoscopy | 15 | 12 (11–57) | 1/24 |

*Note:* CCS, cancer specific survival.

## OUTCOMES

Excellent midrange oncologic efficacy of both cryoablation and RFA has now been demonstrated. Gill et al. (9) showed a 98% cancer-specific survival in 51 patients undergoing laparoscopic CA for a unilateral sporadic renal tumor. In a subset of patients with a median follow-up of 6 years, they demonstrated a 5-year overall survival of 80%. Low tumor recurrence rates have also been shown in multiple other series of laparoscopic CA, yet these had shorter follow up (Table 127.2). With a mean follow-up of 25 months, Park et al. (10) demonstrated a 98.5% cancer-specific survival and a 92.3% overall survival in 78 patients (94 renal masses) treated with percutaneous and laparoscopic RFA. Stern et al. (11) compared the intermediate-term outcomes of patients with clinical T1a renal tumors who were treated with NSS by partial nephrectomy or RFA. All patients had at least 2 years of follow-up (the mean [range] follow-up for the partial nephrectomy and RFA groups was 47 [24–93] and 30 [18–42] months, respectively). The overall actuarial disease-free probability for the partial nephrectomy and RFA groups, respectively, was 95.8% and 93.4% ($p = 0.67$). This initial 3-year actuarial analysis showed that RFA for cT1a renal tumors has comparable oncologic outcomes to partial nephrectomy; however, longer-term data are not yet available. It is notable that tumor seeding in surgical incisions or puncture sites has not occurred in any of the series published to date.

## COMPLICATIONS

Current evidence indicates that both renal RFA and CA have low morbidity and are associated with few complications, most of which are minor. In a multi-institutional study, Johnson et al. (16) found a complication rate of 11.1% in 271 patients undergoing renal RFA and CA. Complications occurred after 14.4% of CA cases and 7.6% of RFA cases, with the most common being paresthesia or pain at the percutaneous probe insertion site for both modalities. Major complications in the RFA group included ileus, ureteropelvic junction obstruction requiring a delayed nephrectomy, and a urinary leak. Significant hemorrhage necessitating a transfusion and an open conversion were the major complications of CA. One patient with poor overall health, obstructive pulmonary disease, congestive heart failure, and pulmonary histoplasmosis died following RFA secondary to aspiration pneumonia. The death was not attributable to the ablation technique, but rather to the patient's overall poor health. In the subgroup of 90 laparoscopic procedures, 3.3% of the complications were attributable to the laparoscopic technique, 4.4% were attributable to the ablation procedure, and one was iatrogenic.

Clinical experience with CA has also shown low complication rates and minimal morbidity. In 56 patients undergoing laparoscopic CA, Gill et al. (17) reported two major and two minor complications. The major complications included a splenic hematoma managed conservatively in one patient and heart failure in another. A pleural effusion and herpetic esophagitis were the minor complications. CA had a minimal impact on renal function. The preoperative and postoperative creatinines were comparable in both the entire study group and the subset of patients with a solitary kidney. Even in 13 patients with a pre-existing renal insufficiency, no significant change in renal function occurred following CA.

In a series of 37 patients undergoing laparoscopic CA, three patients were found to have bleeding complications secondary to renal fracture (12). Perinephric hematomas were seen in two patients and gross hematuria developed in one; all three patients were managed conservatively. Interestingly, this was the first series to show delayed ureteropelvic junction obstruction resulting from CA. This patient was treated successfully with a pyeloplasty at 8 months after CA.

Cryoinjury to the pancreas has been reported in a single patient undergoing retroperitoneal laparoscopic CA (18). The injury was not apparent intraoperatively, and the patient had a delayed presentation with abdominal pain and guarding. Computerized tomography revealed cryoinjury to the pancreas. Abdominal exploration showed no bowel injury, and drains were placed around the pancreas. The patient recovered without further morbidity.

Laparoscopic RFA and CA are promising technologies and can be utilized effectively to treat small renal masses. They require less technical expertise than laparoscopic partial nephrectomy and appear to have lower morbidity and adequate cancer control in the intermediate term. Careful patient selection and meticulous technique are critical to achieving oncologic results comparable to those of partial nephrectomy, which remains the gold-standard therapy for small renal masses. Prospective long-term results of ablative therapy for renal masses are eagerly awaited.

## *References*

1. Uzzo RG. Renal cell carcinoma: urologists in a new era. *J Urol* 2005; 174(5):1723–1724.
2. Fergany AF, Hafez KS, Novick AC. Long-term results of nephron sparing surgery for localized renal cell carcinoma: 10-year followup. *J Urol* 2000; 163(2):442–445.
3. Lane BR, Gill IS. 5-year outcomes of laparoscopic partial nephrectomy. *J Urol* 2007;177(1):70–74.
4. Miller DC, Hollingsworth JM, Hafez KS, et al. Partial nephrectomy for small renal masses: an emerging quality of care concern? *J Urol* 2006; 175(3 Pt 1):853–858.
5. Anderson JK, Matsumoto E, Cadeddu JA. Renal radiofrequency ablation: technique and results. *Urol Oncol* 2005;23(5):355–360.
6. Rehman J, Landman J, Lee D, et al. Needle-based ablation of renal parenchyma using microwave, cryoablation, impedance- and temperature-based monopolar and bipolar radiofrequency, and liquid and gel chemoablation: laboratory studies and review of the literature. *J Endourol* 2004; 18(1):83–104.
7. Baust JG, Gage AA. The molecular basis of cryosurgery. *BJU Int* 2005; 95(9):1187–1191.
8. Woolley ML, Schulsinger DA, Durand DB, et al. Effect of freezing parameters (freeze cycle and thaw process) on tissue destruction following renal cryoablation. *J Endourol* 2002;16(7):519–522.
9. Moinzadeh A, Spaliviero M, Gill IS. Cryotherapy of renal masses: intermediate-term follow-up. *J Endourol* 2005;19(6):654–657.
10. Park S, Anderson JK, Matsumoto ED, et al. Radiofrequency ablation of renal tumors: intermediate-term results. *J Endourol* 2006;20(8):569–573.
11. Stern JM, Svatek R, Park S, et al. Intermediate comparison of partial nephrectomy and radiofrequency ablation for clinical T1a renal tumours. *BJU Int* 2007;100(2):287–290.
12. Cestari A, Guazzoni G, dell'Acqua V, et al. Laparoscopic cryoablation of solid renal masses: intermediate term followup. *J Urol* 2004;172(4 Pt 1): 1267–1270.
13. Stein RJ, Kaouk JH. Renal cryotherapy: a detailed review including a 5-year follow-up. *BJU Int* 2007;99(5 Pt B):1265–1270.
14. Wen CC, Nakada SY. Energy ablative techniques for treatment of small renal tumors. *Curr Opin Urol* 2006;16(5):321–326.
15. Hwang JJ, Walther MM, Pautler, et al. Radio frequency ablation of small renal tumors: intermediate results. *J Urol* 2004;171(5):1814–1818.
16. Johnson DB, Solomon SB, Su LM, et al. Defining the complications of cryoablation and radio frequency ablation of small renal tumors: a multi-institutional review. *J Urol* 2004;172(3):874–877.
17. Gill IS, Remer EM, Hasan WA, et al. Renal cryoablation: outcome at 3 years. *J Urol* 2005;173(6):1903–1907.
18. Lee DI, McGinnis DE, Feld R, et al. Retroperitoneal laparoscopic cryoablation of small renal tumors: intermediate results. *Urology* 2003;61(1):83–88.
19. Ogan K, Jacomides L, Dolmatch BL, et al. Percutaneous radiofrequency ablation of renal tumors: technique, limitations, and morbidity. *Urology* 2002;60(6):954–958.

# CHAPTER 128 ■ DONOR NEPHRECTOMY: LAPAROSCOPIC TECHNIQUES

ERIK P. CASTLE, RAFAEL NUNEZ, COSTAS D. LALLAS, AND PAUL E. ANDREWS

Renal transplantation represents one of the most significant developments in surgery. It has had a markedly positive effect on the survival of patients with end-stage renal disease. The limiting factor has continued to be the number of organs available for transplantation. Deceased donor donation rates have remained relatively stable, and the waiting list has continued to grow—from 47,830 in 2001 to 70,501 in 2006, according to the United Network of Organ Sharing Data Registry (2007).

Living kidney donation stands as an immediate solution to the organ deficiency. The disincentives of living renal donation can be attributed, in part, to concerns by the donor regarding the operation, the length of hospitalization, the prolonged recuperation period, morbidity, and mortality. Laparoscopic donor nephrectomy (LDN) offers better cosmesis, decreased length of stay, and shortened convalescence, decreasing the disincentives of living donation.

## DIAGNOSIS

Individual candidates for living donation are usually between 18 and 70 years of age, without an absolute upper age limit (1). A medical and surgical evaluation is mandatory to accept a living kidney donor (1). The report by the Amsterdam Forum on the care of the live kidney donor set a standard for the evaluation of potential kidney donors (2,3). This report details the following variables that are important for donation: renal function, blood pressure, obesity, dyslipidemia, urine analysis of protein and blood, presence of diabetes, stone disease, malignancy, urinary tract infections, determination of cardiovascular risk, assessment of pulmonary issues, smoking cessation, and alcohol abstinence. A three-dimensional computerized tomography (CT) scan is also necessary to evaluate the vascular and collecting system anatomy of the living kidney donor candidate (1).

## INDICATIONS FOR SURGERY

LDN places healthy individuals at risk of morbidity and mortality to benefit the recipient; however, these risks must be minimized. This distinct practice raises ethical concerns and confers a special character to the indications of surgery. The growth of related and unrelated living kidney donation increases the concerns regarding a variety of issues that are unique to organ donation. Such issues include donor psychological status, motivation, and social aspects (4). Ethical issues of emotional and financial rewards must be addressed. In a recent study, Rodrigue et al. (5) found that in 132 programs across the United States, the presence of financial reward, active substance abuse, and active mental health problems presented complete psychosocial contraindications to donation. To identify healthy and stable individuals, social and psychological evaluation of live kidney donors is needed. Guidelines for such evaluations had been an issue, until recently when they were standardized by the United Network for Organ Sharing, the American Society of Transplant Surgeons, and the American Society of Transplantation (4).

## ALTERNATIVE THERAPY

Open-flank nephrectomy and hand-assisted donor nephrectomy are alternative approaches (6). The procedures are essentially the principles of donor nephrectomy described below, combined with the early use of the hand port as described for laparoscopic hand-assisted nephrectomy (Chapter 125). Less morbid open techniques such as the "mini-nephrectomy" and "mini-incision nephrectomy" use a smaller incision (an average of 10.5 cm) and can reduce morbidity and hospital length of stay compared to a more traditional open approach (6–8). Preliminary work has also been performed using single-port transumbilical access for donor nephrectomy.

## SURGICAL TECHNIQUE

### Patient Preparation and Positioning

Patients undergo standard workup and clearance by the transplant nephrology team. All donors undergo rigorous medical and psychological evaluation. In addition to standard laboratory evaluations, CT is obtained in all patients. Contemporary imaging hardware and software allow for complete evaluation of the urinary tract within prospective donors. The renal parenchyma, collecting system, and vascular structures are evaluated in axial, coronal, and sagittal planes. Three-dimensional reconstructive applications can also provide 360-degree rotational views of the vascular and collecting systems.

The kidneys are inspected carefully for nephrolithiasis, masses, cysts, aberrant vasculature, and variant anatomic formations. Although single arteries, veins, and ureters are desirable, it is not uncommon to encounter multiple arteries, early branching of vessels, circumaortic and preaortic renal veins, duplicated collecting systems, and renal calcifications. The three-dimensional reconstructive CT allows us to determine the optimal kidney for donation. We do not hesitate to utilize the right kidney if there is a contraindication for the left. Many times the right side offers the transplant surgeons better arterial anatomy.

All patients are given standard preoperative intravenous antibiotics 30 to 60 minutes before incision. Aggressive volume infusion of normal saline is started in the preoperative area, with most patients receiving between 3.5 and 4.0 liters of fluids by the time they arrive to the operative suite. Patients are induced under a general anesthetic with endotracheal intubation. An orogastric tube and urethral catheter are inserted.

Patients are positioned using a "modified flank" technique (Fig. 128.1A). A 10-pound sandbag or "bump" is placed under the mattress on the anticipated operative side. The hips are turned and the "bottom" leg is bent at the knee, with the

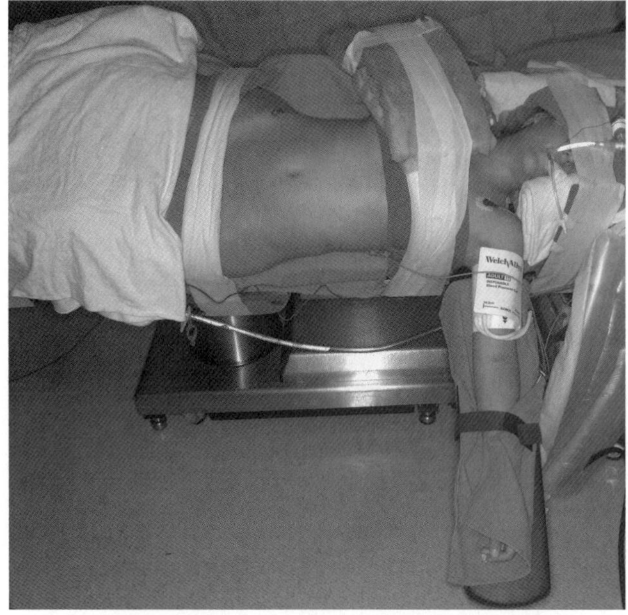

A

B

FIGURE 128.1 A: Positioning for a laparoscopic donor nephrectomy using a modified flank technique. B: "Sling position" of the ipsilateral arm for a right-sided donor.

"top" leg kept relatively straight. The arm on the contralateral, nonoperative side (down side) is placed on an arm board with standard orientation 90 degrees to the table. An axillary roll is not used or needed with this modified positioning as the patient is not in "full flank" and stress is not placed on the contralateral axillary neurologic or vascular structures. The patient is secured to the bed with copious use of 3-inch silk tape wrapped around the patient and bed circumferentially at the level of the nipples, hips, and knees. This secure taping is done before the ipsilateral (up side) arm is positioned.

The ipsilateral arm is finally positioned on the patient's chest using the "sling position" (Fig. 128.1B). This is a natural ergonomic orientation as one might encounter in patients wearing slings following clavicular fracture. The elbow is flexed to 30 degrees, almost as if placing the hand on the patient's heart. This allows for the arm to be cephalad to the costal margin. The arm is placed on soft foam and taped only mildly to prevent movement either into the anesthetic or operative fields. It is important not to overly adduct the shoulder with this arm as one might see when using an arm board across the field. Let the upper arm stay in line with the ipsilateral, axillary side of the body. The overadduction may seem optimal but it actually allows for the arm to end up in a less natural state and can even be intrusive to the surgeon by being a bulky structure in the cephalad portion of the operative field.

## General Technique

Utilizing a transperitoneal technique, access can be obtained one of two ways. A Veress needle or Hasson technique can be used. Alternatively, if the kidney is to be removed via an infraumbilical incision (midline or Pfannenstiel), then a hand port may be used from the beginning (dashed lines in Figs. 128.2 and 128.3). Although we use a GelPort for kidney extraction, we employ conventional pure laparoscopic techniques during dissection. The hand port can be placed at the start of the operation to obtain the pneumoperitoneum if desired and may allow rapid placement of ports. Instruments can also be passed through the GelPort as another working site (Table 128.1). Basic laparoscopic techniques are presented in Chapter 122.

**TABLE 128.1**

**RECOMMENDED INSTRUMENTS FOR LAPAROSCOPIC DONOR NEPHRECTOMY**

- Harmonic scalpel
- Suction irrigator
- One nonlocking atraumatic grasper
- One locking atraumatic grasper
- GelPort
- Laparoscopic articulating endovascular stapler (2.5-mm vascular loads)
- Laparoscopic camera and lens (0 and 30 degrees)
- Laparoscopic clip applier (10 mm)
- Laparoscopic ports, dilating (12 mm × 2, 5 mm × 2)

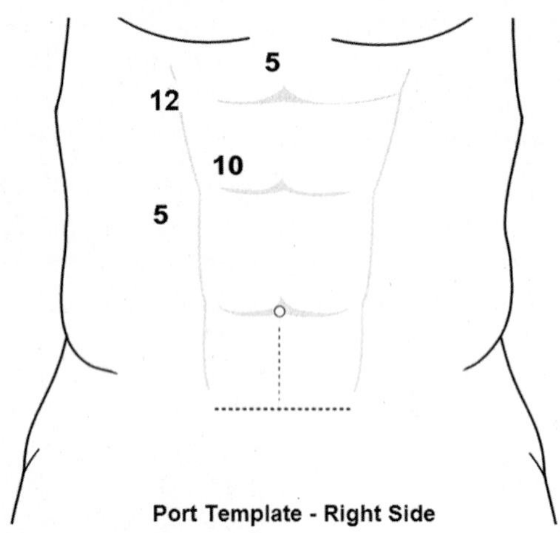


FIGURE 128.2 Port placement for right-sided laparoscopic donor nephrectomy. *Dotted lines* represent the extraction incisions.

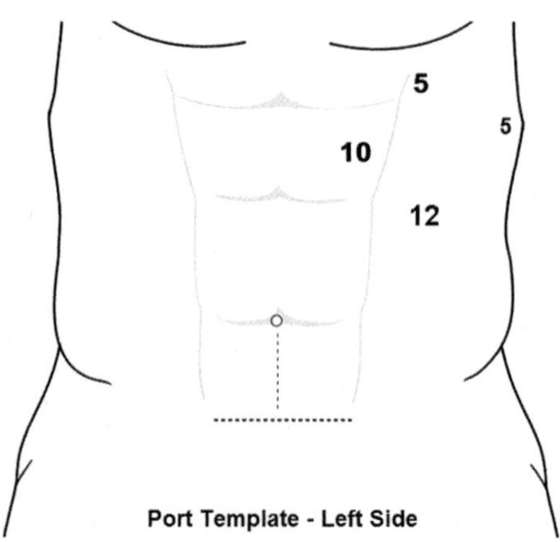


FIGURE 128.3 Port placement for left-sided laparoscopic donor nephrectomy. *Dotted lines* represent the extraction incisions.

Port positioning for the primary three ports (camera and two working ports) is similar for both the right (Fig. 128.2) and left (Fig. 128.3) sides. The two working ports are placed in a subcostal position in the midclavicular line. The camera port is placed 5 cm medial to the midclavicular line between the two working ports. All ports are above the level of the umbilicus, with medial-to-lateral triangulation. A fourth accessory port is often used and placement is dependent on which side is being operated on. On the right side the accessory port is placed in the epigastric/subxiphoid region as a standalone liver retractor (Fig. 128.2). On the left side (Fig. 128.3), we place the accessory port in a more flank orientation to serve as a bowel retractor and retract the left colon medially for optimal medial dissection of the renal vein, adrenal vein, renal artery, and preaortic area. An alternative placement of this retraction port is to utilize a trocar through the GelPort.

## Medications

One of the goals during LDN is to maximize diuresis of the donor renal unit, as volume status and diuresis are generally felt to be associated with better early function of the transplanted kidney. As was discussed above, patients are infused with large volumes of intravenous fluids to expand the intravascular space and maximize renal perfusion. Healthy donors should be able to tolerate the 3- to 4-liter volume load preoperatively and should be diuresing once they arrive to the operating room. To continue the aggressive filtration and diuresis, two separate doses of mannitol are given throughout the laparoscopic dissection. The first dose of 12.5 g is given once the pneumoperitoneum is established. The second dose is given 30 minutes into the dissection. Furosemide is also given (20 mg) toward the end of the renal dissection. In most cases, the hope is to achieve a urinary output of 300 to 500 mL per hour during surgery.

Although not a part of every transplant protocol, we use heparin prior to extraction. The patient is given a 3,000-unit dose of heparin 5 minutes before anticipated stapling of the hilum and extraction. Once the kidney is removed and passed off to the receiving transplant team, 30 mg of protamine sulfate can be infused to reverse the anticoagulant effect of heparin if desired. The use of heparin and protamine has been part of our protocol for over 500 cases and we have yet to experience a deleterious effect attributable to either drug.

## Left-Sided Donor Nephrectomy

Once the pneumoperitoneum is established, the procedure is begun by incising 2 to 3 cm lateral to the left colon. The incision is carried caudal to the pelvic brim, with care taken to avoid the gonadal vessels and internal ring in male patients. The cephalad incision is carried toward the ipsilateral shoulder lateral to the spleen. Incising lateral to the spleen allows the splenic flexure of the left colon and spleen to fall medially as a unit (Fig. 128.4). This provides excellent exposure of the upper pole. Once the colon is freed from its lateral attachments, the atraumatic locking retractor is inserted via the flank port or GelPort to retract the colon medially. Blunt dissection should be used to identify the gonadal vein and ureter as a package and they are retracted anterolaterally. The gonadal vein should be retracted along with the ureter, as it orients the surgeon to the location of the hilum and renal vein. Utilizing a combination of blunt and careful harmonic scalpel dissection, the dissection is carried cephalad toward the renal hilum. Most of the medial attachments, lymphatics, and areolar tissue can be divided with the harmonic scalpel.

The dissection should be kept medial along the lateral border of the aorta to allow for medial exposure of the renal hilum. With the gonadal vein retraction, the medial aspect of the renal vein can be easily identified and lumbar tributaries can be identified. The lumbar vein(s) should be bluntly dissected and divided with a single endovascular staple load. With the lumbar vein(s) taken, the renal artery can be exposed and better visualized. Blunt dissection with the suction irrigator will expose the takeoff of the left renal artery.

The dissection can then be carried to the superior margin of the renal vein. The bowel grasper can be moved more cephalad on the left colon, exposing the superior border of the renal vein and the adrenal gland. If more venous length is desired, the adrenal vein can be bluntly dissected and divided with another endovascular staple load. Care must be taken to work in a medial-to-lateral orientation to avoid inadvertent injury to the superior mesenteric artery, as now the dissection is being performed cephalad to the renal vein and renal artery. Blunt and harmonic scalpel dissection can be used to mobilize the fascia of Gerota on the superomedial aspect of the kidney. By dissecting the fascia of Gerota medially at this point, the adrenal gland and its attachments should fall medially off the kidney. The dissection is then carried around the upper pole of the kidney.

Once the inferior, medial, and upper-pole attachments are dissected free from the kidney, the kidney is attached only by the renal vasculature, the lateral attachments, and the ureter. Any remaining dissection of the renal hilum can be performed to maximize vascular length. The lateral attachments of the kidney are divided within the fascia of Gerota. The dissection is begun at the inferior margin of the kidney and lateral to the ureter. The periureteral tissue is not violated so as to preserve all vascularity of the gonadal vein and ureteral complex. The dissection is carried along the lateral border of the kidney within the fascia of Gerota, resulting in a defatting of the kidney if possible. The dissection is carried cephalad to the incised attachments superiorly. The gonadal vein can then

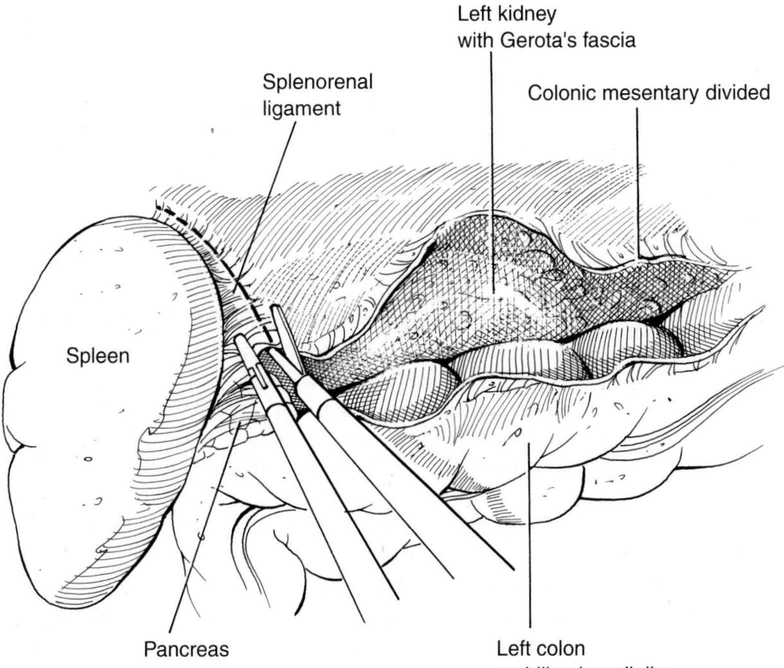


FIGURE 128.4 The cephalad incision is carried to the ipsilateral shoulder. Dividing the colonic mesentery to rotate the colon medially will develop a plane between the spleen and the fascia of Gerota. The line of dissection is carried between the two organs to allow the colon, spleen, and pancreas to fall medially. The incision of this plane continues cephalad and medial until the stomach is visualized.

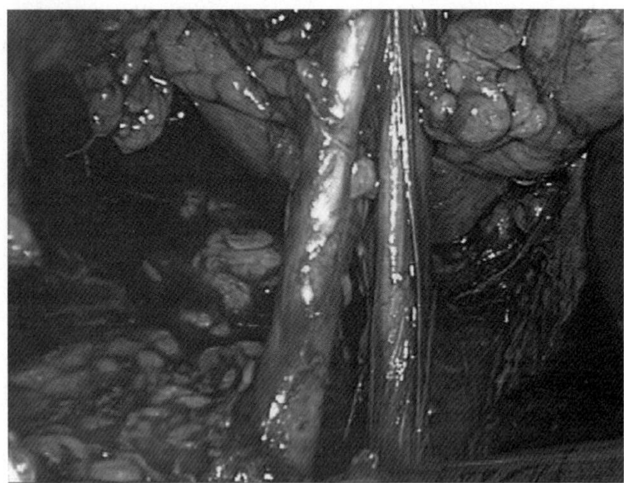

FIGURE 128.5 A goal of laparoscopic donor nephrectomy is to provide a good length of artery and vein on the kidney side.

be dissected and ligated at the pelvic brim. The vein is ligated with laparoscopic clips and divided. The ureter is also ligated and divided, usually at the level of the iliac vessels. The goal is to maximize the length of the artery and vein to assist the transplanting surgeon in a successful vascular anastomosis (Fig. 128.5).

After 3,000 units of heparin have been infused for 3 minutes, the renal artery is taken with a single endovascular staple load. The renal vein can then be similarly taken with an endovascular staple load. In cases of a wide vein, a 45-mm-long staple load can be employed. In most cases, optimal retraction is achieved with pure laparoscopic instruments; in other cases, a hand can be placed in the abdomen through the hand port for retraction. Once the kidney is extracted and passed off, 30 mg of protamine sulfate can be infused. The renal fossa and staple lines are inspected. The adrenal gland should also be inspected, as in some cases there can be some venous ooze from its lateral edge. Hemostatic maneuvers with tissue sealant, clips, or pressure can be employed if needed.

The ports can be removed under direct vision with the pneumoperitoneum down to 5 mm Hg. The extraction is closed with running suture of the surgeon's choice. The ports can be closed with an endoscopic closing device if desired. If dilating ports are used, these can be left open. In our series, we close the 10-mm and 12-mm dilating ports at the external fascial level with a 0 Vicryl UR-6 needle and S-retractors, as herniation has been reported in the literature. Skin edges can be closed based on the surgeon's preference. Wounds can be infiltrated with a local anesthetic of the surgeon's choice, typically lidocaine or bupivacaine.

## Right-Sided Donor Nephrectomy

Pneumoperitoneum is established and ports are placed in the previously described orientation. It is noted that the right colon is not as intrusive and falls medially much more easily than on the left side. The liver is retracted superiorly by placing a locking grasper through the epigastric/subxiphoid port and clamping the underside of the right upper abdomen. The locking retractor should allow for the liver to be maintained in a cephalad fashion without the need to hold the retractor.

The dissection is begun by incising 3 cm lateral to the right colon. This dissection is carried caudal to the pelvic brim. Care is taken to avoid the gonadal vein in men and the possibility of encountering a retrocecal appendix. The dissection is then turned cephalad and along the superomedial surface of the kidney. The duodenum will be encountered and can be bluntly dissected in a medial direction. Often it is easier to "kocherize" the duodenum after the ureter is retracted anterolaterally.

The ureter and its surrounding attachments should be retracted anterolaterally. It is very important to identify the gonadal vein and dissect it medially away from the ureteral package so as not to inadvertently avulse it from the vena cava. With the ureteral retraction, the dissection is carried superiorly toward the hilum along the lateral border of the vena cava. During this portion of the dissection, the duodenum may need to be bluntly dissected medially and its superior attachments incised with the harmonic scalpel. With the renal vein identified, the dissection is carried posterior to the vena cava and renal vein. With careful blunt dissection, the right renal artery should be dissected, and it should be carried as far behind the vena cava as possible. If any lumbar veins are encountered, they can be clipped and divided to allow for greater "rolling" of the vena cava. The dissection is then carried along the cephalad border of the renal vein following the superolateral margin of the right kidney.

The lateral attachments of the kidney can be divided with the harmonic scalpel starting at the inferolateral margin of the lower pole. Once again, care is taken to preserve all the periureteral tissue. With the kidney completely dissected, the ureter can be clipped and divided distally as for the right-sided procedure. When taking the renal vessels, the same endovascular stapler can be used. It has been our experience that adequate venous length can be obtained with articulation of the stapler and lateral retraction of the kidney. The kidney is extracted and passed off and protamine is given as described earlier for the left side. Closure is the same as the left side.

## Key Points

1. It is the authors' practice to avoid using clips near or around the hilum unless necessary. If a vessel cannot be taken with the harmonic scalpel, then we take it with a stapler. Staples can cross other staple lines. If clips are caught within a stapler, the results can be disastrous!
2. The gonadal vein should be retracted with the ureter on the left side. It is a "pathway" to the left renal vein.
3. The lumbar veins should be divided on the left side to give additional length. These should be taken with a stapler to avoid problems with clips at the hilum and the use of staplers.
4. There is often a tendency to work too lateral and not close enough to the aorta or vena cava. Staying close to the great vessels allows for maximizing vascular length and facilitates hilar dissection.
5. A standard articulating endovascular stapler will suffice for both sides. Avoiding heroic measures to obtain 2 to 3 mm of venous length will prevent complications for an otherwise healthy patient such as a kidney donor.

6. We recommend attempting to close 12- and 10-mm ports at the fascial level in patients whose body habitus is amenable, even if dilating ports are used.

# OUTCOMES

A major point of contention is the comparison of open versus laparoscopic donor nephrectomy. In a recent review, Shokeir (9) evaluated 69 studies referent to LDN and open donor nephrectomy (ODN). Within this comprehensive review, seven reports were randomized controlled trials (RCTs). All RCTs concluded that LDN provides equal graft function at 1 year, equal rejection rate, equal urologic complications, and equal patient and graft survival. Analgesic requirements, pain data, hospital stay, and time to return normal activities favored the laparoscopic approach significantly. This report also compares reported mortalities. A total of 11 deaths in the LDN cohorts and 10 deaths in the ODN cohorts were reported. A trend toward higher estimated blood loss was found in the open group. Reports of postoperative complications were also reviewed. Gastrointestinal problems (bowel injury, bowel obstruction, internal hernia, and pancreatitis) were more common with LDN, while pulmonary complications (atelectasis, pneumothorax, pulmonary congestion, and hypoxia) as well as thrombotic complications (deep vein thrombosis, thrombophlebitis, and pulmonary embolism) were more common with ODN. Another aspect to be considered when taking into account outcomes and complications of LDN is the absence of a uniform system to classify them. In order to best address this concern, it is necessary to develop a standardized classification and a nationwide donor registry to determine global complications and long-term outcomes rather than short reports at single institutions (10).

Also important is the report of 15 graft losses directly related to the technical aspect of LDN. It is difficult to say, but this may be related to the learning curve of LDN over the years, and long-term outcomes will have to be compared. It is important to consider that the complications and outcomes in LDN have a tendency to be experience-dependent. Through the analysis of the learning curve, different studies have shown that the incidence of complications tends to diminish as the surgeon becomes more experienced (9–12).

In our own series of over 500 LDNs, we have carefully followed our early and long-term patient and graft outcomes. We have previously reported our results after our initial 200 patients (13,14). Overall complication rates have ranged between 12% and 14%, with only 1.5% of the complications being major complications. Our technique and experience have evolved since 1999, when we were doing the dissection with conventional laparoscopic technique and placing the kidney in a specimen retrieval bag. Since then, we have developed a technique of pure conventional laparoscopic dissection with kidney extraction through a hand port as described previously.

We have found that having the hand port in place before actual extraction has decreased our extraction time to a mean of 1.16 minutes. With a short extraction time, the overall warm ischemia time is kept to a minimum. We continue to do pure laparoscopic dissection as techniques have allowed us to be ready to extract and pass off the specimen in under 50 minutes. With our mean operative times down to under 90 minutes, we are able to keep the anesthesia time short for our healthy donor patients.

Another concern with LDN is the manner in which the vessels are ligated and divided. There are numerous reports of ways to "maximize" venous and arterial length. We have been using the laparoscopic articulating endovascular GIA in all 500 patients (left- and right-sided) without direct technical consequence to our transplant colleagues. We feel that the stapler is a reliable, safe, and efficient way to manage the artery and vein. By eliminating extra steps and tools such as clips and/or directly cutting on a clamp requiring vascular suturing, we feel donor safety is preserved. One must remember that the kidney donor patient is an otherwise healthy person, and his or her well-being and best interests should be of the utmost importance.

## Complications

With an estimated 12% to 14% overall complication rate and a major complication rate of approximately 1.5%, patients must be fully informed of all possible outcomes. As with any surgery, there are risks of bleeding, pain, infection, incisional hernia, deep venous thrombosis, pulmonary embolus, pneumonia, and cardiac risks. These have the same incidence as one would expect in any healthy patient undergoing general anesthesia and laparoscopic renal surgery. Table 128.2 outlines the specific risks of laparoscopic donor nephrectomy.

As with any laparoscopic procedure, there is always the possibility of open conversion. The decision to convert most often reflects good judgment and in and of itself is not a complication. The act of converting should not be considered a complication, as open surgery is the standard to fall back to and not an adverse approach. The surgeon always has the option to convert to open nephrectomy and should have all instruments necessary for open surgery. The incision most often made is a subcostal incision connecting two or more ports if possible. In most cases conversion is due to ongoing hemorrhage or failure to progress secondary to adhesions.

In addition to open conversion, other potential complications inherent to the laparoscopic nature of the operation include pneumothorax, port herniation, and trocar injuries. These should be managed in the standard fashion. The pneumothorax is often not associated with an air leak, so observation or immediate percutaneous drainage is all that is often needed. Port herniation should be treated with return to the operating room for laparoscopic reduction. Trocar injuries to underlying structures should be identified and repaired immediately. In the event of bowel injury during access to the abdominal cavity, the standard of teaching has been to abort the procedure. Although ileus is rare with laparoscopic surgery, it is most often treated with simple bowel rest, ambulation, and observation.

One of the more devastating complications is a vascular complication within the renal hilum. With the U.S. Food and Drug Administration having recalled the Weck Hem-O-Lok L Polymer Ligating Clips (Weck Closure Systems, Research Triangle Park, NC), it is a contraindication for its use in renal hilar control. Nevertheless, failure of the endovascular stapler

**TABLE 128.2**

**RISKS SPECIFIC TO LAPAROSCOPIC DONOR NEPHRECTOMY**

- Need for open conversion
- Pneumothorax
- Port herniation
- Trocar injuries
- Ileus
- Stapler malfunction resulting in hemorrhage
- Clip malfunction
- Injury to the spleen or liver
- Lymphocele
- Degloving injury to the kidney
- Testicular pain/epididymitis

is a rare but possible event, as well as with clips. This complication is usually identified immediately as significant hemorrhage will be encountered. Venous bleeding can often be controlled with direct compression (laparoscopic or digital through the GelPort), increase of the pneumoperitoneum to 20 mm Hg, and laparoscopic suturing techniques. Arterial bleeding from the main renal artery due to stapler or clip malfunction is particularly difficult to control laparoscopically. Simply put, if vascular control cannot be obtained with laparoscopic maneuvers, one should convert and use standard open techniques. The same applies to injuries to surrounding structures such as the spleen. Although newer hemostatic glues and sealants are available, some splenic lacerations and injuries will not stop bleeding. If use of hemostatic agents fails, splenectomy may be needed and can be performed laparoscopically or open, depending on the surgeon. Injuries to the liver are often minimal and most often can be managed with hemostatic applications of glues, sealants, or even argon beam coagulation.

Lymphocele is a known complication of donor nephrectomy. This is often due to the disruption of lymphatic channels within the hilum as well as injury to the cisterna chyli. Although rarely seen with donor nephrectomy as it is often performed transperitoneally, it is still a reported complication. If an area walls off and does not communicate with the peritoneum, it can result in a lymphocele even in transperitoneal cases. Often drainage, percutaneous or open, is all that is needed. If it results in chylous ascites, then diet modification to medium-chain fatty acids is required. Management would be similar to retroperitoneal lymph node dissection patients who suffer this complication.

Degloving injuries to the transplanted renal unit are possible. This usually occurs in cases where there is very adherent perinephric fat and a hand is being used in the dissection. This can be avoided if direct incision of surrounding attachments, splenorenal ligaments, and overlying fat is done directly with pure laparoscopic techniques. It is easy to get "heavy-handed" during manual dissection to expedite an operation. If this degloving injury does occur, it has little consequence for the donor but will have to be addressed by the recipient team, as it can increase the risk of bleeding in the recipient. Often backtable repair of stripped renal capsule or intraoperative application of tissue sealants is used.

Finally, in male patients undergoing left LDN, left testicular pain and/or left epididymitis/orchitis has been reported postoperatively. This is a consequence of taking the left gonadal vein during the procedure. The patients will report an "ache" and fullness in the left hemiscrotum. This is usually self-limiting and should be managed with anti-inflammatories and scrotal elevation. In cases where an infectious etiology is suspected due to urethral catheterization, antibiotic treatment for 3 to 4 weeks is appropriate.

## References


1. Mandelbrot DA, Pavlakis M, Danovitch GM, et al. The medical evaluation of living kidney donors: a survey of US transplant centers. *Am J Transplant* 2007;7:2333–2343.
2. Delmonico F; Council of the Transplantation Society. A report of the Amsterdam Forum on the care of the live kidney donor: data and medical guidelines. *Transplantation* 2005;27(79):S53–66.
3. Delmonico FL, Dew A. Living donor kidney transplantation in a global environment. *Kidney Int* 2007;7:608–614.
4. Dew MA, Jacobs CL, Jowsey SG, et al.; United Network for Organ Sharing (UNOS); American Society of Transplant Surgeons; American Society of Transplantation. Guidelines for the psychosocial evaluation of living unrelated kidney donors in the United States. *Am J Transplant* 2007;7:1047–1054.
5. Rodrigue JR, Pavlakis M, Danovitch GM, et al. Evaluating living kidney donors: relationship types, psychosocial criteria, and consent processes at US transplant programs. *Am J Transplant* 2007;7:2326–2332.
6. Morrissey PE, Monaco AP. Living kidney donation: evolution and technical aspects of donor nephrectomy. *Surg Clin North Am* 2006;86:1219–1235.
7. Shenoy S, Lowell JA, Ramachandran V, et al. The ideal living donor nephrectomy "mini-nephrectomy" through a posterior transcostal approach. *J Am Coll Surg* 2002;194:240–246.
8. Kok NF, Alwayn IP, Lind MY, et al. Donor nephrectomy: mini-incision muscle-splitting open approach versus laparoscopy. *Transplantation* 2006;81:881–887.
9. Shokeir AA. Open versus laparoscopic live donor nephrectomy: a focus on the safety of donors and the need for a donor registry. *J Urol* 2007;178:1860–1866.
10. Kocak B, Koffron AJ, Baker TB, et al. Proposed classification of complications after live donor nephrectomy. *Urology* 2006;67:927–931.
11. Chin EH, Hazzan D, Herron DM, et al. Laparoscopic donor nephrectomy: intraoperative safety, immediate morbidity, and delayed complications with 500 cases. *Surg Endosc* 2007;21:521–526.
12. Martin GL, Guise AI, Bernie JE, et al. Laparoscopic donor nephrectomy: effects of learning curve on surgical outcomes. *Transplant Proc* 2007;39:27–29.
13. Lallas CD, Castle EP, Schlinkert RT, et al. The development of a laparoscopic donor nephrectomy program in a de novo renal transplant program: evolution of technique and results in over 200 cases. *JSLS* 2006;10:135–140.
14. Lallas CD, Castle EP, Andrews PE. Hand port use for extraction during laparoscopic donor nephrectomy. *Urology* 2006;67:706–708.

# CHAPTER 129 ■ LAPAROSCOPIC AND ROBOTICALLY ASSISTED PYELOPLASTY IN ADULTS

KRISTOFER R. WAGNER AND THOMAS W. JARRETT

After the first successful reconstructive procedure was performed by Kuster in 1891, a variety of procedures (open and minimally invasive surgeries) have been described for management of the obstructed ureteropelvic junction (UPJ). Laparoscopic pyeloplasty was first described in 1993 by Schuessler et al. (1) as a less invasive means of reconstructing the UPJ under direct visualization. This approach preserves the principles of open pyeloplasty and offers maximal flexibility in reconstruction without the associated morbidity of a large flank incision. The learning curve for laparoscopic suturing and prolonged operative times initially prevented more widespread utilization of the technique. More recently, use of robotic technology has facilitated the transition for some surgeons and may lead to decreased operative time.

## DIAGNOSIS

The diagnosis of UPJ obstruction in general can be made by intravenous urogram or diuretic renal scan. Preoperative computerized tomography may be helpful in identifying patients with a crossing vessel who are being considered for an endopyelotomy procedure. Retrograde pyelography has an important role in confirmation of the diagnosis and for exact delineation of the obstruction. This can usually be performed in conjunction with the procedure.

## INDICATIONS FOR SURGERY

Laparoscopic pyeloplasty is effective for all types of UPJ obstruction but should be strongly considered in instances where a less invasive procedure is less likely to be successful. Such situations include severe hydronephrosis, crossing vessels, strictures >2 cm in length, failed previous endoscopic procedures, concomitant renal stones, renal ptosis, and poor renal function.

## ALTERNATIVE THERAPY

Open pyeloplasty has been considered the gold-standard intervention for correcting UPJ obstruction, with a success rate exceeding 90% (2,3), but it is associated with significant postoperative morbidity related with open flank surgery. Several minimally invasive endoscopic procedures for treatment of UPJ obstruction have been developed to minimize the postoperative morbidity. Direct-vision endopyelotomy via percutaneous antegrade or retrograde approaches yields a lower early success rate of 66% to 90% when compared to open pyeloplasty and may have even lower long-term success rates (4–6). We do not use the fluoroscopic cautery-wire (Acucise, Applied Medical, Rancho Santa Margarita, CA) technique for UPJ repair.

## SURGICAL TECHNIQUE

The patient is admitted the same day of surgery. After antibiotic administration and induction of general anesthesia, an orogastric tube is inserted and sequential compression devices are placed on the lower extremities. The patient is initially positioned supine (frog-leg position for women and supine for men). Using a flexible cystoscope, angle-tipped glide wire, and 5Fr open-ended catheter, a retrograde pyelogram is performed with C-arm fluoroscopy to confirm the diagnosis and demonstrate the exact site and nature of the obstruction. A 7Fr 28-cm (double-pigtail) stent is placed and correct position confirmed with fluoroscopy. A longer-than-usual stent is used to minimize the possibility of stent displacement out of the bladder during surgical manipulation of the UPJ. In men, the glide wire can be resheathed and prepared into the operative field. The stent can then be placed later with the flexible cystoscope after the back wall of the anastomosis is completed. This avoids the interference with the proximal stent curl while suturing the back wall. In women, access to the urethra is problematic, and it is preferable to place the stent preoperatively. A Foley catheter is inserted before the patient is placed in a 45-degree lateral decubitus position. This position minimizes potential neuromuscular complications that may occur with the 90-degree flank position and is illustrated in previous chapters. A roll is placed under the ipsilateral shoulder and down to the ipsilateral pelvis to keep the operative side elevated and stable. It is not necessary to place an axillary roll, flex the operating table, or elevate the kidney rest. The ipsilateral arm is placed across the chest and the contralateral arm is placed on an arm board abducted 90 degrees from the table with stacked pillows and folded blankets between the arms. Care is taken to protect all pressure points with foam. The lower knee is bent slightly, and the ipsilateral leg is kept almost straight with pillows or foam placed between them to prevent pressure ulcers and neurologic injury. Foam and wide cloth tape are placed across the upper shoulder and arm and across the hip to secure the patient to the operating table. The table is tested tilting maximally to the left and right. The entire abdomen and flank from the xiphoid to the pubis is shaved carefully and then scrubbed.

## Trocar Placement

Laparoscopic pyeloplasty is performed by the transperitoneal approach. Pneumoperitoneum is established by inserting a Veress needle lateral to the rectus border or into the umbilicus. After an insufflation pressure of 15 mm Hg is established, three midline trocars are placed (Fig. 129.1). The umbilical trocar is 10 mm to allow use of a 10-mm 30-degree laparoscope. The remaining trocars are placed two fingerbreadths above the symphysis pubis and 8 cm above the umbilicus. Trocars are either 5 or 12 mm, depending on surgical side (right or left) and dominant hand of the surgeon. The larger trocar would be placed in the dominant hand of the surgeon to allow for passage of the needle driver and/or Endostitch device during the repair of the UPJ.

The surgeon operates from the opposite side of the affected renal unit and uses the supra- and infraumbilical trocars as the working ports. The assistant or the robot arm (AESOP) stands on the same side of the operating table as the surgeon and manipulates the camera by the umbilical port.

The table is rotated with the ipsilateral side up, and the lateral peritoneal reflection overlying the kidney is incised along the white line of Toldt from the upper pole to approximately 3 cm below the lower pole. The renocolic ligaments are then divided sharply and the colon is retracted medially with a sweeping motion, further exposing the retroperitoneum. On the right side, a Kocher maneuver may be necessary to mobilize the duodenum off the medial aspect of the kidney.

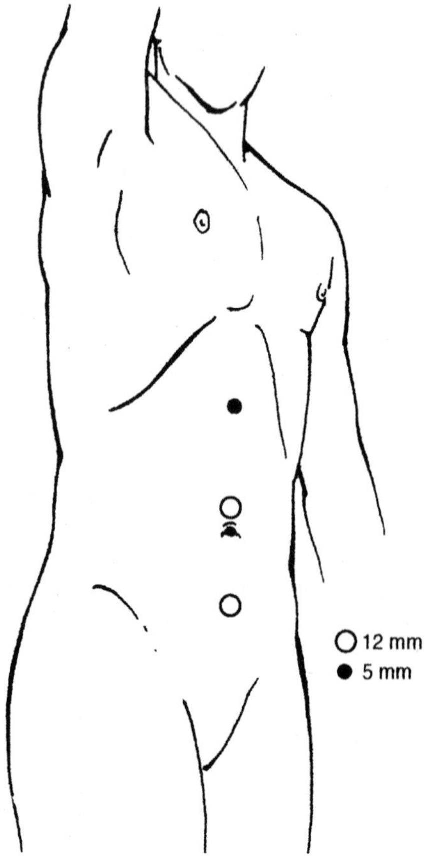

The ureter is identified just medial to the lower pole of the kidney and usually lies lateral and posterior to the gonadal vessels. Gentle palpation of the indwelling stent confirms the structure to be the ureter. A plane between the psoas muscle and the ureter is created using gentle sweeping motions and the ureter is dissected cephalad until the UPJ is identified. It is important to dissect the ureter with its adjacent tissue attached to maximize the blood supply. The ureter should be skeletonized only in the area of the UPJ for delineation of the anatomy.

It is frequently useful to place a 4-0 absorbable suture through the anterior renal pelvis as a stay suture to aid in retraction and fixation during dissection and repair. This suture may be passed through the abdominal wall, renal pelvis, and back through the abdominal wall using a Keith needle. It is secured outside the abdomen using a hemostat to adjust tension on the suture. Extra attention should be made for lower-pole crossing vessels, which can be damaged with overzealous dissection. In the presence of crossing vessels, the renal pelvis and ureter are carefully dissected free so that the ureter can be easily transposed anteriorly as needed. The ureter and renal pelvis are then mobilized as needed to allow for a subsequent tension-free repair. At this point the surgeon must commit to the type of repair to be used depending on the nature of the UPJ obstruction. Any renal calculi can be removed with a combination of direct extraction using forceps through the pyelotomy or with the aid of a flexible cystoscope passed through the upper trocar.

O 12 mm
● 5 mm

FIGURE 129.1 Trocar placement for transperitoneal laparoscopic pyeloplasty.

## Anderson–Hynes Dismembered Pyeloplasty

Dismembered pyeloplasty is our preference in most clinical circumstances (Fig. 129.2). It is especially preferable with crossing vessels and a large redundant renal pelvis. Scissors are used to transect the UPJ, taking care not to damage the ureteral stent. The renal pelvis is first incised circumferentially above the area of stenosis, and the stent is then delivered through this incision. The initial pyelotomy is made on the medial aspect of the renal pelvis and cephalad to the UPJ. This results in a "handle" of tissue that can be used to manipulate the ureter. The posterior wall is transected, thus completely freeing the ureter from the renal pelvis. The proximal ureter is spatulated on the lateral aspect using laparoscopic scissors, with attention not to spiral the incision. When a crossing vessel is present, the ureter must be transposed anteriorly to these vascular structures prior to reanastomosis to the renal pelvis. A reduction pyeloplasty is performed at this point when necessary.

Next, 4-0 absorbable stay sutures are placed at the apex of the spatulated ureter and then through the most dependent portion of the reduced renal pelvis. They are tied using intracorporeal techniques. This suture is then used in a running fashion to approximate the posterior portions of the renal pelvis and ureter. Sutures can be placed using the freehand technique or the Endostitch device (Fig. 129.3) (7). The medial portion of the proximal ureter used as a handle is excised. The proximal curl of the stent is placed back into the renal pelvis or upper pole calyx and the anterior portion of the anastomosis is completed using the same technique. The cephalad portion of the pyelotomy is sutured with

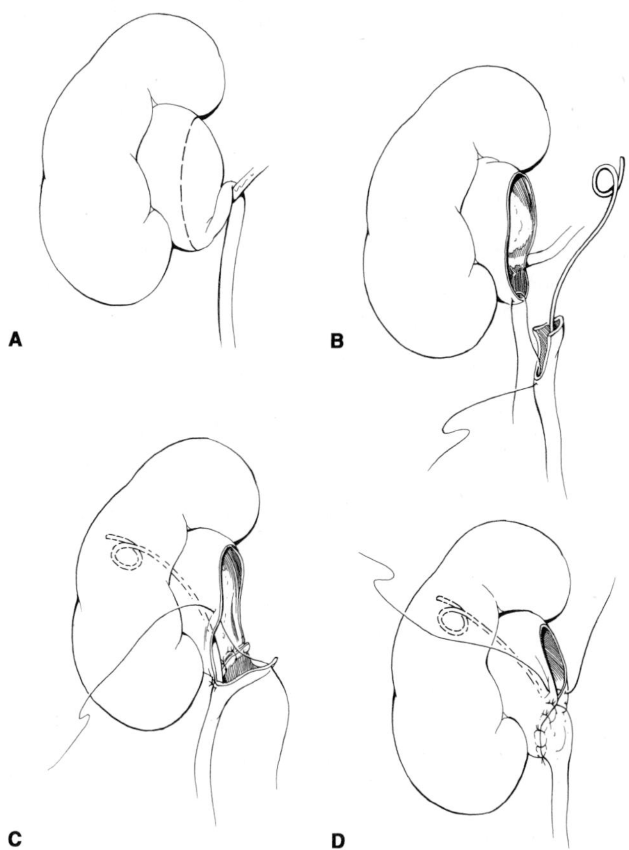


FIGURE 129.2 Anderson–Hynes dismembered pyeloplasty technique.

continuous 4-0 absorbable sutures using the Endostitch or freehand technique. Care is taken to avoid incorporating the stent into the sutures.

## Foley V–V Pyeloplasty

The Foley Y–V pyeloplasty (Fig. 129.4) may be considered in the absence of crossing vessels when there is a small renal pelvis or a high ureteral insertion into the renal pelvis. Using laparoscopic scissors, a wide-based V-shaped flap is constructed from the anterior pelvis. The proximal ureter is spatulated anteriorly. Using 4-0 absorbable sutures, the apex of the V-flap is sutured to the apex of the spatulated ureteral incision and tied intracorporeally with the Endostitch or freehand techniques. The lower wall is completed first using the Endostitch to place the sutures, and the anastomosis is completed with sutures that are placed from the apex out toward the upper pelvis.

## Fenger Nondismembered Pyeloplasty (Heineke–Mikulicz)

The Fenger pyeloplasty (Fig. 129.5) may be considered for a short stenotic segment in the absence of crossing vessels or a high insertion. The principle of this procedure is a longitudinal incision and transverse closure. This technique has the potential advantage of a shorter operative time because fewer intracorporeal sutures are needed. A longitudinal incision is made with laparoscopic scissors from the renal pelvis distally

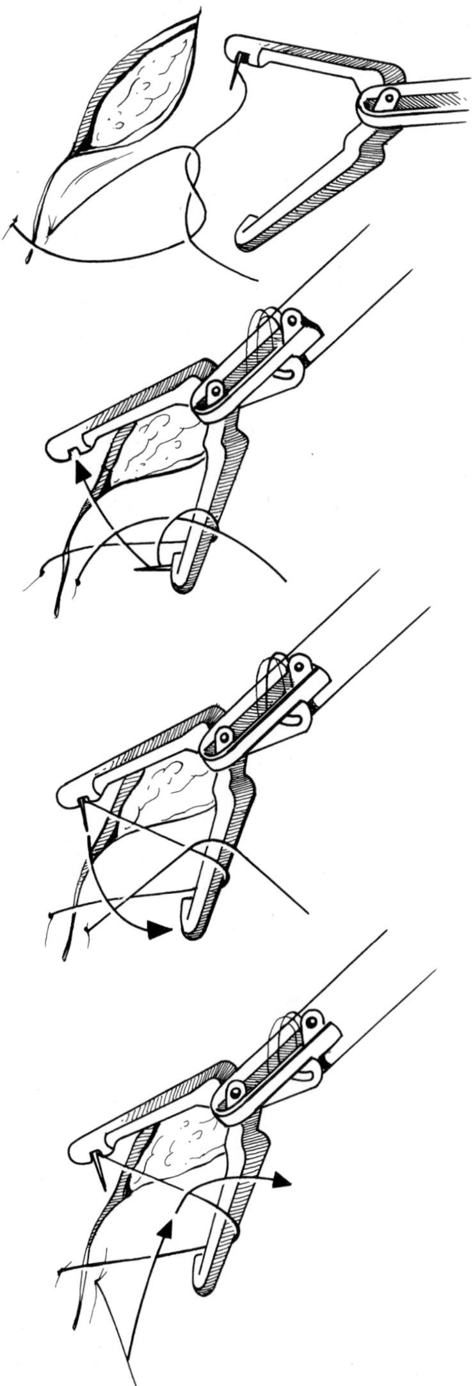

FIGURE 129.3 Endostitch device.

to 1 to 2 cm below the UPJ segment. The initial pyelotomy incision, just above the UPJ, can be made with a laparoscopic knife or scissors. The longitudinal incision is then closed transversely in a Heineke–Mikulicz fashion over the stent using one continuous 4-0 absorbable suture.

## Additional Salvage Maneuvers

Additional maneuvers may be necessary in cases where a long (>2 cm) stricture is present or the anastomosis is under tension. This is more likely in cases of secondary UPJ obstruction

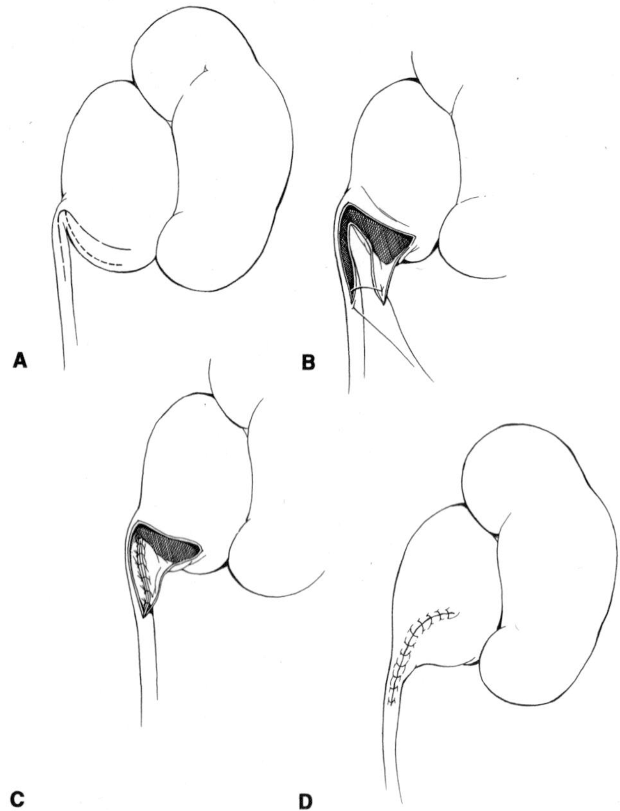


FIGURE 129.4 Foley Y–V pyeloplasty technique.

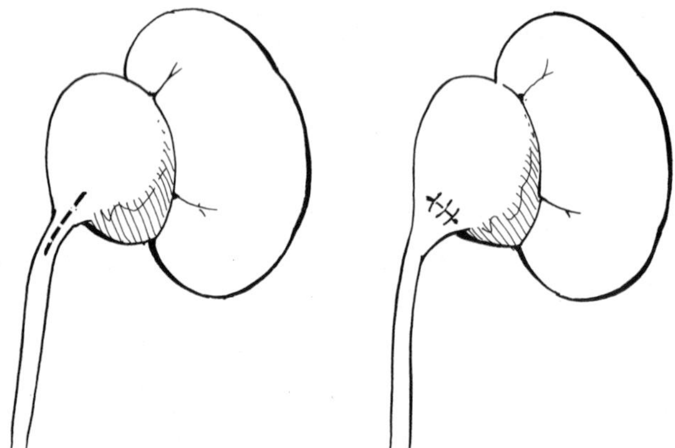

FIGURE 129.5 Fenger nondismembered pyeloplasty (Heineke–Mikulicz) technique.

or those with previous failed treatment. In these cases, it is critical to assess the UPJ and stricture length prior to transecting the UPJ. It may be necessary to create a vertical or spiral flap of renal pelvis to reconstruct the UPJ and gain adequate length. Mobilization of the entire kidney inferiorly may also provide a few centimeters of additional length. In redo salvage situations with a very long stricture, a laparoscopic ureterocalicostomy or ileal ureter might be necessary.

After the chosen anastomosis is completed, fibrin glue may be used to help seal the anastomotic site. Then, the pneumoperitoneum pressure is dropped to 5 mm Hg and the operative sites are examined for bleeding. After hemostasis is adequately obtained, a small closed-bulb suction drain (Jackson–Pratt) is positioned carefully in the retroperitoneum to lie adjacent to the newly completed anastomosis but never in direct contact. The drain is brought out through a small stab incision in the posterior axillary line and then secured with a 3-0 nylon suture. All trocars are then removed under direct vision. The abdominal fasciae of all 10/12-mm port sites are closed with interrupted 0 absorbable sutures using the Carter-Thomason closure device. The $CO_2$ pneumoperitoneum is removed to decrease postoperative shoulder irritation. The drain is connected to bulb suction. The skin incisions are closed with subcuticular 4-0 polyglactin sutures and adhesive skin tape.

## Transmesenteric Approach

The transmesenteric approach may offer advantages of decreased operative time and ileus in appropriately selected cases. This approach is primarily useful in left-sided cases because the splenic flexure lies cephalad to the UPJ (Fig. 129.6A). It is technically feasible in cases with a laterally displaced colon and relatively thin mesentery. This anatomic situation is more frequently encountered in pediatric cases or in thin women. Instead of mobilizing the colon medially, a longitudinal window is created in the mesentery over the UPJ, taking care to avoid mesenteric vessels (Fig. 129.6B). A stay suture through the abdominal wall is most useful to elevate the renal pelvis and UPJ from the mesenteric window. From this vantage point, the proximal ureter and renal pelvis are dissected and the repair of choice is performed as described above.

## Robot-Assisted Laparoscopic Pyeloplasty

The da Vinci robotic surgical system (Intuitive Surgical, Sunnyvale, CA) offers several advantages over standard

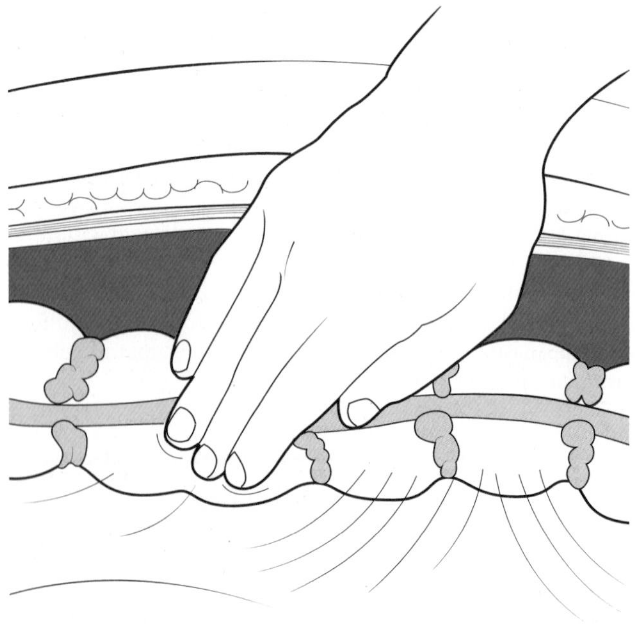

FIGURE 129.6 **A:** Laterally displaced left colon, suitable for transmesenteric approach.

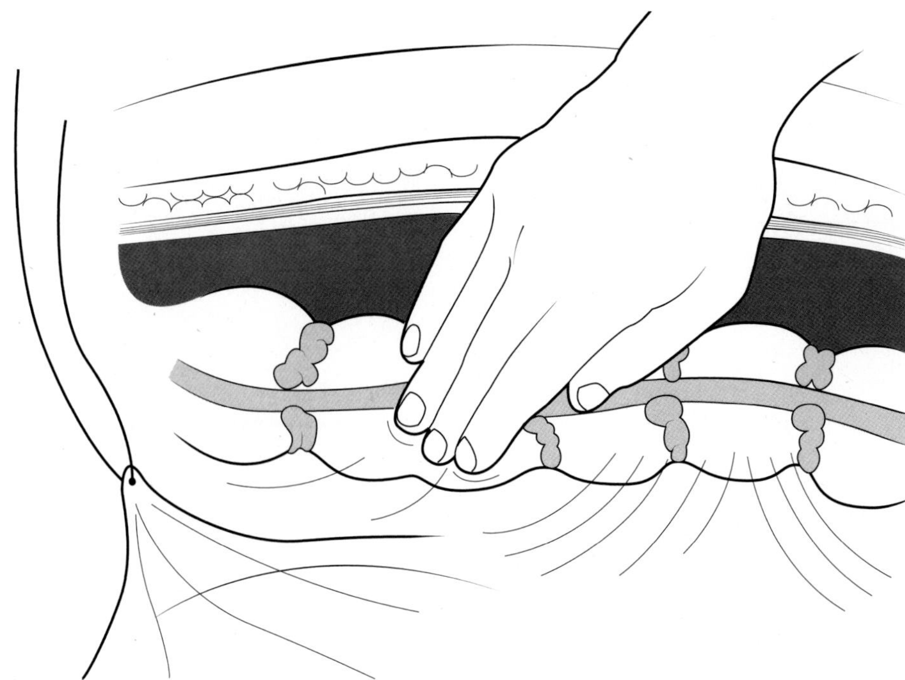

FIGURE 129.6 B: Transmesenteric technique with stay suture through abdominal wall.

laparoscopic pyeloplasty. Additional magnification (10×), three-dimensional stereoscopic vision, motion scaling, and tremor filtering provide an increased level of precision in dissection and reconstruction. In particular, suturing time may be decreased with the use of the da Vinci system. The patient is positioned as described previously for laparoscopic pyeloplasty. Trocar placement includes a 10/12-mm trocar at the umbilicus for the camera and two 8-mm robotic trocars, one in the midline 8 cm above the umbilicus and one in the lower quadrant lateral to the rectus border (Fig. 129.7). An additional 5- or 10-mm port is placed in the lower midline to allow the assistant to pass suture and provide suction and retraction. Mobilization of the colon and exposure of the UPJ are performed using standard laparoscopic instrumentation as described previously. The robot is then docked, with the patient side cart approaching the patient's back at a 45-degree angle from the ipsilateral shoulder toward the umbilicus (Fig. 129.8). The camera arm and two working arms reach across the patient's abdomen and angle back toward the ipsilateral upper quadrant. The 30-degree down-angled da Vinci scope is connected to the camera arm. The Maryland forceps and Potts scissors are used to transect the UPJ. The articulating Potts are particularly useful to precisely spatulate the ureter and tailor the renal pelvis. The robotic needle drivers are then used to perform the reconstruction as described previously. Robotic surgeons should be familiar with standard laparoscopic suturing techniques to avoid open conversion in the event of a robot malfunction.

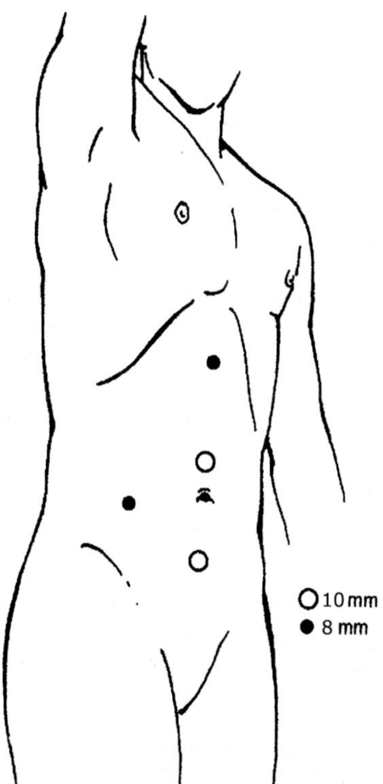


FIGURE 129.7 Trocar placement for right-sided robot-assisted laparoscopic pyeloplasty.

## Postoperative Care

The orogastric tube is removed just before extubation. On the ward, vigilant records of outputs must be kept to dictate drain management. The Foley catheter is removed on postoperative day 1 or 2 if the drain fluid output is consistently <30 to 50 cc per 8 hours. A drain fluid creatinine is obtained if output is greater than this. Following removal of the Foley, the retroperitoneal drain outputs must be monitored for increased output. If the outputs increase, the Foley should be replaced until they drop to acceptable levels. The retroperitoneal drain may be removed when the drainage is negligible after the Foley removal, which is usually postoperative day 2. In some cases, patients are sent home with the drains in place if they have met all other criteria for discharge.

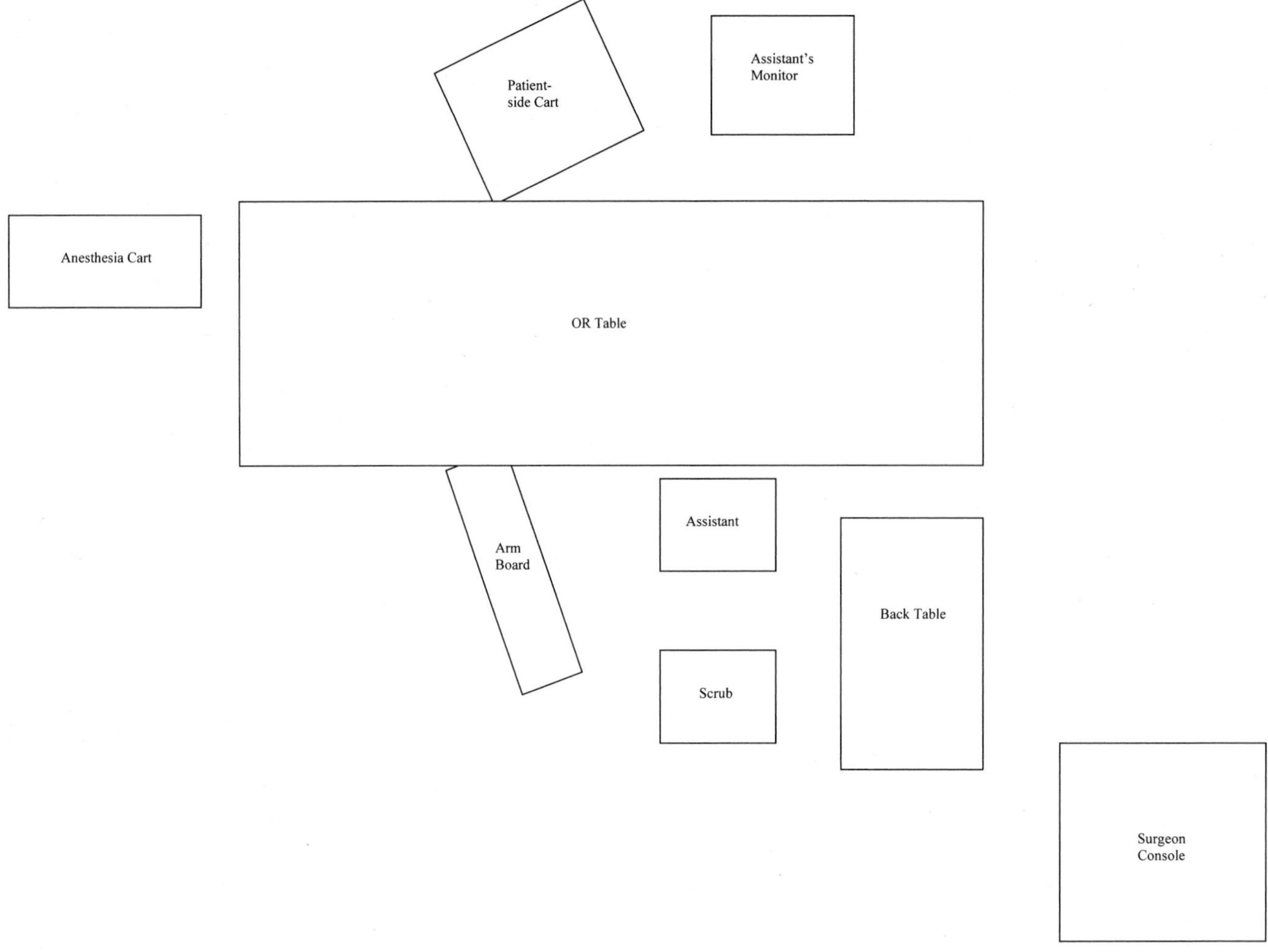


FIGURE 129.8 Room setup for left-sided robot-assisted laparoscopic pyeloplasty.

A clear liquid diet is started on postoperative day 1 and advanced following the passage of flatus. The intravenous antibiotics are continued for 24 hours, and then switched to an oral agent. The ureteral stent is removed in the office in 6 weeks. The anastomosis is then radiologically re-evaluated with an intravenous urogram or renal nuclear scan 6 weeks after stent removal unless the patient has recurrent symptoms. A follow-up diuretic renal scan is obtained at 6 months postoperatively and compared with the previous study. Thereafter, an intravenous urogram or a renal scan is obtained at yearly intervals.

## OUTCOMES

Laparoscopic pyeloplasty retains the benefits of open pyeloplasty while minimizing the morbidity of incisional trauma. This approach should be considered especially in those instances where endopyelotomy is contraindicated or has compromised results. Such situations include severe hydronephrosis, renal ptosis with renal kinking, poor renal function, strictures longer than 2 cm, concomitant nonobstructing renal stones, and crossing lower-pole vessels. The major disadvantage of the laparoscopic approach is the learning curve. The technique requires not only laparoscopic expertise but also experience with intracorporeal suturing and tying.

Results have been excellent and are comparable to open pyeloplasty. In a series of 100 consecutive laparoscopic pyeloplasty cases from the Johns Hopkins Hospital, 96% were successful with a mean radiographic follow-up of 2.2 years (8). Fifty-six of 100 patients were found intraoperatively to have lower-pole crossing vessels and thus underwent dismembered pyeloplasty. In patients with calculi, concomitant laparoscopic pyeloscopy with extraction of the stones was performed. A French multicenter study examined 55 retroperitoneal laparoscopic pyeloplasty cases and found that 95% of cases were successfully completed laparoscopically; all patients were pain-free and radiographically unobstructed by 3 months (9). The overall complication rate was 12.7%. Complications in seven patients included hematoma in three, urinoma in one, severe pyelonephritis in one, and anastomotic stricture in two, requiring open pyeloplasty at 3 weeks and delayed balloon incision at 13 months, respectively.

The largest comparative series between laparoscopic and open pyeloplasties was reported on a retrospective series of 42 patients who underwent laparoscopic pyeloplasty and 35 who underwent open repair with regard to outcome and complications (10). Follow-up was up to 22 months in the laparoscopic group and 58 months in the open series. The complication rate for the laparoscopic group was 12% (five patients) while the open group had 11% (four patients). No significant difference in pain-free rates between both groups was observed (laparoscopic 62%, open 60%). Objective success was based on radiographic findings. Radiologic failure was observed in one patient in the laparoscopic group (within 24 hours after the stent was removed) and in two patients in the open group.

Gettman et al. (11) reported the first robot-assisted laparoscopic pyeloplasty series in six patients and compared them to a control group of six standard laparoscopic pyeloplasties. Operative time and suturing time were significantly decreased in the robotic group and the objective success rate was 100%. A recent multi-institutional series from several hospitals in New York City included 35 patients, with mean operative time of 216 minutes and suture time of 63 minutes (12). Mean hospital stay was 2.9 days, and objective success rates were likewise excellent (94%) with mean follow-up of 7.9 months.

Laparoscopic pyeloplasty is a feasible but technically demanding procedure. This surgical technique maintains the advantages of open reconstruction of the UPJ while decreasing the morbidity due to a large flank incision. The increased availability of laparoscopic training and robot-assisted technology has led to acceptable procedure times. Moreover, longer follow-up has shown durable success rates comparable to open surgery.

## Complications

All complications of abdominal laparoscopy are possible, and injury to adjacent organs should be considered when the clinical situation is deteriorating. The most common complications are usually due to persistence of urinary leak or urinoma. The possibility of urinoma requiring revision of drains can be minimized with vigilant placement at the time of surgery. Most controlled urinary leaks can be managed as an outpatient with continued suction drainage with or without a Foley catheter. Most will close with time. Failure to drain the urine or urinoma requires either percutaneous or surgical drainage.

## *References*


1. Schuessler WW, Grune MT, Tecuanhuey LV, et al. Laparoscopic dismembered pyeloplasty. *J Urol* 1993;150:1795–1799.
2. Notley RG, Beaugie JM. The long-term follow-up of Anderson-Hynes pyeloplasty for hydronephrosis. *Br J Urol* 1973;45:464–467.
3. Persky L, Krause JR, Boltuch RL. Initial complications and late results in dismembered pyeloplasty. *J Urol* 1977;118:162–165.
4. Dimarco DS, Gettman MT, McGee SM, et al. Long-term success of antegrade endopyelotomy compared with pyeloplasty at a single institution. *J Endourol* 2006;20:707–712.
5. Motola JA, Badlani GH, Smith AD. Results of 221 consecutive endopyelotomies: an eight-year follow-up. *J Urol* 1993;149:453–456.
6. Nakada SY, Johnson M. Ureteropelvic junction obstruction: retrograde endopyelotomy. *Urol Clin North Am* 2000;27:677–684.
7. Adams JB, Schulam PG, Moore RG, et al. New laparoscopic suturing device: initial clinical experience. *Urology* 1995;46:242–245.
8. Jarrett TW, Chan DY, Charambura TC, et al. Laparoscopic pyeloplasty: the first 100 cases. *J Urol* 2002;167:1253–1256.
9. Soulié M, Salomon L, Patard JJ, et al. Extraperitoneal laparoscopic pyeloplasty: a multicenter study of 55 procedures. *J Urol* 2001;166:48–50.
10. Bauer JJ, Bishoff JT, Moore RG, et al. Laparoscopic versus open pyeloplasty: assessment of objective and subjective outcome. *J Urol* 1999; 163:692–695.
11. Gettman M, Peschel R, Neururer R, et al. A comparison of laparoscopic pyeloplasty performed with the da Vinci robotic system versus standard laparoscopic techniques: initial clinical results. *Eur Urol* 2002;42:453–458.
12. Palese M, Stifelman M, Munver R, et al. Robot-assisted laparoscopic dismembered pyeloplasty: a combined experience. *J Endourol* 2005;19(3): 382–386.


# CHAPTER 130 ■ LAPAROSCOPIC ADRENALECTOMY

ARVIN K. GEORGE AND LOUIS R. KAVOUSSI

Since Gagner et al. first described laparoscopic adrenalectomy in 1992, this approach has become the preferred technique in the surgical management of most adrenal lesions (1). Laparoscopic adrenalectomy demonstrates the classical benefits of minimally invasive surgery, with multiple studies supporting reduction in postoperative pain, analgesia requirements, and postoperative morbidity with equivalent functional outcome when compared with traditional open surgery. Advances in minimally invasive surgical techniques have generated the development of multiple approaches to adrenalectomy, including transperitoneal, retroperitoneal, transthoracic/transdiaphragmatic, and most recently robot-assisted surgery. The benign nature of the majority of adrenal disease, combined with the deep retroperitoneal location of the adrenal gland, has lent itself ideally to the laparoscopic removal of lesions.

## INDICATIONS

Laparoscopic adrenalectomy is a definitive surgical treatment modality for the broad spectrum of adrenal disease. It has been proven safe and effective in the management of benign functioning and nonfunctioning adrenal conditions as well as the majority of malignant neoplasms (Table 130.1). As surgeon experience has increased, the contraindications to the laparoscopic approach have decreased. In the hands of a proficient and practiced surgeon, contraindications have

**TABLE 130.1**

**INDICATIONS FOR LAPAROSCOPIC ADRENALECTOMY**

| *Benign* | *Malignant* |
|---|---|
| Primary aldosteronism (adenoma/hyperplasia) | Adrenocortical carcinoma |
| Cushing disease or Cushing adenoma | Solitary adrenal metastases |
| Pheochromocytoma | |
| Adrenal cyst | |
| Myelolipoma | |
| Incidentaloma/adenoma with >3 cm of growth over time with serial imaging | |

**TABLE 130.2**

**CONTRAINDICATIONS TO LAPAROSCOPIC ADRENALECTOMY**

| *General* | |
|---|---|
| Poor cardiopulmonary status | |
| Uncorrected coagulopathy | |
| *Specific* | |
| *Relative contraindications* | *Absolute contraindications* |
| Tumor size >6 cm | Tumor with local invasion |
| Obesity | Tumor with venous thrombus |
| Previous abdominal/ retroperitoneal surgery | Regional nodal involvement |
| | Malignant/uncontrolled pheochromocytoma |

become relative, and the advantages of minimally invasive techniques have afforded urologists the opportunity of a more aggressive approach in treatment (Table 130.2).

## DIAGNOSIS

Evaluation generally begins with serum and urine chemistry to distinguish between functioning and nonfunctioning tumors. More specific investigations, combined with the clinical presentation, assist in isolation of a specific pathology when present (Table 130.3). Imaging with computerized tomography (CT) or magnetic resonance imaging (MRI) is an integral step in preoperative assessment, as it provides detailed characterization of adrenal lesions. The presence of significant retroperitoneal and periadrenal fat allows for ready identification of the gland. CT may help delineate malignant versus benign lesions based on their attenuation characteristics, with accuracy approaching 90% in suspected adrenal disease. MRI has a reported sensitivity and specificity of 89% and 99%, respectively, with adenomas exhibiting a lipid-rich composition in distinction to the lipid-depleted nature of nonadenomatous lesions. Intraoperative ultrasound can elicit detailed information regarding internal acoustic appearance, tumor size, extent of invasion if present, and adjacent anatomy. Its use is a defined element in adrenal-sparing surgery and can assist in cases where it is difficult to distinguish the periadrenal fat from the gland proper. Progress in imaging techniques and their interpretation has increased diagnostic accuracy and they are an essential adjunct in determining diagnosis, operability, and surgical approach.

## ALTERNATIVE THERAPY

Alternative treatment for adrenal lesions include conventional open surgery via a transabdominal or retroperitoneal approach, radiofrequency ablation (RFA), and cryoablation (2).

RFA provokes local ion agitation and heat, inducing coagulative tissue necrosis. In one recent study Mayo-Smith and Dupuy (3) demonstrated the successful treatment of hormonally active tumors and small (5 cm) solitary adrenal metastases/adrenocortical carcinoma. RFA's use is currently limited to patients who are not surgical candidates. Munver et al. (4) described the first case of cryoablation as an adrenal-sparing procedure for hyperaldosteronism, with subsequent reduction in the need of antihypertensives postoperatively. RFA and

**TABLE 130.3**

**DIAGNOSIS OF ADRENAL LESIONS**

| | |
|---|---|
| Primary aldosteronism | Plasma aldosterone concentration (PAC) >15 ng/dL<br>Plasma renin activity (PRA) <1 ng/mL/hr<br>Aldosterone-to-renin ratio >20–30 (PAC:PRA)<br>Sodium loading with 24-hour urine aldosterone >12 μg/24 hr<br>Adrenal vein sampling with lateralizing ratio >5 |
| Cushing syndrome | 24-hour urine free cortisol<br>Low-/high-dose dexamethasone suppression with cortisol >5 μg/dL<br>Plasma ACTH level >50 pg/mL is ACTH-dependent |
| Pheochromocytoma | 24 hour serum/urine catecholamines<br>Plasma fractionated metanephrines<br>$^{131}$I methiodylbenzylguanidine (MIBG)/octreotide scintigraphy |
| Radiologic imaging with CT/MRI is essential in the diagnosis of all adrenal lesions. | |

adrenal cryoablation show potential as less invasive surgical alternatives for small lesions and adrenal-sparing procedures in patients who are not ideal surgical candidates (4). The current experience as described in the literature is limited and further evaluation of such alternative therapies is needed.

## SURGICAL TECHNIQUES

The transperitoneal approach is preferred by most surgeons due to the greater working space and familiarity of anatomic landmarks. Retroperitoneoscopic adrenalectomy is generally considered by the more experienced surgeon but may prove useful in patients with adhesions and/or obesity. Thoracoscopic adrenalectomy was described by Gill et al. (5) for the treatment of select patients with adrenal pathology and significant abdominal and retroperitoneal scarring from previous surgery through access via the virgin thoracic cavity and transdiaphragmatic approach. The introduction of robotic technology in the minimally invasive arena has proven to be a successful alternative to other surgeries with specific benefits. Robotic systems aid in eliminating surgeon fatigue, tremor and provide a three-dimensional visualization of the operative field. However, they represent a more costly option to the healthcare system and additional training by the surgeon. A prospective trial of laparoscopic versus robot-assisted adrenalectomies failed to show significant benefit in the latter (6). The study demonstrated that robot-assisted adrenalectomy is a feasible alternative to standard laparoscopic surgery with appropriate robotic experience. Further studies of robotic adrenalectomies are needed to show functional advantage or demonstrate cost-effectiveness. Ultimately the choice of surgical technique is dependent on surgeon experience, the patient's past surgical history, and preoperative findings.

### Preoperative Considerations

Prior to operative intervention, metabolic abnormalities associated with hormonally active tumors must be addressed to optimize the patient for surgery. Hypertension and hypokalemia seen with aldosteronomas are managed with spironolactone. The patient should be maintained normoglycemic with cortisol-secreting adenomas, and stress-dose steroid administration must occur perioperatively. The preoperative management of pheochromocytomas requires special consideration, as inadequate blockade of circulating catecholamines can trigger hypertensive crises secondary to anesthesia or intraoperative manipulation. Patients should receive 14 days of blockade with phenoxybenzamine hydrochloride titrated to control blood pressure. Additional blockade may be indicated if arrhythmias persist or prior treatment proves insufficient.

A mechanical bowel preparation is recommended the night prior to surgery. Parenteral intravenous antibiotic prophylaxis is given prior to incision. Invasive monitoring via arterial lines and central venous lines is performed as indicated. A urinary Foley catheter allows for bladder decompression and intraoperative urine output assessment. Pneumatic compression stockings are placed on the lower extremities bilaterally to help prevent deep venous thrombosis.

### Transperitoneal Laparoscopic Adrenalectomy

The patient is placed in the 45-degree modified flank position and secured with silk tape; all bony pressure points are padded prior to the initial incision. The ipsilateral arm can be folded across the chest or placed in an arm rest (Fig. 130.1).

Three or four ports may be used for laparoscopic instrumentation. Initial access is obtained at the lateral margin of the ipsilateral rectus at the level of the umbilicus. A Veress needle is inserted and with $CO_2$ insufflation, intra-abdominal pressure is increased to 20 mm Hg. This is replaced with a 12-mm laparoscopic port into which a 30-degree lens laparoscope is introduced. The remaining trocars are placed under direct vision at the ipsilateral rectus and costal margin, and anterior axillary line and costal margin. An additional 2-mm port just below the xiphoid process allows for use of locking graspers that assist with cephalad retraction of the liver on the right side (Fig. 130.2). Pneumoperitoneum can be subsequently reduced to 15 mm Hg for the remainder of the operation.

### Transperitoneal Left Adrenalectomy

Adrenal exposure begins with incising the line of Toldt with endoscopic scissors/electrocautery, which allows for medial mobilization of the splenic flexure and descending colon

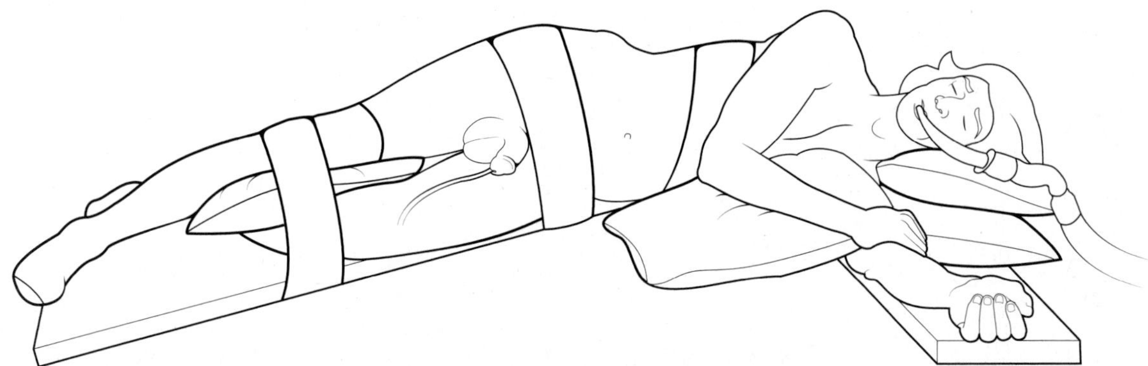

FIGURE 130.1 Laparoscopic transperitoneal adrenalectomy. Patient is positioned in the modified or full flank position for transperitoneal and retroperitoneal approaches respectively. All bony pressure points are adequately cushioned and the patient is secured in position with silk tape.

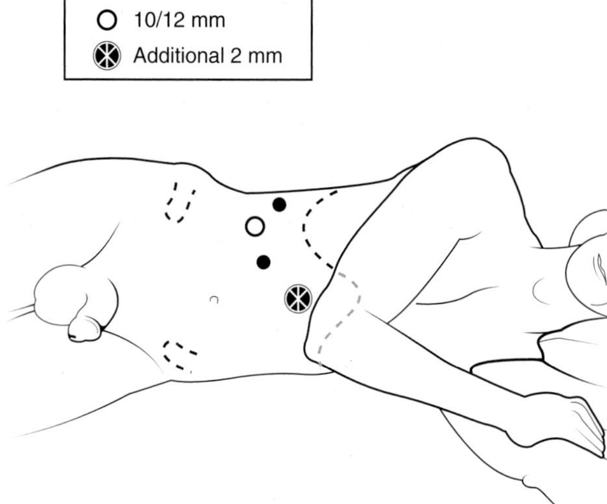


FIGURE 130.2 Laparoscopic transperitoneal adrenalectomy. The primary port site is located at the lateral margin of the ipsilateral rectus muscle at the level of the umbilicus. Secondary ports are placed in the anterior axillary line/ipsilateral rectus near the costal margin. An auxiliary port may be necessary at the xiphoid for retraction of the liver on the right side, as illustrated.

(Fig. 130.3). The splenocolic and lienorenal ligaments are divided and the spleen is mobilized medially to expose the adrenal in the retroperitoneal space (Fig. 130.4). The fascia of Gerota is opened at the upper pole of the kidney and the periadrenal fat is visualized. Dissection is continued to develop the plane between the tail of the pancreas and the renal hilum. The adrenal vein is identified emptying into the renal vein. The adrenal vein is clipped and divided with a minimum of two clips on the medial aspect (Fig. 130.5). Early ligation prevents systemic insult of catecholamines associated with adrenal manipulation and limits the potential for tumor micrometastases. Superiorly, care is taken to control contributions of the inferior phrenic artery to the adrenal. Larger vessels may be clipped and transected or coagulated with the harmonic scalpel. The adrenal gland is freed from its lateral and inferior attachments with gentle inferior traction on the kidney, at which point renal artery branches to the adrenal can been seen and controlled (Fig. 130.6). The adrenal gland and periadrenal fat are then placed in a laparoscopic retrieval bag and delivered through the largest port site (Fig. 130.7). The surgical field is examined at 5 mm Hg for adequate hemostasis. Finally, the fascial layer of the 12-mm port site is repaired with absorbable suture and laparoscopic exit is completed in standard fashion.

## Transperitoneal Right Adrenalectomy

Initial exposure of the adrenal gland begins with cephalad elevation of the liver, which may be completed with a fan retractor or self-retaining locking graspers. The peritoneum is incised at the upper pole of the kidney, close to the liver edge, and the peritoneotomy is extended medially toward the inferior vena cava. At this stage the adrenal gland should be readily visible and retracted laterally to expose the renal vein (Fig. 130.8). It is clipped proximally and distally with two clips on the caval side and divided. Dissection is completed with lateral retraction and elevation of the adrenal to allow mobilization of its superior, medial, and inferior attachments. Careful control of supplying vessels is achieved with hemostatic clips or the harmonic scalpel. The free specimen is then placed in a laparoscopic retrieval bag and delivered through the largest port site. The final steps are completed as described with the left side.

## Retroperitoneal Laparoscopic Adrenalectomy

The patient is positioned in the lateral decubitus position, stabilized with an inflatable beanbag, and secured and protected

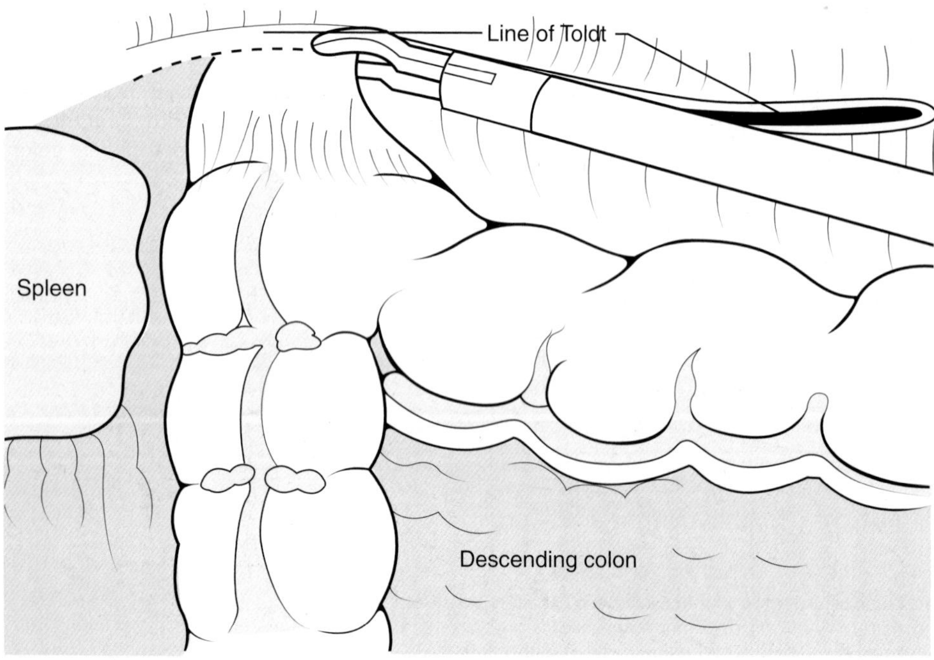


FIGURE 130.3 Transperitoneal left adrenalectomy. Initial exposure begins with incising the white line of Toldt with endoscopic scissors/electrocautery, which allows for gravity-assisted medial mobilization of the splenic flexure and descending colon.

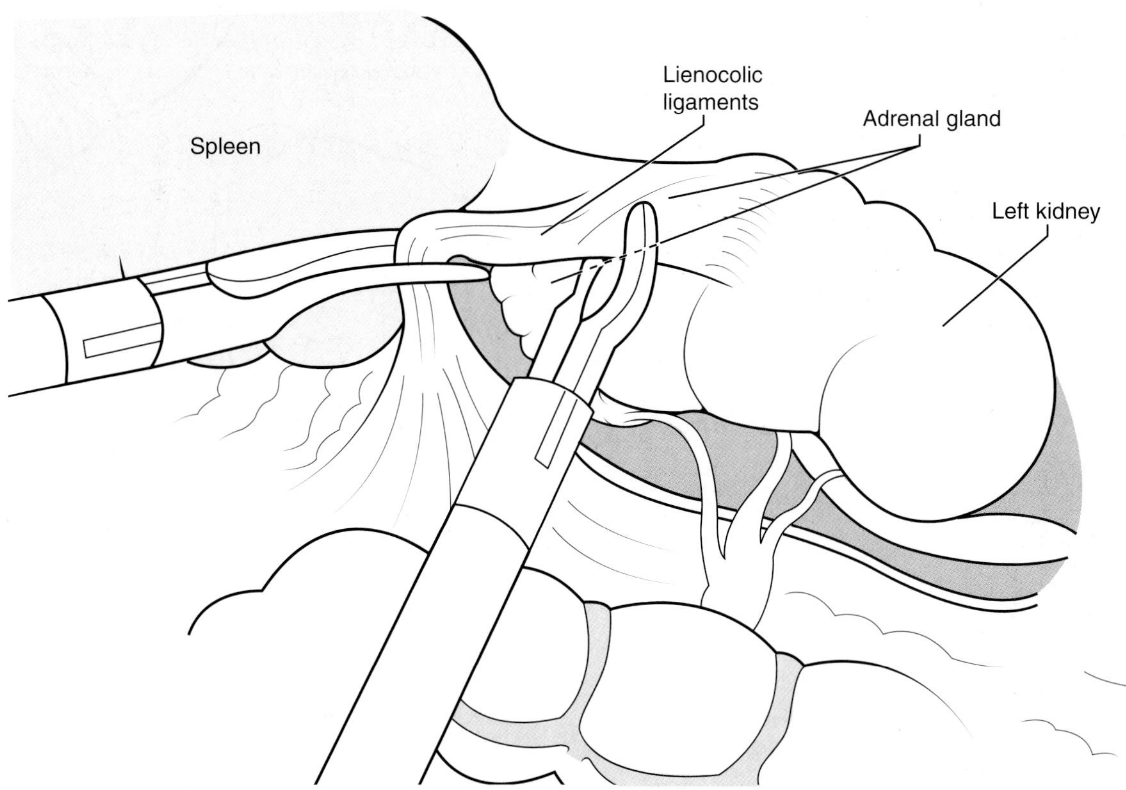


FIGURE 130.4 Transperitoneal left adrenalectomy. The lienocolic and lienorenal ligaments are divided to expose the adrenal in the retroperitoneal space.

as described for the transperitoneal approach. The table is flexed to maximize the operative working space.

A 12-mm transverse skin incision is made at the tip of the twelfth rib. The flank muscles are split until the thoracolumbar fascia can be palpated (Fig. 130.9). The fascia is opened and a finger is inserted to allow digital dissection and to develop the retroperitoneal space. A balloon dilator is introduced into the retroperitoneum and inflated to 800 cc. The dilator may then be repositioned more cephalad and reinflated to enable access/vision between the posterior adrenal outside the fascia of Gerota and the diaphragm (Fig. 130.10). The dilator is replaced with a balloon-tipped trocar and sealed against the abdominal wall, and $CO_2$ pneumoretroperitoneum is created to 15 mm Hg. Under direct laparoscopic visualization with a

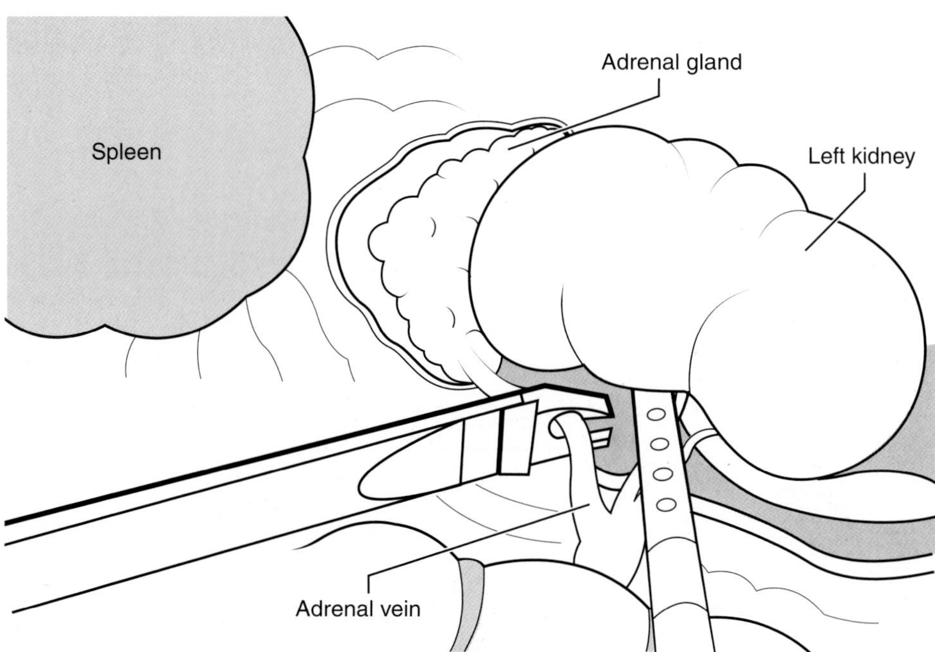


FIGURE 130.5 Transperitoneal left adrenalectomy. The left adrenal vein is ligated with two clips on the side of the renal vein and sharply divided.

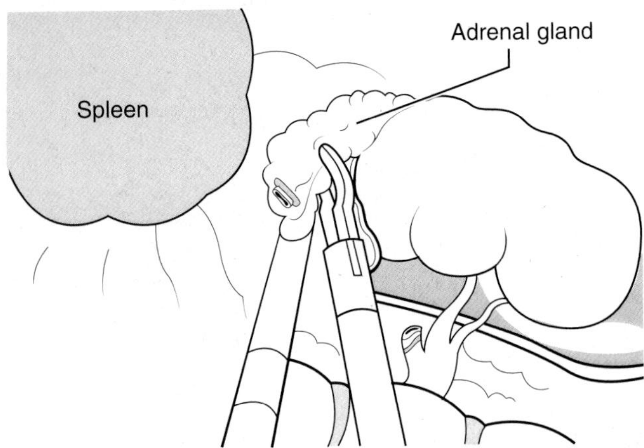


FIGURE 130.6 Transperitoneal left adrenalectomy. The avascular plane between the adrenal and renal upper pole is developed, and care is taken to control the arterial contributions from the aorta, renal, and inferior phrenic arteries.

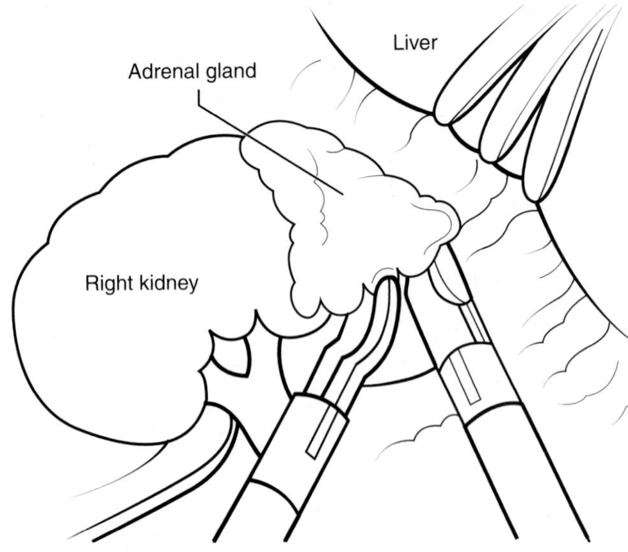


FIGURE 130.8 Transperitoneal right adrenalectomy. After identification of the renal hilum, superior dissection along the inferior vena cava will demonstrate the short, horizontally lying adrenal vein.

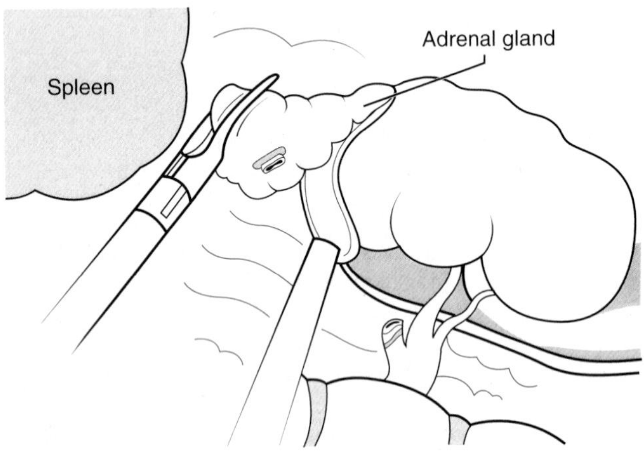


FIGURE 130.7 Transperitoneal left adrenalectomy. The freed specimen is placed in a laparoscopic retrieval bag and removed via the primary port site.

30-degree lens laparoscope, an additional port is placed above the iliac crest in the midaxillary line. The final port is placed at the inferior border of the twelfth rib where it meets the paraspinal musculature. The anatomic landmarks are identified to ensure localization of the adrenal before mobilization is begun. These include the psoas muscle posteriorly, the fascia of Gerota anteriorly, and the diaphragm superiorly (Fig. 130.11). On the left side the pancreas lies medially, whereas in the right it is the liver. Pneumoretroperitoneum is subsequently maintained at 12 mm Hg for the remainder of the operation.

## Retroperitoneoscopic Left Adrenalectomy

An initial 1.5-cm incision is made transversely along the fascia of Gerota toward the renal upper pole with hook cautery. The perirenal fat is cleaned from the adjacent structures. The plane between the upper pole and adrenal gland is identified and developed with superior retraction of the adrenal and inferior

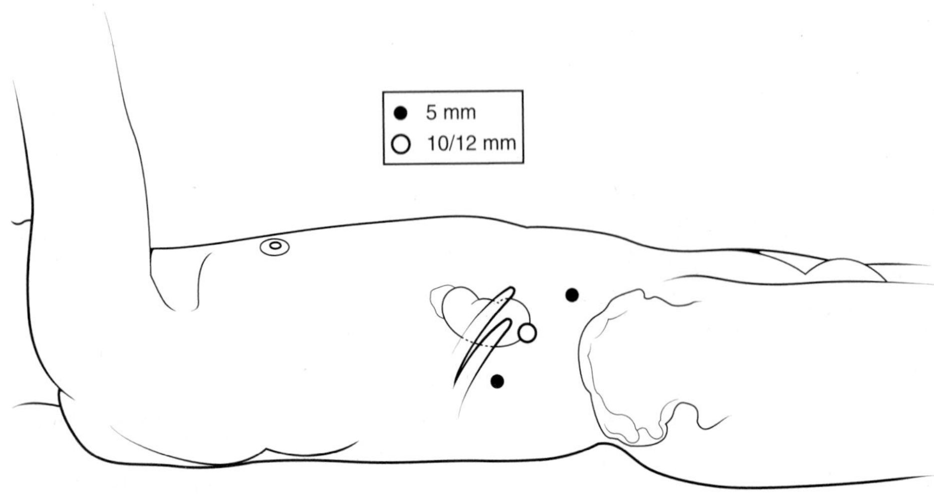


FIGURE 130.9 Laparoscopic retroperitoneal adrenalectomy. Primary port placement is at the tip of the twelfth rib. Additional ports are placed under direct laparoscopic vision in the midaxillary line above the iliac crest and the inferior border of the twelfth rib, where it meets the paraspinal musculature.

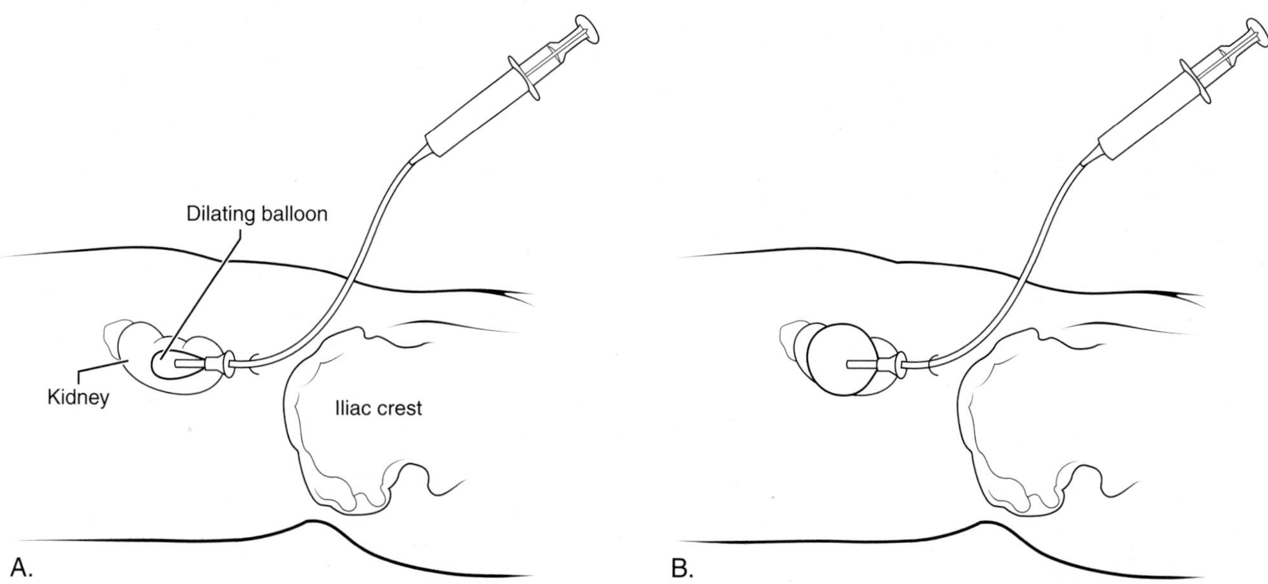


FIGURE 130.10. Laparoscopic retroperitoneal adrenalectomy. A balloon dilator is inserted into the retroperitoneum and inflated to 800 cc. It may be repositioned superiorly and reinflated to maximize exposure and working space before creation of $CO_2$ pneumoretroperitoneum.

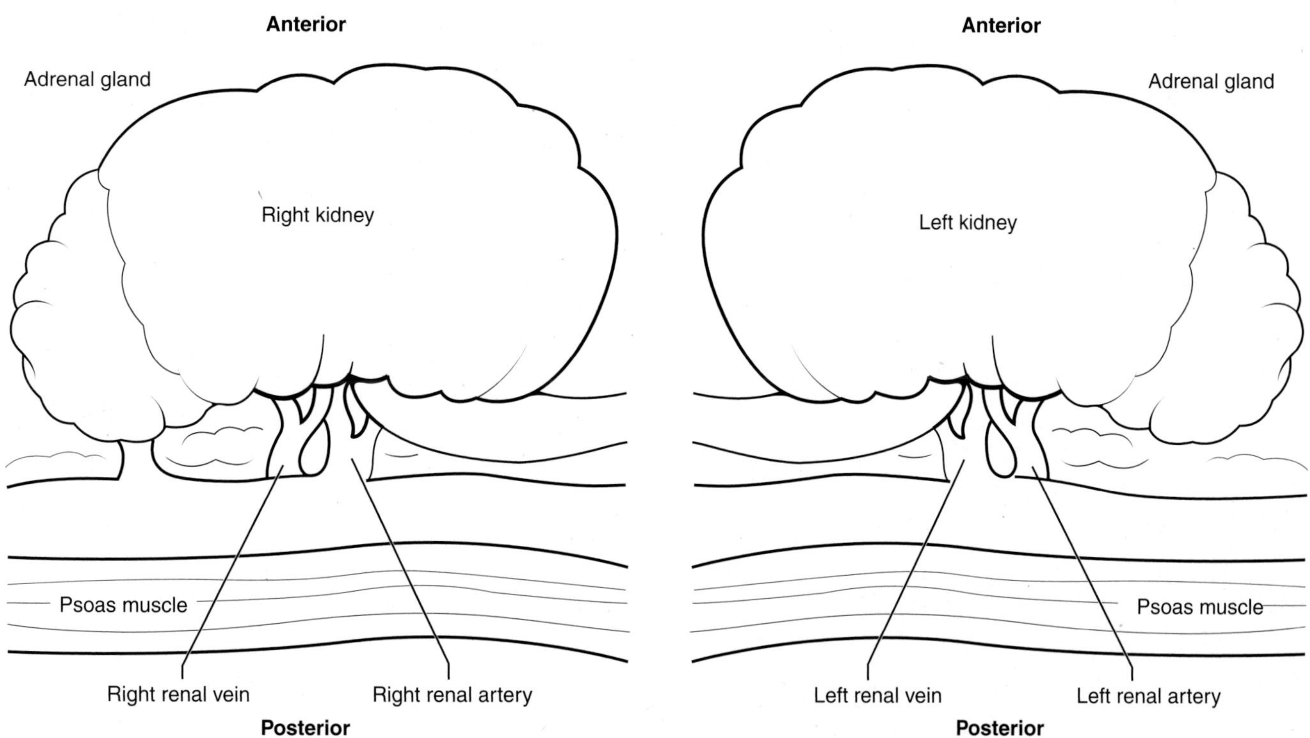


FIGURE 130.11. Laparoscopic retroperitoneal adrenalectomy. Prior to incision of the fascia of Gerota, identification of the anatomic landmarks confirms adequate localization and access to the adrenal. On the right the liver lies medially, whereas on the left it is the tail of the pancreas.

retraction of the kidney. Dissection is continued medially toward the renal hilum, and exposure of the left renal vein facilitates isolation of the adrenal vein arising from the inferomedial border of the gland. The adrenal vein is clip-ligated with two clips on the side of the renal vein and divided. The adrenal is dissected free from the psoas posteriorly and the diaphragm superiorly with ligation of adrenal branches of the inferior phrenic vessels, which may obscure the operative field if not controlled appropriately. Aortic branches arising medially are controlled in a similar fashion with the harmonic scalpel or hemostatic clips. The anterior surface of the adrenal is mobilized from the overlying peritoneum, and the free specimen can then be placed in a laparoscopic retrieval bag for removal via the primary port site.

### Retroperitoneoscopic Right Adrenalectomy

Initial access in retroperitoneal right adrenalectomy is similar to the left side. After incision of the fascia of Gerota and clearance of perirenal fat, the vena cava is readily visualized. Dissection is continued superiorly along the cava until the adrenal vein is encountered. The adrenal vein draining from the posteromedial portion of the gland is shorter and more horizontal than its left-sided counterpart and consequently should be approached with caution to avoid tearing. The vein is ligated and divided as previously described. The adrenal is then freed from its remaining attachments with meticulous control of multiple supplying vessels from the aorta, renal hilum, and inferior phrenic artery. Adrenalectomy is then completed as described on the left side.

## OUTCOMES

Numerous studies have illustrated the dafety and efficacy of Endoscopic adrenal surgery. Laparoscopic surgery has produced excellent outcomes in hormonally active lesions. Adrenalectomy for aldosteronomas effectively reduces blood pressure in the majority of patients, with long-term cure in 33% to 60% of patients. Patients with subclinical Cushing syndrome showed improvement in glucose control, blood pressure, and obesity following laparoscopic adrenalectomy. Initial concerns regarding laparoscopic treatment of pheochromocytoma and complications which have potential to increase catecholamine release including pneumoperitoneum have been dismissed; one study even described a reduction in intraoperative hypertensive events (35% versus 63%) has been described (7). Controversy also exists regarding the laparoscopic treatment of adrenal malignancy. The increased incidence of malignant tumors >6 cm requires careful consideration in surgical approach. Small organ-confined lesions (<6 cm in size) are amenable to laparoscopic excision, but case reports in the literature have even described the feasibility of radical adrenalectomy with en bloc adrenal vein tumor thrombectomy. The current role of laparoscopic adrenalectomy must be tailored to each individual patient without compromising patient safety and ensuring optimal surgical technique with minimal complications (8).

There are several clinical benefits of performing laparoscopic versus open adrenalectomy. Assalia and Gagner (9) demonstrated reduced blood loss (154 versus 309 mL), complication rate (10.9% versus 35.8%), and hospital stay (2.9 versus 7.2 days) when comparing laparoscopic and open surgeries. Additionally this study demonstrated that laparoscopic surgery utilized less analgesia and had improved cosmesis. These key characteristics translate into increased patient satisfaction as compared to open surgery. Operative times for laparoscopic adrenalectomy are generally longer; this is largely dependent on surgeon experience and has been shown to equilibrate with increased number of cases completed (10). The transperitoneal approach is more often employed by urologists due to familiarity with laparoscopic technique and anatomic landmarks. A prospective randomized study by Rubenstein et al. (11) showed no significant disparity in perioperative morbidity or operative time, emphasizing that the choice of laparoscopic approach lies primarily with the surgeon's comfort with the procedure coupled with the clinical characteristics of the individual case.

### Complications

The largest meta-analysis of complications in laparoscopic and open adrenalectomy, by Brunt (12), reported overall complication rates of 10.9% and 25.2%, respectively. Bleeding was the most common complication associated with laparoscopic surgery. Organ injury, including splenic injury requiring splenectomy and pancreatic, diaphragmatic, and large bowel injury, was also decreased. The greatest reduction in morbidity was seen in the incidence of wound (0.6% versus 3.1%), pulmonary, and infectious complications. Thromboembolic phenomena were predominant in obese patients and those with prolonged operative times. The mean conversion rate to open surgery was 3.6%; conversion was most often secondary to intraoperative bleeding, although large tumor size, adhesions, and malignancy with local invasion were also commonly cited reasons. The mean combined mortality rate for laparoscopic adrenalectomy in an analysis of 2,550 cases was 0.2%, and though slightly less than open surgery, the difference has not proven significant. Patients undergoing adrenalectomy for hormonally active tumors must be followed carefully postoperatively, as contralateral adrenal suppression can result in metabolic derangements requiring replacement of electrolytes, mineralocorticoids, or glucocorticoids.

## *References*


1. Gagner M, Lacroix A, Bolté E. Laparoscopic adrenalectomy in Cushing's syndrome and pheochromocytoma. *N Engl J Med* 1992;327:1033.
2. Micali M, Peluso G, De Stefani S, et al. Laparascopic adrenal surgery: new frontiers. *J Endourol* 2005;19(3):272–278.
3. Mayo-Smith WW, Dupuy DE. Adrenal neoplasms: CT-guided radiofrequency ablation-preliminary results. *Radiology* 2004;231(1):225–230.
4. Munver R, Del Pizzo JJ, Sosa RE. Adrenal-preserving minimally invasive surgery: the role of laparascopic partial adrenalectomy, cryosurgery, and radiofrequency ablation of the adrenal gland. *Curr Urol Rep* 2003;4:87–92.
5. Gill IS, Meraney AM, Thomas JC, et al. Thoracoscopic transdiaphragmatic adrenalectomy: the initial experience. *J Urol* 2001;165:1875–1881.
6. Morino M, Beninca G, Giraudo G, et al. Robot-assisted vs. laparoscopic adrenalectomy. *Surg Endosc* 2004;18:1742–1746.
7. Toniato A, Boschin IM, Opocher G, et al. Is the laparoscopic adrenalectomy for pheochromocytoma the best treatment? *Surgery* 2007;141(6):723–727.
8. Cobb WS, Kercher KW, Sing RF, et al. Laparoscopic adrenalectomy for malignancy. *Am J Surg* 2005;189:405-411.
9. Assalia A, Gagner M. Laparoscopic adrenalectomy. *Br J Surg* 2004;91: 1259–1274.
10. Vargas HI, Kavoussi LR, Bartlett DL, et al. Laparoscopic adrenalectomy: a new standard of care. *Urology* 1997;49:673–678.
11. Rubinstein M, Gill IS, Aron M, et al. Prospective, randomized comparison of transperitoneal versus retroperitoneal laparoscopic adrenalectomy. *J Urol* 2005;174:442–445.
12. Brunt LM. The positive impact of laparoscopic adrenalectomy on complications of adrenal surgery. *Surg Endosc* 2002;16:252–257.

# CHAPTER 131 ■ LAPAROSCOPIC AND ROBOTIC RADICAL PROSTATECTOMY

COSTAS D. LALLAS AND EDOUARD J. TRABULSI

The driving force behind the development of a minimally invasive radical prostatectomy was certainly patient satisfaction and quality of life. Accordingly, the first laparoscopic radical prostatectomy (LRP) was performed in 1991 (1). Although the benefits to the patient were readily apparent for LRP, the technical challenges and difficult learning curve were also broadly recognized, paving the way for a facilitator for this procedure: robotic technology.

Robotically assisted laparoscopic (radical) prostatectomy (RALP) has made an enormous, albeit controversial, impact on the treatment of prostate cancer. Although different robotic platforms have been described in the literature, the da Vinci Surgical System (Intuitive Surgical, Sunnydale, CA) has quickly monopolized the market. Like other robotic surgical systems, the da Vinci system operates in a master-slave relationship with the surgeon, with motions being translated in a filtered, nonparadoxical fashion. The surgeon sits remotely from the surgical field but does require an assistant at the bedside for instrument changes, retraction, and suction. The setup is ergonometric, and unlike with the physically taxing LRP, most surgeons can easily accomplish multiple RALPs in a given day. Other direct advantages of RALP over LRP include more degrees of freedom of motion, enabled by wristed instruments, as well as nonparadoxical versus paradoxical movements and three-dimensional versus planar, two-dimensional visualization. To date, four different generations of the da Vinci system have been released, with the latter three having four arms (as opposed to three) and the latest model boasting telestration, which aids in teaching and proctoring, and high-definition visualization.

Opponents to RALP consistently cite the market- and patient-driven acceptance of this procedure without any long-term follow-up. Additionally, some maintain that the lack of tactile feedback afforded by the minimally invasive prostatectomy is disadvantageous when evaluating for induration, palpable nodules, and delineation of the proximity or involvement of the neurovascular bundles by cancer. Finally, several believe that the cost of RALP places it at a distinct disadvantage relative to other, more traditional approaches. At our institution, we have completely converted over from LRP, the last of which we performed 3 years ago, to RALP, with the relative ease and consistently positive patient outcomes of the latter procedure being the main reasons. Since RALP stands firmly on the shoulders of LRP, we describe both procedures, with particular focus on our technique and published outcomes of RALP.

## DIAGNOSIS

Adenocarcinoma of the prostate is typically diagnosed through routine medical screening, which includes a digital rectal examination and a test for serum prostate specific antigen (PSA). An abnormal digital rectal examination, elevated PSA level, or PSA velocity should prompt a transrectal ultrasound–guided biopsy of the prostate. Once the diagnosis of cancer is made, the patient should undergo appropriate staging preoperative counseling, and treatment options should be thoroughly discussed.

A computerized tomography of the abdomen and pelvis and a radioisotope bone scan are traditionally performed on all patients who are evaluated for prostate cancer. These studies have been questioned for patients with low-risk features. MRI with endorectal coil is performed in some centers for local staging but is not widely used.

## INDICATIONS FOR SURGERY

Men with clinically localized prostate cancer who choose surgical treatment are candidates for this procedure. All patients who are evaluated for prostate cancer at our institution are evaluated in a multidisciplinary setting with urologic oncology, radiation oncology, and medical oncology (2). Preoperative tumor parameters are inputted into the Kattan preoperative nomogram to evaluate for risk of extracapsular extension, seminal vesicle invasion, and metastatic disease. Once patients have chosen RALP, they are medically cleared if deemed necessary and their bladder outlet and ureteral orifice location is evaluated by cystoscopy. Patients are excluded if their life expectancy is <10 years or their American Society of Anesthesiologists (ASA) score is >4, indicating that they have severe comorbidities. Morbid obesity (Body Mass Index >45) is a relative contraindication, as these patients may not be able to tolerate Trendelenburg positioning with pneumoperitoneum for an extended period of time. Previous radiotherapy for pelvic malignancy is a contraindication for RALP or LRP. Prior intra-abdominal surgery is not a contraindication, but patients who have undergone prior pelvic procedures or extensive intra-abdominal surgery are counseled that their likelihood of conversion to standard open radical retropubic prostatectomy is elevated. Nerve-sparing or non–nerve-sparing technique is based on the surgeon's preference, which is based on the clinical parameters of the individual patient.

## ALTERNATIVE THERAPY

Treatment options for clinically localized prostate cancer include observation, brachytherapy, external beam or proton radiation therapy, cryotherapy, and radical prostatectomy. Radical prostatectomy includes retropubic, perineal, laparoscopic, and robotically assisted laparoscopy.

## SURGICAL TECHNIQUE

The steps involved in the pure laparoscopic and robotically assisted radical prostatectomy employing the more popular transperitoneal approach are quite similar. One of the most significant differences is the use of robotic instrumentation versus the use of standard laparoscopic instruments. Critical to the success of these procedures is a well-trained and coordinated operating room staff with familiarity of the instruments and devices needed for these complex procedures.

On the day prior to surgery, patients are placed on a clear liquid diet and are given a gentle mechanical bowel preparation with one bottle of oral magnesium citrate as well as a Fleet enema per rectum. Two large-bore intravenous lines and an arterial line, if necessary, are placed. A broad-spectrum intravenous antibiotic (cephalosporin such as Ancef) is given 1 hour prior to incision, and all patients receive Lovenox 40 mg subcutaneously prior to surgery for venous thromboembolism (VTE) prophylaxis. Once intubated in the operating room, patients are placed in a low lithotomy position using Allen stirrups. The arms are tucked at the patient's side using 3-in. cloth tape, and the patient's shoulders, elbows, wrists, and neck are padded (Fig. 131.1). An orogastric tube is placed, and the anesthesia staff are also instructed to limit the intravenous fluids given, to avoid overresuscitation. Typically, we recommend 7 mL per kg intravenous fluids per hour for the entire case (approximately 500 mL per hour or 1.0 to 1.5 L per case.

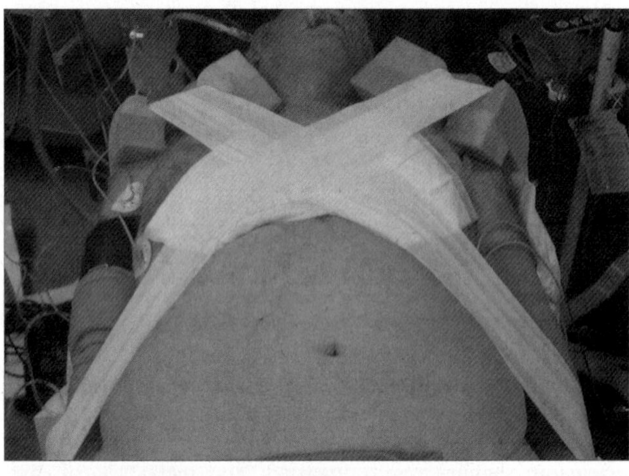

A

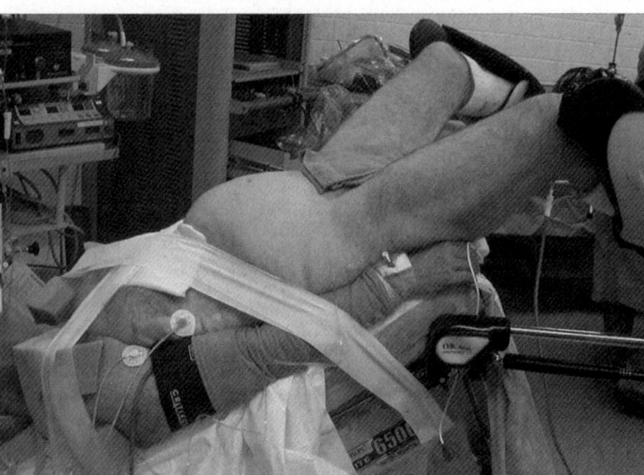

B

FIGURE 131.1 A and B: Proper positioning and padding for laparoscopic or robotically assisted prostatectomy.

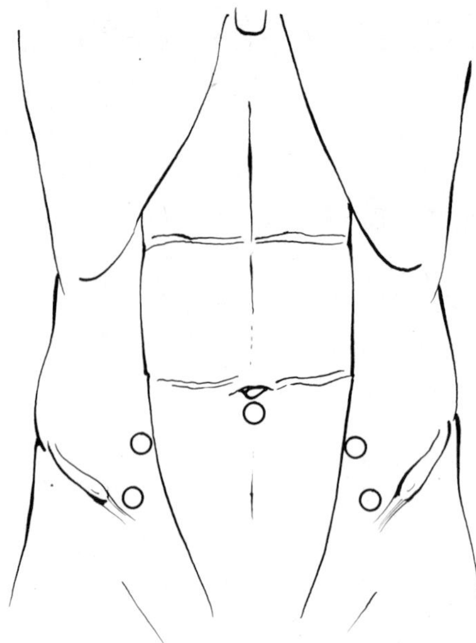

FIGURE 131.2 Port placement for laparoscopic prostatectomy. Five ports are utilized.

### Laparoscopic Prostatectomy (LRP)

After a pneumoperitoneum has been established, five trocars are placed. The first 12-mm trocar is placed at the level of the umbilicus (Fig. 131.2). This can be placed by using an optical port, employing an open technique, or gently applying pressure to the 12-mm trocar and introducing it into the abdomen. We use a 0-degree lens throughout the procedure and inspect the abdominal cavity after placement of our first trocar. Our next two 12-mm trocars are placed just lateral to the rectus on the right-hand and left-hand sides, respectively. These 12-mm trocars are placed 2 to 4 cm inferior to the umbilicus. Finally, two 5-mm trocars are placed off the anterior iliac spine on the right-hand and left-hand sides, respectively. Thus a total of five ports are utilized throughout the procedure (Fig. 131.1). The patient is now placed into extreme Trendelenburg position.

If available, the Aesop (Computer Motion, Inc., Goleta, CA) is placed on the right side of the table and controls the 0-degree laparoscope and camera through the umbilical port. Otherwise the assistant holds the camera. The assistant stands on the right side and the surgeon stands on the left. A fan retractor is useful in the right 12-mm port to retract the bowel. The cul-de-sac and the vas deferens are identified on both the

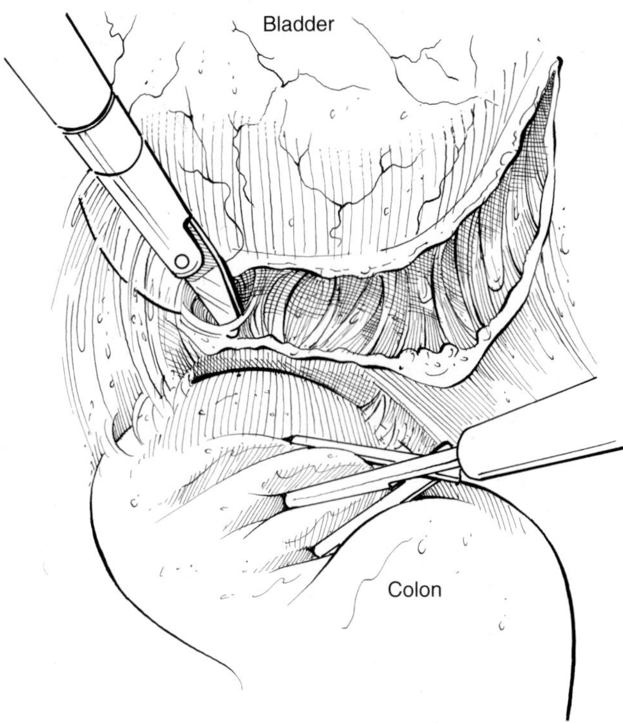


FIGURE 131.3 Scoring the peritoneum along the vas deferens into the cul-de-sac.

right- and left-hand sides at the level of the internal ring. The peritoneum is scored in a line along the vas deferens down to the cul-de-sac (Fig. 131.3). This incision is carried down to the second peritoneal fold in the cul-de-sac, and the vas deferens is skeletonized bilaterally down to the seminal vesicles. The vas is pulled anteriorly with a grasper through the 5-mm right-sided port (Fig. 131.4), and the assistant uses the irrigator-aspirator through the 12-mm right-sided port. The seminal vesicles are dissected using a combination of sharp and blunt dissection to their tips (Fig. 131.4). With retraction on the seminal vesicles, the Denonvilliers fascia is incised to create a plane between the prostate and rectum. The perirectal adipose tissue should be clearly identified. A rectal bougie can be manipulated to confirm the exact location of the rectum.

The bladder is filled with 200 cc of saline, and using the bipolar cautery and laparoscopic scissors through the left-sided ports, the lateral aspect of the bladder is dissected off the anterior abdominal wall by connecting the points between the incised median and umbilical ligaments and the lateral peritoneal reflection (Fig. 131.5). The bladder is emptied and now has been mobilized. The endopelvic fascia is incised bilaterally, the fatty tissue overlying the prostate is dissected with bipolar cautery, and the superficial dorsal vein is cauterized using the bipolar forceps (Fig. 131.5). The puboprostatic ligaments are sharply divided. The deep dorsal vein complex is ligated with a CT-1 needle loaded with 0 Vicryl suture. The needle is slightly straightened before being passed through the right 12-mm port on a laparoscopic needle driver. A laparoscopic grasper is used from the left 12-mm port site. The dorsal vein complex is identified, and a suture is passed around it with a figure-of-eight suture passed anterior to the urethra and posterior to this deep venous dorsal complex (Fig. 131.6). The suture is tied intracorporeally, and the dorsal vein complex is secured but not divided at this point.

The prostatic base is divided from the bladder neck and is a more challenging part of the procedure. A coagulating scissor

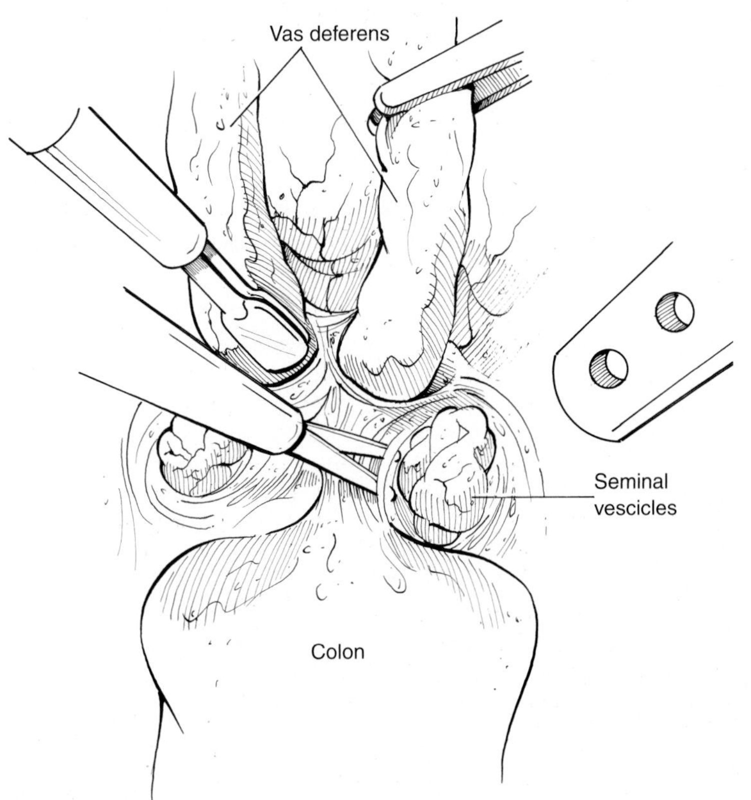


FIGURE 131.4 The vas deferens is lifted anteriorly by the assistant and the seminal vesicles are dissected free.

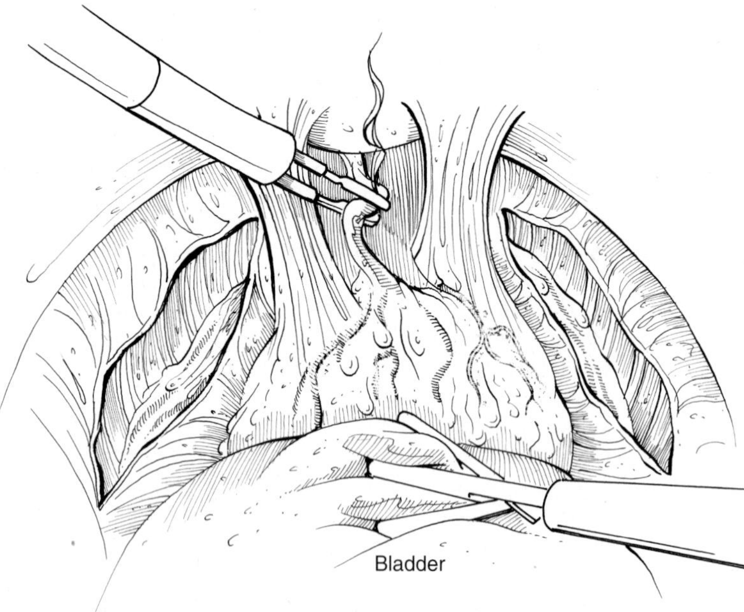


FIGURE 131.5 The bladder is freed off the anterior abdominal wall by incising the umbilical ligaments and lateral attachments.

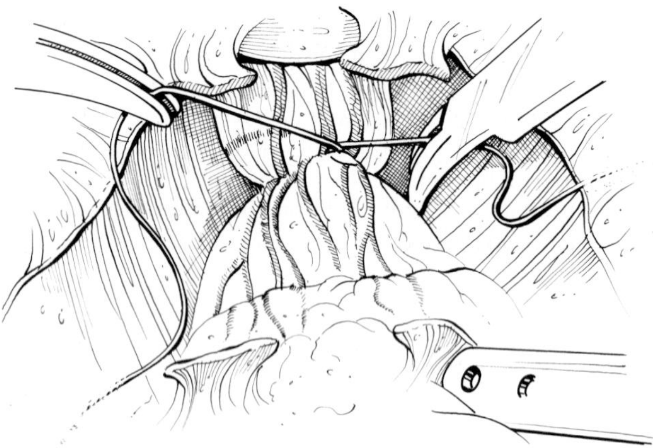

FIGURE 131.6 The endopelvic fascia is incised and the dorsal vein complex identified. The deep dorsal vein complex is ligated using a 0 Vicryl suture on a CT-1 needle.

or curved harmonic scalpel can be used. The assistant retracts the bladder from the right 12-mm port and, using a 5-mm irrigator-aspirator, outlines the Foley catheter balloon down toward the level of the prostatic base. The prostatic base is divided from the bladder neck (Fig. 131.7). The detrusor fibers are often seen, and bladder is entered and the Foley identified. The balloon is deflated, and the assistant retracts the Foley catheter cephalad using a grasper from the right 5-mm port site (Fig. 131.8). The posterior bladder mucosa is scored and carried through the posterior surface of the prostate (Fig. 131.9). The seminal vesicles and vas previously dissected are brought anteriorly and grasped by the assistant using the laparoscopic 5-mm grasper.

If a nerve-sparing approach is attempted, a right-angled dissector with sharp dissection as needed can be used through the right 12-mm port site to free the neurovascular bundle on the lateral surface of the prostate prior to dividing the dorsal venous complex. The assistant lifts the seminal vesicle anteriorly, and the vascular pedicle can be divided with the harmonic

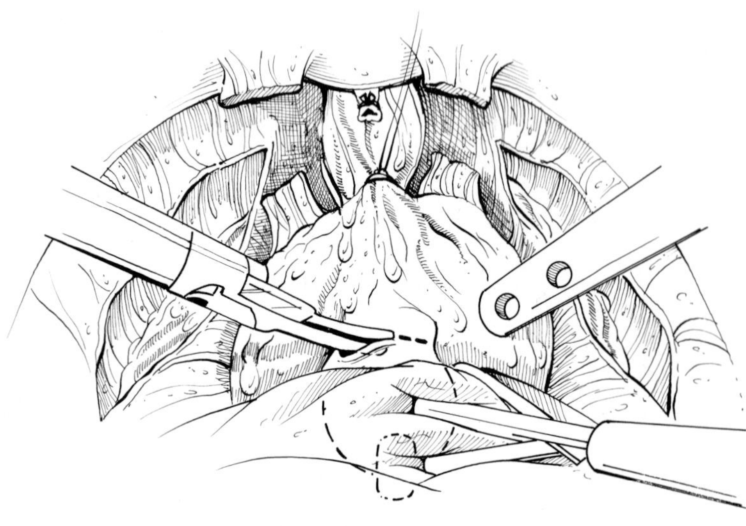

FIGURE 131.7 Division of the anterior bladder neck and prostatic base using the harmonic scalpel.

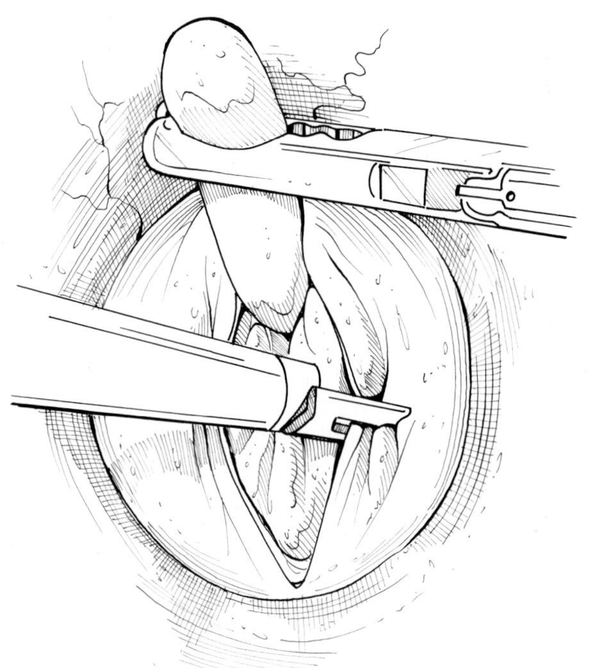

FIGURE 131.8 The Foley catheter is grasped and the dissection of the bladder neck continues posteriorly.

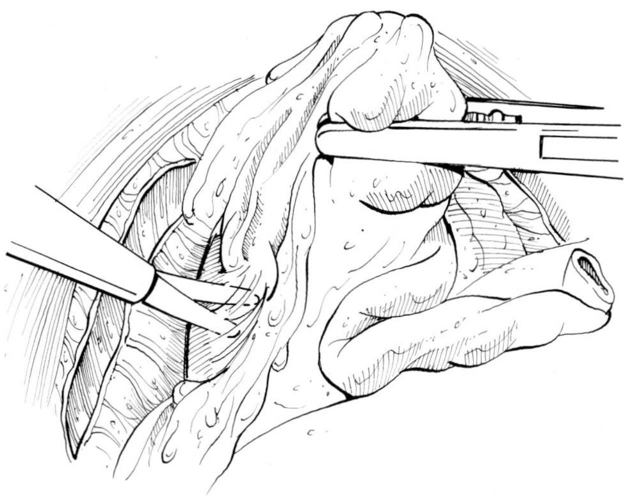

FIGURE 131.9 Division of the posterior bladder neck and identification of the previously dissected seminal vesicles and vas deferens.

scalpel or locking clips. Sharp dissection frees the remaining reflection of endopelvic fascia of the prostate laterally (Fig. 131.10).

With a non–nerve-sparing technique, the assistant grasps the seminal vesicle, lifting anteriorly, and the surgeon divides the entire vascular pedicle and neurovascular bundle with the harmonic scalpel, working toward the apex of the prostate.

The prostate is attached posteriorly by the rectourethralis muscle and the urethra. The dorsal vein complex is sharply incised and the apical notch of the prostate developed. The anterior urethra is now sharply divided, exposing the catheter, which is retracted, and the posterior urethra is divided (Fig. 131.11). The assistant provides cephalad retraction by grasping the base of the prostate in order to allow maximum exposure of the urethra. The rectourethralis muscle is sharply incised, and the prostate can be rolled to both the left- and right-hand sides to facilitate the exposure. The specimen having been placed into the left lower quadrant, the pelvis is irrigated and any bleeding controlled.

If there are concerns about the location or injury to the rectum, a rectal bougie is useful. If necessary, a 20Fr Foley catheter can be placed in the rectum and the pelvis filled with saline. Air is injected into the Foley catheter to identify any injury.

The bladder neck is identified, and the ureteral orifices are observed for efflux of urine. A urethral sound is placed, and apical margins may be sent for frozen section if needed. The urethrovesical anastomosis is begun (Fig. 131.12). Bladder neck reconstruction can be performed anteriorly using a 2-0 Vicryl suture on a UR-6 needle, and the bladder neck can be reconstructed by placing a suture through the anterior portion of the bladder neck in interrupted fashion.

Using a 2-0 Vicryl suture on a UR-6 needle through the right 12-mm port, the anastomosis is begun by placing a stitch through the posterior bladder neck from outside the bladder. The needle is grasped, and, using the right 12-mm port, the

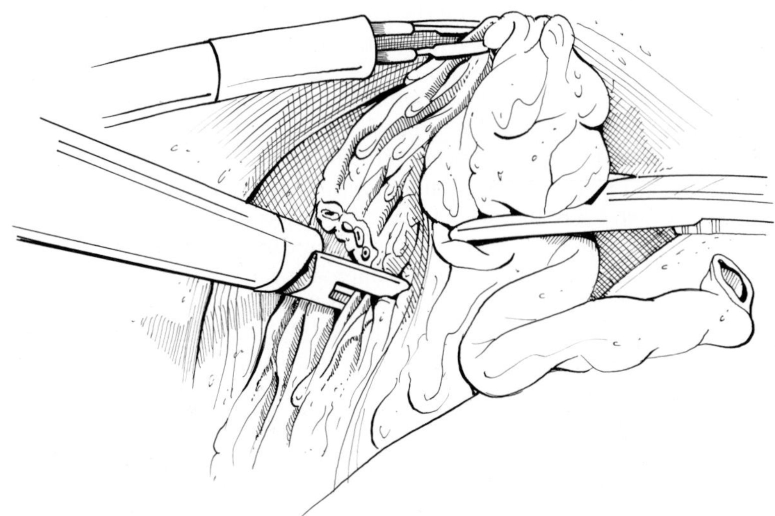

FIGURE 131.10 Sharply dissecting the neurovascular bundle of the lateral aspect of the prostate.

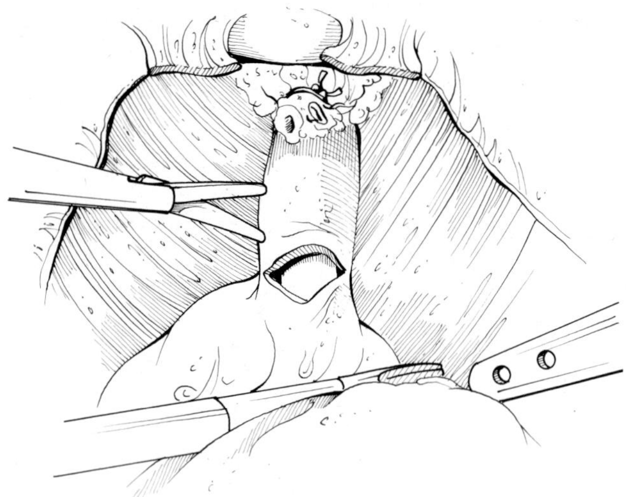

FIGURE 131.11 Division of the anterior urethra.

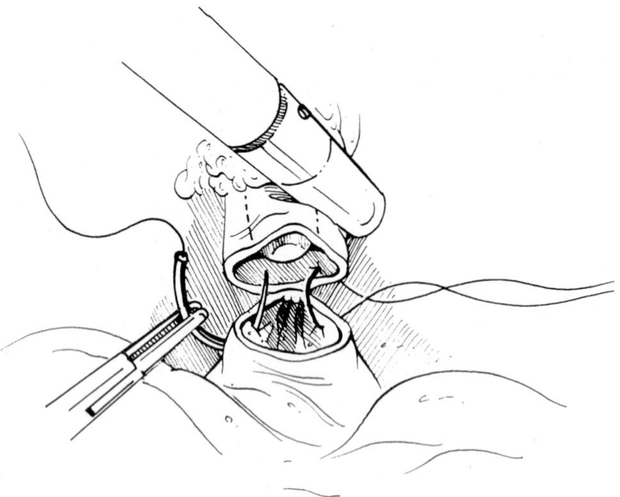

FIGURE 131.12 Urethral anastomosis beginning with the posterior sutures.

posterior stitch on the right side of the urethra is placed. Next, a second suture is introduced through the left 12-mm port, and, in similar fashion, the posterior bladder neck is sutured outside-in followed by the posterior urethra inside-out. Thus the knots are tied on the outside of the bladder. Alternatively, the two-armed suture technique as described for robotic prostatectomy using two 3-0 Monocryl sutures tied together can be used (see below). The table is reflexed and the bladder is reapproximated to the urethra. The posterior bladder can be grasped from the right side and held in place while the sutures are tied intracorporeally.

The anastomosis is completed. Using the 2-0 Vicryl suture, the sutures are placed circumferentially from either the right or left 12-mm port as determined by the patient's anatomy. Occasionally, it is necessary to place a back-handed suture from the left-sided 12-mm port. The sutures are tied intracorporeally. The remaining anterior sutures can be placed. Typically, the left-sided anterior bladder neck and the urethral sutures are placed through the right 12-mm port and vice versa. This allows more effective needle positioning. A new 18Fr to 20Fr Foley catheter is placed under direct visualization prior to completing the anastomosis, and the final anterior sutures are tied intracorporeally. The bladder is tested by instilling 60 cc of saline, and if a leak is detected, another suture can be placed. Generally seven to eight sutures are used for the urethrovesical anastomosis. The right 5-mm port site incision is extended to accompany a 10-mm Endocatch device (Auto Suture, Norwalk, CT). After the Endocatch is deployed, the accompanying needles and prostate with accompanying seminal vesicles and vas deference are delivered into the bag. The bag is closed and brought through the right 5-mm port site. The external oblique fascia and muscle are incised with electrocautery and the bag removed. This small incision is closed, the abdomen is reinsufflated, and then a Jackson-Pratt drain is placed through the left 5-mm port. Ports are closed in standard fashion and the Foley is left to gravity.

## Robotically Assisted Laparoscopic Prostatectomy (RALP)

Pneumoperitoneum is established up to a pressure of 15 mm Hg in a midline supraumbilical location, and a 12-mm trocar is placed at this site. After blind placement of the midline camera trocar (12 mm), an additional 12-mm, three 8-mm, and one 5-mm port are placed under direct vision in the patient's lower abdomen and pelvis. The initial 12-mm port is always placed 1 to 2 cm cephalad to the umbilicus. Two 8-mm robotic working ports are placed at the apex of a triangle that is 10 cm lateral to the top of the umbilicus and 15 cm from the pubic symphysis. The third 8-mm robotic working port is placed at least 8 cm laterally from the one on the patient's left-hand side, and it must be at least two fingerbreadths off of the anterior superior iliac spine. The 12-mm assistant port is placed at least 8 cm laterally from the 8-mm robotic working port on the patient's right-hand side, and it must be at least two fingerbreadths off of the anterior superior iliac spine, mirroring the 8-mm port on the contralateral side. The 5-mm assistant port is placed 5 to 6 cm directly cephalad to the 8-mm robotic working port (Fig. 131.13). Prior to docking the robot, the patient is placed in a steep Trendelenburg position.

Once the robot is docked, instruments are next inserted into the patient and connected to the robot (Fig. 131.14). Both a monopolar and a bipolar electrocautery instrument are used concomitantly, and the fourth arm (if available on the robot) is equipped with a grasping forceps. A 0-degree lens is used for the entire procedure.

The initial report of LRP described an intraperitoneal approach, with the surgeon first dissecting the vasa deferentia and seminal vesicles through the pouch of Douglas (Fig. 131.15). Next attention was turned anteriorly, incising the urachus and medial umbilical ligaments to enter the space of Retzius, and proceeding in an antegrade fashion (Fig. 131.16) (1). This intraperitoneal approach was advocated by surgeons at the Montsouris Institute in Paris, who also used an initial dissection posterior to the bladder (3). As experience with LRP grew, the posterior approach was abandoned by some surgeons who discovered that the vasa and seminal vesicles could be adequately dissected once the bladder neck had been divided. Once surgeons were comfortable with dissection of the vasa and seminal vesicles at this point of the operation, some turned to an extraperitoneal approach.

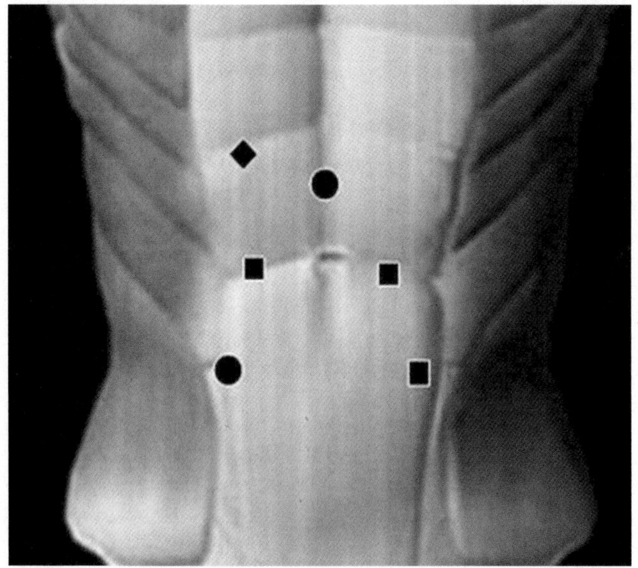

A

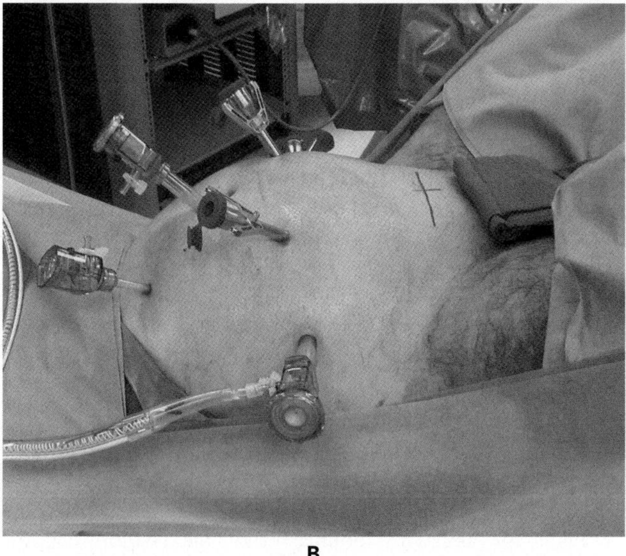

B

FIGURE 131.13 **A:** Port position for RALP: 12-mm ports for camera and assistant, 8-mm robot port for the three robotic arms; and 5-mm port for the assistant. **B:** Ports in position. Note the line indicating the pubis and midline for orientation and placement of the ports.

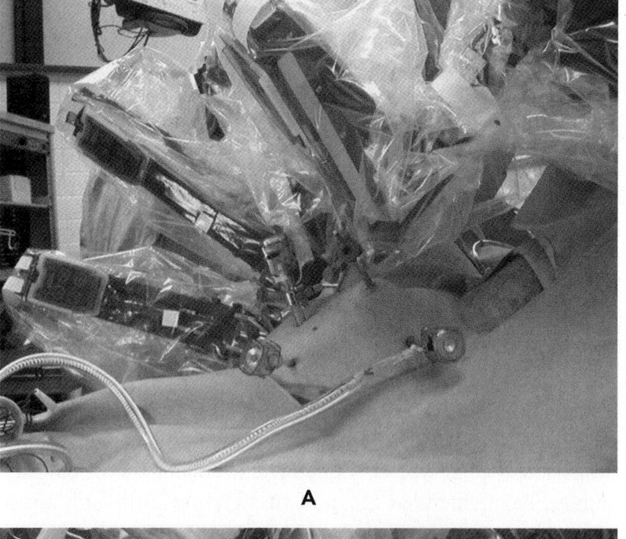

A

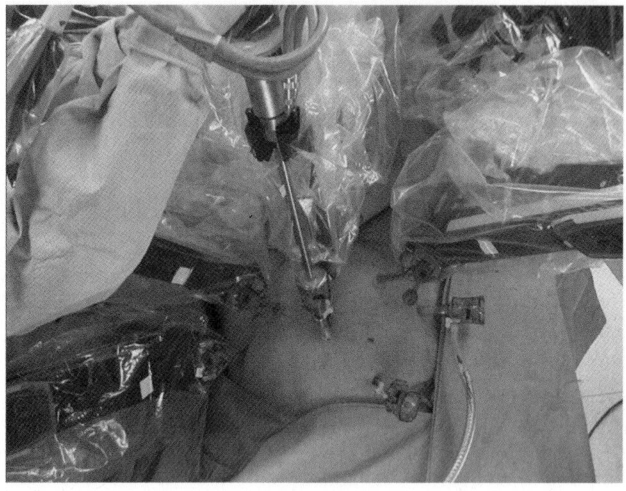

B

FIGURE 131.14 Port placement for RALP once the robot has been docked.

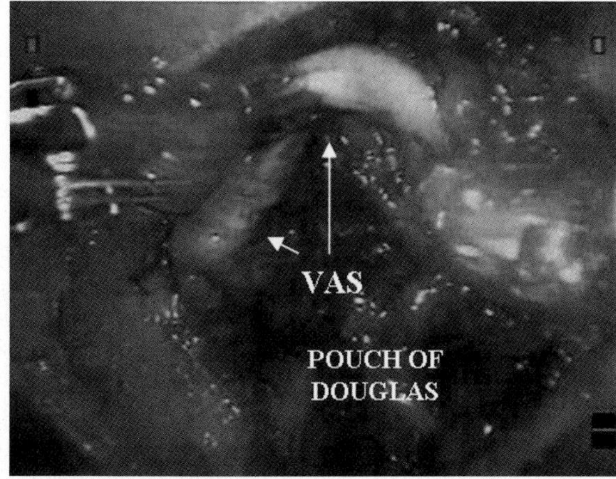


FIGURE 131.15 Posterior dissection.

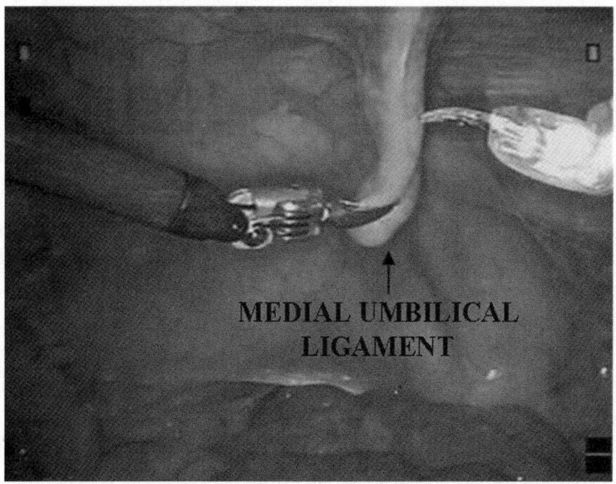


FIGURE 131.16 Beginning intraperitoneal anterior dissection.

The extraperitoneal approach in LRP or RALP places the urologic surgeon who is used to the anatomy of the radical retropubic prostatectomy (RRP) in familiar territory. In this procedure, the preperitoneal space is first bluntly dissected with either a finger or a balloon prior to insufflation. By staying out of the peritoneum altogether, theoretical risks such as small bowel injury from trocar placement, traction, or electrocautery are avoided, and the concerns of bowel stasis or ileus due to a urine leak are minimized. Additionally, this approach would have a hypothetical advantage in those patients who have undergone prior intra-abdominal surgery. Head-to-head comparisons between the two approaches show little difference with regard to intraoperative and postoperative parameters, and it is our opinion that the approach ultimately should be determined by the surgeon. At the Jefferson Kimmel Cancer Center, we use exclusively an intraperitoneal approach and, as we become more comfortable with the procedure, have extended our patient selection to include those individuals who have undergone prior intra-abdominal procedures; these patients currently represent 5% of our overall experience. We have had no small bowel injuries in these patients, nor have we had to convert any of these procedures to an open radical retropubic prostatectomy. Residents and fellows actively participate in the robotic program.

## Posterior Dissection

The original description of the LRP and subsequent RALP included dissection posterior to the bladder to identify the vasa deferentia and seminal vesicles prior to dissecting the bladder off of the anterior wall (1,3). As noted, this approach has become less popular with RALP as the procedure has evolved. However, this initial posterior approach remains an important innovation and can be utilized in patients in whom the posterior dissection of the bladder neck may pose a challenge. Such patients are those who have had a prior transurethral prostatectomy (TRUP) or other procedure for benign disease, those with a very large (>80 g) or small (<20 g) prostate, or those with a large median lobe. By dissecting posterior to the seminal structures and exposing the posterior surface of the prostate, the rectum is released posteriorly, thus minimizing one of the main concerns of this part of the procedure. In fact, we regularly teach this approach to our trainees so that it will be in their armamentarium for a RALP.

## Incising the Endopelvic Fascia

Another derivation of the radical retropubic prostatectomy that has been incorporated into both the LRP and RALP is incision of the endopelvic fascia prior to ligating the dorsal venous complex and dissecting the neurovascular bundle and apex of the prostate. With regard to this portion of the procedure, Stolzenburg et al. (4) have recently reported on 1,300 cases of a completely extrafascial endoscopic prostatectomy, with intermediate follow-up showing oncologic and functional results equivalent to most laparoscopic and robotic large series. In this technique, the endopelvic fascia is left intact and dissected with the neurovascular bundle. The dorsal venous complex is taken at the end of the procedure, prior to dividing the urethra. This method has anatomic merit, given the fact that the endoscopic prostatectomy (both LRP and RALP) is an antegrade procedure, and theoretically the endopelvic fascia, which is intimately related to the apex of the prostate, does not have to be violated until the end of the procedure. Additionally, this approach may have positive implications on nerve sparing, given the fact that a healthy amount of tissue is left over the neurovascular bundle, limiting the possibility of thermal spread and traction injury.

There are situations, however, when early dissection of the endopelvic fascia can be beneficial. Especially for the novice, after the endopelvic fascia has been divided, the lateral margin of the prostate becomes evident. This can be of particular use when identifying the margins of the bladder neck, which is one of the more challenging portions of the RALP. Additionally, in a patient with a large pubic osteophyte or an anteriorly positioned prostate, incision of the endopelvic fascia and the adjacent puboprostatic ligaments can drop the prostate into the pelvis, facilitating the apical dissection and the vesicourethral anastomosis.

## Bladder Neck Dissection

Antegrade division of the bladder neck in LRP and RALP remains one of the most frustrating parts of this procedure for trainers and trainees alike. At Jefferson, there are several points that we reinforce with our residents and fellows in order to guide them through this part of the procedure:

1. Use the posterior dissection for those patients in whom the posterior bladder neck may pose a problem (see above).
2. Always incise the endopelvic fascia in order to visualize the lateral borders of the prostate as they form the bladder neck.
3. Place the bladder on tension using either the fourth arm or an assistant to see where the bladder drapes over the prostate (the prostatovesical junction).
4. Have the assistant "bounce" the Foley balloon on the bladder neck to help identify the area for initial dissection.
5. Limit the use of electrocautery during dissection so that the tissue planes do not become obscured by char.
6. After incising the anterior bladder neck to reveal the Foley, deflate the balloon and raise the catheter anteriorly with either the fourth arm of the da Vinci or an assistant.
7. When initially dividing the posterior bladder neck, incise full thickness through the detrusor muscle.

In patients whose biopsy indicates minimal disease at the prostatic base, a bladder neck–preserving procedure can be performed by peeling the bladder off of the prostate anteriorly (an *anterior peel*) (Fig. 131.17). The resulting bladder neck can be well approximated to the distal urethra for the anastomosis. Additionally, this method can be employed to dissect out a median lobe and still keep the bladder neck diameter adequate for the anastomosis without having to taper it. In contrast, patients at high risk for involvement of the base of the prostate with cancer should have a wide excision of the bladder neck with circumferential frozen section biopsies when indicated. In this subset of patients, reconstruction of the bladder neck is necessary (Fig. 131.18).

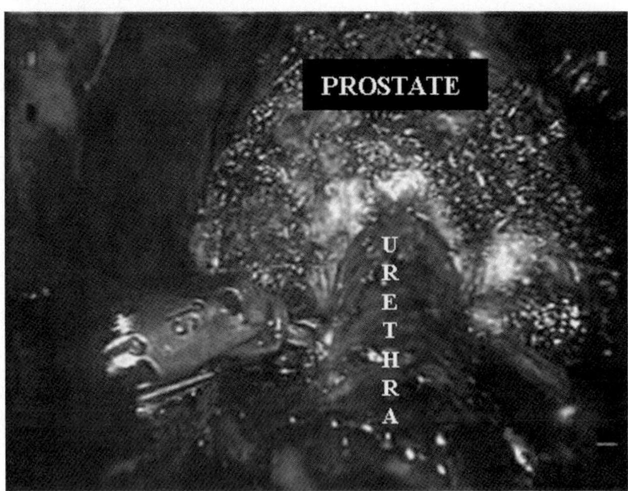


FIGURE 131.17 Demonstration of anterior peel.

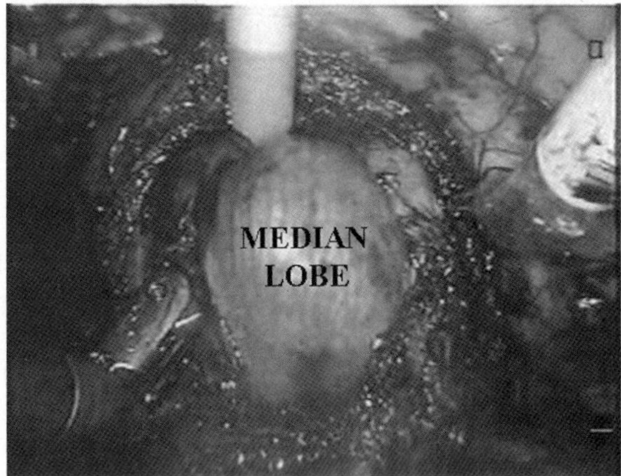


FIGURE 131.18 Dissection posterior to the median lobe.

## Dissection of the Vasa Deferentia and Seminal Vesicles

Recent evidence from cadaveric dissections has demonstrated the intimate proximity of the tips of the seminal vesicles and the pelvic plexus ganglions that feed the neurovascular bundles (NVB) (5). This report stated that the NVB may be particularly vulnerable to thermal, electrical, and/or crush injury during dissection of these structures. For this reason, we believe it prudent to avoid excessive traction or gratuitous electrocautery during dissection in this region.

## Prostatic Pedicles and Neurovascular Bundles

Since the advent of minimally invasive prostatectomy, there has been a new interest in the anatomy and, more importantly, the preservation of the NVB. One of the more pioneering of these innovations is the contention by Menon et al. (6) that the nerves responsible for erections are not only located at the posterolateral border of the prostate but also course through the lateral prostatic fascia toward the anterior surface of the prostate. Menon contends that men who undergo the preservation of these nerves, in addition to the traditionally described NVB, are at a distinct advantage when being evaluated for long-term erectile function after nerve-sparing RALP.

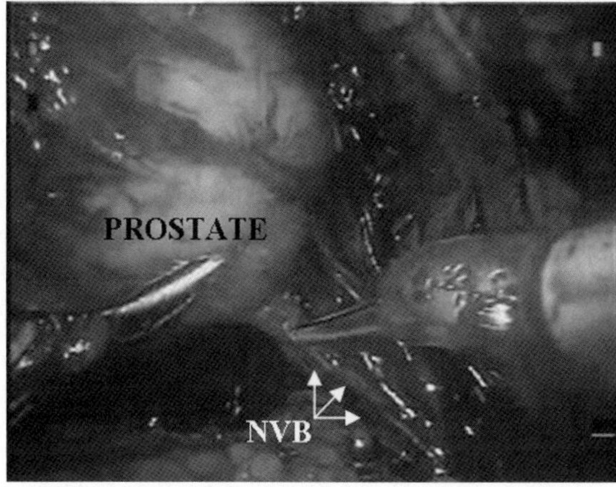


FIGURE 131.19 Athermal nerve sparing. *NVB*, neurovascular bundle.

To set up the NVB for dissection, we first incise the posterior Denovilliers fascia to expose perirectal fat and the posterior surface of the prostate. To preserve the NVB, we adhere to traditional tenets: avoidance of electrocautery and minimization of traction (Fig. 131.19). Vascular pedicles are thus controlled in an athermal fashion. One tool that we have found useful for this is the robotic Hem-O-Lock (Weck, Research Triangle Park, NC) clip applier. This instrument contains Endowrist technology and therefore can articulate in the pelvis with 6 degrees of freedom, allowing the surgeon to place clips at difficult angles and minimizing the importance of the assistant (Fig. 131.20).

In contrast to nerve-sparing procedures, there has been some controversy as to the efficacy of minimally invasive prostatectomy in treating patients with high-risk disease. By stratifying our patients according to the D'Amico classification (7), we preoperatively counsel those patients who are high risk to undergo a wide prostate dissection, including removing all tissue enveloped by the lateral prostatic fascia, including bilateral NVB, and taking a wide bladder neck, as well as an extended lymph node dissection at the end of the procedure. In such patients, vascular pedicles are controlled with bipolar electrocautery.

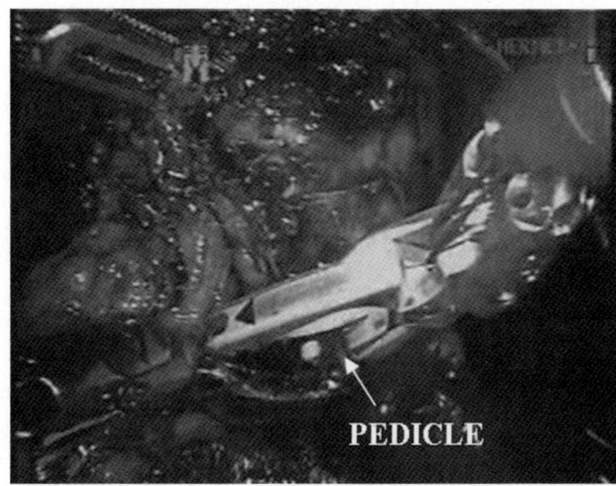


FIGURE 131.20 Placing robotic Hem-O-Lock clip.

## Dorsal Venous Complex and Distal Urethra

We routinely ligate the dorsal venous complex (DVC) at the end of the procedure, after releasing the NVB and prior to dividing the last attachments, the distal urethra and rectourethralis muscle. A 2-0 Vicryl suture on an SH needle is used to ligate the DVC in either a simple or figure-of-eight fashion. We changed our timing of ligating the DVC from the beginning until the end of the procedure for two principal reasons. The first is the fact that RALP is an antegrade, as opposed to retrograde, procedure. We believe that one of the reasons urologists are quick to ligate the DVC early is a holdover from the retropubic procedure. Since converting to the end of the case, we have not seen an increase in blood loss or transfusion rates. Our most important reason for switching, however, was that we wanted to change our apical dissection in the hope of minimizing positive apical margins in our pT2 specimens. After reviewing the margin status of our first 130 cases, we noted a positive margin rate of 14% on pT2 specimens (15 out of 109), with the majority of those being apical (60%). We analyzed a video of these cases and noted that when we ligated the DVC at the beginning of the procedure, the apex of the prostate was not completely mobile, and we frequently placed the suture too proximal and close to the prostate. When we divided the DVC, at the end of the case, we were precariously close to the prostatic apex, leading to a positive margin. By ligating the DVC at the end of the case, we have already separated all other attachments, making the prostate extremely mobile, and we can clearly visualize the DVC in its entirety as we place the suture (Fig. 131.21). Additionally, we divide both puboprostatic ligaments, thus functionally lengthening the DVC so that the suture can be set more distally. With these adjustments, we have realized a significant decrease in our overall pT2 positive margin rate and our incidence of positive apical margins.

After dividing the DVC, the last attachments are the distal urethra and rectourethralis muscle. We leave a Foley catheter in place when approaching the distal urethra to help identify it better. When dividing the urethra, we do so without electrocautery and enter it approximately 2 to 3 mm distal to the apex of the prostate (Fig. 131.22). This technique prevents us from inadvertently entering the apex, another modification that we believe has improved our margin rate. Fortunately, this modification has not compromised continence rates in our patient population.

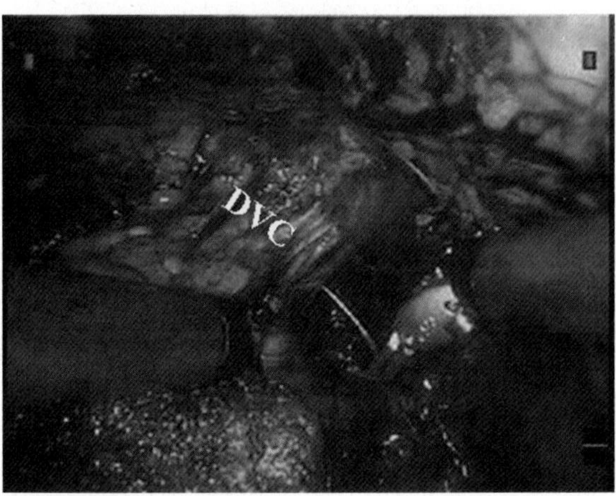


FIGURE 131.21 Placing the dorsal venous complex (DVC) suture.

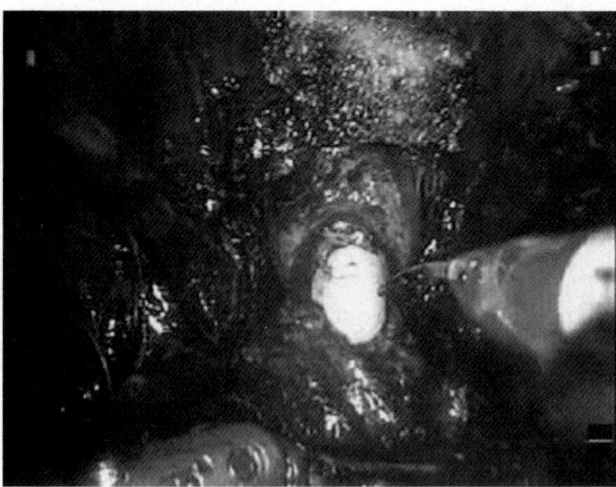

FIGURE 131.22 Dividing the distal urethra.

After the remaining attachments are divided, the prostate is placed in a laparoscopic entrapment bag and brought to the extreme lateral aspect of the field.

## Pelvic Lymph Node Dissection

All patients who undergo a RALP at our institution also receive a bilateral pelvic lymph node dissection. We feel that this represents a sound oncologic practice with prognostic and treatment implications that is standard for RRP but has been deleted by many robotic surgeons. It adds approximately 5 to 10 minutes to the operation, and morbidity is minimal. Our dissection is within the obturator fossa, using the external iliac vein as our superior landmark with the obturator nerve posterior and the pelvic sidewall lateral. We routinely take the Cloquet node and leave accessory obturator vessels intact. For high-risk patients, we extend the superior limit of our dissection to the bifurcation of the common iliac artery. All vessels are neatly skeletonized. We have found that the exceptional visualization provided by minimally invasive technology clearly identifies the anatomy and lymphatic tissue in this area. All lymphatics are secured with bipolar electrocautery. We have had no symptomatic lymphoceles and no complications related to this portion of the procedure. Each lymphatic packet is sent separately to surgical pathology for permanent analysis.

## Vesicourethral Anastomosis

The one portion of RALP in which there appears to be relative uniformity in technique is the vesicourethral anastomosis. Prior to the anastomosis, the bladder neck is tapered to approximate the diameter of the urethral aperture using 2-0 Vicryl suture in figure-of-eight knots. We prefer to perform this anteriorly *and* posteriorly, administering indigo carmine intravenously to help identify the ureteral orifices.

Like others, we have adopted the Van Velthoven one-knot, two-suture method (8). We use two 3-0 Monocryl sutures, one dyed and one undyed, on SH needles and tie them to one

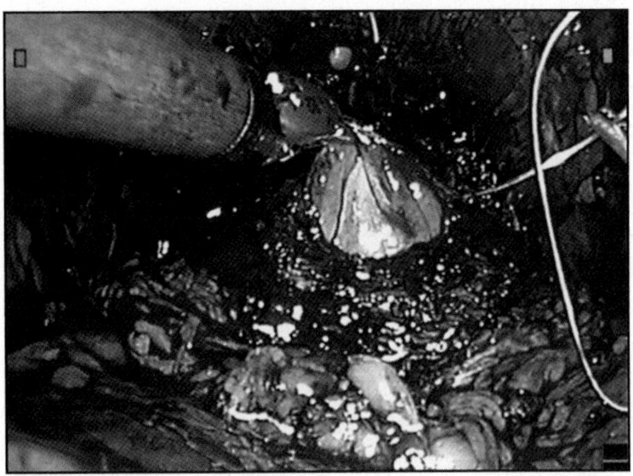

FIGURE 131.23 Starting the anastomosis at the bladder neck.

another, leaving 7 in. of suture length on each. Both sutures are started on the bladder neck at 5 o'clock (Fig. 131.23), and one is placed to the side while the other is run from urethra to bladder neck in a counterclockwise direction in an in-to-out, out-to-in fashion, respectively, to provide mucosal apposition. The assistant slides the catheter along the distal urethra and provides perineal pressure as needed. After three suture throws are placed in the bladder neck, the bladder is parachuted down with constant tension on the suture to seat the posterior plate of the anastomosis. At this point, the catheter should be able to passively slide into the bladder. This suture is then continued in a running fashion to the 12 o'clock position, and then is held on tension by the fourth arm or by the assistant. The other suture is next run in a mirror-image fashion clockwise around the bladder neck. The ultimate bladder neck stitch on both sides is placed in-to-out to end on the outside of the bladder. Ten to 11 passes are made in total. Prior to tying the two sutures together, a fresh 18Fr Foley catheter is placed under direct vision (Fig. 131.24) and 10 cc of sterile water placed in the balloon. This technique is notably different from what has been described with the LRP, in which interrupted sutures are typically placed. Many believe that the colossal challenge and frustration of intracorporeal suturing and tying deep in the pelvis is the reason that many surgeons have converted to RALP. The anastomosis is tested after tying the sutures using 180 cc saline to ensure its integrity.

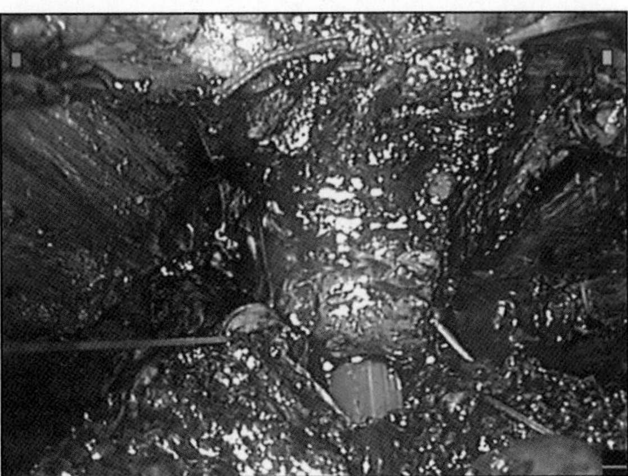

FIGURE 131.24 Visualization of catheter before final completion of urethral anastomosis.

### Retrieval of Specimen and Completion of Surgery

A suction drain is placed under direct vision at the end of the procedure through the fourth arm port. The robot is next undocked and the specimen bag delivered through the camera port, which is opened at the fascial level as needed. This incision is closed in three layers, and all other incisions are closed with a subcuticular suture.

### Postoperative Care and Discharge

Patients are sent to the recovery room on intravenous fluids, antibiotics, and pain medication. A 1-L fluid bolus is typically given intravenously at the end of the procedure because of the fluid restriction during the case. Patients are encouraged to ambulate the night of surgery and are started on oral liquids the first night after surgery. During the first postoperative day, patients receive a clear liquid diet for breakfast and regular food for lunch, and they are aggressively ambulated. The majority of patients are then discharged after lunch on the first postoperative day. The catheter is removed the week after surgery (7 to 10 days), depending on the quality of the anastomosis.

## OUTCOMES

Perioperative, oncologic, and functional outcomes of large (≥200 patients) published series of RALP are listed in Tables 131.1 to 131.4. In each table, the benchmark LRP experience of the first 1,000 patients treated at the Montsouris institute is also included (3,9). (Table 131-4 includes potency data from this group which were reported in a separate manuscript). The major advantage of minimally invasive prostatectomy in the perioperative period appears to be a decreased blood loss, which is directly or indirectly related to most of the parameters listed in Table 131.1. Decreased blood loss to the patient leads to fewer transfusions and shorter convalescence, but decreased blood loss to the surgeon means improved visualization in a relatively dry field, which can have short- and long-term implications on outcomes. Long-term data, however, remain lacking with regard to this procedure, although early indicators, such as surgical margin status, are promising. The ultimate role of RALP in the surgical treatment of prostate cancer and its relationship to the standard of care remain to be seen, although the early impact of this technology has been significant.

## COMPLICATIONS

Reported complications and rates for both LRP and RALP are similar and range from 1.5% to -20.0% in large series for major perioperative complications (e.g., hemorrhage, bowel injury, urine leak, and deep venous thrombosis/pulmonary embolus/myocardial infarction (DVT/PE/MI)) (9,10). At our institution, we have found our complication rates to be similar to what has been reported for RALP in the literature. Of note, of our first 400 pure robotic cases, we have documented 5 cases of hemorrhage requiring blood transfusion (1.3%), 3 bowel injuries (0.8%), 6 clinical urine leaks (1.5%), and 3 DVTs (0.8%), for an overall major perioperative complication rate of 3.5%.

TABLE 131.1

PERIOPERATIVE PARAMETERS OF PUBLISHED LAPAROSCOPIC PROSTATECTOMY SERIES

| Author | Year | # (Type) of cases | Or time (min) | EBL (ml) | Transfusion rate (%) | Conversion rate (%) | Complication rate (%) | In-hospital stay (days) | Catheter removal (days) |
|---|---|---|---|---|---|---|---|---|---|
| Menon (11) | 2003 | 200 (RALP) | 160 | 153 | 0 | 0 | 8 | 1.2 | 7 |
| Patel (12) | 2007 | 500 (RALP) | 130 | 10–130 | 0 | 0 | 1.5 | 1.0 | 6.9 |
| Bhandari (13) | 2005 | 300 (RALP) | 177 | 109 | 0 | 0 | 5.7 | 1.2 | 6.9 |
| Hu (14) | 2006 | 322 (RALP) | 186 | 250 | 1.6 | 0.6 | 17.2 | nr | nr |
| Joseph (15) | 2006 | 325 (RALP) | 130 | 196 | 1 | 0 | 9.6 | 1 | nr |
| Menon (16) | 2007 | 2,652 (RALP) | 154 | 142 | 0 | nr | 2.3 | 1.14 | nr |
| Guillonneau (3) | 2000 | 1,000 (LRP) | 239 | 402 | 10 | 5.8 | 3 | nr | 6.6 |

EBL, estimated blood loss; RALP, robotically assisted laparoscopic prostatectomy; LRP, laparoscopic radical prostatectomy; nr, not reported.
Adapted from Ficarra V, et al. Evidence from robot-assisted laparoscopic radical prostatectomy: a systematic review. *Eur Urol* 2007;51(1):45–55; discussion 56.

TABLE 131.2

SURGICAL MARGIN STATUS OF PUBLISHED ROBOTIC LAPAROSCOPIC PROSTATECTOMY SERIES

| Author | Year | # (Type) of cases | Pathologic stage (%) | | | Overall PSM Rate (%) | PSM Rate (%) | | |
|---|---|---|---|---|---|---|---|---|---|
| | | | pT2 | pT3a | pT3b | | pT2 | pT3a | pT3b |
| Menon (11) | 2003 | 200 (RALP) | 86.8 | 6.8 | 6.3 | 6 | nr | nr | nr |
| Patel (12) | 2007 | 500 (RALP) | 88 | 15 | 5 | 9.4 | 2.5 | 23 | 46 |
| Joseph (15) | 2006 | 325(RALP) | 81 | 14 | 5 | 13 | 9.9 | 37.1 | 273% |
| Menon (16) | 2007 | 2,652 (LRP) | 77.7 | 16.9 | 5.1 | 13 | nr | nr | nr |
| Guillonneau (3) | 2000 | 1,000 (RALP) | nr | nr | nr | 19.2 | 15.5 | 30 | 32 |

RALP: robotically assisted laparoscopic prostatectomy; LRP, laparoscopic radical prostatectomy; nr, not reported.

Adapted from Ficarra V, et al. Evidence from robot-assisted laparoscopic radical prostatectomy: a systematic review. *Eur Urol* 2007;51(1):45–55; discussion 56.

TABLE 131.3

CONTINENCE DATA OF PUBLISHED LAPAROSCOPIC PROSTATECTOMY SERIES

| Author | Year | # (Type) of cases | Continence definition | Method of data collection | Continence rates (%) | | |
|---|---|---|---|---|---|---|---|
| | | | | | 3-mo | 6-mo | 12-mo |
| Menon (11) | 2003 | 200 (RALP) | 0–1 pad ("safety pad") | Interview | nr | 96 | nr |
| Patel (12) | 2007 | 500 (RALP) | No pad | Questionnaire | 89 | 95 | 97 |
| Joseph (15) | 2006 | 325 (RALP) | No pad | Questionnaire | 93 | 96 | nr |
| Menon (16) | 2007 | 2,652 (LRP) | 0–1 pad ("safety pad") | Interview | nr | nr | 95.2 |
| Guillonneau (3) | 2000 | 1,000 (RALP) | 0–1 pad ("safety pad") | Interview/ questionaire | nr | nr | 88.3 |

PSM, positive surgical margin; RALP, robotically assisted laparoscopic prostatectomy; nr, not reported.

Adapted from Ficarra V, et al. Evidence from robot-assisted laparoscopic radical prostatectomy: a systematic review. *Eur Urol* 2007;51(1):45–55; discussion 56.

**TABLE 131.4**

POTENCY DATA OF PUBLISHED LAPAROSCOPIC PROSTATECTOMY SERIES

| Author | Year | # (Type) of cases | Potency definition | Data collection | Potency rates (%) | | |
|---|---|---|---|---|---|---|---|
| | | | | | 3-mo | 6-mo | 12-mo |
| Menon (11) | 2003 | 200 (RALP) | Sexual intercourse | IIEF-5 | 25 (<60 yr)<br>10 (>60 yr) | 64 (<60 yr)<br>38 (>60 yr) | |
| Patel (12) | 2007 | 200 (RALP) | Sexual intercourse | IIEF-5 | | | 85 |
| Joseph (15) | 2006 | 325 (RALP) | IIEF > 21 | IIEF-5 | 46 | | |
| Menon (16) | 2007 | 884 (RALP) | Sexual intercourse | SHIM | | | 70[a] |
| Guillonneau (17) | 2005 | 550 (LRP) | Sexual intercourse | | | | 66 |

[a]100% of patients reported to achieve potency at 48 months of follow-up.

RALP, robotically assisted laparoscopic prostatectomy; IIEF, international index of erectile function; SHIM, sexual health inventory for men; LRP, laparoscopic radical prostatectomy.

Adapted from Ficarra V, et al. Evidence from robot-assisted laparoscopic radical prostatectomy: a systematic review. *Eur Urol* 2007;51(1):45–55; discussion 56.

## *References*


1. Schuessler WW, et al. Laparoscopic radical prostatectomy: initial short-term experience. *Urology* 1997;50(6):854–857.
2. Valicenti RK, Gomella LG, El-Gabry EA, et al. The multidisciplinary clinic approach to prostate cancer counseling and treatment. *Semin Urol Oncol* 2000;18(3):188–191.
3. Guillonneau B, Vallancien G. Laparoscopic radical prostatectomy: the Montsouris experience. *J Urol* 2000;163(2):418–422.
4. Stolzenburg JU, Rabenalt R, Do M, et al. Endoscopic extraperitoneal radical prostatectomy: the University of Leipzig experience of 1,300 cases. *World J Urol* 2007; 25(1):45–51.
5. Tewari A, Peabody JO, Fischer M, et al. An operative and anatomic study to help in nerve sparing during laparoscopic and robotic radical prostatectomy. *Eur Urol* 2003; 43(5):444–454.
6. Savera AT, Kaul S, Badani K, et al. Robotic radical prostatectomy with the "Veil of Aphrodite" technique: histologic evidence of enhanced nerve sparing. *Eur Urol* 2006;49(6):1065–1073; discussion 1073–1074.
7. D'Amico AV, Whittington R, Malkowicz SB, et al. Predicting prostate specific antigen outcome preoperatively in the prostate specific antigen era. *J Urol* 2001;166(6):2185–2188.
8. Van Velthoven RF, Ahlering TE, Peltier A, et al. Technique for laparoscopic running urethrovesical anastomosis: the single knot method. *Urology* 2003;61(4):699–702.
9. Trabulsi EJ, Guillonneau B. Laparoscopic radical prostatectomy. *J Urol* 2005;173(4):1072–1079.
10. Ficarra V, Cavalleri S, Novara G, et al. Evidence from robot-assisted laparoscopic radical prostatectomy: a systematic review. *Eur Urol* 2007; 51(1):45–55; discussion 56.
11. Menon M. Robotic radical retropubic prostatectomy. *BJU Int* 2003;91(3): 175–176.
12. Patel VR, Thaly R, Shah K. Robotic radical prostatectomy: outcomes of 500 cases. *BJU Int* 2007;99(5):1109–1112.
13. Bhandari A, McIntire L, Kaul SA, et al. Perioperative complications of robotic radical prostatectomy after the learning curve. *J Urol* 2005; 174(3):915–918.
14. Hu JC, Nelson RA, Wilson TG, et al. Perioperative complications of laparoscopic and robotic assisted laparoscopic radical prostatectomy. *J Urol* 2006;175(2):541–546; discussion 546.
15. Joseph JV, Rosenbaum R, Madeb R, et al. Robotic extraperitoneal radical prostatectomy: an alternative approach. *J Urol* 2006;175(3, Pt 1): 945–950; discussion 951.
16. Menon M, Shrivastava A, Kaul S, et al. Vattikuti Institute prostatectomy: contemporary technique and analysis of results. *Eur Urol* 2007;51(3):648-657; discussion 657–658.
17. Guillonneau B, et al. Laparoscopic radical prostatectomy: assessment after 550 procedures. *Crit Rev Oncol Hematol* 2002; 43:123–133.


# CHAPTER 132 ■ LAPAROSCOPIC MANAGEMENT OF LYMPHOCELES

SEAN P. HEDICAN AND STEPHEN Y. NAKADA

Lymphoceles are localized encapsulated collections of lymphatic fluid created by disruption of lymphatic vessels that can occur following renal transplantation or other procedures during which lymphatic channels are transected in the pelvis or retroperitoneum. The incidence of asymptomatic lymphoceles following renal transplantation or combined kidney pancreas transplantation has been reported to be as high as 20% (1). Contributing factors in transplant patients include episodes of rejection, cytomegalovirus infections, and post-transplantation reoperations (2,3).

Disruption of the lymphatics in the closed space of the pelvis following limited extraperitoneal pelvic lymph node dissections has also led to localized lymphoceles in patients being treated for prostate cancer, with a reported incidence of 0.5 to 10% (2,4,5). Significant contributing factors to the formation of the lymphoceles include the administration of low-dose heparin (6), prior radiation, presence of metastases, surgical technique, and the extent of the dissection (5). The majority of these pelvic lymphoceles remain clinically asymptomatic. Lymphoceles have also been described following retroperitoneal procedures such as nephrectomy, retroperitoneal lymph node dissections for testis cancer, or aortic surgery.

## DIAGNOSIS

Asymptomatic lymphoceles are usually discovered incidentally at the time of renal allograft ultrasound (Fig. 132.1) or computerized tomographic (CT) imaging of the abdomen and pelvis (Fig. 132.2) performed for unrelated indications. They appear as a single or septated chamber with Hounsfield unit characteristics and echotexture consistent with fluid located in the region of the renal allograft or adjacent to the iliac vessels.

These structures can be difficult to differentiate from a urinoma unless an ongoing urine leak can be documented via contrast or radionuclide imaging. In the case of a urinoma, aspiration and analysis of the fluid will demonstrate a creatinine value elevated above corresponding serum values (7). The creatinine value on the fluid aspirated from a lymphocele will be equivalent to serum. Hematomas and abscesses usually contain fluid with a higher echogenicity on ultrasound

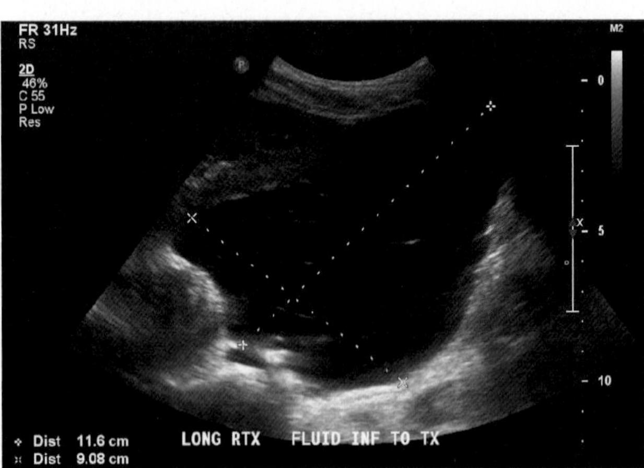


FIGURE 132.1. Ultrasound images of a large lymphocele containing low echogenic fluid extending below and medial to the transplant kidney.

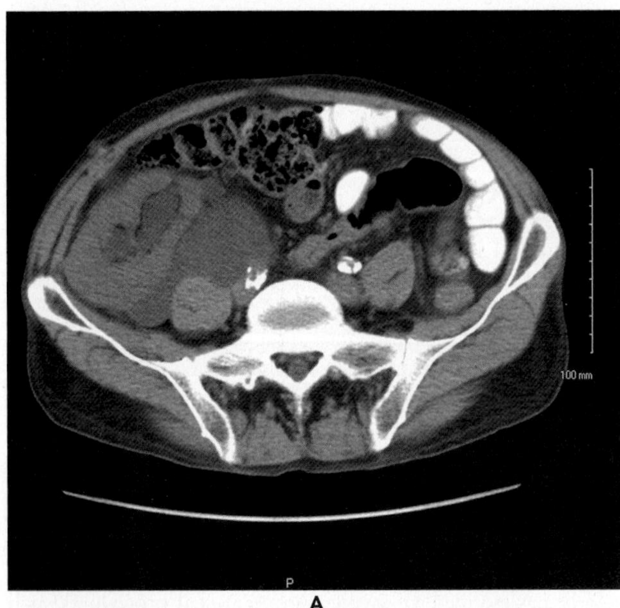


A

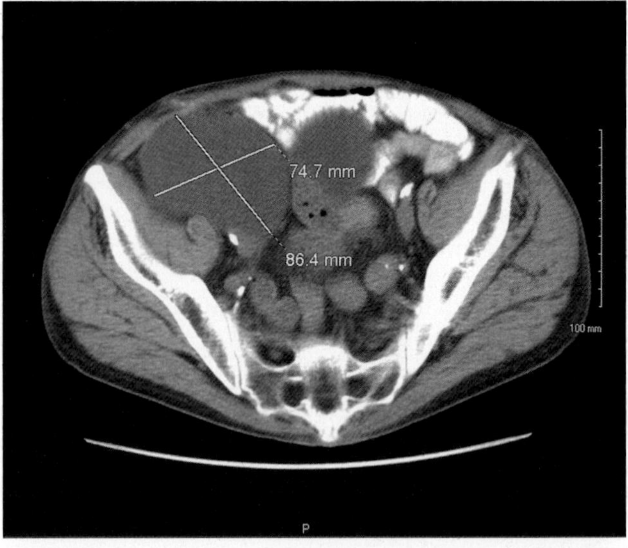


B

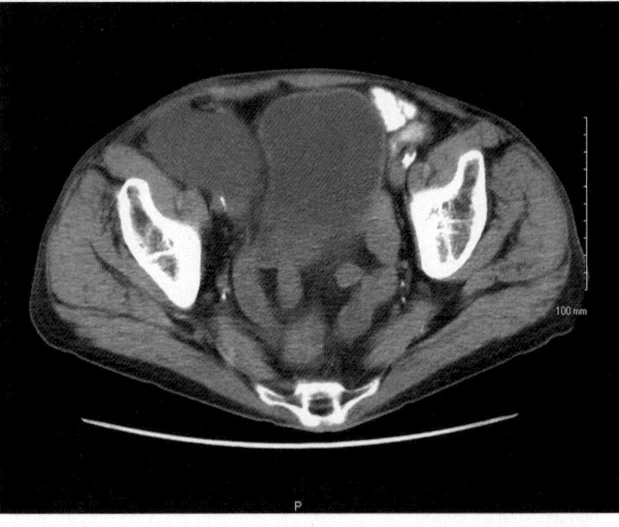


C

FIGURE 132.2. Computerized tomographic images demonstrating the transplant kidney in the right lower quadrant and the inferior and medial location of lymphocele **A:** Note the close proximity of the adjacent iliac vessels containing calcified atherosclerotic plaque. **B:** Extension of the lymphocele at its greatest dimension and the cephalad extent of the bladder appearing medially. **C:** Compression of the lateral wall of the bladder by the medial extent of the lymphocele.

examination, with an increased nonenhanced density on CT imaging (8). The presence of signs and symptoms of an infection in association with a high-density fluid collection, often with mild enhancement of thickened walls or surrounding tissue stranding, usually denotes an abscess. The diagnosis is confirmed and therapeutic intervention often begins with percutaneous drainage or aspiration of purulent material (2).

## INDICATIONS FOR SURGERY

The primary indication for a lymphocelectomy (surgical unroofing or marsupialization of a lymphocele) is symptoms related to its mass effect. The reported incidence of symptomatic lymphoceles following renal transplantation ranges from 3%

to 7% (9,10). Symptomatic lymphoceles after pelvic lymphadenectomy following radical retropubic prostatectomy are rare, and the majority remain asymptomatic and resolve spontaneously. Symptoms necessitating surgical drainage and unroofing include labial, scrotal, or lower extremity swelling, deep venous thrombosis with or without pulmonary embolism, a sensation of pelvic fullness, and irritative voiding complaints due to compressive effects on the bladder or rectum (5). Renal transplant dysfunction secondary to ureteral obstruction with associated hydronephrosis versus direct compressive effects on the allograft has also been reported. A review of indications for surgery in transplant recipients demonstrated that 69% were performed for local symptoms, 14% for graft dysfunction, and 17% for both (9). Ureteral obstruction following pelvic lymphadenectomy for prostate cancer is extremely rare (5).

## ALTERNATIVE THERAPY

Prior to the first reported case of laparoscopic lymphocelectomy in 1991 by McCullough et al. (11), the treatment of choice for a symptomatic lymphocele was open transperitoneal marsupialization, with a reported complication rate of 4% and a recurrence rate of 15% on review of 129 patients undergoing open lymphocelectomy (10). This method is still utilized for complex lymphoceles that are multiseptated and lying in a difficult-to-access lateroposterior or lateroinferior position relative to the allograft. Lymphoceles located in these locations have also been shown to be associated with a higher incidence of conversion from a laparoscopic to open surgery as a result (12). Infected lymphoceles requiring extensive evacuation and washout of purulent debris, excision of all septations, and drain placement also support the use of an open extraperitoneal approach (2,3).

Similar to symptomatic renal cysts, aspiration of lymph fluid alone via a percutaneous approach is associated with a 75% to 100% incidence of lymphocele recurrence. These results are not significantly improved by insertion of a percutaneous drain. The use of sclerosing agents instilled into the lymphocele cavity has been reported to increase the likelihood of successful ablation to approximately 85% to 90% (3). Sclerosing agents vary depending upon the series, but the use of alcohol, tetra- or doxycycline, povidone-iodine, and fibrin sealant have all been reported (3,13). It should be noted that this treatment usually requires multiple instillations that can last as long as 45 days (3). The use of this approach is contraindicated for complex multiseptated lymphoceles due to incomplete drainage and inability to introduce sclerotic agent into all chambers (13). Sclerotic agents are also best avoided when the ureter contacts one of the walls of the lymphocele due to the concern that the inflammatory response induced could result in periureteral fibrosis and ultimate transplant ureteral obstruction. Infected lymphoceles likewise should not be treated with aspiration and sclerosis even when utilizing antibiotic agents, as this can lead to persistence and even aggravation of the infection.

Adani et al. (14) utilized an outpatient technique for draining persistent lymphoceles into the peritoneal cavity in seven patients via intraperitoneal placement of a two-cuff Tenckhoff dialysis catheter with the fenestrated end in the peritoneum and the other end in the lymphocele cavity, with the body of the catheter tunneled subcutaneously with the cuff secured to the fascia. This approach was felt to be especially applicable for lymphoceles in locations not readily accessible to transperitoneal window creation. The catheters were removed 6 months later, with no signs of recurrence after removal in two patients with at least 1 year of follow-up.

## SURGICAL TECHNIQUE

### Preoperative Preparation

Patients are placed on a clear liquid diet beginning at noon the day prior to their procedure and are also instructed to drink a bottle of magnesium citrate in an effort to cleanse the bowel. Decompression of the bowel aids in visualization during the operation and improves the speed of bowel recovery. On call to the operating room, the patient is administered a single dose of an appropriate intravenous broad-spectrum antibiotic. Patients on long-term steroid immunosuppressive therapy may require supplemental stress dosing per the anesthesia team. Compressive knee or thigh-high stockings (TED hose) and sequential compression devices are applied to the lower extremities to reduce the risk of deep venous thrombosis formation. Hair is removed from the area of the operative field, including the pubic region and lower abdomen, using an electric shear.

### Patient Positioning

The operating table should be equipped with a kidney rest and allow flexion/deflection and full Trendelenburg positioning. A 3-inch foam pad mattress is placed on the operating table, followed by a full-size gel pad to aid in securing the patient. Prior to transferring the patient from the transport bed to the operating table, 70% isopropyl alcohol can be used to cleanse the back to remove body oils and debris to establish secure traction between the patient and the gel pad without the use of shoulder bars, chest tape, or straps. Alternatively, any of the other aforementioned securing methods can be utilized. Following intubation of the patient, an orogastric tube is inserted to decompress the stomach, and nitrous oxide should be avoided to prevent bowel distention and to reduce the risk of creating a combustible environment when electrocautery is being utilized. The patient should be positioned with the umbilicus at the region of the kidney rest to allow flexion of the table with slight kidney rest elevation to increase the distance between the umbilicus and the pubic symphysis, assisting in spacing of the trocars.

The Foley catheter should be inserted on the operative field after preparing and draping to allow access for filling and decompressing the bladder, which may assist in localization of the lymphocele. Male patients are placed supine on the operating table. Female patients should be positioned in low lithotomy using Allen stirrups to allow adequate access to the urethral meatus. Alternatively, slight frog-leg positioning can be utilized in nonobese female patients. If the legs are not secured in stirrups, tape can be placed across the upper thighs and a strap across the lower legs to secure them in position.

The arms are protected in eggcrate foam and tucked at the sides using either a split draw sheet or Plexiglas arm sleds. When arm sleds are utilized, care must be taken to avoid disruption of the securing Velcro on their insertion, as this holds the 3-inch foam mattress in place and can lead to its dislodgement and inadvertent patient movement on deep Trendelenburg positioning. Although it is rarely required, the security of the patient's position should be tested in full Trendelenburg tilt prior to preparation and draping. A wide surgical skin preparation should be performed to include the genitals for sterile Foley catheter insertion and adequate exposure to allow adequate trocar spacing and conversion to an open operation if necessary. A standard wide-aperture laparoscopic drape can be utilized when patients are not placed in stirrups; otherwise, standard cystoscopy legging and aperture drapes are utilized after four-towel draping of the abdominoperineal region. The aperture can be enlarged to give adequate exposure to the lower abdomen.

## Establishing Peritoneal Access and Trocar Configuration

Access to the peritoneum can be obtained utilizing a closed needle (Veress) puncture technique or an open direct vision (i.e., Hasson cannula) method. A 1-cm supraumbilical incision is made through the skin and the underlying dermis using a combination of scalpel and electrocautery incision for insertion of the initial port. If the lymphocele is extremely large, extending to or above the level of the umbilicus, this centrally located port can be moved in a cephalad direction to ensure that the port enters approximately a hands-breadth above the upper extent of the lymphocele. Transabdominal ultrasound can be used to assist in port placement or the extent of the lymphocele estimated by counting CT scan slices above and below the umbilicus to predict its location. The underlying soft tissues are bluntly dissected down to fascia using a sharp clamp.

Initial pneumoperitoneum is created as described in Chapter 123. The insufflation pressure set point should be placed at 15 mm Hg, and once this pressure level is obtained, a visual introducing trocar (e.g., Optiview, Ethicon Endo-Surgery, Cincinnati, OH) is used to insert a 10/12-mm port via the previously made periumbilical incision. The 0-degree 10-mm laparoscope is inserted into the Optiview and can be used to visualize each layer of the abdominal wall as it is traversed using a back-and-forth twisting motion until full entry into the peritoneal cavity is confirmed. Once the visual introducing port has been inserted, the 0-degree lens is exchanged for a 30-degree lens to allow a greater range of visualization angles.

Two additional working ports are then placed, adjusting their position depending upon the location of the lymphocele. In general, a 5-mm working port is inserted a hands-breadth down from the supraumbilical port just lateral to the midline on the side contralateral to the lymphocele. If the distance between the umbilicus and the pubic symphysis is sufficient to allow placement of two ports separated by a hands-breadth without entry into the bladder, the third port (5 mm) can be placed below the second port in the midline. This also requires that the lymphocele is not exceptionally large and that the patient is not morbidly obese (Body Mass Index <35). In general, placement of this port a hands-breadth lateral to the midline just below the level of the umbilicus on the side ipsilateral to the lymphocele is preferred. In the standard trocar arrangement, a 10-mm port can be utilized to allow lateral camera positioning if desired during the case (Fig. 132.3). Alternatively, a 5-mm port can be utilized if a 5-mm laparoscope is available.

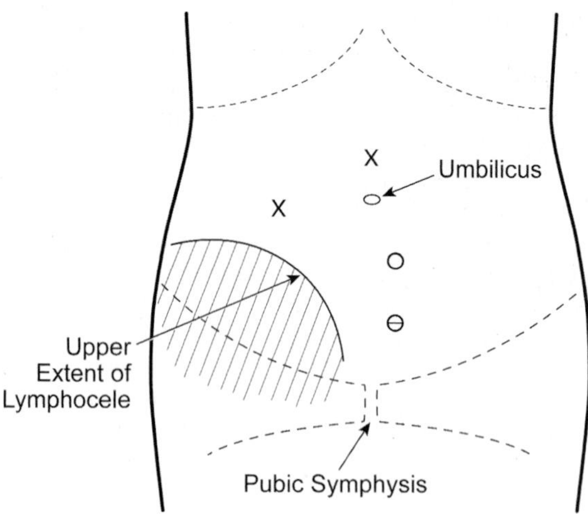


FIGURE 132.3. Recommended port configuration for right laparoscopic lymphocelectomy. X, 10/12-mm port; O, 5-mm port; Θ, alternative 5-mm port.

The surgeon stands on the side opposite the lymphocele and the assistant and scrub personnel stand on the ipsilateral side across from the primary surgeon. The monitor and tower or boom arm containing the insufflation unit, light, and camera source are positioned at the foot of the patient. The patient is placed in Trendelenburg positioning to the extent necessary to liberate the bowel off the area of dissection, and the table is airplaned slightly toward the operating surgeon.

## Identification of the Lymphocele

After release of any overlying bowel or omental adhesions to the lower quadrant of interest, the lymphocele can be identified as a bluish-black pelvic structure if thin-walled. The overall appearance can vary significantly, and when the wall is thickened, differentiation from the bladder can be difficult (Fig. 132.4A). Depending upon its location, other surrounding vital structures, such as the transplant or native ureter or iliac vessels, can also be incorporated into one or more of the walls of the lymphocele. Methods to assist in identification and differentiation from the bladder have been described, including distention followed by decompression of the bladder with sterile saline. The bladder can also be filled with indigo carmine or methylene blue–stained saline and a laparoscopic aspirating needle can be inserted into the identified structure presumed to be the lymphocele (Fig. 132.4B). This is confirmed to be the lymphocele if the aspirated fluid does not contain blue-tinged fluid (15).

A similar but opposite method to assist in the identification of the lymphocele has also been described. This involves outlining the lymphocele using transabdominal ultrasound and percutaneous needle puncture with aspiration followed by injection of the lymphocele with dilute methylene blue–tinged saline. This results in staining of the walls of the lymphocele, allowing confirmation of the structure prior to unroofing by laparoscopic needle aspiration with return of blue–tinged fluid (2,15). Once the lymphocele is entered, the blue staining of the chamber assists in identification of its extent and the amount of unroofing required.

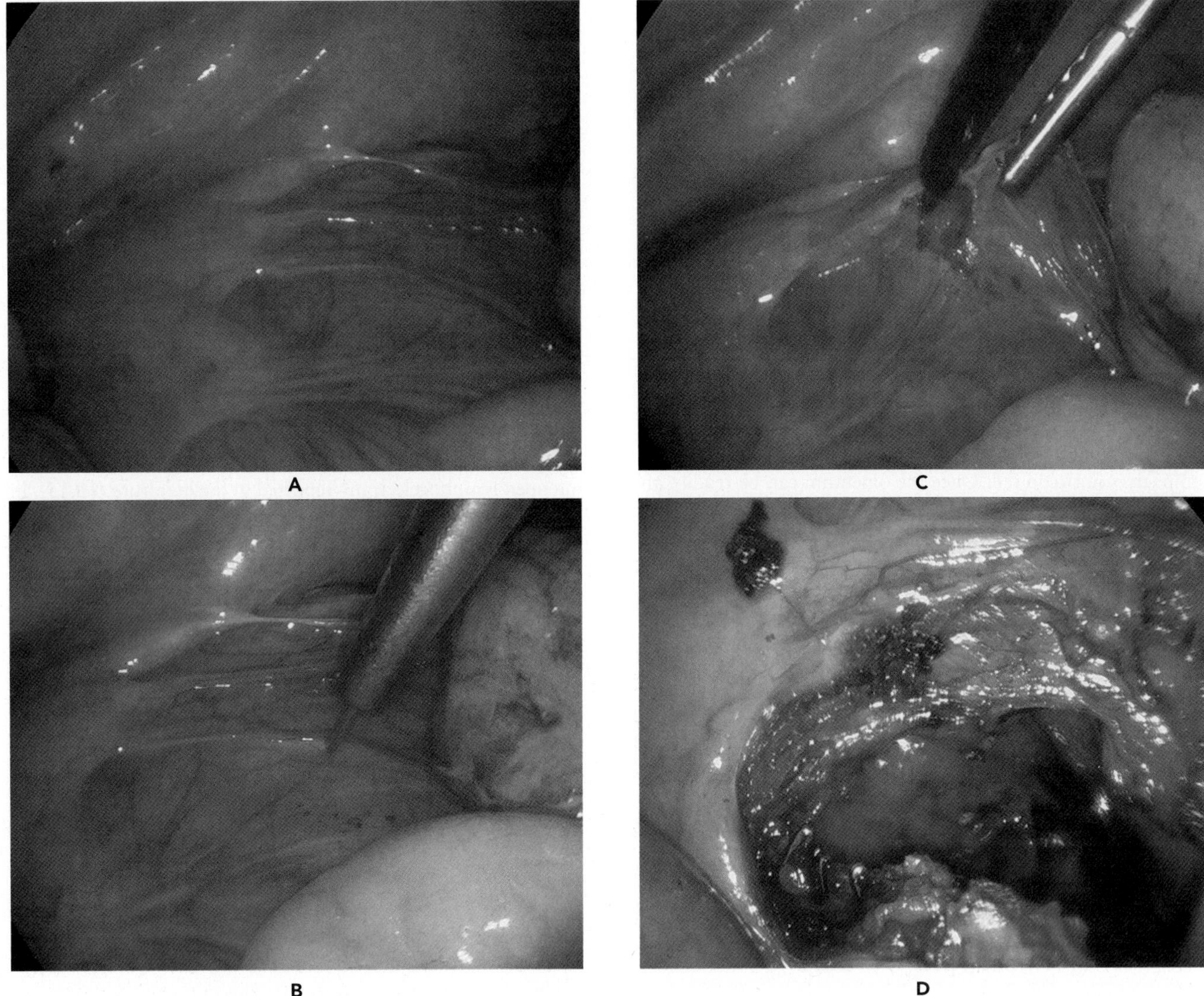


FIGURE 132.4. Laparoscopic view of right lower quadrant lymphocele adjacent to a renal transplant. **A:** Thick-walled appearance making differentiation between the indigo carmine–containing bladder and lymphocele difficult. **B:** Laparoscopic aspiration needle inserted into the lymphocele, yielding clear fluid. **C:** Lymphocele unroofing begins utilizing an electrocautery hook. **D:** Final appearance of wide-mouthed peritoneal aperture created in the lymphocele.

## Excision of the Lymphocele

Once the lymphocele is identified, cold or cautery shears, a cautery hook (Fig. 132.4C), or a harmonic scalpel can be utilized to unroof the lymphocele, incising through the area of the wall that appears to be the thinnest portion of the structure in a direction parallel to the presumed course of the transplant ureter. After the initial incision, care should be taken to inspect the wall to make sure that structures such as the renal allograft ureter or pelvis, native ureter, or bladder are not injured in the process. In general, only the portion of the wall in contact with the peritoneum is excised, and any of the contained loculations are disrupted bluntly and the walls excised. Although stenting of the transplant ureter can be performed to help in its identification, this can be technically challenging. In a large multi-institutional retrospective study, 81 patients underwent laparoscopic marsupialization, and none of the ureters were stented prior to the laparoscopic surgery, yet no ureteral injuries occurred (3). The wall of the lymphocele can then be excised from the central incision to the edge of the thin region of the wall using the laparoscopic instruments to ballot the area to help judge its thickness and the likely involvement of surrounding structures. The excision is then carried out circumferentially until the entire exposed region of the lymphocele is excised (Fig. 132.4D). Once the segments are excised, they can be removed via the 10/12-mm port or cut into strips prior to removal if they are too large to fit through the port. The specimen is visually inspected, and if any concerning elements are identified, such as portions of ureter, these can be confirmed via frozen section analysis, allowing intraoperative management. If the excised region of the lymphocele is small (<4 cm) due to the presence of surrounding vital structures, and this results in a deep-chambered cavity with a narrow aperture, then consideration should be given for placement of an omental wick.

### Placement of Omental Wick

Hsu et al. (3), in their large multi-institutional review of laparoscopic lymphocelectomy, reported that omental interposition was utilized in only 14% of the 81 reported cases and "was not considered to be an essential pre-requisite for long-term success." It was the reported practice of the lead author of the study to utilize an omental tag only if it could be "readily transposed and affixed to the lymphocele window." In theory, use of native vascularized tissues to maintain patency of the unroofed portion of the lymphocele will facilitate continued patency and peritoneal drainage of the lymphatic fluids.

The omental interposition graft is usually established using the most distal tip of the omentum, which is isolated; if necessary the omentum can be divided in a craniocaudad direction to facilitate mobilization. Major vasculature should be left in place, and typically extensive dissection to the margin of the stomach is not required. Once the omentum can be readily affixed to one of the internal walls of the fenestrated lymphocele, several sutures on a small (e.g., RB-1) needle or tacking titanium clips are placed to secure the tip of the mobilized omentum near the base of the lymphocele. Needles for laparoscopic suturing should be introduced and removed via one of the 10/12-mm trocars to prevent their entrapment in the valve mechanism of the port. If the camera port is the only 10/12-mm trocar being utilized for the procedure, this may require switching to a 5-mm laparoscope to use via one of the working ports to allow needles to be introduced into the peritoneal cavity.

In more complex cases of difficult-to-reach lymphoceles, where an omental wick may not be expected to maintain durable patency, laparoscopic marsupialization with placement of peritoneal dialysis catheters cabled together has been utilized to maintain continued lymphoperitoneal flow (16).

### Postoperative Care

The patient's postoperative diet is advanced as tolerated and the Foley catheter is removed once the patient is able to ambulate. In male patients with a history of voiding dysfunction, the Foley catheter is left indwelling until the first postoperative day, and several scanned postvoid residual volumes are evaluated following its removal to ensure adequate bladder emptying. Intravenous pain medication is transitioned rapidly to oral analgesics once the patient is tolerating clear liquids. Laboratory studies are kept to a minimum and individualized depending upon the patient's clinical condition. In general, hemoglobin/hematocrit levels as well as a blood urea nitrogen (BUN) and creatinine (Cr) testing are performed the morning following the operation. If significant lower extremity edema or transplant ureteral obstruction occurred preoperatively due to the lymphocele, then more careful postoperative electrolyte and fluid management may be required.

Discharge criteria include toleration of a regular diet, passage of flatus, and pain adequately controlled on oral analgesics. Typically patients are ready for discharge within 24 hours of the procedure; however, the mean hospital stay in a large reported review series was 1.5 days (3).

## OUTCOMES

In a multi-institutional study of 81 patients, Hsu et al. (3) noted a lymphocele recurrence rate of 6% over an average of 27 months of follow-up after laparoscopic marsupialization. This compares favorably to the 0% to 15% recurrence rate following open lymphocelectomy reported in the literature (10,15). In a comparison of a group of patients treated with laparoscopic lymphocelectomy to a contemporary group of patients treated via an open approach, Gill et al. (2) reported a statistically significant reduction in blood loss (34.6 versus 117.3 mL), more rapid resumption of oral intake (0.9 versus 2.5 days), shorter hospital stay (2 versus 6.1 days), and more rapid convalescence (2.2 versus 6.9 weeks), respectively. A $7,400 reduction in total hospital costs has also been reported for laparoscopic versus open lymphocelectomy, largely due to the significant reduction in hospital stay (12). It is important to note that more contemporary case series would likely reflect trends toward shorter hospital stays for both of these approaches.

### Complications

The reported incidence of complications in one of the largest series of laparoscopic lymphocelectomy was 5% intraoperatively and 4% postoperatively (3). This compares favorably to the 0% to 12% complication rate reported following open lymphocelectomy (2,12,15). One of the most frequently occurring intraoperative complications noted by Melvin et al. (15) was division of the transplanted ureter, which occurred in 7% of their cases. Several methods have been employed to prevent this complication, including ureteral stent placement and insertion of a lighted fiberoptic stent.

The reported incidence of open conversion was shown to be 0% to 36% (12,15). Risk factors for conversion of a laparoscopic to an open approach include prior operations, multiple fluid collections, and unfavorable location of the lymphocele.

## *References*


1. Doehn C, Fornara P, Fricke L, et al. Laparoscopic fenestration of posttransplant lymphoceles. *Surg Endosc* 2002;16:690–695.
2. Gill IS, Hodge EE, Munch LC, et al. Transperitoneal marsupialization of lymphoceles: a comparison of laparoscopic and open techniques. *J Urol* 1995;153:706–711.
3. Hsu THS, Gill IS, Grune MT, et al. Laparoscopic lymphocelectomy: a multi-institutional analysis. *J Urol* 2000;163:1096–1099.
4. McCullough DL, McLaughlin AP, Gittes RF. Morbidity of pelvic lymphadenectomy and radical prostatectomy for prostate cancer. *J Urol* 1977; 117:206–207.
5. Patel A. Complications of lymphadenectomy. In: Taneja SS, Smith RB, Ehrlich RM, eds. *Complications of Urologic Surgery: Prevention and Management.* 3rd ed. Philadelphia: WB Saunders, 2001:370–386.
6. Catalona WJ, Kadmon D, Crane DB. Effects of mini-dose heparin on lymphocele formation following extraperitoneal pelvic lymphadencectomy. *J Urol* 1980;123:890–892.
7. Hamza A, Fischer K, Koch E, et al. Diagnostics and therapy of lymphoceles after kidney transplantation. *Transplant Proc* 2006;38:701–706.
8. Gazelle GS, Mueller PR. Abdominal abscess. Imaging and intervention. *Radiol Clin North Am* 1994;32:913–932.
9. Bailey SH, Mone MC, Holman JM, et al. Laparoscopic treatment of post renal transplant lymphoceles. *Surg Endosc* 2003;17:1896–1899.
10. Fuller TF, Kang SM, Hirose R, et al. Management of lymphoceles after renal transplantation: laparoscopic versus open drainage. *J Urol* 2003;169: 2022–2025.

11. McCullough CS, Soper NJ, Clayman RV, et al. Laparoscopic drainage of a posttransplant lymphocele. *Transplantation* 1991;51:725–727.
12. Gruessner RWG, Fasola C, Benedetti E, et al. Laparoscopic drainage of lymphoceles after kidney transplantation: indications and limitations. *Surgery* 1995;117:288–295.
13. Chin AI, Ragavendra N, Hilorne L, et al. Fibrin sealant sclerotherapy for treatment of lymphoceles following renal transplantation. *J Urol* 2003; 170:380–383.
14. Adani GL, Baccarani U, Risaliti A, et al. Treatment of recurrent symptomatic lymphocele after kidney transplantation with intraperitoneal Tenckhoff catheter. *Urology* 2007;70:659–661.
15. Melvin WS, Bumgardner GL, Davies EA, et al. The laparoscopic management of post-transplant lymphocele. A critical review. *Surg Endosc* 1997; 11:245–248.
16. Matin SF, Gill IS. Laparoscopic marsupialization of the difficult lymphocele using internalized peritoneal dialysis catheter. *J Urol* 2000;163: 1498–1500.

# CHAPTER 133 ■ LAPAROSCOPIC BLADDER PROCEDURES: RADICAL CYSTECTOMY, PARTIAL CYSTECTOMY, URACHAL EXCISION, DIVERTICULECTOMY

SEBASTIEN CROUZET, GEORGES-PASCAL HABER, AND INDERBIR S. GILL

## LAPAROSCOPIC RADICAL CYSTECTOMY

Radical cystectomy is the treatment of choice for high-risk, recurrent, superficial, and invasive cancer of the urinary bladder. This procedure is traditionally performed through an open midline incision. Radical cystectomy is curative for most patients who have localized disease, with 5- and 10-year recurrence-free survival rates approaching 70% (1,2).

Laparoscopic radical cystectomy (LRC) is an attractive minimally invasive alternative to conventional open radical cystectomy, as it faithfully duplicates technical aspects of open surgery yet is associated with decreased blood loss (3,4). In reconstructing the ileal conduit or neobladder, an open-assisted approach is preferable to a purely intracorporeal technique for the following reasons: the operating time is shorter than a pure laparoscopic approach, bowel-related complications are fewer, and the advantages of a laparoscopic approach to cystectomy are preserved and it is technically simpler to perform (5,6).

### Diagnosis

The diagnosis and staging of muscle-invasive bladder cancer are addressed elsewhere in this book.

### Indications

Patients with organ-confined high-risk superficial or invasive bladder cancer are candidates for LRC. Our current contraindications include computerized tomographic evidence of bulky primary tumors, extravesical spread, or gross lymphadenopathy, frozen pelvis due to previous surgery or inflammatory pathology, fixation of the bladder to surrounding structures and pelvic wall on bimanual palpation, and uncorrected bleeding diathesis. Morbid obesity and previous pelvic radiation can significantly complicate the technical performance of LRC. Previous aortoiliac vascular surgery and endovascular stenting can make the ureteric dissection challenging.

### Alternative Therapy

Bladder-preserving protocols utilizing external beam and chemotherapy are available for those who may not be considered for radical cystectomy.

### Surgical Technique

#### Patient Preparation

A thorough preoperative evaluation is necessary, including cardiac and medical clearance. Antiplatelet agents should be discontinued at least 1 week before surgery. Anticoagulant discontinuation may necessitate bridging to heparin perioperatively. Mechanical bowel preparation includes a clear liquid diet and 4 L of polyethylene glycol on the afternoon before surgery. A stoma site is marked before LRC for all patients by a stoma therapist. Broad-spectrum intravenous antibiotics (usually a third-generation cephalosporin and metronidazole) are administered at induction. As such, the patient preparation is the same as for open surgery.

#### Procedure

The patient is secured on the operating table in the low lithotomy position, with both arms adducted and secured to the table, thus allowing access to the patient's perineal area and rectum. All pressure points are meticulously padded. Sequential compressing stockings are applied. The operating table is placed in a steep Trendelenburg position and the patient is prepared from the nipples down to the midthighs, including the genitalia. A warming blanket covers the upper chest and shoulders. The patient is draped in a sterile fashion using leggings and a special laparoscopy drape. An 18Fr Foley catheter is inserted from the operative field after sterile preparation and draping of the patient.

The surgeon stands on the left side of the patient, while the first assistant stands opposite the surgeon on the right side of the patient. The scrub nurse/technician stands between the legs of the patient and has the instrument table behind him or her. If necessary, a second assistant stands to the left of the surgeon. Two camera monitors are positioned 20 to 30 cm above each outstretched foot of the patient, in direct line of sight of the surgeon and the first assistant. Other laparoscopic essentials such as the insufflator, light source, camera console, recording equipment, and electrocautery are located on a ceiling-mounted boom that is situated behind and to the left of the first assistant. A suction unit is placed just below the boom. An ultrasonic scalpel and bipolar electrocautery unit is placed behind the second assistant.

A 1.5-cm vertical incision is made in the midline about 2.5 cm above the umbilicus; this incision will later be incorporated into the midline incision for the open bowel work. A 2-mm Miniport (Autosuture, Norwalk, CT) is inserted into the abdomen through this incision and $CO_2$ pneumoperitoneum is created to 15 mm Hg. We prefer to use a 2-mm Miniport to obtain initial access rather than a Veress needle, as it allows a higher gas flow rate and occasional direct inspection of the peritoneal cavity with a 2-mm laparoscope in case of doubt.

A 12-mm primary port is placed through the supraumbilical incision, and a 10-mm 0-degree laparoscope is introduced. Four secondary ports are inserted under vision. A 12-mm right upper port is placed at the previously marked stoma site and is inserted through the belly of the right rectus muscle, carefully avoiding the right inferior epigastric vessels under clear visualization. For ileal conduit diversion, the stoma will be constructed at this site during the "open" part of the operation. Three other secondary ports are placed: a 5-mm left upper port at the lateral edge of the left rectus muscle just below the level of the umbilicus, and a 5-mm port placed 2.5 cm medial and cephalad to each anterior superior iliac spine.

The surgeon typically uses the right-hand 12-mm port and the left pararectal 5-mm port. The first assistant drives the camera through the midline 12-mm port and simultaneously uses the 5-mm right lateral port for suction and/or retraction.

If a patient has had previous abdominal surgery, we prefer initial access through the spatially most distant quadrant, often the left upper quadrant, as most patients with previous surgery have scars either in the midline or in the right half of the abdomen.

Upon initial inspection the surgeon must identify five important landmarks:

1. The medial umbilical ligaments
2. The peritoneal folds overlying the ureters close to the bladder
3. The vasa on each side
4. The posterior cul-de-sac of the rectovesical pouch
5. The iliac vessels

These allow precise orientation during the procedure and expeditious dissection.

## Mobilization and Division of the Ureters

We first identify the peristaltic right ureter as it crosses the iliac vessels at the pelvic brim. Using J-hook electrocautery, the peritoneum is incised along the anterior aspect of the ureter and dissected linearly and distally to the visible peritoneal fold overlying the ureter as it enters the bladder. When circumferentially mobilizing the ureter from the pelvic brim down to the vesicoureteric junction, it is important to maintain an adequate cover of periureteric fatty tissue. Close to the vesicoureteric junction, the superior vesical artery and the vas deferens are visualized crossing the ureter. These are mobilized away from the ureteric surface to obtain maximum ureteric length and do not routinely need division at this point. If antegrade ureteric dissection proves difficult, the peritoneum of the ureteric fold can be incised closer to the bladder and the incision continued in a cephalad direction up to the pelvic brim.

The right ureter is clipped with Hem-O-Lok clips at the vesicoureteric junction and divided such that there are two clips on the bladder side and one on the distal ureter. The two clips on the bladder side of the transected ureter serve as critical landmarks during the subsequent dissection, as they provide a readily identifiable visual clue during transection of the lateral pedicles. The single clip on the cut end of the proximal ureter allows its hydrodistention, which facilitates later ureteroenteric anastomosis. A terminal ureteric biopsy is sent for frozen section analysis. The left ureter is mobilized similarly. Some patients have significant sigmoid adhesions, which might require lysis to allow identification of the left ureter.

## Retrovesical Dissection

The retrovesical space is now dissected. To achieve this, it is essential to tautly retract the sigmoid colon proximally out of the pelvis to facilitate visualization of the cul-de-sac. We use a 2-0 polypropylene suture on a straight Keith needle inserted into the abdomen directly through the skin in the left hypochondrium. This suture is anchored through two selected appendices epiploicae of the most prominent part of the sigmoid colon and brought back out through the abdominal wall in the left hypochondrium, where it is held taut with a hemostat. This simple maneuver efficiently and tautly retracts the sigmoid colon out of the pelvis, obviates the need for an assistant to do so, and provides an excellent view of the operative field.

The ureters have already been mobilized and transected, and the lateral peritoneum of the rectovesical pouch is already divided. The two lateral peritoneotomies are now joined across the midline. It is important that the peritoneotomy across the cul-de-sac be created quite distally, such that it is only 1 to 2 cm anterior to the surface of the rectum. Often there is a subtle transverse peritoneal fold at this location (we refer to it as the "second peritoneal fold"). This plane is now developed between the vasa and seminal vesicles anteriorly, and the anterior surface of the rectum posteriorly. The vessels supplying the seminal vesicles are controlled, and bilateral vasa and vesicles are maintained en bloc with the bladder. Continued dissection brings the posterior layer of the

Denonvilliers fascia into view, which is incised with cold Endo-shears to reveal the yellow prerectal fat posterior to the prostate. This is an important landmark guiding the posterior dissection, the plane of which must remain between the prostate anteriorly and the prerectal fat posteriorly to minimize chances of rectal injury.

### Lateral Dissection and Control of Vascular Pedicles

The parietal peritoneum lateral to the medial umbilical ligaments is incised from the vas deferens as it crosses the pelvic brim toward the peritoneotomy across the rectovesical cul-de-sac. The vasa are clipped and divided at the pelvic brim. The space between the bladder and the lateral pelvic wall is now developed bluntly, retracting the bladder medially away from the iliac vessels and the obturator nerve. As the bladder is still anteriorly attached to the abdominal wall, this allows the lateral pedicles to be clearly identified bilaterally. The lateral pedicles are now divided with a laparoscopic stapler. Once again, the two clips on the bladder end of the transected juxtavesical ureters serve as critical landmarks for the anteromedial limit of resection; the laparoscopic stapler is deployed just posterolateral to these clips. Usually two or three cartridge firings are necessary on each side to control the entire width of the lateral pedicles down to the endopelvic fascia on either side.

The posterior pedicles are now visualized coursing from just lateral to the rectum toward the urinary bladder (Fig. 133.1). These are controlled with the stapler or divided between sequentially applied Hem-O-Lok clips. Usually only the cephalad part of the posterior pedicles can be controlled at this stage; their caudal aspect is addressed after releasing the bladder from the anterior abdominal wall and completing the anterior dissection. At this point the dissection is close to the anterolateral surface of the rectum. An assistant's finger in the rectum can provide guidance in avoiding rectal injury.

### Anterior Dissection

A liberal inverted-U incision is made with the J-hook electrocautery, starting lateral to each medial umbilical ligament, with the limbs of the U joined anteriorly across the midline at the umbilicus. The urachus and medial umbilical ligaments are divided just caudal to the umbilicus. The bladder is released from the anterior abdominal wall; care is taken to protect the inferior epigastric vessels as they course up from the external iliac vessels to enter the posterior rectus sheath.

The space of Retzius is developed behind the pubic bone. Areolar tissue is dissected away to expose the anterior surface of the prostate and the endopelvic fascia on each side. The endopelvic fascia is incised down to the region of the dorsal venous complex. The superficial dorsal vein is coagulated and divided with the bipolar forceps. Fat overlying the anterior surface of the prostate is cleared off with the bipolar forceps. The puboprostatic ligaments are divided with cold Endo-shears.

### Transection of Dorsal Vein Complex and Membranous Urethra, Specimen Entrapment

The dorsal venous complex (DVC) is now transected with a laparoscopic stapler. Often an additional suture of 2-0 polyglactin on a CT-1 needle is necessary to secure complete hemostasis of the DVC. The membranous urethra is transected with cold Endo-shears, the catheter is removed, and the urethra at the prostate apex is immediately occluded with a 2-0 polyglactin suture on a CT-1 needle to prevent local spillage of urine. The remaining posterior pedicles are clipped and divided. The remaining posterior attachments of the prostate apex are divided and the freed specimen is entrapped in an Endocatch II bag. The mouth of the bag is transiently retrieved outside a port site, double-ligated to prevent any spillage, and returned into the abdomen.

### Modifications for Cystectomy in Women

Once the ureters are clipped and divided, the uterus is anteverted by the RUMI uterine manipulator (Cooper Surgical, Trumbull, CT) and the sigmoid is retracted as described above (Figs. 133.2 and 133.3). The infundibulopelvic ligaments are transected with a laparoscopic stapler. With the uterus still anteverted and the adnexa retracted anteriorly, the peritoneum over the apex of the posterior fornix is scored transversely with the laparoscopic J-hook. The cervical cup aids in identifying the posterior fornix. The remaining posterior dissection and the vaginal incision are made after preparing the DVC.

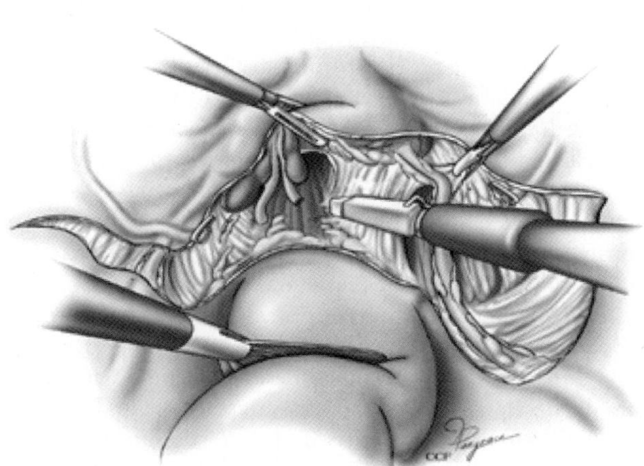

FIGURE 133.1 Stapling of the bladder pedicles.

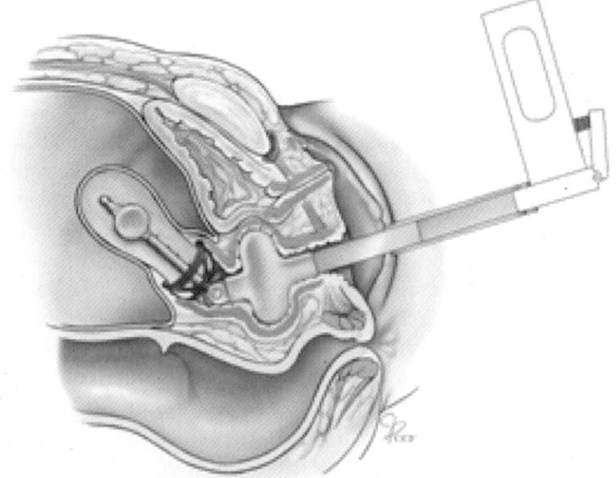

FIGURE 133.2 Modification for cystectomy in the female patient.

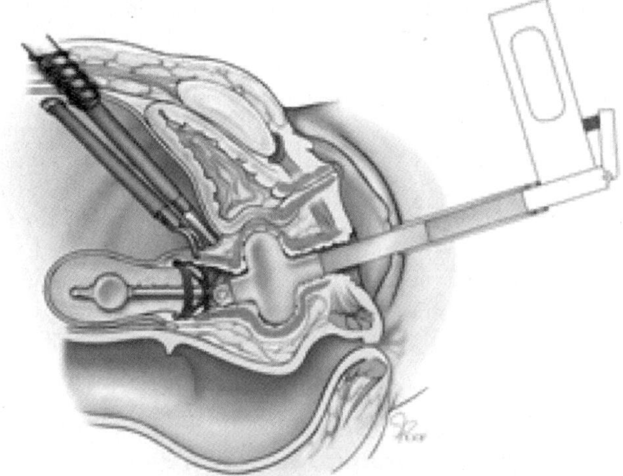

FIGURE 133.3 Modification for cystectomy in the female.

The lateral pedicles are transected with laparoscopic staplers and the bladder is dropped in the usual fashion. The DVC is suture-ligated with a 2-0 polyglactin suture on a CT-1 needle.

Attention is now returned to the posterior dissection. With the uterus anteverted, a transverse incision of the posterior vaginal fornix is completed at the previously scored site. The vaginal incision is extended distally on either side of the urethra, excising a narrow central strip of vagina en bloc with the bladder specimen.

Using a perineal approach, the external meatus and distal urethra are circumferentially cored out using electrocautery. After removing the RUMI manipulator, the distal urethra and an underlying strip of anterior vaginal wall are dissected free by the transvaginal approach. The specimen is delivered en bloc through the vagina. The vagina is reconstructed by combined perineal and laparoscopic suturing before proceeding with urinary diversion (7).

## Modifications for Nerve-Sparing Cystectomy in Men

Once the ureters are divided and posterior dissection commences, care is taken to stay closely along the surface of the seminal vesicles, as the neurovascular bundles run lateral to the apical tip of the vesicles distally toward the prostatovesicular junction. Thermal energy is avoided in the vicinity of the bundles. The plane of dissection is closer to the bladder and further from the rectum. The bundle on either side is dissected away with cold Endo-shears, and hemostasis is secured with Hem-O-Lok clips. This is in contrast to the non–nerve-sparing technique, in which a laparoscopic stapler is used for en masse transection of the lateral pedicle more posterolaterally, closer to the rectum, and at a considerable distance from the bladder. During the anterior dissection, the endopelvic fascia is maintained intact, and the lateral pelvic fascia is incised high on the prostate to drop the bundles posteriorly. The DVC is divided with a laparoscopic stapler, exposing the membranous urethra. The bundles on either side are released from the prostate apex using cold Endo-shears, and the urethra is divided. The remainder of the operation proceeds in the usual fashion. Intraoperative real-time transrectal ultrasound guidance is of help during nerve-sparing cystectomy, as it can confirm the location of and blood flow in the neurovascular bundles during and after the procedure (8).

## Modifications for Reproductive Organ–Sparing Cystectomy in Women

In carefully selected, sexually active young women with low-grade organ-confined disease, a more limited approach can be used. Precise dissection of the bladder away from the uterus and vagina is critically important. The uterus is retroverted, the bladder is identified, and the peritoneum on the anterior surface of the uterus is incised transversely using a J-hook. With the bladder now retracted anteriorly, dissection is performed along and close to the anterior surface of the uterus, developing this avascular plane. Typically dissection proceeds smoothly until the cervix is reached, where adhesions are often dense. At this point extreme care is taken not to thin the vaginal wall or the bladder. This dissection is carried distally down to the bladder neck, which is the end point of posterior dissection. Anterior dissection is now performed and the lateral pedicles are divided with a stapler. The urethra is prepared in the usual fashion. As the vagina is not opened, the specimen is entrapped in an Endocatch II bag.

## Extended and High-Extended Lymphadenectomy

We perform pelvic lymph node dissection after the LRC. The lateral limit of the dissection is the genitofemoral nerve and the medial limit is the obturator nerve. The distal limit is the inguinal ligament and the proximal limit is the aortic bifurcation. The technique mimics the "split-and-roll" technique used during open surgery. Right lymphadenectomy is performed first. The fibroareolar tissue lateral to the genitofemoral nerve is divided, exposing the iliopsoas muscle. The tissue packet is dissected en bloc off the surface of the iliopsoas muscle and swept medially, dissecting behind the iliac vessels down to the obturator nerve. Tissue anterior to the external iliac artery and vein is then individually split longitudinally using the J-hook, skeletonizing the vessels circumferentially. The external iliac vein typically appears flat at standard pneumoperitoneum pressures. Occasionally, pneumoperitoneum pressure might need to be decreased to 5 mm Hg to facilitate identification of the external iliac vein.

Cephalad dissection along the common iliac artery is facilitated by the fact that the transected ureter has already been mobilized away during the LRC procedure. The circumferentially mobilized common iliac artery is retracted with a vessel loop to retrieve the posterior fibrofatty lymphatic tissue distal to the aortic bifurcation. The internal iliac artery is carefully mobilized, taking care to avoid injury to the internal iliac vein. The released tissue packet is rolled medially posterior to the mobilized iliac vessels, delivering it into the pelvis. Dissection along the medial aspect of the packet separates it from the previously identified obturator nerve. Distally, the tissue packet is clipped and transected at the inguinal ligament (Fig. 133.4).

More recently, we have performed a high-extended pelvic lymph node dissection by dissecting the anterior surface of the aorta and vena cava up to the inferior mesenteric artery; the para-aortic, preaortic, interaortocaval, precaval, and pericaval lymphatic fatty tissue is excised. The aortic bifurcation and the presacral area are also dissected.

Care must be taken to avoid cutting into any enlarged lymph nodes to minimize the risk of tumor spillage. The

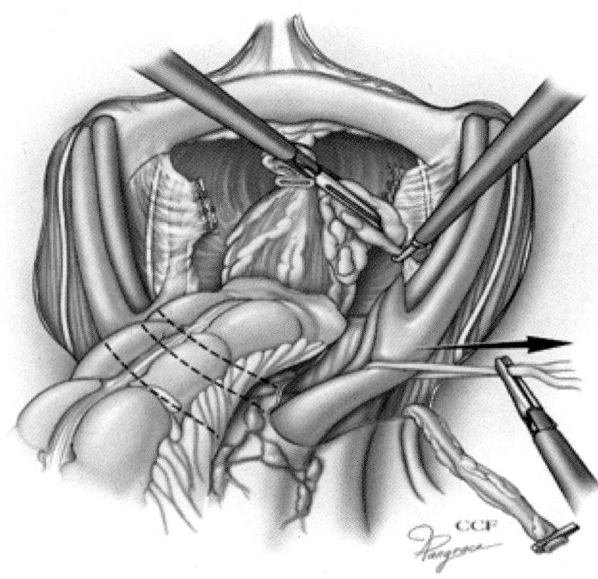

FIGURE 133.4 Extended node dissection.

lymphadenectomy specimen is immediately entrapped in an Endocatch bag, avoiding contact with adjacent tissues. Lymphadenectomy is then performed on the left side in similar fashion (9).

## Urinary Diversion

As mentioned previously, our current preference is to perform this part of the procedure through a 6- to 8-cm midline incision. The three specimens (bladder and two lymphadenectomy specimens) in their separate bags are removed through this incision. The pelvis is carefully inspected to confirm good hemostasis. An ileal conduit or ileal neobladder is fashioned in the usual manner, essentially at or near skin level.

If an ileal conduit is made, the stoma is fashioned at the site of the right-sided 12-mm port. This port site is further expanded and a stoma is fashioned in the usual manner. A 10-mm Jackson–Pratt drain is placed in the pelvis and a 24Fr Foley catheter is placed in the pelvis through the urethra. The balloon of this catheter is inflated to 50 mL and placed on traction for 24 to 48 hours. The abdominal incision is then closed in layers using looped polydioxanone sutures for the fascial layer and 4-0 subcuticular polyglactin for the skin. The 5-mm port sites are closed with 4-0 subcuticular polyglactin.

For the ileal neobladder, the pouch is completed and closed, and the most dependant aspect is defined and a small enterotomy made. This site is tagged with a polyglactin suture and later used for the urethral anastomosis. The ureteric stents and suprapubic tube are brought through separate openings in the anterior wall of the pouch and secured with chromic gut pursestring sutures. The pouch is irrigated to confirm watertight integrity. It is then dropped into the pelvis, one port is reinserted under direct vision, and the abdominal wall is closed in layers as described above. The pneumoperitoneum is then re-established and the other laparoscopic ports are reinserted. The urethroneovesical anastomosis is completed laparoscopically using a running preknotted double-arm suture of 2-0 poliglecaprone 25 and 2-0 polyglytone 6211 on a UR-6 needle over a 22Fr Foley catheter, akin to the technique used for urethrovesical anastomosis during laparoscopic radical prostatectomy. Two 10-mm Jackson–Pratt drains are placed in the pelvis through the left and right lateral 5-mm port sites. The ureteric stents are brought out through the left pararectal 5-mm port site. The suprapubic tube draining the pouch is brought out through the right 12-mm port site. The abdominal cavity is extensively irrigated before closure, and this can be done efficiently using this combined approach.

## Pure Laparoscopic Ileal Conduit and Orthotopic Neobladder

The technique for the pure laparoscopic ileal conduit replicates the open procedure with a few minor modifications (6). A 15-cm segment of ileum is isolated using two applications of an Endo-GIA stapler, and the mesentery is also divided with this stapler. The isolated segment is dropped posteriorly. Ileoileal continuity is restored intracorporeally using an application of the Endo-GIA stapler, followed by another application of the Endo-GIA stapler to close the defect. The proximal end of the conduit is imbricated using a running absorbable suture and the mesenteric window is closed with interrupted suture. The stoma is then fashioned, allowing the conduit to be stretched by gravity, thereby improving exposure of the proximal end in preparation for anastomotic suturing. The left ureter has been brought through a mesenteric defect to the right side of the retroperitoneum. The distal ends of the ureters are spatulated and two separate "Bricker" anastomoses are performed using interrupted sutures.

Briefly, 55 to 65 cm of ileum is isolated and ileoileal continuity is restored intracorporeally as described above. The excluded segment is irrigated and detubularized along its antimesenteric border, keeping the proximal 10 cm intact as an isoperistaltic afferent limb. The posterior neobladder plate is created by continuous intracorporeal suturing and the apex of the posterior neobladder plate is circumferentially sutured to the posterior urethra to complete the urethroileal anastomosis. The anterior neobladder wall is then closed and a 22Fr Foley catheter is placed. Finally, the ureters are implanted into the afferent segment using a technique identical to that for the ileal conduit anastomoses (Fig. 133.5).

## Postoperative Care

The neobladder is gently irrigated with 50 mL of saline every 4 hours to prevent mucous plugging of the catheters. Intravenous fluids and antibiotics are continued until bowel function is regained. Diet is gradually advanced and antibiotics are switched to the oral route. The ileoureteric stents are removed in 1 week after a negative intravenous urogram. The Jackson–Pratt drains are removed sequentially, as per the decrease in their output. The urethral Foley catheter and suprapubic catheter are removed at 10 to 12 days after a normal cystogram.

## Outcomes

In the past consecutive 50 LRC procedures (38 men, 12 women) with a urinary diversion performed extracorporeally through a 5- to 6-cm minilaparotomy at our center, the mean operative time was 6.3 hours and mean blood loss was 363 mL. Twelve percent of patients required blood transfusion, time for first oral intake was 3.4 days, and time to ambulation was 3.0 days (Table 133.1).

This group was compared to a contemporary cohort of 50 open radical cystectomy procedures (34 men, 16 women)

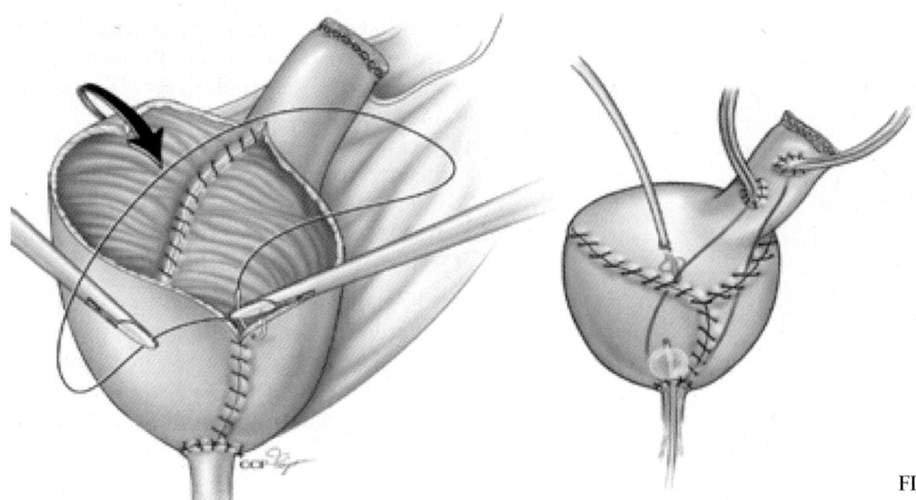

FIGURE 133.5 Pure laparoscopic orthotropic neobladder.

with urinary diversion. There were no significant differences between the groups with respect to mean patient age (66 versus 67; $p = 0.61$), Body Mass Index (27 versus 26; $p = 0.50$), comorbidities, history of prior abdominal surgery and operative indications. Tumor was organ-confined (≤ pT2N0), non–organ-confined (pT3-4N0), and lymph node positive (pTanyN+) in 66%, 28%, and 6% of the LRC patients and 62%, 20%, and 18% of the open surgery patients, respectively, with no significant differences between the groups ($p = 0.15$) (see Table 133.1) (10,11).

## PARTIAL CYSTECTOMY, URACHAL EXCISION

The urachus is a vestigial fibrous cord derived from involution of the allantois that extends from the bladder apex to the umbilicus and forms the median umbilical ligament. Urachal remnant is a rare congenital anomaly, with an incidence of 2:300,000 in infants and 1:5,000 in adults. Traditional surgical management of benign urachal disease involves the radical excision of all anomalous tissue with or without a cuff of bladder tissue via the open approach (12). Urachal carcinoma accounts for <0.5% to 2% of all bladder tumors and approximately 40% of vesical adenocarcinomas.

Patients with resectable tumors traditionally underwent en bloc cystoprostatectomy and wide excision of the urachus and umbilicus. Extended partial cystectomy and umbilectomy provide survival rates comparable to those of radical cystectomy (13). The surgical approach has leaned more toward bladder sparing because published reports have not shown an advantage compared to radical surgery (14).

### Surgical Techniques

#### Urachal Adenocarcinoma

Patient preparation, positioning, and port placement are similar to those previously described for LRC. The only variation is the placement of the camera port 3 cm above the umbilicus.

The peritoneal and preperitoneal tissue between the medial umbilical ligaments is dissected free of the transversalis fascia. The dissection must include an extensive resection of the peritoneum lateral to the two medial umbilical ligaments, which defined the lateral limits, the posterior sheath of the rectus muscle of the abdomen to the arcuate line and the muscle

**TABLE 133.1**

**CLEVELAND CLINIC EXPERIENCE WITH LAPAROSCOPIC RADICAL CYSTECTOMY**

| | Laparoscopic radical cystectomy | Open radical cystectomy | $p$ |
|---|---|---|---|
| Operative time (hr) | 6.3 ± 0.26 | 5.3 ± 0.28 | 0.01 |
| Blood loss (cc) | 363 ± 259 | 801 ± 684 | 0.0004 |
| Transfusion | 12% | 40% | 0.001 |
| Ileus | 18% | 28% | 0.21 |
| Oral intake (days) | 3.4 ± 1.1 | 4.2 ± 2.1 | 0.05 |
| Minor postop complications | 18% | 22% | 0.62 |
| Major postop complications | 8% | 6% | 0.69 |
| Ambulation (days) | 3.0 ± 1.6 | 3.4 ± 3.3 | 0.63 |
| Hospital stay (days) | 8.0 ± 3.2 | 8.7 ± 2.9 | 0.27 |
| Lymph nodes on final pathology ($n$) | 14.8 ± 7.0 | 15.8 ± 7.1 | 0.58 |
| Positive surgical margins | 2% | 6% | 0.29 |

fibers of the rectus muscle below it, the extraperitoneal fat in the space of Retzius as the anterior limit, the urachus up to the umbilicus superiorly, sparing the umbilical skin.

The bladder is distended with 200 mL normal saline to facilitate the mobilization and dissection. The junction of the solid tumor with the bladder is determined on the anterior aspect by inflating and deflating the bladder, and a cystotomy is made. The excision of the bladder dome is performed with a 2-cm margin of normal mucosa. The specimen is enclosed within the Endocatch bag and placed in the right iliac fossa. The bladder is closed in two layers using absorbable sutures.

Bilateral extended pelvic lymphadenectomy is performed as described in the laparoscopic cystectomy section. The three specimens (the resected tumor and two lymphadenectomy specimens) are removed in separate bags through the supraumbilical port.

### Urachal Remnants

The patient is placed in a supine position and a Foley catheter is inserted in the bladder. Three trocars are generally used: the 12-mm camera port is placed in the midline above the umbilicus and two trocars (5 and 12 mm) are placed on either side, lateral to the rectus muscle. There are several other possible trocar placements as well (15).

The medial umbilical ligaments are clipped and divided. The peritoneal and preperitoneal tissue between the medial umbilical ligaments is dissected free of the transversalis fascia. Dissection is carried along the preperitoneal plane toward the umbilicus, surrounding the cyst. The cephalic side of the lesion is ligated at the umbilicus and divided. The umbilicus is usually not excised. The bladder is filled via the urethral catheter and the cuff is removed. The specimen is placed in a laparoscopic bag and removed by the 12-mm port site. The bladder defect is closed with laparoscopic suturing using 4-0 and 3-0 suture.

## BLADDER DIVERTICULECTOMY

A bladder diverticulum is a herniation of the bladder mucosa as a result of bladder outlet obstruction. The surgical treatment of benign prostatic hyperplasia associated with a symptomatic bladder diverticulum classically consists of diverticular ablation by open surgery and relief of the prostatic obstacle (16). An endolaparoscopic approach combining laparoscopic diverticulectomy with transurethral resection of the prostate (TURP) is statistically superior to open surgery in terms of blood loss, postoperative hospital stay, and analgesic requirement.

### Surgical Technique

The patient is first placed in the lithotomy position and a standard TURP is performed with meticulous hemostasis. A holmium laser TURP is preferred because of its hemostatic properties. A ureteral catheter is inserted if the diverticulum is close to the ureter. A 10Fr Foley catheter is placed in the diverticulum and the balloon is inflated with 20 to 25 mL normal saline. The neck of the diverticulum is occluded with a gentle traction. Another 14Fr irrigation catheter is placed in the bladder. The patient is moved into the supine position with 15-degree Trendelenburg. A 10-mm supraumbilical midline incision is made for the camera port. An extraperitoneal space is created by using an atraumatic laparoscopic balloon. The preperitoneal space is inflated up to 12 mm Hg. Two 5-mm working ports are inserted in both iliac fossae and a 12-mm port is placed in the suprapubic area. The bladder is mobilized anterolaterally, and the diverticulum is identified after inflating it selectively with normal saline through a Foley catheter. The diverticulum is then circumferentially dissected until its neck is identified. Sharp transection of the diverticulum directly at its neck is performed over the Foley catheter. The neck is then closed in two layers with 3-0 absorbable running sutures, and a watertightness test is performed with bladder irrigation. The resected diverticulum is removed through the 10-mm port. A 14Fr suction catheter is placed in the perivesical space through the 5-mm port.

The laparoscopic procedure can also be carried out via a transperitoneal approach. The drain is removed postoperatively after 48 hours of dryness. The bladder catheter is removed on the 10th postoperative day after confirmation of watertight healing with a negative cystogram.

## *References*


1. Dalbagni G, Genega E, Hashibe M, et al. Cystectomy for bladder cancer: a contemporary series. *J Urol* 2001;165:1111–1116.
2. Stein JP, Lieskovsky G, Cote R, et al. Radical cystectomy in the treatment of invasive bladder cancer: long-term results in 1,054 patients. *J Clin Oncol* 2001;19:666–675.
3. Haber GP, Gill IS, Rozet F, et al. International registry of laparoscopic radical cystectomy: first report on 392 patients. *J Urol* 2006;175(Supp.):394.
4. Basillote JB, Abdelshehid C, Ahlering TE, et al. Laparoscopic assisted radical cystectomy with ileal neobladder: a comparison with the open approach. *J Urol* 2004;172:489–493.
5. Fergany AF, Gill IS, Kaouk JH, et al. Laparoscopic intracorporeally constructed ileal conduit after porcine cystoprostatectomy. *J Urol* 2001;166: 285–288.
6. Haber GP, Campbell SC, Colombo JR Jr, et al. Perioperative outcomes with laparoscopic radical cystectomy: "pure laparoscopic" and "open-assisted laparoscopic" approaches. *Urology* 200770(5):910–915.
7. Kaouk JH, Gill IS, Desai MM, et al. Laparoscopic orthotopic ileal neobladder. *J Endourol* 2001;15:131–142.
8. Moinzadeh A, Gill IS, Desai M, et al. Laparoscopic radical cystectomy in the female. *J Urol* 2005;173(6):1912–1917.
9. Lane BR, Finelli A, Moinzadeh A, et al. Nerve-sparing laparoscopic radical cystectomy: technique and initial outcomes. *Urology* 2006;68(4): 778–783.
10. Finelli A, Gill IS, Desai MM, et al. Laparoscopic extended pelvic lymphadenectomy for bladder cancer: technique and initial outcomes. *J Urol* 2004;172(5, Pt 1):1809–1812.
11. Haber GP, Gill IS. Laparoscopic radical cystectomy for cancer: oncological outcomes at up to 5 years. *BJU Int* 2007;100(1):137–142.
12. Berman SM, Tolia BM, Laor E, et al. Urachal remnants in adults. *Urology* 1988;31:17–21.
13. Weiss RE, Fair WR. Urachal anomalies and urachal carcinoma. *AUA Update Series* 1998;17:298–303.
14. Ashley RA, Inman BA, Sebo TJ, et al. Urachal carcinoma: clinicopathologic features and long-term outcomes of an aggressive malignancy. *Cancer* 2006;107:712–720.
15. Okegawa T, Odagane A, Nutahara K, et al. Laparoscopic management of urachal remnants in adulthood. *Int J Urol* 2006;13(12):1466–1469.
16. Champault G, Riskalla H, Rizk N, et al. Laparoscopic resection of a bladder diverticulum. *Prog Urol* 1997;7:643–646.

# CHAPTER 134 ■ LAPAROSCOPIC BLADDER NECK SUSPENSION

RICHARD W. GRAHAM

The first modern advance in the surgical treatment of female urinary incontinence was described by Dr. Victor Marshall along with his colleagues Drs. Marchetti and Krantz (1). The Marshall-Marchetti-Kranz procedure was based on the concept that the loss of the angle of bladder neck juncture combined with the bladder neck protruding through the pelvic floor muscles was the cause of stress urinary incontinence (SUI). His idea was to place stitches next to the bladder neck and sew these stitches to the periosteum. This would elevate the bladder neck and might provide a permanent solution for the incontinence from the scar formation. The initial results were excellent, though complications included osteitis pubis and some patients with permanent retention. Most of Dr. Marshall's patients did not void for weeks; he often stated that if the patient voided before 6 weeks that the procedure would not last (private communication). Subsequent procedures and modifications have been tried, none with perfect results.

In the early 1990s we started to investigate laparoscopic surgery as a minimally invasive technique in urology. The initial strategy was to copy open techniques, improving them by using higher magnification with more light and $CO_2$ insufflation to lift the abdominal wall and compress the bowel at the same time.

Our initial experience was very encouraging, and later experience of over 600 cases seems to echo this success (2). In a head-to-head trial with open sling procedures at our institution, the laparoscopic procedure showed superior outcomes and fewer adverse outcomes.

## DIAGNOSIS

The evaluation and selection of patients for any type of treatment for stress urinary incontinence is key to the outcome. The group of patients we want to focus on are the female patients with hypermobility of the bladder neck who have good sphincter control.

The patient's history is one of the most important parts of the preoperative and diagnostic evaluation, which should assess the duration of the problem, time of onset, and cofactors such as whether the problem occurred after pregnancy or at the beginning of menopausal symptoms. In the latter group medical management is usually tried first, and watchful waiting may be appropriate. Other important factors include whether the woman is sexually active, whether the incontinence is mixed, how many pads she is wearing, what induces the leakage, and whether there are signs of intrinsic sphincter deficiency. In considering surgery, it is important to know if there are other pelvic problems associated with the incontinence (cystocele, rectocele, other forms of vaginal prolapse) and whether the patient is obese or has other risk factors for surgery, including chronic bronchitis, prior radiation, extensive varicose veins (we have seen large venous plexi in the space of Retzius), neurologic issues, or diabetes.

The physical examination should be detailed. Often associated with SUI are vaginal defect issues that need to be repaired at the time of surgery. Is there good estrogenation of the vagina and perivaginal areas? What is the status of her uterus? We perform the Marshall test. (We have patients cough with a full bladder and then watch their urinary leakage. Next we apply digital pressure to the periurethral tissue to watch the leakage stop; if it does not, then we re-evaluate the situation.) We check the rectal tone as well.

Cystoscopy is performed in all patients to assess the urethra and bladder. It is important to note urethral length and angulation of the bladder, urethra, and possible cystocele. (We have noted that releasing the veins at the midline of the bladder neck may increase the length of the urethra by a small portion without a laparoscopic bladder neck suspension [LBNS], as Dr. Marshall noted in his experience with open procedures.) Additionally, the estrogenation of the urethra provides us clues to proper treatment. The cotton-tipped swab test may be of some benefit here as well.

Finally, we feel that urodynamics can be a major help in ascertaining the patient's overall incontinence picture and profile. Her leak point pressures, volume capacity, and other measures help guide our decisions to her care. Videourodynamics are now part of our evaluation as well in helping determine the three-dimensional anatomy and function of the patient.

## INDICATIONS FOR SURGERY

The indication for surgery for us is based on a paradigm of clinical evaluations and is based on what we feel will work best for the individual. We like to begin with medical therapy. We start with local estradiol therapy if the patient can tolerate it and there are no contraindications. Our experience has shown us that a poorly estrogenized patient can have excellent responses to the cream alone. We tend to limit the local treatment to <4 g a week (one fingertip of cream). Other noninvasive treatments will include biofeedback, begun a month after starting local estrogen. Failure to respond to noninvasive management in a patient with diagnosed SUI is the primary indication for surgery.

We have found that prior pelvic surgery may restrict the available space for suturing retropubically, so we may perform an LBNS using a ProTac (Tyco Healthcare Group, Norwalk,

CT) and polypropylene mesh system to achieve our goal of suspension as opposed to using permanent Gore-Tex (WL Gore and Associates, Flagstaff, AZ) sutures. If other procedures are necessary at the same time, and these are open procedures (total abdominal hysterectomy), then we will opt for open techniques, often using a ProTac and mesh again.

If the patient has morbid obesity, a previous kidney transplant, history of radiation, significant bronchitis, or requires vaginal surgery at the same time, we may decide to use a transobturator sling instead of an LBNS, as this patient may require more support. We have had fairly good experience with this procedure as well as with the TVT and feel most comfortable with this direction. We have seen two erosions with the TVT, and the chance of urinary retention or the need of later urethrolysis may be higher with a sling, but that is the balance we use (3).

## ALTERNATIVE THERAPY

There have been many operations described for SUI. The anterior colporrhaphy by H. A. Kelly was felt to be a significant achievement in its day for SUI and was subsequently improved upon by others. The initial success rate quoted of 92% was not able to be reproduced over time, and subsequent years showed a reduction in success rates. This seems to be the trend in many operations for the treatment of SUI.

Each technique has its own inherent advantages and disadvantages. There are many studies quoted as alternative surgical techniques with superior success rates, often with small numbers of patients with fewer than 5 years' experience (4). Many of the larger series of composite studies are with numerous surgeons at multiple institutions with variable skills and experience. So sorting out what is the best technique and alternatives can be a challenge in itself. The standard operations through the years have been primarily retropubic procedures with excellent results initially that tend to have a percentage of failing over time. Additionally, suburethral slings of variable materials seem to be mentioned throughout the literature at this time, first described by Goebel in 1910 using a piece of pyramidalis muscle. Now various ways of placement are being used, and the way these materials are now attached appears to be the latest trend.

Nonsurgical options include adult diapers, which are more popular worldwide than surgery. The cost is enormous, and the satisfaction with this alternative is dependent upon the user.

Biofeedback and behavioral modification have had great success in some series as well. One can never rule this approach out as a primary option in the patient's health care. It does require constant attention even after the initial therapy has been taught, as the muscles will atrophy if not stimulated and the problem will return (5). In a similar physical therapy realm, electrical stimulation of the nerves and muscles, both directly through vaginal devices and indirectly through nerve stimulation products, has been used with mixed results (6).

Sometimes the best alternative is the placement of a permanent Foley catheter to keep the bladder empty. There are a significant group of patients with macerated skin who are not candidates for corrective repairs of their condition, either because surgery won't help or for other reasons.

## SURGICAL TECHNIQUE

The patient is prepared and draped in the lithotomy position, arms by her side, with the vagina prepared as well. Needed materials are listed in Table 134.1. A 16Fr Foley catheter is placed in the bladder after the patient is draped, and 30 cc of water is placed in the balloon. The surgeon stands at the patient's side, on the left side if the surgeon is right-handed. A 1.0- to 1.5-cm incision is made lateral to the umbilicus. With a pair of Metzenbaum scissors, the fat is split down to the external oblique fascia. Using 1-cm "S" retractors, the fat is held back and the fascia grasped with a Kocher clamp, and a 1.0- to 1.5-cm cut is made in the external oblique fascia superior to the clamp. This cut is in a medial/lateral direction. Using a 0 Vicryl UR-6 needle, the stitch is placed on the inferior edge of the fascia and the clamp removed. Next the muscle fibers are split in a longitudinal direction and the "S" retractors placed deeper into the wound to hold back the muscle fibers. The posterior sheath is exposed. Next a Tyco/US Surgical PDB 1000 dissecting balloon is lubricated and placed into the space (Tyco Healthcare, Norwalk, CT). The balloon is gently slid to the posterior sheath, and the retractors are then removed.

Using a zero-degree 10-mm laparoscope inside the dissector, the apparatus is carefully slid into the space of Retzius (Fig. 134.1). One should see muscle above the balloon and fascia below. If bowel is seen, then the peritoneum has been violated and there is no need to expand the balloon. If all is intact, the balloon is slowly expanded with about 45 pumps with the hand pump (Fig. 134.2). The apparatus is removed after all the air in the balloon has been released.

Then a Tycos blunt port is placed into the wound (Fig. 134.3). The tip is gently placed such that it abuts the posterior fascia. Then 25 cc is placed in the balloon port and the foam cuff brought down to the skin. The retroperitoneal space is then

**TABLE 134.1**

**MATERIALS NEEDED FOR LAPAROSCOPIC BLADDER NECK SUSPENSION**

- 16Fr Foley catheter
- Two 1-cm "S" retractors
- One Kocher clamp
- Metzenbaum scissors
- One 0 Vicryl suture UR-6
- AutoSuture PDB 1000 dissecting balloon
- AutoSuture 10-mm blunt/balloon port
- AutoSuture ProTac 5 mm
- 5-mm laparoscopic port/10-mm laparoscopic port
- One dissector 5 mm
- Polypropylene fine woven mesh—need two pieces cut 1 cm by 10 cm
- 30 cc sterile water to fill balloon
- 4-0 Monocryl suture
- One ampule of Dermabond
- 5-mm clip applier on standby
- Suction irrigator on standby
- Preoperative antibiotics; we usually use Ancef
- Zero-degree 10-mm laparoscope

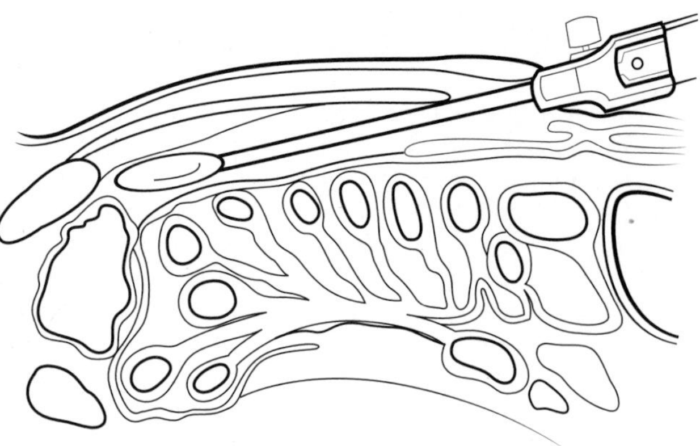

FIGURE 134.1 From the periumbilical incision, the balloon dissector is passed into the space of retzius over the posterior fascia.

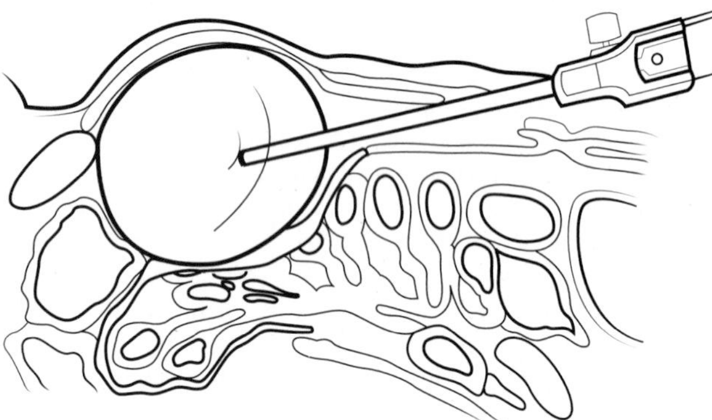

FIGURE 134.2 The balloon dissector is insuflated with the pump for 45 compressions in order to create the space for $CO_2$ infusion.

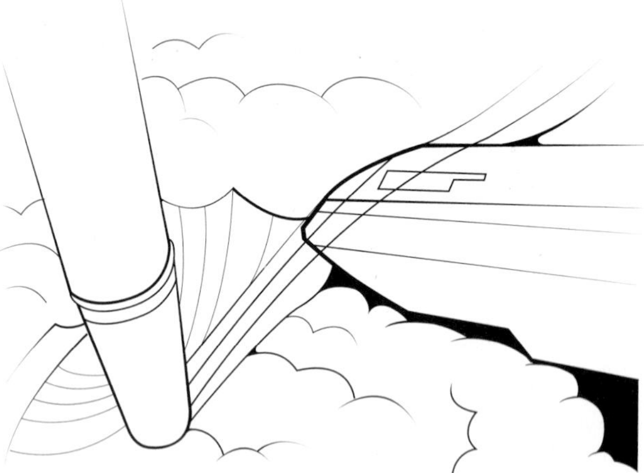

FIGURE 134.3 The blunt port is placed in the periumbilical incision, above the posterior fascia when the balloon dissector is removed. The space of Retzius is then insufflated to a pressure of 15 mmhg.

inflated with $CO_2$ to a pressure of 15 cm. The 10-mm scope is placed in the port. One uses the scope to follow the posterior fascia to the space of Retzius. Sometimes one needs to point the end of the scope up to go over the posterior sheath.

Once into the space, the surgeon looks for signs of bleeding, injuries, and so forth. If all is clear, a 5-mm port is placed below the pubic hair line, midline into the space of Retzius. Since the bladder has been decompressed, this should enter into the space easily. If there has been prior surgery, the port can be placed laterally to midline, being careful not to hit the subumbilical artery just below the lateral rectus muscle.

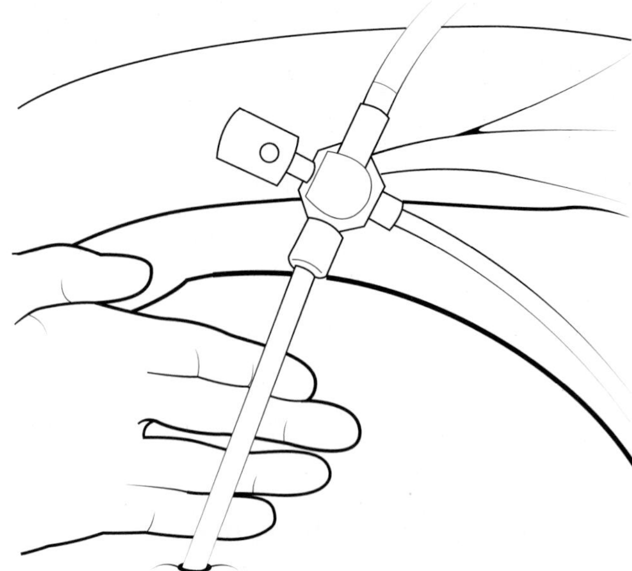

FIGURE 134.4 The clip applier is introduced to clip the vesssels above the anterior bladder neck. This allows some lengthening of the bladder neck once these vessels are cut, and helps to better identify the bladder neck urethral junction.

Using the surgeon's dissector of choice through the 5-mm port, the fat must be dissected off the bladder neck, the Cooper ligament, and the fascia lateral to the bladder neck. Once the fat has been removed, it is critical that the bladder neck be exposed. If there is a small vessel midline above the bladder neck extending from the anterior wall toward the bladder, it should be clipped with a small clip so the bladder neck is truly exposed (Fig. 134.4). With 30 cc in the balloon, one can see where the bladder neck joins the urethra.

The surgeon's left hand is placed into the vagina (right hand if the surgeon is left-handed), and the balloon is palpated. Under the scope one ought to be able to see the fascia lift up where the surgeon's finger is. Then using a piece of polypropylene fine woven mesh, a 10-cm by 1-cm strip is attached to a dissector (Fig. 134.5). The camera is removed and cleaned while the piece of mesh is gently placed down the camera port into the space of Retzius. Note: one has to aim somewhat anteriorly so as not to perforate the posterior fascia.

The camera is placed back in the trochar. A dissector is placed in the 5-mm port. The mesh is identified, and one end of the rectangular piece is laid down on the fascia lateral to the left bladder neck, where the surgeon's finger is waiting. The dissector is removed and a ProTac is placed in the 5-mm port. Five tacs are used to secure the mesh to the fascia (Fig. 134.6). The ProTac is removed and a dissector placed in the 5-mm port. The mesh is pulled toward the left Cooper ligament, the ProTac is reintroduced, and while the mesh is held under some tension the ProTac fires 5 tacs, attaching the mesh to the Cooper ligament. The procedure is repeated on the right side, such that there is a piece of mesh on either side of the bladder neck attached to the sides of the pelvis (Fig. 134.7).

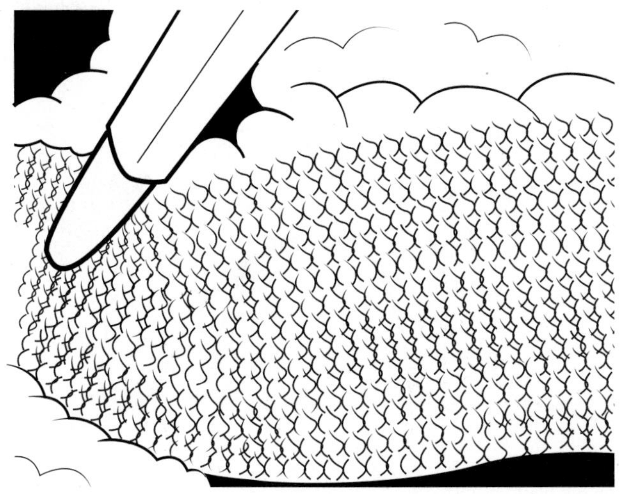

FIGURE 134.5 While the index finger is placed at the bladder neck, the pro tac is used to fire 5 tacs on top of the mesh toward the underlying finger engaging the periurethral fascia. Then the other end of the mesh is placed on Coopers ligament where 3 tacs are fired through the mesh into Cooper's ligament, securing the suspension.

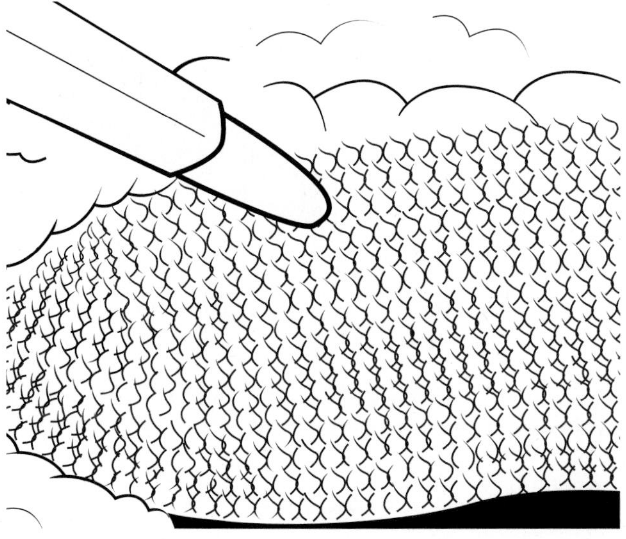

FIGURE 134.6 The mesh is then placed on Cooper's ligament and attached with 3–5 protacs.

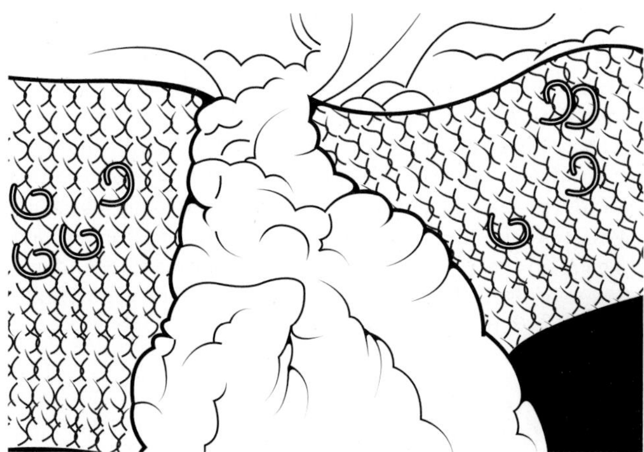

FIGURE 134.7 Here mesh has been attached on both sides with stabilization of bladder neck.

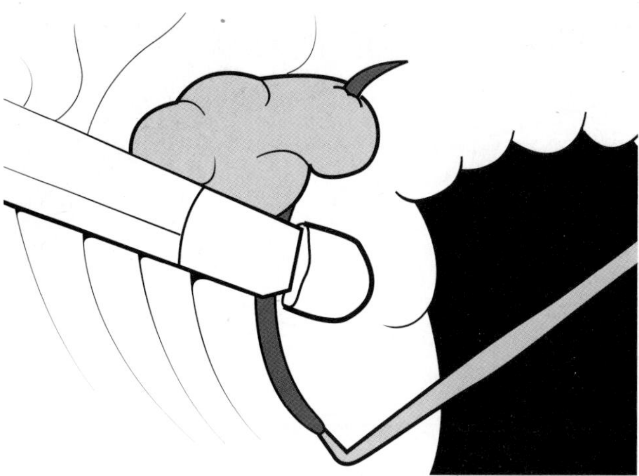

FIGURE 134.8 A bladder neck suspension here with Gortex suture being sewn into the periurethral fascia at the level of the bladder neck.

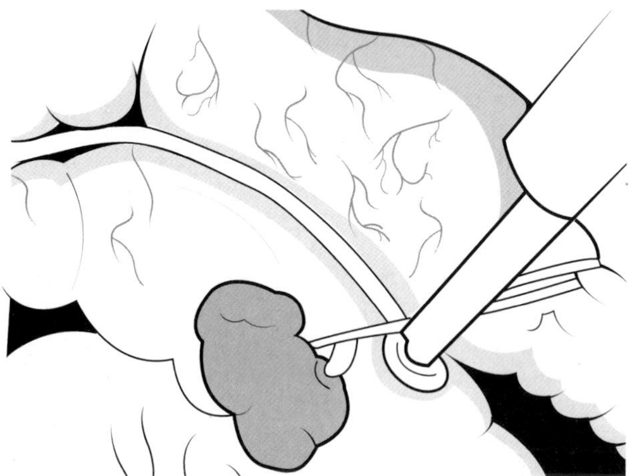

FIGURE 134.9 The gortex suture is first placed in the bladder neck then sewn to Cooper's ligament.

If there is no bleeding or any complications, the gas is emptied out of the pelvis after the 5-mm port is removed under direct vision. Next, the blunt port is removed after deflating its balloon. The fascia is closed with the 0 Vicryl and the wound infiltrated with 0.5% Marcaine without epinephrine. The skin edges are closed with 4-0 Monocryl, and Dermabond is placed over the two small incisions. The Foley balloon is deflated and then refilled with 5 cc of sterile water.

The alternative to using the ProTac system is to use Gore-Tex sutures (Figs. 134.8 and 134.9). Multiple sutures are placed in the same location as the tackers and mesh (Fig. 134.10). The advantage of the Gore-Tex suture is that there is no postneuralgia syndrome from the tacs (in over 600 procedures, we have had 4 cases in which we replaced the mesh and tacs with suture).

The patient is usually discharged the same day or 23 hours postoperatively. The Foley catheter is left in for 2 days. The patient is advised against vaginal intercourse or heavy lifting for 6 weeks.

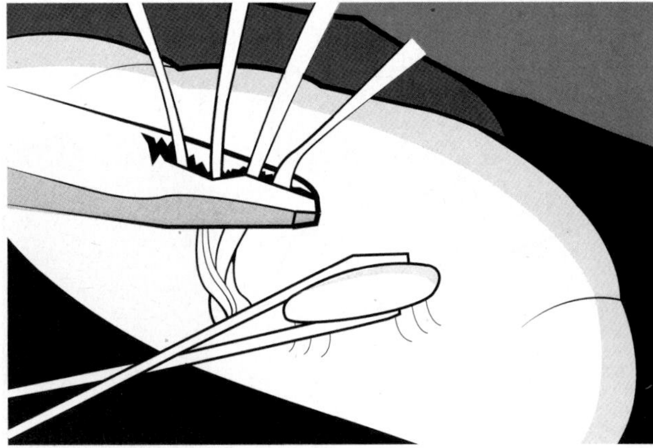

FIGURE 134.10 Usually multiple gortex sutures are used on both sides.

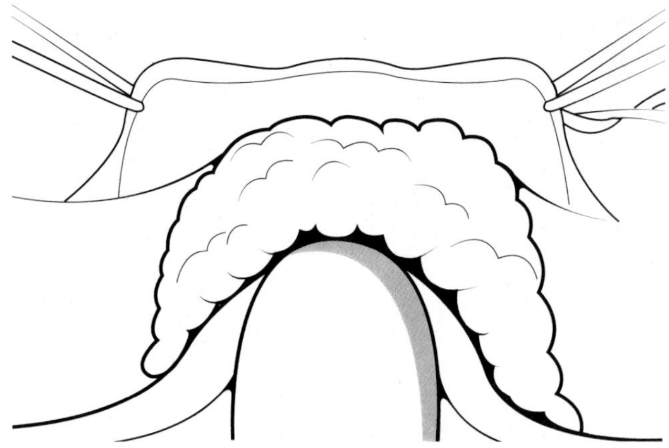

FIGURE 134.11 After the bladder neck is suspended, one can examine the bladder with a flexible cystoscope to inspect the work.

# OUTCOMES

## Complications

Intraoperative complications happen in a very small percentage of people in our experience and in other series (9). The most obvious would be bleeding from the dissection balloon, which has never been an issue for us.

Over 40% of our patients have had previous surgery in the area, and the bladder is encased in significant scar. Our experience is that sometimes the dome of the bladder is densely adhered to the symphysis pubica, and in the process of freeing up the bladder neck, the bladder can be opened. The key for repair of such an opening is to free up the entire area prior to repairing the hole. We place a 2-0 Vicryl suture at each lateral edge of the wound and alternate working the sutures to the middle. This is especially helpful when there is a lot of adipose tissue on the bladder as well. We leave the Foley catheter in for 5 days.

With this technique our experience has been that postoperative retention is rare (<1%). Our Foley catheters are left in for 48 hours to be sure that the patients do not have to return in the middle of the night with urinary retention. If the retention continues, we instruct the patient on intermittent catheterization till the problem resolves. Urethrolysis is a very rare occurrence, and in the few people we explored we found that the mesh was not attached to the sidewall at all. Interestingly, the scar reaction was around the bladder neck. The bladder neck was elevated and suspended by the scar itself (Fig. 134.11). So we lysed the scar, not the mesh.

We have had one erosion of the sidewall mesh into the bladder, which happened several years after the surgery. This was removed laparoscopically and the bladder closed without sequelae.

We expect that some of the patients will develop some urinary frequency, which usually resolves in a few weeks, though some may have prolonged overactivity and should be treated medically.

**TABLE 134.2**

**RESPONSE TO QUESTION "DO YOU LEAK WHEN YOU COUGH, LAUGH, OR SNEEZE?"**

| Follow-Up Interval | Laparoscopic Bladder Neck | Raz |
|---|---|---|
| 1 Month | 140/158 (89%) | 70/83 (84%) |
| 6 Months | 121/144 (84%) | 41/66 (62%) |
| 12 Months | 104/129 (81%) | 40/67 (60%) |
| 24 Months | 47/69 (68%) | 22/43 (51%) |
| 36 Months | 23/34 (68%) | 4/17 (24%) |
| 48 Months | 4/6 (67%) | 1/5 (20%) |

## Results

Our initial success rate for the surgery was 93% to 94% as assessed by patient questionnaires. Long-term follow-up (>2 to 4 years) shows stabilization in the 68% range. We performed a prospective head-to-head study comparing 330 LBNSs versus 200 open sling procedures and found a significant superiority in success and complication rate with the LBNS in a 4-year period.

The LBNS appears to be a viable alternative in the quest for continence control in women with SUI. There are other procedures available, each with its advantages and disadvantages. With the very low complication risk, extremely low sling erosion rate, and minimal bladder hyperactivity and misery rate of the LBNS in our hands, we have returned to it and turned away from suburethral slings.

## *References*

1. Kaufman JM. Operative management of . . . *Surg Gynecol Obstet* 1949;88: 509. 2.
2. Yang SC, Park DS, Lee JM, et al. Laparoscopic extraperitoneal bladder neck suspension (LEBNS) for stress urinary incontinence. *J Korean Med Sci* 1995;10(6):426–430.
3. Burch JC. Cooper's ligament urethrovesical suspension for stress . . . *Gynecology* 1961;81:281–290.
4. Mitrani A, Sharp M, Zilberman A, et al. Urethral length in urinary stress incontinence. *BJOG: Int J Obstet Gynaecol* 78(7):664–666.
5. The Q-tip test correlation with urethroscopic findings in urinary stress incontinence. *BJOG: Int J Obstet Gynaecol* 78(7):664–666.
6. Stein M, Discippio W, Davia M, et al. Biofeedback for the treatment of stress and urge incontinence. *J Urol* 153(3):641–643.
7. Scarpero H, Dmochowski R, Nitti V. Repeat urethrolysis after failed urethrolysis for iatrogenic obstruction. *J Urol* 169(3):1013–1016.
8. Schultheiss D, Brödel M, Kelly HA. Urogynecology and the birth of modern medical illustration. *Eur J Obstet Gynecol Reprod Biol* 86(1):113–115.
9. McDougall E, Heidorn C, Portis A, et al. Laparoscopic bladder neck suspension fails the test of time. *J Urol* 162(6):2078–2081.
10. Ztsch F. Goebel-Stoeckel sling operation. In: Mattingly RF, Thompson JD, eds. *Telinde's operative gynecology... Gynak U Urol* 1910;2:187.
11. Luber K, Wolde-Tsadik G. Efficacy of functional electrical stimulation in treating genuine stress incontinence: a randomized clinical trial. *J Urol* 160(6):2305–2305.

# CHAPTER 135 ■ MISCELLANEOUS LAPAROSCOPIC UROLOGIC PROCEDURES: CALCULUS, VARICOCELE, URETEROLYSIS

GORDON L. FIFER AND RAJU THOMAS

## CALCULUS DISEASE

One can duplicate the traditional open surgical approaches in appropriately selected patients using laparoscopic techniques. One should, however, gain experience with the common laparoscopic procedures and be comfortable with these prior to tackling these less common or unusual procedures.

The advent of endourology in the late 1970s has transformed the practice of urology. U.S. Food and Drug Administration approval of extracorporeal shock wave lithotripsy (ESWL) in 1984 marked a significant paradigm shift in the treatment of urinary tract calculus disease, moving away from open surgery to less invasive techniques. In modern urologic practice, open stone surgery now accounts for <5% of all procedures performed to treat urolithiasis (1,2).

### Diagnosis

Imaging with computerized tomography (CT) is the standard today for the identification of urolithiasis. Less commonly, excretory urography, retrograde pyelography, or ureteroscopy is the diagnostic method.

### Indications

Technologic advances in the design of endourologic instruments, including ureteroscopes, nephroscopes, baskets, and lithotriptors, including the holmium laser, have all contributed to the great success of minimally invasive stone therapy. Yet infrequent cases exist in which endoscopic or ESWL treatment either has failed or has low expectations for success, and in such cases surgical stone removal remains a viable option.

Since the introduction of laparoscopic surgery in the early 1990s, urologists have recreated virtually every open stone surgical procedure using laparoscopic techniques. Appropriate patient selection is crucial to ensure that a given patient is amenable to laparoscopic management of such calculi. The presence of a large impacted stone is one indication for a laparoscopic approach (3). Although laparoscopy is infrequently utilized for management of urolithiasis, this technique is invaluable when really indicated, providing a minimally invasive approach to managing select cases of urolithiasis (2,4,5).

### Alternative Therapy

As noted, ESWL, ureteroscopic, or percutaneous techniques are the preferred standard for the management of urolithiasis. Open ureterolithotomy is another alternative to the laparoscopic approach.

### Surgical Technique

The precise location of the stone must certainly be identified with preoperative imaging. Helical CT scanning provides detailed anatomic information. The planned approach for appropriate trocar placement will depend on the location of the stone and can be categorized as either *upper*, which includes

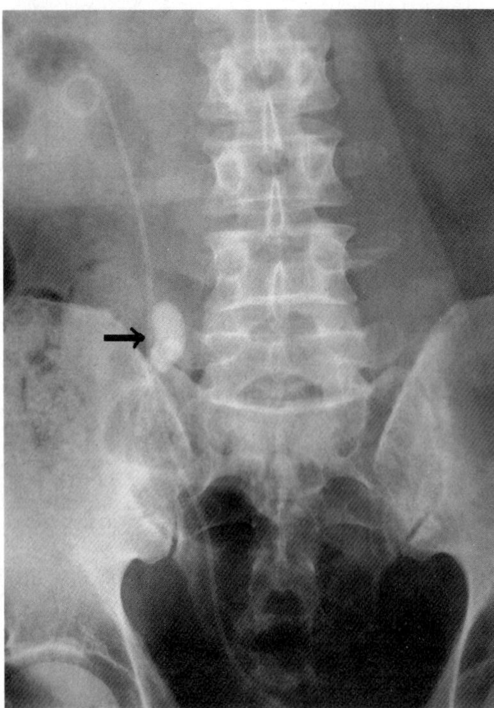

FIGURE 135.1 X-ray shows a very large calculus (*arrow*) impacted in the upper portion of the right ureter.

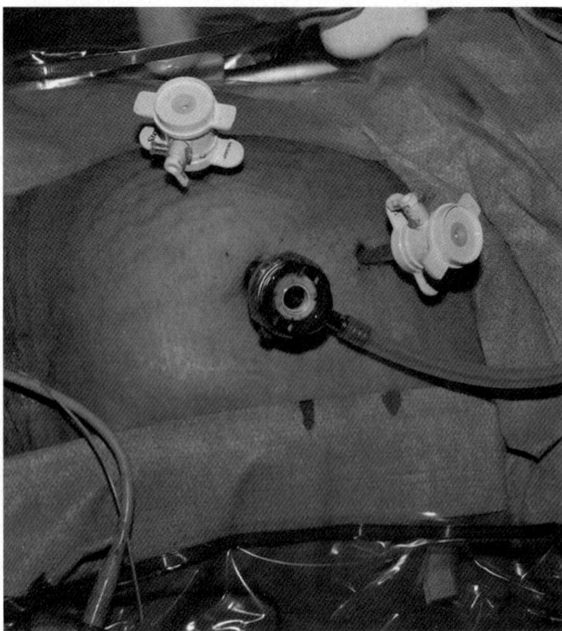

FIGURE 135.2 Patient positioned for right laparoscopic ureterolithotomy. The camera is placed in the umbilical trocar. This configuration can also be used for laparoscopic right ureterolysis, also described in this chapter.

calculi in the renal pelvis and the upper ureter (above the pelvic brim) (Fig. 135.1), or *lower*, for calculi in the ureter distal to the pelvic brim.

Placement of a ureteral stent is often required to manage large or impacted stones. To facilitate intraoperative placement of a ureteral stent, cystoscopy with ureteral catheterization should be performed at the onset of the case. If a guide wire can be manipulated past the stone, this will aid the stent placement; if a wire cannot bypass the stone, an open-ended ureteral catheter is advanced up to the level of the stone. This provides a conduit for passing a wire after the stone is removed and may help identify the ureter during the laparoscopic dissection portion of the procedure. A urethral Foley catheter is placed to drain the bladder and a suture used to secure the ureteral catheter, both of which are prepared into the operative field during laparoscopy.

### For Upper Stones

The patient is placed in a modified lateral recumbent position with the ipsilateral side elevated with a bean bag or kidney rest. The patient is secured to the operating room table with 3-inch silk tape across the chest, waist, and legs. A test airplane roll of the table is performed to ensure the patient is adequately secured. The abdomen is entered with either the Veress needle or the Hasson method, at the surgeon's discretion. Port placement is similar to that used for pyeloplasty, with the camera port placed at the umbilicus. The two operating ports can be placed either in the midline, superior and inferior to the umbilical port, or lateral to the midline and 45 degrees to either side of a "line" from the camera port toward the renal pelvis or ureteral stone location (1). The axis of balance is a line joining the camera trocar to the location of the calculus. The accessory or working trocars are placed with this axis in mind (Fig. 135.2).

The colon is reflected along the white line of Toldt and is allowed to fall medially, aided by airplane rolling the bed, if needed. The ureter is identified and traced to the renal pelvis or until the stone is encountered. For a ureteral stone, since the proximal ureter is usually dilated or tortuous, placement of vascular tape or a vessel loop around the ureter proximal to the stone can help prevent proximal stone migration. The ureter or renal pelvis is opened with either shears or a laparoscopic scalpel handle (Aesculap, Center Valley, PA). The stone should be removed in one piece when possible and may have to be extracted with the use of an Endocatch bag at the end of the procedure. A guide wire can be placed retrograde through the preplaced ureteral 5Fr open-ended catheter, followed by placement of a double-pigtail ureteral stent. The incision in the ureter or pelvis is closed laparoscopically with a 4-0 polyglactin suture (continuous or interrupted) and a closed suction drain is left in place until output subsides.

### For Lower Stones

For stones in the lower portions of the ureter, the patient may be left in a supine position. The peritoneum is again entered at the choice of the surgeon with the camera port placed at the umbilicus. The axis between the camera trocar and the stone is marked, and the two operating ports are then placed under direct vision on either side of the body just lateral to the rectus muscles. The surgeon stands on the contralateral side of the patient and begins the dissection at the level of the bifurcation of the common iliac vessels. The ureter is followed proximally or distally until the stone is located. The surgical procedure proceeds in a similar fashion as described above. For stones located in the midureter, the colon may need to be mobilized for exposure, which may be assisted by a gentle airplaning of the table to the contralateral side.

### Postoperative Management

The Foley catheter is left in place for 48 hours to maintain a low-pressure drainage of the urinary tract. This will expedite removal of the peri-incisional drain. The ureteral stent can be removed with the use of a cystoscope in 2 to 4 weeks.

## Outcomes

This procedure is not commonly performed and is practiced more commonly outside the United States. Success rates of over 94% are reported (6).

### Complications

All standard laparoscopic surgical complications are possible, including infection, bleeding, and conversion to an open surgical procedure. Prolonged urinary leakage and urinary stricture are possible.

# LAPAROSCOPIC VARICOCELE LIGATION

Dilation of the pampiniform plexus of veins draining from the testicles is encountered in up to 15% of the general male population and in 40% to 70% of men undergoing evaluation for infertility. Laparoscopic varicocele ligation closely resembles the retroperitoneal approach first described by Palomo in 1948 (7).

## Indications for Surgery

Indications for surgical correction include infertility with poor-quality semen, decrease in testicular size, and chronic pain or discomfort from a large varicocele. A failed previous attempt at retroperitoneal repair is a contraindication to laparoscopic varicocele ligation. The ultimate choice of varicocele ligation method is determined by surgeon preference and experience as well as patient-specific factors.

## Alternative Therapy

Several different surgical techniques have been described with inguinal (Ivanissevitch), subinguinal microscopic (Marmar–Goldstein), and open retroperitoneal or high ligation techniques (Palomo) approaches. Microscopic techniques are becoming more commonly used to reap the benefits of a less invasive procedure and reduced incidence of hydrocele. Embolization of the dilated veins is sometimes utilized.

## Surgical Technique

Most surgeons utilize the transperitoneal approach, with some reports of successful laparoscopic extraperitoneal varix ligation. The patient is placed in a supine position and the peritoneum entered at the umbilicus with either the Veress needle or Hasson technique. After creation of pneumoperitoneum, the table is rotated, and the additional operative trocars are placed under direct vision.

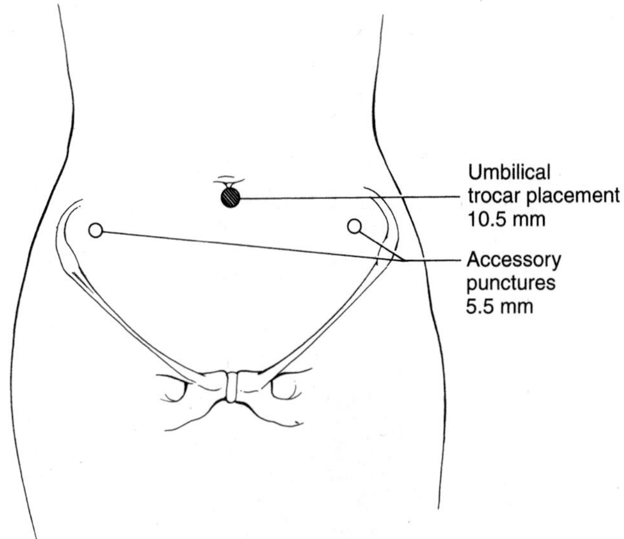


FIGURE 135.3 Appropriate position of trocars for varix ligation. The array of trocars is used in either left or bilateral varix ligation. The subumbilical trocar is either a Hasson cannula for open laparoscopy or a standard trocar inserted following Veress needle insufflation. The operating trocars are 5.5 mm when a 5-mm clip applier is available or 10 mm when one must rely upon a 10.5-mm hemoclip applier.

Two separate trocar templates exist. The first places one port just inferior to the umbilicus and lateral to the rectus muscle on the ipsilateral side, with the second port infraumbilical in the midline. The second template places both operative trocars just lateral to either edge of the rectus muscle and slightly inferior to the umbilicus. The latter allows for bilateral procedures to be performed if necessary (Fig. 135.3).

Once the ports are placed, attention is turned to the internal inguinal ring, and the nearby iliac vessels, vas deferens, and medial umbilical ligament are all identified (Fig. 135.4). If the colon obscures the internal ring, it should be mobilized by incising the line of Toldt or placing the patient in slight Trendelenburg position. The magnification afforded by the laparoscope aids in the visualization of the spermatic vessels running beneath the peritoneum.

The peritoneum is incised lateral to the spermatic cord (Fig. 135.4) and the testicular artery and veins are dissected free. If identified, the testicular artery should be preserved. Use of electrocautery should be restricted so as not to cause thermal injury to the artery. The use of papaverine liquid over the vessels will assist in dilation of the artery, subsequent pulsations, and easier identification of the artery. The intraoperative laparoscopic Doppler probe is helpful to identify the artery. Arterial preservation is not a requirement. The cremasteric and deferential collateral circulations are not jeopardized by the laparoscopic approach and are usually sufficient to maintain the viability of the testicle. The dissection and ligation is described in Figures 135.5 to 135.7. The vessels may be ligated with titanium clips, the endovascular stapler, or intracorporeal knot tying. After ligation, they are transected, completing the procedure. Alternatively, a bulk ligation of the cord with a 2-0 silk or stapler can be performed without regard to preserving the artery. It may be useful to divide the cord into smaller packets without regard to the spermatic artery preservation.

If scrotal emphysema is present, we eliminate it with brief compression before final port removal. Standard laparoscopic

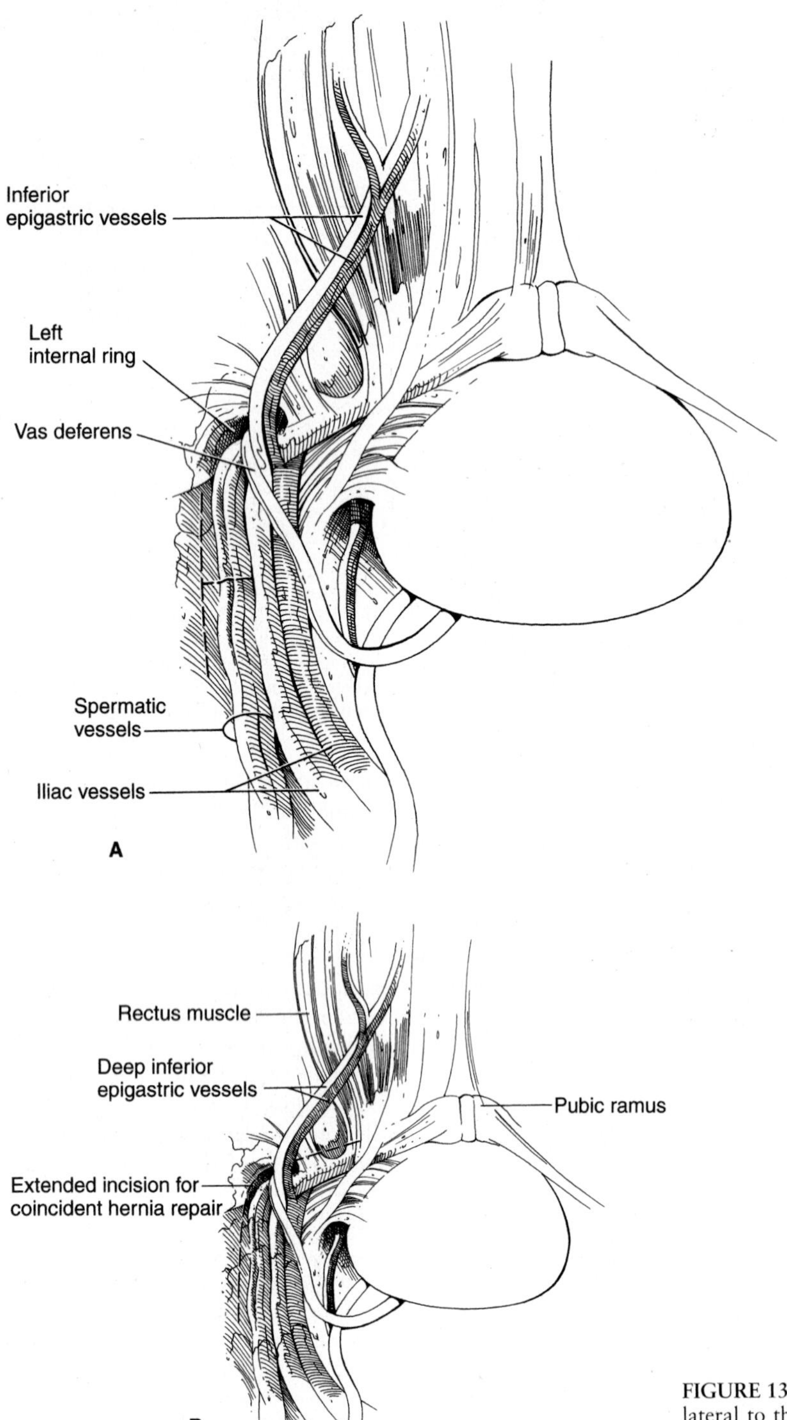


FIGURE 135.4 A 3- to 5-cm incision through the peritoneum is made lateral to the spermatic vascular bundle; it extends cephalad from a point 3 to 5 cm above the internal ring.

closure techniques are followed. Patients are discharged on the day of surgery without restrictions in physical activity.

## Outcomes

Operative times vary based upon extent of operation (unilateral or bilateral), complexity of repair (artery sparing takes longer than artery sacrifice), and laparoscopic experience (novice takes longer than expert). With experience, non–artery-sparing procedures will last 15 to 30 minutes and artery-sparing procedures will last 45 to 60 minutes. A randomized trial comparing open to laparoscopic varix ligation revealed similar outcomes in terms of efficacy and complications, but advantages in terms of pain and recovery time (8). Results indicate that spermatic arterial ligation did not influence response and did not result in testicular atrophy.

### Complications

Due to the age group involved, perioperative complications are very rare. Potential complications include bleeding, a need

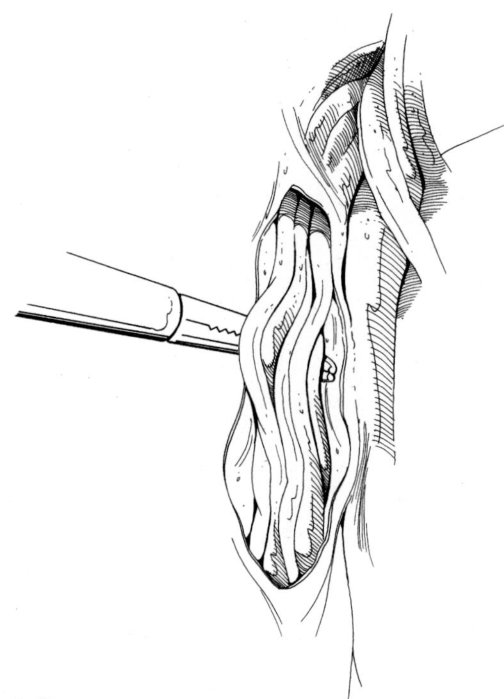

FIGURE 135.5 The entire spermatic vascular bundle is mobilized from the underlying psoas muscle. A combination of sharp and blunt dissection facilitates separation of the spermatic vessels from surrounding tissues. One should avoid deep dissection in order to spare the underlying genitofemoral nerve crossing anterior to the psoas muscle.

to convert to an open procedure, infection, testis atrophy or loss, and failure to correct the varicocele. Even with successful correction of the varicocele (i.e., absence of a palpable varix at 6 months following surgery), signs and/or symptoms that prompted the operation (orchalgia, oligoasthenospermia) may persist.

# LAPAROSCOPIC URETEROLYSIS

Ureteral stenosis or strictures can be caused by a variety of intrinsic as well as extrinsic causes. Thus, ureteral strictures can be caused iatrogenically, such as post-ureteroscopy or following other surgical procedures in close proximity to the ureter. Stenosis may also be secondary to conditions such as retroperitoneal fibrosis (RPF) or extrinsic tumors. The clinical features include flank pain, abdominal pain, renal failure, as well as signs and symptoms of urinary tract obstruction, bacteremia, etc.

RPF is an inflammatory process involving the retroperitoneum that results in excessive fibrosis and often causes ureteral entrapment, compression, and obstruction leading to hydronephrosis. The primary, idiopathic etiology accounts for 70% of the cases, with the remainder of cases occurring secondarily in response to numerous conditions, including vascular aneurysm with or without grafting; radiation exposure; inflammatory bowel disease; malignancy; or drug exposure, including use of beta-adrenergic blockers or ergot alkaloids.

The most common presentation is colicky flank pain from ureteral obstruction; however, the fibrosis may be so extreme as to entrap the great vessels or renal vasculature, so that lower extremity edema, hypertension, or hematuria may also occur. On the other hand, ureteral strictures may be asymptomatic and can present with painless hydronephrosis (6,9,10).

## Diagnosis

Preoperative imaging may consist of intravenous pyelography or CT scans, typically demonstrating hydronephrosis and medial deviation of the course of the ureter, either unilaterally or bilaterally. Retrograde pyelograms performed just prior to ureterolysis may provide updated information regarding the course of the ureter and help identify the extent (length) of ureteral entrapment.

## Indications for Surgery

Ureterolysis can be both diagnostic, allowing for biopsy of the retroperitoneal mass, and therapeutic, allowing release of the ureters.

## Alternative Therapy

Traditionally, ureterolysis is performed by the open surgical approach. Many centers will attempt a trial of steroids empirically before surgical correction. Malignant RPF can sometimes be managed primarily by chemotherapy without the need for ureterolysis (6,9).

## Surgical Technique

### Ureterolysis

Laparoscopic ureterolysis begins with cystoscopy and retrograde placement of either a double-pigtail stent or a ureteral catheter to aid in identification of the ureter during laparoscopy. Either a regular 5Fr open-ended or lighted catheter may be used. To further aid ureteral delineation from the surrounding dense fibrotic tissue, a super-stiff guide wire may also be placed inside a ureteral catheter (10). Similar to laparoscopic pyeloplasty positioning, the patient is placed in a lateral decubitus position with the ipsilateral side elevated to allow gravity retraction of the bowels. If a bilateral ureterolysis (6,9,10) is planned, the patient may either be left supine or repositioned (this is recommended) after completion of the first side.

The template for port placement will vary depending on the extent of fibrosis and the levels of the ureter involved. A standard pyeloplasty template (see earlier under calculus management) may be sufficient for isolated upper ureteral involvement, but additional ports may be necessary to free the entire ureter.

After creating pneumoperitoneum and rotating the patient, the colon is mobilized along the white line of Toldt and allowed to fall medially. When necessary, this incision is extended over the iliac vessels to allow exposure of the full course of the ureter. Depending on the extent of RPF, the ureters are often retracted medially and may be overlying the great vessels entrapped in dense fibrous scars, making localization difficult.

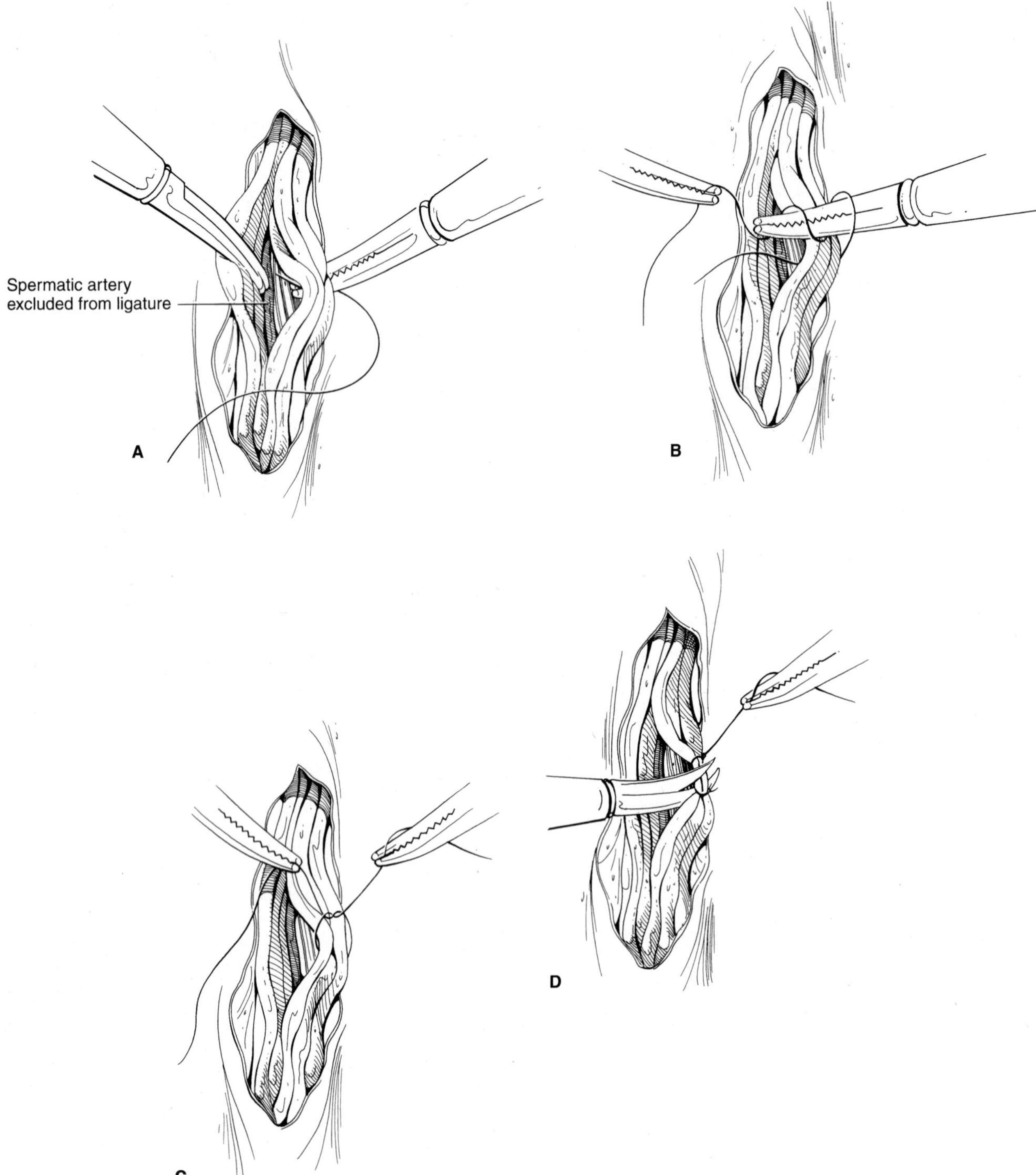


FIGURE 135.6 **A:** When performing an artery-sparing varix ligation, the vascular bundle that does not contain the spermatic artery is ligated and then divided. For small venous aggregates or single spermatic veins, the 5-mm reusable clip or suture ligature is utilized based on surgeon preference. A 5- to 10-cm ligature is passed into the abdominal cavity. One end is passed from right to left under the vessels to be ligated, extending only 1 cm beyond the vessels. The other end is long to facilitate instrument tie. **B.** The long end is grasped by the left-hand instrument, allowing sufficient slack to permit easy wrapping around the tip of the right-hand instrument. The instrument tie can be accomplished with two curved dissectors with tips rotated up. Alternatively, instruments specifically designed for laparoscopic suture and ligation may be used. **C:** The nonarterial vascular bundle is ligated. **D:** The spermatic veins are divided between ligatures.

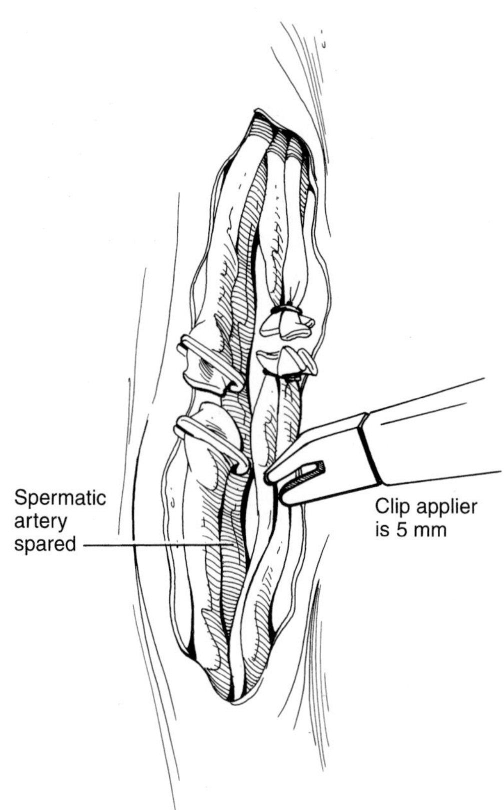


FIGURE 135.7 Upon completion of the procedure, all spermatic veins have been ligated and divided by either clip or suture. Only the spermatic artery or arteries remain, and arterial patency is documented by Doppler.

If a ureteral catheter was placed, gentle manipulation may help locate the ureter. Alternatively, the distal ureter may be encountered medial to the medial umbilical ligament and traced proximally, or the proximal ureter may be isolated at the ureteropelvic junction and dissected distally. Once positively identified, a window is created around the ureter and vascular tape or a vessel loop is placed around to allow retraction without undue manipulation of the ureter. Combinations of blunt, sharp, and electrocautery dissection are necessary to liberate the ureter from surrounding fibrosis, although the latter should be used sparingly to avoid vascular compromise. For patients with RPF, after the ureter is mobilized, it should be intraperitonealized, and after this is accomplished, the posterior peritoneum is closed with clips or preferably with sutures. If a ureteral catheter was placed at the onset, it should be exchanged for an indwelling self-retaining ureteral stent at this time. Special efforts must be made to rule out malignancy as the underlying cause of the fibrosis, and multiple biopsies are taken from periureteral tissues and sent for both frozen and permanent analysis.

Laparoscopic ureterolysis is also amenable to hand-assisted laparoscopic approaches and has also been reported using robotic techniques. The principles of ureterolysis can be followed with the use of the intra-abdominal hand to assist in identification and dissection of the ureter (9).

### Management of Ureteral Strictures

For benign, iatrogenic or idiopathic ureteral strictures, the strictured ureteral segment is excised. Caution should be exercised around the iliac vessels and the inferior vena cava so as to prevent vascular injury. The ureteral ends are then spatulated. The posterior walls of the ureteral ends are anastomosed using 4-0 polyglactin sutures. A ureteral stent is then placed in a retrograde fashion utilizing the 5Fr open-ended ureteral catheter, which is removed after a guide wire is placed through it. The anterior end-to-end anastomosis of the ureteral ends is now completed. A closed-suction drain is placed. A Foley catheter drains the bladder postoperatively to maintain a low-pressure urinary drainage system.

If the ureteral stricture is long, and if the anastomosis is under tension, then the management strategy may involve further laparoscopic ureterolysis to ensure a tension-free anastomosis. Rarely, one may have to utilize procedures such as nephropexy to enable a tension-free end-to-end ureteroureterostomy.

### Postoperative Management

The Foley catheter is usually left indwelling for 48 hours. The drain is kept in place for another day or two, then removed. The indwelling stent is removed using a flexible cystoscope 4 to 6 weeks postoperatively. Postoperative imaging is recommended to evaluate for any residual or silent recurrence of the hydronephrosis.

## Outcomes

A recent multicenter review indicated overall success rates of 83% per renal unit (6). This was confirmed by follow-up imaging in these cases. Other institutional series are also favorable (6,9,11).

### Complications

Any complication that can be associated with laparoscopy, including conversion to an open procedure, has been reported. One series reported a conversion rate to open of 17.6% (11).

## *References*


1. Matlaga BR, Assimos DG. Changing indications of open stone surgery. *Urology* 2002;59:490–493.
2. Paik ML, Wainstein MA, Spirnak JP, et al. Current indications for open stone surgery in the treatment of renal and ureteral calculi. *J Urol* 1998; 159:374–379.
3. Gaur DD. Retroperitoneal laparoscopic ureterolithotomy. *World J Urol* 1993;11:175–177.
4. Goel A, Hamal AK. Upper and mid-ureteric stones: a prospective unrandomized comparison of retroperitoneoscopic and open ureterolithotomy. *BJU Int* 2001;88:679–682.
5. Micali S, Moore RG, Averch TD, et al. The role of laparoscopy in the management of renal and ureteral calculi. *J Urol* 1997;157:463–466.
6. Duchene DA, Winfield HN, Cadeddu JA, et al. Multi-institutional survey of laparoscopic ureterolysis for retroperitoneal fibrosis. *Urology* 2007; 69(6):1017–1021.
7. Palomo A. Radical cure of varicocele by a new technique: preliminary report. *J Urol* 1948;61:604–607.
8. Podkamenev VV, Stalmakhovich VN, Urkov PS, et al. Laparoscopic surgery for pediatric varicoceles: randomized controlled trial. *J Pediatr Surg* 2002;37:727–729.

9. Brown JA, Garlitz CJ, Hubosky SG, et al. Hand-assisted laparoscopic ureterolysis to treat ureteral obstruction secondary to idiopathic retroperitoneal fibrosis: assessment of a novel technique and initial series. *Urology* 2006;68(1):46–49.
10. Kavoussi LR, Clayman RV, Brunt LM, et al. Laparoscopic ureterolysis. *J Urol* 1992;147:426–429.
11. Srinivasan AK, Richstone L, Permpongkosol S, et al. Comparison of laparoscopic with open approach for ureterolysis in patients with retroperitoneal fibrosis. *J Urol* 2008;179(5):1875–1878.
12. Atug F, Woods M, Burgess S, et al. Robotic pyeloplasty in children. *J Urol* 2005;174:1440–1442.
13. Clayman RV, Kavoussi LR, Soper MJ, et al. Laparoscopic nephrectomy. Initial case report. *J Urol* 1991;146:278–282.
14. Elashry OM, Nakada SY, Wolf JS Jr, et al. Ureterolysis for extrinisic ureter obstruction: a comparison of laparoscopic and open surgical techniques. *J Urol* 1996;156(4):1403–1410.
15. Fugita OE, Jarrett TW, Kavoussi P, et al. Laparoscopic treatment of retroperitoneal fibrosis. *J Endourol* 2002;16:571–574.
16. Gad El-Moula M, Abdallah A, El-Anany F, et al. Laparoscopic ureterolithotomy: our experience with 74 cases. *Int J Urol* 2008;15(7): 593–597.
17. Puppo B, Carmiginani G, Gallucci M, et al. Bilateral laparoscopic ureterolysis. *Eur Urol* 1994;25(1):82–84.
18. Soper MJ, Barteau JA, Clayman RV, et al. Comparison of early postoperative results for laparoscopic versus standard open cholecystectomy. *Surg Gynecol Obstet* 1992;174:114–118.

# CHAPTER 136 ■ TISSUE-ENGINEERING STRATEGIES FOR UROGENITAL REPAIR

ANTHONY ATALA

Congenital disorders, cancer, trauma, infection, inflammation, iatrogenic injuries, or other conditions of the genitourinary system can lead to organ damage or complete loss of function. Most of these situations require eventual reconstructive procedures. These procedures can be performed with native nonurologic tissues (skin, gastrointestinal segments, or mucosa), homologous tissues from a donor (cadaver or living donor kidney), heterologous tissues or substances (bovine collagen), or artificial materials (silicone, polyurethane, Teflon). However, these materials often lead to complications after reconstruction. The implanted tissue is sometimes rejected, and often the inherently different functional aspects of the different tissues or materials used in the reconstruction cause a mismatch in the system. As an example, current methods of replacing bladder tissue with gastrointestinal segments can be problematic due to the opposite ways in which these two tissues handle solutes; urologic tissue normally excretes materials, but gastrointestinal tissue generally absorbs the same materials, and this type of mismatch can lead to metabolic complications as well as infection. The replacement of lost or deficient urologic tissues with functionally equivalent ones would improve the outcome of reconstructive surgery in the genitourinary system. This may soon be possible with novel tissue-engineering techniques.

## TISSUE-ENGINEERING BASICS

Tissue engineering uses the principles of cell transplantation, materials science, and biomedical engineering to develop biological substitutes that can restore and maintain the normal function of damaged or lost tissues and organs. It can involve injection of functional cells into a nonfunctional site to stimulate regeneration, or it may involve the use of biomaterials. These are natural or synthetic matrices, often termed scaffolds, that encourage the body's natural ability to repair itself and assist in determination of the orientation and direction of new tissue growth. Often, tissue engineering uses a combination of both of these techniques. For example, biomaterial matrices seeded with cells can be implanted into the body to encourage the growth or regeneration of functional tissue.

### Biomaterials Used in Genitourinary Tissue Construction

Biomaterials in genitourinary tissue engineering function as an artificial extracellular matrix (ECM) and are used to replace biologic and mechanical functions of native ECM found in tissues in the body. They may serve as simple cell carriers, or they can provide structural support for tissue formation. Biomaterials can be fabricated from synthetic materials, naturally derived substances, or both combined, and they can be configured into liquid, gel, or solid forms depending on the specific needs. These substances facilitate the localization and delivery of cells to desired sites in the body as well as define a three-dimensional space for the formation of new tissues with appropriate structure. They also serve as a guide for the development of new tissues with appropriate function (32,33). Direct injection of cell suspensions without a biomaterial carrier has been attempted, but without this specialized scaffold function, it is difficult to control the localization of transplanted cells (13,55). Furthermore, bioactive signals, such as cell-adhesion peptides and growth factors, can be incorporated along with cells to help regulate cellular function (33). Cell behavior in the newly formed tissue can be regulated by multiple interactions of the cells with their microenvironment, including interactions with cell-adhesion ligands and with soluble growth factors (29). Some materials are designed to carry these factors into the body and release them at a specified rate to assist the cells in the organizational process.

The ideal biomaterial should be biocompatible, promote cellular interaction and tissue development, and possess similar mechanical and physical properties to the tissue to be generated so that the nascent tissue will be able to withstand *in vivo* forces. Generally, three classes of biomaterials have been used for the engineering of genitourinary tissues: naturally derived materials, such as collagen and alginate; acellular tissue matrices, such as bladder submucosa and small intestinal submucosa; and synthetic polymers, such as polyglycolic acid (PGA), polylactic acid (PLA), and polylactic (PLGA). While synthetic polymers can be produced reproducibly on a large scale with controlled properties of strength, degradation rate, and microstructure, naturally derived materials and acellular tissue matrices have the potential advantage of biologic recognition, which can lessen host-versus-graft reactions.

### Cells for Urogenital Tissue-Engineering Applications

Often, when cells are used for tissue engineering, donor tissue is removed and dissociated into individual cells, which are either implanted directly into the host or expanded in culture, attached to a support matrix, and then implanted. The implanted tissue can be heterologous, allogeneic, or autologous. Ideally, this approach allows lost tissue function to be restored or replaced in toto with limited complications (1–4,6,7).

Autologous cells are the ideal choice, as their use circumvents many of the inflammatory and rejection issues associated with a nonself donor. However, one limitation of cell-based tissue-engineering techniques has been the difficulty of growing specific cell types in large quantities. Even when certain organs, such as the liver, have a high regenerative capacity in vivo, in vitro expansion of cells derived from these organs has proved to be difficult. However, the discovery of privileged sites for committed precursor cells in specific organs and extensive study of the conditions that promote precursor cell maintenance and differentiation within these sites have begun to overcome some of the limitations associated with cell expansion in vitro. Urothelial cells that are present in the bladder, for instance, have been grown in culture in the past, but only with limited success. However, several novel culture protocols have been developed over the past two decades that allow the maintenance of urothelial precursor cells in an undifferentiated state. As these cells can remain in the growth phase, the ability to expand urothelial cultures is vastly improved (18,42,58,62). These studies suggest that it may be possible to collect autologous urothelial cells from human bladders, expand them in culture, and return them to the donor in sufficient quantities for reconstructive purposes (18,23,42,43,48,58). In addition to urothelial cells, methods to induce the in vitro expansion of a variety of primary human cells have been developed, making the use of autologous cells for clinical applications a real possibility, though there are still hurdles to overcome.

Another major concern has been that, in cases where cells must be expanded from a diseased organ, there may no longer be enough normal cells present in that organ to begin the process. Recent research suggests that this may not be the case, however. For example, one study has shown that cultured neuropathic bladder smooth muscle cells possess and maintain different characteristics than normal smooth muscle cells in vitro, as demonstrated by growth assays, contractility, and adherence tests in vitro (44). Despite these differences, when neuropathic smooth muscle cells were cultured in vitro and then seeded onto matrices and implanted in vivo, the tissue-engineered constructs showed the same properties as the constructs engineered with normal cells (37). It is now known that genetically normal progenitor cells, which are the reservoirs for new cell formation, are present even in diseased tissue. These normal progenitors are programmed to give rise to normal tissue, regardless of whether they reside in a normal or diseased environment. Therefore, the stem cell niche and its role in normal tissue regeneration remains a fertile area of ongoing investigation.

## Stem Cells and Other Pluripotent Cell Types

Most current strategies for tissue engineering depend upon a sample of autologous cells from the diseased organ of the host. In some instances, primary autologous human cells cannot be expanded from a particular organ, such as the pancreas. In these situations, pluripotent human stem cells are envisioned to be an ideal source of cells, as they can differentiate into nearly any replacement tissue in the body.

Embryonic stem (ES) cells exhibit two remarkable properties: the ability to proliferate in an undifferentiated but still pluripotent state (self-renewal), and the ability to differentiate into a large number of specialized cell types (14). They can be isolated from the inner cell mass of the embryo during the blastocyst stage, which occurs 5 days after fertilization. These cells have been maintained in the undifferentiated state for at least 80 passages when grown using current published protocols (69). In addition, many protocols for differentiation into specific cell types in culture have been published. However, many uses of these cells have been controversial in the United States due to the ethical dilemmas that are associated with the manipulation of embryos in culture.

Adult stem cells have the advantage of avoiding some of the ethical issues associated with embryonic cells, and, unlike embryonic cells, they do not transdifferentiate into a malignant phenotype, so there is a diminished risk of teratoma formation should the cells be implanted in vivo. However, adult stem cells are limited for clinical use because expansion to the large quantities needed for tissue engineering is difficult.

Fetal stem cells derived from amniotic fluid and placentas have recently been described and represent a novel source of stem cells (19,20). The cells express markers consistent with human ES cells, such as octamer-4 (OCT4) and stage-specific embryonic antigen-4 (SSEA-4), but they do not form teratomas. The cells are multipotent and are able to differentiate into cells from all three germ layers. In addition, the cells have a high replicative potential and could be stored for future use, without the risks of rejection and without ethical concerns.

Nuclear transfer, or cloning, can serve as another source of pluripotent "stem" cells that could possibly be used for regenerative medicine therapies. Two types of cloning procedures exist: reproductive cloning and therapeutic cloning. Banned in most countries for human applications, reproductive cloning is used to generate an embryo that has identical genetic material as its cell source. This embryo is then implanted into the uterus of a pseudopregnant female to give rise to an infant that is a clone of the donor. While therapeutic cloning also produces an embryo that is genetically identical to the donor nucleus, this process is used to generate blastocysts that are explanted and grown in culture, rather than in utero, to produce ES cell lines. These autologous stem cells have the potential to become almost any type of cell in the adult body, and thus would be useful in tissue and organ replacement applications (25). Therefore, therapeutic cloning, which has also been called somatic cell nuclear transfer, may provide an alternative source of transplantable cells that are identical to the patient's own cells.

Recently, exciting reports have been published of the successful transformation of adult cells into pluripotent stem cells through a type of genetic "reprogramming." Reprogramming is a technique that involves dedifferentiation of adult somatic cells to produce patient-specific pluripotent stem cells, without the use of embryos. Cells generated by reprogramming would be genetically identical to the somatic cells (and thus, the patient who donated these cells) and would not be rejected. Takahashi and Yamanka were the first to discover that mouse embryonic fibroblasts (MEFs) and adult mouse fibroblasts could be reprogrammed into an "induced pluripotent state (iPS)" (67). Takahashi and Yamanaka were the first to discover 24 genes that were thought to be important for ES cells and identified 4 key genes that were required to bestow ES cell–like properties on fibroblasts: Oct3/4, Sox2, c-Myc, and Klf4. Mouse embryonic fibroblasts and adult fibroblasts were co-transduced with retroviral vectors, each carrying one of the 4 genes, and transduced cells were selected via drug resistance. The resultant iPS cells possessed the immortal growth characteristics of self-renewing ES cells, expressed genes specific for ES cells, and generated embryoid bodies in vitro and teratomas in vivo. When iPS cells were injected into mouse blastocysts, they contributed to a variety of cell types. However, although iPS cells selected in this way were pluripotent, they were not identical to ES cells. Unlike ES cells, chimeras made from iPS cells did not result in full-term pregnancies. Gene expression profiles of the iPS cells showed that they possessed a distinct gene expression signature that was different from that of ES cells. In addition, the epigenetic state of the iPS cells was somewhere between that found in somatic cells and that found in ES cells, suggesting that the reprogramming was incomplete.

These results were improved significantly by Wernig and Jaenisch in July 2007 (70). Fibroblasts were infected with retroviral vectors and selected for the activation of endogenous Oct4 or Nanog genes. Results from this study showed that DNA methylation, gene expression profiles, and the chromatin state of the reprogrammed cells were similar to those of ES cells. Teratomas induced by these cells contained differentiated cell types representing all three embryonic germ layers. Most importantly, the reprogrammed cells from this experiment were able to form viable chimeras and contribute to the germ line like ES cells, suggesting that these iPS cells were completely reprogrammed. Wernig et al. (70) observed that the number of reprogrammed colonies increased when drug selection was initiated later (day 20 rather than day 3 post-transduction). This suggests that reprogramming is a slow and gradual process and may explain why previous attempts resulted in incomplete reprogramming.

It has recently been shown that reprogramming of human cells is possible (66,78). Takahashi and Yamanaka (67) showed that retrovirus-mediated transfection of Oct3/4, Sox2, Klf4 and c-MYC generates human iPS cells that are similar to human embryonic stem (hES) cells in terms of morphology, proliferation, gene expression, surface markers, and teratoma formation. Thomson's group (78) showed that retroviral transduction of Oct4, Sox2, Nanog, and LIN28 could generate pluripotent stem cells without introducing any oncogenes (c-MYC). Both studies showed that human iPS cells were similar but not identical to hES cells.

Another concern is that these iPS cells contain three to six retroviral integrations (one for each factor), which may increase the risk of tumorigenesis. Okita et al. (52) studied the tumor formation in chimeric mice generated from Nanog-iPS cells and found that 20% of the offspring developed tumors due to the retroviral expression of c-myc. An alternative approach would be to use a transient expression method, such as adenovirus-mediated system, since both Jaenisch and Yamanaka showed strong silencing of the viral-controlled transcripts in iPS cells (47,52). This indicates that these viral genes are only required for the induction, not the maintenance, of pluripotency.

Another concern is the use of transgenic donor cells for reprogrammed cells in the mouse studies. In both mouse studies, iPS cells were isolated by selecting for the activation of a drug-resistant gene inserted into endogenous Fbx15, Oct3/4, or Nanog. The use of genetically modified donors hinders its clinical applicability for humans. To assess whether iPS cells can be derived from genetically unmodified donor cells, murine embryonic fibroblast (MEF) and adult skin cells were retrovirally transduced with Oct3/4, Sox2, c-Myc, and Klf4 and ES–like colonies were isolated by morphology, without the use of drug selection for Oct4 or Nanog (47). iPS cells from unmodified donor cells formed teratomas and generated live chimeras. This study suggests that genetically modified donor cells are not necessary to generate iPS cells.

Although this is an exciting phenomenon, it is unclear why reprogramming of adult fibroblasts and reprogramming of mesenchymal stromal cells have similar efficiencies (67). It would seem that cells that are already multipotent could be reprogrammed with greater efficiency, since the more undifferentiated the donor nucleus, the better somatic cell nuclear transfer (SNCT) performs (12). This further emphasizes our limited understanding of the mechanism of reprogramming, yet the potential for this area of study is exciting.

# APPLICATION OF TISSUE ENGINEERING TO SPECIFIC UROLOGICAL PROBLEMS

## Injectable (Cell) Therapies

### Injectable Chondrocytes

Vesicoureteral reflux (VUR) and stress urinary incontinence (SUI) are two urologic conditions that can result from dysfunction of a specific sphincter muscle. When severe, these conditions are repaired surgically. However, cell-based therapies for both VUR and incontinence would be an important alternative to surgical repair of these conditions. Ideally, such a therapy would be easily administered by injection and well tolerated by the patient. Currently, the injection of bulking agents such as Teflon paste is used clinically to treat VUR in particular, but the biocompatibility of synthetic bulking agents over the long term is a concern. The ideal substance for endoscopic treatment of reflux and incontinence should be injectable, nonantigenic, nonmigratory, volume-stable, and safe for human use.

Toward this goal, long-term studies were conducted to determine the effects of injectable chondrocytes for the treatment of VUR in vivo (3). Chondrocytes were chosen because the use of autologous cartilage for the treatment of VUR in humans would satisfy all of the requirements for an ideal injectable cell-based therapy. Chondrocytes derived from an ear biopsy can be readily grown and expanded in culture. Neocartilage formation can be achieved in vitro and in vivo using chondrocytes cultured on synthetic biodegradable polymers. In the VUR experiments, chondrocytes were suspended in an alginate matrix and injected around the vesicoureteral sphincter. In time, normal cartilage replaced the alginate as the alginate slowly degraded. This system was then adapted for the treatment of VUR in a porcine model (6). These studies show that chondrocytes can be easily harvested and combined with alginate in vitro, that the suspension can be easily injected cystoscopically, and that the elastic cartilage tissue formed is able to correct VUR without any evidence of obstruction.

Two multicenter clinical trials were conducted using this engineered chondrocyte technology. First, patients with VUR were treated at ten centers throughout the United States. The patients had a similar success rate as with other injectable substances in terms of cure. Cartilage formation was not noted in patients with treatment failure. Patients who were cured probably had a biocompatible region of engineered autologous tissue present (22). Secondly, patients with urinary incontinence were treated endoscopically with injected chondrocytes at three different medical centers. Phase 1 trials showed an approximate success rate of 80% at 3 and 12 months postoperatively (9).

### Injectable Muscle Cells

The potential use of injectable, cultured myoblasts for the treatment of SUI has been investigated (15,73). In one study, labeled myoblasts were directly injected into the proximal urethra and lateral bladder walls with a microsyringe in an open surgical procedure. Tissue harvested up to 35 days postinjection contained the labeled myoblasts, as well as evidence of differentiation into regenerative myofibers. This study shows that a significant portion of the injected myoblast population survived and remained in vivo. Similar techniques of sphincter-derived muscle cells have been used for the treatment of urinary incontinence in a pig model (64). The fact that cultured myoblasts survive after injection and mature into muscle tissue supports the feasibility of using culture-expanded cells of muscular origin as an injectable bioimplant.

The use of injectable muscle precursor cells has also been investigated for use in the treatment of urinary incontinence due to irreversible urethral sphincter injury or developmental defects. Muscle precursor cells are the quiescent satellite cells found in each myofiber that can proliferate to form myoblasts and eventually myotubes and new muscle tissue. Intrinsic muscle precursor cells have previously been shown to play an active role in the regeneration of injured striated urethral sphincter (71). In a subsequent study, autologous muscle precursor cells were injected into a rat model of urethral sphincter injury, and both replacement of mature myotubes and restoration of functional motor units were noted in the regenerating sphincter muscle tissue (72). This is the first demonstration of the replacement of both sphincter muscle tissue and its innervation by the injection of muscle precursor cells. This suggests the possibility that muscle precursor cells may be a minimally invasive solution for urinary incontinence in patients with irreversible urinary sphincter muscle insufficiency.

In addition, injectable muscle-based gene therapy and tissue engineering were combined to improve detrusor function in a bladder injury model, and this may be a novel treatment option for urinary incontinence (26).

### Injectable Leydig Cells

Patients with testicular dysfunction require androgen replacement for somatic development. Conventional treatment for testicular dysfunction consists of periodic intramuscular injections of chemically modified testosterone or application of a transdermal testosterone patch. However, long-term nonpulsatile testosterone therapy is not optimal and can cause multiple problems, including erythropoiesis and bone density changes.

A system was designed wherein Leydig cells were microencapsulated for controlled testosterone replacement. Purified Leydig cells were isolated and encapsulated in an alginate-poly-L-lysine solution. The encapsulated Leydig cells were injected into castrated animals, and serum testosterone was measured serially; the animals were able to maintain testosterone levels in the long term (45). These studies suggest that microencapsulated Leydig cells may be able to replace or supplement testosterone in situations where anorchia or testicular failure is present.

## Tissue Therapy: Engineering Complete Structures in the Genitourinary Tract

### Urethra

Various strategies have been proposed over the years for the regeneration of urethral tissue. Woven meshes of PGA (Dexon) have been used to reconstruct urethras in dogs (53). Also, PGA has been used as a cell transplantation vehicle to engineer tubular urothelium in vivo (7). Small intestinal submucosa (SIS) without cells was used as an onlay patch graft for urethroplasty in rabbits (35). Finally, a homologous graft of acellular urethral matrix was also used in a rabbit model (63).

Bladder-derived acellular collagen matrix has proven to be a suitable graft for repair of urethral defects in rabbits. In the rabbit model, the neourethras created with these matrices demonstrated a normal urothelial luminal lining and organized muscle bundles shortly after repair (35,63). These results were confirmed clinically in a series of patients with a history of failed hypospadias reconstruction, wherein the urethral defects were repaired with human bladder acellular collagen matrices (Fig. 136.1) (5,16). One of the advantages

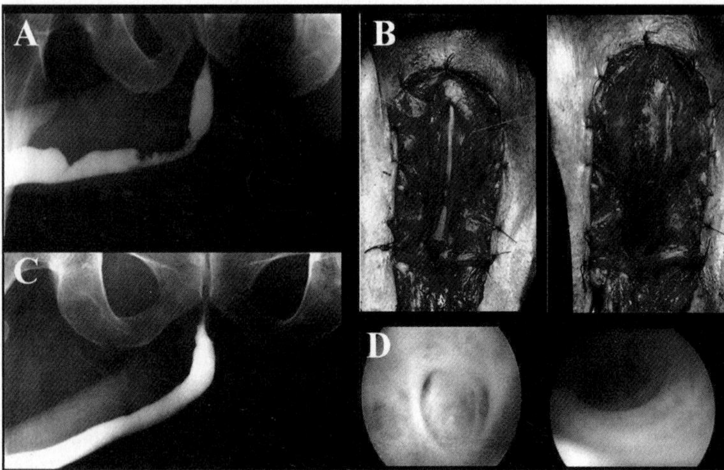


FIGURE 136.1 Tissue engineering of the urethra using a collagen matrix. **A:** Representative case of a patient with a bulbar stricture. **B:** Urethral repair. The strictured tissue is excised, preserving the urethral plate (left), and the matrix is anastomosed to the urethral plate in an onlay fashion on the right. **C:** Urethrogram 6 months after repair. **D:** Cystoscopic view of urethra before surgery (left) and 4 months after repair (right).

of this material over nongenital tissue grafts currently used for urethroplasty (e.g., buccal mucosa) is that the material is "off the shelf." This eliminates the necessity of additional surgical procedures for graft harvesting, which may decrease operative time, as well as the potential morbidity due to the harvest procedure.

The previous techniques, using nonseeded acellular matrices, were successfully applied experimentally and clinically for onlay urethral repairs. However, when tubularized urethral repairs were attempted experimentally, adequate urethral tissue regeneration was not achieved and complications ensued, such as graft contracture and stricture formation (41). Tubularized collagen matrices seeded with cells have performed better in animal studies. In a rabbit model, entire urethral segments were resected and urethroplasties were performed with tubularized collagen matrices either seeded with autologous cells or without cells. The tubularized collagen matrices seeded with autologous cells formed new tissue that was histologically similar to native urethral tissue (59). The tubularized collagen matrices without cells led to poor tissue development, fibrosis, and stricture formation.

## Bladder

Currently, gastrointestinal segments are commonly used for bladder replacement or repair. However, gastrointestinal tissues are designed to absorb solutes that urinary tissue excretes, and due to this difference in function, multiple complications may ensue, such as infection, metabolic disturbances, urolithiasis, perforation, increased mucus production, and malignancy (30,31,46). Because of the problems encountered with the use of gastrointestinal segments, numerous investigators have attempted alternative reconstructive procedures for bladder replacement or repair. The use of tissue expansion, seromuscular grafts, matrices for tissue regeneration, and tissue engineering with cell transplantation has been investigated.

**Tissue Expansion for Bladder Augmentation.** A system of progressive dilation for ureters and bladders has been proposed as a method of bladder augmentation but has not yet been attempted clinically. Augmentation cystoplasty performed with dilated ureteral segments in animals has resulted in an increased bladder capacity ranging from 190% to 380% (38,61). A system for the progressive expansion of native bladder tissue has also been used for augmenting bladder volumes in animals. Within 30 days after progressive dilation, the neoreservoir volume was expanded at least tenfold. Urodynamic studies showed normal compliance in all animals, and microscopic examination of the expanded neoreservoir tissue showed a normal histology. A series of immunocytochemical studies demonstrated that the dilated bladder tissue maintained normal phenotypic characteristics (61).

**Seromuscular Grafts and De-epithelialized Bowel Segments.** Seromuscular grafts and deepithelialized bowel segments, either alone or over a native urothelium, have also been attempted (10,11,17,24,51,60). Keeping the urothelium intact avoids the complications associated with use of bowel in continuity with the urinary tract (11,24). An example of this strategy is the combination of the techniques of autoaugmentation with those of enterocystoplasty. An autoaugmentation is performed and the diverticulum is covered with a demucosalized gastric or intestinal segment.

**Matrices for Bladder Regeneration.** Nonseeded allogeneic acellular matrices have served as scaffolds for the ingrowth of host bladder wall components. The matrices are prepared by mechanically and chemically removing all cellular components from bladder tissue (54,57,65,75). The matrices serve as vehicles for partial bladder regeneration, and relevant antigenicity is not evident. One example is SIS, a biodegradable, acellular, xenogeneic collagen-based tissue matrix. SIS was first used in the early 1980s as an acellular matrix for tissue replacement in the vascular field. It has been shown to promote regeneration of a variety of host tissues, including blood vessels and ligaments (8). Animal studies have shown that the nonseeded SIS matrix used for bladder augmentation is able to regenerate in vivo (34,36).

In multiple studies using various materials as nonseeded grafts for cystoplasty, the urothelial layer was able to regenerate normally, but the muscle layer, although present, was not fully developed (36,57,65,75). Often the grafts contracted to 60% to 70% of their original size with little increase in bladder capacity or compliance (39,56). Studies involving acellular matrices that may provide the necessary environment to promote cell migration, growth, and differentiation are being conducted. Recently, bladder regeneration has been shown to be more reliable when the SIS was derived from the distal ileum (34). With continued research in this area, these matrices may have a clinical role in bladder replacement in the future.

**Bladder Replacement Using Tissue Engineering.** Cell-seeded allogeneic acellular bladder matrices have been used for bladder augmentation in dogs. A group of experimental dogs underwent a trigone-sparing cystectomy and were randomly assigned to one of three groups. One group underwent closure of the trigone without a reconstructive procedure, another underwent reconstruction with a nonseeded bladder-shaped biodegradable scaffold, and the last underwent reconstruction using a bladder-shaped biodegradable scaffold that was seeded with autologous urothelial and smooth muscle cells (50).

The cystectomy-only and nonseeded controls maintained average capacities of 22% and 46% of preoperative values, respectively. However, an average bladder capacity of 95% of the original precystectomy volume was achieved in the cell-seeded tissue-engineered bladder replacements (Fig. 136.2). The subtotal cystectomy reservoirs that were not reconstructed and the polymer-only reconstructed bladders showed a marked decrease in bladder compliance (10% and 42% total compliance, respectively). The compliance of the cell-seeded tissue-engineered bladders was almost no different from preoperative values (106%). Histologically, the nonseeded scaffold bladders presented a pattern of normal urothelial cells with a thickened fibrotic submucosa and a thin layer of muscle fibers. The retrieved tissue-engineered bladders showed a normal cellular organization consisting of a trilayer of urothelium, submucosa, and muscle (50).

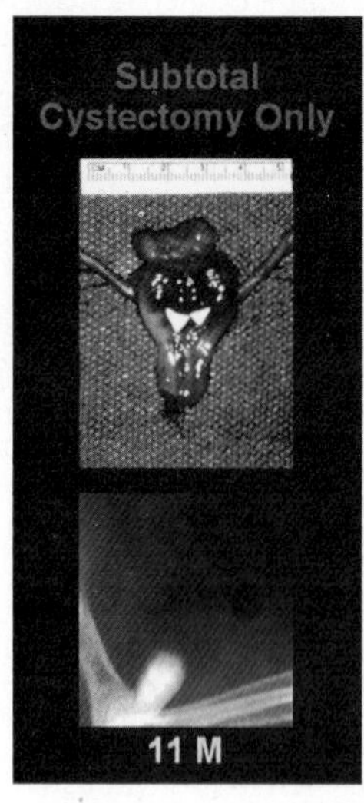

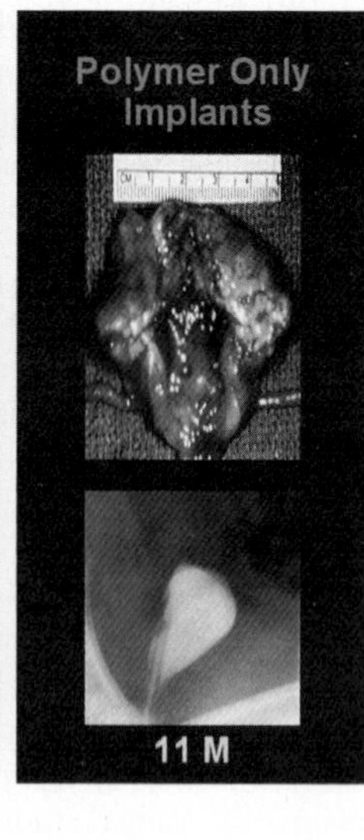

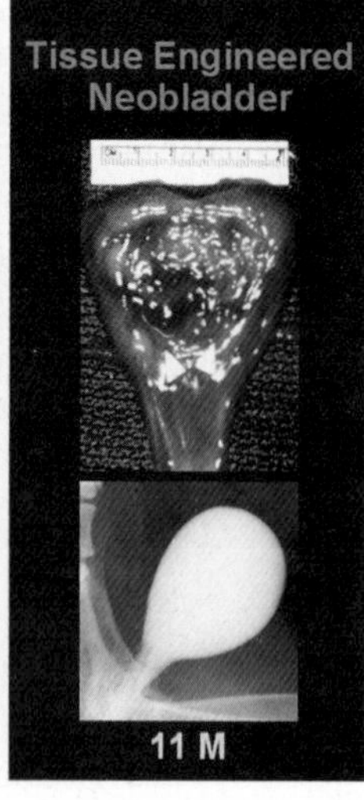


FIGURE 136.2 Gross specimens and cystograms at 11 months of the cystectomy-only, nonseeded controls, and cell-seeded tissue-engineered bladder replacements in dogs. The cystectomy-only bladder had a capacity of 22% of the preoperative value and a decrease in bladder compliance to 10% of the preoperative value. The nonseeded controls showed significant scarring with a capacity of 46% of the preoperative value and a decrease in bladder compliance to 42% of the preoperative value. An average bladder capacity of 95% of the original precystectomy volume was achieved in the cell-seeded tissue-engineered bladder replacements, and the compliance showed almost no difference from preoperative values that were measured when the native bladder was present (106%).

A clinical experience involving engineered bladder tissue for cystoplasty reconstruction was conducted starting in 1999. A small pilot study of seven patients was reported, using a collagen scaffold seeded with cells either with or without omentum coverage, or a combined PGA-collagen scaffold seeded with cells and omental coverage (Fig. 136.3). The patients reconstructed with the engineered bladder tissue created with the PGA-collagen cell-seeded scaffolds showed increased compliance, decreased end-filling pressures, increased capacities, and longer dry periods (2). Although the experience is promising in terms of showing that engineered tissues can be implanted safely, it is just a start in terms of accomplishing the goal of engineering fully functional bladders. Further experimental and clinical work is being conducted.

## Kidney

The kidney is the most challenging organ in the genitourinary system to reconstruct because of its extremely complex structure and function. Concepts for a bioartificial kidney are currently being explored. Some investigators are pursuing the replacement of isolated kidney function parameters using extracorporeal units, while others are aiming to replace total renal function with tissue-engineered bioartificial renal structures.

**Ex Vivo Functioning Renal Units.** Dialysis is currently the most common form of renal replacement therapy. However, the relatively high morbidity and mortality resulting from this process have spurred investigators to seek alternative solutions. In an attempt to assess the viability and physiologic functionality of a cell-seeded device to replace the filtration, transport, metabolic, and endocrinologic functions of the kidney, a synthetic hemofiltration device and a device that contained tissue-engineered porcine renal tubules were incorporated into an extracorporeal perfusion circuit, and this was introduced into acutely uremic dogs. Levels of potassium and blood urea nitrogen (BUN) were controlled during treatment with the device. The fractional reabsorption of sodium and water was possible. Active transport of potassium, bicarbonate, and glucose, as well as a gradual ability to excrete ammonia, was observed. These results demonstrated the feasibility of an extracorporeal assist device that is reinforced by the use of proximal tubular cells (27).

Using similar techniques, the development of a tissue-engineered bioartificial kidney consisting of a conventional hemofiltration cartridge in series with a renal tubule assist device containing human renal proximal tubule cells was used in patients with acute renal failure in the intensive care unit. The initial clinical experience with this bioartificial kidney suggests that renal tubule cell therapy may provide a dynamic

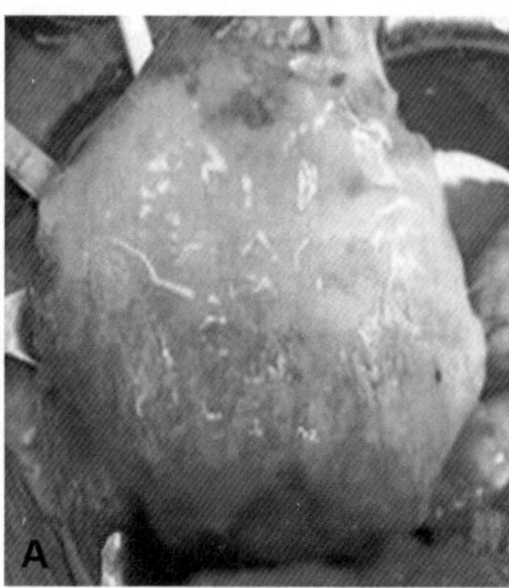

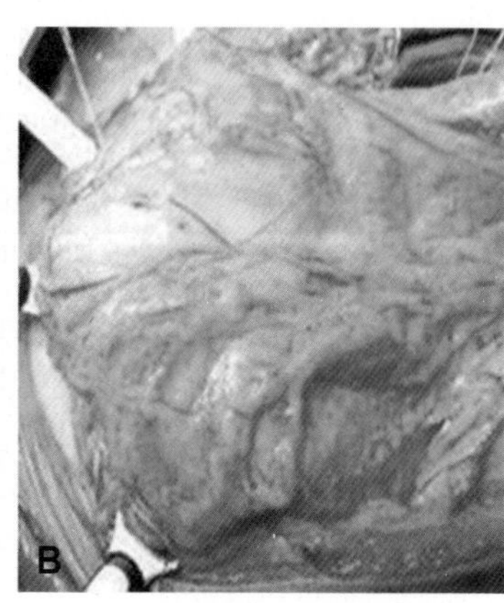


FIGURE 136.3 Construction of an engineered human bladder. **A:** The engineered bladder anastomosed to native bladder tissue with running 4-0 polyglycolic sutures. **B:** Implanted bladder covered with fibrin glue and omentum.

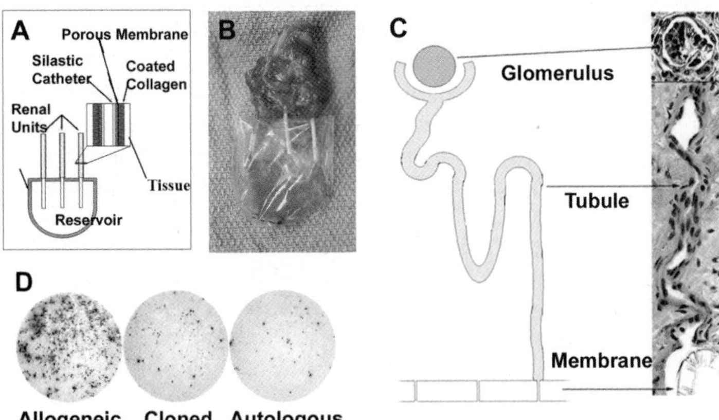


FIGURE 136.4 Combining therapeutic cloning and tissue engineering to produce kidney tissue. **A:** Illustration of the tissue-engineered renal unit. **B:** Renal unit seeded with cloned cells, 3 months after implantation, showing the accumulation of urine-like fluid. **C:** There was a clear unidirectional continuity between the mature glomeruli, their tubules, and the polycarbonate membrane. **D:** Elispot analyses of the frequencies of T cells that secrete IFN-gamma after primary and secondary stimulation with allogeneic renal cells, cloned renal cells, or nuclear donor fibroblasts.

and individualized treatment program as assessed by acute physiologic and biochemical indices (28).

**Creation of Functional Renal Structures in Vivo.** Another approach to improve renal function involves the augmentation of renal tissue with kidney cells expanded in vitro and used for subsequent autologous transplantation. Most recently, an attempt was made to reconstitute renal epithelial cells for the generation of functional nephron units. Renal cells were harvested and expanded in culture. The cells were seeded onto a tubular device constructed from a polycarbonate membrane, which was connected at one end to a Silastic catheter that terminated in a reservoir. The device was implanted in athymic mice. Histologic examination of the implanted devices over time revealed extensive vascularization with formation of glomeruli and highly organized tubulelike structures. Immunocytochemical staining confirmed the renal phenotype. Additionally, yellow fluid was collected from inside the implant, and its creatinine and uric acid concentrations were consistent with the makeup of dilute urine. Further studies have shown the formation of renal structures in cows using nuclear transfer techniques (Fig. 136.4) (40). The expansion of this system to larger, three-dimensional structures is the next challenge awaiting researchers in the urogenital tissue-engineering field.

## Penis

**Reconstruction of Corporal Smooth Muscle.** One of the major components of the phallus is corporal smooth muscle. The creation of autologous functional and structural corporal tissue de novo would be beneficial in cases of congenital abnormality of the genitals and in other situations where reconstruction is functionally and aesthetically necessary. In order to look at the functional parameters of engineered corpora, acellular corporal collagen matrices were obtained from donor rabbit penile tissue, and autologous corpus cavernosal smooth muscle and endothelial cells were harvested, expanded, and seeded on the matrices. The entire rabbit corpora was removed and replaced with the engineered structures. The experimental corporal bodies demonstrated intact structural integrity by cavernosography and showed similar intracorporal pressures by cavernosometry when compared to the normal controls. Rabbits that received scaffolds without cells failed to achieve normal erectile function throughout the study period. However, mating activity in the animals with the cell-seeded corpora appeared normal by 1 month after implantation. The presence of sperm was confirmed during mating, and sperm was present in all rabbits with the engineered corpora. The female rabbits that mated with the animals implanted with engineered corpora conceived and delivered healthy pups. Animals implanted with the matrix alone were unable to demonstrate normal mating activity and failed to ejaculate into the vagina (74,76).

**Engineered Penile Prostheses.** Although silicone is an accepted biomaterial for penile prostheses, biocompatibility is a concern (49,68). Use of a natural prosthesis composed of autologous cells may be advantageous. In a recent study, the feasibility of applying engineered cartilage rods in situ was investigated (77). Autologous chondrocytes were harvested from rabbit ear and expanded in culture. The cells were seeded onto biodegradable poly-L-lactic acid–coated polyglycolic acid polymer rods and then implanted into the corporal spaces of rabbits. Examination at retrieval showed the presence of well-formed, milky-white cartilage structures within the corpora at 1 month, and the polymer scaffolding had degraded by 2 months. There was no evidence of erosion or infection in any of the implantation sites. Subsequent studies were performed to assess the long-term functionality of the cartilage penile rods in vivo. To date, the animals have done well and can copulate and impregnate their female partners without problems.

## Female Genital Tissues

Congenital malformations of the uterus may have profound implications clinically. Patients with cloacal exstrophy and intersex disorders may not have sufficient uterine tissue present for future reproduction. We investigated the possibility of engineering functional uterine tissue using autologous cells. Autologous rabbit uterine smooth muscle and epithelial cells were harvested and expanded in culture. These cells were seeded onto preconfigured uterine-shaped biodegradable polymer scaffolds, and these were used for subtotal uterine tissue replacement in the corresponding autologous animals. Upon retrieval 6 months after implantation, histological, immunocytochemical, and Western blot analyses confirmed the presence of normal uterine tissue components. Biomechanical analyses and organ bath studies showed that the functional characteristics of these tissues were similar to those of normal uterine tissue. Breeding studies using these engineered uteri are currently being performed.

Similarly, several pathologic conditions, including congenital malformations and malignancy, can adversely affect normal vaginal development or anatomy. To investigate tissue-engineering methods of generating vaginal tissue for use in these situations, vaginal epithelial and smooth muscle cells of female rabbits were harvested, grown, and expanded in culture. These cells were seeded onto biodegradable polymer scaffolds, and the cell-seeded constructs were then implanted into nude mice for up to 6 weeks. Immunocytochemical, histological, and Western blot analyses confirmed the presence of vaginal tissue phenotypes. Electrical field stimulation studies in the tissue-engineered constructs showed similar functional properties to those of normal vaginal tissue. When these constructs were used for autologous total vaginal replacement, patent vaginal structures were noted in the tissue-engineered specimens, while the non–cell-seeded structures were noted to be stenotic (21).

## SUMMARY

Tissue-engineering efforts are currently being undertaken for every type of tissue and organ within the urinary system. Most of the effort expended to engineer genitourinary tissues has occurred within the last decade. While some tissue-engineering applications are beginning to enter clinical practice, many of the new tissue-engineering techniques described must be studied further before they can be applied to human disorders. However, recent progress suggests that engineered urologic tissues and cell therapy may have clinical applicability, particularly in reconstruction of this system in children.

## ACKNOWLEDGMENTS

The author would like to thank Dr. Jennifer Olson for editorial assistance with this manuscript.

## *References*


1. Atala A. Tissue engineering, stem cells, and cloning for the regeneration of urologic organs. *Clin Plast Surg* 2003;30:649–667.
2. Atala A, Bauer SB, Soker S, et al. Tissue-engineered autologous bladders for patients needing cystoplasty. *Lancet* 2006;367:1241–1246.
3. Atala A, Cima LG, Kim W, et al. Injectable alginate seeded with chondrocytes as a potential treatment for vesicoureteral reflux. *J Urol* 1993; 150:745–747.
4. Atala A, Freeman MR, Vacanti JP, et al. Implantation in vivo and retrieval of artificial structures consisting of rabbit and human urothelium and human bladder muscle. *J Urol* 1993;150:608–612.
5. Atala A, Guzman L, Retik AB. A novel inert collagen matrix for hypospadias repair. *J Urol* 1999;162:1148–1151.
6. Atala A, Kim W, Paige KT, et al. Endoscopic treatment of vesicoureteral reflux with a chondrocyte-alginate suspension. *J Urol* 1994;152:641–643; discussion 644.
7. Atala A, Vacanti JP, Peters CA, et al. Formation of urothelial structures in vivo from dissociated cells attached to biodegradable polymer scaffolds in vitro. *J Urol* 1992;148:658–662.
8. Badylak SF, Lantz GC, Coffey A, et al. Small intestinal submucosa as a large diameter vascular graft in the dog. *J Surg Res* 1989;47:74–80.
9. Bent AE, Tutrone RT, McLennan MT, et al. Treatment of intrinsic sphincter deficiency using autologous ear chondrocytes as a bulking agent. *Neurourol Urodynam* 2001;20:157–165.
10. Blandy JP. Ileal pouch with transitional epithelium and anal sphincter as a continent urinary reservoir. *J Urol* 1961;86:749–767.
11. Blandy JP. The feasibility of preparing an ideal substitute for the urinary bladder. *Ann Royal Coll Surg Engl* 1964;35:287–311.
12. Blelloch R, Wang Z, Meissner A, et al. Reprogramming efficiency following somatic cell nuclear transfer is influenced by the differentiation and methylation state of the donor nucleus 1. *Stem Cells* 2006;24:2007–2013.
13. Brittberg M, Lindahl A, Nilsson A, et al. Treatment of deep cartilage defects in the knee with autologous chondrocyte transplantation [see comment]. *N Engl J Med* 1994;331:889–895.
14. Brivanlou AH, Gage FH, Jaenisch R, et al. Stem cells. Setting standards for human embryonic stem cells [see comment]. *Science* 2003;300: 913–916.
15. Chancellor MB, Yokoyama T, Tirney S, et al. Preliminary results of myoblast injection into the urethra and bladder wall: a possible method for the treatment of stress urinary incontinence and impaired detrusor contractility. *Neurourol Urodynam* 2000;19:279–287.
16. Chen F, Yoo JJ, Atala A. Acellular collagen matrix as a possible "off the shelf" biomaterial for urethral repair. *Urology* 1999;54:407–410.
17. Cheng E, Rento R, Grayhack JT, et al. Reversed seromuscular flaps in the urinary tract in dogs. *J Urol* 1994;152:2252–2257.
18. Cilento BG, Freeman MR, Schneck FX, et al. Phenotypic and cytogenetic characterization of human bladder urothelia expanded in vitro. *J Urol* 1994;152:665–670.
19. De Coppi P, Bartsch G Jr, Siddiqui MM, et al. Isolation of amniotic stem cell lines with potential for therapy [see comment]. *Nat Biotechnol* 2007; 25:100–106.
20. De Coppi P, Callegari A, Chiavegato A, et al. Amniotic fluid and bone marrow derived mesenchymal stem cells can be converted to smooth muscle cells in the cryo-injured rat bladder and prevent compensatory hypertrophy of surviving smooth muscle cells. *J Urol* 2007;177:369–376.
21. De Filippo RE, Yoo JJ, Atala A. Engineering of vaginal tissue in vivo. *Tissue Eng* 2003;9:301–306.
22. Diamond DA, Caldamone AA. Endoscopic correction of vesicoureteral reflux in children using autologous chondrocytes: preliminary results. *J Urol* 1999;162:1185–1188.
23. Freeman MR, Yoo JJ, Raab G, et al. Heparin-binding EGF-like growth factor is an autocrine growth factor for human urothelial cells and is synthesized by epithelial and smooth muscle cells in the human bladder. *J Clin Invest* 1997;99:1028–1036.
24. Harada N, Yano H, Ohkawa T, et al. New surgical treatment of bladder tumours: mucosal denudation of the bladder. *Br J Urol* 1965;37:545–547.
25. Hochedlinger K, Rideout WM, Kyba M, et al. Nuclear transplantation, embryonic stem cells and the potential for cell therapy. *Hematol J* 2004; 5[Suppl 3]:S114–S117.
26. Huard J, Yokoyama T, Pruchnic R, et al. Muscle-derived cell-mediated ex vivo gene therapy for urological dysfunction. *Gene Ther* 2002; 9:1617–1626.
27. Humes HD, Buffington DA, MacKay SM, et al. Replacement of renal function in uremic animals with a tissue-engineered kidney [see comment]. *Nat Biotechnol* 1999;17:451–455.
28. Humes HD, Weitzel WF, Bartlett RH, et al. Renal cell therapy is associated with dynamic and individualized responses in patients with acute renal failure. *Blood Purif* 2003;21:64–71.
29. Hynes RO. Integrins: versatility, modulation, and signaling in cell adhesion. *Cell* 1992;69:11–25.
30. Kaefer M, Hendren WH, Bauer SB, et al. Reservoir calculi: a comparison of reservoirs constructed from stomach and other enteric segments [see comment]. *J Urol* 1998;160:2187–2190.
31. Kaefer M, Tobin MS, Hendren WH, et al. Continent urinary diversion: the Children's Hospital experience. *J Urol* 1997;157:1394–1399.
32. Kim BS, Baez CE, Atala A. Biomaterials for tissue engineering. *World J Urol* 2000;18:2–9.
33. Kim BS, Mooney DJ. Development of biocompatible synthetic extracellular matrices for tissue engineering. *Trends Biotechnol* 1998;16:224–230.
34. Kropp BP, Cheng EY, Lin HK, et al. Reliable and reproducible bladder regeneration using unseeded distal small intestinal submucosa. *J Urol* 2004;172:1710–1713.
35. Kropp BP, Ludlow JK, Spicer D, et al. Rabbit urethral regeneration using small intestinal submucosa onlay grafts. *Urology* 1998;52:138–142.
36. Kropp BP, Rippy MK, Badylak SF, et al. Regenerative urinary bladder augmentation using small intestinal submucosa: urodynamic and histopathologic assessment in long-term canine bladder augmentations. *J Urol* 1996;155:2098–2104.
37. Lai JY, Yoon CY, Yoo JJ, et al. Phenotypic and functional characterization of in vivo tissue engineered smooth muscle from normal and pathological bladders. *J Urol* 2002;168:1853–1857; discussion 1858.

38. Lailas NG, Cilento B, Atala A. Progressive ureteral dilation for subsequent ureterocystoplasty. *J Urol* 1996;156:1151–1153.
39. Landman J, Olweny E, Sundaram CP, et al. Laparoscopic mid sagittal hemicystectomy and bladder reconstruction with small intestinal submucosa and reimplantation of ureter into small intestinal submucosa: 1-year followup. *J Urol* 2004;171:2450–2455.
40. Lanza RP, Chung HY, Yoo JJ, et al. Generation of histocompatible tissues using nuclear transplantation [see comment]. *Nat Biotechnol* 2002;20: 689–696.
41. le Roux PJ. Endoscopic urethroplasty with unseeded small intestinal submucosa collagen matrix grafts: a pilot study. *J Urol* 2005;173:140–143.
42. Liebert M, Hubbel A, Chung M, et al. Expression of mal is associated with urothelial differentiation in vitro: identification by differential display reverse-transcriptase polymerase chain reaction. *Differentiation* 1997;61: 177–185.
43. Liebert M, Wedemeyer G, Abruzzo LV, et al. Stimulated urothelial cells produce cytokines and express an activated cell surface antigenic phenotype. *Semin Urol* 1991;9:124–130.
44. Lin HK, Cowan R, Moore P, et al. Characterization of neuropathic bladder smooth muscle cells in culture. *J Urol* 2004;171:1348–1352.
45. Machluf M, Orsola A, Boorjian S, et al. Microencapsulation of Leydig cells: a system for testosterone supplementation. *Endocrinology* 2003;144: 4975–4979.
46. McDougal WS. Metabolic complications of urinary intestinal diversion. *J Urol* 1992;147:1199–1208.
47. Meissner A, Wernig M, Jaenisch R. Direct reprogramming of genetically unmodified fibroblasts into pluripotent stem cells 1. *Nat Biotechnol* 2007; 25:1177–1181.
48. Nguyen HT, Park JM, Peters CA, et al. Cell-specific activation of the HB-EGF and ErbB1 genes by stretch in primary human bladder cells. *In Vitro Cell Dev Biol Anim* 1999;35:371–375.
49. Nukui F, Okamoto S, Nagata M, et al. Complications and reimplantation of penile implants. *Int J Urol* 1997;4:52–54.
50. Oberpenning F, Meng J, Yoo JJ, et al. De novo reconstitution of a functional mammalian urinary bladder by tissue engineering [see comment]. *Nat Biotechnol* 1999;17:149–155.
51. Oesch I. Neourothelium in bladder augmentation. An experimental study in rats. *Eur Urol* 1988;14:328–329.
52. Okita K, Ichisaka T, Yamanaka S. Generation of germline-competent induced pluripotent stem cells 1. *Nature* 2007;448:313–317.
53. Olsen L, Bowald S, Busch C, et al. Urethral reconstruction with a new synthetic absorbable device. An experimental study. *Scand J Urol Nephrol* 1992;26:323–326.
54. Piechota HJ, Dahms SE, Nunes LS, et al. In vitro functional properties of the rat bladder regenerated by the bladder acellular matrix graft. *J Urol* 1998;159:1717–1724.
55. Ponder KP, Gupta S, Leland F, et al. Mouse hepatocytes migrate to liver parenchyma and function indefinitely after intrasplenic transplantation. *Proc Natl Acad Sci U S A* 1991;88:1217–1221.
56. Portis AJ, Elbahnasy AM, Shalhav AL, et al. Laparoscopic augmentation cystoplasty with different biodegradable grafts in an animal model. *J Urol* 2000;164:1405–1411.
57. Probst M, Dahiya R, Carrier S, et al. Reproduction of functional smooth muscle tissue and partial bladder replacement. *Br J Urol* 1997;79:505–515.
58. Puthenveettil JA, Burger MS, Reznikoff CA. Replicative senescence in human uroepithelial cells. *Adv Exp Med Biol* 1999;462:83–91.
59. Roger EDF, James JY, Anthony A. Urethral replacement using cell seeded tubularized collagen matrices. *J Urol* 2002;168:1789–1793.
60. Salle JL, Fraga JC, Lucib A, et al. Seromuscular enterocystoplasty in dogs. *J Urol* 1990;144:454–456; discussion 460.
61. Satar N, Yoo JJ, Atala A. Progressive dilation for bladder tissue expansion. *J Urol* 1999;162:829–831.
62. Scriven SD, Booth C, Thomas DF, et al. Reconstitution of human urothelium from monolayer cultures. *J Urol* 1997;158:1147–1152.
63. Sievert KD, Bakircioglu ME, Nunes L, et al. Homologous acellular matrix graft for urethral reconstruction in the rabbit: histological and functional evaluation. *J Urol* 2000;163:1958–1965.
64. Strasser H, Berjukow S, Marksteiner R, et al. Stem cell therapy for urinary stress incontinence. *Exp Gerontol* 2004;39:1259–1265.
65. Sutherland RS, Baskin LS, Hayward SW, et al. Regeneration of bladder urothelium, smooth muscle, blood vessels and nerves into an acellular tissue matrix. *J Urol* 1996;156:571–577.
66. Takahashi K, Tanabe K, Ohnuki M, et al. Induction of pluripotent stem cells from adult human fibroblasts by defined factors. *Cell* 2007;131: 861–872.
67. Takahashi K, Yamanaka S. Induction of pluripotent stem cells from mouse embryonic and adult fibroblast cultures by defined factors 2. *Cell* 2006; 126:663–676.
68. Thomalla JV, Thompson ST, Rowland RG, et al. Infectious complications of penile prosthetic implants. *J Urol* 1987;138:65–67.
69. Thomson JA, Itskovitz-Eldor J, Shapiro SS, et al. Embryonic stem cell lines derived from human blastocysts [see comment][erratum appears in Science 1998 Dec 4;282(5395):1827]. *Science* 1998;282:1145–1147.
70. Wernig M, Meissner A, Foreman R, et al. In vitro reprogramming of fibroblasts into a pluripotent ES-cell-like state 1. *Nature* 2007;448:318–324.
71. Yiou R, Lefaucheur JP, Atala A. The regeneration process of the striated urethral sphincter involves activation of intrinsic satellite cells. *Anat Embryol* 2003;206:429–435.
72. Yiou R, Yoo JJ, Atala A. Restoration of functional motor units in a rat model of sphincter injury by muscle precursor cell autografts. *Transplantation* 2003;76:1053–1060.
73. Yokoyama T, Huard J, Chancellor MB. Myoblast therapy for stress urinary incontinence and bladder dysfunction. *World J Urol* 2000;18:56–61.
74. Yoo JJ, Atala A. Tissue engineering of genitourinary organs. *Ernst Schering Research Foundation Workshop* 2002;35:105–127.
75. Yoo JJ, Meng J, Oberpenning F, et al. Bladder augmentation using allogenic bladder submucosa seeded with cells. *Urology* 1998;51:221–225.
76. Yoo JJ, Park HJ, Atala A. Tissue-engineering applications for phallic reconstruction. *World J Urol* 2000;18:62–66.
77. Yoo JJ, Park HJ, Lee I, et al. Autologous engineered cartilage rods for penile reconstruction. *J Urol* 1999;162:1119–1121.
78. Yu J, Vodyanik MA, Smuga-Otto K, et al. Induced pluripotent stem cell lines derived from human somatic cells. *Science* 2007;318:1917–1920.


# CHAPTER 137 ■ IMAGE-GUIDED THERAPY: CURRENT PRACTICE AND FUTURE DIRECTIONS

PETER PINTO AND HAL B. HOOPER

The use of imaging technology to guide urologic therapy has traditionally found itself limited to one of three modalities: direct visualization, ultrasound, and fluoroscopy. For many urologic conditions these technologies form the bedrock of detection and therapy. For instance, cystoscopy remains the gold standard in the detection, surveillance of, and treatment for superficial bladder cancer. Although other techniques may be employed, none have yet gained wide acceptance.

The declining cost and ever-increasing resolution of advanced imaging devices such as computerized tomography (CT) and magnetic resonance imaging (MRI) scanners has led to their increased availability. Whereas such devices were once quite limited in the quality of the data they could provide and were available sporadically at best, their increasing use as a first-line diagnostic tool, along with current medicolegal requirements, has revolutionized a wide variety of diagnostic algorithms across the field of medicine.

The above factors, combined with the increasing interest of both patient and practitioner in reducing the potential morbidity associated with highly invasive interventions, has fueled the investigation of a wide variety of less invasive techniques for the treatment of a variety of urologic diseases. In addition, circumstances beyond the realm of control of the practitioner, both fiscal and patient-driven, incentivize reducing the number of hospital days for the therapy of a given condition. These conditions have given rise to the nascent field of image-guided therapy.

We will discuss image-guided therapy in the broadest sense, including ultrasound, endoscopy, and fluoroscopy, as well as therapeutic techniques guided in real time by CT and MRI scanners.

## URINARY TRACT ENDOSCOPY

Endoscopy, primarily the management of urinary calculi, represents the historical forefront of image-guided therapy in the field of urology.

Bozzini of Frankfort is credited with the first endoscopic investigations, popularly dated to 1805 (1). Fisher and Segalas also described the construction and use of cystoscopic apparatuses for urethral visualization in the 1820s (2). These early efforts were quickly abandoned, however, as reflected candlelight was insufficient to adequately illuminate the urinary tract sufficient to facilitate adequate examination or manipulation. It was left to Desmoreaux in 1853 to claim the mantle of "Father of Cystoscopy" and to describe the urethral and vesicular mucosa of a living patient. With the aid of petroleum-fired lamps, reflecting mirrors, and a refinement of Bozzini's design of two nested metal tubes, he was able to overcome the technical challenges that had stymied his forebears and to perform detailed examination of the lower urinary tract (3).

Technology has, of course, propelled the management of urinary calculi, urothelial tumors, and other urinary tract pathology beyond the imagination of the earliest investigators. A series of technologic evolutions—the use of fiberoptics for light and image transmission, wire-guided flexible metal instruments, laser lithotripsy, and high-definition closed-circuit television picture reproduction—has produced the ability to perform any number of manipulations for a wide variety of conditions. The indications for and details of these therapies are discussed elsewhere in this text, but endoscopy of the urinary system bears mention as the forebear of all other image-guided therapies in the field of urology.

## IMAGE-GUIDED THERAPY IN THE MANAGEMENT OF RENAL TUMORS

Although there is wide variability between reported series as to the percentage of incidentally detected renal masses (25% to 84% in a review of several recent series [4–6]), the widespread use of imaging technologies for the diagnosis of routine complaints ensures that this trend will continue.

Many of these masses will be <4 cm in diameter at the time of detection (7), and thus their management choices are varied. Treatment has recently focused on sparing as much renal parenchyma as possible. Nephron-sparing procedures are also essential in the management of the cohort of patients with heritable kidney cancers such as von Hippel-Lindau (VHL) disease, Birt-Hogg-Dube (BHD) syndrome, and hereditary papillary renal cell carcinoma (HPRCC). Many of these patients will require multiple interventions for their renal tumors.

The development of minimally invasive surgical (MIS) techniques utilizing image guidance is often an excellent option for both subsets of patients. Several of the more widely available options, including their relative benefits and risks, are discussed below.

### Laparoscopic Partial Nephrectomy with Intraoperative Ultrasound

Although the reported complication rate of laparoscopic partial nephrectomy (LPN) varies widely and is highly operator-dependent, recent literature reviews suggest these rates to be comparable with those of open partial nephrectomy (OPN). A recent review of the available published series undertaken by Porpiglia et al. (8) suggests that while the overall rate of hemorrhage is slightly higher in LPN series than in OPN series (mean of 5% versus 3.2%, respectively), the overall rate of surgical complications with LPN is roughly equivalent (4.1% to 38.6% in OPN versus 9% to 33% in reviewed LPN series). Furthermore, recently published data indicate that increased experience with LPN will reduce complication rates to that of OPN (9). Finally, LPN potentially offers shorter length of stay (5.7 versus 2.9 days) and reduced cost when compared with the open approach, making this option attractive to provider and patient alike (10).

Although preoperative imaging is essential for operative planning and choice of port location, tumor location and nature (endophytic versus exophytic) often make definitive laparoscopic lesion identification and determination of margin difficult. Intraoperative ultrasound is thus often employed to assist in tumor location and adequate resection while minimizing the amount of normal parenchyma removed. Additionally, the relationship of the tumor to structures deeper within the renal sinus may be more readily appreciated. In situations where the presence of venocaval thrombus is equivocal by preoperative imaging, intraoperative ultrasound will assist in definitive diagnosis and in-field management and extirpation (11).

In a National Cancer Institute (NCI) published series of patients with hereditary renal carcinoma, intraoperative ultrasound identified tumors that were undetectable by the surgeon in 25% of cases, some as large as 4 cm, of which 50% were pathologically proven renal cell carcinoma (RCC) (12). Campbell et al. (13) report that although the use of intraoperative ultrasound is no more accurate in the detection of tumors than the combination of preoperative CT imaging and direct inspection for multifocal disease, the detection of small endophytic tumors and of the intrarenal extent of deep tumors was enhanced by its use.

## Cryotherapy

Cryotherapy has emerged as a viable and widely accepted alternative to surgical management of small renal tumors. In most commercially available systems, tissue cooling is created via a heat-sink effect due to the vaporization of a cryogenic liquid, typically liquid nitrogen or argon, between an inner and outer probe lumen. This rapid cooling is alternated with either a rapid thawing mediated by a separate cryogenic liquid or passive thawing. This process is repeated at least twice in most described techniques, although some groups advocate additional cycles (14). Direct tissue destruction by ice crystal formation, local vascular disruption, induction of apoptotic signals, and immunologically mediated destruction of cells within the ablated area that survive the initial freeze-thaw cycles provide for a highly effective ablative modality (7).

Adequacy of treatment has been shown in a porcine model to require cooling cells to −19.4°C, though clinical practice commonly chills tissue to −40°C to ensure adequate tissue destruction. This equates to a roughly 0.5- to 1.0-cm extension of the ice-ball beyond the tumor margin (15). Although widely investigated as a laparoscopic ablative technology, several examples in the available literature support the efficacy and safety of percutaneous cryotherapeutic ablation (PCA) as an image-guided technique (14,16–20).

As mentioned above, PCA techniques vary widely depending upon the chosen imaging modality. The importance of proper probe placement, lesion location and thus accessibility, and the use of an adequate number of probes to generate a sufficient ablative margin must be considered in preoperative planning. Serial imaging throughout treatment to monitor ice-ball margin and its proximity to adjacent structures is essential for both safety and efficacy. The choice of general anesthesia versus sedation varies, with most MRI-based techniques opting for a general approach due to procedure length and the ability to more tightly regulate diaphragmatic excursion. All protocols, however, must take into account the location of adjacent organs and structures, especially in the treatment of anterior renal lesions. Patient positioning, external compression, and needle-based methods such as "hydrodissection" (the introduction of sterile saline between adjacent viscera and the lesion to be ablated), have all been described as safe and effective methods of reducing collateral damage during ice-ball formation (17,19,21).

Gupta et al. (16) describe a series of 27 enhancing tumors treated in 20 patients by a CT-guided, percutaneous approach under conscious sedation. Tumors were located both centrally and peripherally and ranged in size from 1.0 to 4.6 cm. Ice-ball formation was tracked by intermittent, intraprocedural CT, with a margin of over 1.2 cm obtained in all cases through two freeze-thaw cycles and only one major complication (two-unit transfusion) reported. Only one lesion demonstrated enhancement on follow-up CT, with a mean follow-up interval of 5.9 months.

An MRI-guided percutaneous approach in 23 patients is described by Silverman et al. (19). A special procedure room was required due to the presence of a high-field magnet and the choice of general anesthesia. Tumors in this series also measured from 1.0 to 4.6 cm and were located centrally and peripherally. Two major complications were noted (one 1-unit transfusion and one abscess due to involvement of an adjacent bowel loop). Ice-ball formation was tracked by serial MRIs, and a 5-mm overlap was considered sufficient through two freeze-thaw cycles. Twenty-four of 26 tumors were considered ablated by the first treatment on serial follow-up MRI (mean follow-up of 14 months). A subsequent report by this same group noted that external manual compression of adjacent bowel loops was safe and efficacious at displacing the interested organ from the treatment field in 14 patients, further improving the safety profile of this intervention (17).

The most commonly reported complications of the percutaneous approach are operative site pain and parasthesias, although more serious complications, such as renal fracture, ureterocalyceal injury, hemorrhage, and bowel injury, are certainly possible and have been reported.

As with any percutaneous ablative interventions, the lack of histologic confirmation of complete tumor destruction remains problematic (15). Many centers make use of follow-up imaging with either contrast-enhanced CT or MRI imaging and an interval of 1 to 6 months from treatment to the initial scan. Contrast enhancement in the bed of ablation is most often cited as sufficient evidence of local recurrence and should recommend expeditious biopsy to rule out local recurrence.

Shingleton and Sewell (18) report no radiographic evidence of local tumor recurrence in their MRI-guided PCA cohort of four patients with a median follow-up of 14 months; only one patient required retreatment. Although data from the Cleveland Clinic (22) indicate an excellent short-term correlation between radiographic imaging and pathological analysis with laparoscopic cryoablation, poor correlation was seen in their percutaneous radiofrequency ablation cohort (six patients with a positive posttreatment biopsy and no enhancement on MRI or CT).

## Radiofrequency Ablation (RFA)

FDA approved in the treatment of soft tissue lesions and long used for the treatment of bone and liver tumors, RFA generates direct tissue damage by the controlled delivery of alternating current. Hyperthermic protein denaturation and membrane destruction result in coagulative necrosis with extensive local tissue destruction. Energy delivery from the generator is controlled by measuring temperature or local tissue impedance at the probe tip, with temperatures in excess of 70°C for 1 minute often considered adequate, although many protocols have been published that differ by institution (4–6,21,23,24). The infusion of hypertonic saline at the probe tip is often employed to decrease impedance, resulting in larger RFA lesions, referred to as "wet" RFA (15).

Of particular concern in RFA is the presence of nearby major vascular structures or tumors more centrally located. Highly vascularized areas suffer from a "heat-sink" effect that will produce temperature variations within the supposed field of ablation. Although long used for focal ablation of the liver, the kidney's high vascular flux, containing 5 times as much blood per gram as the liver, presents special challenges for successful RFA (25). Such features may prevent tissues from reaching the requisite temperature, preventing adequate tumor destruction. Although this phenomenon has become less pronounced with the introduction of higher-powered generators, medullary and corticomedullary lesions demonstrate persistently higher failure rates than exophytic cortical lesions (26). Some authors recommend renal artery occlusion to circumvent this effect and have described the execution of such in the laparoscopic literature, although a percutaneous approach would prohibit this precaution (15,27).

RFA also proves challenging when trying to monitor the zone of ablation achieved. Unlike cryotherapy, which generates a clearly demarcated barrier between the involved and spared tissues, RFA generates a lesion that resists easy immediate characterization. As ablated tissues fail to enhance with intravascular contrast, intraprocedural contrast-enhanced imaging may help estimate the amount of cellular destruction achieved. For patients with deranged renal function, however, this may prove problematic, particularly with CT-guided modalities.

A series by Fotiadis et al. (23) has been published in which the ablative properties of ethanol, long used in the treatment of hepatic lesions, was combined with CT-guided percutaneous RFA in the ablation of small renal lesions (mean diameter <3 cm, range 0.8 to 6.0 cm). Animal studies suggest that this approach may cause extensive local thrombosis, thereby diminishing the "heat-sink" effect described above. The amount of ethanol administered centrally within the tumors was quite small, 1.7 mL on average, but the need for reablation was small, with only 6 of 28 patients requiring additional treatment as a result of follow-up imaging, somewhat below the rate of 27.5% cited elsewhere (7,23).

An excellent review of the available literature on percutaneous RFA was recently conducted by Park and Cadeddu (28). They reviewed series performed under ultrasound, CT, and MRI guidance using all widely available commercial electrode systems. Lesion size both in this review and within individual series was noted to be an independent predictor for single-session failure, with 3 cm commonly noted as the breakpoint for retreatment (5,15). They noted a combined minor/major complication rate of 5% to 10%, with pyelocalyceal injuries (stricture and urinoma) and hemorrhage requiring surgical intervention the most common major complications (28). Although the risk of injury to adjacent viscera is low, techniques to further minimize these undesired outcomes have also been successfully explored in light of previous experience with RFA of hepatic lesions, including the interposition of carbon dioxide gas or sterile fluid (21). This review also notes that deliberate RFA of tumors located immediately adjacent to the collecting system should be discouraged due to the high risk of stricture creation and persistent urine leak.

Cancer-specific survival was noted to be excellent, with an aggregate cancer-specific survival of around 95% at a mean follow-up of 19.5 months across series. Salvage nephrectomy or partial nephrectomy was performed in only 1.1% of cases. However, definitive histologic demonstration of complete tumor ablation is lacking in this percutaneous technique. Although previously published reports of skip lesions and incomplete tumor ablation after RFA exist, contrary work indicates that oncologic control with RFA may well be adequate (29,30). Radiologic demonstration of lack of tumor growth or enhancement on CT or MRI at follow-up is typically deemed adequate, with initial scans typically performed at 1 month. Unfortunately, the presence of enhancement on follow-up imaging does not definitively indicate recurrence, as granulomatous reactions or infection in the ablated bed may also enhance, and absence of enhancement also does not signify complete tumor ablation. Salvage treatment should therefore proceed with deliberation and only after definitive rebiopsy (4,13).

## Other Ablative Technologies

Although PCA and RFA have both garnered FDA approval for the treatment of small renal lesions, multiple other image-guided ablative modalities are under investigation. Although few of these methods have been evaluated to date beyond modest initial clinical trials, preliminary investigation in animal models and with selected patients continues apace.

Most promising among these emerging technologies is that of high-intensity focused ultrasound (HIFU). By combining a parabolic reflector with a piezoceramic element within an external transducer, highly focused ultrasound waves can be delivered precisely to lesions of interest, quickly (<1 second) raising tissue temperatures in a sharply circumscribed area and producing focal coagulative necrosis via thermal effects and mechanical disruption of membranes via microbubble cavitation (32). Although this phenomenon was realized in the 1940s, advances in technology have decreased the size and power demands of HIFU transducers, thus reviving interest in their use.

Hacker et al. (33) performed transcutaneous HIFU on 19 patients and 24 dogs under general anesthesia prior to radical nephrectomy using in-line ultrasound guidance and a handheld transducer. Although the technique was generally safe, two grade III skin burns were reported in the human arm at higher power settings. The quality of ablation was variable and did not seem to correlate with increases in delivered energy (from 200 to 1,600 W) or pulse duration (1 to 5 seconds). Indeed, some hyperechoic areas visualized during ablation showed no histologic evidence of necrosis, although delayed nephrectomy specimens in the canine arm of the study showed more reliable tissue ablation. Furthermore, the use of in-line ultrasound for intraprocedural guidance was noted as a major limitation. Backscatter during sonication caused by microbubble formation prevented real-time visualization of lesion formation, impairing consistent energy delivery.

Tumor heterogeneity, respiratory motion, and the absorptive and reflective properties of intervening tissues may all contribute to reduce the power applied to the tissue of interest from that generated at the transducer. The transducer has been mounted on a mechanical arm to minimize potential operator error, and the employment of MRI has been hypothesized as a technique for improving guidance (34–36). Major technical hurdles still exist to the successful and widespread deployment of HIFU for the ablation of small renal tumors, but investigation continues at many centers.

There are also several other potential techniques. The use of laparoscopic microwave antennas to induce coagulative necrosis has been successfully tested in a rabbit model and may be adaptable to an image-guided probe-based technique in the future (37). MR-guided laser interstitial therapy, involving the placement of laser fibers directly into malignant tissue, has been investigated under MR guidance, although no published human trials exist at this time (15). Similarly, a number of catheter-based techniques for the delivery of ablative agents have been reported, but none have yet gained widespread acceptance.

## Image-Guided Therapy in the Management of Prostate Cancer (PCa)

Asymptomatically elevated PSA levels drive many to choose biopsy, with the detection of small amounts of low-risk disease often being the result. Although early, definitive, whole-gland therapy for these patients offers them a high likelihood of disease-free survival, the potential morbidities involved with the currently available options are significant. Impotence, urinary incontinence, proctitis, and, for those who choose surgical excision, perioperative complications such as deep venous thromboses and injury to adjacent organs are reported risks of whole-gland therapy.

Although it is likely that many men with low-risk disease will die with, rather than of, their PCa, which individuals fall into which category cannot currently be determined prospectively. The impact of whole-gland therapeutic morbidities may potentially produce a profound diminishment in quality of life. Many groups have initiated the investigation of novel focal therapies or the modification of existing treatment modalities in the treatment of PCa to minimize potential intervention-related adverse outcomes.

### Image-Guided Prostate Biopsy

As prostate biopsy remains the gold standard for cancer diagnosis, increased screening has predictably increased the annual number of biopsies performed. Biopsy is typically performed with TRUS guidance in a sextant fashion, and the yield of the most optimistic reported extended biopsy schema (performed exclusively based on elevated PSA) was only 44% (39). For individuals undergoing repeat biopsy, this rate can be expected to fall, with rates as low as 4% to 12% on the fourth attempt and a higher attendant complication rate (40). Many image-guided techniques have been reported that seek to address the shortcoming with this extant biopsy paradigm.

Investigations into the use of MRI, in particular endorectal coil MRI (erMRI), for the detection of prostate cancer has become increasingly widespread. The use of an endorectal coil to reduce the signal-to-noise ratio increases image resolution, particularly of T-2 weighted images, and reduces the amount of time needed to perform spectroscopic and contrast-enhanced studies. Signal-to-noise is also reduced by the use of higher field magnets, and 3-tesla (3-T) devices are increasingly available. Although published results for specificity and sensitivity vary widely across studies and between the widely used modalities, MRI remains the most sensitive available imaging technique for the detection of prostate cancer (41).

Anastasiadis et al. (42) report on their experience with an in-gantry biopsy system guided by erMRI. Twenty-seven men with one prior negative biopsy were sampled in a 1.5-T closed-bore magnet under local anesthetic using an MRI-compatible template, needle guide, and biopsy needles based on T-2 weighted images. The reported yield of 55% was well above that reported in the literature for biopsies performed with TRUS guidance alone.

The NCI group (41) have reported their initial experience with the use of both 1.5- and 3.0-T MRI instruments to improve the yield of ultrasound-guided transrectal prostate biopsy in a cohort of men at increased risk for PCa. Through a proprietary arrangement with Phillips USA they have developed a system for the registration of previously acquired MRI images with real-time TRUS onto a single platform. Although their initial reported clinical data do not indicate a statistically significant increase in cancer yields, they acknowledge that a number of improvements in their platform have yet to be realized.

A subsequent report by the NCI/Phillips group (43) details the development of a motion-compensation system via the use of closed-loop magnetic tracking for the above-mentioned image fusion platform. *Ex vivo* phantom studies indicate that an accuracy of 2 to 3 mm can be achieved with this refinement in place. Ongoing investigation will determine if this increased accuracy can equate to increased biopsy yield.

### Permanent Prostate Seed Implantation Brachytherapy (PPI)

Available data for the use of intraprostatic radionucleotide-containing seeds (I-125 or Pd-103) in the treatment of PCa suggests a durable oncologic outcome as measured by biochemical relapse, whether this treatment modality is used as monotherapy for low-risk disease or is used in combination with external beam radiation therapy (EBRT) for intermediate- and high-risk patients (44).

Treatment planning to ensure that the low-energy photons used in brachytherapy sufficiently cover the prostate volume while minimizing the dose to adjacent structures, particularly the urethra and rectum, is critical. Planning has traditionally consisted of preoperative imaging of the prostate in contiguous segments using a TRUS probe and correlation of these images with biopsy results. This evaluative study is subject to the vagaries of patient positioning, probe angle and attitude, and change in anatomic relationships in the conscious versus the anesthetized patient. The above factors may conspire to produce either "hot" or "cold" spots, adversely affecting either oncologic efficacy or toxicity profiles (44).

Several groups have reported their experience with the use of MRI guidance in both the planning and execution of PPI to improve dosimetric coverage. Researchers have reported on the use of a real-time interventional 0.5-T open-configuration MRI system for preoperative dosimetric planning, probe tracking, and "on the fly" plan modification based on seed deployment as measured by T-2 weighted imaging (45). They used a specially designed MRI-compatible perineal template for the introduction of I-125 sources with the patient in the lithotomy position under general anesthesia. All the required probes and other equipment were also MRI-compatible. In a series of ten patients, they report median seed misplacement at 3 mm, which corresponded to underdosing of 1% to 13%. With the use of online MRI guidance, they were able to recover as much as 12% of this lost coverage with the addition of a median of eight seeds (46).

A collaborative group from Johns Hopkins University and the NCI/NIH (47) describe the use of a closed-bore 1.5-T system for the guided transperineal delivery of high-dose-rate Ir-192 sources in four patients. They constructed an MRI-compatible device combining the endorectal coil and perineal template and placed the patient in the lateral decubitus position for improved access. Three-dimensional reconstructions indicate that this approach delivered the desired radiation dose to over 90% of the gland, averaging approximately 2-mm needle placement accuracy, with <5% urethral toxicity. Total required time for imaging and therapy was an average of 6 hours.

Muntener et al. (48) have developed a pneumatically actuated, MRI-compatible, fully automated robot for the delivery of PPI. By eliminating the use of electrical circuitry in this device, they report successful use of the device in magnets up to 7 T with no evidence of field perturbation. Furthermore, the device is highly accurate, with a step size of 0.05 mm. Use of this device for the placement of PPI implants in a tissue mockup suggest submillimeter accuracy, with a mean error of 0.72 mm reported in the automated placement of a group of 125 seeds. Although no clinical results are, as yet, reported in this series, continued research is planned.

## Image-Guided Focal Ablation in the Management of PCa

The downward stage migration of PCa in the PSA era has created a situation in which many men may be receiving overtreatment for their disease. As fewer than a third of men diagnosed in this country chose to defer therapy for their disease, according to the NCI SEER database from 1995 to 1999, the evidence suggests that almost 50% of men treated with whole-gland extirpation or irradiation may have died with, rather than of, their disease (49).

This discrepancy, combined with recently published data regarding favorable oncologic-specific survival results with isolated treatment of PCa index lesions, has promoted a widespread and aggressive investigation of subtotal therapeutic modalities for the treatment of PCa (50). Many image-guided focal ablation methods are under investigation, including focal brachytherapy, laser interstitial ablation, cryotherapy, HIFU, and gamma-knife. However, oncologic outcomes data remain sparse at this time for most of these platforms, with the exception of HIFU and cryotherapy. Yet even in these cases, studies involving their use in concert with sophisticated image guidance are currently quite limited.

Regardless of the modality chosen, the decision of who should receive focal therapy continues to be elusive. Clearly these patients should have organ-confined disease, although there the consensus ends. Despite the fact that PCa is a multifocal disease, data suggest that for clinically relevant tumors, the index lesion, that is to say, the largest focus of PCa found at resection, is of the most interest. Published retrospective data indicate that the overall Gleason score, risk of extracapsular extension, and disease-free survival as a function of tumor volume can be determined with the index lesion in >90% of cases (49).

Though PSA screening and the aforementioned stage migration have consistently reduced the size of this index lesion over the past two decades, the mean size of 2.4 cc is well above the detection limits reported in the literature for erMRI. Reports exist in the literature citing >85% sensitivity for the detection of lesions >1 cm by T-2 weighted eMRI combined with spectroscopy (49,51). Despite these preliminary successes, MRI remains to be validated as a stand-alone method for the detection and staging of PCa.

## *References*


1. Kumar P, Nargund V. Samuel Pepys: a patient perspective of lithotomy in 17th century England. *J Urol* 2006;175:1221–1224.
2. Tromponkis C, Giannakaparlias S, Tonlonpidis S. Lithotomy by empirical doctors in the 19th century: a traditional surgical technique that lasted through the centuries. *J Urol* 2007;178:2284–2286.
3. Luys G. *A treatise on cystoscopy and urethroscopy*. St. Louis: Mosby, 1918.
4. Park SM, Cadeddu JA. Outcomes of radiofrequency ablation for kidney cancer. *Cancer Control* 2007;14(3):205–210.
5. Mayo-Smith WW, Parikh PM, Pezzullo JA, et al. Imaging-guided percutaneous radiofrequency ablation of solid renal masses: techniques and outcomes of 38 treatment sessions in 32 consecutive patients. *Am J Roentgenol* 2003;180:1503–1508.
6. Shuvro H, Roy-Choudhury JEIC, Cooksey G, et al. Early experience with percutaneous radiofrequency ablation of small solid renal masses. *Am J Roentgenol* 2003;180:1055–1061.
7. Mouraviev V, Van Poppel H, Polascik TJ. Current status of minimally invasive ablative techniques in the treatment of small renal tumours. *Eur Urol* 2007;51:328–336.
8. Porpiglia F, Billia M, Scarpa RM. Laparoscopic versus open partial nephrectomy: analysis of the current literature. *Eur Urol* 2008; 53(4): 732–742.
9. Simmons MN, Gill IS. Decreased complications of contemporary laparoscopic partial nephrectomy: use of a standardized reporting system. *J Urol* 2007; 177:2067–2073.
10. Park S, Pearle S, Cadeddu JA, et al. Laparoscopic and open partial nephrectomy: cost comparison with analysis of individual parameters. *J Endourol* 2007;21(12):1449–1454.
11. Choyke PL, Daryanani K. Intraoperative ultrasound of the kidney. *Ultrasound Q* 2001;17(4):245–253.
12. Choyke PL, Daryanani KD, Hewitt SM, et al. Intraoperative ultrasound during renal parenchymal sparing surgery for hereditary renal cancers: a 10-year experience. *J Urol* 2001;165:397–400.
13. Cambell EA. Intraoperative evaluation of renal cell carcinoma: a prospective study of the role of ultrasonography and histopathological frozen sections. *J Urol* 1996;155:1191–1195.
14. Shingleon WB, Sewell PE. Percutaneous renal tumor cryoablation with magnetic resonance imaging. *J Urol* 2001;165: 773–776.
15. Aron M. Minimally invasive nephron-sparing surgery (MINSS) for renal tumours Part II: probe ablative therapy. *Eur Urol* 2007;51:348–357.
16. Gupta A, Kavoussi LR, Jarrett TW, et al. Computerized tomography guided percutaneous renal cryoablation with the patient under conscious sedation: initial clinical experience. *J Urol* 2006;175:447–453.
17. Tuncali K, Tatli S, Silverman SG. MRI-guided percutaneous cryoablation of renal tumors: use of external manual displacement of adjacent bowel loops. *Eur J Radiol* 2006;59:198–202.
18. Shingleton WB, Sewell PE. Percutaneous renal cryoablation of renal tumors in patients with von Hippel-Lindau disease. *J Urol* 2002;167:1268–1270.
19. Silverman SG, Tuncali K, vanSonnenberg E, et al. Renal tumors: MR imaging–guided percutaneous cryotherapy—initial experience in 23 patients. *Radiology* 2005;236:716–724.
20. Moinzadeh A, Spaliviero M, Gill IS. Cryotherapy of renal masses: intermediate follow-up. *J Endourol* 2005;9(6):654–657.
21. Kam AW, Littrup PJ, Walther MM, et al. Thermal protection during percutaneous thermal ablation of renal cell carcinoma. *J Vasc Intervent Radiol* 2004;15:753–758.
22. Weight CJ, Kaouk JH, Hegarty NJ, et al. Correlation of radiographic imaging and histopathology following cryoablation and radio frequency ablation for renal tumors. *J Urol* 2008;179(4):1277–1281.
23. Nicos I, Fotiadis TS, Morales JP, et al. Combined percutaneous radiofrequency ablation and ethanol injection of renal tumours: midterm results. *Eur Urol* 2007;52:777–784.
24. Wood BJ, Locklin JK, Viswanathan A, et al. Technologies for guidance of radiofrequency ablation in the multimodality interventional suite of the future. *J Vasc Intervent Radiol* 2007;18: 9–24.
25. Stone MJ, Locklin J, Pinto P, et al. Radiofrequency ablation of renal tumors. *Techniques Vasc Intervent Radiol* 2007;172:132–139.
26. Hwang JJ, Pautler SE, Coleman JA, et al. Radio frequency ablation of small renal tumors: intermediate results. *J Urol* 2004;171:1814–1818.
27. Cowin EA. Laparoscopic radiofrequency ablation of renal tissue with and without hilar occlusion. *J Urol* 2001;166:281–284.
28. Park S, Cadeddu JA. Outcomes of radiofrequency ablation for kidney cancer. *Cancer Control* 2007;14(3):205–210.
29. Park S, Saboorian H, Cadeddu JA. No evidence of disease after radiofrequency ablation in delayed nephrectomy specimens. *Urology* 2006;68(5): 964–967.

30. Bastide C, Anfossi E, Ragni E, et al. Histologic evaluation of radiofrequency ablation in renal cancer. *Eur J Surg Oncol* 2006;32:980–983.
31. Roarke MC, Nguyen BD. Indolent enterococcal abscess mimicking recurrent renal cell carcinoma on MR imaging and PET/CT after radiofrequency ablation. *J Vasc Intervent Radiol* 2006;17(11, Pt 1):1851–1854.
32. Chan DY, Solomon S, Kim FJ, et al. Image-guided therapy in urology. *J Endourol* 2001;15(1):105–110.
33. Hacker A, Marlinghaus E, Kohrmann KU, et al. Extracorporeally induced ablation of renal tissue by high-intensity focused ultrasound. *Br J Urol* 2006;97:779–785.
34. Klingler HC. Kidney cancer: energy ablation. *Curr Opin Urol* 2007;17: 322–326.
35. Marberger M. Ablation of renal tumors with extracorporeal high-intensity focused ultrasound. *Br J Urol* 2007;99(5, Pt B):1273–1276.
36. Hafron J, Kaouk JH. Ablative techniques for the management of kidney cancer. *Nat Clin Pract* 2007;4(5):261–269.
37. Eichel L, Uribe C, Khonsari S, et al. Third prize: comparison of radical nephrectomy, laparoscopic microwave thermotherapy, cryotherapy, and radiofrequency ablation for destruction of experimental VX-2 renal tumors in rabbits. *J Endourol* 2005;19(9):1082–1187.
38. Presti JC, Miller MC, et al. Extended peripheral zone biopsy scheme increases cancer detection rates and minimizes variance in prostate specific antigen and age-related cancer rates: results of a community multi-practice study. *J Urol* 2003;169:125–129.
39. Djavan VR, Zlotta A, Dobronski P, et al. Prospective evaluation of prostate cancer detected on biopsies 1, 2, 3, and 4: when should we stop. *J Urol* 2001;166:1679–2683.
40. Lattouf J-B, Lee SJ, Bjurlin MA, et al. Magnetic resonance imaging-directed transrectal ultrasonography-guided biopsies in patients at risk of prostate cancer. *Br J Urol* 2007;99:1041–1046.
41. Anastasiadis AG, Nagele U, Kuczyk MA, et al. MRI-guided biopsy of the prostate increases diagnostic performance in men with elevated or increasing PSA levels after previous negative TRUS biopsies. *Eur Urol* 2006; 50:738–749.
42. Xu S, Kruecker J, Guion P, et al. Closed-loop control in fused MR-TRUS image-guided prostate biopsy. *Med Image Comput Comput Assist Interv Int Conf Med Image Comput Comput Assist Interv* 2007;10(Pt 1): 128–135.
43. Sahgal A. Permanent prostate seed brachytherapy: a current perspective on the evolution of the technique and its application. *Nat Clin Pract Urol* 2008;4(12):658–670.
44. Tempany C, Straus S, Hata N, et al. MR-guided prostate interventions. *J Magn Reson Imag* 2008;27:356–367.
45. Cormack RA, D'Amico AV. Optimizing target coverage by dosimetric feedback during prostate brachytherapy. *Int J Radiat Oncol Biol Phys* 2000;48(4):1245–1249.
46. Susil RC, Choyke P, et al. System for prostate brachytherapy and biopsy in a standard 1.5 T MRI scanner. *Magn Reson Med* 2004;52:683–687.
47. Muntener M, Petrisior D, Mazilu D, et al. Magnetic resonance imaging compatible robotic system for fully automated brachytherapy seed placement. *Urology* 2006;68:1313–1317.
48. Eggener SE, Scardino PT, Carroll PR, et al. International Task Force on Prostate Cancer and the Focal Lesion Paradigm. Focal therapy for localized prostate cancer: a critical appraisal of rationale and modalities. *J Urol* 2007;178:2260–2267.
49. Polascik TJ. Focal therapy for prostate cancer. *Curr Opin Urol* 2008;18(3): 269–274.
50. Kirkham AP, Allen C. How good is MRI at detecting and characterizing cancer within the prostate? *Eur Urol* 2006;50:1163.


# CHAPTER 138 ■ ROBOTIC SURGERY

DAVID CANES AND MIHIR M. DESAI

Robotic-assisted laparoscopic prostatectomy is now a routine procedure at many academic and community hospitals worldwide. The next leap forward in robotic technology will likely incorporate technology that is now just on the horizon, including flexible robotics, intraluminal minirobots, haptic feedback integration, and image overlay, to name just a few. Surgical robotic systems will continue to enhance our dexterity and will integrate into our daily operative practice in ways we can scarcely conceive. As Yogi Berra famously said, "It's tough to make predictions, especially about the future."

## NOMENCLATURE

An understanding of general robotic nomenclature is essential for the practicing urologist. A partial list is presented in Table 138.1. Purists may argue that the term *robot* is misleading and that *computer-assisted surgery* is more accurate in the current context. However, marketing pressures are likely to retain the terms *robotics* and *robotic surgery* in common usage.

The two broad categories of surgical robotic systems are as follows:

1. Computer-integrated: The operator defines a surgical task that the robot then carries out automatically.
2. Operator-driven: The robot is continuously under surgeon control in a master-slave environment.

## HISTORY OF SURGICAL ROBOTICS

The history of surgical robotics is still in its infancy. The curious reader can find excellent chronologies of the evolution of surgical robotics, both within and outside the urologic arena (1–5). The first fields to incorporate surgical robots were neurosurgery and orthopedics (6), possibly because their anatomy consists of fixed targets readily adaptable to robotic assistance. Minerva, a robotic system for neurosurgery (Integrated Surgical Systems, Davis, CA), is an active powered robot in which CT images are registered with a stereotactic frame encompassing the patient's head (7). Another system for stereotactic neurosurgery for tumor excision or biopsy is NeuroMate, which includes a 5-degree-of-freedom robotic arm (also developed by Integrated Surgical Systems) (8). ROBODOC (Integrated Surgical Systems) consists of a high-speed rotary cutter fitted with a force sensor to precisely bore a channel in the femoral head to house the implant for hip replacement (9). The femur is fixed in space using a rigid metal frame, with pins in the femoral head.

Although the transition to soft tissue surgery was more challenging, urologic applications subsequently emerged. The prostate is relatively fixed in the pelvis, and since transurethral resection consists of a series of repetitive motions, robotics applications were attempted. The PROBOT, introduced in 1989 from the Imperial College in London, was the first surgical

TABLE 138.1

ROBOTICS: NOMENCLATURE, TERMS, DEFINITIONS

| Term | Definition |
|---|---|
| Actuator | Modifies the state of the environment (motorized by electrical, pneumatic, or hydraulic systems). |
| Degrees of freedom (dof) | Number of possible motions at a joint. One joint = 1 dof. Movement is either translational or rotational. The human wrist has 3 dof, and the human palm has 7. Conventional laparoscopic instruments have 4 dof. Complete freedom requires a minimum of 6 degrees. |
| End effector | Instrument with which the robot accomplishes a task. The end effector may be the tool itself, or a grasping tool that is holding another instrument. |
| Envelope | Arc of space the robot occupies with all of its movements. |
| Fiducial | A fixed basis of reference, often used for calibration during surgical navigation or image overlay. |
| Haptics | Tissue contact forces experienced by the surgeon. |
| Robot | From the Czechoslovakian word *robota,* meaning "worker"; originated by Karel Capek's 1921 play, *Rossums Universal Robots.* One definition: a powered computer-controlled manipulator with artificial sensing that can be reprogrammed to move and position tools to carry out a range of surgical tasks. |
| Manipulator | The more common geometry, a robotic arm, consisting of a base, a series of joints, and an end effector. |
| On-line | Category of robotic design in which each movement is dictated by the operator. An example is a *master-slave* system, in which movements at a joystick are translated to the end effector. Surgeon remains in control. |
| Off-line | Preprogrammed autonomous robotic systems, such as those used in the automotive manufacturing industry. |
| Registration | Three-dimensional mapping between the robot, patient, and/or imaging data, such that special relations between robot end effectors are defined. Coordinates are matched such that a point on an image corresponds to an actual point in space. |
| Remote center of motion (RCM) | Fixed point along a robotic arm or instrument with minimal motion. Designed to coincide with the entry portal into a patient's body, for instance, at the trocar or fascia level for transabdominal robotic laparoscopic surgery. Applies to surgical rather than industrial robots. |
| Sensor | Detects the state of the environment by responding to a physical stimulus. |
| Telemedicine | Using telecommunications technology to provide medical services from a remote location (62). |

robotic system used in urology (10–12). The PROBOT was a computer-integrated surgical system in which the robot carried out a predefined task. Ultrasound images were obtained, and the desired resection area was outlined by the surgeon. Cutting trajectories for the robot were computed and then carried out autonomously, followed by electrical diathermy for hemostasis by the surgeon. A safety frame limited motion to 4 degrees of freedom, allowing the resectoscope to move in a conical motion. The robot was first manipulated manually to endure safety, and later powered as an active robot. After this pioneering work in 5 patients, and subsequently in an additional 30 (13), this application did not achieve widespread use.

Transrectal ultrasound–guided prostate biopsy is equally suited to robotic assistance, and such applications soon followed (14,15). Ultrasound images registered the anatomy of the prostate, and transperineal biopsy was performed to within 1 to 2 mm of the desired targets. The ultrasound images were coregistered with patient position coordinates from video cameras. The system did not gain momentum, but other robotic systems have been developed, with renewed interest of late both for biopsy (Fig. 138.1) (16) and for brachytherapy seed placement (17).

Percutaneous needle access to the kidney is another attractive target for robotics, since precision and experience are

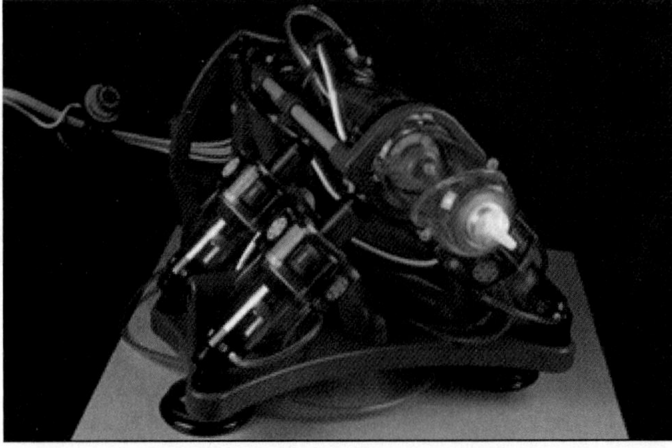

FIGURE 138.1 MrBot, designed for image-guided prostate needle based procedures, is constructed entirely of nonmagnetic materials for MRI compatibility. (Courtesy of Dr. Dan Stoianovici, urobotics laboratory, Johns Hopkins University.)

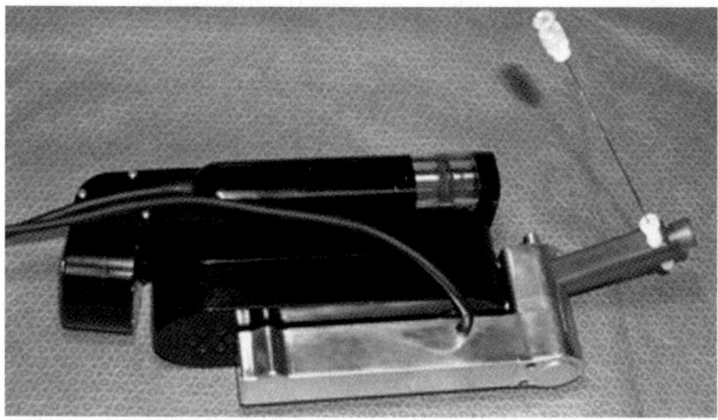

FIGURE 138.2 The PAKY robot, with an active injector for percutaneous access. (Courtesy of Dr. Dan Stoianovici, urobotics laboratory, Johns Hopkins University.)

required to translate two-dimensional (2-D) images into a 3-D trajectory, and a robot system would remove the operator from a radiation source when fluoroscopy is used. The first system was developed in London (18), followed thereafter by the Johns Hopkins group using the PAKY (percutaneous access to the kidney) robot (19). The PAKY system originally consisted of a mechanical manipulator, integrating images from biplanar fluoroscopy. In the porcine kidney, the desired calyx was targeted in only 50% of cases due to needle deflection and interference from ribs. The system was modified into PAKY-RCM, consisting of a passive manipulator (7 degrees of freedom), with an active translational needle injector system (Fig. 138.2). When tested clinically, the PAKY robot achieved 87% success in obtaining access in the desired calyx (20).

Another class of surgical robots includes laparoscopic camera robots, of which AESOP (Automated Endoscopic System for Optimal Positioning, Computer Motion, Inc.) achieved the largest commercial success. AESOP was the first active robotic device to garner FDA approval. It used voice control to permit surgeon control of the laparoscope, and it consisted of a 6-degrees-of-freedom (4 active, 2 passive) table-mounted manipulator that has been shown to be steadier than human camera

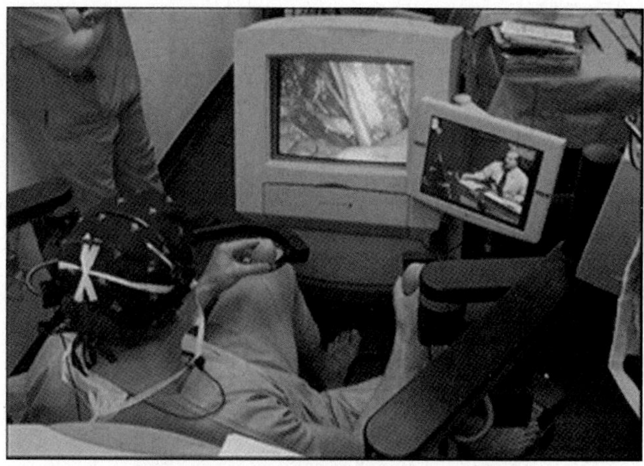

FIGURE 138.3 Surgeon manipulates working arms of the ZEUS surgical system in front of a 2-D display monitor. (Courtesy of Dr. Ingolf Tuerk, Lahey Clinic Medical Center, Burlington, MA.)

holders (21). AESOP was widely used in urologic laparoscopy before the advent of more sophisticated master-slave systems (22). The system was hampered by slow response during critical situations and by variability in voice-control response, so that an experienced assistant would occasionally need to take over its operation. More recent innovations have allowed eye gaze tracking for AESOP automation (23).

Operator-driven robotic surgical systems gained momentum with FDA approval of both the da Vinci surgical system in 2000 (Intuitive Surgical, Sunnyvale, CA) and the ZEUS surgical system in 2001 (Computer Motion). Both consist of a series of manipulators, one of which holds an endoscope and the others whose end effectors are interchangeable surgical instruments. The ZEUS system, shown in Fig. 138.3, incorporated AESOP for laparoscopic vision. The working arms, each table-mounted, had 6 degrees of freedom.

In 2003 Intuitive Surgical acquired Computer Motion and became the dominant and currently the only source of a commercially available complete telesurgical system. Components of the system are depicted schematically in Fig. 138.4. Benefits

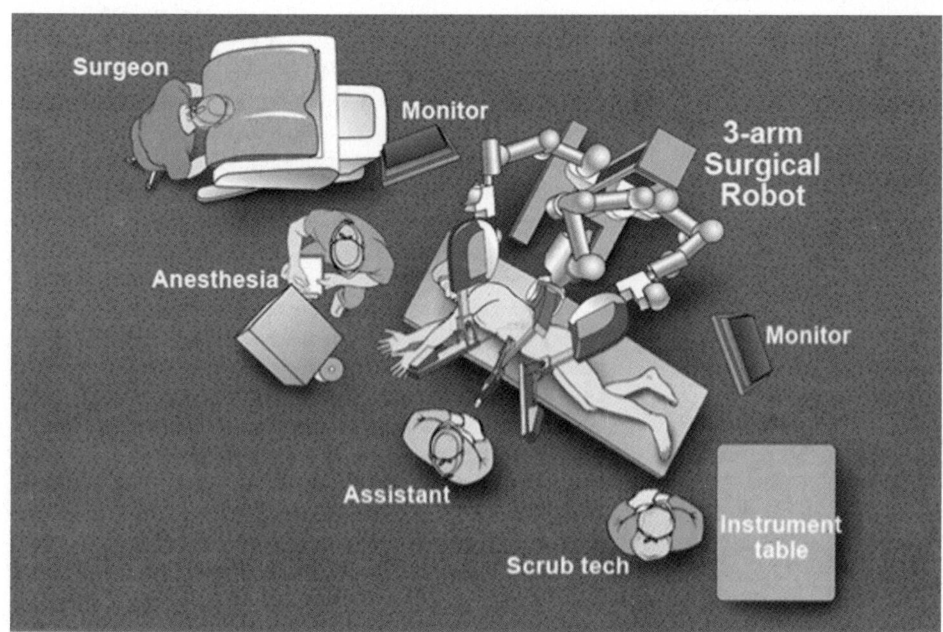


FIGURE 138.4 Cartoon of a typical operating room setup for the da Vinci robot. The surgeon controls the masters at the console, within sight of the bedside assistant. The three to four robotic arms are mounted on a surgical cart.

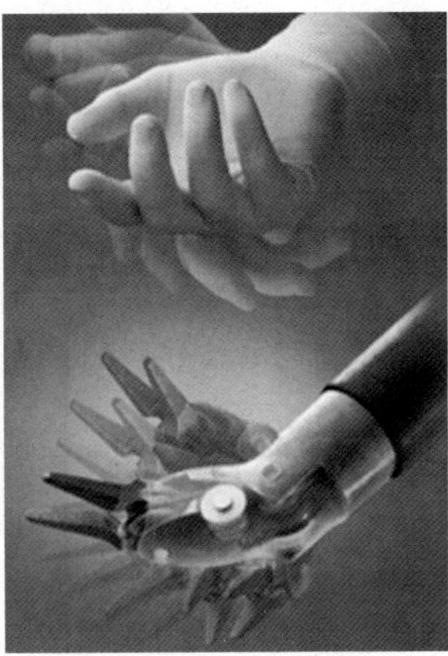

FIGURE 138.5 Wristed instrumentation provides 7 degrees of freedom (left/right, up/down, in/out, rotation, pitch, yaw, open/close).

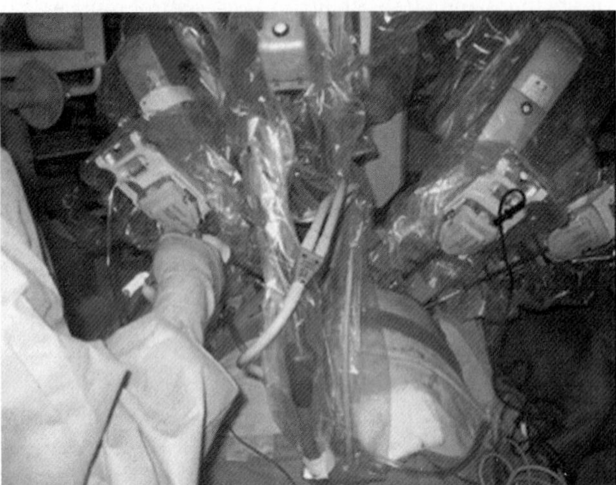

FIGURE 138.6 Bedside assistant's view of the four-arm da Vinci surgical system.

of the da Vinci system include 3-D visualization, wristed instrumentation with 7 degrees of freedom (Fig. 138.5), motion scaling, and incorporation of two to three instrument arms alongside the endoscopic arm (Fig. 138.6). The initial da Vinci system consisted of three arms. The latest upgraded version, the da Vinci-S system, incorporates the option of a fourth arm, high-definition vision, and better range of motion of the instruments. High cost and lack of feedback are commonly cited drawbacks to this system.

# CLINICAL UROLOGY

Just as laparoscopy now pervades urologic practice, robotic counterparts for virtually all procedures are now at least considered feasible (24), and for some procedures they are now standard options in the urologist's armamentarium. Since detailed techniques are presented elsewhere in this text, the evolution and current status for each procedure are briefly summarized in the following sections.

## Robotic-assisted Laparoscopic Radical Prostatectomy

The 2-D vision and 4 degrees of freedom inherent to laparoscopic radical prostatectomy can clearly be overcome in expert hands but may have been too insurmountable for widespread diffusion. After the groundwork was established by early pure laparoscopic pioneers (25,26), robotic technology was primed to be applied to the prostate, enveloped within the restrictive confines of the deep pelvis. The first robotic prostatectomy was performed in 2001 (27). The procedure can be performed using a transperitoneal or extraperitoneal approach, and using the three- or four-arm robot. Although functional data are immature, available evidence suggests acceptable complication rates, equivalent short-term measures of local cancer control (margin status) to open surgery, and promising functional results as regards continence and erectile function (28,29). The largest published series to date comes from Menon's group (30), who reported on 2,766 patients undergoing robotic-assisted prostatectomy (RAP) over 6 years. Console time was under 2 hours, estimated blood loss was 200 mL, and 5-year actuarial biochemical-free survival was 84%. The positive margin rate for pT2 disease in the last 200 patients was 4%. Of preoperatively potent men, 79.2% were able to achieve erections sufficient for intercourse. Continence, defined as the use of no >1 pad per day, was achieved in 93% of patients. These results are encouraging, and longer-term outcomes are awaited.

## Robotic-assisted Laparoscopic Radical Cystectomy

Beecken et al. (31) were the first to report robotic-assisted radical cystectomy and ileal neobladder, in 2003 (31). As with robotic-assisted laparoscopic radical prostatectomy, long-term outcomes with robotic-assisted laparoscopic radical cystectomy are immature, but early indicators are encouraging. Wang et al. (32) prospectively compared 33 patients undergoing robotic cystectomy to 21 patients undergoing open radical cystectomy by a single surgeon. Patients undergoing robotic cystectomy had decreased blood loss, earlier resumption of oral intake, and shorter hospital stay compared to open surgery. Complication rates were equivalent, and operative time was longer in the robotic group. Positive margin rates were statistically equivalent, as were lymph node yields. As is commonly the case, the extirpative portion of the procedure is performed with robotic assistance, and the urinary diversion fashioned with extracorporeal assistance. The robot is redocked for the urethrovesical anastomosis when orthotopic neobladders are chosen. Other groups have confirmed that adequate lymph node yields can be achieved robotically during the course of radical cystectomy, an important factor that will influence the widespread adoption of robotic technology for invasive bladder cancer (33,34).

## Robotic-assisted Laparoscopic Pyeloplasty

The robotic interface may be ideally suited to perform reconstructive procedures, whereas laparoscopic intracorporeal suturing requires dedicated training and perhaps a steeper learning curve. The first report of laparoscopic pyeloplasty was in 1993 (35). Sung et al. (36) demonstrated the technical feasibility of robotic-assisted laparoscopic pyeloplasty in the laboratory. Subsequently, multiple reports have attested to the safety and efficacy of robotic-assisted laparoscopic pyeloplasty. Currently, the robotic procedure is typically performed using a transperitoneal approach. The initial bowel mobilization and dissection of the ureteropelvic junction (UPJ) may be performed laparoscopically with the robotic system used only for dismemberment and suturing, based on initial surgeon preference. The robotic approach has been successfully utilized in performing various types of UPJ repairs, including dismembered, nondismembered, reduction, vessel transposition, and concomitant pyelolithotomy. A large single-center experience in 92 patients demonstrated durable patency rates comparable to acceptable standards, with 96.7% success at 39 months (37).

## Robotic-assisted Laparoscopic Partial Nephrectomy

Laparoscopic partial nephrectomy has become a standard option for the small renal mass at high-volume centers, with outcomes equivalent to that of open surgery at 5 years (38). Robotic assistance may allow more physicians to accomplish minimally invasive partial nephrectomy, during which sutured renorrhaphy is considered technically difficult. Although the technical feasibility of robotic-assisted laparoscopic partial nephrectomy has been demonstrated (39,40), its true advantage over other minimally invasive techniques has not been defined (41).

## Robotic Nephrectomy

The use of robotics for nephrectomy has been infrequently reported, since the standard laparoscopic and hand-assisted nephrectomy have gained widespread acceptance, and adding robotic assistance seems to be of no significant value. Guillonneau and colleagues (42) first reported robotic nephrectomy in 2001 for a hydronephrotic nonfunctioning right kidney using the ZEUS system. The patient-side assistant performed many of the crucial maneuvers required for hilar control. To summarize, the immediate advantages of the robot for radical nephrectomy are less apparent than for other procedures.

## Miscellaneous Robotic Procedures

The first robotic adrenalectomy was reported by Horgan and Vanuno (43), and shortly thereafter by Desai (44). A more recent large series of 30 patients undergoing robotic adrenalectomy for various indications affirmed its safety, efficacy, and cost (45). With laparoscopic adrenalectomy, which is purely extirpative and relatively straightforward, the advantages of robotics remain to be defined. The da Vinci robotic system has been applied to a variety of other urologic applications, including donor nephrectomy (46,47), where feasibility and safety has been demonstrated. Motion scaling and tremor reduction have benefited the field of male infertility, and robotic vasovasostomy has been performed with success (48).

# FUTURE DIRECTIONS AND ALTERNATIVE ROBOTIC PLATFORMS

## Flexible Robotics

Robotics has the potential to revolutionize endoscopy, just as the da Vinci robotic system has facilitated laparoscopic surgery. Flexible robotics was initially designed for interventional cardiology procedures (49). Ureteroscopy was the initial urologic arena in which flexible robotics was investigated. In standard manual ureteroscopy, typically all locations in the collecting system can be accessed, but breathing movements and lack of stability can make controlling subtle movements difficult. Robotics may potentially allow a level of precision that even the expert ureteroscopist might have difficulty duplicating.

Hansen Medical System (Mountain View, CA) (50) has adapted a robotic catheter system for ureteroscopy. The Sensei robotic catheter, a master-slave system, consists of four components: (a) a surgeon console with an LCD display and master input device (MID), (b) a steerable catheter system, (c) a remote table-mounted catheter manipulator, and (d) an electronic rack. At the workstation (Fig. 138.7), three LCD monitors display endoscopic, fluoroscopic, and other procedure-specific imaging. The MID is a joystick that the surgeon manipulates, and these movements are translated to the catheter tip. An outer catheter sheath (14Fr/12Fr) is first manually positioned, followed by an inner catheter guide (12Fr/10Fr) through which the steerable catheter is inserted. The workstation's remote positioning has the secondary advantage of decreasing radiation exposure to the operating surgeon, much the same way as the PAKY robot removes the endoscopist from the radiation source.

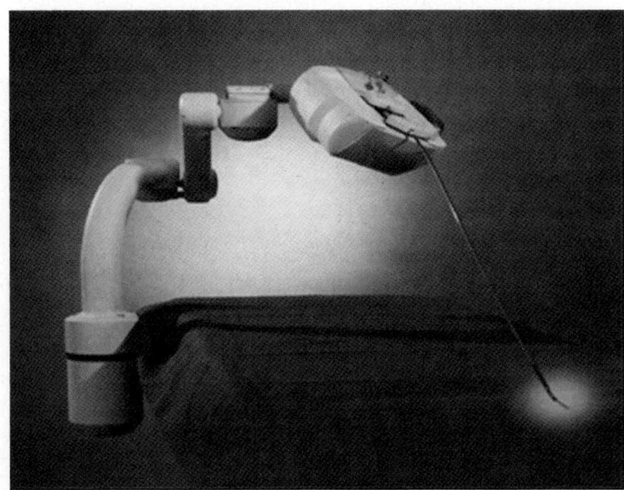

FIGURE 138.7 Table-mounted robotic manipulator for flexible robotics, Hansen Medical System.

The technical feasibility of robotic ureterorenoscopy has been demonstrated in the porcine model (51). The remarkable tip stability and ease of manipulation were acknowledged during this initial experience. The catheter system could be introduced de novo in eight ureters, while two required balloon dilation. The ureteroscope could be successfully manipulated remotely into 83 of the 85 calices (98%). Kidney stones inserted into the collecting system (4 mm) were successfully treated with a holmium laser fiber. The time required to inspect all calices within a given kidney decreased with experience. Clinical trials with robotic ureterorenoscopy are under way and have not yet been reported.

## NOTES and Miniature Robotics

The separate fields of endoluminal surgery (cystoscopy, ureteroscopy) and standard extraluminal surgery (nephrectomy, adrenalectomy) promise to combine in currently unimaginable ways. NOTES (natural orifice transluminal endoscopic surgery) involves traversing intact hollow viscera (stomach, vagina, colon, bladder) to access intra-abdominal targets for ablative or reconstructive surgery (52). The proper instrumentation required, and the reliable entry/exit strategies to effectively accomplish NOTES, have not been determined. NOTES techniques will require even more complex movements in open spaces. It is these limitations that robotic enhancements hope to address. The open environment of the insufflated peritoneal cavity poses significant challenges. Miniature robots deployed in vivo may potentially advance the field (53). Task-specific miniature robots can be used inside the peritoneum without the typical constraints of an externally actuated flexible endoscopic device. While currently available prototypes now perform simple maneuvers, these have the potential to play a role in the future.

Current miniature robotic prototypes are either fixed-base or mobile robots (54). Fixed-base robots are deployed and positioned and cannot self-navigate from their initial position. A pan and tilt camera, fashioned with LEDs for illumination, a 15-mm diameter conical design, spring-loaded tripod "legs," and two independent motors controlling camera movement (pan 360 degrees, tilt 45 degrees). This camera was deployed through an abdominal incision and used in conjunction with standard laparoscopic equipment to facilitate porcine cholecystectomy (55). A second-generation tilting camera has been used in conjunction with a standard laparoscope for canine prostatectomy (54). This initial prototype is a "wired" camera for power input, and wireless prototypes are on the horizon.

In animal studies, a mobile camera has been used to provide sole visualization for abdominal exploration and cholecystectomy (56). In this case, the camera port was therefore unnecessary and the cholecystectomy was performed with two trocars. In another study, the mobile robotic platform has demonstrated the successful biopsy of three samples of hepatic tissue (57). For NOTES applications, successful remote-controlled exploration through a gastrotomy has been performed in the porcine model (58). This was monitored by the endoscopic rather than the robotic camera, but it successfully demonstrated proof of concept. The robot was then retracted into the gastric cavity, and the transgastric incision was closed using two endoclips and one endoloop. Also in pigs, the feasibility of using multiple miniature robots for improving spatial orientation and providing task assistance has been demonstrated (59). Three miniature in vivo robots, shown in Figure 138.8, including a peritoneum-mounted imaging robot, a lighting robot, and a retraction robot, were used in conjunction with a standard upper endoscope to demonstrate various capabilities for NOTES procedures.

## Robotic NOTES

Box et al. (60) reported robotic-assisted NOTES nephrectomy using the da Vinci robotics platform. In this porcine study, a combined transvaginal and transcolonic nephrectomy was performed in 150 minutes. A standard laparoscope was placed through a single 12-mm transumbilical trocar for direct visualization. The specimen was extracted transvaginally. Robotic NOTES was also reported by Haber et al. (61) in ten pigs, in which multiple bilateral upper-tract procedures were performed, including pyeloplasty ($n = 10$), partial nephrectomy ($n = 10$), and radical nephrectomy ($n = 10$). An adjunctive multichannel transumbilical port was employed. The endoscope and one working robotic arm were placed through this port. The second robotic working arm was placed transvaginally. Range of motion was limited by external collision of the robotic arms, but even complex suturing with wristed instrumentation was feasible.

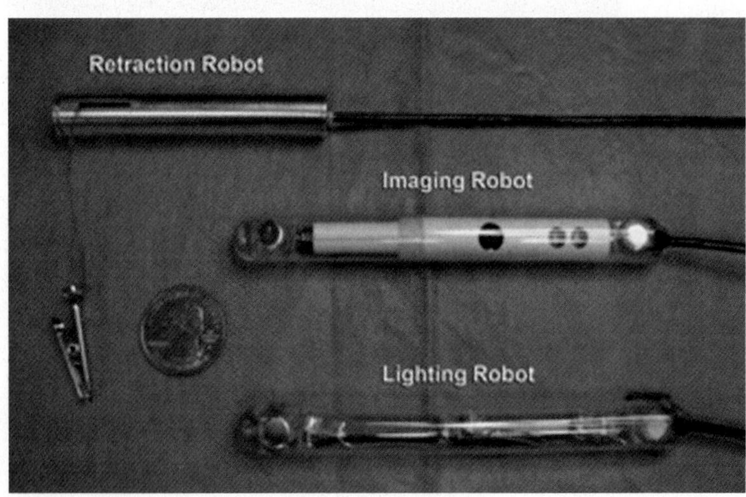


FIGURE 138.8 Retraction, imaging, and lighting minirobots used for hybrid NOTES procedure. (Photo courtesy of Dr. Dmitry Oleynikov, University of Nebraska Medical Center, Omaha, NE.)

Clearly, a task-specific robotic system will ultimately be better suited to the complexity of NOTES procedures in the future. Instrument collision and lack of flexibility are currently limiting factors of the da Vinci system for this application. Robotic systems, including flexible robots, *in vivo* miniature robots, or a combination, may impact intraluminal surgery and NOTES in the future.

## *References*


1. Stoianovici D. Robotic surgery. *World J Urol* 2000;18(4):289–295.
2. Shah J, Mackay S, Rockall T, et al. "Urobotics": robots in urology. *BJU Int* 2001;88(4):313–320.
3. Kim HL, Schulam P. The PAKY, HERMES, AESOP, ZEUS, and da Vinci robotic systems. *Urol Clin North Am* 2004;31(4):659–669.
4. Cadeddu JA, Stoianovici D, Kavoussi LR. Robotic surgery in urology. *Urol Clin North Am* 1998;25(1):75–85.
5. Nguyen MM, Das S. The evolution of robotic urologic surgery. *Urol Clin North Am* 2004;31(4):653–658.
6. Buckingham RA, Buckingham RO. Robots in operating theatres. *BMJ* 19952;311(7018):1479–1482.
7. Glauser D, Fankhauser H, Epitaux M, et al. Neurosurgical robot Minerva: first results and current developments. *J Image Guid Surg* 1995;1(5): 266–272.
8. Li QH, Zamorano L, Pandya A, et al. The application accuracy of the NeuroMate robot: a quantitative comparison with frameless and frame-based surgical localization systems. *Comput Aided Surg* 2002;7(2):90–98.
9. Taylor KS. Robodoc: study tests robot's use in hip surgery. *Hospitals* 1993;67(9):46.
10. Davies BL, Hibberd RD, Coptcoat MJ, et al. A surgeon robot prostatectomy: a laboratory evaluation. *J Med Eng Technol* 1989;13(6):273–277.
11. Harris SJ, Arambula-Cosio F, Mei Q, et al. The Probot: an active robot for prostate resection. *Proc Inst Mech Eng [H]* 1997;211(4):317–325.
12. Ng WS, Davies BL, Timoney AG, et al. The use of ultrasound in automated prostatectomy. *Med Biol Eng Comput* 1993;31(4):349–354.
13. Davies BL, Hibberd RD, Ng WS, et al. The development of a surgeon robot for prostatectomies. *Proc Inst Mech Eng [H]* 1991;205(1):35–38.
14. Rovetta A. Tests on reliability of a prostate biopsy telerobotic system. *Stud Health Technol Inform* 1999;62:302–307.
15. Rovetta A, Sala R. Execution of robot-assisted biopsies within the clinical context. *J Image Guid Surg* 1995;1(5):280–287.
16. Haber GO, Kamoi K, Vidal C, et al. Development and evaluation of a transrectal ultrasound robot for targeted biopsies and focal therapy of prostate cancer. Presented at the Engineering in Urology Society meeting, Orlando, FL, May 2008.
17. Muntener M, Patriciu A, Petrisor D, et al. Transperineal prostate intervention: robot for fully automated MR imaging—system description and proof of principle in a canine model. *Radiology* 2008;247(2):543–549.
18. Potamianos P, Davies BL, Hibberd RD. Intra-operative registration for percutaneous surgery. *Proceedings of the Second International Symposium on Medical Robotics and Computer Assisted Surgery*, Baltimore, 1995, p. 156.
19. Cadeddu JA, Bzostek A, Schreiner S, et al. A robotic system for percutaneous renal access. *J Urol* 1997;158(4):1589–1593.
20. Su LM, Stoianovici D, Jarrett TW, et al. Robotic percutaneous access to the kidney: comparison with standard manual access. *J Endourol* 2002;16(7):471–475.
21. Kavoussi LR, Moore RG, Adams JB, et al. Comparison of robotic versus human laparoscopic camera control. *J Urol* 1995;154(6):2134–2136.
22. Partin AW, Adams JB, Moore RG, et al. Complete robot-assisted laparoscopic urologic surgery: a preliminary report. *J Am Coll Surg* 1995;181(6):552–557.
23. Ali SM, Reisner LA, King B, et al. Eye gaze tracking for endoscopic camera positioning: an application of a hardware/software interface developed to automate Aesop. *Stud Health Technol Inform* 2008;132:4–7.
24. Eichel L, Ahlering TE, Clayman RV. Role of robotics in laparoscopic urologic surgery. *Urol Clin North Am* 2004;31(4):781–792.
25. Schuessler WW, Kavoussi LR, Clayman RV, et al. Laparoscopic radical prostatectomy: initial case report. *J Urol* 1992;147:A246.
26. Guillonneau B, Cathelineau X, Barret E, et al. Laparoscopic radical prostatectomy: technical and early oncological assessment of 40 operations. *Eur Urol* 1999;36(1):14–20.
27. Binder J, Kramer W. Robotically-assisted laparoscopic radical prostatectomy. *BJU Int* 2001;87(4):408–410.
28. Ficarra V, Cavalleri S, Novara G, et al. Evidence from robot-assisted laparoscopic radical prostatectomy: a systematic review. *Eur Urol* 2007; 51(1):45–55.
29. Box GN, Ahlering TE. Robotic radical prostatectomy: long-term outcomes. *Curr Opin Urol* 2008;18(2):173–179.
30. Badani KK, Kaul S, Menon M. Evolution of robotic radical prostatectomy: assessment after 2766 procedures. *Cancer* 2007;110(9):1951–1958.
31. Beecken WD, Wolfram M, Engl T, et al. Robotic-assisted laparoscopic radical cystectomy and intra-abdominal formation of an orthotopic ileal neobladder. *Eur Urol* 2003;44(3):337–339.
32. Wang GJ, Barocas DA, Raman JD, et al. Robotic vs open radical cystectomy: prospective comparison of perioperative outcomes and pathological measures of early oncological efficacy. *BJU Int* 2008;101(1):89–93.
33. Woods M, Thomas R, Davis R, et al. Robot-assisted extended pelvic lymphadenectomy. *J Endourol* 2008;22(6):1467–1470.
34. Pruthi RS, Wallen EM. Robotic-assisted laparoscopic radical cystoprostatectomy. *Eur Urol* 2008;53(2):310–322.
35. Schuessler WW, Grune MT, Tecuanhuey LV, et al. Laparoscopic dismembered pyeloplasty. *J Urol* 1993;150(6):1795–1799.
36. Sung GT, Gill IS, Hsu TH. Robotic-assisted laparoscopic pyeloplasty: a pilot study. *Urology* 1999;53(6):1099–1103.
37. Schwentner C, Pelzer A, Neururer R, et al. Robotic Anderson-Hynes pyeloplasty: 5-year experience of one centre. *BJU Int* 2007;100(4):880–885.
38. Lane BR, Gill IS. 5-Year outcomes of laparoscopic partial nephrectomy. *J Urol* 2007;177(1):70–74.
39. Kaul S, Laungani R, Sarle R, et al. da Vinci-assisted robotic partial nephrectomy: technique and results at a mean of 15 months of follow-up. *Eur Urol* 2007;51(1):186–191.
40. Gettman MT, Blute ML, Chow GK, et al. Robotic-assisted laparoscopic partial nephrectomy: technique and initial clinical experience with DaVinci robotic system. *Urology* 2004;64(5):914–918.
41. Aron M, Koenig P, Kaouk JH, et al. Robotic and laparoscopic partial nephrectomy: a matched-pair comparison from a high-volume centre. *BJU Int* 2008;102(1):86–92.
42. Guillonneau B, Jayet C, Tewari A, et al. Robot assisted laparoscopic nephrectomy. *J Urol* 2001;166(1):200–201.
43. Horgan S, Vanuno D. Robots in laparoscopic surgery. *J Laparoendosc Adv Surg Tech A* 2001;11(6):415–419.
44. Desai MM, Gill IS, Kaouk JH, et al. Robotic-assisted laparoscopic adrenalectomy. *Urology* 2002;60(6):1104–1107.
45. Winter JM, Talamini MA, Stanfield CL, et al. Thirty robotic adrenalectomies: a single institution's experience. *Surg Endosc* 2006;20(1):119–124.
46. Horgan S, Vanuno D, Sileri P, et al. Robotic-assisted laparoscopic donor nephrectomy for kidney transplantation. *Transplantation* 2002;73(9): 1474–1479.
47. Hubert J, Renoult E, Mourey E, et al. Complete robotic-assistance during laparoscopic living donor nephrectomies: an evaluation of 38 procedures at a single site. *Int J Urol* 2007;14(11):986–989.
48. Fleming C. Robot-assisted vasovasostomy. *Urol Clin North Am* 2004; 31(4):769–772.
49. Saliba W, Cummings JE, Oh S, et al. Novel robotic catheter remote control system: feasibility and safety of transseptal puncture and endocardial catheter navigation. *J Cardiovasc Electrophysiol* 2006;17(10):1102–1105.
50. Aron M, Haber GP, Desai MM, et al. Flexible robotics: a new paradigm. *Curr Opin Urol* 2007;17(3):151–155.
51. Desai MM, Aron M, Gill IS, et al. Flexible robotic retrograde renoscopy: description of novel robotic device and preliminary laboratory experience. *Urology* 2008 [Epub ahead of print].
52. Kaloo AN, Singh VK, Jagannath SB, et al. Flexible transgastric peritoneoscopy: a novel approach to diagnostic and therapeutic interventions in the peritoneal cavity. *Gastrointest Endosc* 2004; 60(1):114–117.
53. Rentschler ME, Oleynikov D. Recent in vivo surgical robot and mechanism developments. *Surg Endosc* 2007;21(9):1477–1481.
54. Rentschler ME, Platt SR, Dumpert J, et al. In vivo laparoscopic robotics. *Int J Surg* 2006;4(3):167–171.
55. Oleynikov D, Rentschler M, Hadzialic A, et al. Miniature robots can assist in laparoscopic cholecystectomy. *Surg Endosc* 2005;19(4):473–476.
56. Rentschler ME, Dumpert J, Platt SR, et al. Mobile in vivo camera robots provide sole visual feedback for abdominal exploration and cholecystectomy. *Surg Endosc* 2006;20(1):135–138.
57. Rentschler ME, Dumpert J, Platt S, et al. An *in vivo* mobile robot for surgical vision and task assistance. *ASME J Med Devices* 2007;1(1):23–29.
58. Rentschler ME, Dumpert J, Platt SR, et al. Natural orifice surgery with an endoluminal mobile robot. *Surg Endosc* 2007;21(7):1212–1215.
59. Lehman AC, Berg KA, Dumpert J, et al. Surgery with cooperative robots. *Comput Aided Surg* 2008;3(2):95–105.
60. Box GN, Lee HJ, Santos RJS, et al. Rapid communications: robot-assisted NOTES nephrectomy: initial report. *J Endourol* 2008;22(3):503–506.
61. Haber GP, Crouzet S, Kamoi K, et al. Robotic NOTES (Natural Orifice Transluminal Endoscopic Surgery) in reconstructive urology: initial animal experience. *Urology* 2008;71(6):996–1000.
62. Bashshur RL. On the definition and evaluation of telemedicine. *Telemed J* 1995;1:19–30.

# CHAPTER 139 ■ ENERGY SOURCES IN UROLOGY

MOSES M. KIM AND RICHARD E. LINK

In urology energy sources have been employed in three broad categories: (a) hemostasis, (b) tissue destruction, and (c) lithotripsy. In all applications, the goal is to precisely focus energy onto the target while minimizing damage to adjacent structures. The advent of feedback-modulated bipolar energy platforms has vastly improved electrosurgical options for open and laparoscopic procedures. Harmonic instruments, utilizing sound waves, are similarly used for hemostasis and tissue division. Electromagnetic energy sources, ranging from low-energy radio waves to high-energy microwaves, are used for tissue ablation of the kidney and prostate. Similarly, cryotherapy uses freeze cycles to destroy prostatic and renal tissue. Lasers of many hues have broad applications in lithotripsy and tissue ablation in both benign and malignant urologic conditions.

Surgical energy sources have made many of today's urologic procedures safer, easier, more effective, and in many cases, less invasive. Future advances in energy technology will likely continue to improve patient care as they become integrated into urologic practice.

## ELECTROSURGERY

### Monopolar

Monopolar cautery uses a high-frequency electric current that passes from a single electrode on the instrument to a second, larger electrode plate beneath the patient. The arcing of current from the first electrode to the point of contact on the tissue leads to coagulation. The resulting local hemostasis decreases blood loss and preserves visibility in the surgical field. Monopolar cautery's limitation is that the current is unregulated as it passes through the body to the second electrode. This can lead to tissue damage distant from the contact point.

With minimally invasive surgery, 90% of the instrument lies outside the visual field and may inadvertently be in contact with vulnerable tissue such as bowel. In the event of insulation failure or capacitive coupling, thermal injury to the viscera may occur. Active electrode monitoring was developed to address this concern. If insulation is damaged, an alarm sounds, alerting the operating room staff. This has greatly decreased the incidence of viscera injury from stray currents in laparoscopic procedures (1).

### Bipolar

Bipolar devices place the first and second electrodes near each other, usually at the working tips of the instrument. This arrangement provides better control of the current and minimizes injury to adjacent tissues. Unlike monopolar cautery, the proximity of the two electrodes allows for coagulation of tissue that is immersed in fluid. Traditional bipolar devices, such as the Kleppinger forceps, provide inconsistent vessel sealing, variable thermal spread (Table 139.1), and charring. Recently, new devices offer more consistent vessel seals and less thermal spread with minimal charring and sticking.

The LigaSure instruments utilize high-current, low-voltage, bipolar radiofrequency (RF) energy combined with a feedback-controlled response system that automatically delivers, and then discontinues, power when tissue sealing is completed. When the Ligasure is activated, denatures collagen and elastin to form a seal. The forceps are fitted with an integral blade that can be utilized efficiently to cut the tissue once it is sealed. The EnSeal has a jaw that contains conductive particles that modulate the energy, minimizing thermal spread and charring. The jaw contains an I-shaped blade that is slowly advanced, thereby simultaneously cutting and sealing the tissue (2).

TABLE 139.1

VESSEL SEALING CAPABILITY AND THERMAL SPREAD OF VARIOUS DEVICES

| DEVICE | SIZE OF VESSEL RELIABLY SEALED | THERMAL SPREAD (REF) |
|---|---|---|
| Traditional bipolar | 1—3 mm | Up to 22 mm (5) |
| Plasmakinetic (Gyrus) | 5 mm | 3.5 mm (6) |
| LigaSure V (5-mm device) | 7 mm | 2.5 mm (7) |
| LigaSure Atlas (10-mm device) | 7 mm | 2 mm (8) |
| EnSeal | 7 mm | <1 mm (2) |
| Harmonic Scalpel LCS-K5 | 3 mm | 1 mm (9) |
| Harmonic ACE | 5 mm | 1 mm (10) |

The Gyrus Plasmakinetic (PK) tissue management system utilizes a pulsatile delivery of bipolar energy, allowing for cooling of tissue between pulsations, thus minimizing thermal spread and adherence of charred tissue to the instrument. An audible signal communicates to the surgeon when the tissue is fully sealed. There are various PK instruments available for open, laparoscopic, and transurethral prostatic resections. Saline irrigation may be used with the last-mentioned, decreasing the risk of hyponatremia while providing a similar resection to the standard monopolar resectoscope loop (3,4).

## ULTRASOUND

### Ultrasonic Surgical Devices

Harmonic and SonoSurg are two ultrasound-based instrument systems. The tips vibrate at 55 kHz, causing denaturation of proteins and formation of a coagulum that seals vessels. Earlier models generated temperatures between 50°C and 100°C, whereas the newer Harmonic ACE consistently generates temperatures over 100°C, with peak temperatures exceeding 200°C (11). It has a faster sealing time when compared to earlier models, has a curved blade, and is hand-activated (10). Dual modes provide a faster pulse to seal smaller vessels and a longer pulse to seal larger vessels. At the completion of the pulse cycle, the sealed tissue is cut (12). Immediately following deactivation, heat surges to over 200C can occur (12). Thus, care must be taken when dissecting with the tips to avoid unintentional tissue injury.

### High-Intensity Focused Ultrasound (HIFU)

HIFU uses an intense beam of ultrasonic waves to heat and destroy tissue. A small, focused sound wave is delivered to deep, targeted tissue, with minimal damage inflicted to the intervening tissue. The acoustic waves are focused and increased in intensity, and the energy imparted to the tissue can heat it to 70°C to 100°C within a few seconds. Additionally, the acoustic waves can create microbubbles that oscillate and collapse, thereby releasing more energy in a process called cavitation. The combination of both processes heats the tissue, leading to tissue coagulation and destruction.

HIFU of the prostate is delivered by a transrectal transducer that is placed abutting the prostate. Real-time imaging with ultrasound is used to monitor treatment. There are two HIFU systems in wide use today for the treatment of prostate cancer. The technologies are similar with a few salient differences. Ablatherm (EDAP TMS SA, France) places both the therapeutic and imaging transducers in a unique probe, with the focus set at 40 mm. The patient lies in a lateral position on a special table while treatment is delivered from the base to the apex in four to six segments. Sonablate (Focus Surgery Inc, Indianapolis, IN) incorporates the therapeutic and imaging transducer into a single probe, and it has several probes at various focal lengths from 25 to 45 mm. The patient is positioned in dorsal lithotomy on a standard operating table. Treatment is delivered in three coronal cuts, from anterior to posterior. Both devices have rectal wall temperature monitors and cooling devices.

HIFU was first reported for the treatment of prostate cancer in 1995 and is widely used in Europe, Asia, and parts of North and South America. However, it has not been approved by the Food and Drug Administration. Recent studies showed that with refinement of technique, local control rates have increased significantly. Blana et al. (13) showed actuarial biochemical failure-free survival rates at 5 and 7 years to be 77% and 69%. At 5 years, 94.3% were continent and 56.8% were potent. Poissonnier et al. (14) reported a 5-year biochemical- and pathological-free rate of 66%, with an inverse relationship with pretreatment PSA levels: 90% for PSA <4, 57% for PSA between 4.1 and 10.0, and 61% for PSA between 10.5 and 15.0. A PSA nadir of >0.2 ng per mL was associated with a fourfold increased risk of treatment failure. There is a 0.3% to 8.6% rate of acute urinary retention (15). Rectoprostatic fistula, more common in the earlier experience, has now dropped to almost zero with the use of an intrarectal cooling device. HIFU can also be repeated in the event of treatment failure, as there is no maximal dose for this modality. Retreatment rates are as high as 40% for the Ablatherm system and 22% for the Sonablate system (15). Rates of incontinence and impotence are significantly higher after the second treatment.

HIFU has also been used for salvage therapy following radiation failure. A study of 118 patients showed local control rates of 84% with a median PSA nadir of 0.18 ng per mL and 5-year actuarial progression-free survival rates of 78.0%, 49.5%, and 14.0% for low-, intermediate-, and high-risk patients. The continence rate was 57%, and rectourethral fistula occurred in 7% (15).

## RADIOFREQUENCY ABLATION

### Radiofrequency Ablation for Small Renal Masses

Radiofrequency ablation (RFA) utilizes a high-frequency alternating wave (375 to 500 kHz), delivered through a probe, that heats the tissue, leading to coagulative necrosis. It was first used for the ablation of nonresectable liver masses. Since then, multiple studies have highlighted the safety and efficacy of this technology for small renal masses. Currently, the use of RFA for the treatment of small renal masses (<4 cm) has been approved by the U.S. Food and Drug Administration. Commonly, the probe is positioned into the renal mass percutaneously under CT guidance, which requires minimal anesthetic and a short time to full convalescence. The probes can also be placed laparoscopically, and the treatment effect can be monitored either by using real-time ultrasound or by placing temperature probes at the periphery of the target lesion. (For patient selection, see section on cryoablation of small renal masses.)

The literature reports excellent cancer control rates. A recent summary of the literature showed cancer-specific survival of 94.8% after RFA of small renal tumors (mean size of 2.4 cm), with a mean follow-up of 19.5 months. Failures can be reablated or resected via partial or radical nephrectomy. The reablation rate was 8.8%, and the rate of extirpative surgery was 1.1% (16).

## Transurethral Needle Ablation

TUNA (transurethral needle ablation) is a minimally invasive procedure used for the treatment of benign prostatic hyperplasia (BPH). Two monopolar needles at 40 degrees from each other are attached to a catheter perpendicular from its longitudinal axis, which is advanced to the prostate via the urethra. The needles are inserted into a lateral lobe of the prostate and low-level radiofrequency energy of 465 kHz is applied. The tissue around the needle is heated to approximately 100°C, leading to coagulative necrosis. Starting from the bladder neck, the needles are advanced 1 cm after each treatment, eventually ablating the entire length of the prostate to the verumontanum (Fig. 139.1). This is usually an outpatient procedure and takes about 30 minutes; it appears to benefit the symptoms of BPH.

A meta-analysis showed significant improvement of BPH symptoms after TUNA as measured by American Urological Association (AUA) symptom scores. At the 3-month follow-up, there was a 57% decrease in the AUA symptom scores, a rate similar to TURP. However, at time points >1 year, there was greater improvement of symptoms in the transurethral resection of prostate (TRUP) group. Additionally, there was a 10% retreatment rate with TUNA, compared to only a 1% retreatment rate with TURP. However, TUNA patients reported significantly fewer complications than TURP patients, including less impact on sexual function (17).

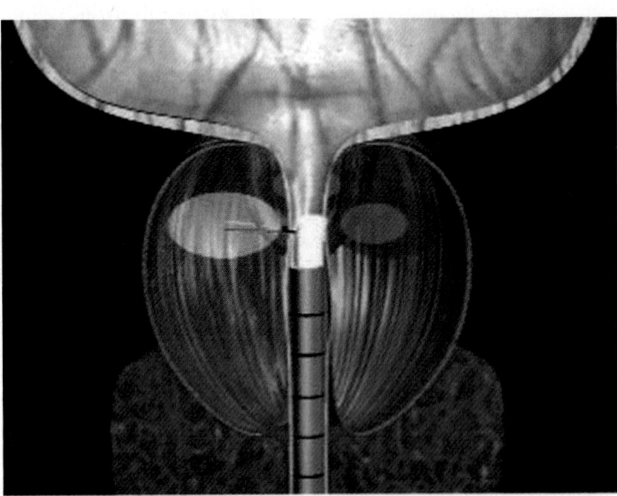

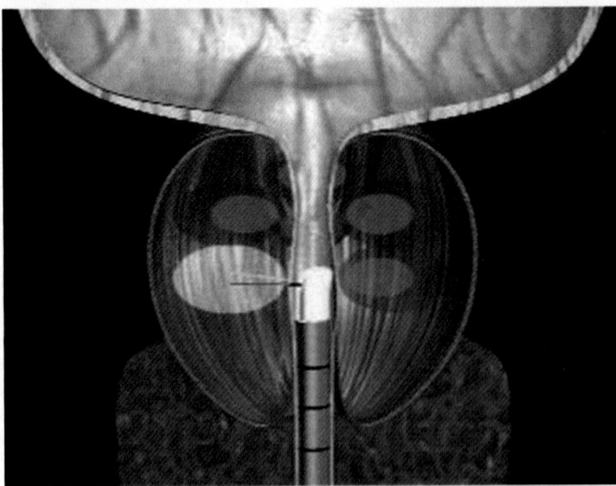

FIGURE 139.1 Transurethral needle ablation (TUNA). Two needles at 40 degrees from each other are attached to a catheter, which is advanced to the prostate via the urethra. The needles are inserted into a lateral lobe of the prostate. Starting from the bladder neck, the needles are advanced 1 cm after each treatment, eventually ablating the entire length of the prostate to the verumontanum. (From www.medtronic.com, with permission.)

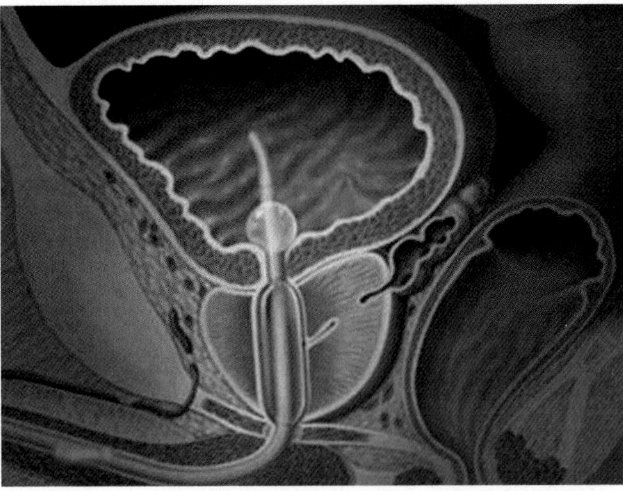

FIGURE 139.2 Transurethral microwave thermotherapy (TUMT). A transurethral catheter containing a microwave antenna is positioned within the prostatic urethra. (From www.bostonscientific.com, with permission.)

## Microwave

Transurethral microwave thermotherapy (TUMT) is a minimally invasive modality for the treatment of BPH. A transurethral catheter containing a microwave antenna is positioned within the prostatic urethra. High-energy microwave power heats the tissue to approximately 70°C, leading to coagulative necrosis. A cooling component to the catheter limits thermal damage to the urethra (Fig. 139.2).

Compared to TURP, microwave procedures have lower complication rates and are usually performed as outpatient procedures. Like TUNA, TUMT is somewhat less effective than TURP in improving urinary symptoms. A recent summary of the literature showed an improvement of the AUA symptom score of 64% (19.4 to 6.7), whereas TURP showed an improvement of 77% (19.6 to 4.5) at 12 months (18). Mattiasson et al. (19) reported in a prospective, randomized study that within 5 years, 10% of the TUMT group required retreatment, whereas in the TURP group, only 4.3% required retreatment. Other studies have shown retreatment rates as high as 30% within 5 years (20). Thus, like TUNA, TUMT seems to have significantly less durability than TURP.

For TUMT, advanced age, small prostate volumes, mild to moderate bladder outlet obstruction, and lower amounts of energy delivered are independent predictors of poor outcome (21). D'Ancona et al. developed a nomogram predicting good and bad responders based on age, prostate volume, degree of bladder outlet obstruction (BOO), amount of energy, international prostate symptom score (IPSS), and maximum flow (Qmax) (22). Additionally, histopathologic findings of lower epithelial-to-stromal ratio and higher vascular density were proposed to decrease efficacy, but studies have not confirmed this (23). The benefit of being able to perform these office-based procedures on nonoperative candidates, coupled with lower morbidity, should be balanced with the somewhat lower efficacy, especially in patients with poor outcome predictive factors.

## CRYOABLATION

### Prostate Cancer

Freezing is also an effective way to ablate unwanted tissue. Cryoablation was first introduced for the treatment of prostate cancer in the 1960s, but it was abandoned due to its high complication rate at that time. Initially, liquid nitrogen was used, but currently argon gas is the cooling agent of choice. Pressurized argon gas (–187°C) is depressurized at the tip of the probe, which allows for cooling at a specific temperature according to the Joule-Thompson effect. Pressurized helium gas (67°C) is used to warm the probes in similar fashion.

Real-time imaging with a transrectal ultrasound and a grid similar to that used for brachytherapy is used to guide the placement of the probes. Six or eight probes are placed percutaneously at the perineum, with additional temperature sensor probes at the rectal wall and external urethral sphincter. A urethral warming catheter is also placed. Standard treatment includes two freeze-thaw cycles to –40°C.

There have been many published studies describing the efficacy of cryotherapy for the primary treatment of prostate cancer. Bahn et al. (24) published a large series of 590 patients showing 7-year actuarial biochemical disease-free survival (bDFS) probabilities in low-, medium-, and high-risk patients of 92%, 89%, and 89%, respectively. Patients were classified as treatment failures according to the American Society of Therapeutic Radiology and Oncology (ASTRO) criteria of three successive increases in PSA. In all patients, the rate of positive biopsy was 13%. Of interest, 94.9% of previously potent patients became impotent following cryotherapy, and 15.9% became incontinent. Other studies report similar results, with rates of erectile dysfunction at 84% to 93% and incontinence at 10%. About 5% of patients required transurethral resection for bladder outlet obstruction (25).

Salvage cryotherapy for recurrent prostate cancer following primary therapy, usually radiotherapy, has been promising. Ng et al. (26) showed that in a series of 187 patients undergoing salvage cryotherapy, patients with pretreatment PSA of <4.0 ng per mL had 5-year and 8-year biochemical recurrence-free rates of 56 and 37%, respectively. For patients with PSA over 10, 5- and 8-year biochemical recurrence-free rates were 14% and 7%. Complication rates are higher for salvage than primary treatment, with incontinence rates up to 20% and rates of rectourethral fistula in the 1% to 3% range (25).

### Small Renal Masses

Cryoablation of small renal masses employs the same pressurized helium-argon system, but with a smaller probe of 1.47 mm. It is a treatment option for peripheral renal lesions measuring <4 cm and can be placed percutaneously or laparoscopically. Similar to RF ablation, cryotherapy is not as effective for tumors around the hilum or major vessels, or those abutting the renal pelvis. The percutaneous approach is equally suitable for inferior pole, lateral, or posterior lesions and can be done under ultrasound, CT, or MRI guidance. With the laparoscopic approach for anterior tumors or lesions abutting vital structures, real-time ultrasound is recommended to monitor the formation of the ice ball.

In human studies, a delayed urine leak has been reported only with RF ablation (48) but not with cryoablation, to date suggesting that the collecting system may be more resilient to cryoablation than to RF ablation.

Several studies demonstrated excellent tumor control following cryoablation. Bandi et al. (27) published a study of 78 patients, 58 who underwent laparoscopic cryoablation and 20 who underwent percutaneous cryoablation. At a mean follow-up of 19 months, the recurrence-free survival rate was 98.7%. In another study, Hegarty et al. (28) reported a 5-year follow-up on 66 patients who underwent cryoablation of a small renal mass. Mean tumor size at treatment was 2.3 cm (range 1.0 to 4.5 cm). Six percent of patients developed a recurrence, and the 5-year cancer-specific survival rate was 98%. Thus, cryoablation should be considered when evaluating treatment options for renal masses smaller than 4 cm.

## LASERS

### Laser Physics

A laser, an acronym for "light amplification by stimulated emission of radiation," is a focused beam of photons. A lasing medium, be it solid, gas, or liquid, emits photons at a specific wavelength when excited by energy (Fig. 139.3). Different mediums emit light at different wavelengths. In a laser, the medium is surrounded by two mirrors, one that is fully reflective, the other partially reflective. These reflected photons collide with excited electrons, releasing an additional photon in the exact same phase, wavelength, and direction. The photons are released through an aperture in the partially reflective mirror. This generates a laser beam with the same wavelength (monochromatic), phase (coherent), and direction (collimated). The

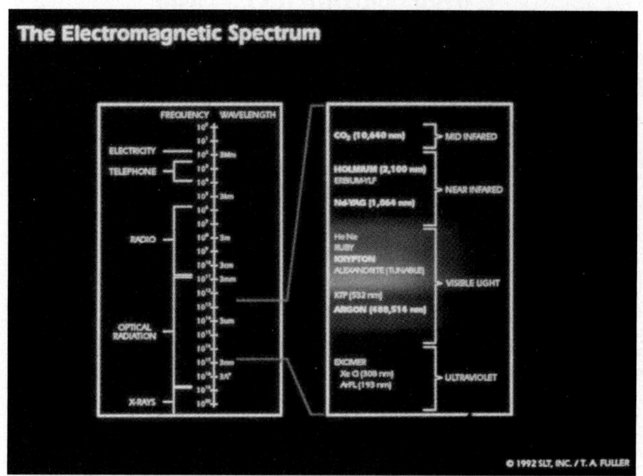


FIGURE 139.3 The electromagnetic spectrum. Each laser emits a very specific wavelength, depending on the substance that is excited (lased).

energy of the laser is expressed in joules (J), and the power is the energy delivered per unit time (1 J per second = 1 W).

## Laser Biophysics

The effect of laser light on tissue is a function of the laser wavelength, tissue absorption characteristics, and power delivered (29). Thermal tissue destruction can be accomplished by either coagulation or vaporization. Capillary coagulation occurs around 60°C to 65°C, and as the tissue temperature increases to 100°C, denaturation of protein and DNA occurs. When the tissue temperature exceeds 100°C, the fluid content of the tissue vaporizes in a plume containing fluid vapor and charred tissue. Following laser treatment, a zone of coagulation necrosis surrounds the site.

By adjusting the wavelength, energy, and time of exposure, tissue effects can be modified to the desired effect. As laser energy is increased, ablation of tissue occurs. At energy levels above the ablation threshold, a focused beam will incise tissue, whereas a lower-power laser causes coagulation and hemostasis. The presence of water will shift the ablation energy to a higher threshold because it cools the tissue. Water also impedes surface ablation and cools the laser fiber to allow a higher-wattage delivery without damage to the fiber. Thus, a higher laser wattage is needed to achieve efficient ablation of the same tissue under water than in air.

The depth of penetration is dependent on both laser and tissue characteristics. In general, a longer wavelength corresponds to greater depth of tissue penetration. Additionally, tissue characteristics that increase laser scatter and energy absorption will decrease penetration. For instance, laser absorption by water or blood will reduce the depth of penetration. These penetration characteristics frequently dictate the type of laser to be used for ablation of tissue in various surgical applications.

## Types of Lasers

The different types of lasers are discussed following see also Manyak and Warner (29).

### Carbon Dioxide ($CO_2$) Laser

The $CO_2$ laser has an invisible infrared wavelength of 10,600 nm and is usually coupled to a visible helium-neon beam to highlight the target area The infrared $CO_2$ beam is absorbed by water, which usually limits its use to surface applications. The $CO_2$ beam can be directed through a waveguide to allow for use through the laparoscope. Depth of tissue penetration is <0.1 mm with a small area of coagulation necrosis. One of the disadvantages of the $CO_2$ laser is the production of a plume with potential vaporization of infectious viral particles. This necessitates the use of a high-filtration mask for all cutaneous applications. In addition, the $CO_2$ laser has poor coagulative properties for vessels over 1.0 mm, and development of oxidized char impedes vaporization of underlying tissue.

### Argon Laser

The argon laser produces wavelengths in the blue-green spectrum (488 to 514 nm) that are absorbed by pigmented molecules such as hemoglobin. The argon beam penetrates 1 to 2 mm in tissue. Advantages include flexible application, minimal plume production, and excellent hemostatic properties. Disadvantages include the need for a dedicated water supply for cooling the laser and the requirement for tinted filters to protect the eyes of operating room staff and patient.

### Neodymium:Yttrium-Aluminum-Garnet (Nd:YAG) Laser

The Nd:YAG laser is a solid-state laser utilizing a crystal seed with neodymium ions to furnish the active medium. The beam is in the near-infrared portion of the light spectrum (1,064 nm) and requires a helium-neon aiming beam for illumination of the target tissue. The Nd:YAG laser is minimally absorbed by water and blood and therefore produces relatively high tissue penetration of 3 to 5 mm with good coagulation. This degree of tissue penetration clearly can be a disadvantage as well. A sapphire tip limits backscatter and enhances the laser cutting properties. Caution is advised due to the extremely high temperatures produced at the tip.

### Potassium Titanyl Phosphate (KTP) Crystal Laser

The KTP crystal laser is generated by passing a rapidly pulsed Nd:YAG beam through a potassium thiophosphate crystal, which doubles the frequency and halves the wavelength to 532 nm. It is strongly absorbed by hemoglobin, and in vascular tissue such as the prostate, the depth of penetration is 1 to 3 mm. There is rapid photothermal vaporization of tissue with excellent hemostasis.

### Holmium:Yttrium-Aluminum-Garnet (Ho:YAG) Laser

Holmium is a rare earth element that, when mixed with YAG, can emit laser radiation at a wavelength of 2,150 nm with a normal pulse duration of 250 ms. This laser operates in the near-infrared portion of the electromagnetic spectrum and is therefore invisible to the human eye. The holmium laser is especially suited for endoscopic procedures because the 2,150-nm wavelength can be transmitted through standard flexible optical fibers. At this wavelength, the pulse is strongly absorbed by water in superficial tissue and provides excellent incisive and tissue ablation properties. Recently, holmium lasers have largely supplanted the use of pulsed dye lasers for lithotripsy of urinary calculi due to their reliability and ease of maintenance.

### Erbium:Yttrium-Aluminum-Garnet (Er:YAG) Laser

Erbium is another rare earth metal used in combination with YAG to produce laser light. This laser emits light at 2,940 nm, which coincides with the water absorption peak in the infrared spectrum. Because of this close approximation with the absorption peak of water, Er:YAG lasers are more efficient in lithotripsy and have more precise tissue ablation with less thermal damage than Ho:YAG lasers. However, the lack of an adequate laser fiber has limited this laser from being more widely used in urology (30).

### Dye Lasers

Dye lasers employ an organic liquid dye as the active medium that is optically excited by another light source. Liquid dyes have complex sets of electronic and vibrational energies, and the wavelength emitted depends on the type of dye used. The wavelength of these lasers can be changed by simply replacing the dye used for excitation, an important advantage of dye lasers. Pulsed dye lasers have been used for lithotripsy of urinary calculi and for photodynamic therapy. The need to change the dye in these lasers at a regular interval makes them more difficult and expensive to maintain than other lasers.

## UROLOGIC LASER PROCEDURES

### Laser Applications for Benign Prostatic Hyperplasia

The Nd:YAG laser was one of the earliest lasers used for the vaporization of BPH. This approach has been largely abandoned due to long catherizations, irritative symtoms, and infections. With the advent of higher-power Ho:YAG and KTP lasers, this technology has become a viable alternate to electroresection and open prostatectomy.

#### Nd:YAG Laser

The Nd:YAG laser was typically used by aiming the laser beam a short distance from the target tissue, called the "free-beam" method. Contact optical fibers, which deliver the laser energy only when the fiber is in contact with the tissue, were used less often. Visual laser ablation of the prostate (VLAP) is the free-beam method of treatment that uses a fiber with a right-angled tip for beam direction. A summary of published studies showed a significant improvement of obstructive symptoms and low rates of perioperative complications (31). However, despite proper patient selection, approximately one-third of patients did not have sufficient symptom relief (32). Many patients remained catheterized for several days post-treatment due to prostatic edema and the potential for urinary retention. Thus, this procedure has been supplanted by newer laser technologies.

#### Ho:YAG Laser

The holmium laser has been used for ablation as well as enucleation of the prostate. HoLAP (holmium laser ablation of the prostate) utilizes a side-fire laser fiber and paints the wall of the prostate, immediately ablating the tissue. This approach allows for immediate visualization of the ablation site, which is an improvement to the invisible deep tissue damage of VLAP. When compared to TURP, HoLAP had similar efficacy in improving AUA symptom scores but with less bleeding, shorter hospital stay, and more consistent next-day catheter removal. The main drawback cited was the length of the procedure with the 60-W laser (31,33). Currently, with the introduction of the 100-W laser, this technique has been mostly superseded by the enucleation technique.

HoLRP (holmium laser resection of the prostate) utilizes the laser to cut small fragments of prostate that can be removed through the resectoscope sheath. This allows for shorter operative time as compared to HoLAP. HoLEP (holmium laser enucleation of the prostate) uses the laser to resect an entire lobe of the prostate in one piece. The laser cuts in the same plane as the index finger would in an open prostatectomy. The adenoma is shelled out and pushed into the bladder. A morcellator is then used to remove the adenoma from the bladder. With this technique, treatment of prostates as large as 300 g has been reported (34). Additionally, a randomized trial comparing HoLEP to TURP showed that the laser was better than TURP at improving symptoms. At a minimum 4-year follow-up, measures of maximal flow, symptom scores, potency rates, and continence rates were similar for HoLRP and TURP. HoLEP had less bleeding and shorter catherization time when compared to TURP or open prostatectomy and had similar retreatment rates at 4 years (31,35).

#### KTP Laser (Green Light)

Photoselective vaporization of the prostate (PVP) with the KTP laser has come into widespread acceptance with the advent of the high-power 120-W laser. PVP provides rapid vaporization of the prostate tissue with limited depth of penetration and a thin rim of coagulation. This leaves a resection site similar to TURP and limits delayed necrosis, minimizing the irritative symptoms seen with the Nd:YAG laser. In contrast to HoLEP, there is no need to morcellate the adenoma. This benefit is also a limitation in that no tissue is obtained for histological analysis.

Te et al. (36) showed in a study with 139 patients from six centers that PVP significantly improved the AUA symptom score from 23.9 to 4.3 at 12 months follow-up. PVP also significantly improved Qmax and decreased the postvoid residual while improving the quality-of-life score. Perioperative morbidity was low, with no patients receiving a blood transfusion and a significant proportion avoiding catherizations. The rates of recatherization, dysuria, infection, urethral stricture, incontinence, and bladder neck contracture were similar to those following TURP or HoLEP. A major advantage of PVP is that it can be performed on patients on anticoagulation, including aspirin, clopidogrel, and even warfarin (37). A disadvantage is that in large prostates, PVP can take several hours and may even need to be performed in stages. PVP with green light KTP laser is now considered a viable alternative to the standard TURP, especially in high-risk patients on anticoagulation.

### Laser Lithotripsy

The most widespread impact of lasers in urology has been in the management of calculi (29). The advent of small rigid and flexible ureteroscopes fitted with holmium lasers has rendered open surgical management of ureteral stones essentially obsolete except in very unusual circumstances.

Laser lithotripsy with pulsed dye lasers is achieved through photoacoustic and photomechanical mechanisms. The discharge of laser energy onto the stone produces a focus of microscopic heating that results in thermal expansion. Further heating leads to ionization of stone material and the formation of plasma, seen as a bright flash of white light (Fig. 139.4). Water is essential for confining the plasma and enhances fragmentation rates approximately tenfold. A cavitation bubble is created that first expands and then collapses, which generates shock waves, causing stone fragmentation (Fig. 139.5). Lithotripsy with the Ho:YAG laser appears to be predominantly a photothermal process that causes chemical decomposition rather than cavitation. This unique mechanism of action allows the holmium laser to be used effectively on all types of stones, including cystine calculi that do not absorb pulsed dye laser energy.

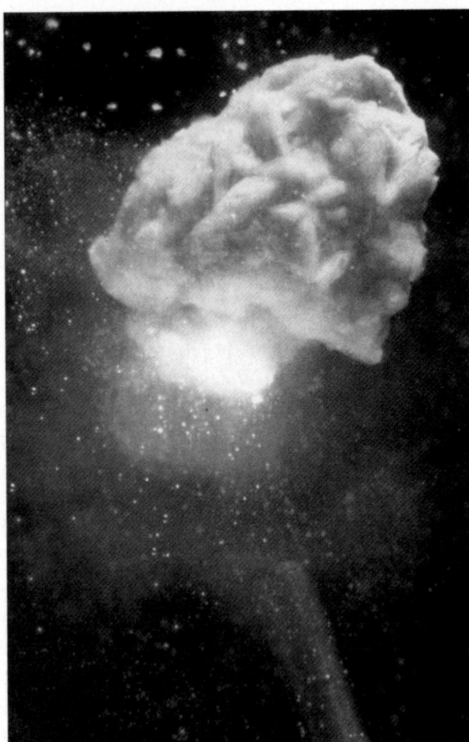

FIGURE 139.4 Plasma formation from holmium:yttrium-aluminum-garnet laser at urinary calculus interface. Plasma propagates shock wave energy from cavitation.

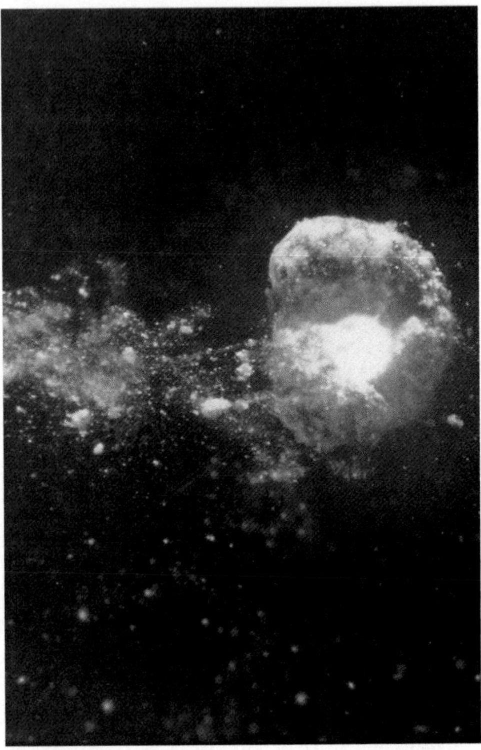

FIGURE 139.5 Photomechanical fragmentation of urinary calculus following plasma formation.

Holmium laser energy can be delivered via fibers of several sizes, with the smaller fibers suitable for both flexible and rigid ureteroscopes. Multiple large series have confirmed both the effectiveness and safety of holmium lithotripsy (38). Stone-free rates after laser lithotripsy of upper urinary calculi are in the 90% range for all ureteral calculi and 85% for renal calculi. The safety profile of holmium laser lithotripsy is well documented, with very low perforation and stricture rates. A further advantage to holmium lithotripsy is its efficacy in morbidly obese patients, whose body habitus precludes effective extracorporeal shock wave lithotripsy or percutaneous nephrostolithotomy. Holmium lithotripsy has also proven successful in cases of failed electrohydraulic lithotripsy and creates significantly smaller stone fragments than pneumatic, pulsed dye laser, or electrohydraulic lithotripsy (39). In addition, pediatric urolithiasis and urolithiasis of pregnancy can be safely treated with this technology.

## Laser Treatment of Transitional Cell Carcinoma of the Renal Pelvis and Ureter

Improvements in endoscopic access to the upper urinary tract have allowed intraluminal laser ablation of papillary transitional cell malignancies. Both the Nd:YAG and Ho:YAG lasers can be delivered via small-diameter optical fibers and have been used for tumor ablation. The Nd:YAG laser is typically set at 20 to 30 W and is activated at a tangential angle, avoiding direct tissue contact, for 2 to 3 seconds. This results in a depth penetration of 5 to 6 mm. The Ho:YAG laser is placed in direct contact with the tumor and set at 1 J and 10 Hz. This laser has a very superficial penetration (0.4 mm) and therefore little risk of perforation, even in the thin-walled ureter. For large tumors (over 1 cm), a tag team approach is often effective: the Nd:YAG laser to first coagulate the bulk of the tumor, followed by the Ho:YAG laser to ablate the residual layers.

Compared to electrofulguration, laser treatment appears to result in less scarring and stricture formation in the upper urinary tract. Local recurrence is reported to be as high as 74% in patients with renal pelvis and ureteral tumors (40). Recurrence and progression of disease correlate closely with higher grade and stage, so laser thermal destruction of tumors is best reserved for lower-grade, superficial lesions. In patients with specific indications for conservative therapy, however, laser ablation of low-grade upper-tract transitional cell carcinoma (TCC) with close ureteroscopic surveillance is now considered a reasonable alternative to surgical removal. This form of treatment may be especially well suited for patients with lesions in a solitary kidney or with bilateral disease.

## Photodynamic Therapy

Photodynamic therapy is an intriguing new treatment modality that has been applied to tumors in multiple anatomic locations, including the bladder, skin, esophagus, head and neck, brain, and peritoneal cavity. This technology utilizes a chemical that is activated by light to trigger a photochemical reaction that causes tissue destruction and cell death (Fig. 139.6). The wavelength of the light source should be that which is maximally absorbed by the photosensitizer.

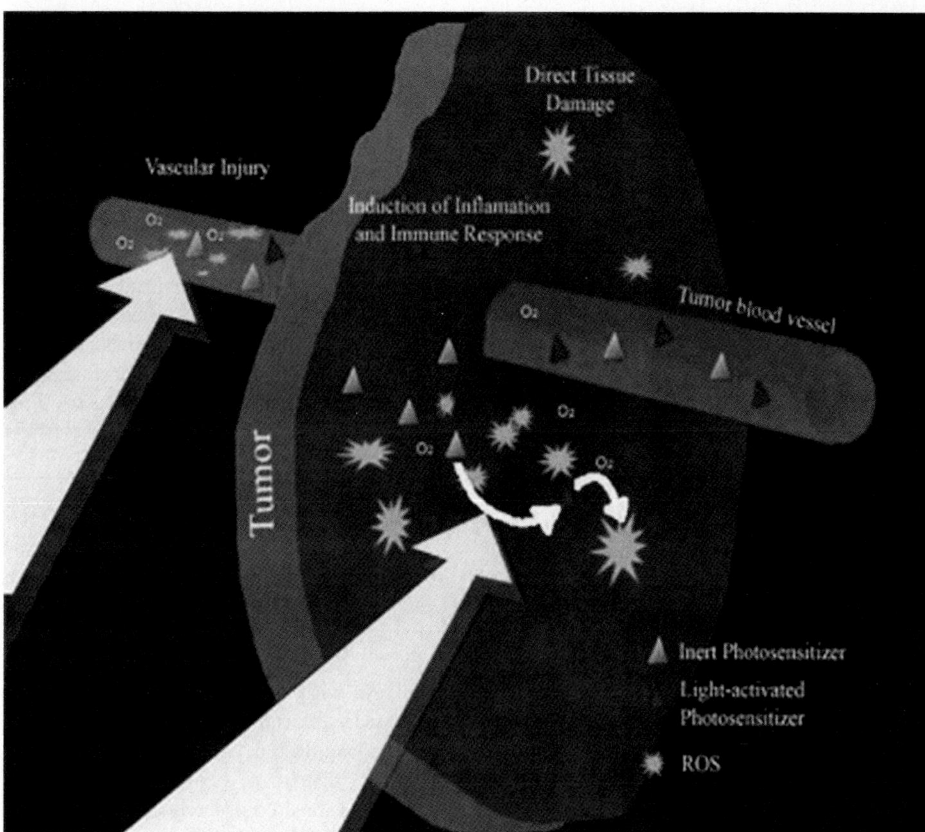


FIGURE 139.6. General concept of photodynamic therapy. Light excitation of photosensitizer in presence of $O_2$ generates reactive oxygen species (ROS), which attack different cellular structures. (From Pinthus JH, Bogaards A, Weersink R, et al. Photodynamic therapy for urological malignancies: past to current approaches. *J Urol* 2006;175:1201, with permission.)

Commonly used photosensitizing agents are derived from porphyrins and chlorophyll. Early experience with Photofrin, a porphyrin-based agent excited at 630 nm, showed efficacy for the treatment of bladder cancer, with response rates of 45% to 80% at 3 months (41). Berger et al. (42) reported the effectiveness of intravesical 5-aminolevulinic acid (5-ALA) in patients with superficial bladder cancer in whom multiple transurethral resections and/or intravesical bacille Calmette-Guérin (BCG) immunotherapy alone had failed. At an average follow-up of 23.7 months (range, 1 to 73), half of the patients were free of tumor. Problems included skin photosensitization, and side-effects included irritative symptoms and bladder shrinkage. However, newer photosensitizers with shorter half-lives and optimization of light doses should improve efficacy and decrease side-effects.

## Laser Treatment of External Genitalia

Lasers are excellent tools for the precise ablation of genital condyloma caused by human papilloma virus (HPV) (29). Excellent therapeutic and cosmetic results have been obtained with the $CO_2$ and Nd:YAG laser treatment of large penile lesions. Magnification with loupes or an operating microscope is required for multiple smaller lesions. HPV particles can remain viable in the laser plume. Safety precautions for operating room personnel are imperative and include charcoal filtration face masks and a dedicated suction apparatus to capture the laser plume. Nd:YAG treatment of condyloma requires irrigation to cool the tissue during treatment. Treatment of urethral condyloma proximal to the meatus is not amenable to $CO_2$ therapy because this laser energy cannot be transmitted via a fiber. Both the Nd:YAG and holmium lasers have been used for urethral condyloma with good results and very few complications.

In addition to benign penile lesions, lasers are currently used for treatment of superficial squamous cell carcinoma of the penis. Successful treatment of premalignant or low-grade penile malignancy (Bowen disease, erythroplasia of Queyrat, bowenoid papulosis) can be achieved using many of the common surgical lasers (Fig. 139.7). Because these lesions are superficial, are often multifocal, and require precise treatment, the $CO_2$ laser in combination with an operating microscope is often considered the ideal approach. The Nd:YAG and $CO_2$

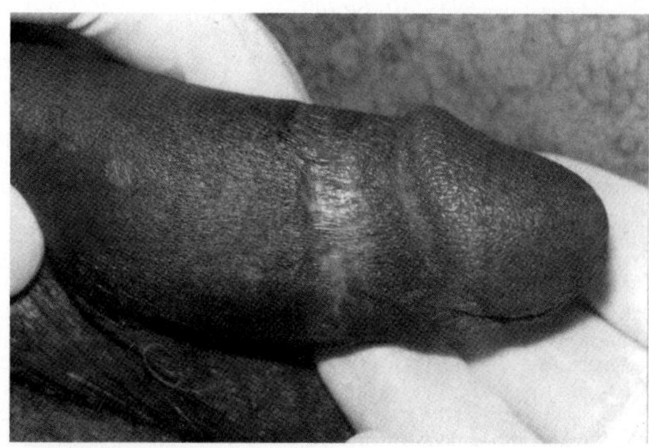

FIGURE 139.7. An excellent cosmetic effect following neodymium: yttrium-aluminum-garnet laser treatment of superficial penile squamous cell carcinoma.

lasers are well suited to treat superficial squamous cell penile lesions with good results reported, but they are not recommended for T1 and T2 squamous cell carcinoma of the penis. Local treatment of Kaposi sarcoma with the Nd:YAG laser has been beneficial for urethral meatal obstruction.

## DIAGNOSTIC USE OF LASERS

Although the most popular application of lasers to date has been for ablation, their use in endoscopic diagnosis has been increasing. The fluorescent properties of tumors in response to photosensitizing agents have long been of interest for the diagnosis of occult malignancy. In urology, the bladder is the primary focus for this application (43). The most common compounds used for fluorescent detection are porphyrins, which produce a characteristic reddish hue in tissue after exposure to ultraviolet or blue-green visible light. The most promising agent, 5-ALA, can be administered directly into the bladder and so avoids the skin reaction associated with most photosensitizers.

In a randomized prospective study involving 102 patients undergoing transurethral resection of a bladder tumor (44), the use of 5-ALA resulted in a more thorough resection of bladder tumors. Six weeks after the initial resection, second-look cystoscopies showed a 16% recurrence in the 5-ALA group versus 41% in the white light group. Sensitivity was 87% to 97% for 5-ALA and 68% to 85% in the white light group. The specificities for both modalities were similar (43% to 76% for 5-ALA and 31% to 89% for white light). Daniltchenko et al. (45) showed that the improvement in bladder cancer detection at the initial cystoscopy significantly decreased the number of recurrences over a 5-year period.

Optical coherence tomography (OCT) uses inexpensive solid-state red diodes to create a cross-sectional tomographic image based on optical scattering within tissue (46). OCT is similar to ultrasound pulse-echo imaging but uses optical rather than acoustic reflectivity. Unlike ultrasound, OCT does not require a conducting medium and can image through air or water and with far greater resolution than ultrasound. In combination with endoscopy, OCT offers imaging of the epithelial surface of internal organs and visualization of tissue beneath the surface. Manyak et al. (47) showed in an evaluation of 87 areas in 24 patients that OCT had a sensitivity of 100% and specificity of 87%. The positive predictive value for invasion was 90%. Though a small study, these results appear very promising and will open the way for further trials to eludicate the usefulness of OCT for bladder cancer staging.

## CONCLUSION

Various energy sources, ranging from cryoablation to microwave to lasers, have been widely adopted into urologic surgery. Bipolar instruments continue to improve electrosurgery, providing better vessel sealing while minimizing current spread. In the treatment of BPH, office-based procedures such as TUNA and TUMT have shown good efficacy in terms of symptom relief, albeit with less durability than TURP. Green light laser has made ablation of the prostate feasible even for patients on anticoagulation. Small renal masses can now be ablated or frozen, instead of being excised. And of course, the holmium laser has completely changed stone surgery, making open surgical removal of stones very rare.

Looking ahead, advances in new technology such as photodynamic therapy or optical coherence tomography will continue to change urologic surgery. In addition, new uses of existing technology, such as in focal therapy for prostate cancer, will continue to make the practice of urologic surgery less invasive with less morbidity and better efficacy.

## *References*


1. Vancaillie TG. Active electrode monitoring: how to prevent unintentional thermal injury associated with monopolar electrosurgery at laparoscopy. *Surg Endosc* 1998;12:1009.
2. Person B, Vivas DA, Ruiz D, et al. Comparison of four energy-based vascular sealing and cutting instruments: a porcine model. *Surg Endosc* 2008; 22(2):534–538.
3. Autorino R, De Sio M, D'Armiento M. Bipolar plasmakinetic technology for the treatment of symptomatic benign prostatic hyperplasia: evidence beyond marketing hype? *BJU Int* 2007;100:983.
4. Seckiner I, Yesilli C, Akduman B, et al. A prospective randomized study for comparing bipolar plasmakinetic resection of the prostate with standard TURP. *Urol Int* 2006;76:139.
5. Kinoshita T, Kanehira E, Omura K, et al. Experimental study on heat production by a 23.5-kHz ultrasonically activated device for endoscopic surgery. *Surg Endosc* 1999;13:621.
6. Pietrow PK, Weizer AZ, L'Esperance JO, et al. PlasmaKinetic bipolar vessel sealing: burst pressures and thermal spread in an animal model. *J Endourol* 2005;19:107.
7. Carbonell AM, Joels CS, Kercher KW, et al. A comparison of laparoscopic bipolar vessel sealing devices in the hemostasis of small-, medium-, and large-sized arteries. *J Laparoendosc Adv Surg Tech A* 2003;13:377.
8. Campbell PA, Cresswell AB, Frank TG, et al. Real-time thermography during energized vessel sealing and dissection. *Surg Endosc* 2003;17:1640.
9. Landman J, Kerbl K, Rehman J, et al. Evaluation of a vessel sealing system, bipolar electrosurgery, harmonic scalpel, titanium clips, endoscopic gastrointestinal anastomosis vascular staples and sutures for arterial and venous ligation in a porcine model. *J Urol* 2003;169:697.
10. Hruby GW, Marruffo FC, Durak E, et al. Evaluation of surgical energy devices for vessel sealing and peripheral energy spread in a porcine model. *J Urol* 2007:178:2689.
11. Bandi G, Wen CC, Wilkinson EA, et al. Comparison of blade temperature dynamics after activation of Harmonic Ace Scalpel and the Ultracision Harmonic Scalpel LCS-K5. *J Endourol* 2008;22:333.
12. Kim FJ, Chammas MF Jr, Gewehr E, et al. Temperature safety profile of laparoscopic devices: Harmonic ACE (ACE), Ligasure V (LV), and plasma trisector (PT). *Surg Endosc* 2008; 22(6):1464–1469.
13. Blana A, Murat FJ, Walter B, et al. First analysis of the long-term results with transrectal HIFU in patients with localised prostate cancer. *Eur Urol* 2008;53(6):1194–1201.
14. Poissonnier L, Chapelon JY, Rouviere O, et al. Control of prostate cancer by transrectal HIFU in 227 patients. *Eur Urol* 2007;51:381.
15. Murat FJ, Poissonnier L, Pasticier G, et al. High-intensity focused ultrasound (HIFU) for prostate cancer. *Cancer Control* 2007;14:244.
16. Park S, Cadeddu JA. Outcomes of radiofrequency ablation for kidney cancer. *Cancer Control* 2007;14:205.
17. Bouza C, Lopez T, Magro A, et al. Systematic review and meta-analysis of transurethral needle ablation in symptomatic benign prostatic hyperplasia. *BMC Urol* 2006;6:14.
18. Hoffman RM, MacDonald R, Monga M, et al. Transurethral microwave thermotherapy vs transurethral resection for treating benign prostatic hyperplasia: a systematic review. *BJU Int* 2004;94:1031.
19. Mattiasson A, Wagrell L, Schelin S, et al. Five-year follow-up of feedback microwave thermotherapy versus TURP for clinical BPH: a prospective randomized multicenter study. *Urology* 2007;69:91.
20. Tan AH, Nott L, Hardie WR, et al. Long-term results of microwave thermotherapy for symptomatic benign prostatic hyperplasia. *J Endourol* 2005;19:1191.
21. D'Ancona FC, Francisca EA, Debruyne FM, et al. High-energy transurethral microwave thermotherapy in men with lower urinary tract symptoms. *J Endourol* 1997;11:285.

22. D'Ancona FC, Francisca EA, Witjes WP, et al. Transurethral resection of the prostate vs high-energy thermotherapy of the prostate in patients with benign prostatic hyperplasia: long-term results. *Br J Urol* 1998;81:259.
23. Gravas S, Laguna MP, De La Rosette JJ. Application of external microwave thermotherapy in urology: past, present, and future. *J Endourol* 2003;17:659.
24. Bahn DK, Lee F, Badalament R, et al. Targeted cryoablation of the prostate: 7-year outcomes in the primary treatment of prostate cancer. *Urology* 2002;60:3.
25. Chin JL, Lim D, Abdelhady M. Review of primary and salvage cryoablation for prostate cancer. *Cancer Control* 2007;14:231.
26. Ng CK, Moussa M, Downey DB, et al. Salvage cryoablation of the prostate: followup and analysis of predictive factors for outcome. *J Urol* 2007;178:1253.
27. Bandi G, Wen CC, Hedican SP, et al. Cryoablation of small renal masses: assessment of the outcome at one institution. *BJU Int* 2007;100:798.
28. Hegarty NJ, Gill IS, Desai MM, et al. Probe-ablative nephron-sparing surgery: cryoablation versus radiofrequency ablation. *Urology* 2006;68:7.
29. Manyak MJ, Warner JW. Lasers in urologic surgery. In: Gillenwater JY, ed. *Glenn's urology,* 6th ed. Philadelphia: Lippincott Williams & Wilkins, 2002:
30. Marks AJ, Teichman JM. Lasers in clinical urology: state of the art and new horizons. *World J Urol* 2007;25:227.
31. Kuntz RM. Current role of lasers in the treatment of benign prostatic hyperplasia (BPH). *Eur Urol* 2006;49:961.
32. Muschter R. Free-beam and contact laser coagulation. *J Endourol* 2003;17:579.
33. Mottet N, Anidjar M, Bourdon O, et al. Randomized comparison of transurethral electroresection and holmium:YAG laser vaporization for symptomatic benign prostatic hyperplasia. *J Endourol* 1999;13:127.
34. Elzayat EA, Elhilali MM. Holmium laser enucleation of the prostate (HoLEP): the endourologic alternative to open prostatectomy. *Eur Urol* 2006;49:87.
35. Westenberg A, Gilling P, Kennett K, et al. Holmium laser resection of the prostate versus transurethral resection of the prostate: results of a randomized trial with 4-year minimum long-term followup. *J Urol* 2004;172:616.
36. Te AE, Malloy TR, Stein BS, et al. Photoselective vaporization of the prostate for the treatment of benign prostatic hyperplasia: 12-month results from the first United States multicenter prospective trial. *J Urol* 2004;172:1404.
37. Sandhu JS, Ng CK, Gonzalez RR, et al. Photoselective laser vaporization prostatectomy in men receiving anticoagulants. *J Endourol* 2005;19:1196.
38. Gould DL. Holmium:YAG laser and its use in the treatment of urolithiasis: our first 160 cases. *J Endourol* 1998;12:23.
39. Teichman JM, Vassar GJ, Bishoff JT, et al. Holmium:YAG lithotripsy yields smaller fragments than lithoclast, pulsed dye laser or electrohydraulic lithotripsy. *J Urol* 1998;159:17.
40. Sowter SJ, Ilie CP, Efthimiou I, et al. Endourologic management of patients with upper-tract transitional-cell carcinoma: long-term follow-up in a single center. *J Endourol* 2007;21:1005.
41. Pinthus JH, Bogaards A, Weersink R, et al. Photodynamic therapy for urological malignancies: past to current approaches. *J Urol* 2006;175:1201.
42. Berger AP, Steiner H, Stenzl A, et al. Photodynamic therapy with intravesical instillation of 5-aminolevulinic acid for patients with recurrent superficial bladder cancer: a single-center study. *Urology* 2003;61:338.
43. Benson RC Jr, Farrow GM, Kinsey JH, et al. Detection and localization of in situ carcinoma of the bladder with hematoporphyrin derivative. *Mayo Clin Proc* 1982;57:548.
44. Riedl CR, Daniltchenko D, Koenig F, et al. Fluorescence endoscopy with 5-aminolevulinic acid reduces early recurrence rate in superficial bladder cancer. *J Urol* 2001;165:1121.
45. Daniltchenko DI, Riedl CR, Sachs MD, et al. Long-term benefit of 5-aminolevulinic acid fluorescence assisted transurethral resection of superficial bladder cancer: 5-year results of a prospective randomized study. *J Urol* 2005;174:2129.
46. Huang D, Swanson EA, Lin CP, et al. Optical coherence tomography. *Science* 1991;254:1178.
47. Manyak MJ, Gladkova ND, Makari JH, et al. Evaluation of superficial bladder transitional-cell carcinoma by optical coherence tomography. *J Endourol* 2005;19:570.
48. Johnson DB, Solomon SB, Su LM, et al. Defining the complications of cryoablation and radio frequency ablation of small renal tumors: a multi-institutional review. *J Urol* 2004;172:874.

# INDEX


## A

Abdominal leak point pressure (ALPP)
  injectable therapies, female incontinence patients, 263
  pubovaginal fascial sling investigation, 272
Abdominal repair, vaginal prolapse, 331, 333f
Abdominal retropubic therapies, incontinence, female patients, 288–291
  alternative therapy, 289
  diagnosis and indications, 288–289
  laparoscopic Burch urethropexy, 290
  open Burch urethropexy, 289–290, 289f–290f
  outcomes and complications, 290–291
Abdominal sacral colpopexy, 349–354
  alternative therapy, 351
  diagnosis, 350–351, 350t
  indications for, 351, 351f
  outcomes and complications, 353–354
  surgical techniques, 351–353, 352f–353f
Abdominal wall reconstruction, triad syndrome, 656, 658, 659f
Ablation technologies
  prostate cancer, image-guided focal ablation, 918
  renal tumors, 915–917
Acute tubular necrosis (ATN), partial nephrectomy and, 7–9, 8f
Adenocarcinoma
  in female urethra, 252–256
  urachal, partial cystectomy for, 890–891
Adrenalectomy
  laparoscopic techniques, 859–866
    alternative therapy, 860–861
    diagnosis, 860, 860t
    indications for, 859–860, 860t
    outcomes and complications, 866
    preoperative considerations, 861
    retroperitoneal approach, 862–864, 864f–865f
    retroperitoneal left adrenalectomy, 864–865
    retroperitoneal right adrenalectomy, 866
    surgical techniques, 861–866
    transperitoneal approach, 861, 861f–862f
    transperitoneal left adrenalectomy, 861–862, 862f–864f
    transperitoneal right adrenalectomy, 862, 864f
  robotic surgical techniques, 923
Adrenal glands
  anatomical relationship, 1, 1f–2f
  contiguous structures, 2–3, 2f
  embryology, 1–2
  vascular anatomy, 2
Advancement flap, female urethra, 223, 223f
Advancement test, transperineal laparoscopy, 803
AESOP surgical robotics, 921
Alloderm, penile reconstruction, 539, 542, 542f
Allograft techniques
  renal transplantation
    allograft positioning and vascular anastomoses, 66–68, 67f–68f
    alternative therapy, 65
    diagnosis, 65
    incision and iliac fossa dissection, 65–66, 66f
    multiple renal vessels, 68
    outcomes and complications, 70–71, 71t
    pediatric patients, 69–70, 69f–70f
    surgical indications, 65
    surgical techniques, 65–70
    ureteral considerations, 68, 69f
    wound closure, 70
  transplant nephrectomy, 32–36
Ambiguous genitalia, corrective surgical techniques, 769–777
Anastomoses
  colonic continent catheterizable reservoir construction, 604–605
  ileal conduit urinary diversion, 547–548, 548f
  ileal neobladder, 568, 570–571, 570f–572f
  microvascular arterial bypass surgery for erectile dysfunction, 512–513, 512f
  neurogenic bladder, 230–232, 231f
  orthotopic urinary diversion, with ileal low-pressure reservoir, afferent tubulary segment
    bladder reconstruction to urethra, 563–564, 563f–564f
    ureteroileal end-to-side anastomosis, 563, 563f
  Padua ileal bladder, 576–577, 576f–577f
  penile replantation, 521
  refluxing ileoureteral anastomosis, 571–573, 572f–573f
  renal allotransplantation, vascular anastomoses, 66–68, 67f–68f
  renovascular disease, saphenous vein grafts, 38–39, 40f
  ureteral complications, renal transplant, 72–75, 75f
  ureterosigmoidostomy, 611–613, 611f–613f
  urethral stricture repair, 240–241, 240f, 242f
  vasoepididymostomy, 383–384
  vasovastostomy procedures, 393, 393f
    special circumstances, 395f, 362596
Anatrophic nephrolithotomy, 45–7–51
  alternative therapy, 46–47
  diagnosis, 45–46
  outcomes and complications, 50
  surgical indications, 47
  surgical technique, 46–50, 47f–50f
Anderson-Hynes dismembered pyeloplasty, robotic techniques, 854–855, 855f
Andrews procedure, hydrocele repair, 529, 529f
Anejaculation, ejaculation induction procedures, 413–418
Angioembolization, renal trauma, 59–60, 60f
Angiotensin receptor agonist (ARB) therapy, renovascular disease, 37
Anterior dissection, laparoscopic radical cystectomy, 887
Anterior exenteration, female radical cystectomy, 106–107, 106f–109f
Anterior urethral valve surgery, 703
Antireflux mechanism
  catherizable reservoir construction, ileal segments, 594–598
  colonic orthotopic bladder substitution, 588–590
  T-pouch ileal neobladder reconstruction, 580–581, 580f, 585
Aortorenal bypass graft, renovascular disease, 37–41, 37f
Appendicovesicostomy, 794–795, 794f–795f
Appendix
  catherizable reservoir construction, ileal segment, 596–597, 597f
  colonic continent catheterizable reservoir, 602, 602f
Arcus tendineus fasciae pelvis (ATFP)
  pelvic floor anatomy, 314, 315f
  vaginal prolapse, 326–327, 326f–327f
Argon laser, 930
Artificial erection, hypospadias surgery, 705
Artificial urinary sphincter (AUS)
  alternative techniques, 293
  basic principles, 292, 292f
  complications and outcomes, 298
  diagnosis, 292–293
  female patients, 297, 297f
  male patients, 293–296
    bladder neck cuff placement, 296
    sling procedures as alternative, 299–304
    synchronous AUS and penile implant insertion, 297
    transcorporeal cuff replacement, 294, 294f
    transverse scrotal incision, 294–296, 295f–296f
  pediatric patients, bladder augmentation with, 297
  preoperative preparation, 293–294
  surgical indications, 293
  surgical technique, 293–297, 293f–297f
Assisted reproduction, sperm retrieval for, 403–406

Augmentation cystoplasty
autoaugmentation techniques, bladder augmentation, 119–120
in pediatric patients, 783–792
alternative therapy, 784
bladder compliance, 120
bladder perforation, 792
caliculi formation and mucus production, 792
"clam" augmentation technique, 785, 785f
diagnosis, 783
gastrocystoplasty, 789, 789f–790f
hematuria-dysuria syndrome, 792
ileocystoplasty, 785–787, 786f, 791
outcomes and complications, 784t, 791–792
right colocystoplasty and Mainz enterocystoplasty, 787, 787f, 791
sigmoidocystoplasty, 787, 788f
surgical indications, 783, 783t
surgical techniques, 784–790, 784t–785t
uretocystoplasty, 789, 790f
urinary and abdominal drainage, 791
urinary tract infection, 792
Autologous fat, injectable therapies, female incontinence patients, 265–266
Autologous materials
autologous cells, genitourinary tissue engineering, 905–906
injectable incontinence therapies, female patients, 265–266
midurethral retropubic slings, 279
Autonomic innervation, bladder anatomy, 89–90, 90f
Autotransplantation, renovascular disease, 43–44, 44f
Autotransplantation, renal
alternative therapy, 76
back-table preparation, 80
diagnosis, 76
flank donor nephrectomy, 78–80, 79f
iliac vessel exposure, 80–81, 81f
midline intraperitoneal approach, doonor nephrectomy, 80
outcomes and complications, 82–83
revascularization, 80–82
surgical indications, 76
surgical instrumentation, 77
surgical techniques, 77–78
ureteroneocystostomy, 82, 82f
wound closure, 82
Avulsion injuries, genitalia, 457–460, 459f
Azoospermia
nonobstructive, 403
vasoepididymyostomy, 379

## B

Bacille Calmette-Guérin, interstitial cystitis management, 151–152
Back-table preparation, renal autotransplantation, 80, 81f
Belt approach, for radical prostatectomy, 196, 197f
Benign prostatic hypertrophy (BPH)
alternative therapies, 167, 167t
bladder histology, 88–89, 88f
diagnosis, 166
epidemiology, 166
laser applications, 168–171, 168t, 169f, 171t, 931–934
minimally invasive therapy, 167
storage reflex, bladder function, 90, 91f
surgical treatment, 166–173, 172–173, 172f–173f
complications, 174
laser ablation, 170–171, 171t
suprapubic prostatectomy, 171–173, 171f–173f, 171t
transurethral incision of the prostate/transurethral resection of the prostate, 167–170, 168t, 169f
transurethral needle ablation, 928, 928f
treatment options, 166–167, 166f, 167t
treatment outcomes, 173–174
Bicycle riding, erectile dysfunction and, 506–507
Bilateral cutaneous ureterostomy, single stoma, 619–620, 619f
Bilateral sacrospinous ligament fixation, 323, 324f
Biomaterials
genitourinary tissue construction, 905
injectable incontinence therapies, female patients, 266
BION device, interstitial cystitis management, 157–158
Biopsy procedures
bladder neck biopsy
colonic continent catheterizable reservoir, 599
orthotopic bladder substitution, 556
prostate
alternative therapy, 176
complications, 177–178
computerized tomography, 178
image-guided techniques, 917–918
magnetic resonance imaging, 178
positron emission tomography, 178
screening and diagnosis, 175
surgical indications, 176
surgical technique, 176–177, 177f
Bipolar cauterization, urologic procedures, 926–927, 926t
Bladder anatomy
augmentation cystoplasty and bladder compliance, 791
blood supply, 89, 89f
contiguous structures, 91
emptying reflex, 91, 91f
female bladder, 85, 85f, 91
histologic structure, 86–88, 87f
innervation, 89–91
ligamentous attachments, 86, 86f–87f
lymphatics, 91
male bladder, 85–86, 86f, 91
micturition reflex, 90
motor innervation, 90
overactive bladder, sacral neurostimulation, 305–306
peritoneal relationships, 85–86, 85f–86f
sensory innervation, 89–90
storage reflex, 90, 90f
ureterovesical junction and trigone, 88–89, 88f
vesical trauma and hemorrhage, 143–149
Bladder augmentation, 118–124. *See also* Augmentation cystoplasty
alternative therapy, 119–120
complications and outcomes, 123–124
diagnosis, 119
indications, 118–119
interstitial cystitis management, 152, 154f, 159t
simultaneous artificial urinary sphincter, pediatric patients, 297
surgical technique, 120–123, 120f–123f
Bladder cancer
histology, 86–88, 87f
laparoscopic pelvic lymph node dissection, 811–813
palliative urinary diversion, 618–622
pelvic lymphadenectomy, limited *vs.* extended lymph node dissection, 184
pelvic lymphadenectomy for
indications for, 183
surgical technique, 183–184
radical cystectomy for, 92–93, 93f
rhabdomyosarcoma, childhood, surgical technique, 663–664
T-pouch ileal neobladder, 579
Bladder cuff techniques, distal ureter management
laparoscopic stapling, 835–836, 835f
transurethral technique, 127
transvesical technique, 126–128, 126f–127f
Bladder diverticulectomy, 739
alternative therapy, 115
diagnosis, 113f–114f, 736
indications for, 114
laparoscopic procedures, 891
outcomes and complications, 117
preoperative assessment, 115
surgical techniques, 115–117, 116f–117f
Bladder exstrophy
epispadias and, 722–730
anatomic reconstruction with, 723–101–102
closure techniques, 725–727, 726f
continence and antireflux procedure, 727–728, 728f–729f
diagnosis, 723
osteotomy, 724–725, 725f–726f
outcomes and complications, 728–730
preoperative preparation, 724
surgical indications, 723
timing and staging, 724
urinary diversion techniques and, 723
inguinal hernias, 720–721
penile/urethral dissection with, 712f–716f, 713–714
postoperative care, 721
primary integrated reconstruction, 711–722
diagnosis, 711–712, 712f
outcomes and complications, 721–722
surgical indications, 712
surgical technique, 712–721
surgical technique
boys, 713–718
girls, 719–720
preoperative care, 712
Bladder flap reconstruction, female urethra, 222, 222f
Bladder hydrodistention, interstitial cystitis management, 152, 152f–153f, 159t
Bladder neck biopsy
colonic continent catheterizable reservoir, 599
orthotopic bladder substitution, 556
Bladder neck closure (BNC)
female, 228–232, 229t, 230f–232f
male, 229, 232–235, 233f–234f

Bladder neck cuff placement, artificial urinary sphincter, male patients, 296
Bladder neck suspension
laparoscopic techniques, 892–896
alternative therapy with, 893
diagnosis, 892
outcomes and complications, 896, 896t
surgical indications for, 892–893
surgical technique, 893–896, 893t, 894f–896f
vesical neck reconstruction, fascial sling technique, 691, 691f
Bladder neck transection and reconstruction
open radical retropubic surgery, 190–191, 190f
robotically assisted laparoscopic (radical) prostatectomy, 874, 875f
Bladder perforation
augmentation cystoplasty and, 792
pubovaginal fascial sling procedure, 277
Bladder substitution, orthotopic, 555–561. *See also* Neobladder, ileal
alternative therapy, 556
bowel function, 556
colonic
alternative therapy, 587–588
diagnostic criteria, 587
goals and function, 586–587
indications for surgery, 587
outcomes and complications, 590–593
surgical technique, 588–590, 589f–593f
continence, 556
diagnostic criteria, 555–556, 555t
hepatic function, 556
intraoperative management, 556–557, 557t
orthotopic urinary diversion, with ileal low-pressure reservoir, afferent tubulary segment, 562–563, 562f
outcomes and complications, 560–561, 560t
paracollicular and bladder neck biopsy, 556
patient agreement and mental status, 555–556
postoperative management, 558–560, 558t
catheter removal, 558–559, 558t
metabolic management, 559–560, 560t
renal function, 556
surgical indications, 556
surgical technique
atraumatic urethral dissection, 557
bladder substitute, 558
pelvic nerve preservation, 557
preoperative period, 556
ureteral dissection, 557, 557f
Bladder tissue engineering, 909–910, 910f
"Bland" thrombus, intracaval tumors, abdominal surgical approaches to, 29–31, 30f
Blind-ending testicular vessels, laparoscopic surgery for, 744, 745f
Blocksom vesicostomy, posterior urethral valves, 698–700, 699f
Blood supply, bladder anatomy, 89
Botulinium toxin, bladder augmentation, 119–120
Bowel function
orthotopic bladder substitution, 556
rectourethral fistula repair and preservation of, 142–143
Brachytherapy, prostate cancer
alternative therapy, 203
diagnosis, 202
hybrid real-time planning and linked seeds approach, 205–207, 205f–207f
isotope selection, 203, 203t
outcomes and complications, 207–208, 208t
postimplant cystoscopy, 207
postimplant dosimetry, 207
real-time planning, 204–205, 205f
surgical indications, 202–203, 202t
surgical techniques, 203–207
Bracka buccal two-stage repair, hypospadias surgery, 708, 710f
Bricker technique, ileal conduit urinary diversion, 547–548, 548f
Broad ligaments, pelvic floor anatomy, 314
Bulbar urethral stricture, 240–241, 248, 248f
Bulbourethral (Cowper) glands, anatomy, 355f, 360
Bulking agents
injectable incontinence therapy, female patients, 263–265
midurethral retropubic slings *vs.*, 278–279
Burch urethropexies, abdominal retropubic therapies, female patients, 289–291, 289f–290f
Burn injury, genitalia, 453, 460, 460f
Buttonhole submucosal implantation technique, colonic orthotopic bladder substitution, 589–590, 592f

## C

Calculi formation
augmentation cystoplasty and, 792
laparoscopic procedures for, 897–899, 898f
Calicoplasty, anatrophic nephrolithotomy, 49–50, 49f–50f
Cantwell-Ransley epispadias repair, 725, 726f, 727, 728f
Carbon-coated zirconium beads (durasphere/durasphere EXP), injectable incontinence therapies, female patients, 267–268
Carbon dioxide laser, 930
Cardiac arrest, intracaval tumors, abdominal surgical approaches to, 29–31
Cardinal-sacrouterine ligament complex, pelvic floor anatomy, 313, 313f, 322f, 323, 324f
Cardiopulmonary bypass, intracaval tumors, abdominal surgical approaches to, 29–31, 30f
Catheterizable reservoir construction
colonic segments
alternative therapy, 599
diagnostic criteria, 599
indications for surgery, 599
outcomes and complications, 605–606, 608–610
surgical technique, 599–609
ileal segments
alternative therapy, 595
outcomes and complications, 598
patient selection and evaluation, 595
postoperative care, 598
surgical indications, 594–595
surgical technique, 595–597, 595f–596f
Catheter removal, orthotopic bladder substitution, 558–559, 558t, 559f
Cauterization
urologic procedures, 926–927, 926t
vasectomy procedures, 374–375, 375f–375f
Cavernostomy, segmental renal tuberculosis, 56
Cesium isotopes, prostate cancer brachytherapy and, 203, 203t
Chemotherapy
laparoscopic retroperitoneal lymph node dissection following, 816
radical cystectomy *vs.*, 98
retroperitoneal lymphadenectomy following, 447
Chondrocytes, injectable, urogenital tissue engineering, 907
Chordee
congenital penile curvature, 534–537, 534f
hypospadias abnormalities, 704, 708, 710, 710f
Circumcision
alternative therapy, 779
diagnosis, 778, 778f
neonatal, 780–782, 781f–782f
outcomes and complications, 782
squamous cell carcinoma of penis, 468–469, 469f
surgical indications for, 778–779, 779f
surgical technique, 779–782, 779f–782f
"Clam" augmentation cystoplasty technique, 785, 785f
Clean intermittent catheterization (CIC), pubovaginal fascial slings, 273
Clitoroplasty, 763, 763f–764f, 771–773, 772f
Cloacal anomalies
alternative therapies, 762
diagnosis, 761–762, 761f
outcomes and complications, 767–768
surgical indications, 762
surgical techniques, 762–764, 763f–768f
Coccygeus muscle, pelvic floor anatomy, 315
Cohen technique, vesicoureteral reflux repair, 672, 672f
Colocystoplasty, bladder augmentation, 787, 791
Colonic segments
continent catheterizable reservoir
alternative therapy, 599
diagnostic criteria, 599
ileocecal pouch (Mainz pouch I), 600–602, 600f–601f
Indiana pouch, 603, 607f
indications for surgery, 599
Mainz pouch III, 603–605, 608f–609f
outcomes and complications, 605–606, 608–610
right colon pouches, intussuscepted/tapered terminal ileum, 603, 607f
surgical technique, 599–609
ureteral implantation, 602, 603f–605f
orthotopic bladder substitution
alternative therapy, 587–588
diagnostic criteria, 587
goals and function, 586–587
indications for surgery, 587
outcomes and complications, 590–593
surgical technique, 588–590, 589f–593f
ureteral implantation, 588–590
renal trauma surgery, 61, 61f

Colonic segments (*continued*)
transperitoneal radical/total nephrectomy, reflection, 820–821, 821f
transverse retubularized colon segments, palliative techniques, 622, 622f
Color test, transperineal laparoscopy, 803
Colpopexy, abdominal sacral, 349–354
alternative therapy, 351
diagnosis, 350–351, 350t
indications for, 351, 351f
outcomes and complications, 353–354
surgical techniques, 351–353, 352f–353f
Colporraphy, posterior, posterior vaginal prolapse repair, 345–346, 346f–347f
Comorbid conditions, female radical cystectomy, 105, 105t
Complete primary repair of exstrophy (CPRE), 712f–718f, 713–719, 722–724
Computerized tomography (CT)
pelvic lymphadenectomy *vs.*, 185
prostatic imaging, 178
Continence. *See* Incontinence
bladder exstrophy/epispadias repair, 727–728, 729f
Continent catheterizable reservoir
colonic segments
alternative therapy, 599
diagnostic criteria, 599
indications for surgery, 599
outcomes and complications, 605–606, 608–610
surgical technique, 599–609
ileal segments
alternative therapy, 595
outcomes and complications, 598
patient selection and evaluation, 595
postoperative care, 598
surgical indications, 594–595
surgical technique, 595–597, 595f–596f
Continent vesicostomy, 797, 798f
Contraceptive techniques, vasectomy, 372
Coroplasty/coroplication procedures, Peyronie disease management, 482–483
Corporo-deep dorsal vein shunt, priapism management, 491
Corporoglandular (Al-Ghorab) shunt, priapism management, 490, 490f
Corporoglandular (Ebbehoj and T-) shunt, priapism management, 490
Corporoglandular (Winter) shunt, priapism management, 489–490, 490f
Corporo-saphenous vein shunt, priapism management, 491
Corporospongiosal shunts, priapism management, 491f, 45931
Cost-benefit analysis, vasovasostomy, 396–397
Costovertebral ligaments, kidney anatomy, 3–4, 4f
Countercurrent heat exchange, testis anatomy, 424
Crossover sling technique, pubovaginal fascial sling procedure, 276, 276f
Crural banding, in penile venous surgery, 503f, 504
Cryoablation
laparoscopic procedures, renal tumors
basic principles, 842
mechanisms, 843–844, 844f
outcomes and complications, 845, 845t
prostate cancer, 929
renal tumors, 915
Cryptorchidism, pediatric, 735–740, 735f
alternative therapy, 736
diagnosis, 736
inguinal orchiopexy, 736–738, 737f–738f
laparoscopic management of
bilateral nonpalpable testes, laparoscopic orchiopexy, 749, 750f–751f
diagnostic assessment, 742
intra-abdominal testis, 745, 745f–746f
outcomes and complications, 750–751
preoperative assessment, 742
second-stage Fowler-Stephens procedure, 749, 750f
single-stage technique, 745–749, 746f–749f
surgical intervention, 114–20–745, 744f–745f
outcomes and complications, 740
scrotal fixation (subdartos pouch), 738–739, 738f–739f
scrotal orchiopexy, 739–740
surgical indications, 736
transperitoneal orchiopexy, 739
Cut-back vaginoplasty, 763
Cystectomy
alternative therapy, 92
extraperitoneal partial, 95–96, 96f
ileal conduit urinary diversion, 545–548
ileal neobladder, 567, 567f
intraperitoneal partial, 96
orthotopic urinary diversion, with ileal low-pressure reservoir, afferent tubulary segment, 562
Padua ileal bladder, 575, 575f–576f
partial cystectomy, 94–97
alternative therapy, 95
indications for, 94–95
interstitial cystitis management, 152–153, 155f
outcomes and complications, 96–97
urachal excision, laparoscopic techniques, 890–891
radical cystectomy, 92
female patient, 104–112
laparoscopic procedures, 885–890
male patient, 97–103
renal, laparoscopic techniques
alternative therapy, 838
diagnosis, 838
outcomes and complications, 839
retroperitoneal approach, 838–839, 838f–839f
surgical indications, 838
transperitoneal approach, 839
robotic procedures, 922
simple cystectomy, 92–94
outcomes and complications, 94
surgical technique, 14–9f, 92–14–9
total, interstitial cystitis management, 153–154
Cystitis
hemorrhagic, 148–149, 148t, 149f
interstitial, 150–159
alternative therapy, 151–152
diagnosis, 150–151
outcomes and complications, 160
surgical indications, 151
surgical techniques, 152–160, 152f–158f, 160t
Cystocele
anterior vaginal prolapse
abdominal repair, 331, 333f
basic principles, 326–327, 326f–327f
diagnosis, 327–328
interposition graft, combination defect repairs, 329–330, 329f
isolated central defects, repair of, 331, 332f
needle suspension, 331
nonsurgical therapies, 328
surgical indications, 328–329, 329t
surgical techniques, 329–334
transobturator approaches, 331–334, 333f–334f
vaginal paravaginal repair, 331
pelvic organ prolapse, 316–317, 317f
Cystoplasty
augmentation cystoplasty, in pediatric patients, 783–792
alternative therapy, 784
bladder compliance, 120
bladder perforation, 792
caliculi formation and mucus production, 792
"clam" augmentation technique, 785, 785f
diagnosis, 783
gastrocystoplasty, 789, 789f–790f
hematuria-dysuria syndrome, 792
ileocystoplasty, 785–787, 786f, 791
outcomes and complications, 784t, 791–792
right colocystoplasty and Mainz enterocystoplasty, 787, 787f, 791
sigmoidocystoplasty, 787, 788f
surgical indications, 783, 783t
surgical techniques, 784–790, 784t–785t
uretocystoplasty, 789, 790f
urinary and abdominal drainage, 791
urinary tract infection, 792
autoaugmentation techniques, bladder augmentation, 119–120
bladder augmentation, 118–123, 120f–123f
interstitial cystitis management, 152–153, 154f–155f
reduction cystoplasty, triad syndrome, 657, 657f
Cystoprostatectomy, radical surgical technique, 99–102, 100f–102f
Cystoprostatourethrectomy, one-stage radical technique, 101
Cystoscopy
postimplant, brachytherapy, prostate cancer, 207
vaginal hysterectomy, for uterine prolapse, 324
Cytolysis, interstitial cystitis management, 159

## D

De novo urge incontinence
midurethral retropubic slings, 279–281
pubovaginal fascial sling procedure, 277
Dermabell device, neonatal circumcision, 780–781, 781f
Dermal fat grafts, penile reconstruction, 538–539, 542
Detrusor hypocontractility, postprostatectomy incontinence, sling procedures, 303

Detrusor striated sphincter dyssynergia (DSD), surgical management, 228–232, 229t, 230f–232f
Dimethyl sulfoxide (DMSO)
  ethylene vinyl alcohol copolymer in, injectable therapies, female incontinence patients, 268
  interstitial cystitis management, 151
Dismembered pyeloplasty technique, 648–649, 648f
Disorders of sexual development (DSD), corrective surgical techniques, 769–777
Distal penile approach, penile prosthetic implantation, 494–495, 494f–495f
Distal ureterectomy, laparoscopic technique
  bladder cuff stapling with, 835–836, 835f
  indications for, 831, 831t
  surgical approaches, 834–836, 834f
Distal urethra, robotically assisted laparoscopic (radical) prostatectomy, 876, 876f
Distal urethrectomy, for female urethral cancer, 254–255, 255f
Diverticulectomy, bladder
  alternative therapy, 115
  diagnosis, 113f–114f, 736
  indications for, 114
  laparoscopic procedures, 891
  outcomes and complications, 117
  preoperative assessment, 115
  surgical techniques, 115–117, 116f–117f
Diverticulum, female urethra, 214–220, 215f
  alternative therapy, 216
  diagnosis, 215–216, 216f
  indications for surgery, 216
  postoperative complications, 219
  postoperative outcomes, 219–220
  surgical technique, 216–219, 216t, 217f–219f
Donor nephrectomy
  laparoscopic techniques, 846–852
    alternative therapy, 847
    diagnosis, 846
    left-sided procedure, 849–850, 849f–850f
    outcomes and complications, 851–852, 852t
    patient preparation and positioning, 847–848, 847f–848f
    right-sided procedure, 850–851
    surgical indications, 846–847
    techniques and instrumentation, 848–849, 848f, 848t
  renal autotransplantation, 78–80, 79f
Dorsal artery dissection, microvascular arterial bypass surgery for erectile dysfunction, 509–510, 509f
Dorsal venous complex
  ileal neobladder, 568, 570–571, 570f–572f
  laparoscopic radical cystectomy, 887
  open radical retropubic surgery, suture ligation and transection, 188–189, 188f–189f
  robotically assisted laparoscopic (radical) prostatectomy, 876, 876f
Drop test, transperineal laparoscopy, 803
Dye lasers, urologic applications, 930–931

E

Echinococcal cyst(s), renal abscesses, 52
  resection, 57
  surgical indications, 54
Ecotopia, scrotal, 733
Ectopic kidney
  alternative therapy, 637
  diagnostic criteria, 635–636, 636f–637f
  epidemiology, 634–635, 635f
  outcomes and complications, 642
  surgical indications, 636–637
  surgical technique, 637, 642
Efferent ducts, anatomy, 426
"Eggplant deformity," penile trauma, 514–515, 515f
Ejaculation induction procedures
  alternative therapies, 413
  diagnosis, 413
  electroejaculation, 415–418, 416f–418f
  indications for, 413
  outcomes and complications, 418–418
  penile vibratory stimulation, 413–415, 414f
Ejaculatory duct, 360f
  diagnostic criteria, 369, 369t
  surgical indications, 369
  surgical technique, 369–371, 370f–371f
    outcomes and complications, 370–371
Elderly patients, female radical cystectomy, 105, 105t
Electroejaculation (EEJ) procedures, 413, 415–418, 416f–418f
Electrosurgery, urologic procedures, 926–927
Eleventh-rib resection, renovascular disease, splenorenal artery bypass, 39, 41f
Embryonic stem (ES) cells, genitourinary tissue engineering, 906–907
Emptying reflex, bladder anatomy, 91
End cutaneous ureterostomy, posterior urethral valves, 701–702, 702f
End-loop stoma formation, ileal conduit urinary diversion, 545–548, 547f
Endo Close fascial closure needle, laparoscopic surgery, 806–807, 806f
Endopelvic fascia incisions
  open radical retropubic surgery, 188, 188f
  robotically assisted laparoscopic (radical) prostatectomy, 874
Endoscopic surgery
  benign prostatic hypertrophy, complications, 174
  interstitial cystitis management, 152
  nephroureterectomy, distal ureter management, 126–129
  seminal vesicles, 368
  ureterocele, 681–683, 681t, 682f–683f
  urinary tract endoscopy, 914
  vesicoureteral reflux, 667
    alternative therapy, 677–678, 678t
    diagnostic criteria, 677
    epidemiology, 676
    outcomes and complications, 679–680
    surgical indications, 677
    surgical technique, 678–679
Endourologic techniques, palliative ureteral obstruction management, 621
Enterocele
  abdominal sacral colpopexy, 352–354, 352f–354f
  transvaginal repair
    alternative therapy, 336
    basic principles, 335–336, 336f
    diagnosis, 336
    enterocele repair, 336–338, 337f–338f
    iliococcygeus fixation, 340–341
    Manchester procedure, 342
    McCall culdoplasty, 338, 339f
    mesh-augmented repairs, 341–342, 341f–342f
    prolapsed uterus preservation, 342
    sacrospinous ligament fixation, 340, 340f
    surgical indications, 336
    uterosacral ligament fixation, 338–340, 339f
  vault suspension, 338
Enterocystoplasty, technique for, 121–123, 122f–123f
Enterovesical fistula, 9179
  alternative therapy, 139
  diagnosis, 138
  etiology, 138t, 9178
  surgical management, 139, 140f
Epididymal orchiectomy, 431–432, 431f
Epididymal sperm aspiration, 407–409
Epididymal tubules, vasoepididymostomy preparation, 381
Epididymectomy, 410–412
Epididymis
  anatomy, 355f–356f, 356–357
  blood supply, 357
  development, 356
  function, 357
  innervation, 357
  obstruction, vasoepididymostomy for, 379–380
  physical examination, 356
Epispadias repair, techniques for, 712–718, 722–730
  anatomic reconstruction with, 723–101–102
  closure techniques, 725–727, 726f
  continence and antireflux procedure, 727–728, 728f–729f
  diagnosis, 723
  osteotomy, 724–725, 725f–726f
  outcomes and complications, 728–730
  preoperative preparation, 724
  surgical indications, 723
  timing and staging, 724
  urinary diversion techniques and, 723
Erbium:yttrium-aluminum-garnet laser, 930
Erectile dysfunction
  alternative therapy, 509
  bicycle riding and, 506
  microvascular arterial bypass surgery, 505–514
    anastomosis, 512–513, 512f–513f
    criteria for, 507, 508f
    diagnostic testing, 507
    dorsal artery dissection, 509–510, 509f
    inferior epigastric artery harvesting, 510–511, 511f
    outcomes and complications, 513
    surgical techniques, 509–513
  open radical retropubic surgery, 192–193
  pathophysiology, 506–507
  penile venous surgery for, 499–504

Erectile dysfunction (*continued*)
physiology, 506
priapism, 487–492
alternative therapy, 489
diagnosis, 488–489, 489f
epidemiology, 487–488, 488f
indications for surgery, 489, 489f
surgical technique, 489–491, 4 90f–491f
corporo-deep dorsal vein shunt, 491
corporoglandular (Al-Ghorab) shunt, 490, 490f
corporoglandular (Ebbehoj and T-) shunt, 490
corporoglandular (Winter) shunt, 489–490, 490f
corporo-saphenous vein shunt, 491
corporospongiosal shunts, 491f, 491
nonischemic priapism, 491
outcomes and complications, 491–492
postoperative management, 491
Ethylene vinyl alcohol copolymer, injectable incontinence therapies, female patients, 268
Exstrophy, bladder
epispadias and, 722–730
anatomic reconstruction with, 723-101-102
closure techniques, 725–727, 726f
continence and antireflux procedure, 727–728, 728f–729f
diagnosis, 723
osteotomy, 724–725, 725f–726f
outcomes and complications, 728–730
preoperative preparation, 724
surgical indications, 723
timing and staging, 724
urinary diversion techniques and, 723
primary integrated reconstruction, 711–722
diagnosis, 711–712, 712f
outcomes and complications, 721–722
surgical indications, 712
surgical technique, 712–721
Extended lymph node dissection
bladder cancer, 184
in prostate cancer, 182–183
External beam radiation therapy (EBRT)
brachytherapy, prostate cancer, 202–207
for prostate cancer, 202–208
hybrid real-time planning and linked seeds approach, 205–207, 206f–207f
isotope selection, 203, 203t
outcomes and complications, 207–208, 208t
postimplant cystoscopy, 207
postimplant dosimetry, 207
real-time intraoperative planning approach, 204–205, 205f
treatment planning, 203–204, 204f
External genitalia, laser therapy, 933–934
Extraanatomic pyelovesical prosthetic bypass, palliative ureteral obstruction management, 621–622, 622f
Extracapsular nephrectomy, technique, 33–34
Extracorporeal shock wave lithotripsy (ESWL), 897–899, 898f
Extraperitoneal approach
laparoscopic pelvic lymph node dissection, 813
partial cystectomy, 95–96, 96f
vesicovaginal fistula surgery, 136
Extraperitoneal ruptures, vesical trauma and hemorrhage, 144, 144f, 147
Extravesical approach
combined intravesical/extravesical bladder diverticulectomy, 115–117, 117f
nephroureterectomy, distal ureter management, 126
*Ex vivo* bench surgery, renovascular disease, 43–44, 44f

F
Fat injections, penile reconstruction, 538, 538f–539f
Female genital tissue engineering, 911–912
Female genitoplasty, corrective surgical techniques, 769–777
Fiberoptics, transverse colonic conduit procedures, 552–553
Fibrin glues, vesicovaginal fistula repair, 131–132
Fine needle aspiration, testis biopsy, 401–403, 404f
Fistula
enterovesical, 9179
female urethra, 220–227, 222f
rectourethral, 139–143
urethroplasty complications, 244–245
vesicovaginal fistula, 130–137
Flap vaginoplasty, 763–764, 766–767, 766f
Flap-valve techniques
colonic orthotopic bladder substitution, 588–589
T-pouch ileal neobladder reconstruction, 580–581, 580f–584f, 585–586
Flexible robotics, surgical applications, 923–924, 923f–924f
Fluoroscopic urodynamic imaging, of myelomeningocele, 273, 273f
Focal endothelial dysfuntion, secondary to trauma-associated erectile dysfunction, 506
Foley V-V pyeloplasty, robotic techniques, 855, 856f
Foley Y-V-plasty, horseshoe kidney repair, 638, 639f
Foramen needle insertion, sacral neurostimulation, 308–309, 308f–309f
Fournier gangrene, 454, 461–462, 463f
Full-thickness bowel flap tube, colonic continent catheterizable reservoir, 602, 603f

G
Gastrocystoplasty, bladder augmentation, 789, 789f–790f, 791
Genitogram, female genitoplasty, 770–771, 771f
Genitourinary tissue engineering, 905
Germ cells, testis anatomy, 425
Gerota's fascia
kidney anatomy, 3–4, 4f
renal trauma surgery, 61, 61f
transperitoneal radical/total nephrectomy dissection and elevation, 822, 822f
Glandular urethra stricture, surgical management, 237–238, 238f–239f
Glans approximation procedure (GAP), hypospadias surgery, 706, 707f
Glans flap meatoplasty, urethral stricture, 237–238, 238f
Glans-sparing surgery, squamous cell carcinoma of penis, 468–469, 469f
Glenn-Anderson procedure, vesicoureteral reflux repair, 671–672, 671f
Glutaraldehyde cross-linked bovine collagen (GAX-collagen), injectable incontinence therapies, female patients, 266
Gomco clamp, neonatal circumcision, 780–781, 781f
Gonadal vein dissection, transperitoneal radical/total nephrectomy, 821–822
Goodwin-Hohenfellner technique, transverse colonic conduit, 551–552, 552f
Graft materials, pubovaginal fascial sling procedure, 276–277
Granulomas, vasectomy complications, 376

H
Halban culdoplasty, vaginal vault repair, 352–353, 353f
Hand-assisted laparoscopy, 809–810, 809f
nephrectomy, 823–824, 823f–824f, 826
donor nephrectomy, 847
nephroureterectomy, 833–834, 833f
Heineke-Mikulicz nondismembered pyeloplasty, robotic techniques, 855, 856f
Hematoma
pubovaginal fascial sling procedure, 277
scrotal, 455–456, 456f
Hematuria-dysuria syndrome, augmentation cystoplasty and, 792
Hemorrhagic cystitis, 148–149, 148t, 149f
Hepatic function, orthotopic bladder substitution, 556
Hepatorenal bypass graft, renovascular disease, 39–41, 41f–42f
Hermaphrodite disorders, corrective surgical techniques, 769–777
Hernia, pediatric, diagnosis and repair, 740–741
Heterogeneous sperm production, 403
High-dose-rate (HDR) brachytherapy, prostate cancer, 202–207
High-intensity focused ultrasound (HIFU), urologic procedures, 927
Holmium laser enucleation of the prostate (HoLEP), benign prostatic hypertrophy, 168–170, 168t, 169f
treatment outcomes, 173–174
Holmium:YAG laser ablation
basic principles, 930
benign prostatic hypertrophy, 170–171, 171t, 931
Hormonal therapy, cryptorchidism, pediatric, 736
Horseshoe kidney
alternative therapy, 637
diagnostic criteria, 635–636, 636f–637f
epidemiology, 634–635, 635f
outcomes and complications, 642
surgical indications, 636–637
surgical technique, 637
ectopic kidney, 642
pyeloplasty, 637–638, 639f, 641f

stone surgery, 642
tumor excision, 638, 641, 641f
ureterocalicostomy, 638, 640f
Hydrocele formation
alternative formation, 528–529
Andrews procedure, 529, 529f
diagnosis, 528
epidemiology, 528
inguinal approach, 530
Jaboulay or Winkleman procedure, 529, 529f
Lord procedure, 529–530, 530f
pediatric patients, diagnosis and repair, 740–741
surgical indications, 528
surgical techniques, 529–530, 529f
varicocelectomy, 400
Hydrodistention implantation technique (HIT), vesicoureteral reflux, endoscopic surgery, 679, 679f
Hypercontinence, orthotopic bladder substitution, 559
Hypoplasia, scrotal, 733
Hypospadias, 703–711
age levels for surgery, 705
artificial erection, 705
diagnostic criteria, 704, 704f
dressings, 705
epidemiology, 703
hemostasis concerns, 705
meatal abnormalities, 704, 704f
nerve block, 705
outcomes and complications, 710–711
outpatient procedures, 705
penile curvature, 704
posterior, 706–707
postoperative problems, 710
preoperative evaluation, 705
repair algorithm, 706f
skin/scrotal abnormalities, 704
surgical techniques, 704–710
Brack buccal two-stage repair, 108–88f, 708
glans approximation, 706, 707f
meatal advancement and glanuloplasty, 706, 707f
onlay island flap, 707, 709f
penile curvature, 708, 710, 710f
tubularized incised plate urethroplasty, 706, 708f
two-stage repair, 707–708, 710f
urethral plate, 706–707
training techniques, 704–705
urinary diversion in children, 705
Hypothalamic-pituitary-gonadal axis, 419, 420f
Hypothermia, intracaval tumors, abdominal surgical approaches to, 29–31
Hypovitaminosis, colonic continent catheterizable reservoir construction, 608
Hysterectomy, vaginal, uterine prolapse, 318–325

I

Ileal bladder, Padua, 574–577
alternative therapy, 575
diagnostic criteria, 575
function and goals, 574–575
outcomes and complications, 577
surgical indications, 575
surgical techniques, 575–576
creation of bladder, 576–577, 576f–577f
cystectomy, 575, 575f–576f
Ileal conduit urinary diversion, 545–549
alternative therapy, 545
diagnostic criteria, 545
laparoscopic radical cystectomy, 889
outcomes and complications, 548–549
palliative techniques, 619, 619f
surgical indications, 545
surgical technique, 545–548, 547f–548f
Ileal neobladder, 566–574
alternative therapy, 567
diagnostic criteria, 566
outcomes and complications, 573–574
surgical indications, 566–567
surgical technique, 567–573
cystectomy, 567
membranous urethra, male patient, 568, 568f–570f
pelvic lymph node dissection, post-laparotomy, 567
refluxing ileoureteral anastomosis, 571–572, 573f
reservoir construction, 568, 570–571, 570f–572f
ureteral mobilization, 567–568, 567f
T-pouch ileal neobladder
alternative therapy, 579
diagnostic criteria, 579
goals and functions, 578–579
outcome and complications, 584–586
surgical indications, 579
surgical technique, 579–584, 579f–584f
Ileal segment preparation
bladder augmentation, 120–123, 120f–123f
catherizable reservoir construction
alternative therapy, 595
outcomes and complications, 598
patient selection and evaluation, 595
postoperative care, 598
right colon pouches, intussuscepted/tapered terminal ileum, 603, 607f
surgical indications, 594–595
surgical technique, 595–597, 595f–596f
orthotopic urinary diversion, with ileal low-pressure reservoir, afferent tubulary segment, 562–563, 562f
Ileocecal reservoir construction
colonic continent catheterizable reservoir, 600–602, 600f–601f
colonic orthotopic bladder substitution, 588–590, 589f–593f
Ileocystoplasty, bladder augmentation, 785–787, 786f, 791
Ileorenal bypass, renovascular disease, 42–43, 43f
Ileovesicostomy, bladder augmentation *vs.*, 119–120
Iliac fossa dissection, renal allotransplantation, 65–66, 66f
Iliac vessel exposure, renal autotransplantation, 80–81
Iliococcygeus fixation, transvaginal enterocele repair, 340–341
Image-guided therapy
overview, 913–914
prostate cancer management, 917–918
renal trauma, 59, 59f
renal tumor management, 914–917
urinary tract endoscopy, 914
Incontinence. *See also* Continent catherizable reservoir; Stress urinary incontinence
artificial urinary sphincter, 292–298
bladder augmentation, 118–124
bladder neck closure
female, 228–232, 229t, 230f–232f
male, 229, 232–235, 233f–234f
female patients
abdominal retropubic therapies, 288–291
alternative therapy, 289
diagnosis and indications, 288–289
laparoscopic Burch urethropexy, 290
open Burch urethropexy, 289–290, 289f–290f
outcomes and complications, 290–291
injectable therapies
autologous material, 265–266
biomaterials, 266
injectable agents, 265
mechanism, 263
periurethral injection, 264
postoperative care, 265
selection criteria, 263–264
synthetic materials, 266–269
transurethral injection, 264
ultrasound guidance, 264–265
midurethral sling, transobturator approach, 282–287
orthotopic bladder substitution, 556, 558–559
postprostatectomy incontinence, male patients, sling procedures for, 299–304
pubovaginal fascial sling, 271–277
severity index, 286t
three incontinence questions (3IQ), 286t
urethral continence mechanisms, 316
urinary, open radical retropubic surgery, 192
Indiana Pouch, 603, 607f
Infected fat, penile reconstruction complications, 541–542, 542f
Inferior epigastric artery harvesting, microvascular arterial bypass surgery for erectile dysfunction, 510–511, 511f
Infertility
ejaculation induction procedures, 412–418
ejaculatory duct obstruction, 369
Infrapubic approach, penile prosthetic implantation, 495–497, 495f–496f
Inguinal approach
hydrocele repair, 530
lymphadenectomy for penile carcinoma
alternative therapy, 475
diagnosis, 474
inguinal reconstruction, 479, 480f
management guidelines, 473–474, 474f
modified inguinal lymphadenectomy, 478–479, 478f
outcomes and complications, 479–480
radical inguinal lymphadenectomy, 476–478, 476f–478f
suprainguinal dissection, 479, 480f
surgical anatomy, 475–479, 476f
surgical indications, 474–475
surgical technique, 475
orchiectomy
alternative therapy, 433
diagnosis, 433

Inguinal approach (*continued*)
outcomes and complications, 434
surgical indications, 433
surgical technique, 433–434, 434f–434f
orchiopexy, 736–738, 737f–738f
varicocele (Ivanissevich) repair, 525, 525f
Inguinal hernia, bladder exstrophy procedures, 720–721
Inguinal reconstruction, after inguinal lymphadenectomy, 479, 480f
Injectable cell therapies, urogenital tissue engineering, 907–908
Injectable therapies, incontinence, female patients
autologous material, 265–266
biomaterials, 266
injectable agents, 265
mechanism, 263
periurethral injection, 264
postoperative care, 265
selection criteria, 263–264
synthetic materials, 266–269
transurethral injection, 264
ultrasound guidance, 264–265
Interposition grafting, vaginal prolapse, 329–330, 329f
InterStim therapy
interstitial cystitis management, 154–155, 157–158, 159t
sacral nerve stimulation, 310, 310f
Interstitial cystitis, 150–159
alternative therapy, 151–152
diagnosis, 150–151
outcomes and complications, 160
surgical indications, 151
surgical techniques, 152–160, 152f–158f, 160t
Intracapsular ligation, transplant nephrectomy, 33–34, 34f
Intracaval tumors
alternative therapy, 25
diagnosis, 24–25, 24f
surgical indications, 25
midline sternotomy, 25, 26f
surgical technique, 25–31
abdominal approaches, 29
thoracoabdominal incision, 25, 26f
Intracytoplasmic sperm injection (ICSI), 380
nonobstructive azoospermia, 403–404
Intraperitoneal approach
donor nephrectomy, renal autotransplantation, 80
partial cystectomy, 95–96, 96f
vesicovaginal fistula repair, 134–136, 134f–136f
Intraperitoneal rupture, vesical trauma and hemorrhage, 144, 144f, 146–147
Intravaginal testicular torsion, 451–452
Intravesical approach
bladder diverticulectomy, 115–117, 116f–117f
for megaureter, 651–653, 651f–653f
nephroureterectomy, distal ureter management, 125–126, 126f
Intrinsic sphincter deficiency (ISD)
injectable therapies, female patients, 263–269
midurethral retropubic slings, 278–281
pubovaginal fascial slings, 271–277
Intussuscepted ileal nipple, colonic continent catheterizable reservoir, 600–602, 600f–601f
right colon pouches, intussuscepted/tapered terminal ileum, 603, 607f
Intussusception, vasoepididymostomy
alternative therapy, 380
diagnostic criteria, 379–380, 379f
indications, 380
outcomes and complications, 386
surgical techniques, 380–386
anastomosis, 383
closure, 383
elongation maneuvers, 383–384
epididymal tubule identification and preparation, 381
long double-armed microsutures, 385–386, 385f
longitudinal intussusception, 381–386, 382f, 384f
single-armed microsutures, 385, 385f
vas preparation, 380, 380f
Iodine isotopes, prostate cancer brachytherapy and, 203, 203t
Isotope selection, brachytherapy, prostate cancer, 203, 203t
Ivanissevich (inguinal) approach, varicocele, 525, 525f

J

Jaboulay procedure, hydrocele repair, 529, 529f

K

Kaliscinski technique, megaureter surgical management, 652, 653f
Kidney. *See also* Renal function; Renovascular disease
anatomical relationship, 3–4, 3f–5f
contiguous structures, 5–6, 6f
lymphatic anatomy, 5
malrotation (*See* Ectopic kidney; Horseshoe kidney; Renal function; Renal fusion)
tissue engineering, 910–911
vascular anatomy, 4–5, 5f
intracaval tumors, radical nephrectomy for, 25–31, 27f–28f
partial nephrectomy and, 7–8, 8f
Kock ileal reservoir, 578–579
Kropp urethral lengthening procedure, vesical neck reconstruction, 693–694, 694f

L

Labia minora pedicle graft, female urethra, 223–224, 225f, 226, 227f
Labioplasty, 764, 765f, 773, 773f
Laparoscopic techniques
adrenalectomy, 859–866
alternative therapy, 860–861
diagnosis, 860, 860t
indications for, 859–860, 860t
outcomes and complications, 866
preoperative considerations, 861
retroperitoneal approach, 862–864, 864f–865f
retroperitoneal left adrenalectomy, 864–865
retroperitoneal right adrenalectomy, 866
surgical techniques, 861–866
transperitoneal approach, 861, 861f–862f
transperitoneal left adrenalectomy, 861–862, 862f–864f
transperitoneal right adrenalectomy, 862, 864f
alternative therapy, 801–802
bladder neck suspension, 892–896
alternative therapy with, 893
diagnosis, 892
outcomes and complications, 896, 896t
surgical indications for, 892–893
surgical technique, 893–896, 893t, 894f–896f
bladder procedures
augmentation, 120
diverteculectomy, 891
partial cystectomy, urachal excision, 890–891
radical cystectomy, 885–890
Burch urethropexy, 290
calculus disease, 897–899, 898f
contraindications, 801
cryptorchidism management
bilateral nonpalpable testes, laparoscopic orchiopexy, 749, 750f–751f
diagnostic assessment, 742
intra-abdominal testis, 745, 745f–746f
outcomes and complications, 750–751
preoperative assessment, 742
second-stage Fowler-Stephens procedure, 749, 750f
single-stage technique, 745–749, 746f–749f
surgical intervention, 742–745, 744f–745f
hand-assisted procedures, 809–810, 809f
indications for, 801
of lymphoceles, 879–884
alternative therapy, 881
diagnosis, 880, 880f
excision, 883
identification, 882–883, 883f
omental wick placement, 884
outcomes and complications, 884
peritoneal access and trochar configuration, 882, 882f
surgical indications, 880–881
surgical techniques, 881–884
nephrectomy/partial nephrectomy, 828–829
alternative therapy, 819
basic principles, 819
diagnosis, 819
donor nephrectomy techniques, 846–852
hand-assisted procedures, 823–824, 823f–824f, 826
outcomes and complications, 827–12–30
patient positioning, 820
patient preparation, 819–820
pediatric patients, 757–760, 758f–759f
postoperative care, 827
retroperitoneal approach, 824–825, 825f
retroperitoneoscopic partial nephrectomy, 827
surgical indications, 819
transperitoneal partial approach, 825–826, 826f
transperitoneal radical or total approach, 820–823, 820f–823f

nephropexy, 840–841, 841f
nephroureterectomy
  alternative therapy, 830–831
  basic principles, 830
  diagnosis, 830, 830f
  distal ureter approaches, 834f–125–134–125–135
  distal ureter excision criteria, 831t
  distal ureter management, extravesical bladder technique, 126
  hand-assisted techniques, 833–834, 833f
  left radical approach, 832–833
  outcomes and complications, 836, 836t
  right radical approach, 833
  stapling of distal ureter and bladder cuff, 835, 835f
  surgical indications, 830
  surgical techniques, 831–836
  transperitoneal radical procedure, 831–832, 832f
  transurethral resection of ureteral orifice (TURUO) (Pluck technique), 836
  transvesical detachment and ligation, 835–836
neuroblastoma management, 625
outcomes and complications, 810–811
patient preparation, 802
pediatric patients, 810
  cryptorchidism, 742–751
  nephrectomy/partial nephrectomy, 757–760, 758f–759f
  pyeloplasty, 638, 752–756, 753f–756f
pelvic extraperitoneal laparoscopy, 808–809, 808f
pelvic lymphadenectomy, in prostate cancer, 182
pelvic lymph node dissection
  alternative therapy, 812
  basic principles, 811
  diagnosis, 811
  extraperitoneal approach, 813
  outcomes and complications, 813
  surgical indications, 811–812
  transperitoneal approach, 812–813, 812f–813f
postoperative management, 810
prostatectomy, radical robotic procedures, 867–879
  alternatives to, 868
  bladder neck dissection, 874, 875f
  diagnosis, 867
  dorsal venous complex and distal urethra, 876, 876f
  endopelvic fascia incision, 874
  outcomes and complications, 877, 878t–879t
  pelvic lymph node dissection, 876
  posterior dissection, 874
  postoperative care and discharge, 877
  specimen retrieval, 877
  surgical indications for, 867
  surgical technique, 868–877
  vasa deferentia/seminal vesicle dissection, 875, 875f
  vesicourethral anastomosis, 876–877, 877f
pyeloplasty, 638, 752–756, 753f–756f
  alternative therapy, 752–753
  diagnosis, 752
  outcomes and complications, 756
  retroperitoneoscopic approach, 753–754, 753f–754f
  robotically assisted techniques, 853–859
  surgical indications, 752
  transperitoneal approach, 755, 755f
radical cystectomy, 885–890
  alternative therapy, 885
  anterior dissection, 887
  diagnosis, 885
  dorsal vein complex transection, 887
  extended/high-extended lymphadenectomy, 888–889, 889f
  ileal conduit and orthotopic neobladder, 889
  modifications for women patients, 887–888, 887f–888f
  nerve-sparing cystectomy in men, 888
  outcomes, 889–890, 890t
  postoperative care, 889
  reproductive organ-sparing cystectomy in women, 888
  retrovesical dissection, 886–887
  surgical indications, 885
  ureter mobilization and division, 886
  urinary diversion, 889
  vascular pedicle dissection and control, 887, 887f
renal abscesses, 55–56
renal biopsy, 839–840, 840f
renal cystectomy
  alternative therapy, 838
  diagnosis, 838
  outcomes and complications, 839
  retroperitoneal approach, 838–839, 838f–839f
  surgical indications, 838
  transperitoneal approach, 839
renal tumor ablation
  basic principles, 842
  cryotherapy mechanisms, 843–844, 844f
  diagnosis, 842
  outcomes and complications, 845, 845t
  radiofrequency ablation, 842–844, 843f, 844t
  surgical indications, 842
renal tumors, image-guided techniques, 914–915
retroperitoneal lymph node dissection
  alternative therapy, 814
  outcomes and complications, 817–818, 818t
  postoperative care, 817
  retroperitoneal approach, 816–817, 817f
  stage II/III post-chemotherapy disease, 816
  surgical indications, 814, 814t
  transperitoneal approach, 814–816, 815f
retroperitoneal techniques, 807–808, 807f–808f
robotic procedures, 922–925, 923f–924f
seminal vesicle surgery, 366–368, 367f
transperitoneal access
  closed technique, 802–803, 803f
  open "Hasson" technique, 805, 805f
transureteroureterostomy, 646
trocar placement
  primary placement, 804–805, 804f
  secondary placement, 805, 806f
trochar removal, 806–807, 806f
ureterolysis, 901, 903
urological procedures, 897–903
varicocele repair, 525
  ligation procedures, 899–901, 900f–903f
  vesicoureteral reflux repair, 674, 675f
  vesicovaginal fistula surgery, 136–137
Laparotomy, ileal neobladder, pelvic lymph node dissection, 567
Laser therapy
  argon laser, 930
  basic physics, 929–930, 929f
  benign prostatic hypertrophy, 170–171, 171t
    enucleation, 168–170, 168t, 169f
  biophysics, 930
  carbon dioxide laser, 930
  diagnostic applications, 934
  dye laser, 930–931
  erbium:yttrium-aluminum-garnet laser, 930
  external genitalia, 933–934
  holmium:yttrium-aluminum-garnet, 930
  neodymium:yttrium-aluminum-garnet laser, 930
  potassium titanyl phosphate crystal, 930
  urologic applications, 931–934
"Le Bag" procedure, colonic orthotopic bladder substitution, 589–590, 591f
Levator ani muscle, pelvic floor anatomy, 315, 315f
Levator hiatus muscle, pelvic floor anatomy, 315, 315f
LEVERA sling system, postprostatectomy incontinence, 304, 304f
Leydig cells
  injectable, urogenital tissue engineering, 908
  testis anatomy, 426
Lichen sclerosis (LS), glandular urethra stricture, 237, 239f
Ligamentous attachments
  bladder anatomy, 86, 86f
  pelvic floor anatomy, 312–314, 312f–314f
Ligation techniques
  intracaval tumors, 29, 29f
  radical nephrectomy, 21–22, 21f
  varicocele, laparoscopic ligation of, 899–901, 900f–903f
Limited lymph node dissection
  bladder cancer, 184
  in prostate cancer, 182–183
Lithotripsy, laser technologies, 931–932, 932f
Long double-armed microsutures, longitudinal intussusception vasoepididymostomy, 385–386, 385f
Longitudinal intussusception vasoepididymostomy (LIVE), 381–386, 382f, 384f
  long double-armed microsutures, 385–386, 385f
  single-armed microsutures, 385, 385f
Lord procedure, hydrocele repair, 529–530, 530f
Low-dose-rate brachytherapy, for prostate cancer, 202–207
Lower-urinary-tract symptoms (LUTS), benign prostatic hypertrophy, 166–167, 167t
Lymphadenectomy
  inguinal, for penile carcinoma
    alternative therapy, 475
    diagnosis, 474
    inguinal reconstruction, 479, 480f

Lymphadenectomy (*continued*)
management guidelines, 473–474, 474f
modified inguinal lymphadenectomy, 478–479, 478f
outcomes and complications, 479–480
radical inguinal lymphadenectomy, 476–478, 476f–478f
suprainguinal dissection, 479, 480f
surgical anatomy, 475–479, 476f
surgical indications, 474–475
surgical technique, 475
laparoscopic radical cystectomy, 888–889, 889f
radical cystectomy, male patient, 98–99, 98f–99f
retroperitoneal, 442–448
alternative therapy, 66–89
diagnosis, 442
dissection templates, 443–444, 445f
nerve-sparing retroperitoneal lymph node dissection, 444–448, 446f–447f
outcomes and complications, 448
postchemotherapy, 447
primary procedures, 443, 444f
surgical indications, 442–443
surgical techniques, 443–447
Lymphatic system, bladder anatomy, 91
Lymph node dissection
laparoscopic pelvic lymph node dissection
alternative therapy, 812
basic principles, 811
diagnosis, 811
extraperitoneal approach, 813
outcomes and complications, 813
surgical indications, 811–812
transperitoneal approach, 812–813, 812f–813f
laparoscopic retroperitoneal lymph node dissection
alternative therapy, 814
outcomes and complications, 817–818, 818t
postoperative care, 817
retroperitoneal approach, 816–817, 817f
stage II/III post-chemotherapy disease, 816
surgical indications, 814, 814t
transperitoneal approach, 814–816, 815f
Lymphoceles, laparoscopic management of, 879–884
alternative therapy, 881
diagnosis, 880, 880f
excision, 883
identification, 882–883, 883f
omental wick placement, 884
outcomes and complications, 884
peritoneal access and trochar configuration, 882, 882f
surgical indications, 880–881
surgical techniques, 881–884

## M

Magnetic resonance imaging (MRI)
pelvic lymphadenectomy *vs.*, 185
prostatic imaging, 178
sacral neurostimulation contraindications, 306
Mainz enterocystoplasty, bladder augmentation, 787, 787f, 791
Mainz pouch techniques
colonic continent catheterizable reservoir
Mainz pouch I, 600–602, 600f–601f
Mainz pouch III, 603–605, 608f–609f
colonic orthotopic bladder substitution, 588–590, 589f
ureterosigmoidostomy, Mainz pouch II, 613–614, 613f–615f
alternative therapy, 611
classical surgical technique, 611–613, 611f–613f
complications and outcomes, 617
diagnostic criteria, 610–611
indications for surgery, 611
serous-lined extramural tunnel ureteral implantation, 614–616, 615f–616f
sigmoid-rectal pouch technique, 613–614, 613f–615f
surgical tricks, 616
Manchester procedure, uterine prolapse, 342
Marshall-Marchetti-Krantz (MMK) procedure, abdominal retropubic therapies, female patients, 288
Martius flap, neurogenic bladder, 34–31–232, 232f
McCall culdoplasty, enterocele repair, 338, 339f
Meatal advancement and glanuloplasty (MAGPI) technique
bladder exstrophy/episadias repair, 727, 728f
hypospadias surgery, 706, 707f
Medications
benign prostatic hypertrophy, 167
donor nephrectomy, 848–849
ejaculation impairment and, 369, 369t
renovascular disease, 37
Megalourethra, surgical reduction, 656–660
Megameatus with intact prepuce (MIP), surgical correction, 660, 661f
Megaureter, 654
alternative therapy, 650
diagnostic criteria, 650
epidemiology, 649
outcomes and complications, 654
surgical indications, 650
surgical technique, 650–653
extravesical approach, 653
intravesical approach, 651–653, 651f–652f
postoperative care, 653
staged approach, 653
Melanoma, in female urethra, 252–256
Mesh-augmented repairs
Perigee mesh placement, vaginal prolapse, 332–333, 333f–334f
transvaginal enterocele repair, 341–342, 341f–342f
Metabolic management
colonic continent catheterizable reservoir construction, 606, 608
orthotopic bladder substitution, 559–560, 560t
Microdissection testicular sperm extraction (MicroTESE), 405–406, 406f
Microdot technique, multilayer microsurgical vasovastostomy procedures, 393–395, 394f–395f
Microscopic epididymal sperm aspiration (MESA), 380
Microsurgical procedures
epididymal sperm aspiration (MESA), 407–409, 408t
multilayer microsurgical vasovastostomy procedures, 393–395, 394f–395f
varicocelectomy, 397–399, 398f–399f, 525–527, 526f–527f
Microvascular arterial bypass surgery, erectile dysfunction, 505–514
anastomosis, 512–513, 512f–513f
criteria for, 507, 508f
diagnostic testing, 507
dorsal artery dissection, 509–510, 509f
inferior epigastric artery harvesting, 510–511, 511f
outcomes and complications, 513
surgical techniques, 509–513
Microwave technologies, radiofrequency ablation therapies, 928–929, 928f
Micturition reflex, bladder anatomy, 90, 91f
Midline dorsal plication technique, hypospadias repair, 708, 710f
Midurethral retropubic sling
contraindications to, 273
failure of, 272
injectable incontinence therapy, female patients, 265
pubovaginal fascial sling alternative to, 273
synthetic slings
alternative therapies, 278–279
basic principles, 468
diagnosis, 278
material selection criteria, 279
outcomes and complications, 280–281, 281f
surgical indications, 278
surgical technique, 279–280, 280f
tension-free vaginal tape, 280
transobturator approach
alternative therapy, 282
basic principles, 282
comparisons, 279
diagnostic criteria, 282–282
outcomes and complications, 285–287, 286t
surgical indications, 282
surgical technique, 282–285, 282f–285f, 284t
"Mini-nephrectomy/mini-incision nephrectomy," 847
Mitrofanoff procedure, urinary tract reconstruction
alternative therapy, 794
appendicovesicostomy, 794–795, 794f–795f
continent vesicostomy, 797, 798f
diagnosis, 793
Monti-Yang ileovesicostomy, 795–797, 796f–797f
outcomes and complications, 799, 799t
surgical indications, 793–794, 793f
surgical techniques, 794–798
ureterovesicostomy, 797–798
Mixed gonadal dysgenesis, corrective surgical techniques, 769–777
Modified inguinal lymphadenectomy, for penile carcinoma, 478–479, 478f
Mogen clamp, neonatal circumcision, 781–782, 782f
Monopolary cauterization, urologic procedures, 926–927
Monti-Yang ileovesicostomy, 795–797, 796f–797f
Motor innervation, bladder anatomy, 89–90

Mucus production, augmentation cystoplasty and, 792
Multifocal carcinoma, colonic continent catheterizable reservoir, 599
Multiple parallel plication, congenital penile curvature, 536, 536f
Muscle cells, injectable, urogenital tissue engineering, 908

## N

Needle placement algorithm, vesicoureteral reflux, endoscopic surgery, 679f
Needle suspension technique, vaginal prolapse, 331
Neobladder, ileal, 566–574
  alternative therapy, 567
  diagnostic criteria, 566
  interstitial cystitis management, 153–154
  laparoscopic radical cystectomy, 889
  outcomes and complications, 573–574
  surgical indications, 566–567
  surgical technique, 567–573
    cystectomy, 567
    membranous urethra, male patient, 568, 568f–570f
    pelvic lymph node dissection, post-laparotomy, 567
    refluxing ileoureteral anastomosis, 571–572, 573f
    reservoir construction, 568, 570–571, 570f–572f
    ureteral mobilization, 567–568, 567f
  T-pouch ileal neobladder
    alternative therapy, 579
    diagnostic criteria, 579
    goals and functions, 578–579
    outcome and complications, 584–586
    surgical indications, 579
    surgical technique, 579–584, 579f–584f
Neodymium:yttrium-aluminum-garnet laser, 930–931
Neoinguinal hiatus, single-stage laparoscopic orchiopexy, 746–747, 747f
Neonatal circumcision, 780–782, 781f–782f
Nephrectomy
  donor nephrectomy
    laparoscopic techniques, 846–852
      alternative therapy, 847
      diagnosis, 846
      left-sided procedure, 849–850, 849f–850f
      outcomes and complications, 851–852, 852t
      patient preparation and positioning, 847–848, 847f–848f
      right-sided procedure, 850–851
      surgical indications, 846–847
      techniques and instrumentation, 848–849, 848f, 848t
    renal autotransplantation, 78–80, 79f
  laparoscopic techniques
    alternative therapy, 819
    basic principles, 819
    diagnosis, 819
    donor nephrectomy, laparoscopic techniques, 846–852
    hand-assisted procedures, 823–824, 823f–824f, 826
    intraoperative ultrasound, 914–915
    outcomes and complications, 827–829
    partial nephrectomy, 828–829
    patient positioning, 820
    patient preparation, 819–820
    pediatric patients, 757–760, 758f–759f
    postoperative care, 827
    retroperitoneal approach, 824–825, 825f
    retroperitoneoscopic partial nephrectomy, 827
    surgical indications, 819
    transperitoneal partial approach, 825–826, 826f
    transperitoneal radical or total approach, 820–823, 820f–823f
  open radical nephrectomy *vs.*, 819
  palliative defunctionalization, contralateral unit, 620
  partial, 6–13
    alternative therapy, 7, 819
    collecting system repair, 12f, 13–12
    diagnosis, 819
    indications, 6–2–7
    outcomes and complications, 12–13, 827–829
    pediatric patients, 757–760, 758f–759f
    renal incision and margin control, 9–11, 9f–11f
    renal preparation, 7–9, 8f
    renal reconstruction, 11, 12f
    renal trauma, 60–63, 62f
    retroperitoneoscopic approach, 827
    surgical technique, 7–8
    transperitoneal approach, 825–826, 826f
  radical
    diagnosis, 14
    indications for, 14
    intracaval tumors, 25–31, 27f
    surgical technique, 15–22
  renal autotransplantation, flank donor, 78–80, 79f
  renal trauma, 62f, 417
  renal tuberculosis, 56–57
  robotic procedures, 923
  subscapular
    renal and retroperitoneal abscess, 55, 55f–56f
    technique, 33–34
  transplant, 32–36
    allograft, 32
    diagnosis, 32
    outcomes and complications, 34–35
    surgical indications, 32
    surgical techniques, 32–34, 33f–35f
  ureterocele, upper-tract/upper pole approach, 683, 683f
Nephrolithogomy, anatrophic, 46–50
  alternative therapy, 46
  diagnosis, 46–47, 47f
  outcomes and complications, 50
  surgical indications, 46
  surgical technique, 46–50, 47f–50f
Nephropexy, laparoscopic, 840–841, 841f
Nephrostomy, palliative applications, 620
Nephroureterectomy
  distal ureter management, 125–129
    combined open/endoscopic technique, 128–129
    diagnosis, 125
    endoscopic techniques, 126
    extravesical approach, 126
    indications for surgery, 125
    intravesical approach, 125–126, 126f
    laparoscopic extravesical bladder technique, 126
    open surgical techniques, 125–126, 126f
    outcomes and complications, 129
    pluck technique, 128
    transurethral bladder cuff technique, 127
    transvesical bladder cuff techniques, 126–128, 126f–127f
    ureteral intussusception (stripping) technique, 128–129, 129f
    ureteral unroofing technique, 128, 128f
  laparoscopic technique
    alternative therapy, 830–831
    basic principles, 830
    diagnosis, 830, 830f
    distal ureter approaches, 834f–125–134–125–135
    distal ureter excision criteria, 831t
    hand-assisted techniques, 833–834, 833f
    left radical approach, 832–833
    outcomes and complications, 836, 836t
    right radical approach, 833
    stapling of distal ureter and bladder cuff, 835, 835f
    surgical indications, 830
    surgical techniques, 831–836
    transperitoneal radical procedure, 831–832, 832f
    transurethral resection of ureteral orifice (TURUO) (Pluck technique), 836
    transvesical detachment and ligation, 835–836
  seminal vesicle surgery and, 364–365
Nerve-sparing procedures
  laparoscopic radical cystectomy, in men, 888
  orthotopic bladder substitution, pelvic nerve preservation, 557
  radical cystoprostatectomy, 101–102
  radical prostatectomy and, 196, 197f
  retroperitoneal lymph node dissection, 444–448, 446f–447f
Nesbitt reduction urethroplasty, megalourethra correction, 659–660, 660f
Neuroblastoma
  diagnostic criteria, 623
  neonatal observation protocol, 624
  outcomes and complications, 625–626, 626f, 627t
  staging systems, 623t–624t
  surgical indications, 623–624
  surgical technique, 624–625
Neurogenic bladder
  female, surgical management, 228–232, 229t, 230f–232f
  male, surgical management, 229, 232–235, 233f–234f
  pubovaginal fascial sling, 272
Neuropathic bladder, catherizable reservoir construction, ileal segments, 594–595
Neurovascular bundles, open radical retropubic surgery
  prophylactic hemostatic suture placement, 189, 189f
  prostate separation from, 190
Nondismembered pyeloplasty, robotic techniques, 855, 856f
No-needle local anesthesia, vasectomy anesthesia protocols, 373–375, 373f
Nonobstructive azoospermia, testicular sperm extraction, 403

No-scalpel vasectomy (NSV), basic techniques, 374–375, 374f–375f
NOTES surgical robotics, 924–925, 924f

O

Obese patients, orthotopic urinary diversion, with ileal low-pressure reservoir, afferent tubulary segment, 564–565, 565f
Obturator anatomy, pelvic organ prolapse, 316
Occlusion therapy, vesicovaginal fistula repair, 131–132
O'Connor technique, vesicovaginal fistula repair, 135
Omental interposition, neurogenic bladder reconstruction, 234, 234f
Omental wick placement, lymphocele laparoscopic management, 884
One-stage cystoprostatourethrectomy, radical technique, 101
Onlay bulbar urethroplasty, 239f, 241, 243f
Onlay island flap, hypospadias surgery, 707, 709f
Open Burch urethropexy, abdominal retropubic therapies, female patients, 289–290, 289f–290f
Open distal ureterectomy, laparoscopic technique, 834–835, 834f
Open-flank nephrectomy, 847
Open nephrectomy, laparoscopic nephrectomy *vs.*, 819
Open nephroureterectomy (ONU), laparoscopic procedure *vs.*, 831
Open surgical drainage, renal and retroperitoneal abscess, 54–55
Open transcolonic ureterosigmoidostomy, 611–613, 611f–613f
Orandi repair, pendulous urethral stricture, 237–240, 239f
Orchiectomy
  inguinal
    alternative therapy, 433–434
    diagnosis, 433
    outcomes and complications, 434
    surgical indications, 433
    surgical technique, 433–434, 434f–434f
  simple procedures, 428–432
    alternative therapy, 428–429
    epididymal orchiectomy, 431–432, 431f
    outcomes and complications, 432
    prostate cancer diagnosis, 428
    scrotal approach, 429, 429f
    subscapular orchiectomy, 431, 431f
    suprapubic approach, 429–431, 430f–431f
Orchiopexy
  cryptorchidism
    bilateral nonpalpable testes, laparoscopic procedure, 749–750, 750f–751f
    inguinal orchiopexy, 736–738, 737f–738f
    laparoscopic techniques, 743–751, 746f–750f
    scrotal orchiopexy, 739–740
    second-stage Fowler-Stephens orchiopexy, 749, 749f
    single-stage laparoscopic orchiopexy, 745–749, 746f–749f
    transperitoneal, 739
  triad syndrome, 656, 658–659
Organ preservation
  penile preservation, urethral carcinoma, 259, 260f
  prostate preservation, radical cystectomy, 102
  reproductive organs, female radical cystectomy, 108, 110
  squamous cell carcinoma of penis, glans-sparing surgery, 468–469, 469f
  testicular tumors, 438–441, 439f–441
  upper-pole preservation, ureterocele, 682–683, 682f–683f
  urethral-sparing technique, female radical cystectomy, 111–112, 111f
  uterine prolapse, transvaginal procedures and preservation of, 342
Orthotopic bladder substitution, 555–561
  alternative therapy, 556
  bowel function, 556
  colonic
    alternative therapy, 587–588
    diagnostic criteria, 587
    goals and function, 586–587
    indications for surgery, 587
    outcomes and complications, 590–593
    surgical technique, 588–590, 589f–593f
  continence, 556
  diagnostic criteria, 555–556, 555t
  hepatic function, 556
  interstitial cystitis management, 153–154
  intraoperative management, 556–557, 557t
  laparoscopic radical cystectomy, neobladder, 889
  outcomes and complications, 560–561, 560t
  paracollicular and bladder neck biopsy, 556
  patient agreement and mental status, 555–556
  postoperative management, 558–560, 558t
    catheter removal, 558–559, 558t
    metabolic management, 559–560, 560t
  radical cystoprostatectomy with, 101
  renal function, 556
  surgical indications, 556
  surgical technique
    atraumatic urethral dissection, 557
    bladder substitute, 558
    pelvic nerve preservation, 557
    preoperative period, 556
    ureteral dissection, 557, 557f
Orthotopic urinary diversion, with ileal low-pressure reservoir, afferent tubulary segment
  alternative therapies, 562
  diagnostic criteria, 561–562
  outcomes and complications, 565
  surgical indications, 562
  surgical technique, 562–565
Osteotomy, bladder exstrophy/epispadias repair, 724–725, 725f–726f
Overactive bladder, sacral neurostimulation, 305–306

P

Padua ileal bladder, 574–577
  alternative therapy, 575
  diagnostic criteria, 575
  function and goals, 574–575
  outcomes and complications, 577
  surgical indications, 575
  surgical techniques, 575–576
    creation of bladder, 576–577, 576f–577f
    cystectomy, 575, 575f–576f
Painful bladder syndrome (PBS), 150–159
  alternative therapy, 151–152
  diagnosis, 150–151
  outcomes and complications, 160
  surgical indications, 151
  surgical techniques, 152–160, 152f–158f, 160t
PAKY surgical robot, 920–921, 921f
Palladium isotopes, prostate cancer brachytherapy and, 203, 203t
Palliative urinary diversion
  alternative therapy, 618
  diagnostic criteria, 618
  indications for surgery, 618
  surgical technique and outcomes, 618–620, 619f
  ureteral obstruction, 620–622, 621f–622f
Palmer test, transperineal laparoscopy, 803
Panurethral stricture, 241
Paquin technique, vesicoureteral reflux repair, 672, 673f–674f, 674
Paracollicular biopsy, orthotopic bladder substitution, 556
Paratestis, rhabdomyosarcoma, childhood, surgical technique, 664
Paravaginal repair, vaginal prolapse, 331
Paravesical approach, seminal vesicle surgery, 364–366
Partial urogenital mobilization (PUM), 766–767
Patent urachus, epidemiology and diagnosis, 684–687, 686f
Patient consent issues, orthotopic bladder substitution, 555–556
Pediatric patients
  artificial urinary sphincter and bladder augmentation, 297
  augmentation cystoplasty in, 783–792
    alternative therapy, 784
    bladder compliance, 120
    bladder perforation, 792
    caliculi formation and mucus production, 792
    "clam" augmentation technique, 785, 785f
    diagnosis, 783
    gastrocystoplasty, 789, 789f–790f
    hematuria-dysuria syndrome, 792
    ileocystoplasty, 785–787, 786f, 791
    outcomes and complications, 784t, 791–792
    right colocystoplasty and Mainz enterocystoplasty, 787, 787f, 791
    sigmoidocystoplasty, 787, 788f
    surgical indications, 783, 783t
    surgical techniques, 784–790, 784t–785t
    uretocystoplasty, 789, 790f
    urinary and abdominal drainage, 791
    urinary tract infection, 792
  bladder exstrophy procedures, 711–722
  cryptorchidism in, 735–740, 735f
    alternative therapy, 736
    diagnosis, 736
    inguinal orchiopexy, 736–738, 737f–738f
    laparoscopic management techniques, 742–751, 810

outcomes and complications, 740
scrotal fixation (subdartos pouch), 738–739, 738f–739f
scrotal orchiopexy, 739–740
surgical indications, 736
transperitoneal orchiopexy, 739
hydrocele/hernia repair in, 740–741
laparoscopic techniques, 742–751, 810
nephrectomy/partial nephrectomy, 757–760, 758f–759f
pyeloplasty, laparoscopic techniques, 752–756
renal allotransplantation, 69, 69f–70f
urinary tract reconstruction, Mitrofanoff procedure, 793–799, 793f
urogenital sinus and cloacal anomalies
alternative therapies, 762
diagnosis, 761–762, 761f
outcomes and complications, 767–768
surgical indications, 762
surgical techniques, 762–764, 763f–768f
Pelvic extraperitoneal laparoscopy, 808–809, 808f
Pelvic floor anatomy, 311–318
bones, 312, 312f
cystocele, 316–317
fascia, 314
ligaments, 312–314, 312f–314f
musculature, 314–316, 315f
obturator anatomy, 316
pelvic diaphragm, 312–316
rectocele, 317–318, 317f
support anatomy, 312–316
urethral continence mechanisms, 316
vaginal prolapse, 326–327, 326f–327f
Pelvic fracture urethral disruption defects (PFUDDs)
alternative therapy, 250t, 251
outcomes and complications, 252
surgical techniques, 249–252, 250f–251f, 250t
Pelvic lymphadenectomy
alternatives to, 185–186
bladder cancer
indications for, 183
limited *vs.* extended lymph node dissection, 184
surgical technique, 183–184
for bladder cancer, 183–184
complications, 184–185, 185t
limited, for prostatectomy, 187–188
outcomes, 184–185, 185t
prostate cancer
laparoscopic and robotic approach, 182
limited *vs.* extended lymph node dissection, 182–183
for prostate cancer, 179–183
indications for, 179–180, 179t
indications for surgery, 179–180
laparoscopic and robotic approach, 182
limited *vs.* extended lymph node dissection, 182–183
surgical technique, 180–183, 180f–181f
techniques for, 180–182, 180f–181f
selection criteria, 179t
Pelvic lymph node dissection
ileal neobladder, standard laparotomy, 567
laparoscopic technique
alternative therapy, 812
basic principles, 811
diagnosis, 811
extraperitoneal approach, 813
outcomes and complications, 813
surgical indications, 811–812
transperitoneal approach, 812–813, 812f–813f
robotically assisted laparoscopic (radical) prostatectomy, 876
Pelvic malignancies, catherizable reservoir construction, ileal segments, 594–595
Pelvic nerve preservation, orthotopic bladder substitution, 557
Pelvic organ prolapse
abdominal sacral colpopexy, 349–354
alternative therapy, 351
diagnosis, 350–351, 350t
indications for, 351, 351f
outcomes and complications, 353–354
surgical techniques, 351–353, 352f–353f
posterior vaginal prolapse repair, 343–349
alternative therapies, 344–345
colporraphy, 345–346, 346f–347f
diagnosis, 344, 345f
outcomes and complications, 348–349
perineal body reconstruction, 347, 347f–348f
postoperative care, 348
site-specific rectocele repair, 346–347
surgical techniques, 345–348
Pelvic organ prolapse (POP). *See also* Uterine prolapse
pelvic floor anatomy, 311–318
support restoration, 317–318, 318f
transvaginal repair
alternative therapy, 336
basic principles, 335–336, 336f
diagnosis, 336
enterocele repair, 336–338, 337f–338f
iliococcygeus fixation, 340–341
Manchester procedure, 342
McCall culdoplasty, 338, 339f
mesh-augmented repairs, 341–342, 341f–342f
prolapsed uterus preservation, 342
sacrospinous ligament fixation, 340, 340f
surgical indications, 336
uterosacral ligament fixation, 338–340, 339f
vault suspension, 338
Pelvioureterostomy-en-Y, posterior urethral valves, 701, 701f
Pendulous urethral stricture, surgical management, 237–240, 239f
Penectomy
with squamous cell carcinoma
circumcision and glans-sparing surgery, 468–469, 469f
diagnosis, 467–468, 467f
outcomes and complications, 471–473
partial penectomy, 469–471, 470f
surgical indications, 468
total penectomy, 471, 472f
urethral tumors, 259, 261f, 262
Penetrating injury
genitalia, 456–457, 458f
penile trauma, 518–519
Penile arterial bypass surgery, erectile dysfunction, 505–514
anastomosis, 512–513, 512f–513f
criteria for, 507, 508f
diagnostic testing, 507
dorsal artery dissection, 509–510, 509f
inferior epigastric artery harvesting, 510–511, 511f
outcomes and complications, 513
surgical techniques, 509–513
Penile prostheses
implantation techniques, 492–499
alternative therapy, 494
available prostheses, 492–493, 492f
diagnosis, 493
distal penile approach, 494–495, 494f–495f
infrapubic approach, 495–497, 495f–496f
outcomes and complications, 498–499
penoscrotal approach, 497–498, 497f–498f
surgical indications, 494
surgical technique, 494–498
synchronous artificial urinary sphincter and, 297
tissue engineering, 911
Penile reconstruction, penile replacement surgical complications, 537–543
alloderm, 539, 542, 542f
dermal fat grafts, 538–539, 542
fat injections, 538
indications and alternative therapy, 539
infected fat, 541–542, 541f–542f
outcomes, 542–543
penile lengthening, 537, 538f
surgical technique, 539–541, 540f–541f
Penile replantation
alternative therapy, 520
diagnosis, 520, 520f
epidemiology, 519–520
outcomes and complications, 522
postoperative management, 522
surgical indications, 520, 520f
surgical technique, 521–522, 521f–522f
Penile trauma. *See also* Urethral trauma
focal endothelial dysfuntion with trauma-associated erectile dysfunction, 506
penetrating injury, 518–519
rupture, 514–516, 515f–516f
skin loss, 516–518, 517f
Penile/urethral dissection, bladder exstrophy and, 712f–716f, 713–714
Penile venous surgery, 499–505
alternative therapy with, 500–501
anatomy of, 499–500, 500f
diagnosis, 499–500
outcomes and complications, 504, 504t
surgical technique in, 501–504, 501f–503f
crural banding and other procedures, 503–504, 503f
Penile vibratory stimulation, 413–415, 414f
Penis. *See also* Circumcision; Hypospadias
anatomy of, 465, 465f–466f
carcinoma of, inguinal lymphadenectomy for, 474–480
alternative therapy, 475
diagnosis, 474
inguinal reconstruction, 479, 480f
management guidelines, 473–474, 474f
modified inguinal lymphadenectomy, 478–479, 478f
outcomes and complications, 479–480
radical inguinal lymphadenectomy, 476–478, 476f–478f
suprainguinal dissection, 479, 480f
surgical anatomy, 475–479, 476f
surgical indications, 474–475
surgical technique, 475

Penis (*continued*)
congenital curvature, 532–537
chordee without hypospadias, 536
diagnosis, 533
incision and plication, 533–535, 534f–535f
multiple parallel plication, 536
penile disassembly, 536
surgical indications, 533
surgical technique, 533–536
Yachia longitudinal plication, 535, 535f
curvature, hypospadias abnormalities, 704, 708, 710, 710f
lymphatic anatomy, 466
outcomes and complications, 536
squamous cell carcinoma of, penectomy for, 467–473
circumcision and glans-sparing surgery, 468–469, 469f
diagnosis, 467–468, 467f
outcomes and complications, 471–473
partial penectomy, 469–471, 470f
surgical indications, 468
total penectomy, 471, 472f
tissue engineering and reconstruction, 911
vascular anatomy, 465–466
webbed penis, 733–734, 733f–734f
circumcision, 778–782
Penoscrotal approach, penile prosthetic implantation, 497–498, 497f–498f
Penoscrotal transposition, 732–733, 732f–733f
Percutaneous drainage, renal and retroperitoneal abscess, 54
Percutaneous epididymal sperm aspiration (PESA), 380, 407–409, 408t
Percutaneous nephrostomy, palliative applications, 620
Percutaneous testicular biopsy, 404
Percutaneous testicular sperm aspiration, 404, 404f
Percutaneous transluminal renal angioplasty (PTRA), renovascular disease, 42–43
Perigee mesh placement, vaginal prolapse repair, 332–333, 333f–334f
Perineal approach, male bladder neck closure, 233–234, 233f–234f
Perineal body
pelvic floor anatomy, 314, 314f
reconstruction, in posterior vaginal prolapse repair, 347, 347f–348f
Perineal prostatectomy, radical, 194–201
alternative therapy, 194–195
diagnosis, 194
outcomes and complications, 200–201, 201t
surgical indications, 194
surgical technique, 195–200, 195f–200f
Perineum, prostatic anatomy, 164, 165f
Peripheral nerve evaluation (PNE), sacral neurostimulation, 306–307, 307t
Peritoneal access, lymphocele laparoscopic management, 882, 882f
Peritoneal folds, bladder anatomy, 85, 85f
Peritoneal pedicle flap, single-stage laparoscopic orchiopexy, 745–746, 747f
Periurethral fascia, pelvic floor anatomy, 314
Periurethral injection, incontinence therapy, female patients, 264
Perivesical fascia, pelvic floor anatomy, 314
Permanent prostate seed implantation (PPI) brachytherapy, prostate cancer, 917–918
Peyronie disease, 481–487
surgical treatment of
alternative therapy, 482
corporoplasty or corporoplication procedures, 482–483
diagnosis, 481, 481f
indications for, 481–482
outcomes and complications, 486–487
plaque excision and grafting, 484, 486f
plaque incision and grafting, 483–484, 483f–486f
postoperative care, 485–486
skin incision, 482, 482f
Photodynamic therapy, urologic applications, 932–933, 933f
Pippi Salle urethral lengthening procedure, vesical neck reconstruction, 694–695, 695f
Plaque excision and grafting, Peyronie disease management, 484, 486f
Plaque incision and grafting, Peyronie disease management, 482f–486f, 483–484
Plastibell device, neonatal circumcision, 781
Pluck technique
nephroureterectomy, distal ureter management, 128
transurethral resection of ureteral orifice (TURUO), 836
Pluripotent cell classification, genitourinary tissue engineering, 906–907
Polar resection technique
partial nephrectomy, 10, 10f
renal trauma surgery, 417
Politano-Leadbetter approach, vesicoureteral reflux repair, 669, 669f–670f, 671
Polomo retroperitoneal approach, varicocele, 524–525, 524f
Polytetrafluoroethylene (Polytef), injectable incontinence therapies, female patients, 266–267
Pontine micturition center (PMC), 90–91, 91f
Positron emission tomography (PET), prostatic imaging, 178
Posterior dissection, robotically assisted laparoscopic (radical) prostatectomy, 874
Posterior tibial nerve modulation, interstitial cystitis management, 158–159, 158f
Posterior urethral valve surgery
alternatives, 697
cutaneous pyelostomy, 700, 700f
diagnostic criteria, 697, 697f
end cutaneous ureterostomy, 701–702, 702f
high cutaneous loop ureterostomy, 701, 701f
indications for, 697, 698f
outcomes and complications, 702–703
pelvioureterostomy-en-Y (Sober loop ureterostomy), 701, 701f
supravesical diversion, 700–702, 702f
transurethral valve ablation, 697–698, 698f
vesicostomy, 698–700, 699f
Posterior vaginal prolapse repair, 343–349
alternative therapies, 344–345
colporraphy, 345–346, 346f–347f
diagnosis, 344, 345f
outcomes and complications, 348–349
perineal body reconstruction, 347, 347f–348f
postoperative care, 348
site-specific rectocele repair, 346–347
surgical techniques, 345–348
Postprostatectomy incontinence, sling procedures
alternative therapy, 299–300
contraindications, 303
detrusor hypocontractility, 303
diagnosis, 299
failure, 49–93
materials for, 303
outcomes and complications, 302
prevalence, 299–49–90
previous surgical procedures, 303
radiation therapy and, 303
severe incontinence, 303
surgical indications, 299
surgical technique, 301–302, 301f, 302t
tensioning sling, 302–303
transobturator approach, 303–304, 304f
Potassium titanyl phosphate (KTP) laser ablation
benign prostatic hypertrophy, 170–171, 171t, 931
urologic applications, 930
Pouch of Douglas, male bladder anatomy and, 86f
Prerectal/pararectal fascia, pelvic floor anatomy, 314
Priapism, 487–492
alternative therapy, 489
diagnosis, 488–489, 489f
epidemiology, 487–488, 488f
indications for surgery, 489, 489f
surgical technique, 489–491, 490f–491f
corporo-deep dorsal vein shunt, 491
corporoglandular (Al-Ghorab) shunt, 490, 490f
corporoglandular (Ebbehoj and T-) shunt, 490
corporoglandular (Winter) shunt, 489–490, 490f
corporo-saphenous vein shunt, 491
corporospongiosal shunts, 491f, 45931
nonischemic priapism, 491
outcomes and complications, 491–492
postoperative management, 491
Prostate
contiguous structures, 164, 165f
imaging and biopsy procedures
alternative therapy, 176
complications, 177–178
computerized tomography, 178
magnetic resonance imaging, 178
positron emission tomography, 178
screening and diagnosis, 175
surgical indications, 176
surgical technique, 176–177, 177f
lymphatic anatomy, 163
neuroanatomy, 164
preservation, radical cystectomy, 102
rhabdomyosarcoma, childhood, surgical technique, 663–664
vascular anatomy, 163, 164f

Prostate cancer. *See also* Orchiectomy
brachytherapy for
alternative therapy, 203
diagnosis, 202
hybrid real-time planning and linked seeds approach, 205–207, 205f–207f
isotope selection, 203, 203t
outcomes and complications, 207–208, 208t
postimplant cystoscopy, 207
postimplant dosimetry, 207
real-time planning, 204–205, 205f
surgical indications, 202–203, 202t
surgical techniques, 203–207
cryoablation therapy for, 929
image-guided therapy for, 917–918
laparoscopic pelvic lymph node dissection for, 811–813
open radical retropubic surgery, control outcome, 192
pelvic lymphadenectomy
indications for, 179–180, 179t
laparoscopic and robotic approach, 182
limited *vs.* extended lymph node dissection, 182–183
surgical technique, 180–183, 180f–181f
Prostatectomy
laparoscopic and robotic techniques, 867–879
alternatives to, 868
bladder neck dissection, 874, 875f
diagnosis, 867
dorsal venous complex and distal urethra, 876, 876f
endopelvic fascia incision, 874
outcomes and complications, 877, 878t–879t
pelvic lymph node dissection, 876
posterior dissection, 874
postoperative care and discharge, 877
specimen retrieval, 877
surgical indications for, 867
surgical technique, 868–877
vasa deferentia/seminal vesicle dissection, 875, 875f
vesicourethral anastomosis, 876–877, 877f
open radical retropubic
alternatives to, 187
bladder neck transection and reconstruction, 190–191, 190f
complications, 193
incisions, 188, 188f
indications for, 186–187
neurovascular bundle separation, 189f, 190
outcomes, 192–193
postoperative care, 192
prophylactic hemostatic suture placement, 189, 189f
prostatic pedicle vascular control and transection, 190, 190f
seminal vesicle and vasa deferentia dissection, 191
surgical technique, 187–192, 188f–191f
suture ligation and dorsal venous complex transection, 188–189, 189f
vesicourethral anastomosis, 190f, 191–192
postprostatectomy incontinence, sling procedures, 299–304
radical perineal, 194–201
alternative therapy, 194–195
diagnosis, 194
outcomes and complications, 200–201, 201t
surgical indications, 194
surgical technique, 195–200, 195f–200f
retropubic, 172–173, 172f–173f
suprapubic, 171–173, 171f–173f, 171t
Prostate-specific antigen (PSA), seminal vesicle tumors, 362
Prostate-specific membrane antigen (PSMA), screening and diagnosis, 175
Prostate stem cell antigen (PSCA), screening and diagnosis, 175
Prostatic pedicles, open radical retropubic surgery
prophylactic hemostatic suture placement, 189, 189f
vascular control and transection, 190, 190f
Prostatic-specific antigen (PSA) assays
benign prostatic hypertrophy, post-treatment changes, 173–174, 174t
pelvic lymphadenectomy *vs.*, 186
screening and diagnosis, 175
Prosthetic grafts, renal artery reconstruction, 43
Prune belly (triad) syndrome, 654–661
alternative therapy, 656
diagnosis, 655
epidemiology, 654
outcomes and complications, 660–661
surgical indications, 655–656
surgical technique, 656–660
abdominal wall reconstruction, 658
distal cutaneous ureterostomy, 657
orchiopexy, 658–659, 659f
reduction cystoplasty, 658, 658f
ureteral reconstruction, 657
urethral reconstruction, 659–660, 660f
vesicostomy, 656
Pseudohermaphroditic disorders, corrective surgical techniques, 769–777
Pubocervical fascia, pelvic floor anatomy, 314
Puboprostatic ligament incision, open radical retropubic surgery, 188, 188f
Pubourethral ligaments, pelvic floor anatomy, 312, 312f
Pubovaginal fascial slings
alternative therapy, 273
basic principles, 271
bladder perforation and hematoma, 277
de novo urge incontinence, 277
diagnostic criteria, 272
erosion, 277
female urethra, 224, 226, 226f
midurethral sling contraindications, 273
outcomes and complications, 277
permanent clean intermittent catheterization, 273
physical examination, 272
prolonged urinary retention, 277
surgical indications, 272–273, 273f
surgical technique, 273–277, 274f–276f
alternative graft material, 276–277
crossover sling, 276, 276f
vesical neck reconstruction, 691, 691f
Pudendal neuromodulation, interstitial cystitis management, 157–158, 158f
Pull-through vaginoplasty, 764–767, 768f
Pyelolithotomy, horseshoe kidney, 642
Pyelonephritis, orthotopic urinary diversion, with ileal low-pressure reservoir, afferent tubulary segment, 565
Pyeloplasty
alternative therapy, 647–648
diagnostic criteria, 647
goals and applications, 647
horseshoe kidney, 637–638, 639f, 641f
indications for, 647
laparoscopic techniques, 752–756
alternative therapy, 752–753
diagnosis, 752
outcomes and complications, 756
retroperitoneoscopic approach, 753–754, 753f–754f
robotically assisted techniques, 853–859
surgical indications, 752
transperitoneal approach, 755, 755f
outcomes and complications, 649
robotically-assisted laparoscopic techniques, 853–859
alternative therapy, 853
Anderson-Hynes dismembered pyeloplasty, 854–855, 855f
complications, 859
diagnosis, 853
Foley V-V pyeloplasty, 855, 856f
nondismembered pyeloplasty (Heineke-Mikulicz), 855, 856f
outcomes, 858–859
postoperative care, 857–858, 858f
salvage maneuvers, 855–856
surgical indications, 853
surgical techniques, 853–854
transmesenteric approach, 856, 856f
trocar placement, 854, 854f
robotic procedures, 923
surgical technique, 648–649, 648f
Pyelostomy, posterior urethral valves, 700, 700f

## Q

Quality-of-life (QOL) score, midurethral retropubic slings and, 278
"Quick prep" cytological evaluation, testis biopsy, 402

## R

Radiation therapy
artificial urinary sphincter outcomes and, 298
postprostatectomy incontinence, sling procedures, 303
radical cystectomy *vs.*, 98
scrotal trauma and, 461, 461f–462f
Radical cystectomy
female patient, 104–112
alternative therapy, 105–106
anterior exenteration, 106–107, 106f–109f
continence issues, 106
indications for, 104–105, 105t
outcome and complications, 112
postoperative care, 112
preoperative care, 106

Radical cystectomy (*continued*)
reproductive organ preservation, 108, 110
retrograde dissection and urethral-sparing technique, 111–112, 111f
sexual function, 106
surgical technique, 106–112
urethrectomy, 107–108, 108f–109f
vaginal reconstruction, 108, 111f
laparoscopic procedures, 885–890
alternative therapy, 885
anterior dissection, 887
diagnosis, 885
dorsal vein complex transection, 887
extended/high-extended lymphadenectomy, 888–889, 889f
ileal conduit and orthotopic neobladder, 889
modifications for women patients, 887–888, 887f–888f
nerve-sparing cystectomy in men, 888
outcomes, 889–890, 890t
postoperative care, 889
reproductive organ-sparing cystectomy in women, 888
retrovesical dissection, 886–887
surgical indications, 885
ureter mobilization and division, 886
urinary diversion, 889
vascular pedicle dissection and control, 887, 887f
male patient, 97–103
alternative therapy, 98
anesthesia and instrumentation, 98
diagnosis, 97
indications, 97
outcomes and complications, 102–103
patient positioning and initial exposure, 98
surgical techniques, 98–102, 98f–102f
Radical cystoprostatectomy, 92
Radical inguinal lymphadenectomy, for penile carcinoma, 476–478, 476f–478f
Radical nephroureterectomy, laparoscopic procedure
comparisons, 830–831
left-handed procedure, 832–833, 832f
right-handed procedures, 833
Radiofrequency ablation (RFA)
laparoscopic procedures, renal tumors
basic principles, 842
outcomes and complications, 845, 845t
techniques, 842–844, 843f, 844t
renal tumors, 915–916
urologic procedures, 927–929, 928f
Rectocele
pelvic organ prolapse, 317–318, 317f
posterior vaginal prolapse repair, 346–347
Rectourethral fistula, 139–143
surgical management, 141–143, 141f–142f
Renal abscesses
alternative treatment, 54
diagnosis, 52–53
echinococcus, 52
resection, 57
surgical indications, 54
epidemiology, 51, 52f, 53t
laparoscopic treatment, 55–56
outcomes and complications, 57–58
renal tuberculosis, 51–52
cavernostomy, 56
nephrectomy, 56–57
surgical indications, 54
surgical indications, 53–54
surgical techniques, 55–57
open surgical drainage, 54–55
percutaneous drainage, 8–55
subscapular nephrectomy, 55, 55f–56f
Renal blood vessels, transperitoneal radical/total nephrectomy, 822–823
Renal cystectomy, laparoscopic techniques
alternative therapy, 838
diagnosis, 838
outcomes and complications, 839
retroperitoneal approach, 838–839, 838f–839f
surgical indications, 838
transperitoneal approach, 839
Renal function. *See also* Renovascular disease
kidney tissue engineering, 910–911
orthotopic bladder substitution, 556
Renal fusion. *See also* Ectopic kidney; Horseshoe kidney
alternative therapy, 637
diagnostic criteria, 635–636, 636f–637f
epidemiology, 634–635, 635f
outcomes and complications, 642
surgical indications, 636–637
surgical technique, 637
ectopic kidney, 642
pyeloplasty, 637–638, 639f, 641f
stone surgery, 642
tumor excision, 638, 641, 641f
ureterocalicostomy, 638, 640f
Renal transplantation
allotransplantation
allograft positioning and vascular anastomoses, 66–68, 67f–68f
alternative therapy, 65
diagnosis, 65
incision and iliac fossa dissection, 65–66, 66f
multiple renal vessels, 68
outcomes and complications, 70–71, 71t
pediatric patients, 69–70, 69f–70f
surgical indications, 65
surgical techniques, 65–70
ureteral considerations, 68, 69f
wound closure, 70
autotransplantation
alternative therapy, 76
back-table preparation, 80
diagnosis, 76
flank donor nephrectomy, 78–80, 79f
iliac vessel exposure, 80–81, 81f
midline intraperitoneal approach, doonor nephrectomy, 80
outcomes and complications, 82–83
revascularization, 81–82
surgical indications, 76
surgical instrumentation, 77
surgical techniques, 77–78
ureteroneocystostomy, 82, 82f
wound closure, 82
donor nephrectomy, laparoscopic techniques, 846–852
alternative therapy, 847
diagnosis, 846
left-sided procedure, 849–850, 849f–850f
outcomes and complications, 851–852, 852t
patient preparation and positioning, 847–848, 847f–848f
right-sided procedure, 850–851
surgical indications, 846–847
techniques and instrumentation, 848–849, 848f, 848t
ureteral complications, 70–75
Renal trauma, 58–64
angioembolization, 59–60, 60f
diagnosis, 58–59
imaging techniques, 59, 59f
management, 59
nephrectomy, 60–63, 62f
outcomes and complications, 63–64, 64f
postoperative care, 63
renal exploration, indications for, 60, 60t
renovascular injuries, 63, 63f–64f
surgical technique, 60–63, 61f–63f
Renal tumors. *See also* Intracaval tumors
cryoablation therapy, 929
image-guided therapy, 914–917
cryotherapy, 915
laparoscopic procedures, 914–915
radiofrequency ablation (RFA), 915–916
laparoscopic ablation
basic principles, 842
cryotherapy mechanisms, 843–844, 844f
diagnosis, 842
outcomes and complications, 845, 845t
radiofrequency ablation, 842–844, 843f, 844t
surgical indications, 842
laparoscopic biopsy techniques, 839–840, 840f
laser therapy, 932
partial nephrectomy
indications for, 6–2–7, 8f
surgical technique, 9–11, 10f
radiofrequency ablation, 927–928, 928f
renal cell carcinoma
intracaval tumors, 23–31
radical nephrectomy, 14–15
Renovascular disease
diagnosis, 36
medical therapies, 37
renal allotransplantation, 68
surgical complications and outcomes, 44
surgical indications, 36–37
surgical technique
additional bypass options, 42
aortorenal bypass graft, 37–41, 37f
autotransplantation and *ex vivo* bench surgery, 43–44, 44f
hepatorenal bypass graft, 39–41 41f–42f
ileorenal bypass, 42, 43f
prosthetic grafts, 43
salvage surgery, 43
saphenous vein graft, 38–39, 38f–40f
saphenous vein procurement, 38, 38f
splenorenal artery bypass, 39, 41f–42f
Renovascular in juries, 63, 63f–64f
Replantation, penile
alternative therapy, 520
diagnosis, 520, 520f
epidemiology, 519–520
outcomes and complications, 522
postoperative management, 522
surgical indications, 520, 520f
surgical technique, 521–522, 521f–522f
Reproductive organ preservation
female radical cystectomy, 108, 110

laparoscopic radical cystectomy, in women, 888
Reservoir construction, ileal neobladder, 568, 570–571, 570f–572f
Rete testis, anatomy, 426
Retrograde dissection, urethral-sparing technique, female radical cystectomy, 111–112, 111f
Retrograde urethrography, anterior urethral trauma, 246–247, 247f
Retroperitoneal abscess
alternative treatment, 53
diagnosis, 52–53
echinococcus, 52
resection, 57
surgical indications, 54
outcomes and complications, 57–58
percutaneous drainage, 54
surgical indications, 53–54
surgical techniques, 54–57, 55f–57f
Retroperitoneal approach
laparoscopic techniques, 807–808, 807f–808f
adrenalectomy, 862–866, 864f–865f
lymph node dissection
alternative therapy, 814
outcomes and complications, 817–818, 818t
postoperative care, 817
retroperitoneal approach, 816–817, 817f
stage II/III post-chemotherapy disease, 816
surgical indications, 814, 814t
transperitoneal approach, 814–816, 815f
nephrectomy, 824–825, 825f
pediatric patients, 759–760, 759f
renal cystectomy, 838–839, 838f–839f
lymphadenectomy, 442–448
alternative therapy, 443
diagnosis, 442
dissection templates, 443–444, 445f
nerve-sparing retroperitoneal lymph node dissection, 444–448, 446f–447f
outcomes and complications, 448
postchemotherapy, 447
primary procedures, 443, 444f
surgical indications, 442–443
surgical techniques, 443–447
varicocele, 524–525, 524f
Retroperitoneoscopic approach
laparoscopic pyeloplasty, 753–754, 753f–754f
partial nephrectomy, 827
Retrovesical approach
laparoscopic radical cystectomy, 886–887
seminal vesicle surgery, 364–366, 365f
Rhabdomyosarcoma, childhood, 662–665
alternative therapy, 663
diagnostic criteria, 662
epidemiology, 662
outcomes and complications, 664–665
postoperative grouping, 662t
staging, 662t
surgical indications, 662–663
surgical technique, 663–664
Robotically assisted laparoscopic (radical) prostatectomy (RALP), 867–879
Robotic techniques
pelvic lymphadenectomy, prostate cancer, 182
prostatectomy, laparoscopic
alternatives to, 868
bladder neck dissection, 874, 875f
diagnosis, 867
dorsal venous complex and distal urethra, 876, 876f
endopelvic fascia incision, 874
outcomes and complications, 877, 878t–879t
pelvic lymph node dissection, 876
posterior dissection, 874
postoperative care and discharge, 877
specimen retrieval, 877
surgical indications for, 867
surgical technique, 868–877
vasa deferentia/seminal vesicle dissection, 875, 875f
vesicourethral anastomosis, 876–877, 877f
pyeloplasty, laparoscopic, 853–859
alternative therapy, 853
Anderson-Hynes dismembered pyeloplasty, 854–855, 855f
complications, 859
diagnosis, 853
Foley V-V pyeloplasty, 855, 856f
nondismembered pyeloplasty (Heineke-Mikulicz), 855, 856f
outcomes, 858–859
postoperative care, 857–858, 858f
salvage maneuvers, 855–856
surgical indications, 853
surgical techniques, 853–854
transmesenteric approach, 856, 856f
trocar placement, 854, 854f
surgical robotics
flexible robotics, 923–924, 923f
history, 919–922, 920f–922f
laparoscopic cystectomy, 922
laparoscopic prostatectomy, 922
miscellaneous procedures, 923
nephrectomy, 923
nomenclature, 919, 920t
NOTES and miniature robotics, 924–925, 924f
pyeloplasty, 923
vesicovaginal fistula surgery, 136–137

## S

Sacral nerve stimulation
alternative therapy, 306
basic principles, 305
diagnostic criteria, 306
foramen needle insertion, 308–309, 308f–309f
InterStim device, 310, 310f
interstitial cystitis management, 154–155, 158f
outcomes and complications, 310–311
overactive bladder, 305–306, 305f
peripheral nerve test stimulation, 307–308, 307f–308f
surgical indications, 306
surgical technique, 307–310, 307f–310f, 307t
tined lead placement, 309–310
urinary retention, 306
Sacrospinous ligaments
pelvic floor anatomy, 314, 314f
transvaginal enterocele repair, fixation of, 340, 340f–341f
Salvage maneuvers, robotically assisted laparoscopic pyeloplasty, 855–856
Saphenous vein graft, renovascular disease
insertion, 38–39, 38f–40f
vein procurement, 38, 38f
Scaphoid megalourethra, diagnostic criteria, 655, 655f
Scrotal approach, simple orchiectomy, 429, 429f
Scrotal fixation, cryptorchidism surgery, subdartos pouch, 738–739, 738f–113–17f
Scrotal orchiopexy, 739–740
Scrotum
anatomy of, 465, 465f–466f
congenital anomalies
alternative therapy, 732
bifid scrotum, surgical technique, 732
diagnosis, 731
outcomes and complications, 734
penoscrotal transposition, 732–733, 732f–733f
scrotal ectopia, 733
scrotal hypoplasia, 733
scrotal inclusion cysts, 734
surgical indications, 731–732
webbed penis, 733–734, 733f–734f
hypospadias abnormalities, 704
lymphatic anatomy, 466
trauma and reconstruction
alternative therapy, 455
avulsion injuries, 457–460, 459f
burn injuries, 460, 460f
diagnosis, 453–455, 454f–455f
Fournier gangrene, 461–462, 463f
hematomas and blunt injury, 455–456, 456f
outcomes and complications, 462–463
penetrating injury, 456–457, 458f
radiation injury, 461, 461f–462f
surgical indications, 455
vascular anatomy, 465–466
Semen analysis, vasectomy follow-up, 375
Seminal vesicles
alternative therapy, 362
anatomy, 358–360, 359f–360f
development, 359
diagnostic criteria, 362
dissection, robotically assisted laparoscopic (radical) prostatectomy, 875, 875f
function, 360
open radical retropubic surgery, dissection, 191
physical examination, 358–359
prostate anatomy, 163, 164f
surgical indications, 362
surgical techniques, 363–368
endoscopic treatment, 368
laparoscopic technique, 366–368, 367f
outcomes and complications, 368, 368t
paravesical approach, 364–366
preoperative preparation, 362–363
retrovesical approach, 364–366, 365f
transcoccygeal approach, 366, 366f
transperineal approach, 363–364, 364f
transurethral resection, 368
transvesical approach, 363, 363f
vascular anatomy, 360

Seminiferous tubules, testis anatomy, 424–425, 425f
Sensory innervation, bladder anatomy, 89–90
Seromuscular grafts
bladder tissue engineering, 909–910
bowel flap tube, colonic continent catheterizable reservoir, 602, 604f
extramural tunnel technique, colonic orthotopic bladder substitution, 589–590, 589f–593f
Serous-lined extramural tunnel ureteral implantation, ureterosigmoidostomy, 614–616, 615f–616f
Sertoli cells, testis anatomy, 425–426
Sexual function, female radical cystectomy, 106
Sigmoid colon conduit, palliative techniques, 619, 619f
Sigmoid colon reservoir construction, colonic orthotopic bladder substitution, 589–590, 593f
Sigmoidocystoplasty, bladder augmentation, 787, 788f
Sigmoid rectal pouch technique, ureterosigmoidostomy, 613–614, 613f–615f
surgical tricks, 616
Silicone polymers (macroplastique, bioplastique), injectable incontinence therapies, female patients, 267
Single-armed microsutures, longitudinal intussusception vasoepididymostomy, 385, 385f
Skin abnormalities, hypospadias, 704
Skin graft, penile trauma, 517–518, 517f
Skin stenosis, colonic continent catheterizable reservoir construction, 605–606
"Sleeve technique," circumcision, 779, 780f
Sling procedures
midurethral retropubic sling
contraindications to, 273
failure of, 272
injectable incontinence therapy, female patients, 265
pubovaginal fascial sling alternative to, 273
synthetic slings, 278–281
transobturator approach, 282–287
postprostatectomy incontinence, male patients
alternative therapy, 299–300
contraindications, 303
detrusor hypocontractility, 303
diagnosis, 299
failure, 49–93
materials for, 303
outcomes and complications, 302
prevalence, 299–49–90
previous surgical procedures, 303
radiation therapy and, 303
severe incontinence, 303
surgical indications, 299
surgical technique, 300–302, 300f, 302t
tensioning sling, 302–303
transobturator approach, 303–304, 304f
pubovaginal fascial slings
female urethra, 224, 226, 226f
vesical neck reconstruction, 691, 691f
Snodgrass tubularized incised plate urethroplasty, 706, 708f
Sober loop ureterostomy, posterior urethral valves, 701, 701f
Somatic innervation, bladder anatomy, 89–90, 90f
Space of Retzius, 86, 87f
Spermatocele
alternative therapy, 530–531
diagnosis, 530
outcomes and complications, 531
surgical indications, 530
surgical technique, 531
Spermatogenesis, testis anatomy, 425
Sperm extraction
epididymal sperm aspiration, 407–409
testicular sperm extraction (TESE), 403–406, 404f
Sperm retrieval techniques, 403–406
Sphincter competence, colonic continent catheterizable reservoir, 599
Sphincterotomy, neurogenic bladder, 228–232, 229t, 230f–232f
Spinal cord injury (SCI), anejaculation, ejaculation induction procedures, 413–418
Splenorenal artery bypass, renovascular disease, 39, 41f–42f
Squamous cell carcinoma, of penis, penectomy
circumcision and glans-sparing surgery, 468–469, 469f
diagnosis, 467–468, 467f
outcomes and complications, 471–473
partial penectomy, 469–471, 470f
surgical indications, 468
total penectomy, 471, 472f
Staged implants, interstitial cystitis management, 155–157, 156f–157f
Starburst XL (RITA) probe, radiofrequency ablation, renal tumors, 844, 844t
Starr plication, megaureter surgical management, 652, 652f
Stem cells, genitourinary tissue engineering, 906–907
Stents, palliative ureteral obstruction management
metallic mesh stents, 621
two double-J stents, 621, 621f
Stoma construction, bilateral cutaneous ureterostomy, 618–620, 619f
Stone surgery. *See* Pyelolithotomy
Storage reflex, bladder anatomy, 90, 90f
Stress urinary incontinence (SUI)
abdominal retropubic therapies, female patients, 288–291
injectable therapies, female patients, 263–269
midurethral retropubic slings, 278–281
transobturator approach, 282–287
postprostatectomy incontinence, sling procedures, 299–304
pubovaginal fascial slings, 271–277
urethral diverticulum with, 215–216
urogenital tissue engineering, 907–908
in women, injectable therapies for, 263–269
Subdartos pouch, cryptorchidism surgery, scrotal fixation, 738–739, 738f–113–17f
Submucosal tunnel technique, colonic orthotopic bladder substitution, 589–590, 589f–593f
Subscapular nephrectomy
renal and retroperitoneal abscess, 55, 55f–56f
technique, 33–34
Subscapular orchiectomy, 431, 431f
Substitution cystoplasty, interstitial cystitis management, 152–153, 155f
Supradiaphragmatic thrombi, intracaval tumors, abdominal surgical approaches to, 29
Suprahepatic thrombi, intracaval tumors, abdominal surgical approaches to, 29
Suprainguinal dissection, in inguinal lymphadenectomy, for penile carcinoma, 479, 480f
Suprapubic orchiectomy, 429–431, 430f
Suprapubic prostatectomy, benign prostatic hypertrophy, 171–173, 171f–173f, 171t
complications, 174
Supravesical urinary diversion
palliative techniques, 618–619, 619f
posterior urethral valves, 700–702, 702f
Synthetic materials
injectable incontinence therapies, female patients, 266–269
calcium hydroxyapatite (Coaptite), 268–269
carbon-coated zirconium beads (durasphere/durasphere EXP), 267–268
ethylene vinyl alcohol copolymer, 268
polytetrafluoroethylene (Polytef), 266–267
silicone polymers (macroplastique, bioplastique), 267
midurethral retropubic slings
alternative therapies, 278–279
basic principles, 278
diagnosis, 278
material selection criteria, 279
outcomes and complications, 280–281, 281f
surgical indications, 278
surgical technique, 279–280, 280f
tension-free vaginal tape, 280
transobturator approach, 282–285, 284t
in posterior vaginal prolapse repair, 347–348
postprostatectomy incontinence, sling procedures, 303

## T

"Table-fixed" ring retraction, urethral stricture surgery, 237
Tension-Free Vaginal Tape (TVT)
midurethral retropubic slings, 280–281
pubovaginal fascial slings, 271–273
Tensioning sling, postprostatectomy incontinence, 302–303
Testicle
bilateral nonpalpable testes, laparoscopic orchiopexy, 749–750, 750f–751f
torsion
alternative therapy, 450–451
appendages, torsion of, 449–450, 450f
in children, adolescents, and adults, 449
epidemiology, 448–449, 449f
outcomes and complications, 451–452
perinatal, 449

surgical indications, 450
surgical technique, 451, 451f–452f
trauma, 455–456, 456f
undescended (cryptorchidism)
additional cord length and fixation, 747, 748f–749f
blind-ending vessels, 744, 745f
internal ring cord structures, 744, 745f
intra-abdominal testis, 745, 746f
laparoscopic management, 743–751, 746f–750f
neoinguinal hiatus, 746–747, 747f–748f
peritoneal pedical flap, 745–746, 747f
second-stage Fowler-Stephens orchiopexy, 749, 749f
single-stage laparoscopic orchiopexy, 745, 746f–749f, 749
Testicular epididymal sperm aspiration (TESA), 380
Testicular ischemia and atrophy, varicocelectomy, 400
Testicular sperm extraction (TESE), 403–406
Testicular tumors
organ-preserving surgery
alternative therapy, 438
diagnosis, 438
outcomes and complication, 441
surgical indications, 438
surgical technique, 438–441, 439f–441f
retroperitoneal lymphadenectomy, 442–448
Testis
anatomy, 419–426
blood supply, 421–424, 422f–423f
blood-testis barrier, 424
capsule, 421, 421f
countercurrent heat exchange, 424
descent, 420–421
development, 420
germ cells and spermatogenesis, 425
germinal epithelium, 425–426
hypothalamic-pituitary-gonadal axis, 419, 420f
innervation, 424
Leydig cells, 426
rete testis and efferent ducts, 426
seminiferous tubules, 424–425, 425f
Sertoli cells, 425–426
biopsy procedures, 401–403, 404f
Thoracoabdominal incision
intracaval tumor surgery, 25, 26f
radical nephrectomy, 16–18, 19f–20f
Three-finger technique, vasectomy procedures, 374–375, 374f
Thrombi formation, intracaval tumors, abdominal surgical approaches to, 29–31
Tibial nerve modulation, interstitial cystitis management, 158–159, 158f
Tiflis pouch, continent catheterizable reservoir construction, 603, 607f
Tissue engineering, urogenital repair
basic principles, 905
biomaterial properties, 905
bladder, 909–910, 910f
cell properties, 905–906
female genital tissue, 911–912
injectable chondrocytes, 907
injectable Leydig cells, 908
injectable muscle cells, 908
kidney, 910–911, 911f
penis, 911
stem cell classification, 906–907
urethra, 908–909, 908f
Torsion, testicular
alternative therapy, 450–451
appendages, torsion of, 449–450, 450f
in children, adolescents, and adults, 449
epidemiology, 448–449, 449f
outcomes and complications, 451–452
perinatal, 449
surgical indications, 450
surgical technique, 451, 451f–452f
Total urogenital mobilization (TUM), 765–767, 766f–117–148f
urogenital sinus repair, 773–775, 774f–776f
Touch prep technique, testis biopsy, 402–403
T-pouch ileal neobladder
alternative therapy, 579
diagnostic criteria, 579
goals and functions, 578–579
outcome and complications, 584–586
surgical indications, 579
surgical technique, 579–584, 579f–584f
suture techniques, 580–585, 580f–584f
Transabdominal approach
radical nephrectomy, chevron/anterior subcostal approach, 18, 20f, 21
vesicovaginal fistula repair, 134–136, 134f–136f
Transanal approach, rectourethral fistula repair, 141, 141f
Transcoccygeal approach, seminal vesicle surgery, 366, 366f
Transcorporeal cuff placement, artificial urinary sphincter, male patients, 294, 294f
Transitional cell carcinoma
female urethra, 252–256
laser therapy, 932
male urethra, 257–262
Transmesenteric approach, robotically assisted laparoscopic pyeloplasty, 856, 856f
Transobturator approach, vaginal prolapse repair, 331–334, 333f–334f
Transobturator route of sling replacement (TOT)
midurethral retropubic sling
alternative therapy, 282
basic principles, 282
comparisons, 279
diagnostic criteria, 282–282
outcomes and complications, 285–287, 286t
surgical indications, 282
surgical technique, 282–285, 282f–283f, 284t
postprostatectomy incontinence, 303–304, 304f
pubovaginal fascial slings, 271
Transperineal approach, seminal vesicle surgery, 363–364, 364f, 367
Transperitoneal approach
laparoscopic techniques, 801–802, 802f
adrenalectomy, 861–862, 861f–864f
nephroureterectomy, 831–832, 832f
open "Hasson" procedure, 805, 805f
partial nephrectomy, 825–826, 826f
pelvic lymph node dissection, 812–813, 812f–813f
radical/total nephrectomy, 820–823, 820f–823f
renal cystectomy, 839
retroperitoneal lymph node dissection
left-sided template, 816
right-sided template, 814–816, 815f
nephrectomy/partial nephrectomy, pediatric patients, 758–759, 758f–759f
orchipexy, for cryptorchidism, 739
Transplant nephrectomy, 32–36
allograft, 32
diagnosis, 32
outcomes and complications, 34–35
surgical indications, 32
surgical techniques, 32–34, 33f–35f
Transrectal ultrasound (TRUS)
brachytherapy, prostate cancer, 202–207
indications for, 176
prostatic screening and diagnosis, 175
seminal vesicles, surgical and diagnostic applications, 361–362
technique, 176–177, 177f
Transtrigonal approach, vesicoureteral reflux repair, 672, 672f
Transureteral cutaneous ureterostomy, palliative applications, 620
Transureteroureterostomy (TUU)
alternative therapy, 643
diagnostic criteria, 643
indications for, 643
laparoscopic approach, 646
outcomes and complications, 646
retroperitoneal approach, 645–646, 645f
surgical technique, 643–646, 644f–645f
transperitoneal approach, 644–645, 644f–645f
Transurethral bladder cuff technique, nephroureterectomy, distal ureter management, 127
Transurethral incision of the prostate (TUIP), benign prostatic hypertrophy, techniques, 167–170, 168t, 169f
Transurethral injection, incontinence therapy, female patients, 264
Transurethral microwave thermotherapy (TUMT), 928–929, 928f
Transurethral needle ablation (TUNA), urologic applications, 928, 928f
Transurethral resection
bladder diverticulectomy, 115
seminal vesicles, 368
of ureteral orifice (TURUO) (Pluck technique), 836
Transurethral resection of the ejaculatory ducts (TURED), 369–371, 370f–371f
Transurethral resection of the prostate (TURP), benign prostatic hypertrophy
complications, 174
outcomes, 166
techniques, 167–170, 168t, 169f
treatment outcomes, 173–174
Transurethral valve ablation, 697–698, 698f
Transvaginal approach
urethral diverticulectomy, 216–219, 216t, 217f–219f
vesicovaginal fistula repair, 132–134, 132f–133f

Transvaginal prolapse repair
alternative therapy, 336
basic principles, 335–336, 336f
diagnosis, 336
enterocele repair, 336–338, 337f–338f
iliococcygeus fixation, 340–341
Manchester procedure, 342
McCall culdoplasty, 338, 339f
mesh-augmented repairs, 341–342, 341f–342f
prolapsed uterus preservation, 342
sacrospinous ligament fixation, 340, 340f
surgical indications, 336
uterosacral ligament fixation, 338–340, 339f
vault suspension, 338
Transverse colonic conduit, 549–554
alternative therapy, 550
diagnostic criteria, 550
outcomes and complications, 553
palliative techniques, 619, 619f
retubularized colon segments, 622, 622f
surgical indications, 550
surgical technique, 550–553, 550f–553f
postoperative care, 553
pyeotransverse pyelocutaneostomy, 552, 554f
Transverse scrotal incision, artificial urinary sphincter, 294–296, 295f–296f
Transvesical approach
bladder diverticulectomy, 115
laparoscopic distal ureterectomy, detachment and ligation, 835–836
nephroureterectomy, distal ureter management
bladder cuff technique, single port, 126–127, 127f
bladder cuff technique, two ports, 127–128
seminal vesical surgery, 363–364
vesicovaginal fistula repair, 136
Trauma
penile trauma
penetrating injury, 518–519
rupture, 514–516, 515f–516f
skin loss, 516–518, 517f
renal trauma, 58–64
angioembolization, 59–60, 60f
diagnosis, 58–59
imaging techniques, 59f, 60
management, 59
nephrectomy, 60
outcomes and complications, 63, 63f–64f
postoperative care, 63
renal exploration, indications for, 60, 60t
renovascular injuries, 63, 63f–64f
surgical technique, 60–63, 61f–63f
scrotum
alternative therapy, 455
avulsion injuries, 457–460, 459f
burn injuries, 460, 460f
diagnosis, 453–455, 454f–455f
Fournier gangrene, 461–462, 462f
hematomas and blunt injury, 455–456, 456f
outcomes and complications, 462–463
penetrating injury, 456–457, 458f
radiation injury, 461, 461f
surgical indications, 455
urethral trauma
anterior injuries, 246–249, 246f
alternative therapy, 247
diagnosis, 246–247, 247f
indications for surgery, 247
outcomes and complications, 248–249
surgical management, 248, 248f
classification, 250t
posterior injuries, 249–36–42
alternative therapy, 251
diagnosis, 249, 250f, 250t
indications for surgery, 250–36–42
outcomes and complications, 251–252
surgical techniques, 251, 251f
surgical management, 245–36–42
vesical trauma and hemorrhage, 143–149
alternative therapy, 146
diagnosis, 144–145, 144f–146f
outcomes and complications, 147
surgical management and technique, 146–147
Triad syndrome (prune belly)
alternative therapy, 656
diagnosis, 655
epidemiology, 654
outcomes and complications, 660–661
surgical indications, 655–656
surgical technique, 656–660
abdominal wall reconstruction, 658
distal cutaneous ureterostomy, 657
orchiopexy, 658–659, 659f
reduction cystoplasty, 658, 658f
ureteral reconstruction, 657
urethral reconstruction, 659–660, 660f
vesicostomy, 656
Trigone, bladder anatomy, 88–89, 88f
Trocar placement
laparoscopic surgery
primary placement, 804–805, 804f
removal, 806–807, 806f
robotically assisted pyeloplasty, 854, 854f
secondary placement, 805, 806f
lymphocele laparoscopic management, 882, 882f
Tube flap reconstructive technique, female urethra, 223, 223f
Tube graft, female urethra, 223–224, 224f
Tubularized incised plate (TIP) urethroplasty, hypospadias surgery, 706, 708f
TUR syndrome, benign prostatic hypertrophy, 174
Two-needle intussusception vasoepididymostomy, 379, 379f

## U

Ulcer fulguration, interstitial cystitis management, 152, 159t
Ultrasound
injectable incontinence therapy, female patients, 264–265
renal biopsy, laparoscopic procedures, 839–840, 840f
urologic procedures, 927
Ultrasound-guided biopsy (USB)
indications for, 176
prostatic screening and diagnosis, 175
technique, 176–177, 177f
Umbilical disorders
diagnostic criteria, 684–687
epidemiology, 684, 685f–686f
indications for surgery, 687
outcomes and complications, 689
surgical technique, 687–689, 688f–689f
Umbrella cells, bladder anatomy, 86–88, 87f
Undescended testicle. *See* Cryptorchidism, pediatric
Upper-pole ablation/preservation
transperitoneal radical/total nephrectomy, 823, 823f
ureterocele, 682–683, 682f–683f
Urachal anomalies
diagnostic criteria, 684–687
epidemiology, 684, 685f–686f
indications for surgery, 687
outcomes and complications, 689
surgical technique, 687–689, 688f–689f
Urachal excision, laparoscopic partial cystectomy, 890–891
Ureter
bladder anatomy, 88–89
distal ureter, nephroureterectomy, 125–129
duplication, vesicoureteral reflux repair, 672, 673f–674f, 674
implantation techniques
colonic continent catheterizable reservoir, 602, 603f–605f
colonic orthotopic bladder substitution, 588–589
ureterocele, 682–683, 682f
ureterosigmoidostomy, 614–616, 615f–616f
megaureter, diagnosis and surgical management, 649–654
mobilization
ileal neobladder, 567, 567f
laparoscopic radical cystectomy, 886
obstruction
palliative treatment, 620–622, 621f–622f
renal transplant complications, 72
orthotopic bladder substitution and resection, 557, 557f
reconstruction, triad syndrome, 657, 657f
renal transplantation
allotransplantation, 68, 69f
complications, 71–75
stricture of, laparoscopic management, 903
transperitoneal radical/total nephrectomy dissection and elevation, 822, 822f
Ureteral carcinoma, laser therapy, 932
Ureteral intussusception technique, nephroureterectomy, distal ureter management, 128–129, 129f
Ureteral unroofing technique, nephroureterectomy, distal ureter management, 128, 128f
Ureterocalicostomy, horseshoe kidney, 638, 640f
Ureteroceles
alternative therapy, 681
diagnostic criteria, 681
epidemiology, 681
indications for surgery, 681
outcomes and complications, 683–684
surgical technique, 681–683, 681f
upper-pole ablation, 683

upper-pole preservation, 682–683, 682f–683f
therapeutic options, 681t
Ureterocystoplasty, bladder augmentation, 789, 790f
Ureteroileal end-to-side anastomosis, orthotopic urinary diversion, with ileal low-pressure reservoir, afferent tubulary segment, 563, 563f
Ureterolysis, laparoscopic techniques, 901, 903
Ureteroneocystostomy
renal allotransplantation, 68, 69f
renal autotransplantation, 82, 82f
Ureteropelvic junction (UPJ) obstruction
alternative therapy, 637
horseshoe kidney, diagnosis, 636
indications for surgery, 636–637
laparoscopic pyeloplasty, 752–756
pyeloplasty, 637–638, 639f, 641f
alternative therapy, 647–648
diagnostic criteria, 647
goals and applications, 647
laparoscopic and robotically assisted techniques, 853–859
surgical technique, 648–649, 648f
robotic surgical techniques, 923
ureterocalicostomy, 638, 640f
Ureterosigmoidostomy, Mainz pouch II technique
alternative therapy, 611
classical surgical technique, 611–613, 611f–613f
complications and outcomes, 617
diagnostic criteria, 610–611
indications for surgery, 611
serous-lined extramural tunnel ureteral implantation, 614–616, 615f–616f
sigmoid-rectal pouch technique, 613–614, 613f–615f
surgical tricks, 616
Ureterostomy
palliative techniques, 618–620, 619f
posterior urethral valves
end cutaneous ureterostomy, 701–702, 702f
high cutaneous loop technique, 701, 701f
pelvioureterostomy-en-Y, 701, 701f
triad syndrome, distal cutaneous, 657
ureteral complications, renal transplant, 72–75, 75f
Ureteroureterostomy/ureteropyelostomy, ureterocele, 683
Ureterovesical junction, bladder anatomy, 88–89, 88f
Ureterovesicostomy, 797–798
Urethra
atraumatic dissection, orthotopic bladder substitution, 557–559, 559f
female urethra
anatomy and innervation, 211–213, 211f–213f
bladder exstrophy procedures, 719–720, 719f–721f
carcinoma, 252–256
contiguous structures, 212–213, 212f–213f
continence mechanisms, 316
gross/microscopic anatomy, 211–212, 211f–212f
innervation, 212
lymphatics, 212
reconstructive surgery, 220–227, 220t, 222f–227f, 227t
trauma and damage, causes of, 220–221, 220t
urethral-sparing technique, female radical cystectomy, 111–112, 111f
vascular anatomy, 212
male urethra
anatomy and innervation, 213–214, 213f
contiguous structures, 214
innervation, 214
lymphatics, 214
membranous urethra, ileal neobladder, 568, 568f–570f
penile/urethral dissection, 712f–716f, 713–714
vascular anatomy, 213
membraneous, laparoscopic radical cystectomy, 887
orthotopic urinary diversion, with ileal low-pressure reservoir, afferent tubulary segment, 563–564, 563f–564f
triad syndrome, reconstruction, 656, 659–660, 660f
urogenital tissue engineering, 908–909, 908f
Urethral cancer
female, 252–256
alternative therapy, 253–254
bladder-sparing surgery, 254
diagnosis, 253
distal urethral tumors, 254
indications for surgery, 253
outcomes and complications, 256
proximal urethral tumors, 256
staging, 253t
surgical technique, 254–256, 255f–256f
male urethra, 257–262
alternative therapy, 258
epidemiology and histology of, 257, 257f
outcomes and complications, 262
proximal urethral tumors, 259–262, 260f–261f
staging, 258t
surgical technique, 258–259
Urethral diverticulum
female urethra, 214–220, 215f
alternative therapy, 216
diagnosis, 215–216, 216f
indications for surgery, 216
surgical technique, 216–219, 216t, 217f–219f
postoperative complications, 219
postoperative outcomes, 219–220
Urethral glands, 355f–356f, 360
Urethral hypermobility, pubovaginal fascial slings, 271–277
Urethral plate, posterior hypospadias surgery, 706–707
Urethral stricture
alternative therapy for, 237
anastomotic urethroplasty, 240–241, 240f
augmented anastomotic urethroplasty, 241, 242f
bulbar stricture repair, 240–241
diagnosis, 236
glandular urethra, 237–238, 238f–239f
one-stage combination urethroplasty, 241, 243
onlay bulbar urethroplasty, 241, 243f
outcomes and complications, 244–245
pendulous urethra, 237–240
staged repair techniques, 243–244, 244f
surgical indications, 236
surgical management, 236–245
surgical outcomes and complications, 244–245
surgical techniques for, 237–244
Urethral trauma
anterior injuries, 246–249, 246f
alternative therapy, 247
diagnosis, 246–247, 247f
indications for surgery, 247
outcomes and complications, 248–249
surgical management, 248, 248f
classification, 250t
posterior injuries, 249–36–42
alternative therapy, 251
diagnosis, 249, 250f, 250t
indications for surgery, 250–251
outcomes and complications, 251–252
surgical techniques, 251, 251f
surgical management, 245–36–42
Urethral valve surgery
anterior valves, 703
posterior valves
alternatives, 697
cutaneous pyelostomy, 700, 700f
diagnostic criteria, 697, 697f
end cutaneous ureterostomy, 701–702, 702f
high cutaneous loop ureterostomy, 701, 701f
indications for, 697, 698f
outcomes and complications, 702–703
pelvioureterostomy-en-Y (Sober loop ureterostomy), 701, 701f
supravesical diversion, 700–702, 702f
transurethral valve ablation, 697–698, 698f
vesicostomy, 698–700, 699f
Urethrectomy
distal procedure, 254–255, 255f–256f
female radical cystectomy, 107–108, 110f
for female urethral cancer, 254–256, 255f–256f
male urethral tumors, 259, 260f
penile preservation and, 259
simple cystectomy with, 14–9f, 92–14–9
Urethropelvic ligament
diverticulum formation, 214–215, 215f
pelvic floor anatomy, 312, 313f
Urethropexies
abdominal retropubic therapies, female patients, 289–291, 289f–290f
injectable incontinence therapy, female patients, 265
Urethroplasty
anastomotic, 240–241, 240f
augmented anastomotic procedure, 241, 242f
failed procedure (panurethral stricture), 241
one-stage combination technique, 241, 243
onlay bulbar, 239f, 241, 243f
outcomes and complications, 244–245

Urethroplasty (*continued*)
staged repair, 243–244
tubularized incised plate urethroplasty, 706, 708f
for urethral stricture, 236–245
urethral trauma, 248–36–42
Urinary Distress Inventory (UDI), 286
Urinary diversion. *See also* Ileal bladder, Padua; Ileal neobladder
catherizable reservoir construction, 595
colonic continent catheterizable reservoir and, 599
exstrophy/epispadias repair, 723
hypospadias surgery, 705
interstitial cystitis management, 153–154
laparoscopic radical cystectomy, 889
orthotopic, with ileal low-pressure reservoir, afferent tubulary segment
alternative therapies, 562
diagnostic criteria, 561–562, 562t
outcomes and complications, 565
surgical indications, 562
surgical technique, 562–565
palliative care techniques
alternative therapy, 618
diagnostic criteria, 618
indications for surgery, 618
surgical technique and outcomes, 618–620, 619f
ureteral obstruction, 620–622, 621f–622f
simple cystectomy, 92
Urinary function. *See also* Incontinence; Stress urinary incontinence
rectourethral fistula repair and preservation of, 142–143
renal transplantation, ureteral complications, 72
Urinary retention
pubovaginal fascial sling procedure, 277
sacral neurostimulation, 306
Urinary tract infection (UTI)
augmentation cystoplasty and, 792
urethral diverticulum, 215–216
Urinary tract reconstruction
Mitrofanoff procedure
alternative therapy, 794
appendicovesicostomy, 794–795, 794f–795f
continent vesicostomy, 797, 798f
diagnosis, 793
Monti-Yang ileovesicostomy, 795–797, 796f–797f
outcomes and complications, 799, 799t
surgical indications, 793–794, 793f
surgical techniques, 794–798
ureterovesicostomy, 797–798
renal transplant complications, 72–75
triad syndrome, 656
Urodynamics, postprostatectomy sling procedures, 302t
Urogenital sinus repair
alternative therapies, 762
diagnosis, 761–762, 761f
high-confluence urogenital sinus, 774–775, 775f–776f
low-confluence urogenital sinus, 773–774, 774f–775f
outcomes and complications, 767–768
surgical indications, 762
surgical techniques, 762–764, 763f–768f
tissue engineering
basic principles, 905
biomaterial properties, 905
bladder, 909–910, 910f
cell properties, 905–906
female genital tissue, 911–912
injectable chondrocytes, 907
injectable Leydig cells, 908
injectable muscle cells, 908
kidney, 910–911, 911f
penis, 911
stem cell classification, 906–907
urethra, 908–909, 908f
Urologic energy sources
cryoablation, 929
electrosurgery, 926–927
lasers, 929–934
radiofrequency ablation, 927–929
ultrasound, 927
Urologic laparoscopic procedures, 897–903
Urologic surgical robotics, 922–925, 923f–924f
Urothelial cancer, radical cystectomy for, 92–93
"Urothelium," bladder anatomy, 86–88, 87f
Uterine prolapse
transvaginal procedures and preservation of, 342
vaginal hysterectomy
alternative therapy, 320
basic principles, 318–319
diagnosis, 320, 320f
outcomes and complications, 324–325
pathophysiology, 319
surgical anatomy, 319
surgical technique, 320–324, 321f–325f
Uterosacral ligament fixation, transvaginal enterocele repair, 338–340, 339f
Uterus, eversion of, 322–323, 323f

## V

Vagina, rhabdomyosarcoma, childhood, surgical technique, 663–664
Vaginal hysterectomy, for uterine prolapse
alternative therapy, 320–321
basic principles, 318–319
diagnosis, 320, 320f
outcomes and complications, 324–325
pathophysiology, 319
surgical anatomy, 319
surgical technique, 321–324, 321f–325f
Vaginal prolapse. *See also* Cystocele
posterior repair techniques, 343–349
alternative therapies, 344–345
colporraphy, 345–346, 346f–347f
diagnosis, 344, 345f
outcomes and complications, 348–349
perineal body reconstruction, 347, 347f–348f
postoperative care, 348
site-specific rectocele repair, 346–347
surgical techniques, 345–348
Vaginal reconstruction
female radical cystectomy, 108, 111f
flap reconstruction, neurogenic bladder, 230–232, 230f–233f
vaginal prolapse, 331
Vaginal vault prolapse (VVP), abdominal sacral colpopexy, 349–354
alternative therapy, 351
diagnosis, 350–351, 350t
indications for, 351, 351f
outcomes and complications, 353–354
surgical techniques, 351–353, 352f–353f
Vaginoplasty, 763–764
Valsalva leak point pressure (VLPP), abdominal retropubic therapies, female patients, 289
Varicocele
alternative therapy, 523–524
diagnosis, 523
epidemiology, 523
laparoscopic ligation of, 899–901, 900f–903f
outcomes and complications, 527
surgical indications, 523
surgical techniques, 524–527, 524f–527f
inguinal (Ivanissevich) approach, 525, 525f
laparoscopic repair, 525
microsurgical varicocelectomy, 525–527, 526f–527f
retroperitoneal (Polomo) approach, 524–525, 524f
Varicocelectomy
alternative therapy, 398
diagnostic criteria, 398
microsurgical technique, 525–527, 526f–527f
outcomes and complications, 400
surgical techniques, 398–400, 399f–400
Vasa deferentia
dissection, robotically assisted laparoscopic (radical) prostatectomy, 875, 875f
open radical retropubic surgery, dissection, 191
vasovastostomy procedures
anastomosis, 393, 393f
exposure, 389–391, 389f–390f
preparation, 391, 391f
Vasal fluid evaluation, vasovastostomy procedures, 391–393, 392f, 392t
Vascular anastomoses, renal allotransplantation, 66–68, 67f–68f
Vascularized interposition, neurogenic bladder reconstruction, 234, 234f
Vascular pedicle dissection and control, laparoscopic radical cystectomy, 887, 887f
Vas deferens
anatomy, 355f–356f, 358
blood supply, 358
development, 358
innervation, 358
physical examination, 357–358
vasectomy anesthesia protocols, 372–373, 373f
vasoepididymostomy preparation, 380–381
Vasectomy
access points, 374–375, 374f–375f
alternative therapy, 372
anesthesia protocols, 372–374, 373f, 374–375
complications, 377–378
diagnostic criteria, 372
follow-up semen analysis, 375
indications for, 372
occlusion techniques, 374–375, 374f–375f
outcomes, 375–376
reversal (*See* Vasovasostomy)
surgical technique, 372

Vasoepididymostomy
alternative therapy, 380
diagnostic criteria, 379–380, 379f
indications, 380
outcomes and complications, 386
surgical techniques, 380–386
anastomosis, 383
closure, 383
elongation maneuvers, 383–384
epididymal tubule identification and preparation, 381
long double-armed microsutures, 385–386, 385f
longitudinal intussusception, 381–386, 382f, 384f
single-armed microsutures, 385, 385f
vas preparation, 380, 380f
Vasovasostomy
alternative therapy, 388
diagnostic procedures, 387
indications for, 387–388
outcomes and complications, 396–397
postoperative care and follow-up, 396
prognostic factors, 387–388
surgical technique, 388–396
anesthesia protocols, 388
closure, 396, 396f
incisions, 388–389, 388f–389f
microdot multilayer microsurgical technique, 393–395, 394f–395f
operating room preparation, 388, 388f
special circumstances, 395–396, 395f
vasa deferentia anastomosis, 393, 393f
vasa deferentia exposure, 389–391, 389f–390f
vasa deferentia preparation, 391, 391f
vasal fluid examination, 391–393, 392f, 392t
Vault suspension, transvaginal enterocele repair, 338–339, 339f
Veress needle, transperineal laparoscopy, 801–802, 802f
Vesical neck reconstruction
alternative therapy, 460, 460f
diagnostic criteria, 689–690
outcomes and complications, 696
surgical indications, 690
surgical technique, 691
fascial sling, bladder neck suspension, 691, 691f
Kropp urethral lengthening procedures, 693–694, 694f
Pippi Salle urethral lengthening procedure, 694–695, 695f
Young-Dees-Leadbetter bladder neck repair, 692–693, 692f–693f
Vesical trauma and hemorrhage, 143–149
alternative therapy, 146
diagnosis, 144–145, 144f–146f
outcomes and complications, 147
surgical management and technique, 146–147
Vesicopelvic ligament
pelvic floor anatomy, 313
vaginal prolapse, 326–327, 326f–327f
Vesicostomy
appendicovesicostomy, 794–795, 794f–795f
continent vesicostomy, 797, 798f
Monti-Yang ileovesicostomy, 795–797, 796f–797f
posterior urethral valves, 698–700, 699f
triad syndrome, 656
ureterovesicostomy, 797–798
Vesicoureteral reflux
alternative therapy, 667
augmentation cystoplasty, 783, 783t
diagnostic criteria, 666, 666f
endoscopic treatment
alternative therapy, 677–678, 678t
diagnostic criteria, 677
epidemiology, 676
outcomes and complications, 679–680
surgical indications, 677
surgical technique, 678–679
epidemiology, 665–666
outcomes and complications, 675–676
postoperative management, 674–675
surgical indications, 666–667
intra-extravesical approach, 672, 673f–674f, 674
surgical technique, 667–675
endoscopic surgery, 667
extravesical approach, 667–669, 667f–669f
intravesical approach, 669, 669f–672f, 671–672
laparoscopic repair, 674
ureteral duplication, 672, 673f–674f, 674
urogenital tissue engineering, 907–908
Vesicourethral anastomosis
open radical retropubic surgery, 191–192, 191f
radical prostatectomy and, 198–199
robotically assisted laparoscopic (radical) prostatectomy, 876–877, 877f
Vesicovaginal fistula, 130–137
alternative therapy, 131–132
diagnosis, 131
etiology, 130, 130t
laparoscopic and robot-assisted repair, 136–137
outcomes and complications, 137
surgical indications, 131
surgical techniques, 132–137
transabdominal (intraperitoneal) approach, 134–136, 134f–136f
transvaginal approach, 132–134, 132f–133f
transvesical (extraperitoneal) approach, 136, 136f
V-Y advancement flap, penile reconstruction, 538–543, 538f–542f

## W

Wallace technique, ileal conduit urinary diversion, 547–548, 548f
Wallstent device, palliative ureteral obstruction management, 621
Watchful waiting, benign prostatic hypertrophy, 167
Water tap enema, anal sphincter function, 611
Webbed penis, 733–734, 733f–734f
circumcision, 778–782
Wedge biopsy, penile lesion, 467–468, 467f
Wedge resection technique, partial nephrectomy, 10, 11f
Wet prep technique, testis biopsy, 403
Wilms tumor, 628–634
bilateral tumors, 631–632
epidemiology and diagnosis, 628–629
horseshoe kidney and, 638, 641, 641f
outcomes and complications, 633–634
postoperative management, 632–633
staging, 629t
surgical indications, 629
surgical technique, 629–632, 630f–632f
therapeutic protocols, 633t
thrombus identification, 630
Window of Deaver, T-pouch ileal neobladder reconstruction, 580, 581f
Winkleman procedure, hydrocele repair, 529, 529f
Wolffian duct, 359
Wound closure, renal allotransplantation, 70

## Y

Yachia longitudinal plication, congenital penile curvature, 535, 535f
Yang-Monti technique, colonic continent catheterizable reservoir, 602, 605f
York-Mason approach, rectourethral fistula repair, 141, 142f
Young-Dees-Leadbetter bladder neck repair
bladder exstrophy/epispadias repair, 727–728, 729f
vesical neck reconstruction, 692–693, 692f–693f
Yttrium-aluminum-garnet lasers, 930–931

## Z

ZEUS surgical robotics, 921, 921f